Critical Care Nursing

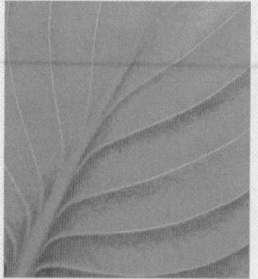

DIAGNOSIS
AND MANAGEMENT
(FORMERLY THELAN'S CRITICAL
CARE NURSING)

Sixth Edition

Critical Care Nursing

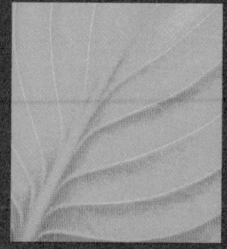

DIAGNOSIS
AND MANAGEMENT

Linda D. Urden, DNSc, RN, CNS, NE-BC, FAAN

Professor and Coordinator
Executive Nurse Leader Graduate Program
University of San Diego
San Diego, California

Kathleen M. Stacy, PhD(c), RN, CNS, CCRN, PCCN, CCNS

Clinical Nurse Specialist–Intermediate Care Unit
Palomar Medical Center
Escondido, California;
Adjunct Faculty Member, School of Nursing, College of Health and Human Services
San Diego State University
San Diego, California

Mary E. Lough, PhD(c), RN, CNS, CCRN, CNRN

Clinical Nurse Specialist, Medical/Surgical/Neuroscience/Trauma ICU
Stanford University Hospital and Clinics
Stanford, California;
Clinical Professor
Department of Physiological Nursing
University of California, San Francisco
San Francisco, California

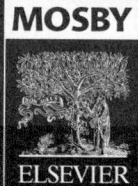

MOSBY

ELSEVIER

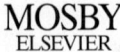

3251 Riverport Lane
St. Louis, Missouri 63043

Critical Care Nursing: Diagnosis and Management ISBN: 978-0-323-05748-6

Notice

Knowledge and best practice in this field are constantly changing. As new research and experience broaden our knowledge, changes in practice, treatment and drug therapy may become necessary or appropriate. Readers are advised to check the most current information provided (i) on procedures featured or (ii) by the manufacturer of each product to be administered, to verify the recommended dose or formula, the method and duration of administration, and contraindications. It is the responsibility of the practitioner, relying on their own experience and knowledge of the patient, to make diagnoses, to determine dosages and the best treatment for each individual patient, and to take all appropriate safety precautions. To the fullest extent of the law, neither the Publisher nor the Authors assume any liability for any injury and/or damage to persons or property arising out of or related to any use of the material contained in this book.

Previous editions copyrighted 2006, 2002, 1998, 1994, 1990

Library of Congress Cataloging-in-Publication Data
Critical care nursing: diagnosis and management / Linda D. Urden, Kathleen M. Stacy, Mary E. Lough. – 6th ed.
    p. ; cm.
  Rev. ed. of: Thelan's critical care nursing / Linda D. Urden, Kathleen M. Stacy, Mary E. Lough [editors]. 5th ed. c2006.
  Includes bibliographical references and index.
  ISBN 978-0-323-05748-6 (hardcover : alk. paper) 1. Intensive care nursing. 2. Emergency nursing. I. Urden, Linda Diann. II. Stacy, Kathleen M. III. Lough, Mary E. IV. Thelan's critical care nursing.
  [DNLM: 1. Critical Care–Nurses' Instruction. 2. Emergency Nursing–methods–Nurses' Instruction. WY 154 C93297 2010]
  RT120.I5C752 2010
  616.02′5–dc22

                                              2009006540

Managing Editor: Maureen Iannuzzi
Senior Developmental Editor: Jennifer Ehlers
Publishing Services Manager: Deborah Vogel
Project Manager: Brandilyn Tidwell
Designer: Jessica Williams

Printed in the United States of America

Last digit is the print number: 9 8 7 6 5 4 3 2

To my friends and colleagues at Palomar Pomerado Health
Thank you for all of your support and encouragement over the past years!

LDU

To the wonderful nursing staff in IMC
Your caring, concern, and compassion for all patients
provides me with daily inspiration and reaffirms why I became a nurse.
To my wonderful family
James and Sherrie-Anne
Roxy and Emma
Thank you for your love, commitment, and support.

KMS

To Jo Ann Schumaker-Watt, RN, BSN, CCRN, and Teri Vidal, RN, BSN, CCRN
For being expert critical care nurses
For being expert teachers who share their knowledge
For your support and friendship

MEL

About the Authors

Linda D. Urden, DNSc, CNS, RN, NE-BC, FAAN

Linda Urden received her diploma in nursing from Barnes Hospital, St. Louis, Missouri; her BSN from Pepperdine University, Malibu, California; her MN, Cardiovascular Clinical Nurse Specialist, from UCLA; and her DNSc from the University of San Diego. She is doubly certified as a clinical nurse specialist and in Executive Nursing by the American Nurses Credentialing Center and is a Fellow in the American Academy of Nursing. Linda has held a variety of clinical and administrative positions, with accountabilities for quality, research, education, advanced practice, and outcomes management and measurement. In her various positions she has striven to create cultures that are sensitive to differentiated practice and to establish mechanisms that promote evidence-based practice and foster professional practice. In addition to this text, Linda coauthored *Priorities in Critical Care Nursing*. Other publications are in the areas of heart failure, ethics, research, outcomes measurement, management and care delivery redesign, executive decision support databases, and collaborative practice models. In addition, she is a member of editorial boards and is a peer reviewer for several nursing journals. Her research is focused on clinical, fiscal, quality, and behavioral outcomes of care delivery and services.

Kathleen M. Stacy, PhD(c), RN, CNS, CCRN, PCCN, CCNS

Kathleen Stacy has been a nurse for 32 years, the majority of which she has spent working in critical care. She graduated in 1978 with a BS in nursing from the State University of New York at Plattsburgh and in 1989 with an MS in critical care nursing from San Diego State University. Kathleen is currently completing her PhD in nursing at the University of San Diego. She has held a variety of positions, including staff nurse, clinical educator, outcomes manager, and nurse manager. Currently Kathleen is the Clinical Nurse Specialist for the Intermediate Care Unit at Palomar Medical Center. As an advanced practitioner, Kathleen collaborates with the health care team to facilitate the achievement of optimal outcomes for the critically ill patient. As a consultant she facilitates change to improve patient care. As an educator Kathleen develops and implements programs to assist the staff with acquisition of the skills and knowledge needed to care for the critically ill patient. As a researcher she facilitates, uses, and conducts nursing research. Kathleen also holds an adjunct faculty position at San Diego State University School of Nursing. In addition to this text, Kathleen coauthored *Priorities in Critical Care Nursing*.

Mary E. Lough, PHD(c), RN, CNS, CCRN, CNRN

Mary Lough is a critical care nurse with more than 30 years of experience as a staff nurse, educator, and Clinical Nurse Specialist. Mary received her BSN from the University of Manchester in England and her MS in cardiovascular nursing from the University of California, San Francisco (UCSF), and she is now pursuing doctoral studies at UCSF. Mary is the Clinical Nurse Specialist for the medical/surgical/neuroscience/trauma ICU at Stanford University Hospital and Clinics in Palo Alto, California. She is also a Clinical Professor in the Department of Physiological Nursing at her alma mater, UCSF.

Mary has been involved with all six editions of *Critical Care Nursing: Diagnosis and Management*, and she also has published many other articles and research abstracts. As a clinician, Mary appreciates the benefits of a clinically grounded textbook because when she began her career as a critical care nurse, so little information was available.

Contributors

Deborah Barnes, MSN, RN, CNS, CCNS
Manager Quality & Patient Safety
Palomar Pomerado Health
Escondido, California
Perianesthesia Management

JJ Baumann, RN, MS, CNS
Stanford University Hospital
Palo Alto, California
Neurologic Anatomy and Physiology, Neurologic Clinical Assessment and Diagnostic Procedures, Neurologic Disorders and Therapeutic Management

Anne Bisch, APRN, PNP, BC
Pediatric Nurse Practitioner
Surgical Services
St. Louis Children's Hospital
St. Louis, Missouri
Burns

Jamie D. Blazek, MPH, APRN, FNP-C
Transplant Nurse Practitioner
Ochsner Multi-Organ Transplant Center
Ochsner Clinic
New Orleans, Louisiana
Organ Donation and Transplantation

Mary Jo Burton, MSN, RN, CCTN
Manager of Clinical Operations
Organ Transplant Unit
Indiana University Hospital
Indianapolis, Indiana
Organ Donation and Transplantation

Beverly Carlson, MS, RN, CNS, CCRN
Lecturer
School of Nursing, College of Health and Human Services,
San Diego State University
San Diego, California
Shock

Diana Clark, RN, MS
President and CEO of LifeCenter Northwest
Bellevue, Washington
Organ Donation and Transplantation

Joni L. Dirks, MS, CCRN
Critical Care Educator
Providence Sacred Heart Medical Center
Spokane, Washington
Cardiovascular Therapeutic Management

Annemarie A. Donjacour, PhD
Lecturer, University of California at San Francisco,
San Francisco, California
Endocrine Anatomy and Physiology

Lorraine Fitzsimmons, DNS, FNP, BC
Chair
Advanced Practice Nursing of Adults and Elderly;
Director
Adult and Geriatric Nurse Practitioner Program
San Diego State University School of Nursing
San Diego, California
Systemic Inflammatory Response Syndrome and Multiple Organ Dysfunction Syndrome

Céline Gélinas, RN, PhD
Assistant Professor
School of Nursing
McGill University
Montreal, Quebec, Canada
Pain and Pain Management

Christine T. Hartley, RN, MS, ACNP
Heart Transplant Nurse Practitioner
Stanford Hospital and Clinics
Stanford, California
Organ Donation and Transplantation

Annette Haynes, RN, MS, CNS, CCRN
Cardiology Clinical Nurse Specialist
Stanford Hospital and Clinics
Stanford, California
Cardiovascular Disorders

Monica Johnson-Tomanka, RN, MS
LifeCenter Northwest
Bellevue, Washington
Organ Donation and Transplantation

Elaine B. Kennedy, EdD
Professor of Nursing
Wor-Wic Community College
Salisbury, Maryland
Concept Maps

Karin T. Kirchhoff, BSN, MSN, PhD
Professor (Emeritus)
University of Wisconsin
Madison, Wisconsin
End-of-Life Issues

Julene B. Kruithof, MSN, RN, CCRN
Nurse Educator
Spectrum Health
Grand Rapids, Michigan
High-Risk and Critical Care in Obstetric Issues

Sheryl E. Leary, MS, RN, CCNS, CCRN, PCCN
Clinical Nurse Specialist
VA San Diego Healthcare System
San Diego State University School of Nursing
San Diego, California
Gastrointestinal Disorders and Therapeutic Management

Cynthia A. Lewis, MS, RN, CNS
Pediatric Clinical Nurse Specialist, Medical/Surgical Unit, Rady
   Children's Hospital San Diego
San Diego, California
The Pediatric Patient in the Adult Critical Care Unit

Mary E. Lough, PhD(c), RN, CNS, CCRN, CNRN
Clinical Nurse Specialist, Medical/Surgical/Neuroscience/
   Trauma ICU
Stanford University Hospital and Clinics
Stanford, California;
Clinical Professor
Department of Physiological Nursing
University of California, San Francisco
San Francisco, California
*Genetics in Critical Care; Sedation, Agitation, Delirium: Assessment and
   Management; Cardiovascular Anatomy and Physiology; Cardiovascular
   Clinical Assessment; Cardiovascular Diagnostic Procedures; Renal
   Disorders and Therapeutic Management; Endocrine Anatomy and
   Physiology; Endocrine Clinical Assessment and Diagnostic Procedures;
   Endocrine Disorders and Therapeutic Management*

Jeanne Maiden, PhD, RN, CNS
Associate Professor
School of Nursing
Point Loma Nazarene University
San Diego, California
Pulmonary Diagnostic Procedures

Barbara Mayer, PhD(c), RN-BC, CNS
Director of Nursing Education
Palomar Pomerado Health
Escondido, California
Hematologic Disorders and Oncologic Emergencies

Colleen O'Leary-Kelley, RN, PhD
Associate Professor
School of Nursing
San Jose State University
San Jose, California
Nutrition Alterations and Management

Karen Garnett Payne, MSN, RN, BC, CCTN
Organ Transplant Unit
University Hospital
Indianapolis, Indiana
Organ Donation and Transplantation

Elizabeth Remsburg-Bell, MSN, RN
Clinical Operations Director
Duke Birthing Center
Duke University Health System
North Durham, North Carolina
High-Risk and Critical Care in Obstetric Issues

Karen L. Rice, DNS, APRN, ACNS-BC, ANP
Program Director
The Center for Nursing Research
Ochsner Medical Center
New Orleans, Louisiana
Gerontologic Alterations and Management; Case Studies

Debra L. Ryan, RN, MN, CCRN
Clinical Nurse Specialist
Spectrum Health
Grand Rapids, Michigan
High-Risk and Critical Care in Obstetric Issues

Mary Schira, PhD, RN, ACNP-BC, CNN-NP
Associate Professor
Associate Dean, MSN Program, The University of Texas at
   Arlington
Arlington, Texas
*Renal Anatomy and Physiology, Renal Clinical Assessment and Diagnostic
   Procedures*

Elizabeth Scruth, RN, MN, MPH, CCNS, CCRN
Critical Care Clinical Nurse Specialist
Kaiser
San Jose, California
Cardiovascular Disorders

Jennifer Seigel, RN, CPNP
Pediatric Nurse Practitioner
St. Louis Children's Hospital
St. Louis, Missouri
Burns

Kara A. Snyder, MS, RN, CCRN
Clinical Nurse Specialist
Surgical Trauma Critical Care
University Medical Center
Tucson, Arizona
Trauma

Kathleen M. Stacy, PhD(c), RN, CNS, CCRN, PCCN, CCNS
Clinical Nurse Specialist–Intermediate Care Unit
Palomar Medical Center
Escondido, California;
Adjunct Faculty Member
School of Nursing
College of Health and Human Services
San Diego State University
San Diego, California
Pulmonary Anatomy and Physiology, Pulmonary Clinical Assessment,
Pulmonary Disorders, Pulmonary Therapeutic Management,
Gastrointestinal Anatomy and Physiology, Gastrointestinal Clinical
Assessment and Diagnostic Procedures, Nursing Management Plans of
Care

Sheila Cox Sullivan, PhD, RN, CNE
Associate Professor
College of Nursing
Harding University
Searcy, Arkansas;
Associate Chief Nurse, Research
Central Arkansas Veterans Healthcare System
Little Rock, Arkansas
Sleep Alterations and Management

Linda D. Urden, DNSc, RN, CNS, NE-BC, FAAN
Professor and Coordinator
Executive Nurse Leader Graduate Program
University of San Diego
San Diego, California
Critical Care Nursing Practice, Ethical Issues, Legal Issues, Patient and
Family Education, Psychosocial Alterations

Christopher Walker, MS, NP, CNS, APRN-BC
Medical Intensive Care Unit
Sharp Memorial Hospital
San Diego, California
Systemic Inflammatory Response Syndrome and Multiple Organ
Dysfunction Syndrome

Carrie M. Wilson, MSN, RN, CPNP
Pediatric Nurse Practitioner
Surgical Services
St. Louis Children's Hospital
St. Louis, Missouri
Burns

Fiona Winterbottom, RGN, RN, BSN, MSN, ACNS-BC,
APRN, CCRN
Clinical Nurse Specialist for Critical Care
Ochsner Health System
New Orleans, Louisiana
Gerontologic Alterations and Management; Case Studies

Reviewers

Anne W. Alexandrov, PhD, RN, CCRN, FAAN
Professor
Department of Neurology Comprehensive Stroke Center
University of Alabama–Birmingham
Birmingham, Alabama

Marie K. Arnone, RN, BSN, MA, CCRN
Swedish Medical Center
Seattle, Washington

Karen Brasel, MD, MPH
Medical College of Wisconsin
Milwaukee, Wisconsin

Marylee Bressie, MSN, RN, CCRN, CCNS, CEN
Instructor
Division of Nursing
Spring Hill College;
PRN Critical Care Clinical Nurse Specialist
Providence Hospital
Mobile, Alabama

Beth Broering, MSN, RN, CEN, CPEN, CCRN
Trauma Program Manager
Vanderbilt Medical Center
Nashville, Tennessee

Diane Byrum, RN, MSN, CCRN, CCNS, FCCM
Presbyterian Hospital
Charlotte, North Carolina

Nita Jane Carrington, EdD, MSN, MBA, MPA
Hawaii Pacific University
Kaneohe, Hawaii

Damon B. Cottrell, MS, RN, CCNS, CCRN, CEN
Washington Hospital Center
Washington, DC

Judy Crewell, PhD, RN, CNE
Assistant Professor
Regis University
Denver, Colorado

Joni Hentzen Daniels, MSN, RN, CEN, CCRN
Clinical Nurse Specialist–Emergency Care
Regional Director, Clinical Services, EmCare, Inc.
Dallas, Texas

Margaret M. Ecklund, MS, RN, CCRN, ACNP-BC
Rochester General Hospital
Rochester, New York

Joyce Foresman-Capuzzi, RN, BSN, CEN, CPN, CCRN
The Lankenau Hospital
Main Line Health Systems
Wynnewood, Pennsylvania

Susan K. Frazier, PhD, RN
University of Kentucky College of Nursing
Lexington, Kentucky

Henry B. GeiterJr., RN, CCRN
Staff Nurse, Critical Care Unit, Tampa General Hospital,
Tampa, Florida;
Critical Care Transport Nurse
Sunstar Critical Care Transport
Largo, Florida

Barbara Konopka, RN, MSN, CCRN, CEN
Instructor of Nursing
Pennsylvania State University–Worthington Scranton
Dunmore, Pennsylvania

Dana Michelle Kyles, RN, BSN
Nurse Manager
Medical Surgical Telemetry
Transfusion Support and Blood Services
Harborview Medical Center;
Clinical Associate
Biobehavioral Nursing and Health Systems
University of Washington School of Nursing
Seattle, Washington

Rosemary Koehl Lee, RN, MSN, CCRN, CCNS
Clinical Nurse Specialist
Critical Care Department
Baptist Hospital
Miami, Florida

Elizabeth A. Mann, RN, MS, CCRN, CCNS
U.S. Army Institute of Surgical Research
Fort Sam Houston
Houston, Texas

Reba McVay, MSN, RN
Clinical Nurse Specialist
Medical Intensive Care Unit
University of Maryland Medical Center
Baltimore, Maryland

Diane J. Mick, PhD, RN, GNP, FNAP
Assistant Director
Clinical Nursing Research Center;
Nurse Practitioner in Gerontology
Critical Care Clinical Nurse Specialist
University of Rochester Medical Center
Rochester, New York

Anne C. Muller, RN, MSN
Clinical Nurse Specialist
Hospital of the University of Pennsylvania
Philadelphia, Pennsylvania

Denise O'Brien, RN, MSN
Clinical Nurse Specialist
UH PACU
Department of Operating Rooms/PACU
University of Michigan Health System;
Adjunct Clinical Instructor
School of Nursing
University of Michigan
Ann Arbor, Michigan

Michaelynn Paul, RN, MS, CCRN
School of Nursing
Walla Walla University
Portland, Oregon

Ellen Peller, RN, BSN, MSN, CNS, PCCN, CCRN
Staff Nurse, CICU, Deaconess Medical Center
Spokane, Washington

Kristine J. Peterson, MS, RN, CCRN, CCNS
Park Nicollet Methodist Hospital
Minneapolis, Minnesota

Cathy Provins-Churbock, RN, PhD, CCRN, CCNS
Grady Health System
Atlanta, Georgia

Hildy Schell, MS, RN, CCRN, CCNS, FAAN
Adult Critical Care Clinical Nurse Specialist
University of California–San Francisco Medical Center
San Francisco, California

Paula Marie Schmidt, RN, MSN
Providence St. Vincent Medical Center
Portland, Oregon

Sandra L. Siedlecki, PhD, RN, CNS
Cleveland Clinic Foundation
Cleveland, Ohio

Diane Vail Skojec, MS, CRNP
Cardiac Transplant Nurse Practitioner
Comprehensive Transplant Center
The Johns Hopkins Hospital
Baltimore, Maryland

Michelle Smeltzer, MSN, RN
Clinical Educator
Emergency Services
Albert Einstein Healthcare Network
Philadelphia, Pennsylvania

Sharon Souter, PhD
University of Mary Hardin Baylor
Belton, Texas

Evangeline N. Veloria, BSN, MS, RN, CCRN, ACNP-BC
Acute Care Nurse Practitioner
Surgical and Cardiothoracic Intensive Care Units
New York Presbyterian–Columbia University Medical Center;
Instructor of Clinical Nursing
Columbia University School of Nursing
New York, New York

Kathleen S. Whalen, PhD, RN
Regis University
Denver, Colorado

Chris Winkelman, RN, PhD, CCRN, ACNP
Frances Payne Bolton School of Nursing
Case Western Reserve University
MetroHealth Medical Center
Cleveland, Ohio

Preface

$\mathcal{W}$e are most grateful to the many students and nurses who made the previous editions of this book successful. This success has validated our commitments to proclaiming the outstanding contributions of critical care nurses and to promoting evidence-based nursing practice in the complex critical care environment. We actively solicited feedback from users of the previous editions and eagerly incorporated their comments and suggestions regarding format, content, and organization. And so, with this sixth edition, we again present to you a book that is thorough in all that is most pertinent to critical care nurses in a format that is organized for clarity and comprehension.

ORGANIZATION

The book's nine units and two appendices are again organized around alterations in dimensions of human functioning that span biopsychosocial realms.

The content of Unit I, "Foundations of Critical Care Nursing," forms the basis of practice, regardless of the physiologic alterations of the critically ill patient. Although chapters in the book may be studied in any sequence, we recommend that Chapter 1, "Critical Care Nursing Practice," be studied first because it clarifies the major assumptions on which the entirety of the book is based. Chapter 2, "Ethical Issues," delineates theories and strategies for dealing with the ethical dilemmas that arise on a daily basis in critical care. Chapter 3, "Legal Issues," provides a base of information to help the critical care nurse be cognizant of practice issues that may have legal implications. Chapter 4, a new chapter titled "Genetics in Critical Care," is discussed in detail below. Teaching and learning theory and strategies to best meet the learning needs of critical care patients are delineated in Chapter 5, "Patient and Family Education." Chapter 6, "Psychosocial Alterations," examines the theoretic basis and nursing process for alterations in self-concept and coping. Chapter 7, "Sleep Alterations and Management," addresses a perennial problem in critical care. Chapter 8, "Nutrition Alterations and Management," examines the nutritional needs of the critically ill patient and provides specific recommendations for different disorders. The concepts of pain management in the critically ill are discussed in Chapter 9, "Pain and Pain Management." "Sedation, Agitation, Delirium: Assessment and Management" are described in Chapter 10. Chapter 11, "End-of-Life Issues," delineates special needs for dealing with end-of-life and palliative care. Unit II, "Special Populations," addresses the needs of the critically ill pediatric, obstetric, and geriatric patient in the critical care unit, as well as the management of the recovery of the perianesthesia patient.

Unit III, "Cardiovascular Alterations," and Unit IV, "Pulmonary Alterations," are each structured with the following chapters:

- Anatomy and Physiology
- Clinical Assessment
- Diagnostic Procedures
- Disorders
- Therapeutic Management

This organization permits easy retrieval of information for students and clinicians and provides flexibility for the instructor to individualize teaching methods by assigning chapters that best suit student needs. Unit V, "Neurologic Alterations"; Unit VI, "Renal Alterations"; Unit VII, "Gastrointestinal Alterations"; and Unit VIII, "Endocrine Alterations," are organized similarly. However, in these units, the assessment parameters, such as clinical and diagnostic procedures, are discussed in one chapter. In addition, disorders and therapeutic management are combined into one chapter.

Unit IX, "Multisystem Alterations," covers disorders that affect multiple body systems and necessitate discussion as a separate category. Unit IX consists of six chapters: "Trauma," "Shock," "Systemic Inflammatory Response Syndrome and Multiple Organ Dysfunction Syndrome," "Burns," "Organ Donation and Transplantation," and "Hematologic Disorders and Oncologic Emergencies."

Appendix A, "Nursing Management Plans of Care," contains management plans organized alphabetically by nursing diagnosis for easy access by students and practitioners.

Finally, Appendix B, "Physiologic Formulas for Critical Care," features commonly encountered hemodynamic, pulmonary, and other calculations and is presented in easily understood formulas. Recommendations for nutritional supplements also are included.

NURSING DIAGNOSIS AND MANAGEMENT

A dominant theme of the book continues to be nursing diagnosis and management, reflecting the strength of critical care nursing practice. Wherever possible, evidence-based critical care practice is incorporated into nursing interventions. To foster critical thinking and decision making, a boxed "menu" of nursing diagnoses complete with specific etiologic or related factors accompanies each medical disorder and major medical treatment discussion and directs the learner to Appendix A, where appropriate nursing management is detailed. To facilitate student learning, the nursing management plans of care incorporate nursing diagnosis definition, etiologic or related factors, clinical manifestations, and interventions with rationale. The nursing management plans are liberally cross-referenced throughout the book for easy retrieval by the reader.

NEW TO THIS EDITION

Chapter 4, **"Genetics in Critical Care,"** has been added to the sixth edition. This field is in its infancy, but over time, as molecular science research is applied to disease treatments, nurses will encounter a range of therapies based on genetic research. To facilitate understanding of the biological basis of genetics, descriptions of the different types of *genetic* and *genomic* studies are included, plus examples of genetic diseases and pharmacogenetic syndromes already encountered in critical care. The genomic arena mandates a new range of clinical and ethical competencies for nursing practice, and this list is included in the chapter.

SPECIAL FEATURES

We've added two new special features to the sixth edition:
- New **Case Studies** promote student learning and critical thinking by illustrating the clinical course of a patient experiencing the history, clinical assessment, diagnostic procedures, and diagnoses discussed in the related unit or chapter. All Case Studies include critical thinking questions to facilitate discussion. Answers to the questions are available on the Evolve website as a special resource for instructors.
- Brand-new **Concept Maps** appear in the disorders chapters. This new feature links pathophysiologic processes and clinical manifestations with medical and nursing interventions for improved comprehension of common disorders, including shock, gastrointestinal hemorrhage, acute renal failure, and many others.

We've also retained many of the special features from the previous edition. The **Evidence-Based Practice** special feature highlights important research-based articles on key topics in critical care nursing. The **Nursing Interventions Classification (NIC)** feature appears in the therapeutic management chapters and lists the important nursing actions for a variety of nursing interventions that would be commonly incorporated in the management of a critically ill patient requiring a specific therapeutic treatment, such as mechanical ventilation. **Pharmacologic Management** tables are also found in the therapeutic management chapters; these tables outline the common medications, along with any special considerations, used in treatment of the different disorders presented in the text. **Patient Education** boxes are placed in the disorders chapters and list the special topics that should be taught to the patient and family to prepare them for discharge. Information that should be included as part of the patient's history has been incorporated into **Data Collection** boxes located in the clinical assessment chapters. Finally, the **Patient Safety** feature highlights special safety issues for the learner, and the **Nursing Diagnoses** feature displays the diagnoses associated with particular disorders.

EVOLVE RESOURCES FOR *CRITICAL CARE NURSING*

We are pleased to offer additional new and updated resources for students and instructors on our companion site, Evolve Resources for *Critical Care Nursing*.

STUDENT RESOURCES

Additional Student Resources are available at http://evolve.elsevier.com/Urden/criticalcare/ and include the following:
- Self-assessment opportunities, including Exercises in Preparation for NCLEX®, Exercises in Preparation for CCRN, and Exercises in Preparation for PCCN
- A selection of assessment animations, audio and video clips, and images
- Heart and lung sounds
- Fifteen procedures from the new edition of *Mosby's Nursing Skills* with corresponding animations
- An interactive Concept Map Creator that allows users to create customized concept maps, from initial diagnoses to interventions to outcomes to completed care plans
- Updated WebLinks organized by chapter, allowing the user the opportunity to explore additional content sources

INSTRUCTOR RESOURCES

Additional Instructor Resources, available at http://evolve.elsevier.com/Urden/criticalcare/, provide a variety of aids to enhance classroom instruction. Instructors have access to all of the Student Resources listed above, as well as the following:
- Instructor's Manual, complete with an overview, objectives, chapter outline, and teaching strategies for each chapter
- Test Bank of approximately 1200 questions
- PowerPoint presentation by chapter, consisting of a total of approximately 1500 lecture slides
- Image Collection containing all of the images from the text
- Answers to all of the Case Study questions appearing in the text

The **Evolve Learning System** is an interactive learning environment that works in coordination with **Critical Care Nursing, sixth edition,** to provide Internet-based course management tools you can use to reinforce and expand concepts. You can use Evolve to
- Publish your class syllabus, outline, and lecture notes.
- Set up "virtual office hours" and e-mail communication.
- Share important dates and information through the online class *Calendar*.
- Encourage student participation through *Chat Rooms* and *Discussion Boards*.

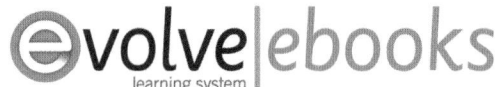

Make the most of your time with **Evolve eBooks.** With easy access from your computer or any Internet browser, you and your students can

- Search across an entire library of Elsevier e-textbooks simultaneously.
- Create focused, customized study documents.
- Make and share notes, highlights, and more.

Evolve eBooks revolutionizes the way your students study and learn. Please contact your Elsevier sales representative for more information, or visit http://evolve.elsevier.com/ebooks.

Critical Care Nursing: Diagnosis and Management, sixth edition, represents our continued commitment to bringing you the best in all things a textbook can offer: the best and brightest in contributing and consulting authors, the latest in scientific research befitting the current state of health care and nursing, an organizational format that exercises diagnostic reasoning skills and is logical and consistent, and outstanding artwork and illustrations that enhance student learning. We pledge our continued commitment to excellence in critical care education.

Linda D. Urden
Kathleen M. Stacy
Mary E. Lough

Acknowledgments

A project of this book's magnitude is never merely the work of its authors. The concerted talent, hard work, and inspiration of a multitude of people have produced *Critical Care Nursing: Diagnosis and Management,* sixth edition, and have helped to make it the state-of-the-science text we affirm it to be. A "tradition of publishing excellence" has been evident throughout our partnership with Elsevier. We deeply appreciate the assistance of Maureen Iannuzzi, Managing Editor, and Jennifer Ehlers, Senior Developmental Editor, who have helped us document and refine our ideas and transform our book into a reality. Their creativity, expertise, availability, and generosity of time and resources have been invaluable to us throughout this endeavor. We are also grateful to Brandi Tidwell, Project Manager, for her scrupulous attention to detail.

Finally, we wish to thank those authors who contributed work to the first five editions of this book. Without the foundation they provided, a sixth edition would not have been born. We would like to acknowledge especially Lynne A. Thelan for her dedication to excellence and for serving as the lead editor for the first three editions of *Critical Care Nursing: Diagnosis and Management.*

Linda D. Urden
Kathleen M. Stacy
Mary E. Lough

Contents

Critical Care Nursing Practice

OVERVIEW

Health care is undergoing dramatic change at a speed that makes it almost impossible to remain current and be proactive. The chaos and many challenges facing health care providers and consumers are evident in critical care, in which new treatment modalities and technology interface with the continuing effort to strive for quality care and positive outcomes. Efficiency and cost-effectiveness in relation to health care services are frequently discussed and are emphasized to all health care practitioners. To some, it appears that quality patient care has taken a back seat to the emphasis on cost containment and that quality and cost-effectiveness are not congruent. It is incumbent on all critical care health care providers to face these challenges from their individual discipline's scope of practice and collectively from collaborative and interdisciplinary approaches.

The ever-changing health care environment creates many challenges for providers and consumers of care. Sensitivity to the appropriate time to eliminate or modify practices and adopt innovations is key to maintaining quality, cost-effective care delivery. Willingness to step outside of traditional structures and roles is the first step in making necessary changes. Change is constant. Flexibility and adaptation to change are essential to maintaining personal and organizational balance and to surviving in today's health care environment.

This chapter provides an overview of the evolution of critical care and describes the trends and current issues affecting the critical care nurse and interdisciplinary team. The information in this chapter serves as the framework for the remainder of the book in the areas of professional nurse decision making, holistic care, and interdisciplinary collaboration.

HISTORY OF CRITICAL CARE

Critical care evolved from the recognition that the needs of patients with acute, life-threatening illness or injury could be better met if the patients were organized in distinct areas of the hospital. In the 1800s, Florence Nightingale described the advantages of placing patients recovering from surgery in a separate area of the hospital. A three-bed postoperative neurosurgical intensive care unit was opened in the early 1900s at Johns Hopkins Hospital in Baltimore. This was soon followed by a premature infant unit in Chicago.[1]

Major societal issues have affected the development of intensive care as a specialty. During World War II, shock wards were established to care for critically injured patients. The nursing shortage after the war forced the grouping of postoperative patients into designated recovery areas so that appropriate monitoring and care could be provided. The technologies and combat experiences of health care providers during the wars of the 20th century also provided an impetus for specialized medical and nursing care in the civilian setting. The 1950s brought the new technology of mechanical ventilation and the need to group patients receiving this new therapy in one location. By 1997, more than 5000 intensive care units were in operation in hospitals in the United States.[1]

CRITICAL CARE NURSING

Critical care nursing was organized as a specialty less than 40 years ago; before that time, critical care nursing was practiced wherever there were critically ill patients.[2] The development of new medical interventions and technology prompted recognition that nursing was important in the monitoring and observation of critically ill patients. Physicians depended on nurses to watch for critical changes in the condition of patients in the physicians' absence, and they sometimes depended on the nurses to initiate emergency medical treatment.

As sophisticated technology began to support more elaborate medical interventions, hospitals began to organize separate units to make more efficient use of equipment and specially trained staff. Postoperative care, once provided by private duty nurses on general nursing wards throughout the hospital, was moved into recovery rooms, where nurses with specialized knowledge regarding anesthesia recovery provided the patient care. Medical and surgical intensive care units segregated the most critically ill patients in locations where they could be cared for by nurses with specialized knowledge in those areas of care. By the 1960s, nurses had begun to consolidate their knowledge and practice into focused areas such as coronary care, nephrology, and intensive care. In the hospital units established for patients needing such specialized care, nurses assumed many functions and responsibilities formerly reserved for physicians, and they assumed a new authority by virtue of their knowledge and expertise.[3]

CONTEMPORARY CRITICAL CARE

Modern critical care is provided to patients by a multidisciplinary team of health care professionals who have in-depth education in the specialty field of critical care. The team consists of physician intensivists, specialty physicians, nurses, advanced practice nurses and other specialty nurse clinicians, pharmacists, respiratory therapy practitioners, other specialized therapists and clinicians, social workers, and clergy. Critical care is provided in specialized units or departments, and importance is placed on the continuum of care, with an efficient transition of care from one setting to another.

Critical care patients are at high risk for actual or potential life-threatening health problems. Those who are more critically ill require more intensive and vigilant nursing care. There are more than 500,000 nurses in the United States who care for critically ill patients. These nurses practice in a variety of settings: adult, pediatric, and neonatal intensive care units; stepdown, telemetry, progressive, or transitional care units; cardiac catheterization laboratories; and postoperative recovery units.[4]

CRITICAL CARE NURSING ROLES

Nurses provide and contribute to the care of critically ill patients in a variety of roles. The most prevalent role for the professional registered nurse is that of direct care provider. The American Association of Critical-Care Nurses has delineated role responsibilities important for the critical care nurse[4] (Box 1-1).

BOX 1-1   AACN CRITICAL CARE NURSE ROLE RESPONSIBILITIES

- Respect and support the right of the patient or patient's designated surrogate to autonomy and informed decision making.
- Intervene when the best interest of the patient is in question.
- Help the patient obtain necessary care.
- Respect the values, beliefs, and rights of the patient.
- Provide education and support help to the patient or patient's designated surrogate to make decisions.
- Represent the patient in accordance with the patient's choices.
- Support the decisions of the patient or patient's designated surrogate or transfer care to an equally qualified critical care nurse.
- Intercede for patients who cannot speak for themselves in situations that require immediate attention.
- Monitor and safeguard the quality of care that the patient receives.
- Act as a liaison between the patient and the patient's family and other health care professionals.

From American Association of Critical-Care Nurses: Fact sheet: about critical care nursing (press room). Available at www.aacn.org (accessed December 2008).

EXPANDED-ROLE NURSING POSITIONS

Expanded-role nursing positions interact with critical care patients, families, and the health care team. Nurse case managers work closely with the care providers to ensure appropriate, timely care and services and to promote continuity of care from one setting to another. Other nurse clinicians, such as patient educators, cardiac rehabilitation specialists, physician office nurses, and infection control specialists, also contribute to the care. The specific types of expanded-role nursing positions are determined by patient needs and individual organizational resources.

ADVANCED PRACTICE NURSES

Advanced practice nurses (APNs) have met educational and clinical requirements beyond the basic nursing educational requirements for all nurses. The most commonly seen APNs in the critical care areas are the clinical nurse specialist (CNS) and the nurse practitioner (NP) or acute care nurse practitioner (ACNP). APNs have a broad depth of knowledge and expertise in their specialty area and manage complex clinical and systems issues. The organizational system and existing resources of an institution determine what roles may be needed and how the roles function.

CNSs serve in specialty roles that use their clinical, teaching, research, leadership, and consultative abilities. They work in direct clinical roles and systems or administrative roles and in various other settings in the health care system. They may be organized by specialty, such as cardiovascular care, or by function, such as cardiac rehabilitation. CNSs also may be designated as case managers for specific patient populations.

NPs and ACNPs manage direct clinical care of a group of patients and have various levels of prescriptive authority, depending on the state and practice area in which they work. They also provide care consistency, interact with families, plan for patient discharge, and provide teaching to patients, families, and other members of the heath care team.[5]

CRITICAL CARE PROFESSIONAL ORGANIZATIONS

Professional organizations support critical care practitioners by providing numerous resources and networks. The Society of Critical Care Medicine (SCCM) is a multidisciplinary, multispecialty, international organization. Its mission is to secure the highest quality, cost-efficient care for all critically ill patients.[1] Numerous publications and educational opportunities provide cutting-edge critical care information to critical care practitioners.

The organization most closely associated with critical care nurses is the American Association of Critical-Care Nurses (AACN). It is the world's largest specialty nursing organization and was created in 1969. The purpose of AACN is "to promote the health and welfare of those experiencing critical illness or injury by advancing the art and science of critical care nursing and promoting environments that facilitate comprehensive professional nursing practice."[6] The top priority of the organization is education of the critical care nurse. AACN publishes numerous documents related to the specialty and is at the forefront of setting professional standards of care.

AACN serves its members through a national organization and many local chapters. The AACN Certification Corporation, a separate company, develops and administers a Critical Care Registered Nurse (CCRN®) certification examination. The certification is valid for a 3-year period and is offered in adult, pediatric, neonatal, and progressive care specialties.

CRITICAL CARE NURSING STANDARDS

AACN has established nursing standards that provide a framework for critical care nurses. Nursing practice varies depending on the setting in which the nurse is employed and the patients cared for in that setting. The standards set forth by AACN describe the practice of the nurse who cares for an acutely or critically ill patient in the health care environment. The standards are authoritative statements that describe the level of care and performance by which the quality of nursing care can be judged. They serve as descriptions of the expected roles and responsibilities, describing the standards of care and the standards of professional practice. Chapter 3 offers an in-depth discussion of critical care standards.

EVIDENCE-BASED NURSING PRACTICE

Much of early medical and nursing practice was based on non-scientific traditions that resulted in variable and haphazard patient outcomes.[8] These traditions and rituals, which were based on folklore, gut instinct, trial and error, and personal preference, were often passed down from one generation of practitioner to another.[8-10] Examples of non–scientific-based critical care nursing practice include suctioning artificial airways every 2 hours, using iced saline injectable when measuring a cardiac output, always using lead II for cardiac monitoring, stripping chest tubes every 2 hours, and limiting visiting hours for all patients.[9]

The dramatic and multiple changes in health care and the ever-increasing presence of managed care in all geographic regions have placed greater emphasis on demonstrating the effectiveness of treatments and practices on outcomes.[11,12] Emphasis is greater on efficiency, cost-effectiveness, quality of life, and patient satisfaction ratings.[13] It has become essential for nurses to use the best data available to make patient care decisions and carry out the appropriate nursing interventions.[13] By using an approach employing a scientific basis, with its ability to explain and predict, nurses are able to provide research-based interventions with consistent, positive outcomes. The content of this book is research-based, with the most current, cutting-edge research abstracted and placed throughout the chapters as appropriate to topical discussions.

The increasingly complex and changing health care system presents many challenges to creating an evidence-based practice. Appropriate research studies must be designed to answer clinical questions, and research findings must be used to make necessary changes for implementation in practice.[14-16] Multiple evidence-based practice and research utilization models exist to guide practitioners in the use of existing research findings. One such model is the *Iowa Model of Evidence-Based Practice to Promote Quality Care,* which incorporates evidence and research as the bases for practice.[17] Inquisitive practitioners who strive for best practices using valid and reliable data will demonstrate quality outcomes-driven care and practices.

HOLISTIC CRITICAL CARE NURSING
CARING

The high technology–driven critical care environment is fast paced and directed toward monitoring and treating life-threatening changes in patients' conditions. For this reason, attention is often focused on the technology and treatments necessary for maintaining stability in the physiologic functioning of the patient. Great emphasis is placed on technical skills and professional competence and responsiveness to critical emergencies. Concern has been voiced about the diminished emphasis on the caring component of nursing in this fast-paced, highly technologic health care environment.[18,19] Nowhere is this more evident than in areas in which critical care nursing is practiced. It has been said that keeping the *care* in nursing care is one of our biggest challenges.[19] The critical care nurse must be able to deliver high-quality care skillfully, using all appropriate technologies, while incorporating psychosocial and other holistic approaches as appropriate to the time and condition of the patient.

The caring aspect between nurses and patients is most fundamental to the relationship and to the health care experience. The literature demonstrates that nurse clinicians focus on psychosocial aspects of caring, whereas patients place more emphasis on the technical skills and professional competence.[20] Physical and emotional absence, inhumane and belittling interactions, and lack of recognition of the patient's uniqueness indicate noncaring. Holistic care focuses on human integrity and stresses that the body, the mind, and the spirit are interdependent and inseparable. All aspects need to be considered in planning and delivering care.[21]

INDIVIDUALIZED CARE

The differences between nurses' and patients' perceptions of caring point to the importance of establishing individualized care that recognizes the uniqueness of each patient's preferences, condition, and physiologic and psychosocial status. It is clearly understood by care providers that a patient's physical condition progresses at fairly predictable stages, depending on the presence or absence of comorbid conditions. What is not understood as distinctly is the effect of psychosocial issues on the healing process. For this reason, special consideration must be given to determining the unique interventions that can positively affect each person and help the patient progress toward the desired outcomes.

An important aspect in the care delivery to and recovery of critically ill patients is the personal support of family members and significant others. The value of patient- and family-centered care should not be underestimated.[22,23] It is important for families to be included in care decisions and to be encouraged to participate in the care of the patient as appropriate to the patient's personal level of ability and needs.

CULTURAL CARE

Cultural diversity in health care is not a new topic, but it is gaining emphasis and importance as the world becomes more accessible to all as the result of increasing technologies and interfaces with places and peoples. Diversity includes not only ethnic sensitivity but also sensitivity and openness to differences in lifestyles, opinions, values, and beliefs. More than 28% of the U.S. population is made up of racial and ethnic minority groups.[24] The predominant minorities in the United States are Americans of African, Hispanic, Asian, Pacific Island, Native American, and Eskimo descent. Significant differences exist among their cultural beliefs and practices and the level of their acculturation into the mainstream American culture.[25]

Unless cultural differences are taken into account, optimal health care cannot be provided. More attention has been directed recently at determining the physiologic differences and those of disease development and progression among various ethnic groups. Death rates from cardiovascular disease are significantly higher for black men and women than for white men and women. The prevalence of coronary heart disease is highest among black women, followed by Mexican American men.[26] An increased sensitivity to the health care needs and vulnerabilities of all groups must be developed by care providers.

Cultural competence is one way to ensure that individual differences related to culture are incorporated into the plan of care.[27,28] Nurses must possess knowledge about biocultural, psychosocial, and linguistic differences in diverse populations to make accurate assessments. Interventions must then be tailored to the uniqueness of each patient and family.

COMPLEMENTARY AND ALTERNATIVE THERAPIES

Consumer activism has increased, and consumers are advocating for quality health care that is cost-effective and humane. They are asking whether options other than traditional Western medical care exist for treating various diseases and disorders. The possibilities of using centuries-old practices that are considered alternative or complementary to current Western medicine have been in demand.[29,30] These types of therapies can be seen in all health care settings, including the intensive care unit. Complementary therapies offer patients, families, and health care providers additional options to assist with healing and recovery.[31]

Two terms, *alternative* and *complementary,* have been in the mainstream for several years. *Alternative* denotes that a specific therapy is an option or alternative to what is considered conventional treatment of a condition or state. The term *complementary* was proposed to describe therapies that can be used to complement or support conventional treatments.[31] The remainder of this section includes a brief discussion about nontraditional complementary therapies that have been used in critical care areas.

Spirituality and Prayer. As persons search for meaning and guidance in critical, emergent, and unexpected tragic circumstances, spirituality becomes more important.[32] Likewise, health care practitioners turn to their own spirituality to manage stress and find answers to the health care issues that they face on an intense, daily basis. Spiritual practices consist of meditation, prayer, and spiritual materials and are based on personal values and beliefs.[33] Holt-Ashley[32] describes how to incorporate prayer into the critical care unit, concentrating on patients, their families, and the nurse. The study author also offers strategies for creating an environment that is conducive to spiritual well-being for patients and staff.

Guided Imagery. One of the most well-studied complementary therapies is guided imagery, a mind-body strategy that is frequently used to decrease stress, pain, and anxiety.[34] Additional benefits of guided imagery are (1) decreased side effects, (2) decreased length of stay, (3) reduced hospital costs, (4) enhanced sleep, and (5) increased patient satisfaction.[34] Guided imagery is a low-cost intervention that is relatively simple to implement. The patient's involvement in the process offers a sense of empowerment and accomplishment and motivates self-care.

Massage. Back massage as a once-practiced part of routine care of patients has been eliminated for various reasons, including time constraints, greater use of technology, and increasing complexity of care requirements. However, there is a scientific basis for concluding that massage offers positive effects on physiologic and psychologic outcomes.

A comprehensive review of the literature revealed that the most common effect of massage was reduction in anxiety, with additional reports of a significant decrease in tension. There was also a positive physiologic response to massage in the areas of decreased respiratory and heart rates and decreased pain. The effects on sleep were inconclusive. The study authors concluded that massage was an effective complementary therapy for promoting relaxation and reducing pain, and they thought it should be incorporated into nursing practice.[35]

Animal-Assisted Therapy. The use of animals has increased as an adjunct to healing in the care of patients of all ages in various settings. Pet visitation programs have been created in various health care delivery settings,[36] including acute care, long-term care, and hospice. In the acute care setting, animals are brought in to provide additional solace and comfort for patients who are critically or terminally ill. Fish aquariums are used in patient areas and family areas, because they humanize the surroundings. Scientific evidence indicates that animal-assisted therapy results in positive patient outcomes in the areas of attention, mobility, and orientation. Other reports have shown improved communication and mood in patients.[37]

NURSING'S UNIQUE ROLE IN HEALTH CARE

Today's health care environment necessitates a nursing framework that is flexible and responsive to the needs of the public that is served. The American Nurses Association has defined nursing as the "protection, promotion, and optimization of health, and abilities, prevention of illness and injury, alleviation of suffering through the diagnosis and treatment of human response, and advocacy in the care of individuals, families, communities, and populations."[38] Although nursing has independent and dependent nursing actions, it is essential that an interdependence with all health care professionals is actualized. It is through such collaborative efforts and exchanges of knowledge and ideas about care delivery that quality patient outcomes are made evident.[38,39]

CRITICAL CARE NURSING PRACTICE

Researchers have studied critical care nurses to better understand their clinical judgment and interventions and the link between the two.[33] They identified two major categories of thought and action and nine categories of practice that illustrate clinical judgment and the clinical knowledge development of critical care nurses. These major categories[40] are delineated in Box 1-2.

THE NURSING PROCESS

The nursing process is a method for making clinical decisions. It is a way of thinking and acting in relation to the clinical phenomena of concern by nurses. The nursing process is a systematic decision-making model that is cyclic, not linear. By virtue of its evaluation phase, the nursing process incorporates a feedback loop that maintains quality control of its decision-making outputs. The nursing process is a method for solving clinical problems, but it is not merely a problem-solving method. Similar to a problem-solving method, the nursing process offers an organized, systematic approach to clinical problems. Unlike a problem-solving method, the nursing process is continuous, not episodic. The six phases constitute a continuous cycle throughout the nurse's moment-to-moment data interpretation and management of patient care (Fig. 1-1).

Nursing Diagnosis. A dynamic thinking process that leads to a hypothesis for explaining clinical states is diagnostic reasoning.[41] By using this process that includes appropriate objective data, more accurate decisions can be made, with appropriate interventions to meet health care needs. Factors affecting diagnostic reasoning include patient factors such as acuity, altered mental status, multisystem disease, and rapidly changing physiologic status and clinician factors such as clinical experience, knowledge, continuous stream of patient data, and uncertainty of data.[41]

The North American Nursing Diagnosis Association (NANDA) has supported the continued development and evolution of research-based nursing diagnoses.[42] With nursing diagnosis as a component of the decision-making method, there is a more systematic collection and interpretation of data. The most essential and distinguishing feature of any nursing diagnosis is that it describes a health condition *primarily resolved by nursing interventions or therapies.*

Nursing Interventions. Also known as *nursing orders* or *nursing prescriptions,* nursing interventions constitute the treatment approach to an identified health alteration. Interventions are selected to satisfy the outcome criteria and prevent or resolve the nursing diagnosis. It is important to link diagnostic labels with interventions and nurse-sensitive outcomes so that a consistent framework is available for evaluating nursing interventions and outcomes.

Intervention strategies that consist solely of monitoring, measuring, checking, obtaining physician orders, documenting, reporting, and notifying do not completely fulfill criteria for the

---

BOX 1-2	CATEGORIES OF CRITICAL CARE NURSING THOUGHT, ACTION, AND PRACTICE

THOUGHT AND ACTION
- Clinical grasp and clinical inquiry: problem identification and clinical problem solving
- Clinical forethought: anticipating and preventing potential problems

PRACTICE
- Diagnosing and managing life-sustaining physiologic functions in unstable patients
- Managing a crisis by using skilled know-how
- Providing comfort measures for the critically ill
- Caring for patients' families
- Preventing hazards in a technologic environment
- Facing death: end-of-life care and decision making
- Communicating and negotiating multiple perspectives
- Monitoring quality and managing breakdown
- Exhibiting the skilled know-how of clinical leadership and the coaching and mentoring of others

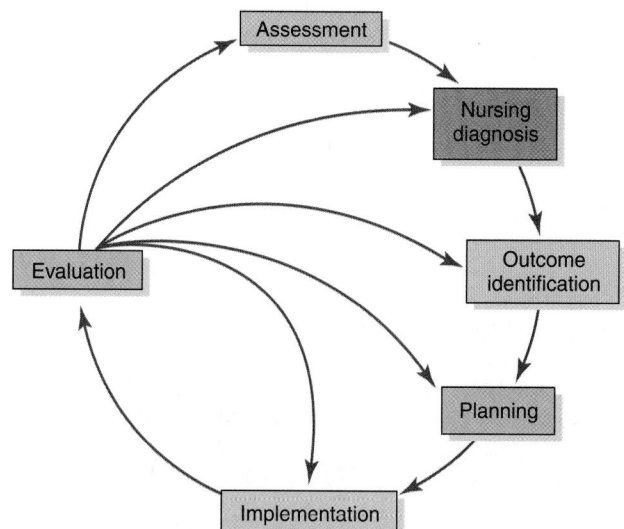

Figure 1-1 Cyclic nature of the nursing process. *(Modified from Fortinash K, Holoday-Worret P: Psychiatric nursing care plans, ed 5, St Louis, 2007, Mosby.)*

treatment of a problem. Nursing interventions for nursing diagnoses designate therapeutic activity that assists the patient in moving from one state of health to another. Medically delegated actions, such as administering medications and initiating ventilator setting changes, are included in the interventions but with the emphasis placed squarely on the assessments and judgments the nurse makes in evaluating their effectiveness, patient tolerance, safety, dosage, titration, and discontinuance.

The Nursing Interventions Classification (NIC) framework contains 542 nursing interventions that are categorized into 30 classes and 7 domains.[43] Many nursing interventions are directly linked with NANDA nursing diagnoses. *Nurse-initiated treatments* are interventions initiated by the nurse in response to a nursing diagnosis. The use of the NIC framework facilitates clinical decision making and provides a standardized language that describes the core of essential nursing interventions. An example of a NIC nursing intervention is presented in the display on surveillance. The research base provides a method to link diagnoses with outcomes in the evaluation of care and services.[43]

Outcomes Evaluation. Evaluation of attainment of the expected patient outcomes occurs formally at intervals designated in the outcome criteria. Informal evaluation occurs continuously. The evaluation phase and the activities that take place within it are perhaps the most important dimensions of the nursing process (see Fig. 1-1). Evaluation of a patient's progress against a standard of nursing management incorporates accountability into the process—accountability to the standard of care. Lack of progress in outcome attainment or lack of progress in problem solving is readily identified and kept in check, and alternate solutions can then be proposed.

The Nursing Outcomes Classification (NOC) is a research-based model of 385 outcomes with definitions, indicators, and measurement scales for use with individual patients, families, and community and population levels.[44] NOC represents one way to standardize terminology for nurse-sensitive outcomes. The outcomes are not nursing assessments or diagnoses and are not prescriptive. The classification does not contain satisfaction outcomes. There are 17 measurement scales that use

---

NIC

Surveillance

Definition
Purposeful and ongoing acquisition, interpretation, and synthesis of patient data for clinical decision making

Activities
Determine patient's health risks, as appropriate
Obtain information about normal behavior and routines
Ask patient for her/his perception of health status
Select appropriate patient indices for ongoing monitoring, based on patient's condition
Ask patient about recent signs, symptoms or problems
Establish the frequency of data collection and interpretation, as indicated by status of the patient
Facilitate acquisition of diagnostic tests, as appropriate
Interpret results of diagnostic tests, as appropriate
Retrieve and interpret laboratory data; contact physician, as appropriate
Explain diagnostic test results to patient and families
Monitor patient's ability to do self-care activities
Monitor neurological status
Monitor behavior patterns
Monitor emotional state
Monitor vital signs, as appropriate
Collaborate with physician to institute invasive hemodynamic monitoring, as appropriate
Collaborate with physician to institute ICP monitoring, as appropriate
Monitor comfort level, and take appropriate action
Monitor coping strategies used by patient and family

Monitor changes in sleep patterns
Monitor oxygenation and initiate measures to promote adequate oxygenation of vital organs
Initiate routine skin surveillance in high-risk patient
Monitor for signs and symptoms of fluid and electrolyte imbalance
Monitor tissue perfusion, as appropriate
Monitor for infection, as appropriate
Monitor nutritional status, as appropriate
Monitor gastrointestinal function, as appropriate
Monitor elimination patterns, as appropriate
Monitor for bleeding tendencies in high-risk patient
Note type and amount of drainage from tubes and orifices and notify the physician of significant changes
Troubleshoot equipment and systems to enhance acquisition of reliable patient data
Compare current status with previous status to detect improvements and deterioration in patient's condition
Initiate or change medical treatment to maintain patient parameters within the limits ordered by the physician using established protocols.
Facilitate acquisition of interdisciplinary services (e.g., pastoral services or audiology), as appropriate
Obtain a physician consult when patient data indicates a needed change in medical therapy
Institute appropriate treatment, using standing protocols
Prioritize actions, based on patient status
Analyze physician orders in conjunction with patient status to ensure safety of the patient
Obtain consultation from the appropriate health care worker to initiate new treatment or change existing treatments

From Bulechek GM et al, editors: *Nursing interventions classification (NIC)*, ed 5, St. Louis, 2008, pp 697-698.
Additional reading sources: Dougherty CM: Surveillance. In Bulechek GM, McCloskey JC, editors: *Nursing interventions: essential nursing treatments*, ed 2, Philadelphia, 1992, pp 500-511, Saunders; Titler MG: Interventions related to surveillance. In Bulechek GM, McCloskey JC, editors: Symposium on nursing interventions. *Nurs Clin N Am* 27(2):495-517, 1992.

5-point Likert-type scale. The model can be used to evaluate the totality of nursing interventions and track effectiveness of nursing on patient outcomes.

INTERDISCIPLINARY PLANNING FOR CARE

The growing managed care environment has placed emphasis on examining methods of care delivery and processes of care by all health care professionals. Collaboration and partnerships have been shown to increase quality of care and services while containing or decreasing costs.[45-50] Early discharge planning and coordination of care in critical care units has been demonstrated to significantly influence patient outcomes.[51,52] It is more important than ever to create and enhance partnerships, because the resulting interdependence and collaboration among disciplines is essential to achieving positive patient outcomes.

INTERDISCIPLINARY CARE MANAGEMENT MODELS

Several models of care delivery and care management are used in health care. An overview of the various terms and models are presented in this chapter, but it is a good idea to seek additional resources and consultation for a more in-depth explanation of the models.

Care Management. *Care management* is a system of integrated processes designed to enable, support, and coordinate patient care throughout the continuum of health care services. Care management takes place in many different settings; care is delivered by various professional health care team members and nonlicensed providers, as appropriate.

Coordination of care and services may be done by the health care staff or the insurance or payer staff. Care management must be patient focused, continuum driven, and results oriented, and it must employ a team approach. Another term associated with this model of care is *disease state management*, which connotes the process of managing a population's health over a lifetime. In disease state management, however, there is a focus on managing complex and chronic disease states, such as diabetes or heart failure, over the entire continuum.

Case Management. *Case management* is the process of overseeing the care of patients and organizing services in collaboration with the patient's physician or primary health care provider. The case manager may be a nurse, allied health care provider, or the patient's primary care provider. Case managers are usually assigned to a specific population group and facilitate effective coordination of care services as patients move in and out of different settings. Ideally, the case manager oversees the care of the patient across the continuum of care. Numerous reports have described the improved patient outcomes, decreased length of hospital stay, reduced readmission rates, and increased continuity of care associated with case management.[53-57]

Outcomes Management. *Outcomes management* refers to a model aimed at managing the outcomes of care by the use of various tools, quality improvement processes, and interdisciplinary team involvement and action. Emphasis is placed on consistent standards of care; measurement of disease-specific clinical outcomes, as well as patient functioning and well-being; and assessment of clinical and outcome data for the specific conditions.[58,59] Outcomes management also takes place in many settings across the continuum of care. Professional nurse outcomes managers ensure that variances from the plan of care are addressed in a timely manner, and they examine aggregate information with the team for quality improvement in the interdisciplinary plan of care.

CARE MANAGEMENT TOOLS

Many quality improvement tools are available to providers for care management. The four tools addressed in this chapter are clinical pathway, algorithm, practice guideline, and protocol.

Clinical Pathway. The *clinical pathway* presents an overview of the entire multidisciplinary plan of care for routine patients. It focuses on the critical elements in the care of certain patient populations and may track variances from the pathway. Pathways are developed by a multidisciplinary team, based on a specific diagnosis or condition, and integrated with the latest research and best practices from the literature. Pathways are ideal for high-volume diagnosis groups that are amenable to standardization. Many pathways are incorporated into the medical record or are computerized, making them a permanent part of the clinical record.

Algorithm. An *algorithm* is a stepwise decision-making flowchart for a specific care process or processes. Algorithms are more focused than clinical pathways and guide the clinician through the "if, then" decision-making process, addressing patient responses to particular treatments. Well-known examples of algorithms are the advanced cardiac life support (ACLS) algorithms published by the American Heart Association.

Algorithms may be used with clinical pathways and are particularly helpful when patients develop variances from the pathway that are amenable to a concise decision-making guide. Whenever bottlenecks in a pathway occur, algorithms are considered an enhancement and serve to facilitate more timely clinical decision making. Weaning, medication selection, medication titration, individual practitioner variance, and appropriate patient placement algorithms have been developed to give practitioners additional standardized decision-making abilities.

Practice Guideline. A *practice guideline* is usually created by an expert panel and developed by a professional organization (e.g., American Association of Critical-Care Nurses, Society of Critical Care Medicine, American College of Cardiology, government agencies such as the Agency for Health Care Research and Quality [AHRQ]).[60] Practice guidelines are generally written in text prose style rather than in the flowchart format of pathways and algorithms. Practice guidelines are used as resources in formulating the pathway or algorithm.

Protocol. A *protocol* is a common tool in research studies. Protocols are more directive and rigid than pathways or guidelines, and providers are not supposed to vary from a protocol. Patients are screened carefully for specific entry criteria before being started on a protocol. There are many national research protocols, such as those for cancer and chemotherapy studies. Protocols are helpful when built-in *alerts* signal the provider to potentially serious problems. Computerization of protocols assists providers in being more proactive regarding dangerous drug interactions, abnormal laboratory values, and other untoward effects that are preprogrammed into the computer.

Order Set. An *order set* consists of preprinted provider orders that are used to expedite the order process after a standard has been validated through analytical review of practice and research. Order sets complement and increase compliance with existing practice standards. They can also be used to represent the algorithm or protocol in order format.

MANAGING AND TRACKING VARIANCES

All variances must be addressed and managed in a timely manner by the health care team members.[61] All of the previously described care management tools provide methods to track variances. Whether variance coding is included on a pathway or is tracked by another quality improvement method, the individual and aggregate data must be assessed and analyzed. Except for protocols, which are more rigid and research based, algorithms, pathways, and guidelines can be used according to the practitioner's discretion. Tracking variances from the expected standard is one method to determine the utility of the tools in particular settings and patient populations. There must be a link between the care management system and the quality improvement program so that changes, as appropriate, can be made to positively affect the outcomes of care and services.

QUALITY, SAFETY, AND REGULATORY ISSUES IN CRITICAL CARE

Patient safety has become a major focus of attention by health care consumers, providers of care, and administrators of health care institutions. The Institute of Medicine publication *Crossing the Quality Chasm: A New Health System for the 21st Century* has been the impetus for debate and actions to improve the safety of health care environments. In this report, information and details were given indicating that health care harms patients too frequently and routinely fails to deliver its potential benefits.[62] Often, the definitions of medical errors and approaches to resolving patient safety issues differ among nurses, physicians, administrators, and other health care providers.[63,64]

Patient safety has been described as an ethical imperative, one that is implied in health care professionals' actions and interpersonal processes.[65] Critical care units are prime examples of where errors may occur because of the hectic, complex environment in which the margins of error are narrow and the demands for safety are crucial.[66] Multiple quality indicators have been developed for critical care.[67] Nurses play a pivotal role in quality monitoring and improvements.[68] In this environment, patients are particularly vulnerable because of their compromised physiologic status, multiple technologic and pharmacologic interventions, and many care providers, who frequently work at a fast pace. Care delivery processes that

minimize the opportunity for errors are essential, and a "safety culture" rather than a "blame culture" must be created.[69] When an injury or inappropriate care occurs, it is crucial that health care professionals promptly give an explanation about how the injury or mistake occurred and the short- or long-term effects to the patient and family. They should be informed that the factors involved in the injury will be investigated so that steps can be taken to reduce or avoid the likelihood of similar injury to other patients.

The AACN has developed practice directives on a variety of topics. Each *Practice Alert* is succinct and evidence based, and it provides an easy reference for critical care nurses and other health care providers to ensure that the most current evidence is used to provide safe, quality care to acutely and critically ill patients. Box 1-3 provides an example.

The Joint Commission (JC) has approved the 2008 National Patient Safety Goals (NPSGs).[70] They are to be implemented in all health care organizations (Box 1-4).

The Safe Medical Device Act (SMDA) requires that hospitals report serious or potentially serious device-related injuries or illness of patients or employees to the manufacturer of the device and, if death is involved, to the U.S. Food and Drug Administration (FDA). Implantable devices must be documented and tracked.[71] This reporting serves as an early warning system so that the FDA can obtain information on device problems. Failure to comply with the act can result in civil action.

In 1996, a landmark law was passed to provide consumers with greater access to health care insurance, promote more standardization and efficiency in the health care industry, and protect the privacy of health care data.[72] The Health Insurance Portability and Accountability Act of 1996 (HIPAA) created additional challenges for health care organizations and providers because of the stringent requirements and additional resources needed to meet the requirements of the law. Most specific to critical care clinicians is the privacy and confidentiality related to protection of health care data. This has implications when interacting with family members and others and the often very close work environment, tight working spaces, and emergent situations. Clinicians are referred to their organizational policies and procedures for specific procedures for their organizations.

HEALTHY WORK ENVIRONMENT

The health care environment is stressful, and increasing challenges in the areas of financial constraints, regulatory requirements, consumer scrutiny, quickly changing technologies and treatment regimens, and workforce diversity contribute to conflicts and difficulties on a daily basis. In this environment, it is essential to offer support for health care providers that can mitigate these challenges and ensure a healthy place to work.

There is an increasing amount of evidence that unhealthy work environments lead to medical errors, suboptimal safety monitoring, ineffective communication among health care providers, and increased conflict and stress among care providers.

BOX 1-3　AACN PRACTICE ALERT: SEVERE SEPSIS

EXPECTED PRACTICE

- Assess all patients, and immediately notify the physician when a patient presents with risk factors for sepsis, which include documented or suspected infection and 2 or more of the following SIRS criteria.
  - Heart rate >90 beats per minute
  - Temperature <36° C (96.8° F) or >38° C (100.4° F)
  - Respiratory rate >20 breaths per minute or Pa_{CO_2} <32 mm Hg or mechanical ventilation
  - White blood cell count >12,000/mm^3 or <4000 mm^3 or <10% mature neutrophils
- Obtain serum lactate measurements.
- Obtain blood cultures and cultures from all potential sites of infection before initiating broad-spectrum antibiotics.
  - Evaluate for and remove other potential sources of infection (i.e., obviously infected invasive devices).
- Administer fluids to maintain mean arterial pressure (MAP) at >65 mm Hg, central venous pressure (CVP) of 8 to 12 mm Hg, and central venous or mixed venous oxygen saturation >70%.
- Administer vasopressors if necessary to achieve a MAP of 65 mm Hg if fluid replacement is not successful.
- Obtain cortisol stimulation test results, and start a continuous low-dose steroid infusion.
- Maintain cardiac output at normal physiologic levels.
- Maintain blood glucose levels at <150 mg/dL.
- Consider administration of human recombinant activated protein C (drotrecogin alfa activated) for patients at risk for dying and presenting with septic shock, sepsis with multiple organ failure, and sepsis-induced acute respiratory distress syndrome.

SUPPORTING EVIDENCE

- More than 750,000 cases of severe sepsis occurred annually (year 2000 data), and mortality rates range from 28% to 50%, with an overall hospital mortality rate of about 30%.[1] Sepsis (infection and 2 of the 4 SIRS criteria) can rapidly progress to severe sepsis (infection + organ dysfunction + SIRS criteria) to septic shock (persistent tissue hypoxia with vasopressors on board) within 24 hours.[1-4] Treatment should be initiated regardless of where the patient is located within the hospital. A prospective, randomized study of 263 emergency department patients diagnosed with severe sepsis or septic shock showed that patients treated aggressively with a goal direction toward tissue oxygenation within the first 6 hours of presentation had a 16% improvement in mortality. Another small, retrospective study showed a decrease in mortality among patients identified with signs of severe sepsis and treated within the first 6 hours.[3,5,6] (Level V)
- Serum lactate levels can be elevated in the setting of a normal or increased cardiac output. The measurement of serum lactate can reflect occult decreases in global tissue perfusion, which may be an indicator of organ dysfunction. The presence and the clearance rate of lactate are associated with increases in patient morbidity and mortality.[3,7] (Level IV)
- Early administration of appropriate antibiotics decreases mortality in patients with gram-positive and gram-negative bacteremias. Empiric, broad-spectrum antibiotics should be initiated before identification of the infecting organism and reassessed after 48 to 72 hours based on culture results and clinical data.[8]
- According to the Surviving Sepsis Campaign guidelines, during the first 6 hours of treatment, the goal is to achieve and maintain a CVP of 8 to 12 mm Hg or 12 to 15 mm Hg for patients receiving mechanical ventilation and a MAP of at least 65 mm Hg with fluid resuscitation.[7] Dobutamine is identified as the medication of choice to increase cardiac output (CO) to normal levels or to improve lactate clearance when cardiac output is not being measured. Two large clinical trials did not show a benefit from increasing CO above normal physiologic levels to increase oxygen delivery to the tissues.[9-11] Available data do not support the use of low-dose dopamine for renal protection.[12] (Level V evidence)
- Colloids have not been shown to be of more benefit than crystalloid for fluid resuscitation. One large, randomized, controlled trial compared 4% albumin with normal saline in the treatment of patients requiring volume resuscitation and found no significant difference in mortality between the groups. Several literature reviews have concluded that choice of fluids does not appear to change outcomes.[13,14] (Level V)
- In the setting of hypotension, fluid replacement should be optimized before vasopressors are started. No high-level evidence exists to identify the most appropriate vasopressor to use for the treatment of septic shock and selection is based on multiple clinical parameters. However, in the Surviving Sepsis Campaign Guidelines for the Management of Severe Sepsis and Septic Shock, norepinephrine or dopamine are identified as the initial vasopressors of choice to increase vascular tone and blood pressure.[7]
- Two meta-analyses concluded that administration of high-dose corticosteroids were of no benefit or may be detrimental to patients with septic shock.[15,16] (Level VI) In vasopressor-dependent shock, the addition of low-dose exogenous cortisol has been shown to improve the uptake of the patients own and the exogenously administered sympathetic stimulants when serum cortisol levels are low.[17] (Level IV)
- Maintaining glucose levels within the normal range (80 to 110 mg/dL) but at least less than 150 mg/dL has been shown to decrease morbidity and morality in a surgical population, but it did not focus on septic patients. Maintaining glucose levels less than 150 mg/dL reduced morbidity but not mortality in critically ill medical patients with sepsis.[18,19] (Level V)
- In a large, double-blind study, human recombinant activated protein C (drotrecogin alfa activated) decreased mortality by 6% for patients with severe sepsis and decreased mortality by 13% for patients at high risk for death (i.e., patients having an APACHE II score of 25 or greater).[20,21] (Level V)

WHAT YOU SHOULD DO

- Educate all nursing staff about the risk factors and clinical signs of sepsis.
- Create an interdisciplinary team, including but not limited to physicians, pharmacist, respiratory care practitioner, nurse, and dietitian, to develop protocols or guidelines for the initial identification and management of the patient presenting with signs of sepsis. Consider development of a rapid response team to facilitate prompt identification and treatment of patients with sepsis.

AACN GRADING OF EVIDENCE SYSTEM

Level I: Manufacturer's recommendations only

Level II: Theory based, no research data to support recommendations; recommendations from expert consensus group may exist

Level III: Laboratory data, no clinical data to support recommendations

Level IV: Limited clinical studies to support recommendations

Continued

BOX 1-3 AACN PRACTICE ALERT: SEVERE SEPSIS—*cont'd*

Level V: Clinical studies in more than one or two patient populations and situations to support recommendations

Level VI: Clinical studies in a variety of patient populations and situations to support recommendations

NEED MORE INFORMATION OR HELP?

Talk with a clinical practice specialist for additional information or assistance at www.aacn.org; select topics as needed.

References

1. Angus DC et al: Epidemiology of severe sepsis in the United States: analysis of incidence, outcome, and associated costs of care, *Crit Care Med* 29: 1303-1310, 2001.
2. Ahrens T, Tuggle D: Surviving severe sepsis: early recognition and treatment, *Crit Care Nurse* 24(suppl):2-13, 2004.
3. Rivers E et al: Early goal-directed therapy in the treatment of severe sepsis and septic shock, *N Engl J Med* 345:1368-1337, 2001.
4. Rivers E et al: Early and innovative interventions for severe sepsis and septic shock: taking advantage of a window of opportunity, *Can Med Assoc J* 173:1054-1065, 2005.
5. McIntyre LA et al: Are delays in the recognition and initial management of patients with severe sepsis associated with hospital mortality? *Crit Care Med* 31(suppl):A75, 2003.
6. Engoren M: The effect of prompt physician visits on intensive care unit mortality and cost, *Crit Care Med* 33:727-733, 2005.
7. Dellinger RP et al: Surviving Sepsis Campaign guidelines for management of severe sepsis and septic shock, *Crit Care Med* 32:858-870, 2004.
8. Bochud P-Y et al: Antimicrobial therapy for patients with severe sepsis and septic shock: an evidence-based review, *Crit Care Med* 32(11 suppl): S495-S512, 2004.
9. Hayes MA et al: Elevation of systemic oxygen delivery in the treatment of critically ill patients, *N Engl J Med* 330:1717-1722, 1994.
10. Gattinoni L et al: A trial of goal-oriented hemodynamic therapy in critically ill patients, *N Engl J Med* 333:1025-1032, 1995.
11. Beale RJ et al: Vasopressor and inotropic support in septic shock: an evidence-based review, *Crit Care Med* 32(11 suppl):S455-S465, 2004.
12. Bellomo R et al: Low-dose dopamine in patients with early renal dysfunction: a placebo-controlled randomized trial, *Lancet* 356:2139-2143, 2000.
13. Finfer S et al: A comparison of albumin and saline for fluid resuscitation in the intensive care unit, *N Engl J Med* 350:2247-2256, 2004.
14. Vincent JL, Herwig G: Fluid resuscitation in severe sepsis and septic shock: an evidence-based review, *Crit Care Med* 32(11 suppl):S451-S454, 2004.
15. Lefering R, Neugebaruer EA: Steroid controversy in sepsis and septic shock: a meta-analysis, *Crit Care Med* 23:1294-1303, 1995.
16. Cronin L et al: Corticosteroid treatment for sepsis: a critical appraisal and meta-analysis of the literature, *Crit Care Med* 1430-1439, 1995.
17. Annane D et al: Effect of treatment with low doses of hydrocortisone and fludrocortisone on mortality in patients with septic shock, *JAMA* 288:862-871, 2002.
18. Van den Berghe G et al: Intensive insulin therapy in the critically ill patients, *N Engl J Med* 345:1359-1367, 2001.
19. Van den Berghe G et al: Intensive insulin therapy in the medical ICU, *N Engl J Med* 354:449-461, 2006.
20. Bernard GR et al: Recombinant human protein C worldwide evaluation in severe sepsis (PROWESS) study group: efficacy and safety of recombinant human activated protein C for severe sepsis, *N Engl J Med* 344:699-709, 2001.
21. Bernard GR et al: Extended evaluation of recombinant human activated protein C United States trial (ENHANCE USA): a single-arm phase 3B multicenter study of drotrecogin alfa (activated) in severe sepsis, *Chest* 125:2206-2216, 2004.

Modified from www.AACN.org/WD/Practice/Content/Practice_Alerts (accessed September 2008).

BOX 1-4 2008 NATIONAL PATIENT SAFETY GOALS

- Improve the accuracy of patient identification.
- Improve the effectiveness of communication among caregivers.
- Improve the safety of using medications.
- Reduce the risk of health care-associated infections.
- Accurately and completely reconcile medications across the continuum of care.
- Reduce the risk of patient harm resulting from falls.
- Encourage the patient's active participation in his or her own care as a patient safety strategy.
- Identify safety risks inherent in the organization's patient population.
- Improve recognition and response to changes in a patient's condition.
- Ensure the organization meets the expectations of the Universal Protocol (preprocedural verification process).

From the Joint Commission Accreditation Program: *Hospital national patient safety goals.* Oak Brook Terrace, II, 2008, The Joint Commission.

Synthesis of research in the area of work environment has demonstrated that a combination of leadership styles and characteristics contributes to the development and sustainability of healthy work environments.[73]

The AACN has formulated standards for establishing and sustaining healthy work environments. The intent of the standards is to promote creation of environments that will have a positive impact on nursing and patient outcomes. Evidence-based and relationship-centered principles were used to create the standards of professional performance. A summary of the six standards is provided in Box 1-5.

Summary

- Sensitivity to appropriate times to eliminate or modify practices and adopt innovations is key to maintaining quality, cost-effective care delivery.
- It is essential for nurses to use the best data available to make patient care decisions and to carry out the appropriate interventions.

BOX 1-5   HEALTHY WORK ENVIRONMENT STANDARDS

STANDARD I: SKILLED COMMUNICATION

Nurses must be as proficient in communication skills as they are in clinical skills.

STANDARD II: TRUE COLLABORATION

Nurses must be relentless in pursuing and fostering true collaboration.

STANDARD III: EFFECTIVE DECISION MAKING

Nurses must be valued and committed partners in making policy, directing and evaluating clinical care, and leading organizational operations.

STANDARD IV: APPROPRIATE STAFFING

Staffing must ensure the effective match between patient needs and nurse competencies.

STANDARD V: MEANINGFUL RECOGNITION

Nurses must be recognized and must recognize others for the value each brings to the work of the organization.

STANDARD VI: AUTHENTIC LEADERSHIP

Nurse leaders must fully embrace the imperative of a healthy work environment, authentically live it, and engage others in its achievement.

From American Association of Critical-Care Nurses (AACN): *Standards for establishing and sustaining healthy work environments.* Aliso Viejo, CA, 2005, AACN.

- The critical care nurse must be able to deliver high-quality care skillfully, using all appropriate technologies while incorporating psychosocial and other holistic approaches as appropriate to the time and condition of the patient.
- Nurses must possess knowledge about biocultural, psychosocial, and linguistic differences in diverse populations to make accurate assessments and plan interventions.
- Although nursing has independent and dependent nursing actions, it is essential that an interdependence with all health care providers is actualized.

- Multiple quality indicators have been developed for critical care; nurses are pivotal in quality monitoring and improvement.
- AACN Practice Alerts are succinct, evidence-based directives for critical care nurses and other health care providers to ensure that the most current evidence is used to provide safe care.
- A healthy work environment is essential for establishing a collaborative, trusting, and safe environment for the delivery of patient care.

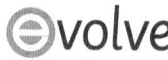 Be sure to check out the bonus material, including free self-assessment exercises, on the Evolve web site at http://evolve.elsevier.com/Urden/.

References

1. Society of Critical Care Medicine: Consumer information, *Brief History of Critical Care.* Available at www.sccm.org (accessed December 2008).
2. Bengco A: The outlook is bright for critical care nurses, *Crit Care Nurse* 20(suppl 1):6, 2000.
3. Melosh B: Doctors, patients, and "big nurse": work and gender in the postwar hospital. In Lagemann E, editor: *Nursing history: new perspectives, new possibilities,* New York, 1983, Teachers College Press.
4. American Association of Critical-Care Nurses: About critical care nursing (press room). Available at www.aacn.org (accessed December 2008).
5. Kleinpell R: Reports of role descriptions of acute care nurse practitioners, *AACN Clin Issues* 9(2):290-295, 1998.
6. American Association of Critical-Care Nurses: Fact sheet (public policy). Available at www.aacn.org (accessed December 2008).
7. American Association of Critical-Care Nurses: Practice resources. Available at www.aacn.org (accessed December 2008).
8. Omery A, Williams RP: An appraisal of research utilization across the United States, *J Nurs Adm* 29(12):50-56, 1999.
9. Wojner AW: Why do we do the things we do? Stop the carnage of nursing research, *AACN News* 17(4):2, 12, 2000.
10. Mick D: Folklore, personal preference, or research-based practice, *Am J Crit Care* 9(1):6-7, 2000.
11. Rosswurm MA, Larrabee JH: A model for change to evidence-based practice, *Image (IN)* 31(4):317-322, 1999.
12. Gawlinksi A: Evidence-based practice changes: measuring the outcome. *AACN Adv Crit Care* 13(3):320-322, 2007.
13. McPheeters M, Lohr KN: Evidence-based practice and nursing: commentary, *Outcomes Manag Nurs Pract* 3(3): 99-101, 1999.
14. Boxer BA, Taylor EM: It starts at home: in-house consulting helps disseminate EBP. *Nurs Manage* 38(9):41-45, 2007.
15. Cannon S et al: Making research come alive at the bedside. *Nurs Manage* 38(10):16-17, 2007.
16. Kleinpell RM: Promoting research in clinical practice. *AACN Adv Crit Care* 19(2):155-161, 2008.
17. Titler MG et al: The Iowa model of evidence-based practice to promote quality care, *Crit Care Nurs Clin North Am* 13(4):497-509, 2001.
18. Panting K: Intensive care/intensive cure: the future of critical care? *Crit Care Nurse* 15(12):100, 1995.
19. Miller KL: Keeping the care in nursing care: our biggest challenge, *J Nurse Adm* 25(11):29-32, 1995.
20. Patistea E, Siamanta H: A literature review of patients' compared with nurses' perceptions of caring: implications for practice and research, *J Prof Nurs* 15(5):302-312, 1999.
21. Mariano C: Holistic ethics, *AJN* 101(1):24A-24C, 2001.
22. Warren NA: The phenomenon of nurses' caring behaviors as perceived by the critical care family, *Crit Care Nurs Q* 17(3):67-72, 1994.
23. Powers PH et al: The value of patient- and family-centered care, *Am J Nurs* 100(5):84-88, 2000.
24. Collins KS, Hall A: *US minority health: a chart book,* 1999, Commonwealth Fund.
25. Bushy A: Social and cultural factors affecting health care and nursing practice. In Lancaster J: *Nursing: issues in leading and managing change,* St Louis, 1999, Mosby.

26. Alspach G: Time for sensitivity training: cultural diversity in cardiovascular disease, *Crit Care Nurse* 20(3):14-24, 2000.

27. Gonzales R et al: Eliminating racial and ethnic disparities in health care, *Am J Nurs* 100(3):56-58, 2000.

28. Leonard B, Plotnikoff GA: Awareness: the heart of cultural competence, *AACN Clin Issues* 11(1):51-59, 2000.

29. Lindquist R, Kirksey K: Preface, *AACN Clin Issues* 11(1):1-3, 2000.

30. Lindquist R et al: Challenges of implementing a feasibility study of acupuncture in acute and critical care settings, *AACN Adv Crit Care* 19(2):202-210, 2008.

31. Kreitzer MJ, Jensen D: Healing practices: trends, challenges, and opportunities for nurses in critical care, *AACN Clin Issues* 11(1):7-16, 2000.

32. Holt-Ashley M: Nurses pray: use of prayer and spirituality as a complementary therapy in the intensive care setting, *AACN Clin Issues* 11(1):60-67, 2000.

33. Eldridge CR. Meeting your patients' spiritual needs. *Am Nurse Today* 2(10):51-52, 2007.

34. Tusek DL, Cwynar RE: Strategies for implementing guided imagery program to enhance patient experience, *AACN Clin Issues* 11(1):68-76, 2000.

35. Richards KC et al: Effects of massage in acute and critical care, *AACN Clin Issues* 11(1):77-96, 2000.

36. McKenney C, Johnson R: Unleash the healing power of pet therapy. *Am Nurse Today* 3(5):29-31, 2008.

37. Cole K, Fawlinski A: Animal-assisted therapy: the human-animal bond, *AACN Clin Issues* 11(1):139-149, 2000.

38. American Nurses Association: *Nursing's social policy statement*, ed 2, Washington, DC, 2003, The Association.

39. White KR, Begun JW: Profession building in the new health care system, *Nurs Adm Q* 20(3):79-85, 1996.

40. Benner P et al: *Clinical wisdom and interventions in critical care*, Philadelphia, 1999, Saunders.

41. Szaflarski NL: Diagnostic reasoning in acute and critical care, *AACN Clin Issues* 8(3):291-302, 1997.

42. North American Nursing Diagnosis Association: *Nursing diagnoses: definitions & classification*, Philadelphia, 2003, The Association.

43. Bulechek GM et al, editors: *Nursing interventions classification (NIC)*, ed 5, St Louis, 2008, Mosby.

44. Moorhead S et al, editors: *Nursing outcomes classification (NOC)*, ed 4, St Louis, 2008, Mosby.

45. Wheelan SA et al: The link between teamwork and patients' outcomes in intensive care units, *Am J Crit Care* 12(6):527-534, 2003.

46. Boyle DK, Kochinda C: Enhancing collaborative communication of nurse and physician leadership in two intensive care units, *J Nurs Adm* 34(2):60-70, 2004.

47. Falise JP: True collaboration: interdisciplinary rounds in nonteaching hospitals—it can be done! *AACN Adv Crit Care* 18(4):346-351, 2007.

48. Golanowski M et al: Interdisciplinary shared decision-making—taking shared governance to the next level. *Nurs Admin Q* 31(4):341-353, 2007.

49. Reina ML et al: Trust: the foundation for team collaboration and healthy work environments, *AACN Adv Crit Care* 18(2):103-107, 2007.

50. Manojlovich M, Antonakos C: Satisfaction of intensive care unit nurses with nurse-physician communication, *JONA* 38(5):237-243, 2008.

51. Knaus W et al: An evaluation of outcome from intensive care in major medical centers, *Ann Intern Med* 104:410-418, 1986.

52. Kleinpell RM: Randomized trail of an intensive care unit-based early discharge planning intervention for critically ill elderly patients, *Am J Crit Care* 13(4):335-345, 2004.

53. Doerge JB: Creating an outcomes framework, *Outcomes Manag Nurs Pract* 4(1):28-38, 2000.

54. Flarey DL: Case management: a system for improving outcomes, *Nurs Leadersh Forum* 3(4):120, 143, 1998.

55. Kee CC, Borchers L: Reducing readmission rates through discharge interventions, *Clin Nurse Spec* 12(5):206-209, 1998.

56. Maljanian R et al: Design and implementation of an outcomes management model, *Outcomes Manag Nurs Pract* 4(1):19-26, 2000.

57. Peters C et al: The process of outcomes management in an acute care facility, *Nurs Adm Q* 24(1): 75-89, 1999.

58. Wojner A: Outcomes management: an interdisciplinary search for best practice, *AACN Clin Issues* 7(1):133-145, 1996.

59. Wojner AW: *Outcomes management*, St Louis, Mosby, 2001.

60. D'Arcy Y: Practice guidelines, standards, consensus statements, position papers: what they are, how they differ, *Am Nurse Today* 2(10):23-24, 2007.

61. Matea M, Newton C: Managing variances in case management, *Nurs Case Manag* 1(1):45-51, 1996.

62. Institute of Medicine: *Crossing the quality chasm: a new health system for the 21st century*, Washington, DC, 2001, National Academy Press.

63. Hurley AC et al: A model of recovering medical errors in the coronary care unit. *Heart Lung* 37(3):219-226, 2008.

64. Cook A et al: An error by any other name, *AJN* 104(6):32-44, 2004.

65. White GB: Patient safety: an ethical imperative, *Nurs Economics* 20(4): 195-197, 2002.

66. Benner P: Creating a culture of safety and improvement: a key to reducing medical error, *Am J Crit Care* 10(4):281-284, 2001.

67. Pyle K, Wavra T: Quality indicators for critical care, *AACN Adv Crit Care* 18(3):229-s243, 2007.

68. Draper DA et al: *The role of nurses in hospital quality improvement.* Research Brief No. 3, March 2008, Center for Studying Health System Change.

69. Smith AP: In search of safety: an interview with Gina Pugliese, *Nurse Economics* 20(1):6-12, 2002.

70. Joint Commission for the Accreditation of HealthCare Organizations: Facts about the 2008 National Patient Safety Goals. Available at www.jcaho.org (accessed December 2008).

71. Jensen JR: FDA's Safe Medical Device Act, *Risk Manag Rep* 1(2):1-4, 1997.

72. Centers for Medicare & Medicaid Services: Health Insurance Portability and Accountability Act (HIPAA)—administrative simplification. Available at www.cms.hhs.gov (accessed December 2008).

73. Pearson et al: Comprehensive systematic review of evidence on developing and sustaining nursing leadership that fosters a healthy work environment in healthcare, *Int J Evidence-Based Health* 5:208-253, 2007.

74. American Association of Critical-Care Nurses (AACN): AACN standards for establishing and sustaining healthy work environments. Available at www.aacn.org (accessed December 2008).

Ethical Issues

*I*t is essential that critical care nurses have an understanding of professional nursing ethics and ethical principles and that they are able to use a decision-making model to guide nursing actions. This chapter provides an overview of principles and professional nursing ethics. An ethical decision-making model is described and illustrated, and recommendations are given concerning methods to use when discussing ethical issues in the critical care setting.

DIFFERENCES BETWEEN MORALS AND ETHICS

Morals are the "shoulds," "should nots," "oughts," and "ought nots" of actions and behaviors, and they are related closely to sexual mores and behaviors in Western society. Religious and cultural values and beliefs largely mold a person's moral thoughts and actions. Morals form the basis for action and provide a framework for the evaluation of behavior.

Ethics are concerned with the basis of the action rather than whether the action is right or wrong, good or bad. Imposition of ethics implies that an evaluation is being made that is based on or derived from a set of standards.

MORAL DISTRESS

Moral distress has been discussed in the literature as a serious problem for nurses. It occurs when a person knows the ethically appropriate action to take but cannot act on it. It also manifests when a nurse acts in a manner contrary to personal and professional values. As a result, there can be significant emotional and physical stress that leads to feelings of loss of personal integrity and dissatisfaction with the work environment.[1] Relationships with coworkers and patients are affected, and the quality of care can be negatively affected. There is also a great impact on personal relationships and family life. It is therefore important that nurses recognize moral distress and actively seek strategies to address the issue through institutional, personal, and professional organizational resources. Knowledge and application of ethical principles and guidelines can assist the nurse in daily practice when ethical dilemmas occur. Box 2-1 provides a position statement on moral distress as promulgated by the American Association of Critical-Care Nurses (AACN). The AACN has created a framework to support nurses who are experiencing moral distress (Fig. 2-1).

ETHICAL PRINCIPLES

Certain ethical principles were derived from classic ethical theories that are used in health care decision making. Principles are general guidelines that govern conduct, provide a basis for reasoning, and direct actions. The six ethical principles that are discussed in this chapter are autonomy, beneficence, non-maleficence, veracity, fidelity, and justice (Box 2-2).

AUTONOMY

The concept of autonomy appears in all ancient writings and early Greek philosophy. In health care, autonomy can be viewed as the freedom to make decisions about one's own body without coercion or interference from others. Autonomy is a freedom of choice or a self-determination that is a basic human right. It can be experienced in all human life events.

The critical care nurse is often "caught in the middle" in ethical situations, and promoting autonomous decision making is one of those situations. As the nurse works closely with patients and families to promote autonomous decision making, another crucial element becomes clear. Patients and families must have all of the information about a particular situation before they can make a decision that is best for them. They should be given all the pertinent information and facts, and they must have a clear understanding of what was presented.[2] This is where the nurse is a most important member of the health care team—as patient advocate, the nurse provides more information as needed, clarifies points, reinforces information, and provides support during the decision-making process.[3] See the Nursing Interventions Classification (NIC) feature on nursing intervention activities that facilitate decision making.

BOX 2-1 AACN POSITION STATEMENT: MORAL DISTRESS

ISSUE

Moral distress is a serious problem in nursing. It results in significant physical and emotional stress, which contributes to nurses' feelings of loss of integrity and dissatisfaction with their work environment. Studies demonstrate that moral distress is a major contributor to nurses' leaving the work setting and profession. It affects relationships with patients and others and can affect the quality, quantity, and cost of nursing care.

DEFINITION

Moral distress occurs when

- You know the ethically appropriate action to take but are unable to act on it.
- You act in a manner contrary to your personal and professional values, which undermines your integrity and authenticity.

EVIDENCE

Compelling evidence indicates that moral distress has a negative impact on the health care work environment. In one study, one in three nurses experienced moral distress.[1] In another, nearly half the nurses studied left their units or nursing altogether because of moral distress.[2]

Additional studies have shown the following:

- Among 760 nurses, nearly 50% had acted against their conscience in providing care to terminally ill patients.[3]
- Nurses lose their capacity for caring, avoid patient contact, and fail to give good physical care as a result of moral distress.[1]
- Nurses experience physical and psychological problems as a result of moral distress.[4-10]
- Nurses physically withdraw from the bedside, barely meeting the patient's basic physical needs, or they leave the profession altogether.[1-2,4-5,11-12]

SUMMARY

Moral distress is a key issue affecting the workplace environment. Research demonstrates that moral distress is a significant cause of emotional suffering among nurses and contributes to loss of nurses from the workforce. Further, it threatens the quality of patient care. In recognition of these harmful effects, the provision of education and tools to address and manage moral distress in the work environment is imperative and will lead to essential improvements in patient care and outcomes.

AACN POLICY POSITION

Moral distress is a critical, frequently ignored, problem in healthcare work environments. Unaddressed, it restricts nurses' ability to provide optimal patient care and to find job satisfaction. AACN asserts that every nurse and every employer is responsible for implementing programs to address and mitigate the harmful effects of moral distress in the pursuit of creating a healthy work environment.

AACN CALLS TO ACTION

For Nurses

Every nurse must

- Recognize and name the experience of moral distress (moral sensitivity).
- Affirm the professional obligation to act and commit to addressing moral distress.
- Be knowledgeable about and use professional and institutional resources to address moral distress, such as
  - ANA Code of Ethics for Nursing
  - ICN Code of Ethics for Nursing
  - AACN 4 A's to Rise Above Moral Distress Facilitator's Toolkit
- Actively participate in professional activities to expand knowledge and understanding of the impact of moral distress.
- Develop skill, through the use of mentoring and resources, to decrease moral distress.
- Implement strategies to accomplish desired changes in the work environment while preserving personal integrity and authenticity.

For Employers

Every organization must

- Implement interdisciplinary strategies to recognize and name the experience of moral distress.
- Establish mechanisms to monitor the clinical and organizational climate to identify recurring situations that result in moral distress.
- Develop a systematic process for reviewing and analyzing the system issues enabling situations that cause moral distress to occur and for taking corrective action.
- Create support systems that include
  - Employee assistance programs
  - Protocols for end-of-life care
  - Ethics committees
  - Critical stress debriefings
  - Grief counseling
- Create interdisciplinary forums to discuss patient goals of care and divergent opinions in an open, respectful environment.
- Develop policies that support unobstructed access to resources such as the ethics committee.
- Ensure nurses' representation on institutional ethics committees with full participation in all decision making.
- Provide education and tools to manage and decrease moral distress in the work environment.

References

1. Redman B, Fry ST: Nurses' ethical conflicts: what is really known about them? *Nurs Ethics* 7(4):360-366, 2000.
2. Millette BE: Using Gilligan's framework to analyze nurses' stories of moral choices, *West J Nurs Res* 16(6):660-674, 1994.
3. Solomon M et al: Decisions near the end of life: professional views on life sustaining treatments, *Am J Public Health* 83:14-25, 1993.
4. Kelly B: Preserving moral integrity: a follow-up study with new graduate nurses, *J Adv Nurs* 28:1134-1145, 1998.
5. Wilkinson JM: Moral distress in nursing practice: experience and effect, *Nurs Forum* 23(1):16-29, 1987-1988.
6. Perkin RM et al: Stress and distress in pediatric nurses: lessons from Baby K, *Am J Crit Care* 6:225-232, 1997.
7. Fenton M: Moral distress in clinical practice: implications for the nurse administrator, *Can J Nurs Adm* 1:8-11, 1988.
8. Davies B et al: Caring for dying children: nurses' experiences, *Pediatr Nurs* 22:500-507, 1996.
9. Krishnasamy M: Nursing, morality, and emotions: phase I and phase II clinical trials and patients with cancer, *Cancer Nurs* 22:251-259, 1999.
10. Anderson SL: Patient advocacy and whistle-blowing in nursing: help for the helpers, *Nurs Forum* 25:513, 1990.
11. Heffernan P, Heilig S: Giving "moral distress" a voice: ethical concerns among neonatal intensive care unit personnel, Cambridge, *Q Healthc Ethics* 8:173-178, 1999.
12. Corley MC: Moral distress of critical care nurses, *Am J Crit Care* 4:280-285, 1995.

From American Association of Critical-Care Nurses: Public Policy Position Statement, Aliso Viejo, California, January 2006, AACN.

NIC

Decision-Making Support

Definition
Providing information and support for a patient who is making a decision regarding health care

Activities
Determine whether there are differences between the patient's view of own condition and the view of health care providers.

Assist patient to clarify values and expectations which may assist in making critical life choices.

Inform patient of alternative views or solutions in a clear and supportive manner.

Help patient identify the advantages and disadvantages of each alternative.

Establish communication with patient early in admission.

Facilitate patient's articulation of goals for care.

Obtain informed consent, when appropriate.

Facilitate collaborative decision making.

Be familiar with institution's policies and procedures.

Respect patient's right to receive or not to receive information.

Provide information requested by patient.

Help patient explain decision to others, as needed.

Serve as a liaison between patient and family.

Serve as a liaison between patient and other health care providers.

Use interactive computer software or Web-based decision aides as an adjunct to professional support.

Refer to legal aid, as appropriate.

Refer to support groups, as appropriate.

From Bulechek GM et al: *Nursing interventions classification (NIC)*, ed 5, St Louis, 2008, Mosby, p. 247.

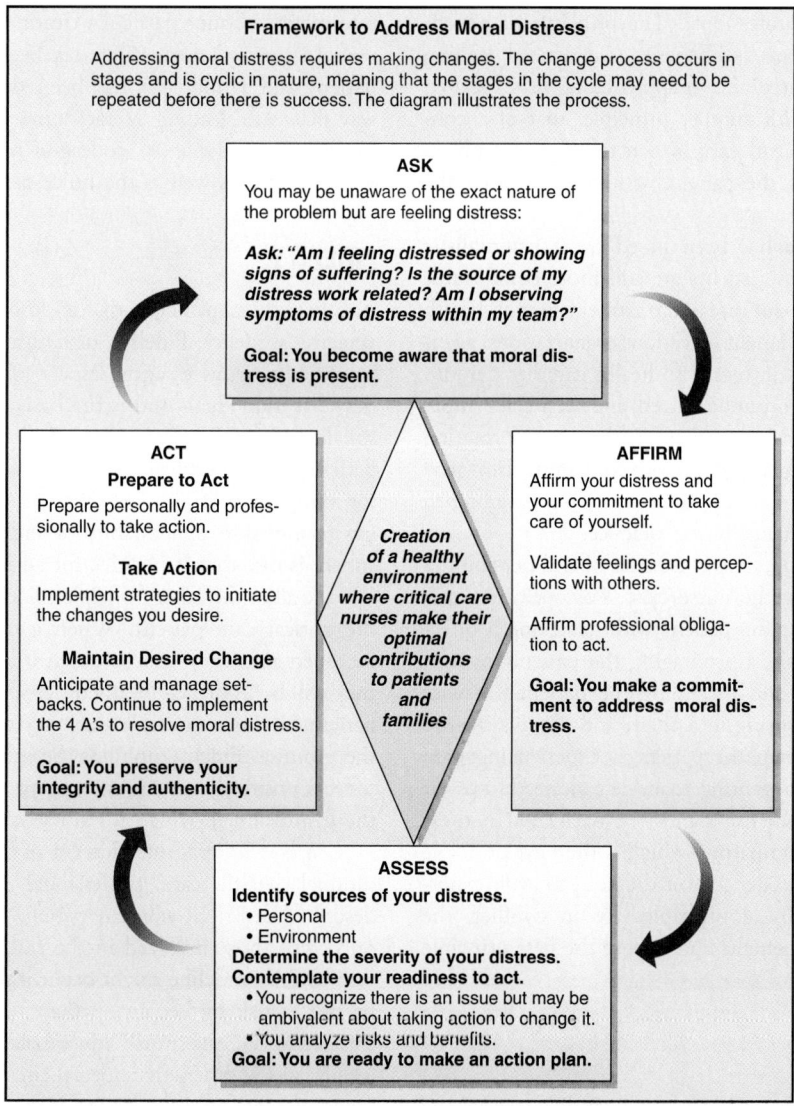

Framework to Address Moral Distress

Addressing moral distress requires making changes. The change process occurs in stages and is cyclic in nature, meaning that the stages in the cycle may need to be repeated before there is success. The diagram illustrates the process.

ASK

You may be unaware of the exact nature of the problem but are feeling distress:

Ask: "Am I feeling distressed or showing signs of suffering? Is the source of my distress work related? Am I observing symptoms of distress within my team?"

Goal: You become aware that moral distress is present.

ACT
Prepare to Act

Prepare personally and professionally to take action.

Take Action

Implement strategies to initiate the changes you desire.

Maintain Desired Change

Anticipate and manage setbacks. Continue to implement the 4 A's to resolve moral distress.

Goal: You preserve your integrity and authenticity.

Creation of a healthy environment where critical care nurses make their optimal contributions to patients and families

AFFIRM

Affirm your distress and your commitment to take care of yourself.

Validate feelings and perceptions with others.

Affirm professional obligation to act.

Goal: You make a commitment to address moral distress.

ASSESS

Identify sources of your distress.
- Personal
- Environment

Determine the severity of your distress.
Contemplate your readiness to act.
- You recognize there is an issue but may be ambivalent about taking action to change it.
- You analyze risks and benefits.

Goal: You are ready to make an action plan.

Figure 2-1 The ACCN 4 A's to Rise Above Moral Distress. *(From American Association of Critical-Care Nurses:* Position statement: moral distress, *Aliso Viejo, California, July 8, 2004, AACN.)*

BENEFICENCE

The concept of doing good and preventing harm to patients is the sine qua non for the nursing profession. However, the ethical principle of beneficence—which requires a nurse to promote the well-being of patients—points to the importance of this duty for the health care professional. The principle of beneficence presupposes that harms and benefits are balanced, leading to positive or beneficial outcomes. In approaching issues related to beneficence, conflict with another principle, that of autonomy, is common. Paternalism exists when the nurse or physician makes a decision for the patient without consulting the patient.

Traditional health care has been based on a paternalistic approach to patients. Many patients are still more comfortable in deferring all decisions about care and treatment to their health care provider. Active involvement by various organizations, agencies, and consumer groups in regard to health care has demonstrated a trend toward the public's need and desire for more information about health care in general and more information about alternative treatments and providers. Paternalism may always be a possibility in the health care setting, but enlightened consumers are causing a change in this practice.

In the critical care setting, many instances of and possibilities for paternalistic actions by the nurse exist. Postoperative care, which is designed to assist the patient with achieving a quick recovery, is a good example. Encouraging the patient to turn, cough, and deep breathe and increasing the patient's activity in the form of dangling, sitting in a chair, and ambulating are all paternalistic actions when the patient is experiencing pain and sleep deprivation and wanting to be left alone. However, the benefits and harms sometimes must be balanced. In these instances, the duty to do no harm—which is the next principle to be discussed—takes precedence over the need to avoid paternalistic actions. When ethical principles are in conflict, the nurse must weigh all the benefits and choose the best principle to follow.

NONMALEFICENCE

The ethical principle of nonmaleficence, which dictates that the nurse prevent harm and correct harmful situations, is a prima facie duty for the nurse. Thoughtfulness and care are necessary, as is balancing risks and benefits, which was discussed earlier. Beneficence and nonmaleficence are on two ends of a continuum and are often adhered to differently, depending on the views of the practitioner.

A practitioner may consider long-term consequences and the good to society as a whole, or the principle and its effect on the single individual in the situation. Such complex problems as quality of life versus sanctity of life are always difficult to analyze in the critical care setting, as well as in noncritical care settings.

VERACITY

Veracity, or truth-telling, is an important ethical principle that underlies the nurse-patient relationship. Veracity is important when soliciting informed consent, because the patient needs to be aware of all potential risks and benefits to be derived from specific treatments or their alternatives.[4,5] The critical care nurse can be in the middle of a situation in which all of the facts and information about a particular treatment option are not disclosed.

Sometimes, information has been given accurately to the patient and family but has been delivered with bias or in a way that is misleading. Veracity must guide all areas of practice for the nurse—that is, colleague relationships and employee relationships, as well as the nurse-patient relationship.

FIDELITY

Another ethical principle that is closely related to autonomy and veracity is fidelity. Fidelity, or faithfulness and promise-keeping to patients, is an essential aspect of nursing. It forms a bond between individuals and is the basis of all professional and personal relationships. Regardless of the amount of autonomy that patients have in critical care areas, they still depend on the nurse for many types of physical care and emotional support. A trusting relationship that establishes and maintains an open atmosphere is one that is positive for all involved.[6]

Like all of the other principles, fidelity extends to the family of the critical care patient. When a promise is made to family members that they will be called if an emergency arises or that they will be informed of any other special events concerning the patient, the nurse must make every effort to follow through on the promise. Fidelity upholds the nurse-family relationship and reflects positively on the nursing profession as a whole and on the institution in which the nurse is employed.

Confidentiality is one element of fidelity that is based on traditional health care professional ethics. Confidentiality is described as a right whereby patient information may be shared only with those involved in the care of the patient. An exception to this guideline might occur if the welfare of others would be put at risk by keeping patient information confidential. In this situation, the nurse must balance ethical principles and weigh risks and benefits. Special circumstances, such as the existence of mandatory reporting laws, guide the nurse in certain situations.[7]

Privacy also has been described as being inherent in the principle of fidelity. It may be closely aligned with confidentiality of patient information and a patient's right to privacy of his or her person, as in maintaining privacy for the patient by pulling the curtains around the bed or making sure that he or she is adequately covered.

JUSTICE

The principle of justice is often used synonymously with the concept of allocation of scarce resources. Contrary to the belief of many people, health care is not a right guaranteed by the Constitution of the United States. Rather, it is the *access* to health care that should be provided to all people. With escalating health care costs, expanded technologies, an aging population with its own special health care needs, and in some instances,) a scarcity of health care personnel, the question of how to allocate health care becomes even more complex.

SCARCE RESOURCES IN CRITICAL CARE

Major factors influencing health care ethics are rapid health care cost inflation and the shrinking allocation of public funds for both primary and secondary care. As health care resources become increasingly scarce, allocation of resources to certain programs and rationing of resources within programs will become more evident.[8] Allocation of resources creates ethical challenges for health care practitioners facing the daily clinical realities.[9] Consulting ethicists and ending life support earlier in the management of some cases have been suggested as approaches to better manage costs.[10]

TECHNOLOGIES AND TREATMENTS

Limitations of resources force society and critical care health professionals to reexamine the goals of critical care for patients. The application of new or experimental treatments and procedures needs to be carefully analyzed for each case, with particular attention paid to the expected outcome.

Quality of life is an issue that should be considered carefully when examining the use of technologies. This issue is personal and value laden; it is different for each individual involved and depends on the various aspects of the case.[11,12] Quality of life has the dual dimensions of objectivity and subjectivity. Objectivity examines the person's ability to function, whereas subjectivity analyzes his or her psychosocial state. Patients' treatment preferences reflect the values they place on various health outcomes.[13]

HEALTH CARE PERSONNEL

Critical care nurses are faced with rationing of critical care beds and nursing staff on a daily basis.[14] Strengths and weaknesses of the staff must be balanced with the needs of the patient.

Orientation and other special circumstances—such as designation of a charge nurse, trauma nurse, or code nurse—must be considered when scheduling staff and making assignments. Any inexperienced staff, float staff, or registry staff must be given appropriate orientation and backup during the shift.

Commonly, a triage system for critical care units is called on when there are more admissions than available beds. The critical care nurse is instrumental in assisting the medical director to determine patient selection for transfer, if appropriate. Hospitals establish a set of standards, criteria, or guidelines for determining patient admission and transfer to and from critical care areas.

WITHHOLDING AND WITHDRAWING TREATMENT

The technologic support of life at all costs has been questioned by health care professionals and health care consumers. Physicians and nurses who are closest to the issues have debated the moral and ethical implications and have looked to ethicists for guidance and legal opinions. Medical and nursing associations have developed guidelines for their practitioners concerning withholding and withdrawing treatments. The decision to not employ aggressive measures or to discontinue treatments that have been in place is always difficult and stressful for all involved in the decision, particularly those who continue to care for the patient on a daily basis.[15]

There appears to be more reluctance to withdraw treatments, reflecting the ethical and moral conflicts within each practitioner. Withholding usually means that there is no hope for success from the onset, whereas withdrawing means surrendering hope. Difficult discussions must take place between the health care professionals and the family, and such communication is especially difficult when families are faced with choices about forgoing life-sustaining treatment. This is a time when families most need timely information, honesty, and care providers who are clear regarding treatment options. Care providers need to listen to the families and be informed about their loved one's wishes.[16]

MEDICAL FUTILITY

The concept of medical futility has resulted in various discussions and proposed criteria or formulas to predict outcomes of care.[17-19] Medical futility has a qualitative and a quantitative basis and can be defined as "any effort to achieve a result that is possible but that reasoning or experience suggests is highly improbable and that cannot be systematically reproduced."[20]

Therapy or treatment that achieves its predictable outcome and desired effect is, by definition, effective, but effect must be distinguished from benefit. If that predictable and desired effect is of no benefit to the patient, the treatment is nonetheless futile. It is suggested that when physicians conclude from personal experience or that of colleagues or from empiric data that a particular treatment has proved to be useless in the most recent 100 cases, the treatment should be considered futile.[20] It is incumbent on health care practitioners to make optimal use of health-related resources in a technically appropriate and effective manner.[21]

ETHICS AS A FOUNDATION FOR NURSING PRACTICE

Traditional theories of professions include a code of ethics on which the practice of the profession is based. It is by adherence to a code of ethics that the professional fulfills an obligation to provide quality practice to society.

A professional ethic is based on three elements: (1) the professional code of ethics, (2) the purpose of the profession, and (3) the standards of practice of the professional. The code of ethics developed by the professionals is the delineation of values and relationships with and among members of the profession and society. The need for the profession and its inherent promise to provide certain duties form a contract between nursing and society. The professional standards describe specifics of practice in a variety of settings and subspecialties. Each element is dynamic, and ongoing evaluations are necessary as societal expectations change, technologies increase, and the profession evolves.

NURSING CODE OF ETHICS

The American Nurses Association (ANA) *Code of Ethics for Nurses*[22] provides the major source of ethical guidance for the nursing profession. The nine statements of the code are found in Box 2-3.

The code was first adopted by the ANA in 1950 and has undergone revisions over the years. It provides a framework for the nurse to follow in ethical decision making and provides society with a set of expectations of the profession. When the requirements of the code are not in concert with the law, it is the nurse's obligation to uphold the code because of the societal commitment inherent in nursing.

ETHICAL DECISION MAKING IN CRITICAL CARE

THE NURSE'S ROLE

Benner[23] described the concept of the relational ethics of comfort, touch, and solace and questioned whether it is an endangered art lost to times past. However, she and her colleagues did find that there are still many examples of such comforting in daily practice, despite the overwhelming emphasis on using technologies in treating critically ill patients. Voice and touch are described as being central for the patient recovering from anesthesia. Critical decisions such as the conservative uses of restraints is another example related to comfort and ethical care of patients.[23] Acknowledging the importance of the nurse-patient relationship and establishing time to listen,

---

NIC

Values Clarification

Definition
Assisting another to clarify her/his own values in order to facilitate effective decision making

Activities
Consider the ethical and legal aspects of free choice, given the particular situation, before beginning the intervention.
Create an accepting, nonjudgmental atmosphere.
Encourage consideration of issues.
Encourage consideration of values underlying choices and consequences of the choice.
Use appropriate questions to assist the patient in reflecting on the situation and what is important personally.
Assist patient to prioritize values.
Use a value sheet clarifying technique (written situation and questions), as appropriate.
Pose reflective, clarifying questions that give the patient something to think about.
Avoid use of cross-examining questions.
Encourage patient to make a list of what is important and not important in life and the time spent on each.
Encourage patient to list values that guide behavior in various settings and types of situations.
Develop and implement a plan with the patient to try out choices.
Evaluate the effectiveness of the plan with the patient.
Provide reinforcement for actions in the plan that support the patient's values.
Help patient define alternatives and their advantages and disadvantages.
Help patient to evaluate how values are in agreement with or conflict with those of family members/significant others.
Support the patient in communicating own values to others.
Avoid use of the intervention with persons with serious emotional problems.

From Bulechek GM, et al: *Nursing interventions classification (NIC)*, ed 5, St Louis, 2008, Mosby, p. 786.

---

explain, and comfort can assist the nurse in determining unmet needs of patients. See the Nursing Interventions Classification (NIC) feature on values clarification.

Ethical conflicts occur frequently in the health care setting. Negative outcomes of such conflicts are in the areas of staff morale, operational and legal costs, and public relations. It is essential that the health care organization have methods in place to address ethical issues.[24]

As discussed earlier, the critical care nurse encounters ethical issues on a daily basis. Because the nurse is on the front line with issues such as do not resuscitate (DNR) orders, response to treatments, and application of new technologies and protocols, he or she may be the one person who best knows the patient's and family's wishes about treatment prolongation or cessation. It is therefore important that the nurse be included as a member of the health care team that determines ethical dilemma resolution.

BOX 2-3   ANA CODE OF ETHICS FOR NURSES

1. The nurse, in all professional relationships, practices with compassion and respect for the inherent dignity, worth, and uniqueness of every individual, unrestricted by considerations of social or economic status, personal attributes, or the nature of health problems.
2. The nurse's primary commitment is to the patient, whether an individual, family, group, or community.
3. The nurse promotes, advocates for, and strives to protect the health, safety, and rights of the patient.
4. The nurse is responsible and accountable for individual nursing practice and determines the appropriate delegation of tasks consistent with the nurse's obligation to provide optimum patient care.
5. The nurse owes the same duties to self as to others, including the responsibility to preserve integrity and safety, to maintain competence, and to continue personal and professional growth.
6. The nurse participates in establishing, maintaining, and improving health care environments and conditions of employment conducive to the provision of quality health care and consistent with the values of the profession through individual and collective action.
7. The nurse participates in the advancement of the profession through contributions to practice, education, administration, and knowledge development.
8. The nurse collaborates with other health professionals and the public in promoting community, national, and international efforts to meet health needs.
9. The profession of nursing, as represented by associations and other members, is responsible for articulating nursing values, for maintaining the integrity of the profession and its practice, and for shaping social policy.

From American Nurses Association: *Code of ethics for nurses*, Washington, DC, 2001, ANA.

BOX 2-4   STEPS IN ETHICAL DECISION MAKING

1. Identify the health problem.
2. Define the ethical issue.
3. Gather additional information.
4. Delineate the decision maker.
5. Examine ethical and moral principles.
6. Explore alternative options.
7. Implement decisions.
8. Evaluate and modify actions.

WHAT IS AN ETHICAL DILEMMA?

In general, ethical cases are not always clear-cut. The most common ethical dilemmas encountered in critical care are forgoing treatment and allocating the scarce resource of critical care, but how does the health care worker know that a true ethical dilemma exists?

Before any decision model is applied, it must be determined whether a true ethical dilemma exists. Criteria for defining moral and ethical dilemmas in clinical practice are threefold: (1) an awareness of the various options; (2) an issue that has options; and (3) two or more options with true or "good" aspects, with the choice of one option compromising the option not chosen.

STEPS IN ETHICAL DECISION MAKING

To facilitate the ethical decision-making process, a model or framework must be used so that all involved will consistently and clearly examine the multiple ethical issues that arise in critical care. Steps in ethical decision making are listed in Box 2-4.

Step One. The major aspects of the medical and health problems must be identified. In other words, the scientific basis of the problem, potential sequelae, prognosis, and all data relevant to the health status must be examined.

Step Two. The ethical problem must be clearly distinguished from other types of problems. Systems problems (i.e., those resulting from failures and inadequacies in the organization and operation of the health care facility and the health care system as a whole) are often misinterpreted as being ethical issues. Occasionally, a social problem that stems from conditions existing in the community, state, or country as a whole is confused with an ethical issue. Social problems can lead to a systemic problem, which can constrain responses to ethical problems.

Step Three. Although categories of necessary additional information vary, whatever is missing in the initial problem presentation should be obtained. If not already known, the health prognosis and potential sequelae should be clarified. Usual demographic data—age, ethnicity, religious preference, and educational and economic status—may be considered in the decision-making process. The role of the family or extended family and other support systems must be examined. It is essential to obtain any desires the patient might have expressed about the treatment decision in writing or in conversation.

Step Four. The patient is the primary decision maker and autonomously makes these decisions after receiving information about the alternatives and sequelae of treatments or lack of treatments. However, in many ethical dilemmas the patient is not competent to make a decision, such as when the patient is comatose or otherwise physically or mentally unable to make a decision. It is in these situations that surrogates are designated or appointed by a court if the urgency of the situation requires a quick decision.

Others who are involved in the decision, such as the family, nurse, physician, social worker, clergy, and members of other disciplines having close contact with the patient, need to be identified at this time. The role of the nurse must be examined. It may not be necessary for the nurse to make a decision at all; rather, the nurse's role may be simply to provide additional information and support to the decision maker.

Step Five. Personal values, beliefs, and moral convictions of all involved in the decision process need to be known. Whether actually achieved through a group meeting or through personal introspection, values clarification facilitates the decision process.

See the Nursing Interventions Classification (NIC) feature on values clarification.

The professional ethical codes of the nurse and physician will serve as a foundation for future decisions. At this time, legal constraints or previous legal decisions regarding circumstances at hand need to be assessed and acknowledged.

General ethical principles must be examined in regard to the case at hand. For instance, are veracity, informed consent, and autonomy being promoted? Beneficence and nonmaleficence should be analyzed as they relate to a patient's condition and desires. Close examination of these principles may reveal any compromise of ethical or moral principles for the patient or the health care provider and can assist in decision making.

Step Six. After the identification of alternative options, the outcome of each action must be predicted. This analysis helps the nurse to select the option with the best fit for the specific situation or problem. The short-range and long-range consequences of each action must be examined, and new or creative actions must be encouraged. Consideration also must be given to the "no action" option, which is another choice.

Step Seven. A decision is reached, usually after much thought and consideration, and the decision is implemented.

Step Eight. Evaluation of an ethical decision assesses the decision at hand and provides a basis for future ethical decisions. If outcomes are not as predicted, it may be possible to modify the plan or to use an alternative that was not originally chosen.

STRATEGIES FOR PROMOTION OF ETHICAL DECISION MAKING

The complexity of health care and ethical dilemmas encountered frequently in clinical practice demand the establishment of mechanisms used to address ethical issues in hospitals and health care facilities. Four types of mechanisms are discussed briefly here: institutional ethics committees, inservice and education programs, nursing ethics committees, and ethics rounds and conferences.

INSTITUTIONAL ETHICS COMMITTEES

Although they are not required by law, many health care facilities have developed institutional ethics committees (IECs) as a way to review ethical cases that are problematic for the practitioner.[25-28] The three major functions of IECs are education, consultation, and recommendation to policy-making bodies. An IEC may function in a variety of ways. The committee may serve as consultants and make recommendations that are not binding. In other situations, health care providers may be required to consult with the committee when there is an ethical problem, with recommendations again not being binding. The third approach requires that ethical dilemmas be presented to the committee and that the recommendations made by the committee must be followed. Regardless of the type of IEC, ethics consultations can help to resolve conflicts that may otherwise prolong unwanted or nonbeneficial treatments.[29]

IECs very often comprise executive medical staff. Membership may include staff physicians, administrators, legal counsel, nurses,

social workers, clergy, and community public volunteers. To fulfill its requirement for consultation, the committee must include members who not only have expertise but also are representative of various groups. Regardless of the type of committee model, the IEC provides consultation and support to the practitioners.

INSERVICE AND EDUCATION PROGRAMS

Basic education about ethical principles and decision making is an important first step in facilitating ethical decision making among nursing staff in the critical care area.[30] It is important for nurses to examine their own values, beliefs, and moral convictions. Nurses need to know and use the ANA *Code for Nurses* in their daily clinical practice. Treatment choices for patients and ethical issues involving patients, nurses, and medical colleagues must be explored and discussed in the classroom setting, where no time constraints or extraneous distractions exist to interrupt the decision-making process. Use of the nursing process as a framework can be a teaching strategy for understanding ethical issues (Box 2-5).

BOX 2-5   ETHICS AND THE NURSING PROCESS

INITIAL STEPS: CLARIFY AND DEFINE THE NATURE OF THE PROBLEM
- What is the crisis (or dilemma) requiring a decision?

ASSESSMENT: IDENTIFY KEY FACTS AND VALUES THAT ARE APPLICABLE
- What are the crucial facts of the case?
- What moral principles are at issue here?
- What decision-making procedure is appropriate?

PLANNING: EXPLORE AVAILABLE AND BEST MEANS TO REACH OUR GOAL
- What is the primary aim or good for which we are acting?
- What objectives, benefits, and moral goals are achievable?
- What previous cases or contingencies should we take into account?

IMPLEMENTATION: TAKE DECISIVE AND EFFECTIVE ACTION TO IMPLEMENT PLAN
- How do we begin, continue, and finish the process of intervention?
- How do we assess costs/benefits of the intervention?
- How do we monitor success/failure in the overall process?

EVALUATION: EVALUATE PROGRESS AND OUTCOMES WITH PLANNED OBJECTIVES
- What means have we set up for debriefing and feedback?
- Have we used the "right" means to a "good" end?
- How do we review the pros/cons for the action taken?

FINAL STEPS: IN RETROSPECT, APPLY THE FOLLOWING TESTS
- Could I/we provide a reasonable ethical justification for the course of action taken?
- Can I/we identify what we have learned from applying this model to decision making?
- How do we integrate this learning into the next decision-making cycle?

NURSING ETHICS COMMITTEES

Nursing ethics committees provide a forum in which nurses can discuss ethical issues that are pertinent to nurses at the individual, the unit, or the department level.[31] Unlike the IEC, which involves treatment choices for patients, the nursing committee may or may not address a patient situation. Depending on the specific goals of the committee, it can also serve as a resource to nursing staff, make recommendations to a policy-making body about a variety of professional issues, or actually formulate policies. It also may serve to educate the department on ethical and professional issues. Membership usually comprises representatives from all major clinical areas or divisions, educators, clinical nurse specialists, administrators, and other specialty staff. Some departments, such as critical care, may have their own unit or division committee.

ETHICS ROUNDS AND CONFERENCES

Ethics rounds at the unit level regarding patients in the unit can be done by nurses on a weekly or other established basis. Rounds educate the staff about problems and can have preventive effects when facilitated appropriately. During the discussion, potential problems may be identified early, and actions may be taken to decrease or prevent the incidence of a problem. An individual patient ethics conference may be scheduled to include only the nursing staff or to include a multidisciplinary group to discuss unit issues. A patient ethics conference may function as a liaison with the IEC or as an end in itself.

Summary

- Ethical dilemmas are encountered daily in the practice of critical care.
- The AACN statement on moral distress and framework to address moral distress provide insight and guidelines for critical care nurses who experience moral distress.
- The critical nature of the situation and the speed that is required to make decisions often prevent practitioners from gaining insight into the desires, values, and feelings of patients.
- By assuming a solely technologic approach, practitioners violate the rights of patients and their professional codes of ethics.
- By using an ethical decision-making process, practitioners protect the rights of the patient, and logical analysis of the case leads to a decision that is made in the best interests of the patient.
- It is through moral reasoning and examining, weighing, justifying, and choosing ethical principles that patient's rights and individuality are upheld.
- The practice of nursing is built on a foundation of moral and ethical caring; the critical care nurse is pivotal in identifying patient situations with an ethical component and can participate in the decision-making process to address the issues.

Case Study: Patient with Ethical Dilemma

⊜volve   Answers to the Case Study Questions can be found on the Evolve web site at http://evolve.elsevier.com/Urden/.

Brief Patient History

Mr. X is a 67 year old obese male. He has a 2 year history of emphysema (100 pack-year history of tobacco abuse in the past) with two recent hospitalizations for pneumonia that required ventilatory support. Mr. X states that he does not want to be placed on a ventilator again but does not want to suffer either. He was involved in a motor vehicular accident (MVA) and sustained blunt trauma to his trunk and lower extremities, with bilateral femur fractures. Although his condition is critical, he is expected to recover. Mr. X received morphine 5 mg by intravenous push in the emergency department, with minimal pain relief; however, he has experienced new-onset confusion. Mr. X's spouse and children express concern about the risk of respiratory depression due to pain medication. They state that they would rather Mr. X experience pain than have him placed on the ventilator again.

Clinical Assessment

Mr. X is admitted to the intensive care unit from the emergency department with blood transfusions in progress. Buck's traction (5 pounds) has been applied to both lower extremities. He is awake, alert, and oriented to person, time, place, and situation. Mr. X is breathing through his mouth, taking shallow breaths. He complains of right upper quadrant abdominal pain when taking a deep breath. His skin is warm and dry. Mr. X is able to move his toes on command, and lower extremity sensation to touch is intact; however, he is complaining of severe bilateral lower extremity pain with restlessness.

Diagnostic Procedures

Arterial blood gases: Pao_2, 55 mm Hg; $Paco_2$, 28 mm Hg; pH, 7.35; HCO_3^-, 24 mEq/L; O_2 saturation, 88%.

  Hematocrit, 24%; hemoglobin, 8 g/dL. Patient reports pain as a 10 on the Baker-Wong Faces Scale. Riker Sedation-Agitation Scale score = 5.

Medical Diagnosis

Mr. X is diagnosed with a hepatic hematoma and bilateral femur fractures from an MVA.

Questions

1. What major outcomes do you expect to achieve for this patient?
2. What problems or risks must be managed to achieve these outcomes?
3. What interventions must be initiated to monitor, prevent, manage, or eliminate the problems and risks identified?
4. What interventions should be initiated to promote optimal functioning, safety, and well-being of the patient?
5. What possible learning needs would you anticipate for this patient?
6. What cultural and age-related factors might have a bearing on the patient's plan of care?

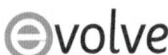 Be sure to check out the bonus material, including free self-assessment exercises, on the Evolve web site at http://evolve.elsevier.com/Urden/.

References

1. American Association of Critical-Care Nurses (AACN): *Position statement: moral distress*, Aliso Viejo, California, July 8, 2004, AACN.
2. Correll N: Identifying patient's needs helps with ethical dilemmas. *AACN News* 17(6):4, 2000.
3. Singleton KA, Dever R: The challenge of autonomy: respecting the patient's wishes, *Dimens Crit Care Nurs* 10(3):160, 1991.
4. Dennis BP: The origin and nature of informed consent: experiences among vulnerable groups, *J Prof Nurs* 15(5):285, 1999.
5. Crow KG et al: Informed consent and truth telling: cultural direction of healthcare providers, *J Nurs Adm* 30(3):148, 2000.
6. Washington G: Trust: a critical element in critical care nursing, *Focus Crit Care* 17(5):418, 1990.
7. Pettrey L: Patient confidentiality: is it ever OK to tell? *AACN News* 17(4):5, 2000.
8. White J: Rationing health care resources, *Nurs Connect* 4(1):22, 1991.
9. Terry P, Rushton CH: Allocation of scarce resources: ethical challenges, clinical realities, *Am J Crit Care* 5(5):326, 1996.
10. Daly G: Ethics and economics, *Nurs Econ* 18(4):194, 2000.
11. Oleson M: Subjectively perceived quality of life, *Image J Nurs Sch* 22(3):187, 1990.
12. Kleinpell RM: Concept analysis of quality of life, *Dimens Crit Care Nurs* 10(4):223, 1991.
13. Patrick DL et al: Validation of preferences for life-sustaining treatment: implications for advance care planning, *Ann Intern Med* 127(10):509, 1997.
14. Byers JF: Apply ethics to the allocation of healthcare resources, *AACN News* 17(2):2, 2000.
15. Dalinis P, Henkelman WJ: Withdrawal of treatment: ethical issues, *Nurs Manage (Crit Care Ed)* 27(9):32AA, 1996.
16. Norton SA et al: Life support withdrawal: communication and conflict, *Am J Critical Care* 12(6):548, 2003.
17. Noland LR: Medical futility: a bedside perspective, *AACN Clin Issues Crit Care Nurs* 5(3):366, 1994.
18. Montague J: A futile-care formula may ease end-of-life issues, *Hosp Health Netw* 8(4):176, 1994.
19. Taylor C: Medical futility and nursing, *Image J Nurs Sch* 27(4):301, 1995.
20. Schneiderman LJ et al: Medical futility: its meaning and ethical implications, *Ann Intern Med* 112(12):949, 1990.
21. Garman ME: Futile care: at what point have we done enough? *AACN News* 17(3):5, 2000.
22. American Nurses Association (ANA): *Code of ethics for nurses*, Washington, DC, 2001, ANA.
23. Benner P: Relational ethics of comfort, touch, and solace—endangered arts? *Am J Crit Care* 13(4):346, 2004.
24. Nelson WA et al: The organizational costs of ethical conflicts, *J Healthc Manag* 53(1):41, 2008.
25. Bushy A, Raub JR: Implementing an ethics committee in rural institutions, *J Nurs Adm* 21(12):18, 1991.
26. Bartels D et al: Ethical committees: living up to your potential, *AACN Clin Issues Crit Care Nurs* 5(3):313, 1994.
27. Bosek MS: A comparison of ethical resources, *Medsurg Nursing* 2(4):332, 1993.
28. Feutz-Harter SA: Ethics committees: a resource for patient care decision-making, *J Nurs Adm* 21(4):11, 1991.
29. Schneiderman LJ et al: Effect of ethics consultations on nonbeneficial life-sustaining treatments in the intensive care setting, *JAMA* 290(9):1166.
30. Corley MC, Selig P: Prevalence of principled thinking by critical care nurses, *Dimens Crit Care Nurs* 13(2):96, 1994.
31. Buchanan S, Cook L: Nursing ethics committees: the time is now, *Nurs Manage* 23(8):40, 1992.

Legal Issues

OVERVIEW

Nursing is defined as (1) the protection, promotion, and optimization of health and abilities; (2) prevention of illness and injury; (3) alleviation of suffering through the diagnosis and treatment of human responses; and (4) advocacy in the care of individuals, families, communities, and populations.[1] Regardless of practice setting, the indicators of minimally competent nursing practice are broadly outlined in this definition. They are further delineated in authoritative statements that are referred to as standards of practice and standards of professional performance. Standards of practice focus on care that is delivered throughout the nursing process to individuals, families, communities, and populations, whereas standards of professional performance articulate what is expected from nurses with regard to quality of care or practice, education, reflective practice, collegiality, ethics, research, resource utilization, and leadership. The standards of practice and standards for professional performance published by the American Nurses Association (ANA)[1] and the American Association of Critical-Care Nurses (AACN)[2] are discussed later in more detail.

Nurses caring for acutely and critically ill patients may be alleged to have acted in a manner that is inconsistent with standards of care or standards of professional practice and may find themselves involved in civil litigation that focuses in whole or in part on the alleged failure. The legal theories on which most of these civil cases are based include the following: negligence, negligence per se, malpractice, wrongful death, defamation, assault and battery, loss of consortium, and emotional distress. These legal theories are considered in this chapter, along with other issues that give rise to civil litigation in acute and critical care settings, including the respiratory management of acutely and critically ill patients and liability associated with blood transfusions, infection control, and informed consent.

NEGLIGENCE

Generally, negligence is failing to act as an ordinarily, prudent person would under similar circumstances. For a negligence-based cause of action to exist, there must have been a duty or obligation to conform to some standard, which was breached. The breach, in turn, must have caused some damage or injury.

Although negligence can occur regardless of whether an individual is acting in a personal or a professional capacity, nurses commit negligence if they act in a manner that deviates from the standard of care and the deviation results in harm to patients for whom they care. Nurses who are found to have acted negligently in their professional capacity are said to have committed *malpractice*. However, for liability to be imposed against a nurse, patient-plaintiffs must prove all four elements of negligence: (1) that the nurse had a duty to care for the patient, (2) that the nurse breached that duty, (3) that the breach caused harm that would not have occurred in the absence of negligence, and (4) that the plaintiff should be compensated for the resulting damages.

DUTY

Nurses assume a duty to provide care for patients in a manner that is consistent with the standard of care when the nurse-patient relationship is established. Providing care that is consistent with the standard of care requires nurses to protect patients from foreseeable injuries.

Cases from a number of states recognize the nurse-patient relationship as a separate and distinct relationship[3] and as a prerequisite for determining whether a nurse owes the patient a duty to provide care in accordance with the requisite standard of care. If a nurse shows that he or she (1) was not assigned to that particular patient on the date that the negligence allegedly occurred or (2) was not working on the day or at the time the negligence allegedly occurred, no duty will be imposed on the nurse. Because no duty is imposed on the nurse, negligence allegations will fail.[4]

Although courts have been willing to construct parameters around a nurse's duty to his or her patient, if the patient establishes that a specific nurse actually rendered care, the nurse will be found to have assumed a duty to provide *reasonable care* for the patient. A nurse's failure to provide reasonable care subjects the nurse to civil liability for negligence, provided the patient proves that the failure caused damage or injury.

Lunsford v Board of Nurse Examiners[5] illustrates this principle. In this case, Donald Wayne Floyd arrived at the emergency department of Willacy County Hospital in Raymondville, Texas, complaining of chest pain and pressure and of pressure that radiated down his left arm. Mr. Floyd arrived at the emergency department accompanied by Francis Farrell. Ms. Farrell attempted to have Mr. Floyd examined by a physician who was sitting at the nurses' station in the emergency department. The physician told Ms. Farrell that Mr. Floyd would need to first be seen by a nurse. On seeing Nurse Lunsford, the physician instructed her to transfer Mr. Floyd to a neighboring hospital located 24 miles away in Harlingen, Texas, because the equipment that would likely be needed to treat Mr. Floyd was already in use by another patient.

Lunsford interviewed Mr. Floyd and suspected cardiac involvement. Because of the transfer instruction that she received from the physician, she instructed Ms. Farrell to drive with her flashers on and to speed to get to the neighboring hospital. Reportedly, Lunsford also asked Ms. Farrell if she knew cardiopulmonary resuscitation (CPR) and suggested that she might need to perform CPR at some point on the way. Unfortunately, within approximately 5 miles of the Harlingen emergency department, Mr. Farrell died from cardiac arrest.

A complaint was subsequently filed with the Texas Board of Nurse Examiners alleging that Lunsford had acted negligently. After a hearing on the matter, the Texas Board of Nurse Examiners suspended the license of Lunsford for 1 year. Lunsford appealed the decision. The appellate court heard the appeal and determined that Lunsford, as well as other nurses who are similarly situated, have a duty to evaluate the status of persons who are ill and seeking professional help. The court also determined that Lunsford, as well as other nurses, have a duty to implement care needed to stabilize a patient's condition and to prevent complications. According to this Texas Court of Appeals, Lunsford failed to act reasonably by breaching her duty to Mr. Floyd when she failed to do the following: assess him, inform the physician of the life-and-death nature of his condition, take appropriate action to stabilize him, and prevent his death. The court also pointed out that hospital policy or physician orders do not relieve a nurse of his or her duty to a patient.

Although the Texas Court of Appeals, as well as other courts throughout the United States, has determined that nurses have a duty to act reasonably when caring for patients, courts have limited the breadth of duties imposed on nurses in a number of specific instances. Nurses have been absolved of duty to assist patients who have no history of impaired mobility and of duty to intervene when a physician exceeds the scope of consent.

What constitutes reasonable care has been the focus of many cases filed against health care professionals and the hospitals in which they practice. For nurses, there seems to be an emerging trend. If the nurse reasonably executes every component of the nursing process by assessing, planning, implementing, and evaluating the care in accordance with the requisite standard of care, reasonable care will have been provided. However, if the nurse fails with regard to a single component of the nursing process, care provided to an acutely or critically ill patient will be deemed insufficient, unreasonable, and negligent.

A nurse's assessment-related failures include failure to assess and analyze the level of care needed by the patient and failure to ascertain the patient's wishes with regard to self-determination. Planning-related failures include failure of the nurse to diagnose appropriately. Implementation failures include failure

to communicate patient findings in a timely fashion; failure to take appropriate action; failure to document assessment findings, interventions, and the responses of the acutely or critically ill patient to those interventions; and failure to preserve patient privacy. Evaluation failures include failure to act as a patient advocate.

ASSESSMENT FAILURES

Failure to Assess and Analyze the Level of Care Needed by the Patient. Nurses caring for acutely and critically ill patients have a duty to assess and analyze the level of care needed by their patient. Where a nurse allegedly fails to fulfill this responsibility, liability for negligence may be threatened. *Brandon HMA, Inc. v Bradshaw*[6] demonstrates how courts handle failure to assess and analyze the level of care needed by acutely and critically ill patients.

In *Brandon,* Dawn Bradshaw contended that, while hospitalized at Rankin Medical Center (RMC) to be treated for bacterial pneumonia, she sustained permanent injuries because of negligence on the part of the nursing staff. The case was tried before a jury, and the jury agreed that Ms. Bradshaw sustained permanent, severe, oxygen deprivation–related brain damage because of the negligence of the nursing staff. They awarded her $9,000,000 in damages.

The alleged failure occurred after a chest tube had been inserted; on the night shift, a nurse allegedly failed to take vital signs between 11:00 PM and 3:30 AM until Ms. Bradshaw's condition had significantly worsened. At 3:30 AM, Ms. Bradshaw was found to be nauseated, disoriented, sweating profusely, and unable to follow verbal commands. Approximately 10 minutes later, she stopped breathing and had no pulse. A code was called, and CPR was administered. The code team arrived, and Ms. Bradshaw was revived. Subsequently, she was transferred to a rehabilitation facility specializing in the treatment of brain injury and filed this negligence cause of action against RMC.

To withstand allegations of failure to assess and analyze, it is important for nurses not only to assess and analyze the level of care needed by patients but also to document their assessment findings, as well as all actions taken to properly care for patients. Failure to assess and analyze the situation and to document the assessment findings, the interventions, and the patient's response to those interventions exposes the nurse and, as in the case of *Brandon,* the hospital to liability for negligence.

Failure to Ascertain a Patient's Wishes with Regard to Self-Determination. Nurses caring for acutely and critically ill patients have a legal and ethical obligation to act in accordance with a patient's wishes with regard to self-determination. This standard was made explicit when the United States Supreme Court issued its opinion in *Cruzan v Director, Missouri Department of Mental Health.*[7] In that case, the Supreme Court Justices ruled that competent adults have the right to decline any and all forms of medical intervention including life-saving or life-prolonging treatment. In the years following the issuance of this opinion, states have codified legislation that governs the creation, execution, and recognition of advanced directives. Nurses caring for the acutely and critically ill must know whether an advanced directive is in place for the patients for whom they are caring. If one is in place, the terms of the directive must be known, so that action consistent with those terms can be taken when and if the need arises.

Failure to abide by the patient's wishes can lead to disciplinary action and civil liability. *Anderson v St. Francis-St. George Hospital*[8] demonstrated how self-determination issues were dealt with in Ohio. In this case, Edward H. Winter was admitted to St. Francis-St. George Hospital because he was having chest pain and was fainting. After George E. Russo, Mr. Winter's treating physician, discussed treatment options with Mr. Winter, the physician entered a "no code" order in Mr. Winter's chart. Three days later, Mr. Winter began having ventricular tachycardia. A nurse defibrillated Mr. Winter, and, after he regained consciousness, he thanked the nurse for saving his life. When Russo was informed of Mr. Winter's condition, he ordered that lidocaine be administered. Two hours later, Mr. Winter experienced another ventricular tachycardia episode, but it resolved spontaneously.

The next day, Russo ordered the discontinuation of lidocaine and heart monitor. The day after that, Mr. Winter suffered a stroke that paralyzed his right side. Mr. Winter was eventually discharged, but his right side paralysis persisted until his death almost 2 years after his admission to St. Francis-St. George Hospital.

Before his death, Mr. Winter sued the hospital, alleging that it was negligent in failing to obey the "no code" order that had been issued. The Ohio Supreme Court eventually heard the case; the justices concluded that the interference in a person's right to die constituted a breach of the health care professional's duty to honor a patient's wishes. Despite that, the court ruled that Mr. Winter was not entitled to damages for the reasonably foreseeable damages associated with the unwanted resuscitation because he did not suffer harm as a result of the defibrillation.

PLANNING FAILURES

Failure to Appropriately Diagnose. Nurses caring for acutely and critically ill patients must plan effective courses of treatment. Such a course of treatment depends on a proper diagnosis. Historically, cases of failure to diagnose have been filed against physicians, rather than nurses. However, nurses who diagnose patient conditions may find themselves the target of a failure to diagnose case and need to be aware that liability may be imposed if the plan of care is based on an erroneous diagnosis.

IMPLEMENTATION FAILURES

Failure to Timely Communicate Patient Findings. Nurses spend more time with patients than any other health care professionals. Nurses caring for acutely and critically ill patients spend even more time with their patients than do nurses in most other specialty settings. As a result, nurses caring for acutely and critically ill patients are in the best position to promptly detect changes in a patient's condition. Detection, however, is only the first step. Nurses caring for acutely and critically ill patients must promptly communicate troublesome patient findings. Failure to properly communicate patient findings can be devastating for patients and can be the reason that patients file malpractice causes of action. *Denesia v St. Elizabeth Community Health Center*[9] exemplifies how courts handle these kinds of cases.

In *Denesia* it was alleged that the death of Lucille Denesia was wrongful and was the result of the nursing staff's administering anticoagulation therapy and then failing to timely notify the physician of an alarmingly high partial thromboplastin time (PTT). Initially, Lucille Denesia was thought to be suffering a transient ischemic attack because of her history of atrial fibrillation. As a result, anticoagulation therapy was ordered. This therapy included an injection of heparin, followed by an intravenous (IV) infusion of that same drug, and the administration of oral Coumadin. After this treatment regimen commenced, a PTT test was ordered, and 1.5 hours later, the laboratory called the results to the nurses' station, reporting that Ms. Denesia's PTT was greater than 200 seconds. The nurse caring for Ms. Denesia called the primary treating physician to report the values, but the answering service the nurse called never contacted the physician. Approximately 1 hour and 10 minutes after the nurse called the answering service, Ms. Denesia started experiencing a headache; the electrocardiogram monitor showed 6 seconds of atrial beats with no corresponding ventricular response. When the nurse entered her room, Ms. Denesia was found to be vomiting but alert. Approximately 7 minutes after that, the nurse called Ms. Denesia's cardiologist. The nurse could not remember what she told the cardiologist but stated that her practice would be to report the patient's headaches, the vomiting, and the results of the PTT test. The cardiologist contended that the nurse only reported that the PTT test had been done and that the nurse was waiting on the primary treating physician to return her call.

Approximately 1 hour and 15 minutes after the telephone conversation with the cardiologist, the nurse spoke with the primary treating physician. Again, she could not remember what she told him but said that her practice would be to report the PTT test result and the nausea and vomiting, as well as the headache Ms. Denesia was having. The primary treating physician testified that he was not informed of the PTT result but that he ordered the IV infusion of heparin to be reduced. Twenty minutes after this conversation, Ms. Denesia vomited again. Antinausea medication was administered, but Ms. Denesia vomited again about 45 minutes later.

After these two vomiting episodes, Ms. Denesia rested comfortably for approximately 2 hours and 5 minutes. When she awoke, she vomited again, became lethargic, could not sit up, and her right hand grasp was found to be stronger than her left. The nurse called the primary treating physician again. The heparin infusion was discontinued. It was at this point, the primary treating physician testified, that he learned of the abnormal PTT result. Twenty-five minutes later, Ms. Denesia was transferred to the intensive care unit because of continuing neurologic impairment. Two hours and 45 minutes later, her PTT was down to 27 seconds. However, Ms. Denesia lapsed into a coma and died from a massive cerebral hemorrhage.

Although a jury initially rendered a decision against the estate of Ms. Denesia, the case was appealed to the Supreme Court of Nebraska, where the justices ordered that the case be retried because prejudicial jury instructions were given during the first trial. For nurses caring for acutely and critically ill patients, it is imperative that interactions with physicians be documented, whether in person or over the telephone, as well as the information conveyed during those interactions. Had the nurse taken the time to document what she told the cardiologist and the primary treating physician, this litigation might have been avoided.

Failure to Take Appropriate Action.

Cases from across the country continue to affirm that it is the nurse's responsibility to take affirmative action when action is indicated. *Brookover v Mary Hitchcock Memorial Hospital*[10] is one such case. In *Brookover,* Ronald Brookover had significant seizure activity that resulted in his need for a corpus callosotomy, a surgical procedure performed in two separate operations. Three days after the second surgery, Mr. Brookover got out of bed, fell, and broke his hip. The medical record indicated that Mr. Brookover was unrestrained and had used his call light to indicate that he needed assistance. Based on this evidence, the hospital was found liable for Mr. Brookover's injury.

Another case of failure to take appropriate action was tried in Colorado. That case was *Garcia v United States.*[11] In *Garcia,* Candido Garcia was admitted to a Veterans Administration Medical Center for removal of a subdural hematoma. After surgery, he began making snorting noises and emitting white bubbles at his mouth. Mr. Garcia's wife reported the occurrence to the nurse caring for him. The nurse, Margaret John, reportedly told the Mrs. Garcia that the extent of her responsibility was to ensure that the surgically inserted drainage tubes were kept clear. Doctors from a neighboring hospital were eventually called but were not informed of the emergency nature of the situation. The result was that Mr. Garcia did not receive proper medical assistance for a period of about 45 to 50 minutes. Following medical intervention, including a return trip to the operating room, Mr. Garcia was quadriplegic. At trial, the hospital was found to be negligent and liable for the damages sustained by Candido Garcia; more than $2.3 million in damages, interest, and the cost of litigation was awarded to Mr. Garcia and his wife. In reaching its decision, the court found that the nursing staff should have recognized the emergency nature of the situation and taken proper steps to notify the attending physician.

Failure to take appropriate action in cases involving acutely and critically ill patients has included not only physician-notification issues but also failure to follow physician orders,[12,13] failure to appropriately administer medication,[14-16] and failure to properly treat.[14] To avoid allegations of failure to take appropriate action, nurses caring for acutely and critically ill patients need to recognize signs and symptoms of complications and patient compromise. Nurses must also ensure that those signs and symptoms are timely communicated to the physician and take other affirmative action that is authorized and appropriate. Patient findings, interventions and actions taken, and patient responses to those interventions must be documented.

Failure to Document.

Nurses caring for acutely and critically ill patients are required not only to take appropriate action but also to accurately document their findings, interventions performed, and patients' response to those interventions. Failure to thoroughly and accurately document any aspect of care gives rise to negligence causes of action. *Haney v Alexander,*[17] a case from North Carolina, demonstrates how courts and juries deal with a nurse's failure to properly document.

In *Haney,* a nurse purportedly failed to take appropriate action and failed to properly document care rendered. Originally, the trial court dismissed the hospital from the case. The physician-defendants later settled with the family. The family appealed the trial court's decision to dismiss the hospital, and, citing the negligence of the nurse, the court of appeals agreed that the hospital should not have been dismissed and that a jury trial should be commenced.

In this case, a nurse caring for a patient who was experiencing atrial fibrillation failed to take, record, and communicate all of the patient's vital signs and failed to properly document the order and administration of Librium. Reportedly, Librium had already been administered, but the on-call physician was told that Librium had not been administered, so the physician again ordered that Librium be given. The nurse gave the medication, and 45 minutes later, the patient was found dead.

In reversing the trial court's previous decision to dismiss the hospital, the court of appeals concluded that the nurse was negligent in several respects. Specifically, the court of appeals observed that the events that led to the double administration of Librium could have prevented the patient from being able to communicate his worsening condition and receiving life-saving medical assistance.

Haney and *Denesia* are indicative of the need for nurses caring for acutely and critically ill patients to thoroughly document the care that is given, interventions and actions taken, and the response of the patient to those interventions and actions. Failure to thoroughly document opens the door for patient-plaintiffs to allege that the absence of documentation signals a breach of the standard of care.

Failure to Preserve Patient Privacy.

Nurses have a duty to preserve patient privacy. State and federal statutes and case law affirm this duty. *Doe v Ohio State University Hospital and Clinics*[18] explores the issue. In *Doe,* a nurse taking care of a patient who was positive for the human immunodeficiency virus (HIV) wrote his HIV status on a laboratory requisition slip in the "other test" section of the form. This was done so that laboratory personnel could be alerted to the patient's HIV status. The patient was to have a complete blood count and potassium level drawn prior to a lithotripsy to remove kidney stones. The laboratory staff interpreted the notation made by the nurse as an instruction to perform an HIV screen, and not a message regarding the patient's HIV status. The patient found out that the HIV screen had been done, and was outraged that the HIV testing had been done without his consent. This facility had a policy that prohibited HIV testing without informed consent being obtained by the physician.

The case was ultimately dismissed, but it serves as a reminder to guard the privacy of every patient. Nurses can ensure that the privacy of acutely and critically ill patients is protected by following privacy-related regulations, policies, and procedures and by refraining from having discussions about specific patients with anyone except other health care professionals involved in the care of the patient. When discussing specific patients with other health care professionals, it is imperative that patient-specific discussions occur in non public settings. Discussions about specific patients are never appropriate in public areas such as elevators, cafeterias, gift shops, and parking lots.

EVALUATION FAILURES

Failure to Act as a Patient Advocate. From admission to discharge, nurses have a duty to act as a patient advocate. For nurses caring for acutely and critically ill patients, this duty imposes the responsibility to evaluate the care that is being given to patients. The landmark failure to advocate case was *Darling v Charleston Community Memorial Hospital,*[19] a case decided by the Illinois Supreme Court in 1965.

In this case, Dorrence Darling II was an 18-year-old athlete who broke his leg playing football. He was taken to Charleston Community Memorial Hospital for treatment. Dorrence was placed in traction, and his broken leg was placed in a plaster cast. A heat cradle was used to dry the cast. Shortly after the cast was applied, Dorrence began to complain of severe pain in the broken leg. Dorrence's toes that protruded from the cast became swollen and dark in color and eventually became cold and insensitive to tactile stimulation.

The day after Dorrence was admitted, his treating physician, John R. Alexander, notched the cast around Dorrence's toes. The next day, Alexander cut the cast approximately 3 inches from the foot toward Dorrence's knee. The day after that, Alexander used a Stryker saw to split the sides of the cast and cut both sides of Dorrence's broken leg. By this time, blood and other drainage had been noted by the nursing staff. The room in which Dorrence was staying became filled with a noxious odor.

Fourteen days after his admission to Charleston Community Memorial Hospital, Dorrence was transferred to Barnes Hospital in St. Louis, Missouri. There he was cared for by surgeon Fred Reynolds. After multiple attempts to save the leg of Dorrence Darling, Reynolds finally had to amputate the lower leg approximately 8 inches below the knee.

Subsequently, Charleston Community Hospital and John R. Alexander were sued. The hospital, through the actions of the nursing staff and John R. Alexander, was alleged to have failed to treat Dorrence consistently with the requisite standard of care. With regard to the nursing staff, Darling alleged that they were negligent in assessing his deteriorating circulatory condition in accordance with hospital policy and procedure and that they failed to report the developments to the medical staff or hospital administration. A settlement was reached with the doctor, John R. Alexander, so the case against the hospital was presented to an Illinois jury. After listening to the evidence, the jury returned a verdict against the hospital for $150,000. The hospital appealed the decision, and the Supreme Court of Illinois eventually heard the appeal. In affirming the jury verdict, the Illinois Supreme Court justices determined that a jury

could have reasonably concluded that the nurses involved in the care and treatment of Dorrence Darling were negligent in assessing his circulatory status. According to the court, if the nursing staff had promptly recognized that circulatory compromise was occurring, steps could have been taken to prevent the irreversible effects of prolonged inadequate circulation. Had they recognized the significance of the symptoms they were seeing, the nursing staff could have exercised their duty to inform hospital authorities so that appropriate action could be taken. Because they failed to act as patient advocate, Dorrence lost his leg, and the hospital was liable for their failure.

Although the *Darling* case was decided in 1965, courts continue to hold that all nurses, including those caring for acutely and critically ill patients, have a nondelegable duty to act as patient advocate. Failure to act as patient advocate exposes the nurse to substantial liability and, more importantly, exposes patients to life-altering and life-ending complications that could have been avoided.

BREACH

Breach is the failure to act consistently with applicable standards of care. For a nurse to be found negligent, the patient-plaintiff must establish that the nurse had a duty to provide care and that the nurse failed to provide care consistent with those standards. Moreover, the nurse's failure, or breach, must have caused the damages about which the patient-plaintiff seeks redress. An Idaho case exemplifies the courts' willingness to conclude that breach did not occur where the actions of nurses met or exceeded the standard of care.

In *Sparks v St. Luke's Regional Medical Center,*[20] the family of Thomas Sparks sued St. Luke's Regional Medical Center and treating physicians, alleging that their negligence resulted in Thomas Sparks' sustaining brain damage after he was extubated and after he experienced cardiac arrest. The trial court granted the motion by St. Luke's to have judgment entered in its favor, and Sparks appealed the matter to the Idaho Supreme Court.

The Idaho Supreme Court reviewed the evidence presented by both parties and concluded that the nurses met the requisite standard of care. Therefore, it found that no breach occurred. In fact, the court pointed out that evidence presented by Thomas Sparks recognized that the standard of care regarding extubation and subsequent hospital care was met by the St. Luke's personnel. As a result, the ruling of the trial court was affirmed.

Sparks demonstrated that courts will consider whether something a nurse did or failed to do provided the requisite standard of care. The applicable Nurse Practice Acts, professional practice standards, job descriptions, and organizational policies, procedures, protocols, and pathways, together with other reference sources including case law, journal articles, textbooks, and other manuscripts, determine the standard of care.

Nurse Practice Acts. Nurse Practice Acts (NPAs) provide statutory authority for the practice of nursing in every state within the United States. Nurses, as licensed and regulated health care professionals, must abide by the requirements of the applicable practice act. Failure to act consistently with NPA requirements exposes a nurse to civil liability in negligence or malpractice causes of action because the statutory standard was breached.

In NPAs, the activities in which a registered nurse may engage are referred to as a nurse's *scope of practice*. Typically, scope of practice activities for registered nurses include assessing the health status of individuals and groups; establishing a nursing diagnosis and goals to meet identified health care needs; creating and implementing a plan of care; prescribing and implementing interventions consistent with the plan of care; delegating nursing interventions to qualified others as the practice act permits; providing for the maintenance of safe and effective nursing care rendered directly or indirectly and evaluating patient responses to interventions; teaching the theory and practice of nursing; and collaborating with other health care professionals in the delivery of health care services.[21]

Professional Practice Standards. Actions that are consistent with professional practice standards will be evidence that the nurse did not breach his or her duty to patients. Therefore, it is important to know what professional practice standards expect of nurses generally, as well as what is expected of nurses practicing in specialty settings. Standards of practice and standards of professional performance for nurses have been issued by the ANA and the AACN. All nurses must practice in a manner that is consistent with the standards issued by the ANA (Box 3-1). Nurses caring for acutely and critically ill patients must also practice in accordance with the practice specialty standards issued by the AACN (Box 3-2). These standards provide guidance for nurses, and they provide definitive guidance in courtrooms. In *Koeniger v Eckrich,*[22] standards promulgated by the ANA were used in a case in which the plaintiff alleged that standards of care were breached.

In *Koeniger,* Winnfred Scoblic was admitted to Dakota Midland Hospital for surgical correction of incontinence. Two days later, J.A. Eckrich performed the surgery. After surgery, Ms. Scoblic had a temperature that fluctuated. On the day of discharge, Ms. Scoblic's temperature was 100.2° F. Despite her temperature, Ms. Scoblic was discharged. Sixteen days after her original surgery, Ms. Scoblic was readmitted because of a fever and severe abdominal pain. She was diagnosed with septicemia. Two days later, Ms. Scoblic was transferred to the University of Minnesota Hospital. She died from multiple organ failure several weeks later.

On behalf of Ms. Scoblic, her daughter Patricia Koeniger filed a malpractice cause of action contending that the care rendered to her mother deviated from the standard of care. An expert retained by Koeniger used the standards published by the ANA and other general nursing treatises to conclude that the nursing staff failed to adhere to standards of care applicable to Ms. Scoblic as a postoperative urologic patient. At the trial court level, the case was dismissed. It was subsequently

---

BOX 3-1   NURSING: SCOPE AND STANDARDS OF PRACTICE

The registered nurse does the following:

STANDARDS OF PRACTICE

Assessment
Collects comprehensive data pertinent to the patient's health or the situation

Diagnosis
Analyzes assessment data to determine the diagnoses or issues

Outcomes Identification
Identifies expected outcomes for an individual patient or situation plan

Planning
Develops a plan that prescribes strategies and alternatives to attain expected outcomes

Implementation
Implements the identified plan, including care coordination, health teaching and health promotion, consultation, prescriptive authority, and treatment and evaluation

Evaluation
Evaluates progress toward outcomes attainment

STANDARDS OF PROFESSIONAL PERFORMANCE

Quality of Practice
Systematically enhances the quality and effectiveness of nursing practice

Education
Attains knowledge and competency that reflects current nursing practice

Professional Practice Evaluation
Evaluates one's own nursing practice in relation to professional practice standards and guidelines, relevant statutes, rules, and regulations

Collegiality
Interacts with and contributes to the professional development of peers and colleagues

Collaboration
Collaborates with patient, family, and others in the conduct of nursing practice

Ethics
Integrates ethical principles in all areas of practice

Research
Integrates research findings into practice

Resource Utilization
Considers factors related to safety, effectiveness, cost, and impact on practice in the planning and delivery of nursing services

Leadership
Provides leadership in the professional practice setting and the profession

From American Nurses Association (ANA): *Nursing: scope and standards of practice,* Washington, DC, 2004, ANA.

BOX 3-2 **STANDARDS FOR ACUTE AND CRITICAL CARE NURSING**

STANDARDS OF CARE FOR ACUTE AND CRITICAL CARE NURSING PRACTICE

Standard 1: Assessment

The nurse caring for the acutely and critically ill patient collects relevant data pertinent to the patient's health or situation.

Measurement Criteria

1. Data are collected from the patient, family, other health care providers, and the community, as appropriate, to develop a holistic picture of the patient's needs.
2. The priority of data collection activities is driven by the patient's characteristics related to immediate condition and anticipated needs.
3. Pertinent and sufficient data are collected using appropriate evidence-based assessment techniques and instruments.
4. Analytical models and problem-solving tools are used.
5. Relevant data are documented.
6. Relevant data are communicated to other healthcare providers.

Standard 2: Diagnosis

The nurse caring for the acutely and critically ill patient analyzes the assessment data in determining diagnosis and care issues.

Measurement Criteria

1. Diagnoses and care issues are derived from the assessment data.
2. Diagnoses and care issues are validated throughout the nursing interactions with the patient, family, other health care providers, the community, and across the healthcare system when possible and appropriate.
3. Diagnoses and care issues are prioritized and documented in a manner that facilitates prioritizing outcomes and developing or modifying the plan.

Standard 3: Outcomes Identification

The nurse caring for the acutely and critically ill patient identifies outcomes for the patient or the patient's situation.

Measurement Criteria

1. Outcomes are derived from actual or potential diagnoses and care issues.
2. Outcomes are formulated in collaboration with the patient, family, and other health care providers, in relation to the level of participation in care and decision making.
3. Outcomes recognize, appreciate, and incorporate differences.
4. Outcomes are attainable in relation to resources available; outcomes consider associated risks, benefits, current evidence, clinical expertise, and cost.
5. Outcomes provide direction for continuity of care.
6. Outcomes are modified on the basis of changes in patient characteristics or evaluation of the situation.
7. Outcomes are documented as measurable goals.

Standard 4: Planning

The nurse caring for the acutely and critically ill patient develops a plan that prescribes interventions to attain outcomes.

Measurement Criteria

1. The plan is individualized and considers patient characteristics and the situation.
2. The plan is developed collaboratively with the patient, family, and healthcare providers in a way that promotes each member's contribution toward achieving the outcomes.
3. The plan reflects current best evidence.
4. The plan provides for continuity of care, matching the nurse's competencies with the patient's characteristics.
5. The plan establishes priorities for care.
6. The plan includes strategies for promotion and restoration of health and prevention of further illness, injury, and disease.
7. The plan considers economic impact and resources available.

Standard 5: Implementation

The nurse caring for the acutely and critically ill patient implements the plan, coordinates care delivery, and employs strategies to promote health and a safe environment.

Measurement Criteria

1. Interventions are delivered in a manner that minimizes complications and life-threatening situations.
2. The patient and family participate in implementing the plan according to their level of participation and decision-making capabilities.
3. Interventions are responsive to the uniqueness of the patient and family and create a compassionate and therapeutic environment, with the aim to promote comfort and prevent suffering.
4. The implemented plan and modifications are documented.
5. Collaboration to implement the plan occurs with the patient, family, healthcare providers, and the healthcare system.
6. The plan facilitates learning for patients, families, nursing staff, other members of the healthcare team, and the community including but not limited to health teaching, health promotion, and disease management according to patient characteristics.

Standard 6: Evaluation

The nurse caring for the acutely and critically ill patient evaluates progress toward attaining outcomes.

Measurement Criteria

1. Evaluation is systematic and ongoing using evidence-based techniques and instruments.
2. The team of patient, family, and healthcare providers is involved in the evaluation process as appropriate.
3. Evaluation of the effectiveness of interventions toward achieving the desired outcome occurs.
4. Evaluation occurs within an appropriate time frame after interventions are initiated.
5. Ongoing assessment data are used to revise the diagnoses, outcomes, and plan as needed.
6. Results of the evaluation are documented.

STANDARDS OF PROFESSIONAL PERFORMANCE

Standard 1: Quality of Practice

The nurse caring for the acutely and critically ill patient systematically evaluates and seeks to improve the quality and effectiveness of nursing practice.

Measurement Criteria

1. The nurse participates in clinical inquiry through quality improvement activities.
2. The nurse uses systems thinking to initiate changes in nursing practice and the healthcare delivery system.
3. The nurse ensures that quality improvement activities incorporate the patient's and family's beliefs, values, and preferences as appropriate.
4. The nurse questions and evaluates practice in an ongoing process, providing informed practice and innovation through research and experiential learning.
5. The nurse identifies organizational systems barriers to quality care and patient outcomes.
6. The nurse collects data to monitor the quality and effectiveness of nursing practice.

Continued

BOX 3-2 STANDARDS FOR ACUTE AND CRITICAL CARE NURSING—*cont'd*

The nurse develops, implements, evaluates, and updates policies, procedures, and/or guidelines to improve the quality and effectiveness of nursing practice.

Standard 2: Professional Practice Evaluation

The nurse caring for the acutely and critically ill patient evaluates his or her own nursing practice in relation to professional practice standards, institutional guidelines, relevant statutes, rules, and regulations.

Measurement Criteria

1. The nurse engages in a self-assessment and/or formal performance appraisal on a regular basis, identifying areas of strength as well as areas where professional development would be beneficial.
2. The nurse seeks and reflects on constructive feedback regarding his or her own competencies from the team of patient, family, and other healthcare providers.
3. The nurse takes action to achieve performance goals.

Standard 3: Education

The nurse acquires and maintains current knowledge and competency in the care of acutely and critically ill patients.

Measurement Criteria

1. The nurse participates in ongoing learning activities to acquire and refine knowledge and skills needed to care for acutely and critically ill patients and their families.
2. The nurse seeks learning opportunities that reflect evidence-based practice in order to maintain clinical skills and competencies needed to care for acutely and critically ill patients and their families.
3. The nurse participates in ongoing learning activities related to professional practice.
4. The nurse maintains professional records that provide evidence of competency and lifelong learning.

Standard 4: Collegiality

The nurse caring for the acutely and critically ill patient interacts with and contributes to the professional development of peers and other healthcare providers as colleagues.

Measurement Criteria

1. The nurse shares knowledge, skills, and experiences with peers and colleagues.
2. The nurse provides peers and colleagues with constructive feedback regarding their practice.
3. The nurse interacts with peers and colleagues to enhance his or her own professional practice and promote optimal patient outcomes.
4. The nurse contributes to a supportive and healthy work environment that is conducive to the education of healthcare professionals.
5. The nurse contributes to a healthy work environment by working with others in a way that promotes mutual respect and meaningful recognition of each person's contribution.

Standard 5: Ethics

The nurse's decisions and actions are carried out in an ethical manner in all areas of practice.

Measurement Criteria

1. The nurse's practice is guided by the ANA *Code of Ethics for Nurses with Interpretive Statements,* the AACN Ethic of Care, and ethical principles.

2. The nurse maintains patient confidentiality within legal and regulatory parameters.
3. The nurse works on another's behalf and represents the concerns of patients, their families, and the community.
4. The nurse delivers care in a nonjudgmental and nondiscriminatory manner that meets the diverse needs, strengths, and weaknesses of the patient and preserves patient autonomy, dignity, and rights.
5. The nurse uses available resources in formulating ethical decisions.
6. The nurse demonstrates a commitment to self-care and self-advocacy.
7. The nurse reports illegal, incompetent, or impaired practices.

Standard 6: Collaboration

The nurse caring for the acutely and critically ill patient uses skilled communication to collaborate with the team, of patient, family, and healthcare providers in providing patient care in a safe, healing, humane, and caring environment.

Measurement Criteria

1. The nurse uses skilled communication to foster true collaboration.
2. The nurse partners with others to effect change and generate optimal outcomes through knowledge of the patient or situation.
3. The nurse commits to establishing and maintaining a healthy work environment.
4. The nurse initiates referrals as appropriate to promote continuity of care.
5. The nurse collaborates with the patient's family and significant others to promote effective transition across care settings.

Standard 7: Research/Clinical Inquiry

The nurse caring for the acutely and critically ill patient uses clinical inquiry and integrates research findings into practice.

Measurement Criteria

1. The nurse continually questions and evaluates practice and uses best available evidence, including research findings, to guide practice decisions.
2. The nurse participates in activities to support clinical inquiry as appropriate to the nurse's skills, knowledge, and experience.

Standard 8: Resource Utilization

The nurse caring for the acutely and critically ill patient considers factors related to safety, effectiveness, cost, and impact in planning and delivering nursing services.

Measurement Criteria

1. The nurse considers factors related to safety, effectiveness, availability, cost, and impact on outcomes when choosing among practice options.
2. The nurse assists the patient and family in identifying and securing appropriate and available services to address health-related needs according to resource availability.
3. The nurse assigns or delegates aspects of care as defined by the state nurse practice acts, based on an assessment of the needs and condition of the patient, the potential for harm, the stability of the patient's condition, the predictability of the outcome, the availability and competence of the healthcare provider, and the availability of resources.
5. The nurse assists the patient and family to become informed consumers by facilitating learning of the options, alternatives, risks, benefits, and costs of treatment and care.

Modified from American Association of Critical-Care Nurses: *Standards for acute and critical care nursing practice,* Aliso Viejo, California, 2008, AACN.

heard and reversed by the South Dakota Supreme Court. The South Dakota Supreme Court ordered that a trial occur so that jurors could have an opportunity to determine whether the defendants' actions caused the alleged wrongful death of Ms. Scoblic.

Job Descriptions and Contracts. Although standards of care are usually derived outside of any single institution, job descriptions and contracts delineating the terms of employment may be institution specific. A nurse's job description or employment contract may contain provisions that require a nurse to act or to refrain from acting in a specific manner and within a specific period of time. Failure to adhere to those provisions could give rise to negligence causes of action wherein the patient-plaintiff asserts that the nurse failed to act in accordance with his or her job description or employment contract. Accordingly, job descriptions and employment contracts must be reflective of the standard of care, and expectations must be articulated in a manner that is reasonable.

Policies, Procedures, Protocols, and Pathways. Nurses caring for acutely and critically ill patients are required to act in a manner that is consistent with organizational policies, procedures, protocols, and clinical pathways. Failure to act consistently with organizational policies, procedures, and protocols may result in liability if a patient is harmed because of the failure. Two cases are illustrative: *Teffeteller v University of Minnesota,*[23] and *Ress v Abbott Northwestern.*[24] In *Teffeteller,* a critically ill pediatric patient died from narcotic toxicity because a nurse failed to follow the applicable protocol. In *Ress,* Randy Ress, an intensive care nurse, contested being terminated. The hospital claimed that he was terminated because he failed to act in a manner consistent with past instruction, warning, and applicable protocols after he lavaged an endotracheal tube with iced, nonsterile saline and subsequently refused to promptly obtain a chest radiograph for a patient with gross hemoptysis. In upholding the termination decision, the Minnesota Supreme Court concluded that Randy Ress had acted with willful disregard for the interests of Abbott Northwestern and that he was disqualified from receiving unemployment benefits.

CAUSATION

In negligence causes of action focusing on care rendered by nurses, patient-plaintiffs must prove that the nurse breached his or her duty to the patient and that the breach caused the patient to sustain injuries or damages for which he or she seeks monetary remuneration. Causation, as an element of negligence, is a pivotal element in civil cases filed against nurses. If causation is not proved by plaintiffs, there can be no recovery.

It should be no surprise that nursing negligence cases focus on causation. If patient-plaintiffs prove that the health care organization, or the nurse practicing in that setting, did or failed to do something that caused an injury, they have met their burden of proof. If, on the other hand, they fail to establish that some act or omission directly resulted in the injuries for which they are seeking compensation, or if the health care organization or the nurse shows that the complained-of injury was the result

of something other than an action or omission falling below the standard of care, recovery will be denied. *McMullen v Ohio State University Hospitals*[25] dealt with the causation issue and was ultimately decided by the Ohio Supreme Court.

In *McMullen,* a patient had been intubated and placed on a ventilator. Three days after she was intubated, her oxygen saturation level suddenly dropped, as did her blood pressure, and she became cyanotic and dyspneic. The patient also developed a squeak, which the nurse thought was a cuff leak on the endotracheal tube. The nurse believed that the patient was dying and made a "stat" page so that on-call physicians would be notified. Before the arrival of the physicians, the nurse removed the patient's endotracheal tube. When the physicians arrived, they attempted to reintubate the patient. It took more than 20 minutes for their reintubation attempts to be successful. The patient never resumed consciousness and died 7 days later.

The patient's estate brought a wrongful death cause of action against the Ohio State University Hospitals. The case went to trial, and damages were awarded to the patient's estate. Ohio State University Hospitals appealed the award to the Franklin County Court of Appeals. The Court of Appeals reversed the award, and the patient's estate then appealed the case to the Ohio Supreme Court. That Court, among other things, concluded that the decision of the Court of Appeals was erroneous and had to be reversed, and that actions of the nurse directly caused the ultimate harm sustained by the patient. According to the Ohio Supreme Court, the nurse's removal of the patient's endotracheal tube was negligent and set into motion a chain of events that directly caused the patient to die.

DAMAGES

The fourth element of negligence is damages. Damages are derived from the harm or injury suffered by the acutely or critically ill patient and are calculated as a dollar amount. In order for liability to be imposed against a nurse caring for an acutely or critically ill patient, that patient must prove that something the nurse did or failed to do was inconsistent with the standard of care and that the inconsistency caused harm or injury for which the patient should be compensated.

The number of nurses being named defendants in these cases is increasing. Accordingly, nurses caring for acutely and critically ill patients need to carefully consider whether to purchase professional liability insurance and, if so, the amount and type of coverage that is needed. Damage trends suggest that nurses caring for acutely and critically ill patients need to consider obtaining substantial insurance coverage.

NEGLIGENCE PER SE

Most courts have ruled that a statutory violation is negligence per se. Negligence per se allows patient-plaintiffs to conclusively establish a presumption of negligence and breach of a nurse's duty to the acutely or critically ill patient. However, a few courts have held that statutory violations give rise to a presumption with regard to the duty and breach components of a negligence cause of action, or that the statutory violation provides only threshold evidence of negligence. Regardless of the jurisdiction, however, statutory violations do assist patient-plaintiffs in proving that negligence occurred. This was the case in *Lama v Borras.*[26] In that case, a patient acquired a postoperative infection, and the nurse failed to recognize the associated signs and symptoms. The court concluded that the nurse was negligent and that the doctrine of negligence per se applied because the nurse's failure was a violation of Puerto Rico Health Regulations.

MALPRACTICE

Malpractice is professional misconduct or the failure to meet the requisite standard of care. Whereas negligence may be committed by anyone, malpractice requires the alleged wrongdoer to have special standing as a professional. If an individual acts negligently in a personal rather than a professional capacity, that individual is subject to liability for negligence rather than malpractice. If the wrongdoer is a nurse caring for acutely and critically ill patients and is accused of acting or failing to act in a manner consistent with the standard of care, that nurse is subject to liability for professional negligence or malpractice.

In civil cases alleging wrongdoing by health care professionals, the terms "malpractice" and "negligence" are used interchangeably, although there are courts that distinguish between the two causes of action. The malpractice-negligence distinction was addressed in *Candler General Hospital Inc. v McNorrill.*[27] In that case, the court concluded that malpractice was merely a professional negligence act. According to the court, when a nurses is acting in their professional capacity, she or he is subject to malpractice causes of action if patients assert that the nurse failed to meet the requisite standard of care.

In *Gould v NY City Health and Hospital,*[28] the court looked at the elements that must be proved in a malpractice case and determined that there were three duties inherent in a malpractice cause of action. They were (1) to possess the requisite knowledge and skill possessed by an average member of the profession; (2) to exercise reasonable and ordinary care in the application of professional knowledge and skill; and (3) to use best judgment in the application of professional knowledge and skill. These duties are consistent with the duties nurses have in traditional negligence-based causes of action.

Griffin v The Methodist Hospital[29] demonstrated that most courts treat malpractice cases like negligence cases. The only difference is that malpractice cases involve individuals with some special standing. In *Griffin,* Sharon Ann Griffin and her husband Dennis Griffin filed a malpractice cause of action against The Methodist Hospital and Sharon's treating physicians. They alleged that Sharon sustained damages because of the negligent treatment of her treating physicians and nursing staff while she was hospitalized at The Methodist Hospital. Specifically, Sharon alleged that her development of an Achilles tendon contraction was the result of negligence. The Methodist Hospital contended that, despite Sharon's development of foot drop,

the staff fully complied with applicable standards of care. As a result, the hospital asked the judge to dismiss the matter. The judge agreed. Sharon and her husband appealed the case to the Court of Appeals. After reviewing the case, the Court of Appeals determined that the case should not have been dismissed and ordered that the matter be slated for trial.

Candler, Gould, and *Griffin* are similar and suggest that professional negligence and malpractice causes of action are treated similarly. Whether sued for professional negligence or malpractice, nurses will be required to defend their actions or alleged failures to act by showing how their actions or inactions were consistent with the standard of care.

WRONGFUL DEATH

Wrongful death causes of action are filed by the survivors of patients who allege that the patient died because of the negligence of health care organizations or health care professionals. *Manning v Twin Falls Clinic & Hospital*[30] provides insight into how courts handle wrongful death cases.

In *Manning,* the trial court determined that the nurse failed to exercise reasonable care, and the nurse was deemed negligent in the death of Daryl Manning, a 67-year-old man. Mr. Manning had been admitted to the hospital in the last stages of chronic obstructive pulmonary disease, hypoxemia, and increased carbon dioxide retention and was receiving continuous supplemental oxygen by a nasal cannula. On his admission to the hospital, Mr. Manning was classified as a "no code." His condition steadily deteriorated, and Virginia L. Anderson, LPN, discontinued Mr. Manning's supplemental oxygen and began to transfer him to a private room. The family requested that oxygen be administered during the move, but the nurse declined to apply it, citing the proximity between the patient's current location and the private room. After the bed had been moved approximately 15 feet, Mr. Manning stopped breathing. Resuscitation was attempted, but when the physician who was aware of Mr. Manning's "no code" status arrived, resuscitative measures were discontinued. The family sued the hospital and two nurses. One nurse, Donna Gay Austin, RN, was relieved of all liability, but the jury determined that Virginia L. Anderson, LPN, was negligent in transferring Mr. Manning without using supplemental oxygen and awarded the Manning family compensatory, emotional distress, and punitive damages.

For families and health care professionals, wrongful death cases are among the most traumatic. It is in these cases that the life-and-death nature of the health care experience is exposed. In reviewing these kinds of cases, one learns that what is at issue is rarely the use, misuse, or malfunction of sophisticated, cutting-edge technology or the miscalculation of a complex formula. On the contrary, a review of wrongful death cases suggests that the alleged failure at issue is typically much more basic and has more to do with paying attention. For instance, failure to thoroughly assess a patient, to take vital signs, to properly administer medication, or to administer portable oxygen to a respiratory-compromised patient has been the focus of most of the wrongful death cases discussed in this chapter. To avoid wrongful death liability, it is imperative that nurses caring for acutely and critically ill patients pay attention, recognize the signs and symptoms of complications and compromise, and take authorized affirmative action to protect the patient.

DEFAMATION

Defamation causes of action can be filed against health care professionals if individuals believe that something the health care professional said or wrote injured the patient's reputation. Any communication may be considered defamatory if it compromises a person's decency, respect for other, integrity, or reputation. If the defamatory communication is in writing, *libel* has been committed. If, on the other hand, the defamatory communication is verbal, *slander* has been committed.

To be successful, individuals alleging that they have been defamed must prove that the defamatory communication came from the defendant and that the defamatory language pertained specifically to the plaintiff. The defamatory communication also must have been published to a third person, and the plaintiff must have suffered damage to his or her reputation. If the case involves a public figure or a matter of public concern, the plaintiff must prove that the defamatory communication was false and was made with malice. *Meuser v Rocky Mountain Hospital*[31] was a case in which a nurse-plaintiff alleged that a hospital administrator had defamed her.

In *Meuser,* Virginia T. Meuser alleged that the hospital administrator, Robert Pierce, defamed her in a letter that was published to other employees and in a statement to employees. In reviewing Meuser's defamation allegations, a Colorado Court of Appeals concluded that she failed to present clear and convincing evidence that the allegedly defamatory statements made by Pierce were false or that the defendant hospital or administrator entertained serious doubts about the truth of the statements. As a result, the trial court did not have jurisdiction to resolve the defamation claims.

ASSAULT AND BATTERY

Assault and battery are two separate torts that can be alleged by patients. Assault is any intentional act that creates reasonable apprehension of immediate harmful or offensive contact with the plaintiff. With assault, no actual contact is necessary. Battery, on the other hand, is any intentional act that brings about actual harmful or offensive contact with the plaintiff. In health care cases, assault occurs if a patient fears harmful or offensive touching. Harmful or offensive touching occurs if the patient has not consented to the touch. Battery occurs if the health care professional actually touches the patient in an unauthorized manner. Sexual misconduct, operating on an unauthorized body part, and removing the wrong limb constitute battery behaviors. In addition to battery, assault may be alleged in these instances if the patient was aware that he or she was going to be touched in a manner not authorized by informed consent.

Historically, assault and battery allegations have been treated differently than traditional negligence-based causes of actions.

Because assault and battery are considered intentional acts, these offenses have not been routinely covered by professional liability insurers. However, two cases recently decided by the Alabama and South Dakota Supreme Courts indicated that some assault and battery cases may be considered malpractice. In Alabama the case was *Mock v Allen,*[32] whereas in South Dakota the case was *Martinmaas v Engelmann.*[33]

LOSS OF CONSORTIUM

In addition to alleging negligence or malpractice, plaintiffs and their family members may allege loss of consortium if their relationships with their spouses, children, or parents have suffered because of the professional negligence of the health care organization or the nurse. Loss of consortium claims are based on the deprivation of an individual's right to enjoy the cooperation, company, affection, love, and aid of others, and they are typically filed by family members of patients who have allegedly been treated negligently by health care professionals.

EMOTIONAL DISTRESS

Like loss of consortium claims, emotional distress claims can be added as causes of action in cases alleging that malpractice or negligence has occurred. Emotional distress claims may be classified as intentional or negligent. Intentional emotional distress claims assert that the defendant acted in a way that intentionally caused emotional distress. Negligent emotional distress claims do not contemplate an intentional act on the part of defendant health care providers.

Regardless of the classification, emotional distress claims are alleged when an act is considered to be outrageous. Outrageous acts are those that are reckless and intolerable and have a tendency to shock the conscience. Because of the extreme nature of emotional distress claims, they are difficult for patients to prove.

OTHER ISSUES GIVING RISE TO CIVIL LITIGATION

Although the issues discussed in this section could have been inserted and discussed as examples of negligence or malpractice, the nature of these cases is such that special attention is warranted. These issues include the respiratory management of acutely and critically ill patients, liability associated with blood transfusions, needlestick injuries, infection control, and informed consent.

RESPIRATORY MANAGEMENT

The management of an acutely or critically ill patient's respiratory status gives rise to more litigation than does the management of any other physiologic system.

In *Allman v Holleman,*[34] Linda Allman was a 28-year-old patient who had been hospitalized because of a ruptured spleen.

After surgery, Ms. Allman's endotracheal tube (ETT) became dislodged, and she was reintubated. Subsequently the ETT became dislodged again, and efforts to revive her were unsuccessful. This case was filed, and a jury returned a verdict in favor of Ms. Allman.

Six years later, *Courteau v Dodd*[35] was published. In *Courteau*, the nasotracheal tube inserted into a nostril of a 20-year-old patient who sustained injury in a diving accident became dislodged. As a result, the patient suffered a myocardial infarction and massive brain damage. This case was filed and then dismissed because of insufficient expert testimony.

In a 1993 case, *Dixon v Taylor*,[36] Willie L. Dixon was admitted to Watauga County Hospital for treatment of pneumonia. Later that day, she was transferred to the intensive care unit because her condition began to deteriorate. In the early morning hours, just after she was transferred to the intensive care unit, a Code Blue was called because Mrs. Dixon was in cardiac and respiratory arrest. During the code, she was intubated and her physiologic condition stabilized. Approximately 17.5 hours after she was intubated, a critical care nurse and respiratory therapist extubated Mrs. Dixon. Nasal prongs were applied initially, but an oxygen mask was needed, so the respiratory therapist left the room to get the mask. When the respiratory therapist returned to the room, he realized that the patient was not breathing normally. The respiratory therapist examined her and found no air movement. Reintubation activities commenced.

However, bed rails had to be removed, the bed rolled down, and the restraints placed on Mrs. Dixon removed. In the process, Mrs. Dixon's heart stopped beating, and a Code Blue was called. During the second code, the nurse recording events on the Code Sheet noted that the respiratory therapist was unsuccessful at attempting to reintubate Mrs. Dixon. The issue was that the laryngoscope blade he was using was too small, and an appropriately sized blade could not be found in the crash cart. The crash cart had not been restocked after the first code, so the blade had to be obtained from the cardiac care unit across the hall.

When the appropriately sized blade was found and taken to her room, Mrs. Dixon was quickly reintubated by a physician. She was placed on a ventilator but never regained consciousness. After the second code, Mrs. Dixon was found to be brain-dead secondary to suffocation. She was eventually discharged from the hospital to a nursing home, where she died approximately 10 months later.

This cause of action was subsequently filed and tried before a jury. The jury returned a verdict in the amount of $900,000 to the estate of Mrs. Dixon, citing that the hospital, because of the actions of the respiratory therapist and nurse, was negligent in failing to adequately assess Mrs. Dixon as a candidate for extubation, failing to communicate concerns about her readiness for extubation to the physician before extubation, failing to stock the crash cart, and failing to properly position Mrs. Dixon after extubation for possible reintubation.

Five years later, *Moon v St. Thomas Hospital*[37] was published. In this case, a portion of Mr. Moon's ETT had to be extricated from his airway after he transected it by biting through it. The family of Mr. Moon alleged that permitting him to bite on the ETT to the extent that it was transected was negligent and that a bite block should have been inserted or the ETT repositioned to avoid the transection.

At the trial court level, the transection of this ETT was determined to be not reasonably foreseeable, and the court dismissed the case. That decision was appealed, and, 1 year later, the appellate court ordered the case to trial, concluding that a jury should determine whether inserting a bite block or repositioning the ETT was consistent with the standard of care.

In *Owensboro Mercy Health System v Payne*,[38] a jury awarded a man $2,270,000 in damages for the negligent transfer of Mr. Payne from the operating room to the critical care unit. Mr. Payne had been involved in a motor vehicle accident and, because of extensive internal injuries, had spent between 8 and 8.5 hours in the operating room. At the conclusion of surgery, he was transferred to the critical care unit without supplemental oxygen's being administered. This failure caused Mr. Payne to sustain a serious brain injury, resulting in a persistent vegetative state. Although this award was appealed, the appellate court affirmed the verdict at the trial court level.

A year after *Owensboro*, a verdict for the defense was rendered in *Martin v St. Vincent Medical Center*.[39] In *Martin*, the family alleged that a certified registered nurse anesthetist (CRNA) punctured Mr. Martin's trachea while inserting an internal jugular line during a quadruple coronary artery bypass graft procedure. After surgery, Mr. Martin developed mediastinitis and died. His family filed this wrongful death cause of action, but the defense verdict was affirmed on appeal, citing in part the inability of Mr. Martin's family to affirmatively establish causation.

As in *Martin*, the patient-plaintiff in *Kent v Baptist Memorial Hospital*[40] was denied a verdict in her favor. The patient in *Kent* was a 16-year-old diabetic who experienced a diabetic seizure and went into septic shock. On arrival at the hospital, she was unresponsive and had to be intubated. After she was intubated, she was transferred to another hospital. She was eventually extubated and filed this cause of action, contending that she sustained vocal cord damage at intubation because the ETT was too large for her height and weight.

In *Miller v Marymount Medical Center*,[41] a 31-year-old pregnant woman, Mrs. Miller, was admitted to Marymount Medical Center to give birth. Two days later, she gave birth via cesarean section to a healthy baby girl. After the C-section, respiratory problems began. A chest radiograph obtained on the morning after the C-section revealed that Mrs. Miller had pneumonia. A blood gas analysis done that same morning indicated that her Po_2 was 64.4 mEq/L. Antibiotic therapy was started, and a nasal canula was applied to improve oxygenation. Mrs. Miller was also treated for pain and stress with Demerol and Vistaril injections. Throughout the day, respiratory distress continued.

At 9:45 PM that same night, her physician told the Miller family that a pulmonologist was going to be called. Five minutes later, the nurse administered Demerol and Vistaril injections. Ten minutes after the injections, Mrs. Miller's physician returned to her room to find Mrs. Miller unresponsive and in respiratory arrest. A code was called, and 5 minutes later Mrs. Miller was intubated, placed on an oxygen bag delivering 100% oxygen, and transferred to the intensive care unit. After she was intubated, another blood gas determination was made, and the Po_2 was 90 mEq/L. Twelve minutes after she was intubated and transferred to the intensive care unit, Mrs. Miller was breathing without assistance. However, she never regained consciousness. She was eventually transferred to a nursing home, where she remains in a comatose state.

Mrs. Miller's family filed this case. With regard to the nursing care rendered to Mrs. Miller, they alleged that the nursing staff failed to furnish treating physicians with up-to-date information about Mrs. Miller's symptoms and to obtain repeat blood gas analyses as required by an order entered by Mrs. Miller's physician. They also contended that the administration of Demerol 10 minutes before her respiratory arrest was negligent, because Demerol accelerates the progression of acute respiratory distress syndrome (ARDS). ARDS is the condition the experts retained by the family concluded that Mrs. Miller had on the morning the chest radiograph was obtained.

The trial lasted 7 days, and the jury returned a defense verdict because they were unable to definitively determine that negligence was the proximate cause of Mrs. Miller's injuries. This verdict was affirmed by the Court of Appeals and the Kentucky Supreme Court.

Regardless of the verdict rendered, these cases serve as a stark reminder of the life-altering and life-ending implications associated with management of the respiratory status of an acutely or critically ill patient. Consequently, nurses caring for patients with respiratory compromise must diligently assess, plan, implement care, and evaluate these patients with laser-like precision. The life of the acutely or critically ill patient depends on it.

BLOOD TRANSFUSIONS

Tobin v Providence Hospital[42] serves as a reminder that blood transfusions carry with them considerable risks. In *Tobin*, Rollin Tobin underwent hip replacement surgery but died from sepsis and disseminated intravascular coagulation. The wife of Mr. Tobin asserted that he died because blood contaminated with *Yersinia* bacteria was administered to him during surgery.

Before surgery, Mr. Tobin donated three units of his own blood, and all three of those units were transfused in the operating room, as well as an additional, allogeneic unit. After Mr. Tobin's death, the American Red Cross and the Centers for Disease Control and Prevention investigated the situation and determined that the fourth unit administered to Mr. Tobin was contaminated with *Yersinia* bacteria.

Mr. Tobin's family filed this wrongful death cause of action, contending that failure to monitor or record his temperature before, during, and after the operation caused his death. This case went to trial, and the jury returned a verdict in the amount of $6,485,681.06 in favor of the estate of Mr. Tobin. However, because there was an absence of testimony asserting failure to monitor or record the patient's temperature before, during, and after the operation and because of other evidentiary errors, the Michigan Court of Appeals ordered a new trial.

Like managing a patient's respiratory status, the administration of blood and blood products, although routine in critical care settings, is a high-risk intervention that can prove to be deadly. *Tobin* is an example. To avoid liability associated with administration of blood and blood products, nurses must carefully follow organizational procedures and protocols that govern these interventions. They must then take the time to thoroughly document the care that was taken to protect the patient.

INFECTION CONTROL

In *Carroll v Sisters of St. Frances Health Services,*[43] Bessie Mae Carroll was visiting her sister, who was a patient in the critical care unit at St. Joseph Hospital when, after washing her hands, she attempted to remove a paper towel from the container located adjacent to the wash basin she was using. She thought the container was a paper towel dispenser and inserted her right hand into the opening at the top of the container. When she did so, three of her fingers were stuck by sharp objects. After she told a nurse that she hurt her fingers on the paper towel dispenser, the nurse told Ms. Carroll that the container was not a paper towel dispenser but a receptacle for contaminated needles.

Ms. Carroll developed a fear of contracting acquired immunodeficiency syndrome (AIDS) and filed this negligence-based cause of action, contending that the container had been placed too close to the wash basin and that a warning should have been placed on the container indicating its purpose and contents.

At the trial court level the case was dismissed, but on appeal a trial was ordered so that the jury could determine whether Ms. Carroll's fear of acquiring AIDS was reasonable.

The case of *Piedmont Hospital v Reddick,*[44] like *Carroll,* arose out of an allegation that appropriate infection control standards were not followed. In *Piedmont,* James Davis died after contracting a fungal infection. His estate filed this cause of action, contending that construction work performed in or near the intensive care unit where Mr. Davis was being treated caused the *Aspergillus* fungus to become airborne and transmitted to him.

The complaint asserted that construction work was performed without proper safeguards and that this failure led to a breach of industry standards. Although a number of issues were addressed by the Georgia Court of Appeals Second Division, the court ordered the case be tried as to the alleged negligence of the construction company and hospital.

Carroll and *Piedmont* demonstrate that infection control issues find their way to courtrooms across America. To minimize risks associated with alleged infection control failures, sharps containers must be clearly labeled and positioned away from wash basins and paper towel dispensers. Before remodeling or other construction begins, the environment must be safeguarded from the airborne spread of deadly microorganisms.

INFORMED CONSENT

Trombley v Starr-Wood Cardiac Group,[45] a case issued from the Alaska Supreme Court, arose from a situation in which a patient undergoing coronary artery bypass graft surgery told her surgeons that she did not want a vein to be harvested from her right leg, because she had a history of phlebitis in that leg. The surgeons agreed to harvest a vein from her left leg and never discussed with her the possibility of having to harvest a vein from her right leg. Despite this conversation and agreement, a vein was harvested from her right leg. After surgery, the right leg incision was lapped over rather than stitched together and became infected, necessitating plastic surgery to remove dead tissue and stitch up the incision.

This malpractice case was subsequently filed but was dismissed at the trial court level. When Mrs. Trombley appealed that decision, the Alaska Supreme Court determined that the decision of the trial court to dismiss her case was in error and ordered a trial. In reversing the decision of the trial court, the Alaska Supreme Court concluded that Mrs. Trombley had a right to insist that her right leg not be used as a harvest site. If, according to the court, her right leg was used without obtaining actual or implied consent, battery may have been committed. If battery occurred, the court observed, Mrs. Trombley would be entitled to damages for that cause of action as well.

Although cases such as *Trombley* have held physicians responsible for obtaining the consent of patients, nurses caring for acutely ill patients should consider obtaining informed consent before performing invasive procedures that she or he is trained and authorized to perform. Failure to obtain informed consent could lead to liability if a patient proves that damages occurred because of the negligence of the nurse in performing the invasive procedure.

A summary of failures to provide reasonable care is shown in Box 3-3.

RIGHT TO ACCEPT OR REFUSE MEDICAL TREATMENT

The right to consent and informed consent includes the right to refuse treatment. In most cases, a competent adult's decision to refuse even life-sustaining treatment is honored.[46-50] The underlying rationale is that the patient's right to withdraw or withhold treatment is not outweighed by the state's interest in preserving life. The right to refuse treatment is *not* honored in some situations, including (but not limited to) the following:

1. The treatment relates to a contagious illness that threatens the health of the public.

BOX 3-3   SUMMARY OF ALLEGED FAILURES TO PROVIDE REASONABLE CARE TO ACUTELY AND CRITICALLY ILL PATIENTS

ASSESSMENT
- Failure to assess and analyze the level of care needed by the patient
- Failure to ascertain the patient's wishes with regard to self-determination

PLANNING
- Failure to diagnose appropriately

IMPLEMENTATION
- Failure to timely communicate patient findings
- Failure to take appropriate action
- Failure to document assessment findings, interventions, and actions taken, as well as the patient's response to those interventions and actions
- Failure to preserve patient privacy

EVALUATION
- Failure to act as patient advocate

---

2. Innocent third parties will suffer (e.g., a parent's wish to refuse blood transfusion for a child most likely would be overruled to save the child's life).
3. The refusal violates ethical standards.
4. Treatment must be instituted to prevent suicide and to preserve life.

When patients refuse treatment, complex ethical, legal, and practical problems arise. Hospitals should have specific policies to guide nurses in these areas, and nurses' participation in hospital or institutional ethics committees is strongly advised.

WITHHOLDING AND WITHDRAWING TREATMENT

As stated earlier, an adult has the right to refuse treatment, even treatment that sustains life. This right means that the critical care nurse may participate in the withholding or withdrawing of treatment. Historically, the distinction between withholding and withdrawing treatment was considered the issue of importance, but this is no longer the case. Health care decisions become most complex when patients lose competency and the capacity to make their own decisions personally.

ADVANCE DIRECTIVES

The U.S. Congress passed landmark legislation known as the Patient Self-Determination Act/Omnibus Budget Reconciliation Act (OBRA) of 1990.[51-59] The statute requires that all adults must be provided written information regarding an individual's rights under state law to make medical decisions, including the right to refuse treatment and the right to formulate advance directives.

The law mandates that providers of health care services under Medicare and Medicaid must comply with requirements relating to patient advance directives, which are written instructions recognized under state law for provision of care when persons are incapacitated. Providers may not be reimbursed for the care they provide unless the requirements of this provision are met.

Providers must have written policies and procedures (1) to inform all adult patients at initiation of treatment of their right to execute an advance directive and of the provider's policies on the implementation of that right, (2) to document in the medical record whether an individual has executed an advance directive, (3) *not* to condition care and treatment or otherwise discriminate on the basis of whether a patient has executed an advance directive, (4) to comply with state laws on advance directives, and (5) to provide information and education to staff and the community on advance directives.

Patients themselves can provide clear direction by preparing in advance written documents that specify their wishes.[60] These documents are termed *advance directives* and include the living will and the durable power of attorney for health care. To be effective in a jurisdiction, both of these directives must be statutorily or judicially recognized. The *living will* specifies that if certain circumstances occur, such as terminal illness, the patient will decline specific treatments, such as cardiopulmonary resuscitation and mechanical ventilation. The living will does not cover all treatments; in some states, for example, nutritional support may not be declined through a living will. The *durable power of attorney for health care* is a directive through which a patient designates an "agent," someone who will make decisions for the patient if the patient becomes unable to do so. Critical care nurses whose patients have executed advance directives must follow state law provisions and the hospital's policies, and they require education regarding advance directives and their important role in patient advocacy.[61]

ORDERS NOT TO RESUSCITATE

Hospital policies that address orders to withhold or withdraw treatment should exist in all critical care units. For example, orders not to resuscitate, typically referred to as do not resuscitate (DNR) orders, should be governed by written policies, including (but not limited to) the following:

1. DNR orders should be entered in the patient's record with full documentation by the responsible physician about the patient's prognosis and the patient's agreement (if he or she is capable) or, alternatively, the family's consensus.
2. DNR orders should require concurrence of another physician as standard policy.
3. Policies should specify that orders are reviewed periodically (some policies require daily review).
4. Patients with capacity must give their informed consent.
5. For patients without capacity, that incapacity must be thoroughly documented, along with the diagnosis, prognosis, and family consensus.
6. Judicial intervention before writing a DNR order is usually indicated when the patient's family does not agree or there is uncertainty or disagreement about the patient's prognosis or mental status. As a general rule, however, in the absence of conflict or disagreement, DNR orders are legal in a majority of jurisdictions if executed clearly and properly.
7. Policies should specify who is to be contacted and notified within the hospital administration.

Other orders to withhold or withdraw treatment may involve mechanical ventilation, dialysis, nutritional support, hydration, and medications such as antibiotics. The legal and ethical implications of these orders for each patient must be carefully considered. Hospitals should have written policies on all orders to withhold and withdraw treatment. Policies must cover how decisions will be made, who will decide, and what roles the patient, family, health care providers, and the institution will play. Policies must be developed that consider state laws and judicial pinions.

Summary

- Protection, promotion, optimization, prevention, and alleviation are action words that convey the dynamic nature of the nurse's responsibility to take affirmative action when caring for the acutely and critically ill.
- Standards of practice and standards of professional performance further delineate expectations of nurses.
- Standards promulgated by the ANA and the AACN provide a framework for critical care nursing practice.
- Legal theories on which civil litigation against nurses is based include negligence, negligence per se, malpractice, wrongful death, defamation, assault and battery, loss of consortium, and emotional distress.
- The risk of liability can be diminished by taking affirmative action that is responsive to the patient's condition.
- Thorough documentation regarding actions taken to protect the patient is essential.
- Nurses can minimize the risk of liability by daily coming to the practice setting focused on the care that must be given and by paying attention to the signs and symptoms of complications and compromise.
- The patient's right to withdraw or withhold treatment is not outweighed by the state's interest in preserving life.
- Providers of health care must comply with requirements relating to patient advance directives.
- DNR orders should be entered into the patient's medical record with full documentation by the responsible physician about the patient's prognosis and the patient's agreement or, alternatively, the family's consensus.

Case Study: Patient with Legal Issues

⊖volve Answers to the Case Study Questions can be found on the Evolve web site at http://evolve.elsevier.com/Urden/.

Brief Patient History

Mr. A is an 87-year-old man. He has a history of aortic stenosis; however, he has been relatively healthy until recent episodes of syncope. Mr. A lives in an assisted living facility because of forgetfulness but was independent in activities of daily living before this hospitalization.

Clinical Assessment

Mr. A. was admitted to the critical care unit yesterday, after undergoing aortic valvuloplasty. Mr. A. has not received any opioids or benzodiazepines since yesterday's interventional procedure. The night nurse reported that Mr. A was confused to place when awakened during the night but commented that this is normal for an 87-year-old. This morning, Mr. A was oriented to person, time, place, and situation. He is easily aroused but dozes off and on when unstimulated. Although Mr. A is able to follow simple commands, he requires repeated instructions. The nurse failed to document or report the patient's mental status change or the abnormal serum electrolyte findings to the physician.

Continued

Case Study: Patient with Legal Issues—*cont'd*

Diagnostic Procedures

Mr. A's baseline vital signs are blood pressure, 110/62 mm Hg; heart rate, 82 beats/min (sinus rhythm); respiratory rate, 18 breaths/min; and temperature, 98.4° F. The chest radiograph is normal; O_2 saturation (pulse oximetry) is 96% on room air. Results from serum electrolyte analysis include the following: sodium, 120 mmol/L; potassium, 4.1 mmol/L; chloride, 95 mmol/L; CO_2, 25 mEq/L; blood urea nitrogen, 60 mg/dL; and creatinine, 2 mg/dL.

Medical Diagnosis

Mr. A is diagnosed with delirium secondary to hyponatremia.

Questions

1. What major outcomes do you expect to achieve for this patient?
2. What problems or risks must be managed to achieve these outcomes?
3. What interventions must be initiated to monitor, prevent, manage, or eliminate the problems and risks identified?
4. What interventions should be initiated to promote optimal functioning, safety, and well-being of the patient?
5. What possible learning needs would you anticipate for this patient?
6. What cultural and age-related factors might have a bearing on the patient's plan of care?

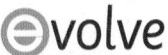 Be sure to check out the bonus material, including free self-assessment exercises, on the Evolve web site at http://evolve.elsevier.com/Urden/.

References

1. American Nurses Association (ANA): *Nursing: scope and standards of practice*, Washington, DC, 2004, ANA.
2. American Association of Critical-Care Nurses (AACN): *Standards for acute and critical care nursing practice*, Aliso Viejo, California, 2008, AACN.
3. For example, California: *Ybarra v Spangard*, 154 P.2d 687 (Cal. 1944); Colorado: *Wood v Rowland*, 592 P.2d 1332 (Colo. 1978); Delaware: *Larrimore v Homeopathic Hospital Association*, 176 A.2d 362 (Del. 1962); Minnesota: *Plutshack v University of Minnesota Hospital*, 316 N.W.2d 1 (Minn. 1982); Montana: *Hunsaker v Bozeman Deaconess Foundation*, 588 P.2d 493 (Mont. 1978); Pennsylvania: *Baur v Mesta Machine Co.*, 176 A.2d 684 (Pa. 1962); Texas: *Childs v Greenville Hospital Authority*, 479 S.W.2d 399 (Tx. 1972); and Washington: *Stone v Sisters of Charity of the House of Providence*, 469 P.2d 229 (Wash. 1970).
4. *Clough v Lively*, 387 S.E.2d 573 (Ga. 1989).
5. *Lunsford v Board of Nurse Examiners*, 648 S.W.2d 391 (Tx. App. 1983).
6. *Brandon HMA, Inc. v Bradshaw*, 809 So.2d 611 (Miss. 2001).
7. *Cruzan v Director, Missouri Department of Mental Health*, 497 U.S. 261 (1990).
8. *Anderson v St. Francis-St. George Hospital*, 671 N.E.2d 225 (Ohio 1996).
9. *Denesia v St. Elizabeth Community Health Center*, 454 N.W.2d 294 (Neb. 1990).
10. *Brookover v Mary Hitchcock Memorial Hospital*, 893 F.2d 411 (1st Cir. 1990).
11. *Garcia v United States*, 697 F.Supp. 1570 (Colo. 1988).
12. *Keyser v Garner*, 922 P.2d 409 (Idaho 1996).
13. *Long v Methodist Hospital of Indiana*, 699 N.E.2d 1164 (Ind. 1998).
14. *Richardson v Miller*, 44 S.W.3d 1 (Tenn. 2000).
15. *Ginsberg v St. Michaels Hospital*, 678 A.2d 271 (N.J. 1996).
16. *G.S. v Dep't of Human Servs., Div. of Youth & Family Servs.*, 723 A.2d 612 (N.J. 1999).
17. *Haney v Alexander*, 323 S.E.2d 430 (1984).
18. *Doe v Ohio State Univ. Hosp. & Clinics*, 663 N.E.2d 1369 (Ohio 1995).
19. *Darling v Charleston Comm. Mem. Hosp.*, 211 N.E. 2d 614 (Ill. 1965).
20. *Sparks v St. Luke's Regional Medical Center*, 768 P.2d 768 (Idaho 1989).
21. *Estate of Reinen v Northern Arizona Othopedics, Ltd.*, 9 P.3d 314 (Ariz. 2000).
22. *Koeniger v Eckrich*.
23. *Teffeteller v University of Minnesota*, 645 N.W.2d 420 (Minn. 2002).
24. *Ress v Abbott Northwestern Hosp., Inc.*, 448 N.W. 2d 519 (Minn. 1989).
25. *McMullen v Ohio State University Hospitals*, 725 N.E.2d 1117 (Ohio 2002).
26. *Lama v Borras*, 16 F.3d 473 (1st Cir. 1994).
27. *Candler General Hospital Inc. v McNorrill*, 354 S.E. 2d 872 (Ga. 1987).
28. *Gould v New York City Health and Hospital Corp.*, 490 NYS.2d 87 (1985).
29. *Griffin v Methodist Hospital*, 948 S.W.2d 72 (Tex. App. 1997).
30. *Manning v Twin Falls Clinic & Hospital*, 830 P.2d 1185 (Id. 1992).
31. *Meuser v Rocky Mountain Hospital*, 685 P.2d 776 (Colo. 1984).
32. *Mock v Allen*, 783 So.2d 828 (Ala. 2000).
33. *Martinmaas v Engelmann*, 612 N.W.2D 600 (S.D. 2000).
34. *Allman v Holleman*, 667 P.2d 296 (Ks. 1983).
35. *Courteau v Dodd*, 773 S.W.2d 436 (Ark. 1989).
36. *Dixon v Taylor*, 431 S.E.2d 778 (N.C. 1993).
37. *Moon v St. Thomas Hospital*, 983 S.W.2d 225 (Tenn. 1998).
38. *Owensboro Mercy Health System v Payne*, 24 S.W.3d 675 (Ky. 1999).
39. *Martin v St. Vincent Medical Center*, 142 Ohio App. 3d 347 (2001).
40. *Kent v Baptist Memorial Hospital*, 853 So.2d 873 (Miss. 2003).
41. *Miller v Marymount Medical Center*, 125 S.W.3d 274 (Ky. 2004).
42. *Tobin v Providence Hospital*, 624 N.W.2d 548 (Mich. 2001).
43. *Carroll v Sisters of St. Francis*, 868 S.W.2d 585 (Tenn. 1993).
44. *Piedmont Hospital, Inc. v Reddick*, 599 S.E.2d 20 (Ga. 2004).
45. *Trombley v Starr-Wood Cardiac Group*, 3 P.3d 916 (Alaska 2000).
46. *Bouvia v Superior Court*, 225 Cal Rptr 297; 179 Cal. App. 3d 1127, review denied (Cal. App. 1986).
47. *In re Farrell*, 529 A.2d 404 (N.J. 1987).
48. *McKay v Bergstedt*, 801 P.2d 617 (Nev. 1990).
49. *State v McAfee*, 385 S.E.2d 651 (Ga. 1989).
50. Wilson-Clayton ML, Clayton MA: Two steps forward, one step back: *McKay v Bergstedt*, *Whittier Law Rev* 12:439, 1991.
51. *Advance directives for health care*, Des Moines, 2003, Iowa Hospital Association, Iowa Medical Society, Iowa State Bar Association.
52. *Put it in writing: questions and answers on advance directives*, Chicago, 2005, American Hospital Association.
53. Cate FH, Gill BA: *The Patient Self-Determination Act: implementation issues and opportunities*, Washington, DC, Annenberg Washington Program, 1991.
54. *Advance directive protocols and the Patient Self-Determination Act: a resource manual for the development of institutional protocols*, New York, Choice in Dying (formerly Society for the Right to Die/Concern for Dying), 1991.
55. Emanuel L, Emanuel E: The medical directive: a new comprehensive advance care document, *JAMA* 261(22):3, 288, 1989.
56. *The Patient Self-Determination Act of 1990: implementation in Iowa hospitals*, Des Moines, Iowa Hospital Association, 1991.
57. *Advance medical directives*, Arlington, Va., National Hospice Organization, 1995.
58. *The patient self-determination directory and resources guide*, Washington, DC, National Health Lawyers Association, 1991.
59. Patient Self-Determination Act/Omnibus Budget Reconciliation Act of 1990, Pub L No. 101-508, Sec. 4206, 42 USC Sec. 1395cc(a)(1) (1990).
60. Douglas R, Brown HN: Patients' attitudes toward advance directives, *J Nurs Scholarsh* 34(1):61, 2002.
61. Ryan CJ et al: Perceptions about advance directives by nurses in a community hospital, *Clin Nurse Spec* 15(6):246, 2001.

Genetics in Critical Care

The field of genetics and genomics continues to expand and affect crucial aspects of medical care. Genetics and genetic testing do not yet have a large role in the critical care unit, but given the exponential growth of knowledge in this field, the day when *personalized health care* will include a genetic screen to tailor treatment to individual biology is on the horizon. This chapter includes an overview of the biologic basis of genetics, a description of the different types of genetic and genomic studies, and the impact of pharmacogenetics. It also incorporates some examples of genetic diseases and pharmacogenetic syndromes in critical care. A glossary of genetic terms is provided at the end of the chapter.

GENETICS AND GENOMICS

Genetics is the study of heredity, particularly as it relates to the ability of genes to transfer heritable physical characteristics. *Genes* are specific sequences of *deoxyribonucleic acid* (DNA) located on chromosomes within the nucleus of each cell (Fig. 4-1). Genes contain the blueprint for protein production that results in the physical characteristics of each individual.

Genomics refers to the study of all of the genetic material within the cell and its impact on biologic and physical characteristics. The *genome* is the complete set of DNA in an organism. Each nucleated somatic cell contains a copy of the genome. Two exceptions are reproductive cells (ovocytes and sperm), which contain only one half of the paired chromosomes. The human genome contains between 20,000 and 25,000 genes.[1]

GENETIC AND GENOMIC STRUCTURE AND FUNCTION

CHROMOSOMES

Human cells contain 23 pairs of chromosomes—22 pairs of autosomes and 1 pair of sex chromosomes—making the total 46. The chromosomes are traditionally arranged in order of size, starting with the largest (chromosome 1) to the smallest (chromosome 22), with the sex chromosomes placed last or to the side. A schematic of this chromosome arrangement to show the variation in size is shown in Figure 4-2A; they are not

arranged this way inside the cell. This number system is used to identify each chromosome to describe the conditions associated with specific DNA sequences on any particular chromosome. A *karyotype* is the arrangement of human chromosomes, as shown in the sequence in Figure 4-2B. Each chromosome consists of an unbroken strand of DNA inside the nucleus of the cell.

It is difficult to imagine how much DNA is packed into the chromosome. One analogy is that if the DNA strand inside chromosome 1 (the largest chromosome) were a cooked spaghetti noodle 1 mm in diameter, it would stretch for 25 miles.[2] To fit all of this genetic material inside the cell nucleus, the DNA is tightly coiled inside the chromosomes in a hierarchical order of compact structures. A specialized class of proteins called *histones* organizes the double-stranded DNA into what looks like a tightly coiled telephone cord (see Fig. 4-1).

Each somatic chromosome is made of two identical strands, called *chromatids*, that are joined near the center (see Fig. 4-1). The central region is called the *centromere*, and the ends of the chromatids are called *telomeres*. The segments of the chromosome separated by the centromere are called *arms*. The shorter arm of each chromosome is called *p* (for *petit*, or small), and the longer arm is called *q*. Differential staining of chromosomes produces alternating dark and light transverse *bands*. The bands are labeled p1, p2, p3, and so forth on the p arm and q1, q2, q3, and so forth on the q arm, counted from the centromere toward the telomeres.

The p and q labels and bands are used to specify the location of specific DNA sections on the chromosome. There are also subbands within the major bands. This series of letters and numbers is the equivalent of an address for the location of a gene on a chromosome. For example, the cystic fibrosis gene *CFTR* (cystic fibrosis transmembrane conductance regulator) is located at 7q31.2, which indicates it is on chromosome 7, q arm, band 3, subband 1, and sub-subband 2.

DNA AND THE DOUBLE HELIX

DNA is foundational to genetics. Within the nucleus of the cell, DNA is arranged like a ladder, with two long strands of subunits twisted around each other to form a double-stranded helix. The subunits of each DNA strand are called *nucleotides* or *bases,* and they form the rungs of the ladder. Four nucleotide

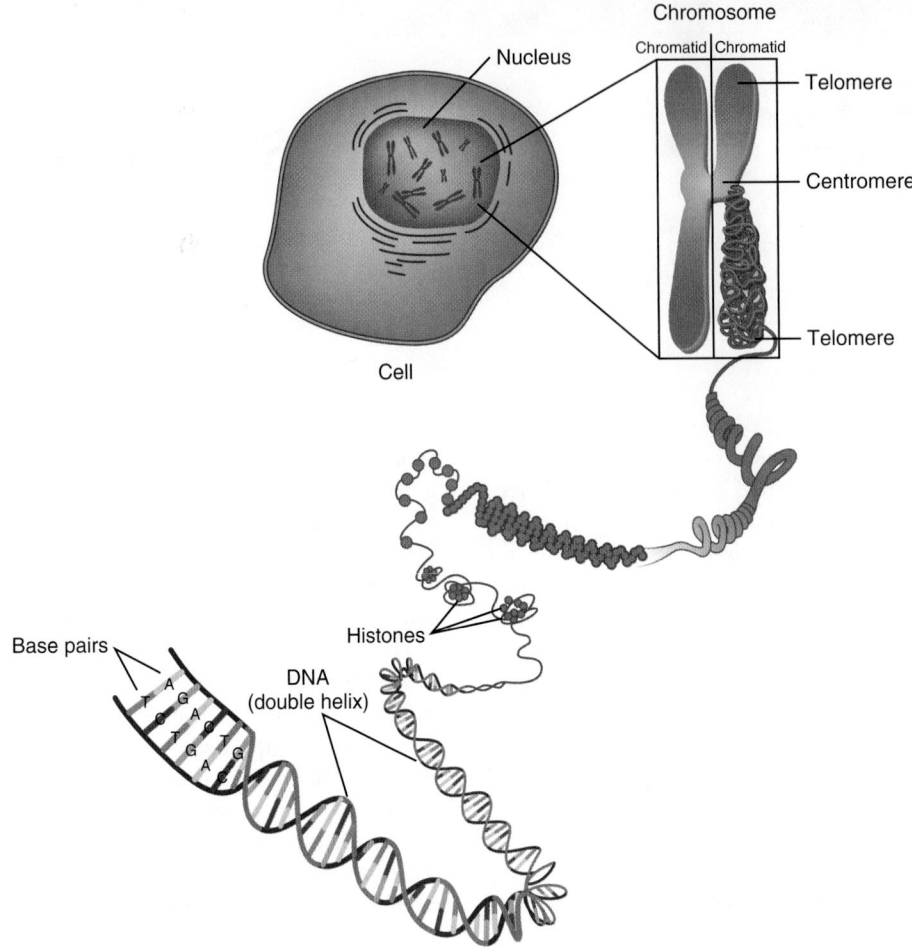

Figure 4-1 Chromosomes are tightly packed with DNA and reside in the nucleus of the cell.

bases—adenine (A), thymine (T), guanine (G), and cytosine (C)—comprise the "letters" in the genetic "alphabet." Each nucleotide base is attached to a phosphorylated molecule of the 5-carbon sugar deoxyribose that forms the backbone of the DNA chain and can be visualized as the two sides of a ladder that have been twisted around (Fig. 4-3). The bases in the double helix are paired T with A and G with C. The nucleotide bases are designed so that only G can pair with C and only T can pair with A to achieve a consistent distance across the width of the DNA strand. The TA and GC combinations are known as *base pairs* (see Fig. 4-3). There are approximately three billion base pairs in the human genome.[1]

The two DNA strands are orientated in opposite directions. Each DNA strand has a specific direction that is labeled as the 3′ end or the 5′ end (pronounced 3 prime, and 5 prime) (see Fig. 4-3). Because the DNA strands face in opposite directions, the 3′ end of one strand is always matched to the 5′ end of the other strand. This fact becomes important for replication (discussed next). The 3′ end is described as the *leading strand* because new nucleotides can be added only at the 3′ end.

DNA Replication. Before a cell divides, it needs to make a second copy of the entire DNA content within the cell. This process is called *DNA replication*. The DNA double helix separates longitudinally, and mirror-image copies are made from the original strands. Stated another way, the original DNA strands provide a template that will be copied and may be called the *parent strands*; the mirror image copies are described as the *daughter strands*. In Figure 4-4 the parent strand is illustrated by the color blue with the 5′ and 3′ ends of each parent strand labeled. The daughter strands are colored in red. The replication process is facilitated by *DNA polymerase*, an enzyme that lengthens the DNA strand by the addition of new nucleotide bases at the 3′ end of the daughter strand (Fig. 4-4). After DNA replication is accomplished, the cell uses a sophisticated mechanism for identifying and fixing errors in the replicated strand.[3] After this procedure, the cell is ready to divide, and each new cell will contain a copy of the original DNA code.

DNA Alphabet. The nucleotides A, T, C, and G can be thought of as "letters" of a genetic alphabet that are combined into three-letter "words" that are transcribed (written) by the intermediary of *ribonucleic acid* (RNA). The RNA translates the three-letter words into the amino acids used to make the polypeptide chains that constitute proteins. This process may be written as DNA → RNA → protein.

Transcription. The process of making an RNA strand from a DNA strand is known as *transcription*. The strand with the genetic code that is to be transcribed is labeled as the *sense* strand or sometimes as the coding strand. The other strand,

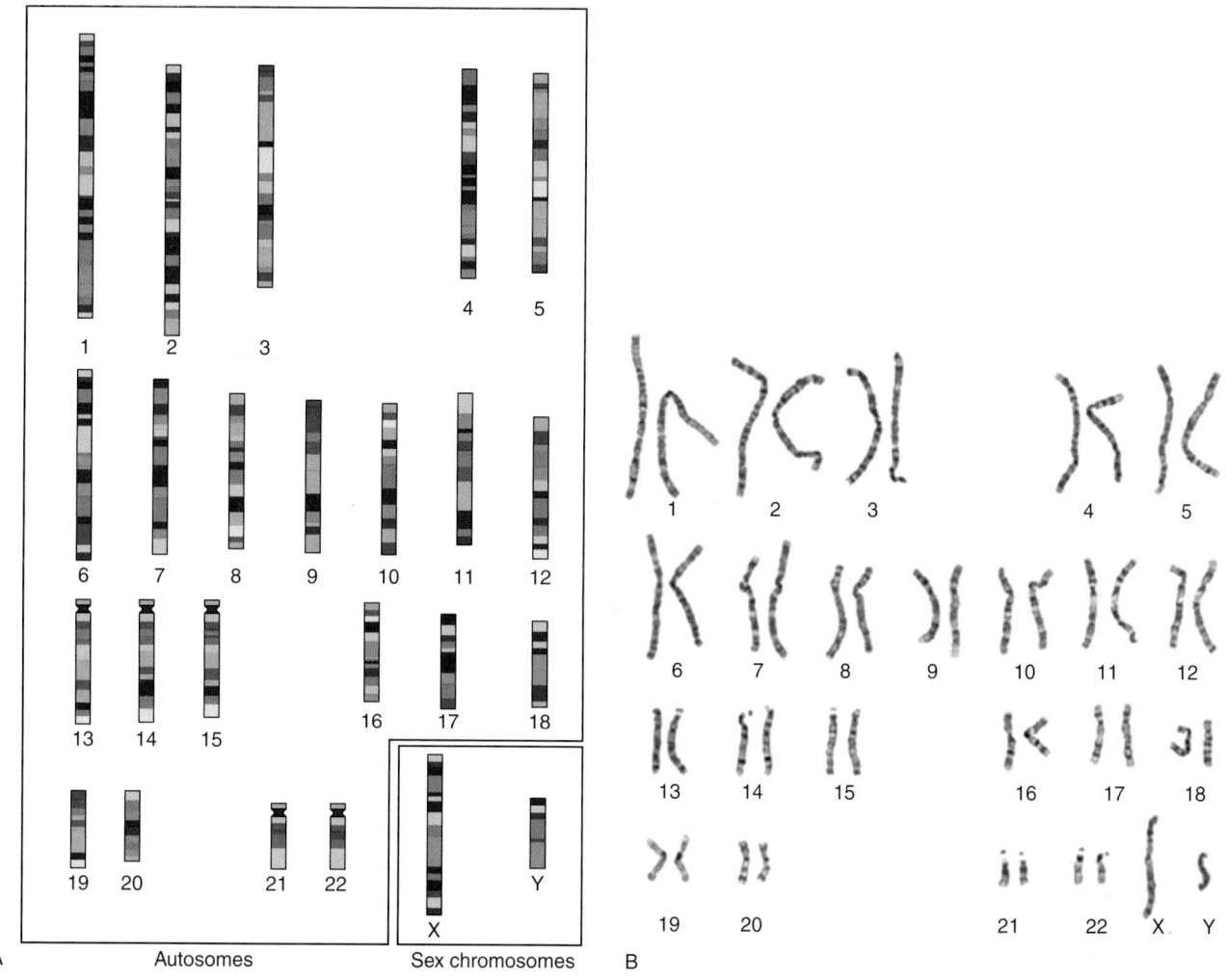

Figure 4-2 *A,* Schematic of the standard chromosomal arrangement used for classification of chromosomes by number, arranged from the largest (chromosome 1) to the smallest (chromosome 22). Chromosomes 1 to 22 are known as autosomes. Autosomal chromosomes are present in two identical copies, which are the same in males and females. The sex chromosomes are X (female) and Y (male). *B,* This is a male karyotype because the sex chromosome arrangement is XY. The striped bands that appear on the chromosomes are achieved by use of specialized staining techniques.

which is the RNA mirror image, is called the *antisense* or non-coding strand (Fig. 4-5). The reason there are two strands orientated in opposite directions is to facilitate replication of a DNA strand during cell division (see Fig. 4-4) or when proteins are needed (see Fig. 4-5) without compromising the original genetic material. To visualize how the process of transcription works, it may be helpful to study Figure 4-5 and locate the names of the different strands; the DNA strand is colored blue, the RNA strand is colored green to make the distinction clear.

To transcribe under the guidance of the enzyme *RNA polymerase,* sections of the DNA double helix unfold and separate into two single strands within the length of the double helix (see Fig. 4-5). The mirror-image DNA strand (shown in red in Fig. 4-4) serves as a template for the synthesis of a complementary, mirror-image strand of RNA (shown in green in Fig. 4-5). The purpose of transcription is to have the RNA mirror strand replicate the genetic code in the original DNA sense strand.

When RNA transcribes DNA nucleotides, it makes one significant change. The adenosine (A) DNA base is paired with a uracil (U) base in the RNA transcript (see Fig. 4-5). Each RNA strand also has a 3′ end (can be conceptualized as a head) and a 5′ end (conceptualized as a tail), and the growing RNA strand adds bases only at the 3′ leading end. The RNA strand, called *messenger RNA,* then leaves the nucleus of the cell, and the next action takes place in the cytoplasm.

Translation. The next step is to translate the RNA bases into three-letter words (e.g., AUC, UGA) called *codons* that can be used to specify an amino acid. The 3-base RNA codons are designed to code for one of 20 amino acids. Some codons signal to stop the sequence; these termination sequences are UAA, UAG, and UGA. The three-letter codons are not unique; for example, both UAU and UUC code for the amino acid *phenylalanine.* Most amino acids can be made from more than one codon. This can be appreciated by an examination of the list of three-letter codons, the corresponding three-letter amino acid abbreviation, the single letter abbreviation, and the name of the amino acid in Table 4-1. The process by which proteins are made from instructions encoded in DNA is called *gene expression.*

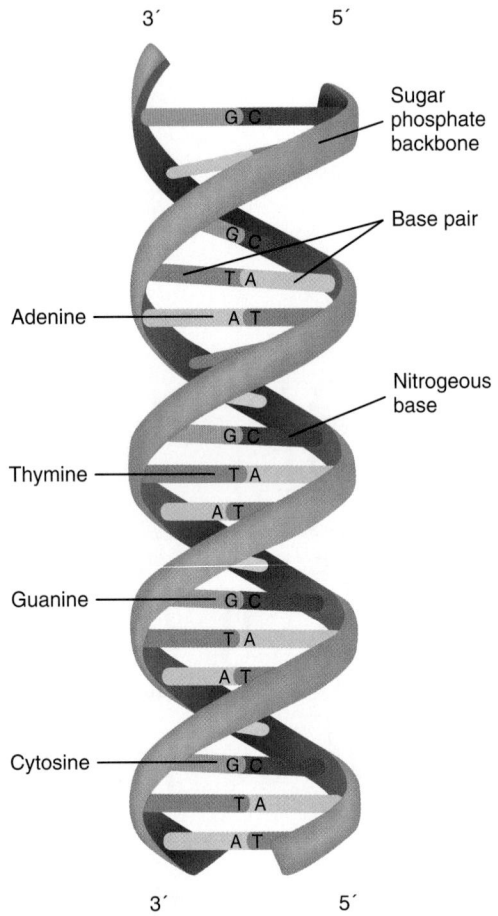

Figure 4-3 Deoxyribonucleic acid (DNA) double helix.

Only a brief review of how DNA contributes to the genetic code is possible in this chapter. The volume of information that underpins genetics and genomics reflects the work of many scientists who performed research to advance this knowledge, and it may take some individual study or additional classes to master the content. An excellent and free online tutorial is available through the Cold Spring Harbor Laboratory Web site.[4] The 41 modules use animation, video interviews, and text to present an interesting and informative introduction to the history and science of genetics.[4]

GENETIC VARIATION, MUTATION AND POLYMORPHISM

Variation. Genetic variation is common to all species. It means that individuals do not have the same nucleotides (A, C, T, G) in exactly the same position on the DNA strand. Some nucleotide differences result in the expression of different proteins and physical traits. Many nucleotide changes produce no visible external alteration, although those that have health-related consequences are of great interest to clinicians, patients, and researchers. Genetic variation can result from a variety of changes. It can be a single-letter substitution of one nucleotide base for another that can produce an inappropriate stop codon or produce a codon for a different amino acid. The amino acid codes are shown in Table 4-1.

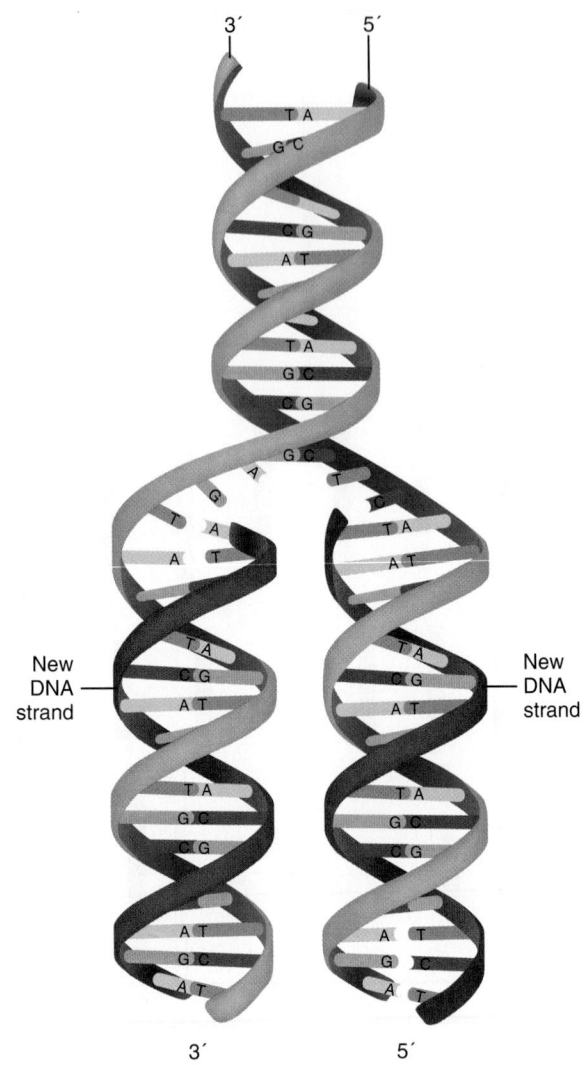

Figure 4-4 DNA replication occurs before the cell divides. The template is provided by the original DNA strand (colored blue). The mirror-image DNA strand (colored red) is adding nucleotides to elongate the new DNA strand.

An example of a single-letter switch that results in an increased risk for disease is the G-to-A substitution at nucleotide 1691 in the coagulation factor V gene. This *single-nucleotide polymorphism* (SNP) alters the protein product and increases the incidence of deep vein thrombosis (DVT), as described in Box 4-1.

Genetic material in the chromosome can also be deleted (Fig. 4-6A), new information from another chromosome can be inserted (Fig. 4-6B), or a *tandem repeat* (multiple repeats of the same sequence) may produce duplicate genetic material within the chromosome (Fig. 4-6C).

Translocation of genetic material describes a process in which chromosomes break and genetic material is moved from one chromosome to another. For example, the *Philadelphia chromosome,* or *Philadelphia translocation,* is a specific chromosomal abnormality associated with chronic myelogenous leukemia (CML). It results from a reciprocal translocation between chromosomes 9 and 22, in which parts of these two chromosomes switch places.[5]

Mutation. The term *genetic mutation* refers to a change in the DNA genetic sequence that can be inherited. The term

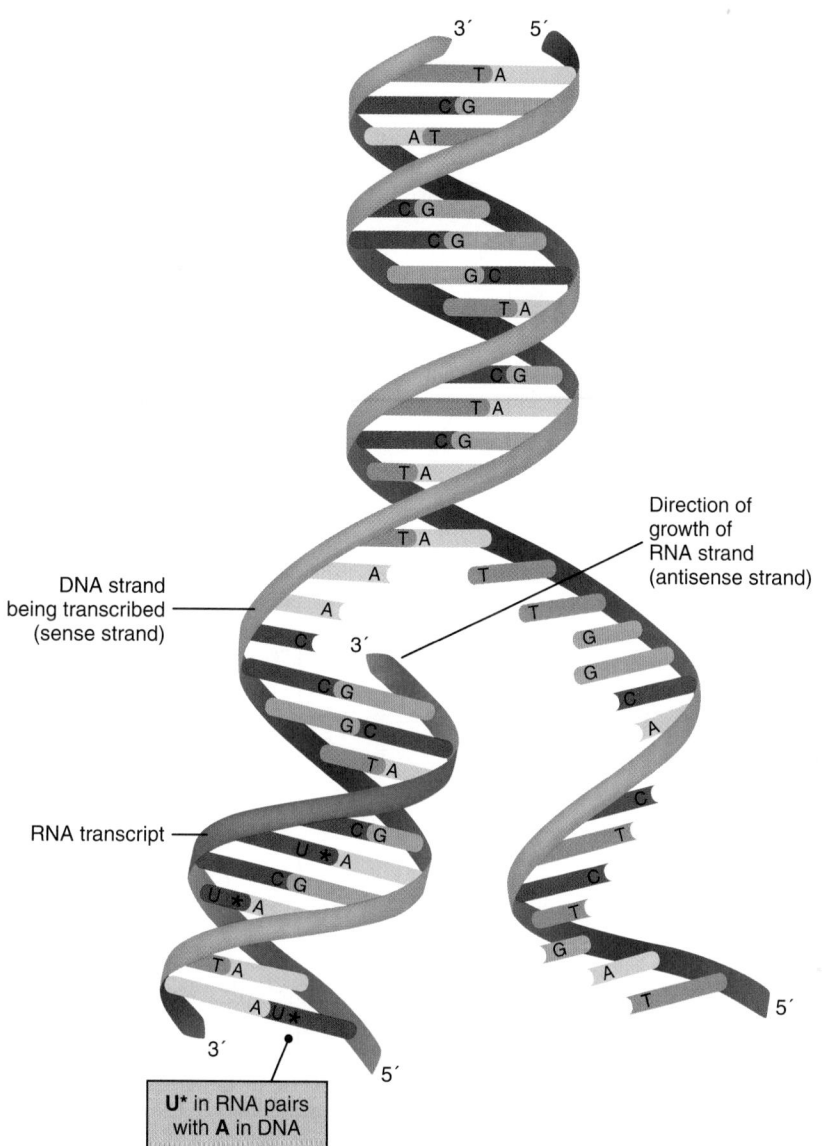

Figure 4-5 DNA transcription and production of a complementary RNA strand. The template DNA strand is colored blue, The RNA nucleotide uracil (U) pairs with the DNA nucleotide adenine (A) in the growing RNA strand (colored green).

mutation typically is used to describe alterations that occur in less than 1% of a population. This use of the word *mutation* does not have the negative connotation of being more deadly than other genetic changes. It just means the incidence is rare.

Single-Nucleotide Polymorphisms. When a genetic variant occurs frequently and is present in 1% or more of the population, it is described as a *genetic polymorphism*. The most common change is the substitution of one single nucleotide base, and this change is referred to as a SNP. When a SNP leads to a change in the amino acid product that is produced, it is called a *non-synonymous SNP*, or *missense SNP*. If a non-synonymous SNP occurs in a coding region, it may affect protein structure and lead to alterations in phenotype (disease manifestation). An example is the G-to-A coding polymorphism at the 1691 site of the factor V gene associated with blood coagulation.[6] This polymorphism leads to the substitution of an arginine (A) by glutamine (G) at amino acid position 506, which alters one of

the cleavage sites for *activated protein C*. Factor Va inactivation is delayed because the cleavage site is atypical. This creates a hypercoagulable state and increases the risk for DVT (see Box 4-1).[7-10]

Alleles. Another name for a variant of a gene that occurs at a single locus is *allele*. Allele symbols consist of the gene symbol, an asterisk, and the italicized allele designation. For example, the apolipoprotein E gene *(APOE)* has three major alleles *(APOE*E2, APOE*E3, APOE*E4)* occurring in the population, and they code for three isoforms of the protein. Apolipoprotein E is one of the apolipoproteins involved with cholesterol metabolism, and expression of the *APOE*E4* allele is associated with the development of hyperlipidemia. *APOE*E4* expression also is associated with late-onset Alzheimer's disease, with a less favorable outcome after traumatic brain injury, and with delirium in the critically ill.[11] Expression of the *APOE*E3* allele appears to protect against the development of these neurologic conditions.

TABLE 4-1 The Genetic Code: Amino Acids*

First nucleotide in codon	Second nucleotide in codon				Third nucleotide
	U	**C**	**A**	**G**	
U	UUU Phe F Phenylalanine	UCU Ser S Serine	UAU Tyr Y Tyrosine	UGU Cys C Cysteine	U
	UUC Phe F Phenylalanine	UCC Ser S Serine	UAC Tyr Y Tyrosine	UGC Cys C Cysteine	C
	UUA Leu L Leucine	UCA Ser S Serine	UAA Termination	UGA Termination	A
	UUG Leu L Leucine	UCG Ser S Serine	UAG Termination	UGG Trp W Tryptophan	G
C	CUU Leu L Leucine	CCU Pro P Proline	CAU His H Histidine	CGU Arg R Arginine	U
	CUC Leu L Leucine	CCC Pro P Proline	CAC His H Histidine	CGC Arg R Arginine	C
	CUA Leu L Leucine	CCA Pro P Proline	CAA Gln Q Glutamine	CGA Arg R Arginine	A
	CUG Leu L Leucine	CCG Pro P Proline	CAG Gln Q Glutamine	CGG Arg R Arginine	G
A	AUU Ile I Isoleucine	ACU Thr T Threonine	AAU Asn N Asparagine	AGU Ser S Serine	U
	AUC Ile I Isoleucine	ACC Thr T Threonine	AAC Asn N Asparagine	AGC Ser S Serine	C
	AUA Ile I Isoleucine	ACA Thr T Threonine	AAA Lys K Lysine	AGA Arg R Arginine	A
	AUG Met M Methionine	ACG Thr T Threonine	AAG Lys K Lysine	AGG Arg R Arginine	G
G	GUU Val V Valine	GCU Ala A Alanine	GAU Asp D Aspartic acid	GGU Gly G Glycine	U
	GUC Val V Valine	GCC Ala A Alanine	GAC Asp D Aspartic acid	GGC Gly G Glycine	C
	GUA Val V Valine	GCA Ala A Alanine	GAA Glu E Glutamic acid	GGA Gly G Glycine	A
	GUG Val V Valine	GCG Ala A Alanine	GAG Glu E Glutamic acid	GGG Gly G Glycine	G

Third nucleotide in codon

Codon

Three-letter and single-letter abbreviations

*Amino acids are the building blocks of proteins. The 20 amino acids are constructed from information contained in the DNA blueprint that is translated and transcribed by RNA. This transfer of information from DNA to amino acids is called the *genetic code*. Triple sets of bases (codons) are transcribed into the 20 amino acids. Sixty-four combinations of codons are possible, and several codons code for the same amino acids. The amino acids are connected in long polypeptide chains that form proteins. Three combinations signal the end of a protein chain: UAA, UAG, and UGA. Each three-letter codon also has a single-letter abbreviation, which is shown in the table.

BOX 4-1 GENETIC CONDITIONS IN CRITICAL CARE: DEEP VEIN THROMBOSIS AND FACTOR V LEIDEN

CLINICAL PRESENTATION

Carriers of the coagulation factor V Leiden polymorphism are at increased risk for venous thromboembolism (VTE), identified by deep vein thrombosis (DVT) or pulmonary embolism (PE). The phenotype (clinical signs and symptoms) is defined by an increased incidence of DVT. Factor V Leiden thrombophilia is suspected in individuals with a history of DVT or PE and in people with first-degree family members who have experienced recurrent thromboemboli. Assessment is warranted for women who experience DVT during pregnancy or a DVT while on oral contraceptives or hormone replacement therapy (HRT).[7-10]

GENETIC EVIDENCE

The factor V *(F5)* gene is located on chromosome 1 on the long arm at position 23 (1q23). The Factor V Leiden polymorphism refers to the specific G-to-A substitution at nucleotide 1691 in the coagulation factor V gene (genotype). This causes a single amino acid replacement at position 506 from arginine to glutamine. The resultant nonfunctional gene protein is called factor V Leiden.

Normal factor V circulates in plasma as an inactive cofactor. Activation by thrombin results in the formation of factor Va, which serves as a cofactor in the conversion of prothrombin to thrombin. To express its anticoagulant function, normal factor Va must be cleaved by activated protein C (APC) at arginine in the 506 position and then at other sites within the factor Va molecule. Factor Va Leiden cannot be cleaved by APC because there is a glutamine at the 506 position. Factor Va Leiden therefore is inactivated more slowly than normal factor Va. This leaves more factor Va available within the prothrombin complex, which increases coagulation because of ongoing generation of thrombin.

The factor V Leiden variant occurs in about 5% of the white U.S. population. The term *Leiden* in the name refers to the town in the Netherlands, where the gene was initially discovered. Factor V Leiden is also the most common cause of APC resistance, which may additively increase the risk of thrombosis.[8,9]

Several large studies have examined the association between factor V Leiden and venous thrombosis. The Longitudinal Investigation of Thromboembolism Etiology (LITE) study was a prospective cohort study involving 335 men and women in the United States who developed a venous thromboembolism during 8 years of follow-up. This was a case-control study nested within a much larger cardiovascular trial. The LITE study evaluated genetic risk factors for future DVT or PE. The occurrence of VTE, adjusted for age, was 3.67-fold higher in carriers of factor V Leiden than in noncarriers.

GENE-ENVIRONMENT INTERACTIONS

The standard risk factors for DVT also apply to patients with factor V Leiden. The risk for DVT is increased by smoking, obesity, immobility, and trauma. Several additional genetic defects in the factor V gene have been identified as possible risk factors for thrombosis. One study identified seven other single nucleotide polymorphisms (SNPs) associated with DVT occurrence. Individuals with two or more genetic risk factors (gene-gene interactions) are at much higher risk for DVT. Studies to more clearly evaluate this risk are ongoing.

INHERITANCE

The factor V Leiden allele is inherited in an autosomal dominant pattern. This means the person needs only one copy of the factor V Leiden gene (heterozygous) to be at increased risk for DVT. People with two copies of the variant gene (one from each parent) have an even greater risk of DVT. In one study, the average age for first venous thrombosis was 44 years for factor V Leiden heterozygotes and 31 years for factor V homozygotes.[9]

WHO SHOULD UNDERGO GENETIC TESTING?

Genetic testing is reserved for those in high-risk groups who have experienced a first DVT before age 50 years; a first, unprovoked (no environmental stimuli) DVT at any age; a history of recurrent DVT; and thromboembolism in unusual venous locations, such as the cerebral, mesenteric, portal, and hepatic veins.[8]

To test for factor V Leiden, the first step is to do an APC-resistance assay. If the blood test shows APC resistance, it is likely the individual carries the factor V Leiden variant, and genetic testing is done as a secondary analysis.

Not all changes in the DNA sequence have deleterious effects. Most SNPs have no effect because they are *synonymous SNPs*, variants that code for the same amino acid (see Table 4-1), or because they are located in noncoding region.

GENETIC INHERITANCE

GENETIC DISORDERS

All genetic disorders do not have the same cause. The major categories of disorders are chromosome disorders, single-gene disorders, complex gene and multifactorial disorders, and mitochondrial disorders.

Chromosome Disorders. In chromosome disorders, the entire chromosome or very large segments of the chromosome are damaged, missing, duplicated, or otherwise altered. Down syndrome (trisomy 21), in which there is an extra copy of chromosome 21, is an example of a chromosome disorder.

Singe-Gene Disorders. In single-gene disorders, a single gene is altered. Single-gene disorders can result from inheritance of one dominant gene or two recessive genes. Cystic fibrosis, sickle cell disease, hemophilia A, and Marfan syndrome are examples of single-gene disorders. Single-gene disorders may also be described as monogenetic or mendelian gene disorders.

Complex Gene and Multifactorial Disorders. In some disorders, many genes interact to produce the condition, or there must be an interaction between vulnerable genes and the environment. Cardiovascular atherosclerotic diseases and type 2 diabetes are examples of complex gene disorders that result from an interaction of genetic and environmental factors. Pharmacogenetic syndromes are caused by the interactions of genes and medications.

Mitochondrial Disorders. Some diseases are caused by alterations in the DNA of the mitochondria, which are intracellular organelles found in the cytoplasm. Mitochondrial DNA is totally different and separate from the double-helix DNA found in the nucleus. Mitochondrial DNA is transferred to offspring by maternal transmission only, because mitochondria occur in oocytes but not in sperm. Most mitochondrial genetic diseases are associated with disorders of enzyme function that disrupts

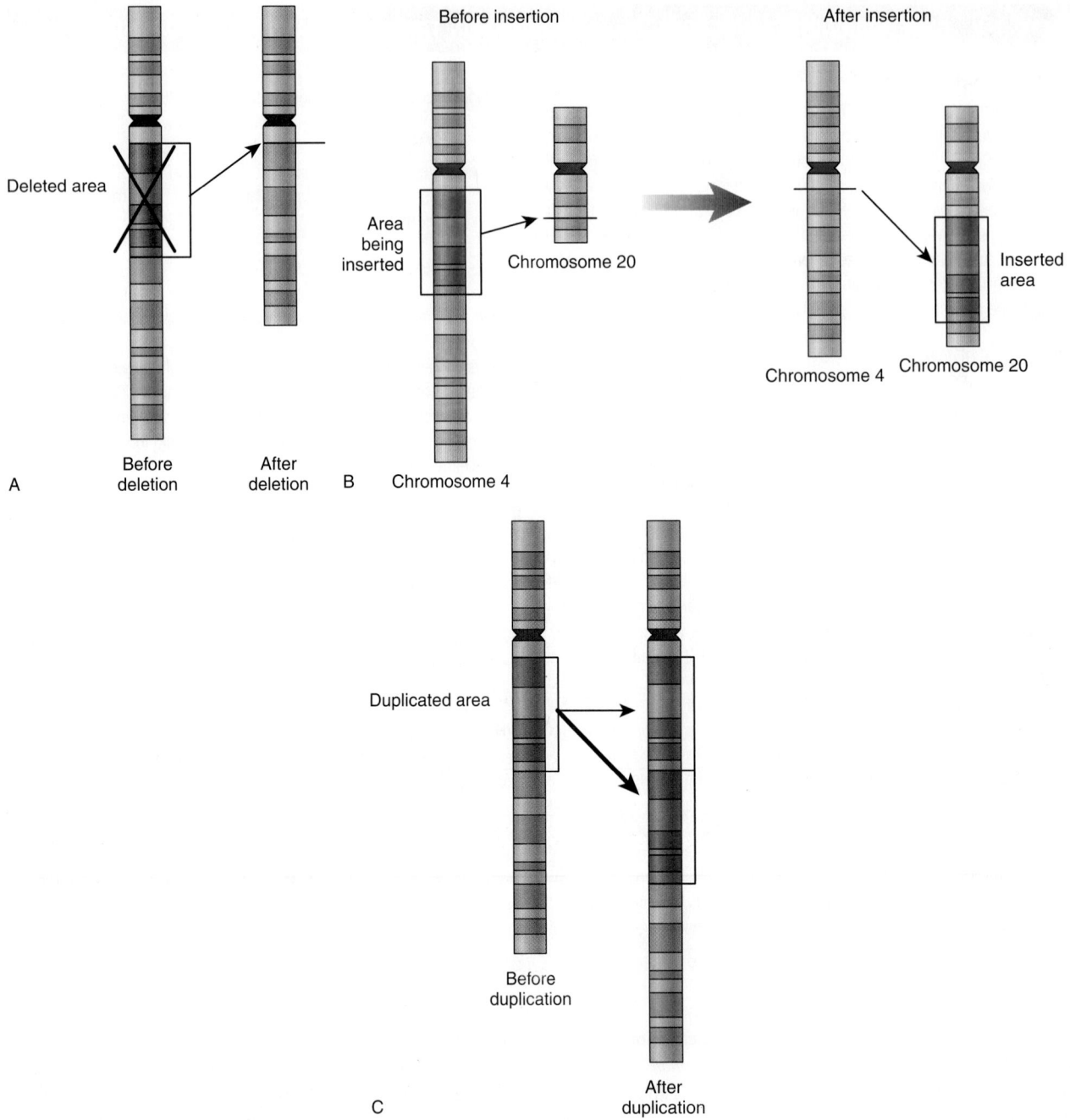

Figure 4-6 *A,* Deletion of chromosomal genetic material. *B,* Insertion of genetic material from one chromosome to another. *C,* Duplication of chromosomal genetic material.

mitochondrial energy production. Tissues and organs that have high-energy requirements such as skeletal muscles, the heart and the central nervous system are most often affected. Although few adult diseases associated with mitochondrial DNA have been identified, this remains an intense area of research.

GENOTYPE AND PHENOTYPE

The *genotype* refers to the genetic makeup at a particular *locus* or location on a specific chromosome within the genome; this is conceptually similar to a unique street address. The *phenotype*

refers to the signs and symptoms that are clinically associated with a particular genetic condition; this is conceptually similar to describing the defining characteristics of the house, apartment, boat, dorm room, or castle at this particular address.

GENETIC HISTORY AND FAMILY PEDIGREE

One of the tools used to determine whether a disease has a genetic component is construction of a family pedigree.[12,13] For nurses, it is important to develop the skills to ask questions to elucidate which family members are affected and which are

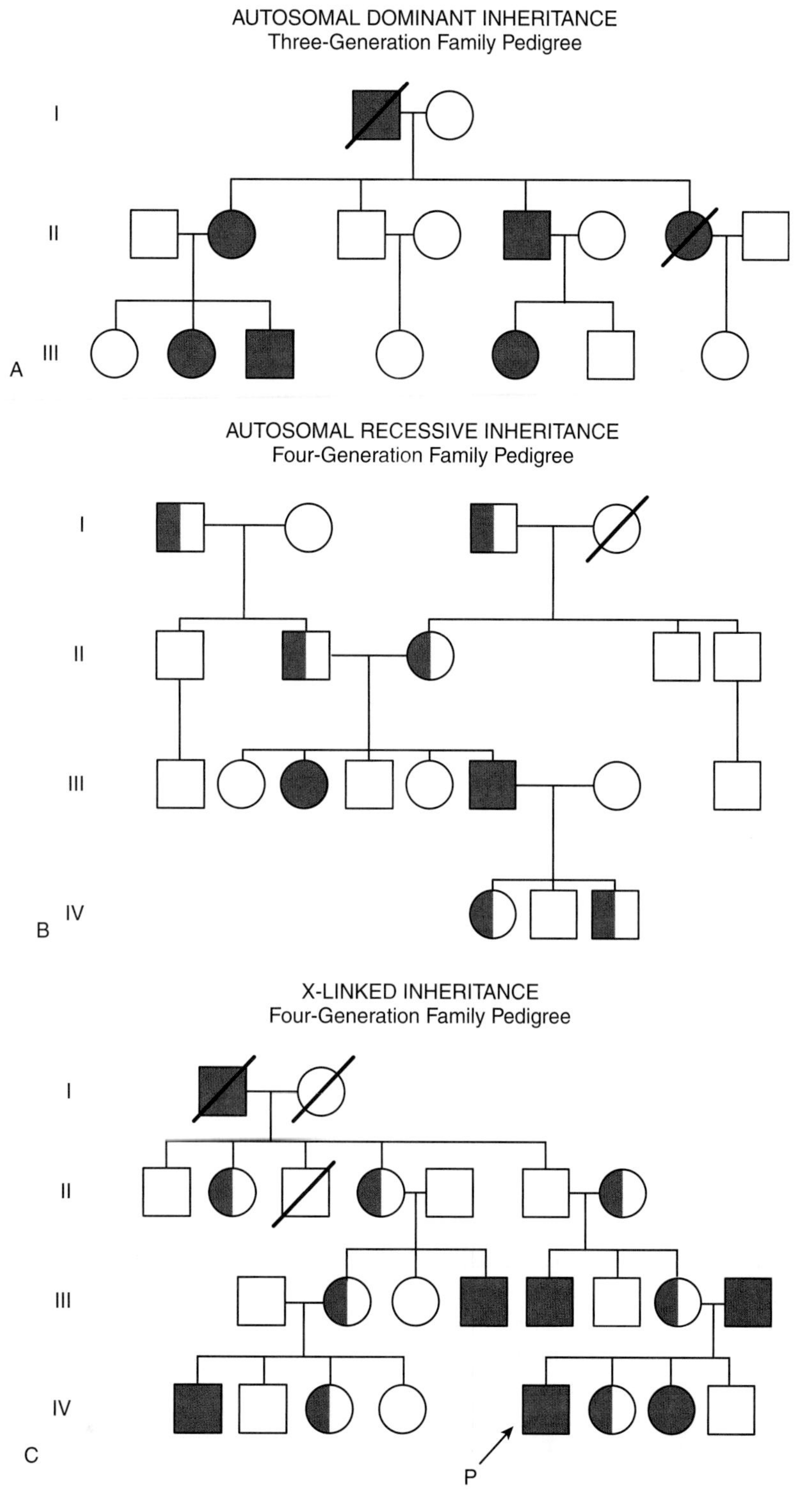

AUTOSOMAL DOMINANT INHERITANCE
Three-Generation Family Pedigree

AUTOSOMAL RECESSIVE INHERITANCE
Four-Generation Family Pedigree

X-LINKED INHERITANCE
Four-Generation Family Pedigree

Figure 4-7 *A,* Pedigree of a dominant mode of inheritance. *B,* Pedigree of a recessive mode of inheritance. *C,* Pedigree of an X-linked mode of inheritance. See text for further information.

(Continued)

unaffected and then to identify the individuals who may carry the gene in question but do not have symptoms (carriers).[14,15] Standardized symbols are used in the construction of a pedigree.[16] The use of a legend to explain what the symbols mean prevents misinterpretation. The *proband* is the name given to the first person diagnosed in the family pedigree. Examples of three simple pedigrees that illustrate the primary modes of genetic disorder inheritance and the symbols used to construct a pedigree are shown in Figure 4-7 with examples described below.

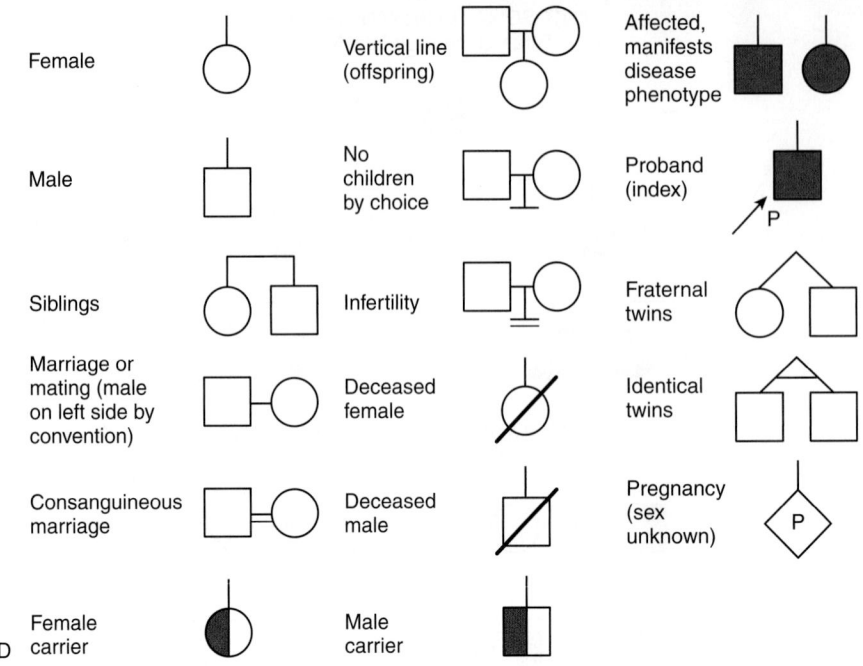

Figure 4-7, cont'd *D,* Symbols used to construct a pedigree.

Homozygous versus Heterozygous. Each individual inherits genetic material from his or her father and mother. If an individual inherits the same gene at a specific locus (genetic address) from both parents, the person is described as *homozygous* for that gene. If the genes donated by the parents differ at that locus, the person is described as *heterozygous* for that gene.

Modes of Inheritance. One of the keys to understanding the genetics literature is to understand the vocabulary. All humans have 23 pair of chromosomes. One pair is sex linked: XX for a woman and XY for a man. The other 22 chromosomes are called *autosomes.* It is from this word that the term *autosomal inheritance* is derived. The differences between some of the major forms of autosomal inheritance are described in the following sections.

Autosomal Dominant Inheritance. Autosomal dominant inheritance is described as a dominant pattern because only one copy of an affected gene is required to transmit the condition. The person has inherited one affected gene from one parent, and one different healthy gene from the other parent, and is described as heterozygous for that gene. Typically, the disease appears in every generation. Each child of an affected parent has a 50% chance of inheriting the condition, depending on whether a parent has transmitted a chromosome with the affected gene or not. Male and female offspring are equally likely to inherit and transmit the condition (see Fig. 4-7A). Examples of conditions with dominant inheritance patterns include familial hypercholesterolemia (FH) and Marfan syndrome.

Autosomal Recessive Inheritance. With an autosomal recessive pattern of inheritance, the disease or condition manifests only if the person has received an affected gene from both parents. The parents are *carriers* of the gene but are not themselves affected. The parents are heterozygous, because they have one copy of a normal gene and one copy of an affected gene. The inheritance pattern for this situation is slightly complex. Any of their children has a 25% chance to inherit in the following combinations: one normal and one affected gene (heterozygous carrier), two normal genes (unaffected), or two affected genes (homozygous affected). Persons who are homozygous for the gene associated with the disease always are affected, which means they demonstrate the phenotype of the disease (see Fig. 4-7B). In autosomal recessive inheritance, the phenotype associated with the condition is seen more often in siblings (sibships) than in the parents. Conditions associated with recessive inheritance include cystic fibrosis and sickle cell disease.

Sex-Linked Inheritance. Traits controlled by genes located on the sex chromosomes are called *sex-linked traits.* Red-green color blindness is an example of an X-linked trait.

Hemophilia A. Some diseases are inherited through an X-linked pattern of inheritance. A classic example is the *F8* gene, which codes for the protein that makes coagulation factor VIII. The *F8* gene is located on the X chromosome. Women always have two X chromosomes (XX), one from the mother and one from the father. Even if the mother carried an affected *F8* gene, the gene on the unaffected chromosome from the father would confer the ability to make coagulation factor VIII and avoid hemophilia. However, men (XY) inherit one X chromosome from their mother and one Y chromosome from their father. If the mother's X chromosome carries the affected *F8* gene, the male offspring will be unable to make sufficient factor VIII, will manifest the bleeding disorder known as hemophilia A, and will be at risk for life-threatening bleeding. In an *X-linked disorder,* each son has a 50% chance of being hemophiliac, and each daughter has a 50% chance of being a carrier. In a family pedigree, the absence of direct male-to-male transmission makes this condition identifiable as an X-linked disorder. Hemophilia A is also an example of a single-gene disorder. Figure 4-7C illustrates an X-linked family pedigree for hemophilia A; a male who is affected (generation I) may pass the X-linked *F8* gene only to his daughters (generation II), who may pass the gene to sons who will be affected, or to daughters who will be carriers (generation III). A female will only be affected if she receives a defective X-linked gene from both her father and mother as occurs in generation IV.

COMPLEX GENE-GENE AND GENE-ENVIRONMENT DISORDERS

Many genetic disorders are complex, and multiple factors are thought to contribute to manifestation of disease phenotypes. They result from *gene-gene* interactions or *gene-environment* interactions. Many patients who are admitted to the critical care unit may exhibit the phenotype of a complex genetic condition if they are obese or have type 2 diabetes.

Obesity and the *FTO* Gene. The pandemic of obesity in the industrialized world has entrained higher rates of cardiovascular atherosclerotic disease and type 2 diabetes. Genome-wide association studies have identified polymorphisms in the *fat mass and obesity-associated gene (FTO)* on chromosome 16 that are linked to obesity.[17] A patient who is overweight or obese may blame it on "my bad genes," and this raises the question of whether the presence of an altered *FTO* gene automatically means the individual will be obese. A study of Amish adults with and without the *FTO* gene who lived a traditional pastoral lifestyle reported that the effect of the gene was blunted by 3 to 4 hours of physical activity each day.[18] This supports current knowledge about risk factor reduction and the importance of regular physical activity, but 3 hours of physical activity per day is rarely recommended. Individuals may be influenced to increase their physical activity if they know they carry the *FTO* gene.

HOW INFORMATION ABOUT GENETICS IS OBTAINED

Genetic information can be collected in many ways. Often, when a gene is selected, all of the methods described here may be used to link the phenotype, genotype, and environmental effects.

GENETIC EPIDEMIOLOGY

Genetic epidemiology represents the fusion of epidemiologic studies and genetic research methods. Before a gene can be mapped (genotyped), it is essential to have a reliable phenotype that can be consistently measured.[19] One of the challenges in applying genetics to the critical care arena is that the genotype is stable but the phenotype is dynamic. Phenotypes are different at different stages of a disease and are influenced by medications, environmental factors, and gene-gene interactions.[19,20] It is helpful to discuss the methods used outside of the critical care unit as a way of understanding the challenges in the application of genetics in this arena.

Family-Based Genetic Studies. In genetic epidemiologic research of a rare disease, it can be a challenge to find enough people to study. One method is to work with large, extended families, known as *kinships*, which have several family members affected with the disease. Genetic testing is done to construct a genetic linkage map of the area close to the polymorphic gene found in that family. Family-based studies can identify a significant phenotype-genotype relationship.[21] Subsequently, it is important to do studies of other groups to determine whether the original finding is unique to the kinship or can be generalized to people outside the family.

Twin Studies. Studies of identical twins offer a unique opportunity to investigate the association of genetics, environment, and health. Identical twins are *monozygotic* and share an identical genome. Twin studies to compare the effects of genetics versus environment have been conducted by studying identical twins separated at birth. This situation occurs much less frequently today because tremendous efforts are made to keep siblings together when they are adopted.

Genetic Association Studies. Genetic association studies are usually conducted in large, unrelated groups based on demonstration of a phenotype (disease trait or symptoms) and associated genotype. In genetic association studies, it is important to recruit a diverse group of individuals to determine whether a trait is universal or found only in selected groups. Genetic studies can be conducted in isolated populations, in which *population stratification* is expected, or in highly mixed groups. It is important to collect information about ancestral and racial heritage to enable linkage of phenotypic and genotypic data. Diverse populations are sometimes called *admixed populations*, indicating that many different heritage groups have been included in the mix of people. The purpose of these different kinds of studies is to make a clear phenotype-genotype match and to identify which genetic conditions are associated with specific racial or ethnic groups and which genetic conditions are universal.

Case-Control Studies. In case-control studies, individuals are identified with the phenotypic and genotypic traits of a disease (cases). Theses cases are then matched to nonrelated controls by age, race, sex, and sometimes other associated disease factors.

Candidate Gene Studies. Candidate gene studies usually are exploratory studies in which a gene is suspected as a contributor to a phenotype or disease. Unrelated individuals with the phenotype are then tested for presence of the gene. These usually are smaller studies, and there is a strong biologic rational for investigating the association between genotype and phenotype.

Genome-Wide Association Studies. Genome-wide association studies (GWAS) examine the breadth of the human genome and typically use very large samples. The intent is to use genetic microarray technology and statistical computational power to find SNPs associated with a disease. Some GWAS are conducted with the intent of finding additional genes. However, one of the strengths of the GWAS model is that it does not have to begin with a biologic model in mind as long as the disease of interest is sufficiently common in the population, and by testing thousands of SNPs, the researchers may find associations that have not been detected by other methods.

An example is a GWAS of 14,000 individuals (cases) with 3000 shared controls genotyped to find SNPs associated with seven common diseases.[22] Significant new SNPs were found for five of seven diseases: type 1 diabetes, type 2 diabetes, rheumatoid arthritis, Crohn's disease, and coronary artery disease.[22] New GWAS are published every month, and the National Human Genome Research Institute (NHGRI) maintains a catalog of published studies that can be searched by disease trait, chromosomal region, gene, or SNP.[23]

GENE MAPPING PROJECTS

The Human Genome Project. The Human Genome Project was a huge, internationally collaborative project that began in 1990 with the goal of making a map of all the human genes (the genome). The final genome sequence was published in 2003. Big discoveries came out of the Human Genome Project, including a map of the human genome and a wealth of new clinical and computational tools that could be used for future studies.

The human genome map was created from the DNA of only a few people. One of the surprising discoveries was that the number of genes possessed by humans was not as large as expected. The number of genes in the chromosome is estimated to be between 20,000 and 25,000.[1] Although researchers were initially surprised that the gene number was not higher, it has become apparent than many posttranscriptional alterations occur to actively change the protein product. The ongoing research agenda is to understand all of these additional sequence elements.

ENCODE Project. The *Encyclopedia of DNA Elements* (ENCODE) pilot project published a detailed analysis of 1% of the human genome using cell lines.[24] The goal is to elucidate all of the functional elements that enable relatively few human genes to produce such a wide variety of biologic products (e.g., proteins). One area of investigation has been to understand the regulatory role of RNAs in modulating cellular functions directly as biologically active molecules or indirectly by encoding other active molecules.[24] Another area of research is focused on the transcriptional regulatory elements that control the expression of each regulatory transcript, such as genetic promoters, enhancers, silencers, insulators, and locus control regions.

HapMap Project. The International HapMap Project database[25] displays genetic linear loci on short sections of the same chromosome in patterns known as *haplotypes* or *haplotype blocks*. Loci are grouped as a haplotype if they are close to each other on a chromosome and are inherited as a linear group. Genetic epidemiologists call this grouped pattern *linkage disequilibrium*. It means that the loci are linked in a nonrandom manner due to shared ancestry, where genetic information was inherited by offspring in "chunks" or "blocks" rather than as individual genes. The mixing of sections of different chromosomes that are inherited from each parent is called *recombination*. The resultant linked genetic loci are called *haplotypes*. The edges of the haplotypes are conceptualized as recombination "hotspots," where little ancestral relationship remains. An example of the expected change over 150,000 years from African ancestral chromosomes to modern chromosomes is shown in Figure 4-8. The biologic rationale for recombination is to increase genetic diversity.

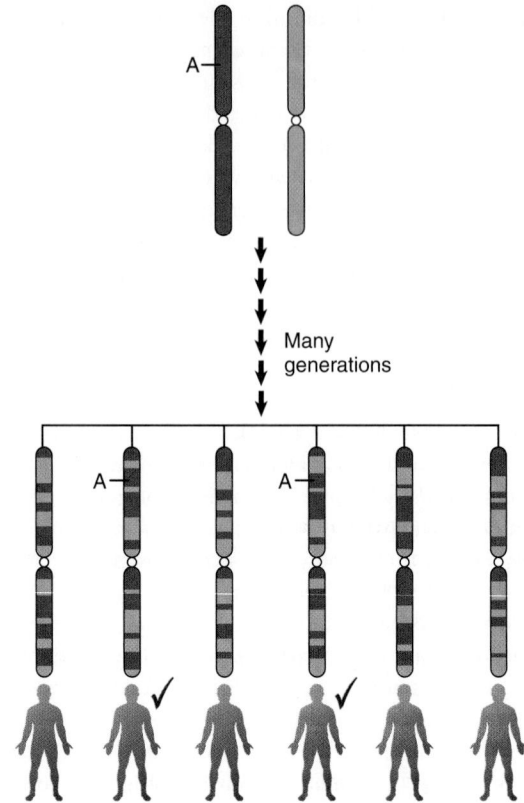

Figure 4-8 Effect of recombination on ancestral chromosomes. A gene is labeled **A** on the red ancestral chromosome. It is an example of a gene that has been conserved in modern chromosomes in one-third of cases. The gene (A) is associated with a specific phenotype or trait (shown as a checkmark). Because of recombination of chromosomes over thousands of generations, two-thirds of modern chromosomes no longer carry this gene.

The initial HapMap phase I database was constructed between 2002 and 2005, and it genotyped approximately 1 million SNPs at an average spacing of 5 kilobases (kb). A kilobase represents 10^3 nucleotide base pairs.[2] One of the goals was to identify haplotype tags, or *tag SNPs,* that identified major haplotypes to reduce the number of SNPs needed for genetic association studies.[26] This was a highly successful strategy, and thousands of tag SNP *candidate gene* studies have been conducted.

An updated HapMap phase II database (2005-2008)[25] contains 3.1 million SNPs from 270 individuals representing four populations: African (Yoruba, Nigerian), European Americans (Utah), Japanese, and Han Chinese.[27] The HapMap phase II database has revealed new information about untaggable SNPs and recombination hotspots. More than 32,000 hotspots have been identified. More than 50% of all untaggable SNPs lie within 1 kb of the center of a recombination hotspot, and more than 90% are within 5 kb.[27] Hotspots account for approximately 60% of recombination in the human genome and represent about 6% of the genomic sequence.[27]

HapMap phase III is just beginning, and one of the significant advances will be to increase the diversity of the number of specific populations who donate DNA. Over time, this will make the HapMap database more representative of the diversity of human populations.

1000 Genomes Project. The scientific goals of the *1000 Genomes Project* are to produce a database of variants that occur at 1% or greater frequency in the human population across most of the genome and down to 0.5% or lower within genes. This study will not collect any health-related phenotypic information. It will produce a catalog of human genome variation.

The Human Microbiome Project. In the healthy human body, microbial cells are estimated to outnumber human cells by a factor of 10 to 1. The human body is host to many microbial communities (human microbiome) located on the skin and in the nose, mouth, gastrointestinal, and urogenital tracts. The spectrum of these microbial communities is almost entirely unknown. The Human Microbiome Project (HMP) is designed to determine whether individuals share a core human microbiome, and to determine whether changes in the human microbiome can be correlated with changes in human health. The HMP is highly relevant to critical care because so many patients are admitted with sepsis or experience disruption of the gastrointestinal tract with diarrhea. The interaction of host bacteria, pathologic bacteria, critical care environment, and pharmacogenetics has the potential to bring novel insights to the ongoing battle against iatrogenic infection in the critically ill.[28]

GENETIC DIVERSITY

The oldest human genetic lineages originate from the continent of Africa. The migration of a subset of humans out of Africa resulted in loss of genetic diversity. Numerous studies have shown higher levels of nucleotide and haplotype diversity of nuclear and mitochondrial genomes in Africans than in non-Africans.[29] Large-scale autosomal studies of African genetic diversity are being conducted.

Copy Number Variation. A study[30] of eight human genomes focused on the topic of copy number variation (CNV), including insertions, deletions, and inversions of DNA. It is not yet clear which copy number variants are benign or are associated with disease. CNV will add an additional layer of variation and understanding to the human genome.[30]

Individual Genome Sequences. It is stratospherically expensive to sequence the genome of an individual. However, two individual genomes of white men have been sequenced and publicly identified: J. Craig Venter[31] and James D. Watson.[31,32] One of the challenges, other than the expense, is how to use all of the data provided by genome analysis. Another issue is personal privacy. Although both of these individuals allowed their genetic information to be published, James Watson requested that information related to the *APOE* gene, with its known risk for Alzheimer's disease, not be analyzed. Such privacy issues are understandable and will require serious thought and discussion on individual and societal levels.

GENETICS IN CRITICAL CARE

The next step in the genomics revolution will be to connect the growing amounts of research data to clinical interventions that may help patients. The areas of clinical practice in which this has received most attention are cancer, cardiovascular disease, and pharmacogenomics.

CANCER GENETICS

Somatic Mutations. The word *somatic* means "related to the body." Somatic mutations are changes within a specific group of body tissues that are not heritable. Often, somatic changes are related to changes in genetic markers associated with cancer or cardiovascular disease.

The Cancer Genome Atlas. There is strong evidence that many forms of cancer are caused by epigenetic alterations; one mechanism is the addition of methyl groups to specific genes to block their effect, a process sometimes referred to as *gene silencing.* Epigenetic changes can disrupt the normal balance in cell proliferation, cell survival, and cell differentiation. The Cancer Genome Atlas (TCGA) pilot project was established to accelerate understanding of the molecular basis of human cancers. The large-scale genome sequencing techniques, first developed in the Human Genome Project, are used to sequence genes associated with lethal and common cancers. The goal is to document all cancer genetic changes from chromosomal rearrangements to DNA mutations to epigenetic changes (chemical modifications of DNA that can turn genes on or off without altering the DNA sequence). TCGA is an international research initiative that has demonstrated it may be more important to identify and target specialized biologic pathways in many lethal cancers than single genes. Biologic pathway disruptions result in multiple gene rearrangements of gene clusters, which at first appear to be unrelated but are connected by cellular signaling systems orchestrated by complex biologic pathways.[33]

CARDIOVASCULAR GENETICS

Genetic markers are being included in many cardiovascular research studies.[34] A classic example is the Framingham Heart Study. This longitudinal, multigenerational study was started in 1948 to identify the common factors that contribute to cardiovascular disease.[35] The researchers have phenotypic and pedigree data for several generations, and they have added genetic markers to their investigation of biologic and epidemiologic factors.[36-38] These genomic research studies have the potential to dramatically improve current knowledge about interactions between genetics and environmental factors.

Long QT Syndrome. Long QT syndrome (LQTS) is a cardiac electrical disorder that can be accurately genotyped to three mutations in about 70% of cases (Box 4-2). Not all patients who have the LQTS genotype are aware of their condition, and if admitted to the critical care unit these patients are at risk of gene-environment or gene-medication interactions that may lengthen their QT interval and increase their risk of torsades de pointes and cardiac arrest.[39-40] Adults with LQTS have a significantly higher risk of sudden cardiac death (SCD) than individuals without the LQTS genotype.[41]

PHARMACOGENETICS

Pharmacogenetics is the study of gene-medication interactions. Pharmacogenetics is likely to be the most visible impact of genetics encountered in the adult critical care unit in the

BOX 4-2 GENETIC CONDITIONS IN CRITICAL CARE: LONG QT SYNDROME

CLINICAL PRESENTATION

Long QT syndrome (LQTS) is a cardiac genetic disorder identified by a prolonged QTc interval, longer than 500 milliseconds on the resting electrocardiogram (ECG). LQTS is estimated to affect 1 in 5000 individuals and is one of the primary causes of sudden cardiac death (SCD) in the young.[39] In children it is often called Congenital LQTS.

Frequently patients are identified following a syncopal episode, a life-threatening dysrhythmia such as torsades de pointes, or SCD. Treatment regimens include beta-blockers. For LQTS patients at high-risk of cardiac arrest insertion of a pacemaker/internal cardioverter defibrillator (ICD) is warranted.

Patients in ICU with undiagnosed LQTS are vulnerable to additional prolongation of their QT interval from a variety of medications. The American Heart Association recommends monitoring of the QT interval.

GENETIC EVIDENCE

Several genes have been identified for LQTS 1-10, and the three most common are listed below.

All encode protein components of the cardiac ion channels, and modulate ionic flow. Sometimes these disorders are described as "channelopathies."

LQTS1 is caused by a mutation in the *KCNQ1* gene (also known as the *KvLQT1* gene), which encodes a potassium channel protein active in phase 3 of the cardiac action potential (the I_{ks} current). It is seen in 35%-50% of LQTS cases. This mutation can be inherited as an autosomal dominant or autosomal recessive gene.

LQTS2 is caused by a mutation in the *KCNH2* gene (also known as the *HERG* gene), which encodes a potassium channel protein that normally terminates the cardiac action potential (the I_{Kr} current). It is seen is 25%-30% of cases.

LQTS3 is caused by a mutation in the *SCN5A* gene, which encodes a sodium channel protein in phase 0 of the cardiac action potential (the NaV15 current). It is seen in 5%-10% of cases.

GENE ENVIRONMENT INTERACTIONS

Gene environment interactions are significant for LQTS patients and vary by genotype and by individual[40,41]:
- LQTS1 have a higher incidence of ventricular dysrhythmias and SCD events during exercise, especially swimming (physical exertion trigger).
- LQST2 have a higher incidence of ventricular dysrhythmias and SCD events during sleep and are very sensitive to sudden loud noises that cause a startle reflex (auditory trigger).
- LQST3 have a higher incidence of ventricular dysrhythmias and SCD events during sleep and rest.

INHERITANCE

Both autosomal dominant and autosomal recessive patterns of inheritance occur.

Not all individuals have the same phenotype even with the same genotype. This is thought to be due to the influence of additional genes acting in concert with the primary gene to alter the cardiac action potential, to cause QT prolongation.

WHO SHOULD UNDERGO GENETIC TESTING?

Clinical Genetic testing is available for LQTS. Genetic testing is very helpful within families of patients with LTQS. If the family member has a prolonged QT interval the reasonable assumption during the cardiac and genetic work-up is that they have the mutation. However, it can be important to test family members with a normal QT interval as well. This is because of a genetic concept termed *penetrance*, where the same gene does not have the same phenotypic effect on everyone who is affected. If a person carries the genetic mutation, but has a normal QT interval at rest, they may still be vulnerable during exercise or physiologic stress.

---

immediate future, particularly in relation to the cytochrome P450 family of enzymes involved in drug metabolism.

Cytochrome P450 Family and Drug Metabolism. The cytochrome P450 (CYP450) enzymes are a superfamily of heme-containing enzymes that are vital for drug metabolism. The CYP450 family is gene regulated, and for many individuals, this pathway determines how well drugs are metabolized.[42] More than 57 CYP enzymes have been identified in humans.[42] The isoenzymes CYP3A4 and CYP3A5 metabolize about 50% of currently marketed drugs, and they constitute approximately 60% of the total hepatic CYP450 enzyme content.[42] The metabolism of more than 90% of the most clinically important medications can be accounted for by seven CYP isozymes: 3A4, 3A5, 1A2, 2C9, 2C19, 2D6, and 2E1.[42]

CYP3A4 can be used to understand what the abbreviations represent. *CYP* represents the symbol for all cytochrome P450 proteins, *3* denotes the gene family, *A* designates the subfamily, and *4* represents the individual gene.[42] The U.S. Food and Drug Administration (FDA) requires that new drugs undergo testing for interactions with the CYP450 pathway before release.

Warfarin. Warfarin (Coumadin) is a frequently prescribed anticoagulant for patents with atrial fibrillation, mechanical cardiac valves, or thrombotic disorders. Variants in the cytochrome P450 enzyme *CYP2C9* gene and in the vitamin K epoxide reductase complex subunit 1 gene *(VKORC1)* contribute to the considerable dose variation seen with this anticoagulant.[43] The vitamin K epoxide reductase (VKOR) enzyme activates the vitamin K–dependent clotting factors (II, VII, IX, X). Warfarin is used to inhibit the VKOR complex to prevent clot formation.

Several prospective studies showed that up to 30% of dose variability during the initiation phase of warfarin anticoagulation could be explained by *CYP2C9* and *VKORC1* polymorphisms. Genetic testing is not currently recommended for everyone who takes warfarin. Laboratory tests to detect the *CYP2C9* and *VKORC1* variants are available only at specialized reference laboratories. In August 2007, the FDA added a warning label on the package to alert clinicians about *CYP2C9* and *VKORC1* polymorphism interactions and their effects on warfarin dosing.[44]

Malignant Hyperthermia. Individuals with polymorphisms in the ryanodine receptor 1 gene *(RYR1)* at chromosome 19q13.1 are at risk for a rare pharmacogenetic condition known as *malignant hyperthermia*.[45,46] In affected individuals, exposure to inhalation anesthetics and depolarizing muscle relaxants during general anesthesia induces life-threatening muscle

BOX 4-3   GENETIC CONDITIONS IN CRITICAL CARE: MALIGNANT HYPERTHERMIA

CLINICAL PRESENTATION

Malignant hyperthermia (MH) is a pharmacogenetic syndrome. MH is a disorder of skeletal muscle calcium regulation. On exposure to inhalation anesthetics and depolarizing muscle relaxants, susceptible patients experience life-threatening symptoms, including sustained muscle contracture with skeletal muscle rigidity, which causes metabolic acidosis, tachycardia, and fever. The symptoms result from an abnormally high release of intracellular calcium in skeletal muscle.

GENETIC EVIDENCE

Genetic linkage studies associated the MH phenotype with the ryanodine receptor 1 gene *(RYR1)* at chromosome 19q13.1 in several families. Calcium transport from muscle sarcoplasmic reticulum through the ryanodine receptor into the sarcoplasm occurs during muscular excitation and contraction. A biologic model also supported *RYR1* as a candidate gene. Other candidate genes exist, but none is as well characterized as the *RYR1* gene variants. The *RYR1* gene is highly polymorphic, with more than 170 polymorphisms, although not all are causative. Currently, 29 *RYR1* mutations are known to cause MH. Presence of any of these mutations is diagnostic for MH susceptibility. A genetic analysis exists to test for causative *RYR1* gene mutations.[43,44]

GENE-ENVIRONMENT INTERACTIONS

MH is an example of a gene-environment interaction. It is not an allergy, and it occurs only under the specific environmental condition of general anesthesia with inhalation anesthetics (e.g., chloroform, desflurane, enflurane, halothane, isoflurane, methoxyflurane, sevoflurane, trichloroethylene) and depolarizing muscle relaxants (e.g., succinylcholine).

INHERITANCE

MH is inherited in an autosomal dominant pattern. This means that only one affected allele is needed to have the condition and that children of an affected person have a 50% chance of inheriting the mutated *RYR1* gene.

WHO SHOULD UNDERGO GENETIC TESTING?

MH crisis under general anesthesia is rare. The genetic test for *RYR1* is not recommended as a general screening test. Genetic testing is recommended only for people who have experienced an MH crisis, those who are first-degree relatives of a person with known MH, or individuals who have had a positive result from a muscle biopsy. The value of the genetic test is that when a mutation is discovered, family members with the same mutation are considered susceptible to MH and can avoid a diagnostic muscle biopsy. The major advantage of being aware of the diagnosis is that high-risk anesthetics can be avoided for general anesthesia in MH-susceptible individuals.[43]

ONLINE RESOURCES

European Malignant Hyperthermia Group: www.emhg.org/
Malignant Hyperthermia Association of the United States: www.mhaus.org/
Online Mendelian Inheritance in Man (OMIM), ryanodine receptor 1 gene *(RYR1):* www.ncbi.nlm.nih.gov/entrez/dispomim.cgi?id=180901

---

contracture with skeletal muscle rigidity, acidosis, and elevated temperature. Malignant hyperthermia is described in more detail in Box 4-3.

GENETICS AND THE HEALTH PROFESSIONS

As genetics exerts more influence in clinical practice, it will have implications for the knowledge base of nurses and other professionals in health care. The addition of genetics also introduces new ethical and legal dilemmas into health care discussions. The learning curve may be steep.

CORE COMPETENCIES FOR HEALTH CARE PROFESSIONALS

Genetics will have a big impact on how health and illness are conceptualized in the future. Essential competencies for nursing practice have been developed and are listed in Table 4-2.[47] It is always demanding to embrace a new model of health care delivery, but that is the challenge for all health care professionals in the coming decades. The tsunami of genetic information that is now flowing into research journals will rapidly make its way into clinical practice, including into critical care. This flood of new and relevant information will mandate that nurses understand genetic terms, incorporate genetic pedigree information into the history and physical examination, and be knowledgeable about pharmacogenetic interventions. Genetics and genomics constitute a complex area of study, made more so by the rapid evolution of scientific knowledge. One way to begin is to look at some of the free, internet-based, interactive educational tutorials listed in Box 4-4 and to become familiar with the vocabulary of genetics as listed in the glossary at the end of the chapter.

ETHICAL AND LEGAL ISSUES IN GENETICS AND GENOMICS

One of the paramount concerns in the genomic era is to protect the privacy of individuals' unique genetic information. Many countries have established biobanks as repositories of genetic material, and many tissue samples are stored in medical center tissue banks. Because all of the genome is contained within the cell, genetic identity or susceptibility to diseases can easily be determined from a small sample. Many ethicists are concerned that technical innovation may have outstripped ethical and legal protections.[48] Key issues are who *owns* the genetic material and *consent* as to who has access to the genetic information.[45] Debate about these issues is expected to continue as new advances push the technical limits of what can be discovered from a few drops of blood, a muscle biopsy sample, or a cheek swab.

The Genetic Information Nondiscrimination Act. The Genetic Information Nondiscrimination Act (GINA) is an essential piece of legislation designed to prevent the use of genetic information in employment and insurance decisions in the United States. The purpose of GINA is to protect

TABLE 4-2 Essential Genetics and Genomics Competencies for Nurses

Domain	Competencies of the Registered Nurse*
Professional Responsibilities	
Competent nursing incorporating genetic and genomic knowledge and skills	Recognizes when one's own attitudes and values related to genetic and genomic science may affect care provided to patients
	Advocates for patients access to desired genetic or genomic services and resources, including support groups
	Examines competency of practice on a regular basis, identifying areas of strength and areas in which professional development related to genetics and genomics would be beneficial
	Incorporates genetic and genomic technologies and information into registered nurse practice
	Demonstrates in practice the importance of tailoring genetic and genomic information and services to patients based on their culture, religion, knowledge level, literacy, and preferred language
	Advocates for the rights of all patients for autonomous, informed genetic and genomic related decision-making and voluntary action
Professional Practice and Assessment	
Application and integration of knowledge	Demonstrates an understanding of the relationship of genetics or genomics to health, prevention, screening, diagnostics, prognostics, selection of treatment, and monitoring of treatment effectiveness
	Demonstrates an ability to elicit a minimum of three generations of family health history information
	Constructs a pedigree from collected family history information using standardized symbols and terminology
	Collects personal, health, and developmental histories that consider genetic, environmental, and genomic influences and risks
	Conducts comprehensive health and physical assessments that incorporate knowledge about genetic, environmental, and genomic influences and risk factors
	Critically analyzes the history and physical assessment findings for genetic, environmental, and genomic influences and risk factors
	Assesses patients' knowledge, perceptions, and responses to genetic and genomic information
	Develops plan of care that incorporates genetic and genomic assessment information
Identification of needed information	Identifies patients who may benefit from specific genetic and genomic information or services based on assessment data
	Identifies credible, accurate, appropriate, and current genetic and genomic information, resources, services, and technologies specific to given patients
	Identifies ethical, ethnic or ancestral, cultural, religious, legal, fiscal, and societal issues related to genetic and genomic information and technologies
	Defines issues that undermine the rights of all patients for autonomous, informed genetic and genomic-related decision making and voluntary action
Assistance with referrals	Facilitates referrals for specialized genetic and genomic services for patients, as needed
Provision of education, care, and support	Provides patients with interpretation of selective genetic and genomic information or services
	Provides patients with genetic and genomic credible, accurate, appropriate, and current information, resources, services, and technologies that facilitate decision making
	Uses health promotion and disease prevention practices that consider genetic and genomic influences on risk with personal and environmental risk factors
	Incorporates knowledge of genetic or genomic risk factors (e.g., patient with a genetic predisposition for high cholesterol levels that can benefit from a change in lifestyle to decrease the likelihood that the genotype will be expressed)
	Uses genetically and genomically based interventions and information to improve patients' outcomes
	Collaborates with health care providers in providing genetic and genomic health care
	Collaborates with insurance providers or payers to facilitate reimbursement for genetic and genomic health care services
	Performs interventions and treatments appropriate to patients' genetic and genomic health care needs

*All registered nurses are expected to engage in activities consistent with the *Nursing: Scope and Standards of Practice*, 2004, by the American Nurses Association.
Modified from Jenkins J, Calzone KA: Establishing the essential nursing competencies for genetics and genomics, *J Nurs Sholarsh* 39(1):10-16, 2007.

BOX 4-4   INTERNET RESOURCES FOR GENETICS

Web Address	Source
Gene Databases	
www.genetests.org/	GeneReviews, University of Washington, Seattle, WA; funded by the National Institutes of Health (NIH)
www.ncbi.nlm.nih.gov/sites/entrez?db=omim	Online Mendelian Inheritance in Man (OMIM), Johns Hopkins University
www.genome.gov/	National Human Genome Resource Institute (NHGRI); catalog of published genome-wide association studies (GWAS) maintained by NHGRI
http://cancergenome.nih.gov/	The Cancer Genome Atlas (TCGA)
www.hapmap.org/	The International HapMap Project
Organizations	
www.isong.org/	International Society of Nurses in Genetics (ISONG)
www.nchpeg.org/	National Coalition of Health Professional Education in Genetics (NCHPEG)
Tutorials and Education	
http://gslc.genetics.utah.edu/	Learn Genetics, The University of Utah
www.genome.gov/Education/	Educational materials about genetics and genomics from the NIH
www.genome.gov/COURSE2008/	Current Topics in Genome Analysis 2008, National Genome Research Institute, NIH
www.dnalc.org/home.html	Cold Spring Harbor Laboratory

individuals who may have the gene for a disorder but do not manifest the phenotype from being penalized. Some people who may be at risk for a disorder will not be tested because they fear that a positive result may affect their employability. When GINA becomes law in 2009, all individuals who undergo genetic testing will be protected.

HUMAN GENETICS GLOSSARY

Allele: one of several alternative gene variants that can exist at a single locus (location) on a chromosome. The term *allele* may also be used when referring to SNP variants. The most frequently found allele in a population is called the *wild-type allele*.

Candidate gene: a gene that is believed to cause or contribute to a disease. This term is typically used when the gene will be included in a research study.

Chromosomes: structures made of DNA and proteins and located in the nuclei of cells. Chromosomes come in pairs, and a normal human cell contains 46 chromosomes: 22 pairs of autosomes and a pair of sex chromosomes. Chromosomes are composed of genes, regulatory sequences, and noncoding DNA segments.

Codon: three-sequence nucleotide bases that code for an amino acid.

Epigenetic: chemical modifications of DNA that can turn genes on or off without altering the DNA sequence. Epigenetic changes are not heritable.

Gene: a unit of inheritance; a working subunit of DNA. Each of the 20,000 to 25,000 genes in the body contains the code for a specific product, typically a protein such as an enzyme, and other specific tissue cells.

Gene expression: the process by which the coded information of a gene is translated into the structures present and operating in the cell (proteins or ribonucleic acid [RNA]).

Gene map: a description of the relative positions of genes on a chromosome and the distance between them.

Genetic linkage maps: DNA maps that assign relative chromosomal locations to genetic locations—either genes for known traits or distinctive sequences of DNA on the basis of how frequently they are inherited together.

Genetics: the scientific study of heredity, which is how particular qualities or traits are transmitted from parents to offspring. Traditionally, the focus has been on individual genes and their impact on uncommon single-gene disorders. Today the study of genetics also involves multi-gene disorders and gene-environment interactions.

Genome: the expansive study of all the genes in the human genome together, including their interactions with each other, the environment, and the influence of other psychosocial and cultural factors.

Genomics: a study of the structure and function of large sections of the genome simultaneously.

Genotype: the genetic code sequence carried by an individual.

Haplotype: closely linked loci on a chromosome. Haplotype blocks denote chromosomal regions where SNPs are in strong linkage disequilibrium, and they are mapped in the HapMap Project database.

HapMap Project: a map of haplotype blocks that researchers use when searching for candidate genes. The HapMap haplotypes are arranged by racial and ethnic groups.

Heterozygous: possessing two different sequences (alleles) of a particular gene, with one inherited from each parent.

Homozygous: possessing two identical sequences of a particular gene, with one inherited from each parent.

Linkage: the association of genes or markers that lie very near each other on a chromosome. Linked genes and markers tend to be inherited together.

Linkage analysis: a gene-mapping technique that finds patterns of heredity in large, high-risk families to locate a disease-causing gene mutation by identifying traits that are co-inherited with the gene.

Linkage disequilibrium (LD): the nonrandom association between alleles at different loci. These alleles at loci occur together on the same section of a chromosome more often than would be predicted by chance alone. This technique has been used to determine which genes are linked and therefore inherited together.

Locus and loci: the place on a chromosome where a specific gene is located, similar in concept to a street address for the gene. The singular term is locus, and the plural is loci.

Mendelian diseases: single-gene disorders that often appear in families in dominant or recessive inheritance patterns.

Mutation: a change, deletion, or rearrangement in an individual's DNA sequence that may lead to the synthesis of an altered protein or the inability to produce the protein. The term *mutation* is used when the variant occurs in less than 1% of the population.

Nucleotide: a building block of DNA or RNA that consists of one nitrogenous base, one phosphate molecule, and one glucose molecule.

Pharmacogenetics: the study of genetically determined responses to drugs or of genetic variation in drug metabolizing enzymes and the effect on drug response.

Pharmacogenomics: the study of the entire spectrum of genes that affect drug metabolism in the genome.

Phenotype: the observable manifestation of a genetic trait that results from a specific genotype or gene-environment interaction. These are physical characteristics such as the signs and symptoms associated with a disease.

Polymorphism: a common variation in the sequence of DNA that occurs in more than 1% of the population. The most frequent sequence is referred to as the *wild type*, and less common variants are called *polymorphisms*.

Proband: the first person diagnosed with a condition in a family pedigree. The proband is usually identified with an arrow in the family pedigree.

Single-nucleotide polymorphism (SNP): a change in the DNA nucleotide sequence caused by replacement of a single nucleotide base. If the change of nucleotide results in a different protein product, it is called a *non-synonymous SNP*. If the protein product is not changed, it is called a *synonymous SNP*.

Somatic cells: all body cells, except the reproductive cells.

Transcription: the process used by DNA to code for messenger RNA.

Translation: the process used by RNA to code for a protein.

Summary

- DNA is arranged inside the nucleus of the cell. DNA resembles a ladder with two long strands twisted around each other to form a double-stranded helix. The rungs of the ladder are made up of nucleotide base pairs. There are 20,000 to 25,000 genes in the human genome.

- Several conditions seen in critical care have a genetic component, including factor V Leiden thrombosis, hemophilia A, cystic fibrosis and LQTS genotype. Pharmacogenetic syndromes represent medication-gene interactions, and examples include malignant hyperthermia owing to *RYR1* polymorphisms and warfarin dosage affected by *CYP2C9* and *VKORC1* polymorphisms.

- The GINA legislation is designed to prevent the use of an individual's genetic risk profile in employment and insurance decisions in the United States.

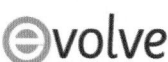 Be sure to check out the bonus material, including free self-assessment exercises, on the Evolve web site at http://evolve.elsevier.com/Urden/.

References

1. International Human Genome Sequencing Consortium: Finishing the euchromatic sequence of the human genome, *Nature* 431(7011):931-945, 2004.
2. Hartl DL, Jones EW: *Genetics: analysis of genes and genomes*, ed 6, Sudberry, MA, 2005, Jones & Bartlett.
3. Caldecott KW: Single-strand break repair and genetic disease. *Nat Rev Genet* 9(8):619-631, 2008.
4. Cold Spring Harbor Laboratory: DNA from the beginning. Available at www.dnaftb.org (accessed December 2008).
5. Nowell PC: Discovery of the Philadelphia chromosome: a personal perspective, *J Clin Invest* 117(8):2033-2035, 2007.
6. Bertina RM et al: Mutation in blood coagulation factor V associated with resistance to activated protein C, *Nature* 369(6475):64-67, 1994.
7. Segers K et al: Coagulation factor V and thrombophilia: background and mechanisms, *Thromb Haemost* 98(3):530-542, 2007.
8. Kujovich JL: Factor V Leiden thrombophilia, from GeneReviews of the University of Washington, Seattle, WA. Available at www.geneclinics.org (accessed December 2008).
9. Bezemer ID et al: Gene variants associated with deep vein thrombosis, *JAMA* 299(11):1306-1314, 2008.
10. Rosendorff A, Dorfman DM: Activated protein C resistance and factor V Leiden: a review, *Arch Pathol Lab Med* 131(6):866-871, 2007.
11. Ely EW et al: Apolipoprotein E4 polymorphism as a genetic predisposition to delirium in critically ill patients, *Crit Care Med* 35(1):112-117, 2007.
12. Laird NM, Lange C: Family-based methods for linkage and association analysis, *Adv Genet* 60:219-252, 2008.
13. Hinton RB Jr: The family history: reemergence of an established tool, *Crit Care Nurs Clin North Am* 20(2):149-158, 2008.
14. Nauman D et al: The family history as a tool to identify patients at risk for dilated cardiomyopathy, *Prog Cardiovasc Nurs* 23(1):41-44, 2008.
15. Ashcraft PF et al: Obtaining family histories from patients with cancer, *Clin J Oncol Nurs* 11(1):119-124, 2007.

16. Bennett RL et al: Recommendations for standardized human pedigree nomenclature. Pedigree Standardization Task Force of the National Society of Genetic Counselors, *Am J Hum Genet* 56(3):745-752, 1995.

17. Loos RJ, Bouchard C: FTO: the first gene contributing to common forms of human obesity, *Obes Rev* 9(3):246-250, 2008.

18. Rampersaud E et al: Physical activity and the association of common *FTO* gene variants with body mass index and obesity, *Arch Intern Med* 168 (16):1791-1797, 2008.

19. Wojczynski MK, Tiwari HK: Definition of phenotype, *Adv Genet* 60: 75-105, 2008.

20. Williams RW: Expression genetics and the phenotype revolution, *Mamm Genome* 17(6):496-502, 2006.

21. Cupples LA: Family study designs in the age of genome-wide association studies: experience from the Framingham Heart Study, *Curr Opin Lipidol* 19(2):144-150, 2008.

22. Wellcome Trust Case Control Consortium: Genome-wide association study of 14,000 cases of seven common diseases and 3,000 shared controls, *Nature* 447(7145):661-678, 2007.

23. Hindorff LA et al: A catalog of published genome-wide association studies. Available at www.genome.gov/26525384 (accessed December 2008).

24. The ENCODE Project Consortium: Identification and analysis of functional elements in 1% of the human genome by the ENCODE pilot project, *Nature* 447(7146):799-816, 2007.

25. International HapMap Project: Project data, information, and publications. Available at www.hapmap.org (accessed December 2008).

26. Barnes MR: Navigating the HapMap, *Brief Bioinform* 7(3):211-224, 2006.

27. The International HapMap Consortium: A second generation human haplotype map of over 3.1 million SNPs, *Nature* 449(7164):851-861, 2007.

28. Frank DN, Pace NR: Gastrointestinal microbiology enters the metagenomics era, *Curr Opin Gastroenterol* 24(1):4-10, 2008.

29. Campbell MC, Tishkoff SA: African genetic diversity: implications for human demographic history, modern human origins, and complex disease mapping, *Annu Rev Genomics Hum Genet* 9:403-433, 2008.

30. Kidd JM et al: Mapping and sequencing of structural variation from eight human genomes, *Nature* 453(7191):56-64, 2008.

31. Levy S et al: The diploid genome sequence of an individual human, *PLoS Biol* 5(10):e254, 2007.

32. Wheeler DA et al: The complete genome of an individual by massively parallel DNA sequencing, *Nature* 452(7189):872-876, 2008.

33. The Cancer Genome Atlas Research Network: Comprehensive genomic characterization defines human glioblastoma genes and core pathways, *Nature* 455(7216), 2008.

34. Arnett DK et al: Relevance of genetics and genomics for prevention and treatment of cardiovascular disease: a scientific statement from the American Heart Association Council on Epidemiology and Prevention, the Stroke Council, and the Functional Genomics and Translational Biology Interdisciplinary Working Group, *Circulation* 115(22):2878-2901, 2007.

35. Framingham Heart Study: Available at www.framinghamheartstudy.org (accessed December 2008).

36. Cupples LA et al: The Framingham Heart Study 100K SNP genome-wide association study resource: overview of 17 phenotype working group reports, *BMC Med Genet* 8(suppl 1):S1, 2007.

37. Florez JC et al: A 100K genome-wide association scan for diabetes and related traits in the Framingham Heart Study: replication and integration with other genome-wide datasets, *Diabetes* 56(12):3063-3074, 2007.

38. Kottgen A et al: Genome-wide association study for renal traits in the Framingham Heart and Atherosclerosis Risk in Communities studies, *BMC Med Genet* 9:49, 2008.

39. Collins KK & Van Hare GF: Advances in congenital long QT syndrome, *Currr Opin Pediatr* 18:497-502, 2006.

40. Schwartz PJ: The congenital long QT syndromes from genotype to phenotype: clinical implications, *Journal of Internal Medicine* 259:39-47, 2007.

41. Sauer AJ et al: Long QT syndrome in adults, *J Am Coll Card* 49:329-337, 2007.

42. Mann HJ: Drug-associated disease: cytochrome P450 interactions, *Crit Care Clin* 22(2):329-345, 2006.

43. Rieder MJ et al: Effect of *VKORC1* haplotypes on transcriptional regulation and warfarin dose, *N Engl J Med* 352(22):2285-2293, 2005.

44. Schwarz UI et al: Genetic determinants of response to warfarin during initial anticoagulation, *N Engl J Med* 358(10):999-1008, 2008.

45. Girard T, Litman RS: Molecular genetic testing to diagnose malignant hyperthermia susceptibility, *J Clin Anesth* 20(3):161-163, 2008.

46. Robinson R et al: Mutations in *RYR1* in malignant hyperthermia and central core disease, *Hum Mutat* 27(10):977-989, 2006.

47. Jenkins J, Calzone KA: Establishing the essential nursing competencies for genetics and genomics, *J Nurs Scholarsh* 39(1):10-16, 2007.

48. Shickle D: The consent problem within DNA biobanks, *Stud Hist Philos Biol Biomed Sci* 37(3):503-519, 2006.

Patient and Family Education

CHALLENGES OF PATIENT AND FAMILY EDUCATION

At no other point in history has the availability of information within the general population been so great. Televisions are practically in every home, computers with wireless access to the Internet are available for use anywhere at anytime, and cell phones are clipped to the waistbands of the young and old. It seems as if this century's population of adults cannot tolerate a lack of information. The ease of access to the world's library of information meets a compulsive need to satisfy a desire for immediate gratification. Gathering information in bits and pieces from various sources allows people to collect information at their own pace and to gather as much or as little information as they desire. These "knowledge bites" are sorted and stored on an individual's "cerebral hard drive." The "file" is retrieved and "opened" whenever the situation warrants.

When alterations in health arise in daily life, people use all available resources to discover information to help them cope and adapt to the new experience. This type of consumerism has developed a populace that is more educated in health matters than ever before. It is our duty as health professionals to assist patients and families with information gathering and self-care management skills so they can lead lives of the best quality possible. According to The Joint Commission, patients must receive "sufficient information to make decisions and to take responsibility for self-management activities related to their needs."[1] The goals of patient and family education are to improve health outcomes by promoting healthy behavior and involvement in care and care decisions.[1]

Admission to an acute care unit usually is an unexpected event in anyone's life. The seriousness of the situation and unfamiliarity of the hospital or unit environment evokes a stress response in patients and their families. Nursing care is focused on improving the patient's physiologic stability and promoting end-organ tissue perfusion. Promoting the most basic human physiologic survival need for cellular oxygenation is the priority. Alterations in normal functioning related to disease-process progression, sedation, assist devices, or mechanical ventilation contribute to the possibility of mental alterations in the patient. Sleep deprivation and sensory overload add to the complexity of the issues that affect the patient's ability to receive and understand medical information. Mental alterations may limit the effectiveness of the teaching-learning encounter. These physical and cognitive limitations prevent patients from receiving or understanding information related to their care and impair their ability to make an informed decision.[2] At these times, critical life-or-death care decisions are transferred to a proxy, usually an immediate family member. The designated proxy has the responsibility to make informed treatment decisions for the patient. These types of situations present the nurse with special challenges in the education of patients and families.

Acute illness disrupts the normal patterns of daily life. Stress and crisis can develop within the family unit and stretch its members' coping resources.[3] These many emotional factors build barriers to the teaching-learning process and can become frustrating for the learner and the nurse. Amid the chaos, how do bedside nurses effectively provide patient and family education that can optimize outcomes and deliver quality, cost-effective care? It is the nurse's responsibility to educate himself or herself about concepts that provide insight into the framework for patient and family education. Adult educational concepts such as adult learning principles, types of educational needs, barriers to learning, stress and coping strategies, and evidence-based interventions must be used to develop an individualized education plan to meet the identified learning needs of the patient and family.

EDUCATION

DEFINITION

Patient education is a process that includes the purposeful delivery of health-related information to promote changes in behavior that will optimize health practices and assist the individual in attaining new skills for living.[4,5] This concept can be overwhelming in the fast-paced, technology-rich setting of the acute care environment. The bedside nurse must incorporate the abundant educational needs of the patient or family into the education plan and be aware of the requirements of regulatory agencies and the legalities of documenting the teaching-learning encounter.

BENEFITS

Studies have documented that quality education shortens hospital length of stay, reduces readmission rates, and improves self-care management skills.[4-6] Complications associated with the physiologic stress response may be prevented if the patient or family perceives the education encounter as positive. Positive encounters decrease the stress response, relieve anxiety, promote individual growth and development, and increase patient and family satisfaction.[4-6] The following are examples of positive outcomes associated with a structured teaching-learning process[7,8]:

- Clarification of patients' understanding and perceptions of their chronic illness and care decisions
- Improved health outcomes relative to self-management techniques, such as symptom management
- Promotion of informed decision making and control over the situation
- Diminished emotional stress associated with an unfamiliar environment and unknown prognosis
- Improved adaptation to stressful situation
- Improved satisfaction with the care received
- Improved relationship with the health care team
- Promotion of self-concept

THE EDUCATION PROCESS

The education process follows the same framework as the nursing process: assessment, diagnosis, goals or outcomes, interventions, and evaluation.[4] Box 5-1 lists the steps in this process.

BOX 5-1   STEPS IN THE EDUCATION PROCESS

STEP 1: ASSESSMENT: INFORMATION GATHERING
- Assess the patient and family in terms of culture and age-specific considerations.
- Evaluate the actual and potential learning needs.
- Consider possible barriers to the teaching-learning process.

STEP 2: EDUCATION PLAN DEVELOPMENT
- Identify needs and write expected outcomes.
- Design interventions for information to be taught and removal of barriers.
- Mobilize resources as needed to remove barriers and enhance communication of information.

STEP 3: IMPLEMENTATION
- Implement interventions for information sharing and learner participation in the education process.
- Use a written plan to structure the teaching encounter, cover essential information, and communicate outcomes between practitioners.

STEP 4: EVALUATION
- Evaluate the learner's response to the encounter and any need for follow-up teaching to attain goals.
- Evaluate the learner's comfort level with information in terms of coping and adaptation.

STEP 5: DOCUMENTATION
- Document the interventions used, resources used, information taught, and outcome of the teaching encounter.

Although this chapter discusses these steps individually, in practice, they may occur simultaneously and repetitively. The teaching-learning process is a dynamic, continuous activity that occurs throughout the entire hospitalization and may continue after the patient has been discharged. This process is often envisioned by the nurse as a time-consuming task that requires knowledge and skills to accomplish. Whereas knowledge and skills can be obtained, time in the acute care unit is a scarce commodity. Many nurses believe they cannot educate unless formal blocks of education time are planned during the shift. Although this type of education encounter is optimal, it is not realistic for contemporary nursing. The nurse must recognize that teaching occurs during every moment of a nurse-patient encounter.[9] Instructions for how to use to the call bell or explanations of events and sensations to expect during a bed bath can be considered an education session. It is the nurse's role to recognize that education, no matter brief or extensive, affects the daily lives of each person with whom they come in contact. By following the nursing process, the physical assessment and education assessment can occur simultaneously.

STEP 1: ASSESSMENT

According to The Joint Commission, education provided should be appropriate to the patient's condition and should address the patient's identified learning needs.[1] The assessment is an important first step to providing need-targeted patient and family education. It begins on admission and continues until the patient is discharged. A formal, comprehensive, initial education assessment produces valuable information; however, it can take the nurse hours to complete. The nurse must focus the initial and subsequent education assessments on identifying gaps in knowledge related to the patient's current health-altering situation. Information must also be gathered on factors that affect the education process and impair the ability of the patient or family to respond. These factors include (1) cultural and religious views of illness or health, (2) emotional barriers, (3) desire and motivation, (4) physical or cognitive limitations, and (5) barriers to effective communication.[1]

EFFECTIVE QUESTIONING

Strategic questioning provides an avenue for the nurse to determine whether the patient or family has any misconceptions about the environment, their illness, self-management skills, or the medication schedule. Health care providers use the term *noncompliant* to describe a patient or family members who do not modify behaviors to the meet the demands of the prescribed treatment regimen, such as following the rules of a low-fat diet or medication dosing. However, the problem behind noncompliance may not be a conscious desire to defy the treatment plan but instead be a misunderstanding of the importance of the medication or how to take the medication. The technique of asking open-ended questions ("Can you tell me what you know about your medication?") can elicit more information about the patient's knowledge base than asking closed-ended questions

("You know this is your water pill, right?"). Open-ended questions provide the nurse an opportunity to assess actual knowledge gaps rather than assume knowledge by obtaining a yes-or-no response. These types of questions also assist the patient and family to tell their story of the illness and communicate their perceptions of the experience,[5] allowing the adult learner to feel respected and involved in the treatment process. Questions that elicit a yes-or-no response close off communication and do not provide an interactive teaching-learning session. Box 5-2 contains sample questions the nurse can use in an assessment to obtain needed information. Generally, with practice and effort, it can be determined what educational information is needed in a brief period without much disruption in the routine care of the patient. Patients and families are multidimensional. Even with good questioning skills, the nurse cannot assess many aspects of the learner during the initial contact or even during the hospital stay.

LEARNER IDENTIFICATION

Identifying learner characteristics benefits the nurse and results in optimal communication and the patient's understanding of information. Certain factors can affect the education process. Culture or ethnicity, age, and adult learning principles influence the manner in which information is presented and concepts are understood.[5,10]

Family. A family can be defined as a group of individuals who are bonded by biologic, legal, and social relationships.[3] The modern family is diverse in ethnic backgrounds, sexual orientation, age, gender, work experience, physical or mental challenges, communication skills, educational backgrounds, work

experience, geographic location, lived experiences, and religious beliefs.[11-13] A picture of the modern family would resemble that of a large patchwork quilt. Patches of different sizes, ethnicities, religions, cultures, attitudes, stages of development, and lived experiences would overlap and occupy their own individual spaces within the quilt framework. Bedside practitioners are expected to provide culturally competent care to each individual in the acute care setting. Culturally competent care is the delivery of sensitive, meaningful care to patients and families from diverse backgrounds.[13] This implies that the practitioner must value diversity and become knowledgeable concerning the cultural strengths and abilities of those for whom they care.[14] Communication and understanding impact the education process. Provision of language-appropriate literature and translation services and recognition of cultural or religious differences in the perception of illness and treatment influence the education encounter.[13]

Age-Specific Considerations. The acute care patient population differs culturally and by age and stages of human development. Older adult patients may have more difficulty reading patient educational materials or the label on the bottle of prescription medication than younger adults. Printed materials with larger fonts may be needed for these patients. Older adults were not exposed to technology during their youth and may find it difficult to navigate the fragmented maze of modern health care. Because of advanced age, this population of adults may have prescriptions for multiple drug therapies. Education to prevent adverse drug reactions may be required because of the prevalence of multiple drug therapies.[15] Older adults may also be coping with end-of-life issues and are in need of information to make informed decisions. Young adults may struggle with the issue of how to incorporate intimacy into their lives without feeling isolated from the mainstream social scene. The need for privacy and peer support may be required to assist the young adult in coping with the current situation. The practitioner must recognize these age-specific issues and incorporate them into the education plan.[1]

Adult Learners. Adults learn in large part through lived experiences. The motivation to learn is internal and problem-oriented, focusing on life events. Malcolm Knowles described these principles of adult learning in a model known as *andragogy*. Adult learning theory stresses concepts of individualism, self-assessment, self-direction, motivation, experience, and autonomy. Adults tend to have a strong sense of self-concept, are goal-oriented learners, and like to make their own decisions.[16] They take responsibility and accountability for their own learning and want to be respected as individuals, as well as recognized for accomplished life experiences. Adults have individualized learning styles and often lack confidence in their ability to learn. Education is resisted when the information given is perceived to be in conflict with the individual's self-image.

The learning process generally involves altering some part of current behavior to produce changes in lifestyle, incorporating the new or chronic illness into daily living. Coping mechanisms such as anger, disbelief, and denial affect the willingness of the patient or family to learn. The unwillingness to change behavior

---

BOX 5-2   ASSESSMENT QUESTIONS

- Why have you come to the hospital today?
- What problem are you having?
- How can we help you today?
- When did these problems start?
- Have you had these problems before?
- Have you been hospitalized for these problems before?
- Who is your doctor for this problem? Who is your family doctor?
- What medications are you taking?
- Can you tell me why you take each medication?
- How do you care for yourself at home? Do you have help?
- Are any family or friends with you today?
- Are these people your main support system?
- Are there any special needs, religious or otherwise, that we need to be aware of while you are in the hospital?
- What is your goal for coming to the hospital today?
- How can we help you reach this goal?
- Is there any information that I can give you right now that would help you understand more about why you are here or about your plan of care?
- What information have you received from other members of the health care team today?

to manage health needs adds to the complexity of the acute care teaching-learning encounter. The nurse must provide need-to-know information in easy, understandable terms and in short bursts. Positive feedback and repetition of information may also be required before health education is incorporated into the patient's or family's bank of experiences.[16] Adults are sensitive about making mistakes and tend to view mistakes as failures. Learning situations that the patient and family interpret as belittling or embarrassing or that are perceived as insurmountable will be avoided or disregarded. The nurse should act more as a coach or facilitator of information instead of a didactic instructor.[10] The teacher can only show the learner to the door; the learner must decide to walk through that door. Learning is an active process that occurs internally over time and cannot be forced. Bedside nurses are obliged to be proactive and to have a good understanding of adult learning theory and to incorporate its concepts into the assessment of learning needs, development of an education plan, implementation of the plan, and evaluation of the outcomes of the education encounter.

EDUCATIONAL NEEDS

Learning needs can be defined as gaps between what the learner knows and what the learner needs to know, such as survival skills, coping skills, and ability to make a care decision. Identification of actual and perceived learning needs directs the health care team to provide need-targeted education. Need-targeted or need-to-know education is directed at helping the learner to become familiar with the current situation. Educational needs of the patient and family can be categorized as (1) information only (environment, visitation hours, get questions answered), (2) informed decision making (treatment plan, informed consent), or (3) self-management (recognition of problems and how to respond).[5,17] Patient education to be included in the education plan should address the plan of care, health practices and safety, safe and effective use of medications, nutrition interventions, safe and effective use of medical equipment or supplies, pain, and habilitation or rehabilitation needs.[1]

Learning needs may change from day to day, shift to shift, or minute to minute. Educational needs are influenced by how the patient or the family perceive or interpret the acute illness.[18] Perceptions of experiences vary from person to person, even if two people are involved in the same event. This intense internal feeling affects the desire to learn and understanding of the current situation. Satisfaction with the learning encounter is often judged to be positive if the nurse meets the expected learning needs of the patient and family. Congruency between nurse-identified needs and patient-identified needs brings about more positive learning experiences and encourages the learner to seek further information. The nurse must actively listen, maintain eye contact, seek clarification, and pay attention to verbal and nonverbal cues from the patient and the family to gather relevant information concerning perceived learning needs. The nurse should seek to first understand the learning need from the patient's point of view and then seek to be understood.

BARRIERS TO THE LEARNING PROCESS

Ability, Willingness, and Readiness. Assessing ability, willingness, and readiness to learn is an essential part of developing and implementing an education plan of care. The ability to learn is the capacity of the learner to understand, pay attention, and comprehend the material being taught. Willingness to learn describes the learner's openness to new ideas and concepts. Readiness to learn is the motivation to try out new concepts and behaviors.[5] Even if the inventive teaching methods, well-considered education materials, and amounts of time are unlimited, learning cannot take place if the patient or family is not ready, willing, and able to learn.[19] Several factors affect the ability, willingness, and readiness to learn, as well as the ability to cope and adapt to the current situation. These factors include physiologic, psychological, sociocultural, financial, and environmental aspects.[5,10]

Physiologic Factors. The need for oxygen and survival predominates over all other human needs. This need is described by a theory known as Maslow's hierarchy of human needs. It is a concept in which lower-level, physiologic needs must be satisfied before an individual can move on to higher-level, self-esteem–building issues. The motivation to meet the need to survive and to feel safe and secure predominates over the need to learn a lifestyle change such as smoking cessation. Only when lower-level needs are met can the patient be open to learning new concepts and skills. There is an instinctive need to decrease the effects of stressors and reestablish a normal daily routine. A physical assessment can supply the nurse with information concerning the patient's response to the stressors.

Physiologic alterations in heart rate and blood pressure can be measured and taken into consideration during the teaching-learning encounter.[3] Sources of physiologic stress in the acutely ill include medications, pain, hypoxia, decreased cerebral and peripheral perfusion, hypotension, fluid and electrolyte imbalances, infection, sensory alterations, fever, and neurologic deficits.[10] Experiencing one or more of these stressors may completely consume all the patient's available energy and thoughts, affecting his or her ability to interact, comprehend, and respond to teaching.

Psychological Factors. When confronted with life-altering situations such as admission to an acute care unit, patients and families may experience anxiety and emotional stress. Anxiety and fear disrupt the normalcy of daily life. Sources of emotional stress include fear of death, uncertain prognosis, role change, self-image change, social isolation, disruption in daily routine, financial concerns, and unfamiliar critical care environment.[3,20] These intense emotions can lead to a crisis situation and alter the ability of the patient and family to cope.[21,22] During the acute illness, an individual's ability to process or retain information and ability to participate in the treatment plan could be altered.[2] If the disease process or physiologic stressors impair the patient's ability to make decisions, the burden of decision making will transfer to the family. Gender differences affect a patient's reaction to stress. For example, women who have experienced a myocardial infarction report higher anxiety levels than men at all points during the hospital stay.[23] Physiologic alterations caused by anxiety negatively impact the recovery process and the long-term prognosis.[23] In acute situations, the nurse may find it necessary to repeat information or limit teaching sessions to short bursts rather than one long encounter. Medical jargon should be limited and replaced by terms that are easy to understand. Provision of honest and accurate disease state information may decrease the effects of stressors and alleviate anxiety and fear.

Adaptation. A stressor can be any condition, situation, or perception that requires an individual to adapt.[20] All situations in an acute care facility may well be considered stressful. The capacity of an individual to adapt is paramount in breaking down emotional barriers that affect willingness and readiness for learning. Culture, beliefs, attitudes, and ability to mobilize resources affect a person's ability to respond to a crisis situation.[24] General characteristics of the stages of adaptation to illness are outlined in Table 5-1 with corresponding applications for the teaching-learning process. Patients and families move through these stages on an individual timeline and at a variable pace. A person may move back and forth between stages and may skip one all together. The patient and each member of the family may be experiencing different stages in the adaptation process at the same time. The education encounter may need to be modified to meet the needs of the patient and family.

Coping. Coping refers to the way a person manages stressful events that are straining or exceeding personal resources.[5,24] The stressful event is appraised according to the level of threat to the individual and is managed by focusing on the problem at hand or the emotions felt at the moment.[25] Acute illness disrupts the normalcy of daily routines. Coping strategies are used

by the patient and family to help maintain control over the situation and encourage hope and stability in life. Disbelief and denial may be present anytime during the hospitalization. Phrases such as "Why me" and "I can't believe this is happening" are common in the acute care setting. Other coping mechanisms, such as denial and anger, hamper the ability of the patient or family to problem solve and cope with the situation. All are barriers to the ability of the patient to receive information and incorporate it into the self-concept. Adults must be physically ready and emotionally willing to learn. Teaching new skills or self-management techniques to the adult learner therefore presents a special challenge to the nurse in acute care. For example, until the patient accepts the diagnosis of heart failure as part of who he or she is, he or she will not make appropriate changes in lifestyle to avoid an exacerbation of the disease.

Sociocultural Factors. Variables such as culture, ethnicity, values, beliefs, lifestyle, and family role influence the way an individual perceives illness, pain, and healing.[13] Culturally sensitive educational strategies should be developed to communicate specific needs to other members of the health care team and achieve optimal learning outcomes.[1]

Financial Factors. Patients and families often worry about financial issues related to the hospitalization and the possibility of long-term disability. Examples of financial concerns are (1) fear of income loss related to time away from work or possible long-term disability, (2) how health care expenses will be paid, and (3) complex insurance coverage issues. Patients may be more concerned with the amount of out-of-pocket expenses they will have to pay for this illness rather than receiving information on symptom management strategies. The nurse must

TABLE 5-1 Teaching-Learning Process in Adaptation to Illness

Stage of Adaptation	Characteristic Patient Response	Implications for Teaching-Learning Process
Disbelief	Denial	Orient teaching to present. Teach during other nursing activities. Reassure patient about safety. Explain all procedures and activities clearly and concisely.
Developing awareness	Anger	Continue to orient teaching to present. Avoid long lists of facts. Continue to foster development of trust and rapport through good physical care.
Reorganization	Acceptance of sick role	Orient teaching to meet patient. Teach whatever patient wants to learn. Provide necessary self-care information; reinforce with written material.
Resolution	Identification with others with same problem; recognition of loss	Use group instruction. Use patient support groups and visits by recovered patients with same problem.
Identifying change	Definition of self as one who has undergone change and is now different	Answer the patient's questions as they arise. Recognize that as basic needs are met, more mature needs will arise.

recognize these issues as patient concerns and mobilize resources to calm financial anxiety. Practitioners in other disciplines, especially social work, are available to assist patients and families obtain community resources to help cover expenses such as medication costs.

Environmental Factors. The acute care environment can be considered a source of stress to the learner. Although sounds, people, and state-of-the-art equipment are familiar and mundane for the nurse, this environment may appear foreign and intimidating to the patient and family. Prior exposure to an acute care unit is a double-edged sword. Depending on whether the outcome of the experience was positive or negative, it may help alleviate or heighten anxiety. The nurse must pay attention to the perceptions of the environment by the patient and family and alter the teaching-learning encounter accordingly. Sleep cycle alterations caused by sleep deprivation or sensory overload related to continuous noise from machines or people affect the patient's ability to concentrate and comprehend information. Allowing frequent uninterrupted rest periods assists the patient in obtaining structured sleep.[20]

For patients and families to value education, they must believe the information source is reliable. The bedside nurse is the most available source of information in the acute care unit. It is important for him or her to develop a rapport and establish a sense of trust within the nurse-patient relationship. These positive characteristics are recommended for a supportive learning environment. Assignment of multiple caregivers may negatively affect the ability of the patient and family to form a trusting relationship with the nursing staff. Arranging consistency in the assigned caregivers can help promote rapport and trust, as well as decrease anxiety and enhance comfort level with the environment.[5,24]

STEP 2: EDUCATION PLAN DEVELOPMENT

Education must be ongoing, interactive, and consistent with the patient's plan of care and education level.[1] The nurse must analyze information gathered from the assessment to prioritize the educational needs of the patient and family. The nursing diagnosis for deficient knowledge and accompanying interventions can be applied to any situation. The nurse must also consider the patient's physical and emotional status when setting education priorities. Ability, willingness, and readiness to learn are factors that impair acceptance of new information and add to the complexity of teaching-learning encounter. These factors should be recognized by the nurse before implementation of teaching. The written teaching plan should identify the learning need, goals or expected outcome of the teaching-learning encounter, interventions to meet that outcome, and appropriate teaching strategies.

Research and accepted national guidelines or standards can be used to assist the practitioner in developing an evidence-based plan for education. Examples of organizations that offer education standards are the American Association of Critical-Care Nurses, American Heart Association Guidelines for Practice, and the Society of Critical Care Medicine. A database for nursing interventions and outcomes has been developed from research that began in the 1980s. This research is known as the IOWA Project. It can be used in daily practice and can be found in two books: *Nursing Interventions Classification (NIC)* and *Nursing Outcomes Classification (NOC)*. These evidence-based interventions and outcomes assist the nurse in providing consistent outcomes and interventions from nurse to nurse, shift to shift, and discipline to discipline.

DETERMINING WHAT TO TEACH

It can be difficult to prioritize the multitude of learning needs that practitioners are required to address during a period in acute care. Learning needs in the intensive care unit (ICU), the progressive care, or the telemetry setting can be separated into four different categories to help set teaching priorities in each phase of the hospitalization (Table 5-2). Learning needs during the initial contact or first hours of hospitalization can be predicted. Education during this time frame should be directed toward the reduction of immediate stress, anxiety, and fear rather than future lifestyle alterations or rehabilitation

TABLE 5-2 Categories of Educational Needs in Acute Care

Phase	Educational Needs
Initial contact or first visit, with a focus on immediate needs	Preparation for the visit: patient representatives or nurses can prepare the family and patient for the first visit What to expect in the environment How long the visit will last What the patient may look like (e.g., tubes, IV lines) Orientation to the unit or environment: call light, bed controls, waiting rooms, unit contact numbers Orientation to unit policies and hospital policies HIPAA, advanced directives, visitation policies Equipment orientation: monitors, IV pumps, pulse oximetry, pacemakers, ventilators Medications: rationale, effects, side effects What to do during the visit: talk to the patient, hold the patient's hand, monitor length of visits (if applicable) Patient status: stable or unstable and what that terminology means

Continued

TABLE 5-2 Categories of Educational Needs in Acute Care—*cont'd*

Phase	Educational Needs
Initial contact or first visit, with a focus on immediate needs—*cont'd*	What treatments and interventions are being done for the patient Upcoming procedures When the doctor visited or is expected to visit Disciplines involved in care and the services they provide Immediate plan of care (next 24 hours) Mobilization of resources for crisis intervention
Continuous care	Day-to-day routine: meals, laboratory visits, doctor visits, frequency of monitoring (VS), nursing assessments, daily weights, and shift routines Explanation of any procedures: expected sensations or discomforts (e.g., chest tube removal, arterial sheath removal) Plan of care: treatments, progress, patient accomplishments (e.g., extubation) Medications: name, why the patient is receiving them, side effects to report to the nurse or health care team Disease process: what it is and how it will affect life, symptoms to report to health care team How to mobilize resources to assist the patient and family in coping with stress and crisis: pastoral care, social workers, case managers, victim assistance, domestic violence counseling Gifts: When a loved one is ill, it is traditional to send flowers, balloons, or cards. If your unit has restrictions on gifts, make the family aware. Begin teaching self-management skills, and discuss aftercare information.
Transfer to a different level of care	**Sending Unit** Acknowledge positive move out of critical care When the transfer will occur Why the transfer is occurring What to expect in the different unit Name of the new caregiver Availability of care provider Visiting hours Directions for how to get there; the new room number and phone number **Receiving Unit** Orientation to environment, visitation policies, visitors Unit routine, meals shift changes, doctor visits Expectations about patient self-care; ADLs Medication and diagnostic testing routine times
Planning for aftercare, discharge planning	Self-care management: symptom management, medication administration, diet, activity, durable medical equipment, tasks or procedures What to do for an emergency What constitutes an emergency or when to call the physician How to care for incisions or procedure sites
Completed throughout the hospital stay	Return appointment: name of physician practice, practice phone numbers and contacts Obtaining medications: prescriptions, pharmacy, special drug ordering information Required lifestyle changes: mobility and safety issues for the paraplegic or stroke victim, activities of daily living issues relative to medications or symptoms Potential risk modifications: smoking cessation, diet modifications, exercise Resources: cardiac rehabilitation, support groups, home care agencies
End-of-life care	End-of-life care: participation in care, services available, mobilizing resources Palliative care Hospice

ADLs, Activities of daily living; *HIPAA,* Health Insurance Portability and Accountability Act; *IV,* intravenous; *VS,* vital signs.

needs. Interventions are targeted to promote comfort and familiarity with the environment and surroundings.[26] The plan should focus on survival skills, orientation to the environment and equipment, communication of prognosis, procedure explanations, and the immediate plan of care.

Three learning domains are considered when developing an individualized education plan: knowledge, attitude, and skills. The knowledge domain is centered on the acquisition of information or facts by the patient about a given topic, such as listing the signs and symptoms of hypoglycemia and knowing what

BOX 5-3 INTERVENTIONS FOR IDENTIFIED PATIENT AND FAMILY NEEDS

- Answer questions openly and honestly.
- Give as much or as little realistic information as the patient and family members need to understand about the situation or the patient's physiologic condition.
- Provide specific facts about the patient's daily or hourly progress.
- Provide information that is understandable and given in simple terms.
- Use short sentences, and incorporate only a couple of pieces of information at one time.
- Provide emotional comfort to reduce anxiety and facilitate the feeling of hope.
- Prepare the patient and family for their first visit to the unit.
- Explain the possible appearance of the patient, purpose of the equipment, the family role in visitation, and the unit environment.
- Keep the family informed and involved in the daily plan of care.
- Explain what procedures will be done, why they are being done, and what information is hoped to be gained from each procedure.

to do if he or she becomes symptomatic. A patient who has had diabetes for years has life experiences with his or her disease process that are different from those of the newly diagnosed patient. Even though two patients have the same diagnosis, educational needs differ. The attitude domain includes the incorporation of new values, beliefs, or attitudes into patients' behavior, such as believing smoking is bad for them and then exerting a conscious effort to stop. The skills domain is involved with the acquisition of skills that enable a person to perform a new technique, such as endotracheal suctioning or dressing changes. The nurse may incorporate one or more of these domains into the education plan.

Patients and their families are attempting to cope with the seriousness of the current situation and need information continually to adapt their behavior accordingly. Leske and Molter's hallmark research in the area of needs of the families of critically ill patients has provided nursing with a scientific body of knowledge for identification of the learning needs of this population. Results of these studies found that families of critically ill patients needed to have their questions answered honestly and to have a feeling of hope.[27] The outcomes of this research can be used in developing interventions for the initial phase in the hospitalization process. Box 5-3 includes a sample listing of interventions that can be used to help meet the needs of the family. During this time of elevated stress, the nurse may have to refocus the patient and family to help concentrate efforts on coping with the present instead of dwelling on possibilities of the future. Not addressing these immediate concerns can result in further anxiety, affect the ability to cope, and prevent open and honest communication.[3]

As the hospital length of stay increases, patients and families begin to adapt to the situation, and learning needs change. The patient and family develop positive feelings of relief and happiness in the fact that survival has been achieved. Because lower-level, physiologic needs are met, the patient's efforts can be

concentrated on modifying behavior to meet higher-level needs, such as self-concept and self-actualization. Teaching during the continuous phase of nursing care is aimed at answering the patient's or family members' questions about the treatment plan or how the acute illness will impact their daily lives. Education on lifestyle modification and self-management skills should be presented during this phase of nursing care.

Discharge planning is also part of the education process and should start with admission to the hospital. Instructions for home care, also known as aftercare, should be accomplished before the day of discharge to avoid decreased retention of education that occurs with information overload.

WRITING GOALS OR OUTCOMES

An outcomes statement helps clarify to the teacher and the learner what is to be taught, what is to be learned, what is to be evaluated, and what is to be documented. When goals or expected outcomes of the education encounter are clearly stated, the teacher and the learner understand the expectations and will do their best to achieve them. These statements differ from interventions in that they reflect what the learner is to accomplish, not what the nurse is to teach.[28] Identifying and writing outcomes may be the most difficult aspect in the development of the education plan of care. The written outcomes provide direction for the teaching-learning process and should be straightforward, attainable, and include one task or learning domain.[28]

The three components in the outcomes statement are (1) the individual who will meet the objective, (2) a measurable or observable verb, and (3) the content to be evaluated or learned. Examples of measurable verbs include define, list, identify, perform, prepare, and demonstrate, whereas nonmeasurable, higher-level verbs include believe, value, and understand. Remember the KISS rule: Keep it simple, Simon. Outcomes should include behavioral lifestyle changes for self-management, psychomotor skill acquisition, and acquisition of knowledge. This is an example of a clearly stated outcome: The patient and family will list the signs and symptoms of postoperative infection.

DEVELOPING INTERVENTIONS

Interventions describe how a nurse will become involved in providing education to the patient or the family. Determining education interventions is part of clinical decision making.[29] Nurse-initiated interventions are based on clinical knowledge and judgment and have a direct impact on the outcome of the teaching encounter.[29] Although physiologic problems occupy most of the nursing plan of care, it is essential to incorporate teaching interventions into the daily plan to create positive patient outcomes. Nurses just entering the profession readily refer to education plans developed by experienced nurses to guide them in their new role of patient educator.[30] Carefully planned and developed interventions support nurses, patients, and families focused on achievable outcomes. Education interventions are targeted toward information to be taught, such as how to care and use oxygen or how to recognize signs and symptoms of an infection. The following is an example of a clearly stated research-based intervention: Instruct the patient and family on proper name of prescribed diet.[29]

STANDARDIZED EDUCATION PLANS

Standardized education plans provide the health care team with consistent outcomes and interventions. Even though standardized plans are easy to implement, they must be individualized to meet the specific needs of the patient or family. Examples of standardized plans of care include patient pathways, traditional nursing care plans for Deficient Knowledge, and Nursing Interventions Classification (NIC). Examples of nursing management plans for Deficient Knowledge are included in Appendix A.

NIC

Teaching: Disease Process

Definition
Assisting the patient to understand information related to a specific disease process

Activities
Appraise the patient's current level of knowledge related to a specific disease process
Explain the pathophysiology of the disease and how it relates to the anatomy and physiology, as appropriate
Describe common signs and symptoms of the disease, as appropriate
Describe the disease process, as appropriate
Identify possible etiologies, as appropriate
Provide information to the patient about condition, as appropriate
Avoid empty reassurances
Provide the family/significant other(s) with information about the patient's progress, as appropriate
Provide information about available diagnostic measures, as appropriate
Discuss lifestyle changes that may be required to prevent future complications and/or control the disease process
Discuss therapy/treatment options
Describe rationale behind management/therapy/treatment recommendations
Encourage the patient to explore options/get a second opinion, as appropriate or indicated
Describe possible chronic complications, as appropriate
Instruct the patient on measures to prevent/minimize side effects of treatment for the disease, as appropriate
Instruct the patient on measures to control/minimize symptoms, as appropriate
Explore possible resources/support, as appropriate
Refer the patient to local community agencies/support groups, as appropriate
Instruct the patient on which signs and symptoms to report to health care provider, as appropriate
Provide the phone number to call if complications occur
Reinforce information provided by other health care team members, as appropriate

From Bulecheck GM et al, editors: *Nursing interventions classification (NIC)*, ed 5, St. Louis, 2008, Elsevier, p. 709.

STEP 3: IMPLEMENTATION

After the assessment is completed and the education plan is developed, need-targeted education can commence. Beginning practitioners differ from experienced practitioners in their skills of implementing the education plan of care. Experienced practitioners use their intuition and knowledge base to anticipate learning needs and form a mental list of interventions and possible outcomes.[30] Those just starting in the profession need the concrete education plan that has been developed to guide the teaching-learning encounter.[30]

SETTING UP THE ENVIRONMENT

The optimal environment for learning is one that is nonthreatening, comfortable, open, and honest. Many factors concerning the acute care environment can be threatening or anxiety producing. The practitioner must assess for these distractions and control them as much as possible. Providing the family with open visitation and access to the patient and health care providers can help decrease their anxiety level and improve satisfaction with care.[3] Current Health Insurance Portability and Accountability Act (HIPAA) requirements for patient confidentiality necessitate a need for privacy during the teaching-learning encounter. Bedside practitioner attention to this detail in open environments such as ICUs, waiting rooms, and emergency departments is important in creating an environment of trust and reassurance. Supportive education promotes behaviors that facilitate motivation to learn and adherence to lifestyle changes.[31] The following is a list of strategies the practitioner can implement to facilitate learning[31]:

- Show empathy and concern. Actively listen to the learner and acknowledge lived experiences and ideas.
- Use language and nonverbal communication to enhance choice and promote problem solving.
- Reduce language that is controlling, criticizing, guilt provoking, judgmental, or punishing.
- Provide rationale for self-management behaviors: the importance of changing lifestyle to manage symptoms.

One example of the difference between supportive education and nonsupportive education is demonstrated by a patient diagnosed with chronic heart failure who is experiencing an exacerbation of symptoms related to dietary salt intake. Suppose the patient states that he or she is doing "okay" at adhering to the low-salt diet, but family members complain that he or she eats too many processed foods and too much take-out fast food. This is an example of a nonsupportive teaching phrase: "You know salt isn't good for you."[31] This phrase is judgmental, critical, and guilt provoking and makes an assumption of the patient's level of knowledge. By revising the wording in the phrase, the meaning of the information is changed. This is an example: "I know it is difficult not to eat all of your favorite foods. Adding salt is up to you. Do you understand that salt will affect your heart condition?"[31] This supportive statement transfers accountability of performing the self-management skill from the nurse to the patient and motivates the patient to make the conscious decision to limit salt intake.

TEACHING STRATEGIES

The nurse may be the first health care provider to initiate patient teaching. Bedside nurses are in a unique position to facilitate, mentor, and coach patients through the endless maze of information presented in the acute care arena. Information overload often occurs, and the information taught can easily be forgotten. Nurses may become frustrated when family members and patients ask the same questions repeatedly. Patience with repeated questioning is essential, because information taught may be lost within minutes after its presentation. Although health care providers would like patients and families to retain 100% of information given, in reality, learning does not take place in one session or may not occur at all. An individual may be able to remember only two to three pieces of information in one education session.

Nurses are continuously interacting with patients and discussing their progress, updating them on treatment plans, and describing procedures. With that in mind, every patient contact can be thought of as a brief teaching-learning encounter. The nurse must use every teachable moment and take advantage of the patient's readiness and willingness to learn. When educating adults, a combination of teaching strategies should be used to facilitate giving and receiving information. Each individual has a different learning style: visual, auditory, or tactile. Common strategies include discussion, demonstration, and use of media.

Discussion. Informal discussion can take place anywhere and at any time. This strategy allows for interaction between the teacher and the learner. Discussion occurs one on one or in groups. Education sessions need to be adapted quickly, as they are occurring, to meet the ever-evolving needs of the patient and family. Although teaching through discussion is informal, the information given should promote the goals of the education plan. Focus on what the patient or family wants or *needs* to know at that moment, rather than on what might be *nice* to know. Obtaining and maintaining the learner's attention during the discussion may be challenging. The nurse must use different teaching strategies and techniques and modify them frequently according to the situation and the patient's or family's response to the education.

Several strategies are used to maintain a positive teaching-learning encounter:
- Addressing the patient and family members by name
- Clearly stating the purpose of the education encounter
- Getting and keeping them involved in the learning process
- Maintaining eye contact during the encounter
- Keeping the encounter brief and to the point
- Giving positive reinforcement
- Communicating with professionals in other disciplines about the progress and additional learning needs of the patient and family[4,5]

Demonstration and Practice. Demonstration and practice are the best strategies for teaching technical skills. Adults learn best when they are able to participate in the learning process. Involving the learner, providing consistent step-by-step instructions, and presenting a visual demonstration of the skill being performed are important strategies to achieve successful task acquisition. By allowing the patient or family to practice the skill in a simulated or real situation, the outcome of the teaching encounter can be evaluated. This strategy allows the nurse to offer positive reinforcement and constructive feedback during the learning encounter, thereby building learner confidence in performing the newly acquired skill. Many demonstration sessions and repetitive practice may be required for the patient or family to acquire and feel comfortable with the new skill.

Audiovisual Media. The use of media in mainstream patient education is becoming more prevalent as a first-line teaching strategy. Media are excellent tools to relay information to persons with any one of the three learning styles. Pamphlets, videos, and anatomic pictures or models are the most common types of audiovisual aids. This teaching strategy supplies the learner with a large amount of information in a relatively short period. Videos and written materials enable different nurses to distribute information that remains consistent from patient to patient and family to family. The use of media can assist practitioners to obtain informed consent and to communicate current and future prescribed treatment plans.

Media are used to educate patients on a variety of educational needs, such as medications, disease processes, procedures, symptom management, weight monitoring, laboratory tests, diet, surgery, and health maintenance issues. Patient education videos require the patient's attention for only a few minutes and supply the learner with "nice-to-know" and "need-to-know" information. Interactive video technology offers on-demand educational and health information video programs, which are delivered to the patient through television. Patients and families are able to access education videos anytime they desire during their hospital stay. The digital video system allows multiple TVs to show the same video at the same time. Bedside call systems are linked to the computer server, and the video is selected from the bedside. These video systems can be customized to meet the needs of specialty patient populations (e.g., cardiac, obstetrics). Individual reports can be generated to list all educational films viewed during the patient's stay. Evaluation of learning can be achieved through the system by administration of a pretest or posttest available on the system.

Viewing a video does not ensure retention of information or knowledge acquisition. Patient education videos should not be used in place of patient-family interaction. After the patient watches the video, the nurse must review the content and reiterate key points of information. This postvideo encounter is also used to evaluate the outcome of the teaching-learning encounter. To review the content with the patient or family, the nurse must also watch the video and choose key points to discuss with the learner in the postvideo discussion. Video presentation should be used to assist the learner in meeting identified educational needs.

Written Materials. Written media, such as brochures, pamphlets, patient pathways, and booklets, are common in outpatient and inpatient areas of health care. They usually are inexpensive and offer opportunities for a wide range of education: disease process education, risk factor modification information, procedure education, medication education, and use of medical equipment in the home setting. Written materials address multiple learning styles and offer learner-centered teaching with concrete, basic information that can be placed at the learner's fingertips for immediate review, as well as future review anytime the learner desires. Several factors should be considered when choosing printed materials for patient education: target patient population, cultural considerations, age-specific considerations, and literacy.[6]

The practitioner must make sure that written materials are appropriate for the patient population as a whole and for a particular individual patient or family. Literacy is the ability to use printed and written information to function in society, to achieve goals, and to develop knowledge and potential.[32] Persons with low literacy levels have trouble functioning in society. They may not be able to read a bus schedule, complete a simple form, or even follow the instructions on a bottle of aspirin. The term *health literacy* refers to the patient's ability to understand and communicate important medical and health information to members of the health care team.[33] Low literacy levels are considered a barrier to successful patient and family education and the teaching-learning process.[9]

If a person with a low literacy level cannot read the material or understand its meaning, he or she cannot perform self-management tasks to maintain health. This sets the patient and the family up for failure and being labeled noncompliant. Inadequate literacy is an independent risk factor for increasing hospital admissions among the elderly.[34] Nearly 20% of the U.S. adult population have low literacy skills and read at or below the fifth-grade reading level.[35] Typical patient educational materials are written at or above the eighth- or ninth-grade reading level and may be out of reach for many readers.[5,36] A common misconception among health care providers is that reading levels are directly related to the level of education; the implication is that someone with a graduate-level education has a higher reading level than someone who completed only grade school. This is not true; education levels do not necessarily correlate with the ability to read and comprehend health care information.

Several tools are available to assist health care professionals to screen for low literary skills. The Rapid Estimate of Adult Literacy in Medicine (REALM) assesses the patient's ability to pronounce medical terms.[4] It takes only a few minutes to complete and is relevant to health care. Another literacy screening tool is the Test of Functional Health Literacy in Adults (TOFHLA). This tool assesses the ability of the individual to read and comprehend directions for taking medications, monitoring blood glucose, and keeping appointments.[37] The only drawback to this tool is it takes approximately 22 minutes to complete and may not be appropriate for the bedside practitioner to use.

Readability is another important factor in the consideration of printed educational materials. *Readability* refers to how easy or hard the literature is to read. Readability formulas are designed to make a quick, easy assessment of the readability level in patient educational materials. Formulas such as the Simplified Measure of Gobbledygook (SMOG), Suitability

Assessment of Materials (SAM), and Fog and Fry assessment tools are available to assist practitioners in determining the readability of health educational materials. Providing written educational materials at the appropriate reading level is important, if the information is to be easily read and understood by most patients and families. To assist the nurse in overcoming literacy-related barriers to health education, it is recommended that patient educational materials be printed at or below the fifth-grade reading level.[35,38] Samples of health-related instructions at different reading levels are provided in Box 5-4.

Patients and families who cannot read and understand the written word provide a special challenge with regard to printed materials. Provision of educational materials with illustrations for those who cannot read or in Braille for the blind can be helpful. The inability of a patient or family to read the English language does not mean they cannot understand directions and treatment regimens. Multilingual, written educational materials are a necessity in any health care institution. Many health education vendors supply ready-made materials for patient education. Examples are HERC publishing, Pritchett and Hall, and Krames. National associations such as the American Cancer Society, the American Lung Association, and the American Heart Association also publish educational materials for patients. Each of these companies has a Web site for easy viewing of sample patient education materials and pricing information. Prices for these materials vary from pennies per pamphlet to several dollars; some pamphlets by national organizations are available free of charge to the consumer. When choosing standardized, printed educational materials, there are several items to consider. Read the entire pamphlet or booklet to determine appropriateness of the material for the desired patient population. Ask the vendor to supply the reading level of the material and the method used to determine it. Inquire about the frequency with which the printed material is updated to ensure that the patient or family members have the most recent edition.

Thoroughly read the document for inconsistent information or information that is incongruent with a specific unit's

---

BOX 5-4   SAMPLES OF READING LEVELS

COLLEGE READING LEVEL
Consult your physician immediately at the onset of chest discomfort, shortness of breath, or increased perspiration.

TWELFTH-GRADE READING LEVEL
Call your physician immediately if you experience chest discomfort, shortness of breath, or increased sweatiness.

EIGHTH-GRADE READING LEVEL
Call your doctor immediately if you start having chest pain or shortness of breath or you feel sweaty.

FOURTH-GRADE READING LEVEL
Call your doctor right away if you start having chest pain, cannot breathe, or feel sweaty.

treatment plan. For example, if the nurse educates the patient on a low-fat diet, but the pamphlet teaches only a low-salt diet, the patient may become confused and frustrated and not be able to determine which diet to follow at home. Another point to consider is whether the material contains information required by the institution and regulatory agencies such as The Joint Commission. Core measures outlined by The Joint Commission include certain items that must be included in discharge education and tracked by the institution. Some materials may not properly fit with a unit's plan for education and therefore are not appropriate for that particular institution. Printed material should be an adjunct to patient and family education and match what is taught and practiced in a specific facility.

When predeveloped educational materials do not meet the need of the institution's patient population, the decision is made to develop internal patient educational materials. Producing home-grown educational materials can be time consuming and difficult.[10] Time must be spent determining content, readability, and design. The practitioner must keep in mind that patients and families may receive a variety of educational materials during their hospital stay. Streamlining educational materials within an organization decreases inconsistency of information, increases the clarity of prescribed treatment, and helps to avoid duplication of efforts between disciplines and shifts. Although providing written materials may seem like a quick and easy educational method, the practitioner must still review the content with the patient or family to determine whether learning has occurred and whether there are any questions about the material.

Computer-Assisted Instruction. Computer-assisted instruction is a relatively new strategy for providing patient and family education. Even though personal computers have become common, they may not be suitable because comfort levels with the technical aspects of the computer vary from person to person. The learner should be able to pay attention to the material being presented and not be preoccupied with learning how to use the computer mouse. The costs of computers and new software development may prohibit institutions from considering them for their patient education programs. Software programs can be accessed through a single hard drive or through a server for multiple computer sites. The use of touch screen technology instead of the standard mouse opens up computer learning to many individuals who do not feel comfortable with standard systems. Touch screen technology is even available in local grocery stores for self-checkout. Computer screens may be placed in every patient's room at the bedside for easy access to education videos or the Internet. Bedside computers provide the patient and family with an avenue to receive education on demand whenever they are ready, willing, and able. Computers offer self-directed learning. Because adults are self-directed individuals, they can go through the program at their own pace and spend as much or as little time as desired in one area of content. Computers stimulate all aspects of the adult learner—visual, auditory, and tactile.

Internet Sites. Patients and families often use Web sites to research information about the illness or condition they are concerned with.[39] Information on the Internet is generally presented on an eighth-grade reading level.[9] Web sites contain a wealth of information. However, the information is not regulated or controlled for reliability or validity,[39] and not all information provided on every Web site is accurate. The nurse must advise the patient and family about this concern and ask them to print out and bring in such material so it can be discussed. Government Web sites and those of professional organizations, reputable health care organizations, and consumer health groups offer trustworthy information for the practitioner and the public.[39]

Communication. Communicating information is essential to obtaining positive outcomes for patient education. Interpreter services should be used if the patient or family is not fluent in the English language. Informational materials should be made available in other languages to facilitate relaying information and for enhancing self-care management skills after discharge.

All patients and families desire to be understood and have their concerns validated. This can be difficult for patients who are critically ill and whose ability to communicate to family and health care providers is impaired. Communication aids such as picture cards, picture boards, or word boards enhance the ability of the nurse to understand educational needs and communicate information. Augmentative and alternative communication (AAC) systems may be considered for temporarily nonspeaking patients in the ICU. Technology that has been available in the outpatient setting to help persons who cannot speak is becoming available in the intensive care environment. This technology is known as an electronic voice output communication aid (VOCA). VOCA is a prerecorded, human or digitalized computer-generated voice message.[40] It can be beneficial for patients who awake and alert but are unable to talk for reasons such as mechanical ventilation through an endotracheal tube or tracheostomy tube. Whole phrases, as opposed to pictures or single words, are communicated to the health care team; for example, "I am having pain."[40] This technology can assist the patient to communicate comfort needs, anxiety, and fears and to ask questions concerning care or progress. Intubated patients describe the inability of families and caregivers to effectively understand their needs as an extremely stressful part of being in the ICU.[20] AACs can also assist the nurse to more effectively evaluate the outcome of education. Use of verbal, whole-sentence communication rather than traditional, nonverbal picture board communication has been found to decrease the guesswork in interpreting patient needs.[40]

CONSCIOUS AND UNCONSCIOUS PATIENTS

Patient education should not be reserved for the conscious and coherent patient only; it should be provided to the unconscious or sedated patient as well. Addressing the learning needs of this critically ill population of patients is challenging. These patients cannot communicate their educational needs, nor can they interact and participate in the learning process. Although it is not known what the unconscious or sedated patient hears or remembers, it is known that some sedated patients undergoing surgery remember discussions that took place among physicians and staff during the procedure. Practitioners frequently tell family members to speak to the unconscious patient even though the patient cannot respond. The nurse therefore should not ignore unconscious or sedated patients during the education process. These patients may not be able to respond or participate, and the effectiveness of the teaching process cannot be evaluated, but providing information regarding environment, procedures, sensations, and time of day is benevolent and may help to decrease immediate physiologic stress.

STEP 4: EVALUATION

Evaluation is the final component in the patient and family education process. The intent of evaluation is to determine the effectiveness of the educational interventions. The nurse must use his or her clinical judgment and knowledge of adult learning principles to determine how well the learner has met the expected outcomes and objectives. The evaluation process is continual and assesses the entire teaching-learning interaction, including the level of learner interest in the session, willingness to learn the content, and level of participation during the encounter. Evaluation should be completed at the end of each teaching-learning encounter. This allows the nurse to immediately present positive and constructive feedback to the patient and family, as well as revise the education plan to accommodate ongoing learning needs. It is also important to assess the response to teaching and determine whether follow-up education is required.

HOW TO EVALUATE

How does the nurse know if learning has occurred? Techniques such as verbalization of information, return demonstration, and physiologic measurement are common evaluation methods to determine the effectiveness of a teaching-learning encounter. Evaluation of knowledge retention can be completed by verbally questioning the learner. Questioning is an interactive process that assists the nurse in determining whether the learner has retained the information taught. The nurse may ask the patient if he or she is able to list signs and symptoms of heart failure. Verbal questioning should occur immediately after the teaching event and throughout the hospitalization to assess knowledge retention. For example, the physician orders a new medication for the patient today, and the nurse educates that patient on the effects and side effects; the next day, the nurse may assess retention by asking the patient if he or she remembers the reason for taking the new medication. Common items that patients and families are asked to verbalize are reportable signs and symptoms, how to manage symptoms at home, when to take medication, how often the medication should be taken, and who to call for questions or concerns.

Changes in attitude, beliefs, or lifestyle are often difficult to evaluate, because learners can say they have changed their attitude when actually they have not. In this learning domain, the nurse must use his or her detective skills to assess whether the individual has accepted the prescribed treatment plan and modified behavior accordingly. Sometimes, the best way to evaluate a change in attitude is by observation and verbal questioning. An example is a patient who has been asked to comply with a low-cholesterol diet; a food diary the patient has kept as requested provides some evidence about what the patient has eaten. A wealth of information can also be obtained from the family concerning the patient's exhibited changes.

Physiologic evidence of the effectiveness of education can also be measured. Indicators such as blood cholesterol levels, blood pressure, heart rate, blood sugars, and weight can lead the practitioner to the conclusion that the patient and family may be having difficulties understanding or following through with the identified plan of care.[31] Adults generally want to comply with new expectations but often cannot for various reasons, such as a lack of money for medications or an inability to understand what is expected of them. These barriers must be explored and included in the education plan.

Observation and return demonstration is the evaluation of choice for the skills learning domain. For the patient and family members to be "checked off" on a particular skill, they should be able to perform it independently, using the nurse only as a resource for questions. Endotracheal suctioning, placing condom catheters, and performing dressing changes are examples of common tasks that patients and families may be asked to learn. Because of the increasingly complex care that patients require at home after discharge, these skills may be the entire focus of teaching before discharge. Not every teaching moment is a success, and the nurse need not feel guilty or like a failure when the learner has not achieved the desired objective. Revisiting and revising the goals and objectives during the teaching-learning session may be necessary to meet the ever-changing needs of the patient or family.

STEP 5: DOCUMENTATION

Documentation of education is necessary to communicate educational efforts to members of the health care team, patients and families, and regulatory agencies. The nurse should recognize that informal teaching at the bedside is education. It is important to record any information given to the patient on formal documents approved for use by each health care institution. In most institutions, formal education records are used to document education rendered by practitioners of any discipline involved in the care of a particular patient and family. These forms are communication tools used to indicate progress in the teaching-learning process from shift to shift, day to day, and discipline to discipline.[41] Documentation should include education from admission to discharge on topics ranging from orientation to the environment to acquisition of self-management skills for home care.

WHAT SHOULD BE DOCUMENTED?

The complexity of information, demand by governing agencies, lawsuits, and the sheer volume of patients in and out of a unit are driving nurses to provide quality documentation of the

BOX 5-5   KNOWLEDGE: DISEASE PROCESS

Definition: Extent of understanding conveyed about a specific disease process

Indicators	None	Limited	Moderate	Substantial	Extensive
Description of disease process	1	2	3	4	5
Description of cause or contributing factors	1	2	3	4	5
Description of risk factors	1	2	3	4	5
Description of effects of disease	1	2	3	4	5
Description of signs and symptoms	1	2	3	4	5
Description of usual disease course	1	2	3	4	5
Description of measures to minimize disease progression	1	2	3	4	5
Description of complications	1	2	3	4	5
Description of signs and symptoms of complications	1	2	3	4	5
Description of precautions to prevent complications	1	2	3	4	5

From Moorhead S et al, editors: *Nursing outcomes classification (NOC),* ed 4, St. Louis, 2008, Elsevier.

education encounter.[41] Documentation of the teaching-learning process is multifaceted. The documentation form should "tell the story" of the education encounter from assessment to evaluation. Documentation of the education assessment should include learning preferences; factors that impair ability, readiness, and willingness to learn; and actual or perceived learning needs. Information should be recorded on the interaction, material taught, supplemental materials distributed, response to the education, achievement of outcome, and any follow-up education or resources needed. The Nursing Outcomes Classification (NOC), clinical pathways, and patient education guides can provide a means of consistent documentation. Box 5-5 contains an example of a NOC evaluation for a disease process.

FACTORS THAT AFFECT THE TEACHING-LEARNING PROCESS

Many factors can produce barriers to a successful teaching-learning process. The physiologic, psychological, sociocultural, financial, and environmental factors previously discussed are known to affect the patient's and family's ability, willingness, and readiness to learn. Physical disabilities, impaired vision, and hearing loss affect the learner's ability to read materials, listen to instructions, or perform a technical task.[42] If a technical task is required, ensure that the patient or family member has the physical ability or manual dexterity to perform the required skill. Provision of eyeglasses and hearing aids is essential to improving participation in learning. Several other factors have an impact on the teaching-learning process[5,10]:

- Lack of an accurate assessment
- Setting unrealistic goals
- Not involving the patient or the family in the process
- Overloading the learner with information
- Relying too heavily on resources
- Haphazard and nondirected teaching; lack of an education plan of care
- Teaching at the wrong time, hurried teaching, not paying attention to the learner

- Lack of trust and rapport between the teacher and learner
- Lack of communication among health care providers
- Language-related communication barriers

Although this list may seem overwhelming, it is important to be proactive and to remove as many of these barriers as possible. It takes less time and fewer resources to start with a structured education plan than it does to start over after the teaching-learning process has begun.

Barriers to the teaching-learning process exist for the patient or family and for the bedside nurse. Time constraints, decreased length of stay, and daily routines interrupt or impair the nurse's ability to communicate information to the patient and the family. Table 5-3 includes common barriers to the education process experienced by nurses. The patient's positive interactions

TABLE 5-3 Nursing Barriers to Education

Barrier	Example	Solution
Interruptions	Daily routines	Use all available teachable moments.
Distractions	Tasks; medication administration Phone calls TV or other noise in patient's room	Turn TV off; minimize noise.
Night shift	Sleeping patients	Plan education before bedtime.
Sedation or pain medications	Narcotic analgesic	Teach before administering the medication.
Nurse unaware of what to teach	Diabetic education	Educate self.

Data from London F: *No time to teach,* Philadelphia, 1999, JB Lippincott; Rankin S, Stallings K: *Patient education: principles and practice,* ed 4, Philadelphia, 2001, JB Lippincott.

and relationships with health care providers, as well as a clear understanding of his or her illness, symptoms, and medications, will promote adherence to the patient education plan.[43]

INFORMATIONAL NEEDS OF FAMILIES IN CRITICAL CARE

Family members and significant others of critically ill patients are integral to the recovery of their loved ones. When planning for the overall care of patients, nurses and other caregivers need to consider the informational and emotional support needs of this group.[44] Families of critically ill patients report their greatest need is for information.[45] Flexible visiting hours and informational booklets regarding the critical care experience are recommended to meet this need (Box 5-6).[46]

PREPARATION OF THE PATIENT AND FAMILY FOR TRANSFER FROM CRITICAL CARE

When patients are more stable, requiring less hemodynamic monitoring and close observation, they are frequently transferred to another level of care in a different geographic hospital setting. They may be transferred to an intermediate care unit (i.e., step-down unit, intermediate care area, or telemetry). While on these units, patients receive optimal care to their level of requirement, a lower nurse-to-patient ratio, and less expensive technologic monitoring in a quieter environment.[47-48]

Transferring a patient from the critical care unit to a step-down unit may result in anxiety and stress. Patients and families have become dependent on the monitors, equipment, constant nursing attention, and abundant information received while in the critical care unit. The patient has become secure knowing that immediate physiologic and emotional needs are being met. A strong bond has often developed between the staff and the family. Many patients and families are reluctant to give up that bond and believe that their needs will not be met as well on a step-down unit. To avoid anxiety and provide the patient and family with some control over the event, nurses need to prepare them for the transfer process.

Preparation for transfer should start after the patient has been stabilized and the life-threatening event that resulted in hospitalization has subsided. The stressor at this point is no longer the critical care environment but has become the unfamiliar step-down environment. Explanations about where the patient will be transferred, the reason for transfer, and the name of the nurse who will be providing care should be offered as soon as known. Before transfer, information about changes in care, expectations for self-care, and visiting hours should be provided to the patient and family. Family members should be contacted concerning exactly when the patient will be transferred so they can be present during the transfer or made aware of the patient's new location (Box 5-7).

The education plan of care and tips learned by the critical care staff about that particular patient and family should be communicated to the step-down unit staff. Most of the patient transfers made from the critical care unit to a step-down unit are planned events. However, unplanned or unexpected transfers sometimes occur, usually when the critical care unit requires bed space for a more seriously ill patient. In this situation, the transfer occurs quickly during the day or often at night. Families may be present in the hospital or may have gone home for the evening. This sudden need to transfer the patient can produce as much anxiety as the initial event, primarily because the patient and family may not feel ready for the transfer or may think they have lost control of the situation. Providing the patient and family with concrete evidence of improvement, such as more favorable vital signs or the need for fewer medications or tubes, can assure them about improvement in the patient's condition before unplanned transfers occur. Increasing communication and providing consistent information to patients and families also increases satisfaction with care and services.[49]

BOX 5-6 INFORMATIONAL REQUIREMENTS FOR FAMILY MEMBERS OF A CRITICALLY ILL PATIENT

- To have questions answered honestly
- To know the facts about the patient's progress
- To know the results of procedures as soon as possible
- To have staff inform family members about the patient's status
- To know why things are being done
- To know about possible complications
- To receive explanations that can be understood
- To know exactly what is being done
- To know about the staff providing care
- To receive directions about what to do during a procedure

Modified from Miracle VA, Hovenkamp G: Am J Crit Care 3(3):155, 1994.

BOX 5-7 EDUCATION COMPONENTS FOR PATIENT TRANSFER TO ANOTHER UNIT

SENDING UNIT

- Acknowledge positive move out of critical care
- When the transfer will occur
- Why the transfer is occurring
- What to expect in the different unit
- Name of the new caregiver
- Availability of care provider
- Visiting hours
- Directions for how to get there; the new room number and phone number

RECEIVING UNIT

- Orientation to environment, visitation policies, visitors
- Unit routine, meals, shift changes, doctor visits
- Expectations about patient self-care, activities of daily living
- Medication and diagnostic testing routine times

Summary

- A collaborative, well-organized, need-targeted education plan of care is essential to improving health outcomes and decreasing lengths of stay.
- The teaching-learning process is a dynamic, continuous activity that occurs throughout the entire hospitalization and may continue after the patient has been discharged.
- Information must be gathered on many factors that may affect the education process: cultural or religious views of illness or death, emotional barriers, desire and motivation, physical or cognitive limitations, and barriers to effective communication.
- The learner's needs can be defined as gaps between what the learner knows and what the learner needs to know (e.g., survival skills, coping skills, ability to make a care decision).
- Standardized education plans provide consistent interventions and outcomes; however, they must be indi-

vidualized to meet the unique needs of the patient and family.
- The optimal environment for learning is one that is nonthreatening, comfortable, open, and honest.
- Determination of an appropriate teaching strategy is essential to meet the needs of the patient.
- Providing information regarding the environment, procedures, sensations, and time of day is important for patients who are unconscious and may help to decrease immediate physiologic stress.
- When planning for the overall care of patients, nurses must consider the informational needs and emotional support of family members.
- It is important to prepare patients and families for transfers to other units to decrease stress and anxiety related to going to a less intensively monitored environment.

Case Study: Patient and Family Education

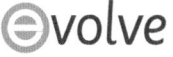 Answers to the Case Study Questions can be found on the Evolve web site at http://evolve.elsevier.com/Urden/.

Brief Patient History

Mr. S is a 30 year-old Vietnamese-American man who is employed as a fisherman. Mr. S is married and has three children younger than 5 years. He was diagnosed a few months earlier with type 1 diabetes mellitus after a 30-pound weight loss and a change in visual acuity. He has had two admissions for diabetic ketoacidosis in the past month.

Clinical Assessment

Mr. S was admitted to the intensive care unit with diabetic ketoacidosis 2 days ago. His condition has been stabilized, and he is ready to be transferred to a nursing unit today. Mr. S states that he does not understand why "this keeps happening" because he takes his insulin if he plans on eating but does not always eat. Mr. S's wife states that his blood sugar seems to be okay when he is at home but that he gets into trouble when offshore.

Diagnostic Procedures

These laboratory results were obtained on admission: blood glucose level of 620 mg/dL, carbon dioxide concentration of 11 mEq/L, and pH of 7.25. Ketones were identified in the urine and blood.

Assessment of learning needs identified a deficit in understanding regarding glucose monitoring and insulin requirements while away from home.

Medical Diagnosis

Mr. S is diagnosed with diabetic ketoacidosis resulting from noncompliance.

Questions

1. What major outcomes do you expect to achieve for this patient?
2. What problems or risks must be managed to achieve these outcomes?
3. What interventions must be initiated to monitor, prevent, manage, or eliminate the problems and risks identified?
4. What interventions should be initiated to promote optimal functioning, safety, and well-being of the patient?
5. What possible learning needs do you anticipate for this patient?
6. What cultural and age-related factors may have a bearing on the patient's plan of care?

Evolve Be sure to check out the bonus material, including free self-assessment exercises, on the Evolve web site at http://evolve.elsevier.com/Urden/.

References

1. The Joint Commission: *2004 Comprehensive accreditation manual for hospitals*, Oakbrook Terrace, IL, 2004, The Joint Commission.
2. Davis N et al: Improving the process of informed consent in the critically ill, *JAMA* 289(15):1963-1968, 2003.
3. Leske J: Comparison of family stresses, strengths, and outcomes after trauma surgery, *AACN Clin Issues Crit Care* 14(1):33-41, 2003.
4. Redman BK: *The practice of patient education*, ed 9, St Louis, 2004, Mosby.
5. Rankin S, Stallings K: *Patient education: principles and practice*, ed 4, Philadelphia, 2001, JB Lippincott.
6. Wei H, Camargo C: Patient education in the emergency department, *Acad Emerg Med* 7(6):710-717, 2000.
7. Briggs L et al: Patient-centered advance care planning in special patient populations: a pilot study, *J Prof Nurs* 20(1):47-58, 2004.
8. Moorhead S et al, editors: *Nursing outcomes classification (NOC)*, ed 4, St Louis, 2008, Mosby.
9. Burkhead V et al: Enter: a care guide for successfully educating patients, *J Nurses Staff Dev* 19(3):143-146, 2003.

10. Phillips LD: Patient education: understanding the process to maximize time and outcomes, *J Intraven Nurs* 22(1):19-35, 1999.

11. Glittenburg J: A transdisciplinary, transcultural model for health care, *J Trans Nurs* 15(1):6-10, 2004.

12. Walsh S: Formulation of a plan of care for culturally diverse patients, *Int J Nurs Terminol Classif* 15(1):17-26, 1999.

13. Leininger M, McFarland M: *Transcultural nursing*, ed 3, New York, 2002, McGraw-Hill.

14. Suh EE: The model of cultural competence through an evolutional concept analysis, *J Transcultural Nurs* 15(2):93-102, 2004.

15. Blount KA, Moore LA: Medications and the elderly, *Crit Care Nurs Clin North Am* 14(1):111-119, 2002.

16. Knowles MS: *The modern practice of adult education: from pedagogy to andragogy*, New York, 1976, Cambridge Books.

17. London F: *No time to teach*, Philadelphia, 1999, JB Lippincott.

18. Gentz C: Perceived learning needs of the patient undergoing coronary angioplasty: an integrative review of the literature, *Heart Lung* 29(3): 161-172, 2000.

19. Ruzicki D: Realistically meeting the educational needs of hospitalized acute and short stay patients, *Nurs Clin North Am* 24(3):629-637, 1989.

20. Thomas L: Clinical management of stressors perceived by patients on mechanical ventilation, *AACN Clin Issues Crit Care* 14(1):73-81, 2003.

21. Leske JS: Protocols for practice: applying research at the bedside, *Crit Care Nurs* 18(4):92-95, 1998.

22. VanHorn E et al: Family interventions during the trajectory of recovery from cardiac event: an integrative literature review, *Heart Lung* 31(3): 186-198, 2002.

23. An K et al: A cross-sectional examination of changes in anxiety early after acute myocardial infarction, *Heart Lung* 33(2):75-82, 2004.

24. Leske JS: Family stresses, strengths, and outcomes after critical injury, *Crit Care Nurs Clin North Am* 12(2):237-244, 2000.

25. Lazarus RS, Folkman S: *Stress, appraisal, and coping*, New York, 1984, Springer.

26. Laubach E: How to communicate with seriously ill patients, *Nurs Manage* 31(4):24H-24J, 2000.

27. Leske J: Overview of family needs after critical illness: from assessment to intervention, *AACN Clin Issues Crit Care* 2(2):220-226, 1991.

28. Saunders R: Constructing a lesson plan, *J Nurses Staff Dev* 19(2):70-78, 2003.

29. Bulechek GM et al, editors: *Nursing interventions classification (NIC)*, ed 5, St. Louis, 2008, Mosby.

30. Benner C et al: *From beginner to expert: excellence and power in clinical nurse practice*, Menlo Park, 1984, Addison-Wesley.

31. Clark P, Dunbar S: Family partnership intervention: a guide for family approach to care of patients with heart failure, *AACN Clinical Issues* 14(4): 467-476, 2003.

32. Kaestle C et al: *Adult literacy and education in America*, Washington, DC, 2001, U.S. Department of Education.

33. Wilson J: The crucial link between literacy and health, *Ann Intern Med* 139(10): 875-878, 2003.

34. Baker DW et al: Functional health literacy and the risk of hospital admission among Medicare managed care enrollees, *Am J Pub Health* 92(8): 1278-1283, 2002.

35. Doak C et al: Improving comprehension for cancer patients with low literacy skills: strategies for clinicians, *CA Cancer J Clin* 38(3):151-162, 1998.

36. Doak C et al: *Teaching patients with low literacy skills*, ed 2, Philadelphia, 1996, JB Lippincott.

37. Quirk P: Screening for literacy and readability: implications for the advanced practice nurse, *Clin Nurse Spec* 14(1):26-32, 2000.

38. Kingbeil C et al: Readability of pediatric patient education materials, *Clin Pediatr* 34(2):96-102, 1995.

39. Jones J: Patient education and the use of the Internet, *Clin Nurs Spec* 17(6): 281-283, 2003.

40. Happ MB et al: Electronic voice-output communication aids for temporarily non-speaking patients in a medical intensive care unit: a feasibility study, *Heart Lung* 33(2):92-101, 2004.

41. Russell C, Freiburghaus M: Heart transplant patient teaching documentation, *Clin Nurs Spec* 17(5):249-257, 2004.

42. Bruccoliere T: How to make patient teaching stick, *RN* 63(2):34-38, 2000.

43. Wu JR et al: Factors influencing medication adherence in patients with heart failure, *Heart Lung* 37(1):8-16, 2008.

44. Doering LV et al: Recovering from cardiac surgery: what patients want to know, *Am J Crit Care* 11(4):333, 2002.

45. Henneman EA et al: An evaluation of interventions for meeting the information needs of families of critically ill patients, *Am J Crit Care* 1(3):85, 1993.

46. Miracle VA, Hovenkamp G: Needs of families of patients undergoing invasive cardiac procedures, *Am J Crit Care* 3(3):155, 1994.

47. White SK, Edwards RJ: Visitation guidelines promote safe satisfying environments, *Nurs Manage* 37(8):21, 2006.

48. Radtke A: Telemetry monitoring: a preferred solution for intermediate care, *Nurs Manage* 37(12):52, 2006.

49. Mages ME: Helping patients, helping families, *Healthc Exec* 11(4):40, 2006.

Chapter 6

Psychosocial Alterations

PSYCHOSOCIAL ALTERATIONS, COPING MECHANISMS, AND MANAGEMENT

Patients who require critical care must cope with a variety of stressors. A patient's response to these stressors depends on individual differences, such as age, gender, social support, cultural background, medical diagnosis, current hospital course, and prognosis. A person's perceptions of self and relationships with others, of spiritual values, and of self-competency in social roles also play a major role in how he or she responds to stress and illness. The purpose of this chapter is to provide a theoretic basis for understanding these various issues and to provide the nurse with additional insight into implementing holistic nursing care.

The human self-concept is a major concern for nurses, because nursing interventions that do not consider the individual in his or her wholeness—including the self-concept—will probably not be effective. The self-concept comprises attitudes about oneself; perceptions of personal abilities, body image, and identity; and a general sense of worth. The stressors imposed by physical illness, trauma, and surgical procedures can cause disturbances in the self-concept. A person's response to these stressors depends on a variety of individual differences.

The following discussions address the nursing diagnoses related to self-concept disturbances imposed by critical stages of illness (i.e., Disturbed Body Image, Situational Low Self-Esteem, Ineffective Role Performance, Ineffective Coping, and Compromised Family Coping) as developed by the North American Nursing Diagnosis Association (NANDA).[1] Stuart's stress adaptation conceptual model[2] is presented as a means to address coping mechanisms and holistic methods of care. Some of the stressors experienced in the critical care setting are depicted in Box 6-1.

The selected diagnoses presented relate to the major concerns and problems that are common to the critical care setting. Customary responses to stress, such as anxiety and depression, are described, as well as the risks for spiritual distress, powerlessness, hopelessness, and self-directed violence (suicide). The psychosocial needs of specific populations, including chronically ill people with acute exacerbations, people with suppressed immune systems, and transplant recipients, are also discussed. Ways to enhance patient coping mechanisms and support family and friends with an attitude of care, openness, and warmth are presented. These interpersonal skills lead to effective interventions.

HOLISTIC NURSING PRACTICE

Holistic nursing care requires consideration of all individual and environmental factors that affect the patient's well-being and the ability to cope with crises such as an acute or chronic illness. The nurse must have a sound knowledge of anatomy and physiology, disease processes, remedial measures, and human responses. The critical care nurse not only should be able to work with technology but also needs to "know the patient" in order to humanize and individualize the care. The value of "presence," being attuned to the patient's needs, represents the caring aspect of nursing and can assist in early identification of patient problems.[3,4] Decisions to implement interventions are then based on an understanding of the patient's experiences, cultural beliefs, behavior patterns, feelings, and preferences (Table 6-1).[5-9]

Research conducted by Jenny and Logan[10] asked patients to provide examples of nurse caring behaviors. Positive comments included alleviating discomfort, caring attitudes and behaviors, advocacy, encouragement, and respect for the individual. Comments regarding noncaring behaviors were related to task-oriented behaviors and impersonal communication. The art of caring requires skills in communication and interpersonal relationships, a personal commitment, and the ability to create a sense of trust.

EFFECTS OF STRESS ON MIND-BODY INTERACTIONS

Stress of any type—whether positive or negative, biologic, psychological, or social—elicits the same physical responses.[11] Extensive literature exists describing the relationship between mind-body interactions and the immune response to stress. All personal resources can be depleted by exposure to severe or prolonged stress. Several studies have shown the effects of life events such as an acute illness that is perceived to be a threat to personal integrity.[12-14] The effects of an illness that requires hospitalization can be further compounded if admission to an intensive care unit (ICU) becomes necessary.

The ICU environment can be frightening. Technologic equipment can control one's breathing and prevent speaking. Invasive procedures, abrupt or continual noises, loss of privacy,

BOX 6-1 STRESSORS IN THE CRITICAL CARE SETTING

Although the experience of critical illness and care varies, each patient must cope with at least some of the following stressors:

- Threat of death
- Threat of survival with significant residual problems related to the illness or injury
- Pain or discomfort
- Lack of sleep
- Loss of autonomy over most aspects of life and daily functioning
- Loss of control over one's environment, such as loss of privacy and exposure to light, noise, and general activity of the critical care unit, including the care of other patients
- Daily hassles or common frustrations
- Loss of usual role and, with that, the arena in which usual coping mechanisms serve the patient

- Separation from family and friends
- Loss of dignity
- Boredom broken only by brief visits, threatening stimuli, and frightening thoughts
- Loss of ability to express oneself verbally when intubated

Effects of and responses to stressors depend on the individual's perception of the intensity of the stress and the following factors:

- Acute and chronic duration of stressors
- Cumulative effect of simultaneous stressors
- Sequence of stressors
- Individual's previous experience with stressors and coping effectiveness
- Amount of social support

---

sleep interruptions, pain, medications, isolation, and minimal contact with significant support people all create feelings of powerlessness and loss of control. Disorientation, which is common for patients in the ICU, is influenced by several factors, including the severity of the physical problem, chemical imbalances, sensory overload or deprivation, and previous experiences with the health care system. In addition to these factors are personal variables such as biologic factors, social roles, and the individual's emotional responses of anxiety, confusion, or depression.[5,13] However, for some people, the ICU is perceived as a safe environment where life-saving procedures are immediately at hand and administered by highly competent caregivers.

Three of the principal stress theories proposed by scientists describe stress in terms of a stimulus, a response, and a transaction.[11,15-17] Hans Selye's pioneering work[11] portrayed the body's responses to the stress stimulus as the general adaptation syndrome (GAS). Stimulation of the sympathetic nervous division of the autonomic nervous system (ANS) and the release of neurotransmitters and endocrine hormones occur in the initial stage, which is commonly referred to as the *fight or flight response*. Elevations in blood pressure, tachycardia, increased muscle tone, increased alertness, and "free-floating" anxiety are some of the responses. After all reserves have been depleted, a stage of exhaustion occurs, leading to further complications or death. Reversal of these processes can be accomplished by restoration of reserves through the use of medications, nutrition, stress reduction measures, and psychotherapy. Selye's work continues to be the primary framework for stress and coping theories.

Nuerberger[15] was the first to propose that a person's emotional response to stress (or a perceived threat), described as "shutting down," is the result of overstimulation of the parasympathetic nervous system. He labeled this survival tactic the general inhibition syndrome (GIS), or the "possum response." Defense mechanisms such as withdrawal, avoidance, and detachment are typical behaviors associated with this type of response.[2,17] Both ANS responses are protective measures. Imbalances of either system can be detrimental.

The extensive work of Lazarus and others[16,17] provides the framework for transactional theories of stress that suggest that the ways in which people cope with stress may be more important to overall morale, social function, and health or illness states than the frequency and severity of stress episodes. The patient confronted by stress first makes a *cognitive appraisal* of its intensity. Response to the stressor depends on the perceived degree of threat imposed. A *secondary appraisal* determines what the response will be or what coping method will be used to minimize the threat.

Coping, or adaptation, is an ongoing process that involves cognitive and physiologic neurochemical and endocrine processes. The individual's sensitivity and vulnerability to the stressor are the determining factors of emotional and behavioral responses.[17,18] What may be an acutely stressful event to one individual is not necessarily perceived as stressful by another. A person may employ different coping mechanisms in response to various stressors or to the same stressor at different times. A mechanism that is ineffective in one situation may be appropriate in another. Each patient comes to an illness with a history and knowledge of the particular situation and its impact on life. Interpretation of the event and responses to it depend on this history. The history changes with each new encounter.[2,11,12,17]

The Stuart stress adaptation model[2] addresses nursing interventions for persons whether they are sick or well. Concepts depicting biologic and psychological responses to stress parallel those of the stress theories presented. Precipitating stressors may arise from the individual's internal or external environment; adaptation may depend on the number of stressors and the timing of their occurrence, as well as the degree of change that is represented. The accumulation of daily hassles can often influence a person's response to a major stressor. Personal characteristics that facilitate constructive adaptation to stress include hardiness, resilience, hope, a positive self-concept and internal locus of control, a sense of belonging, and the presence of social support.[19-21] Use of maladaptive or destructive measures may temporarily minimize anxiety but do not resolve the personal conflicts. There are four stages of nursing activities: (1) stabilizing the patient

TABLE 6-1 Assessment, Nursing Actions, and Expected Outcomes of Holistic-Centered Care

Assessment	Nursing Actions	Expected Outcomes
Person **Biologic Characteristics** Age, gender, developmental phase Body functions (balance or imbalance), including internal environmental factors	Focus all actions toward total strengths and needs of the patient, including aspects related to environment and health status; use theoretic knowledge base for comparison purposes.	Continuity of care will be provided.
Psychological Characteristics Self-concept components Spiritual beliefs or values Locus of control Coping mechanisms Role competency or role conflict Perception of current illness Intellect	Identify the patient's perception of the current illness, control of events, and availability of appropriate support system. Identify coping mechanisms used with previous stressors. Assess and support ability to learn new self-care techniques.	Patient will have realistic expectations of outcomes from current illness and its impact on physical and mental health. Patient will use effective coping mechanisms in response to illness-related stressors. Patient will participate in self-care and learn new psychomotor skills to achieve confidence in skill performance.
Social Aspects Interrelationships Availability of support system	Provide positive, honest feedback. Establish trust.	Patient will place trust in caregivers and verbalize satisfaction with care or express need for changes.
Environment Cultural, ethnic, and societal influences Area of residence, condition of living quarters or workplace Access to available community resources (transportation, food, sanitation, support services) Access to recreation facilities Membership, attendance at religious or social functions Availability of significant others in social support system	Identify factors in the external environment that influence (facilitate or inhibit) patient's coping with current health problem. Collaborate with the health care team members in providing holistic care. Provide a safe, comfortable environment that is as stress-free as possible during hospitalization. Encourage positive interactions with significant others.	Inhibiting factors will be minimized; facilitative factors will be enhanced. Collaborative team efforts will promote a holistic approach to decision making; family will be included in decisions. Hospital environment will be modified to provide a safe, secure atmosphere. Significant others will have a central role in providing social support; patient will not be isolated.
Health Current and past mental, spiritual, and physical health status Lifestyle practices Types of coping mechanisms Attitude toward life	Encourage positive interactions with significant others. Instruct the patient and family on self-care activities. Involve the family in patient-centered activities as early as possible; support family members.	Patient and family will have knowledge about illness and prognosis and can plan realistically for the future. Patient can implement a balanced plan of care for self. Family caregivers will recognize their own limits and seek help.

in a time of crisis, (2) providing symptomatic relief and assessment of the patient's coping responses, (3) reinforcing adaptive behaviors and improved patient functioning, and (4) implementing strategies for health promotion and optimal quality of life.

ANXIETY AS A RESPONSE TO STRESS

Anxiety is a normal subjective human response to a perceived or actual threat to self-integrity, which can range from a vague, generalized feeling of discomfort to a state of panic and loss of control. Anxiety is the most common of all mental illnesses.[22] Symptoms of anxiety closely parallel the biologic stress responses described earlier. The initial emotional responses of excitement and heightened awareness diminish as anxiety levels increase, the individual's perceptual field narrows, and problem-solving and coping skills are lost. Prolonged stress can exhaust available resources.

Experiencing an acute or chronic illness, facing a real or anticipated loss, being hospitalized, or any other event that is perceived as stressful can be a trigger for anxiety. The nature of the stressor and the biopsychosocial conditioning of the person being stressed are the determining factors of a response.[7,17,23,24] Individuals who possess an anxiety trait may have poorer coping mechanisms and may respond quite differently to an anxiety-producing situation than do individuals who do not possess this trait (see Appendix A).

Anxiety elicits changes in the neurohumoral release patterns involving the neurotransmitters—including acetylcholine, norepinephrine, dopamine, and serotonin—and their corresponding receptors. The complex and elusive integration of these responses within the central nervous system relies on communication among the cerebral cortex, the limbic system, the thalamus, the hypothalamus, the pituitary gland, and the reticular activating system. The cortex is involved with cognition, attention, and alertness, whereas emotional responses to stress are located in the limbic system. Corticotropin-releasing factor (CRF) controls the endocrine response and the norepinephrine pathway that is active in regulating the sympathetic branch of the ANS. It is suggested that a positive feedback system between the CRF and the ANS occurs when the increased activation in one system influences an increased activation in the other system. It is also proposed that large amounts of circulating CRF can accelerate behavioral responses (i.e., anxiety and hypersensitivity) to stressful stimuli.[25,26]

ANXIETY AND PAIN

A cyclic relationship exists between levels of anxiety and perceptions and tolerance of pain. This relationship varies according to whether pain is produced by disease processes or invasive procedures, is acute or chronic, or is anticipatory. Pain affects the whole person. It has been defined as "an unpleasant sensory and emotional experience associated with actual and potential damage, or described in terms of such damage."[25] Pain also is multidimensional in nature, necessitating comprehensive assessment and management. In conditions of high acuity, pain can be caused by a variety of sources, such as injured tissues, imposed immobility, intubation, lighting, noise, and interrupted sleep.

When an illness or pain is severe enough, the person experiencing it is forced to conserve all energies and focus inward to gain control of anxiety feelings. He or she may startle easily, become irritable, display anger and rage, be vigilant and wary of caregivers, or be demanding. There is a tendency to blame others, to be confused, and to be indecisive. The patient may withdraw from interpersonal contact and may indicate that the situation is overwhelming.[2,22] It is crucial for the nurse to identify the cause of the patient's pain, validate observations with the patient, and identify a plan for pain management. (For detailed information on pain management, see Chapter 9.)

Once pain management has been addressed, the nurse evaluates for ongoing anxiety. Again, the nurse needs to identify the cause of a patient's anxiety and to validate observations with the patient. Medications frequently administered in the ICU can contribute to anxiety feelings; they include theophylline, anticholinergics, dopamine, levodopa, salicylates, and steroids.[22,25,26] Whether the causes of anxiety are biochemically induced, related to genetic

factors, or secondary to a threat imposed in an emergency or a crisis situation, the nurse must take all factors into consideration for interventions to be effective. Panic attacks (outcomes of severe anxiety), which are frequent occurrences in the ICU, can also produce physiologic symptoms such as tachycardia, hyperventilation, and dyspnea.[2]

SELF-CONCEPT

THEORETIC BASIS

The terms *self-concept* and *self-esteem* have often been used synonymously. No clear-cut distinctions have been made. However, theoretic models used in the development of measurements refer to the self-concept as the "self-schema," or knowledge of abilities, beliefs, and values that influence behavior during interactions with others in the social and cultural environments, whereas self-esteem is most closely linked to one's sense of self-worth.[2,27,28] Although the self-concept is relatively stable, it can be modified by the developmental phases and social roles a person experiences over a lifetime.[2,29] The nursing discipline has chosen the multidimensional construct of self-concept, because it is useful for understanding individuals in regard to regulating health and illness behaviors and for distinguishing the importance of the environment in relation to these behaviors.[29]

GENERAL DISTURBANCES IN SELF-CONCEPT

Any event with unpredictable body changes and effects on functions requires adjustments in the self-concept as well as a realistic readjustment to the role limitations that are imposed. These adjustment stages are complex and highly individualized.

A person faced with an intolerable situation may panic, may display behavior that distorts reality, and may exhibit excessive demands or be suspicious of the motives and methods of caregivers. Depression and anxiety are common reactions as the patient experiences a loss of control and worries over outcomes.[30] The illness experience may have different meanings for people from different cultures and ethnic groups. Assessment of their needs can be elicited through use of tools that include questions that are sensitive to cultural values.[9] Patients in critical care units usually do not have time to adjust to their illness conditions; they may exhibit signs of shock, numbness, and avoidance of reality and may be unable to clearly understand the implications of the situation.[2,11,31-34] The patient is usually transferred to an intermediate unit before a true acknowledgment phase occurs. However, establishing rapport, repeating information as needed, and reassuring the patient of her or his immediate safety are appropriate interventions. As patients begin to deal with what has happened to them, active listening, conveyance of validation, empathy, warmth, and reassurance help patients understand that they are being heard by a caring professional.

DISTURBED BODY IMAGE

Body image is the mental picture an individual has of his or her body and its physical functioning at a given time. It includes attitudes and feelings about one's body in reference to appearance, build, health, performance ability, and gender-related concepts.[2,14,34-36] The body image develops over time from postural changes sensed internally, contact with people and objects in the environment, emotional experiences, and fantasies.[22,35] Stein[27] suggested that the ability to project possible images of one's self in the future that are highly desirable or feared can play a powerful role in motivating and regulating goal-directed behavior.

Disturbances in body image arise when the person fails to perceive or adapt to the changes that are imposed by age, disease, trauma, or surgery. In some instances, the person may feel betrayed by the body, which no longer seems normal. Body image may also be altered by the need to incorporate a prosthetic device or a donated body part.[37-40] Although the disease or problem may be corrected by surgery and medical treatments, whenever the result is visible to the patient and others, the change in body image can arouse intense feelings of anger, frustration, depression, and powerlessness.[14,38] The critical care nurse often begins the process of helping the patient live with this permanent alteration. Interventions by the nurse and others on the health care team focus on helping the patient manage the physical changes and the psychosocial alterations.

DISTURBANCES IN SELF-ESTEEM

Self-esteem, or self-measurement of one's worth, develops as a part of self-concept through the perceived appraisals of significant others.[41] The need for self-esteem is a part of the hierarchy of human needs postulated by Maslow.[42] Having high self-esteem helps one deal with the environment and face the maturational and situational crises of life more easily. Persons with well-developed self-esteem are at less risk for disturbances of self-esteem than those with poorly developed self-esteem.[20,35]

Self-esteem has been studied often in a variety of contexts. Because nurses have a significant impact on ill patients, self-esteem is an important concept for them to understand.[6,28,43] Illness can rob the person of perspective, and it shrinks the familiar world and the one of possibility, often leading to low self-esteem and feelings of powerlessness, helplessness, and depression.[44,45] A low self-regard impairs one's ability to adapt. The patient may refuse to participate in self-care, exhibit self-destructive behavior, or be too compliant—asking no questions and permitting others to make all decisions.[23,41,45] For the critical care nurse who values a holistic approach to treatment, it is essential to request psychological or psychiatric consultation and ongoing treatment if patients jeopardize their own safety or the safety of others. Ideally, this type of comprehensive approach to recovery includes the provision of ongoing supportive and adjustment psychotherapy.

DISTURBANCES IN PERSONAL IDENTITY OR SELF-IDENTITY

"Self-identity is different from self-concept in that it refers to a feeling of distinctness from others."[27,33] It represents a whole picture of the self, or "who I am," through a combination of conscious and unconscious perceptions. When behaviors are in accordance with the self-concept, the self-identity is confirmed or reinforced. Ego-identity is developed throughout the life span and is influenced by sociocultural norms, gender roles, and interpersonal relationships.

Personal identity disturbance is the inability to differentiate the self as a unique and separate human being from others within a social environment, and this sense of depersonalization engenders a high level of anxiety.[41] This problematic aspect of the self-concept is most often seen during maturational or situational crises and in mental illnesses including anxiety disorders. Additional causes of personal identity disturbance are use of psychoactive drugs; biochemical imbalances in the brain; organic brain disorders of dementia, amnesia, or delirium; and traumatic insult to the brain. A careful nursing assessment and appropriate interventions, such as psychiatric referral, are needed because of the varied causes of identity disturbances.

INEFFECTIVE ROLE PERFORMANCE

Roles are sets of socially expected behavior patterns that individuals fulfill throughout the life span.[2,29] Interactions with others that create and modify these roles are an important part of the self-concept. Primary roles are those associated with gender, age, and developmental stage. Secondary roles include membership in a family, and tertiary roles are those assumed by choice, such as an occupation. Illness, when it occurs, disrupts secondary and tertiary roles, and responses can be affected by primary role characteristics. The rapid and potentially drastic changes that accompany critical illness may seriously interfere with role relationships, expectations, or abilities in role performance. Role performance alterations often are referred to as *role strain, role stress,* or *role insufficiency*. In helping patients with disruption of roles, it is important to explore their feelings, generate and explore alternatives, and identify available resources that would allow them to resume a relatively normal life as soon as possible.

POWERLESSNESS

Powerlessness, as a nursing diagnosis, is defined as the perception of the individual that his or her own action will not significantly affect an outcome.[41] Unrelieved powerlessness may result in hopelessness, which is discussed in the next section.

The causes of powerlessness include factors in the health care environment, interpersonal interactions, cultural and religious beliefs, illness-related regimen, and a lifestyle of helplessness. The range in levels of powerlessness varies and depends on the person's perceived sense of control, the amount of loss experienced, and the availability of social support. Powerlessness can be manifested by delayed decision making or refusal to make decisions or by expressions of self-doubt in role performance. Frustration, anger, and resentment over being dependent on others often occur and are exhibited as verbal expressions regarding dissatisfaction with care.[44]

Individuals vary in the amount of control they prefer.[45] The routines of the critical care unit may oppose or preclude any control by the patient. The person for whom control is important should be helped to continue to control as many areas of his or her life as possible. On the other hand, a patient must be given the opportunity to choose not to control.

Rotter's early research[46] on human behavior and perception of control has been particularly helpful in explaining the variability of responses people have in similar situations. He proposed the major concept of internal versus external locus of control. Individuals who have an internal locus of control perceive themselves to be responsible for the outcome of events. Individuals with an external locus of control believe that their actions will have no effect on the outcome of a situation. The scale to measure locus of control developed by Rotter is useful in assessing this personality trait. However, later, situation-specific measures are better predictors than the original global scale.

Another aspect of powerlessness is *learned helplessness,* or *excessive dependence.*[45] A person who repeatedly experiences uncontrollable situations loses the motivation for making decisions about life events. Some people assume a martyr role and accept the illness state as their fate, doing nothing to improve their status. Some find the sick role a gratifying means for gaining control over others by using their symptoms to gain attention.[47] Setting limits on these behaviors, encouraging independence and participation in self-care, counseling, and involving family members in establishing realistic goals are helpful strategies to assist a patient to diminish this manipulative behavior. However, for patients who have a premorbid mental health history of excessive dependence, limit-setting may aggravate an already difficult situation. These patients may become very angry or withdrawn. These patients require a comprehensive mental health assessment, a carefully considered treatment plan, and ongoing psychotherapy. Therapy begins with the development of trust, open dialogue, and a discussion of realistic expectations that encourages small, measurable improvements in self-care over time. It is essential that the critical care nurse work in concert with the mental health professionals to ensure continuity of care. Working together with the patient will set a nonthreatening tone and aid in beginning to diminish these dependent behaviors.

Critically ill patients generally have experienced a rapid onset of illness without having had time to acquire the illness role. If control is defined as the ability to determine the use of time, space, and resources, admission to a critical care unit strips away this power. On admission, persons lose their independent status. They become patients. Choice of clothing and use of other personal belongings are usually restricted in a critical care unit. Patients cannot decide who enters the room, who provides personal care, or who intrudes with painful treatments. Hospital rules are usually not open to modification. Patients may feel anxious because they are separated from a familiar environment and have restrictions on who may visit them.

Poor interactions with health care providers can make the situation worse. Patients may react aggressively, may try bargaining, or may refuse to comply with diagnostic and treatment regimens. They may resent the close scrutiny of the nurses and physicians and the invasion of their privacy. By virtue of their experiences

with critical illness and care, people may lose sight of areas of influence they still do retain over themselves because so much control has been taken from them. Nurses can emphasize the patient's influence or control and thereby help to preserve it.[3,44]

HOPELESSNESS

Hopelessness is a subjective state in which an individual sees limited or no alternatives or personal choices available and is unable to mobilize energy on his or her own behalf.[41] In 1996, Boling[48] proposed a nursing diagnosis for this situation, entitled Defect in Hope. To help clarify hopelessness, the following definition of hope is included: a feeling that provides comfort while enduring life threats and personal challenges; a feeling that what is wanted will happen; a desire that is accompanied by anticipation or expectation. Most people agree that an element of hope must be maintained, no matter how hopeless things appear. Hope is a force that helps one survive.[18,49] An interdisciplinary concept analysis of hope and hopelessness in the literature from theology, medicine, nursing, and psychology revealed that absolute hopelessness is viewed as incompatible with life. Hope often arises in the presence of crisis and instills vigorous resistance to giving up. The help of others in the situation supports the patient's belief.[3,19] Hope wards off despair, mental anguish, disorganization, and helplessness.[49]

When people expect something to happen, they usually act in ways that increase the likelihood that the expectation will be met.[27] The expectation, whether positive or negative, becomes stronger the more times the "reinforcing circle" occurs. This process is defined as a *self-fulfilling prophecy.*

The critically ill patient is a multiproblem patient. Nurses and physicians are tempted to focus on the crisis and the use of technical equipment and to overlook the patient in his or her totality. The health care team may stereotype patients and underestimate their individual strengths.[4,34] The very nature of the critical care unit is frightening and increases a patient's sense of vulnerability and fear of death. Therefore, it is important to foster a realistic sense of hope in the patient.[41,50] The critical care nurse can project an attitude of hope; identify some aspect of the situation in which hope is warranted, no matter how grave the situation; and attempt to channel feelings toward some positive outcome.

When the situation moves from hopeful to hopeless in the critical care unit, the decision to write a "do not resuscitate" order must be carefully considered.[51,52] It must be recognized that members of the health care team and the family may reach this decision at varying times.[9,53] However, it is important to not avoid difficult conversations and to keep patients and families informed. Careful medical and nursing assessments, use of family and team conferences to foster communication, and enlisting the assistance of a spiritual counselor can make these situations less frustrating for all concerned.

Families also need hope. Nursing strategies for supporting the family include clarifying any distorted thinking, providing opportunities for the family to be with the patient,

BOX 6-2 STRATEGIES TO INSPIRE HOPE IN FAMILIES OF CRITICALLY ILL PATIENTS

RESPONDING TO FAMILY CONCERNS

- Explore one's own feelings about interacting with families of critically ill patients and end-of-life issues.
- Use active listening, therapeutic communication skills, and touch (when appropriate); allow the family to share concerns; avoid giving messages that convey false hope.
- Establish mutually trusting relationships with the patient and family.
- Provide comfort and pain relief care to the patient; demonstrate a caring attitude.
- Provide adequate and appropriate information regarding the patient's condition and progress; clarify misinformation.
- Express empathy; consider the impact of the patient's illness on roles within the family; respect membership in nontraditional family structures.
- Assess ability to cope; recognize that family members may use defense mechanisms to cope with anxiety or a crisis situation; accept individual responses to stress (which typically are not characteristic of usual behavior).
- Be sensitive to reactions to adverse changes in the patient's condition; observe for expressions of anticipatory grief, helplessness, hopelessness, and depression.
- Address spiritual needs through facilitating contacts with a chaplain or spiritual counselor; notify the family about areas available for privacy or meditation.
- Support processes that are meaningful to the family and congruent with their cultural beliefs and values.

RESPONDING TO THE FAMILY'S PHYSICAL NEEDS

- Encourage family members to attend to their own health and physical needs—nutrition, rest, and sleep.
- Provide information about available community resources for personal needs.

FAMILY PARTICIPATION

- Prepare the family regarding the patient's condition and behaviors; instruct them about the environment of the intensive care unit before their first visit; monitor family interactions with the patient; discourage confrontations; remove overemotional persons from the unit, and provide support until they can gain control of their emotions.
- Involve the family in decision making and in participation in basic patient care activities (they can be a patient's major support system).
- If possible, have the family select one person to serve as liaison at interdisciplinary team planning sessions and to be the contact for scheduling visits and receiving updates of information to decrease uncertainties the family may have.
- Use the expertise of the interdisciplinary team to provide social support, explore the meaning of the crisis, expand the coping repertoire, and help maintain caring relationships among family members.

Modified from Wheeler RW: Helping families cope with death and dying, *Nursing* 98(7):25-30, 1996; Czerwiec M: When a loved one is dying: families talk about nursing care, *Am J Nurs* 96(5):32-36, 1996; Durhan E: How patients die, *Am J Nurs* 97(12):41-46, 1997; Powers P et al: The value of patient- and family-centered care, *Am J Nurs* 100(5):84-88, 2000; and Barry P: *Psychosocial nursing: assessment and intervention in care of the physically ill*, ed 3, Philadelphia, 1996, JB Lippincott.

presenting realistic patient outcome expectations, and expanding the coping repertoire of the family.[9,51,52,54] See Box 6-2 for additional strategies.

SPIRITUAL DISTRESS

Spiritual distress has been defined as a disruption in the life principle that pervades a person's entire being and that integrates and transcends one's biologic and psychosocial nature.[41] Adherence to a particular philosophic, psychological, sociologic, or political belief may provide a sense of one's value and of life's meaning. Threats imposed by any physiologic or psychological illness or prolonged pain and suffering can challenge a person's spirituality.[33] Life-threatening illness causes a person to face his or her own mortality. The provision of holistic nursing care is not limited to meeting a patient's religious needs; it also encompasses all that provides meaning to life.

An individual who is in spiritual distress may question the meaning of suffering and death in relation to his or her personal belief system. Anger toward God or a supreme being, feelings of self-blame, or regret over inability to practice belief rituals may be expressed. Individuals may even question the necessity for the therapeutic regimen. Spiritual care has been described as

health-promoting interventions to relieve responses to stress that affect the spiritual perspectives of individuals or groups.[41] Creating an environment of compassion in which patients feel that their emotional and spiritual needs are met is at the heart of holistic care.[55] Listening to the patients' concerns, offering support, and enlisting the support of a spiritual counselor can promote the healing process.

THE MENTAL STATUS EXAMINATION

The Mental Status Examination (MSE) is a full, criteria-based assessment of a patient's cognitive function and thought processes. Although the examination is rarely conducted in its entirety in the critical care setting, knowledge of its main components enhances the nurse's effectiveness in collecting data, improves the nurse's use of accepted terminology in documentation of findings, and helps the nurse identify issues that require further assessment. This tool can be useful in evaluating the nursing diagnoses of Deficient Knowledge, Disturbed Sensory Perception, and Disturbed Thought Processes.

Categories of the MSE are (1) general description of appearance, speech, motor activity, and behaviors noted during the interview process; (2) emotional state, covering mood and

BOX 6-3   COMPONENTS OF THE MENTAL STATUS EXAMINATION

Documentation of the assessment of mental status is indicative of the person's mental status at the specific time of the interview or observation.

ASSESSMENT CRITERIA

- *Orientation and level of awareness:* A common means of assessing confusion is asking patients if they know who they are and where they are and asking them to state the day of the week, the month, or the year.
- *Appearance and behavior:* General observations include the patient's appearance and behaviors in terms of their consistency with a normal range for the patient's age, station in life, general health, and nutritional status.
- *Speech and communication:* Speech may be garbled, slurred, distinct, rapid or slow, loud or soft. The patient may remain mute. Nonverbal communications (e.g., eye contact, gestures, posture) are indicators of the patient's mood, thought formation, and content. It is important to evaluate the match between verbal and nonverbal communication patterns.
- *Mood or affect:* Communication with caregivers and family may be normal, or there may be wide mood swings. Anxiety, fear, or apathy; lethargic or agitated behaviors; and unusual gestures may be demonstrated.
- *Thinking process:* Illogical statements, rapid speaking with quick shifts from one idea to another (flight of ideas), disconnected mixture of unrelated words (word salad), delusions, hallucinations, or obsessive behaviors may be present at various times. Memory impairment may be masked by the patient's attempts to "fill in the gaps" with false statements.
- *Memory:* Recent memory is the first to be impaired and is most often seen in patients with chronic organic mental disorder (which is irreversible), acute organic mental disorders, or depression. Recent memory refers to recall of events that occurred within the recent past.

This is assessed by assessing the patient's orientation to person, time, and place. Long-term memory is assessed by asking patient to describe childhood events. Questions can be asked conversationally without causing patient to feel she or he is being "cross-examined."

- *Perception:* Perception of self, environment, and interpersonal relationships is derived through the senses of vision, hearing, touch, and smell. Defense mechanisms used during times of stress or illness can distort the perception of reality. Visual, auditory, or tactile hallucinations are frequently experienced by patients in intensive care. Hypnagogic hallucinations are false sensory perceptions that occur during the twilight period between wakefulness and sleep. (This can be a common occurrence for well persons, especially during times of severe stress or fatigue.)
- *Abstract thinking and judgment:* Differences between concrete and abstract thinking include logical reasoning in problem solving and providing a solution to a hypothetical problem.

PSYCHOSOCIAL CRITERIA

- *Stressors:* Stressors may be internal (e.g., mental or physical illness, perceived loss) or external (e.g., actual loss of something significant to the person).
- *Coping skills:* These are the methods used in adaptation to stressors.
- *Relationships:* The type of interrelationships should be congruent with developmental stage (including sexual relationships).
- *Cultural:* Cultural criteria refers to the ability to adapt as appropriate to norms for an identified group.
- *Spiritual:* Spiritual criteria are values or beliefs that are considered to be satisfying, worthwhile, and comforting.
- *Occupational:* Occupational criteria include involvement in useful, rewarding activity (e.g., work, school, recreation) that is congruent with the patient's developmental stage.

Modified from Stuart G: A stress adaptation model of psychiatric nursing care. In Stuart GW, Laraia MT, editors: *Principles and practices of psychiatric nursing,* ed 6, St. Louis, 2005, Mosby; Hollinger-Smith L: The elderly. In Fortinash K, Holoday-Worret P, editors: *Psychiatric mental health nursing,* ed 3, St. Louis, 2004, Mosby.

affect; (3) perceptions of experiences; (4) thought content and process; (5) level of consciousness; and (6) cognitive abilities (i.e., memory, level of concentration and calculation ability, judgment, and insight). Refer to Box 6-3 for categories of measurement, which are organized around theoretic concepts.[2,29,56] Several shorter instruments to assess mental function have been developed. The so-called Mini-Mental State Examination (MMSE)[57] is particularly useful in evaluating the elderly. Each item is tied to a score that, when totaled, provides an estimate of function depending on age, education, and language origin. Another rapid assessment tool by Pfeiffer[58] registers the person's orientation, memory, thought processes, and attention span.

MAJOR DEPRESSIVE EPISODE

A major depressive episode is a mood disorder of at least 2 weeks' duration that is characterized by depressed mood, diminished interest or pleasure in usual activities, insomnia,

poor appetite, psychomotor retardation or agitation, and loss of energy. Patients with this disorder also may report feelings of hopelessness, worthlessness, and guilt. Recurrent thoughts of death, loss of interest in life, and recurrent suicidal ideation may be present.[59] Major depression may complicate a patient's underlying physical illnesses; for example, asthma, headaches, ulcers, arthritis, or coronary heart disease may be exacerbated to the point of a life-threatening situation.[2,59] Depression deepens and suicide ideation frequently resurfaces after surgery if a life-threatening diagnosis is confirmed.

The nurse who suspects that a patient is severely depressed can assess thought content by using the MSE. The nurse can listen empathetically and convey to the patient that recovery from the depression is expected, while understanding that the patient's depression cannot be overcome by cheerfulness or reassurance. If the patient is on suicide precautions, the nurse safeguards the patient according to department policy and procedure and alerts all members of the health care team and the family. The nurse also informs the patient that precaution measures are being taken as a safeguard until his or her mood improves. Requesting a comprehensive mental health assessment by a mental health professional would provide the means for giving proper attention to the patient's mind-body experience.

SUICIDE

Depression is mentioned as a causal factor in 30% to 70% of suicide attempts among the high-risk groups of youth (ages 15 to 24 years), the elderly population (>65 years), and individuals with psychiatric disorders. The suicide rate for persons with acquired immunodeficiency syndrome (AIDS) has been reported to be 66 times greater than that of the general population.[34] Suicide has been described as a self-destructive response to a stimulus resulting from an undesirable, unacceptable, or overwhelming event; as a response to overcome high anxiety feelings about abandonment by God or significant others; as a hostility toward self; and as the only solution for ending a helpless or hopeless situation. Suicide is the eighth-leading cause of death in the United States, statistically represented by 30,000 deaths annually that result from more than 1 million reported suicide attempts, although the actual number may be underreported.[2,60]

Etiologic factors in the suicide risk profile include biopsychological and sociologic circumstances. Biopsychological events may involve living within the limits of a chronic disease or facing an acute, life-threatening illness and pain such as that produced by cancer or end-stage renal failure.[34] Depression is associated with irregularities in the levels of serotonin, dopamine, norepinephrine, and γ-aminobutyric acid (GABA), the neurotransmitters in the brain that regulate mood. Genetic predisposition toward suicidal and antisocial behavior also may play a role. Frontal lobe dysfunction has been associated with the feelings of hopelessness and worthlessness that contribute to depression. Other psychological factors are negative thinking patterns and reduction of positive reinforcement. Comorbidity with a psychiatric disorder is the highest indicator in the risk profile. "The common emotions of suicide are helplessness and hopelessness. The common consistency in suicide is lifelong patterns of failure, stress, duress, and threats to self-esteem."[60]

Nurses in high acuity and emergency settings will be challenged by patients who have attempted suicide or are at risk for doing so. Persons with cognitive impairment resulting from delirium effects of medications, fluid and electrolyte imbalances, anoxia, surgery, or trauma are at greatest risk for attempting suicide. Hallucinations may compel their self-destructive behavior.[61]

A primary focus for care of the person with self-destructive behavior is protection from harm.[2,61,62] Nurses also must consider their own responses to patients' self-destructive behaviors, which can enhance or inhibit their interactions with patients. Interventions may include removal of harmful objects; consistent supervision; active listening; contracting with the individual to cease harmful activities; promoting the person's self-esteem and self-control in regulating emotions and behaviors, which frequently includes administration of anxiolytic medications as well as mobilizing social support systems; and providing mental health education.

When a person commits suicide, nurses also can be involved with providing care for the survivors, who may be at increased risk for similar actions. Feelings of guilt or anger over why the suicide occurred need to be expressed by the survivors, and they need to learn how to deal with the stigma that is frequently associated with the suicide event.[2,60-62]

Clark's suicide risk factor inventory[62] provides a useful assessment tool. Each of the six dimensions contains items related to high-risk behaviors. The presence of an illness, pain, or a crisis situation of a developmental or situational nature; the person's age; the types of coping skills used; daily activities; level of self-concept; expressions of hopelessness and suicidal intent; and history of recent trauma are some of the areas that are covered. Identified risk factors can be used to design appropriate interventions.

COPING

Patients who require critical care must cope with a variety of stressors (see Box 6-1). Each patient's response to these stressors is unique and depends on a variety of environmental factors and individual differences. The nurse's knowledge of assessment, diagnosis, and effective coping strategies also affects how well the patient copes. The uncomfortable effects of a situation (e.g., anxiety, grief, loss of control) can lessen the effectiveness of coping mechanisms when people are faced with serious problems that they cannot overcome using familiar behaviors.

Coping is a dynamic process involving cognitive and behavioral efforts to manage specific internal or external demands that are perceived to exceed the person's resources.[16,17] Aquilera[63] stated that coping activities encompass all the diverse behaviors that people use to meet actual or potential demands. The available coping mechanisms are those behaviors that a person draws on that have been found to be effective in the past. The key to effective coping is using the best strategy or mix of strategies in a given situation.

NANDA[1] defines *Ineffective Coping* as "the impairment of adaptive behaviors and problem-solving abilities of a person meeting life's demands and roles." The defining characteristics of Ineffective Coping usually associated with critical illness include verbalization of an inability to cope or to ask for help and being unable to meet personal basic needs. The patient exhibits inappropriate use of defense mechanisms and cannot problem-solve. The patient may display destructive behavior toward self and others.

COPING MECHANISMS

When a patient copes effectively, what he or she is doing to cope often goes unnoticed. Emotionally, the patient seems relatively comfortable, is a cooperative recipient of care, and exhibits nonproblematic behavior. The patient may be using multiple appropriate coping mechanisms that help to manage a problem or a stressful situation. The following discussion covers several coping mechanisms that may or may not be effective, depending on the degree to which they are used. Some authors differentiate between coping mechanisms that relate to adjusting, adapting, and successfully meeting a challenge and defense mechanisms that are automatic self-protective measures developed in response to an internal or external stressor.[12,34,64] Examples of the latter include denial, acting-out behavior, avoidance, hypochondriasis, passive-aggressive behavior, and projection.

Regression. Regression is an unconscious defense mechanism that involves a retreat, in the face of stress, to behavior characteristic of an earlier developmental level.[65] Regression allows the patient to give up his or her usual role, autonomy, and privacy to become the passive recipient of medical and nursing care. In fact, the patient who does not regress jeopardizes his or her own care. However, the patient who becomes too regressed presents another problem. Regression is a normal reaction to severe burns. The person may become childlike in interactions with staff. Behaviors such as whining, clinging to staff, and attempting to keep the nurse constantly at the bedside are not uncommon. In both cases, the patient must know the limits set on behavior if he or she is to receive essential care. The patient is best served when limits are set in a supportive manner.

Although the behavior of these patients can provoke confrontations or reprimands, they should be avoided. Such responses from staff may only worsen a situation in which the patient is already struggling with issues of dependence and autonomy.

Suppression. Suppression is a conscious, intentional process in which patients push ideas, problems, or desires out of their conscious thoughts.[64] Patients often use suppression when their problems are overwhelming and they are in no position to resolve them. For example, before becoming ill, an individual might have been struggling to meet financial obligations, but she or he now uses suppression to postpone dealing with this concern until further along in the recovery phase.

Denial. According to NANDA, denial includes conscious and unconscious attempts to disavow knowledge or the meaning of an event.[1] This text uses the psychoanalytic definition of denial—"an unconscious defense mechanism that reduces anxiety by eliminating or reducing the seriousness of the perceived threat"—to allow for the distinction between denial and suppression. When used by a critically ill patient, denial reduces the anxiety and the perceived threat level of the illness.[65] The degree to which denial is used varies among patients and may vary in the same patient at different times.

Patients also may deny various aspects of their illness. Some deny the probable medical significance of symptoms, as in the case of the 55-year-old cardiologist who interprets severe substernal chest pain as indigestion or the quadriplegic who cheerfully insists that he will be back on his feet in no time. Other patients cannot recognize signs of illness that are obvious to others, as in the case of the patient who cannot "see" the gangrenous foot requiring amputation.[65]

Other people cannot readily influence the beliefs of a patient using denial. For example, the patient who is denying a myocardial infarction will not be convinced of its occurrence by being shown the cardiogram interpretation or laboratory reports. This patient is best served by a nurse who recognizes his need to deny at the present time but who watches for cues from the patient that indicate readiness to accept the reality of the medical diagnosis. A patient with a tracheostomy may refuse to look at her body, avoid mirrors, and fear rejection by others because of her appearance. Forcing her to look at herself before she is ready can be extremely detrimental.

Trust. Trust manifests itself in the critical care patient as a belief that the staff will get him or her through the illness, managing any untoward event that might occur. Trust is an unconscious process in which the patient transfers the trust learned in early significant relationships onto caregivers in the present.[2,47] For example, a patient with severe burns must learn to trust her caregivers. Intense fear of pain or of falling when being moved from a stretcher to a Hubbard tank can affect other coping skills as well.

Hope. Although hope has long been recognized as a significant factor in patient recovery and survival, the phenomenon receives little attention until the patient comes to feel hopeless. Hope is the expectation that a desire will be fulfilled. It can exist even in the face of a realistic appraisal of a grim situation.[52] Hope supports the patient and helps the patient endure the physical and psychological insults that are a part of the daily experience. Hope is central to resilience and spiritual strength.[30]

Hardiness and Resilience. Hardiness and resilience are multidimensional concepts that depict an individual's capacity for mastering stressful situations and viewing adverse circumstances as challenges; they are attributed to persons who have an internal locus of control. Individuals who are resilient view themselves as "overcomers" rather than just "survivors"; they feel stronger for persevering. A "self-healing personality" is often ascribed to a person of resilience. Resilience has been associated with strength of the human spirit and the will to survive.[20,33,66-68]

Spiritual Beliefs and Practices. Spiritual beliefs and practices may provide the patient with some measure of acceptance of an illness, a sense of mastery and control, a source of hope and trust beyond the limits of what the staff can provide, and strength to endure the current stress. A patient may discuss personal beliefs and concerns openly or may view the subject as a private and personal matter.[6,69-74]

Use of Family Support. The patient can use the presence of a supportive family to cope with critical illness. The patient with a supportive family knows that family members share a past and hope for a future with the patient. They love the patient as a person and as a member of the family. The patient also realizes that family members know him or her in ways the staff cannot. With family, the patient may know that his or her experience is truly understood, even when little is said. Family members also can be involved in the patient's personal care and can attend to practical problems the patient cannot take care of, such as managing finances.[75] Family members can help the nurse to understand and know the patient, especially patients who are unable to communicate.

NIC

Family Support

Definition
Promotion of family values, interests, and goals

Activities
Assure family that best care possible is being given to patient.
Appraise family's emotional reaction to patient's condition.
Determine the psychological burden of prognosis for family.
Foster realistic hope.
Listen to family concerns, feelings, and questions.
Facilitate communication of concerns or feelings between patient and family or between family members.
Promote trusting relationship with family.
Accept the family's values in a nonjudgmental manner.
Answer all questions of family members or assist them to get answers.
Orient family to the health care setting, such as hospital unit or clinic.
Provide assistance in meeting basic needs for family, such as shelter, food, and clothing.
Identify nature of spiritual support for family.
Identify congruence between patient, family, and health professional expectations.
Reduce discrepancies in patient, family, and health professional expectations through use of communication skills.
Assist family members in identifying and resolving a conflict in values.
Respect and support adaptive coping mechanisms used by family.
Provide feedback for family regarding their coping.

Counsel family members on additional effective coping skills for their own use.
Provide spiritual resources for family, as appropriate.
Provide the family with information about the patient's progress frequently, according to the patient preference.
Teach the medical and nursing plans of care to family.
Provide necessary knowledge of options to family that will assist them to make decisions about patient care.
Include family members with patient in decision making about care, when appropriate.
Encourage family decision making in planning long-term patient care affecting family structure and finances.
Acknowledge understanding of family decision about postdischarge care.
Assist family to acquire necessary knowledge, skills, and equipment to sustain their decision about patient care.
Advocate for family, as appropriate.
Foster family assertiveness in information seeking, as appropriate.
Provide opportunities for visitation by extended family members, as appropriate.
Introduce family to other families undergoing similar experiences, as appropriate.
Give care to patient in lieu of family to relieve them and/or when family is unable to give care.
Arrange for ongoing respite care, when indicated and desired.
Provide opportunities for peer group support.
Refer for family therapy, as appropriate.
Tell family members how to reach the nurse.
Assist family members through the death and grief processes, as appropriate.

From Bulechek GM et al, editors: *Nursing interventions classification (NIC)*, ed 5, St. Louis, 2008, Mosby, pp. 356-357.

Sharing Concerns. Sharing concerns with a caring and understanding listener can relieve some of the patient's spiritual and emotional distress. The patient is consoled knowing that he or she is not alone and that someone knows and cares about what is being experienced (as mentioned earlier in the discussion of suicidal ideation).[4,34,60] Although the patient may share concerns with family members, she or he may be reluctant to upset loved ones further or may have a family among whom such communication is not the norm. A patient who relies on this coping mechanism will benefit from a nurse who recognizes when the patient needs to talk and who knows how to listen.

COPING ASSESSMENT

Ineffective coping may be suggested by patient behaviors. Overt hostility, severe regression, or noncompliance with treatment may suggest ineffective coping. The patient may also report such problems as severe anxiety, despondence, or despair. The nurse who suspects that coping is ineffective should consider a number of factors before questioning the patient directly.[34]

It is not always clear whether the patient's coping is truly ineffective or whether intervention by the nurse is indicated. Witnessing problematic behavior can be very uncomfortable, especially when that behavior is directed at the caregiver. Careful evaluation of one's reaction to the behavior is needed to discover whether patient care can continue to be provided objectively by the nurse alone or whether consultation with others on the team is needed to alleviate the problem.[4,44]

ENHANCING THE COPING PROCESS
SUPPORTING THE PATIENT

Attention to the total patient is an ultimate goal of nursing care. Nightingale believed that it was "unthinkable to consider sick humans as mere bodies who could be treated in isolation from their minds and spirits."[72] Essential techniques for effective interventions include an attitude of caring; openness and warmth; and withholding judgment until you "know" the patient (have an understanding of the individual's self-perception), the current illness or problem, and the type of social support available. Assessment skills are essential, as is a willingness to become involved when the potential or actual use of ineffective coping mechanisms exists.

Teaching the patient new coping skills may be impossible, because individuals have a repertoire of conscious and unconscious defense and coping mechanisms that automatically come into play when they are facing a stressful situation. A person who is experiencing extreme psychological stress cannot learn new methods to manage these defense mechanisms. However, the nurse may help to reduce the level of anxiety by employing active listening, by encouraging support from family members and other caregivers, and by introducing changes in the environment as appropriate. In doing so, the nurse can facilitate the changes the patient must make. It is extremely important that the patient express an interest in learning and recognize a personal need for help.[2,74]

A patient's trust in the nurse's competence in the physical and technical aspects of care aids in the patient's participation. Hope is instilled when the nurse and other caregivers display a sense of realistic optimism regarding the patient's progress. It is essential that patients receive honest feedback, for patients are keen observers of their caregivers and read them well. Trust and hope are easily lessened when inappropriate information is given.

SUPPORTING FAMILY MEMBERS

Patient-centered care is also family-centered care. Consideration of nonbiologic or nonlegal partners of the patient as members of the patient's support system is also necessary in providing holistic care. The nurse's support of family members at the bedside can enhance the value of the visits for the patient. Patients often look to the family for love, understanding, and support and for care of matters to which they cannot attend themselves. Although the nurse cannot perform full family assessment or give ongoing support to all family members, the critical care nurse can observe the quality of the patient-family interaction and formulate interventions that will aid the family in supporting the patient.[4,37,43]

An illness of a family member can be a hardship on the total family. The illness (or death) of a patient can affect the health of other family members—particularly an elderly spouse.[51,75] Reactions to the stress are similar to the emotions experienced by the patient. The extended waiting time between visits with the patient, lack of information or misinterpretation of information, disruption in family roles and routines, being in an unfamiliar and challenging environment, and worry over outcomes, finances, and additional responsibilities can be overwhelming. Disorganization and emotional turmoil may result. Sleep deprivation is a frequent experience leading to confusion and inability to make decisions.

Family members also may react to the crisis with expressions of anger and hostility toward the patient or staff, or they may be immobilized.[6,52] The family member may be at a loss for what to say or do during visits with the patient. The nurse might find some words to put the family member at ease and offer a suggestion for what to say to his or her loved one.

If the family member is so upset that he or she completely loses composure, a brief attempt at supporting this family member away from the bedside may be an adequate intervention. In doing so, the nurse may determine that the family member needs the assistance of a consistent outside source of support

and therefore may consult with another member of the health care team such as a psychiatric nurse consultant, pastor or chaplain, or social worker.

Family members need understanding, respect, and emotional support. A study of patients' perspectives on health care revealed that their definition of patient-centered care included early involvement of families in the patient's care and decision making; support, accommodation, and respect for the family and friends; and accurate, updated information.[38,52]

Families often must deal with the impending death of a loved one when the patient's condition deteriorates despite all efforts. Anticipatory grief is a process that is filled with emotional upheaval and can be as intense as when the loved one actually dies.[51,53,76] At such times, family members are particularly sensitive to the nurse's words and actions and may misinterpret them as signs of indifference. This may be particularly true for the nontraditional family members. It is essential that the health care team convey understanding and acceptance of the patient and his or her family. Some interventions that are meaningful to the family are reassurance that the patient is receiving adequate pain medication, telling the family what to expect as the dying process progresses, and helping them to comfort the patient with their presence. After the death, allow the family members to spend some time alone with the patient; be supportive of them as they work through their grief. Recognizing cultural and religious factors and incorporating them into the plan of care are also beneficial to the family.[9,52]

A study by Powers and colleagues[54] revealed that nurses did discuss care plans with patients and their families; however, they did not inquire whether the plans were acceptable. The majority of the respondents wanted to be more involved. A pilot program in patient- and family-centered care was initiated that included the families in ongoing planning sessions. The program received very positive responses from everyone. Because of the success of this program, hospital-wide planning sessions were implemented. The nurse-patient relationship was strengthened. Patients and families reported that anxieties were decreased and expressed satisfaction with their increased participation in the plan of care.

SUPPORTING SPIRITUAL CARE

Spiritual needs assessment is often inadequate when patients are asked only about their religious affiliation. If no affiliation is mentioned, no further questions are asked of the patient regarding spiritual matters. The right to receive care that respects individual spiritual values was added to The Joint Commission standards in 1998.[69] Spirituality is a basic human phenomenon that helps create meaning in the world and can be experienced before any awareness of religious beliefs.[30,77] Separation from philosophical and religious rituals and ties, together with intense suffering, can induce spiritual distress for patients and their families. Probing questions such as "How can a caring God let this happen?," "Why me?," or "Am I being punished for some wrong that I have done?" are common indicators of spiritual distress. Some individuals may question their very existence and may even display anger toward religious representatives.

Others may accept their illness as fate or just punishment and resist help, give up, and wait to die.[78]

Philosophical belief practices can directly affect caregiving practices such as diet and hygiene and rituals surrounding birth, death, and medical interventions. The nurse should have a basic understanding of the various religious tenets of Eastern and Western philosophies and how they may affect a patient's plan of care.[2,71,72]

Patients easily succumb to feelings of helplessness and powerlessness in the technologic, impersonalized environment of the ICU. Including a pastor or chaplain on the health care team is also an important aspect of holistic care. The chaplain may be the best person to assess spiritual needs and to assist patients and their families to cope with the crisis. Providing access to religious rituals, prayer, and scriptures and readings are meaningful strategies in alleviating stress. The patient, with the help of the agency chaplain, pastor, or counselor, can identify inner resources of strength, meaning, and purpose to help cope with the crisis event. The spiritual leader is also valuable in ethical decisions such as termination of life support. Moreover, the spiritual advisor can be of great assistance to the health care team as their own personal resources are drained as a result of the sustained or cumulative assistance they have provided to others in crisis.[72]

Spiritual health has been found to be associated with hardiness, a composite measure composed of commitment, challenge, a sense of control, and a mark of psychological health.[9,72,77] Spiritual well-being also can refer to one's valuing of goodness, love, and relatedness to others or a general feeling of having a purposeful and fulfilled life.

SUPPORTING COMPLEMENTARY THERAPIES

The field of complementary therapies is evolving. The purpose of these therapies and practices is to help maintain wellness and, when necessary, to facilitate the body's own healing responses to restore balance and harmony. Integrative health care implies blending conventional health care with complementary therapies, accompanied by open communications among practitioners and conscious recognition of the possible synergy. Integrative health care, like nursing, holds a holistic philosophy.

Interest in complementary therapies has increased dramatically in the past decade, and the national demand for these services has reached unprecedented levels. The most recent utilization study, in 2001, studied time trends and found that almost 70% of adults in the United States had used at least one complementary therapy in their lifetime.[79] The number of hospitals providing complementary therapies is also growing. Nursing, in turn, is returning to those holistic roots with an increased awareness and integration of complementary therapies. Today, nursing combines biomedical understanding of disease and treatment with the caring behaviors and treatments that have been part of holistic nursing practice throughout history.[80]

The importance of complementary therapies in modern health care has been recognized at the national level. In 1998, Congress established the National Center for Complementary and Alternative Medicine to facilitate the evaluation of alternative medical treatment modalities and to provide a public information clearinghouse and a research training program. Music therapy, relaxation, guided imagery, art therapy, therapeutic massage, and mindfulness meditation are a few of the complementary therapies currently being evaluated by nurses. Smith and colleagues examined the effects of therapeutic massage on pain, sleep, symptom distress, and anxiety in hospitalized cancer patients.[81] Significant decreases in pain and symptom distress were attributed to therapeutic massage. Bauer-Wu[82] performed a study examining the feasibility of mindfulness meditation in patients undergoing bone marrow transplantation. At the completion of the intervention, patients reported improved psychological functioning, decreased symptom distress, and subjective benefits of improved coping and quality of life.[82] Although more research is needed to support the value of complementary therapies on selected outcomes related to the symptoms of critically ill hospitalized patients, early studies are supporting their potential as therapeutic nursing interventions.

CARE OF SPECIFIC POPULATIONS

CHRONICALLY ILL PERSONS IN THE INTENSIVE CARE UNIT

Chronic illnesses have a direct effect on successful outcome of a critical illness incident. The typical length of stay in the ICU is 2 to 4 days; however, this time may be extended to 1 week or longer for a chronically ill patient who becomes acutely ill.[83] Usually, this type of patient is older; has multiple system problems such as cardiac, respiratory, and renal disturbances; has nutritional deficits; and has diminished reserves resulting from the prolonged stress of coping with the primary problem. These individuals are at high risk for developing episodes of mental confusion or delirium. They often have difficulty adjusting to the ICU environment, the isolation from family, and their reactions to medications. Sensory deficits in hearing and vision also may complicate their course of recovery. If possible, patients should be allowed to wear their hearing aids and glasses.

Care of chronically ill patients can be very costly, and fewer than 50% live to be discharged. Two similar longitudinal studies[84,85] compared the effects of care provided for the critical condition of chronically ill patients in traditional ICUs with that provided in low-technology special care units (SCUs). Outcomes of complications, length of stay, costs, recovery and survival rates, and patient and family satisfaction were examined. Patients were carefully selected for placement in the two groups. The average age of the participants was 64 years, and respiratory and cardiac illnesses were the common chronic problems. The average hospital stay was 32.2 days.

In the study by Douglas and coworkers,[84] SCUs were designed with private rooms to ensure privacy and to promote sleep, and a nursing care management model, including experienced staff, was used. The family-oriented units allowed unlimited visiting hours and arrangements for overnight stays by family members, if desired. Care in the ICUs followed the traditional protocols, limited visits with family, and used a primary care model under the supervision of physicians. Few significant outcome differences were found in the Douglas or the Fisher and Hegge study.[84,85] However, costs were drastically lower in the SCUs, primarily because of the reduction in diagnostic costs and the minimal use of high-technology equipment other than mechanical ventilators.

According to Rudy and associates,[83] chronically ill patients survive one complication only to succumb to another. When complications do occur, the patient and family must make difficult decisions regarding whether to extend further aggressive treatment or to restrict treatment (e.g., making "do not resuscitate" decisions). The frequent and close contact with the health care team and the friendlier environment of the SCU would facilitate making those decisions.

Both studies demonstrated that the efficacy of care in the SCU was equal to the care provided in the ICU. Satisfaction with care was implied. These studies contributed to the early body of knowledge that carefully selected, highly vulnerable patients can be appropriately cared for outside the ICU. These studies also supported the social support theories by including the patients and their families in making treatment choices.

Nurses caring for these patients should be especially aware of the patients' particular needs, watch for early signs of disorders, and act promptly to avoid major complications. Patience, excellent therapeutic communication skills, and a solid foundation in geriatric nursing are valuable attributes.[30]

PATIENTS WHO REQUIRE TRANSPLANTS

Advances in technology have contributed to the belief that any organ can be replaced. People often have unrealistic expectations about what can or cannot be done to help them.[7,86] Statistics reported by the scientific registry of the United Network for Organ Sharing (UNOS)[87] revealed that more than 100,500 persons were on the national waiting list for donor organs in 2008. (This number includes those who are waiting for more than one organ.)

Waiting for a donor organ can be an emotional drain on the recipient. The recipient may experience guilt, knowing that a sacrifice is being requested from a living donor or that someone else must die so that the recipient can live. At the same time, the recipient realizes that his or her own death may come before an organ is available. These patients and their families experience a gamut of emotions. Concerns include worry over the financial burden, stress on the family, anxiety over the possible rejection of the transplanted organ, and the consequences of taking immune-suppressant drugs for the remainder of one's life. The fear of infections is ever present, because becoming ill may delay or deny a recipient's eligibility for the operation.[88]

Persons receiving bone marrow transplants experience a complex process involving repeated hospital stays of various lengths. Coping with prolonged isolation and the side effects of immune-suppressant drugs and body radiation can be very taxing. The fear of rejection is a major concern. The donor, who often is a family member, may experience guilt feelings if the graft fails. The nurse's role is critical in maintaining hope during these periods. Demonstrating patience and empathy with the patient's and the family's array of emotions is very important.[87]

Psychological evaluation is an essential component of the preoperative workup to determine the patient's ability to cope with the necessary lifelong medical regimen and the ability to accept the donated organ as a part of the body. Postsurgical quality-of-life perceptions may be affected by internal and external environmental factors and gender differences regarding self-image, self-esteem, and functioning ability, as well as social support and cultural and religious values.[88] Emotions also can be exacerbated by the presence of steroid medications.[89]

Living donors also are evaluated psychologically. A donor must offer the kidney freely, without coercion, and must fully understand the possible risks and benefits of the procedure. Most kidney transplant patients experience at least one episode of rejection. The threat of rejection can cause much anxiety. Although a second kidney transplant may be possible if a suitable organ can be found, progression of the disease process may preclude the patient's chances of survival during the waiting period. Psychosocial nursing care for these patients is challenging, because they face the wide-ranging emotions of hope or hopelessness, anxiety, despair, grief, helplessness, and depression.[40,86]

Annually, national statistics have reported more than 4000 individuals awaiting heart transplants; however, only half of the needed hearts have been available. During each year, approximately 222 people need heart-lung transplants, and fewer than one third of these double-transplant operations can be performed. Roark[90] indicated that the average waiting period for donor organs in the year 2000 was 1 to 2 years. Stressors are increasing as the number of potential recipients increases, and 24% to 30% of these individuals die before a heart becomes available.[89]

Patients and families have much information to process concerning the uncertain future of a transplant recipient and the prediction of an average survival rate of 1 year. Average costs are $250,000 during the first year and $20,000 for annual follow-up.[87] Many ethical issues surround the people involved in the process of procuring donor organs. A multidisciplinary health care team consisting of nurse, chaplain, psychiatric consultant, social worker, patient, and family is extremely helpful in resolving these issues and in making decisions.[38,89] Regulations initiated in 1998 require the education of a "designated requestor" to approach families of potential organ donors. These changes offer new opportunities for nurses to educate families regarding their options and individuals regarding their own decision to be a donor. It is estimated that the donor supply could be increased by 20% through such education.[90] The patient and family experience a variety of emotional responses postoperatively; these range from the initial euphoria that comes from receiving a second chance at life to anguish felt about the death of the donor. They also must deal with acceptance of another person's heart, dependence on immune-suppressants, and the ever-present fear of organ rejection. The nurse can be a valuable resource for individuals learning to cope with these emotions.

It is predicted that hospitals will become more specialized and organ transplants will become more common. Rejection of human and animal transplants will most likely be conquered. By 2020, most hospitalized patients will be older, will experience multisystem failures, and will have major trauma injuries or complex operations. A major challenge then will be addressing the many moral and ethical issues involved in balancing the rights of individuals and the rights of society. Advanced knowledge, decision making, and expertise in technologic skills will be required; however, caring attitudes and interpersonal and therapeutic communication skills will still be essential components of the nursing role.

Summary

- It is paramount that nurses consider the mind-body links in providing holistic nursing care to patients who are critically ill.
- A person's perceptions of self and relationships with others, of spiritual values, and of self-competency in social roles also play a major role in how he or she responds to stress or illness.
- Anxiety is a normal subjective response to a perceived or actual threat to self-integrity, which can range from a vague, generalized feeling of discomfort to a state of panic and loss of control.

- A cyclic relationship exists between levels of anxiety and perceptions and tolerance of pain.
- Depression and anxiety are common reactions as the person experiences a loss of control and worries over outcomes.
- Disturbances in body image arise when a person fails to perceive or adapt to the changes that are imposed by disease, trauma, or surgery.
- Unrelieved powerlessness may result in hopelessness.
- Patients requiring critical care must cope with a variety of stressors; each patient's response is unique and depends on a variety of environmental factors and individual differences.
- Spiritual beliefs and practices may provide the patient with some measure of acceptance of an illness, a sense of mastery and control, a source of hope and trust beyond what staff can provide, and the strength to endure current stress.
- The patient can use the presence of a supportive family to cope with critical illness.
- Complementary therapies may be used to enhance or support technologies and pharmacologic therapies in critical care.

Case Study: Patient with Psychosocial Needs

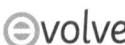 Answers to the Case Study Questions can be found on the Evolve web site at http://evolve.elsevier.com/Urden/.

Brief Patient History

Ms. T is a 17-year-old woman who took an acetaminophen overdose after her boyfriend broke up with her. She states that she did not want to kill herself but just wanted to scare her boyfriend because of what he did. Ms. T is having difficult facing the need for a psychiatric evaluation and the fact that she may need a liver transplant. An emergency physician's psychiatric commitment is in place with a sitter at the bedside.

Clinical Assessment

Ms. T was admitted to the intensive care unit from the emergency department in stable condition with a 24-hour attendant. She is awake, alert, and oriented to person, time, place, and situation. She is irritable and is demanding that she be left alone. Her parents are at the bedside and are unable to hide their emotions about the potential poor prognosis resulting from Ms. T's overdose.

Diagnostic Procedures

A psychiatric evaluation was completed and suggested Ms. T has a histrionic personality disorder and denial regarding the consequences of her actions.

Medical Diagnosis

Ms. T is diagnosed with acetaminophen toxicity and risk for fulminant hepatic failure.

Questions

1. What major outcomes do you expect to achieve for this patient?
2. What problems or risks must be managed to achieve these outcomes?
3. What interventions must be initiated to monitor, prevent, manage, or eliminate the problems and risks identified?
4. What interventions should be initiated to promote optimal functioning, safety, and well-being of the patient?
5. What possible learning needs do you anticipate for this patient?
6. What cultural and age-related factors may have a bearing on the patient's plan of care?

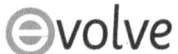 Be sure to check out the bonus material, including free self-assessment exercises, on the Evolve web site at http://evolve.elsevier.com/Urden/.

References

1. North American Nursing Diagnosis Association (NANDA): *Nursing diagnosis: definitions & classification 2007-2008*, Philadelphia, 2007, NANDA.
2. Stuart G: A stress adaptation model of psychiatric nursing care. In Stuart GW, editor: *Principles and practices of psychiatric nursing*, ed 6, St. Louis, 2004, Mosby.
3. Radwin LE, Alster K: Individualized nursing care: an empirically generated definition, *Int Nurs Rev* 49(1):54-63, 2002.
4. Snyder M et al: Use of presence in the critical care unit, *AACN Clin Issues* 11(1):27-33, 2000.
5. Benner P et al: *Expertise in nursing practice*, New York, 1998, Springer.
6. Phillips S, Benner P, editors: *The crisis of care: affirming and restoring caring practices in helping professions*, Washington, DC, 1994, Georgetown University.

7. Gordon S et al, editors: *Caregiving: readings in knowledge, practice, ethics, and politics*, Philadelphia, 1996, University of Pennsylvania.

8. Down J: Therapeutic nursing and technology: clinical supervision and reflective practice in a critical care setting. In Freshwater D, editor: *Therapeutic nursing: improving patient care through self awareness and reflection*, London, 2002, Sage.

9. Spector R: *Cultural diversity in health and illness*, ed 6, Upper Saddle River, NJ, 2003, Prentice-Hall Health.

10. Jenny J, Logan J: Caring and comfort metaphors used by patients in critical care, *Image J Nurs Sch* 28(4):349-352, 1996.

11. Selye H: *Stress in health and disease*, Boston, 1976, Butterworth.

12. Bauer S: Psychological and immunological correlates of surviving breast cancer, dissertation, Chicago, 1997, Rush University.

13. Motzer SA et al: Natural killer cell function and psychological distress in women with and without irritable bowel syndrome, *Biol Res Nurs* 4(1):31-42, 2002.

14. Dropkin MJ: Anxiety, coping strategies, and coping behaviors in patients undergoing head and neck cancer surgery, *Cancer Nurs* 24(2):143-148, 2001.

15. Neurberger P: *Freedom from stress: a holistic approach*, Honesdale, PA, 1981, The Himalayan International Institute of Yoga Science and Philosophy.

16. Lazarus R, Folkman S: *Stress, appraisal, and coping*, New York, 1984, Springer.

17. Lazarus R, Lazarus B: *Passion and reason: making sense of emotions*, New York, 1994, Oxford University.

18. Morse J: Responding to threats to integrity of self, *Adv Nurs Sci* 19(4):21-36, 1999.

19. Morse J, Penrod J: Linking concepts of enduring, uncertainty, suffering, and hope, *Image J Nurs Sch* 31(2):145-150, 1999.

20. Tusaie K, Dyer J: Resilience a historical review of the construct, *Holistic Nurs Pract* 18(1):3-8, 2004.

21. Wagnild G, Young H: Development of psychometric evaluation of the resilience scale, *J Nurs Meas* 1(2):165-178, 1993.

22. Doenges ME, Moorhouse MF: *Nurse's pocket guide: diagnoses, interventions, and rationales*, ed 7, Philadelphia, 2004, FA Davis.

23. Bulechek GM et al, editors: *Nursing interventions classification (NIC)*, ed 5, St. Louis, 2008, Mosby.

24. Marcus PE: Anxiety and related disorders. In Fortinash K, Holoday-Worret P, editors: *Psychiatric mental health nursing*, ed 3, St. Louis, 2004, Mosby.

25. Porth C: *Pathophysiology: concepts of altered health states*, ed 5, Philadelphia, 1998, JB Lippincott.

26. O'Leary A et al: Stress and immune function. In Miller T, editor: *Clinical disorders and stressful life events*, Madison, Conn, 1997, International Universities.

27. Stein K: Schema model of the self-concept, *Image J Nurs Sch* 27(3):187-192, 1995.

28. Coopersmith S: *The antecedents of self-esteem*, San Francisco, 1967, WH Freeman.

29. Fortinash KM: The nursing process. In Fortinash KM, Holoday-Worret PA, editors: *Psychiatric mental health nursing*, ed 3, St. Louis, 2004, Mosby.

30. O'Neill D, Kenny E: Spirituality and chronic illness, *Image J Nurs Sch* 30(3):275-280, 1998.

31. Giarelli E: Spiraling out of control one case of pathologic anxiety as a response to a genetic risk of cancer, *Cancer Nurs* 22(5):327-339, 1999.

32. Keough V, Letizia M: Perioperative care of elderly trauma patients, *AORN J* 63(5):932-937, 1996.

33. Pettie D, Triolo A: Illness as evolution the search for identity and meaning in the recovery process, *Psych Rehab J* 22(3):255-262, 1999.

34. Minarik P: Psychosocial intervention with ineffective coping responses to physical illness: depression-related. In Barry P, editor: *Psychosocial nursing*, ed 3, Philadelphia, 1996, JB Lippincott.

35. Byrne B: *Measuring self-concept across the life span*, Washington, DC, 1996, American Psychiatric Association.

36. Price B: A model for body-image care, *J Adv Nurs* 15:585, 1995.

37. Johnson C et al: Racial and gender differences in quality of life following kidney transplantation, *Image J Nurs Sch* 30(2):125-129, 1998.

38. DePalma J, Townsend R: Ethical issues in organ donation and transplantation are we helping a few at the expense of many, *Crit Care Nurs Q* 19(1):1-9, 1996.

39. Hunter A, Chandler G: Adolescent resilience, *Image J Nurs Sch* 31(3):243-247, 1999.

40. Juneau B: Psychologic and psychosocial aspects of renal transplantation, *Crit Care Nurs Q* 7(4):62-66, 1995.

41. McFarland G, McFarland E: *Nursing diagnosis and interventions*, ed 3, St. Louis, 1997, Mosby.

42. Maslow H: *Motivation and personality*, New York, 1954, Harper & Row.

43. Carroll RG: Psychosocial foundations. In Black JM, Hawks JH, editors: *Medical-surgical nursing*, ed 8, St. Louis, 2009, Saunders.

44. Nield-Anderson L et al: Responding to difficult patients, *Am J Nurs* 99(12):27-33, 1999.

45. Hollinger-Smith L: Growth and development across the life span. In Fortinash K, Holoday-Worret P, editors: *Psychiatric mental health nursing*, ed 3, St. Louis, 2004, Mosby.

46. Rotter JB: Generalized expectancies for internal versus external control of reinforcement, *Psychol Monogr* 80(1):1-28, 1966.

47. Beyea S: Collaboration in health practice. In Blais K et al: *Professional nursing practice: concepts and perspectives*, ed 4, Menlo Park, CA, 2001, Addison Wesley.

48. Boling A: *Defect in hope*, Presented at the Joint Southern California STTI Chapters Research Conference, October 10-12, 1996.

49. Herth K: Abbreviated instrument to measure hope development and psychometric evaluation, *J Adv Nurs Res* 17:1251-1259, 1992.

50. Morse J, Doberneck B: Delineating the concept of hope, *West J Nurs Res* 27(4):277-278, 1995.

51. Wheeler RW: Helping families cope with death and dying, *Nursing* 98(7):25-30, 1996.

52. Czerwiec M: When a loved one is dying families talk about nursing care, *Am J Nurs* 96(5):32-36, 1996.

53. Durhan E: How patients die, *Am J Nurs* 97(12):41-46, 1997.

54. Powers P et al: The value of patient and family-centered care, *Am J Nurs* 100(5):84-88, 2000.

55. Nussbaum GB: Spirituality in critical care patient comfort and satisfaction, *Crit Care Nurs Q* 26(3):214-220, 2003.

56. Barry P: *Psychosocial nursing: assessment and intervention in care of the physically ill*, ed 3, Philadelphia, 1996, JB Lippincott.

57. Folstein MF et al: "Mini-mental state" a practical method for grading the cognitive state of patients for the clinician, *J Psychiatr Res* 12(3):189-198, 1975.

58. Pfeiffer E: A short portable mental status questionnaire for the assessment of organic brain deficit in elderly patients, *J Am Geriatr Soc* 23(10):433-441, 1975.

59. Hagerty B, Patusky KL: Mood disorders: depression and mania. In Fortinash K, Holoday-Worret P, editors: *Psychiatric mental health nursing*, ed 3, St. Louis, 2004, Mosby.

60. Marcus P: Suicide. In Fortinash K, Holoday-Worret P, editors: *Psychiatric mental health nursing*, ed 3, St. Louis, 2004, Mosby.

61. Badger J: Reaching out to the suicidal patient, *Am J Nurs* 95(3):24-31, 1995.

62. Rabie D et al: Suicide prevention control, *Am J Nurs* 99(12):53-57, 1999.

63. Aquilera DC: *Crisis intervention: theory and methodology*, ed 7, St. Louis, Mosby, 1998.

64. Holoday-Worret P: Foundations of psychiatric mental health nursing. In Fortinash K, Holoday-Worret P, editors: *Psychiatric mental health nursing*, ed 3, St. Louis, 2004, Mosby.

65. Beyers M: The new reality, *J Nurs Adm* 20(6):5-6, 1996.

66. Coward D: Facilitation of self-transcendence in a breast cancer support group: II, *Oncol Nurs Forum* 30(2):291-300, 2003.

67. Mynatt S: Increasing resiliency to substance abuse in recovering women with comorbid depression, *J Psychosoc Nurs Ment Health Serv* 36(1):28-36, 1998.

68. Tolsma AN: Evaluation of theoretical model of resilience and salient predictors of resiliency in a sample of community based elderly, dissertation, Ann Arbor, 1995, University of Michigan.

69. Sumner C: Recognizing and responding to spiritual distress, *Am J Nurs* 98(1):26-30, 1998.

70. Armentrout D: Heart cry a biblical model of depression, *J Psychol Christianity* 14(2):101-111, 1995.

71. Dossey B, Dossey L: Holistic modalities and healing moments, *Am J Nurs* 98(6):44-47, 1998.

72. Gillman J: Religious perspectives on organ donation, *Crit Care Nurs Q* 22(3):19-29, 1999.

73. Holt-Ashley M: Nurses pray use of prayer and spirituality as complementary therapy in the intensive care setting, *AACN Clin Issues* 11(1):60-67, 2000.

74. Lougren G et al: A care policy and its implementation, *Int J Nurs Practice* 7(2):92-103, 2001.

75. Johnson S et al: Perceived changes in adult family members' roles and responsibilities during critical illness, *Image J Nurs Res* 27(3):238-243, 1995.

76. Buchanan H et al: Trauma bereavement program review of development and implementation, *Clin Care Nurs Q* 19(1):35-44, 1996.

77. Frankl V: *Man's search for meaning*, New York, 1959, Washington Square Press.

78. Shelly J: *Spiritual care: a guide for caregivers*, Downers Grove, IL, 2000, Intervarsity Press.

79. Kessler R et al: Long-term trends in the use of complementary and alternative medical therapies in the United States, *Ann Intern Med* 135(4):262-268, 2001.

80. Libster M: *Demonstrating care: the art of integrative nursing*, Independence, KY, 2001, Thompson Delmar Learning.

81. Smith M et al: Outcomes of therapeutic massage for hospitalized cancer patients, *J Nurs Scholarship* 34(3):257-262, 2002.

82. Bauer-Wu S: *Facing the challenges of stem cell/bone marrow transplantation with mindfulness mediation*, Cambridge, MA, 2004, Dana Farber/Harvard Cancer Center, unpublished manuscript.

83. Rudy E et al: Patient outcomes for the chronically critically ill special care unit versus intensive care unit, *Nurs Res* 44(6):324-331, 1996.

84. Douglas S et al: Survival experience of chronically critically ill patients, *Nurs Res* 45(2):73-77, 1996.

85. Fischer C, Hegge M: The elderly woman at risk, *Am J Nurs* 100(6):54-59, 2000.

86. Decker W: Psychosocial considerations for bone marrow transplant recipients, *Crit Care Nurs Q* 17(4):67-73, 1995.

87. United Network for Organ Sharing: National patient waiting list. Available at www.unos.org (accessed December 2008).

88. Bartucci MR: Kidney transplantation state of the art, *AACN Clin Issues* 10(2):153-163, 1999.

89. AACN Cardiopulmonary Nursing Update. Part III. Wyeth-Ayerst Nursing Fellows program Supplement to *AJN* 99(5): 1999. Also available at www.nursingcenter.com/ce/test/article.

90. Roark D: Overhauling the organ donation system, *Am J Nurs* 100(6): 45-48, 2000.

Sleep Alterations and Management

Sleep is the only medication that gives ease.—**Sophocles**

$\mathcal{N}$urses who have an appreciation of the importance of sleep place a higher priority on protection of patients' sleep.[1] Health care providers interrupt patients' sleep for assessment, treatments, or interventions, and environmental noise, pain, or anxiety can also disturb it.[2] Although prioritizing care is essential, the consequence of sleep interruptions is not merely sleep-deprived patients; alterations in sleep patterns can delay physical and mental healing.[1] To facilitate sleep and healing, critical care nurses need to understand the essentials of sleep and chronobiology, the effect of pharmacologic therapy on sleep, and the consequences of disrupted sleep. The purpose of this chapter is to acquaint nurses with the characteristics of normal human sleep and chronobiology, changes in sleep associated with aging and pharmacologic treatment, and abnormal sleep patterns that may affect critically ill patients. Evidence-based nursing care for critically ill patients with sleep disturbances is discussed.

NORMAL HUMAN SLEEP

SLEEP PHYSIOLOGY

Humans spend about one third of their lives engaged in a process known as *sleep*. Although little is now known about the physiologic process or the depths to which it affects us, researchers are learning more about sleep every day. The behavioral definition of sleep is a reversible behavioral state of perceptual disengagement from and unresponsiveness to the environment.[3] Sleep is a basic human need, just as food and water are. For patients to regain and maintain their optimal physical and emotional health, they must be able to get adequate amounts of quality sleep. To help patients obtain their optimal amount of sleep, a nurse must first understand what constitutes normal sleep and how the nursing plan of care can contribute to accomplishing this goal.

Polysomnography (PSG) is the collection of multiple channels of physiologic data to assess sleep and its disorders using various electrodes.[4] Electroencephalographic (EEG) electrodes are attached to the patient's scalp to measure brain waves. Changes in the EEG frequency (number of waveforms) and amplitude (height of waveform) over the course of the study allow the sleep

to be scored into stages. Sleep stages are distinguished primarily by the EEG waveforms they produce. Sleep is scored by each 30-second epoch or segment of the tracing. The criteria for scoring sleep in infants differ from those used for adults.

Electrooculography (EOG) measures eye movement activity. The study can help to determine when the patient is in rapid eye movement (REM) sleep; it also can establish when sleep onset occurs as reflected by slow, rolling eye movements. Electromyography (EMG) involves leads placed over various muscle groups. When placed over the chin, the leads can help detect muscle atonia associated with REM sleep. Intercostal leads detect respiratory effort, whereas leads over the anterior tibialis detect leg movements that may be causing the patient to arouse. The electrocardiogram (ECG) shows any cardiac abnormalities, oximetry monitors the oxygen saturation levels, and piezoelastic bands around the chest and abdomen detect respiratory disorders such as apnea. Thermocouples are used to monitor airflow through the nose and mouth.

SLEEP STAGES

Non–Rapid Eye Movement Sleep. Humans experience three states of being. They are awake (Fig. 7-1), in REM sleep, or in non–rapid eye movement (NREM) sleep. NREM sleep can be further divided into stages 1 through 4, with each stage being a progressively deeper sleep state. Adults usually enter sleep through NREM stage 1 sleep (Fig. 7-2), which is a transitional, lighter sleep state from which the patient can be easily aroused by light touch or by softly calling his or her name. Stage 1 comprises 2% to 5% of a night's sleep and is demonstrated by an EEG pattern of low-voltage, mixed-frequency waveforms with vertex sharp waves. The EOG during stage 1 may demonstrate slow, side-to-side eye movements. A patient with severely disrupted sleep may experience an increase in the amount of stage 1 sleep throughout the sleep cycle. As a patient makes the transition from awake to asleep, a brief memory impairment may occur.[5] As a result, the patient may not remember educational or care instructions given by the nurse during the transition between sleep and wake states. Patients sometimes may

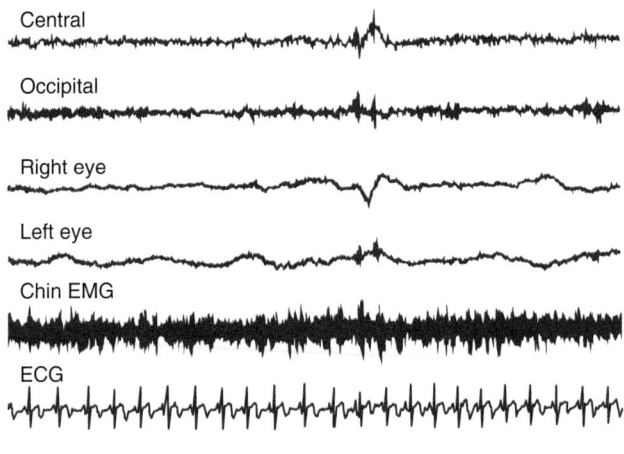

Figure 7-1 Awake.

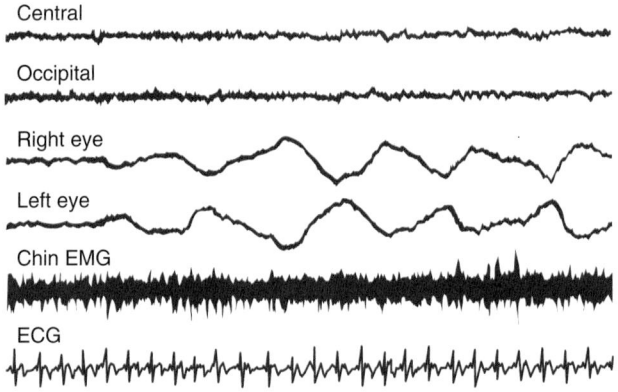

Figure 7-2 Non–rapid eye movement (NREM) stage 1 sleep.

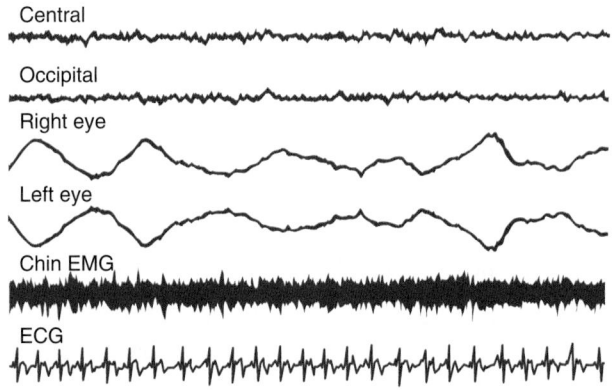

Figure 7-3 Non–rapid eye movement (NREM) stage 2 sleep.

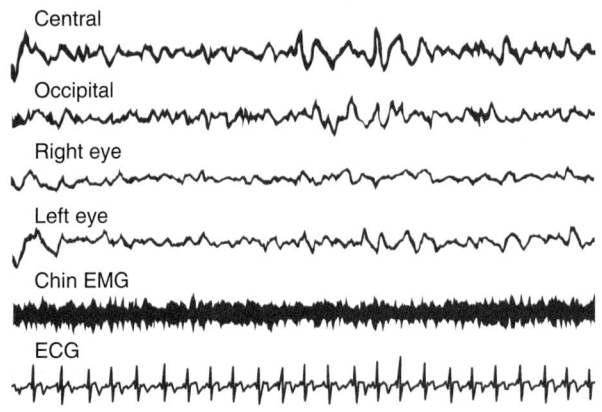

Figure 7-4 Delta sleep: non–rapid eye movement (NREM) stage 3.

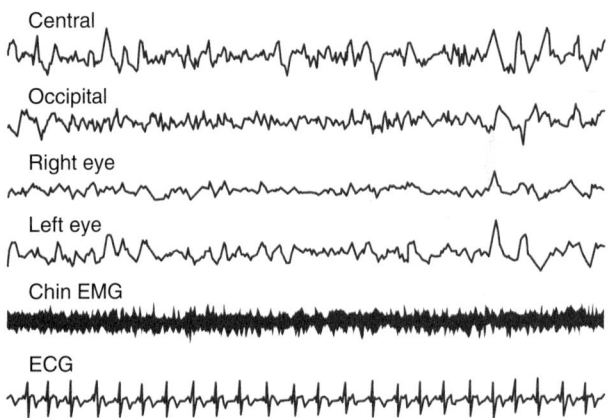

Figure 7-5 Delta sleep: non–rapid eye movement (NREM) stage 4.

experience muscle jerks and recall vivid images on awakening. This is called *hypnic myoclonia;* although not pathologic, it can cause the patient to awaken feeling frightened.

Stage 2 NREM sleep (Fig. 7-3) occupies about 45% to 55% of the night, with sleep deepening and a higher arousal threshold being required to awaken the patient. Changes seen in the EEG pattern include sleep spindles and K complexes. As stage 2 continues, high-voltage, slow-wave activity begins to appear. When these slow waves represent 20% of the EEG activity

per page, the criteria are met for stage 3 sleep, which constitutes 3% to 8% of the cycle. In stage 3 NREM (Fig. 7-4) sleep, slow waves continue to develop until 50% of the EEG waveforms are slow wave; this is called stage 4 sleep. Stage 4 (Fig. 7-5) comprises 10% to 15% of the cycle. Stages 3 and 4 often are combined and referred to as *slow-wave sleep,* or *delta sleep.* Delta sleep has the highest arousal threshold. NREM sleep usually occupies 70% to 75% of the sleep cycle, with REM sleep comprising 20% to 25%.

NREM sleep is dominated by the parasympathetic nervous system. The body tries to maintain a homeostatic regulation, and this causes a decreased level of energy expenditure. Blood pressure, heart and respiratory rates, and the metabolic rate return to basal levels. EMG levels are lower in NREM as opposed to wake states but not as low as in REM sleep. Sweating or shivering that a patient may experience with temperature extremes occurs during NREM sleep but ceases during REM sleep.[3]

During slow-wave sleep, 80% of the total daily growth-stimulating hormone is released, which works to stimulate protein synthesis while sparing catabolic breakdown. The release of other hormones, such as prolactin and testosterone, suggests that anabolism is occurring during slow-wave sleep. Cortisol release peaks during early morning hours, whereas melatonin is released only during darkness, and thyroid-stimulating hormone is

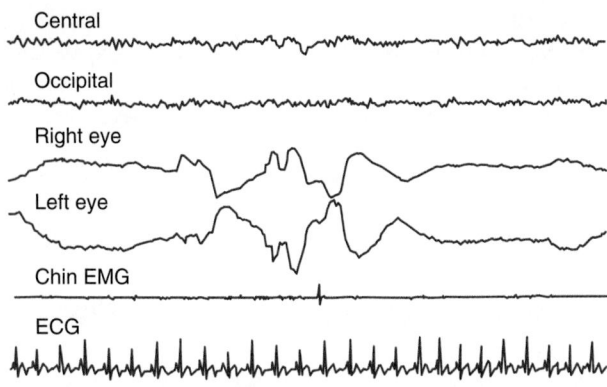

Figure 7-6 Rapid eye movement (REM) sleep.

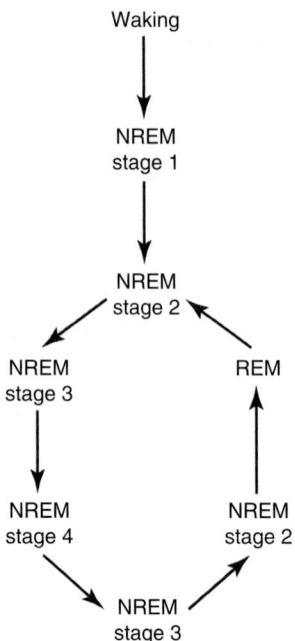

Figure 7-7 The cyclic nature of sleep.

inhibited during sleep. The activities associated with stage 4 NREM sleep (see Fig. 7-5) include protein synthesis and tissue repair, such as the repair of epithelial cells and specialized cells of the brain, skin, bone marrow, and gastric mucosa.[6] Some theorize that NREM sleep is a restorative period that relieves the stresses of waking activities, whereas REM sleep serves to refuel creative brain stores.

Rapid Eye Movement Sleep. REM sleep occupies about 20% to 25% of the night in healthy young adults and is sometimes known as the *dream stage*. However, dreaming is not the exclusive property of any one stage. REM can be viewed as a highly active brain in a paralyzed body and is frequently referred to as a *paradoxic sleep*. The paradox is that some areas of the brain remain very active, whereas others are suppressed. EEG waveforms (Fig. 7-6) are relatively slow voltage, and sawtooth waves are present. Increased cortical activity occurs, with the EEG pattern resembling those of the wake state. Synchronized bursts of rapid, side-to-side eye movements with suppressed EMG activity (muscle atonia) are seen, indicating functional paralysis of the skeletal muscles. Infants enter sleep onset through REM and spend about 50% of their night in REM sleep.

The sympathetic nervous system predominates during REM sleep.[6] Oxygen consumption increases, and blood pressure, cardiac output, and respiratory and heart rates become variable. The body's response to decreased oxygen levels and increased carbon dioxide levels is lowest during REM sleep. Cardiac efferent vagus nerve tone is generally suppressed during REM sleep, and irregular breathing patterns can lead to oxygen reduction, particularly in patients with pulmonary or cardiac disease. An increase in premature ventricular contractions and tachydysrhythmias may be associated with respiratory pauses during REM sleep.[6] Arterial pressure surges and increases in heart rate, coronary arterial tone, and blood viscosity may cause the combination of plaque rupture and hypercoagulability in persons with cardiac disease.[7]

SLEEP CYCLES

NREM and REM sleep cycles alternate (Fig. 7-7) throughout the night. Sleep onset usually occurs in stage 1 sleep, progressing

through stages 2 to 4 and then going back to stage 2, at which time the person usually enters REM. This first cycle typically takes about 70 to 100 minutes, with later cycles lasting 90 to 120 minutes. Four to five cycles are completed during normal adult sleep. NREM sleep predominates during the first third of the night, whereas REM is more prominent during the last third. Brief episodes of wakefulness (usually less than 5%) tend to intrude later into the night and are usually not remembered the next morning.

The amount of sleep required is uncertain. No set number of hours has been established, and sleep length may be determined by many factors, including genetic predisposition. A sufficient amount of sleep has been achieved when one awakens without external stimuli and gets through the day without feeling sleepy.

SLEEP CHANGES IN AGING

Important changes in sleep occur with aging, and critical care nurses must consider these changes when planning care for elderly patients. Assessment for sleep disturbances in the elderly is essential, because lack of sleep can compromise daytime function, thereby lowering quality of life.[8]

Elders most commonly complain about excessive sleepiness or insomnia, and current research offers justification for both of these complaints.[9] Sleep pattern changes in older adults include fewer episodes of stages 3 and 4 NREM and REM sleep.[10] Elders also report that they do not sleep as soundly or feel as rested after awakening.[11] One reason for this may be that elders do not consolidate their sleep into one session. They may go to bed, awake 4 hours later, stay awake for an extended period, and then go back to sleep, resulting in fragmented sleep patterns.[8] Many of the diseases associated with aging may contribute to these

---

Evaluating Excessive Sleepiness in the Older Adult

Recommendations for Assessment

1. Obtain a sleep history, including family input.
2. Use validated scales to evaluate excessive sleepiness, such as Epworth Sleepiness Scale or Pittsburgh Sleep Quality Index.
3. Assess the patient's use of sleep hygiene principles.
4. Assess for signs and symptoms of sleep disorders such as snoring, excessive leg movement during sleep, or difficulty staying awake during the day.

Nursing Care Strategies

1. Ensure the patient understands medical conditions and is compliant with treatment regimen.
2. Individualize the treatment plan, including
   a. Treatment of any identified sleep disorders
   b. Education regarding sleep hygiene
3. Evaluate the appropriateness and consistency in use of continuous positive airway pressure (CPAP) devices or oral appliances.
4. Ensure that patients with unresolved symptoms are seen by a board-certified sleep health care provider.

Modified from Chasens ER, Williams LL, Umlauf MG. (2008). Excessive sleepiness. *National Guidelines Clearinghouse.* Available at: www.guidelines.gov/summary/summary.aspx?ss=15&doc_id=12263&string=sleep+AND+hygiene (accessed April 2009).

---

nocturnal arousals, including diabetes, nocturia, cardiovascular symptoms, chronic pain, and depression.[8,12,13] Sleep-related respiratory disorders and increased incidence of periodic leg movements in elders may further disrupt their sleep.[14] Increasing age brings many physical and social changes with which elders must cope. Assessment of elder patients must always include sleep history as an indicator of mental health, because depression is a common struggle for the elderly.[15]

One common misconception is that elders require less sleep than younger adults do. Because their sleep is not as consolidated as that of younger adults, elders often take daytime naps to satisfy their sleep needs. In a study involving 45 healthy subjects at least 78 years of age and 33 healthy adults aged 20 to 30 years, Buysse and coworkers[11] found that their elder subjects napped an average of 3.4 times in 14 days, as opposed to 1.1 times for young controls ($n = 33$). The elders went to bed earlier, slept less time, and did not sleep through the night as well as the control group. These findings are consistent with those of other investigators reviewed by Bliwise.[12]

Ancoli-Israel[10] believed that elders lose the ability to sustain a sleep state because of alterations in their circadian rhythms. Their internal clocks reset, causing them to become sleepy during the early evening and to awaken during the early morning. Combined with fragmented sleep, this change in the internal clock leads to increased daytime sleepiness and napping. Elders who are constantly battling fatigue are less involved socially and mentally, resulting in decreased quality of life, and they may be at higher risk for mortality.[16]

In critical care areas, nurses need to identify these altered sleep patterns as well as other impediments to adequate rest and methods to minimize acute disruption of sleep while accommodating age-related changes in sleep patterns. Authorities on sleep[17] recommend the use of nonpharmacologic means to promote sleep, such as control of environmental noise and light, use of white noise, music, massage, and allowing specified blocks of time for sleep. It is also important for nurses to educate patients about the changes in sleep that result from aging and to teach sleep hygiene practices such as adhering to regular bedtimes and rising times and avoiding napping.

CHRONOBIOLOGY

Sleep is not merely a response to fatigue. A complex group of interacting systems determines the timing and depth of sleep. The following section reviews circadian and homeostatic processes and theories of sleep regulation.

CIRCADIAN SYSTEM

Many body systems cycle with approximately a 24-hour period, hence the name *circadian rhythm* (from *circa* ["about"] and *dia* ["day"]).[18] Among these systems is the sleep-wake rhythm. A bundle of cells in the anterior hypothalamus, known as the *suprachiasmatic nucleus,* functions as the pacemaker for these rhythms. The circadian system facilitates cycling of the prescribed functions within a predictable period, but the functions are also influenced by other conditions, such as social activity, posture, and physical environment.[18] Rhythms can be seasonal or ultradian (less than a day). One example of an ultradian rhythm is the pattern of sleep during one night's sleep, in which the sleeper cycles between stages.

Under normal conditions, a person's rhythms interact and influence one another. For example, when body temperature is becoming lower, a person is more likely to sleep, and as the body temperature rises in early morning hours, people awaken.[19] Another example is the melatonin cycle, which tends to run in synchrony with the sleep-wake cycle.[20,21]

External influences such as posture, exercise, and light also influence the sleep circadian rhythm.[22] These external influences, known as *zeitgebers,* can shift the rhythm, causing it to peak at different times, or fragment it. Light is the most influential zeitgeber for sleep[23,24]; critical care nurses therefore need to limit the light in the environment during nocturnal hours to facilitate sleep and circadian continuity in their patients.

HOMEOSTATIC MECHANISM

The recent history of the sleep obtained by an individual also influences timing and depth of sleep. Known as the *homeostatic process of sleep regulation,* this determinant of sleep is linked to how much sleep the individual has had previously. Essentially, someone who is sleep-deprived will sleep more readily, regardless of circadian phase, whereas someone who is well rested will not fall asleep readily.[25] The amount of slow-wave sleep (stages 3 and 4 NREM sleep) reflects sleep intensity,[24,25] and individuals recovering from sleep deprivation have increased amounts of slow-wave sleep.

CIRCADIAN AND HOMEOSTATIC INTERACTION

Circadian and homeostatic processes function together to ensure optimal sleep for an individual. However, researchers can study each process separately using desynchrony protocols. These protocols isolate the circadian process from the homeostatic process by imposing a set sleep-wake routine that is not 24 hours in length. This allows the emergence of the subject's intrinsic circadian rhythm, which is usually slightly longer than 24 hours long.[26] In essence, these studies have shown that homeostatic processes primarily regulate slow-wave activity and that the ratio of REM to NREM sleep is primarily regulated by the interaction of circadian and homeostatic processes.[25]

MODELS OF SLEEP REGULATION

A variety of models for sleep regulation exist, and research to determine the adequacy of these explanations is ongoing. The two-process model suggests that sleep in humans is controlled by an interaction of the circadian process (C) and the homeostatic process (S). The interplay of these two processes sets the timing for sleep and wake.[25,26] As the sleep circadian rhythm wanes, it intersects the homeostatic rhythm, and the sleeper awakens (Fig. 7-8).

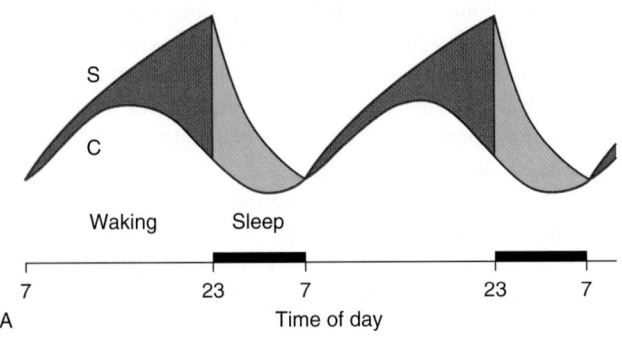

Figure 7-8 Two-process model of sleep regulation shows the time course (A) of the homeostatic process (S) and the circadian process (C). S rises during waking and declines during sleep. The intersection of S and C defines the time of wake-up. *(Modified from Borbely AA: A two-process model of sleep regulation,* Hum Neurobiol *1:195, 1982.)*

A second model is the two-oscillator model.[27] This theory suggests the existence of two separate circadian modulators, *x* and *y*. The *x* is a strong oscillator that controls body temperature, REM sleep, and cortisol levels, whereas the weaker *y* oscillator controls sleep. A variant of this model considers temperature as factor *x* and deems the thermoregulatory mechanism to be the most important factor in sleep regulation.[28] This model does not acknowledge the role of homeostasis in sleep regulation.

SUMMARY OF CHRONOBIOLOGY

In the critical care environment, light is often needed to facilitate assessment or nursing actions. Frequent interruptions to sleep that are associated with bright light and social interaction may cause circadian disruption and result in sleep loss and slowed healing. Interventions that assist in maintaining patient orientation, such as the use of natural light, putting clocks and updated calendars where patients can see them, and facilitating the patient's normal schedule and sleep rituals, are important methods of supporting circadian processes.

PHARMACOLOGY

It is essential that nurses understand the relationship between various medications and the sleep of patients in the critical care unit. Pathophysiology and age may profoundly affect not only medication absorption and elimination but also how patients cope with their illness and their ability to maintain health.

Hypnotic benzodiazepines remain the drugs of choice to treat insomnia. Insomnia is a patient complaint of inability to initiate or maintain sleep, and prescriptions for treatment of insomnia cost more than 1 billion dollars annually.[29] Acute stress, such as admission to a critical care unit, may cause some patients to experience acute sleep-onset insomnia. Hypnotics tend to promote lighter sleep stages and have a higher lipophilicity, which can cause the elderly to experience an increased drug half-life.[30] Care should be used in the administration and dosage of hypnotics in the elderly. This age group may experience night terrors, nightmares, and increased agitation. The metabolism of hypnotics in elderly patients can be inhibited by the use of steroids, or it can be accelerated in those who smoke. Hypnotics may also produce anterograde amnesia, which is a memory failure of information processed after the drug is consumed. Patients with normal ventilation should not be affected by the mild respiratory depression caused by hypnotics, although patients with chronic obstructive pulmonary disease (COPD) or sleep-disordered breathing may be affected.

Wake-promoting medications produce increased arousal, behavioral activation, and alertness. They can be divided into three classes: direct-acting sympathomimetics (e.g. phenylephrine), indirect-acting sympathomimetics (e.g., methylphenidate, amphetamine, mazindol), and stimulants that are not sympathomimetics (e.g., caffeine). Common side effects can include irritability and sweating, with talkativeness, anorexia, gastrointestinal complaints, dyskinesias, insomnia, and palpitations occurring less frequently.[31] Wake-promoting medications can be used for patients who experience disabling symptoms of sleepiness resulting from narcolepsy, idiopathic central nervous system hypersomnia, or sleep deprivation. Wake-promoting medications should be used only when sustained alertness is required for the individual or for reasons of public safety.

Wake-promoting medications possess a high abuse potential. A sequence of euphoria, dysphoria, paranoia, and psychosis can occur after a single exposure, and sustained use can lead to cognitive and behavioral disorders. Proper dosing and a structured management plan are recommended for wake-promoting medication use. This includes providing patient education with treatment goals, beginning with low doses, emphasizing good sleep hygiene such as naps, and adjusting the dosage according to clinical information.[32] Wake-promoting medications should be included as part of a treatment plan only to decrease excessive somnolence. Sustained use of high-dose wake-promoting medications can lead to cognitive and behavioral disorders.[32] Effective sleep hygiene and attention to other substances or medications that can affect sleep may be beneficial for patients who want to avoid the abuse potential.

Many people use alcohol to assist them in falling asleep. Alcohol is a central nervous system sedative and will cause suppression of REM sleep. More than two alcoholic drinks may cause an increase in NREM stages 1 and 2 and decrease the onset of slow-wave sleep. Alcohol also may cause shallow, fragmented sleep and may precipitate or aggravate an existing obstructive sleep apnea (OSA) condition. In the 2008 National Sleep Foundation survey, 8% reported self-medicating for insomnia with alcohol.[33] Of those polled, 20% reported using alcohol, over-the-counter medications (7%), prescription sleep medications (3%), or alternative therapy or herbal supplements (2%).

Some persons who suffer from sleep problems have turned to alternative therapies or herbs for treatment. Because these are not considered prescription drugs, patients do not always inform their caregivers that they are using them. Some herbs are considered effective hypnotics, whereas others may be used as stimulants. It is the responsibility of the nurse to inquire about all medications used, whether prescription or over-the-counter.

Patients with illness may respond differently to medications than do healthy patients. Patients may come to the critical care unit with impaired sleep or poor cognitive function. Beta-blockers, a commonly used class of drugs in critical care, are known to produce nightmares and have disruptive effects on sleep quality in some individuals.[34] The effects of various drug combinations are not well known.

For patients requiring continuous sedation, propofol (Diprivan) is a common choice. It is unclear whether sedation is an adequate replacement for natural sleep; however, investigators have shown that rats injected with higher doses of propofol experienced decreased sleep latency as well as increases in NREM and total sleep time.[35] The adequacy of this sleep in humans remains an area of concern.

The critical care nurse should assess the patient's need for sedative and analgesic medications. The nurse has a responsibility to administer these medications in the most efficient manner to promote sleep and to monitor effectiveness. This can be achieved through assessment, including a drug history, diagnostic test results, and review of the patient's medical history. Information from that assessment assists the nurse in formulating a nursing diagnosis with outcome criteria and interventions. Evaluation of the patient ensures attainment of the desired outcomes. Drugs that disrupt sleep and wakefulness are discussed in Table 7-1.

ABNORMAL SLEEP

SLEEP PATTERN DISTURBANCE IN CRITICALLY ILL PATIENTS

Definition. Sleep disturbance in critically ill patients is defined as insufficient duration or stages of sleep that results in discomfort and interferes with quality of life. When ill, most people need more sleep than usual, and sleep seems to promote recovery. Studies have demonstrated that the nocturnal sleep of patients in critical care units is severely disturbed, even though many receive medications to promote sleep.[36,37] Few studies have examined the effectiveness or the side effects of sedative-hypnotics in vulnerable populations such as elderly and critically ill patients. Studies in younger, healthy populations show that some sedative-hypnotics may produce disturbances in sleep architecture, diminished daytime performance, residual daytime fatigue, dependence, tolerance, and REM suppression and rebound.[30]

Etiology and Pathophysiology. Normal sleep is a period of decreased physiologic workload for the cardiovascular system. Insufficient sleep in acutely and critically ill patients has been associated with physiologic and psychological exhaustion and may delay recovery from illness. These effects include mental status change, also known as *intensive care unit psychosis*.[7]

Patient Education: Sleep Hygiene

- Establish a bedtime routine.
- Use the bed only for sleeping or sex.
- Avoid daytime napping.
- Avoid stimulants such as caffeine or nicotine after noon.
- Avoid consuming more than three drinks containing alcohol.
- Avoid eating a large meal or exercising within 3 to 4 hours of bedtime.
- Do exercise vigorously in the morning or in the late afternoon.
- Ensure that the sleep environment is pleasant, relaxing, and cool.
- Try to wake up and go to sleep at the same time every day.

Modified from Thorpy M: Ask the sleep expert: sleep hygiene. *National Sleep Foundation.* 2003. Available at www.sleepfoundation.org/site/c.huIXKjM0IxF/b.2422637/k.5B7E/Ask_the_Sleep_Expert_Sleep_Hygiene.htm (accessed December 2008); and Avidan AY: Sleep disorders in the older patient. *Prim Care* 32: 563-586, 2005.

TABLE 7-1 Pharmacologic Management: Drugs That Affect Sleep and Wakefulness

MEDICATION CLASS AND DRUG GROUP	EXAMPLES	EFFECTS	COMMENTS
Hypnotics[29]			
Benzodiazepines		↓ SWS, ↑ TST, ↓ WASO, ↓ stage 1 sleep, mild REM suppression	↑ Apnea, ↑ daytime residual sedation, mild respiratory depression, ↓ psychomotor function
Immediate-acting	Quazepam	Half-life of 20-120 hr	
	Temazepam	Half-life of 8-20 hr	
Long-acting	Flurazepam, HCl	Half-life of 40-250 hr	
Rapid-acting	Triazolam	Half-life of 2-6 hr	Rebound insomnia
	Estazolam	Half-life of 8-24 hr	
Nonbenzodiazepines		No effect on REM or SWS	
Rapid-acting	Zolpidem	Half-life of 1 hr	
	Zaleplon	Half-life of 1 hr	No cognitive or performance impairment; ↓ abuse potential; may be taken in middle of night
Intermediate-acting	Eszopiclone	Half-life of 5-7 hr	May cause impairment of activities the next day
Wake-Promoting Medications[32]			
Nicotine		↑ SL, ↓ TST, ↓ REM	
Amphetamines		↓ REM, ↓ SWS, ↓ TST, ↑ WASO	Less daytime fatigue
Nonsympathomimetics	Xanthine derivatives: coffee, chocolate, tea; scopolamine; strychnine; pentylenetetrazol; modafinil	↓ TST, ↓ REM, ↓ SWS, ↑ SL, ↑ WASO	
Direct sympathomimetics	Isoproterenol, epinephrine, norepinephrine, phenylephrine, phenylpropanolamine, apomorphine	↑ Wakefulness, ↑ REM onset, ↓ fatigue, ↓ sleepiness	↑ Blood pressure, ↓ heart rate
Indirect sympathomimetics	Amphetamine, methamphetamine, cocaine, piperacillin (Pipradol), methylphenidate, tyramine	↑ WASO, ↑ daytime SL, ↓ sleepiness	Narcolepsy treatment, ↑ cognitive tasks
	Pemoline		Possible liver damage
Antihypertensives[34]			
β-Antagonists	Propranolol, metoprolol	↑ Wakefulness, TWT, SL, ↓ REM	Insomnia, nightmares
α₂-Agonists	Atenolol, clonidine	↓ REM, ↓ TST in hypertensives, ↑ TST in normal subjects	Nightmares, sedation, ↓ concentration, mental slowing
Methyldopa		↑ REM, ↑ TST	Sedation, insomnia, nightmares
Diuretics	Hydrochlorothiazide, chlorthalidone, indapamide	No data	CNS effects unlikely
Vasodilators	Hydralazine	No data	Depression, insomnia, anxiety
Catecholamine depletors	Reserpine	↑ REM and stage shifts	
Calcium antagonists	Verapamil, nifedipine, diltiazem, amlodipine, felodipine, nisoldipine	No data	Insomnia, nightmares, depression, sedation, difficulty concentrating

TABLE 7-1 Pharmacologic Management: Drugs That Affect Sleep and Wakefulness—*cont'd*

MEDICATION CLASS AND DRUG GROUP	EXAMPLES	EFFECTS	COMMENTS
Antihistamines[34]			
H$_1$ antihistamines (*chem. class:* selective histamine H$_1$-receptor antagonist)	Diphenhydramine, hydroxyzine, triprolidine	↑ Drowsiness, ↓ SL	Impaired daytime performance
H$_1$ antihistamines (*chem. class:* ethanolamine derivative H$_1$-receptor antagonist)	Loratadine, terfenadine	No sedation effects	
H$_2$ antagonists	Cimetidine, ranitidine	May cause insomnia or somnolence	Drowsiness in patients; renal impairment
Antidepressants[34]			
Tricyclic antidepressants	Amitriptyline, doxepin, imipramine (Trimipramine), clomipramine, desipramine, nortriptyline, protriptyline	↑ TST, ↓ wakefulness	↓ Psychomotor and cognitive performance and daytime drowsiness
Selective serotonin reuptake inhibitors	Fluoxetine	↑ TST, ↑ wakefulness, ↑ stage 1, ↑ SEM	Mild ↑ in psychomotor performance
	Paroxetine	↑ Wakefulness, ↓ TST, ↑ stage 1, ↑ SL	
	Sertraline	No data	Insomnia 7-16%
	Fluvoxamine	↓ TST, ↑ wakefulness, ↑ stage 1, ↑ SL	
	Citalopram	No change	Insomnia, no impairment in performance
	Trazodone	Variable, may ↑ TST, ↓ SL	↓ Cognitive performance in elderly
Monoamine oxidase inhibitors	Phenelzine, tranylcypromine, moclobemide, brofaromine	↑ Daytime sleepiness because of ↓ TST, ↑ wakefulness	Some improved psychomotor performance
Other Compounds Used for Insomnia[71]			
Melatonin (hormone)		↓ SL, ↑ TST	Study results are mixed, nonaddictive
Valerian (plant extract)		↓ SL, ↓ WASO	Side effects include headache and rare morning drowsiness

REM, Rapid eye movement; SEM, slow eye movement; SL, sleep latency; SWS, slow-wave sleep; TST, total sleep time; TWT, total wakefulness time; WASO, wakefulness after sleep onset.

In another study, sleep debt was found to produce the following effects: decreased glucose tolerance, decreased thyrotropin concentration, increased evening cortisol production, and increased nervous system activity.[38] A general consensus among sleep experts and researchers is that sleep deprivation results in psychological alterations such as changes in mood and performance, fatigue, increased irritability, and feelings of persecution.

The intensification of pain related to sleep disturbance is a significant problem in acutely and critically ill patients. Sunshine and colleagues[39] related a potential theory for pain alleviation from massage therapy that is linked to quiet or restorative sleep.

During deep sleep, somatostatin is normally released. Without this substance, pain is experienced. Substance P is released when an individual is deprived of deep sleep, and substance P is noted for causing pain. When people are deprived of deep sleep, they may have less somatostatin and increased substance P, which results in greater pain and more sleep disruption.

Sleep disturbance in critically ill patients may stem from psychological stress associated with critical illness and the critical care environment, surgical stress, noise, interruptions for care, painful procedures or physiologic processes, excessive bright light, and muscular and joint discomfort that result from bed rest.

Of 84 patients' recollections about sleep-disturbing factors in the critical care unit, the most frequently mentioned factors included an inability to get comfortable or lie comfortably (recalled by 70% of patients), inability to perform one's usual routine before going to sleep (57%), anxiety (55%), and pain (54%).[40] The stressful nature of the critical care environment and uncertainty and worry regarding the outcomes of a critical illness may explain why some patients have such difficulty sleeping while hospitalized. These concerns are not culturally isolated. A Swedish study identified pain, anxiety, and environmental noise among factors that interfered with sleep.[41] However, perhaps because of staffing issues and general work flow, nurses tend to provide labor-intensive tasks during early morning hours.[2] This trend is clearly counterproductive and should be discouraged.

Another source of sleep disturbance in critically ill patients is surgical stress. A general inflammatory response caused by the heart-lung machine or the incisions, altered endocrine neurometabolism control, and the effects of medications such as benzodiazepines, barbiturates, scopolamine, and systemic opioids may disturb sleep.[42]

Bright nocturnal light, excessive noise, and frequent interruptions for care procedures also may disturb sleep in critically ill patients. In a study of light and sound levels and interruptions to sleep in medical and respiratory critical care units, light levels maintained a day-night rhythm, with peak levels dependent on window orientation. Peak sound levels were extremely high in all areas and exceeded recommendations of the Environmental Protection Agency as acceptable for a hospital. Patient interruptions for care procedures tended to be variable but ubiquitous, leaving little time for condensed sleep.[2,43] However, one group determined that noise and nursing interventions explained fewer than 30% of sleep interruptions.[44] Identifying additional factors that create these sleep disruptions remains an area of potential research.

In a study of the sleep of 38 male patients before and after coronary artery bypass grafting, the investigators found that there was a decrease in sleep at night and an increase in daytime sleep in the immediate postoperative period.[45] Nocturnal sleep was reduced to a mean of 253.6 minutes, and the minutes of stages 3 and 4 NREM sleep also were decreased. However, daytime sleep increased. The total sleep times during the 24-hour period before surgery, the first 24-hour period after surgery, and the second 24-hour period after surgery were 421.1, 483.2, and 433.2 minutes, respectively. This study suggests the need for daytime napping immediately after coronary artery bypass graft surgery.

Not surprisingly, mechanical ventilation and the required care associated with it contribute to sleep disturbances. Cooper and colleagues[46] studied 20 subjects who were receiving mechanical ventilation and classified as critically ill; based on PSG-accepted criteria, none of these patients had normal sleep. Twelve did not experience sleep at all, and the remaining eight demonstrated PSG findings consistent with severely disrupted sleep. The magnitude of sleep disruption found in the latter group was similar to the excessive daytime sleepiness and cognitive impairment of patients with untreated OSA. Ventilatory modes may also influence sleep patterns. Bosma and associates[47]

compared the effects of pressure support and proportional assist ventilation (PAV) on sleep. PAV resulted in greater patient-ventilator synchrony and therefore improved sleep. A comparison of assist control ventilation (AC) and low levels of pressure support also found that use of AC improved sleep quality. The authors suggested that ventilating patients at night may improve weaning outcomes.[48] However, additional evidence suggests that sleep disturbances associated with prolonged mechanical ventilation do not resolve with extubation and discharge.[49,50] These findings emphasize the nursing responsibility to promote and protect the sleep of all patients in the critical care environment.

Assessment and Diagnosis. Assessment of the patient on admission to the critical care unit includes a description of multiple sleep-related factors: the normal sleep pattern, including awakenings, naps, normal bedtime, and waking time; customary habits that enhance sleep (e.g., number of pillows, extra blankets, bedtime rituals, medications); any recent changes in the patient's normal sleep pattern resulting from the acute illness; recent history of difficulty falling asleep or staying asleep, snoring, gasping for breath at night, stopping breathing at night, or excessive daytime sleepiness; frequency and duration of daytime naps; and the severity, duration, and history of chronic illnesses and disturbances that may disrupt sleep, such as COPD, arthritis, nocturnal angina, reflux esophagitis, or nocturia.

The patient's psychological response to admission to the critical care unit needs to be assessed, along with the noise level in the patient's immediate environment. The critical care nurse needs to elicit any history of snoring because of its relationship to sleep apnea and sleep disturbances. One effective way to assess the quality of the patient's sleep is for the nurse to ask the patient how his or her sleep in the hospital compares with sleep at home. Because individuals differ in their sleep behaviors and requirements, a flexible, individualized plan of care must be formulated to promote rest and sleep.

Compiling a record of a patient's sleep for 48 to 72 hours may assist in assessing actual quantity of sleep as well as necessary and unnecessary awakenings. The sleep record includes the date and time, whether the patient was awake or asleep, and any procedures that necessitated waking the patient. A 24-hour flow sheet, commonly used in critical care units, could include an area for documentation of sleep.

Just as nurses document other data relevant to the patient's recovery, sleep periods of more than 90 minutes in duration, number and length of awakenings, and total possible sleep time should be recorded and evaluated.

Medical Management. Medical management of sleep pattern disturbance in critically ill patients consists of sedative-hypnotics. The nonbenzodiazepine, short-acting hypnotics zolpidem and zaleplon have few side effects and little effect on sleep architecture. Because of their short half-life, they may be repeated once during the night. Although hypnotics may assist the patient in falling asleep, it is a nursing responsibility to provide an environment and care procedures that promote sleep and allow patients to stay asleep.

Nursing Management. If one of the primary causes of the sleep pattern disturbance for a patient hospitalized in the critical care unit is a state of heightened anxiety and discomfort, nursing interventions, such as massage, that promote relaxation and comfort may be effective. In a review of 22 articles investigating the effects of massage on relaxation, comfort, and sleep, massage consistently reduced anxiety and pain.[51] Another research-based intervention is playing audio of ocean sounds or other relaxing auditory sounds. Williamson[52] found that an audiotape of the ocean or the rain significantly increased sleep quality in patients in a progressive care unit. Providing a relaxed, caring environment that encourages confidence in care providers may also assist the patient to relax. Allowing close family members to sit quietly at the bedside while the patient rests may comfort the family and the patient and allow the patient to rest better. Stanchina and colleagues found that white noise machines in patient rooms decreased the variance in peak noises and increased arousal thresholds for patients.[53]

Nurses should limit interruptions for care procedures and should coordinate the care among other disciplines to allow patients time for consolidated nocturnal sleep and a daytime nap. Draperies or blinds should be opened during the day to allow patients to receive bright natural light and to help orient them to time of day, with lights dimmed at night. Noise from staff, squeaky carts, alarms, televisions, slamming doors, and ringing phones should be minimized. Offering the patient earplugs may help decrease noise and promote sleep. Outcomes of these nursing interventions can be assessed and documented on the 24-hour flow sheet. One group reported that an enforced afternoon quiet time resulted in benefits for patients as well as the multidisciplinary team.[54]

It is important for nurses to instruct patients who have had coronary artery bypass graft surgery about sleep disturbance, which commonly persists for up to 1 year after the operation. In a study of the sleep patterns of 22 women over a 6-month period using a wrist-worn Actigraph, sleep gradually became less fragmented and more consolidated over time.[42]

Often nurses have influence on the design of critical care units. Critical care units should be designed with private rooms and acoustical features that limit noise.[55]

SLEEP APNEA SYNDROME

Sleep apnea syndrome, sometimes called *sleep-disordered breathing,* occurs when airflow is absent or reduced. Apnea during sleep can be divided into three types: (1) obstructive, (2) central, and (3) mixed. In obstructive apnea, the absence of airflow is caused by an obstruction in the upper airway. Complete obstruction lasting 10 seconds or longer is referred to as an *obstructive apnea,* whereas a partial obstruction is known as a *hypopnea* (Fig. 7-9). In central apnea, airflow is absent because of lack of ventilatory muscle effort. The third type of sleep apnea syndrome, mixed apnea, occurs when a combination of obstructive and central patterns occurs in a single apneic event. An apnea-hypopnea index (the number of apneas and hypopneas per hour divided by the hours of sleep) of 5 or greater is diagnostic of sleep apnea syndrome. With new understandings of alterations in ventilatory effort, researchers have developed the respiratory distress index (RDI). To calculate the index, the total number of apneas and hypopneas plus the number of respiratory effort–related arousals (RERAs) or other respiratory events is divided by the hours of sleep. An RDI greater than 5 in addition to reports of daytime sleepiness supports a diagnosis of sleep apnea.[56]

All types of sleep apnea syndrome are accompanied by arterial desaturation and potentially by hypoxemia, which may cause pulmonary vasoconstriction and an increased systemic vascular resistance. However, desaturation and hypoxemia are most severe in the obstructive type. Although the pathophysiology of OSA is unclear, hypotheses suggest that the various types of sleep apnea are all part of a disease continuum. Failure of the central respiratory rhythm control center to generate a stable rhythm is thought to be the basic defect responsible for sleep apnea syndrome. Cyclic oscillations occur with greater frequency at night and are further exacerbated by mouth breathing.[57]

OBSTRUCTIVE SLEEP APNEA

Definition, Etiology, and Pathophysiology. OSA syndrome occurs when at least five apnea or hypopnea events per hour of sleep occur as the result of an obstruction in the upper airway. In the general population, between 3% and 7% of people have severe OSA.[58] The incidence of OSA is believed to increase with age. Consequences include chronic hypoventilation syndrome, arousals that fragment sleep, cardiovascular changes such as hypertension, stroke, ischemic heart disease, insulin resistance, ventricular hypertrophy, and nocturnal angina.[59] Because of the cardiovascular complications and accidents caused by sleepiness, OSA is a significant condition that should be effectively evaluated.

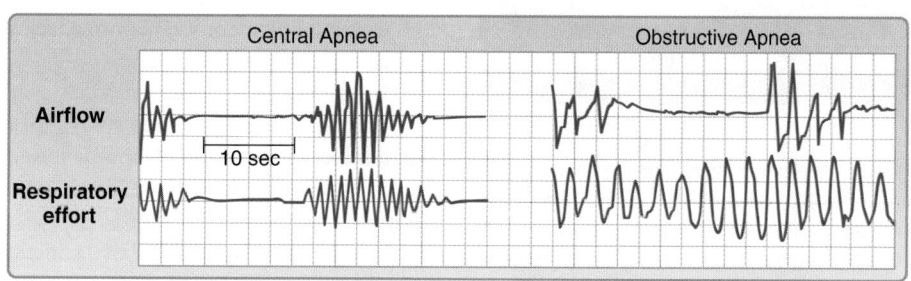

Figure 7-9 Comparison of airflow and respiratory effort in obstructive sleep apnea (OSA) and central sleep apnea (CSA). *(From Kryger MH et al, editors: Principles and practice of sleep medicine, ed 4, Philadelphia, 2005, Saunders, p. 970.)*

The cause of OSA is not entirely understood; however, upper airway structure, hormonal balance, and neural control are implicated. Factors that contribute to OSA are (1) anatomic narrowing of the upper airway, (2) increased compliance of the upper airway tissue, (3) reflexes affecting upper airway caliber, and (4) pharyngeal inspiratory muscle function.[60] Computed tomographic studies of awake subjects have shown that patients with OSA have narrower airways than normal subjects do. The narrower the airway, the more easily it may become obstructed (Fig. 7-10).

Upper airway patency is also affected by upper airway function, which is under the control of the respiratory motor neurons. During sleep, this control varies and causes decreased neural activity, thereby narrowing the airway. This effect is especially prevalent during REM sleep, when the motor neurons are hypotonic. Unstable control of the respiratory nerves of the diaphragmatic, intercostal, and upper airway muscles can cause sleep apneas.[57] Hypothyroidism can alter respiratory controls and thereby contribute to OSA. Other contributing disorders are exogenous obesity, kyphoscoliosis, and autonomic dysfunction.

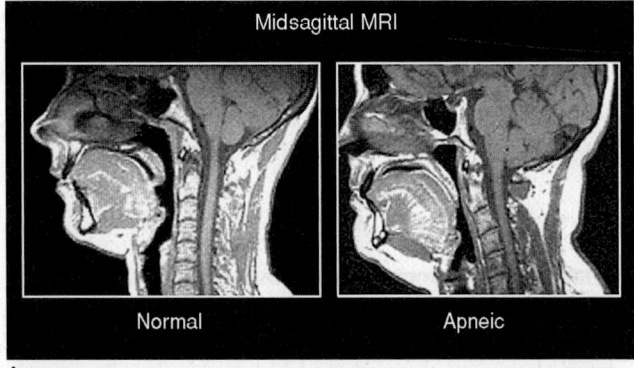

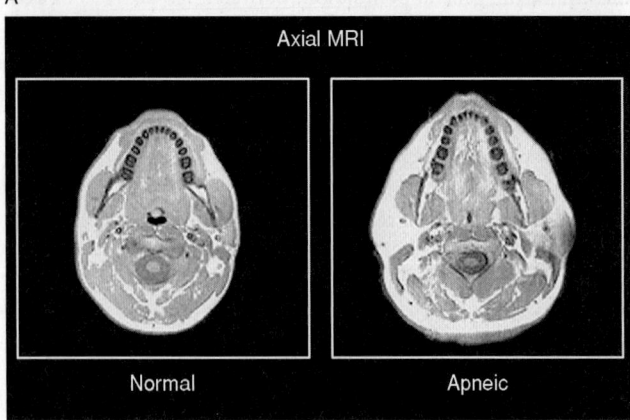

Figure 7-10 *A*, Midsagittal magnetic resonance imaging of a normal subject *(left)* and a subject with sleep apnea *(right)*. Notice the narrowing of the trachea and the elongated soft palate. *B*, Axial image of a normal subject *(left)* and a subject with sleep apnea *(right)*. Notice the diameter of the trachea in the subject with sleep apnea. *(From Kryger MH et al, editors: Principles and practice of sleep medicine, ed 4, p. 990, Philadelphia, 2005, Saunders.)*

The patient with OSA develops cycles of hypoxemia, hypercapnia, and acidosis with each episode of apnea until he or she is aroused and airflow resumes. Alveolar hypoventilation accompanies each episode of apnea and results in hypercapnia. Between episodes, alveolar ventilation improves so that overall there is no retention of carbon dioxide (CO_2).

With obstruction, inspiratory subatmospheric intrathoracic pressures are abnormally elevated. This leads to a tendency for airways to collapse, resulting in hemodynamic and electrocardiographic changes. The extremely elevated pressures that occur in individuals with OSA who have apneic episodes in REM and NREM stages cause systemic and pulmonary hypertension. Systemic pressures of 200/120 mm Hg (awake control: 130/80 mm Hg) and pulmonary artery pressures of 80/54 mm Hg (awake control: 30/20 mm Hg) have been reported.[61] Cardiac dysrhythmias associated with obstructive apnea include bradycardias, sinus arrest, and occasionally, second-degree heart blocks. After resumption of airflow, tachycardias commonly occur. Bradycardia-tachycardia syndrome is associated with OSA.[62]

Assessment and Diagnosis. Careful monitoring of oxygen saturation and breathing patterns can help the critical care nurse identify patients with this syndrome and assist in its diagnosis and treatment. Patients at risk for OSA may have the following symptoms: snoring; obesity; short, thick neck circumference; cardiovascular disease; systemic hypertension; pulmonary hypertension; sleep fragmentation; gastroesophageal reflux; and an impaired quality of life. Apneas may occur in people whose throats are abnormally small or collapsible. Muscles that would normally hold the throat open relax while the patient is asleep. Snoring is caused when those soft tissues in the throat vibrate. Snoring often precedes the complaint of daytime sleepiness, and the intensity increases with weight gain and alcohol ingestion.[60] Men with a collar size of 17 or greater and women with a size 16 or greater are thought to have an increased incidence of apnea. Friedman and others showed a clinical correlation between Modified Mallampati grade (MMP), tonsil size, body mass index, and the severity of apnea. These assessments are used by anesthesiologists to determine intubation difficulty.[60] There is an increased incidence of sleep apnea among African Americans as well as Mexican Americans, and an increased incidence is observed among those with metabolic syndrome.

OSA episodes frequently end in brief EEG arousals. Patients may experience hundreds of arousals and not even realize they awaken hundreds of times during the night. These arousals cause sleep fragmentation and daytime sleepiness, which can lead to irritability, poor job performance, troubled relationships, depression, and impaired quality of life.

The definitive diagnosis of OSA syndrome is made with PSG during an overnight sleep study. PSG is used to determine the number and length of apnea episodes and sleep stages, number of arousals, airflow, respiratory effort, and oxygen desaturation.

Medical Management. For patients with mild OSA (apnea-hypopnea index of 5 to 10), weight loss, sleeping on the side if apneas are associated with sleeping on the back, avoidance of sedative medications and alcohol before bedtime,

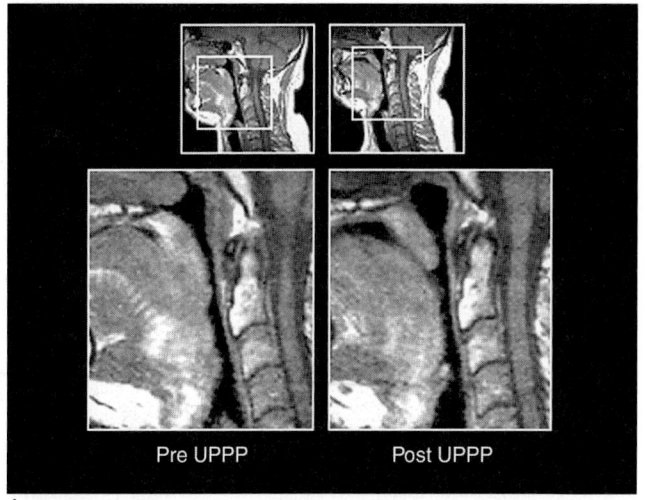

Pre UPPP   Post UPPP

A

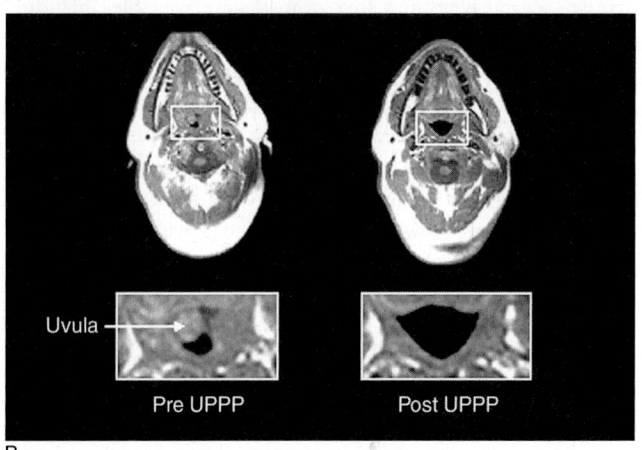

Uvula

Pre UPPP   Post UPPP

B

Figure 7-11 *A,* Midsagittal images of a patient before and after uvulopalatopharyngoplasty (UPPP). Notice the shortened uvula. Because the soft palate was not resected, the tracheal lumen remains narrow. *B,* Axial images at the level of the uvula; notice the significant increase in the diameter of the airway. *(From Kryger MH et al, editors: Principles and practice of sleep medicine, ed 4, p. 996, Philadelphia, 2005, Saunders.)*

and avoidance of sleep deprivation may be all that is necessary. Oral appliances may be prescribed to stabilize the jaw or retain the tongue. These devices must be fitted by a dentist and are not always as effective as continuous positive airway pressure (CPAP). Moderate to severe levels of apnea may be treated with mechanical, surgical, or pharmacologic therapy. Treatment can vary depending on the type and severity of illness.

CPAP via nasal mask is the treatment of choice. CPAP machines are simply pressure generators with the effective pressure being determined during the titration part of the PSG. This holds the airway open and prevents collapse. The patient wears a small, triangle-shaped mask over the nose or uses nasal pillows if the mask is not tolerated. CPAP treats the obstruction and the snoring, choking, and gasping that accompany it, and it provides cardiovascular benefits. Although CPAP is the treatment of choice, is effective only if the patient is compliant with therapy. Regular attendance at CPAP clinics can improve patient compliance.[63] If a patient cannot tolerate the continuous pressure of CPAP, bimodal positive airway pressure (BiPAP), which provides separate pressures for inspiration and expiration, may be tried.

Various surgical interventions are available for the treatment of apnea and snoring. Patients with mild OSA or snoring alone may undergo an outpatient procedure called *laser uvulopalatopharyngoplasty (LAUP),* which uses lasers to remove excess tissue at the soft palate level. For patients who snore but do not have apnea, somnoplasty may provide relief. Somnoplasty involves inserting a small electrode into the soft palate and heating the tissue, causing the area to shrink and tighten.[64]

Uvulopalatopharyngoplasty (UPPP) was one of the earlier surgeries used to treat OSA. Essentially, a large tonsillectomy is performed and all redundant tissue is removed (Fig. 7-11). Reports of success from UPPP vary widely, with 40% to 80% of patients experiencing sleep apnea improvement.[64,65] Complications include speech impairment, inability to eat, postoperative bleeding, and infection. Severe pain after UPPP is documented and may continue well into the postoperative period.[65] Although tracheostomy was the original surgery procedure used to treat OSA, it is now used only in the most severe cases of apnea that do not respond to other treatments. Bariatric surgery is an effective means to facilitate weight loss and subsequent improvement in OSA.[66]

Treatment of OSA with medication is usually a last resort and has proved to be very disappointing. Protriptyline has been shown to decrease apnea and reduce excessive daytime sleepiness by decreasing sleep apnea frequency that increases during REM sleep. Oxygen may be used to lower hypoxemia and nocturnal desaturations.

Nursing Management. The nurse's role in the management of sleep apnea includes educating the patient and family about the syndrome and the consequences of noncompliance with treatment regimens. This education may also include preoperative teaching for any surgery procedures such as UPPP. Monitoring of patients with OSA while in critical care should include assessment of the breathing patterns, hours of sleep, and pulse oximetry. Cautious administration of narcotics to patients with sleep apnea is suggested because of the potential for respiratory depression, although the concern regarding adequate pain relief is not well studied.

Nasal CPAP is most effective when patients are properly fitted with the nasal mask and have clear instructions regarding its use. Several types and sizes of masks are available, including one type called a *nasal pillow,* which does not cover the nose but instead fits into the nostrils. If patients are admitted to the critical care unit with a history of OSA, they need to use their home CPAP mask and equipment as part of their regular sleep routine. The nurse can enhance compliance with the CPAP system. Nursing care includes ensuring proper fit of the CPAP mask, with no air blowing into the patient's eyes, correct airway pressure, no pressure sores from the mask, and no gastric insufflation.

UPPP patients are not usually admitted to critical care areas, because the postoperative recovery does not require intensive care.[67] Postoperative monitoring after UPPP includes risk of aspiration, pain management, anxiety relief, patient education, and monitoring for respiratory complications, hemorrhage, infection, impaired speech, nutritional concerns, and sleep disturbance (see the Nursing Diagnoses feature).

CENTRAL SLEEP APNEA

Definition, Etiology, and Pathophysiology. Central sleep apnea (CSA) can be seen on PSG as an absence of airflow and respiratory effort for at least 10 seconds. A complete loss of electromyographic activity by the respiratory muscles would be expected, because since CSA is defined as a pause in respiration without ventilatory effort.[68]

A chemoreceptor sensitive to the levels of CO_2 resides within the brain. When CO_2 levels become excessive, ventilatory efforts are increased to blow off the excess CO_2. This negative-feedback loop exists to provide a homeostatic balance in the carbon dioxide and oxygen levels of the body. Whereas OSA results from an obstructed or collapsed airway, patients with CSA suffer from a lack of ventilatory effort. This can be observed in patients with cardiopulmonary disease (e.g., COPD) or heart failure, because their chemoreceptors have become adjusted to an increased CO_2 level. Javaheri[69] studied patients with congestive heart failure and found that as many as 40% had CSA. CSA includes numerous manifestations, such as idiopathic CSA and Cheyne-Stokes breathing. However, the uniting factor is cessation of breathing momentarily during sleep due to the transient withdrawal of central nervous system

drive to the muscles of respiration.[70] It is not uncommon for a patient who experiences CSA to also have some obstructive events.

CSA may result from many physiologic or pathophysiologic events.[70] Possible causes of nonhypercapnic CSA include periodic breathing at high altitude, renal or metabolic disturbances, and idiopathic central apnea seen at sea level. Hypercapnic CSA can occur in many neuromuscular conditions such as spinal cord or brain injury, encephalitis, brainstem neoplasm or infarcts, muscular dystrophy, myasthenia gravis, bulbar poliomyelitis, and postpolio syndrome.

Assessment and Diagnosis. Clinical characteristics of hypercapnic CSA include respiratory failure, cor pulmonale, peripheral edema, polycythemia, daytime sleepiness, and snoring. Patients with nonhypercapnic CSA have clinical features very similar to those of OSA. Nonhypercapnic CSA characteristics include daytime sleepiness, insomnia or poor sleep, mild or intermittent snoring, and awakenings accompanied by choking or feeling short of breath; frequently, the patients are of normal body weight. Diagnosis is made by overnight PSG or sleep study, which will determine the respiratory and sleep patterns of the patient.

Medical Management. Because there are two types of CSA, there are two therapeutic approaches depending on the cause of the apnea. The hypercapnic patient who has worsening hypoventilation during sleep is best served by nocturnal ventilation. Most such patients experience some respiratory muscle failure. One treatment for the nonhypercapnic or heart failure patients is nasal CPAP, which also may provide a beneficial cardiovascular effect. Nocturnal oxygen supplementation may be effective as well. If CPAP is not tolerated, pharmacologic management may be tried. Medroxyprogesterone, a respiratory stimulant, may improve ventilation in selected patients.[68] Acetazolamide, a carbonic anhydrase inhibitor that can result in metabolic acidosis, also may decrease the frequency of apneic episodes. Several studies have reported the development of obstructive apnea in patients successfully treated for central apnea.[69]

Nursing Management. For the nurse caring for a patient with CSA, patient and family education about the patient's condition and treatment regimen can help to ensure patient compliance. The nurse needs to address any fear or anxiety about going to sleep. Nurses also need to caution patients to avoid alcohol and sedative medications. Weight loss is recommended if the patient is obese. The nurse needs to carefully monitor and assess the respiratory status of the patient. For more information, see the Case Study on Sleep Alterations.

Summary

- Sleep plays an important role in human homeostasis that remains underappreciated by the public.

- The development of good sleep hygiene habits at an early age may help prevent cardiovascular disease, cerebrovascular disease, and type 2 diabetes.
- Sleep patterns are altered with aging.
- Exercise and exposure to adequate levels of light help entrain circadian rhythms to facilitate the sleep-wake cycle. If sleep patterns are disturbed, guided use of light and activity may help retrain the sleeper.
- Numerous medications can interrupt the sleep cycle. Because many of these medications are used to treat cardiovascular conditions, health care providers need to monitor the sleep of patients with those conditions.
- Sleep apnea is a common disorder that is readily treated but has dire consequences if not addressed.

Case Study: Patient with Sleep Alterations

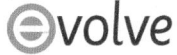 Answers to the Case Study Questions can be found on the Evolve web site at http://evolve.elsevier.com/Urden/.

Brief Patient History

Mr. D is a 43-year-old, severely obese, self-employed man. His medical history includes excessive daytime sleepiness, hypertension, and sinus dysrhythmia. He received a diagnosis of obstructive sleep apnea (OSA) 2 years ago, and his health care provider prescribed nasal continuous positive airway pressure (CPAP) for use at night. However, Mr. D has been, for the most part, noncompliant because of reported discomfort and interference with his sex life. Mr. D's hypertension has required increasing medication, and he has begun to develop cardiomegaly. His business suffers from his inability to stay awake and focus. He and his wife have started sleeping in separate rooms because of his snoring. These circumstances have prompted Mr. D's physician to recommend surgical correction of Mr. D's airway. He refused to consider a tracheostomy but agreed to uvulopalatopharyngoplasty (UPPP) despite the 50% chance of success. Mr. D and his spouse understand that endotracheal intubation may be necessary for 24 to 48 hours because of the severity of his condition.

Clinical Assessment

Mr. D is admitted to the surgical intensive care unit after a very complicated surgical procedure with an oral endotracheal tube connected to supplemental oxygen with spontaneous respiration. He is awake and follows commands; however, he is having periods of restlessness and pulling at tubes.

Diagnostic Procedures

Mr. D's vital signs include blood pressure of 160/72 mm Hg, heart rate of 120 beats/min (sinus tachycardia), respiratory rate of 20 breaths/min, and temperature of 97.8° F. The chest radiograph is clear. Arterial blood gases were obtained: pH of 7.38, Pao_2 of 90 mm Hg, $Paco_2$ of 35 mm Hg, HCO_3^- level of 24%, and O_2 saturation of 98%. Mr. D indicates that his pain is a 5 on the Baker-Wong faces scale by pointing. The Riker Sedation-Agitation Scale score is 5.

Medical Diagnosis

Mr. D is diagnosed with OSA.

Questions

1. What major outcomes do you expect to achieve for this patient?
2. What problems or risks must be managed to achieve these outcomes?
3. What interventions must be initiated to monitor, prevent, manage, or eliminate the problems and risks identified?
4. What interventions should be initiated to promote optimal functioning, safety, and well-being of the patient?
5. What possible learning needs do you anticipate for this patient?
6. What cultural and age-related factors may have a bearing on the patient's plan of care?

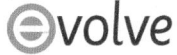 Be sure to check out the bonus material, including free self-assessment exercises, on the Evolve web site at http://evolve.elsevier.com/Urden/.

References

1. Evans JC, French DG: Sleep and healing in intensive care settings, *Dimens Crit Care Nurs* 14(4):189-199, 1995.
2. Celik S et al: Sleep disturbance: the patient care activities applied at the night shift in the intensive care unit. *J Clin Nurs* 14:102-106, 2005.
3. Carskadon MA, Dement WC: Normal human sleep: an overview. In Kryger MH et al, editors: *Principles and practice of sleep medicine*, ed 4, Philadelphia, 2005, Saunders.
4. Rechtschaffen A, Kales A: *A manual of standardized terminology, techniques, and scoring system for sleep stages of human subjects*, Bethesda, MD, 1968, U.S. Department of Health, Education, and Welfare.

5. Douglas NJ: Respiratory physiology: control of ventilation. In Kryger MH et al, editors: *Principles and practice of sleep medicine*, ed 4, Philadelphia, 2005, Saunders.

6. Davidhizar RE et al: What nurses need to know about sleep, *J Nurs Sci* 1:61-67, 1995.

7. Krachman SL et al: Sleep in the intensive care unit, *Chest* 107(6):1713-1720, 1995.

8. Vitiello MV: Normal versus pathologic sleep changes in aging humans. In Kuna ST, editor: *Sleep and respiration in aging*, St Louis, 1991, Mosby.

9. Ancoli-Israel S et al: Identification and treatment of sleep problems in the elderly, *Sleep Med Reviews* 1:3-17, 1997.

10. Ancoli-Israel S: Sleep problems in older adults: putting myths to bed, *Geriatrics* 52(1):20-30, 1997.

11. Buysse DJ et al: Napping and 24-hour sleep/wake patterns in healthy elderly and young adults, *J Am Geriatr Soc* 40(8):779-786, 1992.

12. Bliwise DL: Normal aging. In Kryger MH et al, editors: *Principles and practice of sleep medicine*, ed 4, Philadelphia, 2005, Saunders.

13. Bliwise DL et al: Habitual sleep durations and health in a 50-65 year old population, *J Clin Epidemiol* 47(1):35-41, 1994.

14. Sloan E, Flint A: Circadian rhythms and psychiatric disorders in the elderly, *J Geriatr Psychiatry Neurol* 9(4):164-170, 1996.

15. Arbelaez JJ et al: Depressive symptoms, inflammation, and ischemic stroke in older adults: a prospective analysis in the cardiovascular health study. *J Am Geriatr Soc* 55(11):1825-1830, 2007.

16. Foley DJ et al: Sleep complaints among elderly persons: an epidemiologic study of three communities, *Sleep* 18(6):425-432, 1995.

17. Richards KC: Sleep promotion, *Crit Care Nurs Clin North Am* 8(1):39-52, 1996.

18. Schwartz W: A clinician's primer on the circadian clock: its localization, function, and resetting, *Adv Intern Med* 38:81-106, 1993.

19. Carrier J et al: Amplitude reduction of the circadian temperature and sleep rhythms in the elderly, *Chronobiol Int* 13(5):373-386, 1996.

20. Haimov I, Lavie P: Potential of melatonin replacement therapy in older patients with sleep disorders, *Drugs Aging* 7(2):75-78, 1995.

21. Scheer VA et al: Melatonin in the regulation of sleep and circadian rhythms. In Kryger MH et al, editors: *Principles and practice of sleep medicine*, ed 4, Philadelphia, 2005, Saunders.

22. Czeisler CA et al: The human circadian timing system and sleep-wake regulation. In Kryger MH et al, editors: *Principles and practice of sleep medicine*, ed 4, Philadelphia, 2005, Saunders.

23. Warman VL et al: Phase advancing human circadian rhythms with short wavelength light. *Neurosci Lett* 342(1-2):37-40, 2003.

24. Dijk DJ, Czeisler CA: Contribution of the circadian pacemaker and the sleep homeostat to sleep propensity, sleep structure, electroencephalographic slow waves, and sleep spindle activity in humans, *J Neurosci* 15(5 Pt 1):3526-3538, 1995.

25. Borbely AA, Achermann, P: Sleep homeostasis and models of sleep regulation. In Kryger MH et al, editors: *Principles and practice of sleep medicine*, ed 4, Philadelphia, 2005, Saunders.

26. Borbely AA, Achermann P: Sleep homeostasis and models of sleep regulation, *J Biol Rhythms* 14(6):557-568, 1999.

27. Kronauer RE et al: Mathematical model of the human circadian system with two interacting oscillators, *Am J Physiol* 242(1):R3-R17, 1982.

28. Nakao M et al: Dynamical features of thermoregulatory model of sleep control, *Jpn J Physiol* 45(2):311-326, 1995.

29. Mendelson WB: Hypnotic medications: Mechanisms of action and pharmacologic effects. In Kryger MH et al, editors: *Principles and practice of sleep medicine*, ed 4, Philadelphia, 2005, Saunders.

30. Walsh JK et al: Pharmacologic treatment of primary insomnia. In Kryger MH et al, editors: *Principles and practice of sleep medicine*, ed 4, Philadelphia, 2005, Saunders.

31. Nishino S, Mignot E: Wake-promoting medications: basic mechanisms and pharmacology. In Kryger MH et al, editors: *Principles and practice of sleep medicine*, ed 4, Philadelphia, 2005, Saunders.

32. Mitler MM, O'Malley, MB: Wake-promoting medications: efficacy and adverse effects. In Kryger MH et al, editors: *Principles and practice of sleep medicine*, ed 4 Philadelphia, 2005, Saunders.

33. National Sleep Foundation: 2008 Sleep in America Poll. Washington, DC, National Sleep Foundation, 2008. Available at www.sleepfoundation.org/ (accessed December 2008).

34. Schweitzer PK: Drugs that disturb sleep and wakefulness. In Kryger MH et al, editors: *Principles and practice of sleep medicine*, ed 4, Philadelphia, 2005, Saunders.

35. Tung A et al: The hypnotic effect of propofol in the medial preoptic area of the rat, *Life Sci* 69:855-862, 2001.

36. Nicolas A et al: Perception of nighttime sleep by surgical patients in an intensive care unit, *Nurs Crit Care* 13(1):25-33, 2008.

37. Ugras GA, Oztekin SD: Patient perception of environmental and nursing factors contributing to sleep disturbances in a neurosurgical intensive care unit. *Tohoku J Exp Med* 212:299-308, 2007.

38. Spiegel K et al: Impact of sleep debt on metabolic and endocrine function, *Lancet* 354:1435-1439, 1999.

39. Sunshine W et al: Massage therapy and transcutaneous electrical stimulation effects on fibromyalgia, *J Clin Rheumatol* 2:18-22, 1997.

40. Simpson T et al: Patients' perceptions of environmental factors that disturb sleep after cardiac surgery, *Am J Crit Care* 5(3):173-181, 1996.

41. Frisk, U Nordstrom G: Patients sleep in an intensive care unit: patients' and nurses' perception, *Intens Crit Care Nurs* 19:342-349, 2003.

42. Redeker NS et al: Sleep patterns in women after coronary artery bypass surgery, *Appl Nurs Res* 9(3):115-122, 1996.

43. Meyer TJ et al: Adverse environmental conditions in the respiratory and medical ICU settings, *Chest* 105(4):1211-1216, 1994.

44. Gabor JY et al: Contribution of the intensive care unit environment to sleep disruption in mechanically ventilated patients and health subjects, *Am J Respir Crit Care Med* 167:708-715, 2003.

45. Edell-Gustafsson UM, Hetta JE: Anxiety, depression, and sleep in male patients undergoing coronary artery bypass surgery, *Scand J Caring Sci* 13(2):137-143, 1999.

46. Cooper AB et al: Sleep in critically ill patients requiring mechanical ventilation, *Chest* 117:809-818, 2000.

47. Bosma K et al: Patient-ventilator interaction and sleep in mechanically ventilated patients: pressure support versus proportional assist ventilation. *Crit Care Med* 35(4):1048-1054, 2007.

48. Toublan B et al: Assist-control ventilation vs. low levels of pressure support ventilation on sleep quality in intubated ICU patients. *Intensive Care Med* 33(7):1148-1154, 2007.

49. Combes A et al: Morbidity, mortality, and quality-of-life outcomes of patients requiring >14 days of mechanical ventilation, *Crit Care Med* 31(5):1373-1381, 2003.

50. Chisti A et al: Sleep-related breathing disorders following discharge from intensive care, *Int Care Med*, 26:426-433, 2000.

51. Richards KC et al: Effects of massage in acute and critical care, *AACN Clin Issues* 11(1):77-96, 2000.

52. Williamson JW: The effects of ocean sounds on sleep after coronary artery bypass graft surgery, *Am J Crit Care* 1(1):91-97, 1992.

53. Stanchina JL et al: The influence of white noise on sleep in subjects exposed to ICU noise. *Sleep Med* 6:423-428, 2005.

54. Lower J et al: High-tech high-touch: mission possible? *Dimens Crit Care Nurs*, 21(5):201-205, 2002.

55. Fontaine DK et al: Designing humanistic critical care environments. *Crit Care Nurs Q* 24(3):21-34, 2001.

56. Guilleminault C, Bassiri A: Clinical features and evaluation of obstructive sleep apnea-hypopnea syndrome and upper airway resistance syndrome. In Kryger MH et al, editors: *Principles and practice of sleep medicine*, ed 4, Philadelphia, 2005, Saunders.

57. Hudgel DW: Mechanisms of obstructive sleep apnea, *Chest* 101(2):541-549, 1992.

58. Punjabi NM: The epidemiology of adult obstructive sleep apnea. *Proc Am Thorac Soc* 5(2):136-143, 2008.

59. Krieger S, Caples SM: Obstructive sleep apnea and cardiovascular disease: implications for clinical practice. *Cleve Clin J Med* 74(12):853-856, 2007.

60. Friedman M et al: Clinical predicators of obstructive sleep apnea, *Sleep* 23: A268, 2000.

61. Young T, Javaheri S: Systemic and pulmonary hypertension in obstructive sleep apnea. In Kryger MH et al, editors: *Principles and practice of sleep medicine*, ed 4, Philadelphia, 2005, Saunders.

62. Somers VK, Javaheri S: Cardiovascular effects of sleep-related breathing disorders. In Kryger MH et al, editors: *Principles and practice of sleep medicine*, ed 4, Philadelphia, 2005, Saunders.

63. Neumeyer DA et al: Compliance of CPAP in patients with obstructive sleep apnea who are enrolled in a CPAP clinic, *Sleep* 12:A257, 2000.

64. Krug P: Snoring and obstructive sleep apnea, *AORN J* 69:792-797, 1999.

65. Carpenter JM, LaMear WR: Uvulopalatopharyngoplasty: results of a patient questionnaire. *Ann Otol Rhinol Laryngol* 117(1):24-26, 2008.

66. Buchwald H et al: Bariatric surgery: a systematic review and meta-analysis. *JAMA* 292:1724-1737, 2004.

67. Mickelson SA, Hakim I: Is postoperative intensive care monitoring necessary after uvulopalatopharyngoplasty? *Otolaryngol Head Neck Surg* 119(4): 352-356, 1998.

68. White DP: Central sleep apnea. In Kryger MH et al, editors: *Principles and practice of sleep medicine*, ed 4, Philadelphia, 2005, Saunders.

69. Javaheri S: A mechanism of central sleep apnea in patients with heart failure, *N Engl J Med* 341(13):949-954, 1999.

70. Ekhert DJ et al: Central sleep apnea: Pathophysiology and treatment. *Chest* 131:595-607, 2007.

71. Buysse DJ et al: Clinical pharmacology of other drugs used as hypnotics. In Kryger MH et al, editors: *Principles and practice of sleep medicine*, ed 4, Philadelphia, 2005, Saunders.

Nutrition Alterations and Management

Chapter 8

NUTRIENT METABOLISM

ENERGY-YIELDING NUTRIENTS

The energy-yielding nutrients are carbohydrates, proteins, and fats. They are composed mostly of carbon, hydrogen, and oxygen. For proper metabolic functioning, adequate amounts of vitamins, electrolytes, minerals, and trace elements also must be supplied to the human body. The process by which nutrients are used at the cellular level is known as *metabolism*. The major purposes of metabolism of the energy-yielding nutrients are the production of energy and the formation and preservation of lean body mass.

Carbohydrates. Through the process of digestion, carbohydrates are broken down into glucose, fructose, and galactose. After absorption from the intestinal tract, fructose and galactose are converted to glucose, the primary form of carbohydrate used by the cells. Glucose provides the energy needed to maintain cellular functions, including transport across cell membranes, secretion of specific hormones, muscle contraction, and synthesis of new substances. Most of the energy produced from carbohydrate metabolism is used to form adenosine triphosphate (ATP), the principal form of immediately available energy within all body cells. One gram of carbohydrate provides approximately 4 kcal of energy.

One form of carbohydrate that is poorly digested by most of the world's adults is lactose, or milk sugar. In lactose intolerance, the individual lacks lactase, the intestinal enzyme required for digestion of lactose. Consumption of lactose causes abdominal cramping, bloating, and diarrhea. The individual with lactose intolerance may tolerate cheeses, yogurt, acidophilus milk, and buttermilk, because these products contain less lactose than unmodified milk. Lactase enzyme supplements are available to be taken orally, and many markets now sell milk that has been treated with lactase.

Inside the cell, glucose is stored as glycogen (the storage form of carbohydrate) or lipid (fat), or it is metabolized for the release of energy. Liver and muscle cells have the largest glycogen reserves. In addition to glucose obtained from glycogen, glucose can be formed from lactate, amino acids, and glycerol. This process of manufacturing glucose from nonglucose precursors is called *gluconeogenesis*. Gluconeogenesis is carried out at all times, but it becomes especially important in maintaining a source of glucose in times of increased physiologic need and limited supply. Only the liver and, to a lesser extent, the kidney are capable of producing significant amounts of glucose for release into the blood for use by other tissues.

Proteins. Proteins are made up of chains of amino acids. Each amino acid consists of carbon, hydrogen, and oxygen, and nitrogen in the form of one or more amine groups ($-NH_2$). Amino acids are the protein components that can be used by cells.

Proteins have important structural and functional duties within the body. Proteins provide the structural basis of all lean body mass, such as the vital organs and skeletal muscle. Proteins are important for visceral (cellular) functions, such as initiation of chemical reactions (e.g., hormones, enzymes), transportation of other substances (e.g., apoproteins, albumin), preservation of immune function (e.g., antibodies), and maintenance of osmotic pressure (e.g., albumin) and blood neutrality (e.g., buffers). Some amino acids are used for energy, providing approximately 4 kcal/g.

Proteins are synthesized continuously, broken down into amino acids, and then resynthesized into new protein. This three-step process is called *protein turnover*. The rate of turnover is fastest (often only a few hours) in enzymes and hormones involved in metabolic activities. In very active tissues—such as those of the liver, kidney, and gastrointestinal mucosa—protein turnover occurs every few days. If necessary, 90% of the amino acids released by tissue breakdown can be reused, with the diet providing the remaining 10% of the amino acids needed for protein synthesis. In the injured or undernourished individual, many of the amino acids released by tissue breakdown may be used for gluconeogenesis. To preserve lean body mass, adequate energy must be supplied by the diet so that most of the amino acids from the diet and from tissue breakdown can be used for tissue synthesis, rather than gluconeogenesis.

Proteins, which often consist of hundreds or thousands of amino acids, are too large to be absorbed intact under normal circumstances. Through digestion, the proteins are broken down into amino acids and dipeptides or tripeptides (composed of two or three amino acids, respectively) that can be absorbed across the intestinal wall. Certain amino acids are *essential*; they cannot be produced by the body and must be supplied through the diet. Essential amino acids include valine, leucine, isoleucine, lysine, phenylalanine, tryptophan, threonine, and methionine, as well as histidine and arginine in infants. Other amino acids are nonessential and can be manufactured by the body under normal circumstances if the essential amino acids are in adequate supply. Some amino acids that may be nonessential in healthy adults become essential during illness. For example, histidine is an essential amino acid for adults with renal failure, and glutamine may be essential for individuals with trauma, sepsis, or other physiologic types of stress.

The amine group is essential for protein synthesis, but the nonamine portion of the molecule (ketoacid) is used in gluconeogenesis. If a ketoacid is used for gluconeogenesis, the amine group can be excreted in the urine as ammonia or urea. If the rate of gluconeogenesis rises, urinary nitrogen excretion also increases. In assessing protein nutrition, it is common to measure nitrogen balance, or the amount of nitrogen excreted compared with that consumed. Normally, most of the body's nitrogen losses are in the urine, and in determining nitrogen balance, urinary nitrogen excretion is measured (preferably over a 24-hour period). Nitrogen (protein) intake is recorded over the same period, and losses of nitrogen from feces and other routes (e.g., sloughing of skin cells) are usually estimated.

Most healthy adults are in *nitrogen equilibrium*, meaning that they excrete the same amount of nitrogen that they consume. Individuals who excrete less nitrogen than they consume are said to be in *positive nitrogen balance;* this occurs during growth, pregnancy, and healing. Individuals who excrete more nitrogen than they consume are in *negative nitrogen balance*. Negative nitrogen balance is common in the early period after trauma or surgery. When the rate of gluconeogenesis is high, as may occur in the trauma patient who is initially too unstable to be fed, extensive loss of body proteins can occur. Losses include structural (e.g., muscle) and visceral proteins. Visceral proteins, including immunoglobulins, albumin, and complement, are critical for survival. Preservation of body protein is therefore a key goal of nutritional support of critically ill patients.

Fat (Lipids). Lipids include fatty acids, triglycerides (three fatty acids bound to a glycerol backbone), phospholipids (lipids containing phosphate groups), cholesterol, and cholesterol esters. Aside from their involvement in functions such as the maintenance of cell membranes and the manufacture of prostaglandins, lipids—primarily in the form of triglycerides—provide a stored source of energy. They are calorically dense molecules, providing more than twice the amount of energy per gram (9 kcal) as protein and carbohydrates.

Most dietary lipids—consisting primarily of triglycerides—are too large to be absorbed intact and are partially broken down (hydrolyzed) in the intestine to form monoglycerides and diglycerides, which contain one or two fatty acids, respectively, bound to glycerol.

Bile salts produced in the liver are detergents, and they promote the formation of micelles, which are emulsions of fatty acids, monoglycerides, and bile salts. Long-chain fatty acids, which contain more than 12 carbon atoms, are very insoluble in water; they are found mainly in the interior of the micelle. The external portion of the micelle, which includes the glycerol part of the triglycerides, is more water soluble than the interior portion. This allows the micelle to cross the unstirred water layer that coats the intestinal absorptive surface.

Inside the intestinal cells, monoglycerides and long-chain fatty acids rejoin to form triglycerides, and they are surrounded by specific proteins to form chylomicrons. These chylomicrons are transported out of the intestine through the lymphatic system, finally entering the blood circulation through the thoracic duct. Some of the chylomicrons are taken up by the liver, but most are directly transported to other tissues. Short-chain fatty acids (less than 8 carbon atoms long) and medium-chain fatty acids (8 to 12 carbon atoms long) are more water soluble than longer fatty acids; triglycerides containing these fatty acids can be absorbed without hydrolysis and are soluble enough to be transported to the liver through the portal vein, without chylomicron formation. Short- and medium-chain fatty acids have advantages in nutritional care of patients who have insufficient bile salt formation or inadequate intestinal surface area for absorption of long-chain fatty acids.

With the aid of the enzyme lipoprotein lipase, triglyceride-containing chylomicrons are broken down outside the cell and enter the cell as fatty acids and glycerol. (Heparin stimulates lipoprotein lipase, and low doses of heparin are sometimes given to patients receiving intravenous lipid emulsions to improve lipid use.) Insulin also stimulates the cellular uptake of triglycerides. Inside the cell, the fatty acids are oxidized (metabolized for energy) or reformed into triglycerides for storage. During an overnight fast, prolonged starvation, or metabolic stress when the carbohydrate supply is limited, the blood glucose level declines, and consequently, insulin levels decrease. In response, a process called *lipolysis* causes the breakdown of intracellular triglycerides, which provides fatty acids for energy production and glycerol for gluconeogenesis.

The fatty acids released from adipose tissue can be used by the liver, heart, or other tissues. In the liver, fatty acids are broken down to ketones (beta-hydroxybutyrate, acetoacetate, and acetone). In the absence of glucose, fatty acid breakdown and ketone production are increased. Ketones can be directly oxidized by skeletal muscle and used for energy. During prolonged starvation, the brain—which normally uses glucose—converts to using ketones as its primary energy source. This is a body defense mechanism to ensure a supply of energy when carbohydrate intake is low.

ENERGY DEFICIENCY

Protein-Calorie Malnutrition. Malnutrition results from the lack of intake of necessary nutrients or improper absorption and distribution of them, as well as from excessive intake of some nutrients. Malnutrition can be related to any essential nutrient or nutrients, but a serious type of malnutrition found frequently among hospitalized patients is protein-calorie malnutrition (PCM). Poor intake or impaired absorption of protein and energy from carbohydrate and fat worsens the debilitation that may occur in response to critical illness. In PCM, the body proteins are broken down for gluconeogenesis, reducing the supply of amino acids needed for maintenance of body proteins and healing. Malnutrition can be caused by simple starvation—the inadequate intake of nutrients (e.g., in the patient with anorexia related to cancer). It also can result from an injury that increases the metabolic rate beyond the supply of nutrients (hypermetabolism). In the seriously ill patient, if malnutrition occurs, usually it is the result of the combined effects of starvation and hypermetabolism.

Metabolic Response to Starvation and Stress. To understand the development of malnutrition in the hospitalized patient, the nurse must understand the metabolic response to starvation and physiologic stress. Changes in endocrine status and metabolism together determine the onset and extent of malnutrition. Nutritional imbalance occurs when the demand for nutrients is greater than the exogenous nutrient supply. The major difference between a person who is starved and one who is starved and injured is that the latter has an increased reliance on tissue protein breakdown to provide precursors for glucose production to meet increased energy demands. Although carbohydrate and fat metabolism are also affected, the main concern is about protein metabolism and homeostasis.

During an acute, nonstressed fast, blood levels of glucose and insulin fall, and glucagon levels rise. Glucagon stimulates the liver to release glucose from its glycogen reserves, which become exhausted within a few hours. Glucagon also stimulates gluconeogenesis, and skeletal muscle provides a large amount of the substrates required for gluconeogenesis. As fasting progresses, fat becomes the primary source of fuel, and the blood ketone levels begin to increase. After the circulating ketone level rises, the brain is able to use ketones for 70% of its energy, thereby decreasing the total body's reliance on glucose as an energy source. As gluconeogenesis from protein precursors decreases, protein breakdown and nitrogen excretion also slow. Some tissues, such as red blood cells, the renal medulla, and 30% of brain cells, are obligatory glucose users, and they continue to require a small amount of amino acids for gluconeogenesis. However, endogenous protein stores are spared from use for gluconeogenesis to a major extent, and protein homeostasis is partially restored.

Critically ill patients are at risk for a combination of starvation and the physiologic stress resulting from injury, trauma, major surgery, or sepsis. Starvation occurs because the person must have nothing by mouth (NPO) for surgical procedures, is unable to eat because of disease-related factors, or is hemodynamically too unstable to be fed. The physiologic stress causes an increased metabolic rate (hypermetabolism) that results in increased oxygen consumption and energy expenditure.

The hypermetabolic process results from increased catabolic hormone changes caused by the stressful event. The sympathetic nervous system is stimulated, causing the adrenal medulla to release catecholamines (epinephrine and norepinephrine). Other hormones released in response to stress include glucagon, adrenocorticotropic hormone (ACTH), antidiuretic hormone (ADH), and glucocorticoids and mineralocorticoids (e.g., cortisol, aldosterone). Cytokines are peptide messengers secreted by macrophages as part of the inflammatory response, and they serve as hormonal regulators of the immune system. Cytokine levels increase in response to sepsis and trauma. Important cytokines include tumor necrosis factor (TNF), cachectin, interleukin 1 (IL-1), and interleukin 6 (IL-6). All of these hormonal changes cause nutrient substrates, primarily amino acids, to move from peripheral tissues (e.g., skeletal muscle) to the liver for gluconeogenesis.

Unfortunately, this mobilization of substrates occurs at the expense of body tissue and function at a time when the needs for protein synthesis (e.g., wound healing, acute-phase proteins) also are high. Hyperglycemia results from the effects of increased catecholamines, glucocorticoids, and glucagon. The body relies on its protein stores to provide substrates for gluconeogenesis, because glucose becomes the major fuel source. Loss of protein results in a negative nitrogen balance and weight loss. Catabolism may be unresponsive to nutrient intake.

IMPLICATIONS OF UNDERNUTRITION FOR THE SICK OR STRESSED PATIENT

As many as 12% to 50% of hospitalized patients are at risk for malnutrition.[1-5] Although illness or injury is the major factor contributing to development of malnutrition, other possible contributing factors are lack of communication among the nurses, physicians, and dietitians responsible for the care of these patients; frequent diagnostic testing and procedures, which lead to interruption in feeding; medications and other therapies that cause anorexia, nausea, or vomiting and thereby interfere with food intake; insufficient monitoring of nutrient intake; and inadequate use of supplements, tube feedings, or total parenteral nutrition (TPN) to maintain the nutritional status of these patients.

Nutritional status tends to deteriorate during hospitalization unless appropriate nutrition support is started early and continually reassessed. Malnutrition in hospitalized patients is associated with a wide variety of adverse outcomes. Wound dehiscence, pressure ulcers, sepsis, infections, respiratory failure requiring ventilation, longer hospital stays, and death are more common among malnourished patients.[6-8] Decline in nutritional status during hospitalization is associated with higher incidences of complications, increased mortality rates, increased length of stay, and higher hospital costs.

ASSESSING NUTRITIONAL STATUS

A nutrition screening should be conducted on every patient. A brief questionnaire to be completed by the patient or significant other, the nursing admission form, or the physician's admission note usually provides enough information to determine whether the patient is at nutritional risk (Box 8-1). Any patient judged to be nutritionally at risk needs a more thorough nutrition assessment.

Nutrition assessment involves collection of four types of information: (1) anthropometric measurements, (2) biochemical (laboratory) data, (3) clinical signs (physical examination), and (4) diet and pertinent health history. This information provides a basis for (1) identifying patients who are malnourished or at risk of malnutrition, (2) determining the nutritional needs of individual patients, and (3) selecting the most appropriate methods of nutrition support for patients with or at risk of developing nutritional deficits. Nutrition support is the provision of specially formulated or delivered oral, enteral, or parenteral nutrients to maintain or restore optimal nutrition status.[9] The nutrition assessment can be performed by or under the supervision of a registered dietitian or by a nutrition care specialist (e.g., nurse with specialized expertise in nutrition). Figure 8-1 shows the route of administration of specialized nutrition support.

BOX 8-1   PATIENTS WHO ARE AT RISK FOR MALNUTRITION

ADULTS WHO EXHIBIT ANY OF THE FOLLOWING:

- Involuntary loss or gain of a significant amount of weight (>10% of usual body weight in 6 months, >5% in 1 month), even if the weight achieved by loss or gain is appropriate for height
- Chronic disease
- Chronic use of a modified diet
- Increased metabolic requirements
- Illness or surgery that may interfere with nutritional intake
- Inadequate nutrient intake for >7 days
- Regular use of three or more medications
- Poverty

INFANTS AND CHILDREN WHO EXHIBIT ANY OF THE FOLLOWING:

- Low birth weight
- Small for gestational age
- Weight loss of 10% or more
- Weight-for-length or weight-for-height <5th percentile or >95th percentile
- Increased metabolic requirements
- Impaired ability to ingest or tolerate oral feedings
- Inadequate weight gain or a significant decrease in an individual's usual growth percentile
- Poverty

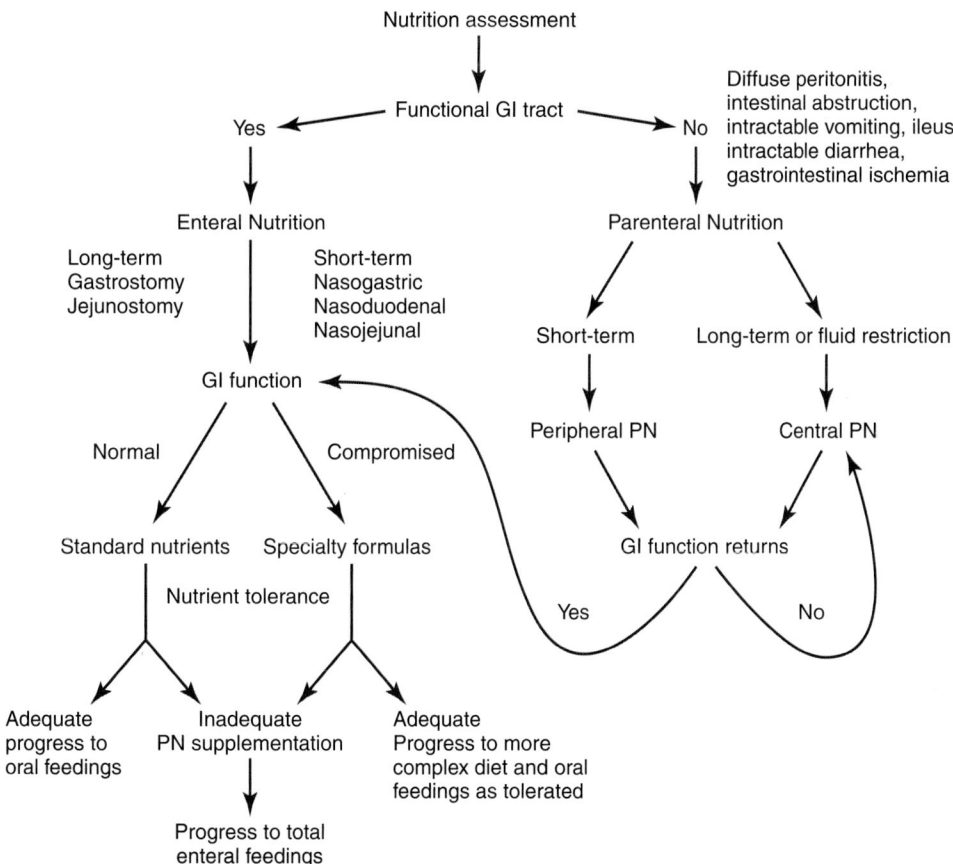

Figure 8-1 Route of administration of specialized nutrition support. *(From ASPEN, Board of Directors, and the Clinical Guidelines Task Force: Guidelines for the use of parenteral and enteral nutrition in adult and pediatric patients,* JPEN J Parenter Enter Nutr *26[suppl 1]:8SA, 2002.)*

ANTHROPOMETRIC MEASUREMENTS

Height and current weight are essential anthropometric measurements, and they should be measured rather than obtained through a patient or family report. The most important reason for obtaining anthropometric measurements is to be able to detect changes in the measurements over time (e.g., response to nutritional therapy). The patient's measurements may be compared with standard tables of weight-for-height or standard growth charts for infants and children. Another simple and reliable tool for interpreting appropriateness of weight for height for adults and older adolescents is the body mass index (BMI).

$$BMI = weight \div height^2$$

Weight is measured in kilograms and height in meters. A chart is available for estimating BMI and classifying it without

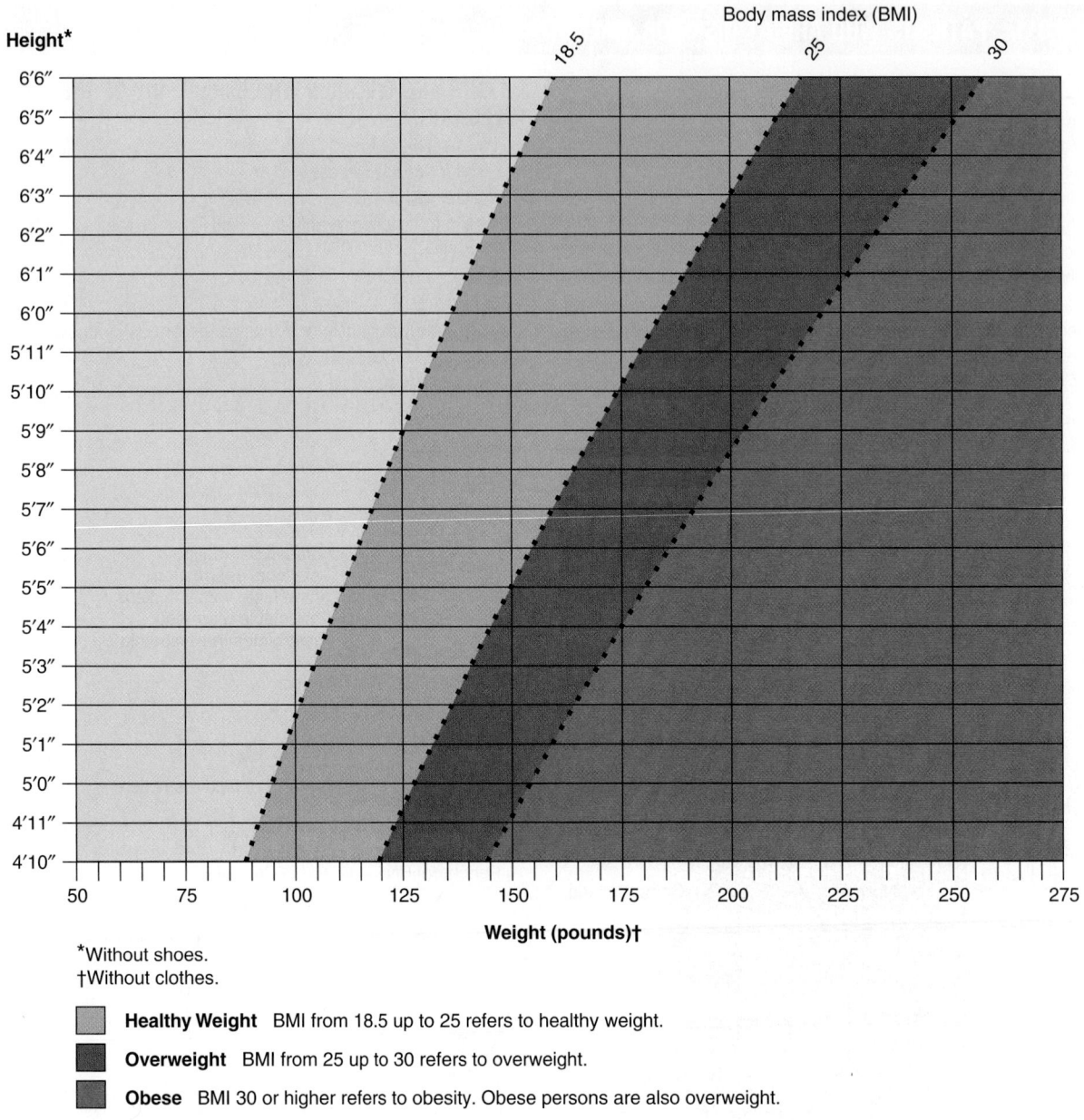

*Without shoes.
†Without clothes.

Healthy Weight BMI from 18.5 up to 25 refers to healthy weight.

Overweight BMI from 25 up to 30 refers to overweight.

Obese BMI 30 or higher refers to obesity. Obese persons are also overweight.

Figure 8-2 Chart for estimating and categorizing body mass index (BMI). To use, find the point where body weight and height intersect. *(Modified from Departments of Health and Human Services (HHS) and Agriculture (USDA): Report of the Dietary Guidelines Advisory Committee on the dietary guidelines for Americans, Washington, DC, 2000, USDA and DHHS.)*

performing any calculations (Fig. 8-2). The BMI can be classified as follows: (1) underweight, less than 18.5; (2) desirable, 18.5 to 24.9; (3) overweight, 25 to 29.9; and (4) obese, 30 or greater.[10]

It may be impossible to measure the height of some patients accurately. Total height can be estimated from knee height.[11] To measure knee height, bend the knee 90 degrees, and measure from the base of the heel to the anterior surface of the thigh.

For men:

$$\text{height (cm)} = 6419.0 - (0.04 \times \text{age in years}) + (2.02 \times \text{knee height [cm]})$$

For women:

$$\text{height (cm)} = 84.88 - (0.24 \times \text{age in years}) + (1.83 \times \text{knee height [cm]})$$

During critical illness, changes in anthropometric measures such as weight are more likely to reflect changes in body water and its distribution. Good judgment must be used in interpreting anthropometric data. For example, edema may mask significant weight loss or underweight. Despite these limitations, weight remains an important measure of nutritional status, and any recent weight change must be evaluated. A woman who was obese 4 months earlier and has lost 15 kg (33 lb) since then may be at nutritional risk even if her current weight is appropriate for her height.

In addition to height and weight data, other measurements such as arm muscle circumference, skin fold thickness, and body composition (proportion of fat and lean tissue, determined by bioelectric impedance or other methods) are sometimes performed, but these measurements are of limited use in assessing critically ill patients.[12]

BIOCHEMICAL DATA

A wide range of laboratory tests can provide information about nutritional status. Those most often used in the clinical setting are described in Table 8-1. No diagnostic tests for evaluation of nutrition are perfect, and care must be taken in interpreting the results of the tests.[13]

CLINICAL OR PHYSICAL MANIFESTATIONS

A thorough physical examination is an essential part of nutrition assessment. Box 8-2 lists some of the more common findings that may indicate an altered nutritional state. It is especially important for the nurse to check for signs of muscle wasting, loss of subcutaneous fat, skin or hair changes, and impairment of wound healing.

DIET AND HEALTH HISTORY

Information about dietary intake and significant variations in weight is a vital part of the history. Dietary intake can be evaluated in several ways, including a diet record, a 24-hour recall,

| BOX 8-2 | CLINICAL MANIFESTATIONS OF NUTRITIONAL ALTERATIONS |

MANIFESTATIONS THAT MAY INDICATE PROTEIN-CALORIE MALNUTRITION

- Hair loss; dull, dry, brittle hair; loss of hair pigment
- Loss of subcutaneous tissue; muscle wasting
- Poor wound healing; decubitus ulcer
- Hepatomegaly
- Edema

MANIFESTATIONS OFTEN PRESENT IN VITAMIN DEFICIENCIES

- Conjunctival and corneal dryness (vitamin A)
- Dry, scaly skin; follicular hyperkeratosis, in which the skin appears to have gooseflesh continually (vitamin A)
- Gingivitis; poor wound healing (vitamin C)
- Petechiae; ecchymoses (vitamin C or K)
- Inflamed tongue, cracking at the corners of the mouth (riboflavin [vitamin B_2], niacin, folic acid, vitamin B_{12}, or other B vitamins)
- Edema; heart failure (thiamine [vitamin B_1])
- Confusion; confabulation (thiamine [vitamin B_1])

MANIFESTATIONS OFTEN PRESENT IN MINERAL DEFICIENCIES

- Blue sclerae; pale mucous membranes; spoon-shaped nails (iron)
- Hypogeusia, or poor sense of taste; dysgeusia, or bad taste; eczema; poor wound healing (zinc)

MANIFESTATIONS OFTEN OBSERVED WITH EXCESSIVE VITAMIN INTAKE

- Hair loss; dry skin; hepatomegaly (vitamin A)

TABLE 8-1 Common Blood and Urine Tests Used in Nutrition Assessment

Test	Comments and Limitations
Serum Proteins	
Albumin or prealbumin	Levels decrease with protein deficiency and in liver failure. Albumin levels are slow to change in response to malnutrition and repletion. Prealbumin levels fall in response to trauma and infection.
Hematologic Values	
Anemia	
Normocytic (normal MCV, MCHC)	Common with protein deficiency
Microcytic (decreased MCV, MCH, MCHC)	Indicative of iron deficiency (can be from blood loss)
Macrocytic (increased MCV)	Common in folate and vitamin B_{12} deficiency
Lymphocytopenia	Common in protein deficiency

MCH, Mean corpuscular hemoglobin; MCHC, mean corpuscular hemoglobin concentration; MCV, mean corpuscular volume.

and a diet history. The diet record, a listing of the type and amount of all foods and beverages consumed for some period (usually 3 days), is useful for evaluating the patient's intake in the critical care setting if the adequacy of intake is questionable. However, such a record reveals little about the patient's habitual intake before the illness or injury. The 24-hour recall of all food and beverage intake is easily and quickly performed, but it also may not reflect the patient's usual intake and has limited usefulness. The diet history consists of a detailed interview about the patient's usual intake, along with social, familial, cultural, economic, educational, and health-related factors that may affect intake. Although the diet history is time consuming to perform and may be too stressful for the acutely ill patient, it does provide a wealth of information about food habits over a prolonged period and provides a basis for planning individualized nutrition education if changes in eating habits are desirable. Other information to include in a nutrition history is listed in Box 8-3.

EVALUATING NUTRITION ASSESSMENT FINDINGS

It is rare for a patient to exhibit a lack of only one nutrient. Nutritional deficiencies usually are combined, with the patient lacking adequate amounts of protein, calories, and possibly vitamins and minerals. A common form of combined nutritional

BOX 8-3 NUTRITION HISTORY INFORMATION

INADEQUATE INTAKE OF NUTRIENTS
- Alcohol abuse
- Anorexia, severe or prolonged nausea or vomiting
- Confusion, coma
- Poor dentition
- Poverty

INADEQUATE DIGESTION OR ABSORPTION OF NUTRIENTS
- Previous gastrointestinal operations, especially gastrectomy, jejunoileal bypass, and ileal resection
- Certain medications, especially antacids and histamine H_2-receptor antagonists (reduce upper small bowel acidity), cholestyramine (binds fat-soluble nutrients), and anticonvulsants

INCREASED NUTRIENT LOSSES
- Blood loss
- Severe diarrhea
- Fistulas, draining abscesses, wounds, decubitus ulcers
- Peritoneal dialysis or hemodialysis
- Corticosteroid therapy (increased tissue catabolism)

INCREASED NUTRIENT REQUIREMENTS
- Fever
- Surgery, trauma, burns, infection
- Cancer (some types)
- Physiologic demands (pregnancy, lactation, growth)

deficit among hospitalized patients is PCM. Two types of PCM are kwashiorkor and marasmus.

Kwashiorkor results in low levels of the serum proteins *albumin, transferrin*, and *prealbumin;* low total lymphocyte count; impaired immunity; loss of hair or hair pigment; edema resulting from low plasma oncotic pressure caused by a loss of plasma proteins; and an enlarged, fatty liver. Marasmus is recognizable by weight loss, loss of subcutaneous fat, and muscle wasting. In the marasmic person, creatinine excretion in the urine is low, an indication of reduced muscle mass. Because PCM weakens muscles, increases vulnerability to infection, and can prolong hospital stays, the health care team should diagnose this serious disorder as quickly as possible so that an appropriate nutrition intervention can be implemented.

DETERMINING NUTRITIONAL NEEDS

A variety of methods can be used in clinical practice to estimate caloric requirements. Indirect calorimetry, a method by which energy expenditure is calculated from oxygen consumption ($\dot{V}O_2$) and carbon dioxide production ($\dot{V}CO_2$), is the most accurate method for determining caloric needs.[14] Indirect calorimetry is useful in those patients suspected to have a high metabolic rate. This test can also analyze substrate use, which can be extrapolated from $\dot{V}O_2$ and $\dot{V}CO_2$ during a steady state of respiration. The respiratory quotient (RQ) is equal to the $\dot{V}CO_2$ divided by the $\dot{V}O_2$. Fat, protein, and carbohydrates each have a unique RQ (0.7, 0.8, and 1.0, respectively). The RQ identifies which substrate is being preferentially metabolized and may provide target goals for calorie replacement.[14] The test can be performed on spontaneously breathing patients and on those who require mechanical ventilation. Some ventilators are constructed so that they can perform indirect calorimetry. However, for most patients, indirect calorimetry requires the use of a metabolic cart, which is not available in all institutions. To maintain accuracy and reliability of measurement, several testing criteria must be met.[15] Information received from the metabolic cart is limited; measurements are conducted over a relatively brief period (often 20 to 30 minutes) and may not be representative of energy expenditure over the whole day.

TABLE 8-2 Estimating Energy Needs

Category	Description	Calories/kg	Calories/lb
Obese	More than 40% over ideal body weight or BMI >30	21	9.5
Sedentary	Relatively inactive individual without regular aerobic exercise; hospitalized patient without severe injury or sepsis	25-30	11-13.5
Moderate activity or injury	Individual obtaining regular aerobic exercise plus routine activities; patient with trauma or sepsis	30-35	13.5-16
Very active or severe injury	Manual laborer or athlete in very active training; patient with major burns or trauma	40	18

Calorie and protein needs of patients are often estimated using formulas that provide allowances for increased nutrient use associated with injury and healing. Although indirect calorimetry is considered the most accurate method to determine energy expenditure, estimates using formulas have demonstrated reasonable accuracy.[16,17] Commonly used formulas can be found in Appendix B. Some rules of thumb are available to provide a rough estimate of caloric needs so that nurses and other caregivers can quickly determine if patients are being seriously overfed or underfed (Table 8-2).

ANTHROPOMETRIC MEASUREMENTS
- Overweight or obesity; underweight (cardiac cachexia)
- Abdominal fat: increased risk of cardiovascular disease with waist measurement >102 cm (>40 inches) for men and >88 cm (>35 inches) for women

BIOCHEMICAL (LABORATORY) DATA
- Elevated total serum cholesterol, low-density lipoprotein (LDL) cholesterol, and triglycerides

CLINICAL FINDINGS
- Wasting of muscle and subcutaneous fat (cardiac cachexia)

DIET OR HEALTH HISTORY
- Sedentary lifestyle
- Excessive intake of saturated fat, cholesterol, salt, or alcohol
- Angina, respiratory difficulty, or fatigue during eating
- Medications that impair appetite (e.g., digitalis preparations, quinidine)

The goal of nutrition assessment is to obtain the most accurate estimate of nutritional requirements. Underfeeding and overfeeding must be avoided during critical illness. Overfeeding results in excessive production of carbon dioxide, which can be a burden in the person with pulmonary compromise. Overfeeding increases fat stores, which can contribute to insulin resistance and hyperglycemia. Hyperglycemia increases the risk of postoperative infections in diabetic and nondiabetic individuals.[18-20] Hyperglycemia is a complication to be avoided if possible.

NUTRITION AND CARDIOVASCULAR ALTERATIONS

Diet and cardiovascular disease may interact in a variety of ways. Excessive nutrient intake—manifested by overweight or obesity and a diet rich in cholesterol and saturated fat—is a risk factor for development of arteriosclerotic heart disease. However, the consequences of chronic myocardial insufficiency can include malnutrition.

NUTRITION ASSESSMENT IN CARDIOVASCULAR ALTERATIONS

A nutrition assessment provides the nurse and other members of the health care team the information necessary to plan the patient's nutrition care and education. Common findings in the nutrition assessment of the cardiovascular patient are summarized in Box 8-4. The major nutritional concerns relate to appropriateness of body weight and the levels of serum lipids and blood pressure. Guidelines for more extensive nutrition assessment are provided on pp. 113-114.

NUTRITION INTERVENTION AND EDUCATION IN CARDIOVASCULAR ALTERATIONS

Myocardial Infarction

Short-Term Interventions. In the early period after a myocardial infarction (MI), nutrition interventions and education are designed to reduce angina, cardiac workload, and risk of dysrhythmia. Meal size, caffeine intake, and food temperatures are some of the dietary factors that are of concern. Small, frequent snacks are preferable to larger meals for patients with severe myocardial compromise or postprandial angina.

If caffeine is included in the diet, its effects should be monitored. Because caffeine is a stimulant, it may increase heart rate and myocardial oxygen demand. In the United States and in most industrial nations, coffee is the richest source of caffeine in the diet, with about 150 mg of caffeine per 180 mL (6 fluid oz) of coffee. In comparison, the caffeine content of the same volume of tea or cola is approximately 50 mg or 20 mg, respectively. Very hot or very cold foods should be avoided because they can potentially trigger vagal or other neural input and cause cardiac dysrhythmias.

Long-Term Changes. The focus of nutritional and lifestyle interventions for the person who has had one MI or is at increased risk for heart disease are directed at primary and secondary prevention strategies. These strategies include weight reduction if the person is overweight and control of cholesterol, fat, and saturated fat intake. Most of the education regarding these changes takes place in the rehabilitation period. However, during the acute phase of recovery, the patient and family may have an interest in learning more about risk reduction.

For the individual who is overweight or obese, gradual loss of weight (0.45 to 0.9 kg [1 to 2 lb] per week) is the goal.[10] Weight loss can be achieved through moderate exercise (with the physician's approval) and reduction of dietary intake by 500 to 1000 kcal/day. A balanced low-fat, low-calorie diet is recommended. There is insufficient evidence to support the efficacy and safety of low-carbohydrate diets for weight loss.[21] The most recent guidelines for the National Cholesterol Education Program (NCEP) Adult Treatment Panel III (ATP III) support lipid-lowering therapy through adoption of a low-saturated-fat and low-cholesterol diet, maintenance of a healthy weight, and regular physical activity.[22] New features include recommendations of low-density lipoprotein (LDL) cholesterol levels of 100 mg/dL as optimal, and increased focus on the metabolic syndrome.[23,24]

Metabolic syndrome, or insulin resistance syndrome, is associated with increased risk for cardiovascular disease and has been recognized as a secondary target of lipid-lowering therapy after LDL cholesterol reduction and recommended use of weight reduction and increased physical activity.[25]

Elevated plasma levels of homocysteine, derived from the essential amino acid *methionine*, are a risk factor for heart disease. Homocysteine can damage the endothelium of the blood vessels, cause proliferation of smooth muscle in the vessel walls, and activate platelets and the coagulation cascade, contributing to thrombus formation. Adequate amounts of folic acid, vitamin B_{12} and B_6 are known to reduce homocysteine levels. Although elevated homocysteine levels remain a risk marker for heart disease, current research does not support treatment with folic acid, B_{12} and B_6 in lowering homocysteine levels to prevent risk of death from cardiovascular disease.[26]

For hypertensive cardiac disease, sodium chloride restriction is recommended. Some individuals have been shown to be more salt sensitive than others, and this salt sensitivity contributes to hypertension. Adoption of a healthy lifestyle is critical for the prevention of high blood pressure and is an indispensable part of the management of those with hypertension.[27] Weight loss of as little as 10 pounds reduces blood pressure. Adoption of the Dietary Approaches to Stop Hypertension (DASH)[28] eating plan also benefits blood pressure. DASH comprises a diet rich in fruits, vegetables, and low-fat dairy products with a reduced content of dietary cholesterol and reduced levels of saturated and total fat. It is rich in potassium and calcium content. Dietary sodium should be reduced to no more than 100 mmol per day (2.4 g of sodium). Alcohol intake should be limited to no more than 1 ounce (30 mL) of ethanol per day in men and no more than 0.5 ounce of ethanol in women.

Heart Failure. Nutrition intervention in heart failure is designed to reduce fluid retained within the body and therefore reduce the preload. Because fluid accompanies sodium, limitation of sodium is necessary to reduce fluid retention. Specific interventions include limiting salt intake, usually to 5 g a day or less, and limiting fluid intake as appropriate. If fluid is restricted, the daily fluid allowance is usually 1.5 to 2 L/day, which includes fluids in the diet and those given with medications and for other purposes (see "Heart Failure" in Chapter 19).

Cardiac Cachexia. Malnutrition is common in patients with heart failure. The term *cachexia* is derived from the Greek words *kakos*, meaning "bad," and *hexis*, meaning "condition." It is characterized by weight loss, anorexia, weakness, early satiety, and edema.[29] Cachexia is seen in a variety of disorders, including cancer and cardiac failure. It is well recognized as an independent predictor of higher mortality in patients with heart failure.[30] Sodium and fluid restriction are appropriate interventions. It is important to concentrate nutrients into as small a volume as possible and to serve small amounts frequently, rather than three large meals daily, which may overwhelm the patient. The individual should be encouraged to consume calorie-dense foods and supplements.

Because the patient is likely to tire quickly and to suffer from anorexia, enteral tube feeding may be necessary. Most commonly used tube feeding formulas provide 1 calorie per milliliter, but more concentrated products are available to provide adequate nutrients in a smaller volume. The nurse must monitor the fluid status of these patients carefully when they are receiving nutrition support. Assessing breath sounds and observing for presence and severity of peripheral edema and changes in body weight are performed daily or more frequently. A consistent weight gain of more than 0.11 to 0.22 kg (0.25 to 0.5 lb) per day usually indicates fluid retention rather than gain of fat and muscle mass.

NUTRITION AND PULMONARY ALTERATIONS

Malnutrition has extremely adverse effects on respiratory function, decreasing surfactant production, diaphragmatic mass, vital capacity, and immunocompetence. Patients with acute respiratory disorders find it difficult to consume adequate oral nutrients and can rapidly become malnourished. Individuals who have an acute illness superimposed on chronic respiratory problems are also at high risk. Nearly three fourths of patients with chronic obstructive pulmonary disease (COPD) have had weight loss.[31] Patients with undernutrition and end-stage COPD, however, often cannot tolerate the increase in metabolic demand that occurs during refeeding. They also are at significant risk for development of cor pulmonale and may fail to tolerate the fluid required for delivery of enteral or parenteral nutrition support. Prevention of severe nutritional deficits, rather than correction of deficits after they have occurred, is important in nutritional management of these patients (see "Acute Respiratory Failure" and "Long-Term Mechanical Ventilator Dependence" in Chapter 24).

NUTRITION ASSESSMENT IN PULMONARY ALTERATIONS

Common findings in nutrition assessment related to pulmonary alterations are summarized in Box 8-5. Guidelines for more extensive nutrition assessment are provided on pp. 113-114. The patient with respiratory compromise is especially vulnerable to the effects of fluid volume excess and must be assessed continually for this complication, particularly during enteral and parenteral feeding.

NUTRITION INTERVENTION AND EDUCATION IN PULMONARY ALTERATIONS

Prevent or Correct Undernutrition and Underweight. The nurse and dietitian work together to encourage oral intake in the undernourished or potentially undernourished patient who

---

BOX 8-5 **COMMON FINDINGS IN THE NUTRITION ASSESSMENT OF THE PATIENT WITH PULMONARY DISEASE**

ANTHROPOMETRIC MEASUREMENTS
Underweight

BIOCHEMICAL (LABORATORY) DATA
Elevated P_{CO_2} related to overfeeding

CLINICAL FINDINGS
Edema, dyspnea, signs of pulmonary edema related to fluid volume excess

DIET OR HEALTH HISTORY
Poor food intake related to dyspnea, unpleasant taste in the mouth from sputum production or bronchodilator therapy; endotracheal intubation preventing oral intake

is capable of eating. Small, frequent feedings are especially important, because a very full stomach can interfere with diaphragmatic movement. Mouth care should be provided before meals and snacks to clear the palate of the taste of sputum and medications. Administering bronchodilators with food can help to reduce the gastric irritation caused by these medications.

Because of anorexia, dyspnea, debilitation, or need for ventilatory support, however, many patients will require enteral tube feeding or TPN. It is especially important for the nurse to be alert to the risk of pulmonary aspiration in the patient with an artificial airway. To reduce the risk of pulmonary aspiration during enteral tube feeding, keep the patient's head elevated at least 45 degrees during feedings, unless contraindicated; keep the cuff of the artificial airway inflated during feeding, if possible; monitor the patient for increasing abdominal distention; and check tube placement before each feeding (if intermittent) or at least every 4 to 8 hours if feedings are continuous.

Avoid Overfeeding. Overfeeding of total calories or of carbohydrate or lipid alone can impair pulmonary function. The production of carbon dioxide ($\dot{V}CO_2$) increases when carbohydrate is relied on as the primary energy source. This is unlikely to be significant in the patient who is eating foods. Instead, it is an iatrogenic complication of TPN, in which glucose is often the predominant calorie source, or occasionally of tube feeding in a patient with a very high carbohydrate formula. Excessive calorie intake can raise $PaCO_2$ sufficiently to make it difficult to wean a patient from the ventilator. A balanced regimen with lipids and carbohydrates providing the nonprotein calories is optimal for the patient with respiratory compromise, and the patient needs to be reassessed continually to ensure that caloric intake is not excessive.[9]

Excessive lipid intake can impair capillary gas exchange in the lungs, although this is not usually sufficient to produce an increase in $PaCO_2$ or decrease in PaO_2.[32] However, the patient with severe respiratory alteration may be further compromised by lipid overdose. If lipid intake is maintained at no more than 2 g/kg/day, lipid excess is rarely a problem. Serum triglyceride levels greater than 400 mg/dL may indicate inadequate lipid clearance and a need to decrease the lipid dosage.

Prevent Fluid Volume Excess. Pulmonary edema and failure of the right side of the heart, which may be precipitated by fluid volume excess, further worsen the status of the patient with respiratory compromise. Maintaining careful intake and output records allows for accurate assessment of fluid balance. Usually the patient requires no more than 35 to 40 mL/kg/day of fluid. For the patient receiving nutrition support, fluid intake can be reduced by using 20% lipid emulsions as a source of calories, by using tube feeding formulas that provide at least 2 calories/mL (the dietitian can recommend appropriate formulas), and by choosing oral supplements that are low in fluid. Some examples are cottonseed oil (Lipomul [Upjohn]), an oral lipid supplement providing 6 calories/mL, and powdered glucose polymers, which increase caloric intake without increasing volume. The nurse plays a valuable role in continually reassessing the patient's state of hydration and alerting other team members to changes that may indicate the need for an increase or decrease in fluid intake.

NUTRITION AND NEUROLOGIC ALTERATIONS

Because neurologic disorders such as stroke and closed head injury tend to be long-term problems, they necessitate good nutritional care to prevent nutritional deficits and promote well-being.

NUTRITION ASSESSMENT IN NEUROLOGIC ALTERATIONS

Nutrition-related assessment findings vary widely in the patient with neurologic alterations, depending on the type of disorder present. Some common assessment findings are listed in Box 8-6. Guidelines for more extensive nutrition assessment are provided on pp. 113-114.

NUTRITION INTERVENTION AND EDUCATION IN NEUROLOGIC ALTERATIONS

Prevention or Correction of Nutritional Deficits

Oral Feedings. Patients with dysphagia or weakness of the swallowing musculature often experience the greatest difficulty in swallowing foods that are dry or thin liquids, such as water, that are difficult to control. For these patients, the nurse, the dietitian, and the speech therapist can work together to plan suitable meals and evaluate patient acceptance and tolerance (see "Stroke" in Chapter 28).

Soft, moist foods are usually easier to swallow than dry ones. An upright sitting position is preferable during meals, if possible, to allow gravity to facilitate effective swallowing. Water and other thin liquids may be especially difficult for the person with swallowing dysfunction to manage. Beverages may be thickened with commercial thickening products, with infant cereal, or with yogurt if the patient has difficulty swallowing thin fluids. Fruit nectars may be better tolerated than thinner juices.

BOX 8-6   COMMON FINDINGS IN THE NUTRITION ASSESSMENT OF THE PATIENT WITH NEUROLOGIC ALTERATIONS

BIOCHEMICAL (LABORATORY) DATA
- Hyperglycemia (with corticosteroid use)

CLINICAL FINDINGS
- Wasting of muscle and subcutaneous fat related to disuse or to poor food intake

DIET OR HEALTH HISTORY
- Poor food intake related to altered state of consciousness, dysphagia or other chewing or swallowing difficulties, or ileus resulting from spinal cord injury or use of pentobarbital
- Hypermetabolism resulting from head injury
- Pressure ulcers

The patient should not be rushed while eating because this may increase the risk of pulmonary aspiration. Providing small amounts of food at frequent intervals rather than larger amounts only at mealtimes may help the patient feel less need to hurry. Suction equipment should be kept available in case aspiration occurs. Dysphagia is frustrating and frightening for the patient and requires much understanding and patience by the family and caregivers.

Tube Feedings or Total Parenteral Nutrition. Patients who are unconscious or unable to eat because of severe dysphagia, weakness, ileus, or other reasons require tube feedings or TPN. Prompt initiation of nutrition support must be a priority in the patient with neurologic impairments. Needs for protein and calories are increased by infection and fever, as may occur in the patient with encephalitis or meningitis. Needs for protein, calories, zinc, and vitamin C are increased during wound healing, as occurs in the trauma patient and the patient with pressure ulcers.

Patients with neurologic deficits are at increased risk for certain complications (particularly pulmonary aspiration) during tube feeding and therefore require especially careful nursing management. Patients of most concern are (1) those with an impaired gag reflex, such as some patients with cerebral vascular accident; (2) those with delayed gastric emptying, such as patients in the early period after spinal cord injury and patients with head injury treated with barbiturate coma; and (3) patients likely to experience seizures. To help prevent pulmonary aspiration, the patient's head is kept elevated, if not contraindicated; when elevation of the head is not possible, administering feedings with the patient in the prone or lateral position allows free drainage of emesis from the mouth and decreases the risk of aspiration (see "Aspiration Pneumonitis" in Chapter 24).

Administering phenytoin with enteral formulas decreases the absorption of the drug and the peak serum level achieved. A problem arises when a patient is receiving continuous enteral feedings and requires anticonvulsant therapy. One way to deal with the problem is stop the feeding for 1 to 2 hours before and after phenytoin administration.[33] Even when this practice is followed, the patient may require a higher phenytoin dosage than normal to maintain therapeutic serum concentrations. When continuous feedings are discontinued and the patient resumes eating meals or receives intermittent enteral feedings, the phenytoin dosage must be adjusted appropriately. Phenytoin levels should be monitored carefully in patients receiving enteral feedings. The infusion rate may need to be increased to account for the time that the enteral feeding is held for phenytoin administration.

Hyperglycemia is a common complication in patients receiving corticosteroids. Regular monitoring of blood glucose levels is an important part of care of such patients. They may require insulin to control the hyperglycemia.

Prompt use of nutrition support is especially important for patients with head injuries because head injury causes marked catabolism, even in patients who receive barbiturates, which should decrease metabolic demands. Head-injured patients rapidly exhaust glycogen stores and begin to use body proteins to meet energy needs, a process that can quickly lead to PCM.

The catabolic response is partly a result of corticosteroid therapy in head-injured patients. However, the hypermetabolism and hypercatabolism are also caused by dramatic hormonal responses to this type of injury.[34] Levels of cortisol, epinephrine, and norepinephrine increase as much as seven times normal. These hormones increase the metabolic rate and caloric demands, causing mobilization of body fat and proteins to meet the increased energy needs. Head-injured patients undergo an inflammatory response and may be febrile, creating increased needs for protein and calories. Improvement in outcome and reduction in complications have been observed in head-injured patients who receive adequate nutrition support early in the hospital course[34,35] (see "Traumatic Brain Injuries" in Chapter 38).

Prevention of Overweight and Obesity. Many stable patients with neurologic disorders are less active than their healthy counterparts and require fewer calories. They may become overweight or obese if given normal amounts of calories for their age and gender. Within 1 or 2 months after spinal cord injury, substantial amounts of muscle atrophy and loss of body mass begin to occur as a result of denervation and disuse. Consequently, body weight and caloric needs decline. Ideal body weights for paraplegics and quadriplegics are less than those for healthy adults of the same height.[36] Stable, rehabilitating paraplegics need approximately 27.9 calories/kg/day, and quadriplegics need approximately 22.7 calories/kg/day.[36,37] Patients with dysphagia or extreme swallowing musculature weakness may rely on very soft, easy-to-chew foods that are usually more dense in calories than are bulky, high-fiber foods. They also may gain unneeded weight that will hamper their care and impede mobility. For these reasons, nutrition education of the patient and family coping with a spinal cord injury should include instruction about prevention of undesirable weight gain. Decreased use of high-fat foods (e.g., milk—such as shakes, ice cream, butter, margarine, pastries) can help to reduce calorie intake. Fruits and vegetables without added fat or sauces are good choices because they are generally low in fat and supply fiber needed to help maintain regular bowel habits.

NUTRITION AND RENAL ALTERATIONS

Providing adequate nutrition care for the patient with renal disease can be extremely challenging. Although renal disturbances and their treatments can markedly increase needs for nutrients, necessary restrictions in intake of fluid, protein, phosphorus, and potassium make delivery of adequate calories, vitamins, and minerals difficult. Thorough nutrition assessment provides the basis for successful nutrition management in patients with renal disease.

NUTRITION ASSESSMENT IN RENAL ALTERATIONS

Some common assessment findings in individuals with renal disease are listed in Box 8-7. Guidelines for more extensive nutrition assessment are provided on pp. 113-114.

BOX 8-7   COMMON FINDINGS IN THE NUTRITION ASSESSMENT OF THE PATIENT WITH RENAL FAILURE

ANTHROPOMETRIC MEASUREMENTS
- Underweight (may be masked by edema)

BIOCHEMICAL (LABORATORY) DATA
- Electrolyte imbalances
- Hypoalbuminemia related to protein restriction and amino acid losses in dialysis
- Anemia related to inadequate erythropoietin production and blood loss with hemodialysis

- Hypertriglyceridemia related to use of glucose as osmotic agent in dialysis and use of carbohydrates to supply needed calories

CLINICAL FINDINGS
- Wasting of muscle and subcutaneous tissue (may be masked by edema)

DIET OR HEALTH HISTORY
- Poor dietary intake related to protein and electrolyte restrictions and alterations in taste

---

NUTRITION INTERVENTION AND EDUCATION IN RENAL ALTERATIONS

Nutritional needs of patients with renal disease are complex. The goal of nutrition intervention is to balance adequate calories, protein, vitamins, and minerals, while avoiding excesses of protein, fluid, electrolytes, and other nutrients with potential toxicity.

Protein. The kidney is responsible for excreting nitrogen from amino acids or proteins in the form of urea. When urinary excretion of urea is impaired in renal failure, blood levels of urea rise. Excessive protein intake may worsen uremia. However, the patient with renal failure often has other physiologic stresses that increase protein or amino acid needs: losses because of dialysis, wounds, and fistulas; use of corticosteroid drugs that exert a catabolic effect; increased endogenous secretion of catecholamines, corticosteroids, and glucagon, all of which can cause or aggravate catabolism; metabolic acidosis, which stimulates protein breakdown; and catabolic conditions, such as trauma, surgery, and sepsis.[38] Patients with acute renal failure need adequate amounts of protein to avoid catabolism of body tissues. Patients with acute renal failure who are malnourished should receive approximately 1.5 to 1.8 g of protein/kg/day to limit catabolism.[9]

Patients with stable acute renal failure without evidence of fluid overload or electrolyte or acid-base disturbances can often be managed conservatively without dialysis. However, when renal function worsens, some form of renal replacement therapy (RRT) is required to maintain homeostasis and prevent metabolic complications. Types of RRT include peritoneal dialysis, intermittent hemodialysis, and continuous arteriovenous (AV) hemofiltration.[38] During hemodialysis, amino acids are freely filtered and lost, but proteins such as albumin and immunoglobulin are not. Proteins and amino acids are removed during peritoneal dialysis, creating a greater nutritional requirement for protein.[39,40] Protein needs are estimated at approximately 1.1 to 1.4 g/kg/day for stable patients receiving hemodialysis or hemofiltration and 1.2 to 1.5 g/kg/day for those receiving peritoneal dialysis.[41] Protein needs may be higher, depending on the level of stress.[42]

Fluid. The patient with renal insufficiency usually does not require a fluid restriction until urine output begins to diminish.

Patients receiving hemodialysis are limited to a fluid intake resulting in a gain of no more than 0.45 kg (1 lb) per day on the days between dialysis. This generally means a daily intake of 500 to 750 mL plus the volume lost in urine. With the use of continuous peritoneal dialysis, hemofiltration, or hemodialysis, the fluid intake can be liberalized.[41] This more liberal fluid allowance permits more adequate nutrient delivery by oral, tube, or parenteral feedings. Enteral formulas containing 1.5 to 2 calories/mL or more provide a concentrated source of calories for tube-fed patients who require fluid restriction. Intravenous lipids, particularly 20% emulsions, can be used to supply concentrated calories for the TPN patient. Intradialytic TPN can be given during hemodialysis sessions to some malnourished patients; it supplies an additional source of nutrients at a time when the fluid can be rapidly removed in dialysis.[39]

Energy (Calories). Energy needs are not increased by renal failure, but adequate calories must be provided to avoid catabolism.[38,41] It is essential that the renal patient receive an adequate number of calories to prevent catabolism of body tissues to meet energy needs. Catabolism reduces the mass of muscle and other functional body tissues, and it releases nitrogen that must be excreted by the kidney. Adults with renal insufficiency need about 30 to 35 calories/kg/day to prevent catabolism and ensure that all protein consumed is used for anabolism rather than to meet energy needs.[41] After renal transplantation, when the patient usually receives large doses of corticosteroids, it is especially important to ensure that caloric intake is adequate (usually 25 to 35 calories/kg/day) to prevent undue catabolism.

Glucose in the peritoneal dialysate may be a significant calorie source and a contributing factor in hypertriglyceridemia. Approximately 70% of the glucose instilled during peritoneal dialysis to serve as an osmotic agent may be absorbed, and this must be considered part of the patient's carbohydrate intake. The glucose monohydrate used in intravenous and dialysate solutions supplies 3.4 calories/g. If the patient receives 4.25% glucose (4.25 g glucose/100 mL solution) in the dialysate, he or she receives the following:

$$42.5 \text{ g/L} \times 70\% \times 3.4 \text{ calories/g} = 101 \text{ calories/L of dialysate}$$

To help control hypertriglyceridemia, only about 30% to 35% of the patient's calories should come from carbohydrates, including glucose from the dialysate, with the major portion of dietary carbohydrate coming from complex carbohydrates.

Consuming at least 20 to 25 g of fiber daily can help to control triglyceride levels. Sources of dietary fiber include cooked dried beans and peas (5 to 7 g of fiber/0.5 cup); cereals containing whole grains (not 100% bran); berries, apples, oranges, pears, corn, and peas (3 to 5 g/serving); whole-grain breads; and most fruits and vegetables other than those listed previously (1 to 2 g/serving). Wheat bran is a good source of fiber (5 to 10 g/oz), but it is also a good source of phosphorus and therefore may cause renal failure to progress more rapidly. For the tube-fed patient, a formula containing dietary fiber can be chosen. To help control hypertriglyceridemia and to provide concentrated calories in minimal fluid, fat may need to supply as much as 40% of the patient's calories.

Hypercholesterolemia is commonly found in patients with renal failure, and unsaturated fats and oils (corn, soybean, sunflower, safflower, cottonseed, canola, and olive) are preferred over saturated fats (primarily from meats and dairy products), which tend to raise cholesterol levels. The necessary restriction of meat, milk, and other protein foods in the diet helps lower intake of cholesterol and saturated fat. Intravenous lipids and the long-chain fats found in most commercial enteral formulas are primarily polyunsaturated. Avoiding alcohol or limiting alcohol intake to occasional small servings also helps to reduce hypertriglyceridemia.

Other Nutrients. Certain nutrients such as potassium and phosphorus are restricted because they are excreted by the kidney. The patient has no specific requirement for the fat-soluble vitamins A, E, and K, because they are not removed in appreciable amounts by dialysis and restriction generally prevents development of toxicity. Patients with end-stage renal disease may have decreased clearance of vitamin A, and levels should be monitored.[9] The needs for several water-soluble vitamins and trace minerals are increased in the dialysis patient because they are small enough to pass freely through the dialysis filter. Vitamin and minerals should be supplemented as necessary.[41]

NUTRITION AND GASTROINTESTINAL ALTERATIONS

Because the gastrointestinal (GI) tract is inherently related to nutrition, it is not surprising that impairment of the GI tract and its accessory organs has a major impact on nutrition. Two of the most serious GI-related illnesses seen among critical care patients are hepatic failure and pancreatitis, and the following discussion focuses on these disorders.

NUTRITION ASSESSMENT IN GASTROINTESTINAL ALTERATIONS

Some common assessment findings in individuals with GI disease are listed in Box 8-8. Guidelines for more extensive nutrition assessment are provided on pp. 113-114.

BOX 8-8   COMMON FINDINGS IN THE NUTRITION ASSESSMENT OF THE PATIENT WITH GASTROINTESTINAL DISEASE

ANTHROPOMETRIC MEASUREMENTS
- Underweight related to malabsorption (from inadequate production of bile salts or pancreatic enzymes), anorexia, or poor intake (because of pain caused by eating)

BIOCHEMICAL (LABORATORY) DATA
- Hypoalbuminemia (may result primarily from liver damage and not malnutrition)
- Hypocalcemia related to steatorrhea
- Hypomagnesemia related to alcohol abuse
- Anemia related to blood loss from bleeding varices

CLINICAL FINDINGS
- Wasting of muscle and subcutaneous fat
- Confusion, confabulation, nystagmus, or peripheral neuropathy related to thiamine deficiency caused by alcohol abuse (Wernicke-Korsakoff syndrome)

DIET OR HEALTH HISTORY
- Steatorrhea

NUTRITION INTERVENTION AND EDUCATION IN GASTROINTESTINAL ALTERATIONS

Hepatic Failure. The liver is the most important metabolic organ, and it is responsible for carbohydrate, fat and protein metabolism, vitamin storage and activation, and detoxification of waste products. Hepatic failure is associated with a wide spectrum of metabolic alterations. Because the diseased liver has impaired ability to deactivate hormones, levels of circulating glucagon, epinephrine, and cortisol are elevated. These hormones promote catabolism of body tissues and cause glycogen stores to be exhausted. Release of lipids from their storage depots is accelerated, but the liver has decreased ability to metabolize them for energy. Moreover, inadequate production of bile salts by the liver results in malabsorption of fat from the diet. Body proteins are used for energy sources, producing tissue wasting. The branched-chain amino acids (BCAAs)—leucine, isoleucine, and valine—are especially well used for energy, and their levels in the blood decline. Conversely, levels of the aromatic amino acids (AAAs)—phenylalanine, tyrosine, and tryptophan—increase as a result of tissue catabolism and impaired ability of the liver to clear them from the blood. BCAAs are not as dependent on liver metabolism as the AAAs are.[43] The AAAs are precursors for neurotransmitters (serotonin and dopamine) within the central nervous system. Rising levels of AAAs cause encephalopathy by promoting synthesis of false neurotransmitters that compete with endogenous neurotransmitters. The damaged liver cannot clear ammonia from the circulation adequately, and ammonia accumulates in the brain. The ammonia may contribute to the encephalopathic symptoms and to brain edema.[9,43]

Monitoring Fluid and Electrolyte Status. Ascites and edema are caused by a combination of factors. Colloid osmotic pressure in the plasma decreases because of the reduction of production of albumin and other plasma proteins by the diseased liver, increased portal pressure caused by obstruction, and renal sodium retention from secondary hyperaldosteronism. To control the fluid retention, restriction of sodium (usually 2000 mg) and fluid (1500 mL or less daily) usually is necessary in conjunction with the administration of diuretics. Patients are weighed daily to evaluate the success of treatment. Physical status and laboratory data must be closely monitored for deficiencies of potassium, phosphorus, zinc, and vitamins A, D, E, and K.[9]

Provision of a Nutritious Diet and Evaluation of Response to Dietary Protein. PCM and nutritional deficiencies are common in patients with hepatic failure. The causes of malnutrition are complex and usually are related to decreased intake, malabsorption, maldigestion, and abnormal nutrient metabolism. Nutrition intervention is individualized and based on these metabolic changes. A diet with adequate protein helps to suppress catabolism and promote liver regeneration. Stable patients with cirrhosis usually tolerate 0.8 to 1 g of protein/kg/day. Patients with severe stress or nutritional deficits have increased needs—as much as 1.2 to 2 g/kg/day.[43] Aggressive treatment with medications, including lactulose, neomycin, or metronidazole, is considered first-line therapy in the management of acute hepatic encephalopathy. In a minority of patients, pharmacotherapy may not be effective, and protein restriction to as little as 0.5 g/kg/day or less may be necessary for brief periods. Chronic protein restriction is not recommended as a long-term management strategy for patients with liver disease.[9,43]

Anorexia may interfere with oral intake, and the nurse may need to provide much encouragement to the patient to ensure intake of an adequate diet. Prospective calorie counts may need to be instituted to provide objective evidence of oral intake. Small, frequent feedings are usually better tolerated by the anorexic patient than are three large meals daily. Soft foods are preferred because the patient may have esophageal varices that may be irritated by high-fiber foods. If patients are unable to meet their caloric needs, they may require oral supplements or enteral feeding. Small-bore nasoenteric feeding tubes can be used safely without increasing risk of variceal bleeding.[43] TPN should be reserved for patients who are absolutely unable to tolerate enteral feeding.[9] Diarrhea from concurrent administration of lactulose should not be confused with feeding intolerance.

A diet adequate in calories (at least 30 calories/kg daily) is provided to help prevent catabolism and to prevent the use of dietary protein for energy needs.[44] In cases of malabsorption, medium-chain triglycerides (MCTs) may be used to meet caloric needs. Pancreatic enzymes may also be considered for malabsorption problems.

BCAA-enriched products have been developed for enteral and parenteral nutrition of patients with hepatic disease. These products may be used in patients with acute hepatic encephalopathy who do not tolerate standard diets or enteral formulas or who are unresponsive to lactulose. However, no substantial evidence exists showing BCAAs are superior to standard formulas in regard to nitrogen balance or as treatment for encephalopathy.[9,43] The patient who undergoes successful liver transplantation is usually able to tolerate a regular diet with few restrictions. Intake during the postoperative period must be adequate to support nutritional repletion and healing; 1 to 1.2 g of protein/kg/day and approximately 30 calories/kg/day are usually sufficient. Immunosuppressant therapy (corticosteroids and cyclosporine or tacrolimus) contributes to glucose intolerance. Dietary measures to control glucose intolerance include (1) obtaining approximately 30% of dietary calories from fat, (2) emphasizing complex sources of carbohydrates, and (3) eating several small meals daily. Moderate exercise often helps to improve glucose tolerance.

Pancreatitis. The pancreas is an exocrine and endocrine gland required for normal digestion and metabolism of proteins, carbohydrates, and fats. Acute pancreatitis is an inflammatory process that occurs as a result of autodigestion of the pancreas by enzymes normally secreted by that organ. Food intake stimulates pancreatic secretion, increasing the damage to the pancreas and the pain associated with the disorder. Patients usually present with abdominal pain and tenderness and with elevations of pancreatic enzymes. A mild form of acute pancreatitis occurs in 80% of patients requiring hospitalization, and a severe form of acute pancreatitis occurs in the other 20%.[45] Patients with the mild form of acute pancreatitis do not require nutrition support and generally resume oral feeding within 7 days. Chronic pancreatitis may develop, and it is characterized by fibrosis of pancreatic cells. This results in loss of exocrine and endocrine function because of the destruction of acinar and islet cells. The loss of exocrine function leads to malabsorption and steatorrhea. In chronic pancreatitis, the loss of endocrine function results in impaired glucose intolerance.[45]

Prevention of Further Damage to the Pancreas and Preventing Nutritional Deficits. Effective nutritional management is a key treatment for patients with acute pancreatitis or exacerbations of chronic pancreatitis. The concern that feeding may stimulate the production of digestive enzymes and perpetuate tissue damage has led to the widespread use of TPN and bowel rest. Recent data suggest that enteral nutrition infused into the distal jejunum bypasses the stimulatory effect of feeding on pancreatic secretion and is associated with fewer infectious and metabolic complications compared with TPN.[46,47]

The results of randomized studies comparing TPN with total enteral nutrition (TEN, or enteral tube feeding) indicate that TEN is preferable to TPN in patients with severe acute pancreatitis, reducing costs and the risk of sepsis and improving clinical outcome.[46-48] Patients unable to tolerate TEN should receive TPN, and some patients may require a combination of TEN and TPN to meet nutritional requirements.[49,50] Low-fat enteral formulas and those with fat provided by MCTs are more readily absorbed than formulas that are high in long-chain triglycerides (e.g., corn oil, sunflower oil).

When oral intake is possible, small, frequent feedings of low-fat foods are least likely to cause discomfort.[47] Alcohol intake should be avoided because it worsens the tissue damage and the pain associated with pancreatitis. Guidelines for the treatment of diabetes (discussed later) are appropriate for the care of the person with glucose intolerance or diabetes related to pancreatitis.

NUTRITION AND ENDOCRINE ALTERATIONS

Endocrine alterations have far-reaching effects on all body systems and affect nutritional status in a variety of ways. One of the most common endocrine problems in the general population and among critically ill patients is diabetes mellitus.

NUTRITION ASSESSMENT IN ENDOCRINE ALTERATIONS

The nutrition assessment process is summarized on pp. 113-114. Because of the prevalence of patients with non–insulin-dependent diabetes mellitus (type 2 diabetes) among the hospitalized population and the association of type 2 diabetes with overweight, the nutritional problems most commonly identified in patients with endocrine alterations are overweight and obesity. Hyperglycemia and hyperlipidemia are other common findings in the individual with diabetes.

NUTRITION INTERVENTION IN ENDOCRINE ALTERATIONS

Nutrition Support and Blood Glucose Control. Patients with insulin-dependent diabetes mellitus (type 1 diabetes) or endocrine dysfunction caused by pancreatitis often have weight loss and malnutrition as a result of tissue catabolism because they cannot use dietary carbohydrates to meet energy needs. Although patients with type 2 diabetes are more likely to be overweight than underweight, they also may become malnourished as a result of chronic or acute infections, trauma, major surgery, or other illnesses.[51] Nutrition support should not be neglected simply because a patient is obese, because PCM can develop in these patients. When a patient is not expected to be able to eat for at least 5 to 7 days or inadequate intake persists for that period, initiation of tube feedings or TPN is indicated. No disease process benefits from starvation, and development or progression of nutritional deficits may contribute to complications, such as pressure ulcers, pulmonary or urinary tract infections, and sepsis, which prolong hospitalization, increase the costs of care, and may even result in death.

Blood glucose control is especially important in the care of surgical patients. Poorly controlled diabetes reduces immune function by impairing granulocyte adherence, chemotaxis, and phagocytosis.[18,19] In surveys of critically ill patients undergoing a variety of elective operations and coronary artery surgery,[18] glucose levels of 206 to 220 mg/dL or higher during the first 24 to 36 postoperative hours were associated with higher rates of nosocomial infection than lower glucose levels.[18,52] To maintain tight control of blood glucose, glucose levels are monitored regularly, usually several times a day, until the patient is stable. Patients unable to tolerate oral diets or enteral feeding may require TPN to meet nutritional requirements during acute illness.[53] Regular insulin added to the solution is a common method of managing hyperglycemia in the patient receiving TPN. The dosage required may be larger than the patient's usual dose because some of the insulin adheres to glass bottles and plastic bags or administration sets. Multiple injections or, preferably, a continuous infusion of regular insulin may be used to maintain tight control of blood glucose in the enterally fed patient.[54] Although further study is needed, the following glucose goals are recommended: 80 mg/dL to 120 mg/dL in critically ill patients in the intensive care unit (ICU) and 100 mg/dL to 150 mg/dL for stable patients on the wards.[53]

In patients receiving enteral tube feedings, the postpyloric route (through a nasoduodenal, nasojejunal, or jejunostomy tube) may be the most effective, because gastroparesis may limit tolerance of intragastric tube feedings.[55] Postpyloric feedings are given continuously because dumping syndrome and poor absorption may occur if feedings are given rapidly into the small bowel. Continuous enteral infusions are associated with improved control of blood glucose. Fiber-enriched formulas may slow the absorption of the carbohydrate, producing a more delayed and sustained glycemic response. Most standard formulas contain balanced proportions of carbohydrate, protein, and fats appropriate for diabetic patients. Specialized diabetic formulas have not shown improved outcomes compared with standard formulas.[54]

Severe Vomiting or Diarrhea in the Patient with Type 1 Diabetes Mellitus. When insulin-dependent patients experience vomiting and diarrhea severe enough to interfere significantly with oral intake or result in excessive fluid and electrolyte losses, adequate carbohydrates and fluids must be supplied. Nausea and vomiting should be treated with antiemetic medication.[55] Delayed gastric emptying is common in diabetes and may improve with administration of prokinetic agents.[55] Small amounts of food or liquids taken every 15 to 20 minutes usually are the best tolerated by the patient with nausea and vomiting. Foods and beverages containing approximately 15 g of carbohydrate include 1/2 cup of regular gelatin, 1/2 cup of custard, 3/4 cup of regular ginger ale, 1/2 cup of a regular soft drink, and 1/2 cup of orange or apple juice. Blood glucose levels should be monitored at least every 2 to 4 hours.

NUTRITION EDUCATION IN DIABETES

Optimal control of blood glucose in type 1 and type 2 diabetes is associated with a decreased risk of development of retinopathy, neuropathy, and other long-term complications.[51] Self-monitoring of blood glucose is essential in maintaining diabetic control, and nutrition is considered the most critical component of diabetes care in achieving blood glucose goals.[56] Meals are based on heart-healthy diet principles, according to which saturated fat and cholesterol are limited and protein accounts for 15% to 20% of total calories. Instead of focusing on the type of carbohydrate, the emphasis is on the total amount of carbohydrate in each meal. Most carbohydrate foods should be whole grains, fruits, vegetables, and low-fat milk; some sucrose-containing foods can be included as part of the total carbohydrate allowance.[57] Evidence-based medical nutrition therapy supports a consistent carbohydrate meal plan for diabetic patients.[20] The meal plan is based on the amount of carbohydrate that is consistent from meal to meal each day. Although exact calorie levels are not specified, a typical daily menu provides approximately 1500 to 2000 calories with a range of three to five carbohydrate foods at each meal, each containing 15 g of carbohydrate.[57]

Careful monitoring of dietary intake and blood glucose levels are essential during critical illness to meet nutritional needs and maintain glucose control. Avoidance of overfeeding limits hyperglycemia and associated complications. Insulin can be adjusted to maintain blood glucose control based on frequent monitoring. Intensive insulin therapy has been shown to reduce mortality rates for critically ill surgical patients.[18] However, it is unknown whether the reduction in mortality is a result of lower blood glucose, the administration of insulin, or a combination of both. It is vital for the dietitian to work closely with the interdisciplinary team to determine feeding methods, appropriate enteral formulas, and the amounts of protein, lipid, and carbohydrate supplied in parenteral nutrition.[20]

ADMINISTERING NUTRITION SUPPORT
NURSING MANAGEMENT OF NUTRITION SUPPORT

Nutrition support is an important aspect of the care of critically ill patients. Maintenance of optimal nutritional status may prevent or reduce the complications associated with critical illness and promote positive clinical outcomes.[58] Critical care nurses play a key role in the delivery of nutrition support and must work closely with dietitians and physicians in promoting the best possible outcomes for their patients.

Nutrition support is the provision of oral, enteral, or parenteral nutrients. It is an essential adjunct in the prevention and management of malnutrition in critically ill patients.[9] The goal of nutrition support therapy is to provide enough support for body requirements, to minimize complications, and to promote rapid recovery. Critical care nurses must have a broad understanding of nutrition support, including the indications, prevention, and management of associated complications.

When possible, the enteral route is the preferred method of feeding. The proposed advantages of enteral nutrition over TPN include lower cost, better maintenance of gut integrity, and decreased infection and hospital length of stay.[9] A review of the literature comparing TEN and TPN indicates that enteral nutrition is less expensive than TPN and is associated with a lower risk of infection.[59] However, other research in a variety of patient populations found no difference in risk of infection between TEN and TPN.[60-62] The GI tract plays an important role in maintaining immunologic defenses, which is why nutrition by the enteral route is thought to be more physiologically beneficial than TPN. Some of the barriers to infection in the GI tract include neutrophils; the normal acidic gastric pH; motility, which limits GI tract colonization by pathogenic bacteria; the normal gut microflora, which inhibit growth of or destroy some pathogenic organisms; rapid desquamation and regeneration of intestinal epithelial cells; the layer of mucus secreted by GI tract cells; and bile, which detoxifies endotoxin in the intestine and delivers immunoglobulin A (IgA) to the intestine. A second line of defense against invasion of intestinal bacteria is the gut-associated lymphoid tissue (GALT).[63] The systemic immune defenses in the GI tract are stimulated by the presence of food within it. In animal models, resting the GI tract by providing TPN contributes to *bacterial translocation*, whereby bacteria normally found in the GI tract cross the intestinal barrier, are found in the regional mesenteric lymph nodes, and give rise to generalized sepsis. However, there is insufficient evidence in humans that TPN causes atrophy of the intestinal mucosa or that enteral nutrition prevents bacterial translocation.[64,65]

Oral Supplementation. Oral supplementation may be necessary for patients who can eat and have normal digestion and absorption but cannot consume enough regular foods to meet caloric and protein needs. Patients with mild to moderate anorexia, burns, or trauma sometimes fall into this category. To improve intake and tolerance of supplements, there are several steps for the critical care nurse to take:

1. Collaborate with the dietitian to choose appropriate products and allow the patient to participate in the selection process, if possible. Milk shakes and instant breakfast preparations are often more palatable and economical than commercial supplements. However, lactose intolerance is common among adults. Many disease processes (e.g., Crohn's disease, radiation enteritis, human immunodeficiency virus [HIV] infection, severe gastroenteritis) can cause lactose intolerance. Individuals with this problem require commercial lactose-free supplements or milk treated with lactase enzyme.

2. Serve commercial supplements well chilled or on ice, because this improves flavor.

3. Advise patients to sip formulas slowly, consuming no more than 240 mL over 30 to 45 minutes. These products contain easily digestible carbohydrates. If formulas are consumed too quickly, rapid hydrolysis of the carbohydrate in the duodenum can contribute to dumping syndrome, characterized by abdominal cramping, weakness, tachycardia, and diarrhea.

4. Record all supplement intake separately on the intake-and-output sheet so that it can be differentiated from intake of water and other liquids.

Enteral Nutrition. Enteral nutrition or tube feedings are used for patients who have at least some digestive and absorptive capability but are unwilling or unable to consume enough by mouth. Patients with profound anorexia and those experiencing severe stress that greatly increases their nutritional needs (caused by major surgery, burns, or trauma) often benefit from tube feedings. Individuals who require elemental formulas because of impaired digestion or absorption or the specialized formulas for altered metabolic conditions (Table 8-3) usually require tube feeding because the unpleasant flavors of the free amino acids, peptides, or protein hydrolysates used in these formulas are very difficult to mask.

Immune-enhancing formulas (IEFs) have emerged as a means to protect and stimulate the immune system. Some of the enterally delivered nutrients that may benefit critically ill patients include fiber, the amino acids glutamine and arginine, the omega-3 fatty acids, and the nucleotide ribonucleic acid (RNA).[66] Fiber is not digested by humans but can be metabolized by gut bacteria to yield short-chain fatty acids, the primary

TABLE 8-3 Enteral Formulas

Formula Type	Nutritional Uses	Clinical Examples	Examples of Commercial Products (Manufacturer)
Formulas Used When GI Tract is Fully Functional			
Polymeric (standard): Contains whole proteins (10%-15% of calories), long-chain triglycerides (25%-40% of calories), and glucose polymers or oligo-saccharides (50%-60% of calories); most provide 1 calorie/mL	Inability to ingest food Inability to consume enough to meet needs	Oral or esophageal cancer Coma, stroke Anorexia resulting from chronic illness Burns or trauma	Ensure (Ross) NuBasics (Nestlé) IsoSource (Novartis) Pediasure (Ross), for children 1-10 years old Boost (Mead Johnson)
High-nitrogen: Same as polymeric except protein provides >15% of calories	Same as polymeric plus mild catabolism and protein deficits	Trauma or burns Sepsis	IsoSource HN (Novartis) Osmolite HN (Ross) Ultracal (Mead Johnson)
Concentrated: Same as polymeric except concentrated to 2 calorie/mL	Same as polymeric but fluid restriction needed	Heart failure Neurosurgery COPD Liver disease	Deliver 2.0 (Mead Johnson) TwoCal HN (Ross) Nutren 2.0 (Nestlé)
Formulas Used When GI Function is Impaired			
Elemental or predigested: Contains hydrolyzed (partially digested) protein, peptides (short chains of amino acids), and/or amino acids, little fat (<10% of calories) or high MCT, and glucose polymers or oligosaccharides; most provide 1 calorie/mL	Impaired digestion and/or absorption	Short bowel syndrome Radiation enteritis Inflammatory bowel disease	Criticare HN (Mead Johnson) Vital High Nitrogen (Ross) Reabilan HN (Nestlé)
Diets for Specific Disease States*			
Renal failure: Concentrated in calories; low sodium, potassium, magnesium, phosphorus, and vitamins A and D; low protein for renal insufficiency; higher protein formulas for dialyzed patients	Renal insufficiency Dialysis	Predialysis Hemodialysis or peritoneal dialysis	Suplena (Ross) Renalcal (Nestlé) Nepro (Ross) Magnacal Renal (Mead Johnson)
Hepatic failure: Enriched in BCAA; low sodium	Protein intolerance	Hepatic encephalopathy	NutriHep (Nestlé) Hepatic-Aid II (B Braun/ McGaw)
Pulmonary dysfunction: Low carbohydrate, high fat, concentrated in calories	Respiratory insufficiency	Ventilator dependence	NutriVent (Nestlé) Pulmocare (Ross)
Glucose intolerance: High fat, low carbohydrate (most contain fiber and fructose)	Glucose intolerance	Individuals with diabetes mellitus whose blood sugar is poorly controlled with standard formulas	Glucerna (Ross) Choice dm (Mead Johnson) Diabeti Source (Novartis) Glytrol (Nestlé)
Critical care, wound healing: High protein; most contain MCT to improve fat absorption; some have increased zinc and vitamin C for wound healing; some are high in antioxidants (vitamin E, betacarotene); some are enriched with arginine, glutamine, and/or omega-3 fatty acids	Critical illness	Severe trauma or burns Sepsis	Immun-Aid (B Braun/McGaw) Impact (Novartis) Perative (Ross) Crucial (Nestlé) TraumaCal (Mead Johnson)

*These diets may be beneficial for selected patients; costs and benefits must be considered.
BCAA, Branched chain–enriched amino acid; COPD, chronic obstructive pulmonary disease; GI, gastrointestinal; MCT, medium-chain triglyceride.

fuel of the colon cells. Glutamine is the major fuel of the small intestinal cells. It is considered a nonessential amino acid, but it becomes conditionally essential in illness. It has been shown to improve mortality and infectious morbidity in critically ill patients.[67-69] Arginine is involved in protein synthesis and is a precursor of nitric oxide, a molecule that stimulates vasodilation in the GI tract and heart and mediates hepatic protein synthesis during sepsis.[66] The omega-3 (n-3) fatty acids, derived primarily from fish oils, are involved in synthesis of eicosanoids (molecules with hormone-like activity)—prostaglandins, prostacyclin, and leukotrienes—and may modulate the inflammatory response.

There are a variety of commercial enteral feeding products, some of which are designed to meet the specialized needs of the critically ill. Products designed for the stressed patient with trauma or sepsis are usually rich in glutamine, arginine, branched amino acids (a major fuel source, especially for muscle), and antioxidant nutrients, such as selenium and vitamins C, E, and A.[70] The antioxidants help to reduce oxidative injury to the tissues (e.g., from reperfusion injury). Despite the fact that IEFs may reduce the incidence of infectious complications, the efficacy and safety of these formulas in critically ill patients has not been clearly demonstrated.[71-74]

Early enteral nutrition, administered with the first 24 to 48 hours of critical illness, has been advocated as a way to reduce septic complications and improve feeding tolerance in critically ill patients. Although studies[75] have shown a lower risk of infection and decreased length of stay with early enteral nutrition, the benefit of early enteral nutrition compared with enteral nutrition delayed a few days remains controversial.[9,76] Current guidelines support the initiation of nutrition support in critically ill patients who will be unable to meet their nutrient needs orally for a period of 5 to 10 days.[9] To avoid complications associated with intestinal ischemia and infarction, enteral nutrition must be initiated only after fluid resuscitation and adequate perfusion have been achieved.[77,78]

Critically ill patients may not tolerate early enteral feeding because of impaired gastric motility, ileus, or medications administered in the early phase of illness. This is particularly true for patients receiving gastric enteral feeding.[79] The assessment of enteral feeding tolerance is an important aspect of nursing care. Monitoring of gastric residual volume is a method used to assess enteral feeding tolerance. However, evidence suggests that gastric residuals are insensitive and unreliable markers of tolerance to tube feeding.[58,80] There is little evidence to support a correlation between gastric residual volumes and tolerance to feedings, gastric emptying, and potential aspiration. Except in selected high-risk patients, there is little evidence to support holding tube feedings in patients with gastric residual volumes less than 400 mL.[80] The gastric residual volume should be evaluated within the context of other gastrointestinal symptoms. Prokinetic agents, including metoclopramide and erythromycin, have been used to improve gastric motility and promote early enteral nutrition in critically ill patients.[81-83]

Enteral Feeding Access. Achievement of enteral access is the cornerstone of enteral nutrition therapy. Several techniques can be used to facilitate enteral access. These include surgical methods, bedside methods, fluoroscopy, endoscopy, air insufflation, and prokinetic agents.[9] Placement of feeding tubes beyond the stomach (postpyloric) eliminates some of the problems associated with gastric feeding intolerance. However, placement of postpyloric feeding tubes is time-consuming and may be costly. Tubes with weights on the proximal end are available; they were originally designed for postpyloric feeding in the belief that that they would be more likely than unweighted tubes to pass spontaneously through the pyloric sphincter. However, randomized trials with the two types of tubes have shown that unweighted tubes are more likely to migrate through the pylorus than weighted tubes.[84] The weights sometimes cause discomfort while being inserted through the nares. Unweighted tubes therefore may be preferable.

After the tube is placed, correct location must be confirmed before feedings are started and regularly throughout the course of enteral feedings. Radiographs are the most accurate way of assessing tube placement, but repeated radiographs are costly and can expose the patient to excessive radiation. After correct placement has been confirmed, marking the exit site of the tube to check for movement is helpful. Alternative methods for confirming tube placement have been researched that attempt to verify placement in the stomach or small intestine. An inexpensive and relatively accurate alternative method involves assessing the pH of fluid removed from the feeding tube; some tubes are equipped with pH monitoring systems. Assessing the pH and the bilirubin concentration in fluid aspirated from the feeding tube is a new method for confirming tube placement.[85]

Location and Type of Feeding Tube. Decisions regarding enteral access should be determined based on gastrointestinal anatomy, gastric emptying, and aspiration risk.[9] Nasal intubation is the simplest and most commonly used route for enteral access. This method allows access to the stomach, duodenum, or jejunum. Tube enterostomy—a gastrostomy or jejunostomy—is used primarily for long-term feedings (6 to 12 weeks or more) and when obstruction makes the nasoenteral route inaccessible. Tube enterostomies may also be used for the patient who is at risk for tube dislodgment because of severe agitation or confusion. A conventional gastrostomy or jejunostomy is often performed at the time of other abdominal surgery. The percutaneous endoscopic gastrostomy (PEG) tube has become extremely popular because it can be inserted at the bedside without the use of general anesthetics. Percutaneous endoscopic jejunostomy (PEJ) tubes are also used.

Postpyloric feedings through nasoduodenal, nasojejunal, or jejunostomy tubes are commonly used when there is a high risk of pulmonary aspiration, because the pyloric sphincter theoretically provides a barrier that lessens the risk of regurgitation and aspiration.[86] However, some studies have demonstrated that gastric feeding is safe and not associated with an increased risk of aspiration.[87-89] Postpyloric feedings have an advantage over intragastric feedings for patients with delayed gastric emptying, such as those with head injury, gastroparesis associated with uremia or diabetes, or postoperative ileus. Delivery of enteral nutrition into the small bowel is associated with improved tolerance,[90] higher calorie and protein intake,[91] and fewer gastrointestinal complications.[79] Small bowel motility returns more quickly than gastric motility after surgery, and it is often possible to deliver transpyloric feedings within a few hours of injury or surgery.[86] Figure 8-3 shows the locations of tube feeding sites.

Assessment and Prevention of Feeding Tube Complications. Nursing care of patients receiving enteral nutrition involves prevention and management of complications associated with the use of feeding tubes. Nursing management of these problems is summarized in Table 8-4. The skin around the feeding tube should be cleaned at least daily and the tape

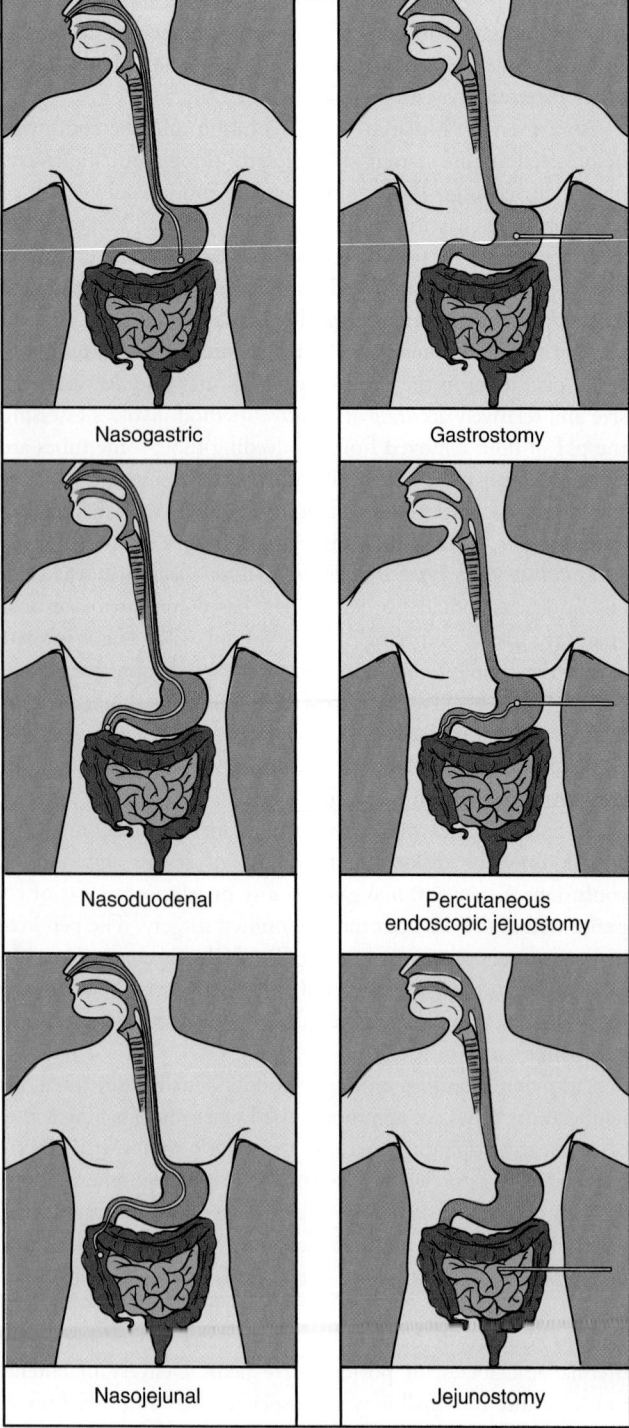

Nasogastric

Gastrostomy

Nasoduodenal

Percutaneous endoscopic jejuostomy

Nasojejunal

Jejunostomy

Figure 8-3 Tube feeding sites.

around the tube replaced whenever loosened or soiled. Secure taping helps to prevent movement of the tube, which may irritate the nares or oral mucosa or result in accidental dislodgment. The tube must be taped in the dependent position to prevent unnecessary pressure and prevent necrosis. Commercially available attachment devices may be used to avoid inadvertent dislodgment.

To prevent mouth dryness, the patient is encouraged to breathe through the nose as much as possible. Frequent mouth care can clear the palate of unpleasant flavors from the formula and clean the teeth, tongue, and oral mucous membranes.

Dressings are used initially around gastrostomy insertion sites. The dressing is changed daily and the skin cleansed with soap and water. If leakage of gastric fluid occurs around a gastrostomy tube, the integrity of the gastrostomy balloon should be evaluated.[92] Karaya powder can be used to protect the peristomal skin from leakage. Fever, redness, purulent drainage, foul odor, or pain at the insertion site may indicate infection. Treatment may include application of a topical antibiotic ointment and daily cleansing with soap and water. Buried bumper syndrome may occur when the gastrostomy device disk, or bumper, is pulled tight against the abdominal wall. To prevent this, it is necessary to minimize tension on the disk. The tube may also become dislodged. A new gastrostomy tube needs to be reinserted within hours to prevent closure of the stoma.

Feeding Tube Occlusion. Regular irrigation helps to prevent feeding tube occlusion. Usually, 20 to 30 mL of warm water every 3 to 4 hours during continuous feedings and before and after intermittent feedings and medication administration can maintain patency.[9] The volume of irrigant may have to be reduced for fluid restriction. Automatic enteral flush pumps are also available. Although cranberry juice or cola beverages are sometimes used in an effort to reduce the incidence of tube occlusion, water is the preferred irrigant because it has been shown to be superior in maintaining tube patency.[93] Tube occlusion may occur as a result of stagnant formula, inadequately crushed pills, or medication interactions with formula. Enteral infusion pumps should be used, and tubes should be flushed before feeding infusions are paused. Liquid medications or elixirs should be used when possible to avoid tube occlusion with pill fragments. The use of pancreatic enzymes in the feeding tube appears to reduce the risk of tube clogging and may be successful in removing a clog after it has formed.[93,94]

Aspiration. Pulmonary aspiration of enteral formulas and subsequent pneumonia is a serious complication of enteral feeding in critically ill patients. Risk factors for aspiration of enteral feeding include decreased level of consciousness, supine position, and swallowing disorders.[95] Figure 8-4 shows the risk factors for aspiration. To reduce the risk of pulmonary aspiration of formula during enteral feeding, the nurse must keep the head of the bed elevated unless contraindicated; temporarily stop feedings when the patient must be supine for prolonged periods; position the patient in the right lateral decubitus position when possible to encourage gastric emptying; use postpyloric feeding methods; keep the cuff of the endotracheal tube inflated as much as possible during enteral feeding, if applicable; and be alert to any increase in abdominal distention.

TABLE 8-4 Nursing Management of Enteral Tube Feeding Complications

Complication	Contributing Factors	Prevention or Correction
Pulmonary aspiration	Feeding tube positioned in esophagus or respiratory tract	Check tube placement before intermittent feeding and every 4-6 hr during continuous feedings by checking the pH of fluid aspirated from the tube (usually gastric juice pH is <3.5).
	Regurgitation of formula	Elevate head to 45 degrees during feedings unless contraindicated; if the head cannot be raised, position the patient in lateral (especially right lateral, which facilitates gastric emptying) or prone position to improve drainage of vomitus from the mouth. Keep cuff of endotracheal or tracheostomy tube inflated during feedings, if possible.
		Metoclopramide may improve gastric emptying and decrease the risk of regurgitation.
		Evaluate feeding tolerance every 2 hr initially, then less frequently as condition becomes stable. Intolerance may be manifested by bloating, abdominal distention and pain, lack of stool and flatus, diminished or absent bowel sounds, tense abdomen, increased tympany, nausea and vomiting, residual volume >200 mL aspirated from an NG tube or >100 mL aspirated from a gastrostomy tube, although a high residual volume in the absence of other abnormal findings may not be grounds for stopping feedings (measuring residual volumes is a controversial practice; see the section on tube occlusion that follows). If intolerance is suspected, abdominal radiographs may be done to check for distended gastric bubble, distended loops of bowel, or air-fluid levels.
Diarrhea	Medications with GI side effects (e.g., antibiotics, digitalis, laxatives, magnesium-containing antacids, quinidine, caffeine, many others)	Evaluate the patient's medications to determine their potential for causing diarrhea, and consult the pharmacist if necessary.
	Hypertonic formula or medications (e.g., oral suspensions of antibiotics, potassium, other electrolytes), which cause dumping syndrome	Evaluate formula administration procedures to ensure that feedings are not being given by bolus infusion; administer the formula continuously or by slow intermittent infusion. Dilute enteral medications well.
	Bacterial contamination of the formula	Use scrupulously clean technique in administering tube feedings; prepare formula with sterile water if there are any concerns about the safety of the water supply or if the patient is seriously immunocompromised; keep opened containers of formula refrigerated, and discard them within 24 hr; discard enteral feeding containers and administration sets every 24 hr; hang formula no more than 4-8 hr unless it comes prepackaged in sterile administration sets.
	Fecal impaction with seepage of liquid stool around the impaction	Perform a digital rectal examination to rule out impaction; see guidelines for prevention of constipation that follow.
Constipation	Low-residue formula, creating little fecal bulk	Consult with the physician regarding the possibility of using a fiber-containing formula.
Tube occlusion	Medications administered by tube that physically plug the tube or coagulate the formula, causing it to clog the tube	If medications must be given by tube, avoid use of crushed tablets; consult with the pharmacist to determine whether medications can be dispensed as elixirs or suspensions. Irrigate tube with water before and after administering any medication; never add any medication to the formula unless the two are known to be compatible.
	Sedimentation of formula. Aspirating gastric contents to measure residual volumes (acidified protein from the formula clots in the tube)	Irrigate tube every 4 hr during continuous feedings and after every intermittent feeding. It has been suggested that aspiration of gastric residuals be avoided with small-bore feeding tubes (8 Fr) and that patient tolerance be assessed by physical examination. If residuals are measured, flush the tube thoroughly after returning the formula to the stomach.
Gastric retention	Delayed gastric emptying related to head trauma, sepsis, diabetic or uremic gastroparesis, electrolyte balance, or other illness	The cause must be corrected if possible. Consult with the physician about use of postpyloric feedings or metoclopramide to stimulate gastric emptying. Encourage the patient to lie in the right lateral position frequently, unless contraindicated.

GI, Gastrointestinal; NG, nasogastric.
Modified from Moore MC: *Pocket guide to nutritional assessment and care*, ed 5, St Louis, 2005, Mosby.

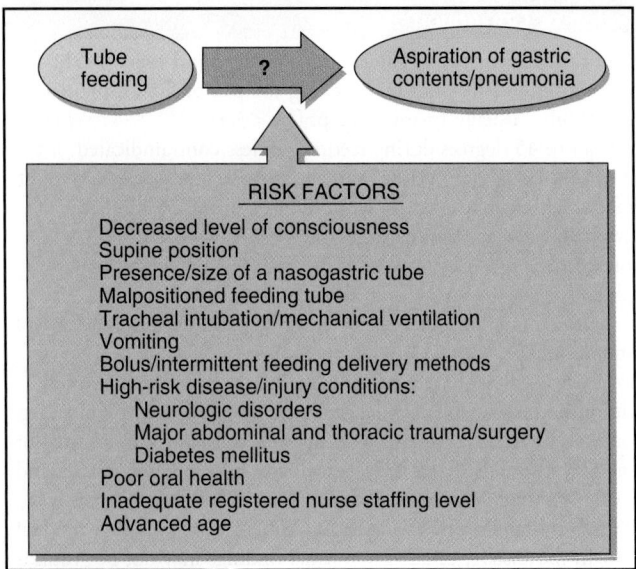

Figure 8-4 Factors that influence aspiration. *(From Metheny NA: Risk factors for aspiration,* JPEN J Parenter Enteral Nutr *26(6 suppl):S26-S33, 2002.)*

Two bedside methods have been used to detect pulmonary aspiration of enteral feeding. One is the addition of blue dye to the enteral formula and observation of the patient for any dye-tinged tracheal secretions, and the other is glucose testing of tracheal secretions to detect the presence of the glucose-containing enteral formula. The glucose oxidase method may cause false-positive reactions if blood is present. It has a low sensitivity when low-glucose formulas are used, and it has questionable specificity.[96] There is no established protocol for blue dye testing. Although it has been used routinely in clinical practice for several years, there is no evidence to support its efficacy or safety. It lacks sensitivity and specificity in ruling out aspiration. Numerous clinical reports of systemic absorption of blue dye and adverse outcomes have been described.[97,98] Glucose oxidase testing and blue food coloring are not recommended as appropriate methods for detecting aspiration of enteral feedings.[97,99]

Gastrointestinal Complications. Diarrhea is common in patients receiving enteral nutrition, with an incidence of 2% to 70%.[100] No single definition has been established for diarrhea. Current definitions include various stool frequencies, volumes, and weights.[101] Diarrhea in enterally fed critically ill patients has many factors. Common causes include medications, malabsorption, formula contamination, or low-fiber formulas. While the cause of diarrhea is being determined, nurses must provide adequate fluid and electrolyte replacement, maintain skin integrity, and administer antidiarrheal agents. To prevent complications, stool must be checked for infection, especially *Clostridium difficile*, before antidiarrheal drugs can be administered.[102] Constipation is a complication of enteral feeding that may result from dehydration, bed rest, opioid administration, or lack of adequate fiber in enteral formulas. Pasty stools are normal in enterally fed patients. Bowel movements should be assessed daily. The nurse must ensure adequate fluid and fiber intake, promote optimal mobility, and administer laxatives and stool softeners as necessary.[103]

Formula Delivery. Careful attention to administration of tube feedings can prevent many complications. Very clean or aseptic technique in the handling and administration of the formula can help prevent bacterial contamination and a resultant infection. When using cans of formula transferred to a feeding container, wash hands and tops of cans before opening, hang enough formula for just 8 hours of infusion, and do not add new formula to formula already hanging. Closed systems that use a prefilled sterile container that can be spiked with the enteral tube are also available.

Tube feedings may be administered intermittently or continuously. Bolus feedings, which are intermittent feedings delivered rapidly into the stomach or small bowel, are likely to cause distention, vomiting, and dumping syndrome with diarrhea. Instead of using bolus feedings, nurses can gradually drip intermittent feedings, with each feeding lasting 20 to 30 minutes or longer, to promote optimal assimilation. The question of which feeding schedule—continuous or intermittent—is superior for critically ill patients remains unanswered.

Adequacy of Enteral Nutrition. Critically ill patients have so many needs for care that it is easy to overlook the importance of nutrition. Many studies have shown that critically ill patients receive considerably less enteral nutrition than required.[104-107] This is a complication unique to enteral nutrition not observed with TPN. The discrepancy in nutritional intake has a variety of causes, including patient factors (e.g., high residual volumes, emesis, abdominal distention), tube-related factors (e.g., occlusion, malposition), and treatment-related factors (e.g., interruptions caused by procedures, airway management, and medications).[105] Inadequate enteral nutrition delivery is also related to physicians' prescribing practices in the ICU.[107] The enteral delivery practices in the ICU and clinicians' concerns about aspiration may lead to inappropriate and prolonged interruptions in enteral feeding. Chest physiotherapy, suspicion of formula in the tracheobronchial secretions, and excessive gastric retention of formula are examples of appropriate reasons for stopping feedings. Enteral nutrition delivery practices that are evidence based are necessary for optimal nutritional outcomes in critically ill patients.

Total Parenteral Nutrition. TPN refers to the delivery of all nutrients by the intravenous route. It is used when the GI tract is not functional or when nutritional needs cannot be met solely through the GI tract. Likely candidates for TPN include patients who have a severely impaired absorption (e.g., short bowel syndrome, collagen vascular diseases, radiation enteritis), intestinal obstruction, peritonitis, or prolonged ileus. Some postoperative, trauma, or burn patients may need TPN to supplement the nutrient intake that they are able to tolerate by the enteral route.

Types of Parenteral Nutrition. TPN involves administration of highly concentrated dextrose (25% to 70%), providing a rich source of calories. These highly concentrated dextrose solutions are hyperosmolar, as much as 1800 mOsm/L, and therefore must be delivered through a central vein.[108] Peripheral parenteral nutrition (PPN) has a glucose concentration of 5% to 10% and may be delivered safely through a peripheral vein. PPN solution delivers nutrition support in a large volume that cannot be tolerated by patients who require fluid restriction. It provides short-term nutrition support for a few days to less than 2 weeks.

Regardless of the route of administration, PPN and TPN provide glucose, fat, protein, electrolytes, vitamins, and trace elements. Although dextrose–amino acid solutions are commonly thought of as good growth media for microorganisms, they actually suppress the growth of most organisms usually associated with catheter-related sepsis, except yeasts. However, because the many manipulations required to prepare solutions increase the possibility of contamination, TPN solutions are best used with caution. They should be prepared under laminar flow conditions in the pharmacy, with avoidance of additions on the nursing unit. Solution containers need to be inspected for cracks or leaks before hanging, and solutions must be discarded within 24 hours of hanging. An in-line 0.22-μm filter, which eliminates all microorganisms but not endotoxins, may be used in the administration of solutions. Use of the filter, however, cannot be substituted for good aseptic technique.

Nursing Management of Potential Complications. Nursing management of the patient receiving TPN includes catheter care, administration of solutions, prevention or correction of complications, and evaluation of patient responses to intravenous feedings. Table 8-5 describes nursing management of TPN complications. Evaluation of the patient's response is discussed later in this chapter.

Because TPN requires an indwelling catheter in a central vein, it carries an increased risk for sepsis and potential insertion-related complications such as pneumothorax and hemothorax. Air embolism is also more likely with central vein TPN. Patients requiring multiple intravenous therapies and frequent blood sampling usually have multilumen central venous catheters, and TPN is often infused through these catheters.

Some clinical studies have reported that catheter-related sepsis is higher with multilumen catheters; others have found no difference compared with single-lumen catheters.[109] Patients requiring multilumen catheters are likely to be very ill and immunocompromised, and scrupulous aseptic technique is essential in maintaining their multilumen catheters. The manipulation involved in frequent changes of intravenous fluid and obtaining blood specimens through these catheters increases the risk of catheter contamination. Peripherally inserted central catheters (PICCs) allow central venous access through long catheters inserted in peripheral sites. This reduces the risk of complications associated with percutaneous cannulation of the subclavian vein and provides an alternative to PPN.[110]

The indwelling central venous catheter provides an excellent nidus for infection. Catheter-related infections arise from endogenous skin flora, contamination of the catheter hub, seeding of the catheter by organisms carried in the bloodstream from another site, or contamination of the infusate. Good hand washing and scrupulous aseptic technique in all aspects of

---

TABLE 8-5 Nursing Management of Total Parenteral Nutrition Complications

Complication	Clinical Manifestations	Prevention or Correction
Catheter-related sepsis	Fever, chills, glucose intolerance, positive blood culture	Use aseptic technique when handling catheter, IV tubing, and TPN solutions. Hang a bottle of TPN no longer than 24 hr, lipid emulsion no longer than 12-24 hr. Use an in-line 0.22-μm filter with TPN to remove microorganisms. Avoid drawing blood, infusing blood or blood products, piggybacking other IV solutions into TPN IV tubing, or attaching manometers or transducers through the TPN infusion line, if possible. If catheter-related sepsis is suspected, remove the catheter or assist in changing the catheter over a guidewire and administer antibiotics as ordered.
Air embolism	Dyspnea, cyanosis, apnea, tachycardia, hypotension, "millwheel" heart murmur; mortality estimated at 50% (depends on quantity of air entering)	Use Luer-Lok connections; use an in-line air-eliminating filter. Have the patient perform a Valsalva maneuver during tubing changes; if the patient is on a ventilator, change tubing quickly at end expiration. Maintain occlusive dressing over catheter site for at least 24 hr after removing catheter to prevent air entry through catheter tract. If an air embolism is suspected, place the patient in left lateral decubitus and Trendelenburg positions (to trap air in the apex of the right ventricle, away from the outflow tract) and administer oxygen and CPR as needed; immediately notify physician, who may attempt to aspirate air from the heart.
Pneumothorax	Chest pain, dyspnea, hypoxemia, hypotension, radiographic evidence, needle aspiration of air from pleural space	Thoroughly explain the catheter insertion procedure to the patient, because when a patient moves or breathes erratically, he or she is more likely to sustain pleural damage. Perform x-ray examination after insertion or insertion attempt. If pneumothorax is suspected, assist with needle aspiration or chest tube insertion, if necessary.

Continued

TABLE 8-5 **Nursing Management of Total Parenteral Nutrition Complications—*cont'd***

Complication	Clinical Manifestations	Prevention or Correction
Central venous thrombosis	Edema of neck, shoulder, and arm on same side as catheter; development of collateral circulation on chest; pain in insertion site; drainage of TPN from the insertion site; positive findings on venography	Follow measures to prevent sepsis; repeated or traumatic catheterizations are most likely to result in thrombosis. If thrombosis is confirmed, remove the catheter, and administer anticoagulants and antibiotics, as ordered.
Catheter occlusion or semi-occlusion	No flow or a sluggish flow through the catheter	If the infusion is stopped temporarily, flush the catheter with saline or heparinized saline. If the catheter appears to be occluded, attempt to aspirate the clot; if this is ineffective, the physician may order a thrombolytic agent such as streptokinase or alteplase (tPA) instilled in the catheter.
Hypoglycemia	Diaphoresis, shakiness, confusion, loss of consciousness	Infuse TPN within 10% of the ordered rate; monitor blood glucose until stable after discontinuance of TPN. If hypoglycemia is present, administer oral carbohydrate; if the patient is unconscious or oral intake is contraindicated, the physician may order an IV bolus of dextrose.
Hyperglycemia	Thirst, headache, lethargy, increased urinary output	Administer TPN within 10% of the ordered rate; monitor blood glucose level at least daily until stable. The patient may require insulin added to the TPN if hyperglycemia is persistent; sudden appearance of hyperglycemia in a patient who was previously tolerating the same glucose load may indicate the onset of sepsis.

CPR, Cardiopulmonary resuscitation; *IV,* intravenous; *TPN,* total parenteral nutrition.
Modified from Moore MC: *Pocket guide to nutritional assessment and care,* ed 5, St Louis, 2005, Mosby.

catheter care and TPN delivery are the primary steps for prevention of catheter-related infections. Other measures to reduce the incidence of catheter-related infections include using maximal barrier precautions (e.g., cap, mask, sterile gloves, sterile drape) at the time of insertion, tunneling the catheter underneath the skin, use of a 2% chlorhexidine preparation for skin cleansing, no routine replacement of the central venous catheter for prevention of infection, and use of antiseptic- or antibiotic-impregnated central venous catheters.[111]

Metabolic complications associated with parenteral nutrition include glucose intolerance and electrolyte imbalance. Slow advancement of the rate of TPN (25 mL/hr) to goal rate allows pancreatic adjustment to the dextrose load. Capillary blood glucose should be monitored every 4 to 6 hours. Insulin can be added to the TPN solution or can be infused as a separate drip to control glucose levels. Rapid cessation of TPN may not lead to hypoglycemia; however, tapering the infusion over 2 to 4 hours is recommended.[112]

Serum electrolytes are obtained on starting TPN. During critical illness, levels should be monitored and corrected daily and then weekly or twice weekly after the patient is more stable. The refeeding syndrome is a potentially lethal condition characterized by generalized fluid and electrolyte imbalance. It occurs as a potential complication after initiation of oral, enteral, or parenteral nutrition in malnourished patients. During chronic starvation, several compensatory metabolic changes occur. The reintroduction of carbohydrates and amino acids leads to increased insulin production. This creates an anabolic

environment that increases intracellular demand for phosphorus, potassium, magnesium, vitamins, and minerals.[113] These metabolic demands result in severe shifts from the extracellular compartment. Increased insulin levels also result in fluid retention. Severe hypophosphatemia, hypokalemia, and hypomagnesemia result in altered cardiac, gastrointestinal, and neurologic function. In particular, hypophosphatemia causes a decrease in 2,3-diphosphosoglycerate (2,3-DPG) and limits the many reactions that require ATP. Hypophosphatemia and other electrolyte deficiencies may lead to respiratory failure, congestive heart failure, and dysrhythmias.

It is important to anticipate refeeding syndrome in patients who may be at risk. Patients with chronic malnutrition or underfeeding, chronic alcoholism, or anorexia nervosa or those maintained NPO for several days with evidence of stress are at risk for refeeding syndrome.[114] In high-risk patients, nutrition support should be started cautiously at 25% to 50% of required calories and slowly advanced over 3 to 4 days as tolerated. Close monitoring of serum electrolytes before and during feeding is essential. Normal values do not always reflect total body stores. Correction of preexisting electrolyte imbalances are necessary before initiation of feeding. Continued monitoring and supplementation with electrolytes and vitamins is necessary throughout the first week of nutrition support.[114]

Lipid Emulsion. Lipids or fat emulsions provide calories for energy and prevent essential fatty acid depletion. In contrast to dextrose–amino acid solutions, intravenous lipid emulsions provide a rich environment for the growth of bacteria and fungi, including *Candida albicans.* Lipid emulsions cannot be filtered through an in-line 0.22-μm filter, because some particles in the emulsions have larger diameters than this. Lipids may be infused into the TPN line downstream from the filter. No other drugs should be infused into a line containing lipids or TPN. Lipid emulsions are handled with strict asepsis, and they must be discarded within 12 to 24 hours of hanging. There is a trend toward mixing lipid emulsions with dextrose–amino acid TPN solutions; these are called 3-in-1 solutions or total nutrient admixtures (TNAs). Consolidating the nutrients in one container is more economical and saves nursing time, although TNA solutions may be less stable.[108]

EVALUATING RESPONSE TO NUTRITION SUPPORT

A multidisciplinary approach is required in evaluating the effects of nutrition support on clinical outcomes. Assessment of response to nutrition support is an ongoing process that involves anthropometric measurements, physical examination, and biochemical evaluation. Daily monitoring of nutritional intake is an important aspect of critical care and is a key element in preventing problems associated with underfeeding and overfeeding. Daily weights and the maintenance of accurate intake-and-output records are crucial for evaluating nutritional progress and the state of hydration in the patient receiving nutrition support. Serum levels of electrolytes, calcium, phosphorus, and magnesium serve as a guide to the amount of these nutrients that must be supplied; blood urea nitrogen and creatinine levels reflect the adequacy of renal function to handle nutrition support; blood glucose is an indicator of the patient's tolerance of the carbohydrate; prealbumin is an indicator of the adequacy of nutrition support; and serum triglyceride concentrations (in patients receiving intravenous lipid emulsions) reflect the ability of the tissues to metabolize the lipids.

It is within the scope of practice for critical care nurses to calculate caloric requirements and analyze daily caloric delivery, advocate for early nutrition support, and minimize feeding interruptions through careful patient assessment and interruption analysis. In addition to monitoring changes in weight and laboratory values, the nurse is the health care team member who has the most constant contact with the patient and who is therefore uniquely qualified to evaluate feeding tolerance and adequacy of delivery.

Summary

Nutrient Metabolism

- The major purposes of metabolism of the energy-yielding nutrients are the production of energy and the formation and preservation of lean body mass.
- Malnutrition can be related to any essential nutrient or nutrients, but a serious type of malnutrition found frequently among hospitalized patients is protein-calorie malnutrition (PCM). It is usually the result of the combined effects of starvation and hypermetabolism.

- The hypermetabolic process results from increased catabolic changes caused by a stressful event.
- Malnutrition is associated with a variety of adverse outcomes: wound dehiscence, pressure ulcers, infections, respiratory failure requiring ventilation, longer hospital stays, and death.

Nutrition and Cardiovascular Alterations

- In the early period after an MI, interventions are aimed at reducing angina, cardiac workload, and the risk of dysrhythmia; meal size, caffeine intake, and food temperatures are monitored closely.
- Interventions in heart failure are designed to reduce fluid retention, thereby reducing the preload.
- Calorie-dense foods and supplements are provided to the patient with cardiac cachexia.

Nutrition and Pulmonary Alterations

- Malnutrition has adverse effects on respiratory function, decreasing surfactant production, diaphragmatic mass, vital capacity, and immunocompetence.
- Because of anorexia, dyspnea, debilitation, or the need for ventilatory support, many patients require tube feeding or TPN.
- It is especially important to be alert to the risks of pulmonary aspiration in the patient with an artificial airway, keeping the hob elevated 45 degrees during feedings, unless contraindicated, and keeping the cuff of the artificial airway inflated during feedings.

Nutrition and Neurologic Alterations

- Patients with dysphagia or weakness of the swallowing musculature often experience the greatest difficulty in swallowing foods that are dry or thin liquids, such as water, that are difficult to control.
- Beverages may be thickened with commercial thickening products, infant cereal, or yogurt; fruit nectars may be better tolerated than fruit juices.
- Prompt use of nutrition support is important for patients with head injuries because head injuries cause marked catabolism, and patients undergo an inflammatory response and may be febrile, increasing the need for proteins and calories.

Nutrition and Renal Alterations

- The goal of intervention is to balance adequate calories, protein, vitamins, and minerals while avoiding excesses of proteins, fluid, electrolytes, and other nutrients with potential toxicities.
- Patients with acute renal failure need adequate amounts of protein to avoid catabolism of body tissues.
- With the use of continuous peritoneal dialysis, hemofiltration, or hemodialysis, the fluid intake can be liberalized. This allows for more adequate nutrient delivery through oral, tube, or parenteral feedings.
- The need for several water-soluble vitamins and trace minerals is increased in dialysis patients because these nutrients are small enough to pass through the dialysis filter.

Nutrition and Gastrointestinal Alterations

- Ascites and edema in the patient with hepatic failure have many causes. There is decreased colloid osmotic pressure in the plasma because of reduced production of albumin and other plasma proteins; increased portal pressure caused by obstruction; and renal sodium retention from secondary hyperaldosteronism.
- Causes of malnutrition in hepatic failure are complex and related to decreased intake, malabsorption, maldigestion, and abnormal nutrient metabolism.
- In the patient with pancreatitis, concern that feeding may stimulate the production of digestive enzymes and perpetuate liver damage has led to the use of TPN and bowel rest.

Nutrition and Endocrine Alterations

- Blood glucose control is especially important in the care of surgical patients.

- Poorly controlled diabetes reduces immune function by impairing granulocyte adherence, chemotaxis, and phagocytosis.

Nursing Management of Nutrition Support

- Whenever possible, the enteral route is the preferred method of feeding because of lower cost, better maintenance of gut integrity, and decreased infection and hospital stay.
- Oral supplementation may be necessary for patients who can eat and have normal digestion and absorption.
- Early enteral nutrition (within the first 24 to 48 hours of critical illness) reduces septic complications and improves feeding tolerance in critically ill patients.
- It is essential to check tube placement before feedings and regularly throughout the course of enteral feedings.
- Continued oral care is provided during the course of the enteral feedings.

Case Study: Patient with Nutritional Issues

⊖volve   Answers to the Case Study Questions can be found on the Evolve web site at http://evolve.elsevier.com/Urden/.

Brief Patient History

Mrs. S is a 49-year-old woman with end-stage cardiomyopathy. She and her husband have been restaurant owners for many years. She is anorexic and finds it difficult to eat solid foods, which is emotionally distressing for her and her family. She has lost 10 pounds in the past month. Mrs. S was placed on the heart transplant list 6 months ago. She has agreed to hospitalization to optimize her medical management and nutritional status.

Clinical Assessment

Mrs. S is admitted to the critical care unit. A central line has been inserted for dobutamine therapy. A nutritional assessment has been completed by the dietician that includes recommendations for frequent, small, calorie-dense, low-sodium feedings.

Diagnostic Procedures

Mrs. S is 5 feet 2 inches tall and weighs 90 pounds. Her vital signs are as follows: blood pressure of 100/60 mm Hg, heart rate of 80 beats/min (sinus rhythm), respiratory rate of 20 breaths/min, and temperature of 98.2° F.

Serum laboratory findings are as follows: hemoglobin level of 8.3 g/dL, prealbumin level of 14 mg/dL, sodium level of 125 mmol/L, potassium level of 3.3 mmol/L, chloride level of 94 mmol/L, carbon dioxide concentration of 26 mEq/L, calcium level of 8 mg/dL, magnesium level of 1.5 mg/dL, and B-type natriuretic peptide concentration of 500 pg/mL.

Medical Diagnosis

Mrs. S is diagnosed with cachexia resulting from end-stage cardiomyopathy.

Questions

1. What major outcomes do you expect to achieve for this patient?
2. What problems or risks must be managed to achieve these outcomes?
3. What interventions must be initiated to monitor, prevent, manage, or eliminate the problems and risks identified?
4. What interventions should be initiated to promote optimal functioning, safety, and well-being of the patient?
5. What possible learning needs do you anticipate for this patient?
6. What cultural and age-related factors may have a bearing on the patient's plan of care?

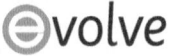 Be sure to check out the bonus material, including free self-assessment exercises, on the Evolve web site at http://evolve.elsevier.com/Urden/.

References

1. Huang YC et al: Nutritional status of mechanically ventilated critically ill patients: comparison of different types of nutrition, *Clin Nutr* 19(2): 101-107, 2000.
2. Kelly IE et al: Still hungry in hospital: identifying malnutrition in acute hospital admissions, *Q J Med* 93:93, 2000.
3. Waitzberg DL et al: Hospital malnutrition: the Brazilian national survey (IBRANUTRI): a study of 4000 patients, *Nutrition* 17(7):573-580, 2001.
4. Pirlich M et al: Prevalence of malnutrition in hospitalized medical patients: impact of underlying disease, *Dig Dis* 21(3):245-251, 2003.
5. Kyle UG et al: Prevalence of malnutrition in 1760 patients at hospital admission: a controlled population study of body composition, *Clin Nutr* 22(5):473-481, 2003.

6. Braunschweig C et al: Impact of declines in nutritional status on outcomes in adult patients hospitalized for more than 7 days, *J Am Diet Assoc* 100:1316-1322, 2000.

7. Mathus-Vliegen EMH: Nutritional status, nutrition and pressure ulcers, *Nutr Clin Pract* 16: 286-291, 2001.

8. Rubinson L et al: Low caloric intake is associated with nosocomial bloodstream infections in patients in the medical intensive care unit, *Crit Care Med* 32:350-357, 2004.

9. August D et al: Guidelines for the use of parenteral and enteral nutrition in adult and pediatric patients, *JPEN J Parenter Enteral Nutr*26: 33SA–41SA, 65SA–70SA, 78SA–81SA, 90SA–91SA, 18SA-19SA, 2002.

10. National Heart, Lung, and Blood Institute: *Clinical guidelines on the identification, evaluation, and treatment of overweight and obesity in adults,* Washington, DC, 1998, NIH.

11. Gianino S, St John RE: Nutritional assessment of the patient in the intensive care unit, *Crit Care Nurs Clin North Am* 5:1-16, 1993.

12. Ravasco P et al: A critical approach to nutritional assessment in critically ill patients, *Clin Nutr* 21(1):73-77, 2002.

13. Raguso C et al: The role of visceral proteins in the nutritional assessment of intensive care unit patients, *Curr Opin Nutr Metab Care* 6:211-216, 2003.

14. Fung EB: Estimating energy expenditure in critically ill adults and children, *AACN Clin Issues* 11(4):480-497, 2000.

15. McCarthy MS: Use of indirect calorimetry to optimize nutrition support and assess physiologic dead space in the mechanically ventilated ICU patient: a case study approach, *AACN Clin Issues* 11(4):619-630, 2000.

16. Cheng CH et al: Measured versus estimated energy expenditure in mechanically ventilated critically ill patients, *Clin Nutr* 21(2):165-172, 2002.

17. Alberda CL et al: Energy requirements in critically ill patients: how close are our estimates? *Nutr Clin Pract* 17(1):38-42, 2002.

18. Van den Berghe, G et al: Intensive insulin therapy in critically ill patients, *N Engl J Med* 345:1359-1367, 2001.

19. Rassias AJ et al: Insulin increases neutrophil count and phagocytic capacity after cardiac surgery, *Anesth Analg* 94:1113-1119, 2002.

20. Clement S et al: Management of diabetes and hyperglycemia in hospitals, *Diabetes Care* 27:553-591, 2004.

21. Bravata DM et al: Efficacy and safety of low-carbohydrate diets: a systematic review, *JAMA* 289:1837-1850, 2003.

22. Executive summary on the third report of the National Cholesterol Education Program (NCEP) expert panel on detection, evaluation, and treatment of high blood cholesterol in adults (Adult Treatment Panel III), *JAMA* 285:248-2497, 2001.

23. Lipsy RJ: The National Cholesterol Education Program Adult Treatment Panel III guidelines, *J Managed Care Pharm* 9(1 suppl):2-5, 2003.

24. Brewer HB: New features of the National Cholesterol Education Program Adult Treatment Panel III lipid-lowering guidelines, *Clin Cardiol* 26: 19-24, 2003.

25. Ginsberg HN: Treatment for patients with the metabolic syndrome, *Am J Cardiol* 91(7):29-39, 2003.

26. Ebbing M et al: Mortality and cardiovasculuar events in patients treated with homocysteine-lowering B vitamins after coronary angiography, *JAMA* 300:795-804, 2008.

27. Chobanian AV et al: Seventh report of the Joint National Committee on Prevention, Detection, Evaluation, and Treatment of High Blood Pressure, *Hypertension* 42(6):1206-1252, 2003.

28. Sacks FM et al: Effects of blood pressure of reduced dietary sodium and the dietary approaches to stop hypertension (DASH) diet, *N Engl J Med* 344(1):3-10, 2001.

29. Barber MD: The pathophysiology and treatment of cancer cachexia, *Nutr Clin Pract* 17:203-209, 2002.

30. Gerasimos S et al: Leptin levels in cachectic heart failure patients, *Int J Cardiol* 76:117-122, 2000.

31. Cochrane WU, Afolabi OA: Investigation into the nutritional status, dietary intake and smoking habits of patients with chronic obstructive pulmonary disease, *J Hum Nutr Diet* 17(1):3-11, 2004.

32. Driscoll DF: Intravenous lipid emulsions: 2001, *Nutr Clin Pract* 16: 215-218, 2001.

33. Dickerson RN et al: Adverse effects from inappropriate medication administration via a jejunostomy feeding tube, *Nutr Clin Pract* 18:402-405, 2003.

34. Donaldson J et al: Nutrition strategies in neurotrauma, *Crit Care Nurs Clin North Am* 12(4):465-475, 2000.

35. Taylor SJ et al: Prospective, randomized, controlled trial to determine the effect of early enhanced enteral nutrition on clinical outcome in mechanically ventilated patients suffering head injury, *Crit Care Med* 27(11): 2525-2531, 1999.

36. Cox SA et al: Energy expenditure after spinal cord injury: an evaluation of stable rehabilitating patients, *J Trauma* 25:419, 1985.

37. Aquilani R et al: Energy expenditure and nutritional adequacy of rehabilitation paraplegics with asymptomatic bacteriuria and pressure sores, *Spinal Cord* 39:437-441, 2001.

38. Kapadi FN et al: Special issues in the patient with renal failure, *Crit Care Clin* 19:233-251, 2003.

39. Charney P, Charney D: Nutrition support in renal failure, *Nutr Clin Pract* 17:226-236, 2002.

40. Case KO et al: Nutrition support in the critically ill patient, *Crit Care Nurs Q* 22(4):75-89, 2000.

41. Wiggins KL, Harvey KS: A review of guidelines for nutrition care of renal patients, *J Renal Nutr* 12(3):190-196, 2002.

42. Scheinkestel CD et al: Prospective randomized trial to assess caloric and protein needs of critically ill, anuric, ventilated patients requiring continuous renal replacement therapy, *Nutrition* 19:909-916, 2003.

43. Patton KM, Aranda-Michel J: Nutritional aspects in liver disease and liver transplantation, *Nutr Clin Pract* 17:332-340, 2002.

44. Florez DA, Aranda-Michel J: Nutritional management of acute and chronic liver disease, *Semin Gastrointest Dis* 13(3):169-178, 2002.

45. Khokhar AS, Seidner DL: The pathophysiology of pancreatitis, *Nutr Clin Pract* 19:5-15, 2004.

46. Avgerinos C et al: Nutritional support in acute pancreatitis, *Dig Dis* 21(3): 214-219, 2003.

47. Russell MK: Acute pancreatitis: a review of pathophysiology and nutrition management, *Nutr Clin Pract* 19:16-24, 2004.

48. Al-Omran M et al: Enteral versus parenteral nutrition for acute pancreatitis, *Cochrane Database Syst Rev* 1:CD002837, 2003.

49. Dejong CH et al: Nutrition in patients with acute pancreatitis, *Curr Opin Crit Care* 7(4):251-256, 2001.

50. Abou-Assi S, O'Keefe SJ: Nutrition support during acute pancreatitis, *Nutrition* 18:938-943, 2002.

51. Woolf SH et al: Controlling blood glucose levels in patients with type 2 diabetes mellitus: an evidence-based policy statement by the American Academy of Family Physicians and American Diabetes Association, *J Fam Pract* 49(5):453-460, 2000.

52. Umpierrez GE et al: Hyperglycemia: an independent marker of in-hospital mortality in patients with undiagnosed diabetes, *J Clin Endocrinol Metab* 87:978-982, 2002.

53. McMahon MM: Management of parenteral nutrition in acutely ill patients with hyperglycemia, *Nutr Clin Pract* 19:120-128, 2004.

54. Charney P, Hertzler SR: Management of blood glucose and diabetes in the critically ill patient receiving enteral feeding, *Nutr Clin Pract* 19:129-136, 2004.

55. Jones MP: Management of diabetic gastroparesis, *Nutr Clin Pract* 19:145-153, 2004.

56. Paul E: New interventions in diabetes with medical nutrition therapy, *Case Manager* 13(2):78-81, 2002.

57. American Diabetes Association: Evidence-based nutrition principles and recommendations for the treatment and prevention of diabetes and related complications [position statement], *Diabetes Care* 26(suppl 1):S51-S61, 2003.

58. Swanson RW, Winkelman C: Special feature: exploring the benefits and myths of enteral feeding in the critically ill, *Crit Care Nurs Q* 24(4):67-74, 2002.

59. Braunschweig CL et al: Enteral compared with parenteral nutrition: a meta-analysis, *Am J Clin Nutr* 74(4):534-542, 2001.

60. Bozzetti F et al: Perioperative total parenteral nutrition in malnourished, gastrointestinal cancer patients: a randomized, clinical trial, JPEN *J Parenter Enteral Nutr* 24:7-14, 2000.

61. Braga ML et al: Early postoperative enteral nutrition improves oxygenation and reduces costs compared with parenteral nutrition, *Crit Care Med* 29(2):242-248, 2001.

62. Woodcock NP et al: Enteral versus parenteral nutrition: a pragmatic study, *Nutrition* 17(1):1-12, 2001.

63. Langkamp-Henken B: If the gut works, use it: but what if you can't? *Nutr Clin Pract* 18:449-450, 2003.

64. Jeejeebhoy KN: Total parenteral nutrition: potion or poison? *Am J Clin Nutr* 74(2):160-163, 2001.

65. Alpers DH: Enteral feeding and gut atrophy, *Curr Opin Nutr Metab Care* 5:679-683, 2002.

66. Schloerb PR: Immune-enhancing diets: products, components, and their rationales, *JPEN J Parenter Enteral Nutr* 25(2):S3-S7, 2001.

67. Kelly D, Wischmeyer PE: Role of L-glutamine in critical illness: new insights, *Curr Opin Nutr Metab Care* 6:217-222, 2003.

68. Wernerman J: Glutamine and acute illness, *Curr Opin Crit Care* 9:279-285, 2003.

69. Boelens PG et al: Glutamine alimentation in the catabolic state, *J Nutr* 131:2569S-2577S, 2001.

70. Preiser J-C et al: Enteral feeding with a solution enriched with antioxidant vitamins A, C, and E enhances the resistance to oxidative stress, *Crit Care Med* 28(12):3828-3832, 2000.

71. Heyland DK et al: Should immunonutrition become routine in critically ill patients? A systematic review of the evidence, *JAMA* 286(8):944-953, 2001.

72. Heyland DK: Immunonutrition in the critically ill patient: putting the cart before the horse? *Nutr Clin Pract* 17:267-272, 2002.

73. Montejo JC et al: Immunonutrition in the intensive care unit: a systematic review and consensus statement, *Clin Nutr* 22(3):221-233, 2003.

74. Stechmiller JK et al: Arginine immunonutrition in critically ill patients: a clinical dilemma, *Am J Crit Care Nurs* 13(1):17-23, 2004.

75. Marik PE, Zaloga GP: Early enteral nutrition in acutely ill patients: a systematic review, *Crit Care Med* 29(12): 2264-2270, 2001.

76. Jeejeebhoy KN: Enteral feeding, *Curr Opin Clin Nutr Metab Care* 5: 695-698, 2002.

77. Zaloga GP, Roberts PR, Marik PE: Feeding the hemodynamically unstable patient: a critical evaluation of the evidence, *Nutr Clin Pract* 18: 285-293, 2003.

78. Moore FA, Weisbrodt NW: Gut dysfunction and intolerance to enteral nutrition in critically ill patients, *Nestle Nutr Workshop Ser Clin Perform Programme* 8:149-170, 2003.

79. Montejo JC et al: Multicenter, prospective, randomized, single-blind study comparing the efficacy and gastrointestinal complications of early jejunal feeding with early gastric feeding in critically ill patients, *Crit Care Med* 30(4):796-800, 2002.

80. McClave SA, Snider HL: Clinical use of gastric residual volumes as a monitor for patients on enteral tube feeding, *JPEN J Parenter Enteral Nutr* 26(suppl 6):S43-S50, 2002.

81. Berne JD et al: Erythromycin reduces delayed gastric emptying in critically ill trauma patients: a randomized, controlled trial, *J Trauma* 53(3): 422-425, 2002.

82. Booth CM et al: Gastrointestinal promotility drugs in the critical care setting: a systematic review of the evidence, *Crit Care Med* 30(7): 1429-1435, 2002.

83. Doherty WL, Winter B: Prokinetic agents in critical care, *Crit Care* 7(3): 206-208, 2003.

84. Lord LM et al: Comparison of weighted vs. unweighted enteral feeding tubes for efficacy of transpyloric intubation, *JPEN J Parenter Enteral Nutr* 17(3):271-273, 1993.

85. Metheny NA et al: pH and concentration of bilirubin in feeding tube aspirates as predictors of tube placement, *Nurs Res* 48:189, 1999.

86. Heyland DK et al: Effect of postpyloric feeding on gastroesophageal regurgitation and pulmonary microaspiration: results of a randomized controlled trial, *Crit Care Med* 29(8):1495-1501, 2001.

87. Esparza J et al: Equal aspiration rates in gastrically and transpylorically fed critically ill patients, *Intensive Care Med* 27:660-664, 2001.

88. Neumann DA, DeLegge MH: Gastric versus small-bowel tube feeding in the intensive care unit: a prospective comparison of efficacy, *Crit Care Med* 30(7):1436-1438, 2002.

89. Marik PE, Zaloga GR: Gastric versus post-pyloric feeding: a systematic review, *Crit Care* 7(3):R46-R51, 2003.

90. Davies AR et al: Randomized comparison of nasojejunal and nasogastric feeding in critically ill patients, *Crit Care Med* 30(3):586-590, 2002.

91. Kearns PJ et al: The incidence of ventilator-associated pneumonia and success in nutrient delivery with gastric versus small intestine feeding: a randomized clinical trial, *Crit Care Med* 28(6):1742-1746, 2000.

92. Grant MJC, Martin S: Delivery of enteral nutrition, *AACN Clin Issues* 11(4):507-516, 2000.

93. Lord LM: Restoring and maintaining patency of enteral feeding tubes, *Nutr Clin Pract* 18:422-426, 2003.

94. Bourgault AM et al: Prophylactic pancreatic enzymes to reduce feeding tube occlusions, *Nutr Clin Pract* 18:398-401, 2003.

95. Metheny NA: Risk factors for aspiration, *JPEN J Parenter Enteral Nutr* 26(6 suppl):S26-S33, 2002.

96. Metheny NA et al: A survey of bedside methods used to detect pulmonary aspiration of enteral formula in intubated tube-fed patients, *Am J Crit Care* 8:160-169, 1999.

97. Maloney JP, Ryan TA: Detection of aspiration in enterally fed patients: a requiem for bedside monitors of aspiration, *JPEN J Parenter Enteral Nutr* 26(6):S34-S41, 2002.

98. Lucarelli MR et al: Toxicity of food drug and cosmetic blue no. 1 dye in critically ill patients, *Chest* 125(2):793-795, 2004.

99. McClave SA et al: North American summit on aspiration in the critically ill patient: consensus statement, *JPEN J Parenter Enteral Nutr* 26(6): S80-S85, 2002.

100. Eisenberg P: An overview of diarrhea in the patient receiving enteral nutrition, *Gastroenterol Nurs* 25(3):95-104, 2002.

101. Wiesen P et al: Diarrhoea in the critically ill, *Curr Opin Crit Care* 12(2): 149-154, 2006.

102. Bernard AC et al: Defining and assessing tolerance in enteral nutrition, *Nutr Clin Pract* 19(5):481-486, 2004.

103. Mostafa SM et al: Constipation and its implications in the critically ill patient, *Br J Anaesth* 91(6):815-819, 2003.

104. Elpern EH et al: Outcomes associated with enteral tube feedings in a medical intensive care unit, *Am J Crit Care* 13:221-227, 2004.

105. Engel JM et al: Enteral nutrition practice in a surgical intensive care unit: what proportion of energy expenditure is delivered enterally? *Clin Nutr* 22(2):187-192, 2003.

106. Krishnan JA et al: Caloric intake in medical ICU patients: consistency of care with guidelines and relationship to clinical outcomes, *Chest* 124:297-305, 2003.

107. DeJonghe B et al: A prospective survey of nutritional support practices in intensive care unit patients: What is prescribed? What is delivered? *Crit Care Med* 29(1):8-12, 2001.

108. Worthington P et al: Parenteral nutrition for the acutely ill, *AACN Clin Issues* 11(4):559-579, 2000.

109. Dobbins BM et al: Each lumen is a potential source of central venous catheter-related bloodstream infection, *Crit Care Med* 31(6):1688-1690, 2003.

110. Orr ME: The peripherally inserted central catheter: what are the current indications for its use? *Nutr Clin Pract* 17:99-104, 2002.

111. O'Grady NP et al: Guidelines for the prevention of intravascular catheter-related infections, *Infect Control Hosp Epidemiol* 23(12):759-769, 2002.

112. Speerhas R et al: Maintaining normal blood glucose concentrations with total parenteral nutrition: is it necessary to taper total parenteral nutrition? *Nutr Clin Pract* 18:414-416, 2003.

113. Crook MA et al: The importance of the refeeding syndrome, *Nutrition* 17:632-637, 2001.

114. Hearing SD: Refeeding syndrome, *BMJ* 328(7445):908-909, 2004.

Pain and Pain Management

Despite national and international efforts, guidelines, standards of practice, position statements, and many important discoveries in the field of pain management in the past 3 decades, pain remains a major stressor for patients in critical care settings.[1] Because many sources of pain are present in critical care settings, such as acute illness, surgery, trauma, invasive equipment, and nursing and medical interventions,[2,3] it is not surprising that more than 50% of critically ill patients experience moderate to severe pain.[4-6] In a large, international study involving 5957 critically ill adults, the Thunder Project II sponsored by the American Association of Critical-Care Nurses (AACN), turning, drain removal, wound care, and endotracheal suctioning were described as painful procedures of moderate to severe intensity.[5] Despite these findings, pain remains undertreated in most critically ill patients.[4,6-9] In the Thunder Project II, less than 20% of critically ill adults received opiates before and during painful procedures.[9] Poor treatment of acute pain may lead to the development of serious complications[10,11] and chronic pain syndromes,[12,13] which may seriously impact the patient's functioning, quality of life, and well-being. Such evidence reinforces the importance of providing attention to pain in this specific context of care.

IMPORTANCE OF PAIN ASSESSMENT

Pain is an important problem in critical care, and its detection is a priority. To detect pain, it has to be adequately assessed. Because pain is recognized as a subjective experience,[14] the patient's self-report is the most valid measure for pain and should be obtained as often as possible. Unfortunately in critical care, many factors alter verbal communication with patients: the administration of sedative agents, mechanical ventilation, and the patient's change in level of consciousness.[2,3,15] These obstacles make pain assessment more complex. Nevertheless, except for being unable to speak, many mechanically ventilated patients can communicate that they are in pain by using head nodding, grimacing, or hand motions or by seeking attention with other movements.[4,16]

Pain scales have been used with postoperative mechanically ventilated patients who were asked to point on the pain intensity scale to communicate their pain.[5,17,18] However, in a study of mechanically ventilated adults with various diagnoses

(trauma, surgical, or medical), only one third of mechanically ventilated patients were able to use a pain intensity scale.[19] With a greater degree of critical illness, providing a pain intensity self-report becomes more difficult because it requires concentration and energy. When the patient is unable to express himself or herself in any way, observable, clustered behavioral and physiologic indicators become unique indices for pain assessment and are part of clinical guidelines and recommendations developed in North America.[20-23] Many health care agencies have increased their vigilance regarding the patient's pain and its management, including designating pain assessment as the fifth vital sign, as stated by the American Pain Society in 1995. Pain is a frequent diagnosis in critical care, and there is increased emphasis on the professional responsibility to manage the patient's pain effectively. The critical care nurse must understand the mechanisms, assessment process, and appropriate therapeutic measures for managing pain.

This chapter provides nurses with a better understanding of the physiology of pain. It also demonstrates indicators that can be used for pain assessment and pain management in critically ill patients.

DEFINITION AND DESCRIPTION OF PAIN

Pain is described as an unpleasant sensory and emotional experience associated with actual or potential tissue damage.[14] This definition emphasizes its subjective and multidimensional nature. Its subjective characteristic implies that pain is whatever the person experiencing it says it is and that pain exists whenever he or she says it does.[24] This definition implies that the patient is able to self-report. In the critical care context, many patients are unable to self-report.

Infants represent a unique group of vulnerable patients who cannot self-report their pain and therefore communicate by behaviors. Clinicians must be attuned to infant's behaviors for pain-related clinical assessment.[25] This same principle applies to any nonverbal population, for whom behavioral alterations caused by pain are valuable forms of self-report and should be considered as alternative measures of pain.[25] Based on this idea, pain assessment must be designed to conform to the patient's communication capabilities, and this is consistent with the fact that pain is multidimensional.

COMPONENTS OF PAIN

The experience of pain includes sensory, affective, cognitive, behavioral, and physiologic components[26,27]:

The sensory component is the perception of many characteristics of pain, such as intensity, location, and quality.

The affective component includes negative emotions such as unpleasantness, anxiety, and fear that may be associated with the experience of pain.

The cognitive component refers to the interpretation of pain by the person who experiences it.

The behavioral component includes the strategies used by the person to express, avoid, or control pain.

The physiologic component refers to nociception and the stress response.

TYPES OF PAIN

Pain can be acute or chronic, with different sensations related to the origin of the pain.

Acute Pain. Acute pain has a short duration, and it usually corresponds to the healing process (30 days) but should not exceed 6 months. It implies tissue damage that is usually from an identifiable cause. If undertreated, acute pain can become chronic pain.[12,13]

Chronic Pain. Chronic pain persists for more than 3 to 6 months after the healing process from the original injury, and it may or may not be associated with an illness.[28,29] It develops when the healing process is incomplete or when there is permanent damage to the nervous system. It has also been associated with a prolonged stress response.[27]

Nociceptive Pain. Acute and chronic types of pain can have a nociceptive or neuropathic origin.[30] Nociceptive pain refers to the nociception mechanism, and it can be somatic or visceral. Somatic pain involves superficial tissues, such as the skin, muscles, joints, and bones. Its location is well defined.

Visceral Pain. Visceral pain involves organs such as the heart, stomach, and liver. Its location is diffuse, and it can be referred to a different location in the body.

Neuropathic Pain. Neuropathic or deafferentation pain is described as an abnormal sensory process caused by changes in the excitability of nerve cells.[31] These changes are associated with the acute inflammatory process or with nociceptive nerve damage that can be caused by surgery or an illness process.[32-34] The origin of the pain may be peripheral or central. Neuralgia and phantom pain are peripheral deafferentation pains. Patients can experience central deafferentation pain after a stroke. Neuropathic pain can be difficult to manage and frequently requires a multimodal approach.

Pain in Critical Care. Pain in the critical care setting is a subjective and multidimensional experience. Its components are sensory, affective, cognitive, behavioral, and physiologic. Pain experienced by critical care patients is mostly acute and has multiple origins. An understanding of the physiology of pain provides a foundation for assessment and treatment.

PHYSIOLOGY OF PAIN

Nociception. Nociception represents the neural and the brain activity necessary, but not sufficient, for pain. Pain is the conscious experience that emerges from nociception, especially from brain activity.[35] Four processes are involved in nociception[30]:

1. Transduction
2. Transmission
3. Perception
4. Modulation

The four processes are shown in Figure 9-1, which integrates pain assessment with nociception, and in Figure 9-2.

Transduction. Transduction refers to mechanical (e.g., surgical incision), thermal (e.g., burn), or chemical (e.g., toxic substance) stimuli that damage tissues. In critical care, many nociceptive stimuli exist, including the patients' acute illness or condition, technology used for patients, and multiple interventions that have to be done for them. These stimuli, also called stressors, stimulate the liberation of many chemical substances, such as prostaglandins, bradykinin, serotonin, histamine, glutamate, and substance P. These neurotransmitters stimulate peripheral nociceptive receptors and initiate nociceptive transmission.

Transmission. As a result of transduction, an action potential is produced and is transmitted by nociceptive nerve fibers in the spinal cord that reach higher centers of the brain. This is called transmission, and it represents the second process of nociception. The principal nociceptive fibers are the Aδ and C fibers. Large-diameter, myelinated Aδ fibers transmit well-localized, sharp pain. Small-diameter, unmyelinated C fibers transmit diffuse, dull, and aching pain. These fibers transmit the noxious sensation from the periphery through the dorsal root of the spinal cord. With the liberation of substance P, these fibers then synapse with ascending spinothalamic fibers to the central nervous system (CNS). These spinothalamic fibers are clustered into two specific pathways: neospinothalamic (NS) and paleospinothalamic (PS) pathways. Generally, the Aδ fibers transmit the pain sensation to the brain within the NS pathway, and the C fibers use the PS pathway.[36]

Through synapsing of nociceptive fibers with motor fibers in the spinal cord, muscle rigidity can appear because of a reflex activity.[10] Muscle rigidity can be a behavioral indicator associated with pain. It can contribute to immobility and decrease diaphragmatic excursion. This can lead to hypoventilation and hypoxemia. Hypoxemia can be detected by a pulse oximeter (SpO$_2$) and by oxygen arterial pressure (PaO$_2$) monitoring. A ventilated patient's interaction with the machine (e.g., activation of alarms, fighting the ventilator) also may indicate the presence of pain.[37]

Perception. The pain message is transmitted by the spinothalamic pathways to centers in the brain, where it is perceived. Pain sensation transmitted by the NS pathway reaches the thalamus, and the pain sensation transmitted by the PS pathway reaches brainstem, hypothalamus, and thalamus.[36] These parts of the CNS contribute to the initial perception of pain. Projections to the limbic system and the frontal cortex

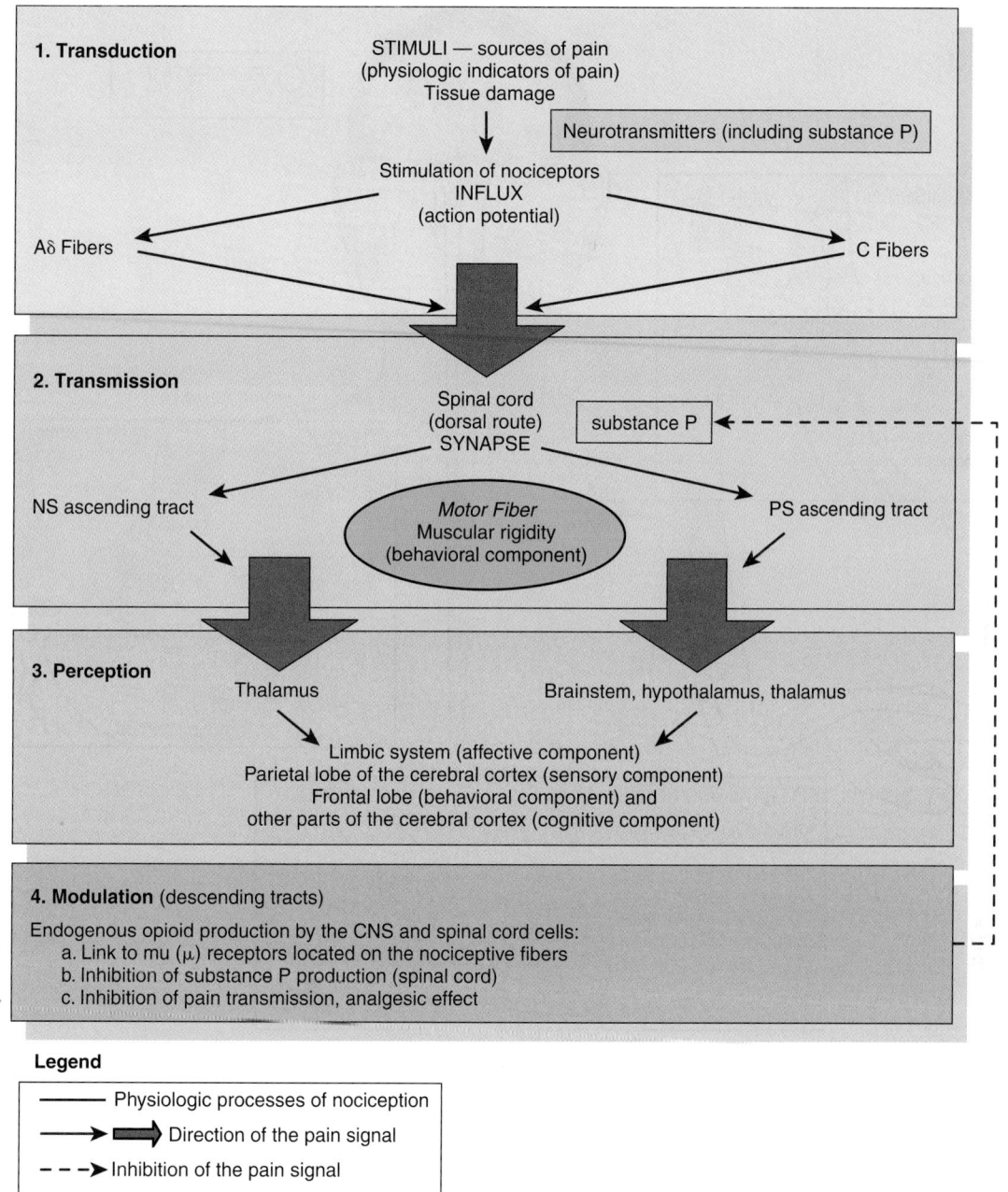

Figure 9-1 Integration of pain assessment in the four processes of nociception. CNS, central nervous system; NS, neospinothalamic pathway; PS, paleospinothalamic pathway. *(Courtesy Céline Gélinas, School of Nursing, McGill University, Canada.)*

allow expression of the affective component of pain.[38-40] Projections to the sensory cortex located in the parietal lobe allow the patient to describe the sensory characteristics of his pain, such as location, intensity, and quality.[38-42] The cognitive component of pain involves many parts of the cerebral cortex and is complex. These three components (affective, sensory, and cognitive) represent the subjective interpretation of pain. Parallel to this subjective process, certain facial expressions and body movements are behavioral indicators of pain occurring as a result of pain fiber projections to the motor cortex in the frontal lobe.

Modulation. Modulation is the liberation of endogenous opioids, such as β-endorphins, enkephalins, and dynorphins, by the CNS. Endogenous opioids inhibit through the descending pathways the transmission of pain sensation in the spinal cord and produce analgesia. These substances link to mu (μ) receptors located on nociceptive fibers, inhibiting the liberation of substance P and blocking the transmission of the pain sensation.

In summary, nociception is an important physiologic mechanism of pain that can integrate many components of pain for its assessment. In transduction, stimuli are sources of pain that can be considered as physiologic indicators for pain assessment. In transmission, muscle rigidity is a reflex activity and can be observed as a behavioral indicator associated with pain. In

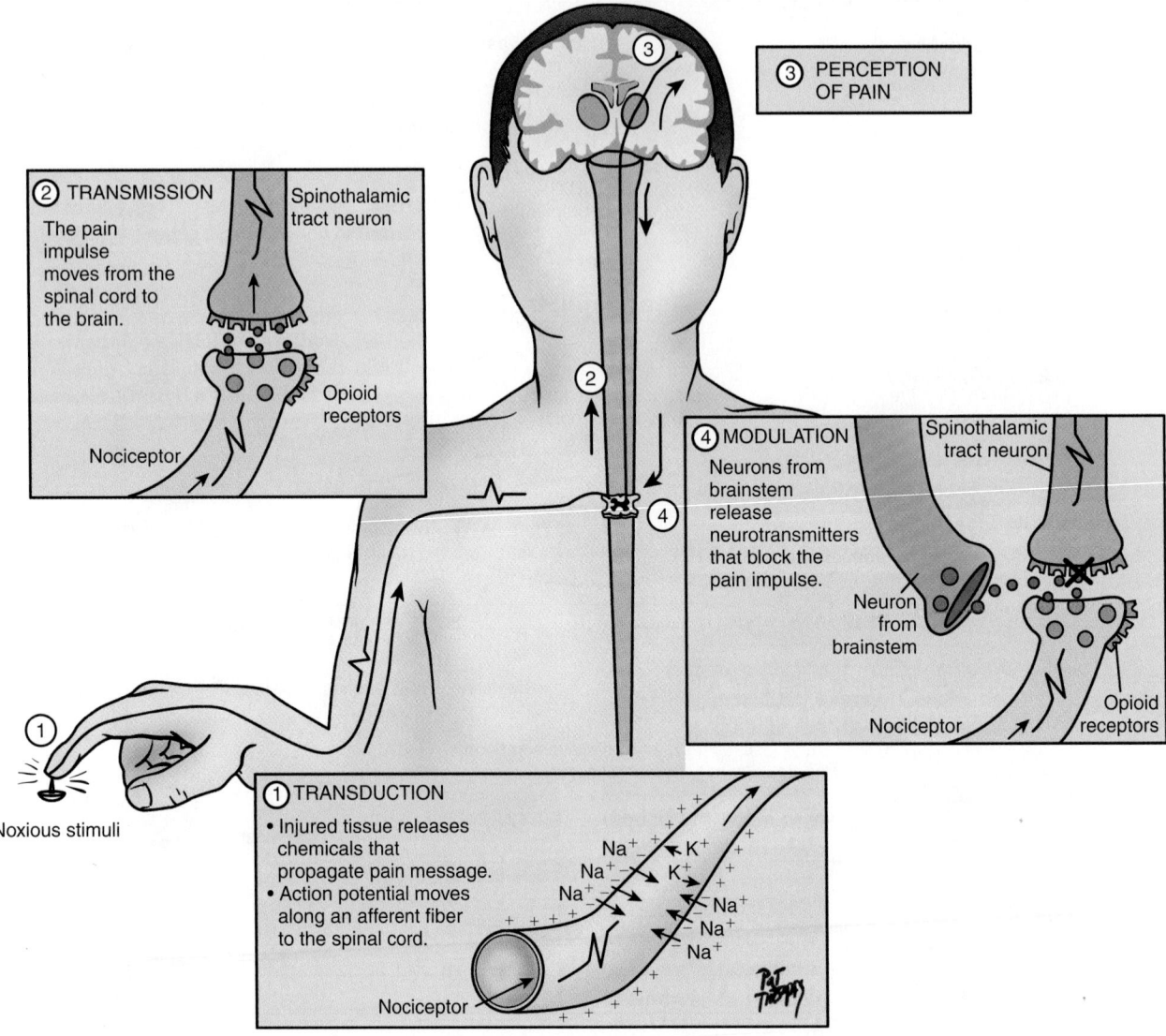

Figure 9-2 The four processes of nociception. *(From Jarvis C: Physical examination & health assessment, ed 5, Philadelphia, 2008, Saunders.)*

perception, the patient's self-report of affective, sensory, and cognitive information can be obtained, and behavioral responses to pain also may be observed.

BIOLOGIC STRESS RESPONSE

A biologic stress response is activated by pain, an obvious stressor.[10,11] This stress response involves the nervous, endocrine, and immune systems in the hypothalamic-pituitary-adrenal axis (HPA).[43,44] The biologic stress response includes a short-term direct response, a midterm response, and a long-term indirect response. Stress mechanisms are depicted in Figure 9-3.

Short-Term Direct Response. In the presence of pain, the hypothalamus releases corticotropin releasing factor (CRF), which activates the sympathetic nervous system (SNS). Norepinephrine is then released from the terminals of sympathetic nerves, and epinephrine is released from the adrenal cortex. This mechanism constitutes the short-term direct stress response. The effects of these stress hormones allow observation of physiologic responses associated with activation of SNS. For instance, increased blood pressure and increased heart rate are common signs of acute pain.[19,45,46] Moreover, increased respiratory rate, perspiration, and pupil dilation can be observed.[46]

If pain persists over time or injuries are located in the bladder or the intestines, the parasympathetic nervous system (PNS) may be dominant. The blood pressure and heart rate may decrease rather than increase. Different responses to stressors involving PNS or SNS patterns have been documented.[47] The absence of pain-related indicators related to the activation of the SNS does not necessarily imply an absence of pain sensation.[37,46]

Midterm Indirect Response. At midterm, the CRF released from the hypothalamus stimulates the anterior pituitary to release adrenocorticotropic hormone (ACTH) and the posterior pituitary to release vasopressin, the antidiuretic hormone. ACTH activates the adrenal cortex to release aldosterone and cortisol. Vasopressin and aldosterone increase sodium and water retention. This increases intravascular volume and decreases diuresis and increases blood pressure and cardiac preload. Cortisol also

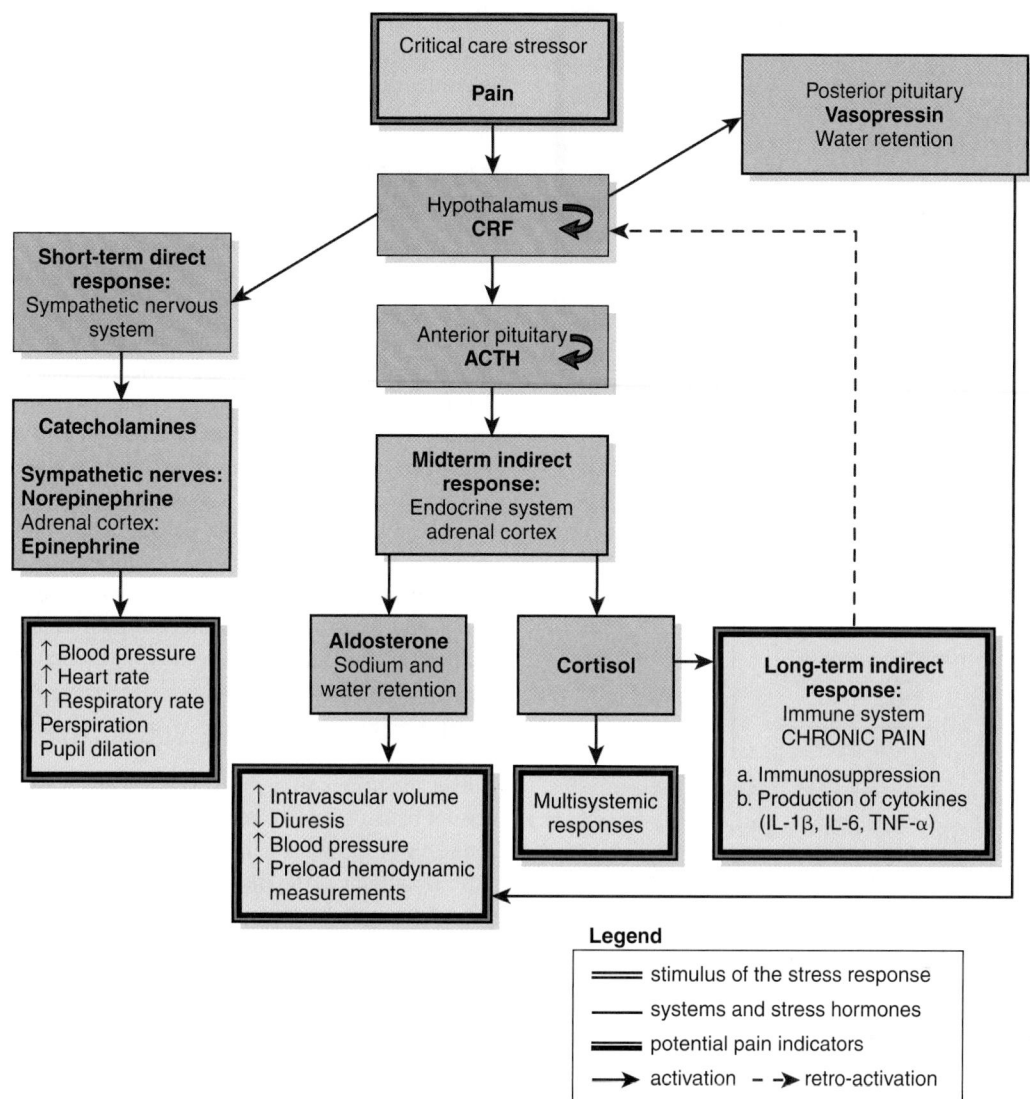

Figure 9-3 Integration of potential physiologic pain indicators in the biologic stress response. ACTH, adrenocorticotropic hormone; CRF, corticotropin-releasing factor; IL, interleukin, TNS, tumor necrosis factor. *(Courtesy Céline Gélinas, School of Nursing, McGill University, Canada.)*

may contribute to systemic responses such as infection and hyperglycemia.

At midterm, pain may be associated with decreased diuresis, increased blood pressure, increased central venous pressure (CVP), and increased pulmonary artery capillary occlusion pressure (PAOP). However, changes in these parameters are not specific to pain, and their correlations with pain are not supported by empirical data.

Long-Term Indirect Response. Long term, the stress hormones, specifically cortisol, influence the immune system in two ways: immunosuppression and release of cytokines.[48] However, these mechanisms have not been associated with acute pain. Their potential role in the chronic pain process is still being investigated. Cytokines may prolong by retroactivation the release of cortisol, which may exacerbate tissue damage, contributing to the chronic pain process.[27,49] The long-term indirect response of stress therefore does not seem to be relevant to acute pain.

In summary, the biologic stress response activated by pain allows observation of relevant physiologic signs that may be associated with pain and that represent a source of stress. The short-term signs are related to SNS activation. Other signs, such as decreased diuresis and increased CVP and PAOP, relate to the midterm indirect stress response. The immune system is involved in the long-term indirect response of stress. No acute pain indicators have been associated with this process. All the indicators identified within the biologic stress response are not specific to pain because they can be they can be attributed to other distress conditions, homeostatic changes, and medications.[21] Moreover, some of them have not yet been studied empirically within the context of pain in critically ill patients.

FRAMEWORK FOR PAIN ASSESSMENT AND DEFINITION

Melzack[27] developed a multidimensional theory and framework that provides a relevant operational definition of pain and an appropriate model for pain assessment. This theory integrates the

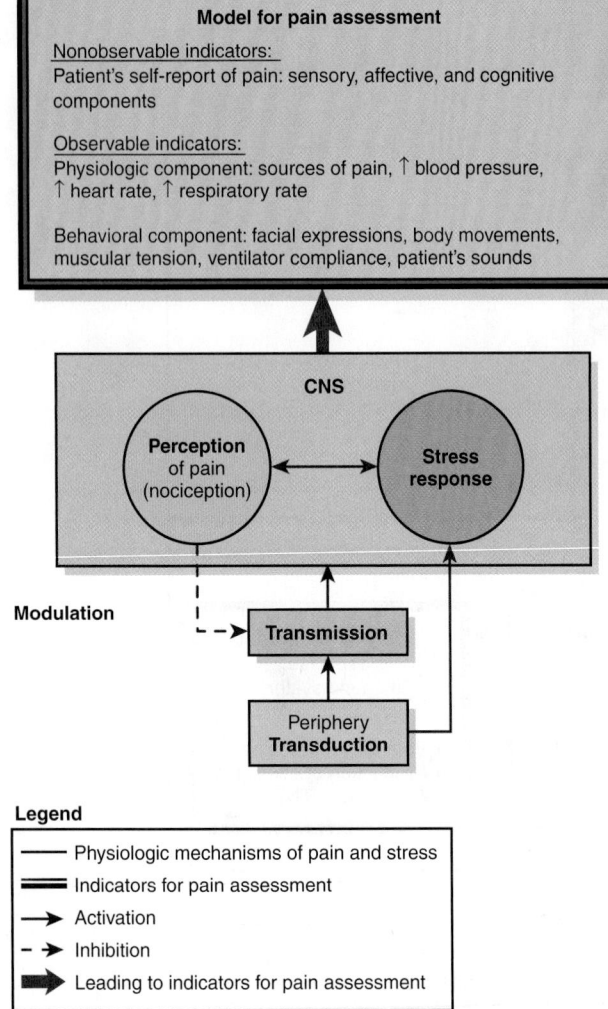

Figure 9-4 Adaptation of the multidimensional theory of Melzack. CNS, central nervous system. *(From Melzack R: Pain and stress: a new perspective. In Gatchel RJ, Turk DC, editors: Psychological factors in pain, p. 98, New York, 1999, Guilford Press.)*

physiologic mechanism of pain (nociception) with the stress response. It also includes components of pain relevant for assessment.

The model for pain assessment proposed by Melzack can be adapted for clinical use (Fig. 9-4). Pain indicators can be clustered into nonobservable or subjective and observable or objective categories. Nonobservable indicators constitute subjective information, such as the patients' self-report of pain, including the sensory, emotional, and cognitive components of pain. Observable indicators include physiologic and behavioral indicators that can be detected by health professionals to document pain assessment. Physiologic indicators (i.e., vital signs) can be easily documented in critical care settings because of their continuous monitoring. Some measurable components are blood pressure, heart rate, respiratory rate, and oxygen saturation. These physiologic indicators are common to every critical care setting. However, vital signs should be used with caution in the pain assessment process; this is discussed subsequently in "Pain Assessment." Behavioral indicators, such as the patient's facial expression, body movements, and rigid posture, can be

observed and documented by nurses. By using a model such as the one presented here, nurses can conduct a systematic assessment of pain in critically ill patients.

PAIN ASSESSMENT

Pain assessment is a vital part of nursing care. It is a prerequisite for adequate pain control and relief. Pain is a subjective, multidimensional concept that requires complex assessment. Many factors may alter verbal communication in critically ill patients, making pain assessment more difficult. This situation should not discourage nurses from assessing pain in these patients because acute pain is a stressor, and critically ill patients frequently have sources of pain that further stress their conditions.

Pain assessment has two major components: nonobservable or subjective and observable or objective. The complexity of pain assessment requires the use of multiple strategies by critical care clinicians. In the following sections, patient, health professional, and organizational barriers to pain assessment and management are addressed, and recommendations are proposed.

PAIN ASSESSMENT: THE SUBJECTIVE COMPONENT

Pain is an entirely subjective experience. The subjective component of pain assessment refers to the patient's self-report of pain about his or her sensorial, affective, and cognitive experience of pain. Because it is the most valid measure of pain, the patient's self-report must be obtained whenever possible.[21] A simple yes or no (presence versus absence of pain) is considered a valid self-report. Mechanical ventilation should not be a barrier for nurses to document patients' self-reports of pain. Many mechanically ventilated patients can communicate that they have pain or can use pain scales by pointing to numbers or symbols on the scale.[4,5,17-19] Before concluding that a patient is unable to self-report, three attempts to ask the patient about pain are recommended.[3] Sufficient time should be allowed for the patient to respond with each attempt.

If sedation and cognition levels allow the patient to give more information about pain, a multidimensional assessment can be documented. Multidimensional pain assessment tools, including the sensorial, emotional, and cognitive components, are available (e.g., Brief Pain Inventory,[50] Initial Pain Assessment Tool,[30] McGill Pain Questionnaire–Short Form[51]). Because of the administration of sedative and analgesic agents in mechanically ventilated patients, the tool must be short enough to be completed. For instance, the McGill Pain Questionnaire–Short Form takes 2 to 3 minutes to complete and has been used to assess mechanically ventilated patients who were in a stable condition.[5,17,18]

The patient's self-report of pain can also be obtained by questioning the patient using the mnemonic PQRSTU[52]:

P: provocative and palliative or aggravating factors
Q: quality
R: region or location, radiation
S: severity and other symptoms
T: timing
U: understanding

P: Provocative and Palliative or Aggravating Factors. The P in the mnemonic indicates what provokes or causes the patient's pain, what he or she was doing when the pain appeared, and what makes the pain better or worse. Deep breathing intensifying chest pain because of pericarditis is an illustration of an aggravating factor. Moderating factors that reduce the pain or discomfort are also important findings. Knowledge of any alleviation activities contributes to the patient's plan of care throughout the continuum of care.

Q: Quality. The Q in the mnemonic refers to the quality of the pain or the pain sensation that the patient is experiencing. For instance, the patient may describe the pain as dull, aching, sharp, burning, or stabbing. This information provides the nurse with data regarding the type of pain the patient is experiencing (i.e., somatic or visceral). The differentiation between types of pain may contribute to the determination of cause and management. A patient who has had open-heart surgery may complain of chest pain that is shooting or burning.[4] This information can lead the nurse to investigate for cutaneous or bone injuries as a result of a sternotomy. Another patient may describe a sharp thoracic pain that may lead the nurse to consider visceral pain as a result of pulmonary embolism. A verbal description of pain is important because it provides a baseline account, allowing the critical care nurse to monitor changes in the type of pain, which may indicate a change in the underlying pathology.

R: Region or Location, Radiation. R usually is easy for the patient to identify, although visceral pain is more difficult for the patient to localize.[30] If the patient has difficulty naming the location or is mechanically ventilated, ask that the patient to point to the location on himself or herself or on a simple anatomic drawing.[53]

S: Severity and Other Symptoms. S, the severity or intensity of pain, is a measurement that has undergone much investigation. Many visual analog scales are available, as are the descriptive and numeric pain rating scales often used in the critical care environment (Fig. 9-5). Numeric and descriptive pain rating scales have been used to assess in mechanically ventilated patients.[5,19,46] The Faces Pain Rating Scale was identified as the easiest pain intensity scale by adults in acute and critical care settings.[54,55] To have a faces scale more specific to adults, Gelinas[56] developed and validated the Faces Pain Thermometer (FPT) for critically ill patients.

Many critical care units use a specific pain intensity scale. The use of a single tool provides consistency of assessment and documentation. Employment of a pain intensity scale is useful in the critical care environment. Asking the patient to grade his or her pain on a scale of 0 to 10 is a consistent method and aids the nurse in objectifying the subjective nature of the patient's pain. However, the patient's tool preference should be considered.

The S in the mnemonic also refers to other symptoms accompanying the patient's pain experience, such as shortness of breath, nausea, and fatigue. Anxiety and fear are common emotions associated with pain.

T: Timing. The T in the mnemonic refers to documenting the onset, duration, and frequency of pain. This information

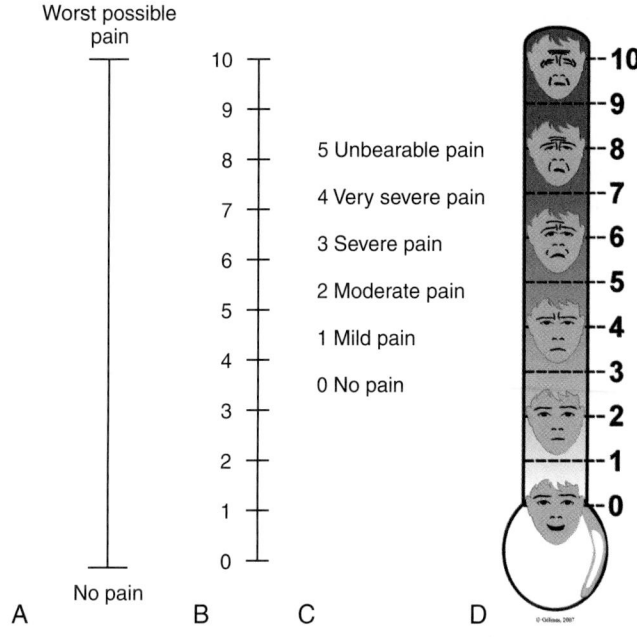

Figure 9-5 Pain intensity scales (vertical format). *A,* Visual analog scale (VAS). *B,* Numeric Rating Scale (NRS). *C,* Descriptive Rating Scale (DRS). *D,* Faces Pain Thermometer. *(Courtesy Céline Gélinas, School of Nursing, McGill University, Canada.)*

can help to determine whether the origin of the pain is acute or chronic. Duration of pain can indicate the severity of the problem. For instance, chest pain of less than 15 minutes' duration may be angina, and pain lasting more than 15 minutes may indicate a myocardial infarction.

U: Understanding. The U in the mnemonic is the patient's perception of the problem or cognitive experience of pain. Patients with known cardiac problems can tell the nurse whether their pain is the same as they had during myocardial infarction. Patients with a cerebral hemorrhage often describe experiencing the worst headache they have ever had.

Because of the patient's change in communication, lack of concentration due to sedation therapies, and the life or death immediacy of most actions in the critical care environment, pain assessment is often reduced to minimal information. Begin by asking, "Do you have pain?" The use of a simple yes or no question allows the patient to answer verbally or to indicate his or her response by nodding the head or by other signs.[3] It is easier for mechanically ventilated patients to communicate with clinicians in this way because they cannot express themselves verbally. Pain intensity and location also are necessary for the initial assessment of pain.[53]

PAIN ASSESSMENT: THE OBSERVABLE OR OBJECTIVE COMPONENT

When the patient's self-report is impossible to obtain, nurses can rely on observation of behavioral and physiologic indicators that are strongly emphasized in clinical recommendations and guidelines for pain management in nonverbal patients.[20-22]

Pain-related behaviors have received attention in critical care and were also studied in the AACN Thunder Project II.[57] Patients who experienced pain during nociceptive procedures were three times more likely to have increased behavioral responses such as facial expressions, muscle rigidity, and vocalization than patients without pain. Similar observations were found in a study of 257 mechanically ventilated intensive care unit (ICU) adults. Patients who experienced pain during turning showed significantly more intense facial expressions (e.g., grimacing), muscle rigidity, and less compliance with the ventilator (e.g., fighting the ventilator) compared with patients without pain.[58] Behavioral indicators are strongly recommended for pain assessment in nonverbal patients,[21,25] and several tools have been developed and tested in critically ill adults: Behavioral Pain Scale (BPS),[45] Critical-Care Pain Observation Tool (CPOT),[59] Postanesthesia Care Unit Behavioral Pain Rating Scale (PACU-BPRS),[60] and Pain Assessment and Intervention Notation (PAIN) algorithm.[46] The BPS and the CPOT are supported by experts as appropriate for use with uncommunicative critically ill adults[61,62] and by the clinical practice recommendations of a Task Force of the American Society for Pain Management Nursing (ASPMN).[21]

Behavioral Pain Scale. The BPS shown in Table 9-1 was tested exclusively in mechanically ventilated, unconscious patients.[45,63,64] Its validity was supported with significantly higher BPS scores during nociceptive procedures (e.g., turning, endotracheal suctioning) compared with rest or nonnociceptive procedures (e.g., central venous catheter dressing change, compression stocking applications, eye care). The BPS can be used quickly (2 to 5 minutes). Most clinicians were satisfied with its ease of use, but some expressed concerns about its relative complexity.[45] For instance, scores of 3 and 4 for compliance with the ventilator may be ambiguous, and movements with upper limbs may be confused with muscle tension.

TABLE 9-1 Behavioral Pain Scale (BPS)

Item	Description	Score
Facial expression	Relaxed	1
	Partially tightened (e.g., brow lowering)	2
	Fully tightened (e.g., eyelid closing)	3
	Grimacing	4
Upper limbs	No movement	1
	Partially bent	2
	Fully bent with finger flexion	3
	Permanently retracted	4
Compliance with ventilation	Tolerating movement	1
	Coughing but tolerating ventilation for most of the time	2
	Fighting ventilator	3
	Unable to control ventilation	4
Total		3 to 12

From Payen JF, et al: Assessing pain in the critically ill sedated patients by using a behavioral pain scale. *Crit Care Med* 29 (12):2258-2263, 2001.

Critical-Care Pain Observation Tool. The CPOT shown in Table 9-2 was tested in verbal and nonverbal, critically ill adult patients.[19,59] Content validity was supported by ICU expert clinicians, including nurses and physicians.[65] Validity of the CPOT was supported with significantly higher CPOT scores during a nociceptive procedure (e.g., turning with or without other care) compared with rest or a nonnociceptive procedure (e.g., taking blood pressure). Significant associations were found between the CPOT scores and the patient's self-report of pain (the gold standard).[66] Feasibility and clinical utility of the CPOT were positively evaluated by ICU nurses.[67] Nurses agreed that the CPOT was quick enough to be used in the ICU, simple to understand, easy to complete, and helpful for nursing practice. The CPOT identifies patients with severe pain very well. For patients with mild to moderate pain, the cutoff seems to be between 2 and 3, depending on the diagnosis of the patient.[68] Head injury patients seemed to react differently to the nociceptive procedure.[19] They were less likely to show frowning, brow lowering, and grimacing. Compared with other patients, a higher proportion of head injury patients showed tearing and open eyes when exposed to the nociceptive procedure.[58]

Behaviors represent valid information for pain assessment in the critically ill patient, but they present some limitations. They are impossible to monitor in paralyzed patients receiving neuromuscular blocking agents, and their presence may be blurred by the use of sedative agents such as propofol or midazolam.[19] Minimal behavioral responses to painful procedures were found in unconscious mechanically ventilated ICU adults who were more heavily sedated compared with conscious patients.[58] Similar results were found in previous studies in which patients who received a higher dose of midazolam obtained a lower score on the BPS.[45,64] In those difficult situations, the only possible clues left for the detection of pain are physiologic indicators.

Physiologic Indicators. Physiologic vital signs as indicators of pain have received little attention in critically ill adults. Although vital sign values generally increase during painful procedures,[19,45,58,64] they are not consistently related to the patient's self-report of pain, nor are they predictive of pain.[19,58] For example, none of the monitored vital signs (heart rate, mean arterial pressure [MAP], respiratory rate, transcutaneous oxygen saturation [SpO_2], and end-tidal CO_2) predicted the presence of pain in ICU patients.[58]

The ASPMN recommendations emphasize that vital signs should not be considered as primary indicators of pain because they can be attributed to other distress conditions, homeostatic changes, and medications.[21] Changes in vital signs should rather be considered a cue to begin further assessment of pain or other stressors.[69] Physiologic measures other than vital signs can support the clinicians in detecting the presence of pain in critically ill, nonverbal patients, especially when behavioral indicators are no longer available.

Cerebral Monitoring and Pain Assessment. Other than vital signs, human brain reactivity has been studied using cerebral hemodynamic methods such as positron emission tomography (PET) and functional magnetic resonance imaging (fMRI)

TABLE 9-2 Critical Care Pain Observation Tool (CPOT)

Indicator	Score		Description
Facial expression Relaxed, neutral 0 Tense 1 Grimace 2	Relaxed, neutral	0	No muscle tension observed
	Tense	1	Frowning, brow lowering, orbit tightening, and levator contraction or any other change (e.g., opening eyes or tearing during nociceptive procedures)
	Grimacing	2	All previous facial movements plus eyelids tightly closed (the patient may present with mouth open or biting the endotracheal tube)
Body movements	Absence of movements or normal position	0	Does not move at all (does not necessarily mean absence of pain) or normal position (movements not aimed toward the pain site or not made for the purpose of protection)
	Protection	1	Slow, cautious movements, touching or rubbing the pain site, seeking attention through movements
	Restlessness	2	Pulling the tube, attempting to sit up, moving limbs or thrashing, not following commands, striking at staff, trying to climb out of bed
Compliance with the ventilator (mechanically ventilated patients)	Tolerating ventilator or movement	0	Alarms not activated, easy ventilation
	Coughing but tolerating	1	Coughing, alarms may be activated but stop spontaneously
	Fighting ventilator	2	Asynchrony: blocking ventilation, alarms frequently activated
or Vocalization (nonventilated patients)	Talking in normal tone or no sound	0	Talking in normal tone or no sound
	Sighing, moaning	1	Sighing, moaning
	Crying out, sobbing	2	Crying out, sobbing
Muscle tension Evaluation by passive flexion and extension of upper limbs when patient is at rest or evaluation when patient is being turned	Relaxed	0	No resistance to passive movements
	Tense, rigid	1	Resistance to passive movements
	Very tense or rigid	2	Strong resistance to passive movements, incapacity to complete them
Total		___/8	

Directions for Using the CPOT

1. The patient is observed at rest for 1 minute to obtain a baseline value of the CPOT.
2. The patient is observed during nociceptive procedures (e.g., turning, endotracheal suctioning, wound dressing) to detect any changes in the patient's behavioral responses to pain.
3. The patient is evaluated before and at the peak effect of an analgesic agent to assess whether the treatment was effective in relieving pain.
4. For the rating of the CPOT, the patient should be given the highest score observed during the observation period.
5. Muscle tension is evaluated last, especially when the patient is at rest, because the stimulation of touch (passive flexion and extension of the arm) may lead to behavioral reactions.
6. The patient is given a score for each behavior included in the CPOT.

Modified from Gélinas C et al: Validation of the Critical-Care Pain Observation Tool (CPOT) in adult patients. *Am J Crit Care,* 15(4):420-427, 2006.
Figure courtesy Caroline Arbour, RN, BSc, MScA(c), McGill University, Canada.

in healthy individuals and in patients with clinical pain conditions.[70] Many regions of the brain are involved in the perception of pain, including the somatosensory cortex, the frontal cortex, and the thalamus. The anatomic connections between these regions suggest that they function in an interactive way in encoding the different aspects of pain (sensory and affective components of pain). For instance, the somatosensory cortex plays a major role in processing the sensory component of pain, whereas the frontal cortex appears to reflect the affective component of pain.[38-42] A closer look into brain activity may elucidate how pain inputs are first received and processed within the cerebral cortex, offering a direct and more precise indicator of pain. Brain activation by a sensory stimulation is accompanied by changes in vascular resistance and blood flow in specific areas of the brain.[71]

Near-Infrared Spectroscopy. Near-infrared spectroscopy (NIRS) is used to noninvasively measure change in regional cerebral oxygenation in a specific cortical region. Its primary utility is the detection of neurologic complications during surgery. The NIRS electrodes are placed on the frontal region unless the patient is bald. The research field related to NIRS and pain perception in humans is new, and many avenues remain be explored. NIRS has been used in three studies that documented cortical pain responses in critically ill infants[72-74] and in one study of adult patients undergoing cardiac surgery.[75]

In the study with 40 adult patients undergoing cardiac surgery,[75] significant increases in regional cerebral oxygenation (rSo_2) were found when patients were exposed to nociceptive procedures during conscious (awake) and unconscious (anesthetized) states. While patients were awake, higher but mild levels of pain-related behaviors using the CPOT (<1.5/8) and pain intensity rating (≤3/10) were obtained during the insertion of the intravenous line and the arterial line.[75] In this study, 29 patients received morphine as a premedication 1 hour before data collection, which might have contributed to the low pain levels reported. Such a result is consistent with the result of a previous study in which behavioral displays of pain were more often observed in adults with more severe pain than those with mild pain.[68]

Other studies found positive and strong correlations among cortical activity, facial expressions, and the nociceptive procedure used.[74] For example, a heel lance is known to cause moderate to severe pain in infants.[76,77] Although further research is needed in critically ill adults undergoing more painful procedures, the NIRS appears to be a promising technique in the pain assessment process.

Bispectral Index. Another innovative technology, the Bispectral Index (BIS), is being explored for its relevance in the pain assessment process of critically ill, sedated patients.[62] The primary utility of the BIS is as an objective measure of sedation levels during surgery in the operating room or during neuromuscular blocking in the ICU. This noninvasive monitor uses electrodes placed on the forehead, and displays a signal-processed electroencephalogram (EEG) with a digital number that relates to the depth of sedation. An electromyographic (EMG) sensor that reflects muscle stimulation of the forehead is included to identify EMG artifact.

A study of 48 mechanically ventilated and sedated ICU patients after cardiac surgery[78] reported that the BIS value significantly increased when patients were exposed to a noxious stimulation (endotracheal suctioning or turning) instead of a nonnoxious procedure (gentle touch). However, the most commonly reported pain-related behaviors (e.g., facial expressions, body movements, tense posture, ventilator asynchrony) were not induced by the noxious stimulation in deeply sedated patients.[78] These results highlight the limitation of the use of behaviors for pain assessment in sedated ICU patients and support the need for using other indicators in those patients to detect the presence of pain and provide appropriate treatment.

Fifth Vital Sign. Because pain is considered the fifth vital sign, including pain assessment with other routinely documented vital signs may help ensure that pain is assessed and controlled for in all patients on a regular basis. This approach can ensure that pain is detected and treatment implemented before the patient develops complications associated with unrelieved pain. The use of a pain flow sheet in critical care settings allows for a visible and on-going pain assessment before and after an intervention for pain that is accessible to all clinicians involved in the assessment and management of pain.[79,80]

PATIENT BARRIERS TO PAIN ASSESSMENT AND MANAGEMENT

Communication. The most obvious patient barrier to the assessment of pain in the critical care population is an alteration in the ability to communicate. The patient who is mechanically ventilated cannot verbalize a description of the pain. If the patient can communicate in any way, such as by head nodding or pointing, he or she may report the pain in that manner. If writing is possible, the patient may be able to thoroughly describe the pain. With nonverbal patients, the nurse relies on behavioral and physiologic clues to assess the presence of pain.

The patient's family can contribute significantly in the assessment of pain. The family is intimately familiar with the patient's normal responses to pain and can assist the nurse in identifying clues. A family member's impression of a patient's pain should be considered in the pain assessment process of the critically ill patient.[21]

Altered Level of Consciousness. The unconscious patient presents a dilemma for all clinicians. Because pain relies on cortical response to provide recognition, the belief that the patient without higher cortical function has no perception of pain may persist. Conversely, the inability to interpret the nociceptive transmission does not negate the transmission. Interviews by Lawrence[81] with 100 patients, who recalled their experiences from a time when they were unconscious in critical care, revealed that they could hear, understand, and respond emotionally to what was being said. Experts recommend assuming that unconscious patients have pain and that they be treated the same way as conscious patients are treated when they are exposed to sources of pain.[21] Studies[19,45] have demonstrated that behavioral and physiologic indicators of pain can be observed in reaction to a painful procedure in critically ill patients, no matter what their level of consciousness. Knowing this, the critical care nurse can initiate a discussion with the other members of the health care team to formulate a plan of care for the patient's comfort.

Elderly Patients. Many elderly patients do not complain much about pain. Some misconceptions, such as believing that pain is a normal consequence of aging or being afraid to disturb the health care team, are barriers to pain expression for the elderly.[30] Cognitive deficits or delirium present additional pain assessment barriers. Many elderly patients with mild to moderate cognitive impairments and even some with severe impairment are able to use pain intensity scales.[82,83] Vertical pain intensity scales are more easily understood by this group of patients and are recommended[84] (see Fig. 9-5). Elderly patients with cognitive deficits should receive repeated instructions and be given sufficient time to respond.[28] When the self-report of pain is impossible to obtain, direct observation of pain-related behaviors is highly recommended in this population.[21,83] More than 24 behavioral tools have been developed for elderly patients with cognitive deficits.[82,85,86] The Pain Assessment Checklist for Seniors with Limited Ability to Communicate (PACSLAC)[87] and Doloplus-2[88,89] are promising tools that are recommended by experts.[83,85,86]

Delirium is a form of transient cognitive impairment that is highly prevalent among elderly patients in the ICU.[90] A major challenge with delirium is that there is overlap between delirium behaviors and pain-related behaviors. It remains unclear whether pain behavioral tools may assist the nurse in the detection of pain of elderly patients during episodes of delirium. Because pain is a modifiable factor of delirium, it can be controlled with adequate pain management.[91]

Neonates and Infants. Two-way verbal communication is impossible with critically ill infants, and this remains an important barrier to pain assessment. The misconception that preterm neonates were incapable of pain sensation has persisted for a long time. Evidence supports that term and preterm neonates have the anatomic and functional capacity for pain sensation at birth.[92] One critical review examined more than 35 instruments used to assess pain in neonates and infants.[93] The Premature Infant Pain Profile (PIPP)[94] is the most recommended valid tool for pain assessment of infants, and it has been implemented in many clinical settings. The PIPP includes behavioral and physiologic indicators. The emphasis in pain assessment should be on behavioral indicators. Physiologic indicators should be interpreted with caution because they are also affected by disease, medications, and physiologic status.[95]

Cultural Influences. Another barrier to accurate pain assessment is cultural influences on pain and pain reporting. Cultural influences are compounded when the patient speaks a language other than that of the health team members. To facilitate communication, the use of a pain intensity scale in the patient's language is vital. The 0 to 10 numeric pain scales have been translated into many different languages.[30]

Although this chapter does not address specific cultural groups and their typical responses to pain, a few generalizations can be made. First, when assessing a patient from a cultural group different from your own, do not assume the patient will have a specific response to pain or exhibit a particular behavior because of his or her culture. Patients have individual responses to pain. The health care practitioner may unjustly assign or expect behaviors that a patient will not exhibit. A second consideration that is commonly overlooked is the role of pain in the life of the patient. The nurse must communicate with the patient or the family to ascertain what that role is.

Some cultures believe that God's test or punishment takes the form of pain. Persons with these cultural backgrounds do not necessarily believe that the pain should be relieved. Other cultures perceive pain as being associated with an imbalance in life. Persons from these cultures believe they need to manipulate the environment to restore balance to control pain.[96]

The complexities and intricacies of cultural beliefs require more extensive discussion than is possible here. It is important for the nurse to support, whenever possible, the special beliefs and needs of the patient and his family to provide the most therapeutic environment for healing to occur.

Lack of Knowledge. A relatively overlooked patient barrier to accurate pain assessment is the public knowledge deficit regarding pain and pain management. Many patients and their families are frightened by the risk of addiction to pain medication. They fear that addiction will occur if the patient is medicated frequently or with sufficient amounts of opiates necessary to relieve the pain. This concern is so powerful for some that they will deny or deliberately underreport the frequency or intensity of pain. Another misconception held by some patients is the expectation that unrelieved pain is simply part of a critical illness or procedure.[97] Many patients have no memory of receiving an explanation of their pain management plan.[98] With that in mind, it is important that the critical care nurse teach the family and the patient about the importance of pain control and the use of opioids in treating pain in the critically ill.

HEALTH PROFESSIONAL BARRIERS TO PAIN ASSESSMENT AND MANAGEMENT

The health professional's beliefs and attitudes about pain and pain management are frequently a barrier to accurate and adequate pain assessment. This can lead to poor management practices. Misconceptions or lack of knowledge regarding addiction, physiologic dependence, drug tolerance, and respiratory depression remain. Addiction rates for patients in acute pain who receive opioid analgesics are less than 1%. Some of the false beliefs that surround addiction result from a lack of knowledge about addiction and tolerance, and other concerns are related to the possible side effects of opioids.

Addiction and Tolerance. Addiction is defined by a pattern of compulsive drug use that is characterized by an incessant longing for an opioid and the need to use it for effects other than pain relief.

Tolerance is defined as a diminution of opioid effects over time. Physical dependence and tolerance to opioids may develop if the drug is given over a long period. Physical dependence is manifested by withdrawal symptoms when the opioid is abruptly stopped. If this is an anticipated problem, withdrawal may be avoided by weaning the patient from the opioid slowly to allow the brain to reestablish neurochemical balance in the absence of the opioid.[30]

Respiratory Depression. Another concern of the health care professional is the fear that aggressive management of pain with opioids will cause critical respiratory depression. Opioids can cause respiratory depression, but in the critically ill, this is a rare phenomenon. The incidence of respiratory depression is less than 2%.[99] Respiratory depression from the administration of opioids can be managed with diligent assessment practices, which are discussed later.

ORGANIZATIONAL BARRIERS TO PAIN ASSESSMENT AND MANAGEMENT

The organizational system influences pain and pain management practices as well as associated outcomes. Failure to make pain management a priority is the initial barrier. Failure to adopt standard pain assessment tools or to provide staff with sufficient time to assess and document pain, and a lack of accountability for pain management practices are observed in some organizations.[23] Evidence continues to demonstrate the lack of documentation of pain assessment and the undertreatment of pain in critical care settings.[8,9,100] The lack of collaboration between physicians and nurses is still identified as a barrier to effective pain management.[37,101]

Because unrelieved pain is harmful to patients and increases the cost of care, it needs to be a priority for the health organization. Every organization must analyze their pain management issues and practices; and provide education about pain and pain management to staff. Now that pain is considered as the fifth vital sign, pain assessment must be included in documentation systems as a standard. Pain has to be assessed in all critically ill patients, regardless of their clinical condition or their level of consciousness.[59] The implementation of pain assessment tools is essential so that the health care team can establish a common language of communication. This facilitates interprofessional collaboration. There is an increased commitment to clinical practice guidelines and standards for pain assessment and management by organizations such as The Joint Commission (www.jointcommission.org) that have considerable influence in healthcare institutions. In addition, strategies to enhance collaboration among health professionals may include interdisciplinary care rounds or case reviews. Patients have the right to be consulted about their pain care plan, and should be involved in making decisions.[102] The organization must continually evaluate outcomes and work to improve the quality of pain management.

PAIN MANAGEMENT

The management of pain in the critically ill patient is as multidimensional as the assessment. It is a multidisciplinary task. The control of pain can be pharmacologic, nonpharmacologic, or a combination of the two therapies. Pharmacologic pain management is predominantly used in critical care.

PHARMACOLOGIC CONTROL OF PAIN

Pharmacologic management of pain has infinite variety in the critical care unit. Although this chapter is not an in-depth discussion of pharmacology, some commonly administered agents are discussed. Pain pharmacology is divided into three categories of action: opioid agonists (morphine, fentanyl, hydromorphone, meperidine, codeine, methadone, and more potent drugs), nonopioids (acetaminophen, nonsteroidal antiinflammatory drugs [NSAIDs]), and adjuvants (anticonvulsants, antidepressants, and local anesthetics). Elements of the 2002 clinical guidelines[22] of the Society of Critical Care Medicine (SCCM) for pharmacologic interventions in the critically ill adult are presented for each drug discussed (updated guidelines are planned for publication in 2010). The algorithm from the current SCCM guidelines for sedation and analgesia management is shown in Figure 10-1 in Chapter 10. How pain is approached and managed is a progression or combination of the available agents, the type of pain, and the patient response to the therapy. Figure 9-6 illustrates the analgesic action sites in relation to nociception.

Opioid Analgesics. The opioids most commonly used and recommended as first-line analgesics are the agonists. These opioids bind to mu (μ) receptors (transmission process; see Fig. 9-6), which appear to be responsible for pain relief. Additional pharmacologic information is presented in Table 9-3. In the SCCM guidelines, scheduled opioid doses or a continuous infusion is preferred over an as-needed regimen to ensure consistent analgesia in critically ill patients.[22]

Morphine. Morphine is the most commonly prescribed opioid in the critical care unit. Because of its water solubility, morphine has a slower onset of action and a longer duration compared with the lipid-soluble opioids (e.g., fentanyl). This makes it and hydromorphone preferred opioids for intermittent therapy in the SCCM guidelines.[22] Morphine has two main metabolites: morphine-3-glucuronide (M3G, inactive) and morphine-6-glucuronide (M6G, active). M6G is responsible for the analgesic effect but may accumulate and cause excessive sedation in patients with renal failure or hepatic dysfunction.[103] Morphine is available in a variety of delivery methods. It is the standard by which all other opioids are measured. It is also the agent that most closely mimics the endogenous opioids in the human pain modification system.

Morphine is indicated for severe pain. It has additional actions that are helpful for managing other symptoms. Morphine dilates peripheral veins and arteries, making it useful in reducing myocardial workload. Morphine is also viewed as an antianxiety agent because of the calming effect it produces.

Many side effects have been reported with the use of morphine (see Table 9-3). The hypotensive effect can be particularly problematic in the hypovolemic patient. The vasodilation effect is potentiated in the volume-depleted patient, and the hemodynamic status must be carefully monitored. Volume resuscitation restores blood pressure in the event of a prolonged hypotensive response.

A more serious side effect requiring diligent monitoring is the respiratory depressant effect. Opioids may cause this complication

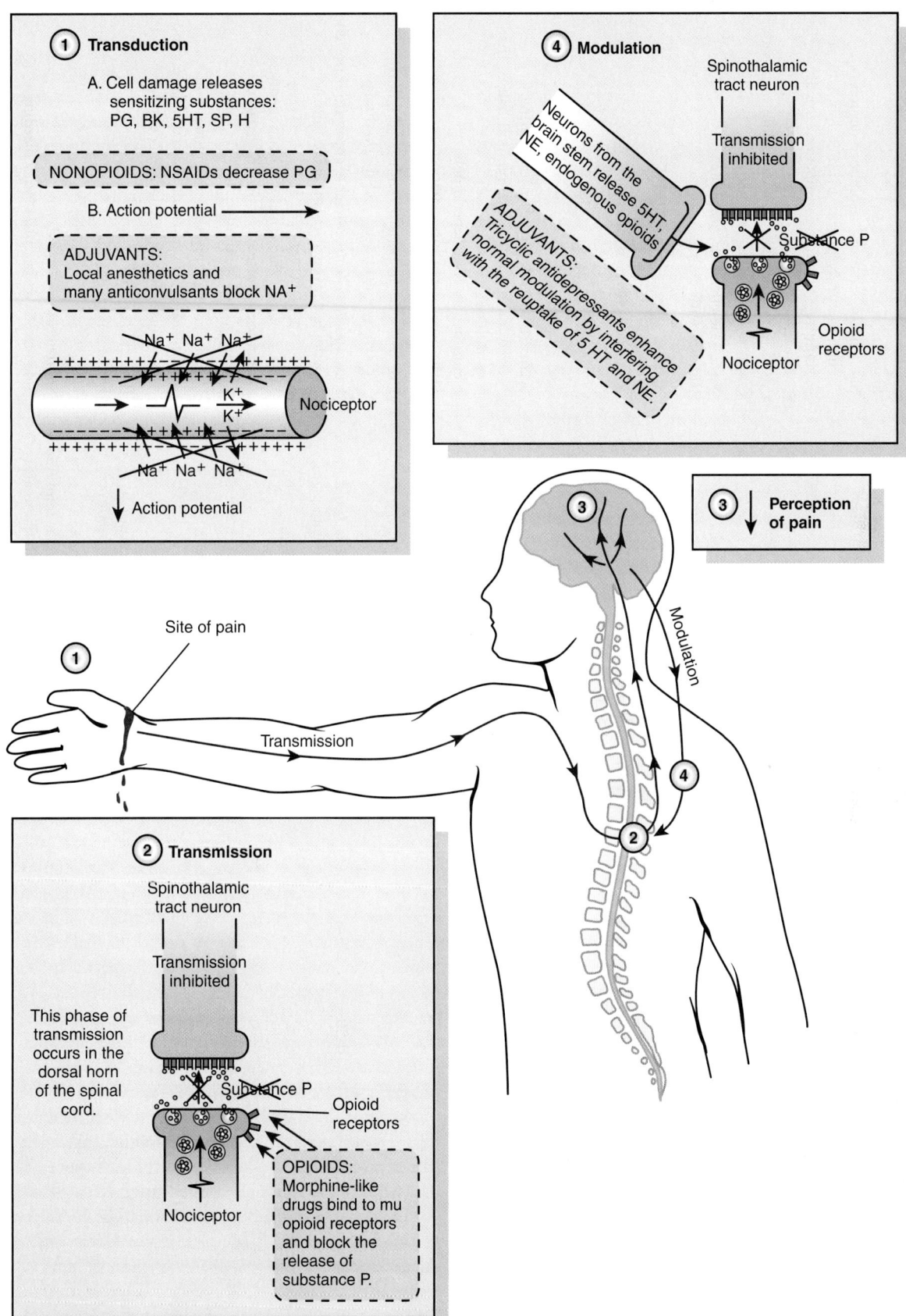

Figure 9-6 Nociception and analgesic action sites. BK, bradykinin; H, histamine; PG, prostaglandins; SP, substance P; 5HT, serotonin. *(From McCaffery M, Pasero C: Pain: clinical manual for nursing practice, ed 2, p 107, St. Louis, 1999, Mosby.)*

TABLE 9-3 Pharmacologic Management: Pain

DRUG	DOSAGE	ONSET (MIN)	DURATION (HR)	AVAILABLE ROUTES	PROPERTIES	SIDE EFFECTS AND COMMENTS
Morphine	1-4 mg IV bolus 1-10 mg IV infusion	5-10	3-4	PO, SL, R, IV, IM, SC, EA, IA	Analgesia, antianxiety	Standard for comparison Side effects: sedation, respiratory depression, euphoria or dysphoria, hypotension, nausea, vomiting, pruritus, constipation, urinary retention M6G can accumulate in renal failure or hepatic dysfunction patients.
Fentanyl	25-100 µg IV bolus 25-200 µg IV infusion	1-5	0.5-4	OTFC, IV, IM, TD, EA, IA	Analgesia, antianxiety	Same side effects as morphine Rigidity with high doses
Hydromorphone (Dilaudid)	0.2-1 mg IV bolus 0.2-2 mg IV infusion	5	3-4	PO, R, IV, IM, SC, EA, IA	Analgesia, antianxiety	Same side effects as morphine
Meperidine (Demerol)	75-100 mg IM	5-10	2-4	PO, IV, IM, SC, EA, IA	Analgesia	Seems to cause less constipation, urinary retention, pruritus, sedation, and nausea than morphine Neurotoxicity (normeperidine) High doses may cause agitation, muscle jerking, seizures, or hypotension. Use with care in patients with renal failure, convulsive disorders, and dysrhythmias.
Codeine	15-30 mg IM, SC	10-20	3-4	PO, IM, SC	Analgesia (mild to moderate pain)	Lacks potency (unpredictable absorption; not all patients convert it to an active form to achieve analgesia) Most common side effects: light-headedness, dizziness, shortness of breath, sedation, nausea, and vomiting
Methadone (Dolophine)	5-10 mg IV	10	4-8	PO, SL, R, IV, SC, IM, EA, IA	Analgesia	Usually less sedating than morphine, but repeated doses can result in accumulation and can cause serious sedation (2-5 days).
Acetaminophen	650 mg Maximum of 4 g/day	20-30	4-6	PO, R	Analgesia, antipyretic	Rare side effects Hepatotoxicity
Ketorolac (Toradol)	15-30 mg IV	<10	6-8	PO, IM, IV	Analgesia, minimum antiinflammatory effect	Short-term use (<5 days) Side effects: gastric ulceration, bleeding, exacerbation of renal insufficiency Use with care in elderly and renal failure patients.

EA, epidural analgesia; IA, intrathecal analgesia; IM, intramuscular; IV, intravenous; M6G, morphine-6-glucuronide; OTFC, oral transmucosal fentanyl citrate; PO, oral; R, rectal; SC, subcutaneous; SL, sublingual; TD, transdermal.

because they reduce the responsiveness of carbon dioxide chemoreceptors in the respiratory center located in the medulla.[104] Although infrequent, this effect can have significant sequelae for the critically ill patient. A subset of patients is at greater risk for respiratory depression after morphine administration. This subset includes newborns (younger than 6 months), elderly patients with chronic obstructive pulmonary disease (COPD) or known obstructive sleep apnea syndrome, patients who are opiate naïve (receiving opiates for less than a week), and patients with kidney failure.[99] The critical care nurse must monitor the patient intensively to prevent this complication. Monitoring of patients receiving opioid analgesics is discussed in more detail later in this chapter. In addition to side effects common to all opioids, morphine may stimulate histamine release from mast cells, resulting in cardiac instability and allergic reactions.

Fentanyl. Fentanyl is a synthetic opioid preferred for critically ill patients with hemodynamic instability or morphine allergy. It is a lipid-soluble agent that has a more rapid onset than morphine and a shorter duration.[103] The metabolites of fentanyl are largely inactive and nontoxic, which makes it an effective and safe opioid. The use of fentanyl in the critical care unit is growing in popularity, and it is the preferred agent for acutely distressed patients. Fentanyl or hydromorphone are also recommended in hemodynamically unstable or renal impaired patients in the SCCM guidelines.[22] It is available in intravenous, intraspinal, and transdermal forms. The transdermal form is commonly referred to as the *Duragesic patch* or the *72-hour patch.*

Because the side effects of fentanyl are similar to those of morphine, the nurse must monitor carefully the hemodynamic and respiratory response. When fentanyl is given by rapid administration and at higher doses, it has been associated with the additional hazard of bradycardia and rigidity in the chest wall muscles.[22,103] The use of transdermal fentanyl is indicated rarely in the critically ill patient. The customary use of the "fentanyl patch" is for those experiencing chronic pain or cancer pain, and in critical care, it is used for the patient who requires extended pain control. Transdermal delivery requires 12 to 16 hours for onset of action, and it has a duration of 72 hours.[30] If this delivery method is used, the patient will require other opioid management until the transdermal fentanyl takes effect.

Hydromorphone. Hydromorphone is a semisynthetic opioid that has an onset of action and a duration similar to those of morphine.[103] It is an effective opioid with multiple routes of delivery. It is more potent than morphine. Hydromorphone should be used with caution in renal or hepatic failure patients because its metabolite, hydromorphone-3-glucuronide, accumulates and can cause CNS toxicity. Studies have shown that some side effects (e.g., pruritus, sedation, nausea, vomiting) may occur less with hydromorphone than morphine.[105]

Meperidine. Meperidine (Demerol) is a less potent opioid with agonist effects similar to those of morphine. It is considered the weakest of the opioids, and it must be administered in large doses to be equivalent in action to morphine. Because the duration of action is short, dosing is frequent. A major concern with this drug is the metabolite *normeperidine,* which is a CNS neurotoxic agent. At high doses in patients with kidney failure or liver dysfunction or in elderly patients, it may induce CNS toxicities, including irritability, muscle spasticity, tremors, agitation, and seizures.[30] Research has shown that meperidine can cause delirium in postoperative patients of all ages.[106] Although meperidine is useful in short-term specific conditions (e.g., treating postoperative shivering), it should be avoided in patients who require longer periods of analgesia. Any patient receiving meperidine for pain control must be carefully monitored for signs of toxicity. The Agency for Healthcare Research and Quality (AHCPR) guidelines suggest its use be limited to patients with a documented sensitivity or allergic response to other μ-agonists.[20]

Codeine. Codeine has limited use in the management of severe pain. It is rarely used in the critical care unit. It provides analgesia for mild to moderate pain. It is usually compounded with a non-opioid (e.g., acetaminophen). To be active, codeine must be metabolized in the liver to morphine.[30] Codeine is available only through oral, intramuscular, and subcutaneous routes, and its absorption can be reduced in the critical care patient by altered gastrointestinal motility and decreased tissue perfusion.[107]

Methadone. Methadone is a synthetic opioid with morphine-like properties but less sedation. It is longer acting than morphine and has a long half-life. This makes it difficult to titrate in the critical care patient. Methadone lacks active metabolites, and routes other than the kidney eliminate 60% of the drug. This means that methadone does not accumulate patients with kidney failure.[108] Methadone is recommended as a second-line opioid analgesic.[109] It is a good alternative for the patient who has a long recovery ahead with an anticipated prolonged wean from mechanical ventilation.[103]

More Potent Opioids: Remifentanil and Sufentanil. Remifentanil and sufentanil are agonist opioids. The use of these potent drugs has been studied in critically ill patients.

Remifentanil is 250 times more potent than morphine, and it has a rapid onset and predictable offset of action. For this reason, it allows a rapid emergence from sedation, facilitating the evaluation of the neurologic state of the patient after stopping the infusion.[110,111]

Sufentanil is 7 to 13 times more potent than fentanyl and 500 to 1000 times more potent than morphine. It has more pronounced sedation properties than fentanyl and other opioids. Patients under sufentanil require minimal sedative agent doses to achieve an adequate sedation level. It has a rapid distribution and a high clearance rate, preventing accumulation when given for a long period.[112] Sufentanil has a longer emergence from sedation compared with remifentanil, but it allows a longer analgesic effect after stopping its administration.[111]

These drugs appear to have many advantages for use in critical care. They have not yet been included in evidence-based guidelines.

Preventing and Treating Respiratory Depression. Respiratory depression is the most life-threatening opioid side effect. The risk of respiratory depression increases when other drugs with CNS depressant effects (e.g., benzodiazepines, antiemetics, neuroleptics, antihistamines) are concomitantly administered to the patient.[104] Respiratory depression is defined as a decrease in the rate or depth of respirations, not necessarily a specific number of respirations per minute. This means that a patient breathing deeply but less than 10 times per minute may not have respiratory depression. A change in the patient's level of consciousness or an increase in sedation normally precedes respiratory depression.

Monitoring. Patients should be monitored before the administration of the opioid agent and at its peak effect. Monitoring for the following parameters at least every 2 hours for the first 24 hours and every 4 hours thereafter in stable patients[113] is recommended to prevent respiratory depression:

- Pain intensity (using a valid pain scale)
- Respiratory rate and depth (be cautious with loud snoring)
- Sedation level (using a valid sedation scale; see Chapter 10, Table 10-1)

Loud snoring does not necessarily indicate that the patient has a comfortable status. Loud snoring is frequently a sign of respiratory depression associated with airway obstruction by the tongue, leading to hypoxemia and possibly to cardiorespiratory arrest. A patient snoring after the administration of an opioid requires the critical care nurse to observe closely. Monitoring oxygen saturation (SpO_2) is recommended to detect a deterioration in the patient's respiratory condition.[114] The use of capnography, which is becoming more available in critical care settings, should be considered for high-risk patients with parenteral therapy.[113]

Opioid Reversal. Critical respiratory depression can be readily reversed with the administration of the opiate antagonist *naloxone*. The usual dose is 0.4 mg, which is mixed with 10 mL of normal saline (for a concentration of 0.04 mg/mL). Naloxone is normally given intravenously very slowly while the patient is carefully monitored for reversal of the respiratory signs. Naloxone administration can be discontinued as soon as the patient is responsive to physical stimulation and able to take deep breaths. However, the medication should be kept nearby. Because the duration of naloxone is shorter than most opioids, another dose of naloxone may be needed as early as 30 minutes after the first dose. The nurse must monitor sedation and respiratory status and remind the patient to breathe deeply every 1 to 2 minutes until he or she becomes more alert. The benefits of reversing respiratory depression with naloxone must be carefully weighed against the risk of a sudden onset of pain and the difficulty achieving pain relief. To prevent this from occurring, it is important to provide a nonopioid medication for pain management.[115] Moreover, the use of naloxone is not recommended after prolonged analgesia, because it can induce withdrawal and may cause nausea and cardiovascular complications (e.g., dysrhythmias).[22]

Nonopioid Analgesics. In the SCCM guidelines, the use of nonopioids in combination with an opioid is recommended in selected critical care patients.[22] This may reduce the opioid requirement and provide greater analgesic effect through action at the peripheral and central levels.[23] Pharmacologic information is presented in Table 9-3.

Acetaminophen. Acetaminophen is an analgesic used to treat mild to moderate pain. It inhibits the synthesis of neurotransmitter prostaglandins in the CNS, and this is why it has no antiinflammatory properties.[116] Acetaminophen is metabolized by two pathways: major (nontoxic metabolite) and minor (toxic metabolite that is rapidly converted into a nontoxic form by glutathione). In an acetaminophen overdose, a larger amount is processed by the minor pathway, and this results in a larger quantity of toxic metabolites and may cause damage to the liver. Side effects are rare at therapeutic doses (total daily dose should not exceed 4 g in 24 hours).[30] Nonopioids are rarely used alone in critical care patients. The nurse must consider the other products containing acetaminophen that the patient may receive when calculating the total daily dose of acetaminophen. Special care must be taken for patients with liver dysfunction, malnutrition, or a history of excess alcohol consumption, and their acetaminophen total dose should not exceed 2 g/day.[22]

Nonsteroidal Antiinflammatory Drugs. The use of NSAIDs in combination with opioids is indicated in the patient with acute musculoskeletal and soft tissue inflammation.[30] The mechanism of action of NSAIDs is to block the action of cyclooxygenase (COX, which has two forms: COX-1 and COX-2), the enzyme that converts arachidonic acid to prostaglandins. This inhibits the production of prostaglandins (transduction process; see Fig. 9-6). This action occurs in the PNS and the CNS components of pain. NSAIDs can be grouped as first-generation (COX-1 and COX-2 inhibitors, such as aspirin, ibuprofen, naproxen, and ketorolac) or second-generation (COX-2 inhibitors, such as celecoxib) agents. The inhibition of COX-1 is thought to be responsible for many of the side effects, such as gastric ulceration, bleeding due to platelet inhibition, and acute renal failure. In contrast, the inhibition of COX-2 is responsible for the suppression of pain and inflammation.[116] Second-generation NSAIDs are associated with minimal risks of serious adverse effects, but their role in critically ill patients remains unknown.[22]

Ketorolac is the most appropriate NSAID for use in the critical care setting. Research has shown that it is a safe and effective agent for postoperative pain.[117] Patients who received ketorolac in conjunction with an opioid had more effective pain relief and fewer side effects than patients who received just an opioid.[118] Not all critically ill patients are candidates for ketorolac therapy because of its side effects. Caution is advised for using ketorolac in the elderly or patients with kidney dysfunction because of their slower clearance rates. Because ketorolac is an NSAID, monitoring for clumping of platelets is of primary importance. Laboratory data should be evaluated for an increase in bleeding time, and the patient should be assessed for any signs of abnormal bleeding. Of particular concern is any evidence of gastrointestinal bleeding.[119] Moreover, prolonged use of ketorolac for more than 5 days has been associated with an increase in kidney failure and bleeding.[120,121] It is important to consider the concurrent use of opioids and NSAIDs to affect pain modification at both areas of transmission. This combination of agents often significantly reduces the amount of opioids required for effective pain management.

Other pharmacologic agents are used in the critical care unit. The most important factor to be considered in the management of pain with any pharmacologic agent is the careful assessment and reassessment of the patient's pain status during the administration of the drug. The need to adjust the dosage, increase the frequency, or change the agent is based on assessment findings. The use of a pain flow sheet allows on-going pain assessment and complete documentation of pain and pain management in the critical care setting.

Adjuvants. Although not widely mentioned in the critical care literature, adjuvants can be helpful for pain relief in patients with complex pain syndromes such as neuropathic pain or for other specific purposes (e.g., procedural pain). Anticonvulsants (e.g., carbamazepine, phenytoin, gabapentin) are first-line analgesics for lancing neuropathic pain. Even if the specific mechanism for pain relief is unknown, analgesia probably results from the suppression of sodium ion (Na^+) discharges, reducing the neuronal hyperexcitability (action potential) in the transduction process[30] (see Fig. 9-6). Antidepressants (e.g., amitriptyline, imipramine, desipramine) are also considered as analgesics in a variety of chronic pain syndromes, such as headache, arthritis, low back pain, neuropathy, central pain, and cancer pain. The analgesic dose is often lower than that required to treat depression. The mechanism of analgesia most widely accepted is the ability of antidepressants to block the reuptake of neurotransmitters serotonin and norepinephrine in the CNS. This increases the activity of the modulation process[30] (see Fig. 9-6).

Ketamine. Anesthetics may be used to treat pain in the critical care setting. Ketamine is a dissociative anesthetic agent that has analgesic properties. It was traditionally used intravenously for procedural pain in burn patients. It is also available in enteral routes. Compared with opioids, ketamine has the benefit of sparing the respiratory drive, but it has many side effects related to the release of catecholamines and the emergence of delirium. For this reason, ketamine is not recommended for routine therapy in critically ill patients.[103,117] Before administering ketamine, the dissociative state should be explained to the patient. *Dissociative state* refers to the feelings of separateness from the environment, loss of control, hallucinations, and vivid dreams. The use of benzodiazepines (e.g., midazolam) can reduce the incidence of this unpleasant effect.[30]

Lidocaine. Lidocaine is another anesthetic that can be used for procedural and acute pain or for some patients with chronic neuropathic pain.[30] When used locally, anesthetics act through the transduction process (see Fig. 9-6).

DELIVERY METHODS

The most common route for drug administration is the intravenous route by means of continuous infusion, bolus administration, or patient-controlled analgesia (PCA). Traditionally, the choice has been intravenous bolus administration. The benefits of this method are the rapid onset of action and the ease of titration. The major disadvantage is the rise and fall of the serum level of the opioid, leading to periods of pain control with periods of breakthrough pain[116] (Fig. 9-7).

Continuous infusion of opioids with an infusion pump provides constant blood levels of the ordered opioid. This promotes a consistent level of comfort. It is a particularly helpful method of administration during sleep because the patient awakens with an adequate level of pain relief. It is important that the patient be given the loading dose that relieves the pain and raises the circulating dose of the drug. After the basal rate is established, the patient maintains a steady state of pain control unless there is additional pain from a procedure, an activity, or a change in the patient's condition. In this situation, physician orders to administer additional boluses of opioid need to be available.

Patient-Controlled Analgesia. PCA is a method of drug delivery that uses the intravenous route and an infusion pump. It allows the patient to self-administer small doses of analgesics.

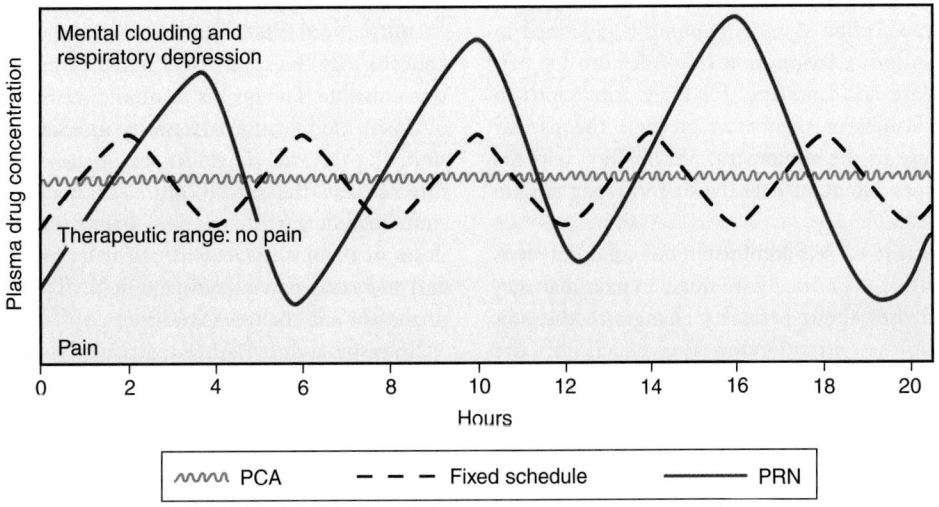

Figure 9-7 Fluctuations in opioid blood levels seen with three dosing procedures. PCA, patient-controlled analgesia; PRN, as required. *(From Lehne RA: Pharmacology for nursing care, ed 5, p. 243, St Louis, 2004, Saunders.)*

NIC

Patient-Controlled Analgesia Assistance

Definition
Facilitating patient control of analgesic administration and regulation

Activities
Collaborate with physicians, patient, and family members in selecting the type of narcotic to be used.

Recommend administration of aspirin and nonsteroidal antiinflammatory drugs in conjunction with narcotics, as appropriate.

Avoid use of meperidine (Demerol).

Ensure that patient is not allergic to the analgesic to be administered.

Teach patient and family to monitor pain intensity, quality, and duration

Teach patient and family to monitor the respiratory rate and blood pressure.

Establish nasogastric, venous, subcutaneous, or spinal access, as appropriate.

Validate that the patient can use a patient-controlled analgesia (PCA) device: is able to communicate, comprehend explanations, and follow directions.

Collaborate with patient and family to select appropriate type of patient-controlled infusion device.

Teach patient and family members how to use the PCA device.

Assist patient and family to calculate appropriate concentration of drug to fluid, considering the amount of fluid delivered per hour by the PCA device.

Assist patient or family member to administer an appropriate bolus loading dose of analgesic.

Teach patient and family to set an appropriate basal infusion rate on the PCA device.

Assist patient and family to set the appropriate lockout interval on the PCA device.

Assist patient and family in setting appropriate demand doses on the PCA device.

Consult with patient, family members, and physician to adjust lockout interval, basal rate, and demand dosage, according to the patient responsiveness.

Teach patient how to titrate doses up or down, depending on respiratory rate, pain intensity, and pain quality.

Teach the patient and family members the action and side effects of pain-relieving agents.

Document patient's pain, amount and frequency of drug dosing, and response to pain treatment in a pain flow sheet.

Recommend a bowel regimen to avoid constipation.

Consult with clinical pain experts for a patient who is having difficulty achieving pain control.

From Bulechek GM et al: *Nursing interventions classification (NIC)*, ed 5, 2008, St Louis, Mosby.

Different opioids can be used, but the most extensively used is morphine.[116] This method of medication delivery allows the patient to control the level of pain and sedation and to avoid the peaks and valleys of intermittent dosing by the health care professional (see Fig. 9-7). The patient can self-administer a bolus of medication the moment the pain begins, acting preemptively. Nursing management for the patient receiving analgesia medication via a PCA pump is described in the Nursing Interventions Classification (NIC) feature.

Certain patients are not candidates for PCA. Alterations in the level of consciousness or mentation preclude the patient understanding the use of the equipment. Very elderly patients or patients with kidney failure or liver dysfunction may require careful screening for PCA.

Allowing the patient to self-administer opioid doses does not diminish the role of the critical care nurse in pain management. The nurse advises about necessary changes to the prescription and continues to monitor the effects of the medication and doses. The patient is closely monitored during the first 2 hours of therapy and after every change in the prescription. If the patient's pain does not respond within the first 2 hours of therapy, a total reassessment of the pain state is essential. The nurse monitors the number of boluses the patient delivers. If the patient is pressing the button to bolus medication more often than the prescription, the dose may

be insufficient to maintain pain control. Naloxone must be readily available to reverse adverse opiate respiratory effects. Ideally, the patient undergoing an elective procedure requiring opioid analgesia postoperatively is instructed in the use of PCA during preoperative teaching. This allows the patient to become comfortable with the concept of self-medication before use.

Intraspinal Pain Control. Intraspinal anesthesia uses the concept that the spinal cord is the primary link in nociceptive transmission. The goal is to mimic the body's endogenous opioid pain modification system by interfering with the transmission of pain and providing an opiate receptor binding agent directly into the spinal cord. The benefits of the intraspinal route include good to excellent pain control with typically lower doses of opioids, increased patient mobility, minimal sedation, and increased patient satisfaction.[122] The hemodynamic status of the patient changes very little.

Intraspinal anesthesia is particularly appropriate for pain in the thorax, upper abdomen, and lower extremities. The two intraspinal routes are intrathecal and epidural (Fig. 9-8). Regardless of the route, the effects of the opioid agonist used is the same, and assessment parameters are the same as those used for other routes. Nursing management of the patient receiving intraspinal analgesia is described in the Nursing Interventions Classification (NIC) feature.

NIC

Analgesic Administration: Intraspinal

Definition
Administration of pharmacologic agents into the epidural or intrathecal space to reduce or eliminate pain

Activities
Check patency and function of the catheter, port, and pump.

Ensure that intravenous access is in place at all times during therapy.

Label the catheter, and secure it appropriately.

Ensure that the proper formulation of the drug is used (e.g., correct concentration, preservative-free).

Ensure narcotic antagonist availability for emergency administration, and administer per physician order, as necessary.

Start continuous infusion of analgesic agent after correct catheter placement has been verified, and monitor rate to ensure delivery of the prescribed dosage of medication.

Monitor temperature, blood pressure, respirations, pulse, and level of consciousness at appropriate intervals, and record on flow sheet.

Monitor level of sensory blockade at appropriate intervals, and record on flow sheet.

Monitor catheter site and dressings to check for a loose catheter or wet dressing, and notify appropriate personnel per agency protocol.

Administer catheter site care according to agency protocol.

Secure needle in place with tape, and apply appropriate dressing according to agency protocol.

Monitor for adverse reactions, including respiratory depression, urinary retention, undue somnolence, itching, seizures, nausea, and vomiting.

Monitor orthostatic blood pressure and pulse before the first attempt at ambulation.

Instruct patient to report side effects, alterations in pain relief, numbness of extremities, and need for assistance with ambulation if weak.

Follow institutional policies for injection of intermittent analgesic agents into the injection port.

Provide adjunct medications as appropriate (e.g., antidepressants, anticonvulsants, nonsteroidal antiinflammatory agents).

Increase the intraspinal dose based on a pain intensity score.

Instruct and guide the patient through nonpharmacologic measures (e.g., simple relaxation therapy, simple guided imagery, biofeedback) to enhance pharmacologic effectiveness.

Instruct patient about proper home care for external or implanted delivery systems, as appropriate.

Remove or assist with removal of catheter according to agency protocol.

From Bulechek GM et al: *Nursing interventions classification (NIC)*, ed 5, St Louis, 2008, Mosby.

Intrathecal Analgesia. Intrathecal (subarachnoid) opioids are placed directly into the cerebral spinal fluid and attach to spinal cord receptor sites. Opioids introduced at this site act quickly at the dorsal horn. The dural sheath is punctured, eliminating the barrier for pathogens between the environment and the cerebral spinal fluid. This creates the risk of serious infections. The intrathecal route is usually reserved for intraoperative use. Single-bolus dosing provides short-term relief for pain that is short lived (the pain of labor and delivery is well managed using this regimen).[119] Side effects of intrathecal pain control include postdural puncture headache and infection.

Epidural Analgesia. Epidural analgesia is commonly used in the critical care unit after major abdominal surgery, nephrectomy, thoracotomy, and major orthopedic procedures. Certain conditions preclude the use of this pain control method: systemic infection, anticoagulation, and increased intracranial pressure. Epidural delivery of opiates provides longer-lasting pain relief with less dosing of opiates. When delivered into the epidural space, 5 mg of morphine may be effective for 6 to 24 hours, compared with 3 to 4 hours when delivered intravenously. Opioids infused in the epidural space are more unpredictable than those administered intrathecally. The epidural space is filled with fatty tissue and is external to the dura mater. The fatty tissue interferes with uptake, and the dura acts as a barrier to diffusion, making diffusion rate difficult to predict.

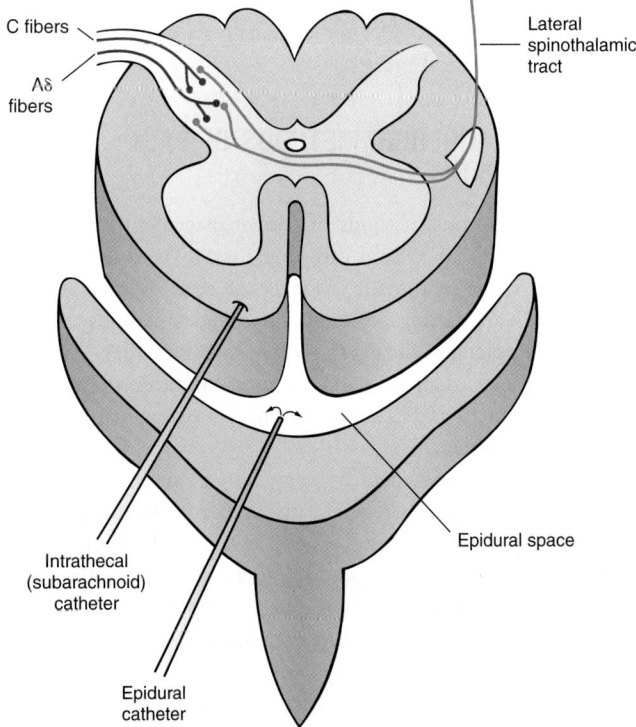

C fibers

Aδ fibers

Lateral spinothalamic tract

Intrathecal (subarachnoid) catheter

Epidural space

Epidural catheter

Figure 9-8 Intraspinal catheter placement in a spinal cord cross section.

The type of drug used determines the rapidity of drug diffusion. Drugs are *hydrophilic* or *lipophilic*. Hydrophilic drugs are water soluble and penetrate the dura slowly, giving them a longer onset and duration of action. Morphine is hydrophilic. Lipophilic drugs are lipid soluble; they penetrate the dura rapidly and therefore have a rapid onset of action and a shorter duration of action. Fentanyl is lipophilic.

The dura acts as a physical barrier and causes delay in diffusion of the drug. Compared with the intrathecal route, it allows more drug to be absorbed in the systemic circulation, requiring greater doses for pain relief.[122] Drugs delivered epidurally may be administered by bolus or continuous infusion. Epidural analgesia is being used more often in the critical care environment, and it requires careful monitoring.

The nurse must assess the patient for respiratory depression. This phenomenon may occur early in the therapy or as late as 24 hours after initiation. The epidural catheter also puts the patient at risk for infection. The efficiency of this pain control method and the increased mobility of the patient does not diminish the nurse's responsibility to monitor and evaluate the outcomes of the pain management protocol in use.

Equianalgesia. When a modification of opioid is considered, the nurse must be aware of equianalgesic dosages. In doing any conversion, the goal is to provide equal analgesic effects with the new agents. This concept is referred to as *equianalgesia.* Morphine is the standard for the conversion of opioids. Prescribed dosages must take into account the patient's age and health status.[30] The critical care nurse must have access to a chart for easy referral on the unit to administer the correct dosages of opioids to critically ill patients. Because of the variety of agents and routes, the professional pain organizations have developed equianalgesia charts for use by the health care professional. All critical care units need to have a chart posted for easy referral. Table 9-4 provides the equianalgesia dose for different drugs used in clinical practice.

NONPHARMACOLOGIC METHODS OF PAIN MANAGEMENT

Although numerous methods of pain management other than drugs appear in the critical care literature,[123] very few studies have been done to provide evidence of their effectiveness in the critical care settings. Nonpharmacologic methods can be used to supplement analgesic treatment, but they are not intended to replace analgesics.[124] In most instances, these therapies may augment and enhance the pharmacologic management of the patient's pain.

Critical care nurses identify many barriers to the use of nonpharmacologic methods for pain management, including a lack of knowledge, training, and time.[125] Despite these problems, more than 60% of them are willing to use the methods to relieve their patients' pain. It is crucial that critical care nurses be provided with the appropriate training and equipment

required to apply nonpharmacologic methods for pain management in the critically ill.

Transcutaneous Electrical Nerve Stimulator. Stimulating other non–pain sensory fibers (Aβ) in the periphery modifies pain transmission. These fibers are stimulated by thermal changes as in the application of heat or cold, by simple massage, or by the action of the transcutaneous electrical nerve stimulator (TENS). The use of massage has been a mainstay in the nursing management of the patient in acute pain.[126]

The use of TENS has some contraindications in the critical care unit. Because the device is controlled by the patient, mentation must be intact. TENS is also contraindicated in patients with pacemakers or automatic implantable defibrillators because these devices may recognize and erroneously interpret the TENS electrical signal. TENS therapy is efficient, patient-controlled pain management for orthopedic, obstetric, and some postoperative pain states.[127]

COGNITIVE TECHNIQUES

Using the cortical interpretation of pain as the foundation, several interventions can reduce the patient's pain report. These modalities include cognitive techniques: patient teaching, relaxation, distraction, guided imagery, music therapy, and hypnosis.

Relaxation. Relaxation is a well-documented method for reducing the distress associated with pain. Although not a substitute for pharmacology, relaxation is an excellent adjunct for controlling pain.[128,129] Relaxation decreases oxygen consumption and muscle tone, and it can decrease heart rate and blood pressure. Relaxation gives the patient a sense of control over the pain and reduces muscle tension and anxiety. Not all patients are interested in relaxation therapy. For those patients, deep-breathing exercises may be helpful, and they frequently lead to relaxation.[130] Excellent references for thorough techniques in relaxation therapy are available.[30]

Guided Imagery. Guided imagery is a technique that uses the imagination to provide control over pain. It can be used to distract or relax. Guiding a patient to a place that is pain free and relaxing takes a considerable time commitment on the part of the nurse. Although this may be difficult in the critical care environment, guiding a patient to a place in his or her imagination that is free from pain may be beneficial.[123]

Music Therapy. Music therapy is a commonly used intervention for relaxation. Music that is pleasing to the patient may have soothing effects, but its effects on reducing pain are controversial.[131] Ideally, the music should be supplied by a small set of headphones. It is important to educate the patient and family regarding the role of music in relaxation and pain control and to provide music of the patient's choice.

The patient and family may provide information about other sources of distraction for the patient. Determining what distraction therapies the patient normally uses may provide a clue to which one may work during the illness. Some persons are distracted by television; for others, television is a source of

TABLE 9-4 Equianalgesic Chart: Approximate Equivalent Doses of Opioids for Moderate-to-Severe Pain

Analgesic	Parenteral (IM, SC, IV) Route[1,2] (mg)	PO Route[1] (mg)	Comments
Mu Opioid Agonists			
Morphine	10	30	Standard for comparison; multiple routes of administration; available in immediate-release and controlled-release formulations; active metabolite M6G can accumulate with repeated dosing in renal failure
Codeine	130	200 NR	IM has unpredictable absorption and high side effect profile; used PO for mild-to-moderate pain; usually compounded with nonopioid (e.g., Tylenol No. 3)
Fentanyl	100 mcg/hr parenterally and transdermally $\cong$ 4 mg/hr morphine parenterally; 1 mcg/hr transdermally $\cong$ 2 mg/24 hr morphine PO	—	Short half-life, but at steady state, slow elimination from tissues can lead to a prolonged half-life (up to 12 hr); start opioid-naïve patients on no more than 25 mcg/hr transdermally; transdermal fentanyl NR for acute pain management; available by oral transmucosal route
Hydromorphone (Dilaudid)	1.5	7.5	Useful alternative to morphine; no evidence that metabolites are clinically relevant; shorter duration than morphine; available in high-potency parenteral formulation (10 mg/mL) useful for SC infusion; 3 mg rectal $\cong$ 650 mg aspirin PO; with repeated dosing (e.g., PCA), it is more likely than 2-3 mg parenteral hydromorphone = 10 mg parenteral morphine
Levorphanol (Levo-Dromoran)	2	4	Longer-acting than morphine when given repeatedly; long half-life can lead to accumulation within 2-3 days of repeated dosing.
Meperidine	75	300 NR	No longer preferred as a first-line opioid for the management of acute or chronic pain due to potential toxicity from accumulation of metabolite, normeperidine; normeperidine has 15-20 hr half-life and is not reversed by naloxone; NR in elderly or patients with impaired renal functions; NR by continuous IV infusion
Methadone (Dolophine)	10	20	Longer-acting than morphine when given repeatedly; long half-life can lead to delayed toxicity from accumulation within 3-5 days; start PO dosing on PRN schedule; in opioid-tolerant patients converted to methadone, start with 10%-25% of equianalgesic dose
Oxycodone	—	20	Used for moderate pain when combined with a nonopioid (e.g., Percocet, Tylox); available as single entity in immediate-release and controlled-release formulations (e.g., OxyContin); can be used like PO morphine for severe pain
Oxymorphone (Numorphan)	1	10 rectal	Used for moderate to severe pain; no PO formulation

[1]Duration of analgesia is dose dependent; the higher the dose, usually the longer the duration.

[2]IV boluses may be used to produce analgesia that lasts approximately as long as IM or SC doses. However, of all routes of administration, IV produces the highest peak concentration of the drug, and the peak concentration is associated with the highest level of toxicity, e.g., sedation. To decrease the peak effect and lower the level of toxicity, IV boluses may be administered more slowly, e.g., 10 mg of morphine over a 15-minute period, or smaller doses may be administered more often, e.g., 5 mg of morphine every 1-1.5 hours.

FDA, U.S. Food and Drug Administration; IM, intramuscular; IV, intravenous; M6G, morphine-6-glucuronide; MCG, micrograms; MG, milligrams; NR, not recommended; PCA, patient-controlled analgesia; PO, by mouth; PRN, pro re nata (as needed); SC, subcutaneous.

Continued

TABLE 9-4   Equianalgesic Chart: Approximate Equivalent Doses of Opioids for Moderate-to-Severe Pain—*cont'd*

Analgesic	Parenteral (IM, SC, IV) Route[1,2] (mg)	PO Route[1] (mg)	Comments
Agonist-Antagonist Opioids:	Not recommended for severe, escalating pain. If used in combination with mu agonists, may reverse analgesia and precipitate withdrawal in opioid-dependent patients.		
Buprenorphine (Buprenex)	0.4	—	Not readily reversed by naloxone; NR for laboring patients
Butorphanol (Stadol)	2	—	Available in nasal spray
Dezocine (Dalgan)	10	—	
Nalbuphine (Nubain)	10	—	
Pentazocine (Talwin)	60	180	

Selected references for more information: Pasero C, Portenoy RK, McCaffery M: Opioid analgesics, pp. 161-299. In McCaffery M, Pasero C: *Pain: clinical manual,* St Louis, 1999, Mosby, pp 241-243; American Pain Society (APS): *Principles of analgesic use in the treatment of acute and cancer pain,* ed 3, Glenview, IL, 1992, APS; Lawlor P et al: Dose ratio between morphine and hydromorphone in patients with cancer pain: a retrospective study, *Pain* 72(1,2):79-85, 1997; Manfredi PL et al: Intravenous methadone for cancer pain unrelieved by morphine and hydromorphone: clinical observations, *Pain* 70:99-101, 1997; Portenoy RK: Opioid analgesics. In Portenoy RK, Kanner RM, editors: *Pain management: theory and practice,* pp 249-276, Philadelphia, 1996, FA Davis.

Eqiuianalgesic Chart **Approximate equivalent doses of PO nonopioids and opioids for mild to moderate pain**	
ANALGESIC	**PO DOSAGE (mg)**
Nonopioids	
Acetaminophen	650
Aspirin (ASA)	650
Opioids*	
Codeine	32-60
Hydrocodone[†]	5
Meperidine (Demerol)	50
Oxycodone[‡]	3-5
Propoxyphene (Darvon)	65-100

*Often combined with acetaminophen; avoid exceeding maximum total daily dose of acetaminophen (4000 mg/day).
[†]Combined with acetaminophen (e.g., Vicodin, Lortab).
[‡]Combined with acetaminophen (e.g., Percocet, Tylox); also available alone as controlled-release OxyContin and immediate-release formulations.

A Guide to Using Equianalgesic Charts

- Equianalgesic means approximately the same pain relief.
- The equianalgesic chart is a guideline. Doses and intervals between doses are titrated according to the individual's response.
- The equianalgesic chart is helpful when switching from one drug to another or when switching from one route of administration to another.
- Dosages in the equianalgesic chart for moderate to severe pain are not necessarily starting doses. The doses suggest a ratio for comparing the analgesia of one drug with another.
- For elderly patients, initially reduce the recommended adult opioid dose for moderate to severe pain by 25% to 50%.
- The longer the patient has been receiving opioids, the more conservative the starting dose of a *new* opioid.

Selected references for more information: McCaffery M, Portenoy RK: Nonopioids: acetaminophen and nonsteroidal antiinflammatory drugs, p 133. In McCaffery M, Pasero C, editors: *Pain: clinical manual,* St Louis, 1999, Mosby; American Pain Society (APS): Principles of analgesic use in the treatment of acute pain and cancer pain, ed 3, Glenview, IL, 1992, APS; Kaiko R et al: Analgesic efficacy of controlled-release (CR) oxycodone and CR morphine, *Clin Pharmacol Ther* 59:130, 1996. Modified from McCaffery M, Pasero C: *Pain: clinical manual,* St Louis, 1999, Mosby.

Increased anxiety. Do not assume that the patient does or does not want to watch television until you determine whether it will be beneficial or harmful to the patient.

The key to success with any of these therapies is a comprehensive understanding of their mechanism of action so that the therapy matches the needs of the patient. Most of the previously mentioned interventions require the patient's cooperation. There must be some commitment to the treatment on the part of the patient. When handled effectively, nonpharmacologic methods can assist in pain management.

Case Study: Patient with Pain

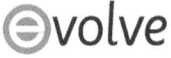 Answers to the Case Study Questions can be found on the Evolve web site at http://evolve.elsevier.com/Urden/.

Brief Patient History

Ms. X is a woman with type 2 diabetes mellitus and peripheral arterial occlusive disease with neuropathy. Ms. X is disabled because of limited mobility and chronic pain associated with lower extremity claudication and neuropathic pain. She has been admitted for an elective right femoral to distal tibial bypass. Ms. X's chronic pain has been effectively managed with gabapentin (600 mg three times daily) and a 75-μg fentanyl patch every third day. Ms. X reports that her pain patch is due to be changed the next day. Her diabetes mellitus has been effectively managed with diet and a combination of oral agents. Postoperatively, orders for pain management include her home regimen of gabapentin and fentanyl patch and an order for morphine for breakthrough pain.

Clinical Assessment

Ms. X is admitted to the intensive care unit from the perianesthesia recovery room after an 8-hour surgical revascularization of the right lower extremity. She is awake, alert, and oriented to person, time, place, and situation. Ms. X is breathing through her mouth and taking shallow breaths. She complains of right lower extremity and bilateral foot pain. Her skin is warm and dry. Ms. X is able to move her toes on command, and lower extremity sensation to touch is intact; however, she is complaining of severe burning both feet.

Diagnostic Procedures

Ms. X reports that her pain is a 10 on the Baker-Wong Faces Scale. The Riker Sedation-Agitation Scale score is 5.

Medical Diagnosis

The diagnosis is acute postoperative incisional pain superimposed on chronic neuropathic pain involving both lower extremities. Neuropathic pain is likely worsened because of missed doses of gabapentin.

Questions

1. What major outcomes do you expect to achieve for this patient?
2. What problems or risks must be managed to achieve these outcomes?
3. What interventions must be initiated to monitor, prevent, manage, or eliminate the problems and risks identified?
4. What interventions should be initiated to promote optimal functioning, safety, and well-being of the patient?
5. What possible learning needs do you anticipate for this patient?
6. What cultural and age-related factors may have a bearing on the patient's plan of care?

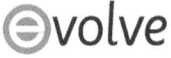 Be sure to check out the bonus material, including free self-assessment exercises, on the Evolve web site at http://evolve.elsevier.com/Urden/.

Summary

- Pain in the critically ill patient is difficult to assess and manage. There are many sources of pain in the critical care setting, and the effects of unrelieved acute pain can have a significant impact on the patient's recovery.
- When possible, the patient's self-report of pain must be obtained. A simple yes or no communicated by head nodding from a mechanically ventilated patient is considered a valid self-report of pain.
- When the patient's self-report is not available, behavioral indicators represent alternative measures of pain assessment, and assessment tools (e.g., BPS, CPOT) have been developed for assessment of pain in the critically ill mechanically ventilated population.
- In some situations, behavioral indicators may be impossible to assess accurately. The use of physiologic indicators is then crucial. However, vital signs do not represent valid information for pain assessment. Innovative physiologic measures (e.g., NIRS, BIS) are being explored and may support the clinicians in the pain assessment process.
- The critical care nurse must collaborate with the multidisciplinary team to ensure a plan of care for management of the patient's pain is developed. To fully participate, the critical care nurse must have extensive knowledge of nonpharmacologic and pharmacologic therapies designed to achieve effective pain relief.

References

1. Rotondi AJ et al: Patients' recollections of stressful experiences while receiving prolonged mechanical ventilation in an intensive care unit, *Crit Care Med* 30:746, 2002.
2. Hamill-Ruth RJ, Marohn L: Evaluation of pain in the critically ill patient, *Crit Care Clin* 15:35, 1999.
3. Kwekkeboom KL, Herr K: Assessment of pain in the critically ill, *Crit Care Nurs Clin North Am* 13:181, 2001.
4. Gélinas C: Management of pain in cardiac surgery ICU patients: have we improved over time? *Intensive Crit Care Nurs* 23:298, 2007.
5. Puntillo KA et al: Patients' perceptions and responses to procedural pain: results from Thunder Project II, *Am J Crit Care* 10:238, 2001.
6. Stanik-Hutt J et al: Pain experiences of traumatically injured patients in a critical care setting, *Am J Crit Care* 10:252, 2001.
7. Desbiens NA et al: Pain and satisfaction with pain control in seriously ill hospitalized adults: findings from the SUPPORT research investigations, *Crit Care Med* 24:1953, 1996.
8. Gélinas C et al: Pain assessment and management in critically ill intubated patients: a retrospective study, *Am J Crit Care* 13:126, 2004.

9. Puntillo KA et al: Practices and predictors of analgesic interventions for adults undergoing painful procedures, *Am J Crit Care* 11:415, 2002.

10. Carr DB, Goudas LC: Acute pain, *Lancet* 353:2051, 1999.

11. Kehlet H: Surgical stress and postoperative outcome—from here to where? *Reg Anesth Pain Med* 31:47, 2006.

12. Joshi GP, Ogunnaike BO: Consequences of inadequate postoperative pain relief and chronic persistent postoperative pain, *Anesth Clin North Am* 23:21, 2005.

13. Kehlet H et al: Persistent postsurgical pain: risk factors and prevention, *Lancet* 367:1618, 2006.

14. International Association for the Study of Pain (IASP) Subcommittee on Taxonomy: Pain terms: a list with definitions and notes on usage, *Pain* 6:249, 1979.

15. Shannon K, Bucknall T: Pain assessment in critical care: what have we learnt from research, *Intensive Crit Care Nurs* 19:154, 2003.

16. Puntillo KA: Pain experience of intensive care unit patients, *Heart Lung* 19:526, 1990.

17. Puntillo KA: Dimensions of procedural pain and its analgesic management in critically ill surgical patients, *Am J Crit Care* 3:116, 1994.

18. Puntillo KA, Weiss SJ: Pain: its mediators and associated morbidity in critically ill cardiovascular surgical patients, *Nurs Res* 43:31, 1994.

19. Gélinas C, Johnston C: Pain assessment in the critically ill ventilated adult: validation of the Critical-Care Pain Observation Tool and physiological indicators, *Clin J Pain* 23:497, 2007.

20. Agency for Health Care Policy and Research (AHCPR): *Clinical Practice Guideline Acute pain management: operative or medical procedures and trauma*, Rockville, MD, Department of Health and Human Services, Public Health Service, 1992, AHCPR.

21. Herr K et al: Pain assessment in the nonverbal patient: Position statement with clinical practice recommendations, *Pain Manag Nurs* 7:44, 2006.

22. Jacobi J et al: Clinical practice guidelines for the sustained use of sedatives and analgesics in the critically ill adult, *Crit Care Med* 30:119, 2002.

23. Joint Commission on Accreditation of Healthcare Organizations (JCAHO): *Pain: current understanding of assessment, management, and treatments*, Oakbrook Terrace, IL, 2001, JCAHO.

24. McCaffery M: *Nursing management of the patient with pain*, ed 2, Philadelphia, 1979, JB Lippincott.

25. Anand KJS, Craig, KD: New perspectives on the definition of pain, *Pain* 67:3, 1996.

26. McGuire D: Comprehensive and multidimensional assessment and measurement of pain, *J Pain Symptom Manage* 7:312, 1992.

27. Melzack R: Pain and stress: a new perspective. In Gatchel RJ, Turk DC, editors: *Psychological factors in pain*, New York, 1999, Guilford Press.

28. American Geriatrics Society (AGS) Panel on Persistent Pain in Older Persons: The management of persistent pain in older persons, *J Am Geriatr Soc* 50:S205, 2002.

29. International Association for the Study of Pain (IASP) Task Force on Taxonomy: *Classification of chronic pain*, Seattle, 1994, IASP Press.

30. McCaffery M, Pasero C: *Pain: clinical manual for nursing practice*, ed 2, St Louis, 1999, CV Mosby.

31. Dworkin RH et al: Advances in neuropathic pain: diagnosis, mechanisms, and treatment recommendations, *Arch Neurol* 60:1524, 2003.

32. Hayes C, Molloy AR: Neuropathic pain in the perioperative period, *Int Anesthesiol Clin* 35:67, 1997.

33. Siddall PJ, Cousins MJ: Neurobiology of pain, *Int Anesthesiol Clin* 35:1, 1997.

34. Woolf CJ, Mannion RJ: Neuropathic pain: aetiology, symptoms, mechanisms, and management, *Lancet* 353:1959, 1999.

35. Charlton JE: *Core curriculum for professional education in pain*, ed 3, Seattle, 2005, IASP Press.

36. Melzack R, Wall PD: *The challenge of pain*, ed 2, London, 1996, Penguin Books.

37. Gélinas C et al: Les indicateurs de la douleur en soins critiques [Pain indicators in critical care], *Perspect Infirm* 2:12, 2005.

38. Hofbauer RK et al: Cortical representation of the sensory dimension of pain, *J Neurophysiol* 86:402, 2001.

39. Rainville P: Brain mechanisms of pain affect and pain modulation, *Curr Opin Neurobiol* 12:195, 2002.

40. Rainville P et al: Pain affect encoded in human anterior cingulate but not somatosensory cortex, *Science* 277:968, 1997.

41. Derbyshire SW, Osborn J: Modeling pain circuits: how imaging may modify perception, *Neuroimaging Clin N Am* 17:485, 2007.

42. Treede RD et al: The cortical representation of pain, *Pain* 79:105, 1999.

43. Selye H: *Stress without distress*, Philadelphia, 1974, JB Lippincott.

44. McCance KL, Huether SE: *Pathophysiology: the biologic basis for disease in adults and children*, ed 5, St. Louis, 2006, Mosby.

45. Payen JF et al: Assessing pain in the critically ill sedated patients by using a behavioral pain scale, *Crit Care Med* 29:2258, 2001.

46. Puntillo KA et al: Relationship between behavioral and physiological indicators of pain, critical care self-reports of pain, and opioid administration, *Crit Care Med* 25:1159, 1997.

47. Hurwitz BE et al: Differential patterns of dynamic cardiovascular regulation as a function of task, *Biol Psychol* 36:75, 1993.

48. Rabin BS et al: Bidirectional interaction between the central nervous system and the immune system, *Crit Rev Immunol* 9:279, 1989.

49. Sapolsky RM: Stress, glucocorticoids, and damage to the nervous system: the current state of confusion, *Stress* 1:1, 1996.

50. Daut RL, Cleeland CS: The prevalence and severity of pain in cancer, *Cancer* 50:1913, 1982.

51. Melzack R: The short form McGill Pain Questionnaire, *Pain* 30:191, 1987.

52. Jarvis C: *Physical examination & health assessment*, ed 5, Philadelphia, 2008, Saunders.

53. Puntillo KA: Pain management. In Schell HM, Puntillo KA, editors: *Critical care nursing secrets*, ed 2, Philadelphia, 2006, Hanley & Belfus.

54. Carey SJ et al: Improving pain management in an acute care setting: the Crawford Long Hospital of Emory University Experience, *Orthopaed Nurs* 16:29, 1997.

55. Stuppy DJ: The Faces Pain Scale: reliability and validity with mature adults, *Appl Nurs Res* 11:84, 1998.

56. Gélinas C: Le thermomètre d'intensité de douleur: un nouvel outil pour les patients adultes en soins critiques [The Faces Pain Thermometer: a new tool for critically ill adults], *Perspect Infirm* 4:12, 2007.

57. Puntillo KA et al: Pain behaviors observed during six common procedures: results from Thunder Project II, *Crit Care Med* 32:421, 2004.

58. Gélinas C, Arbour C: Behavioral and physiological indicators during a nociceptive procedure in conscious and unconscious mechanically ventilated adults: similar or different? *J Crit Care* 2009 (in press).

59. Gélinas C et al: Validation of the Critical-Care Pain Observation Tool (CPOT) in adult patients, *Am J Crit Care* 15:420, 2006.

60. Mateo OM, Krenzischek DA: A pilot study to assess the relationship between behavioral manifestations and self-report of pain in postanesthesia care unit patients, *J Post Anesth Nurs* 7:15, 1992.

61. Li D et al: A review of objective pain measures for use with critical care adult patients unable to self-report, *J Pain* 9:2, 2008.

62. Sessler CN et al: Evaluating and monitoring analgesia and sedation in the intensive care unit, *Crit Care* 12(suppl 3):S2, 2008.

63. Aïssaoui Y et al: Validation of a behavioral pain scale in critically ill sedated, and mechanically ventilated patients, *Anesth Analg* 101:1470, 2005.

64. Young J et al: Use of a Behavioral Pain Scale to assess pain in ventilated, unconscious and/or sedated patients, *Intensive Crit Care Nurs* 22:32, 2006.

65. Gélinas C et al: Item selection and Content validity of the Critical-Care Pain Observation Tool: an instrument to assess pain in critically ill non-verbal adults, *J Adv Nurs* 65(1):203, 2009.

66. Gélinas C: Theoretical, psychometric, and pragmatic issues in pain measurement, *Pain Manag Nurs* 9:120, 2008.

67. Gélinas C, Hammond L: Nurses' evaluations of the Critical-Care Pain Observation Tool, 2009 (unpublished).

68. Gélinas C et al: Sensitivity and specificity of the Critical-Care Pain Observation Tool for the detection of pain in intubated adults following cardiac surgery, *J Pain Symptom Manage* 37(1):58, 2009.

69. Foster RL: Nursing judgment: the key to pain assessment in critically ill children, *J Soc Pediatr Nurs* 6:90, 2001.

70. Apkarian AV et al: Human brain mechanisms of pain perception and regulation in health and disease, *Eur J Pain*, 9:463, 2005.

71. Bartocci M: *Brain functional near infrared spectroscopy in human infants* [PhD thesis], Solna, Sweden, 2006, Karolinska Institute.

72. Bartocci M et al: Pain activates cortical areas in the preterm newborn brain, *Pain* 122:109, 2006.

73. Slater R et al: Cortical pain responses in human infants, *J Neurosci* 26:3662, 2006.

74. Slater R et al: How well do clinical pain assessment tools reflect pain in infants? *PLoS Med* 5:928, 2008.

75. Gélinas C et al: Towards a new approach for the detection of pain in adults undergoing cardiac surgery: the near-infrared spectroscopy (NIRS)—a pilot study, *Pain* 2009 (in press).

76. Huang CM et al: Comparison of pain responses of premature infants to the heelstick between containment and swaddling, *J Nurs Res* 12:31, 2004.

77. Simons SHP et al: Do we still hurt newborn babies? A prospective study of procedural pain and analgesia in neonates, *Arch Pediatr Adolesc Med* 157:1058, 2003.

78. Li DT et al: Physiologic and behavioral responses associated with noxious procedures in sedated critically ill patients, *J Crit Care* 2009 (in press).

79. Gordon DB et al: American Pain recommendations for improving the quality of acute and cancer pain management, *Arch Intern Med* 165:1574, 2005.

80. Miaskowski C et al: *Guidelines for the management of cancer pain in adults and children*, Clinical Practice Guidelines Series, no 3, Glenville, IL, 2005, American Pain Society.

81. Lawrence M: The unconscious experience, *Am J Crit Care* 4:227, 1995.

82. Bjoro K, Herr K: Assessment of pain in the nonverbal or cognitively impaired older adult, *Clin Geriatr Med* 24:237, 2008.

83. Hadjistavropoulos T et al: An interdisciplinary expert consensus statement on assessment of pain in older persons, *Clin J Pain* 23:S1, 2007.

84. Herr KA, Mobily PR: Comparison of selected pain assessment tools for use with the elderly, *Appl Nurs Res* 6:39, 1993.

85. Aubin M et al: L'évaluation systématique des instruments pour mesurer la douleur chez les personnes àgées ayant des capacités réduites à communiquer, *Pain Res Manag* 12:195, 2007.

86. Zwakhalen SM et al: Pain in elderly people with severe dementia: a systematic review of behavioral pain assessment tools, *BMC Geriatr* 6:1, 2006.

87. Fuchs-Labelle S, Hadjistavropoulos T: Development and preliminary validation of the Pain Assessment Checklist for Seniors with Limited Ability to Communicate (PACSLAC), *Pain Manag Nurs* 5:37, 2004.

88. Wary B, Doloplus C: Doloplus-2, a scale for pain measurement, *Soins Gerontol* 19:25, 1999.

89. Wary B et al: Doloplus 2: validation d'une échelle d'évaluation comportementale de la douleur chez la personne âgée, *Douleurs* 1:35, 2001.

90. McNicoll L et al: Delirium in the intensive care unit: occurrence and clinical course in older patients, *J Am Geriatr Soc* 51:591, 2003.

91. Graf C, Puntillo KA: Pain in the older adult in the intensive care unit, *Crit Care Clin* 19:749, 2003.

92. Anand KJS: The applied physiology of pain. In Anand KJS, McGrath PJ, editors: *Pain in neonates*, Amsterdam, 1993, Elsevier.

93. Duhn LJ, Medves JM: A systematic integrative review of infant pain assessment tools, *Adv Neonatal Care* 4:126, 2004.

94. Stevens B et al: Premature Infant Pain Profile: development and initial validation, *Clin J Pain* 12:13, 1996.

95. Foster RL: Physiologic correlates of comfort in healthy children, *Pain Manag Nurs* 4:23, 2003.

96. Bozeman M: Cultural aspects of pain management. In Salerno E, Willens J, editors: *Pain management handbook: an interdisciplinary approach*, St Louis, 1996, Mosby.

97. Ulmer J: Identifying and preventing pain mismanagement. In Salerno E, Willens J, editors: *Pain management handbook: an interdisciplinary approach*, St Louis, 1996, Mosby.

98. Carroll KC et al: Pain assessment and management in critically ill postoperative and trauma patients: a multisite study, *Am J Crit Care* 8:105, 1999.

99. Smith LH: Opioid safety: is your patient at risk for respiratory depression? *Clin J Oncol Nurs* 11:293, 2007.

100. Idvall E, Ehrenberg A: Nursing documentation of postoperative pain management, *J Clin Nurs* 11:734, 2002.

101. Kirkchhoff LT, Beckstrand RL: Critical care nurses perceptions of obstacles and helpful behaviors in providing end-of-life care to dying patients. *Am J Crit Care* 9:96, 2000.

102. Wild LR: Pain management: an organizational perspective, *Crit Care Nurs Clin North Am* 13:297, 2001.

103. Liu LL, Gropper MA: Postoperative analgesia and sedation in the adult intensive care unit: a guide to drug selection, *Drugs* 63:755, 2003.

104. Pasero CL, McCaffery M: Avoiding opioid-induced respiratory depression, *Am J Nurs* 94(4):24-30, 1994.

105. Sarhill N et al: Hydromorphone: pharmacology and clinical applications in cancer patients, *Support Care Cancer* 9:84, 2001.

106. Marcantonio ER et al: The relationship of postoperative delirium with psychoactive medications, *JAMA* 272:1518, 1994.

107. McGory R: Pharmacokinetic and pharmacodynamic concerns in the critically ill. In Hamill RJ, Rowlingson RC, editors: *Handbook of critical care pain management*, New York, 1994, McGraw-Hill.

108. Davis MP, Walsh D: Methadone for relief of cancer pain: a review of pharmacokinetics, pharmacodynamics, drug interactions and protocols of administration, *Support Care Cancer* 9:73, 2001.

109. World Health Organization (WHO): *Cancer pain relief*, Geneva, 1986, WHO.

110. Cavalière F et al: A low-dose remifentanil infusion is well tolerated for sedation in mechanically ventilated, critically ill patients, *Can J Anaesth* 49:1088, 2002.

111. Soltész S et al: Recovery after remifentanil and sufentanil for analgesia and sedation of mechanically ventilated patients after trauma or major surgery, *Br J Anaesth* 86:763, 2001.

112. Ethuin F et al: Pharmacokinetics of long-term sufentanyl infusion for sedation in ICU patients, *Intensive Care Med* 29:1916, 2003.

113. Pasero C et al: IV opioids range orders for acute pain management, *Am J Nurs* 107:62, 2007.

114. Yantis MA: Obstructive sleep apnea syndrome, *Am J Nurs* 102:83, 2002.

115. Pasero C, McCaffery M: Reversing respiratory depression with naloxone. *Am J Nurs* 100:26, 2000.

116. Lehne RA: *Pharmacology for nursing care*, ed 6, Philadelphia, 2007, Saunders.

117. Summer GJ, Puntillo KA: Management of surgical and procedural pain in a critical care setting, *Crit Care Nurs Clin North Am* 13:233, 2001.

118. Ready LB et al: Evaluation of intravenous ketorolac administered by bolus of infusion for treatment of postoperative pain, *Anesthesiology* 80:1277, 1994.

119. American Society of Hospital Pharmacists: *American hospital formulary service drug information* 99, Bethesda, MD, 1999, The Association.

120. Feldman HI et al: Parenteral ketorolac: the risk for acute renal failure, *Ann Intern Med* 126:193, 1997.

121. Strom BL et al: Parenteral ketorolac and risk of gastrointestinal and operative site bleeding, *JAMA* 275:376, 1996.

122. Dyble K: Epidural and intrathecal methods of analgesia in the critically ill. In Puntillo K, editor: *Pain in the critically ill: assessment and management*, Gaithersburg, MD, 1991, Aspen.

123. Gujol M: A survey of pain assessment and management practices among critical care nurses, *Am J Crit Care* 3:123, 1994.

124. Pasero C et al: Postoperative pain management in the older adult. In Gibson D, Weiner D, editors: *Pain in older persons. Progress in pain research and management*, vol 35, pp 377-401, Seattle, 2005, IASP Press.

125. Tracy MF et al: Nurse attitudes towards the use of complementary and alternative therapies in critical care, *Heart Lung* 32:197, 2003.

126. Richards KC et al: Effects of massage in acute and critical care, *AACN Clin Issues* 11:77, 2000.

127. Rakel B, Herr K: Assessment and treatment of postoperative pain in older adults, *J PeriAnesthesia Nurs* 19:194, 2004.

128. Houston S, Jesurum J: The quick relaxation technique: effect on pain associated with chest tube removal, *Appl Nurs Res* 12:196, 1999.

129. Miller KM, Perry PA: Relaxation technique and postoperative pain in patients undergoing cardiac surgery, *Heart Lung* 19:136, 1990.

130. Good M et al: Relief of postoperative pain with jaw relaxation, music and their combination. *Pain* 81:163, 1999.

131. Biley FC: The effects on patient well-being of music listening as a nursing intervention: a review of the literature, *J Clin Nurs* 9:668, 2000.

Sedation, Agitation, Delirium: Assessment and Management

$\mathcal{O}$ne of the challenges facing clinicians is how to provide a therapeutic environment for patients in the alarm-filled, emergency-focused critical care unit. Rest and relaxation can be difficult to find. Up to 74% of critical care patients demonstrate some degree of agitation during their critical care hospitalization.[1] Patients often report upsetting dreams, hallucinations, nightmares, and flashbacks once they are recovered. The many causes of this agitation include painful procedures, invasive tubes, sleep deprivation, fear, anxiety, and the stress associated with critical illness. Some patients experience a posttraumatic stress disorder (PTSD) syndrome after prolonged hospitalizations.[2]

Clinical practice guidelines were developed under the auspices of the Society of Critical Care Medicine (SCCM) to increase awareness of these issues in the critically ill.[3] When the sedation assessment, pain assessment, and delirium assessment are recognized as having equal importance with blood pressure and heart rate, clinicians may be able to decrease the incidence of agitation and delirium in critically ill patients.[1,4]

The need for analgesics and sedatives to maintain patient safety and comfort is important, but it is increasingly recognized that excessive sedation can prolong the duration of mechanical ventilation, create physical and psychological dependence, and increase the length of the hospital stay.[5] The goal is to find a balance between providing compassionate patient care and avoiding oversedation.

SEDATION

SEDATION SCALES

The use of scoring systems to assess and record levels of sedation and agitation is now strongly recommended.[3] Four frequently used scales are the Ramsay Scale,[6] the Riker Sedation-Agitation Scale (SAS),[7] the Motor Activity Assessment Scale (MAAS),[8] and the Richmond Agitation-Sedation Scale (RASS)[9,10] (Table 10-1). Other sedation scales are designed to identify specifics of patient comfort, such as the Adaptation To The Intensive Care Environment (ATTICE) scale.[11] Because individuals do not metabolize sedative medications at the same rate,[12] the use of a standardized scale can ensure that continuous infusions of sedatives such as propofol or lorazepam are titrated to a specific goal. Collaboratively, the critical care team must decide which level of sedation is most appropriate for each individual patient.[3]

Sedative levels may also be categorized by the descriptors *light*, *moderate*, and *deep* to describe the level of sedation (Box 10-1).[3,13] *Light sedation*, or minimal sedation, is used when the goal of sedative therapy is to relieve anxiety and ensure patient comfort while allowing the patient to remain responsive to the environment. In one research survey of critical care nurses, most were found to believe that treating patient's anxiety is both beneficial and important.[14] *Moderate sedation*, also called conscious or procedural sedation, is used in conjunction with analgesia to ensure patient comfort during a painful or invasive procedure (e.g., bronchoscopy). *Deep sedation* is used when the patient must be unresponsive so that care may be delivered safely. For example, in the management of acute respiratory distress syndrome (ARDS), deep sedation and analgesia may be required to achieve ventilator synchrony.[3] By contrast, when a patient is weaning from the ventilator, only light sedation may be necessary. During ventilator-weaning trials, it is more reasonable to limit sedation so that the patient is comfortable and arousable to voice while avoiding the twin perils of agitation and oversedation.

The first step in assessing the agitated patient is to rule out any sensations of pain.[3] Clinical assessment is more challenging when the patient is obtunded or has an artificial airway in place. If the patient can communicate, the verbal pain scale of 0 to 10 is very useful. If the patient is intubated and cannot vocalize, pain assessment becomes considerably more complex. After medication for pain has been provided, the next step is to determine the minimum level of sedation required. If deep or moderate sedation is being applied, it is essential that all individuals be qualified and have appropriate credentials to manage these medications and any potential patient complications that arise.[3,13]

CONTINUOUS CEREBRAL FUNCTION MONITORING

One of the challenges with deep sedation is recognizing whether a patient is effectively sedated and pain free. Two clinicians evaluating the same patient may not agree about whether the level of applied sedation and analgesia is appropriate; one may describe the patient as "oversedated," and the other may describe the patient as "inadequately sedated." Clinical parameters such as heart rate and blood pressure are not always reliable, because they can be changed by other conditions.

TABLE 10-1 Sedation Scales

Score	Description	Definition
Riker Sedation-Agitation Scale (SAS)*		
7	Dangerously agitated	Pulls at endotracheal tube (ETT), tries to remove catheters, climbs over bed rail, strikes at staff, thrashes side to side
6	Very agitated	Does not calm despite frequent verbal reminding of limits, requires physical restraints, bites ETT
5	Agitated	Anxious or mildly agitated, attempts to sit up, calms down to verbal instructions
4	Calm and cooperative	Calm, awakens easily, follows commands
3	Sedated	Difficult to arouse, awakens to verbal stimuli or gentle shaking but drifts off again; follows simple commands
2	Very sedated	Arouses to physical stimuli but does not communicate or follow commands; may move spontaneously
1	Unarousable	Minimal or no response to noxious stimuli; does not communicate or follow commands
Motor Activity Assessment Scale (MAAS)†		
6	Dangerously agitated	No external stimulus required to elicit movement; is uncooperative, pulls at tubes or catheters, thrashes side to side, strikes at staff, tries to climb out of bed, does not calm down when asked
5	Agitated	No external stimulus required to elicit movement; attempts to sit up or move limbs out of bed, does not consistently follow commands (e.g., will lie down when asked but soon reverts back to attempts)
4	Restless and cooperative	No external stimulus required to elicit movement; picks at sheets or tubes or uncovers self; follows commands
3	Calm and cooperative	No external stimulus required to elicit movement; adjusts sheets or clothes purposefully; follows commands
2	Responsive to touch or name	Opens eyes, raises eyebrows, or turns head toward stimulus; or, moves limbs when touched or when name loudly spoken
1	Responsive only to noxious stimulus	Opens eyes, raises eyebrows, or turns head toward stimulus; or, moves limbs with noxious stimulus
0	Unresponsive	Does not move with noxious stimulus
Ramsey Scale‡		
1	Awake	Anxious; agitated and/or restless
2		Cooperative, oriented, and tranquil
3		Responds only to commands
4	Asleep	Brisk response to light glabellar tap or loud auditory stimulus
5		Sluggish response to light glabellar tap or loud auditory stimulus
6		No response to light glabellar tap or loud auditory stimulus

Richmond Agitation-Sedation Scale (RASS)§,¶

Score	Term	Description	
+4	Combative	Overtly combative, violent, immediate danger to staff	
+3	Very agitated	Pulls or removes tube(s) or catheter(s); aggressive	
+2	Agitated	Frequent non-purposeful movement, fights ventilator	
+1	Restless	Anxious but movements not aggressive vigorous	
0	Alert and calm		
−1	Drowsy	Not fully alert, but has sustained awakening (eye-opening/eye contact) to *voice* (**≥10 seconds**)	Verbal Stimulation
−2	Light sedation	Briefly awakens with eye contact to *voice* (**<10 seconds**)	
−3	Moderate sedation	Movement or eye opening to *voice* (**but no eye contact**)	
−4	Deep sedation	No response to voice, but movement or eye opening to *physical* stimulation	Physical Stimulation
−5	Unresponsive	No response to *voice or physical* stimulation	

*Riker RR et al: Prospective evaluation of the Sedation-Agitation Scale for adult critically ill patients, *Crit Care Med* 27:1325-1329, 1999.

†Devlin JW et al: Motor Activity Assessment Scale: a valid and reliable sedation scale for use with mechanically ventilated patients in an adult surgical intensive care unit, *Crit Care Med* 27:1271-1275, 1999.

‡Ramsey MA et al: Controlled sedation with alphaxalone-alphadolone, *Br Med J* 2:656-659, 1974.

§Sessler CN et al: The Richmond Agitation-Sedation Scale: validity and reliability in adult intensive care unit patients, *Am J Respir Crit Care Med* 166:1338-1344, 2002.

¶Ely EW et al: Monitoring sedation status over time in ICU patients: reliability and validity of the Richmond Agitation-Sedation Scale (RASS), *JAMA* 289: 2983-2991, 2003.

BOX 10-1   LEVELS OF SEDATION

LIGHT SEDATION (MINIMAL SEDATION, ANXIOLYSIS)

Drug-induced state during which patients respond normally to verbal commands. Although cognitive function and coordination may be impaired, ventilatory and cardiovascular functions are unaffected.

MODERATE SEDATION WITH ANALGESIA (CONSCIOUS SEDATION, PROCEDURAL SEDATION)

Drug-induced depression of consciousness during which patients respond purposefully to verbal commands, alone or accompanied by light tactile stimulation. No interventions are required to maintain a patent airway, and spontaneous ventilation is adequate. Cardiovascular function is usually maintained.

DEEP SEDATION AND ANALGESIA

Drug-induced depression of consciousness during which patients cannot be easily aroused but respond purposefully after repeated or painful stimulation. The ability to maintain ventilatory function independently is impaired. Patients require assistance in maintaining a patent airway, and spontaneous ventilation may be inadequate. Cardiovascular function is usually maintained.

GENERAL ANESTHESIA

Drug-induced loss of consciousness during which patients are not arousable, even by painful stimulation. The ability to maintain ventilatory function independently is impaired, and assistance to maintain a patent airway is required. Positive-pressure ventilation may be required because of depressed spontaneous ventilation or drug-induced depression of neuromuscular function. Cardiovascular function may be impaired.

Data from Joint Commission on Accreditation of Healthcare Organizations: *Comprehensive accreditation manual for hospitals,* Oakbrook Terrace, IL, 2000, The Joint Commission; and Jacobi J et al: Clinical practice guidelines for the sustained use of sedatives and analgesics in the critically ill adult, *Crit Care Med* 30:119-141, 2002.

In an attempt to clarify the clinical assessment of depth of consciousness, some hospitals use continuous monitoring of the electroencephalogram (EEG) for sedated, mechanically ventilated patients. The U.S. Food and Drug Administration (FDA) has approved two continuous EEG monitoring systems. The first and most widely used system in critical care units is the Bispectral Index (BIS; Aspect Medical Systems, Norwood, MA). The BIS system uses sensor electrodes on a single band placed on the patient's forehead.[15-18] The other continuous EEG monitoring system is the Patient State Index (PSI; Hospira, Lake Forest, IL), which monitors cerebral function through an electrode array placed on the forehead.[19] Both systems analyze the patient's EEG signals to detect the effect of sedatives and anesthetics on the brain. These technologies have been successfully used in the operating room for patients under general anesthesia and are increasingly used in the critical care unit for ventilated patients who are deeply sedated or sedated and pharmacology paralyzed.[16,17,20] Both systems calculate a number on a scale of 0 to 100. A value greater than 95 indicates wakefulness, and a value less than 50 to 60 indicates that the patient is unconsciousness or deeply sedated with a low

probability of mental recall of events. A value lower than 20 denotes an extremely deep level of sedation sufficient to cause brain wave suppression. Unless the goal is to achieve a level of sedation equivalent to a barbiturate coma, brain wave suppression is not desirable. Both systems incorporate an electromyelogram (EMG) sensor to filter out erroneous muscle movement that may distort the numerical sedation value.

Continuous nervous system monitoring by EEG may have a role for the most severely critically ill patients who are deeply sedated, receiving opiate analgesia, and pharmacologically paralyzed, although research outside the operating room is limited.[17,18]

It is recommended that all critically ill, intubated, mechanically ventilated patients have a stated goal for analgesia and sedation (Fig. 10-1). After the sedation goal is articulated and documented, the ongoing use of a validated assessment scale is recommended to facilitate consistency among the various health care practitioners[3] (see Table 10-1).

COMPLICATIONS OF SEDATION

Oversedation is recognized as a state of unintended patient unresponsiveness in which the patient resides in a state of suspended animation resembling general anesthesia. Prolonged deep sedation is associated with significant complications of immobility, including pressure ulcers, thromboemboli, gastric ileus, nosocomial pneumonia, and delayed weaning from mechanical ventilation.

Too little sedation is equally hazardous. Most nurses have experienced the challenge of caring for a patient who unexpectedly removes the endotracheal or nasogastric tube. Unplanned extubation in restless, anxious, agitated patients occurs in 8% to 10% of intubated patients after an average of 3.5 days in the critical care unit. Six percent of self-extubations cause significant complications, including aspiration, dysrhythmias, bronchospasm, and bradycardia.[21]

PHARMACOLOGIC MANAGEMENT OF SEDATION

Several categories of sedatives are commercially available. None of these medications has any analgesic properties. If the patient is experiencing pain, analgesia must be administered in addition to any sedative agents. Sedative agents include the benzodiazepines, anesthetic agents such as propofol, and the central alpha agonists (Table 10-2).[3]

BENZODIAZEPINES

Benzodiazepines are sedative-hypnotics with powerful amnesic properties that inhibit reception of new sensory information.[3,21] Benzodiazepines do not have analgesic properties. The most frequently used critical care benzodiazepines are *diazepam* (Valium), *midazolam* (Versed), and *lorazepam* (Ativan). Midazolam is recommended for control of acute short-term agitation because its intravenous onset of action is less than 3 minutes (see Fig. 10-1). However, when midazolam is administered for longer than 24 hours as a continuous infusion, the sedative effect is prolonged by active metabolites.[3,22]

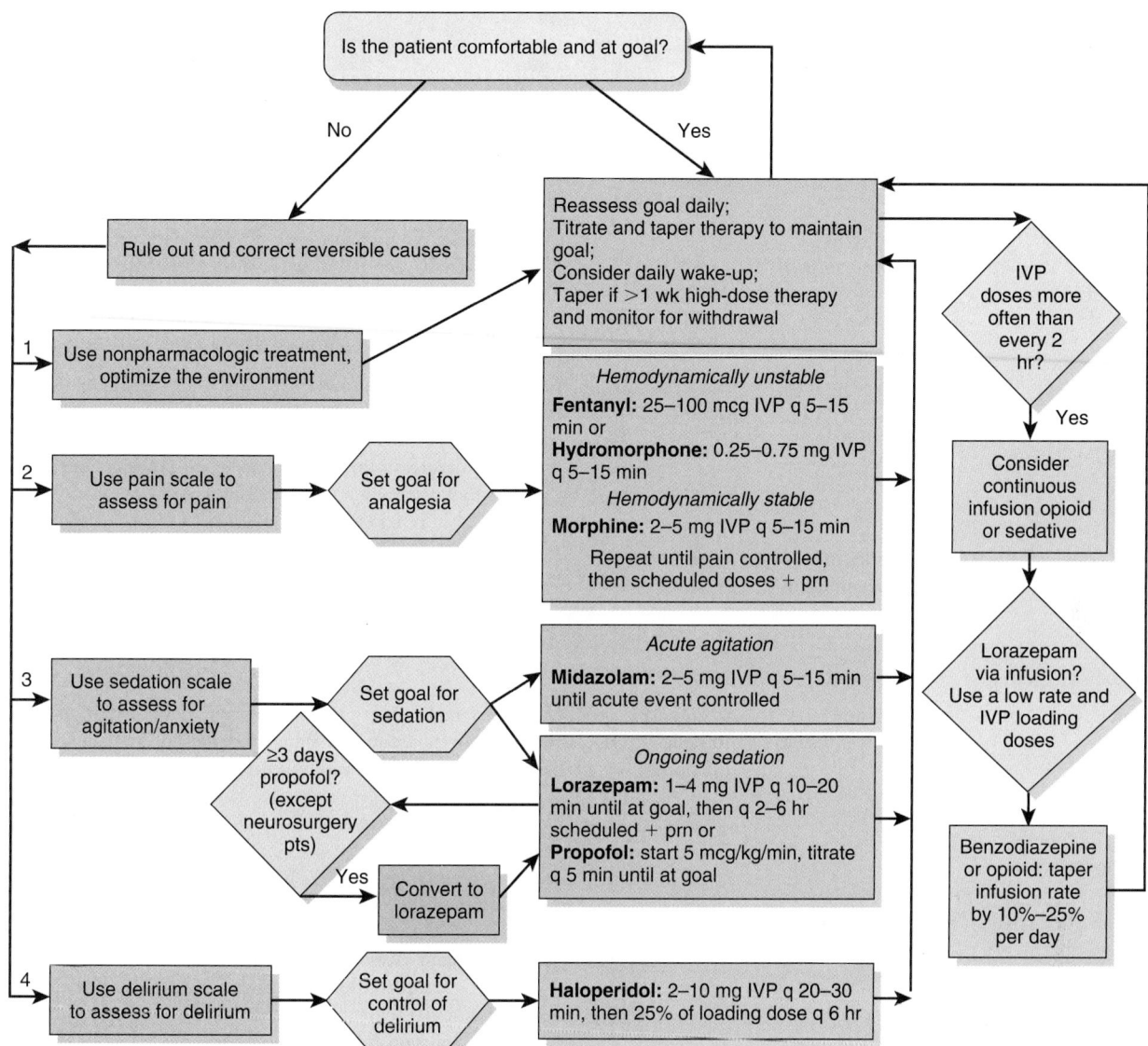

Figure 10-1 The algorithm provides guidelines for the use of analgesics and sedatives in mechanically ventilated patients. The text describes clinical and pharmacologic issues that dictate optimal drug selection, recommended assessment scales, and precautions for patient monitoring. Doses are approximate for a 70-kg (154-pound) adult. IVP, intravenous push; q, every; prn, as needed. *(From Jacobi J et al: Clinical practice guidelines for the sustained use of sedatives and analgesics in the critically ill adult,* Crit Care Med *30:119-141, 2002.)*

TABLE 10-2	Pharmacologic Management: Sedation		
DRUGS	**DOSAGE**	**ACTIONS**	**SPECIAL CONSIDERATIONS**
Benzodiazepines			
Diazepam	0.03-0.1 mg/kg every 0.5-6 hr (slow IV intermittent doses)	Anxiolysis Amnesia Sedation	*Onset:* 2-5 min after IV administration *Side effects:* hypotension, respiratory depression *Half-life of parent compound:* long (20-120 hr); active sedative metabolites also contribute to prolonged sedative effect *Drug tolerance:* physical tolerance develops with prolonged use, and more drug is required to achieve the same effect over time; slow wean required from diazepam after continuous prolonged use Phlebitis occurs with peripheral IV administration.

Continued

TABLE 10-2 Pharmacologic Management: Sedation—*cont'd*

DRUGS	DOSAGE	ACTIONS	SPECIAL CONSIDERATIONS
Lorazepam	0.02-0.06 mg/kg every 2-6 hr (slow IV intermittent doses)	Anxiolysis Amnesia Sedation	*Onset:* 5-20 min after IV administration *Side effects:* hypotension, respiratory depression *Half-life of parent compound:* relatively long (8-15 hr); sedative effect is also prolonged
	0.01-0.1 mg/kg/hr (continuous infusion)		*Drug tolerance:* physical tolerance develops with use, and higher drug dosage is required to achieve the same effect over time; slow wean required from lorazepam after continuous prolonged use Solvent-related acidosis and renal failure occur at high doses.
Midazolam	0.02-0.08 mg/kg every 0.5-2 hr (slow IV intermittent doses)	Anxiolysis Amnesia Sedation	*Onset:* 2-5 min after IV administration *Side effects:* hypotension, respiratory depression *Half-life of parent compound:* 3-11 hr; sedative effect is prolonged when midazolam infusion has continued for many days, due to presence of active sedative metabolites; sedative effect is also prolonged in renal failure
	0.04-0.2 mg/kg/hr (continuous infusion)		*Drug tolerance:* physical tolerance develops with prolonged use, and higher drug dosage is required to achieve the same effect over time; slow wean required from midazolam after prolonged use

Anesthetic Agents

DRUGS	DOSAGE	ACTIONS	SPECIAL CONSIDERATIONS
Propofol	5-50 mcg/kg/min (continuous infusion)	Anxiolysis Amnesia Sedation	*Onset:* very rapid onset (1-2 min) after IV administration *Side effects:* hypotension, respiratory depression (patient must be intubated and mechanically ventilated to eliminate this complication) *Half-life of parent compound:* 2-8 min when used as a short-term agent *Sedative effect:* range of 26-32 hr with prolonged continuous IV infusion; effective short-term anesthetic agent, useful for rapid "wake-up" of patients for assessment; if continuous infusion is used for many days, emergence from sedation can take hours or days; sedative effect depends on dose administered, depth of sedation, and length of time sedated Change IV infusion tubing every 12 hr. Requires a dedicated IV catheter and tubing (do not mix with other drugs). Monitor serum triglyceride levels.

Neuroleptic Agents

DRUGS	DOSAGE	ACTIONS	SPECIAL CONSIDERATIONS
Haloperidol	0.03-0.15 mg/kg every 0.5-6 hr (IV intermittent doses)	Antipsychotic Antidelirium	*Onset:* 3-20 min after IV administration *Half-life of parent compound:* 18-54 hr Used in management of delirium; sedation is an unintended side effect.
	0.04-0.15 mg/kg/hr (continuous infusion)		Measure QT interval at baseline and periodically during haloperidol infusion. Active metabolites may cause extrapyramidal symptoms (EPS); anticholinergic agent may be administered if EPS occur.

α-Adrenergic Receptor Agonists

DRUGS	DOSAGE	ACTIONS	SPECIAL CONSIDERATIONS
Dexmedetomidine	1 mcg/kg initial loading dose over 10 min	Anxiolysis Analgesia Sedation	*Half-life:* ≈ 2 hr Duration of infusion is up to 24 hr only. Bolus dosing is not recommended. Maintenance infusion is adjusted to achieve desired level of sedation.
	0.2-0.7 mcg/kg/hr (continuous infusion)		

The 2002 SCCM clinical guidelines[3] recommend a continuous infusion of lorazepam if long-term sedation is needed for a mechanically ventilated patient (see Fig. 10-1). One advantage of lorazepam for long-term sedation is that it does not have active metabolites that contribute to the overall sedative effect.[22] Lorazepam has a slow onset, which makes it unsuitable for the treatment of acute agitation. As would be expected, the recovery time from a sedated state takes longer after infusion of lorazepam compared with midazolam; the higher the dose infused, the longer the recovery time for both drugs.[23] Mechanically ventilated patients who were sedated with a continuous infusion of lorazepam for 72 hours emerged from light sedation in 11.9 hours, whereas recovery from deep sedation took 31.1 hours. By contrast, in the same research study, patients who were sedated with a continuous midazolam infusion emerged from light sedation in 3.6 hours and from deep sedation in 14.9 hours.[23] Not unexpectedly, compared with other sedative drugs, lorazepam is associated with more days on the ventilator.[24,25] The dose of lorazepam is also important to consider, because the higher the dose of lorazepam in a 24-hour period, the greater the risk of transition into delirium for the mechanically ventilated patient.[26,27]

Because benzodiazepines have been associated with a longer duration of mechanical ventilation than either propofol or dexmedetomidine, some clinicians now recommend that benzodiazepines be limited to patients with symptoms of anxiety, seizures, or alcohol withdrawal and patients whose clinical condition necessitates mechanical ventilation and a deeper level of sedation or therapeutic paralysis.[28] Therapeutic use of benzodiazepines requires that the sedative agent be selected carefully, anticipating how long the patient will be sedated, the dose of drug required, and how long it will take to recover from the sedative state.

The major unwanted side effects associated with the benzodiazepines are dose-related respiratory depression and hypotension. If needed, *flumazenil* (Romazicon) is the antidote used to reverse benzodiazepine overdose in symptomatic patients.[21] Flumazenil should be avoided in patients with benzodiazepine dependence, because rapid withdrawal can induce seizures.[21,29]

SEDATIVE-HYPNOTIC AGENTS

Propofol is classified as a sedative-hypnotic. It is also used as an intravenous general anesthetic agent. At high doses (>100 to 200 mcg/kg/min), propofol is intended to produce a state of general anesthesia in the operating room.[30] In the critical care unit, propofol is prescribed as a continuous infusion at lower doses (5 to 50 mcg/kg/min) to induce a state of deep sedation.[30] The clinical advantage of propofol is its rapid onset of action (about 30 seconds), very short half-life with initial use (2 to 4 minutes), and rapid elimination from the body (30 to 60 minutes).[30,31] It does not have active metabolites.[30] This drug is especially suitable for management of the agitated neurologic patient with brain injury. Propofol quickly crosses the blood-brain barrier, slows cerebral metabolism, and decreases elevated intracranial pressure.[30]

With short-term administration, the patient can be fully alert within 30 minutes after the drug infusion is turned off. The half-life is 2 to 4 minutes with short-term use.[30] If propofol is infused for several days, the wake-up time becomes prolonged.[32,33] If propofol is infused for more than 10 days, the half-life extends to 1 to 3 days.[30] Propofol is not a reliable amnesic, and patients sedated with only propofol can have vivid recollections of their experiences. It is therefore important to add an opiate, such as fentanyl, to ensure adequate amnesia.[32]

Significant disadvantages of propofol are mainly related to the high lipid content. It comes packaged in a glass container and has the appearance of milk. Propofol is emulsified in a soybean Intralipid emulsion that delivers 1.1 kcal/mL as fat. These calories must be taken into account when assessing nutritional intake.[30] Propofol can elevate serum triglyceride levels and has been associated with pancreatitis. Triglyceride levels should be checked after 48 hours of propofol infusion.[3] The lipid emulsion can also act as a potential medium for bacterial growth. Administration requires a dedicated intravenous line, and all intravenous solutions and tubing must be changed every 12 hours.[30] Propofol shares with other sedatives the propensity for hypotension when delivered rapidly.[30,32] Propofol is prescribed only for intubated patients.

Propofol infusion syndrome (PIS) is a rare complication of prolonged high-dose propofol administration.[31,34] It occurs more commonly in children than in adult critically ill patients. The syndrome includes cardiac arrest, myocardial failure, metabolic acidosis, rhabdomyolysis, and hyperkalemia and occurs after 48 hours of high-dose propofol infusion.[31,34] Clinicians are advised not to administer dosages greater than 4 mg//kg/hr for longer than 48 hours.[31] The cause of PIS is not known but is hypothesized to involve inhibition of enzymes in the mitochondrial respiratory chain, impaired fatty acid oxidation, diversion of carbohydrate metabolism to fat substrates, or the production of unidentified toxic metabolites.[34] If PIS develops, the propofol infusion must be stopped immediately and a different sedative started; volume resuscitation with crystalloid 0.9% saline to treat hypotension is initiated, and vasopressors are added if shock is refractory. Sodium bicarbonate may be administered if the acidosis is severe; cardiac pacing may be required if bradycardia occurs; and some patients may require hemodialysis if acute renal failure develops.[31]

CENTRAL ALPHA AGONISTS

Two central α-adrenergic agonists are available for sedation. Clonidine is often prescribed as a Catapres patch and dexmedetomidine (Precedex) as a continuous infusion. *Clonidine* is prescribed for patients experiencing withdrawal syndromes. *Dexmedetomidine* is a newer α_2-agonist that is approved for use as a short-term sedative (<24 hours) in mechanically ventilated patients. Several studies have demonstrated that dexmedetomidine confers sedation and analgesic effects without respiratory depression.[35] This has made it useful in weaning patients from short-term ventilation after cardiac surgery.[36] Dexmedetomidine has also been used for patients on noninvasive mask ventilation.[37]

Dexmedetomidine is prescribed with a loading dose of 1.0 mcg/kg over 10 minutes, followed by a continuous infusion of 0.2 to 0.7 mcg/kg/hr.[35] This drug has a short half-life

(6 minutes) and is eliminated from the body in about 2 hours.[35] It is metabolized in the liver by oxidative metabolism through the cytochrome P450 enzyme system and direct glucuronidation in the liver; 95% of inactive dexmedetomidine metabolites are excreted by the kidneys.[35,38] Elimination from the body is dramatically slowed if the patient has liver failure. One retrospective analysis showed that when dexmedetomidine was prescribed in critical care as adjunctive therapy in combination with other sedatives (propofol or lorazepam) and analgesics (fentanyl), it reduced sedative dose requirements but did not alter analgesic dosage requirements.[39] Other researchers have reported lower analgesic dose requirements when dexmedetomidine was added to the regimen.[40]

The choice of sedative is highly specific to the patient and the situation. If the need is for *short-term* sedation (<24 hours), the most frequently used sedative is midazolam or propofol.[3,23] Both drugs may be combined with a short-acting opioid analgesic (e.g., fentanyl). If the need is for *intermediate-term* sedation (1 to 3 days), the most frequently prescribed drugs again are propofol and midazolam, plus an opiate. If the need is for *long-term* sedation, the recommended agent is lorazepam.[3] Research using continuous EEG monitoring has shown that patients who receive continuous sedative infusions are more deeply sedated than patients who are given sedatives as an intravenous bolus; patients receiving continuous infusions are also more likely to be oversedated.[41]

PREVENTING SEDATIVE DEPENDENCE AND WITHDRAWAL

The question of which drugs to use for prolonged sedation is complex. Some critically ill patients are mechanically ventilated and seriously ill for weeks or months. To tolerate the ventilator and other procedures, patients must receive sedation and analgesia. By the time sedation can be decreased, many patients have become physically and psychologically dependent; as the drug dosage is reduced, they become highly agitated. Agitation may result in the use of soft wrist restraints that may further increase agitation.[42,43]

Physical symptoms of agitation include increased heart rate, blood pressure, and respiratory rate. Other notable symptoms are lack of self-awareness, unawareness of surroundings, very-short-term memory for information, irritability, anxiety, confusion, delirium, and even seizures.[3] Patients may pull at the tubes, attempt to climb out of bed, and represent a danger to themselves, the nurse, and family visitors. The temptation to resedate is powerful, because it is painful to watch a patient experience the stages of withdrawal. During this period, the patient does not sleep well, even when sedation provides the appearance of sleep.

SEDATION VACATION

One innovative strategy to avoid the pitfalls of sedative dependence and withdrawal is a planned strategy to turn off the sedative infusions once each day. This intervention has been given several names, including *drug holiday, sedation vacation,* and *spontaneous awakening trial.* At a scheduled time, all sedative drugs (sometimes analgesic drugs are also turned off, depending on the hospital's protocol) are stopped, and the patient is allowed to awaken for clinical assessment using a standardized instrument such as the RASS (see Table 10-1).[44-47] The patient is carefully monitored, and when consciousness and awareness are attained, an assessment of level of consciousness and neurologic function is performed. When protocols that incorporate daily interruption of sedative infusions are used, it is imperative that accurate assessment be performed and documented during the wake-up period. If the patient becomes agitated, it is essential that a protocol be in place for the nurse to restart the sedatives, plus opiates if applicable.[45,46,48] One protocol scheduled the daily interruption of sedatives in the morning and recommended, after a full assessment, restarting the sedative and opiate infusions at 50% of the previous morning dose and adjusting upward until the patient was comfortable.[45,48] Initially, it was assumed that patients would be highly agitated during each interruption. However, because patients have less accumulation of sedative and opiate medications, they may be less restless in the wake-up period. The intubated patients who were woken up daily by turning off the sedative infusions (either propofol or midazolam) experienced a lower rate of medical complications and lower levels of posttraumatic stress disorder.[25,44]

An important nursing responsibility is to prevent the patient from coming to harm during sedative or analgesic drug withdrawal (Table 10-3). Some movement in bed is expected, but

TABLE 10-3 Signs and Symptoms of Sedative or Analgesic Drug Withdrawal*

System	Opiate Withdrawal	Benzodiazepine Withdrawal[†]
Neurologic	Delirium, tremors, seizures	Agitation, anxiety, delirium, tremors, myoclonus, headache, seizures, fatigue, paresthesias, sleep disturbances
Hemodynamic	Tachycardia, hypertension (sympathetic nervous system stimulation)	Tachycardia, hypertension (sympathetic nervous system stimulation)
Sensory	Dilation of pupils, teary eyes, irritability, increased sensitivity to pain, sweating, yawning	Increased sensitivity to light/sound, sweating
Musculoskeletal	Cramps, muscle aches	Muscle cramps
Gastrointestinal	Vomiting, diarrhea	Nausea, diarrhea
Respiratory	Tachypnea	Tachypnea

*Data on propofol is limited, but withdrawal symptoms after prolonged use are similar to those of the benzodiazepines.[3]

[†]Not all symptoms are seen in all patients.[3,67]

extreme restlessness increases myocardial oxygen consumption and work of breathing and activates the sympathetic nervous system. If the patient is seriously agitated, it is vital to consult with the physician and pharmacist to establish an effective treatment plan that will allow weaning from sedative drugs without harm. The approach to avoidance of drug dependence and withdrawal symptoms is not yet fully delineated but clearly requires a multidisciplinary effort with ongoing evaluation using an established assessment scale (see Table 10-1).

DELIRIUM

Delirium represents a global impairment of cognitive processes, usually of sudden onset, coupled with disorientation, impaired short-term memory, altered sensory perceptions (i.e., hallucinations), abnormal thought processes, and inappropriate behavior. Delirium is more prevalent than generally recognized; it is difficult to diagnose in the critically ill patient and represents acute brain dysfunction caused by sepsis, critical illness, or dysfunction of other vital organs (Box 10-2).[49] The incidence of delirium ranges from 60% to 85% among mechanically ventilated patients.[49] Delirium increases hospital stay and mortality rates for patients who are mechanically ventilated.[50,51] The increased mortality remains even after controlling for associated variables such as coma and administration of sedatives and analgesics.[51]

When patients are agitated, restless, and pulling at tubes and lines, they are often identified as being delirious. In this scenario, delirium may be described as "ICU psychosis" or "sundowner syndrome." However, the delirious patient is not always agitated, and it is much more difficult to detect delirium when the patient is physically calm.[3,52] Provision of adequate analgesia is an essential component of delirium prevention.[3]

Specific scoring instruments are available to assess delirium, and two have been validated for use with mechanically ventilated critical care patients (Fig. 10-2 and Tables 10-4 and 10-5).[53,54] They are the *Confusion Assessment Method for the Intensive Care Unit* (CAM-ICU)[55-57] and the *Intensive Care Delirium Screening Checklist* (ICDSC).[58-60] Both instruments are used in tandem with the RASS to identify hyperactive delirium (see Table 10-1). A difference between the scales is that the CAM-ICU assessment is focused on a specific point in time, whereas the ICDSC assessment includes information form the previous 24 hours. Both instruments provide a structured format with which to evaluate delirium in nonverbal and mechanically ventilated patients.

PHARMACOLOGIC MANAGEMENT OF AGITATION AND DELIRIUM

The medications typically prescribed for sedation (benzodiazepines) may exacerbate symptoms of delirium. Lorazepam, the benzodiazepine that is recommended for longer-term sedation in critical care, has been associated with an increased incidence of delirium.[26] Sedatives make delirious patients confused, less responsive, and more obtunded.[25] If the patient becomes agitated, the neuroleptic drug haloperidol (Haldol) is frequently prescribed.[61] This antipsychotic agent stabilizes cerebral function by blocking dopamine-mediated neurotransmission at the cerebral synapses and in the basal ganglia. Delirium is reduced, but the patient tends to have a flat affect and diminished interest in surroundings; with higher doses, the patient becomes sedated. Electrocardiographic (ECG) monitoring is recommended, because neuroleptic agents such as haloperidol

---

BOX 10-2	CAUSES OF DELIRIUM IN CRITICALLY ILL PATIENTS

METABOLIC CAUSES
- Acid-base disturbance
- Electrolyte imbalance
- Hypoglycemia

INTRACRANIAL CAUSES
- Epidural or subdural hematoma
- Intracranial hemorrhage
- Meningitis
- Encephalitis
- Cerebral abscess
- Tumor

ENDOCRINE CAUSES
- Hyperthyroidism or hypothyroidism

- Addison's disease
- Hyperparathyroidism
- Cushing's syndrome

ORGAN FAILURE
- Liver encephalopathy
- Uremic encephalopathy
- Septic shock

RESPIRATORY CAUSES
- Hypoxemia
- Hypercarbia

DRUG-RELATED CAUSES
- Alcohol withdrawal
- Drug-induced delirium
- Heavy metal poisoning

Modified from Szokol JW, Vender JS: Anxiety, delirium, and pain in the intensive care unit, *Crit Care Clin* 17(4):821-842, 2001.

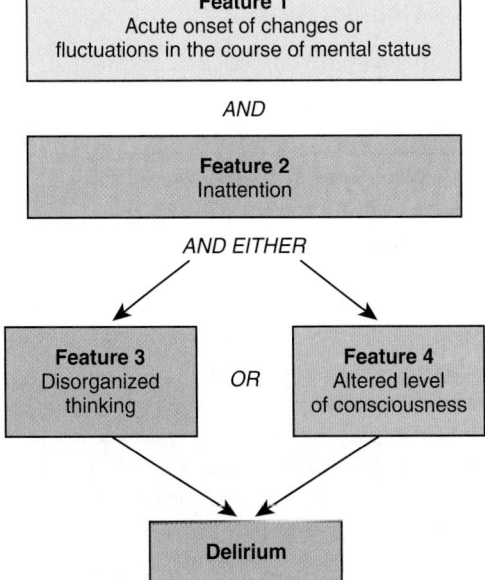

Figure 10-2 The Confusion Assessment Method for the ICU (CAM-ICU).

TABLE 10-4 Confusion Assessment Method for the Intensive Care Unit (CAM-ICU)* RASS and CAM-ICU Worksheet

<u>**Step One:**</u> **Sedation Assessment**

The Richmond Agitation and Sedation Scale: The RASS[†]

Score	Term	Description	
+4	Combative	Overtly combative, violent, immediate danger to staff	
+3	Very agitated	Pulls or removes tube(s) or catheter(s); aggressive	
+2	Agitated	Frequent non-purposeful movement, fights ventilator	
+1	Restless	Anxious but movements not aggressive vigorous	
0	Alert and calm		
−1	Drowsy	Not fully alert, but has sustained awakening (eye-opening/eye contact) to *voice* (≥**10 seconds**)	Verbal Stimulation
−2	Light sedation	Briefly awakens with eye contact to *voice* (<**10 seconds**)	
−3	Moderate sedation	Movement or eye opening to *voice* (**but no eye contact**)	
−4	Deep sedation	No response to voice, but movement or eye opening to *physical* stimulation	Physical Stimulation
−5	Unresponsive	No response to *voice or physical* stimulation	

Procedure for RASS Assessment

1. **Observe patient**
   a. Patient is alert, restless, or agitated. (score 0 to +4)
2. **If not alert, state patient's name and *say* to open eyes and look at speaker.**
   a. Patient awakens with sustained eye opening and eye contact. (score −1)
   b. Patient awakens with eye opening and eye contact, but not sustained. (score −2)
   c. Patient has any movement in response to voice but no eye contact. (score −3)
3. **When no response to verbal stimulation, physically stimulate patient by shaking shoulder and/or rubbing sternum.**
   a. Patient has any movement to physical stimulation. (score −4)
   b. Patient has no response to any stimulation. (score −5)

If RASS is −4 or −5, then **Stop** and **Reassess** patient at later time
If RASS is above −4 (−3 through +4) then **Proceed to Step 2**

[†]Sessler, et al. AJRCCM 2002; 166:1338–1344. Ely, et al. JAMA 2003; 289:2983–2991.

<u>**Step Two:**</u> **Delirium Assessment**

See Figure 10-2 on p. 167 for delirium assessment.

	Positive	Negative
Feature 1: Acute Onset or Fluctuating Course Positive if you answer 'yes' to either 1A or 1B.	**Positive**	**Negative**
1A: Is the pt different than his/her baseline mental status? Or **1B:** Has the patient had any fluctuation in mental status in the past 24 hours as evidenced by fluctuation on a sedation scale (e.g. RASS), GCS, or previous delirium assessment?	**Yes**	**No**
Feature 2: Inattention Positive if either score for 2A *or* 2B is less than 8. Attempt the ASE letters first. If pt is able to perform this test and the score is clear, record this score and move to Feature 3. If pt is unable to perform this test *or* the score is unclear, then perform the ASE Pictures. If you perform both tests, use the ASE Pictures results to score the Feature.	**Positive**	**Negative**

TABLE 10-4 Confusion Assessment Method for the Intensive Care Unit (CAM-ICU)*
RASS and CAM-ICU Worksheet—*cont'd*

2A: ASE Letters: record score (enter NT for not tested) Directions: Say to the patient, *"I am going to read you a series of 10 letters. Whenever you hear the letter 'A', indicate by squeezing my hand."* Read letters from the following letter list in a normal tone. **S A V E A H A A R T** Scoring: Errors are counted when patient fails to squeeze on the letter "A" and when the patient squeezes on any letter other than "A."	Score (out of 10): _____	
2B: ASE Pictures: record score (enter NT for not tested)	Score (out of 10): _____	

Feature 3: Disorganized Thinking Positive if the combined score is less than 4	**Positive**	**Negative**

3A: Yes/No Questions
 	
(Use either Set A *or* Set B, alternate on consecutive days if necessary):
 	
   Set A   **Set B**
  1. Will a stone float on water?   1. Will a leaf float on water?
  2. Are there fish in the sea?   2. Are there elephants in the sea?
  3. Does one pound weigh more than   3. Do two pounds weigh more
    two pounds?   than one pound?
  4. Can you use a hammer to pound   4. Can you use a hammer to cut
    a nail?   wood?
 	
Score ___ (Patient earns 1 point for each correct answer out of 4)
 	
3B: Command
 	
Say to patient: "Hold up this many fingers" (Examiner holds two fingers in front of patient)
"Now do the same thing with the other hand" (Not repeating the number of fingers).
If pt is unable to move both arms, for the second part of the command ask patient "Add one more finger."
 	
Score ___ (Patient earns 1 point if able to successfully complete the entire command)
	Combined Score (3A+3B):
	  _____ (out of 5)	

Feature 4: Altered Level of Consciousness Positive if the Actual RASS score is anything other than "0" (zero)	**Positive**	**Negative**
Overall CAM-ICU (Features 1 and 2 and either Feature 3 or 4):	**Positive**	**Negative**

*Refer to *The Confusion Assessment Method for the ICU Training Manual* (2005 updated version), which can be downloaded from www.ICUdelirium.org/delirium/
CAM-ICUTraining.html for more detailed information on how to use the CAM-ICU. The training manual has worksheets that explain how to use the RASS
(Table 10-1) and the CAM-ICU in tandem. The www.ICUdelirium.org Web site has the information needed to complete the Attention Screening Examination
(ASE) under section II "Inattention" of the CAM-ICU. The Web site also contains video demonstrations to show how to use the CAM-ICU.
Data from Ely EW et al: Delirium in mechanically ventilated patients: validity and reliability of the confusion assessment method for the intensive care unit (CAM-
ICU), *JAMA*; 286:2703-2710, 2001; Ely EW et al: Evaluation of delirium in critically ill patients: validation of the Confusion Assessment Method for the Intensive
Care Unit (CAM-ICU), *Crit Care Med.* 29:1370-1379, 2001; and Ely EW, Pum BT: *The Confusion Assessment Method for the ICU Training Manual* (2005 updated
version). Available at www.ICUdelirium.org/delirium/CAM-ICUTraining.html under section on delirium assessment (accessed December 2008).

produce dose-dependent QTc-interval prolongation, with an increased incidence of ventricular dysrhythmias.[62]

NONPHARMACOLOGIC INTERVENTIONS TO PREVENT DELIRIUM

Agitation and delirium are common in critically ill patients.[3] The nonpharmacologic strategies used to prevent agitation and delirium are similar to those used as adjuncts to minimize pain.[3] These methods include back massage, music therapy, noise reduction in the environment, decreasing lights at night to promote sleep, clustering of nursing care to provide some uninterrupted rest periods, and speaking in a calm, quiet, and gentle voice. Some prehospital patient conditions increase the likelihood that a patient will experience delirium, including preexistent dementia, alcohol use disorder, and sedative use dependence.[63,64] Knowledge of these conditions may be helpful when developing a plan of care for sedation management and delirium prevention.

Causes of delirium are multifactorial, but *sleep deprivation* is a universal experience that may contribute.[65] Even when patients

TABLE 10-5A The Intensive Care Delirium Screening Checklist (ICDSC)

1. **Altered level of consciousness**
   (A) No response or (B) the need for vigorous stimulation in order to obtain any response signified a severe alteration in the level of consciousness precluding evaluation. If there is coma (A) or stupor (B) most of the time period, then a dash (—) is entered and there is no further evaluation for that period.
   (C) Drowsiness or response to a mild to moderate stimulation implies an altered level of consciousness and scores 1 point.
   (D) Wakefulness or sleeping state that could easily be aroused is considered normal and scores zero points.
   (E) Hypervigilance is rated as an abnormal level of consciousness and scores 1 point.

2. **Inattention**
   Difficulty in following a conversation or instruction, easily distracted by external stimuli, or difficulty in shifting focus all score 1 point.

3. **Disorientation**
   Any obvious mistake in time, place or person scores 1 point.

4. **Hallucination, delusion or psychosis**
   The unequivocal clinical manifestation of hallucination or of behaviour probably due to hallucination (e.g., trying to catch a non-existent object) or delusion, or gross impairment in reality testing all score 1 point.

5. **Psychomotor agitation or retardation**
   Hyperactivity requiring the use of additional sedative drugs or restraints in order to control potential danger (e.g., pulling out IV lines, hitting staff), hypoactivity or clinically noticeable psychomotor slowing all score 1 point.

6. **Inappropriate speech or mood**
   Inappropriate, disorganized or incoherent speech, inappropriate mood related to events or situation all score 1 point.

7. **Sleep/wake cycle disturbance**
   Sleeping less than four hours or waking frequently at night (do not consider wakefulness initiated by medical staff or loud environment), or sleeping during most of the day all score 1 point.

8. **Symptom fluctuation**
   Fluctuation of the manifestation of any item or symptom over 24 hours (e.g., from one shift to another) scores 1 point.

Source: Bergeron N, Dubols MI, Dumont M, Dial S, Skrobk Y. Intensive Care Delirium Screening Checklist: evaluation of a new screening tool. Intensive Care Med 2001;27(5):859–64. Copyright notice of Springer-Verlag.

TABLE 10-5B How to Calculate a Score for the ICDSC*

Patient Evaluation	Day 1	Day 2	Day 3	Day 4	Day 5
Altered level of consciousness (A-E)*					
Inattention					
Disorientation					
Hallucination, delusion, psychosis					
Psychomotor agitation or retardation					
Inappropriate speech or mood					
Sleep-wake cycle disturbance					
Symptom fluctuation					
Total Score (0–8)					

*Level of Consciousness	Score
A: no response	–
B: response to intense and repeated stimulation (loud voice and pain)	–
C: response to mild or moderate stimulation	1
D: normal wakefulness	0
E: exaggerated response to normal stimulation	1
If **A** or **B**, do not complete patient evaluation for the period.	

Scoring System
The scale is completed based on information collected from each 8-hour shift or from the previous 24 hours. Obvious manifestation of an item = 1 point. No manifestation of an item or no assessment possible = 0 points. The score of each item is entered in the corresponding space and is 0 or 1. A total score of ≥4 on any given day has a 99% sensitivity for correlation with a psychiatric diagnosis of delirium.

*The ICDSC is also used in tandem with the RASS (see Table 10-1) to assess sedation-agitation in addition to delirium.
From Bergeron N et al: Intensive Care Delirium Screening Checklist: evaluation of a new screening tool, *Intensive Care Med* 27:859-864, 2001.

are apparently sleeping, if the sleep is induced by sedatives, opiates, neuromuscular blockade, or neuroleptics, it is unlikely that it represents true rapid eye movement (REM) sleep. Circadian rhythms are disrupted by mechanical ventilation and by the lack of a recognizable day-night pattern in the intensive care unit.[66] As with pain assessment, self-report of sleep deprivation is considered to be the most accurate measure. Clustering of nursing care interventions to minimize sleep fragmentation may be helpful.

COLLABORATIVE MANAGEMENT

Collaborative management of anxiety, agitation, sedation, and delirium is a responsibility shared by all members of the health care team (see the Evidence-Based Practice feature on Sedation in the Critically Ill). Recognition of the problem is the first step toward a solution to establish a more effective standard of patient care in sedation, analgesia, and delirium management.

Evidence-Based Practice: Collaborative

Sedation in the Critically Ill

The key recommendations from the clinical practice guideline for the sustained use of sedatives and analgesia in the critically ill adult, based on research and expert panel opinion, are as follows.

Assessment, Communication, and Documentation
1. Frequent assessment of critically ill patients is mandated to determine whether sedation and analgesia are required and appropriate as part of the plan of care.
2. A sedation goal or end point should be established for each patient at the beginning of therapy; for example, "a calm patient that can be easily aroused with maintenance of the normal sleep-wake cycle." Some patients may require deep sedation to facilitate synchrony with mechanical ventilation.
3. Need for sedation should be re-evaluated on a frequent basis as the clinical condition of the patient changes.
4. Sedation regimens should be written with the flexibility to allow titration to the desired end point, anticipating fluctuations in sedation requirements throughout the day.
5. Use of a validated sedation assessment scale to standardize assessment among clinicians and document the patient's level of sedation and response to sedatives is recommended. Vital signs such as blood pressure or heart rate are not sufficiently specific or sensitive to serve as indicators of sedation effectiveness.
6. Sedation and analgesia goals must be communicated to all caregivers and to the patient and family.
7. Because of insufficient research, use of sedation monitors that interpret EEG data is not endorsed for monitoring of critical care patients.

Agitation
8. Sedation of agitated critically ill patients should be started only after adequate analgesia and treatment for reversible physiologic causes of agitation have been provided.
9. Cautious use of sedatives is warranted for patients who are not yet intubated, because of the risk of respiratory depression.

Drug Therapy
10. Midazolam or diazepam should be used for rapid sedation of acutely agitated patients.
11. Propofol is the preferred sedative when rapid awakening for neurologic assessment or extubation is important.
12. Midazolam is recommended for short-term use only, because it provokes unpredictable awakening and time to extubation when infusions continue longer than 48 to 72 hours.
13. Lorazepam is the recommended sedative when prolonged mechanical ventilation is required and is given by intermittent intravenous administration or continuous infusion.

Avoidance of Complications
14. Titration of the sedative dose to a defined end point is recommended, with systematic tapering of the dose or daily interruption with retitration to minimize prolonged sedative effects.
15. Triglyceride concentrations should be monitored after 2 days of propofol infusion, and the total caloric intake from lipids should be included in the nutrition support prescription.
16. The potential for opioid, benzodiazepine, and propofol withdrawal should be considered after high doses of more than approximately 7 days of continuous therapy. Doses should be tapered systematically to prevent withdrawal symptoms.

Delirium
17. Routine assessment for the presence of delirium is recommended. The CAM-ICU is a promising assessment tool for delirium.
18. Haloperidol is the preferred agent for the treatment of delirium in critically ill patients.
19. ECG monitoring for detection of potential QT interval prolongation and dysrhythmias is recommended when haloperidol is administered.

Sleep
20. Sleep promotion should include optimization of the environment and nonpharmacologic methods to promote relaxation with adjunctive use of hypnotics.

CAM-ICU, Confusion Assessment Method–ICU instrument; ECG, electrocardiogram; EEG, electroencephalogram.
Data from Jacobi J et al: Clinical practice guidelines for the sustained use of sedatives and analgesics in the critically ill adult, *Crit Care Med* 30:119-141, 2002.

Summary

- Use a validated sedation instrument, and titrate sedation medications to achieve a clinically agreed-on level of sedation.
- Sedatives for short-term use are well delineated, but no ideal agent is available for long-term sedation.
- Long-term infusion of sedatives is associated with iatrogenic complications, including more days on the ventilator, delirium, symptoms of withdrawal when the sedatives are stopped, and ventilator-associated pneumonia (VAP).

- Sedation vacation is a procedure used with mechanically ventilated patients. The sedatives are stopped temporarily until the patient becomes more alert. When alert, the patient is assessed for readiness to wean from the ventilator. If the patient is not ready to be weaned from mechanical ventilation (i.e., fails a spontaneous breathing trial or other measure), the sedatives are restarted per hospital protocol.
- Delirium is a frequent complication of critical illness. Delirium can be hypoactive (withdrawn) or hyperactive (with agitation).
- Use a validated delirium assessment instrument to identify delirium.

Case Study: Patient with Delirium

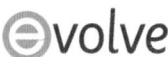 Answers to the Case Study Questions can be found on the Evolve web site at http://evolve.elsevier.com/Urden/.

Brief Patient History

Mr. K is a 42-year-old, Asian, out-of-town businessman in your city. He is transported to your facility from his hotel because of a witnessed grand mal seizure. Paramedics administered lorazepam in the field. Mr. K's wife reports by phone that he is in good health and that she is not aware that he takes any medications regularly. However, she states that he recently quit drinking alcohol because of pressure from the family. She also comments that she thinks he takes alprazolam to calm his nerves once in a while.

Clinical Assessment

Mr. K is admitted to the intensive care unit from the emergency department with hypertension, restlessness, mental confusion, paranoid ideations with rambling speech, and visual and auditory hallucinations. Mr. K's skin is warm and moist. Intravenous administration of thiamine, folic acid, multivitamins, and magnesium was begun in the emergency department. Physician orders were written for lorazepam every 6 hours and clonidine every 4 hours as needed for delirium-related symptoms.

Diagnostic Procedures

Mr. K's baseline vital signs are as follows: blood pressure of 190/92 mm Hg, heart rate of 130 beats/min (sinus tachycardia), respiratory rate of 26 breaths/min, and temperature of 98.8° F. Pulse oximetry O_2 saturation is 90% on 4 L/min oxygen using a nasal cannula. Confusion

Assessment Method indicates presence of acute and fluctuating change in mental status, inattention, and disorganized thinking. The Riker Sedation-Agitation Scale score is 5. Serum and urine toxicology studies are negative for ethyl alcohol, cannabis, and opioids; urine is strongly positive for benzodiazepines. The sodium level is 135 mmol/L, potassium level is 4.3 mmol/L, chloride level is 84 mmol/L, carbon dioxide level is 26 mEq/L, calcium level is 8 mg/dL; magnesium level is 2.0 mg/dL, and γ-glutamyl transpeptidase (GGT) level is 80 IU/L.

Medical Diagnosis

Mr. K is diagnosed with delirium tremens caused by alcohol and benzodiazepine withdrawal.

Questions

1. What major outcomes do you expect to achieve for this patient?
2. What problems or risks must be managed to achieve these outcomes?
3. What interventions must be initiated to monitor, prevent, manage, or eliminate the problems and risks identified?
4. What interventions should be initiated to promote optimal functioning, safety, and well-being of the patient?
5. What possible learning needs do you anticipate for this patient?
6. What cultural and age-related factors may have a bearing on the patient's plan of care?

Evolve Be sure to check out the bonus material, including free self-assessment exercises, on the Evolve web site at http://evolve.elsevier.com/Urden/.

References

1. Fraser GL, Riker RR: Monitoring sedation, agitation, analgesia, and delirium in critically ill adult patients, *Crit Care Clin* 17:967-987, 2001.
2. Fraser GL, Riker RR: Sedation and analgesia in the critically ill adult, *Curr Opin Anaesthesiol* 20:119-123, 2007.
3. Jacobi J et al: Clinical practice guidelines for the sustained use of sedatives and analgesics in the critically ill adult, *Crit Care Med* 30:119-141, 2002.
4. Flaherty JH et al: Delirium is a serious and under-recognized problem: why assessment of mental status should be the sixth vital sign, *J Am Med Dir Assoc* 8:273-275, 2007.
5. Fraser GL, Riker RR: Comfort without coma: changing sedation practices, *Crit Care Med* 35:635-637, 2007.
6. Ramsay MA et al: Controlled sedation with alphaxalone-alphadolone, *Br Med J* 2:656-659, 1974.
7. Riker RR et al: Prospective evaluation of the Sedation-Agitation Scale for adult critically ill patients, *Crit Care Med* 27:1325-1329, 1999.
8. Devlin JW et al: Motor Activity Assessment Scale: a valid and reliable sedation scale for use with mechanically ventilated patients in an adult surgical intensive care unit, *Crit Care Med* 27:1271-1275, 1999.
9. Ely EW et al: Monitoring sedation status over time in ICU patients: reliability and validity of the Richmond Agitation-Sedation Scale (RASS), *JAMA* 289:2983-2991, 2003.

10. Sessler CN et al: The Richmond Agitation-Sedation Scale: validity and reliability in adult intensive care unit patients, *Am J Respir Crit Care Med* 166:1338-1344, 2002.

11. Schweickert WD, Kress JP: Strategies to optimize analgesia and sedation, *Crit Care* 2008;12(suppl 3):S6, 2008.

12. Masica AL et al: Clinical sedation scores as indicators of sedative and analgesic drug exposure in intensive care unit patients, *Am J Geriatr Pharmacother* 5:218-231, 2007.

13. Joint Commission on Accreditation of Healthcare Organizations: Standards and intents for sedation and analgesia care in the revisions to anesthesia care standards. In *Comprehensive accreditation manual for hospitals*, Oakbrook Terrace, IL, 2000, Joint Commission.

14. Frazier SK et al: Critical care nurses' beliefs about and reported management of anxiety, *Am J Crit Care* 12:19-27, 2003.

15. Arbour R: Continuous nervous system monitoring, EEG, the bispectral index, and neuromuscular transmission, *AACN Clin* Issues 14:185-207, 2003.

16. Arbour RB: Using the Bispectral Index to assess arousal response in a patient with neuromuscular blockade, *Am J Crit Care* 9:383-387, 2000.

17. Olson DM et al: Perspectives on sedation assessment in critical care, *AACN Adv Crit Care* 18:380-395, 2007.

18. Sessler CN et al: Evaluating and monitoring analgesia and sedation in the intensive care unit, *Crit Care* 12(suppl 3):S2, 2008.

19. Schneider G et al: Patient State Index (PSI) measures depth of sedation in intensive care patients, *Intensive Care Med* 30:213-216, 2004.

20. Sessler CN, Varney K: Patient-focused sedation and analgesia in the ICU, *Chest* 133:552-565, 2008.

21. Young CC, Prielipp RC: Benzodiazepines in the intensive care unit, *Crit Care Clin* 17:843-862, 2001.

22. Olkkola KT, Ahonen J: Midazolam and other benzodiazepines, In Olkkola KT, Ahonen J (eds): *Handbook of Experimental Pharmacology* 182:335-360, 2008.

23. Barr J et al: A double-blind, randomized comparison of I.V. lorazepam versus midazolam for sedation of ICU patients via a pharmacologic model, *Anesthesiology* 95:286-298, 2001.

24. Fong JJ et al: Propofol associated with a shorter duration of mechanical ventilation than scheduled intermittent lorazepam: a database analysis using Project IMPACT, *Ann Pharmacother* 41:1986-1991, 2007.

25. Carson SS et al: A randomized trial of intermittent lorazepam versus propofol with daily interruption in mechanically ventilated patients, *Crit Care Med* 34:1326-1332, 2006.

26. Pandharipande P et al: Lorazepam is an independent risk factor for transitioning to delirium in intensive care unit patients, *Anesthesiology* 104:21-26, 2006.

27. Pandharipande PP et al: Effect of sedation with dexmedetomidine vs lorazepam on acute brain dysfunction in mechanically ventilated patients: the MENDS randomized controlled trial, *JAMA* 298:2644-2653, 2007.

28. Devlin JW: The pharmacology of oversedation in mechanically ventilated adults, *Curr Opin Crit Care* 2008;14:403-407, 2008.

29. Betten DP et al: Antidote use in the critically ill poisoned patient, *J Intensive Care Med* 21:255-277, 2006.

30. Whitcomb JJ et al: The use of propofol in the mechanically ventilated medical/surgical intensive care patient: is it the right choice? *Dimens Crit Care Nurs* 22:60-63, 2003.

31. Zaccheo MM, Bucher DH: Propofol infusion syndrome: a rare complication with potentially fatal results, *Crit Care Nurse* 28:18-26, 2008.

32. Angelini G et al: Use of propofol and other nonbenzodiazepine sedatives in the intensive care unit, *Crit Care Clin* 17:863-880, 2001.

33. Barr J et al: Propofol dosing regimens for ICU sedation based upon an integrated pharmacokinetic-pharmacodynamic model, *Anesthesiology* 95:324-333, 2001.

34. Corbett SM et al: Propofol-related infusion syndrome in intensive care patients, *Pharmacotherapy* 28:250-258, 2008.

35. Lam SW, Alexander E: Dexmedetomidine use in critical care, *AACN Advanced Critical Care* 19:113-120, 2008.

36. Dasta JF et al: Addition of dexmedetomidine to standard sedation regimens after cardiac surgery: an outcomes analysis, *Pharmacotherapy* 26:798-805, 2006.

37. Akada S et al: The efficacy of dexmedetomidine in patients with noninvasive ventilation: a preliminary study, *Anesth Analg* 107:167-170, 2008.

38. Szumita PM et al: Sedation and analgesia in the intensive care unit: evaluating the role of dexmedetomidine, *Am J Health Syst Pharm* 64:37-44, 2007.

39. MacLaren R et al: Adjunctive dexmedetomidine therapy in the intensive care unit: a retrospective assessment of impact on sedative and analgesic requirements, levels of sedation and analgesia, and ventilatory and hemodynamic parameters, *Pharmacotherapy* 27:351-359, 2007.

40. Gerlach AT, Dasta JF: Dexmedetomidine: an updated review, *Ann Pharmacother* 41:245-252, 2007.

41. de Wit M, Epstein SK: Administration of sedatives and level of sedation: comparative evaluation via the Sedation-Agitation Scale and the Bispectral Index, *Am J Crit Care* 12:343-348, 2003.

42. Micek ST et al: Delirium as detected by the CAM-ICU predicts restraint use among mechanically ventilated medical patients, *Crit Care Med* 33:1260-1265, 2005.

43. Martin B, Mathisen L: Use of physical restraints in adult critical care: a bicultural study, *Am J Crit Care* 14:133-142, 2005.

44. Kress JP et al: The long-term psychological effects of daily sedative interruption on critically ill patients, *Am J Respir Crit Care Med* 168:1457-1461, 2005.

45. Kress JP et al: Daily interruption of sedative infusions in critically ill patients undergoing mechanical ventilation, *N Engl J Med* 2000;342:1471-1477, 2005.

46. Girard TD et al: Efficacy and safety of a paired sedation and ventilator weaning protocol for mechanically ventilated patients in intensive care (Awakening and Breathing Controlled trial): a randomised controlled trial, *Lancet* 371:126-134, 2008.

47. Mehta S et al: A randomized trial of daily awakening in critically ill patients managed with a sedation protocol: a pilot trial, *Crit Care Med* 36:2092-2099, 2008.

48. Schweickert WD et al: Daily interruption of sedative infusions and complications of critical illness in mechanically ventilated patients, *Crit Care Med* 32:1272-1276, 2004.

49. Pun BT, Ely EW: The importance of diagnosing and managing ICU delirium, *Chest* 132:624-636, 2007.

50. Ely EW et al: The impact of delirium in the intensive care unit on hospital length of stay, *Intensive Care Med* 27:1892-1900, 2001.

51. Ely EW et al: Delirium as a predictor of mortality in mechanically ventilated patients in the intensive care unit, *JAMA* 291:1753-1762, 2004.

52. Roberts BL et al: Patients' dreams in ICU: recall at two years post discharge and comparison to delirium status during ICU admission. A multicentre cohort study, *Intensive Crit Care Nurs* 22:264-273, 2006.

53. Devlin JW et al: Delirium assessment in the critically ill, *Intensive Care Med* 33:929-940, 2007.

54. Plaschke K et al: Comparison of the confusion assessment method for the intensive care unit (CAM-ICU) with the Intensive Care Delirium Screening Checklist (ICDSC) for delirium in critical care patients gives high agreement rate(s), *Intensive Care Med* 34:431-436, 2008.

55. Ely EW et al: Evaluation of delirium in critically ill patients: validation of the Confusion Assessment Method for the Intensive Care Unit (CAM-ICU), *Crit Care Med* 29:1370-1379, 2001.

56. Ely EW et al: Delirium in mechanically ventilated patients: validity and reliability of the confusion assessment method for the intensive care unit (CAM-ICU), *JAMA* 286:2703-2710, 2001.

57. Pun BT et al: Large-scale implementation of sedation and delirium monitoring in the intensive care unit: a report from two medical centers, *Crit Care Med* 33:1199-1205, 2005.

58. Bergeron N et al: Intensive Care Delirium Screening Checklist: evaluation of a new screening tool, *Intensive Care Med* 27:859-864, 2001.

59. Ouimet S et al: Subsyndromal delirium in the ICU: evidence for a disease spectrum, *Intensive Care Med* 33:1007-1013, 2007.

60. Roberts B et al: Multicentre study of delirium in ICU patients using a simple screening tool, *Aust Crit Care* 18:6, 8-9, 11-14, 2005.

61. Milbrandt EB et al: Haloperidol use is associated with lower hospital mortality in mechanically ventilated patients, *Crit Care Med* 33:226-229, 2005.

62. Riker RR, Fraser GL: Adverse events associated with sedatives, analgesics, and other drugs that provide patient comfort in the intensive care unit, *Pharmacotherapy* 25:8S-18S, 2005.

63. Girard TD et al: Delirium in the intensive care unit, *Crit Care* 12(Suppl 3): S3, 2008.

64. de Wit M et al: Drug withdrawal, cocaine and sedative use disorders increase the need for mechanical ventilation in medical patients, *Addiction* 103:1500-1508, 2008.

65. Ozsancak A et al: Sleep and mechanical ventilation, *Crit Care Clin* 24: 517-531, 2008.

66. Olofsson K et al: Abolished circadian rhythm of melatonin secretion in sedated and artificially ventilated intensive care patients, *Acta Anaesthesiol Scand* 48:679-684, 2004.

67. Szokol JW, Vender JS: Anxiety, delirium, and pain in the intensive care unit. *Crit Care Clin* 17:821-842, 2001.

End-of-Life Issues

$\mathcal{E}$nd of life has become an important clinical topic in critical care, although requisite improvements in end-of-life care have been slow to follow. Because the primary purpose of admission of patients to a critical care unit is to provide aggressive, life-saving care, the death of a patient is generally regarded as a failure. Because the culture emphasizes saving lives, the language that describes the end of life employs negative terms, such as forgoing life-sustaining treatments, do not resuscitate (DNR), and withdrawal of life support. Sometimes, the phrase *withdrawal of care* is used—imagine the impact on families when they hear that phrase! This lack of end-of-life language has hampered literature searches until recently. The medical subject headings (MeSH) term for withdrawal of life support is *passive euthanasia*. Content on the end of life in medical[1] and nursing[2] critical care textbooks is minimal. The first textbook on end of life in critical care was published in 1998[3] and the second in 2001.[4]

More attention is being given to the quality of the end-of-life experience of the critically ill, with recognition of the numbers of patients who die in critical care units. This chapter focuses on the evidence available for the care we are rendering to the dying critical care patient and his or her family and on care that is recommended by evidence, research reports, and summaries of research and guidelines.

One such report is from the National Consensus Project and the National Quality Forum,[5] in which the preferred practices of the imminently dying are discussed. This type of report can be used to make a checklist of indicators for quality improvement in end-of-life care. Other such reports which are specific to the ICU have been written by groups headed by Teno,[6] Nelson,[7] Glavan,[8] Beckstrand,[9] and Mularski.[10] The American Association of Critical-Care Nurses published a Protocol for Practice for Palliative Care and End-of-Life Issues.[11] Curtis and Rubenfeld[4] have provided a "how to" guide for critical care quality improvement to outline the process that can be used with these indicators.

END-OF-LIFE EXPERIENCE IN CRITICAL CARE

Attention to the end of life of hospitalized patients has increased since the publication of the Study to Understand Prognoses and Preferences for Outcomes and Risks of Treatments

(SUPPORT).[12] In this major report, more than 9000 seriously ill patients in five medical centers were studied. Despite an intervention to improve communication, shortcomings were found, aggressive treatment was common, only one half of physicians knew their patients' preferences to avoid cardiopulmonary resuscitation (CPR), more than one third of patients who died spent at least 10 days in a critical care unit, and for 50% of conscious patients, family members reported moderate to severe pain at least one half of the time.

Following closely after the publication of the SUPPORT study, the Institute of Medicine (IOM) released a report, *Approaching Death: Improving Care at the End of Life*.[13] The group detailed deficiencies in care and gave seven recommendations to improve care:

1. Patients with fatal illnesses and their family should receive reliable, skillful, and supportive care.
2. Health professionals should improve care for the dying.
3. Policymakers and consumers should work with health professionals to improve quality and financing of care.
4. Health profession education should include end-of-life content.
5. Palliative care should be developed, possibly as a medical specialty.
6. Research on end of life should be funded.
7. The public should communicate more about the experience of dying and options available.

In SUPPORT and in the IOM report, critical care patients were not distinguished from other hospitalized patients, preventing distinctions to be made between types of units. To describe the number of deaths in critical care units, Angus and colleagues[14] reviewed hospital discharge data from six states and the National Death Index. Of the more than 500,000 deaths studied, 38.3% were in hospitals, and 22% (59% of all hospital deaths) occurred after admission to the critical care unit. Terminal admissions associated with critical care accounted for 80% of all terminal hospitalization costs.[14] The likelihood of dying in the hospital increased from age 25 to 74 years, and the likelihood of dying after critical care unit admission remained at 25% of all deaths for each age category. Although 90% of people would prefer to die in their own homes,[13] more than 20% of those who died in this review received high-tech, aggressive care before they died.

ADVANCE DIRECTIVES

Although advance directives, also known as a *living will* or a *health care power of attorney*, were intended to ensure that patients received the care they desired at end of life, their enactment has been less than desired. Like other preventive measures, advance directives are underused, even though they are inexpensive and potentially effective.[15] Most patients have expressed a desire to avoid "general life support" if dying or permanently unconscious, and few have expressed preferences regarding specific life-sustaining treatments.[16] Cook and others[17] found that factors differed for determining the establishment of directives for advance life support more than for informing a decision to limit or withdraw that support after admission to an ICU. Care providers also reported discomfort because they believed interventions were excessive and not compatible with an acceptable future quality of life. Even when advance directives are present, the question arises about whether they are applicable for current care decisions; in other words, is this a terminal illness?

ADVANCE CARE PLANNING

Cultural influences in the United States discourage discussion of death. Planning for decisions to be made at a later date if one is deemed incompetent is a difficult process, but this knowledge helps the family members left to make the treatment decisions. Advance care planning for those with chronic illness is advantageous for all involved.[18] When surrogates hear the patient's wishes for end-of-life care, they can be more congruent and knowledgeable about those wishes in future decision making.

Communication of the patient's wishes between primary care providers and intensivists is critical. If patients have stated desires, they should be communicated when patients are transferred out of the ICU. If the patient has not specified his or her preferences, that information also is important and should be communicated to new health care providers; the level of care patients desire should be offered as appropriate. Families and care providers should be informed if patients decline aggressive care, so their families will not be left with difficult decisions in emergency situations. Emotional support for the patient and the family is important as they discuss advance care planning in the critical care setting and is described in the Nursing Interventions Classification (NIC) feature on Family Support.

ETHICAL AND LEGAL ISSUES

Legal and ethical principles guide many of our decisions in caring for the dying patient and the family. The patient is respected as autonomous and able to make his or her own

---

NIC

Family Support

Definition
Promotion of family values, interests, and goals

Activities
Assure the family that the best care possible is being given to the patient.
Appraise family's emotional reaction to patient's condition.
Determine the psychological burden of prognosis for family.
Foster realistic hope.
Listen to family concerns, feelings, and questions.
Facilitate communication of concerns or feelings between patient and family or between family members.
Promote trusting relationship with family.
Accept the family's values in a nonjudgmental manner.
Answer all questions of family members, or assist them to get answers.
Orient family to the health care setting, such as the hospital unit or clinic.
Provide assistance in meeting basic needs of family, such as shelter, food, and clothing.
Identify nature of spiritual support for family.
Identify congruence between patient, family, and health professional expectations.
Reduce discrepancies patient, family, and health professional expectations through use of communication skills.
Assist family members in identifying and resolving any conflict in values.
Respect and support adaptive coping mechanisms used by the family
Provide feedback for the family regarding their coping.
Counsel family members on additional effective coping skills for their own use.

Provide spiritual resources for family, as appropriate.
Provide family with information about patient's progress frequently, according to patient preference.
Teach the medical and nursing plans of care to family.
Provide necessary knowledge of options to family that will assist them to make decisions about patient care.
Include family members with patient in decision making about care, when appropriate.
Encourage family decision making in planning long-term patient care affecting family structure and finances.
Acknowledge understanding of family decisions about postdischarge care.
Assist family to acquire necessary knowledge, skills, and equipment to sustain their decision about patient care.
Advocate for family, as appropriate.
Foster family assertiveness in information seeking, as appropriate.
Provide opportunities for visitation by extended family members, as appropriate.
Introduce family to other families undergoing similar experiences, as appropriate.
Give care to patient in lieu of family to relieve them or when family is unable to give care.
Arrange for ongoing respite care, when indicated and desired.
Provide opportunities for peer group support.
Refer for family therapy, as appropriate.
Tell family members how to reach the nurse.
Assist the family members through the death and grief processes, as appropriate.

From Bulechek GM et al: *Nursing interventions classification (NIC)*, ed 5, St Louis, 2008, Mosby.

decisions. When the patient is unable to make decisions, however, the same respect should be accorded to surrogates. These wishes might have been put in writing by the patient as an advance directive and preferably discussed with the surrogate. The Patient Self-Determination Act supports the patient's right to control future treatment in the event the individual cannot speak for himself or herself.

Two of the basic principles underlying the provision of health care are beneficence and nonmaleficence. *Beneficence* is the principle of intending to benefit the other through one's actions. *Nonmaleficence* means to do no harm. Sometimes at end of life, these two principles are in conflict, such as when resuscitation is attempted under beneficence but does cause harm to the patient, especially if resuscitation was not desired by the patient.

COMFORT CARE

The decision to withdraw life-sustaining treatments and switch to comfort care at end of life should be made with as much involvement of the patient as possible, including physical presence of the patient in decision making or procuring paper documents if the patient is not able to be present. If neither is available, the patient's intent as understood from discussions or knowledge of the patient should guide the decision about whether to withdraw treatment. Withholding and withdrawing care are considered to be morally and legally equivalent.[19] However, because families experience more stress in withdrawing treatments than in withholding them,[20] treatments are not started that the patient would not want or that would not benefit him or her.

The goal of withdrawal of life-sustaining treatments is to remove treatments that are not beneficial and may be uncomfortable. Any treatment in this circumstance may be withheld or withdrawn. After the goal of comfort has been chosen, each procedure should be evaluated to see if it is necessary or causes discomfort. Treatments that cause discomfort do not need to be continued. When disagreements arise, ethics consultations have been found to resolve conflicts regarding inappropriately prolonged, nonbeneficial, or unwanted treatments in the ICU, shifting the focus to more appropriate comfort care.[21]

Forgoing life-sustaining treatments is not the same as active euthanasia or assisted suicide. Killing is an action causing another's death, whereas allowing a person to die by withholding or withdrawing life-sustaining treatment is avoiding any intervention that interferes with a natural death after illness or trauma.[3]

CARDIOPULMONARY RESUSCITATION

CPR was originally developed for those with coronary artery disease, and they are the most likely to survive resuscitation to discharge, as well as those who suffer cardiac arrest in the critical care unit.[22] The benefits of resuscitation may be overestimated for survival and for the more relevant outcome of resumption of baseline functional status. In a meta-analysis of 51 studies, Ebell and colleagues[22] found that the rate of overall survival to discharge after in-hospital CPR was 13.4%. A decreased rate of immediate survival was found for patients with acquired immune deficiency syndrome, those with a hematocrit above 35%, and patients who were male. Decreased survival to discharge was related to sepsis on the day before resuscitation, cancer with or without metastasis, dementia, elevated serum creatinine level, African American race, and dependent status. Brindley and colleagues[23] found the same rate for overall survival to hospital discharge (13.4%) in a retrospective study of hospital charts for inpatients who had undergone or experienced resuscitation. A study from Norway found that only 17% of elderly patients older than 75 years survived resuscitation to return home.[24]

FitzGerald and others[25] found that functional status among almost half of the survivors of in-hospital CPR had deteriorated compared with their condition 2 months before the event. After 6 months, 30% of those patients had died, and two thirds continued to lose function. Despite these dismal statistics, CPR is offered as an option without fully informing patients or families of the low possibility of survival, the pain and suffering involved during and after the procedure, and the potential for decline in functional status.

Family members typically are asked to leave the room during resuscitation. The American Association of Critical-Care Nurses (AACN)[26] and the Emergency Nurses Association (ENA)[27] have issued position statements recommending that families be allowed to be present during CPR and invasive procedures. Family presence is a significant source of support for the patient, and there may be a benefit to the family in observing the resuscitation that can aid in the grieving process when resuscitation is not successful by knowing that all was done that could be done.

IMPACT OF DO NOT RESUSCITATE ORDERS

As death approaches, the decision to initiate a DNR order is frequently delayed.[28] A DNR order is intended to prevent the initiation of life-sustaining measures such as endotracheal intubation or CPR. In a review of the literature covering the 25 years since the DNR was established, Burns and colleagues[29] found that those with a DNR order sometimes received less care and that some treatments were withheld[30] without those changes being specified in the DNR order. Although acuity of illness and organ dysfunction consistently predicted mortality, only the medical history was positively associated with a DNR order for critically ill surgical patients.[31] Documentation of consent conversations for DNR is less than ideal because the reasons for the DNR order were documented in only 55% of cases, and a consent conversation was documented in only 69%.[32]

DNR is sometimes perceived to mean "do not care," but that is not the intent. Families should be assured that patients will continue to receive care, including pain and symptom management, but that aggressive measures to extend life will not be employed. DNR orders should be written before withdrawal of life support is initiated; this documentation ensures that the patient is not subjected to unwanted interventions during the period between initiation of withdrawal and death.

PROGNOSTICATION AND PROGNOSTIC TOOLS

Why patients who are dying would have received life-prolonging therapy shortly before their death can be explained in part by a series of studies. It was found that physicians' ability to prognosticate the length of time before death is limited[33,34] and that the time to death usually is overestimated. Patients' wishes are usually not known, can be vague even when they are known,[35] or change over the course of an illness.[36] Care is often not in accord with patients' wishes, and this discrepancy is more prevalent when comfort care is desired over aggressive care.[37] Skills in communication and end-of-life care that would enable providers to better assess patient and family wishes are poorly developed and are not emphasized in medical curricula.[38,39]

Severity scoring systems belong to one of four classes: prognostic, single-organ failure, trauma scores, and organ dysfunction.[40] Two common tools for estimating critical care unit mortality are the Acute Physiology and Chronic Health Evaluation (APACHE) and multiple organ dysfunction score (MODS).[41] However, when these tools were compared with physicians' estimates of ICU survival of less than 10%, the physicians' estimates were associated with subsequent life-support limitation. A physician's estimate was more powerful in predicting mortality than illness severity, organ dysfunction, and use of inotropes or vasopressors.[42]

Despite this information and these tools, uncertainty remains a major issue in decision making for physicians, patients, and families.[36] Because of uncertainty and because a few patients who were never thought likely to survive actually return to visit a critical care unit, professionals are not confident about issues of survivability. Moreover, many families cling to small hopes of survival and recovery.

COMMUNICATION AND DECISION MAKING

Communication with the patient and family is critical. White and colleagues[43] found that shared decision making about end-of-life treatment choices in physician-family conferences was often incomplete, especially among less educated families. Higher levels of shared decision making were associated with greater family satisfaction. Families were found to go through a process in their decision making in which they considered the personal domain (rallying support and evaluating quality of life), the ICU environment domain (chasing the doctors and relating to the health care team), and the decision domain (arriving at a new belief and making and communicating the decision).[44] Focusing on improving ICU communication when patients are dying reduces lengths of stay and resource use.[45]

PATIENT COMMUNICATION

Patients' capacity for decision making is limited by illness severity; they are too sick or are hampered by the therapies or medications used to treat them.[46] When decision making is required, the patient is the first person to be approached. Information that can assist the clinical team to facilitate and support health-related decision making is provided in the NIC feature on Decision-Making Support in Chapter 2. When the patient is not able to safely make health care decisions because of disease progression or the therapy used for treatment, written documents such as a living will or a health care power of attorney should be obtained when possible. Additional information on power of attorney for health care can be found in the section on "Advance Care Planning" earlier in this chapter. Without those documents, wishes of the patient should be ascertained from those closest to the patient. Some states have a legal order of priority for surrogates. Some patients have neither capacity nor surrogates to assist in decision making, accounting for up to 27% of deaths in one study.[47]

FAMILY COMMUNICATION

How questions are asked of surrogates is extremely important. The question is not "What do you want to do about (patient's name)?" but rather "What would (patient's name) want if he knew he were in this situation?" These two questions have vastly different meanings and consequences for the patient and the family. The former question has a greater likelihood of engendering guilt over "pulling the plug." The latter question provides a sense of fulfilling the patient's wishes and respecting choices. Sometimes, this discussion is held during the family meeting, in which a general sense of goals can be discussed. As families make decisions, they appreciate support for those decisions, because the support can reduce the burden they experience. There is some evidence from a French study that families are reluctant to participate in decision making.[48] This evidence reinforces the need to support families who are highly stressed and possibly exhausted while they are trying to make the most difficult decisions they have ever faced.

Family members have reported dissatisfaction with communication and decision making.[49] Increasing the frequency of communication and sharing concerns early in the hospitalization will make subsequent discussions easier for the patient, family, and health professional. Having the entire critical care unit team present for morning rounds is one method of improving communication.[50] Family members who understood the communication of staff were acknowledged and comforted by them; those who had difficulties drew back and received less adequate communication.[51] Families who reported increased understanding when communicating with staff also reported greater acknowledgment and comfort from staff members, whereas families who experienced a lack of understanding when communicating with staff tended to withdraw, further limiting the effectiveness in communication with the hospital staff. Having to focus on understanding the professional is an unacceptable burden.

A publication from the Society of Critical-Care Medicine (SCCM) recommends supporting the families of ICU patients.[52] Forty-three recommendations are presented, including an endorsement of a shared decision-making model, family care conferencing, culturally appropriate requests for truth-telling and informed refusal, spiritual support, staff education and debriefing, family presence at rounds and resuscitation, open and flexible visitation, family-friendly signs, and family support before, during, and after a death. One use of this guideline is to assess the level of family support for each ICU so that the most deficient recommendations could be addressed with quality-improvement actions. The categories used in this guideline are for general support of ICU families. When cross-indexed with seven end-of-life domains,[53] the needs of a family with a dying patient are decision making; spiritual and cultural support; emotional and practical support of families, including visitation and family preparation for death; and continuity of care.[54]

CULTURAL AND RELIGIOUS INFLUENCES ON COMMUNICATION

Cultural and religious influences on attitudes and beliefs about death and dying differ dramatically. The cultures of the predominant religions commonly seen in the surrounding community should be familiar to the local health care team. These differences may affect how the health care team is viewed, how decisions are made, whether aggressive treatment is preferred, how death is met, and how grieving will occur.[55,56] Satisfaction with ICU care has been associated with the extent to which the family is satisfied with their spiritual care, especially when the patient is near death.[57] Staff members own attitudes about the specific practices of a culture should be carefully assessed[58] and should be tempered with respect and humility. Interpreters are necessary when the patient or the family members do not speak English. A cultural and religious assessment is warranted in all situations, because cultural or religious affiliation does not imply that patients or families follow all of the tenets of that group.

HOSPICE INFORMATION

Although hospice care has been available for many years, patients and families often consider this method of care only in the last weeks or months of a patient with end-stage illness, and they frequently view hospice care as "giving up." Health professionals can assist patients and families by providing information about the hospice benefit. Some hospices are offering to partner with critical care units in the provision of end-of-life care and in the process of withdrawal of ventilatory support. Hospice care is an option that should be considered, especially in end-stage illness.

WITHDRAWAL OR WITHHOLDING OF TREATMENT

Discussions about the potential for impending death are never held early enough. Usually, the first discussion about prognosis occurs in conjunction with the topic of the discontinuation of life support. The late timing of that first discussion is an issue, particularly because some families have arrived at the notion of withdrawal before physicians.[46,59] Physicians should give families time to adjust to this information and make preparations by providing discussions early about prognosis, goals of therapy, and the patient's wishes.[4]

PROACTIVE APPROACH

After a poor prognosis is established, a period can elapse before end-of-life treatment goals are determined. Campbell and Guzman[60] recommended a proactive case-finding approach by palliative care personnel to decrease hospital length of stay for patients with multiorgan system failure and global cerebral ischemia. They shortened the time between identifying the poor prognosis and establishing comfort care goals, decreased length of critical care unit stay for patients with multisystem organ dysfunction, and reduced the cost of care. Proactive palliative care should occur when admission diagnoses trigger a consultation instead of after several avenues of treatment have been exhausted. When patients are admitted with serious illnesses and are likely to die. a proactive approach to palliative care has been found to shorten ICU stays without a significant difference in mortality rates or discharge disposition.[61] The use of nonbeneficial resources decreased, and prolonged dying was avoided.[60]

DISAGREEMENT AND DISTRESS FOR CAREGIVERS

Nurses and doctors frequently disagree about the futility of interventions. Sometimes, nurses consider withdrawal before physicians and patients do, and they then feel the care they are giving is unnecessary and possibly harmful. Nurses in one study were found to be more pessimistic but more often correct than physicians about the prognoses of dying patients, but the nurses also proposed treatment withdrawal for some very sick patients who survived.[62] This issue is a serious one for critical care nurses, because emotional and ethical distress can lead to burnout. Meltzer found that the score on the emotional exhaustion subscale of the Maslach Burnout Inventory and the score on the frequency subscale on the Moral Distress Scale correlated for a group of 60 critical care nurses.[63]

BARRIERS TO DYING

Ellershaw and Ward[64] identified a number of barriers to diagnosing dying: hope for the patient to improve, unclear diagnosis, pursuance of futile interventions, disagreement about the patient's condition, failure to recognize key signs and symptoms, poor ability to communicate, fears about foreshortening life, concerns about withdrawal and withholding, and medicolegal issues. Prognostic models are used to predict mortality rates for groups of critical care patients, not to guide specific decisions to forgo treatment.[65]

STEPS TOWARD COMFORT CARE

If a series of interventions is to be withdrawn, dialysis usually is discontinued first along with diagnostic tests and vasopressors.

Next, intravenous fluids, monitoring, laboratory tests, and antibiotics are stopped.[65] Withdrawal of specific treatments may have effects necessitating symptom management. Withdrawal of dialysis may cause dyspnea from volume overload, which may necessitate the use of opioids or benzodiazepines. Efforts to discontinue artificial feeding may be met with concern from the family, because offering food has great social significance.

PALLIATIVE CARE

Patients who are identified as being near the end of life require aggressive care for their symptom management that is provided by a team of health professionals. The most relevant clinical goal is to palliate these unpleasant situations by assessing for them and implementing appropriate interventions.[3] Palliative care guidelines have been released by a consortium of organizations concerned with palliative care and end-of-life care, and they may provide guidance when the usual first-line treatments do not promote comfort for critically ill patients who are near death.[66] Palliative care has been thought of as desirable only when the patient nears death or when several interventions have been tried for management of symptoms without success. However, publications such as these guidelines and the IOM report, *Improving Palliative Care for Cancer*[67] have stated that palliative care ideally begins at the time of diagnosis of a life-threatening illness and continues through cure or until death and into the family's bereavement period.

PAIN MANAGEMENT

Because many critical care patients are not conscious, assessment of pain and other symptoms becomes more difficult.[68] Gélinas and colleagues[69] recommended using signs of body movements, neuromuscular signs, facial expressions, or responses to physical examination for pain assessment in patients with altered consciousness (see Chapter 9). Foley,[70] while acknowledging the usual three-step approach of the World Health Organization, admitted that in critical care units, step 3 is frequently used because of the intensity of the pain.

Nonopioid drugs are the first-line approach, followed by adding an opioid for additional analgesia when relief is not obtained. Because opioids provide sedation, anxiolysis, and analgesia, they are particularly beneficial in the ventilated patient. Morphine is the drug of choice, and there is no upper limit in dosing.[3] In nonventilated patients, sedation may cause respiratory depression,[70] and nonopioids or specific anesthetic agents may be more appropriate. Jacobi and others[71] published a guideline for the sustained use of sedatives and analgesia (see Chapter 10); it is also available on the SSCM's Web site (www.sccm.org).

SYMPTOM MANAGEMENT

Campbell,[3] in her book chapter titled "Usual Care Requirements for the Patient Who Is Near Death," listed the following symptoms as necessary parts of the assessment: dyspnea, nausea and vomiting, edema and pulmonary edema, anxiety and delirium, metabolic derangements, skin integrity, and anemia and hemorrhage.

Dyspnea. Campbell published a review of terminal dyspnea and respiratory distress.[72] Dyspnea is best managed with close evaluation of the patient and the use of opioids, sedatives, and nonpharmacologic interventions (oxygen, positioning, and increased ambient air flow). Morphine reduces anxiety and muscle tension and increases pulmonary vasodilatation. Benzodiazepines may be used in patients who are not able to take opioids or for whom the respiratory effects are minimal. Benzodiazepines and opioids should be titrated to effect. Treatment efforts should be aimed at the patient's expression of dyspnea rather than at respiratory rates or oxygen levels.[73]

Nausea and Vomiting. Nausea and vomiting are common and should be treated with antiemetics. The cause of nausea and vomiting may be intestinal obstruction. Treatment for decompression may be uncomfortable in dying patients, and its use should be weighed using a benefit-to-burden ratio.

Fever and Infection. Fever and infection necessitate assessment of the benefits of continuing antibiotics so as not to prolong the dying process.[3] Management of the fever with antipyretics may be appropriate for the patient's comfort, but other methods such as ice or hypothermia blankets should be balanced against the amount of distress the patient may experience.

Edema. Edema may cause discomfort, and diuretics may be effective if kidney function is intact. Dialysis is not warranted at the end of life. The use of fluids may contribute to the edema when kidney function is impaired and the body is slowing its functions. In a Database of Abstracts of Reviews of Effectiveness (DARE) report,[74] little relationship was found between thirst and fluid therapy or fluid status.

Anxiety. Anxiety should be assessed verbally, if possible, or by changes in vital signs or restlessness. Benzodiazepines, especially midazolam with its rapid onset and short half-life, are frequently used.

Delirium. Delirium is commonly observed in the critically ill and in those approaching death. Haloperidol is recommended as useful, and restraints should be avoided. In a review of the available literature, Kehl[75] concluded that despite the recommendations of most study authors to use neuroleptic medications as a treatment for restlessness, several studies demonstrated the effectiveness of other medications, such as benzodiazepines (notably midazolam and lorazepam) or phenothiazines, alone or in combination.

Metabolic Derangement. Treatments for metabolic derangements, skin problems, anemia, and hemorrhage should be tempered with concerns for the patient's comfort. Only interventions promoting comfort should be performed. Patients do not necessarily feel better "when the laboratory values are right."

Providing Comfort. The nursing interventions at end of life should focus on the provision of comfort care as an active, desirable, and important service. Unnecessary checks of vital signs, laboratory work, and any treatment that does not promote comfort should be avoided. Positioning the patient who is actively dying has as its purpose only comfort, not the schedule to promote skin integrity. Coordinating this care with the many members of the critical care team is important to ensure consistency across disciplines and across shifts. When symptom management is not successful in ensuring comfort, the services of the pain team or the palliative care service may be required.

NEAR-DEATH AWARENESS

Two hospice nurses have described a phenomenon of near-death awareness.[76] The same behaviors may be seen in conscious critical care patients near death. Having an awareness of the phenomenon enables more careful assessment of behaviors that may be interpreted as delirium, acid-base imbalance, or other metabolic derangements. These behaviors include communicating with someone who is not alive, preparing for travel, describing a place they can see, or even knowing when death will occur.[77] Family members may find these behaviors disturbing but find comfort in understanding the phenomenon and in sharing these experiences with their loved one.

FAMILY MEETINGS

Although family meetings should be held within 72 hours of an admission,[78] they are frequently held to formulate a decision to withdraw life support. Lilly and colleagues[78] found that an earlier meeting led to shorter ICU stays for patients who eventually died and allowed them earlier access to palliative care. These results held up in a 4-year evaluation of this intervention, and they found that they were providing advanced life support to patients with the potential to survive and an earlier withdrawal when ineffective.[79]

WITHDRAWAL OF MECHANICAL VENTILATION

A dramatic geographic variation in the prevalence of withdrawal of life-sustaining therapies has been found. Some evidence suggests this variation may be driven more by physicians' attitudes and biases than by factors such as patients' preferences or cultural differences.[80] This inconsistency in care further complicates a difficult process.

During the family meeting in which a decision to withdraw life support is made, a time to initiate withdrawal is usually established. For example, a distant family member may need to arrive, and then the procedure will occur. When appropriate, the patient should be moved to a separate or special room. It is helpful if other staff members are alerted to the fact that a withdrawal is occurring. A neutral sign hung on the door or use of a special room may caution staff to avoid loud conversations and laughter, which is quite upsetting to grieving families.

After the decision to remove ventilatory support is made and the family is gathered, the family should be told what the impending death will be like. When the patient is dependent on ventilatory support or vasopressors and that support is removed, death typically follows in minutes. The patient appears as if sleeping, and the usual signs of color and skin temperature changes will not be seen before death. The opposite is true if the patient is not ventilator dependent. When the patient will be extubated at the beginning of the withdrawal process, the family should be prepared for respiratory noises and gasping respirations. These signs are less likely when the endotracheal tube is removed near the end of the withdrawal process, as is more commonly done. When assessing how prepared family members felt for what would happen during withdrawal of life support, Kirchhoff and colleagues[81] found that families who did not receive preparatory information before the withdrawal of life support requested this information during interviews 2 to 4 weeks after the patient's death. Family members who received this recommended information felt significantly more prepared. Providing information to families for the experience of withdrawal alerts them to what the patient may exhibit as death approaches, reducing the distress families may feel during the withdrawal process.

Pacemakers or implantable cardioverter-defibrillators should be turned off to prevent patient distress from their firing[82] and to avoid interfering with the pronouncement of death.[65] Wiegand and Kalowes[83] provide detailed information about the conversations that should be held with the patient[84] and how each of the specific devices are deactivated. Neuromuscular blocking agents should be discontinued, because paralysis precludes the assessment of the patient's discomfort and the means of the patient to communicate with loved ones. Time for clearance of the medication should be carefully considered in planning the withdrawal process.[65]

The removal of monitors is usually recommended.[85] However, physicians and nurses may use the monitor to assess the distress of the patient during the withdrawal process and to adjust the amount of medication needed for symptom management. Families may glance at the monitor to verify that electrical activity has ceased, because the appearance of death may be too subtle to detect. If not needed, monitors should be removed to make the room appear as normal as possible. It is important, however, to include family members in the decision-making process.

OPIOIDS AND SEDATIVES

Opioids and benzodiazepines are the most commonly administered medications, because dyspnea and anxiety are the usual symptoms related to ventilator withdrawal. Campbell[86] stated that brain-dead patients do not require sedation and that patients with brainstem activity only may not show signs of distress or need sedation. Von Gunten and Weissman[87] recommended sedating all patients, even those who are comatose. They recommend a bolus dose of morphine (2 to 10 mg IV) and a continuous morphine infusion at 50% of the bolus dose per hour. Midazolam (1 to 2 mg IV) is given, followed by an infusion at 1 mg/hr. The intent is to provide good symptom control so that doses accelerate until the patient's comfort is achieved. Additional medication should be available at the bedside for immediate administration if discomfort is observed in the patient. In one study, the use of narcotics or benzodiazepines to treat discomfort after the withdrawal of life support did not hasten death in critically ill patients.[88]

VENTILATOR SETTINGS

After the patient's comfort is achieved, ventilator settings are reduced. An experienced physician, a respiratory therapist, and a nurse should be present during this time. Ventilator alarms should be turned off. The method of withdrawal adopted is usually determined by the clinician's preference. The choice of terminal wean as opposed to extubation is based on considerations of access for suctioning, appearance of the patient for the family, how long the patient will survive off the ventilator, and whether the patient has the ability to communicate with loved ones at the bedside.

If terminal wean is used, positive end-expiratory pressure (PEEP) is reduced to normal, and then the mode is set to patient control. Next, the F_{IO_2} is reduced to 0.21 (21%). All of these steps are taken slowly while observing the patient for distress or anxiety. If extubation is performed immediately rather than at the end of the terminal wean, the family should be prepared for airway compromise and the appearance of the patient.

All patients do not require the same ventilator weaning or extubation protocols. For example, Campbell[86] recommended turning off the ventilator and extubating patients who are brain dead, placing patients who have brainstem-only injuries on a T-piece, and using terminal weaning for those with altered consciousness or those who are conscious. The terminal wean offers the most control over secretions, respiratory noises, and gasping.

PROFESSIONAL ISSUES
HEALTH CARE SETTINGS

Professional issues surround the provision of palliative care within traditional acute and clinical settings. In critical care units, care may be managed by an intensivist or by a committee of specialists, but seldom by the family physician who knows the patient. The use of consultants may be limited. Palliative care specialists may be available at certain times, but they are often considered "outsiders" and are infrequently invited. How the consultation is arranged may vary by institution. Turf issues should not compromise patient care. Having a clear plan for withdrawal and better preparation of the family may assist the professionals involved in feeling more comfortable with the care provided.[89] Expert nurses should advocate for vulnerable patients by communicating the patient's wishes and presenting a realistic picture to family members.[90]

Some interventions have been found helpful for health professionals in improving patient care. Although it did not improve nurses' assessment of patients' dying experience, a standardized order form for withdrawal was found to increase the amount of medications nurses administered for sedation.[91] Death rounds for ICU residents were well received and recommended to be included in future rotations.[92]

EMOTIONAL SUPPORT FOR THE NURSE

Nurses who care for the dying patient need to have their work as valued as other high-tech functions in the critical care unit. Critical care units usually have several nurses who are looked to by other staff to provide end-of-life care or to assist with withdrawal of life support. When several deaths occur close together, those nurses may be called on frequently. Some consideration in assignment should be given when a nurse has more than one death in a shift or a week. Taking a new admission is also difficult immediately after a death, and it can occur before the family has left the unit. Nurse administrators can provide some additional resources, debriefing, or time off when the burden has been high. Hearing supportive words from colleagues has been reported by critical care nurses as helpful in coping with the death of a patient.[93]

Nurses experience moral distress when aggressive care is offered to patients who are not expected to benefit from it. These levels of distress are high and have implications for retention of highly skilled nurses.[94] The experience of moral distress and a negative ethical environment is more severe than that of their physician colleagues.[95] Developing a consensus about care was found to be the most helpful approach.[96] Nurses had a number of suggestions when questioned about what could be done to improve end-of-life care, such as facilitating dying with dignity, having someone with patients who are dying, managing patients' symptoms, knowing and then following patients' wishes for end-of-life care, and promoting earlier cessation of treatment or not initiating aggressive treatment at all.[9]

ORGAN DONATION
LEGAL ISSUES

The Social Security Act Section 1138 requires that hospitals have written protocols for the identification of potential organ donors.[97] The Joint Commission (TJC) has a standard on organ donation.[98] Although an impending death marks a difficult time for family members, the nurse must notify the organ procurement official to approach the family with a donation request. These individuals have training to make a supportive request and are the ones to decide whether a family should not be approached based on the patient's disease. Although organ donation may not be appropriate in some cases, tissue donation remains a consideration. More information is available in Chapter 42.

BRAIN DEATH

Death may be pronounced when the patient meets a list of neurologic criteria. However, there are differences among hospital policies for certification of brain death, which may permit differences in the circumstances under which patients are pronounced dead in different U.S. hospitals.[99] Families do not understand the meaning of brain death, and they are less likely to donate organs when they believe the patient will not be dead until the ventilator is turned off and the heart stops.[100] How these conversations are held will determine families' understanding and positively affect donation. Campbell[3] recommended not suggesting that the organs are alive while the brain is dead, but rather that the organs are functioning as a result of the machines used. Chapter 42 provides more information on the specifics of brain death.

FAMILY CARE

In this chapter, the term *family* means whatever the patient states is the family. An integral part of the patient-family dyad, families expect a cure for any condition the patient may have; they do not expect to receive bad news. They look for the good news in any message received from caregivers and are surprised when told that death is the only outcome possible.[93] Families need assistance in forming their expectations about outcomes. Ongoing communication about the patient's progress is preferable to waiting until the patient is near death and then communicating with the family. Most studies of families at this time are descriptive, and interventions need to be developed to help them.[101]

One intervention used with families at the end of life is the use of a grieving cart. In one ICU,[102] the cart has a top drawer with English and Spanish versions of the Bible, Koran, and Book of Mormon and pamphlets about grief and bereavement. The lower portion of the cart holds paper cups, napkins, and condiments. Fresh coffee and tea are brewed on the unit and served with muffins and cookies from the cafeteria. Family responses have been positive because they do not want to leave the bedside despite their hunger.

COMMUNICATION NEEDS

Families have complained about infrequent physician communication,[103] unmet communication needs in the shift from aggressive to end-of-life care,[104] and lacking or inadequate communication.[105] Sometimes, families are not ready to receive the prognosis and engage in decision making.[106] Communication seems to be the most common source of complaints in families across studies and should be at the center of efforts to improve end-of-life care.

The health care team can reinforce the legitimacy of the family expressing feelings of disappointment, sadness, and loss. It is important that the family is made aware that the patient was more than a clinical disease and that he or she was recognized as an individual while in the critical care unit. When relatives of ICU patients were provided with a brochure on bereavement and received a proactive communication, they had lower negative scores on the Impact of Event Scale and on the Hospital Anxiety and Depression Scale. Ways to address the cultural, social, and emotional issues surrounding the expression of grief are given in the NIC feature on Grief Work Facilitation.

WAITING FOR GOOD NEWS

Patients and families do not come to the critical care unit with the expectation of death. Even those who have had previous admissions expect to be "saved." They tend to listen to imparted information looking for good news; even when bad news is given, they may initially deny it or have great difficulty taking it in.[105] Having this in mind while talking to families may assist professionals in interpreting families' responses.

Preparing families for changes in the patient as the health condition deteriorates helps them make plans. They need to know if other family members should be called, if someone should spend

---

NIC

Grief Work Facilitation

Definition
Assistance with the resolution of a significant loss

Activities
Identify the loss.
Assist the patient to identify the nature of the attachment to the lost object or person.
Assist the patient to identify the initial reaction to the loss.
Encourage expression of feelings about the loss.
Listen to expression of grief.
Encourage discussion of previous loss experiences.
Encourage the patient to verbalize memories of losses, past and current.
Make empathetic statements about grief.
Encourage identification of greatest fears concerning the loss.
Instruct in the phases of the grieving process, as appropriate.
Support progression through personal grieving stages.

Include significant others in discussions and decisions, as appropriate.
Assist patient to identify personal coping strategies.
Encourage patient to implement cultural, religious, and social customs associated with the loss.
Communicate acceptance of discussing loss.
Answer children's questions associated with the loss.
Use clear words, such as *dead* or *died*, rather than euphemisms.
Encourage children to discuss feelings.
Encourage expression of feelings in ways comfortable to the child, such as writing, drawing, or playing.
Assist the child to clarify misconceptions.
Identify sources of community support.
Support efforts to resolve previous conflict, as appropriate.
Reinforce progress made in the grieving process.
Assist in identifying modifications needed in lifestyle.

From Bulechek GM et al: *Nursing interventions classification (NIC)*, ed 5, St Louis, 2008, Mosby.

the night, or if financial arrangements should be changed before an impending death (e.g., to enable the widow to have access to funds). Anticipated changes can be described to prepare families.

Families may refuse to forgo life-supporting treatments and want "everything done" because of mistrust of health professionals, poor communication, survivor guilt, or religious or cultural reasons.[46] Effective communication throughout the hospitalization and information provided throughout the stay predispose the family to better acceptance of news as the patient deteriorates. Family satisfaction is increased when they feel supported during their decision making[107,108] or hear more empathic statements from physicians.[109]

FAMILY MEETINGS

Families may experience a sense of crisis as emergencies occur or as the patient deteriorates and dies. Responses to the news of the death vary. Family members may show anger or be quiet, exhibit emotions or stoicism. Culture or religious beliefs may affect their response to news. It is helpful to ask if they would like to see a chaplain or a social worker. Quiet and calm, some privacy, and support are always appreciated.

Family meetings in the presence of the critical care team have been one method used to arrive at a common understanding of the patient's prognosis and goals for future care.[110,111] An analysis of the amount of opportunity families had to speak in these meetings revealed that when families had greater opportunity to talk, their satisfaction with physician communication increased and their ratings of conflict with the physician decreased. Abbott and colleagues[112] discussed families' descriptions, 1 year after decisions about withdrawal of life support, of conflict centering on communication and the behavior of the staff. After the patient's death, greater family satisfaction with withdrawal of life support was associated with the following measures[113]:

- The process of withdrawal of life support being well explained
- Withdrawal of life support proceeding as expected
- Patient appearing comfortable
- Family and friends being prepared
- Appropriate person initiating discussion
- Adequate privacy during withdrawal of life support
- A chance to voice concerns

Curtis and colleagues[111] have been studying the process of family meetings and how to improve them to promote better end-of-life care for ICU patients and their families. They found that the missed opportunities that occur during these meetings were occasions to listen to family, to acknowledge and address emotions, and to pursue key tenets of palliative care, such as patient preferences, surrogate decision making, and nonabandonment.[114]

FAMILY PRESENCE DURING CARDIOPULMONARY RESUSCITATION

To be helpful, the family's presence during procedures or resuscitative attempts[27] should be coupled with staff support. Critical care nurses and emergency nurses have taken family members to the bedside for resuscitation or invasive procedures, but most did not have written policies for the family's presence.[115] Sometimes, these experiences provide opportunities for the family to be supportive of the patient. At other times, the family may become more aware of what is involved in decisions they have made on behalf of the patient. Seeing the steps of resuscitation may make clearer the impact of decisions made or delayed.

VISITING HOURS

Visiting in ICU continues to be restricted,[116] despite national calls for increases in patient or family control over the care.[117] Restricting visiting for dying ICU patients seems to be unconscionable. Providing the visiting time to help family members say good-bye is an important function. Family members may have difficulty in seeing the person they knew among all the tubes. Coaching can be provided about how to approach the patient and about how the patient may still be able to hear despite appearing to be nonresponsive. Visitors should be permitted to the extent possible, while not interfering with other patients' privacy or rest. Children, unless they represent a significant source of infection, should be allowed to say good-bye, but they may need adult assistance in understanding the situation. Families may have religious or cultural ceremonies that are important for them to perform before the patient dies or experiences withdrawal of life support. These practices should be encouraged and facilitated as much as possible.

Continuity of care by the same nurse is important. As the patient nears death, nurses have sometimes stayed with the family after the end of a shift when death was imminent so they would not need to adjust to another person at this difficult time.[93]

AFTER DEATH

After the death, the family may wish to spend time at the bedside. The family members' time with the body should be unhurried and private. They need adequate room to sit and spend time. They can be asked if they need assistance or resources and whether they wish to be alone or have someone nearby. Frequently, the bed is needed for another patient, and juggling is required to ensure that the family has sufficient time even as another patient needs to be admitted. Supporting families after a death involves immediate bereavement support, information on what to do about the death, bereavement support for the future, contact with the family after death, and assessment of the quality of care the patient experienced.[118] Having material already prepared with the necessary after-death information is quite helpful at this time. Nurses need to be aware of their own judgment on what is an appropriate response, because individuals respond differently to the same news, even within the same family.

COLLABORATIVE CARE

The ability to provide collaborative, compassionate end-of-life care is the responsibility of all clinicians who work with the critically ill. Interdisciplinary collaborative efforts are associated with improvement in care.[119] In 2008, the SCCM published a revised guideline, "Recommendations for End-of-Life Care in the Intensive Care Unit," to provide guidance for end-of-life care for the team.[120] The Evidence-Based Practice feature on End-of-Life Care provides a summary of the topics included. The Robert Wood Johnson Foundation (RWJF) Critical Care End-of-Life Peer Workgroup[53] identified seven end-of-life care domains for use in the ICU:

1. Patient- and family-centered decision making
2. Communication
3. Continuity of care
4. Emotional and practical support
5. Symptom management and comfort care
6. Spiritual support
7. Emotional and organizational support for ICU clinicians

Individuals[121] and groups[122] have developed Web sites for online tools to improve end-of-life care. Critical care unit staff will be able to assess the quality of their care by assessing perceptions of families and staff, auditing documentation,[123] or making observations of care. The same attention should be placed on improving end-of-life care that is placed on skills of electrocardiogram interpretation or hemodynamic monitoring.

Summary

- End-of-life care requires knowledge and skill, similar to any other aspect of ICU care.
- Patient- and family-centered decision making is key.
- Family presence during procedures or resuscitative attempts should be coupled with staff support.
- Extended visiting times are needed to help family members say good-bye.
- Proactive control of symptoms is vital for the patient's comfort.

Evidence-Based Practice: Collaborative

End-of-Life Care

The key topics of the guidelines for end-of-life care in the intensive care unit, based on research and expert panel review, are categorized.

Patient- and Family-Centered Care and Decision Making: The Comprehensive Ideal for End-of-Life Care
- Use the legal standards for decision making.
- Resolve conflict.
- Communicate with families.

Ethical Principles Related to Withdrawal of Life-Sustaining Treatment
- Withholding versus withdrawing
- Killing versus allowing to die
- Intended versus merely foreseen consequences

Practical Aspects of Withdrawing Life-Sustaining Treatments in the Intensive Care Unit
- The procedure
- Specific issues

- Use of paralytics

Symptom Management in End-of-Life Care
- Pain and dyspnea
- Delirium
- Medications used

Considerations at the Time of Death
- Notification of death
- Brain death
- Organ donation
- Bereavement and support
- Needs of the interdisciplinary team

Research, Quality Improvement, and Education
- Develop interventions likely to improve the quality of care.
- Develop education programs.

Data from Truog RD et al: Recommendations for end-of-life care in the intensive care unit: a consensus statement by the American Academy of Critical Care Medicine, *Crit Care Med* 36(3):953-963, 2008.

Case Study: Patient at the End of Life

⊝volve   Answers to the Case Study Questions can be found on the Evolve web site at http://evolve.elsevier.com/Urden/.

Brief Patient History

Mr. C is a 17-year-old, African American boy who was involved in a motor vehicle accident. He sustained a cervical fracture at the level of C2 that transected his spinal column and both vertebral arteries. Rescue breathing was begun in the field by bystanders, and he was intubated by paramedics enroute to the hospital. Mr. C's parents state that they want everything possible done and that they have faith that God will heal their son.

Clinical Assessment

Mr. C is admitted to the critical care unit from the emergency department. He is ventilator dependent. His skin is warm and dry. He is unresponsive to

Continued

Case Study: Patient at the End of Life—cont'd

verbal or painful stimuli, and there is no physical movement. Mr. C's family remains at the bedside 24 hours each day throughout the week. They converse with Mr. C, speaking about all the things they are going to do when he gets home.

Diagnostic Procedures

Mr. C's vital signs are as follows: blood pressure of 120/72 mm Hg, heart rate of 120 beats/min (sinus tachycardia), no spontaneous respiration, temperature of 97.8° F, and Glasgow Coma Scale score of 3. Computed tomography of the head showed a global ischemic infarct involving both ventricles, and electroencephalography revealed no detectable cortical activity.

Medical Diagnosis

Mr. C is diagnosed with brain death.

Questions

1. What major outcomes do you expect to achieve for this patient?
2. What problems or risks must be managed to achieve these outcomes?
3. What interventions must be initiated to monitor, prevent, manage, or eliminate the problems and risks identified?
4. What interventions should be initiated to promote optimal functioning, safety, and well-being of the patient?
5. What possible learning needs do you anticipate for this patient?
6. What cultural and age-related factors may have a bearing on the patient's plan of care?

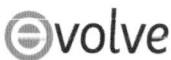 Be sure to check out the bonus material, including free self-assessment exercises, on the Evolve web site at http://evolve.elsevier.com/Urden/.

References

1. Rabow MW et al: End-of-life care content in 50 textbooks from multiple specialties, *JAMA* 283(6):771-778, 2000.
2. Kirchhoff KT et al: Analysis of end-of-life content in critical care nursing textbook, *J Prof Nurs* 19(6):372-381, 2003.
3. Campbell ML: *Forgoing life-sustaining therapy: how to care for the patient who is near death*, Aliso Viejo, CA, 1998, AACN.
4. Curtis JR, Rubenfeld GD, editors: *Managing death in the intensive care unit: the transition from cure to comfort*, Oxford, 2001, Oxford University Press.
5. Lynch M, Dahlin C: The national consensus project and national quality forum preferred practices in care of the imminently dying: implications for nursing, *J Hosp Palliat Nurs* 9(6):316-322, 2007.
6. Teno JM et al: Bereaved family member perceptions of quality of end-of-life care in U.S. regions with high and low usage of intensive care unit care, *J Am Geriatr Soc* 53(11):1905-1911, 2005.
7. Nelson JE et al: End-of-life care for the critically ill: a national intensive care unit survey, *Crit Care Med* 34(10):2547-2553, 2006.
8. Glavan BJ et al: Using the medical record to evaluate the quality of end-of-life care in the intensive care unit, *Crit Care Med* 36(4):1138-1146, 2008.
9. Beckstrand RL et al: Providing a "good death": critical care nurses' suggestions for improving end-of-life care, *Am J Crit Care* 15(1):38-45, 2006.
10. Mularski RA et al: Quality of dying in the ICU: ratings by family members, *Chest* 128(1):280-287, 2005.
11. Medina J, Puntillo K, editors: *AACN protocols for practice: palliative care and end-of-life issues in critical care*, Boston, 2006, Jones & Bartlett.
12. SUPPORT Investigators: A controlled trial to improve care for seriously ill hospitalized patients. The study to understand prognoses and preferences for outcomes and risks of treatments (SUPPORT), *JAMA* 274(20): 1591-1598, 1995.
13. Field MJ, Cassell CK, editors: *Approaching death: improving care at the end of life*, Washington, DC, 1997, National Academy Press.
14. Angus DC et al: Use of intensive care at the end of life in the United States: an epidemiologic study, *Crit Care Med* 32(3):638-643, 2004.
15. Gillick MR: Advance care planning, *N Engl J Med* 350(1):7-8, 2004.
16. Nishimura A et al: Patients who complete advance directives and what they prefer, *Mayo Clin Proc* 82(12):1480-1486, 2007.
17. Cook D et al: Levels of care in the intensive care unit: a research program, *Am J Crit Care* 15(3):269-279, 2006.
18. Briggs LA et al: Patient-centered advance care planning in special patient populations: a pilot study, *J Prof Nurs* 20(1):47-58, 2004.
19. Rubenfeld GD: Principles and practice of withdrawing life-sustaining treatments, *Crit Care Clin* 20(3):435-451, 2004.
20. Tilden V et al: Family decision-making to withdraw life-sustaining treatments from hospitalized patients, *Nurs Res* 50(2):105-115, 2001.
21. Gilmer T et al: The costs of nonbeneficial treatment in the intensive care setting, *Health Aff (Millwood)* 24(4):961-971, 2005.
22. Ebell MH et al: Survival after in-hospital cardiopulmonary resuscitation: a meta-analysis, *J Gen Intern Med* 13(12):805-816, 1998.
23. Brindley PG et al: Predictors of survival following in-hospital adult cardio-pulmonary resuscitation, *CMAJ* 167(4):343-348, 2002.
24. Elshove-Bolk J et al: In-hospital resuscitation of the elderly: characteristics and outcome, *Resuscitation* 74(2):372-376, 2007.
25. FitzGerald JD et al: Functional status among survivors of in-hospital cardiopulmonary resuscitation. SUPPORT investigators study to understand progress and preferences for outcomes and risks of treatment, *Arch Intern Med* 157(1):72-76, 1997.
26. American Association of Critical-Care Nurses: Family presence during CPR and invasive procedures, 2004. Available at www.aacn.org/WD/Practice/Docs/Family_Presence_During_CPR_11-2004.pdf (accessed January 2009).
27. Emergency Nurses Association: Family presence at the bedside during invasive procedures and cardiopulmonary resuscitation, 2005. Available at www.ena.org/about/position/PDFs/5F118F5052C2479C848012F5BCF87F7C.PDF (accessed January 2009).
28. Covinsky KE et al: Communication and decision-making in seriously ill patients: findings of the SUPPORT project. The study to understand prognoses and preferences for outcomes and risks of treatments, *J Am Geriatr Soc* 48(5 suppl):S187-S193, 2000.
29. Burns JP et al: Do-not-resuscitate order after 25 years, *Crit Care Med* 31(5):1543-1550, 2003.
30. Keenan CH, Kish SK: The influence of do-not-resuscitate orders on care provided for patients in the surgical intensive care unit of a cancer center, *Crit Care Nurs Clin North Am* 12(3):385-390, 2000.
31. Bacchetta MD et al: Factors influencing DNR decision-making in a surgical ICU, *J Am Coll Surg* 202(6):995-1000, 2006.

32. Sulmasy DP et al: The quality of care plans for patients with do-not-resuscitate orders, *Arch Intern Med* 164(14):1573-1578, 2004.

33. Christakis NA, Lamont EB: Extent and determinants of error in doctors' prognoses in terminally ill patients: prospective cohort study, *BMJ* 320 (7233):469-472, 2004.

34. Lynn J et al: Prognoses of seriously ill hospitalized patients on the days before death: implications for patient care and public policy, *New Horiz* 5(1):56-61, 1997.

35. McDonald DD et al: Communicating end-of-life preferences, *West J Nurs Res* 25(6):652-666; discussion 667–675, 2003.

36. Fried TR, Bradley EH: What matters to seriously ill older persons making end-of-life treatment decisions? A qualitative study. *J Palliat Med* 6(2): 237-244, 2003.

37. Teno JM et al: Medical care inconsistent with patients' treatment goals: association with 1-year Medicare resource use and survival, *J Am Geriatr Soc* 50(3):496-500, 2002.

38. Mularski RA et al: Educational agendas for interdisciplinary end-of-life curricula, *Crit Care Med* 29(2 suppl):N16-N23, 2001.

39. Wood EB et al: Enhancing palliative care education in medical school curricula: implementation of the palliative education assessment tool, *Acad Med* 77(4):285-291, 2002.

40. Strand K, Flaatten H: Severity scoring in the ICU: a review, *Acta Anaesthesiol Scand* 52(4):467-478, 2008.

41. Marshall JC et al: Multiple organ dysfunction score: a reliable descriptor of a complex clinical outcome, *Crit Care Med* 23(10):1638-1652, 1995.

42. Rocker G et al: Clinician predictions of intensive care unit mortality, *Crit Care Med* 32(5):1149-1154, 2004.

43. White DB et al: Toward shared decision making at the end of life in intensive care units: opportunities for improvement, *Arch Intern Med* 167(5):461-467, 2007.

44. Limerick MH: The process used by surrogate decision makers to withhold and withdraw life-sustaining measures in an intensive care environment, *Oncol Nurs Forum* 34(2):331-339, 2007.

45. Ahrens T et al: Improving family communications at the end of life: implications for length of stay in the intensive care unit and resource use, *Am J Crit Care* 12(4):317-323; discussion 324, 2003.

46. Prendergast TJ, Puntillo KA: Withdrawal of life support: intensive caring at the end of life, *JAMA* 288(21):2732-2740, 2002.

47. White DB et al: Decisions to limit life-sustaining treatment for critically ill patients who lack both decision-making capacity and surrogate decision-makers, *Crit Care Med* 4(8):2053-2059, 2006.

48. Azoulay E et al: Half the family members of intensive care unit patients do not want to share in the decision-making process: a study in 78 French intensive care units, *Crit Care Med* 32(9):1832-1838, 2004.

49. Baker R et al: Family satisfaction with end-of-life care in seriously ill hospitalized adults, *J Am Geriatr Soc* 48(5 suppl):S61-S69, 2000.

50. Curtis JR: Communicating about end-of-life care with patients and families in the intensive care unit, *Crit Care Clin* 20(3):363-380, 2004.

51. Soderstrom IM et al: Interactions between family members and staff in intensive care units—an observation and interview study. *Int J Nurs Stud* 43(6):707-716, 2006.

52. Davidson JE et al: Clinical practice guidelines for support of the family in the patient-centered intensive care unit: American College of Critical Care Task Force 2004-2005, *Crit Care Med* 35(2):605-622, 2007.

53. Clarke EB et al: Quality indicators for end-of-life care in the intensive care unit, *Crit Care Med* 31(9):2255-2262, 2003.

54. Kirchhoff KT, Faas AI: Family support at end of life, *AACN Adv Crit Care* 18(4):426-435, 2007.

55. Degenholtz HB et al: Race and the intensive care unit: disparities and preferences for end-of-life care, *Crit Care Med* 31(5 suppl):S373-S378, 2003.

56. Lipson JG et al: *Culture and nursing care: a pocket guide*, San Francisco, 1996, UCSF Nursing Press.

57. Wall RJ et al: Spiritual care of families in the intensive care unit, *Crit Care Med* 35(4):1084-1090, 2007.

58. Crawley LM: Racial, cultural, and ethnic factors influencing end-of-life care, *J Palliat Med* 8(suppl 1):S58-S69, 2005.

59. Breen CM et al: Conflict associated with decisions to limit life-sustaining treatment in intensive care units, *J Gen Intern Med* 16(5):283-289, 2001.

60. Campbell ML, Guzman JA: Impact of a proactive approach to improve end-of-life care in a medical ICU, *Chest* 123(1):266-271, 2003.

61. Norton SA et al: Proactive palliative care in the medical intensive care unit: effects on length of stay for selected high-risk patients, *Crit Care Med* 35(6):1530-1535, 2007.

62. Frick S et al: Medical futility: predicting outcome of intensive care unit patients by nurses and doctors-a prospective comparative study, *Crit Care Med* 31(2):456-461, 2003.

63. Meltzer LS, Huckabay LM: Critical care nurses' perceptions of futile care and its effect on burnout, *Am J Crit Care* 13(3):202-208, 2004.

64. Ellershaw J, Ward C: Care of the dying patient: the last hours or days of life, *BMJ* 326(7379):30-34, 2003.

65. Faber-Langendoen K, Lanken PN: Dying patients in the intensive care unit: forgoing treatment, maintaining care, *Ann Intern Med* 133(11): 886-893, 2000.

66. National Consensus Project: Clinical practice guidelines for quality palliative care, 2004. Available at www.nationalconsensusproject.org (accessed January 2009).

67. Institute of Medicine: *Improving palliative care for cancer: summary and recommendations*, Washington, DC, 2001, National Academy Press.

68. Mularski RA: Pain management in the intensive care unit, *Crit Care Clin* 20(3):381-401, 2004.

69. Gélinas C et al: Pain assessment and management in critically ill intubated patients: a retrospective study, *Am J Crit Care* 13(2):126-135, 2004.

70. Foley KM: Pain and symptom control in the dying ICU patient. In Curtis JR, Rubenfeld GD, editors: *Managing death in the intensive care unit: the transition from cure to comfort*, Oxford, 2001, Oxford University Press.

71. Jacobi J et al: Clinical practice guidelines for the sustained use of sedatives and analgesics in the critically ill adult, *Crit Care Med* 30(1):119-141, 2002.

72. Campbell ML: Terminal dyspnea and respiratory distress, *Crit Care Clin* 20(3):403-417, 2004.

73. Fabbro ED et al: Symptom control in palliative care, part III: dyspnea and delirium, *J Palliat Med* 9(2):422-436, 2006.

74. Viola RA et al: The effects of fluid status and fluid therapy on the dying, 2003 Database of Abstracts of Reviews of Effectiveness (DARE), NHS Centre for Reviews and Dissemination, University of York. Available at www.crd.york.ac.uk/CRDWeb/ShowRecord.asp?ID=11998005105 (accessed January 2009).

75. Kehl KA: Treatment of terminal restlessness: a review of the evidence, *J Pain Palliat Care Pharmacother* 18(1):5-30, 2004.

76. Callanan M, Kelley P: *Final gifts: understanding the special awareness, needs, and communications of the dying*, New York, 1997, Bantam Books.

77. Marchand L: Fast fact and concept #118: near death awareness, 2004. Available at www.eperc.mcw.edu/FastFactPDF/Concept%20118. pdf (accessed January 2009).

78. Lilly CM et al: An intensive communication intervention for the critically ill, *Am J Med* 109(6):469-475, 2000.

79. Lilly CM et al: Intensive communication: four-year follow-up from a clinical practice study, *Crit Care Med* 31(5 suppl):S394-S399, 2003.

80. Curtis JR: Interventions to improve care during withdrawal of life-sustaining treatments, *J Palliat Med* 8(suppl 1):S116-S131, 2005.

81. Kirchhoff KT et al: Preparing ICU families for withdrawal of life support: a pilot study, *Am J Crit Care* 17(2):113-121, 2008.

82. Mueller PS et al: Ethical analysis of withdrawal of pacemaker or implantable cardioverter-defibrillator support at the end of life, *Mayo Clin Proc* 78(8):959-963, 2003.

83. Wiegand DL, Kalowes PG: Withdrawal of cardiac medications and devices, *AACN Adv Crit Care* 18(4):415-425, 2007.

84. Goldstein NE et al: Management of implantable cardioverter defibrillators in end-of-life care, *Ann Intern Med* 141(11):835-838, 2004.

85. Rubenfeld GD, Crawford SW: Withdrawal of life-sustaining treatment. In Curtis JR, Rubenfeld GD, editors: *Managing death in the intensive care unit: the transition from cure to comfort*, Oxford, 2001, Oxford University Press.

86. Campbell ML: How to withdraw mechanical ventilation: a systematic review of the literature, *AACN Adv Crit Care* 18(4):397-403, 2007.

87. von Gunten C, Weissman DE: Fast fact and concept #034: symptom control for ventilator withdrawal in the dying patient (part II), 2001. Available

at www.eperc.mcw.edu/FastFactPDF/Concept%20034.pdf (accessed January 2009).

88. Chan JD et al: Narcotic and benzodiazepine use after withdrawal of life support: Association with time to death? *Chest* 126(1):286-293, 2004.

89. Rocker GM et al: Canadian nurses' and respiratory therapists' perspectives on withdrawal of life support in the intensive care unit, *J Crit Care* 20(1):59-65, 2005.

90. Robichaux CM, Clark AP: Practice of expert critical care nurses in situations of prognostic conflict at the end of life, *Am J Crit Care* 15(5):480-489, 2006.

91. Treece PD et al: Evaluation of a standardized order form for the withdrawal of life support in the intensive care unit, *Crit Care Med* 32(5):1141-1148, 2004.

92. Hough CL et al: Death rounds: End-of-life discussions among medical residents in the intensive care unit, *J Crit Care* 20(1):20-25, 2005.

93. Kirchhoff KT et al: Intensive care nurses' experiences with end-of-life care, *Am J Crit Care* 9(1):36-42, 2000.

94. Elpern EH et al: Moral distress of staff nurses in a medical intensive care unit, *Am J Crit Care* 14(6):523-530, 2005.

95. Hamric AB, Blackhall LJ: Nurse-physician perspectives on the care of dying patients in intensive care units: collaboration, moral distress, and ethical climate, *Crit Care Med* 35(2):422-429, 2007.

96. Badger JM: Factors that enable or complicate end-of-life transitions in critical care, *Am J Crit Care* 14(6):513-521, 2005.

97. Social Security Administration: Hospital protocols for organ procurement and standards for organ procurement agencies, 2004: compilation of the Social Security laws. Available at www.ssa.gov/OP_Home/ssact/title11/1138.htm (accessed January 1, 2009).

98. The Joint Commission: Approved: revisions to Standard LD.3.1.10, Element of Performance 12, for critical access hospitals and hospitals. *Joint Commission Perspectives* 27(6):14, 2007.

99. Powner DJ et al: Variability among hospital policies for determining brain death in adults, *Crit Care Med* 32(6):1284-1288, 2004.

100. Siminoff LA et al: Families' understanding of brain death, *Prog Transplant* 13(3):218-224, 2003.

101. Wiegand DL: Families and withdrawal of life-sustaining therapy: state of the science, *J Fam Nurs* 12(2):165-184, 2006.

102. Whitmer M et al: Caring in the curing environment. *J Hosp Palliat Nurs* 9(6):329-333, 2007.

103. Heyland DK et al: Family satisfaction with care in the intensive care unit: results of a multiple center study, *Crit Care Med* 30(7):1413-1418, 2002.

104. Norton SA et al: Life support withdrawal: communication and conflict. *Am J Crit Care* 12(6):548-555, 2003.

105. Kirchhoff KT et al: The vortex: families' experiences with death in the intensive care unit, *Am J Crit Care* 11(3):200-209, 2002.

106. Murphy PA et al: Under the radar: contributions of the SUPPORT nurses, *Nurs Outlook* 49(5):238-242, 2001.

107. Gries CJ et al: Family member satisfaction with end-of-life decision making in the ICU, *Chest* 133(3):704-712, 2008.

108. Stapleton RD et al: Clinician statements and family satisfaction with family conferences in the intensive care unit, *Crit Care Med* 34(6):1679-1685, 2006.

109. Selph RB et al: Empathy and life support decisions in intensive care units, *J Gen Intern Med* 23(9):1311-1317, 2008.

110. Ambuel B, Weissman D: Fast fact and concept #016: conducting a family conference, 2001. Available at www.eperc.mcw.edu/fastFact/ff_016.htm (accessed January 2009).

111. Curtis JR et al: The family conference as a focus to improve communication about end-of-life care in the intensive care unit: opportunities for improvement, *Crit Care Med* 29(2 suppl):N26-N33, 2001.

112. Abbott KH et al: Families looking back: one year after discussion of withdrawal or withholding of life-sustaining support, *Crit Care Med* 29(1):197-201, 2001.

113. Keenan SP et al: Withdrawal of life support: how the family feels, and why, *J Palliat Care* 16(suppl):S40-S44, 2000.

114. Curtis JR et al: Missed opportunities during family conferences about end-of-life care in the intensive care unit, *Am J Respir Crit Care Med* 171(8):844-849, 2005.

115. MacLean SL et al: Family presence during cardiopulmonary resuscitation and invasive procedures: practices of critical care and emergency nurses, *Am J Crit Care* 12(3):246-257, 2003.

116. Kirchhoff KT, Dahl N: American association of critical-care nurses' national survey of facilities and units providing critical care, *Am J Crit Care* 15(1):13-28, 2006.

117. Berwick DM, Kotagal M: Restricted visiting hours in ICUs: time to change, *JAMA* 292(6):736-737, 2004.

118. Shannon S: Helping families cope with death in the ICU. In Curtis JR, Rubenfeld GD, editors: *Managing death in the intensive care unit: the transition from cure to comfort*, Oxford, 2001, Oxford University Press.

119. Baggs JG et al: The dying patient in the ICU: role of the interdisciplinary team, *Crit Care Clin* 20(3):525-540, 2004.

120. Truog RD et al: Recommendations for end-of-life care in the intensive care unit: a consensus statement by the American Academy of Critical Care Medicine, *Crit Care Med* 36(3):953-963, 2008.

121. Curtis JR: End of life care research program, 2008. Available at http://depts.washington.edu/eolcare/currentprojects/ (accessed January 2009).

122. Promoting Excellence in End of-Life Care: Innovative models and approaches for palliative care. Available at www.promotingexcellence.org (accessed January 2009).

123. Kirchhoff KT et al: Documentation on withdrawal of life support in adult patients in the intensive care unit, *Am J Crit Care* 13(4):328-334, 2004.

Chapter 12

The Pediatric Patient in the Adult Critical Care Unit

Some of the developmental and physiologic differences between adults and children older than 1 month are discussed in this chapter. Although children may experience medical conditions similar to those of adults, they are assessed and managed differently. During periods of stress, children can maintain physiologic stability for a period, but they can then decompensate quickly. Children are not small adults. Box 12-1 describes the differences between children and adults. Many of the laboratory values, medications, blood product dosages and methods of administration, and other therapeutic modalities are different from those used with adults.

Regardless of the anticipated outcome, admission to a critical care unit is stressful for families. Critical care nurses who successfully deal with pediatric patients see the child and the family as an integral unit and are perceptive to the needs of the entire family.[1] A knowledge of normal growth and development and the ability to assess the child's developmental level are important for working with children and their parents. Nurses who take care of pediatric patients can conceptualize using a developmental perspective as the ideal norm.[1] The developmental stages include the different age groups: infancy (0 to 12 months), toddlers (1 to 3 years), preschoolers (3 to 5 years), school-age children (6 to 12 years), and adolescents (12 to 18 years).

Even though some critically ill children can be managed in adult critical care units, there are certain situations in which children need the services of various pediatric subspecialists or pediatric intensivists, and they must be transferred to a tertiary care pediatric intensive care unit (PICU). This also is true for pediatric trauma patients. There is a significantly lower risk of death for patients receiving care in a facility with a designated trauma center.[2] Conditions that may require transfer to a hospital with a PICU include the need for high-frequency ventilation, extracorporeal membrane oxygenation (ECMO), or cardiac surgery and treatment for some neurologic conditions that require intracranial pressure monitoring. Transfer is considered for children who do not respond to treatment.

RESPIRATORY SYSTEM

ANATOMY AND PHYSIOLOGY

Upper Airway. The upper airway of the infant and child is different from that of the adult. The epiglottis is located at the level of the cervical spine. It is located at C1 in the newborn, at C3 in the older infant, and at C4 to C5 in the adult.

The infant's epiglottis is large and floppy, and because of its high placement, it can press against the pharyngeal soft palate on inspiration. The infant's tongue is large relative to its head size. The tongue fills most of the oral cavity. Because of this anatomy, the infant usually is an obligate nose breather until between 4 and 6 months of age, after which the larynx descends with growth.[1] Oral breathing is a very complex process for an infant, and it never occurs alone. Oronasal breathing is possible, but only up to 30% to 40% of ventilation can be provided orally. During sleep, oronasal breathing can occur spontaneously and last for about 20 seconds.

The larynx of the infant and young child, unlike that of the adult, is a funnel-shaped structure, with the narrowest portion at the cricoid ring.[3] The larynx is pliable because the cartilage is less developed, making it easier to collapse on inspiration or expiration. With changes in intrathoracic pressure, collapse can occur even with crying.[3] By 8 to 10 years of age, the larynx has grown cylindric, has assumed the narrowest portion at the glottic opening, and has increased in length, width, and internal diameter. By 12 years of age, the diameter has grown to 1.8 cm.[3]

The submucosal layer of the larynx is also looser in the infant and young child, and fluid can accumulate more easily in that space.[3] Within the airway's relatively rigid confines, any accumulation of fluid encroaches into the airway space. Along with a shorter and narrower airway, any decrease in airway radius leads to an exponential increase in airflow resistance, which increases the work of breathing. Turbulent airflow, as occurs with crying, doubles the already increased airflow resistance.[4] Figure 12-1 illustrates the changes in airway diameter and airflow resistance with obstruction from edema in an adult and in an infant. The infant or child with an abnormally small jaw and low-set ears should be considered as having a potentially difficult airway to manage and must have a consultation with an anesthesiologist if airway management is required.

Lower Airway. Alveolar collapse is more likely in the infant and young child because of the smaller alveolar size. Infants and young children are at greater risk for ventilation-perfusion mismatch and atelectasis without this collateral ventilation.

Infants and children have a higher metabolic rate than adults; therefore, oxygen consumption per kilogram is higher.

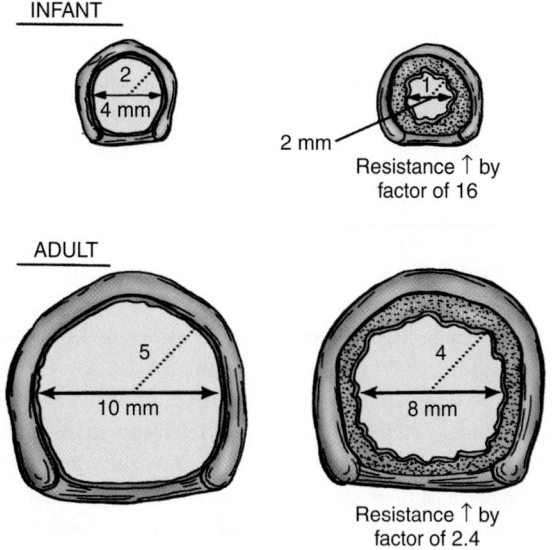

Figure 12-1 Effects of edema on airway resistance are shown by proportional increases in airflow resistance with 1 mm of circumferential edema in the infant versus the adult. *(From Zander J, Hazinski MF: Pulmonary disorders. In Hazinski MF, editor: Manual of pediatric critical care, St Louis, 1999, Mosby.)*

Hypoxemia develops more rapidly in the context of respiratory compromise in young children than in adults.[3]

Chest Mechanics. The respiratory structure and mechanics of infants and young children are very different from those of mature adults. In the infant and young child, the chest wall is more compliant because the bones are smaller and more cartilaginous. The ribs are more horizontally placed, providing less

of a bellowing action on inspiration. Accessory muscles are less developed, and the external intercostals do not contribute to pulling the ribs up on inspiration. The diaphragm is the principal muscle for inspiration. The diaphragm is more horizontal in the chest in the infant and tends to pull the lower ribs inward on inspiration.[5] Because of these mechanics, the infant and toddler depend almost totally on diaphragmatic contraction for lung expansion. Anything that impedes diaphragmatic contractions can result in respiratory compromise. The intracostal muscles are inadequately developed before school age, and they are unlikely to help with effective ventilation if the diaphragm is impaired.[3] With any decrease in lung compliance, as with lung disease, diaphragmatic contractions, which cause decreased intrathoracic pressure, produce intercostal and substernal retractions rather than inflation of the lungs.[5] The greater the chest wall retractions, the more the diaphragm must contract to offset the changes in intrathoracic pressure to generate an adequate tidal volume for the child. The compliant chest wall of the infant or young child should expand easily outward with positive-pressure ventilation. If the chest wall does not expand bilaterally during the positive-pressure ventilation, either the ventilation effort is inadequate or the airway is obstructed.[3]

ASSESSMENT AND OXYGEN DEVICES

The infant or child usually experiences respiratory failure more often than primary cardiac failure. Unlike the older adult who may have underlying cardiovascular disease, the infant and child tend to demonstrate bradycardia and apnea in cardiopulmonary failure and not ventricular dysrythmias.[4] For the infant or child who is conscious and needs supplemental oxygen, the device of comfort must be selected.[3] Minimizing anxiety and fear in the child is paramount to decrease the work of breathing. Table 12-1 outlines the assessment areas for the infant or child at risk for respiratory failure.[3]

Airway Positioning. Knowledge of childhood anatomy is necessary to establish a patent airway. The infant or toddler younger than 2 years of age, because of their large occiput, needs to have a small roll or towel placed under the upper shoulders, with the jaw slightly extended into a "sniffing" position.[4] Optimal positioning of the head should assist in maintenance of a patent airway or help when bag-mask ventilation is required.[37] This head positioning displaces the tongue and lines up the posterior pharynx and tracheal opening for a clear airway. For the infant younger than 6 months, correct head positioning still may not prevent the large tongue from falling back into the posterior pharynx. Oral airways must not be used unless the infant is unconscious, because the airway tip can stimulate laryngospasm as a result of the higher placement of the larynx. Side-lying placement, with the neck in a neutral position, should be attempted.[3] The older child needs to have a folded towel placed under the head, with the neck in an extended position to maintain a patent airway.[3] Figure 12-2 illustrates proper head positioning for the infant and child. The conscious child must be allowed to assume a position of choice for airway maintenance.

TABLE 12-1 Significant Findings for the Infant or Child at Risk for Respiratory Failure

Assessment Area	Physical Findings	Discussion Points
Respiratory rate	Infant: >60/min Child: >40/min Slow or irregular	Tachypnea usually first sign of distress in an infant; fatigue is a common contributing factor in respiratory failure
Mechanics	Retractions (intercostal, supraclavicular, substernal) Paradoxic movements (chest in and abdomen out) Grunting Stridor Wheezing	 Closing of the glottis to create "auto-PEEP" to keep alveoli open at end-expiration Sign of upper airway obstruction Sign of lower airway obstruction
Air entry	Changes in pitch rather than volume of breath sounds	Chest expansion sometimes is barely perceptible in a normal, spontaneously breathing infant. The small, thin chest wall causes breath sounds from any area of the lungs to be easily referred throughout the chest, even over fluid or atelectasis. Listen for bilateral breath sounds high in the axillae, because these are the two most separated points.
Color or temperature Heart rate	Central coolness, pallor, or cyanosis <5 years: <60 or >180 beats/min 5-10 years: <60 or >160 beats/min >10 years: <50 or >140 beats/min	Peripheral changes may be normal in the infant or child. The infant and child have a limited ability to increase stroke volume; therefore, with hypoxemia, the heart rate increases to improve cardiac output. If bradycardia occurs with cardiorespiratory distress, arrest may be imminent.
Neurologic status	Infant: hypotonia Child: irritability Decreased level of consciousness	Sign of hypoxia for infants An early sign of hypoxia, often manifested as a decreased responsiveness to parents or to pain

PEEP, positive end-expiratory pressure.

Supplemental Oxygen Devices. Many of the oxygen devices used for adults also are used for children. Some additions include oxygen hoods for infants up to 1 year old. The hoods are clear plastic boxes that envelop the head and allow full vision of the head and access to the body. Other oxygen devices include oxygen tents, which are used less often, and oxygen "blow-by," which uses oxygen tubing or a hose to blow oxygen toward the child's face without touching him or her. Oxygen masks can aggravate and upset the child and often are not tolerated well by the child. One option in older infants and children is to use nasal prongs or cannula.[6] This method allows the child to talk and eat without a facial obstruction. Another method to deliver oxygen to the child is for the parent to hold the blow-by tubing by the child's face. The amount of oxygen can be titrated according to the patient's oxygen saturation readings.

An adult-sized, self-inflating resuscitation bag can be carefully used on an infant, providing only the force needed to cause appropriate chest expansion is used.[3] An appropriately sized bag minimizes the potential for overinflating the lungs and causing injury. Resuscitation bag sizes, along with other supplemental oxygen devices and oxygen administration, are summarized in Table 12-2. There must be no leaf-flap outlet valves when a self-inflating bag is used to assist spontaneous ventilation in an infant, because the infant cannot generate enough negative inspiratory pressure to open the valve.[3]

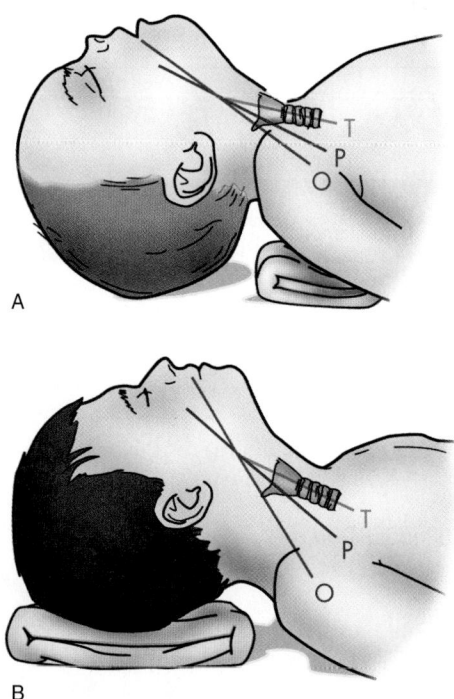

Figure 12-2 Correct airway positioning for ventilation is shown for an infant *(A)* and a child *(B)*. Better airflow is provided with a straight alignment of the oropharynx (O), pharynx (P), and trachea (T).

TABLE 12-2 Supplemental Oxygen Devices and Oxygen Administration in Infants and Children

Device	Administration	Discussion Points
Nasal cannula	Infant	Minute volume, inspiratory/expiratory times, and amount of mouth breathing affects infant FIO_2 by a nasal cannula differently from an adult given the same gas flow and O_2 percent
	Child	Low-flow O_2 devices are inaccurate for FIO_2 delivery. Titrate to patient's O_2 saturation readings.
Oxygen hood	10-15 L/min = nearly 100% O_2	Use with infants <1 year old.
Oxygen blow-by	10-15 L/min	Better tolerated than oxygen masks Short-term method of O_2 delivery Titrated to child's O_2 saturation Allows child or parent to hold tubing
Simple mask	0.4-0.5 FIO_2	Entrains room air. FIO_2 does not correlate with high flow rates.
Non-rebreather mask	0.9-0.95 FIO_2	There is no entrainment of room air. O_2 flow is determined by child's minute ventilation.
Self-inflating resuscitation bag	Infant <3 mo old: 0.25-L bag 3 mo-4 yr old: 0.5-L bag Child 5-10 yr old: 1-L bag >10 yr old: 1.5-L bag	Do not use bags with leaf-flap outlet valves or with spring-loaded PEEP valves.
Anesthesia bag	Spontaneously breathing Flow rate 3 × minute ventilation Not spontaneously breathing 8-10 L/min flow rate	Set the O_2 flow rate at a level necessary to achieve the desired level of ventilation.
Peak inspiratory pressure	≤20-30 cm H_2O	
Ventilatory mask size	<6 mo old: 0 6 mo-3 yr old: 1 3-6 yr old: 2 >6 years old: 3	Fit and placement on face same as for adult

PEEP, positive end-expiratory pressure.

BOX 12-2   ENDOTRACHEAL TUBE MEASUREMENT

SIZE
- For children >2 years old: (age in years + 16) ÷ 4
- For infants and toddlers: size based on age
- For any age: compare the circumference of the child's little finger with the external diameter size of the endotracheal tube (ETT)
- Cuffed tube: external diameter one-half size smaller than appropriate-sized uncuffed tube

DEPTH OF INSERTION
- From the teeth to midtrachea: internal diameter of ETT × 3

CUFF PRESSURE
- Allow for a barely sealed air leak

Resuscitation bags equipped with spring-loaded, positive end-expiratory pressure (PEEP) valves to provide constant positive airway pressure (CPAP) must not be used with the spontaneously breathing child for the same reason previously discussed.[3]

Anesthesia ventilation bags have no flow valves that require opening on inspiration and therefore can be used to provide supplemental oxygen, PEEP, or CPAP to the spontaneously breathing infant or child.[3] Pressure manometers can be attached to the ventilation bags to measure peak inspiratory pressure. Ventilatory masks are measured in the child as in the adult— from the bridge of the nose to before the end of the chin. The correctly sized mask for the infant or child is critical for adequate oxygenation and ventilation of the patient.

ENDOTRACHEAL INTUBATION

Procedure. Endotracheal tube (ETT) placement and management for the pediatric patient is an important intervention to maintain an airway in a patient with respiratory failure.[4] Preoxygenation of the child before intubation is very important. Bag-mask ventilation is an effective way to assist the child's ventilation. Intubation attempts need to be no longer than approximately 30 seconds per attempt to prevent a drop in the child's heart rate or oxygen saturation. Box 12-2 provides formulas as a guideline for ETT measurements in the pediatric patient. To ensure that the correct intubation equipment is selected for the different sizes and ages of pediatric patients, many hospitals are using length-based/color-coded resuscitation tapes, such as the Broselow system.[4,7] This tape gives an estimate of the child's body weight based on the crown-heel length and can be used to determine the appropriate size of resuscitation equipment and medication dosages for the child. Figure 12-3 provides an example of a Broselow tape.

When correctly placed, the tip of the ETT should be 1 to 2 cm above the carina, no higher than the first rib.[3] After the child is intubated, bilateral breath sounds should be assessed high in the axillae along with bilateral chest expansion. The easy transmission of sounds in the chest of the child can be mistaken for breath sounds if there is an accidental esophageal intubation. Confirmation of the tube placement after assessment of bilateral breath sounds is to obtain a chest radiograph. Additional confirmation of the correct placement of the endotracheal tube can be obtained by using a device to monitor exhaled carbon dioxide (CO_2) by a colorimetric device.[4] This device will turn gold in color when CO_2 is being exhaled.[4]

ETT dislodgment can occur easily in the infant or young child. The tip of the ETT is pulled upward with neck extension or when the head is turned completely to the side. Conversely, the ETT moves downward with neck flexion. With the existing short trachea of the young child, an ETT placed higher or lower can become dislodged or intubate the bronchus. ETT obstruction can occur with high placement, neck flexion, or head rotation, which can cause the bevel of the ETT to press against the tracheal wall, occluding the lumen. Secretions and mucus plugs may more easily occlude the lumen of a small-diameter ETT.

The nurse must ensure that the child's ETT remains patent and in correct placement to maintain correct oxygenation and ventilation. Causes of acute deterioration in the intubated pediatric patient can be recalled by using the mnemonic DOPE[3]:

D: displacement of the tube
O: obstruction of the tube
P: pneumothorax (or other air leak)
E: equipment failure

Suction and bag-valve-mask needs to be readily available for resuscitation if any of the above intubation complications occurs.

Securing Endotracheal and Nasotracheal Tubes.
The small infant or child has less facial area for tape adherence for securing the tubes. A method with a low incidence of accidental extubation uses two pieces of cloth tape, split halfway down the middle, creating a Y shape. Figure 12-4 shows this technique. The skin of the child is more fragile than that of an adult. Cloth tape can be irritating. A DuoDERM dressing can be applied to the cheeks, with the securing tape attached on top of the Duo-DERM, or a zinc oxide–based "pink tape" can be used. Auscultate breath sounds before and after tubing taping or re-taping to ensure that the ETT position has not changed.[3]

Mechanical Ventilation.
Many types of unconventional mechanical ventilation (e.g., high-frequency, oscillation, jet ventilation) are used, but for most infants and children standard means of positive-pressure ventilation support using volume- or pressure-controlled ventilators. The type of ventilation chosen depends on the child's size, minute ventilation requirements, and lung compliance. Newer ventilators have flow and pressure triggers that are sensitive enough to ventilate infants and children.[8]

For the older child, noncontinuous-flow, volume-limited ventilation in synchronized intermittent mandatory ventilation (SIMV) mode is used most often. Pressure support ventilation is also used in the child in conjunction with other modes to assist with spontaneous breathing, especially during the weaning process. Currently used ventilators have flow triggering designed for infants. Some type of synchronized ventilation mode is used almost exclusively for the ventilation of infants and children. Table 12-3 outlines ventilator settings for initiating positive-pressure ventilation for the infant and child.

Ventilator-patient asynchrony can have several causes. The Hering-Breuer reflex is a vagal reflex in which the child's sensing of positive lung inflation sets off immediate expiration, and lung deflation stimulates inspiration. Apnea, or active expiration during the ventilator's inspiratory cycle, also can cause asynchrony. The use of adult ventilators not appropriately adapted for the infant or child can cause asynchrony. In the small child, decreased tidal volume and increased respiratory rates occur to deal with respiratory compromise. Adult ventilators may not sense rapidly enough, if at all, any spontaneous respiratory efforts, which leads to increased work of breathing in the child.

Asynchrony can lead to poor oxygenation or volutrauma. Significant asynchrony may require sedation or sedation with neuromuscular blockade. Criteria for weaning and extubation are much more extensive for the adult than for the child, but there are some guidelines for these procedures. SIMV with pressure support ventilation (PSV) is used to wean from positive-pressure ventilation. PSV allows the child to have greater control over breathing, and asynchrony is not a problem. Table 12-4 outlines guidelines for weaning and extubation.[8] Supplemental oxygen may be supplied after extubation by a nasal cannula, ventilation mask, or oxygen hood. Nasal or facial CPAP can be given, but if the child cannot be managed on CPAP, he or she may need to be reintubated.

Extubation Complications.
A postextubation croup can occur in the small child. Manifestations arising from airway edema include hoarseness, stridor, or a crowing cough that begins immediately or up to 3 hours after extubation. Initial treatment consists of keeping the child calm. Procedures must be withheld if possible, and crying must be averted to avoid increasing airway resistance. The nurse can hold supplemental humidified oxygen at the child's mouth immediately after extubation and continue to provide a cool mist. More severe symptoms can be treated with racemic epinephrine and with intravenous or inhaled steroid therapy. Intubation equipment and personnel qualified to intubate should be available for 24 hours after extubation.

TRACHEOSTOMIES

Over the past three decades, the tracheostomy in children has become an increasingly common procedure. The primary reasons for having a tracheotomy performed include upper airway

Equipment	PINK Newborn/Small Infant (3-5 kg)	RED Infant (6-9 kg)	PURPLE Toddler (10-11 kg)	YELLOW Small Child (12-14 kg)	WHITE Child (15-18 kg)	BLUE Child (19-22 kg)	ORANGE Large Child (24-28 kg)	GREEN Adult (30-36 kg)
Resuscitation bag O$_2$ mask Oral airway	Child Newborn Infant/small child	Child Newborn Infant/small child	Child Pediatric Small child	Child Pediatric Child	Child Pediatric Child	Child Pediatric Child/small adult	Child/adult Adult Child/small adult	Adult Adult Medium adult
Laryngoscope blade (size)	0-1 straight	1 straight	1 straight	2 straight	2 straight or curved	2 straight or curved	2-3 straight or curved	3 straight or curved
Tracheal tube (mm)	Premature infant 2.5 Term infant 3.0-3.5 uncuffed	3.5 uncuffed	4.0 uncuffed	4.5 uncuffed	5.0 uncuffed	5.5 uncuffed	6.0 uncuffed	6.5 cuffed
Endotracheal tube length (cm at lip)	10-10.5	10-10.5	11-12	12.5-13.5	14-15	15.5-16.5	17-18	18.5-19.5
Stylet (F)	6	6	6	6	6	14	14	14
Suction catheter (F)	6-8	8	8-10	10	10	10	10	12
BP cuff	Newborn/infant	Newborn/infant	Infant/child	Child	Child	Child	Child/adult	Adult
IV catheter (G)	22-24	22-24	20-24	18-22	18-22	18-20	18-20	16-20
Butterfly (G)	23-25	23-25	23-25	21-23	21-23	21-23	21-22	18-21
Nasogastric tube (F)	5-8	5-8	8-10	10	10-12	12-14	14-18	18
Urinary catheter (F)	5-8	5-8	8-10	10	10-12	10-12	12	12
Defibrillation/cardioversion external paddles	Infant paddles	Infant paddles until 1 yr or 10 kg	Adult paddles when ≥1 yr or ≥10 kg	Adult paddles	Adult paddles	Adult paddles	Adult paddles	Adult paddles
Chest tube (F)	10-12	10-12	16-20	20-24	20-24	24-32	28-32	32-40

Figure 12-3 Broselow pediatric color-coded resuscitation tape (2002 Broselow Pediatric Resuscitation Tape, Armstrong Medical Industries). *(Modified from Hazinski MF, editor: Manual of pediatric critical care, St Louis, 1999, Mosby).*

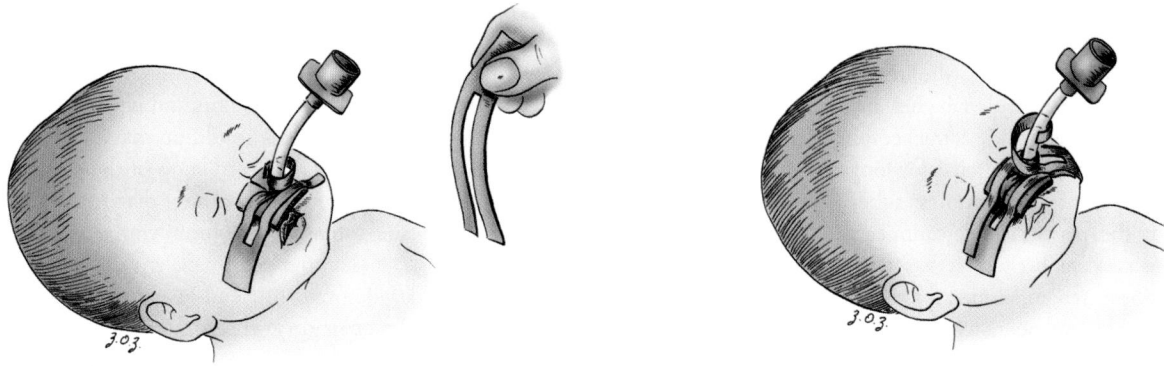

Figure 12-4 Securing an endotracheal tube with split taping. *(Modified from Zander J, Hazinski MF: Pulmonary disorders. In Hazinski MF, editor:* Nursing care of the critically ill child, *ed 2, St Louis, 1992, Mosby.)*

TABLE 12-3 Initiating Positive-Pressure Ventilation in the Infant or Child

Parameter	Setting	Discussion Points
Rate of F_{IO_2}	Age-based to maintain PaO_2 >70 mm Hg	
Tidal volume	5-7 mL/kg for infants 10-15 mL/kg for children	Includes compressibility of ventilator circuit tubing and dead space
I:E	Age-specific, usually 1:2	Increase expiratory time with obstruction disease
Inspiratory time	0.3-0.5 sec for infants 0.75-1.5 sec for children	
PEEP or CPAP	Starts at 3 cm H_2O and increases by 2-3 cm increments	Maintain PaO_2 >70 mm Hg with nontoxic O_2 (0.40-0.50) without causing circulatory depression; PEEP >15 cm warrants a pulmonary artery catheter to measure circulatory status; volutrauma must be addressed with pneumothorax suspicions

CPAP, constant positive airway pressure; I:E, inspiratory to expiratory: PEEP, positive end-expiratory pressure.

TABLE 12-4 Guidelines for Discontinuing Positive-Pressure Ventilation in the Infant or Child

Weaning Ventilatory Mode	Ventilatory Parameter	Discussion Points
Non-PSV	Rate: decrease by 2-5 breaths/min (may be 1 breath/min in chronic conditions) Infant: down to minimum of 4 breaths/min Child: possibly down to spontaneous breathing with CPAP trials PEEP/CPAP: decrease by 2-3 cm H_2O Infant: down to 2-3 cm H_2O Child: down to <5 cm H_2O F_{IO_2}: decrease by 5%-10%, to <0.40-5.0	Rapidity of each change can be variable, from hourly to long-term, difficult-to-wean patients; for infants, rates must not go fewer than 4 breaths/min just before extubation, because ETT creates airway resistance and the work of breathing may be increased too much with total spontaneous breathing

To maintain PaO_2 >70 mm Hg or SaO_2 >93% |
| PSV | With SIMV: decrease to a low rate Pressure: to achieve tidal volume of 5-7 mL/kg for infants and 10-15 mL/kg for children; then decrease to 5 cm H_2O | See previous guidelines for rate and pressure changes |
| Extubation | Vital capacity: Infant/toddler: >15 mL/kg when crying Older child: >10-15 mL/kg Minute ventilation doubled PaO_2 >60-70 mm Hg at an F_{IO_2} <0.4 $PaCO_2$ 35-45 mm Hg | Positive gag/cough reflex Can tolerate own secretions |

CPAP, constant positive airway pressure; ETT, endotracheal tube; PEEP, positive end-expiratory pressure; PSV, pressure support ventilation; SIMV, synchronized intermittent mandatory ventilation.

obstruction caused by anatomic abnormalities, the anticipated need for prolonged ventilation, or the need for effective pulmonary toilet.[9] Most children who require a tracheostomy are younger than 1 year, and a higher incidence is seen among boys.[9] For the older child, a tracheotomy is recommended if the child is to remain intubated for longer than 2 to 3 weeks.

Several types of tracheostomy tubes are available for the child, with the plastic, single-cannula type the most popular for in-hospital care because it has few complications. Silastic tubes have been recommended for the infant and child because they are pliable and bend with tracheal movement. Uncuffed tubes usually are preferred for the pediatric patient to prevent subglottic stenosis.[10] The diameter of the tracheostomy tube should be selected to avoid any damage to the tracheal wall, to minimize the work of breathing, and to promote translaryngeal airflow when possible. Table 12-5 describes tracheostomy tube sizes for infants and children.

Complications with a tracheostomy can be categorized as those occurring early or late. Early complications can occur intraoperatively and up to the first tracheostomy tube change. Studies have shown that a cannula obstruction is the most common early complication.[9] Late complications can occur after the first tube change. Some of the most significant late complications include recurrent tracheitis, accidental decannulation, cannula obstruction, subglottic stenosis, suprastomal obstruction, and tracheal ulceration.[10]

If accidental decannulation occurs in a new tracheostomy, replacing the tube may be a difficult procedure. However, in the child who has had a long-term tracheostomy, reinserting a tracheal tube after accidental decannulation should be relatively easy because the stoma is well established. An extra tracheostomy tube and obturator of the child's size should be kept at the bedside in case of emergency. Tracheomalacia with cricoid cartilage collapse can develop, resulting in upper airway obstruction after the tube is no longer in place. In some cases, an airway can be reestablished only surgically. In other children, an ETT that is a size smaller can be inserted into the stoma; otherwise, the child may have to be orally or nasally intubated.

BRONCHIOLITIS

Acute viral bronchiolitis is one of the most common conditions caused by respiratory viruses in infants and children.[11] *Bronchiolitis* is a term used to describe a condition that affects the lower respiratory tract that results in obstruction of the small airways. Bronchiolitis is one of the most common diagnoses in children who present in the intensive care unit with respiratory failure.[40] The disease is characterized by tachypnea, hyperinflation of the check, and widespread fine end-inspiratory crackles heard on auscultation. An expiratory wheeze may also be heard. This clinical pattern can be seen for the first year of life, with most hospital admissions occurring within the first 6 months of life.[11] Respiratory syncytial virus (RSV) is the most common cause of viral bronchiolitis, and it infects almost all children by the age of 2 years.[12] The peak incidence for viral bronchiolitis occurs during midwinter and into early spring. RSV is highly contagious and can be spread by close contact through droplets. Meticulous hand washing by clinical staff is the most important step to prevent nosocomial infections of other patients or staff members.[13]

Pathophysiology. RSV infection has an overall low mortality rate, but infected infants with congenital heart disease have a mortality rate of 37%. Those with cystic fibrosis or bronchopulmonary dysplasia or who are immunocompromised are also at greater risk for more serious disease and for occurrence beyond 1 year of age. The chance of recovery from RSV can be excellent, but reactive airway disease residual effects may be seen several years after infection.[14] RSV involves inflammation of respiratory epithelium, leading to necrosis. The epithelium is replaced with nonciliated tissue. Submucosal edema forms with lymphocytic infiltrates and other alveolar debris. Obstruction occurs from mucus secretions and debris not being cleared because of the lack of ciliated epithelium. Pathologic pulmonary dynamics involve lung hyperinflation almost two times normal. Obstruction occurs in a patchy distribution with complete obstruction, leading to atelectasis and partial obstruction, which results in hyperinflation. Inspiratory resistance and

TABLE 12-5 Approximate Sizes of Intubation Equipment and Tracheostomy Tubes for Infants and Children

	EQUIPMENT CHOICES BASED ON AGE AND WEIGHT							
Factors	3 mo 6 kg	6 mo 8 kg	1 yr 10 kg	3 yr 15 kg	6 yr 20 kg	8 yr 25 kg	12 yr 40 kg	16 yr 60 kg
ETT size (mm)	3.0-3.5	3.5-4.0	4.0-4.5	4.5-5.0	5.0-5.5	6.0 c/u	7.0 c	7.0-8.0 c
Laryngoscope blade	0-1 s	0-1 s	1 s	2 s	2 s	2 s/c	3 s/c	3 s/c
Stylet (Fr)	6	6	6	6	14	14	14	14
Suction catheter (Fr)[†]	6-8	8	8	8-10	10	10-12	12-14	12-14
Shiley Tracheostomy								
Shiley size (mm)	0	1	1-12	4	4	4	6	6
Internal diameter (mm ID)	3.4	3.7	3.7-4.1	5	5	5	7	7
Length (cm)	4	4.1	4.1-4.2	4.6	4.6	4.6	6.7	6.7

†Catheter size twice the internal diameter size of any tracheal tube.

c/u, cuffed or uncuffed; ETT, endotracheal tube; Fr, French; ID, internal diameter; s/c, straight or curved.

expiratory resistance are present, along with ventilation perfusion mismatch, which leads to hypoxemia and some degree of CO_2 retention. The probable mechanism in addition to the ventilation-perfusion mismatch is hypoventilation that results from a marked increase in the work of breathing in the infant.[14]

Clinical Assessment. The first symptoms to appear are those of an upper respiratory tract infection—sneezing and rhinorrhea. In many cases, a family member has had a respiratory illness. After 2 to 3 days, respiratory distress ensues with increased respirations, coughing, nasal flaring, chest retractions, wheezing, irritability, and feeding difficulties. Fever and lung rhonchi may or may not occur. After bronchiolar obstruction has occurred, these patients present with increased work of breathing. This can lead to muscle fatigue and respiratory failure if the work of breathing exceeds the capacity of the patient's respiratory muscles. Infants tolerate respiratory loads poorly and are susceptible to fatigue due to the immature pattern of their muscle fibers.[15]

Treatment. The overall treatment goal with bronchiolitis is supportive. Oxygen continues to be the primary therapy to decrease work of breathing and oxygen demands. Depending on the severity of illness, the infant can receive supplemental humidified oxygen by mask, tent, nasal CPAP (despite lung hyperinflation), or mechanical ventilation.[5,16] RSV causes airway obstruction, and no therapy has demonstrated the ability to rapidly reduce this obstruction.

Suctioning of the airways will be required to help alleviate the signs and symptoms of airway obstruction from mucus secretions. The mucus will be thick and initially cause the infant to be suctioned frequently. Inhaled β_2-agonists, anticholinergic agents, and corticosteroids during the acute or recovery phase have been tried with various degrees of success.[11]

The current recommendation from the American Academy of Pediatrics for the prevention of RSV is the administration of the monoclonal antibody palivizumab (Synagis, MedImmune). Clinicians may administer palivizumab prophylactically to selected infants and children with chronic lung disease or a history of prematurity (<35 weeks' gestation) or with congenital heart disease.[13] Palivizumab is administered in five monthly doses during the RSV season, usually beginning in November or December, at a dose of 15 mg/kg per dose administered intramuscularly.[13]

STATUS ASTHMATICUS

Pathophysiology. Asthma is a chronic inflammatory disorder of the airways in which many cells and cellular elements play a role, including mast cells, eosinophils, T lymphocytes, neutrophils, and epithelial cells.[17] An acute asthma exacerbation is an event of progressive wheezing, cough, chest tightness, shortness of breath, or a combination of all these symptoms. Asthma is identified as the disease with a triad of physiologic processes, airway inflammation, edema, and airway hyperactivity. Inflammation has been recognized as the primary underlying cause in the pathogenesis of this disease.[17] The treatment for asthma is aimed at decreasing and reducing airway inflammation.

The universal feature of the inflammatory response in asthma includes the activation and infiltration of the airway by cells. The early phase in the inflammation reaction is caused by a trigger and this can be different with each child. The immediate response to this trigger is bronchospasm and smooth muscle contraction caused by the mediators from the various inflammatory cells in the airway. If this early phase is not responsive to β_2-agonists, a late phase will occur about 6 to 9 hours after the initial exposure to the trigger.[17] This will lead to increased release of the mediator cells in the airway and produce cellular infiltration, airway edema, mucus secretions, bronchospasm, and smooth muscle contraction. Without treatment, atelectasis and mucus plugging can occur in the child.

Clinical Assessment. Assessing severe asthma in the infant is different compared with that in the older child because of the anatomic and physiologic differences between them. Physiologic changes can progress rapidly to respiratory failure in the infant. Table 12-6 outlines guidelines for classifying the severity of an asthma exacerbation. A moderate asthma episode requires hospitalization with close monitoring. A severe episode requires intensive care with intubation equipment readily available.[5]

Treatment. Standard treatment for the pediatric patient who has asthma includes receiving oxygen, β-adrenergic therapy, corticosteroids, and anticholinergic medications, as indicated.[5,17] Pharmacologic therapy is based on the concept of reducing airway inflammation. β-Adrenergic agonists are the first-line agents in the treatment of asthma. β-Agonist medications that are selective for β_2 receptors on airway smooth muscle (e.g., albuterol, levalbuterol) are preferred to avoid the stimulation of the β_1 cardiac receptors.[17] These medications are given by nebulation intermittently or continuously. Anticholinergic medications in conjunction with β-agonists improve pulmonary function in children, especially school-age patients.[17] These medications can decrease bronchomotor tone and secretions. The most commonly administered inhaled anticholinergic is ipratropium bromide. This medication works synergistically with β-agonists to improve and prolong bronchodilation. Ipratropium bromide should be administered with albuterol in a nebulizer and not given alone. Corticosteroids are also an important part of the treatment for airway inflammation. Corticosteroids can be administered enterally or parenterally. Both methods are equally efficacious in the treatment of asthma.[17] The peak effect for corticosteroids is virtually the same with either route. Treatment for asthma does not have to be held up because of a lack of intravenous access in the pediatric patient. The corticosteroid of choice is a glucocorticoid (e.g., prednisone, prednisolone, methylprednisolone). Intravenous magnesium sulfate is administered to pediatric patients who are resistant to standard bronchodilating treatments.[18] Magnesium is a physiologic calcium antagonist that has a direct effect on the calcium uptake in the muscle, causing smooth muscle relaxation.[5] Magnesium sulfate (12 to 50 mg/kg) is administered intravenously, usually over 20 minutes.[36]

Intensive care management of the child with status asthmaticus involves humidified oxygen to maintain an oxygen saturation of more than 95%, combined with the pharmacologic therapies. Heliox is a mixture of 80% helium and 20% oxygen, which makes this mixture lighter than air. Administration of

TABLE 12-6 Guidelines for Assessing Severe Asthma in Infants and Children

Assessment Area	PHYSICAL FINDINGS		Discussion Points
	Infant	Child	
Respiratory rate	Increase of >50% above normal	Can range from normal to >95th percentile for age	Sleeping rates in infants and resting rates in children are good measures of obstruction; awake or activity rates are too variable.
Level of consciousness	Decreased	May be decreased	Assess response to parents and pain.
Accessory muscle use	Retractions in less-than-severe states	Severe intercostal, tracheosternal, and sternocleidomastoid retractions and nasal flaring	In infants, compliant chest wall produces retractions earlier in course. In children, retractions and flaring correlate well with degree of obstruction and with PEFR <50% of predicted for age.
Color	Pallor, grayness, or cyanosis	Possible cyanosis	
Dyspnea		Can speak only single words or short phrases; cannot count to 10 in one breath	
Quality of cry	Softer and shorter as FEV_1 decreases		
O_2 saturation	<90% in less-than-severe states	<90% on room air	Infants have greater ventilation-perfusion mismatch. In children, hypoxemia correlates well with degree of obstruction.
Breath sounds	Wheezing; then becoming inaudible because of decreased air movement	Same as in infant	Presence and volume of wheezing is the least-sensitive predictor of obstruction.
$PaCO_2$	If >50 mm Hg or if rising 5-10 mm Hg/hr, consider mechanical ventilation	Can range from <40 mm Hg with respiratory distress to >40 mm Hg as air movement significantly decreases	$PaCO_2$ is best measure of ventilation in infants. A continually rising $PaCO_2$ of >40 mm Hg in a child occurs when PEFR is <20% of predicted for age.
PEFR			It is contraindicated in cases of severe asthmatic exacerbation. This is used after asthma is under control.
Feeding/sucking ability	Decreased or absent		

FEV_1, forced expiratory volume over 1 second; PEFR, peak respiratory flow rate.

heliox is effective in decreasing airway resistance and decrease the work of breathing. The use of heliox does not appear to have adverse effects, and its administration may improve the status of the child.[17] The use of noninvasive positive-pressure ventilation by means of nasal prongs or a facemask may avoid the need to be intubated. Some of the indications for considering mechanical ventilation are respiratory muscle fatigue, markedly diminished or absent breath sounds, pulsus paradoxus greater than 2040 mm Hg, deterioration in mental status, and PaO_2 less than 70 mm Hg on 100% FIO_2.[17] The child and family should be informed of the management approach and plan of care. Pediatric patients who have status asthmaticus, if properly and effectively treated, can return to their usual state of

health but will require close follow-up by their pediatrician or pulmonologist.[17]

APPARENT LIFE-THREATENING EVENT

Pathophysiology. An apparent life-threatening event (ALTE) is an episode that is characterized by a combination of apnea, change in skin color, marked changes in muscle tone, and choking or gagging, as defined by the National Institutes of Health Consensus Development Conference on Infant Apnea in 1986.[19] An ALTE is an apneic event combined with pallor or cyanosis and a loss of muscle tone that requires vigorous stimulation all the way to full cardiopulmonary resuscitation

(CPR).[20] Many abnormalities have been found through detailed investigation and reported in the literature. They include relationships among gastroesophageal reflux disease (GERD), apnea, and sleep-related impairment of respiratory control when the infant sleeps in the prone position.[20]

In one study, GERD was documented in 55% of the infants with ALTE.[20] The next highest documented condition (30%) related to ALTE was chronic gastric volvulus.[20] Chronic gastric volvulus is a condition in which all or part of the stomach has rotated over the physiologic range. In infants, this condition can occur easily because of weak ligaments around the stomach. This can cause a large amount of gas to accumulate and push the stomach upward, resulting in worsening of the volvulus and causing vomiting and apnea.[20] Vagally induced fainting spells can occur in specific circumstances, such as after vomiting, feeding, crying, bathing, and pain. Vagal overstimulation is probably an underestimated condition in ALTE infants.[20]

Some of the infants with ALTE that required resuscitation ultimately pass away and may be classified as sudden infant death syndrome (SIDS), raising the possibility that ALTE and SIDS are the same disease.[21] Although there are some similarities in the clinical presentation, ALTE and SIDS should not be considered different manifestations of the same disease process. ALTE and SIDS are disorders of the first year of life; there is a difference in age when each event occurred, with ALTE manifesting 10 weeks earlier than SIDS on average.[21]

Monitoring. One of most widely used diagnostic tests for ALTE is the use of a continuous recording of cardiorespiratory patterns, a pneumocardiogram.[6] The four channels can monitor heart rate, respiratory rate, nasal airflow, and oxygen saturation. Some infants who have normal results may still have subsequent apneic episodes. The critical care nurse can be a major source of support for families in terms of education, observation of the infant's status, and immediate intervention during an apneic episode. The appropriately sized resuscitation equipment should be available at the bedside of these infants.

Treatment. Episodes of apnea must first be treated with gentle shaking of the infant or tapping the bottoms of the infant's feet while observing for return of effective respirations. Slight extension of the neck to reopen the airway can be attempted. If recovery does not occur, manual ventilation with bag and mask at the infant's normal respiratory rate for age should be performed. This manual ventilation should continue until the infant's normal respiratory pattern and heart rate return. For frequent episodes (i.e., more than two to three per hour) or for those who require prolonged manual ventilation, other treatments include prone positioning, rocker beds, recurrent cutaneous stimulation, nasal CPAP, or a switch to continuous gavage feedings to help control symptoms of GERD. Treatment may also include the use of respiratory stimulant drugs, such as theophylline or caffeine.[6] The therapeutic ranges are 6-13 µg/mL of theophylline and 10-20 µg/mL of caffeine. These infants are sent home on a continuous home monitor until they have gone at least 3 months without an ALTE requiring intervention. The parents should attend a class on CPR prior to discharge.

CARDIOVASCULAR SYSTEM

ANATOMY AND PHYSIOLOGY

The differences in cardiovascular function between children and adults are related to early physical development and the presence or absence of congenital cardiac disease. Congenital heart defects (CHDs) occur during the embryologic development of the heart, whereas acquired defects occur after birth. Most fetal cardiac development occurs between the fourth and seventh week of fetal life. The heart is most susceptible to teratogenic influences at this time.[3] About 90% of CHDs are caused by a genetic predisposition and an adverse response to environmental teratogens during cardiac development. Environmental factors alone account for only about 1% of all CHDs. Approximately 5% to 8 % of CHDs are associated with genetic anomalies or syndromes.[3] Although there are more than 35 well-recognized cardiac defects, the most common is ventricular septal defect (VSD).[6]

The design of fetal circulation allows prenatal needs to be met and permits the modifications at birth that support the postnatal circulation.[3] Before the child is born, the lungs are essentially nonfunctional, the liver is partially functional, and the brain requires the highest oxygen concentration. The structures that support fetal circulation and bypass the lungs and liver are the foramen ovale, ductus arteriosus, ductus venosus, umbilical arteries, and umbilical vein (Fig. 12-5). After the child is born, the lungs and liver begin normal function, and the structures of fetal circulation are no longer needed. The foramen ovale closes, and the ductus arteriosus, the ductus venosus, and the umbilical vessels become ligaments (Fig. 12-6). During fetal life, the patency of the ductus arteriosus is controlled by the low oxygen content and exogenous prostaglandins. Postnatally, hypoxia maintains patency of the ductus arteriosus. Before repair of some congenital defects, it is essential that the ductus arteriosus remain open and that the newborn receives a pulmonary vasculature vasodilator, such as a prostaglandin E_1 (PGE_1) continuous intravenous drip.[22] At birth, pulmonary resistance is high but quickly falls to 80% and reaches adult levels in the first few weeks of life if the ductus closes normally.[3] In newborns, hypoxia, acidosis, and hypothermia may result in pulmonary vasoconstriction. This can lead to right-to-left (pulmonary-to-systemic) shunting of blood through the ductus arteriosus and foramen ovale. Treatment includes oxygenation, mechanical ventilation with hyperventilation to produce alkalosis, sedation, and keeping the newborn warm.

ASSESSMENT

Assessment of the cardiovascular system in the child requires the complete health history, including birth history and physical assessment. As the pediatric database is completed for the child with cardiac disease, the parents may report any of the following: poor feeding with fatigue noticed during feeding, diaphoresis with feeding, weight loss or inability to gain weight, respiratory problems (e.g., dyspnea, tachypnea), frequent respiratory infections, cyanosis, and fatigue during play. Heart rate and blood pressure should be within normal range for age (Tables 12-7 and 12-8). Measurement of blood pressure is the

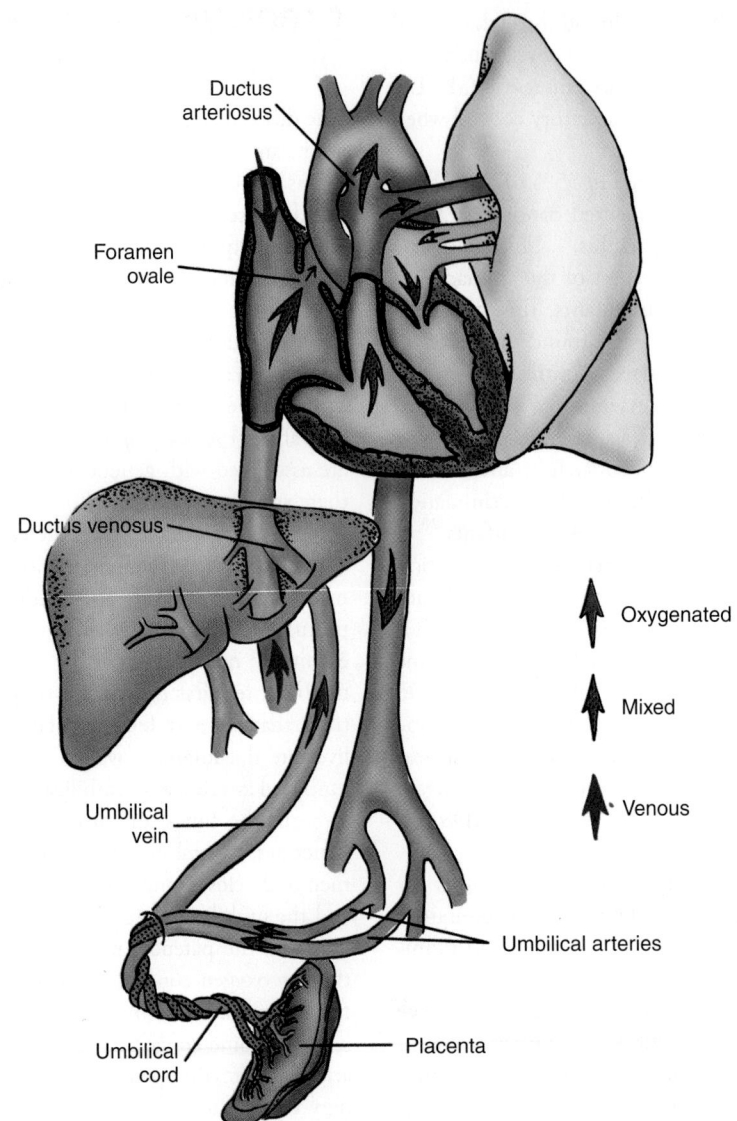

Ductus
arteriosus

Foramen
ovale

Ductus venosus

Umbilical
vein

Umbilical arteries

↑ Oxygenated

↑ Mixed

↑ Venous

Umbilical
cord

Placenta

Figure 12-5 In the fetal circulation, blood is oxygenated in the placenta, which is a less-efficient oxygenator than the lungs. The oxygenated blood enters the fetus through the umbilical vein and enters the ductus venosus, bypassing the hepatic circulation and flowing into the inferior vena cava. When this blood reaches the right atrium, it is diverted by the crista dividens toward the atrial septum and flows through the foramen ovale into the left atrium. The blood then passes through the left ventricle and ascending aorta to perfuse the head and upper extremities. This pathway allows the best-oxygenated blood from the placenta to perfuse the fetal brain. Venous blood from the head and upper extremities returns to the fetal heart through the superior vena cava, enters the right atrium and ventricle, and flows into the pulmonary artery. Because pulmonary vascular resistance is high, this blood is diverted through the ductus arteriosus into the descending aorta. Ultimately, much of this blood returns to the placenta through the umbilical arteries. *(Modified from Hazinski MF: Nursing care of the critically ill child, ed 2, St Louis, 1992, Mosby.)*

most important diagnostic tool in the detection of hypertension in the child.[23] Blood pressure readings should be obtained on all four extremities on admission. If the readings are greater in the upper extremities than the lower ones, the child may have a coarctation of the aorta. Thigh blood pressure readings are equal to the upper extremity readings until a child is 1 year old.[23] Selection of the correct blood pressure cuff size is considered one of the most important factors when measuring blood pressure.[24] Auscultate the heart for extra heart sounds and murmurs. Auscultation may be the most important action in obtaining important information about the diagnosis of acyanotic heart disease. Conversely, auscultation is rarely diagnostic for children with cyanotic CHDs, in which the heart murmur is often absent.[23] Murmurs are heard because of turbulent flow through an abnormal opening or obstructed area. Systolic murmurs are heard between S_1 and S_2. Midsystolic ejection murmurs start after S_1 and end before S_2, usually with a crescendo-decrescendo sound.[23] Diastolic murmurs are heard after S_2 heart sounds. To further monitor perfusion, central and pedal pulses, skin temperature and color, and capillary refill are evaluated hourly. Urine output must be at least 1 mL/kg/hr.

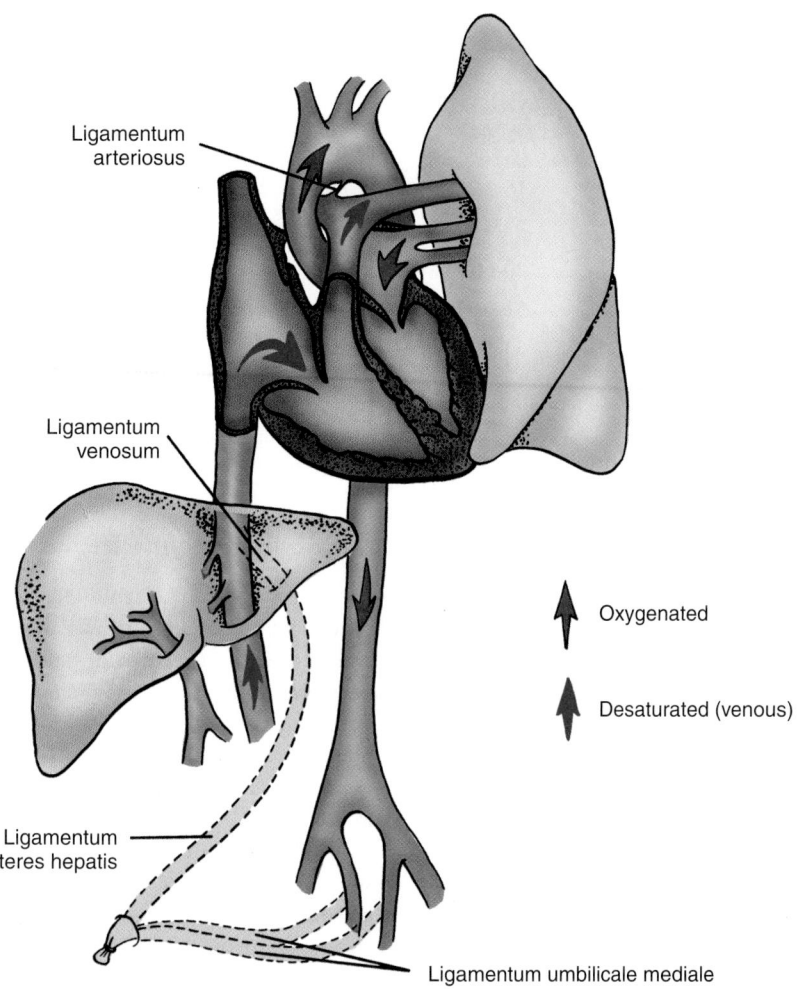

Ligamentum
arteriosus

Ligamentum
venosum

↑ Oxygenated

↑ Desaturated (venous)

Ligamentum
teres hepatis

Ligamentum umbilicale mediale

Figure 12-6 In the postnatal circulation, blood is oxygenated in the lungs, and pulmonary vascular resistance is low. Systemic venous (desaturated) blood returns to the heart through the superior and inferior vena cavae. This blood then flows through the right atrium and right ventricle, into the pulmonary artery, and ultimately into the pulmonary circulation. Oxygenated blood from the lungs returns to the left atrium through the pulmonary veins. This blood passes into the left ventricle and flows into the aorta and systemic arteries to perfuse the body. *(Modified from Hazinski MF: Nursing care of the critically ill child, ed 2, St Louis, 1992, Mosby.)*

HEMODYNAMIC MONITORING

Hemodynamic monitoring may be indicated in the critically ill pediatric patient. Issues in monitoring are related to the smaller size of the pediatric patient; fluid overload and blood loss are concerns. To accurately monitor intake, all fluid used for intravascular hemodynamic monitoring lines must be given by volume infusion pumps. Heparinized fluid is given in each line, and only small volumes of blood are drawn for laboratory tests. Each medical facility that cares for pediatric patients has policies for how much blood to draw for each test. All flush volumes are recorded as intake, an accurate record is kept of the amount of blood lost, and the child periodically receives replacement. Table 12-9 describes pediatric blood volumes.

When continuously monitoring the blood pressure in the child, the arterial reading is preferred when arterial blood sampling or vasoactive medications are in use.[25] A 4- or 5-Fr pulmonary artery catheter is used for the child. The child's vessel must be large enough to accept the 4-Fr catheter to initiate

TABLE 12-7 Normal Heart Rates in Children

Age	Awake Heart Rate (per minute)	Sleeping Heart Rate (per minute)
Neonate	100-180	80-160
Infant (6 mo)	100-160	75-160
Toddler	80-110	60-90
Preschooler	70-110	60-90
School-age child	65-110	60-90
Adolescent	60-90	50-90

From Hazinski MF: *Manual of pediatric critical care,* St Louis, 1999, Mosby.

pulmonary artery monitoring. Because the smaller catheters have smaller balloons, the clinician should refer to the catheter for balloon volume. To limit fluid intake, smaller volumes (usually 3 or 5 mL) of injectant are used for cardiac output studies. Table 12-10 provides cardiac output and stroke

TABLE 12-8 Normal Blood Pressures in Children

Age	Systolic Pressure (mm Hg)*	Diastolic Pressure (mm Hg)*
Birth (12 hr, <1000 g)	39-59	16-36
Birth (12 hr, 3 kg)	50-70	25-45
Neonate (96 hr)	60-90	20-60
Infant (6 mo)	87-105	53-66
Toddler (2 yr)	95-105	53-66
School age (7 yr)	97-112	57-71
Adolescent (15 yr)	112-128	66-80

*Blood pressure ranges are taken from the following sources. *Neonate:* Versmold H et al: Aortic blood pressure during the first 12 hours of life in infants with birth weight 610-4220 g, *Pediatrics* 67:107, 1981. Tenth through ninetieth percentile ranges are used. *Others:* Horan MJ, chairman: Task Force on Blood Pressure Control in Children, report of the Second Task Force on Blood Pressure in Children, *Pediatrics* 79:1, 1987. Fiftieth through ninetieth percentile ranges are indicated.
Modified from Hazinski MF: *Manual of pediatric critical care,* St Louis, 1999, Mosby.

TABLE 12-9 Calculation of Circulating Blood Volume

Age Group	Blood Volume (mL/kg)
Neonates	85-90
Infants	75-80
Children	70-75
Adults	65-70

From Hazinski MF: *Manual of Pediatric Critical Care,* St Louis, 1999, Mosby.

TABLE 12-10 Normal Pediatric Cardiac Output and Stroke Volume

Age	Cardiac Output (L/min)	Heart Rate (beats/min)	Normal Stroke Volume (mL)
Newborn	0.8-1.0	145	5
6 mo	1.0-1.3	120	10
1 yr	1.3-1.5	115	13
2 yr	1.5-2.0	115	18
4 yr	2.3-2.75	105	27
5 yr	2.5-3.0	95	31
8 yr	3.4-3.6	83	42
10 yr	3.8-4.0	75	50
15 yr	6.0	70	85

From Hazinski MF: *Manual of pediatric critical care,* St Louis, 1999, Mosby.

volume values. Left atrial pressure (LAP), central venous pressure (CVP), and pulmonary artery pressure (PAP) in the child are comparable with adult values. Hemodynamic parameters are related to the body surface area of the child. The normal cardiac index for children is 3.5 to 5.5 L/min/m^2, which is higher than that for adults. The stroke volume in adults and children is influenced by cardiac preload, ventricular contractility, afterload, and compliance. Subtle differences exist between pediatric and adult ventricular function. The principles of treatment for shock and the manipulation of stroke volume are the same in all age groups.[3] When evaluating hemodynamic parameters, the numbers should always be related to the clinical condition of the child. If the numbers do not correlate, the calibration and zeroing of the monitoring equipment should be reevaluated.

CONGENITAL HEART DEFECTS

Some CHDs can be diagnosed by ultrasound before birth, and some parents decide to deliver these babies at a tertiary center affiliated with a pediatric cardiac surgery program. Other newborns with cardiac anomalies are diagnosed after birth and transferred to tertiary care centers for further evaluation and, often, for immediate surgery. Certain defects are completely repaired in the first few days of life, other defects are repaired in stages, and some are repaired when the child is older. Infants with CHDs may develop complications after discharge after a surgical procedure or while waiting for surgery, and they may be admitted to an adult critical care unit. Examples of postoperative surgical complications in the pediatric cardiac patient are wound infection, pericardial effusion, pleural effusion, and cardiac arrhythmia.

A useful classification system for CHDs is based on the hemodynamic pathophysiology or movements involved in the circulation of blood. The four defining pathophysiologic characteristics[25] are (1) increased pulmonary blood flow, (2) decreased pulmonary blood flow, (3) mixed blood flow, and (4) obstruction of the flow of blood out of the heart. This classification system is outlined in Figure 12-7.

Using this hemodynamic classification system, the clinical characteristics of each CHD are more uniform and presentable. Cardiac defects that allow the blood to flow from a high-pressure left side of the child's heart to the lower-pressure right side (i.e., left-to-right shunt) cause an increase in pulmonary blood flow and congestive heart failure (CHF). Obstructive defects impede blood flow out of the ventricles. Obstructions on the left side of the heart results in (CHF), whereas obstructions on the right side cause cyanosis. The pediatric patient with mixed lesions presents with variable clinical symptoms that depend on the degree of mixing of the pulmonary blood, hypoxemia, and CHF.[25]

Two major clinical conditions can be seen in a child with a cardiac defect with altered hemodynamics. These conditions are CHF and hypoxemia.[25] Critical care nurses play a critical role with the pediatric patient in early identification and supportive management of these conditions.

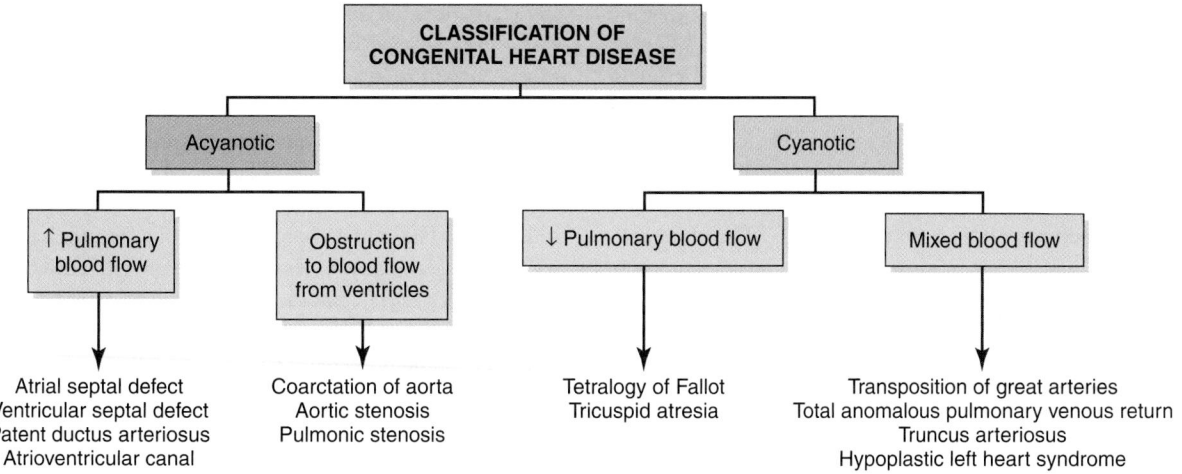

Figure 12-7 Comparison of acyanotic-cyanotic and hemodynamic classification systems of congenital heart disease. *(From O'Brien P, Baker, B: The child with cardiovascular disease. In Hockenberry MF, Wilson D, editors:* Wong's nursing care of infants and children, *ed 8, St Louis, 2007, Mosby.)*

CONGESTIVE HEART FAILURE

CHF is a clinical syndrome in which the heart is unable to pump enough blood to the body to meets its needs, to dispose of systemic or pulmonary venous return adequately, or a combination of both conditions.[23] Common causes of CHF are volume or pressure overload, congenital or acquired heart disease, and myocardial diseases. The most common cause of CHF in infancy is a CHD. Beyond infancy, myocardial dysfunctions have various causes.[23] Symptoms of CHF are related to responses of impaired cardiac function, pulmonary venous congestion, and systemic venous congestion. Infants may exhibit a change in responsiveness and may be lethargic or irritable, have tachypnea with feedings, have poor weight gain, and have a cold sweat on the forehead.[23] Tachycardia is a common and early sign of CHF. Older children may complain of dyspnea, especially with activity, or early fatigue and exhibit puffy eyelids or swollen feet. Crackles and wheezing may be auscultated in the infant.[23] During an abdominal assessment, the liver may be palpated, but hepatomegaly may be absent in early CHF. In children younger than 5 years, the liver is normally palpated at the costal margin to 1 cm below. Cardiomegaly is almost always present. Chest x-ray films are more reliable than a physical examination for determining cardiomegaly.[23]

Treatment of CHF consists of eliminating the underlying causes and getting control of the heart failure state.[23] The three major classes of medications commonly used to treat CHF in children are inotropic agents, diuretics, and afterload reducers. Rapid-acting inotropic agents such as dopamine, dobutamine or milrinone are used in the critically ill child.[23] Diuretics remain the principal therapeutic agent to control pulmonary and systemic venous congestion. Diuretic therapy alters the patient's serum electrolyte levels. Hypokalemia is a common problem and needs to be monitored. Digoxin is the inotropic drug of choice for CHF in pediatric patients. The pediatric dosage of digoxin is much larger than an adult dosage on the basis

of body weight. Pharmacokinetic studies indicate that pediatric patients require a larger dose of digoxin than adults to attain a comparable serum level.[23] When the child is receiving digoxin, the nurse should observe for signs of digitalis toxicity. Digoxin toxicity is best detected by the monitoring of the child's electrocardiogram (ECG), not serum levels for the first 3 to 5 days after digitalization.[23] Any cardiac arrhythmia or conduction disturbance detected may indicate digoxin toxicity. The therapeutic range of serum digoxin for treating CHF is 0.8 to 2 ng/mL.

HYPOXEMIA

Cyanosis is a bluish discoloration of the skin and mucous membranes, and it is observed in children with certain congenital heart defects.[23] Cyanosis is visible when there is 5 g of reduced hemoglobin per 100 mL of blood.[23] Cyanosis associated with desaturation of arterial blood is called *central cyanosis*. Peripheral cyanosis is a condition in which cyanosis exists, but the child has a normal arterial oxygen saturation.[23]

Cyanosis may have a number of causes. Central cyanosis may result from cyanotic CHD, lung disease, or central nervous system depression. Differentiation of cardiac cyanosis from cyanosis caused by pulmonary disease is essential for proper medical management. The Hyperoxitest helps to distinguish the source of the infant's cyanosis[23] by assessing the infant's arterial PO_2 response to the inhalation of 100% oxygen. With pulmonary disease, the arterial PO_2 usually rises to a level greater than 100 mm Hg. If there is a significant intracardiac right-to-left shunt, the arterial PO_2 does not exceed 100 mm Hg, with a rise of usually not more than 10 to 30 mm Hg.[23]

Some children with CHD manifest hypercyanotic spells. This is most common in children with tetralogy of Fallot (TOF). These episodes often are called *Tet spells*. These spells rarely are seen before 2 months of age, occur most often during the first year of life, and occur more often in the morning.[6] During these episodes, the child becomes very cyanotic, hypoxic, and tachypneic and may lose consciousness or develop seizures due to the extreme hypoxemia causing cerebral hypoxia. The persistent hypoxemia as a result of TOF places the infant at risk for neurologic consequences from the development of polycythemia and increased viscosity of the blood.[6] The treatment of hypercyanotic spells includes soothing the child while placing him or her in a knee-chest position and administering oxygen, fluid boluses, and possibly sedation.[25] The child may require intubation, mechanical ventilation, and treatment of metabolic acidosis.

ARRHYTHMIAS

Electrophysiology and electrocardiography principles are similar for adult and pediatric patients (see Chapters 16 and 18). Differences include a faster heart rate in children and the variances in the PR and QT intervals related to the child's rapid heart rate. Table 12-7 provides normal pediatric heart rates. At birth, the right ventricle is thicker than the left ventricle. Right ventricular dominance of the newborn period is replaced by left ventricular dominance in childhood and in adulthood. Anatomic changes are most rapid in the first month, and by 6 months of age, the left ventricle is dominant. With increasing age, the heart rate decreases, and the PR interval, QRS duration, and QT interval increases.

In the pediatric patient, monitoring of respiratory rate and oxygen saturation is done concurrently with cardiac monitoring. It is important to recognize the manifestations of impending respiratory failure in the pediatric patient, because respiratory failure precedes cardiac failure and potential cardiac arrest. ECG monitoring electrodes are placed along the nipple line on the chest to facilitate monitoring the cardiac rate and rhythm and the respiratory rate. To capture and diagnose transient events such as an arrhythmia or conduction disorders, the best method is to use a 24-hour Holter monitor. The Holter monitor uses the modified chest leads that most closely resemble leads V_1 and V_5 for monitoring.[26]

Arrhythmias can result from CHD, surgical correction, hypoxia, electrolyte or acid-base imbalances, drug toxicity, or myocardial injury.[3] Arrhythmias can be symptomatic or asymptomatic, and they have the potential to deteriorate into a symptomatic condition. The three most common types of clinically significant pediatric arrhythmias are bradyarrhythmias, tachyarrhythmias, and those that produce cardiac collapse or loss of pulses.[3,4] Hypoxia and heart block are the most common causes of bradyarrhythmias. Supraventricular tachycardia (SVT) is probably the most common form of pediatric tachyarrhythmias. Sinus tachycardia is not an arrhythmia; it is an indication that an increased heart rate and cardiac output are needed for the child's condition.

Supraventricular Tachycardia. The most common symptomatic tachyarrhythmia in children is SVT. P waves may or may not be seen, and the rate often exceeds 220 beats/min. Wide QRS SVT is uncommon in children, and any wide QRS tachycardia must be treated as ventricular in origin until proved otherwise. If the child in SVT is unstable and shows signs of decreased cardiac output and poor perfusion,

immediate treatment is indicated.[4] If the child has intravenous access readily available, adenosine (0.1 mg/kg) should be administered up to a maximum of a 6-mg rapid bolus. This dose can be doubled up to maximum of 12 mg for a second dose. Adenosine should be given as a rapid intravenous bolus due to the drug's short half-life of about 10 seconds. If intravenous access is not readily available, synchronized cardioversion is indicated.[4] The initial energy dose is 0.5 J/kg to 1 J/kg. If the SVT persists, the dose of electricity is doubled. The child should be sedated if possible, but cardioversion should not be delayed. In a stable child, an initial procedure may include vagal maneuvers, but these should never delay synchronized cardioversion. Consultation with a pediatric cardiologist is advised. If additional treatment is needed, amiodarone (5 mg/kg given intravenously over 20 to 60 minutes) or procainamide (15 mg/kg given intravenously over 30 to 60 minutes) should be considered. These medications should not routinely be given together.[4]

Bradycardias. Bradycardia can result from hypoxia, acidosis, or hypothermia. Bradycardia is defined as a cardiac rate less than 100 beats/min for an infant and less than 60 beats/min for a child.[3] Treatment initially includes adequate oxygenation and ventilation for the pediatric patient. If the bradycardia continues to cause cardiopulmonary compromise despite oxygenation and ventilation, compressions are started for a heart rate of less than 60 beats/min. If the bradycardia continues, the nurse should plan to administer epinephrine (0.01 mg/kg, 1:10,000 concentration) given intravenously or intraosseously) or through the ETT (0.1 mg/kg, 1:1000 concentration). Epinephrine can be repeated every 3 to 5 minutes. The intravenous or intraosseous route is preferred to medications given through the ETT.[4] If increased vagal tone or a primary atrioventricular block is the cause of the bradycardia, atropine (0.02 mg/kg) can be given. This dose can be repeated (minimum dose 0.1 mg to maximum dose of 1 mg for a child and 2 mg for an adolescent).[4] If additional treatment is indicated, consider cardiac pacing. If the child's rhythm develops into pulseless arrest, then proceed to the pulseless arrest resuscitation procedure.

SHOCK IN INFANTS AND CHILDREN

Shock is a critical condition that results from inadequate delivery of oxygen and nutrients to the tissues to meet the metabolic demand.[3] Shock frequently is the end result of severe dehydration, hemorrhage, progressive heart failure, or sepsis. The treatment goal for a child in shock is to prevent end-organ injury and stop the progression from cardiopulmonary failure to cardiac arrest. Shock is typically classified by etiologic mechanism. These classifications include: hypovolemic, distributive or septic, cardiogenic, or obstructive.[4]

Shock can be present in a pediatric patient with normal or abnormal blood pressure. The blood pressure reading may be used to further classify the shock as compensated or hypotensive shock.[4] Compensated shock describes a child with signs of poor perfusion but normal blood pressure. The systolic reading may be normal, but the diastolic pressure may not be normal due to increased systemic vascular resistence.[4] In hypotensive shock, the blood pressure is low, and cardiopulmonary failure may be imminent.[3]

Hypovolemic Shock. Hypovolemic shock is the most common cause of shock in children worldwide.[4] Fluid loss from diarrhea is the leading cause of hypovolemic shock.[4] Causes of volume loss than can lead to hypovolemic shock include diarrhea, hemorrhage, vomiting, inadequate fluid intake, osmotic diuresis, third space losses, and burns.[4] The treatment for hypovolemic shock is fluid resuscitation. Pediatric patients with hypovolemic shock need to receive the appropriate volume of fluid within the first hour of resuscitation to have the best chance of survival and recovery. Fluid resuscitation should start with rapid infusion of isotonic crystalloid in boluses of 20 mL/kg.[4] With severe fluid losses, the child may require up to two to three fluid boluses initially. If blood replacement is required, packed red cells should be considered, starting with 10 mL/kg. The child must be closely monitored and reassessed after each fluid bolus for effectiveness of the fluid resuscitation on end-organ perfusion.

Cardiogenic Shock. Cardiogenic shock is a condition of inadequate tissue perfusion resulting from myocardial dysfunction. This dysfunction can be the result of pump failure, congenital heart disease, or a rhythm abnormalilty.[4] Cardiogenic shock is characterized by decreased cardiac output, marked tachycardia, and a high systemic vascular output. The child has decreased urine output (<0.5 to 1 mL/kg/hr) and changes in mental status as end-organ perfusion is affected. Crackles may be heard on lung auscultation, and frothy sputum may be present. Increased respiratory effort is often what distinguishes cardiogenic shock from hypovolemic shock.[4]

The main treatment objectives are to improve the effectiveness of cardiac function and overall cardiac output by increasing the efficiency of ventricular emptying.[4,25] Many children with cardiogenic shock have a high preload and do not require additional fluids. However, if the child's history is consistent with fluid loss, a fluid bolus of 5 to 10 mL/kg may be cautiously given. Frequent assessments of the child's respiratory function should be performed in anticipation of respiratory failure. Supplemental oxygen should be given, but the nurse should be prepared to assist ventilation with intubation and ventilation[4] and consider establishing central venous access in the child. This approach allows for the measurement of the central venous pressure and provides access for fluid and medication infusion.

Typical pharmacologic support of a child with car diogenic shock includes the use of diuretics and vasodilators. Diuretics are indicated when the child has evidence of pulmonary edema. The vasodilators are given as a continuous infusion. Milrinone is the preferred medication for cardiogenic shock (infusion at 0.5 to 0.75 µg/kg/min).[4]

Laboratory studies should be obtained to assess the impact of the shock on the end organ function. No single laboratory test is specific for cardiogenic shock. Consultation with a pediatric cardiologist should be initiated at the earliest opportunity to help facilitate a diagnosis (using the ECG), guide the therapy, and possibly transfer of the patient for additional care or surgery with a pediatric specialist.[4]

Distributive Shock, Sepsis, and Septic Shock. Septic shock is the most common form of distributive shock. This condition is caused by infectious agents or their endotoxins, which stimulate the child's immune system and trigger release or activation of inflammatory mediators. Septic shock in children typically evolves along a continuum from a systemic inflammatory response in the early stages to septic shock in the later ones.[4] The child exhibits manifestations of systemic inflammatory response syndrome (SIRS) with severe sepsis or septic shock. Instead of temperature elevation, the infant or child may have a low temperature or temperature instability. Along with level of consciousness changes, the child may be irritable, restless, or lethargic. Urine output is decreased, the skin may be warm or mottled, and peripheral pulses may be strong and bounding. The child does not feed well, and decreased fluid intake may precipitate dehydration. Blood pressure is maintained within normal limits from activation of the body's compensatory mechanisms. Parents may remark that the child "does not seem right" or "something is different" with the child. Always listen to the parents' assessment of the child's status.

Treatment of SIRS includes administration of oxygen, fluids, and antibiotics. However, the most effective treatment of SIRS is prevention. Hand washing before and after patient contact is essential. Sterile technique is maintained during suctioning, while managing invasive lines, and during dressing changes and wound care.

Severe sepsis or septic shock is diagnosed when perfusion decreases and the child becomes hypotensive. If the child is receiving inotropic agents, the blood pressure may be normal, but there is a change in perfusion. The patient exhibits metabolic acidosis and hypoxemia. This may require intubation, mechanical ventilation, sedation, fluids, and vasopressor medications. Complications of septic shock include acute respiratory distress syndrome, acute renal failure, disseminated intravascular coagulation, and multiple organ dysfunction syndrome (MODS).

Obstructive Shock. Obstructive shock is a condition of impaired cardiac output caused by some physical obstruction of the blood flow. The physiology of the clinical symptoms varies according to the cause of the obstruction.[4] Four types of obstructive shock occur in children.

One type of obstructive shock is caused by a cardiac tamponade.[4] This occurs when there is an accumulation of fluid, blood, or air in the pericardial space around the heart. This condition is seen after cardiac surgery or a penetrating cardiac injury. Symptoms of a cardiac tamponade include muffled or distant heart sounds, distended neck veins, or pulses paradoxus (i.e., decrease in systolic blood pressure by more than 10 mm Hg during inspiration). The treatment is supportive, including fluids, adequate oxygenation and ventilation, and vasopressors.

A second type of obstructive shock is a tension pneumothorax,[4] which is caused by entry of air into the pleural space. This is most often seen in a pediatric patient when there has been chest trauma or in an intubated child on positive-pressure ventilation that deteriorates suddenly. The signs and symptoms include diminished breath sounds on the affected side, distended neck veins, tracheal deviation, and a rapid deteriorating clinical condition of the child that can result in bradycardia, hypotension, and hypoxemia. The treatment is immediate needle decompression over the third rib at the midclavicular line. The decompression should be accompanied by an escaping of air. The decompression should be followed by an insertion of a chest tube.

A third but rare cause of obstructive shock is a massive pulmonary embolism,[4] which results from partial or total obstruction of the pulmonary artery. The symptoms include signs of cyanosis, hypotension, and right heart failure. Treatment includes adequate oxygenation and ventilation, and fluid therapy is administered if the patient is poorly perfused. Additional diagnostic tests and medications, such as thrombolytic agents, may be required.

A fourth type of obstructive shock is a ductal-dependent congenital heart lesion.[4] Because systemic circulation is supported by the right side of the heart through the ductus arteriosus, these lesions are called ductal-dependent lesions. The affected infant shows signs of severe shock, CHF, hypotension, poor perfusion, lethargy, and acidosis. The infant is treated with PGE_1 to maintain the patency of the ductus arteriosus.

CARDIOPULMONARY ARREST

The pediatric patient must be assessed for manifestations of respiratory failure and sepsis, because not recognizing these problems may result in the development of cardiopulmonary failure and respiratory or cardiac arrest. In the pediatric patient, respiratory arrest usually precedes cardiac arrest. In an arrest situation, oxygen is administered, and an airway established and maintained (see "Assessment and Oxygen Devices"). For a cardiac arrest, compressions are started, and an intravenous or intraosseous line is established. Intraosseous placement is recommended as an alternative means to deliver intravenous fluids and medications in children of all ages when vascular access is not obtained within 90 seconds or after three attempts. Intraosseous access often can be achieved in 30 to 60 seconds and is the preferred route over the endotracheal route for medications. Any drug or fluid that can be administered by a peripheral intravenous line can be given by the intraosseous route.[4] The preferred site is the broad, flat portion of the anteromedial surface of the tibia approximately 1 to 2 cm below the tibial tuberosity. Other interventions are based on the cardiac rhythm and the cause of the arrest.

Pulseless arrest includes the following arrhythmias: asystole, ventricular fibrillation (VF), pulseless ventricular tachycardia (VT), and pulseless electrical activity (PEA).[4] Treatment of asystole starts with CPR (rate of 15 compressions to two breaths), airway maintenance with oxygenation, attachment to a monitor or defibrillator, and obtaining intravenous or intraosseous access. After an advanced airway is in place, chest compressions can continue without pauses for breaths. A child requires 8 to 10 breaths/min. The next step in the treatment algorithm depends on whether the rhythm is shockable.[4] The rhythms of VF or VT are shockable. On a manual defibrillator, the initial dose of electricity is 2 J/kg. If using an Automatic External Defibrillator (AED,) this equipment is be used only

for children older than 1 year.[4] Immediately after the shock, CPR is resumed for 2 minutes (five cycles). The compressions support the heart while it is in a recovery state even if a perfusion rhythm has returned.[4] If the VT or VF persists, another shock is administered at 4 J/kg, CPR is resumed, and epinephrine is given. The first dose of epinephrine is 0.01 mg/kg (1:10,000 at 0.1 mL/kg) given intravenously or intraosseously; if given endotracheally, the dose is 0.1 mg/kg (1:1,000 at 0.1 mL/kg). Subsequent doses may be given every 3 to 5 minutes. Maximum dosage is 1 mg (1 mL). After 2 minutes of CPR, the patient's rhythm should be checked. If the VT or VF rhythm continues, the patient is defibrillated again at 4 J/kg. CPR is resumed immediately, and an antiarrhythmic medication, such as amiodarone (5 mg/kg given intravenously or intraosseously) or lidocaine (1 mg/kg given intravenously or intraosseously), is considered.

If the rhythm is not shockable, as in asystole or PEA, the first action after starting CPR is to give the epinephrine at the same dose listed previously. After five cycles or 2 minutes of CPR, the patient's rhythm is checked, and if asystole or PEA persists, CPR and dosing with epinephrine every 3 to 5 minutes are continued.

The primary goals of postresuscitation management of the pediatric patient include the following[4]:

1. Optimization of the cardiopulmonary function to restore and maintain vital organ perfusion and function, especially the brain
2. Prevention of any secondary organ injury
3. Identification and treatment of the cause of any acute illnesses
4. Initiation of measures to help improve a long-term, neurologically intact survival for the child

The nurse should assess the patient using a systematic approach. In addition to primary assessments, the approach should include review of the patient's history, a thorough physical examination, the use of invasive and noninvasive monitoring techniques, and use of appropriate laboratory testing.[4]

NERVOUS SYSTEM

ANATOMY

The nervous system grows rapidly before birth, and growth continues during infancy and childhood. Compared with the adult, an infant or toddler's head size is proportionally larger than the rest of the body. When infants fall, the head usually leads, and a significant head injury can occur.[3] The skull is more flexible because the skull bones are not fused and are separated by spaces called *fontanelles*. The anterior fontanelle is the junction of the coronal, sagittal, and frontal sutures, whereas the posterior fontanelle is the junction of the parietal and occipital bones. By 3 months of age, the posterior fontanelle is usually closed, and the anterior fontanelle is closed by the age of 20 months.

The brain of a young child has a high water content and contains less myelin than the brain of an adult. This makes the child's brain more homogeneous and less compartmentalized.[3]

Shear hemorrhages and diffuse brain injuries are more common in children than adults.

Spinal cord injuries are less common in children than adults because the spine is elastic and the vertebrae less likely to fracture. In children with head injuries or multisystem trauma, spinal cord injuries should always be suspected until ruled out.[3]

PHYSIOLOGY

Cerebral blood flow and oxygen consumption are increased in childhood in relation to increased metabolic needs. Hyperemia, tissue hypoxia, and acidosis result in cerebral arterial dilation and increased cerebral blood flow. Hyperventilation decreases cerebral blood flow, but severe hypercarbia may result in decreased oxygen consumption and use. The normal cerebral perfusion pressure (CPP) values in children are unknown. It is thought, that CPP should be in the range of 40 to 60 mm Hg, but this figure may vary because perfusion is determined by blood flow and not by blood pressure.[3] CPP must be maintained at a level to maintain blood flow. A patient with a normal CPP does not necessarily have effective cerebral perfusion.

ASSESSMENT

Cognitive function cannot be evaluated until the preschool and early childhood years, but level of consciousness, movement, and pupils can be evaluated in the pediatric patient. The Glasgow Coma Scale (GCS) is used for older children and has been modified for use in infants and younger children (Table 12-11). Survival and recovery of a patient with a GCS score of 5 to 8 are better for children than adults.[3] Evaluation of reflexes in children is comparable to that of adults, with a

couple of exceptions. Although a positive Babinski reflex is an abnormal response in an adult, this response is normal in the child until the age of 1 year.[6] In the first few months of life, grasp is reflexive in the infant. With severe neurologic disease or injury, grasp may revert to a reflex as opposed to a purposeful response, and the grasp response may not indicate improvement of the child's neurologic status.

The pediatric patient's responsiveness needs to be evaluated in regard of the child's age, clinical condition, and changes in responsiveness over time. Infants and children should always respond to their parents or caregivers and to a painful stimuli. A decrease in the responsiveness is abnormal and should be investigated.[3] If the child is older than 2 years, the ability to follow commands can be assessed by asking him or her to hold up two fingers or wiggle the toes. This action is not accomplished by a reflex action.

When a child is unconscious, the most important component of the GCS to assess is the motor function.[3] The patient's central and peripheral responses to a painful stimuli need to be assessed. A central stimulus is applied to the head and trunk, above the nipple line. The peripheral stimulus can be assessed at the medial aspect of each extremity. The patient's best response is the one that is recorded for the GCS score.

Signs of increased intracranial pressure (ICP) in pediatric patients include a change in responsiveness, a deterioration in the ability to follow commands, a change in the response to pain, and pupil dilation with light stimulation.[3] The Cushing triad sign of an increased ICP may only be observed during cerebral herniation and should not be used as an early indicator or ICP. If any neurologic deterioration is detected in the pediatric patient, a complete neurologic assessment is required, including the child's vital signs and consultation with the patient's physician.

TABLE 12-11   Modified Glasgow Coma Scale for Infants and Children

	Child	Infant	Score
Eye opening	Spontaneous	Spontaneous	4
	To verbal stimuli	To verbal stimuli	3
	To pain only	To pain only	2
	No response	No response	1
Verbal response	Oriented, appropriate	Coos and babbles	5
	Confused	Irritable cries	4
	Inappropriate words	Cries to pain	3
	Incomprehensible words or nonspecific sounds	Moans to pain	2
	No response	No response	1
Motor response	Obeys command	Moves spontaneously and purposefully	6
	Localizes painful stimulus	Withdraws to touch	5
	Withdraws in response to pain	Withdraws in response to pain	4
	Flexion in response to pain	Decorticate posturing (abnormal flexion) in response to pain	3
	Extension in response to pain	Decerebrate posturing (abnormal extension) in response to pain	2
	No response	No response	1

Data from Davis RJ et al: Head and spinal cord injury. In Rogers MC, editors: *Textbook of pediatric intensive care,* Baltimore, 1987, Williams & Wilkins; James H et al: *Brain insults in infants and children,* New York, 1985, Grune & Stratton; Morray JP et al: Coma scale for use in brain-injured children *Crit Care Med* 12:1018, 1984.

SEIZURES

Seizures are brief manifestations of the brain's electrical system that result from cortical neuronal discharge. Seizures are the most commonly observed neurologic deficit in children and can occur with a variety of central nervous system conditions (Box 12-3). At least 80% of the general population will experience one or more seizures in their lifetime.[27] The incidence of causative factors that are associated with seizures in children is related to the child's age. In infants, the most common factors are related to birth traumas (i.e., anoxia, congenital defects, and intracranial bleeds).[27] Acute infections are a common cause in late infancy and early childhood but uncommon in the child who is in middle childhood. In children who are older than 3 years, the most common cause of seizures is idiopathic epilepsy.[27] As children enter adolescence, hormonal and metabolic changes may alter the seizure threshold. The child who is in an unconscious state must be evaluated for a history of seizures, because unconsciousness may be the result of a postictal state.

There are many different types of seizures, and each has unique clinical manifestations. Seizures can be classified in three major groups: partial seizures, generalized seizures, and unclassified epileptic seizures.[27] Partial seizures have a local onset and involve a relative small part of the brain. Manifestation of this type of seizure depends on what part of the brain is involved. The initial event may provide the best clue for assessing the type of seizure and the location. Generalized seizures involve both hemispheres of the brain without a focal onset. Loss of consciousness and motor impairment occur from this type of seizure. Unlike the partial seizure, there is no aura, and the seizure can occur at any time of the day or night, with different lengths of time between seizures.[27] Unclassified epileptic seizures are events for which there is insufficient information available to classify them. In addition to seizures, there are several types of epileptic syndromes that display a group of signs and symptoms that characterize a certain condition.

Clinical manifestations of seizures may be subtler in the infant because of immaturity of the central nervous system. Some common behaviors seen with subtle seizures include (1) tonic horizontal deviations of the eyes with or without nystagmoid jerking; (2) repetitive blinking or fluttering of the eyelashes; (3) drooling, sucking, or tongue thrusting; and (4) swimming or rowing movements of the arms with occasional bicycling movements of the legs. Apnea may also occur, and the respiratory status of the infant must be closely monitored. Seizures must be differentiated from jitteriness in infants. With jitteriness, the predominant type of movement is tremors characterized by alternating rhythmic movements of equal rate and magnitude. Jitteriness and seizures may be observed in the infant with asphyxia, hypoglycemia, or hypocalcemia. Laboratory studies can help determine the metabolic status of the infant.

Nursing management of seizures includes monitoring respiratory status and perfusion, assessing for the cause of the seizure, determining methods to prevent additional seizures, providing a safe environment for the child, and documenting the seizure activity. Children admitted to the critical care unit may require intubation for respiratory complications of seizures, for the sedative effects of anticonvulsants, or for status epilepticus. Anticonvulsant therapy may be indicated for prolonged or recurrent seizures. Phenobarbital, phenytoin (Dilantin), and benzodiazepines (lorazepam, diazepam) are some medications that may be ordered for the child.

BOX 12-3   CAUSES OF SEIZURES IN CHILDREN

Nonrecurrent (Acute)	Recurrent (Chronic)
• Febrile episodes	• Idiopathic epilepsy
• Intracranial infection	• Epilepsy resulting from
• Intracranial hemorrhage	• Trauma
• Space-occupying lesions (cyst, tumor)	• Hemorrhage
• Acute cerebral edema	• Anoxia
• Anoxia	• Infections
• Toxins	• Toxins
• Drugs	• Degenerative phenomena
• Tetanus	• Congenital defects
• Lead (encephalopathy)	• Parasitic brain disease
• *Shigella, Salmonella*	• Hypoglycemic injury
• Metabolic alterations	• Epilepsy—sensory stimulus
• Hypocalcemia	• Epilepsy—stimulating states
• Hypoglycemia	• Narcolepsy and catalepsy
• Hyponatremia or hypernatremia	• Psychogenic causes
• Hypomagnesemia	• Tetany from hypocalcemia, alkalosis
• Alkalosis	• Hypoglycemic states
• Disorders of amino acid metabolism	• Hyperinsulinism
• Deficiency states	• Hypopituitarism
• Hyperbilirubinemia	• Adrenocortical insufficiency
	• Hepatic disorders
	• Uremia
	• Allergy
	• Cardiovascular dysfunction or syncopal episodes
	• Migraine

Modified from Bryant R, Schultz R: The child with cerebral dysfunction. In Hockenberry MJ, Wilson D, editors: *Wong's nursing care of infants and children*, 8 ed, St Louis, 2007, Mosby.

STATUS EPILEPTICUS

Status epilepticus is a medical emergency and is characterized by two or more unprovoked seizures that can be caused by a variety of pathologic processes in the brain.[27] Causes can include high fever, meningitis, encephalitis, metabolic disorders, and abrupt cessation of anticonvulsant drugs. There is an increase in cerebral blood flow, metabolic requirements, and oxygen needs when a seizure occurs. An electroencephalogram (EEG) is required to confirm status epilepticus in patients in deep coma or with pharmacologic paralysis. The goal of treatment is to control the seizures or reduce their frequency and severity and to discover the correct the cause of the seizures if possible to help the child live as normal a life as possible.

Treatment includes short-term administration of anticonvulsant medications, such as diazepam, lorazepam, or midazolam. The critical care nurse should assess and evaluate the child to ensure the patient has a patent airway, adequate ventilation effort, and adequate oxygenation and systemic perfusion. Clinical documentation should contain the patient's neurologic assessment, including the seizure manifestation and duration.

BACTERIAL MENINGITIS

Meningitis is an acute inflammation of the meninges, the outer covering of the brain and spinal cord, and the cerebral spinal fluid (CSF). The pathogens usually come from a distant site and colonize. They enter the bloodstream, producing sepsis, and they then invade the meninges.[28] The highest incidence is found among children younger than the age of 1 year. Meningococcal meningitis is readily transmitted by droplet infection from nasopharyngeal secretions. The risk of transmission increases with the number of contacts. This can occur most frequently in school-age children or adolescents.[27]

The causes of meningitis are septic (bacterial or fungal) or aseptic (viral), but the information in this section pertains only to bacterial meningitis. Common causative organisms are *Haemophilus influenzae,* type B; *Streptococcus pneumoniae*; and *Neisseria meningitides.* Other causative organisms are β-hemolytic streptococci, *Staphylococcus aureus, Escherichia coli, Pseudomonas,* and *Listeria monocytogenes.* Invasion of microorganisms triggers a response that causes inflammation, production of purulent exudates, white blood cell accumulation, and various degrees of tissue damage.[27] The brain becomes hyperemic and edematous. The entire surface of the brain is covered in purulent exudates, and this can obstruct the flow of CSF, leading to the development of hydrocephalus.

The clinical manifestations of bacterial meningitis include fever, chills, headache, vomiting, irritability or lethargy, photophobia, nuchal rigidity, and a positive Kernig or Brudzinski sign. In meningococcemia, petechiae and purpura may be observed on the child.[27] The late stages of this disease may produce an increased ICP and cardiovascular collapse. Symptoms in infants are less specific and can include lethargy, vomiting, bulging fontanelles, hypothermia or hyperthermia, diarrhea, and poor feeding.

CSF analysis is the standard for diagnosing bacterial meningitis obtained by a lumbar puncture. The CSF studies show an elevated white blood cell count, increased protein level, decreased glucose concentration, and positive results from the Gram stain and culture of the organism. The CSF may look cloudy or turbid. The child with meningitis is isolated during initial antibiotic treatment and for 24 hours after appropriate antibacterial therapy is started. The appropriate antibiotic therapy is continued for 10 to 14 days. The administration of dexamethasone is recommended in children with *H. influenzae* to prevent hearing loss.[28] Acetaminophen may be given for elevated temperature; aspirin must not be used.

Nursing management must include early recognition and immediate start of therapies to prevent possible disabilities. The initial therapy management includes use of isolation precautions, starting antibiotic therapy, maintenance of ventilation and hydration, reduction of increased ICP, management of systemic shock, control of seizures and temperature, and providing family education and support.[27] The sudden nature of the illness makes emotional support of the child and parents extremely important. Parents frequently feel guilty for not having suspected the seriousness of this disease.[34] They should be kept informed about their child's progress and all procedures and results. The complications of bacterial meningitis may include the development of hearing loss, hydrocephalus, loss of digits or parts of extremities, and possible death. The long-term effect on infants manifests as communicating hydrocephalus, whereas in the older child, the effects are related to the inflammatory process or vasculitis associated with the disease.[34]

HEAD TRAUMA

Unintentional injury is the leading cause of death in children between the ages of 1 and 17 years. More children in this age range die of their injuries than the total number of pediatric patients dying of the next nine leading causes.[2] Current evidence suggests that most injured children are not being treated in pediatric trauma centers. About 47% of pediatric trauma care occurs in nontrauma centers.[29] The best outcome after pediatric trauma occurs when the clinical team is prepared and knowledgeable about the unique aspects of the injured child.[7] Much of the anxiety of taking care of injured pediatric patients can be eliminated by having instruments, equipment, and drug dosages carefully precalculated. One solution practiced by many centers is using a Broselow tape that is colored coded for specific weight groups (see Fig. 12-3).

Head trauma in the pediatric patient results from closed head injuries resulting from motor vehicle accidents, bicycle crashes, falls, or child abuse.[30] Children during infancy and childhood tend to have heads that are proportionally large compared with the remainder of their bodies. As a result, a child can be propelled head first in unrestrained crashes, causing acceleration-deceleration injuries when their head hits an object. Child abuse resulting from blunt trauma to the head or from shaking is the leading cause of head injury among infants and young children.[30]

Diffuse head injury is more likely to result from blunt head trauma, especially in accidents that cause acceleration-deceleration injures, because the pediatric patient's brain is more homogenous than the adult's brain, contains a higher water content, and has less myelinization. The head injury is the primary insult, but hypoxemia and hypotension can be secondary insults that can significantly worsen the outcome of the patient.[7] Secondary insults to the injured brain must be avoided in all phases of the child's care.

Definitions and descriptions of the various types of head injuries in children are similar to those for the adult. Although the pathophysiology of head injury is similar in adults and children, there are variations in the nursing assessment and management for pediatric patients. The most common types of cerebral injuries include concussions, contusions, skull fractures, and vascular injuries, including epidural, subdural, and subarachnoid hematomas.[3] Head injuries are classified based on the GCS score for the patient: 13 to 15 for mild injuries, 9 to 12 for moderate injuries, and less than 8 for severe injuries. Children with severe head injuries need to be admitted to a critical unit for management and treatment of an increased ICP.[30] The treatment goals include measures to ensure adequate cerebral oxygenation and the prevention of secondary brain injury. The child's plan of care includes providing optimal ventilation and oxygenation, maintenance of a normal PCO_2, maintenance of a normal ICP with monitoring and interventions, and maintenance of adequate systemic and cerebral perfusion pressures.[30]

Complications of head injuries include hemorrhage, infections, cerebral bleeding, cerebral edema, seizures, and brain herniation. Treatment is based on what clinical signs are manifested by the patient. Treatment for epidural hematoma is surgical intervention. Subdural hematomas are more common in children, and treatment of subdural hematoma may be a surgical intervention for large hematomas associated with an increased ICP.[3]

Children, especially infants, are at risk for seizures after severe head injury. The child admitted to the critical care unit with a head injury must be constantly monitored for cerebral edema and signs of increased ICP. Two other potential complications of head injury—diabetes insipidus and syndrome of inappropriate antidiuretic hormone (SIADH)—are discussed in Chapter 37.

Nursing interventions include precise neurologic assessment, including using GCS scores and monitoring for signs of increased ICP. The psychological impact of injury on a child cannot be underestimated. Studies have shown that 60% of injured children have posttraumatic stress disorder symptoms immediately after the injury. Thirty-eight percent of children continue to have symptoms 18 months after their injury.[7] Children who survive severe head injury often require extended rehabilitation services to help with long-term outcomes. Involvement the pediatric rehabilitation team in the care of the child should occur while the child is in the critical care unit.

Working with the family of the child with a head injury is challenging. Information given to the parents must be accurate and consistent. The parents may be guilt-ridden, especially if they feel they might have been able to prevent the injury. Parents are encouraged to interact with the child soothingly and gently, even if the child cannot respond. Reading books, making a tape of home activities, and bringing in familiar toys or stuffed animals are ways to involve the family in the care of the child.

If the child is not expected to survive, the parents should be informed. The child should be evaluated for brain death and possible organ donation. Before the tests begin, the parents are offered the opportunity to spend time with the child. If brain death has been determined, the parents are told the test results. Parents may be asked to participate in the decision of when, but not if, to discontinue support. After the decision has been made to discontinue the intensive treatment, the priorities for the critical care nurse include providing comfort and dignity for the child and the family.[31] The most important aspects of care for the families at this time are to show a genuinely caring attitude, to extend kindness and understanding, and to be present with them.[31] Parents must always be approached in a sensitive and compassionate manner. The critical care nurse is typically the member of the team who is closest to the family and the best person to help the family members get ready for the death of the child. Special circumstances, such as the impending arrival of additional family members, may influence the timing of the decision. Parents must be allowed to spend as much time as they desire with the child to see that everything possible has been done for their child.

GASTROINTESTINAL SYSTEM, FLUIDS, AND NUTRITION

ANATOMY AND PHYSIOLOGY

Coordination of sucking, swallowing, esophageal peristalsis, and breathing is established just after birth. Infant sucking, which is also a reflex, can be nutritive or nonnutritive. Nonnutritive sucking involves no swallowing; occurs at a rapid rate; has self-soothing capacities, which can also be used with the intubated infant; and affects the postprandial process. Nutritive sucking involves moving food from the mouth through the small intestines. It involves bursts of about 10 to 30 sucks, interspersed with one to four swallows. The quality of nutritive sucking is one of several indicators of illness in the infant. Sucking involves a considerable amount of motor activity, and when changes in oxygen demand and consumption occur during illness, the infant fatigues more readily, and sucking becomes weaker or even abates.

After birth, growth and maintenance of the small intestine require nutritional components and the stimulation that comes from having food in the gut lumen. The intestinal tracts of infants and young children are larger compared with body weight than the adult's. Sodium and water conservation, which occurs in the large intestine, is an immature process in the infant. For the first 2 years of life, gut immunity is lower, and there is greater mucosal binding for bacterial toxins. With these differences in immunity, sensitivity, and greater potential for fluid loss, the infant and toddler have greater morbidity and mortality rates associated with enteric infections than does the adult.[3]

ASSESSMENT AND TREATMENT

The child's fluid requirements involve replacing output and insensible losses and extra fluid for the production of new intracellular and extracellular fluid during growth. Fluid maintenance for the child with normal renal and cardiac status can be calculated using several formulas, but these account only for basal metabolic needs and growth. The amount of fluid given to a pediatric patient must be determined by the child's clinical condition, fluid balance, and insensible water losses.[3] Table 12-12 provides formulas for normal fluid and electrolyte

TABLE 12-12 Normal Fluid and Electrolyte Maintenance for Infants and Children

Component	Weight of Infant or Child	Total Amount
Fluids	1-10 kg 11-20 kg >20 kg	100 mL/kg/day 1000 mL + 50 mL/each kg over 10 days 1500 mL + 20 mL/each kg over 20 days or 100 mL/100 kcal/day can be used for children of any weight or 1500 mL/m²/day can be used for children >10 g
Sodium		2-4 mEq/kg/day
Potassium		2-3 mEq/kg/day
Hourly fluid maintenance	1-10 kg 11-20 kg >20 kg	4 mL/kg/hr 40 mL + 2 mL/kg over 10 kg 60 mL + 1 mL/kg over 20 kg

Modified from Roberts KE: Fluid and electrolyte regulation. In Curley M, Smith J, Moloney-Harmon P: *Critical care nursing of infants and children*, ed 2, Philadelphia, 2001, Saunders.

BOX 12-4   ADJUSTMENTS TO FLUID MAINTENANCE

- Fever or hypothermia: increases or decreases 12% for each degree greater or less than 37.8° C, rectal
- Tachypnea: increases 25% to 30%
- Humidified mechanical ventilation: decreases 12%
- Activity of noncritically ill resting child: increases 10%
- Restless or active child: increases 30%
- Diaphoresis: increases 10% to 25%
- High-humidity environment: decreases 25% to 40%

---

maintenance for the infant and child. Box 12-4 provides adjustments to fluid maintenance based on level of activity or increased metabolic rate associated with disease.

Pediatric patients with fluid volume deficit may present with vomiting and diarrhea. When considering fluid requirements, the bedside nurse can assess the pediatric patient for signs and symptoms of dehydration. The degree of dehydration can be classified as mild, moderate, or severe[3]:

- Mild dehydration: The child is restless, thirsty, and alert; has a normal pulse rate and strength; and has normal blood pressure, respiratory rate, and fontanelles. The skin readily retracts when pinched; mucous membranes are moist; and urine output is normal. Dehydration accounts for approximately 4% to 5% body weight loss in infants or 3% in children or adolescents.
- Moderate dehydration: The child is thirsty, restless, lethargic, and irritable; has a rapid or weak pulse; has respirations that may be deep and the rate may be rapid; has a sunken fontanelle; and has normal or low blood pressure. The skin retracts slowly when pinched; mucous membranes are dry; and urine is dark and the amount reduced. Dehydration accounts for approximately 10% of body weight loss in infants and 5% to 7% in children and adolescents.
- Severe dehydration: The child is drowsy, limp, cold, and sweaty, and extremities may be cyanotic; has a rapid or feeble pulse that is sometimes difficult to palpate; and has respirations that are deep and a rate that is rapid; signs of hypotensive shock. The fontanelle is very sunken; there is no urine for several hours and no tears; and the eyes are very sunken. Dehydration accounts for approximately 15% body weight loss in infants and 7% to 9% loss in children and adolescents.

Fluid and electrolyte requirements are based on the patient's history, degree of dehydration, and presenting symptoms. The infant and child need more calories per body weight than the adult for energy expenditure because of growth. The information listed in Table 12-12 can also be used for determining normal fluid and electrolyte maintenance for infants and children. Critical illness has a major impact on the nutritional status of a child. If a child is in a critical care unit for longer than 5 to 7 days, the chances of developing a serious nutritional deficiency increases significantly.[32] Nutritional support after the initial nutritional assessment is an essential aspect of care for the child. Critical care nurses play an important role in the feeding of critically ill children. Many procedures, such as placing feeding tubes, checking gastric retentions, performing mouth care, and administering enteral or parenteral nutrition, are within the nursing domain.[32]

Parenteral Nutrition. Providing needed calories in the face of fluid restrictions is a significant problem for the critically ill infant and child if the intestinal tract is nonfunctional. One method that can provide the necessary nutrition is parenteral nutrition. This form of nutrition is given by the intravascular route, and although it does not provide greater nutrition than enteral feedings, it can give support until the enteral route for feeding is possible.[3] Table 12-13 outlines daily dextrose, lipid, and amino acid amounts; administration rates; and intravenous line concentration limits for the infant or child receiving total parenteral nutrition (TPN).

Dextrose solutions initially are titrated up gradually over several days to reach desired caloric levels to prevent hyperglycemia

TABLE 12-13 Total Parenteral Nutrition Administration for Term Infants and Children

	INFANTS AND CHILDREN			
Per 24 hours	10 kg	10-20 kg	>20 kg	Adolescents
Fluids (mL/kg)	100-125	1000 mL: add 50 mL/kg for each extra kg >10 kg		1500 mL: add 20-25 mL for each extra kg >20 kg
Calories (kcal/kg)	75-90	75-90	>40	30-60
Protein (g/kg) Max peripheral: 2 g/kg/day Max central: 3.5 g/kg/day	2-2.5	1.5-2.5	1.5-2.5	1-2
Dextrose (%) Max peripheral: 10%-12.5% Max central: 30%	5-30	5-30	5-30	5-30
Fat (g/kg/day)	1-3	1-3	1-3	1-3

	Infants and Children (>2.5 kg and <11 yr)	Children and Adults (>11 yr)
Vitamins (mL/day) MVI-peds (vit K = 0.2 mg/5 mL) MVI-13 (vit K = 0.15 mg/10 mL)	5 mL/day	10 mL/day
Heparin*	0-0.5 unit/mL	0-0.5 unit/mL
Levocarnitine†	>30 days = 5 mg/kg/day	>30 days = 1-5 mg/kg/day

*Recommended for slow infusion rates.
†Prematurity or TPN dependent.
MVI, multiple vitamins for infusion; PN, parenteral nutrition; TPN, total parenteral nutrition.
Based on the guidelines from American Society for Parenteral and Enteral Nutrition.

and to allow endogenous insulin secretions to adjust. Intravenous fat emulsion may be started at the same time as the amino acid and dextrose solution. The rate of infusion of the fat emulsion is increased in a stepwise manner.[33] The preferred route for parenteral nutrition administration is through a central venous catheter. There are four types of central venous catheters: peripherally inserted central catheter (PICC) and nontunneled, tunneled, and totally implanted venous devices (ports).[3] The administration of parenteral nutrition requires close attention to the administration, nutritional requirements and monitoring, and patient assessments.

Enteral Nutrition. The enteral route is important for providing nutrition to a child.[32] Its advantages are convenience, safety, and low cost. The enteral route also is important in maintaining gastrointestinal mucosal integrity and immunologic function.[32]

Many different formulas are available for the infant and child based on age, host factors, and nutritional requirements. Amounts for formula feeds are based on needed kilocalories per kilogram per day (kcal/kg/day) and tolerance for each child and the clinical condition. For the full term infant younger than 1 year, cow's milk (Enfamil, Similac) or soy-based formulas (Isomil, ProSobee) are most commonly given. Standard dilution for infant formulas is 20 kcal/ounce.[33] Human breast milk is highly recommended for feedings for infants. Feedings designed specifically for children between 1 and 6 years old include infant formulas, pediatric follow-up formulas, pediatric enteral

formulas, various homemade and blenderized feedings, and commercial adult formulas.[35] Adult formulas can be given to children older than 6 years. Osmolite and Isocal are preferred for their isotonicity and caloric and protein content.

Continuous gavage feedings have advantages over bolus feedings. The risk for aspiration is less, particularly for the infant with reflux. In practice, the individual child's tolerance ultimately dictates the method on how the formula is delivered. Feeding pumps are typically used to control the rate of continuous drip-feeding. The important features of the enteral pump for use with children is the ability to provide low delivery rates (<5 mL/hr) and to advance in small increments (1-5 mL/hr).[35]

Gastric and duodenal or jejunal feeding tubes are used to administer enteral feeds in the critically ill child.[32] Gastric feeding tubes can be placed easily at the bedside by the nurse. Determining the insertion length of a nasogastric tube in the child has traditionally been the same as that in the adult—naris to ear to xyphoid process. However, this measurement may not always allow for all the side holes of a feeding tube to be in the stomach. Measuring to a point between the xyphoid and the umbilicus is a safer method. Table 12-14 provides guidelines for gavage feeding tube sizes and feeding rates for infants and children. Nasoduodenal feeding tubes are recommended to reduce the risk of aspiration in the presence of delayed gastric emptying or reflux. Gastric retention, diarrhea, and abdominal distention can limit the use of enteral nutrition. Parenteral

TABLE 12-14 Guidelines for Gavage Feeding in Infants and Children

Parameters	Age and Size Determinations				
Age	3 mo	6 mo	2 yr	5 yr	10 yr
Tube size	6 Fr	8 Fr	10 Fr	12 Fr	14 Fr

Method	Initial Volume and Rate	Advancement Volume and Rate
Bolus	2-5 mL/kg every 3-4 hr over 20 min	2-5 mL/kg every other feeding
Continuous	1-2 mL/kg/hr; initial volume not to exceed 55 mL/hr regardless of child's weight	1-2 mL/kg every 8-12 hr

Fr, French.

nutrition should be considered when it is impossible to obtain enteral access or when enteral nutrition cannot meet the child's nutritional requirements.[32]

PAIN MANAGEMENT

The past 20 years of research has witnessed remarkable growth in pediatric pain management. Research has proven that infants and children do feel pain; when they are not treated, there are increased morbidity and mortality rates and hyperalgesia. There can be a negative impact on development of the infant or child. Pain is defined as an unpleasant sensory and emotional experience associated with actual or potential tissue damage or described in terms of such damage.[41]

PHYSIOLOGY AND PHARMACOKINETICS

Neurotransmitters and peripheral and central neural pathways for pain transmission are developed and are functional before birth, and they continue to mature during the first 2 years of life. After the age of 2 years, the perception of pain is the same for adults and children, but the psychosocial and behavioral expressions of the responses to pain change with the child's growth and developmental stage.[3] The nerve tracks to the brain are myelinated by 30 weeks' gestation, and the thalamocortical tracks are myelinated by 37 weeks' gestation, indicating that neonates can perceive all forms of pain. There is no perfect guide for providing analgesia to a pediatric patient. Children may demonstrate a wide variety in the medications needed, the duration and dosing requirements, and the responses to the medications.[3] Each child must be monitored for his or her response to the pain therapy.

The physiologic effects of untreated pain in the child can result in the following:
- Hyperglycemia from decreased insulin secretion with breakdown of carbohydrate and fat stores
- Metabolic acidosis from increased use of fat
- Increased corticosteroids, growth hormone, and catecholamines
- Increased pulmonary vascular resistance
- Hypoxemia

ASSESSMENT

Pain assessment is the key to good pain management. Many of the factors that influence an adult's pain also influence a child's pain. One difference is the influence of parental anxiety and behavior regarding their child's overall experience of pain. Although most of the pain research has involved procedural pain, it is important to be cognizant of the acute and chronic pain and distress associated with the critical care unit and its repetitive procedures.

The child may not spontaneously express his or her need for pain treatment. Staff members must be vigilant and actively explore a child's level of pain whenever the potential for pain exists. A child's verbal statement of pain is the most reliable indicator in acute pain management. However, this approach may not be possible with the preverbal child, the child who cannot comprehend the request to symbolically identify pain, or the child who has a significantly altered level of consciousness. For the child up to age 3 years, behavioral scales are used as the primary source for pain assessment, and physiologic parameters are used as secondary sources. One such tool is the face, legs, activity, crying, and consolability (FLACC) postoperative pain scale.

For the child at least 6 years old, self-reports are the primary assessment tool, with behavioral scales used as secondary sources. For the child 3 to 6 years old, self-reports can be used but with a caveat. Many self-report scales have been tested as effective with this age group, but the young child 3 to 4 years old may have difficulty using them. Cognitive ability may not be advanced enough, or the child might have regressed in cognitive ability because of the illness. The child's rating may indicate a mood state rather than pain. Within this age group, self-reports and behavioral scales may need to be used together to get a true picture of the child's pain. One of the most valuable clues to pain relief is a change in behavior and vital signs after the administration of pain medication.

Parents often are the primary source of information about how their child exhibits pain. Parents are sensitive to changes in the child's behavior and often want to be involved in efforts for the child's pain relief.[6] Encouraging parents to be involved gives them a sense of control and helping. Parents usually know what comfort measures to take with their children when they are in pain. For most children, having the supportive presence of their parents provides the most comfort. Figure 8-5 in Chapter 8 shows pain-rating scales.

TREATMENT OF PAIN

Some general principles are applied to the management of pain in children:

- *Prevention of pain.* If pain can be anticipated, pain should be treated prophylactically.
- *Adequate assessment.* Developmentally appropriate assessment tools are available.
- *Multimodal approach.* Analgesics; physical strategies such as massage, acupuncture, and hot/cold therapies; and behavioral, cognitive, and psychological approaches are available.
- *Parental involvement.* Parents are the best source of information about their child. They can be taught different strategies to help their child with the pain.
- *Nonnoxious routes.* The route of administration of analgesia should be as painless as possible.
- *Pain control during procedures.* Inadequate pain control during procedures can create an atmosphere of anxiety and increased pain during subsequent procedures.

Nonsteroidal Antiinflammatory Drugs. Nonsteroidal antiinflammatory drugs (NSAIDs) are effective for the management of mild to moderate pain, and they can be used in combination with opioids. They have superior antiinflammatory properties compared with aspirin or acetaminophen.[3] The drawback to NSAIDs is that there is a ceiling effect and that they affect the gastric mucosa, decrease platelet aggregation, and cause peptic ulcer formation and hepatic dysfunction. It is recommended that an H_2-receptor blocker be given concurrently for prolonged use of these medications.[36] The use of NSAIDS should be avoided in children with a history of severe renal disease, dehydration, or heart failure.[36] Examples of NSAIDS

commonly used are ibuprofen and ketorolac (1 mg/kg given intravenously). Ketorolac is the only NSAID that is approved for parenteral use by the U.S. Food and Drug Administration.[37]

Opioid Analgesics. Narcotic analgesics are the single most important class of medications for the relief of moderate to severe pain. Administration of narcotics requires decisions about the route of administration of the medication, the choice of narcotic, and the method of administration.

The most commonly used narcotics for the child are morphine (0.02 to 0.1 mg/kg given intravenously), fentanyl (0.5 to 1.5 µg/kg given intravenously), and hydromorphone (0.005 to 0.2 mg/kg given intravenously). Methadone (0.1 mg/kg) is an extremely long-acting narcotic, but it is not used as commonly for acute pain control. This drug is used for weaning from iatrogenic narcotic dependency or for chronic pain control.[3] Meperidine (0.75 mg/kg) is not a drug of choice because it decreases cardiac output and causes tachycardia. The drug's metabolite lowers the child's seizure threshold, causing hyperexcitability with multiple dosing. Opioids are given by intravenous push (IVP), continuous infusion, patient-controlled analgesia (PCA), or epidurals. Table 12-15 outlines standard dosages of morphine and fentanyl for the infant and child. Ketorolac in combination with morphine PCA in children has provided a very effective combination of analgesia.[37]

Naloxone is an opioid antagonist that is required if the child becomes unresponsive after receiving narcotics, the respirations become shallow and less than eight per minute, and the pupils become pinpoint. The initial dose is 1-2 µg/kg/dose given intravenously over 2 minutes. The patient will need to be observed for the response to the medication. If patient is not responsive, the medication is continued until a total dose of 10 µg/kg/dose has been given.[36]

Topical Anesthetics. The use of topical analgesic ointments reduces the local pain of procedures such as suturing or venipuncture and reduces the child's anticipated pain and anxiety over the upcoming procedure. The use of these agents

TABLE 12-15 Opioid Dosages for Infants and Children

AGENT	AGE	DOSAGE
Morphine		
Intravenous push (IVP)	<6 mo	0.03-0.05 mg/kg/dose
	>6 mo	0.1 mg/kg/dose
Continuous infusion	<6 mo	0.01-0.015 mg/kg/hr + IVP loading dose
	>6 mo	0.02-0.03 mg/kg/hr + IVP loading dose
Patient-controlled analgesia (PCA)		0.02-0.03 mg/kg/hr continuous + boluses
Epidural		0.03-0.1 mg/kg bolus q 6-12 hr
Fentanyl		
Intravenous (short procedure)		2-3 mcg/kg/dose (if sedation used: 1-2 mcg/kg/dose)
Continuous infusion (intubated)		10 mcg/kg loading dose + 2.5 mcg/kg/hr
Epidural		0.2-2 mcg/kg/hr, possibly with bupivacaine

has been expanded to include pain reduction for lumbar punctures or bone marrow aspiration. Some of the ointments take approximately 10-60 minutes to be effective. EMLA cream, a combination of lidocaine and prilocaine, was introduced in the 1990s. It takes at least 1 hour to produce acceptable anesthesia. This ointment should not be used on patients with methemoglobinemia-predisposing conditions.[36] ElaMax is a topical formulation of 4% lidocaine that is encapsulated by liposomes, which create lipid solubility and allow transdermal drug delivery. ElaMax provides anesthesia in about 30 minutes.[36] Lidocaine iontophoresis allows active transdermal delivery of lidocaine under the influence of a low-level electric current. It is available under the name of Numby Stuff. Numby provides topical anesthesia to the child in as little as 10 minutes.

Nonpharmacologic Management of Pain. Nonpharmacologic techniques should be used to supplement, not replace, the use of pain medications. Some of the nonpharmacologic interventions that can be used in children include distraction, relaxation, guided imagery, and cutaneous stimulation.[6] The use of these techniques can decrease the perceived threat of pain, provide a sense of control, enhance the child's comfort, and allow for rest or sleep. These nonpharmacologic techniques are safe, noninvasive, and usually inexpensive, and most are independent nursing functions.[6]

PSYCHOSOCIAL ISSUES OF THE CHILD AND FAMILY

An unplanned admission of a child to a critical care unit, including those with illnesses or injuries, can be a traumatic event for the parents and the child.[6] In a crisis situation, the parents can be overwhelmed and become focused solely on the physiologic well-being of their child. If the child is conscious, he or she desperately needs the continual physical presence and emotional support of the parents; however, this is a time when it can be very difficult for the parents to help their child emotionally. Critical care nurses encounter the child and family at a very emotionally vulnerable time. Parents can view the nurses and physicians as a lifeline, controlling the needs and the life of their child.[3] The critical care nurse needs to be knowledgeable about childhood cognitive and emotional development and about family dynamics to assist the child and the family through this health crisis. The following sections address some common issues that hospitalized children and their families face during hospitalization.

THE ILL CHILD'S EXPERIENCE OF CRITICAL ILLNESS

The term *family-centered care* defines the focus of care for a child because the nursing care of a child not only involves the child but the family as a whole. Family-centered care supports the child's family by prioritizing the family members' needs and values and empowering the family unit.[6] Two basic concepts in family-centered care are *enabling* and *empowering*. The critical care staff can enable the families by creating opportunities and means for family members to display their present abilities. Empowerment describes the interaction of the staff members with the families in a way that allows the families to maintain control or acquire a sense of control over their lives.[6]

The emotional reactions of the child to hospitalization depend on the type and quantity of stress produced by the illness itself, the hospitalization experience, and the notions that the child has about the situation. The final outcome is influenced by the child's age and level of development. A child in the critical care unit experiences significant stress, and the important question is whether the child's capacity to cope physically or emotionally in an age-appropriate fashion is exceeded.

Three elements can help a child cope successfully with a crisis: a resilient personality, a supportive family, and an outside support system.[3] The critical care health team can serve as the outside support system, applying the family-centered concept as they reinforce and strengthen the coping efforts of the child and family. Nurses must take every opportunity to reassure the parents that they are an integral part of the child's care and recovery. When children were asked whom or what helped the most while they were in the PICU, 43% stated their nurses and 29% said their families.[38] This is not a surprising finding considering that the critical care nurse has the most contact with the child in the intensive care unit and provides most of the care to the child.[38]

The critically ill child needs the physical presence of the parents (or primary caretaker) at the bedside. Young children are most frightened by the separation from parents. Unrestricted visitation (i.e., 24 hr/day) for parents is imperative. The parents are the most reassuring persons in the child's eyes and are needed psychologically by the child to believe that he or she will not be abandoned, left to be unsafe, or left in pain and distress. Anxiety and fear are easily heightened when the child recognizes scary words or fills in ambiguities heard with his or her own distorted interpretations. For the child who is very ill and prostrate, anxieties may fester within the child, unknown to staff members. Every member of the health care team should have an understanding of the five phases of development of logical thought to communicate effectively with a child and should understand the basis of a child's perceptions, fears, and misunderstandings.[3]

During infancy, the infant and the primary caregiver bond and develop the ability to signal one another. Oral gratification is very important to infants and can provide them comfort. Touch is also important; infants need to be caressed, cuddled, and comforted by being held close to the body. A major source of fear for the young infant is separation from parents. The critical care environment disrupts the infant's normal sleep cycle and feeding routines and can provide noxious and sometimes painful stimuli. Sleep deprivation or sensory overload can be interpreted as irritability or lethargy.[3]

Toddlers are at high risk for emotional sequelae related to the experiences of hospitalization and separation from parents. The critical care unit can be very frightening because of all the unfamiliar faces routines, sights, and sounds.[3] Any procedure that is painful may be perceived as punishment. If possible, parents should remain with the toddler as much as possible for comfort. Parents should not be asked to participate in painful procedures but should be there to comfort the child afterward. Most of a toddler's time is spent in play. Passive play, such as music, mobiles, toys that make sounds, and movies, can be used in a critical care environment and can involve the family members.

The preschool-age child can tolerate brief separations from parents and is less upset by strangers than the toddler. The major fears of this age group include bodily injury and mutilation, loss of control, the unknown, the dark, and being left alone. This anxiety can be lessened by telling the child that his parents or nurse are close by. The coping style a preschooler uses often is apparent when the child is hospitalized. Withdrawal, projection, aggression, or regression may be observed behaviors.[3] Sleeping is one type of activity that children can use to maintain control when in an environment that allows them very little control.[38] Play is an important aspect of care for a child, and it can help the preschooler cope with the anger and fear about procedures. Preschool children are very verbal, and health care workers may forget how vulnerable and immature these children are.

The school-age years are ones of accomplishment and tremendous intellectual growth. The major crisis of the school years is the resolution of the balance between assuming new knowledge and skills. However, this can cause of sense of inferiority if attempts at tasks or goals are met with repeated failure. This age group enters a period of concrete operational thought. The school-age child can become accustomed to brief separations from family members but takes comfort and strength from their presence. The hospitalized school-age child is forced to depend on others for basic personal care and hygiene, and this can create stress. The health care team needs to respect the child's privacy and modesty and enable the child to make some choices regarding personal care.[3] In addition to the child's parents, members of the child's peer group play an important role in providing comfort and support.

Adolescence is a time of great physical and psychological change. Critical illness or injury may cause a crisis for children in this age group. The major threats of hospitalization for adolescents are loss of control and of identity, change in body appearance or image, and separation from their peer group.[3] It is hard for adolescents to be surrounded by strangers who are discussing their personal information. The adolescent may use a variety of coping strategies while hospitalized, such as denial, regression, withdrawal, intellectualization, projection, and displacement.[3] The critical care staff should support the adolescent's attempt to master the situation and help to provide support. Their questions should be answered honestly, and any misconceptions they may have should be clarified. The adolescent should be allowed to be an integral part of the decision making about their care and to make choices when possible. They should be allowed to maintain contact with their peer group if possible. The nurse should teach the adolescent coping techniques, such as relaxation, deep breathing, and the use of imagery.[3]

THE PARENTS' EXPERIENCE OF A CHILD'S CRITICAL ILLNESS

Parents may experience a staged response not unlike the grief process when their child is admitted to the critical care unit.[3] With a sudden illness or injury, the initial emotions can be shock, disbelief, and denial. These feelings may last for a few hours or a few days. Parents may question the diagnosis or want to prove the physician wrong. The situation can feel unreal, as if it were not happening to them. It may be difficult to grasp the totality of what has happened to their child. They can feel immobile and not know what they should do next. The parents may find it difficult to remember and process explanations given to them about what is happening with their child. This is usually a defense against pain. Forgetting can result in some parents feeling that staff members do not explain much to them. Other parents may feel that this is a sign of their own inadequacy. Explanations about their child's condition may have to be given in small amounts of information with compassion and repetition. Some parents may appear outwardly as competent and composed during the height of the crisis, but this should not be interpreted as the parents being less stressed or anxious.

Parents need to be reunited with their child, if this is their wish, as soon as they have been prepared about what to expect. However, parents may be afraid to see their child. Changes in their child's appearance and in the child's emotional reactions can be very upsetting to parents. If the child is conscious and relatively alert, the parents need to be informed that their child may show some form of regressive behavior, such as withdrawal or anger, which is expected given the stress of the situation and the degree of illness or injury. Parents also can feel frightened about touching or talking to their child, believing this may harm the child. They must be reassured that it is okay to do this and that if there are any concerns, staff will be present in the room.

Intense anxiety can make parents question whether their reactions are normal. They wonder how other parents feel or behave. They can be extremely frightened by the intensity of their feelings and may wonder whether they will have a breakdown. These feelings are common in a crisis, and parents need to hear that their feelings are understandable. Some parents may behave with hostility toward staff or family members. Some may behave quite rigidly, visiting only briefly or not asking questions in an attempt to maintain composure.

Anger is an emotion that usually takes its toll after the crisis period, usually with longer critical care unit stays. Destructive anger occurs when parents seek justification for their anger by blaming others for their child's condition. They are unreasonably critical of the health care team and may make complaints about the child's care as a manifestation of the anger. Parents may become depressed as they realize the severity of their child's condition. At this time, the parents should be given an opportunity to express their feelings and participate in activities such as bathing the child.

The critical care nurse can assist the parents by clarifying information and by helping them to support their child.[3] During crises, communication with the parents must be frequent and clear. Key elements to effective communication include communication at frequent, predictable intervals; use of consistent, understandable terminology; provision of opportunities for parents to ask questions and express opinions; and assistance of support personnel.[3]

Critical care nurses who care directly for the child and their parents have the greatest degree of contact with the family. In addition to the nurse's role in psychological assessment and intervention, other support staff members should be available to assist the family. Clinical nurse specialists can assess parental worries and concerns and, based on the assessment, help the parents to make plans to address their concerns.[39] Social workers can provide the family support and advocacy during their time of crisis. Many intensive care units also have access to child life specialists, chaplains, discharge planners, and ethicists to assist in providing psychosocial support to the families.[31] An important role of the critical care nurse is to mobilize and introduce the families to the support staff available in their institutions for their support. The case study (Pediatric Patient in the Adult Intensive Care Unit) discusses some of these concepts.

Summary

- Children are physically, physiologically, and emotionally immature, and they are different from adults.
- Complete respiratory failure may develop rapidly in a child when respiratory distress is present.
- Bradycardia is an ominous sign in the seriously ill or injured child.
- Hypotension is typically only a late sign of hypotensive shock in children.
- Head injury is a primary insult to the child. Patient outcomes will be comprised if secondary insults such as hypotension or hypoxemia occur.
- Most children in the intensive care unit experience pain and anxiety, and they should be treated accordingly.
- The concept of family-centered care recognizes that the family is the one constant in a child's life.

Case Study: Pediatric Patient in the Adult Critical Care Unit

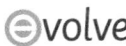 Answers to the Case Study Questions can be found on the Evolve web site at http://evolve.elsevier.com/Urden/.

Brief Patient History
A 2-month-old infant is admitted directly to the intensive care unit with a history of vomiting and diarrhea over the past 24 hours. The mother reports that the infant was irritable yesterday but is more lethargic today. The infant has had three wet diapers over the past 24 hours, and the urine appears dark. She continues not to tolerate any formula or Pedialyte.

Clinical Assessment
Physical assessment reveals the following—weight: 6.84 kg (weight 1 week prior: 7.6 kg), temperature: 38.5° C; pulse: 180; respiratory rate: 46-50; BP: 60/43; pulse oximetry: 93%. The infant's lips and mucous membranes are dry and tacky. Her fontanelle is sunken. Extremities are cool and mottled, nail beds are dusky, and capillary refill is 4 seconds. Pulses are rapid and weak both centrally and peripherially. The infant is lethargic.

Diagnostic Procedures
The infant is placed on oxygen, and IV access is attained. A point-of-care testing glucose reveals a blood sugar of 60.

Medical Diagnosis
This infant presents in the intensive care unit with a diagnosis of hypovolemic, hypotensive shock.

Questions
1. For the bedside nurse, what is the priority in caring for this infant?
2. What category of shock applies to this situation?
3. Describe the pathophysiology of hypovolemic shock in the pediatric patient.
4. What are the two goals of therapy?
5. What level of dehydration does this infant appear to suffer?
6. Describe how and when to treat hypoglycemia in infants.
7. What is the fluid of choice to treat the volume deficit?
8. After the infant has received the initial volume replacement of two normal saline boluses, the infant is aroucable. Vital signs are the following—pulse: 160; BP: 70/40, capillary refill is 3 seconds, blood glucose is 80. What is the next step in the treatment of the infant's hypovolemic shock?

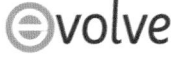 Be sure to check out the bonus material, including free self-assessment exercises, on the Evolve web site at http://evolve.elsevier.com/Urden/.

References

1. Mullen J, Frances, M: Caring for critically ill children and their families. In Slota M, editor: *Core curriculum for pediatric critical care nursing*, ed 2, St Louis, 2006, Mosby.
2. Guice K et al: Traumatic injury and children: a national assessment. *J Trauma* 36:S68-S80 2007.
3. Hazinski MF: *Manual of pediatric critical care*, St Louis, 1999, Mosby.
4. Ralston M et al: *Pediatric Advanced Life Support*, Dallas, *2006.* American Heart Association.
5. Grant M, Webster H: Pulmonary system. In Slota M, editor: *Core curriculum for pediatric critical care nursing*, ed 2, St Louis, 2006, Mosby.
6. Hockenberry M et al: *Wong's nursing care of infants and children*, ed 7, St Louis, 2003, Mosby.
7. Knudson M, McGrath J: Improving outcomes in pediatric trauma care: essential characteristics of the trauma center, *J Trauma* 63:S140-S142, 2007.
8. Kacmarek R et al: *The essentials of respiratory care*, ed 4, St Louis, 2005, Mosby.
9. Amin R: Chronic respiratory failure. In Chernick V et al, editors: *Kendig's disorders of the respiratory tract in children*, ed 7, Philadelphia, 2006, WB Saunders.

10. Frankel L, Kache S: Mechanical ventilation. In Kliegman R et al, editors: *Nelson's textbook of pediatrics*, ed 18, Philadelphia, 2007, WB Saunders.

11. Calogero C, Sly P: Acute viral bronchiolitis: to treat or not to treat—that is the question, *J Pediatr* 151:235-237, 2007.

12. Mansbach J et al: US outpatient office visits for bronchiolitis, 1993-2004, *Ambul Pediatr* 7:304-307, 2007.

13. American Academy of Pediatrics Subcommittee on Diagnosis and Management of Bronchiolitis: Diagnosis and management of bronchiolitis, *Pediatrics*, 118:1774-1793, 2006.

14. Wohl M: Bronchiolitis. In Chernick V et al, editors: *Kendig's disorders of the respiratory tract in children*, ed 7, Philadelphia, 2006, WB Saunders.

15. Cambonie G et al: Clinical effects of Heliox administration for acute bronchiolitis in young infants, *Chest* 129:676-682, 2006.

16. Buckmaster A et al: Continuous positive airway pressure therapy for infants with respiratory distress in nontertiary care centers: a randomized controlled trial, *Pediatrics* 120:509-518, 2007.

17. Marcoux K: Current management of status asthmaticus in the pediatric ICU, *Crit Care Nurs Clin North Am* 17:463-479, 2005.

18. Ciarallo L et al: Higher-dose intravenous magnesium therapy for children with moderate to severe acute asthma, *Arch Pediatr Adolesc Med* 154:979-983, 2000.

19. National Institutes of Health: Consensus Development Conference on Infantile Apnea and Home Monitoring, consensus statement, *Pediatrics* 17:292-299, 1987.

20. Okada K et al: Discharge diagnoses in infants with apparent life-threatening event, *Pediatr Int* 45:560-563, 2003.

21. Kiechl-Kohlendorfer U et al: Epidemiology of apparent life threatening events, *Arch Dis Child* 90:297-300, 2005.

22. Ibsen L, Ungerleider R: Perioperative management of patient with congenital heart disease: a multidisciplinary approach. In Nichols D et al, editors: *Critical heart disease in infants and children*, ed 2, Philadelphia, 2006, Mosby.

23. Park M: *Pediatric cardiology for practitioners*, ed 5, Philadelphia, 2008, Mosby.

24. Schell K: Evidence-based practice: noninvasive blood pressure measurement in children, *Pediatric Nursing* 23:263-266, 2006.

25. Callow L, Suddaby E: Cardiovascular system. In Slota M, editor: *Core curriculum for pediatric critical care nursing*, ed 2, St Louis, 2006, WB Saunders.

26. Finer N et al: Obstructive, mixed, and central apnea in the neonate: physiological correlates, *J Pediatr* 121:943-950, 1992.

27. Bryant R, Schultz R: The child with cerebral dysfunction. In Hockenberry MJ et al, editors: *Wong's nursing care of infants and children*, ed 8, St Louis, 2007, Mosby.

28. Vernon-Levett P: Neurologic system. In Slota M, editor: *Core curriculum for pediatric critical care nursing*, ed 2, St Louis, 2006, WB Saunders.

29. Ochoa C et al: Prior studies comparing outcomes from trauma care at children's hospitals versus adult hospitals, *J Trauma* 63:S87-S91,2007.

30. Pasek TA, Etzel KA: Multisystem issues. In Slota M, editor: *Core curriculum for pediatric critical care nursing*, ed 2, St Louis, 2006, Saunders.

31. Smith J, Martin S: Caring practice: providing developmentally supportive care. In Curley M, Maloney-Harmon P, editors: *Critical care nursing of infants and children*, ed 2, Philadelphia, 2001, WB Saunders.

32. Ista E, Joosten K: Nutritional assessment and enteral support of critically ill children, *Crit Care Nurs Clin North Am* 17:385-393, 2005.

33. Shuman R, Phillips S: Parental nutrition indications, administration, and monitoring. In Baker S et al, editors: *Pediatric nutrition support*, Sudbury, MA, 2007, Jones & Bartlett.

34. Bryant R: The child with cerebral dysfunction. In Hockenberry M et al, editors: *Wong's essentials of pediatric nursing*, ed 7, St Louis, 2005, Mosby.

35. Nevin-Filino N, Miller M: Enteral nutrition. In Samour P, King K, editors: *Handbook of pediatric nutrition*, ed 3, Sudbury, MA, 2003, Jones & Bartlett.

36. Taketomo C et al, editors: *Pediatric dosage handbook*, ed 12, Hudson, OH, 2005, Lexi-Comp.

37. Drain C: *Perianesthesia nursing: a critical care approach*, ed 4, St Louis, 2003, WB Saunders.

38. Board R: School-age children's perceptions of their PICU hospitalization, *Pediatr Nurse* 31:166-175, 2005.

39. McNelis A et al: Concerns with needs of children with epilepsy and their parents, *Clin Nurse Spec* 21:195-202, 2007.

40. Langley J, Bradley J: Defining pneumonia in critically ill infants and children, *Pediatr Crit Care Med* 6:S9-S13, 2005.

41. The International Association for the Study of Pain® (IASP®) www.iasppain.org/AM/Template.cfm?Section=Pain_Definitions&Template=/CM/HTMLDisplay.cfm&ContentID=1728 (accessed March 2009).

Chapter 13

High-Risk and Critical Care in Obstetric Issues

*I*nnovations in technology and advances in treatment options have placed the worlds of critical care and obstetrics on a pathway of collaboration and sometimes of conflict. Traditionally, the two specialties have been separated in part because of the typical normalcy and health-oriented approach of obstetrics and the crisis and illness orientation of critical care. Pregnancy alters the function of virtually every organ system, and the baseline state and patient response to physiologic changes are very different in the pregnant patient. Fetal considerations often are important in designing and leading the clinical approach to the critically ill woman. There are many common conditions in pregnancy that require special medical care with associated complications that have the potential for serious maternal morbidity and mortality. An alarming trend in maternal mortality is race-specific pregnancy-related mortality rates. Analysis of rates has demonstrated that African American women are more than four times as likely to die from pregnancy-related causes as white women.[1] Concern for maternal mortality has caused public health priorities for 2010 to include the goal of reducing maternal mortality to no more than 3.3 maternal deaths per 100,000 live births.[1]

It is important to recognize that critical care obstetrics encompasses two distinct populations: women with preexisting disease who become pregnant and women with normal pregnancies who become compromised by critical illness or injury. The two priorities for the pregnant critically ill woman are supporting fetal growth and development and optimizing the maternal and family experience.

It is impossible to discuss every aspect of management of the critically ill obstetric patient in one chapter. Instead, the focus is to provide a synopsis of the more commonly seen conditions or concerns in the realm of critical care obstetrics and to emphasize the collaborative nature of this emerging field, recognizing that the manifestations and management of critical illness are typically identical in pregnant and nonpregnant patients, although the data value changes associated with pregnancy must be considered. Nursing management, unless unique to the critically ill obstetric patient, is not detailed here.

RISKS TO FETAL DEVELOPMENT

Factors that influence embryonic and fetal development may be intrinsic or extrinsic in nature. Intrinsic factors such as chromosomal abnormalities and congenital anomalies account for 25% of all birth defects.[2] Extrinsic factors such as radiation exposure,

bacterial, fungal, and viral infections, medication exposure, and unknown causes account for those remaining.[2] Exposure to ionizing radiation is usually not a concern until more than a cumulative 100 to 200 mGy (10 to 20 rads) have been exceeded, but some experts express caution for the first 25 weeks due to fetal organogenesis and central nervous system development.[3-6] The radiation dose received by the unshielded fetus is approximately 30% of the dose the mother receives, but as digital technology improves, the amount of radiation required for some studies is decreasing.[3,4] Table 13-1 lists radiation exposures of common radiologic studies, although estimated doses can vary widely from source to source.[4-8]

Medication use in critically ill obstetric patients requires analysis of the risk-benefit ratio. Often, the benefit may outweigh the potential fetal risk when all factors are considered. It is important to consider the influence that drug exposure can have on the developing fetus. Box 13-1 describes the U.S. Food and Drug Administration (FDA) labeling regarding a drug's risk to a fetus.[2,9,10]

Technologic advances, improvements in maternal-fetal diagnostics, and aggressive neonatal interventions have improved the survival of extremely low-birth-weight infants. Research has placed minimal viability parameters between 23 and 24 weeks' gestation and fetal weight between 500 and 1000 g (0.5 and 1 kg). Critical care clinicians may encounter situations in which extrauterine viability, fetal outcomes, and maternal stability are uncertain. Clinical decisions must be made in light of the maternal-fetal risk-benefit ratio. Personal, cultural, spiritual, and social beliefs regarding viability may affect the clinical decision-making process. Parental and family beliefs and desires may conflict with those of the health care team. When confronting the dilemma of viability, the parameters of gestational age, fetal weight, parental desires, and maternal-fetal mortality must be considered.

PHYSIOLOGIC ALTERATIONS IN PREGNANCY

During pregnancy, the woman's body undergoes profound physiologic changes. These changes are necessary to maintain the pregnancy and to allow for fetal growth and development. So dramatic are the changes that they would probably be considered pathologic in the nonpregnant woman. Adaptations occur in nearly every organ system, beginning during the first week of gestation and continuing until up to 6 weeks after

TABLE 13-1 Radiation Doses from Radiologic Studies

Radiologic Study	Estimated Fetal Dose (1 mGy = 0.1 rad)
Conventional X-ray Studies	
Skull	<0.01 mGy (<0.001 rad)
Cervical spine	<0.01 mGy (<0.001 rad)
Thoracic spine	<0.01 mGy (<0.001 rad)
Lumbar spine	1.7 mGy (0.17 rad)
Chest	<0.01 mGy (<0.001 rad)
Abdomen	1.4 mGy (0.14 rad)
Pelvis	1.1 mGy (0.11 rad)
Pelvimetry	0.024 mGy (0.0024 rad)
CT Studies	
Head	<0.005 mGy (<0.0005 rad)
Chest	0.06 mGy (0.006 rad)
Spiral (helical)	0.003-0.02 mGy (0.0003-0.002 rad)
Abdominal	8 mGy (0.8 rad)
Lumbar spine	2.4 mGy (0.24 rad)
Pelvis	25 mGy (2.5 rad)
Fluoroscopic and Nuclear Medicine Studies	
Upper GI tract	1.1 mGy (0.11 rad)
Lower GI tract	6.8 mGy (0.68 rad)
Venography	5 mGy (0.5 rad)
Pulmonary angiography through the femoral vein	2.2-3.7 mGy (0.22-0.37 rad)
Ventilation scan	0.1-0.3 mGy (0.01-0.03 rad)
Perfusion scan	0.4-0.6 mGy (0.04-0.06 rad)

GI, gastrointestinal; Gy, gray; IV, intravenous.

delivery. The only system in which there are no documented characteristic changes is the nervous system. Understanding the physiologic adaptations is important to the management of the critically ill pregnant woman. In the limited space of this chapter, the physiologic changes are summarized, with special attention given to areas that affect or are affected by critical illness or injury. More detailed information can be found in textbooks dedicated to obstetric issues.

ENDOCRINE SYSTEM

Hormonal changes are necessary for the initiation and maintenance of pregnancy. Maintenance of adequate estrogen and progesterone levels is essential (Box 13-2). During pregnancy, estrogen production increases approximately 1000-fold.[11,12]

BOX 13-2 PRIMARY FUNCTIONS AND IMPLICATIONS OF ESTROGEN AND PROGESTERONE

FUNCTIONS AND EFFECTS OF ESTROGEN
- Promote growth and function of the uterus
- Cause uterine musculature hypertrophy and hyperplasia
- Increase blood supply to uteroplacental unit
- Promote breast (ductal, alveolar, nipple) development
- Increase pliability of connective tissue
  - Relax pelvic joints and ligaments
  - Allow cervical softening
- Promote sodium and water retention
- Produce psychological changes leading to emotional lability
- Decrease gastric secretion of hydrochloric acid and pepsin
- Increase sensitivity to carbon dioxide (CO_2) levels in the blood
- Produce integumentary changes
  - Hyperpigmentation
  - Striae gravida
- Affect blood component concentrations
  - Increase fibrinogen (factor 1) concentration
  - Decrease plasma protein concentration
  - Cause leukocytosis

FUNCTIONS AND EFFECTS OF PROGESTERONE
- Decrease maternal smooth muscle contractility
  - Uterus: prevent contractility
  - Gastrointestinal tract: contribute to nausea, heartburn, and constipation
  - Renal system: contribute to urinary dilation leading to urinary stasis
  - Vascular system: dilate vessels and contribute to peripheral edema
- Produce metabolic effects
  - Reset hypothalamus up approximately 0.2° C (0.5° F)
  - Promote fat storage
  - Stimulate respiratory center to decrease CO_2 retention
- Stimulate secretion of sodium in the urine, thereby stimulating aldosterone production
- Promote breast development and inhibit the action of prolactin

BOX 13-1 FDA CATEGORIES OF LABELING FOR DRUG USE IN PREGNANCY

- Category A: Controlled studies in women fail to demonstrate risk to the fetus in the first 12 weeks. Possibility of fetal harm is remote.
- Category B: Animal studies do not indicate a risk to the fetus. Well-controlled studies with pregnant mothers fail to demonstrate a risk to the fetus.
- Category C: Studies have shown teratogenic effects in animal studies. There are no controlled studies in women.
- Category D: Evidence of fetal risk exists, but benefits in life-threatening or serious disease may make it acceptable despite risks.
- Category X: Studies demonstrate fetal abnormalities, or there is evidence of risk from human experience. The risk clearly outweighs the benefit.

Data from Briggs G et al: *Drugs in pregnancy and lactation*, ed 7, Baltimore, 2005, Williams & Wilkins; Riordan J, Auerbach K: *Breastfeeding and human lactation*, ed 3, Boston, 2005, Jones & Bartlett.

Progesterone is essential for maintenance of pregnancy and is first produced by the corpus luteum and then by the placental unit. Human placental lactogen (hPL) promotes maternal breakdown of lipids, causing increased levels and use of free fatty acids, and it has an anti-insulin effect, contributing to hyperglycemia. The hPL also contributes to breast growth and development, preparing the breasts for lactation. Thyroid enlargement and stimulation occur during pregnancy, causing an increase of approximately 25% in the maternal basal metabolic rate.

REPRODUCTIVE SYSTEM

Reproductive organs undergo remarkable changes during pregnancy. The uterus increases in weight 20 times and alters its capacity from 10 mL to 4.5 to 5 L. The uterus grows out of the pelvic cavity, displacing intestines laterally and superiorly. When the pregnant woman assumes a supine position, the gravid uterus may compress the inferior vena cava and aorta, decreasing venous return to the heart.

Uterine blood flow increases dramatically as pregnancy progresses—from 50 mL/min at 10 weeks to 500 mL/min at 40 weeks.[11,12] Major expansion of the uterine vascular bed contributes to the development of decreased systemic vascular resistance.

CARDIOVASCULAR SYSTEM

Pregnancy is characterized as a hyperdynamic (high-flow), low-resistance state. This is facilitated through adaptations in blood volume, cardiac structure, cardiac output, vascular resistance, and heart rate.[11,12]

Blood volume changes are as follows:
- Total blood volume increases approximately 30% to 40%, or 1 to 1.5 L.
- Blood volume maximizes between the 26th and 34th week.
- Red blood cell volume increases approximately 20%.
- Plasma volume increases 45% to 50%.
- Total-body water increases by approximately 6 to 8 L.
- Colloid oncotic pressure (COP) decreases.

Cardiac structural changes are as follows:
- The heart is displaced to the left and upward and rotates slightly anteriorly.
- There are no characteristic electrocardiographic changes.
- Left axis deviation may occur because of mechanical displacement.
- Cardiac volume increases slightly because of increased volume and hypertrophy.

Cardiac auscultatory changes are as follows:
- There is a physiologic S_1 (first heart sound) split.
- S_3 (third sound) development is considered normal.
- Systolic murmurs develop in 90% of all pregnant women.
- Diastolic murmurs develop in 20% of all pregnant women.
- Murmurs are generally physiologic in nature and disappear after delivery.

Blood pressure variations may occur during pregnancy. Blood pressure may decrease slightly during the first trimester, reach a low point in the second trimester, and then return to normal for the duration of the pregnancy. Postural hypotension may occur with sudden position changes or supine positioning.

Cardiac output changes begin early in the first trimester, peak at the end of the second trimester, and remain elevated until term. Cardiac output increases 30% to 50% during pregnancy, with normal levels usually 6 to 7 L/min.[12,14] Changes are attributed to increased blood volume, increased heart rate, and decreases in systemic vascular resistance. Heart rate increases 10 to 15 beats/min during the second trimester and usually returns to normal 6 weeks after delivery. Marked variations in cardiac output depend on maternal position[14] (Table 13-2). The American College of Obstetricians and Gynecologists (ACOG) has defined indications for hemodynamic monitoring in pregnancy[15] (Box 13-3). Table 13-3 summarizes the hemodynamic value changes associated with pregnancy, which are reflected most in the third trimester.[13,14]

PULMONARY SYSTEM

Pulmonary physiologic changes are essential to provide adequate oxygenation for the mother's increased metabolic demands and for the dependent fetus. As the uterus grows, it causes diaphragmatic elevation of approximately 4 cm, decreasing lung length. Compensatory and hormonal changes cause lower rib flaring and thoracic cage enlargement of 5 to 7 cm.[13,16]

TABLE 13-2 Positional Cardiac Output Changes in Pregnancy

Maternal Position	Cardiac Output (L/min)
Knee-chest	6.9 (±2.1)
Right lateral	6.8 (±1.3)
Left lateral	6.6 (+1 4)
Sitting	6.2 (±.0)
Supine	6.0 (±.4)
Standing	5.4 (±2.0)

BOX 13-3 INDICATIONS FOR HEMODYNAMIC MONITORING IN PREGNANCY

- Severe pregnancy-induced hypertension with persistent oliguria or pulmonary edema
- Massive hemorrhage or volume replacement needs
- Adult respiratory distress syndrome
- Shock of unknown cause
- Sepsis with oliguria or refractory hypotension
- Cardiovascular decompression during intrapartum or intraoperative periods
- Chronic disease during labor or intraoperatively (New York Heart Association class III or IV cardiac disease)
- Pulmonary edema, oliguria, or heart failure refractory to treatment or of unknown cause

Oxygen consumption increases approximately 15% to 25% throughout pregnancy. To meet these needs for additional oxygen, ventilatory changes (Fig. 13-1) must occur. Vital capacity remains unchanged during pregnancy; however, there is an increase in tidal volume and slight increase in respiratory rate. Together, these changes account for an increase in minute ventilation by approximately 50% at term.[16,17] Hyperventilation is normal and is mediated primarily by the effects of progesterone on the respiratory center. Hyperventilation causes a normal decrease in $Paco_2$ levels to approximately 28 to 32 mm Hg.[12,16] The resulting alkalosis is compensated by increased renal excretion of bicarbonate. Normal maternal Pao_2 is 101 to 108 mm Hg.[13,16] The maternal oxyhemoglobin dissociation curve shifts to the right, facilitating the exchange of carbon dioxide from the fetus to the mother and the exchange of oxygen from the mother to the fetus.

GASTROINTESTINAL AND GENITOURINARY SYSTEMS

Functional and structural gastrointestinal and genitourinary system changes occur in pregnancy. Physiologic adaptations of the gastrointestinal system are summarized in Table 13-4. Genitourinary structural changes include slight enlargement of the

TABLE 13-3 Hemodynamic Changes Associated with Term Pregnancy

Parameter	Pregnancy Normal Value	Change
Mean arterial pressure (mm Hg)	90 ± 6	No significant change
Central venous pressure (mm Hg)	8 ± 2	No significant change
Pulmonary artery wedge pressure (mm Hg)	4 ± 3	No significant change
Heart rate (beats/min)	83 ± 10	Increase 17%
Cardiac output (L/min)	6.2 ± 1.0	Increase 43%
Systemic vascular resistance (dyn $\cdot$ sec $\cdot$ cm^{-5})	1210 ± 266	Decrease 21%
Pulmonary vascular resistance (dyn $\cdot$ sec $\cdot$ cm^{-5})	78 ± 22	Decrease 34%
Serum colloid oncotic pressure (mm Hg)	18 ± 1.5	Decrease 14%
Left ventricular stroke work index (g-m/m^2)	48 ± 6	No significant change

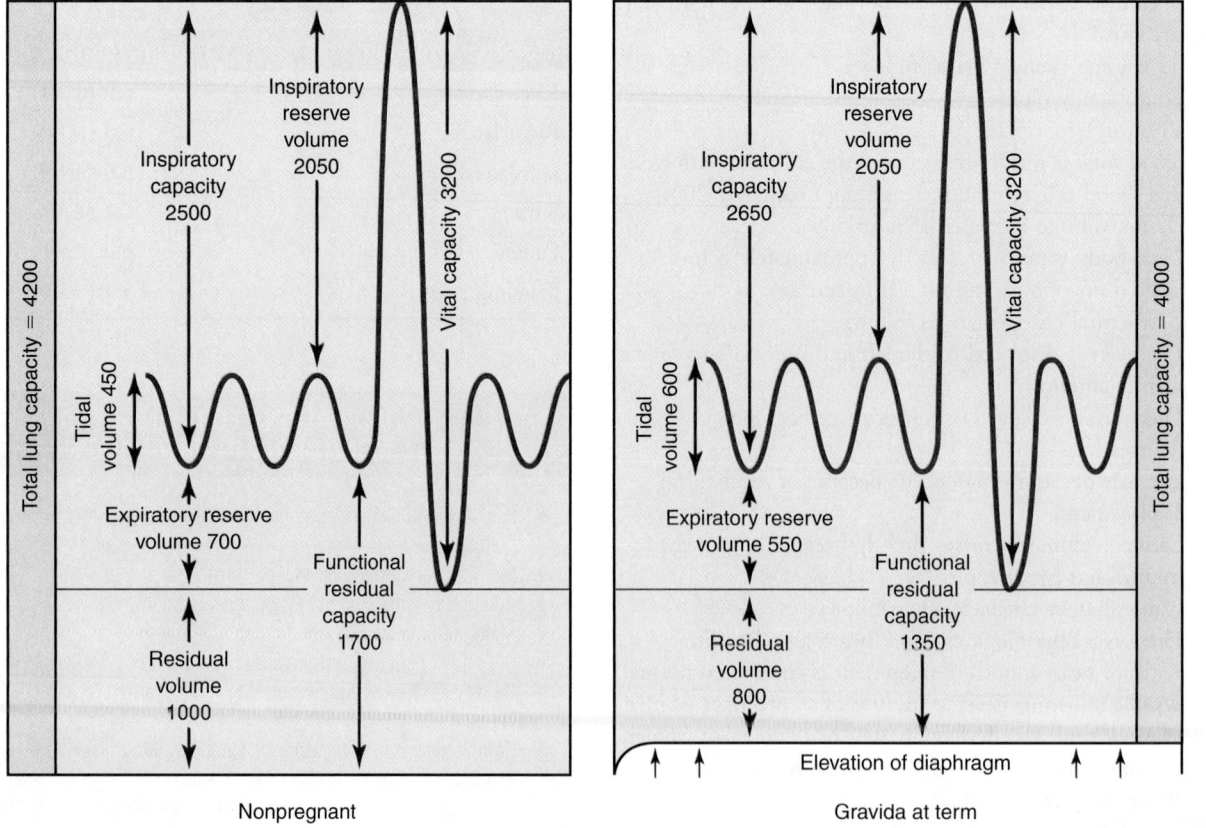

Figure 13-1 Pulmonary volumes and capacities (in milliliters) during pregnancy, labor, and the postpartum period. *(From Bonica JJ: Principles and practice of obstetric analgesia and anesthesia, Philadelphia, 1967, FA Davis.)*

TABLE 13-4 Physiologic Adaptation of the Gastrointestinal System During Pregnancy

Gastrointestinal Function Change	Presumed Cause
Heartburn	Progesterone and estrogen; size of gravid uterus impeding gastroesophageal junction
Bleeding gums	Hyperemia
Constipation	Progesterone, causing decreased motility and intestinal secretion, enhanced water absorption
Hemorrhoids	Hyperemia, pelvic congestion, obstruction of venous return
"Morning sickness" or nausea	Increased levels of estrogen and human chorionic gonadotropin (hCG)
Risk for aspiration	Displacement of lower esophageal sphincter and reduced gastric motility
Gallstones	Decreased gallbladder activity, impaired emptying

kidneys; dilation of pelvic, caliceal, and ureteral structures; bladder displacement forward and upward; and impaired blood and lymph drainage after the second trimester. Increases in blood volume and cardiac output, lowered systemic vascular resistance, and hormonal effects contribute to the primary physiologic functional changes summarized in Table 13-5.[12,16,18] The greater increase in glomerular filtration rate over renal plasma flow increases the proportion of filtered plasma. This lowers serum plasma protein concentration and colloid oncotic pressure. The increase in filtration also enhances the renal clearance of many substances, causing decreased plasma levels. Urea and creatinine are excreted more efficiently, and normal adult values therefore signify decreased renal function in the pregnant patient. Normal pregnant serum creatinine levels are 0.46 mg/dL, and blood urea nitrogen (BUN) levels are 8.2 mg/dL.[12,18]

Glycosuria and mild proteinuria are common in pregnancy but may indicate underlying pathology. While glomerular filtration is increased, tubular reabsorption of glucose and protein cannot increase proportionately, resulting in glycosuria and proteinuria. Both occurrences in pregnancy warrant further investigation.

TABLE 13-5 Renal Physiologic Changes in Pregnancy

Parameter	Percent Change	Normal Levels in Pregnancy
Renal blood flow	Increase 25%-50%	1250-1500 mL/min
Glomerular filtration rate	Increase 50%	140-170 mL/min
Renal plasma flow	Increase 35%	700-900 mL/min

PHYSIOLOGIC CHANGES DURING LABOR AND DELIVERY

Labor and delivery bring additional stresses to the maternal system, especially as a result of the pain and anxiety associated with labor. The most dramatic requirements are in the cardiopulmonary systems. During labor, uterine contractions produce cyclic autotransfusions of approximately 300 to 500 mL. Delivery of the fetus produces a final autotransfusion of approximately 1000 mL into the maternal vascular system.[16] This occurs because of the contracted uterus shunting its blood, sudden removal of fetal supply demands, and resolution of vena caval compression. Table 13-6 summarizes the cardiac output changes in labor and delivery.[18]

Normal blood loss from a vaginal birth is more than 600 mL; blood loss from cesarean births usually is 1000 mL.[13,16,18] The cardiopulmonary changes occurring during labor and delivery are of significant concern because they occur over a short time and maternal decompensation may occur.

In summary, maternal physiology is profoundly and rapidly affected by pregnancy. Adaptations begin early in the pregnancy and continue through the postpartum period, gradually returning to prepregnant states over 6 weeks. Understanding the physiologic stresses uniquely presented during pregnancy allows the clinician to provide comprehensive care to the pregnant woman experiencing critical illness or injury.

CARDIAC DISEASE

There are several considerations in the care of the pregnant woman with cardiac disease. Cardiac disease during pregnancy may be a result of preexisting conditions, such as congenital diseases, or it may be a result of primary cardiac disease arising during pregnancy. Prepregnancy counseling is highly recommended for women with known cardiac disease. Counseling includes determining the New York Heart Association (NYHA)[19] functional class (see Chapter 18) of the woman and determining the maternal and fetal risks associated with the pregnancy[20] (Table 13-7). Major fetal risks include fetal development of congenital heart disease, prematurity, intrauterine growth restriction (IUGR), and intrauterine fetal demise (IUFD).

TABLE 13-6 Cardiac Output Changes in Labor and Delivery

Stage of Labor or Delivery	Change in Cardiac Output
Early first stage of labor	↑15% plus additional 15% with each contraction
Last first state of labor	↑ 30% plus additional 15% with each contraction
Second stage of labor	↑ 45% plus additional 15% with each contraction
First 5 minutes postpartum	↑ 65% secondary to autotransfusion
First hour postpartum	↑ 40%

TABLE 13-7 Maternal Mortality Risks

Group 1: Mortality <1%
- Atrial septal defect
- Ventricular septal defect
- Patent ductus arteriosus
- Pulmonic tricuspid disease
- Tetralogy of Fallot, corrected
- Bioprosthetic valve
- Mitral stenosis, NYHA classes I and II

Group 2: Mortality 5%-15%
Group 2A
- Mitral stenosis, NYHA classes III and IV
- Aortic stenosis
- Coarctation of aorta, without valvular involvement
- Tetralogy of Fallot, uncorrected
- Previous myocardial infarction
- Marfan syndrome with normal aorta

Group 2B
- Mitral stenosis with atrial fibrillation
- Artificial valve

Group 3: Mortality 25%-50%
- Pulmonary hypertension
- Coarctation of aorta, with valvular involvement
- Marfan syndrome with aortic involvement

NYHA, New York Heart Association.

During the prenatal period, anticoagulant therapy is frequently recommended because of the already hypercoagulable state of pregnancy or preexisting conditions. Anticoagulant therapy using heparin is recommended because of the teratogenic effects of oral agents.[9]

Special consideration must be given to physical assessment during the antepartum period. Normal physiologic changes, such as murmur development or shortness of breath, may mask symptoms of cardiac disease or make diagnosis more challenging.

The method and timing of delivery are decided primarily by obstetric considerations, taking into account the woman's ability to tolerate the labor process and associated physiologic changes. Selection of anesthesia techniques involves weighing risks and benefits of the procedures. As a general rule, most patients tolerate epidural anesthesia more favorably than general anesthesia (see Chapter 15).

PREGNANCY WITH PREEXISTING HEART DISEASE

Much progress has been made during the past 2 decades in managing preexisting cardiac disease in the pregnant woman. Pregnant women in NYHA class I or II usually have a favorable prognosis; however, the dramatic physiologic changes present a significant confounding variable.

Atrial Septal Defect. Atrial septal defect (ASD) is the most common congenital anomaly seen during pregnancy, and most women with ASD tolerate pregnancy, labor, and delivery without complications. The decrease in systemic vascular resistance (SVR) lessens the degree of left-to-right shunt, whereas the hypervolemic state may slightly worsen the shunt and increase right ventricular workload. The most common complications seen with ASD are dysrhythmias, heart failure, and thromboembolism.

Ventricular Septal Defect. The outcome for the pregnant woman with ventricular septal defect (VSD) and resultant left-to-right shunt depends on the size of the defect, with larger defects producing a less favorable prognosis. In the absence of significant symptoms and pulmonary hypertension, pregnancy is typically well tolerated. Therapy is aimed at early recognition and treatment of signs of cardiac failure. Common complications include tachycardias, heart failure, and pulmonary hypertension.

Patent Ductus Arteriosus. In general, patent ductus arteriosus (PDA) is well tolerated during pregnancy, labor, and delivery. Precautions against the risks of infective endocarditis and thromboembolism may be taken. Severe PDA can produce large left-to-right shunts, producing pulmonary hypertension that is associated with significant maternal mortality.

Pulmonic or Tricuspid Disease. Isolated pulmonic or tricuspid valvular disease is uncommon but may be seen during the peripartum period. Because of the right-sided nature of the lesions, pregnancy, labor, and delivery are generally well tolerated despite the hypervolemic state. The mainstay of treatment focuses on cautious fluid administration and balance.

Valve Prosthesis. Management of the pregnant woman with a prosthetic valve focuses on maintenance of adequate anticoagulation to prevent thromboembolism and on infective endocarditis prophylaxis. Pregnant women with biologic valves usually do not require anticoagulation during pregnancy unless evidence of thromboembolic disease or atrial fibrillation is present. Biologic valves are associated with slightly lower mortality risks, because anticoagulation is normally not required with their use.

Mitral Stenosis. The presence of a stenotic mitral valve is the most common rheumatic valve disease. The primary concern with mitral stenosis during pregnancy is the impedance to ventricular filling, which produces a relatively fixed cardiac output. Additional risks include thromboembolism and dysrhythmias, especially atrial fibrillation. Cardiac output in the face of mitral stenosis is determined by two primary factors: length of diastolic filling and left ventricular preload. The length of diastolic filling may be negatively affected because of the normal hypervolemic state of pregnancy. Discomfort or anxiety associated with labor may produce tachycardia, which can drastically impede ventricular filling, producing an even lower cardiac output with resultant cardiac failure and pulmonary edema. Tachycardia is commonly managed with beta-blockade therapy.

Maintenance and management of left ventricular preload is the second important consideration in mitral stenosis. Patients may require high normal or slightly elevated left ventricular filling pressures to maintain adequate flow across the stenotic mitral valve. Caution must be used when employing therapies that decrease preload, such as diuresis or epidural anesthesia. Invasive hemodynamic monitoring may be indicated to carefully tailor therapy (see "Bedside Hemodynamic Monitoring" in Chapter 18).

In the immediate postpartum period, careful monitoring is essential because of the massive fluid shifts and large increases in cardiac output. Authorities recommend that optimal predelivery pulmonary artery occlusion pressures be maintained at 14 mm Hg or less to accommodate the increase in occlusion pressure of up to 16 mm Hg that can be associated in the immediate postpartum period.[13]

Aortic Stenosis. Aortic stenosis often is accompanied by other valvular disease, especially disease affecting the mitral valve. The hallmark of aortic stenosis is decreased left ventricular ejection. Mild aortic stenosis is usually well tolerated during pregnancy because of the natural hypervolemic state. Significant aortic stenosis can produce left ventricular hypertrophy and dilation. Thromboembolic prophylaxis is advised. Critical to successful management is maintenance of cardiac output through prevention of hypovolemia, especially at the time of delivery. Any factor that diminishes venous return or produces hypotension worsens the effects of aortic stenosis and significantly reduces cardiac output. The average mortality rate is 17%.[13]

Tetralogy of Fallot. The four primary lesions associated with tetralogy of Fallot include VSD, overriding aorta, right ventricular hypertrophy, and pulmonary stenosis. Women with corrected tetralogy of Fallot generally can tolerate pregnancy well. Although rare, if the congenital anomalies are not corrected, the maternal mortality rate and fetal complications increase significantly. Cardiopulmonary function must be maximized by measures including the treatment of dysrhythmias and the use of prophylaxis for endocarditis. Considerations during labor and delivery include maintenance of adequate preload and blood pressure.

Prior Myocardial Infarction. The outcome of the pregnant woman with prior myocardial damage depends on many factors. The length of time between the myocardial event and delivery is especially important. Increased myocardial oxygen demands during pregnancy must be considered, and therapy is usually supportive in nature. Careful attention to preload is essential to prevent burdening the heart and producing congestive failure (see "Heart Failure" in Chapter 18).

Marfan Syndrome. Marfan syndrome is characterized by connective tissue weakness that can lead to aortic root and wall weakness. Mitral valve prolapse is commonly seen. Prognosis is based on aortic root diameter, with most authorities citing 4.0 cm as maximal, after which significant increases in mortality occur.[21] Prevention of tachydysrhythmias and hypertension is recommended, along with endocarditis prophylaxis. Beta-blockade therapy may be initiated for cardiac rate control and to decrease pressure on the weakened aortic wall. Goals of management include maintenance of cardiac output to meet physiologic needs without producing undue stress on the aortic wall. Careful blood pressure maintenance is essential. Differential diagnosis of chest and back pain is essential, along with recognition of other signs of aortic dissection (see "Aortic Dissection" in Chapter 19).

Pulmonary Hypertension and Eisenmenger Syndrome. Pulmonary hypertension during pregnancy may be primary or idiopathic. Eisenmenger syndrome develops when, in the presence of a congenital left-to-right shunt caused by ASD, VSD, or PDA, progressive pulmonary hypertension leads to shunt reversal or bidirectional shunting.[11] Regardless of the cause, the risk of sudden death because of pulmonary hypertension in pregnancy is 50%, and deaths have been reported up to 4 to 6 weeks after delivery.[22] Avoidance or termination of pregnancy is commonly recommended. If pregnancy is continued, therapeutic management is directed at avoidance of pulmonary vasoconstrictors, thromboembolism, and hypotension; maintenance of adequate preload and oxygenation; fetal surveillance; and reduction of stress at the time of delivery.

Coarctation of the Aorta. Coarctation of the aorta may occur in isolation or, most often, in combination with valvular or septal anomalies. Patients with uncomplicated coarctation of the aorta who are relatively asymptomatic (NYHA class I or II) have demonstrated good prognosis and minimal risk of complications or death.[13]

Intrapartal management focuses on the prevention of hypertension to avoid aortic wall stress. Careful management of fluid balance and left ventricular function must occur to prevent congestive heart failure and to promote adequate perfusion.

CARDIAC DISEASE ARISING DURING PREGNANCY

Peripartum Cardiomyopathy. Women who have no evidence of previous cardiac disease but have cardiac failure during the last month of pregnancy or within the first 6 months after delivery are considered to have peripartum cardiomyopathy. To confirm the diagnosis, other causes of cardiac failure must be ruled out. Peripartum cardiomyopathy is a relatively rare disorder, occurring in 1 of 4025 deliveries[23] to 1 of 15,000 deliveries,[24] and it carries mortality rate ranging from 3.3% to 50%.[24] Ethnicity appears to be a significant risk factor, with a 2.9-fold higher incidence in African American women.[23] Controversy continues regarding exact causes of peripartum cardiomyopathy, and although viral and immune sources remain as the leading suspected causes, selenium deficiency, cardiac stress, and myocarditis have all been proposed.[25]

Symptoms are identical to those of classic cardiac failure, as is the treatment of diuretics, digoxin, beta-blockade, and afterload reduction. Anticoagulation is commonly employed to prevent thromboembolism and the formation of left ventricular thrombus, which is associated with a worse prognosis for recovery.[26] The clinical course of peripartum cardiomyopathy is quite variable, but 50% to 60% of patients show clinical recovery within the first 6 months after delivery.[27] Prognostic factors for recovery of ventricular function include ejection fraction, small cavity size, left ventricular stroke work index, and troponin T levels.[26,28]

Acute Myocardial Infarction. Although acute myocardial infarction (AMI) is rare during pregnancy, mortality rates range from 37% to 50%,[29] depending on the timing of the myocardial event. Increased mortality is associated with many factors, including occurrence of the event during the third trimester, patients younger than 35 years old, cesarean section delivery, and delivery occurring within 2 weeks of infarction.[30,31] The dramatic physiologic demands throughout pregnancy challenge the woman's cardiovascular system and can cause ischemia, leading to infarction.

Clinical diagnostics are similar to those for standard AMI detection, although diagnosis must be made with consideration of the normal physiologic cardiovascular changes. Treatment of AMI during pregnancy is focused on restoring myocardial blood flow and balancing myocardial oxygen supply and demand. Management may include percutaneous coronary intervention; nitrate or beta-blockade therapy, or both; cardiac monitoring; oxygen therapy; management of pain and anxiety; and afterload reduction. Special consideration is given to the maternal physiologic demands required during the labor and delivery processes. Operative delivery interventions, such as forceps or cesarean section, may be necessary (see "Myocardial Infarction" in Chapter 19).

Shock. Shock is best defined as tissue hypoxia that is a result of decreased perfusion. Because pregnancy is a hyperdynamic, low-resistance state with increased oxygen delivery and consumption requirements, the management of shock in the pregnant patient necessitates a different approach than for the nonpregnant patient. Normal physiologic adaptations that occur during pregnancy alter ranges in vital signs and laboratory values. Frequently, the clinician may be obtaining data from and managing two patients—the mother and fetus. here are causes for shock in pregnancy and immediately postpartum that must be considered in addition to routine causes (see Chapter 39).

Hemorrhagic, septic, and cardiogenic shock are most commonly seen in pregnancy; neurogenic shock occurs infrequently. Causes of hemorrhagic shock unique to pregnancy include abruptio placentae, ectopic pregnancy, placenta previa, and postpartum hemorrhage.[13] Postpartum hemorrhage can be attributed to uterine atony, genital tract lacerations, hematoma formation, retained placenta, and uterine prolapse.[13] Unique causes of septic shock in the pregnant patient include chorioamnionitis, septic abortion, and postpartum pyelonephritis.[11] Cardiogenic shock is most frequently a result of the presence of severe valve disease. Regardless of the cause, whether specific to pregnancy or not, the occurrence of shock requires aggressive intervention with treatment of the underlying cause.

Management of shock in pregnancy focuses on optimizing maternal stability in an effort to provide the most stable in utero environment. Clinical judgments include assessment of the risks and benefits of therapeutic interventions and fetal viability. Consideration must be given to the potential vasoconstrictive nature of some pharmacotherapeutics and the potential for uteroplacental insufficiency.

Resuscitation. The occurrence of cardiopulmonary arrest during pregnancy is uncommon. Successful management of the pregnant patient requires integration of physiologic changes present during pregnancy and adaptations for those from standard resuscitative guidelines. Fetal outcomes are directly related to the mother's condition and well-being. The interrelationship between fetal and maternal well-being may present unique ethical dilemmas for health care providers and family members. Causes, predisposing factors, and accompanying rationales for cardiopulmonary arrest during pregnancy are summarized in Table 13-8.

Basic Cardiac Life Support. American Heart Association recommendations include only minor deviations from usual procedures.[32] Critically important is the facilitation of venous return. This is accomplished by performing chest compressions slightly above the center of the sternum and lateral displacement of the uterus through manual manipulation or through the use of a wedge under the woman's hip.[32] Airway management includes application of cricoid pressure during positive-pressure ventilation for any unconscious pregnant woman to reduce the risk of regurgitation.[32] Physiologic adaptations in pregnancy place the woman at greater risk for complications from cardiopulmonary resuscitation, such as fractured ribs and sternum, hemothorax, hemopericardium, and internal organ damage. Specific organs of concern include the uterus, spleen, and liver.

Advanced Cardiac Life Support. Pharmacologic and electrical therapeutic interventions are carried out as usual, although there are minor considerations in the case of pregnancy. The airway should be secured early with effective preoxygenation and continuous cricoid pressure. Airway edema and swelling may require the use of a smaller endotracheal tube than in a nonpregnant woman.[32] Careful attention to confirmation of tube placement and oxygenation is required because of the enhanced oxygen demands during pregnancy.

Standard advanced cardiac life support (ACLS) recommendations should be followed for administration of resuscitation medications. Use of lower extremity sites or the femoral vein for

TABLE 13-8 Causes of Cardiopulmonary Arrest in Pregnancy

Cause	Discussion
Preexisting cardiac disease	Dramatic volume changes and cardiac output requirements may be greater than the diseased heart's ability to tolerate
Acute cardiac disease	May occur during pregnancy in relation to increased myocardial demands
Pregnancy-induced hypertension	May induce multisystem dysfunction
Anaphylaxis/laryngeal edema	May occur as reaction to medications used to treat urinary infections
Preexisting asthma	Stress induced by pregnancy may compromise maternal ability to maintain adequate oxygenation
Aspiration pneumonia	May occur as a result of gastrointestinal sphincter incompetence
Pulmonary embolism	Hypercoagulable nature of pregnancy, venous stasis
Hypermagnesemia	Therapeutically used for seizure prevention, increased levels depress reflexes and may cause respiratory depression and subsequent arrest
Anesthesia	Complications from local, spinal, epidural, or general anesthesia used to facilitate delivery
Other causes	Sepsis, trauma, amniotic fluid embolism, drug overdose

venous access should be avoided due to the potential of the gravid uterus to impede venous return.[32] Epinephrine may decrease uteroplacental perfusion because of its vasoconstrictive nature; however, the benefits outweigh the risks of administration. Lidocaine crosses the placenta but in therapeutic levels does not have adverse fetal or uteroplacental effects. If maternal toxicity occurs, fetal cardiac and central nervous system depression may occur. Fetal bradycardia is associated with bretylium administration, and careful fetal monitoring is recommended. There are no contraindications for use of atropine in pregnancy. Administration of sodium bicarbonate is to be undertaken cautiously. Maternal acidosis increases uteroplacental adrenergic reactivity and must be avoided, although maternal alkalosis may impair oxygen exchange to the fetus. Electrical therapies such as defibrillation, cardioversion, and pacing are not contraindicated in pregnancy.

Evaluation of fetal tolerance of the mother's condition is essential during cardiopulmonary arrest. Fetal hypoxia may develop because of decreased uteroplacental perfusion. Fetal gestational age is a prime consideration when determining course of action. Before 24 weeks' gestation, resuscitative efforts are focused primarily on maternal outcome. After the 24th week of gestation, evaluation includes maternal and fetal responses to resuscitative efforts. Emergent cesarean section may be undertaken for fetal distress or to improve maternal status, although consideration also must be given to the stress that cesarean section produces. In late pregnancy, survival of the infant is directly proportional to the time interval between death of the mother and delivery of the infant. Infant viability is best if delivery occurs within 5 minutes of cardiac arrest.[29,32]

HYPERTENSIVE DISEASE

Hypertensive disease is a potentially life-threatening complication of pregnancy that affects 4% to 10% of all pregnancies. It is the second leading cause of death in childbearing women, and it contributes to high rates of newborn morbidity and mortality.[11,13,33-38] Maternal complications include pathologic compromise of the cardiovascular, pulmonary, renal, neurologic, and hepatic systems[37-39] (Table 13-9).

TABLE 13-9 Complications of Hypertensive Disease in Pregnancy

Body System	Complication
Cardiovascular	Dysrhythmias, congestive heart failure, severe hypertension
Pulmonary	Pulmonary edema, acute airway obstruction
Renal	Oliguria, renal failure, acute tubular necrosis (ATN)
Neurologic	Cerebral edema, eclampsia, cerebral hemorrhage, coma
Hepatic	Necrosis, rupture, periportal and subcapsular hemorrhage
Hematologic	Disseminated intravascular coagulation (DIC), hemolysis thrombocytopenia

Understanding of hypertensive disease in pregnancy is based on (1) a classification according to manifestations and time of onset in relation to gestation; (2) the fact that pregnancy can induce hypertension in women without a history of high blood pressure; and (3) the fact that elevated blood pressure in pregnancy can occur without the presence of generalized edema or proteinuria (transient hypertension). Proper diagnosis of hypertensive complications is critical and requires in-depth knowledge of disease pathophysiology to prevent or decrease the risk of maternal or fetal compromise.

CLASSIFICATION OF HYPERTENSION

The National Institutes of Health Working Group on High Blood Pressure has endorsed the classification and terminology of ACOG for hypertensive disease in pregnancy.[33,34,39] These definitions have proved useful in establishing consistent guidelines for pregnancy management[40]:

  I. *Chronic hypertension* is hypertension before conception or diagnosed before 20 weeks' gestation
  II. *Preeclampsia and eclampsia* constitute a systemic syndrome of hypertensive disease, with proteinuria diagnosed after 20 weeks' gestation. Eclampsia indicates the additional presence of convulsions.
  III. *Preeclamsia superimposed on chronic hypertension* may occur before 20 weeks' gestation or have a sudden onset.
  IV. *Gestational hypertension* is hypertension without proteinuria.

PREECLAMPSIA

While the etiologic agent remains unknown, preeclampsia is characterized by widespread physiologic changes, including vasospasms in the arterial systems that result in endothelial damage, platelet aggregation, and decreased vascular volume. Research suggests two stages of disease progression: alterations to placental perfusion (stage 1) and a maternal syndrome (stage 2).[41] The widespread arteriolar vasospasms result from abnormal sensitivity to vasoconstrictor substances of vascular smooth muscle, leading to injury of the endothelial lining. These generalized cyclic vasospasms lead to tissue ischemia and eventually end-organ dysfunction[38] (Fig. 13-2).

Patients with preeclampsia or chronic hypertension may have a significant decrease in circulating plasma volume as a result of damage done by vasospasms.[37,38] These vasospasms are the result of an imbalance of sensitivity to vasoconstrictive substances such as angiotensin II, prostacyclin, and thromboxane A_2.[42] It is theorized that patients with hypertensive disease have a higher cardiac output and lower systemic vascular resistance in early pregnancy, which precedes an elevation in blood pressure and the classic manifestations of preeclampsia. This theory suggests that patients progress from a high–cardiac output, low-resistance state to a low-cardiac output, high-resistance state, leading to multisystem organ dysfunction. Approximately 50% of all patients are intravascularly volume depleted, 30% demonstrate normal hemodynamic functioning, and the remaining 20% have intravascular volume overload.

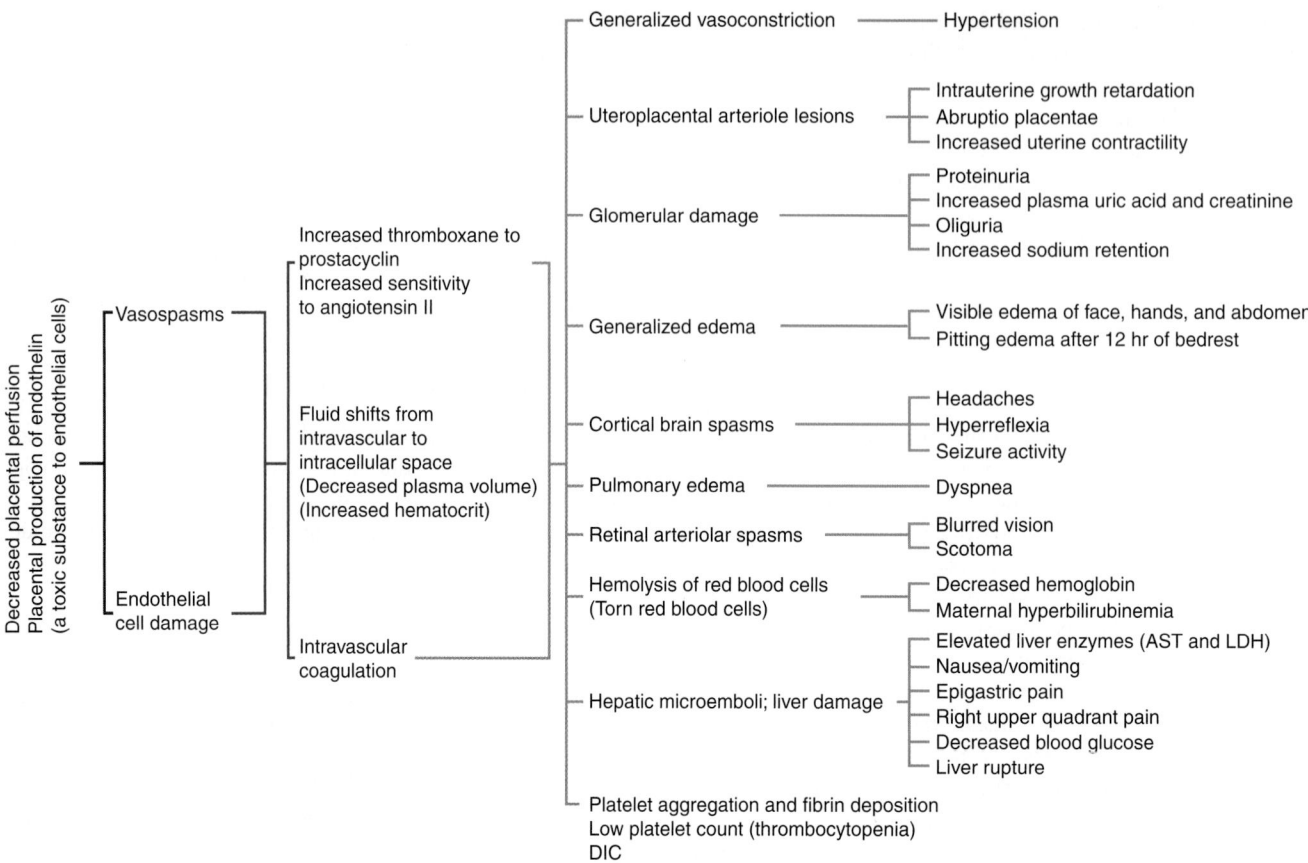

Figure 13-2 Pathophysiologic changes of pregnancy-induced hypertension. AST, aspartate aminotransferase (SGOT); DIC, disseminated intravascular coagulation; LDH, lactate dehydrogenase. *(From Gilbert E, Harmon J: Manual of high risk pregnancy and delivery, ed 4, St Louis, 2007, Mosby.)*

There is a lack of randomized, large trials, but some research shows there may be no clear benefit of antihypertensive treatment for pregnant women with mild to moderate hypertension. Antihypertensive therapy is used to reduce arterial vasospasms and decrease blood pressure, reducing left ventricular workload and enhancing placental and renal perfusion. Hypertensive control also decreases the potential for maternal cerebral vascular accidents. The goal of antihypertensive therapy is to maintain diastolic pressures less than 100 mm Hg.[13,33] Methyldopa is the drug of choice for treating chronic hypertension during pregnancy. Vasodilators, such as hydralazine, are the most common first-line medications used for management of hypertensive crisis. Beta-blockers, such as labetalol, are common second-line drugs when hypertension remains refractory to first-line management. Sodium nitroprusside is rarely used antepartally or intrapartally, but it may be administered to the severely preeclamptic-eclamptic patient when first-line drugs have failed. Its use is considered only when delivery is imminent or during the postpartum period, because thiocyanate is the metabolite. Nifedipine is a calcium channel blocker that must be used cautiously when given concurrently with magnesium sulfate (MgSO$_4$), because exaggerated hypotension may occur.

HEMOLYSIS, ELEVATED LIVER ENZYMES, AND LOW PLATELET SYNDROME

Hemolysis, elevated liver enzymes, and low platelet (HELLP) syndrome affects 4% to 12% of patients with severe preeclampsia or eclampsia.[13,33,38] Maternal mortality ranges from 3.5% to 24%, whereas perinatal mortality ranges from 10% to 60%.[11,38,43] Approximately 10% to 20% of pregnant patients with HELLP syndrome do not have elevated blood pressure diagnostic of hypertensive disease.[44] The clinical manifestations of HELLP syndrome may suggest a multitude of other clinical diagnoses. Misdiagnosis is common and may result in a delay of correct treatment. HELLP syndrome may be confused with acute fatty liver disease of pregnancy and thrombotic thrombocytopenic purpura/hemolytic uremic syndrome (TTP/HUS).[45] Any pregnant woman demonstrating clinical manifestations and showing hemolysis, elevated liver enzymes, and low platelets must be diagnosed with HELLP syndrome. Complications of HELLP syndrome include abruptio placentae, liver hematoma, disseminated intravascular coagulation (DIC), pulmonary edema, liver rupture, and acute renal failure.[13,45]

The treatment goals of severe preeclampsia are to prevent seizures, decrease arterial spasms, and effect prompt delivery of the fetus. MgSO$_4$ is the standard treatment for prevention and control of seizure activity in women with preeclampsia or eclampsia. Typical anticonvulsant therapies such as phenytoin, phenobarbital, or diazepam are not used, because they address primarily neurologic dysfunction rather than vasospastic disease. Serum magnesium levels of 4 to 7 mEq/L are thought to be therapeutic for prevention of seizure activity. A loading dose of 4 to 6 g is given by infusion pump over 15 to 20 minutes, followed by a maintenance infusion of 2 to 3 g/hr.

TABLE 13-10 Conditions Associated with Disseminated Intravascular Coagulation

Obstetric	Obstetric or Nonobstetric	Nonobstetric
Abruptio placentae	Prolonged shock, any cause	Malignancy
Amniotic fluid embolism	Transfusion-incompatible blood	Extensive surgery
Eclampsia, severe eclampsia	Septicemia: bacterial fungal, viral	Collagen vascular disease
Abortion	Septic abortion	Central nervous system trauma
Dead fetus syndrome	Severe chorioamnionitis	Allergic reactions
Hydatidiform mole		Burns
Retained placenta		Vascular malformations
Uterine rupture		Pancreatitis
Maternal hemorrhage		

Control of eclamptic seizures is accomplished through administration of 4 to 6 g of intravenous $MgSO_4$ over 5 to 10 minutes. This bolus is followed by a continuous infusion of 2 to 3 g/hr. If a patient has a recurrent seizure, another bolus of 2 to 4 g can be given over 3 to 5 minutes. Occasionally, a patient has continuing seizure activity despite magnesium therapy, necessitating intubation, ventilatory support, and consideration of delivery.[33,43,46]

Collaborative management for patients with severe preeclampsia or eclampsia or with HELLP syndrome is key to the stabilization of the mother and fetus. Continuous assessment of the cardiovascular, renal, central nervous, and pulmonary systems provides early indications of worsening maternal condition. Fetal surveillance may include continuous fetal monitoring, biophysical profile, and fetal lung maturity testing. Delivery of the fetus may be indicated because of the maternal condition or fetal compromise. The goal of the health care team is to accurately monitor ongoing organ system dysfunction and prevent further damage leading to end-organ failure and maternal-fetal mortality. Research is focusing on angiogenesis and factors such as soluble FMS-like tyrosine kinase 1 (sFLT-1, the soluble form of the vascular endothelial growth factor [VEGF] receptor 1) and placenta-derived growth factor (PLGF), which may serve as diagnostic or predictive markers for preeclampsia.

OBSTETRIC DISSEMINATED INTRAVASCULAR COAGULATION

Obstetric causes of DIC include abruptio placentae, preeclampsia or eclampsia, dead fetus syndrome, septic abortion, and amniotic fluid embolus. Pathophysiologic mechanisms are summarized in Table 13-10.[11,37,38] Primary treatment goals include identification of the underlying disorder, removal of the trigger or initiating event, and volume replacement, including blood component therapy. Secondary treatment may include anticoagulation therapy (see Chapter 39).

ABRUPTIO PLACENTAE

Abruptio placentae is the most common obstetric cause of DIC. Of mothers experiencing abruption, 20% have a significant clotting defect, with 25% of this group experiencing postpartum hemorrhage.[37,47] The basic elements of treatment include delivery, the removal of blood clots from the uterus, blood component therapy, and fluid volume resuscitation.

DEAD FETUS SYNDROME

Dead fetus syndrome is consistent with a chronic DIC condition. Onset occurs gradually over 2 to 4 weeks. Of women who experience fetal demise, 80% will experience spontaneous onset of labor. Treatment of the stable patient is delivery of the fetus. Heparin may be used for women with associated coagulopathy.

SEPTIC ABORTION

Septic abortion is a well-documented cause of obstetric DIC. Bacterial endotoxins are the most likely initiating mechanism. The clinical findings of gram-negative septic shock are applicable to this condition. The severity of the disease correlates well with the degree of coagulopathy. Aggressive antibiotic therapy and evacuation of the uterus are the frontline therapies for patients who are hemodynamically stable. Heparin therapy remains controversial.

PULMONARY DYSFUNCTION

Pulmonary dysfunction carries clinical significance because of the normally slightly hyperoxygenated condition associated with the physiologic changes in pregnancy. Compromise of respiratory function places the mother and fetus at risk for harm. Maternal hypoxia can be the end result of several conditions, including pneumonia, asthma, cystic fibrosis, trauma, acute lung injury (ALI), acute respiratory distress syndrome (ARDS), and pulmonary embolism. Contributing factors (e.g., smoking, drug use, preexisting disease states), manifestations, and management differ very little from those seen in the nonpregnant individual. Common to these respiratory disorders is the issue of maternal-fetal hypoxia. Maternal hypoxia is defined by a PaO_2 less than 100 mm Hg, an SpO_2 less than 95%, a $PaCO_2$ greater than 32 mm Hg, a pH less than 7.40, and an SvO_2 less than 60%. Hyperventilation, shortness of breath, and dyspnea are commonly seen in pregnancy and must be differentiated from the usual maternal complaints.

ASTHMA

Although asthma, which affects 4% to 8% of pregnant women, often can be easily managed, it has been associated with an increased incidence of pneumonia (more than 60% of pneumonias that occur during pregnancy occur in women with asthma), hyperemesis gravidarum, gastroesophageal reflux disease, preeclampsia, chronic hypertension, preterm labor or birth, perinatal mortality, spontaneous abortion, complicated labor, and low birth weight.[49,50] The literature indicates maternal and fetal outcomes are related to the severity of the disease, especially compliance with medical regimens while pregnant for fear of fetal harm, and the degree of control achieved with medical management, although the prevalence, morbidity, and mortality for asthma appear to be increasing.[49-51] It is estimated that approximately one third of patients will experience no change in asthma symptoms, one third will see improvement, and one third will have worsening of symptoms. The peak incidence of asthma exacerbation occurs during the second and early third trimesters; exacerbations during labor are rare because of the natural occurring increase of endogenous epinephrine and steroids.[48,50] The lessening of asthma symptoms during pregnancy is the result of smooth muscle relaxation caused by progesterone. Decreased cell-mediated immunity and an increased level of corticosteroids may assist in diminishing the inflammatory response. Cyclic adenosine monophosphate (cAMP) levels are increased and aid in maintaining an ongoing energy supply to cells. Other factors may contribute to worsening of symptoms. Nasal congestion, decreased functional residual volume, anxiety, noncompliance with medical regimens, stress, exercise, exposure to allergens, environmental irritants, respiratory infections, sinusitis, and smoking can contribute to exacerbation of asthma symptoms.[48,50,51] The decrease in cell-mediated immunity may predispose the mother to viral infections. Pregnancy usually does not change the peak expiratory flow rate (PEFR).

Management recommendations include use of a peak flow meter twice per day to assist in objectively measuring maternal pulmonary function. A decrease in PEFR of more than 20% of the patient's personal best requires a call the to the physician; a decrease to of greater than 50% of the patient's personal best signals the need for a visit to the emergency department and the need for rapid assessment and intervention.[48,51]

CYSTIC FIBROSIS

Cystic fibrosis (CF) is an autosomal recessive, multisystem disease that affects the exocrine glands and epithelial tissues of the pancreas, sweat glands, and mucous glands of the respiratory, digestive, and reproductive tracts.[52,53] Pregnancy can lead to decompensation of the pulmonary and cardiovascular systems and to development of nutritional insufficiency. More women are living to reproductive age and becoming pregnant because of improved pulmonary and pharmacologic therapies and because of the opportunity of lung transplantation. The normal pulmonary changes of pregnancy (e.g., increased resting minute ventilation, upward displacement of the diaphragm with resultant decrease in functional residual volume, widened alveolar-arterial oxygen gradient) lead to pulmonary decompensation and increased morbidity and mortality for the mother

and fetus.[51] In advanced lung disease, pulmonary hypertension may be present, and when combined with the normal pregnancy-related increase in blood volume and consequent inability to increase cardiac output, it can lead uteroplacental insufficiency and cardiovascular collapse (especially during labor and delivery).[51] Management recommendations include ongoing cardiopulmonary assessment (e.g., chest radiographs, pulmonary function studies, SpO_2 monitoring, arterial blood gas determinations, pulmonary artery pressure monitoring), bronchial drainage and chest physiotherapy, ongoing replacement of pancreatic enzymes and supplementation of nutrition by tube feedings or total parenteral nutrition, and antibiotic administration for persistently present organisms such as *Pseudomonas aeruginosa* and *Burkholderia cepacia*.[48,51,52]

PNEUMONIA

Pneumonia can result from a variety of factors and is often associated with asthma. Exacerbations are more common in the second and third trimesters, and they are often associated with other maternal disease processes. Prior respiratory disease, concurrent illness, human immunodeficiency virus (HIV) infection, drug or tobacco use, and anemia have been linked with an increased maternal risk of pneumonia. Physiologic changes of pregnancy decrease the mother's ability to clear secretions and place her at increased risk for gastric aspiration. The severity of aspiration correlates directly to aspirate amount, particulate content, and pH. Typically, the pneumonia is of a bacterial origin; however, a variety of organisms can be seen. Some of the most common pathogens identified are *Streptococcus pneumoniae* (>50% of bacterial pneumonias), *Haemophilus influenzae, Staphylococcus aureus, Legionella pneumophila, Mycoplasma pneumoniae, Chlamydia pneumoniae,* and influenza viruses.[48,51] Pregnant women experiencing a varicella infection have a 45% to 50% chance of developing varicella pneumonia, which carries a 35% to 40% mortality rate. *Pneumocystis jirovecii* (formerly *Pneumocystis carinii*) pneumonia and resistant strains of tuberculosis are a growing concern, because most women who are HIV positive or have acquired immunodeficiency syndrome (AIDS) are in their reproductive years.

ACUTE LUNG INJURY AND ACUTE RESPIRATORY DISTRESS SYNDROME

ALI and ARDS in pregnancy are often the result of a variety of conditions, including pharmacologic agents (e.g., aspirin, tocolytic agents, cocaine), aspiration, preeclampsia or eclampsia, abruptio placentae, postpartum hemorrhage, massive blood transfusions, anaphylactoid syndrome of pregnancy (ASP, formerly known as amniotic fluid embolism), and a variety of other conditions that lead to the development of pulmonary edema. Some of the most common causes of ALI/ARDS in the perinatal patient are sepsis resulting from pyelonephritis, chorioamnionitis, IUFD, septic abortion, and postpartum endometritis. Women at risk for ALI/ARDS need to be assessed for early signs of worsening or changing dyspnea and tachypnea. As ALI/ARDS evolves, pulmonary function rapidly deteriorates over a 24-hour period. Symptoms, including diffuse or basilar rales, bilateral opacities on the chest radiograph, and a deteriorating PaO_2 with increasing FIO_2 demands and declining PF ratio need to be differentiated from other causes, such as fluid overload and cardiac failure, which can sometimes be seen in the last trimester (see "Acute Lung Injury" in Chapter 24).

Management of Respiratory Failure. Management of maternal hypoxia includes restoration and maintenance of the hypervolemic state without inducing fluid overload and further compromising cardiopulmonary function. Because colloidal osmotic pressure is decreased, great care must be taken to prevent the development of pulmonary edema when providing fluid replacement therapy. Oxygen is administered at a high flow rate by mask to achieve an optimal PaO_2 greater than 100 mm Hg and an SpO_2 greater than 95%. Noninvasive mechanical ventilation should be used with caution because of the risk of gastric aspiration. If intubation is required, placement of an orotracheal tube is more desirable than a nasotracheal tube because of

hyperemic nasal passageways. If nasotracheal intubation is required, the smallest tube possible that still allows adequate ventilation is used. Gastric decompression is instituted with a small-bore nasogastric or orogastric tube. When initiating mechanical ventilation, FIO_2 should be maintained at less than 60% if possible, positive end-expiratory pressure (PEEP) should be less than 8 to 15 cm H_2O, and tidal volumes should be set at 10 to 12 mL/kg or 6 to 8 mL/kg if they are experiencing decreased pulmonary compliance.[48,54] Caution must be taken to maintain the maternal $PaCO_2$ of 28 to 32 mm Hg, because respiratory alkalosis can lead to decreased uterine blood flow. Pulmonary compliance should be routinely assessed to evaluate the effectiveness of interventions. Pulmonary compliance may decrease from the normal average of 75 mL/cm H_2O to 20 mL/cm H_2O in severe ARDS.[13] Pharmacologic therapies must consider maternal-fetal risk and benefits. Table 13-11 summarizes obstetric concerns of common drugs used in pulmonary dysfunction.[48,50,51,53]

TABLE 13-11 Pharmacologic Management: Pulmonary Dysfunction During Pregnancy	
DRUG	**CONSIDERATIONS**
Antibiotics	Cephalosporins, erythromycin are generally well tolerated.
	Sulfites should be avoided.
	Vancomycin, aminoglycosides, and tetracycline can lead to fetal toxicity.
	Acyclovir improves maternal morbidity and appears to improve fetal outcomes.
Inhaled corticosteroids	Beclomethasone generally considered safe.
Systemic corticosteroids	Documentation of decreased birth weights and increase in small-for-date babies.
	Most drug is metabolized by placental enzymes before entering the fetal circulation.
	Small amount of steroid may cross into breast milk, but it is still considered safe to breastfeed.
Mast cell stabilizers	Cromolyn and nedocromil are generally considered safe.
	They are not associated with increased risks to the fetus.
Beta adrenergic agonists	Epinephrine and isoproterenol may contribute to maternal-fetal tachycardia.
	Albuterol and terbutaline have fewer side effects and may have the additional benefit of tocolytic actions.
Leukotriene receptor antagonists	They appear to be safe for the management of chronic, mild to moderate asthma.
Inhaled anticholinergics	Ipratropium is beneficial for acute asthma attack.
	They probably are safe for the fetus because they are poorly absorbed by bronchial mucosa, decreasing the risk of fetal exposure.
Theophylline	It is not commonly used because of maternal side effects.
	It is recommended that serum levels be maintained between 5 and 12 mg/mL to prevent complications of toxicity.
Analgesics	Morphine and meperidine should be avoided in active labor because they can worsen bronchospasm
	They will cross the placenta and should be considered when completing a fetal assessment
	Fentanyl may be a better agent to use.
	Epidural analgesia is considered safe.
Beta-mimetic tocolytics	These are contraindicated because they can worsen maternal lung damage.
Labor induction	Oxytocin is the drug of choice.
	Prostaglandin F_2 should be avoided because it is a bronchoconstrictor.
Neuromuscular blockade	They can be administered safely as long as peripheral nerve testing is conducted to monitor drug dosages.
	They will cross the placenta, and this should be considered when assessing fetal activity.

PULMONARY EMBOLISM

Thromboembolic disorders, including pulmonary embolism (PE), result from a variety of causes, many of which are related to the physiologic changes in pregnancy. Other factors to be considered include the increasing frequency of long-term bed rest for high-order multiple pregnancies, premature labor, maternal age older than 35 years, obesity, smoking, cancer, surgery, and a history of venous thromboembolism (VTE) or PE.[55-59] The greatest risk for developing PE is in the immediate postpartum period, especially if a cesarean section was performed. Two thirds of the patients who die of PE do so within 30 minutes of the initial event. Assessment, management, and complications associated with PE are essentially no different from those of the nonpregnant woman; however, differential diagnosis of anaphylactoid syndrome of pregnancy (ASP) must be considered. Heparin is administered initially intravenously and then subcutaneously for the remainder of the pregnancy, because warfarin sodium derivatives are known fetal teratogens that readily cross the placenta. Unfractionated heparin does not cross the placenta or become excreted in breast milk, and low-molecular-weight heparin does not cross the placenta; however, during early and late pregnancy, the maximum concentration and plasma activity are substantially lower.[55,60,61] Heparin-induced thrombocytopenia (HIT) is a serious complication that has been estimated to occur in 1% to 5% of patients receiving heparin.[58,62] A vena cava filter may be implanted, but a suprarenal position is selected to prevent restriction of venous blood coming from the left ovary and draining into the left renal vein (see "Pulmonary Embolism" in Chapter 24).

ANAPHYLACTOID SYNDROME OF PREGNANCY

ASP was previously known as amniotic fluid embolism (AFE). Investigations suggest the process is more comparable to anaphylaxis than embolism, in part because of large-scale mast cell degranulation, independent of typical antigen-antibody–mediated anaphylaxis.[63] ASP/AFE is rare, but it is associated with mortality rates as high as 60% to 70% and is the leading maternal cause of death.[54,64,65] The most common precipitating factors associated with the syndrome are a large fetus, multiparity, premature separation of the placenta, IUFD, tumultuous labor, and small tears in the endocervical veins that may occur during normal labor.[54,63,66,67] Placental abruption is seen in almost half of cases, with fetal death having occurred before the event.[67]

Sudden onset of symptoms during or immediately after delivery can lead to the suspicion of ASP. Acute respiratory distress, hypoxia, hypotension, shock out of proportion to blood loss, coagulopathy or DIC, altered mental status, chills, fever, shivering, and sweating are observed. Pulmonary edema occurs and is followed by acute cardiovascular collapse. Chest pain and bronchospasm are uncommon. In a small percentage of patients, a grand mal seizure may be the initial symptom. More than 25% to 50% of patients die within the first hour, 80% die within the first 9 hours, and 40% of survivors develop DIC.[54,67] There is no specific diagnostic test for ASP, although the presence of fetal squamous cells, lanugo, vernix caseosa,

meconium, and mucin in blood aspirated from the pulmonary artery indicates a possibility of its occurrence.[54,68] Testing should be done to rule out DIC. Chest radiographs may show pulmonary edema, effusions, and cardiac enlargement. Electrocardiograms may show tachycardia, nonspecific ST-wave changes, and right ventricular strain. Lung scans may indicate perfusion defects.

Management consists of maintaining oxygenation and supporting cardiac function. Supportive therapy consists of maintenance of blood pressure through aggressive volume replacement and inotropic support, intubation and mechanical ventilation, and blood component therapy for hemorrhage.[48,64] Other therapies, such as low-dose heparin, bronchodilators, and steroids, may be used.

TRAUMA

Trauma in the pregnant woman is the leading cause of nonobstetric death; the rate has been estimated to be about 6% to 7%, although a precise number is difficult to obtain because injuries can range from minor to life threatening.[65,69,70] The primary cause of trauma is blunt trauma from motor vehicle accidents, especially in the third trimester. Penetrating injuries such as gunshot wounds and stabbings have a lower maternal mortality rate; however, fetal morbidity and mortality rates are higher and are thought to result from the gravid uterus acting as a buffer for maternal organs.[70,71] For domestic violence or intimate partner violence, rates are estimated to be 4% to 17%; exact rates are unknown due to underreporting and differences in methods of data collection. Injuries associated with domestic violence include defensive wounds; multiple blunt trauma injuries; bruises in various stages of healing; injuries to the face, neck, and especially the abdomen; and uterine rupture.[72-75] It may be difficult to differentiate between damage occurring as a result of an accidental fall and that of having been pushed or struck; therefore, the patient should be carefully interviewed. Reports of violence were more likely to be associated with alcohol consumption, smoking, inadequate prenatal care (contributing to low birth weight), and a history of a fetal death and previous induced or spontaneous abortion.[73] Burn injuries are uncommon. The severity of maternal total-body surface area (TBSA) of thermal injury correlates with worsening fetal outcomes related to prolonged hypotension, inadequate volume resuscitation, sepsis, hyponatremia, and carbon monoxide exposure.[69,71,76]

Approximately 10% of traumatic injuries occur in the first trimester, 40% occur in the second trimester, and 50% occur in the third trimester.[77] As women continue to work late into their pregnancies and become involved in higher-risk activities, the type and severity of injuries may begin to increase. Mechanisms that produce injuries in pregnant patients are no different from those that injure nonpregnant women.

Management of trauma during pregnancy and in the first 6 weeks after delivery is, with few exceptions, no different from the management of trauma for any other patient (see Chapter 37).[71,76,78,79] Normal physiologic changes associated with pregnancy may mask assessment findings and therefore affect decisions about interventions that are provided (Table 13-12).

TABLE 13-12 Initial Assessment and Management of Obstetric Trauma

Assessment	Management, Rationale, or Purpose
Primary Survey	
Airway	
Signs of Obstruction	
Same as for nonpregnant patient	Remove visible debris with caution because of increased hyperemia of nasal or oral area.
	Decrease risk of aspiration (because of enlarged uterus and effects of progesterone) by lateral tilt or by inserting an NGT or OGT.
	Emergency cricoid thyrotomy or tracheotomy, if performed, is done above usual site because of upward displacement of thoracic structures.
Breathing	
Signs of Ineffective Respiration	
Same as for nonpregnant patient with exception of the following:	100% oxygen by mask because passages tend to be hyperemic and there is tendency for breathing through mouth
SpO_2 <95	Elevate head of bed if possible to decrease pressure on thoracic structures caused by elevated diaphragm.
PaO_2 <100 mm Hg	Oral intubation using smaller size (5.5 to 7.0 Fr) endotracheal tubes to reduce risk of bleeding caused by increased vascularity of area
$PaCO_2$ >30 mm Hg	Gastric decompression with OGT (or small NGT if patient does not tolerate OGT placement) because prone to ileus and gastric reflux
pH <7.40	Physiologic monitoring (RR, SpO_2, $ETCO_2$)
Tidal volume <800 mL	Obtain ABGs, chest radiograph
Labored respirations	Emergent needle decompression or chest tube insertion for hemopneumothorax; may need to reassess entry point because of upward or outward displacement of thorax
RR <20 breaths/min or >24 beats/min	
Circulation	
Signs of Ineffective Circulation	
Same as for nonpregnant patient with exception of the following:	Diagnostic peritoneal lavage can be performed; open technique is usually preferred.
Systolic blood pressure <110 mm Hg	Assess for possible placental abruption.
Mean arterial pressure <80 mm Hg	Normally hypervolemic skin is warm and slightly moist because of progesterone and may mask signs of hypoperfusion.
Central venous pressure <6 mm Hg	Central venous catheter or large-bore IV access to upper extremity sites because of potential for impeded venous return from lower extremities
Pale, moist, cool skin	Fluid resuscitation
	LR is recommended because it has the potential to metabolize into bicarbonate through intrinsic body pathways; do not administer blood products through same IV line.
	With 0.9 NS, can administer blood products through line; may decrease risk of developing maternal alkalosis (compared with LR).
	O-negative blood can be given until type and cross are done.
	Replace 3 mL per 1 mL of blood lost to compensate for hypervolemia associated with pregnancy.
	Use caution because of increased risk of pulmonary edema caused by decreased colloidal osmotic pressure.
	May apply MAST but *do not* inflate abdominal compartment.
	Tilt the patient to her side, even if on a back board, to maximize venous return.
Secondary Survey	
Focused Obstetric History	
Gestational age	Keep the mother alive.
Single vs. multiple pregnancy	Keep the baby where it is.
Number of pregnancies, live births, abortions	Perform vaginal examination to determine fetal presentation, status of amniotic membrane, and presence of fetal parts or umbilical cord in vagina.
Name of obstetrician	Avoid manipulating cord because of risk of spasms.
Rh factor	Emergent delivery; vaginal vs. cesarean; live vs. perimortem
Prenatal complications	
Past vaginal drainage, bleeding, clots	
Past abdominal pain/uterine contractions	

Continued

TABLE 13-12 Initial Assessment and Management of Obstetric Trauma—*cont'd*

Assessment	Management, Rationale, or Purpose
Maternal Studies	
Unexpected Diagnostic Study Results	
CBC	Insert a urinary Foley catheter with caution because of the risk of bleeding because of increased pelvic vascularity; consider using a smaller size of catheter.
WBC >18,000/mm^3	
RBC <6,500,000/mm^3	Consider significance of positive toxicity results. Is the fetus at risk for issues such as drug withdrawal or fetal alcohol syndrome?
Hg <12 g/dL	
Hct <32%	Hct and Hg values that are below those identified may put the mother and fetus at risk for hypoxia.
Platelets <200,000/mm^3	
Fibrinogen >400 mg/dL	Use caution when performing a rectal examination to assist in determining fetal position or traumatic damage; pelvic vascular congestion contributes to development of hemorrhoids and predisposes the mother to bleeding from this site.
Chemistries:	
BUN <9 mg/dL	
Creatinine >0.5 mg/dL	Obtain radiologic studies as needed; however, implement measures to decrease risk to fetus.
Na$^+$ slightly increased	Left axis deviation may be seen on the 12-lead electrocardiogram as a normal variant.
Glucose slightly decreased	
Fetal Studies	
Signs of Fetal Distress	
Fetal heart rate <100-110	Ultrasound to evaluate fetus
Nonreassuring patterns on fetal monitor	Assess fundal height, firmness, contractions every 30 min.
Fundal height not appropriate for gestational age	Fetal monitoring (with pocket Doppler, ultrasound, or fetal monitor) as allowed based on interventions provided to mother
Vaginal drainage, bleeding, clots present	Differentiate uterine pain or contractions from other sources of abdominal pain.
	Administer tocolytics as needed.
Abdominal pain, uterine firmness or contractions present	L/S ratio and presence of PG to determine fetal lung maturity
Amniocentesis:	Kleihauer-Betke result indicates a break in the integrity of placental circulation if fetal cells are present.
Presence of RBCs	
L/S ratio and presence of PG	
Kleihauer-Betke test to detect presence of fetal blood in maternal bloodstream	
Tertiary Survey	
Aspect of Care	

Administer "follow-up meds"	Prophylactic measures:
	   Choose broad-spectrum antibiotics, nonteratogenic agents.
	   Tetanus toxoid does not cross placenta.
	Rh-negative mothers:
	   Can become Rh immunized within 72 hr
	   Administer Rh immune globulin (300 µg/15 mL of fetal blood or 30 mL of whole blood) if possibility of mother having received Rh-positive blood
	   Breach in integrity of the placenta of an Rh-positive fetus as evidenced by positive Kleihauer-Betke test result

ABGs, arterial blood gas determinations; BUN, blood urea nitrogen; CBC, complete blood cell count; $ETCO_2$, end tidal CO; Hct, hematocrit; Hg, hemoglobin; IV, intravenous; LR, lactated Ringer's solution; L/S, lecithin-to-sphingomyelin ratio; MAST, military antishock trousers; Na$^+$, sodium ion; NGT, nasogastric tube; NS, normal saline; OGT, orogastric tube; PG, phosphatidylglycerol; RBC, red blood cell; RR, respiration rate; WBC, white blood cell.

It is recommended that any pregnant woman beyond 22 to 24 weeks' gestation who experiences trauma should receive at least 4 hours of fetal monitoring. The first priority is to provide the interventions that would normally be provided to the nonpregnant woman, with the goal of keeping the mother alive. Keeping the mother alive is the best thing that can be done for the fetus, even though some of the interventions may produce transient alterations in fetal blood flow. Hesitation in providing necessary interventions increases the risk of harming both mother and fetus. An exception to this situation may occur after the fetus has reached the state of viability and the mother is at risk for immediate demise. In this situation, it may be decided to perform an emergent cesarean section to save the infant. To achieve the most optimal fetal outcome, a perimortem cesarean section should be performed within 5 minutes in a patient who is unresponsive to cardiopulmonary resuscitation (CPR).[13,69,76,77,80,81] Removal of the fetus may also increase the potential survival of the mother by relieving fetal compression of the aorta and vena cava, thereby improving venous return and cardiac output, increasing in intravascular volume by means of uterine autotransfusion, enhancing more effective chest compressions, and improving the functional residual capacity.[80]

TYPES OF INJURIES

Types of injuries can vary with the stage of pregnancy. In the first trimester, injuries are commonly associated with falls resulting from fainting from fatigue, hypoglycemia, and normal physiologic changes. The fetus is usually well protected from external trauma, because the uterus is located within the pelvis and is protected by bony structures. In the second trimester, as the enlarging uterus expands out of the pelvis, maternal abdominal organs are displaced upward and laterally. Some protection is provided to the maternal abdominal organs, because the uterus and fetus now occupy much of the abdominal cavity; however, the growing fetus becomes more vulnerable to injury. By the third trimester, the fetus has begun to settle into the pelvis in preparation for birth. Hyperventilation and fainting are common as the fetus grows and places greater metabolic demands on the mother. As relaxin secretion increases, the end effect of relaxed pelvis ligaments can lead to lordosis and pelvic tilt. This produces a change in gait and in the center of gravity and balance, which can increase the risk of falls.

SPECIFIC BODY SYSTEM INJURIES

Cardiovascular Injuries. Manifestations related to cardiovascular injury may be masked because of normal physiologic changes in pregnancy. The hypervolemic, low systemic-resistance state that occurs during pregnancy can mask shock, because significant blood volume can be lost before the classic manifestations are seen.[13] Lower extremity wounds may bleed more vigorously than expected because of venous congestion of the lower extremities.

Pulmonary Injuries. The most commonly fractured ribs are the middle ribs (5 through 9). The upper ribs (1 through 4) are associated with potential damage to the great vessels and the spine. The lower ribs (10 through 12) are associated with damage to the diaphragm, liver, and spleen. As pregnancy progresses, the anteroposterior diameter of the chest increases, the length decreases, and abdominal organs shift.

Neurologic Injuries. Spinal cord injury (SCI) in pregnancy may be acute (result of recent trauma) or may be chronic (due to preexisting damage). Initial management of acute SCI is the same as for nonpregnant patients, including the administration of steroids. Adequate uterine perfusion can be evaluated by observing for a reassuring fetal heart rate tracing and lack of uterine contractions.[82] SCI patients, as are pregnant women, are at high risk for deep vein thrombosis, which necessitates the provision of prophylactic anticoagulation. Vaginal delivery is possible; however, patients with injuries above T6 are more likely to develop autonomic dysreflexia (ADR) and therefore may require assisted vaginal delivery or a cesarean section.[82-84] Disruption of autonomic nervous system activity is not associated with labor dysfunction. Uterine sensory nerves enter the spinal cord at T11 to L1; women with SCI above T10 are therefore unable to feel uterine contractions. They must rely on uterine palpation and symptoms such as shortness or breath and abdominal or leg spasms. Epidural anesthesia in early labor may be provided, because uterine contractions are associated with ADR. If severe, irreversible traumatic brain injury (TBI) or maternal brain death occurs, the fetus may remain viable and continue to develop in utero. The issue of pregnancy maintenance in an irreversibly brain-damaged or brain-dead mother remains a controversial ethical issue.

Abdominal and Pelvic Injuries. Failure to wear or improper use of seat belts can lead to blunt abdominal injury. Penetrating abdominal injuries are also seen, and gunshot and stab wounds are the most common causes of abdominal injury. The engorgement of pelvic vasculature increases the risk of retroperitoneal hemorrhage after lower abdominal trauma. Because the uterus displaces maternal abdominal structures, the traditional assessment findings and sites of referred pain may be altered. Diagnostic peritoneal lavage (DPL) may be performed; however, a supraumbilical site (if the uterus is palpable above the pubis) using the open technique using direct visualization is preferred. The use of ultrasound to detect intraperitoneal fluid or hematoma can be used in place of DPL. Peritoneal signs such as tenderness, rigidity, and rebound tenderness are unreliable indicators because of stretching of the abdominal wall. Bowel sounds may be absent because pregnant women are prone to ileus. All of these factors can contribute to delayed detection of abdominal injuries. Splenic injuries are seen more commonly in the third trimester, and damage with blood loss may be seen after relatively mild trauma due to vascular engorgement. As the uterus enlarges, the bladder is displaced upward, and damage should be suspected if the patient has hematuria. Pelvic fractures can potentially injure the reproductive and urinary structures, although pelvic injury is not an absolute contraindication to vaginal delivery. Additional studies must be obtained before a final decision is made.

Reproductive System Injuries. Until 12 weeks' gestation, the uterus is a pelvic organ. As the uterus enlarges, it can assist in protecting other organs, but it becomes more vulnerable to injury. Direct trauma to the uterus or placenta reverses protective hemostasis by releasing an increased concentration of placental thromboplastin, a plasminogen activator, from the myometrium. The uteroplacental bed functions as a dilated, passive, low-resistance system that lacks autoregulation and therefore has few or no compensatory mechanisms. The body perceives the uterus as a peripheral or nonvital organ. Because the uteroplacental system receives 20% to 30% of maternal cardiac output, maintenance of adequate circulating blood volume is essential to ensure adequate blood flow. The abdomen must be palpated to assess uterine position, size, and firmness; the presence of contractions; and the fetal position.

Abruptio placentae, commonly seen with blunt abdominal trauma and pelvic fractures, may occur immediately, within 48 hours, or up to 5 days after injury. Uterine damage or rupture is rare, but if it occurs, it is commonly at the fundus or the site of a previous cesarean section and usually results in fetal death. Even if there was no identifiable damage to the reproductive system, there may be an increased risk for premature rupture of membranes (PROM), premature labor, fetal or maternal hemorrhage, or fetal damage or demise. It is recommended that pregnant patients with trauma be admitted to the hospital for 24 to 48 hours of fetal monitoring, because there may be latent injuries or the need for tocolytics.

Fetal Injuries. The fetus is usually well cushioned by amniotic fluid, the gravid uterus, and the abdominal wall, which distribute the force of injury. The most common cause of fetal death is maternal death. Placental abruption and fetal skull fracture, resulting from engagement of the fetal head into the pelvis, and intracranial hemorrhage have been identified as leading causes of fetal death. Potential predictors of fetal demise vary, depending on the study. Increased injury severity score (ISS), decreased hemoglobin level, need for blood replacement, presence of DIC, and abruptio placentae have been associated with increased fetal mortality rates.

NEUROLOGIC DYSFUNCTION

No known neurologic changes are associated with pregnancy, but women may have preexisting neurologic conditions. There are many neurologic conditions (see Chapter 27), but only those associated with the potential to place the mother and fetus at risk are discussed in this chapter.

EPILEPSY

Some of the most common maternal neurologic disorders are seizures, although seizures do not appear to increase the risk of pregnancy-induced hypertension (PIH), premature delivery, or other common complications. The frequency of seizures during pregnancy with preexisting epilepsy has been known to increase by 20% to 50%.[84-86] This is thought to be a result of reduced plasma concentrations and altered pharmacokinetics due to impaired absorption. Failure to adjust drug doses to compensate for increased maternal vascular volume, electrolyte changes, increased renal clearance, hormonal changes that alter hepatic enzyme systems responsible for drug metabolism, respiratory alkalosis, sleep deprivation (which lowers the seizure threshold), and noncompliance with medical regimen because of nausea, vomiting, or fear of harming the fetus have been identified as increasing the risk of seizure activity.[84-87] Efforts must be made to differentiate neurologic causes (e.g., epilepsy) from nonneurologic causes (e.g., PIH), because management is significantly different. The major goals in managing the epileptic patient are to prevent seizures in the mother and to minimize the risk of fetal teratogenic effects from anticonvulsant medications. Discontinuing anticonvulsant drugs should be considered if the electroencephalogram shows a lack of ectopic activity and if the patient has been seizure free on long-term, low-dose drugs. Discontinuing medications must be carefully balanced against the potential for development of seizures,

because fetal damage resulting from hypoxia during seizures can occur.

Management focuses on identifying the minimal drug dose required to prevent seizures and drugs that pose the least risk for fetal harm. Status epilepticus can be acutely managed with intravenous benzodiazepines followed by phenytoin or valproic acid. Although most anticonvulsant drugs have been associated with fetal abnormalities, studies have shown that most fetuses are unaffected. Because anticonvulsants interfere with folic acid metabolism, which can lead to maternal macrocytic anemia and fetal neural tube defects, folic acid supplements should be given. Polypharmacotherapy with multiple anticonvulsant agents must be avoided because this practice is associated with an increased risk for fetal damage. During the last month of pregnancy, supplemental vitamin K may be administered to protect the newborn against bleeding caused by vitamin K depletion.[84-86] As maternal physiology gradually returns to the nonpregnant state, drug doses may need to be reduced in the first 2 to 3 weeks after delivery.

INTRACRANIAL HEMORRHAGE

The most common cause of intracranial hemorrhage (ICH) in pregnancy is subarachnoid hemorrhage resulting from a ruptured cerebral aneurysm or arteriovenous malformation.[12,84,87] Cocaine use may lead to an increased incidence of ICH associated with vasospasm. Estimated mortality rates for pregnant patients with ICH are 30% to 40%.[13,84] Although it has been theorized that physiologic changes of pregnancy place increased strain on previously weakened cerebral vessels, clinical data have not supported this.

Management of ICH is only slightly different in the pregnant patient. Hypotensive agents such as sodium nitroprusside are commonly used to maintain the blood pressure within a desired range, but they must be used with great caution if the patient has not yet delivered. Hypotension and the toxic effects of nitroprusside can pose significant risk to the fetus.

MYASTHENIA GRAVIS

The few studies that have been conducted on patients with myasthenia gravis offer conflicting results. Some suggest that patients will experience an improvement in their condition, but others will experience an exacerbation during pregnancy and immediately after delivery.[88,89] Postpartum exacerbations are relatively common, and routine physician follow-up every 2 weeks for the first 6 weeks is recommended. Management during pregnancy should be the same as when the patient is not pregnant, although interventions may be required in the second stage of labor when the abdominal muscles are required for pushing. Physical and emotional stress during delivery should be limited as much as possible, and parental anticholinesterase agents should be administered as needed. Studies have shown that myasthenia gravis is associated with a higher occurrence of delivery complications necessitating interventions such as forceps, vacuum-assisted delivery, and cesarean section if the mother cannot effectively push with contractions.[90] There is increased maternal sensitivity to medications such as narcotics, central nervous system depressants, neuromuscular blockers, some anesthetics, and tocolytic agents. A myasthenic crisis may occur if magnesium sulfate is administered and may require ventilatory support. Epidural medications may be safely used to decrease pain and fatigue during labor. Critical respiratory muscle fatigue is best assessed by measurement of the forced vital capacity. Maternal antibodies to neurotransmitters may cross the placenta and cause the fetus to have transient symptoms of MG, manifested by respiratory depression, poor tone, weak cry, and poor sucking; however, these symptoms spontaneously subside within 6 weeks.[88-90]

Summary

- Optimal care for the critically ill obstetric patient or one who has sustained injuries requires persistent application of physiologic changes of pregnancy to normal adult values.

- Symptoms may be altered because of the pregnant state.
- Understanding the intricate maternal-fetal relationship provides practitioners with a focus of maintaining maternal stability to enhance uteroplacental perfusion and an optimal in utero environment.
- All potential therapeutic interventions must be weighed in light of the risk-benefit ratio to maternal-infant status.
- Critical situations may bring personal, cultural, social, spiritual, and ethical values into conflict.
- Determining the appropriate environment can be challenging. Some institutions have created dedicated obstetric intensive care units, whereas others provide care in the obstetric care unit or critical care unit.
- Decision making must be done in collaboration with family and health care team members, and all options should be considered.
- The key factor is collaboration among specialties to optimize maternal-fetal outcomes and facilitate the family experience.

Case Study: Patient with Obstetric Issues

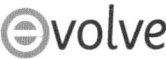 Answers to the Case Study Questions can be found on the Evolve web site at http://evolve.elsevier.com/Urden/.

Brief Patient History

Mrs. S is 33 years old. She delivered a term baby boy by cesarean section this morning. Mrs. S has experienced chills, malaise, and abdominal pain since the operation, and she has been given morphine for pain relief but is still complaining of abdominal pain.

Clinical Assessment

Mrs. S is admitted to the intensive care unit with hypotension, tachypnea, and tachycardia. She is lethargic, curled up in bed, and groaning. She does not follow commands or answer questions. There has been no urine output over the last 4 hours, and when a urinary catheter is placed, there is only 10 mL of dark amber urine.

Diagnostic Procedures

Her admission vital signs are as follows: blood pressure of 60/35 mm Hg, heart rate of 145 beats/min (sinus tachycardia), respiratory rate of 30 breaths/min, temperature of 97.5° F, hemoglobin level of 5 g/dL, and

platelet level of 30,000/μL. Ultrasound reveals a large fluid collection in the abdomen.

Medical Diagnosis

Mrs. S is diagnosed with an intraabdominal bleed.

Questions

1. What major outcomes do you expect to achieve for this patient?
2. What problems or risks must be managed to achieve these outcomes?
3. What interventions must be initiated to monitor, prevent, manage, or eliminate the problems and risks identified?
4. What interventions should be initiated to promote optimal functioning, safety, and well-being of the patient?
5. What possible learning needs do you anticipate for this patient?
6. What cultural and age-related factors may have a bearing on the patient's plan of care?

⊖volve Be sure to check out the bonus material, including free self-assessment exercises, on the Evolve web site at http://evolve.elsevier.com/Urden/.

References

1. Poole J, Long J: Maternal mortality—a review of current trends, *Crit Care Nurs Clin North Am* 16:227-230, 2004.
2. Niebyl J: Teratology and drugs in pregnancy. In Scott JR et al, editors: *Danforth's obstetrics and gynecology*, ed 10, Philadelphia, 2008, Lippincott.
3. Hill C, Pickinpaugh J: Trauma and surgical emergencies in the obstetric patient, *Surg Clin North Am* 88:421-440, 2007.
4. Lowe S: Diagnostic radiology in pregnancy: risks and reality, *Aust N Z J Obstet Gynaecol* 44:191-196, 2004.
5. Valentin J: Pregnancy and medical radiation, ICRP publication no. 84, *Ann ICRP* 30:1-43, 2000.

6. American College of Obstetricians and Gynecologists: *Guidelines for diagnostic imaging during pregnancy*, ACOG committee opinion no 299, Washington, DC, ACOG, 2004.

7. Stabin M: Doses from medical radiation sources, Health Physics Society, June 2008. Available at http//hps.org (accessed January 2009).

8. McCollough C et al: Radiation exposure and pregnancy: when should we be concerned? *Radiographics* 24:909-918, 2007.

9. Briggs G et al: *Drugs in pregnancy and lactation*, ed 7, Baltimore, 2005, Williams & Wilkins.

10. Riordan J, Auerbach K: *Breastfeeding and human lactation*, ed 3, Boston, 2005, Jones & Bartlett.

11. Heppard M, Garite T: *Acute obstetrics—a practical guide*, ed 3, St Louis, 2002, Mosby.

12. Cunningham FG et al: *Williams' obstetrics*, ed 22, New York, 2005, McGraw-Hill.

13. Dildy G et al, editors: *Critical care obstetrics*, ed 4, Malden, MA, 2004, Blackwell.

14. Clark S et al: Central hemodynamic observations in normal third trimester pregnancy, *Am J Obstet Gynecol* 161:1439-1442, 1989.

15. American College of Obstetricians and Gynecologists: *Invasive hemodynamic monitoring in obstetrics and gynecology*, ACOG technical bulletin 121, Washington, DC, ACOG, 1988.

16. Harvey MG: Physiologic changes of pregnancy. In Harvey CJ, editor: *Critical care obstetrical nursing*, Gaithersburg, MD, 1991, Aspen.

17. Gardner M, Doyle N. Asthma in pregnancy. *Obstet Gynecol Clin North Am*, 31:385-413, 2004.

18. Monga M, Creasy R: Cardiovascular and renal adaptation to pregnancy. In Creasy R, Resnik R, editors: *Maternal-fetal medicine*, ed 5, Philadelphia, 2004, Saunders.

19. Criteria Committee of the New York Heart Association: *Nomenclature and criteria for diagnosis of disease of the heart and great vessels*, ed 6, Boston, 1964, Little, Brown.

20. American College of Obstetricians and Gynecologists: *Cardiac disease in pregnancy*, ACOG technical bulletin 168, Washington, DC, ACOG, 1992.

21. Rutherford JD, Hands M: Pregnancy with preexisting heart disease. In Douglas PS, editor: *Cardiovascular health and disease in women*, Philadelphia, 1993, Saunders.

22. Shabetai R: Cardiac disease. In Creasy R, Resnik R, editors: *Maternal-fetal medicine*, ed 5, Philadelphia, 2004, Saunders.

23. Brar S et al: Incidence, mortality, and racial differences in peripartum cardiomyopathy. *Am J Cardiol* DOI: 10.1016/j.amjcard.2007.02.092.

24. Yang H et al: Extracorporeal membrane oxygenation in a patient with peripartum cardiomyopathy. *Ann Thorac Surg* 84.262-264, 2007. DOI: 10.1016/j.athoracsur.2007.02.050.

25. Mulari S, Baldisseri MR: Peripartum cardiomyopathy. *Crit Care Med* 33(10): S340-S346, 2005.

26. Amos A et al: Improved outcomes in peripartum cardiomyopathy with contemporary. *Am Heart J* 152(3):509-513, 2006. DOI: 10.1016/j.ahj.2006.02.008.

27. Mishra T et al: Peripartum cardiomyopathy. *Int J Gynecol Obstet* 95: 104-109, 2006. DOI: 10.1016/j.ijgo.2006.06.013.

28. Hu C et al: Troponin T measurement can predict persistent left ventricular dysfunction in peripartum cardiomyopathy. *Heart* 93:488-490, 2007.

29. Lange S, Jenner M: Myocardial infarction in the obstetric patient. *Crit Care Nurs Clin North Am* 16:211-219, 2004.

30. Klein L, Galan H: Cardiac disease in pregnancy. *Obstet Gynecol Clin North Am* 31:429-459, 2004.

31. Ladner H et al: Acute myocardial infarction in pregnancy and the puerperium: a population based study. *Obstet Gynecol* 105:480-484, 2005.

32. American Heart Association: *2005 American Heart Association guidelines for cardiopulmonary resuscitation and emergency cardiovascular care. Circulation* 112 (suppl IV):IV150-IV153, 2005.

33. Habli M, Sabai B: Hypertensive disorders of pregnancy. In Gibbs RS et al, editors: *Danforth's obstetrics and gynecology*, ed 10, Philadelphia, 2008, Lippincott, Williams & Wilkins.

34. National High Blood Pressure in Pregnancy Education Program Working Group (NHBPEP): *Working Group report on high blood pressure in pregnancy*, Bethesda, MD, 2000, National Heart Lung and Blood Institute.

35. Grimes DA: The morbidity and mortality of pregnancy: still risky business, *Am J Obstet Gynecol* 170(Pt 2):1489-1494, 1994.

36. American College of Obstetricians and Gynecologists: *Invasive hemodynamic monitoring in obstetrics and gynecology*, ACOG technical bulletin 219, Washington, DC, ACOG, 1996.

37. Clark S et al: *Handbook of critical care obstetrics*, Boston, 1994, Blackwell Scientific.

38. Gilbert E, Harmon J: *Manual of high risk pregnancy and delivery*, ed 3, St Louis, 2003, Mosby.

39. Peters RM, Flack JM: Hypertensive disorders of pregnancy, *J Obstet Gynecol Neonatal Nurs* 33(2):209-214, 2004.

40. American College of Obstetricians and Gynecologists: *Hypertension in pregnancy*, ACOG practice bulletin no 29, Washington, DC, 2001, ACOG.

41. National High Blood Pressure Education Working Group on High Blood Pressure in Pregnancy: Report of the National High Blood Pressure Education Working Group on High Blood Pressure in Pregnancy, *Am J Obstet Gynecol* 183(1):S1-S22, 2000.

42. Walsh S: Preeclampsia: an imbalance in placental prostacyclin and thromboxane production, *Am J Obstet Gynecol* 152:335-340, 1985.

43. Sibai B, Mabie C: Hemodynamics of preeclampsia, *Clin Perinatol* 18(4): 727-747, 1991.

44. Sibai BM: Treatment of hypertension in pregnant women, *N Engl J Med* 335:257-264, 1996.

45. Wolf JL: Liver disease in pregnancy. *Med Clin North Am* 80:1167-1187, 1996.

46. Villar M, Sibai B: Eclampsia, *Obstet Gynecol Clin North Am* 15(2): 355-377, 1988.

47. Clark S: Critical care obstetrics. In Gibbs RS et al, editors: *Danforth's obstetrics and gynecology*, ed 10, Philadelphia, 2008, Lippincott, Williams & Wilkins.

48. Powrie R: Respiratory disease. In James D et al, editors: *High risk pregnancy: management options*, ed 3, Philadelphia, 2006, Elsevier Saunders.

49. Montoro M: Pulmonary disorders in pregnancy. In DeCherney A et al, editors: *Current diagnosis and treatment obstetrics and gynecology*, ed 10, New York, 2007, McGraw-Hill.

50. Schatz M: Asthma. In Queenan J, editors: *Management of high-risk pregnancies*, ed 5, Malden, MA, 2007, Blackwell Publishing.

51. Whitty J, Dombrowski M: Respiratory diseases in pregnancy. In Gabbe S, editors: *Obstetrics: normal and problem pregnancies*, ed 5, Philadelphia, 2007, Churchill Livingstone Elsevier.

52. Grossman S, Grossman L: Pathophysiology of cystic fibrosis: implications for critical care nurses, *Crit Care Nurs* 25(4):46-51, 2005.

53. Cunningham G et al: Pulmonary disorders: In Cunningham G et al, editors: *Williams' obstetrics*, ed 22, New York, 2005, McGraw-Hill.

54. Goldberg J, Smith R: Critical care obstetrics. In DeCherney A et al, editors: *Current diagnosis and treatment obstetrics and gynecology*, ed 10, New York, 2007, McGraw-Hill.

55. Laros R: Thromboembolic disease. In Creasy R, Resnik R, editors: *Maternal-fetal medicine: principles and practice*, ed 5, Philadelphia, 2004, Saunders.

56. Pettker C, Lockwood C: Thromboembolic disorders. In Gabbe S et al, editors: *Obstetrics: normal and problem pregnancies*, ed 5, Philadelphia, 2007, Churchill Livingstone Elsevier.

57. Pettker C, Lockwood C: Pathophysiology and diagnosis of thromboembolic disorders in pregnancy. In Queenan J et al, editors: *Management of high-risk pregnancies*, ed 5, Malden, MA, 2007, Blackwell Publishing.

58. Shaughnessy K: Massive pulmonary embolism, *Crit Care Nurs* 27(1):39-50, 2007.

59. Rosenberg V, Lockwood C: Thromboembolism in pregnancy, *Obstet Gynecol Clin North Am* 34:481-500, 2007.

60. American College of Obstetricians and Gynecologists: *Thromboembolism in pregnancy*, ACOG practice bulletin no 19, Washington, DC, ACOG, 2000.

61. Farquharson R, Greaves M: Thromboembolic disease. In James D et al, editors: *High-risk pregnancy: management options*, ed 3, Philadelphia, 2006, Elsevier Saunders.

62. Cooney M: Heparin-induced thrombocytopenia: advances in diagnosis and treatment, *Crit Care Nurs* 26(6):30-36, 2006.

63. Stafford I, Sheffield J: Amniotic fluid embolism, *Obstet Gynecol Clin North Am* 34:545-553, 2007.

64. Perozzi K, Englert N: Amniotic fluid embolism: an obstetric emergency, *Crit Care Nurse* 24(4):54-61, 2004.

65. Naylor DF, Olson MM: Critical care obstetrics and gynecology, *Crit Care Clin* 19(1):127-149, 2003.

66. DeJong MJ, Fausett MB: Anaphylactoid syndrome of pregnancy: a devastating complication requiring intensive care, *Crit Care Nurse* 23(6):42-48, 2003.

67. Dildy GA, Clark SL: Anaphylactoid syndrome of pregnancy (amniotic fluid embolism). In Dildy GA, editor: *Critical care obstetrics*, ed 4, Malden, MA, 2003, Blackwell Scientific.

68. Rudisill P: Amniotic fluid embolism, *Crit Care Nurs Clin North Am* 16(2):221-225 2004.

69. American College of Obstetricians and Gynecologists: *Obstetric aspects of trauma management*, ACOG educational bulletin 251, Washington, DC, ACOG, September 1998.

70. El Kady D: Perinatal outcomes of traumatic injures during pregnancy, *Clin Obstet Gynecol* 50(3):582-591, 2007.

71. Tweedale C: Trauma during pregnancy, *Crit Care Nurs Q* 29(1):53-67, 2006.

72. American College of Obstetricians and Gynecologists: *Domestic violence*, ACOG educational bulletin 257, Washington, DC, ACOG, December 1999.

73. Lipsky S et al: Impact of police reported intimate partner violence during pregnancy on birth outcomes, *Obstet Gynecol* 102(3):557-564, 2003.

74. Lu M et al: Domestic violence and sexual assault. In DeCherney A et al, editors: *Current Diagnosis and treatment obstetrics and gynecology*, ed 10, New York, 2007, McGraw-Hill.

75. Gunter J: Intimate Partner Violence, *Obstet Gynecol Clin North Am* 34:367-388, 2007.

76. Muench MV, Canterino JC: Trauma in pregnancy, *Obstet Gynecol Clin North Am* 34:555-583, 2007.

77. Stallard TC, Burns B: Emergency delivery and perimortem C-section, *Emerg Med Clin North Am* 21:679-693, 2003.

78. Bobrowski R: Trauma. In James D et al, editors: *High risk pregnancy: management options*, ed 3, Philadelphia, 2006, Elsevier Saunders.

79. Constanty P, Cruz D: Trauma and the obstetric patient: Collaboration in care, *Crit Care Nurs Clin North Am* 18:273-278, 2006.

80. Meroz Y et al: Initial trauma management in advanced pregnancy, *Anesthesiol Clin* 24:117-129, 2007.

81. Cusick S, Tibbles C: Trauma in pregnancy, *Emerg Med Clin North Am* 25:861-872, 2007.

82. Pereira L: Obstetric management of the patient with spinal cord injuries, *Obstet Gynecol Surv* 58(10):678-686, 2003.

83. American College of Obstetricians and Gynecologists: *Obstetric management of patients with spinal cord injuries*, ACOG committee opinion 275, Washington, DC, ACOG, 2002.

84. Carhuapoma F et al: Neurologic disorders. In James D et al, editors: *High risk pregnancy: management options*, ed 3, Philadelphia, 2006, Elsevier Saunders.

85. Pennell P: Epilepsy. In Queenan J et al, editors: *Management of high-risk pregnancies*, ed 5, Malden, MA, 2007, Blackwell Publishing.

86. Samuals P, Niebyl J: Neurologic disorders. In Gabbe S et al, editors: *Obstetrics: normal and problem pregnancies*, ed 5, Philadelphia, 2007, Churchill Livingstone Elsevier.

87. Neurologic and psychiatric disorders: In Cunningham G et al, editors: *Williams' obstetrics*, ed 22, New York, 2005, McGraw-Hill.

88. Aminoff M: Neurologic disorders. In Creasy R, Resnik R, editors: *Maternal-fetal medicine: principles and practice*, ed 5 Philadelphia, 2004, WB Saunders.

89. Porter T, Branch D: Autoimmune diseases. In James D et al, editors: *High risk pregnancy: management options*, ed 3, Philadelphia, 2006, Elsevier Saunders.

90. Hoff JM et al: Myasthenia gravis: consequences for pregnancy, delivery, and the newborn, *Neurology* 61:1362-1366, 2003.

Gerontologic Alterations and Management

Chapter

14

$\mathcal{P}$atients in critical care units include an increasing number of older adults. Patients older than 65 years currently account for 42% to 52% of admissions to intensive care units (ICUs) and for almost 60% of all ICU days.[1] This trend is directly related to the aging of America. The total number of older Americans in 2006 was 37.3 million, including 21.6 million women and 15.7 million men. This translates to 12.4% of the American population older than 65 years, with an average life expectancy of 83.7 years. The population of Americans older than 65 years is predicted to increase to 40 million in 2010 and then to 55 million in 2020.[2] Overall, there was a 10% increase in the number of people reaching 65 years of age in the decade from 1996 to 2006. The composition of the elderly population by culture or minority group includes 8.3% African Americans, 6.4% Hispanic, 3.1% Asian or Pacific Islander, and less than 1% American Indian or Native Alaskan.[2]

Statistics from 2005 reflect that 13.2 million persons who were 65 years old or older were discharged from short-stay hospitals, with an average length of stay of 5.5 days. In 2004 through 2005, older persons tended to present with at least one chronic condition. The most common conditions were hypertension (48%), arthritis (47%), all types of heart disease (29%), cancer (20%), diabetes (16%), and sinusitis (14%).[2] More than 35% of older adults reported a severe disability.[2] Older consumers' out-of-pocket health care expenditures averaged $4331, an increase of 57% since 1995, whereas the comparable figure for the total U.S. population was $2766. Older Americans spent 12.4% of their total expenditures on health care, more than twice the proportion spent by all consumers (5.7%).[2] Health care costs included insurance, drugs, medical services, and medical supplies.

The process of senescence (growing old) is characterized by tissue and organ changes. This, in combination with the prevalence of chronic conditions in older adults, contributes to increased morbidity and mortality in the critical care unit. Aging is accompanied by physiologic changes in the cardiovascular, respiratory, renal, gastrointestinal, hepatic, integumentary, immune, and central nervous systems. With advancing age, the incidence of disease increases, with cardiovascular and neoplastic diseases being the most common causes of death.[3] Although physiologic decline and disease processes influence each other, physiologic decline occurs independently of disease and is responsible for the development of symptoms at an earlier stage of disease in older adults than in their younger counterparts.[3] Changes in physiologic function are important to consider when caring for the older adult patient. The purpose of this chapter is to acquaint the critical care nurse with literature and research on the age-associated changes in physiologic function in healthy older adults and to describe implications for this population in critical care.

CARDIOVASCULAR SYSTEM

Advancing age has many effects on the cardiovascular system. With advancing age, a multitude of anatomic and cellular changes in the myocardium and peripheral vascular system alter their functional capability.[4] These changes in age-related effects on cardiovascular structure and function have a significant impact on critical illness in the older adult. Because age is a major risk factor for cardiovascular disease in the older adult, this high-risk population encounters more cardiovascular events when admitted to the critical care unit for noncardiac problems.[5]

AGE-RELATED CHANGES IN MYOCARDIAL STRUCTURE AND FUNCTION

Myocardial collagen content increases with age.[6,7] Collagen is the principal noncontractile protein occupying the cardiac interstitium.[8] Increased myocardial collagen content renders the myocardium less compliant. A decrease in myocardial compliance can adversely affect diastolic filling (through decreased distensibility and dilation) and myocardial relaxation. Consequently, the left ventricle must develop a higher filling pressure for a given increase in ventricular volume. Decreased left ventricular compliance may be evident in the older adult by the presence of an S_4 heart sound.[8,9]

The functional consequence of these changes could be an increase in myocardial oxygen consumption. Under normal physiologic conditions, an increase in myocardial oxygen demand is met with a corresponding increase in coronary artery blood flow. However, in the presence of coronary artery disease, coronary artery blood flow can be limited because of atherosclerotic-mediated narrowing of the coronary arteries. Hence, the older patient is at risk for developing myocardial ischemia or infarction. Clinical manifestations of myocardial ischemia include electrocardiographic (ECG) changes and chest pain. However, the sensation of chest pain may be altered in the older adult. Nadelmann and colleagues[10] found that complaints of chest pain were absent in 50% of older adult patients (>74 years) who sustained a myocardial infarction. Others[11] have reported that chest pain in the older adult is less intense, of shorter duration, and originates in other areas of the chest besides the substernal region. Atypical symptoms, such as dyspnea, confusion, and failure to thrive are frequently the only symptoms associated with myocardial infarction in this high-risk population.[12]

Atypical or unrecognized signs and symptoms of myocardial infarction frequently lead to delays in diagnosis and treatment. Although 60% to 65% of ST-segment–elevated myocardial infarctions occur in patients 65 years old or older, most myocardial infarctions in the elderly are associated with ST-segment depression. Bundle branch blocks and acute heart failure are more commonly seen in patients 85 years old or older. Up to 80% of all myocardial-related deaths occur in persons 65 years old or older.[13]

The aging heart undergoes a modest degree of hypertrophy that is similar to pressure overload–induced hypertrophy. Such hypertrophy entails a thickening of the left ventricular wall without appreciable changes in left ventricular cavity size.[14] Increases in left ventricular cavity size associated with aging occur only in men.[12] The increase in left ventricular wall thickness is a result primarily of an increase in muscle cell size. In older individuals the myocardial hypertrophy may be caused by corresponding increases in aortic impedance and systemic vascular resistance.[15]

Myocardial contractility depends on numerous factors. However, the most important determinants of myocardial contraction are the intracellular level of free calcium and the sensitivity of the contractile proteins for calcium.[15,16] Because peak contractile force in the senescent myocardium is unaltered, this suggests that neither the amount of intracellular free calcium during systole nor the sensitivity of the contractile proteins for calcium is altered. The prolonged duration of contraction (systole) is caused in part by a slowed or delayed rate of myocardial relaxation, which may be an adaptive mechanism to preserve contractile function compromised by age-related increases in afterload.[4,16]

AGE-ASSOCIATED CHANGES IN HEMODYNAMICS AND THE ELECTROCARDIOGRAM

The resting (supine) heart rate decreases with age.[17,18] Cinelli and colleagues[17] reported a decrease in the resting heart rate from 78.8 beats/min in young adults to 62.3 beats/min in older adults. Heart rate is an important determinant of cardiac output (CO), and the normal resting heart beats approximately 70 times each minute. At rest or with minimal activity, the older adult probably will not experience any untoward cardiovascular effect (i.e., a decrease in CO) with a heart rate of 62 beats/min. However, if the heart rate response is attenuated during exercise, the older person's capacity for exercise may be limited.[18] Intrinsic heart rate also decreases with aging.[18] The *intrinsic heart rate* is the heart rate in the absence of parasympathetic and sympathetic influences. In healthy, resting individuals, parasympathetic (cholinergic) influences predominate, causing a heart rate of approximately 70 beats/min.[11] In the absence of parasympathetic and sympathetic influences, the heart rate of young adults averages about 100 beats/min (intrinsic heart rate). Jose[19] found that the intrinsic heart rate (in the presence of sympathetic and parasympathetic blockers) in a 20-year-old person was 100 beats/min, compared with a heart rate of 74 beats/min in an 80-year-old man. This decrease in intrinsic heart rate may in part explain the decrease in the resting (supine) heart rate that occurs with aging.

Resting CO and stroke volume are not changed with advancing age. Rodeheffer and coworkers[20] studied subjects without coronary artery disease or other types of illness over a 30- to 80-year period and found no changes in the resting CO or the cardiac index in participants.[20] At rest, left ventricular end-diastolic volume (preload), end-systolic volume, and the ejection fraction are not affected by age.[21] In the elderly human myocardium, the early diastolic filling period and isovolumic phase of myocardial relaxation are prolonged.[21-23] However, these changes, although suggestive of diastolic dysfunction, do not translate into decreases in end-diastolic volume or stroke volume.[22,23] Aging is associated with a moderate increase in pulmonary artery pressure.[24]

Advancing age produces changes in the ECG. R wave and S wave amplitude significantly decrease in persons older than 49 years, whereas QT duration increases[25] (Table 14-1). The increase in the duration of the QT interval is reflective of the prolonged rate of relaxation.[25] The frontal plane axis shifts downward from 48.93 to 38.83 degrees between the ages of 30 and 49 years, which suggests a modest degree of cardiac enlargement or hypertrophy.[25] The incidence of asymptomatic cardiac dysrhythmias increases in elderly patients.[26] The most common dysrhythmia occurring in older individuals is the premature ventricular contraction (PVC). Carom and associates[27] and Fleg and Kennedy[28] reported that 70% to 80% of all patients older than 60 years experience PVCs. In a healthy

TABLE 14-1 Age-Related Changes in Electrocardiographic Variables

ECG Variable	Age (yr)			
	<30	30–39	40–49	>49
R wave amplitude (mm)	10.43	10.53	9.01	9.25
S wave amplitude (mm)	15.21	14.21	12.22	12.42
Frontal plane axis (degrees)	48.93	48.13	36.50	38.83
PR duration (msec)	15.89	16.23	16.04	16.25
QRS duration (msec)	7.64	7.51	7.36	8.00
QT duration (msec)	37.83	37.50	37.99	39.58
T wave amplitude (msec)	5.21	4.57	4.31	4.42

Data from Bachman S et al: Effect of aging on the electrocardiogram, *Am J Cardiol* 48:513, 1981.

geriatric population (60 to 85 years old) studied with the use of 24-hour ambulatory ECG recordings, 78 of 98 subjects experienced asymptomatic ventricular ectopic beats. Other common types of dysrhythmias are sinus node dysfunction (i.e., atrial fibrillation, atrial flutter, or paroxysmal supraventricular tachycardia) and atrioventricular conduction disturbances.[21,25,26] Because most patients are asymptomatic, the use of antidysrhythmic agents is generally not recommended. The side effects and toxic effects of antidysrhythmic agents impose a greater risk than the risk of mortality or morbidity related to the dysrhythmia.[26,29] However, rate control and anticoagulation are recommended for most patients with atrial fibrillation.

Beta-blockers and calcium channel blockers are recommended for rate control at rest and during exercise. Amiodarone can be effective for acute conversion and maintenance of sinus rhythm after conversion from atrial fibrillation.[30] Aging increases the risk of major hemorrhage in patients with atrial fibrillation, with or without warfarin therapy. Risk factors associated with increased bleeding risk with anticoagulation therapy include polypharmacy, age greater than 75 years, concomitant use of antiplatelet drugs, uncontrolled hypertension, and poorly controlled anticoagulation therapy. Careful monitoring of warfarin therapy is essential for optimizing clinical outcomes in this vulnerable population.[31]

Symptomatic or malignant ventricular dysrhythmias (e.g., sustained ventricular tachycardia or fibrillation) are best managed with the use of pharmacologic therapy.[26,29] Studies support the addition of cardiac-resynchronization therapy rather than pharmacologic therapy alone in patients with advanced heart failure, as a mechanism to further reduce mortality associated with dysrhythmias.[30,32]

AGE-RELATED CHANGES IN BARORECEPTOR FUNCTION

Baroreceptor-reflex function is altered with aging.[33] *Baroreceptors*—mechanoreceptors that respond to stretch and other changes in the blood vessel wall—are located at the bifurcation of the common carotid artery and the aortic arch.[15] Impulses arising in the baroreceptor region project to the vasomotor center (nucleus of tractus solitarius) in the medulla. Abrupt changes in blood pressure caused by increases in peripheral resistance, CO, or blood volume are sensed by the baroreceptors, resulting in an increase in the impulse frequency to the vasomotor center within the medulla. This increase inhibits vasoconstrictor impulses arising from the vasoconstrictor region within the medulla.[15] The result is a decrease in heart rate and peripheral vasodilation; both of these effects return the blood pressure to within normal limits. The baroreflex can be tested by measuring the heart rate response (i.e., increase or decrease in heart rate) after the administration of a pressor or a depressor agent and by changing the patient's position from lying to standing. Yin[54] and Elliott[55] and their colleagues found an attenuated increase in heart rate response in elderly subjects after the infusion of phenylephrine, an α_1-adrenoreceptor agonist that produces vasoconstriction and increases the blood pressure. Likewise, the baroreflex-mediated tachycardia response to

depressor agents is also attenuated in older adults.[34] There are several reports of attenuation in the heart rate response of older adults after changes in position (e.g., supine to standing).[36,37]

When an individual changes his or her position from supine to standing, the distribution of blood volume changes. This can result in a reduction in CO and hence blood pressure.[15] However, simultaneous baroreceptor-mediated increases in the heart rate maintain blood pressure by increasing CO. The baroreceptor-reflex response also mediates changes in peripheral resistance and in the force of myocardial contraction, which likewise serve to offset the drop in blood pressure. It was once thought that postural hypotension occurred more frequently in older adults and was an age-related phenomenon. However, the prevalence of postural hypotension is quite low in older adults.[38,39] The prevalence of orthostatic hypotension is greater in institutionalized geriatric patients who are receiving antihypertensive medications.[37]

LEFT VENTRICULAR FUNCTION DURING EXERCISE IN THE OLDER ADULT

In most individuals, aging is associated with a decline in exercise performance. Exercise performance depends on a multitude of physiologic variables. Cardiac performance and the ability of the heart to increase and maintain CO are critical for increasing oxygen delivery to the peripheral tissues. During exercise, CO is increased by several mechanisms, the most important of which are increased heart rate, increased inotropic state of the myocardium, and decreased aortic impedance.[20] Some reports suggest that changes in exercise performance are related to a decrease in the maximal CO that can be achieved with exercise. However, Rodeheffer and associates[20] reported that this is not the cause of the older adult's diminished ability to exercise. They found no difference in CO response to various levels of exercise in subjects from the Baltimore Longitudinal Study of Aging.[20] With advancing age, the maximal heart rate achieved during exercise is attenuated; however, the decreased heart rate response is accompanied by an increase in left ventricular end-diastolic volume and stroke volume. These augmentations offset the attenuated heart rate response and maintain CO during exercise. Changes in aortic impedance have not been studied in older individuals; however, blood pressure and systemic vascular resistance are increased during exercise in senescent animals, but not in young adult animal models.[40] In summary, in healthy older individuals there is no age-associated decline in CO during exercise; however, other factors, such as neural functioning, skeletal and joint functioning, and pulmonary function, may limit an older individual's ability to exercise.

PERIPHERAL VASCULAR SYSTEM

The effects of aging on the peripheral vascular system are reflected in the gradual but linear rise in systolic blood pressure up until age 80 years, when values tend to plateau.[21,41,42] Diastolic blood pressure is less affected by age and generally remains the same or decreases.[41,42] Important determinants of systolic blood pressure include the compliance of the vasculature and the blood volume within the vascular system. As in the heart, the compliance of the vasculature is determined by its cell type and tissue composition. With advancing age, the intimal layer thickens, principally because of an increase in smooth muscle cells (that have migrated from the medial layer), and the amount of connective tissue (collagen and elastic tissue) increases.[41] These changes occur in the intima of the large and distal arteries. This gradual decrease in arterial compliance, or "stiffening of the arteries," is sometimes referred to as *arteriosclerosis*. Arteriosclerotic changes are also accompanied by changes caused by atherosclerosis, which is the accumulation within a vessel of lipoproteins and fibrinous products such as platelets, macrophages, and leukocytes.[43] The consequences of arteriosclerotic and atherosclerotic processes are that the arteries become progressively less distensible and the vascular pressure-volume relationship is altered. These changes are clinically significant, because small changes in intravascular volume are accompanied by disproportionate increases in systolic blood pressure.[44] The decrease in arterial compliance and disproportionate increase in systolic blood pressure may lead to an increase in afterload and the development of concentric (pressure-induced) ventricular hypertrophy in the older adult.[44]

Increased serum lipoprotein levels are risk factors for the development and progression of atherosclerosis.[43] Lipoprotein levels increase with advancing age. However, innumerable factors can influence serum lipoprotein levels, making it very difficult to determine whether such changes contribute to the aging of the peripheral vascular system.[45,46] Serum lipoproteins are particles that contain various amounts of cholesterol, triglycerides, phospholipids, and apoproteins.[43] The five principal serum lipoproteins are chylomicrons, low-density lipoproteins (LDLs), very-low-density lipoproteins (VLDLs), intermediate-density lipoproteins (IDLs), and high-density lipoproteins (HDLs). The classification of lipoproteins is based on their size and relative concentration of cholesterol, triglycerides, and apoproteins.[43] In men, the serum total cholesterol level (all of the lipoproteins combined) increases progressively from 150 to 200 mg/dL between the ages of 20 and 50 years and remains relatively unchanged until the age of 70 years.[46] As may be predicted, the age-related changes in serum LDL levels parallel the changes in the total serum cholesterol level. All lipoprotein fractions transport cholesterol; however, in healthy people, three fourths of the total cholesterol is transported within the LDL.[43] There are relatively few age-related changes in VLDL and HDL levels in men. In men, serum triglyceride levels peak at approximately age 40 years and then decrease.[45,46]

In women, serum total cholesterol levels are low between the ages of 20 and 50 years.[45,46] However, between the ages of 55 and 60 years, serum total cholesterol levels progressively increase, usually simultaneously with changes in the hormonal production of estrogen.[46] The increase in total serum cholesterol levels is primarily the result of an increase in the LDL fraction and, to a lesser extent, the VLDL and HDL fractions, which do not change appreciably with age in women. In women, serum triglyceride levels progressively increase with age.[46]

Arterial pressure is also governed by the amount of blood volume, which is regulated by plasma levels of sodium and water and the activity of the renin-angiotensin system (RAS).[47] Plasma renin activity declines with age, and aging per se has no appreciable effect on sodium and water homeostasis.[47,48] However, there are age-related changes in tubular function and a decrease in the glomerular filtration rate (GFR), both of which can affect overall sodium and water homeostasis. Circulating levels of sodium-regulating hormones, such as natriuretic hormone, aldosterone, and antidiuretic hormone (ADH), are not appreciably altered by advancing age.[48] However, a delayed natriuretic response after sodium loading and plasma volume expansion and diminished renal response to ADH secretion have been reported in older adults.[48]

PULMONARY SYSTEM

Many of the changes in the pulmonary system that occur with aging are reflected in tests of pulmonary function and include changes in thoracic wall expansion and respiratory muscle strength, morphology of alveolar parenchyma, and decreases in arterial oxygen tension (PaO_2)[49,50] (Tables 14-2 and 14-3). These changes occur progressively as age advances and should not alter the older adult's ability to breathe effortlessly. However, factors such as repeated exposure to environmental pollutants, cigarette smoking, and frequent pulmonary infections can accelerate age-related changes, making it difficult to identify the age-associated changes in pulmonary function.[51] Thurlbeck[52] did not find age-related morphologic changes in the lung tissue of aging mice raised in a pollution- and infection-free environment, suggesting the immense effect of environmental variables on pulmonary function.

THORACIC WALL AND RESPIRATORY MUSCLES

The aging chest wall (i.e., thoracic skeleton) and vertebrae undergo a small degree of osteoporosis. Rib mobility declines because of contractures of intercostal muscles and calcification of costal cartilage. Progressive decreases in chest wall compliance due to structural changes of kyphosis and vertebral collapse lead to deterioration in respiratory function (Fig. 14-1).[49,50,53,54] Maximum inspiratory and expiratory force may decrease by as much as 50% because of decline in respiratory muscle strength.[1] The functional effect is a decrease in thoracic wall excursion. Other factors, such as an increase in abdominal girth and change in posture, also decrease thoracic excursion. These anatomic changes are reflected by an increase in residual volume and decrease in vital capacity (see Table 14-2).

Strength of the diaphragm and the external and internal intercostal muscles decreases with age. The diaphragm is the most important inspiratory muscle because its movement accounts for 75% of the change in intrathoracic volume during quiet respiration.[54] The respiratory muscles are composed of skeletal muscle fibers.[55] During aging, skeletal muscle progressively atrophies, and its energy metabolism decreases, which may partially explain the declining strength of the respiratory

TABLE 14-2   Age-Related Changes in Commonly Performed Pulmonary Function Tests

Pulmonary Function Test	Description	Standard Lung Volume and Capacity (mL)	Age-Related Change (mL)
Total lung capacity (TLC)	Vital capacity plus residual volume	6000	No change
Vital capacity (VC)	Amount of air exhaled after a maximal inspiration	5000	↓ 3750
Tidal volume (V_T)	Amount of air inhaled or exhaled with each breath	500	No change
Residual volume (RV)	Amount of air left in lungs after forced exhalation	1200	↓ 1800
Inspiratory reserve volume (IRV)	Amount of air that can be forcefully inhaled after inspiring a normal V_T	3100	↓ 2800
Expiratory reserve volume (ERV)	Amount of air that can be forcefully exhaled after expiring a normal V_T	1200	↓ 1000
Forced expiratory volume in 1 second (FEV_1)	Volume exhaled in the first second of a single forced expiratory volume; expressed as a percentage of the forced vital capacity	80%	↓ 75%

TABLE 14-3   Progressive Changes in Arterial Oxygen Tension and Carbon Dioxide Tension

Age Group (yr)	Pao_2 (mm Hg)	$Paco_2$ (mm Hg)
≤30	94	39
31–40	87	38
41–50	84	40
51–60	81	39
>60	74	40

$Paco_2$, carbon dioxide tension; Pao_2, arterial oxygen tension.
Data from Sorbini CA et al: Arterial oxygen tension in relation to age in healthy subjects, *Respiration* 25:3, 1968.

muscles.[55,56] There also is an age-associated decrease in the effectiveness of the cough reflex, which is possibly caused by a decrease in ciliary responsiveness and motion.[50,57] These changes underscore the importance of deep breathing and coughing for the bedridden older patient in the critical care unit.

Age-associated changes in pulmonary function do not alter the older adult's ability to breathe effortlessly; however, a decrease in respiratory muscle strength may be a limiting factor during exercise. The accessory inspiratory muscles (i.e., sternocleidomastoid, scalene, and trapezius) facilitate inspiration during exercise. Belman and Gaesser[58] reported that neither submaximal nor maximal exercise tolerance improved, although ventilatory muscle strength improved after elderly men and women received ventilatory muscle training.

ALVEOLAR PARENCHYMA

With advancing age, a diminished recoil (or increased compliance) of the lung occurs.[59] The reduced recoil results from the increase in the ratio of elastin to collagen content that occurs with advancing age.[60] Collagen, elastin, and reticulin are the primary connective tissue proteins of the lung tissue.[61,62] They are responsible for the elasticity and performance of the airways of the lung. Whereas total lung collagen remains unaltered, the amount of elastin increases with age in the interlobular septa and pleura and possibly within the bronchi and their vessels.[61,62] These anatomic changes are reflected by an increase in residual volume and a decrease in forced expiratory volume. An additional anatomic structural change includes an increase in the size of the alveolar ducts, which occurs after 40 years of age.[49] The bronchial enlargement displaces inhaled air volume away from the alveoli that line the alveolar ducts (see Fig. 14-1).[49]

Ventilation and the process of oxygen and carbon dioxide exchange (i.e., diffusion) depend on numerous factors, one of which is the surface area available for diffusion. A displacement of inhaled air volume away from the alveoli limits the surface area available for gas exchange. This may in part explain the progressive and linear decrease in the pulmonary diffusion capacity, which depends on the surface area and capillary blood volume. There are reports that capillary blood volume and surface area decrease with advancing age.[63]

PULMONARY GAS EXCHANGE

Loss of lung elasticity leads to increased alveolar compliance with collapse of the small airways. A ventilation/perfusion ($\dot{V}/\dot{Q}$) mismatch then results from alveolar ventilation with air trapping, causing a decline in arterial oxygen tension of approximately 0.3 mm Hg per year from the age of 30 years.[1] The median Pao_2 for healthy persons older than 60 years is 74.3 mm Hg, compared with 94 mm Hg for younger adults.[64] In contrast, arterial carbon dioxide ($Paco_2$) does not change with advancing age (see Table 14-3).[64]

Control of ventilatory responses to hypoxia and hypercapnia falls by 50% and 40%, respectively, in the older adult, possibly because of declining chemoreceptor function.[1] Decreases in Pao_2 may be the result of an increase in the closing volume

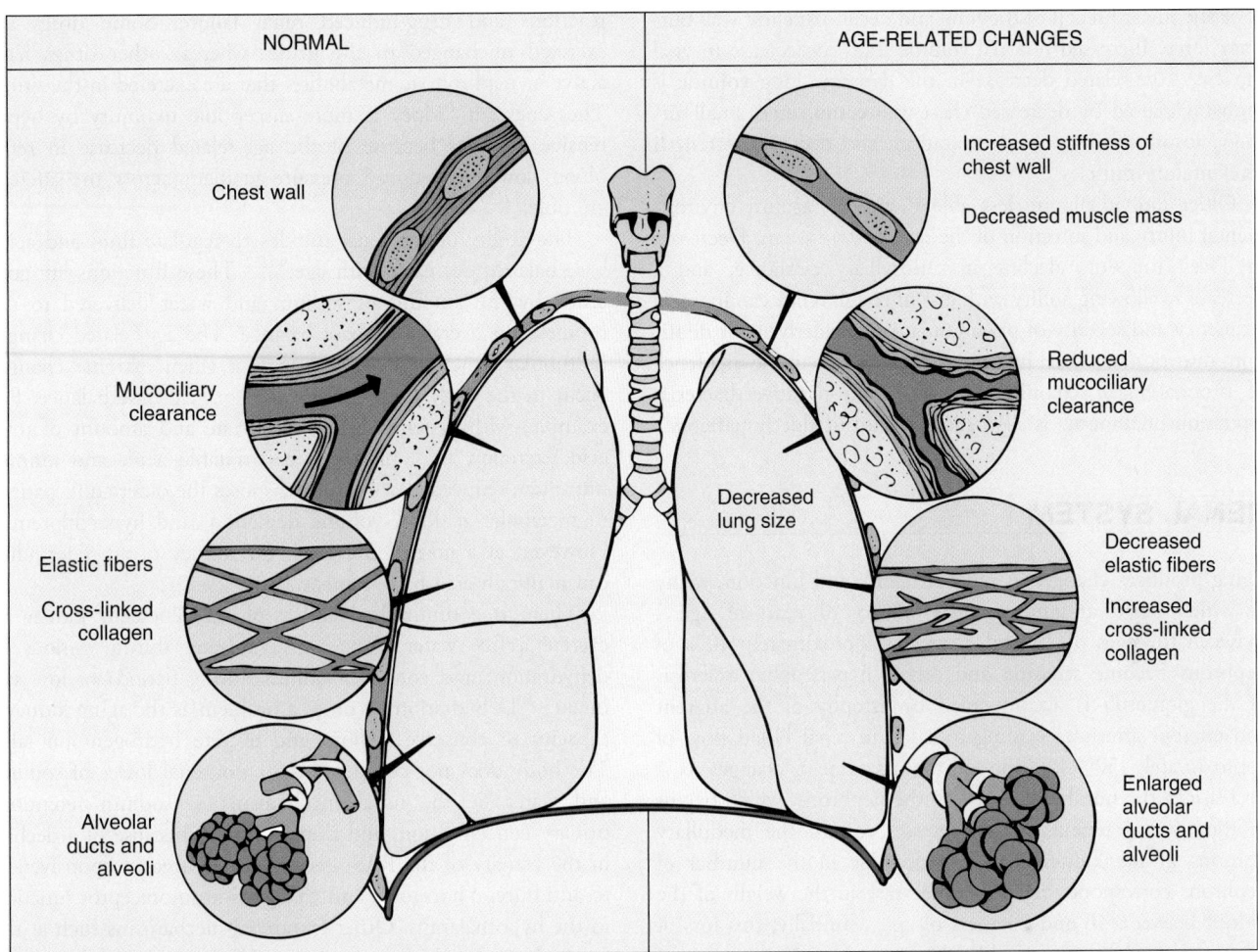

NORMAL	AGE-RELATED CHANGES
Chest wall	Increased stiffness of chest wall Decreased muscle mass
Mucociliary clearance	Reduced mucociliary clearance
	Decreased lung size
Elastic fibers Cross-linked collagen	Decreased elastic fibers Increased cross-linked collagen
Alveolar ducts and alveoli	Enlarged alveolar ducts and alveoli

Figure 14-1 Age-related changes occur in the respiratory system. With advancing age, the compliance of the chest wall and lung tissue changes. There is also a reduced clearance of mucus by the cilia that line the pulmonary tree and an enlargement of the alveolar ducts and alveoli.

in the dependent lung zones during resting tidal breathing in older subjects.[65,66] Consequently, dependent lung zones may be ventilated intermittently, leading to regional differences in ventilation. Alterations in blood volume and vascular resistance within the pulmonary circulation may also contribute to $\dot{V}/\dot{Q}$ mismatching. Other factors, such as smoking and pulmonary disease, also have an impact on the level of arterial oxygenation.

LUNG VOLUMES AND CAPACITIES

Total lung capacity and tidal volume do not change with advancing age[52] (see Table 14-2). Residual volume (RV) increases with age, paralleling the decrease in chest wall compliance and reduced strength of the respiratory muscles (see Table 14-2).[49] The increase in RV may add to the diminished strength of the inspiratory muscles by stretching the diaphragm and altering the tension-length relationship. Results from studies are conflicting with regard to age-related changes in functional residual capacity (FRC), which is the volume of air in the lungs at the normal resting end-expiratory position. There are reports of no change[67] and of decreases[53] in FRC in older adults. The balance of two opposing forces, the elastic recoil of the lung and the

outward recoil of the chest wall, determine the FRC.[54] These factors change in opposite directions with age: the elastic recoil of the lung decreases and the outward recoil of the chest wall decreases. Because these factors change in opposite directions, it could be predicted that FRC would remain unaltered. Knudson and colleagues.[67,68] found no change in FRC in older adults, supporting this prediction.

Other lung volumes that decrease with age include the inspiratory reserve volume (IRV) and the expiratory reserve volume (ERV).[51,53] The decrease in the ERV is the result of an increase in the RV. The decrease in IRV has been found only in studies reporting a corresponding increase in FRC. Table 14-2 and Figure 14-1 summarize age-related changes in pulmonary function.

Dynamic lung volumes and flow rates depend on resistance of airways and chest wall compliance and are limited by collapse of small airways during forced expiration. Forced vital capacity decreases by 14 to 30 mL/yr, and the 1-second forced expiratory volume (FEV_1) decreases by 23 to 32 mL/yr in men. Maximal expiratory flow rate and maximal mid-expiratory flow rate are also decreased. Total lung capacity remains unchanged, and resting lung volume or FRC is slightly increased despite loss of elastic inward recoil of the lung and decline in chest wall outward force. Increased residual volume leads to decrease in vital capacity. Age-related decrease in the dynamic lung volume is probably caused by decreased chest wall compliance, small airways closure during forced expiration, and decreased strength of expiratory muscles.[69,70]

Older individuals are less able to protect against environmental injury and infection of the respiratory system. Decreases in T-cell function, decline in mucociliary clearance, and a decrease swallowing ability with loss of cough reflex can increase frequency and severity of pneumonia in the elderly. Poor dentition, nutrition, and oral hygiene also play a role in the incidence of oropharyngeal colonization with gram-negative bacteria; aspiration pneumonia is a potential hazard in elderly patients.[1]

RENAL SYSTEM

Aging produces changes in renal structure and function, many of which begin at approximately 30 to 40 years of age.[71] Between the ages of 25 and 85 years, approximately 40% of nephrons become sclerotic and others hypertrophy. Sclerosis of the glomeruli is accompanied by atrophy of the afferent and efferent arterioles leading to a fall in renal blood flow of approximately 50%.[72] One of the prominent changes is a decrease in the number and size of the nephrons, which begins in the cortical regions and progresses toward the medullary portions of the kidney.[72,73] The decrease in the number of nephrons corresponds to a 20% decrease in the weight of the kidney between 40 and 80 years of age.[73] Initially, this loss of nephrons does not appreciably alter renal function because of the large renal reserve: the kidney contains approximately 2 to 3 million nephrons, not all of which are needed to maintain adequate fluid and acid-base homeostasis. However, with time, the geriatric patient also loses this renal reserve.[73] Nephron loss is caused by a gradual reduction in blood flow to the glomerular capillary tuft.[74] Total renal blood flow declines after the fourth decade of life[71] because of hyaline arteriosclerosis.[74,75] The cause of this vascular lesion within the glomerular tuft is unknown. By the eighth decade of life, 50% of the glomeruli are lost as a result of arteriolar hyalinization.[73]

FLUID FILTRATION

The GFR, reflected as decreased creatinine clearance (CrCl), declines approximately 45% by age 80 years.[71-73] The GFR, which is the volume of fluid traversing the glomerular membrane in a given period, is an important regulator of water and solute excretion. GFR depends on the permeability of the glomerular capillary and the surface area available for filtration, as well as the balance of pressure gradients between the glomerular capillary and Bowman's space.[71-74] In older adults, the decrease in GFR is most likely caused by the decreased nephron number and reduced renal blood flow.[71,72] Even though the remaining nephrons adapt to the loss of nephrons by glomerular hyperfiltration and increased solute load per nephron, the reduced GFR predisposes the older adult to adverse drug

reactions and drug-induced renal failure. Some drugs are excreted unchanged in the urine, whereas other drugs have active or nephrotoxic metabolites that are excreted in the urine. The senescent kidney is more susceptible to injury by hypotensive episodes because of the age-related decrease in renal blood flow and reduced pressure gradient across the afferent arteriole.[72,75]

The ability of the renal tubules to regulate fluid and acid-base balance decreases with age.[44,72] These functions are governed by the amount of sodium and water delivered to the tubules and overall acid-base balance. The age-related changes in tubular function become apparent when extreme changes occur in the body fluid composition or acid-base balance. For example, with systemic acidosis the rate and amount of total acid excretion (i.e., bicarbonate, titratable acid, and ammonium) are reduced.[71,72] This predisposes the older adult patient to metabolic acidosis, volume depletion, and hyperchloremia. However, at a normal pH level, the kidney of an older adult can maintain acid-base homeostasis.

There is a diminished ability of the senescent kidney to excrete a free water load, conserve water during periods of dehydration, and conserve sodium during periods of low salt intake.[71] Dehydration becomes a problem as the aging kidney's capacity to conserve sodium and excrete hydrogen ion falls. The body does not compensate for nonrenal losses of sodium and water by the usual mechanisms of sodium retention, urinary concentration, and thirst, possibly because of a decline in the activity of the RAS, decreased end-organ responsiveness to antidiuretic hormone, and changes in osmoreceptor function in the hypothalamus. Other extrarenal mechanisms such as the sympathetic nervous system are also important in homeostasis and maintaining blood pressure in response to changes in body position.[45,72]

Age-related changes also occur in extrarenal mechanisms, such as the decreased activity and responsiveness of the senescent kidney to the sympathetic nervous system and renin-angiotensin-aldosterone system, which are important in integrating overall fluid homeostasis and maintaining blood pressure in response to changes in body position.[45,71]

GASTROINTESTINAL SYSTEM
AGE-RELATED CHANGES

The gastrointestinal tract is made up of an epithelium, a mucosal immune system, many bacteria, and the enteric nervous system.[76] The gut is complex and plays a key role in homeostasis. Age-related gastrointestinal changes occur in the processes of swallowing, motility, and absorption.[77,78] Swallowing may be difficult for the older adult because of incomplete mastication of food within the oral cavity.[78] The result of deteriorating dentition, diminished lubrication (from salivary dysfunction), and ill-fitting dentures, and incomplete mastication can put the older adult patient at risk for aspiration.[77,78] The number and velocity of the peristaltic contractions of the older adult's esophagus decreases, and the number of nonperistaltic contractions increases.[78]

These changes in esophageal motility are referred to as *presbyesophagus*. The changes may predispose the patient to erosion of the esophageal wall (i.e., recurrent esophagitis), because food remains in the esophagus longer. Bed rest and reclining in a supine position for a prolonged period can cause esophageal reflux, which also can lead to esophagitis.[79] The aging process produces thinning of the smooth muscle within the gastric mucosa.[78,79] The epithelial layer of the gastric mucosa, which contains the chief and parietal cells, undergoes a modest degree of atrophy, resulting in the hyposecretion of pepsin and acid, respectively.[78-80] However, with aging, gastritis-induced achlorhydria (decreased acid secretion) is prevalent. Mucin secretion from the mucus cells decreases, thereby altering the protective function of the gastric mucosal (bicarbonate) barrier. Because of this, the stomach wall is more susceptible to acid injury, increasing the incidence of gastric ulcerations.[78-81] It remains unknown whether the changes in gastric acid secretion are a result of age-related changes or a disease process such as gastritis. Most duodenal and gastric ulcers arise because of the presence of *Helicobacter pylori*. Ulcers can also be promoted by the use of nonsteroidal antiinflammatory drugs. The combination of *H. pylori* and medication effects can be a significant risk for gastrointestinal bleeding in critically ill elderly.[78,79]

Aging does not appreciably alter gastric emptying of solid foods. However, Moore and associates[82] found a delay in the emptying of liquids from the stomach in older adults. No changes in small intestinal peristalsis or segmental movements with aging have been reported.[83] Alterations within the small intestine include a decrease in intestinal weight after the age of 50 years and a flattening and shortening of jejunal villi.[83] Age produces no change in the small intestine's absorption of fats and proteins; however, decreased carbohydrate absorption has been reported.[79,84,85] A gradual decline in albumin is also evidenced with increased age; however, serum levels generally remain within normal limits in healthy older adults.[85] Although most vitamins and minerals are normally absorbed, calcium absorption is reduced, fat-soluble vitamin A is increased, and there is the potential for impaired absorption of vitamin D.[85] In patients who are not hypochlorhydric, iron is normally absorbed. However, the absorption of zinc and calcium decreases with advancing age.[78,79,85] In summary, age-associated changes in gastrointestinal function occur; however, these changes are not of sufficient magnitude to produce malnutrition in healthy individuals.

LIVER

With advancing age, hepatocyte number and liver weight decrease.[86] Total liver blood flow decreases significantly, such that between 25 and 65 years of age, total liver blood flow decreases by 50%.[86-88] The liver has many complex functions, including carbohydrate storage, ketone body formation, reduction and conjugation of adrenal and gonadal steroid hormones, synthesis of plasma proteins, deamination of amino acids, synthesis and storage of cholesterol, urea formation, and detoxification of toxins and drugs. Age-related changes in hepatic function include a reduction in synthesis of cholesterol,

total bile acid pool, and bile acid from cholesterol.[88] There is also a reduced capacity of the liver for regeneration in response to injury compared with a younger population. However, despite these age-related changes, liver function is not appreciably altered.[88] Several tests of liver function, such as serum bilirubin, alkaline phosphatase, and aspartate aminotransferase (AST) levels, are not altered with advancing age. However, because of the decrease in total liver blood flow, first-pass clearance of drugs is somewhat reduced. The most important age-related change in liver function is the decrease in the liver's capacity to metabolize drugs.[89,90] Although clinical tests of liver function do not reflect this change in metabolism, it is well recognized that drug side effects and toxic effects occur more frequently in older adults than in young adults.[90] This reduced drug-metabolizing capacity is caused by a reduction in the activity of the drug-metabolizing enzyme system, microsomal ethanol oxidizing system, and decrease in total liver blood flow.[87,91] Drugs that depend on the cytochrome P450 group of liver enzymes are the most affected, because age-associated changes cause as much as a 50% decline in enzymatic function.[88]

CENTRAL NERVOUS SYSTEM
COGNITIVE FUNCTIONING AND AGING

Cognitive functioning involves the process of transforming, synthesizing, storing, and retrieving sensory input. Additional components include perception, attention, thinking, memory, and problem solving. For the aging individual, cognition is altered by the speed at which information is processed and retrieved.[92] Performance on timed tests declines slowly past the age of 20 years. Intelligence remains fairly stable past the age of 30 years until a person reaches the mid-80s. Although the rate at which complex tasks are completed may be diminished, these age-related changes are not synonymous with cognitive impairment. Marked deterioration of any component of cognitive functioning is not a normal expectation of the aging process.[93] Although some type of cognitive change, such as mild memory dysfunction, is generally apparent with increasing age, this decline may represent a change in individual need rather than a change in function. However, cognitive impairment in older adults more commonly results from acute and chronic causes.

Acute mental status changes due to problems such as infection, fluid, electrolyte, and metabolic imbalances, or medication-induced events usually are reversible after they are identified. Observable indicators of delirium include an acute change in mental status from baseline, inattention, and disorganized thinking or change in level of consciousness. Although delusions and hallucinations may be present in delirium, they are also evident in other psychiatric disorders. In contrast, long-term chronic impairment develops from more organic causes, such as those associated with neurodegenerative dementias (e.g., Alzheimer's type, Lewy body disease) or nonneurodegenerative types (e.g., multiinfarct dementia, traumatic brain injury). Although dementia is pathology based and not necessarily an expected outcome of aging, there is an increased incidence associated with advanced age, particularly in those older than 85 years.[93] Alzheimer's disease is identified by amyloid-containing neuritic plaques and intraneuronal neurofibrillary tangles in various areas of the cortex.[94] Alzheimer's disease is characterized initially by progressive short-term memory loss, and later by long-term memory loss. Marked decline in memory ultimately leaves the individual functionally impaired and physically dependent. In contrast, nonneurodegenerative dementias, such as multiinfarct types, present as fixed deficits associated with the area of brain injury. In contrast to the Alzheimer's type of dementia, cognitive impairment may be associated with significant impairment following stroke rather than over time.[95]

Baseline dementia, stress of surgery or acute illness, and hospitalization can cause cognitive decline and significantly increase the risk for delirium in the elderly. Sensory perception ameliorates with aging, resulting in difficulties for the older patient in unfamiliar surroundings such as hospitals. This coupled with immobility and deprivation of visual and hearing aids increases the likelihood of dehydration, anorexia, confusion, depression, and disorientation.[72,93]

CHANGES IN STRUCTURE AND MORPHOLOGY

The brain decreases approximately 20% in size between 25 and 95 years of age (Fig. 14-2).[93,96] The reduced brain weight may be related in part to the overall decrease in the number of neurons that occurs with advancing age. Neurons are lost from the hippocampus, the amygdala, and the cerebellum and from areas of the brainstem such as the locus ceruleus, the dorsal motor nucleus of the vagus, and the substantia nigra.[92] In contrast, in areas such as the hypothalamus, very few neurons disappear with advancing age.[96] Portions of the cerebral cortex atrophy, principally the frontal and temporal cortical association areas (the superior frontal gyrus and superior temporal gyrus, respectively).[97]

The cerebral ventricles enlarge and develop an asymmetric appearance.[98] Cerebrospinal fluid (CSF) also accumulates in the ventricles; however, total brain CSF is not increased.[98] Accompanying the loss of neurons are changes in the ultrastructure and intracellular structures of the neuron.[99] The neuron is composed of a cell body, a dendrite, and an axon. Dendrites are long, spiny processes that extend out from the cell body. One of the most ubiquitous changes in the aging brain is a decrease in the number of dendrite spines. Between middle and late old

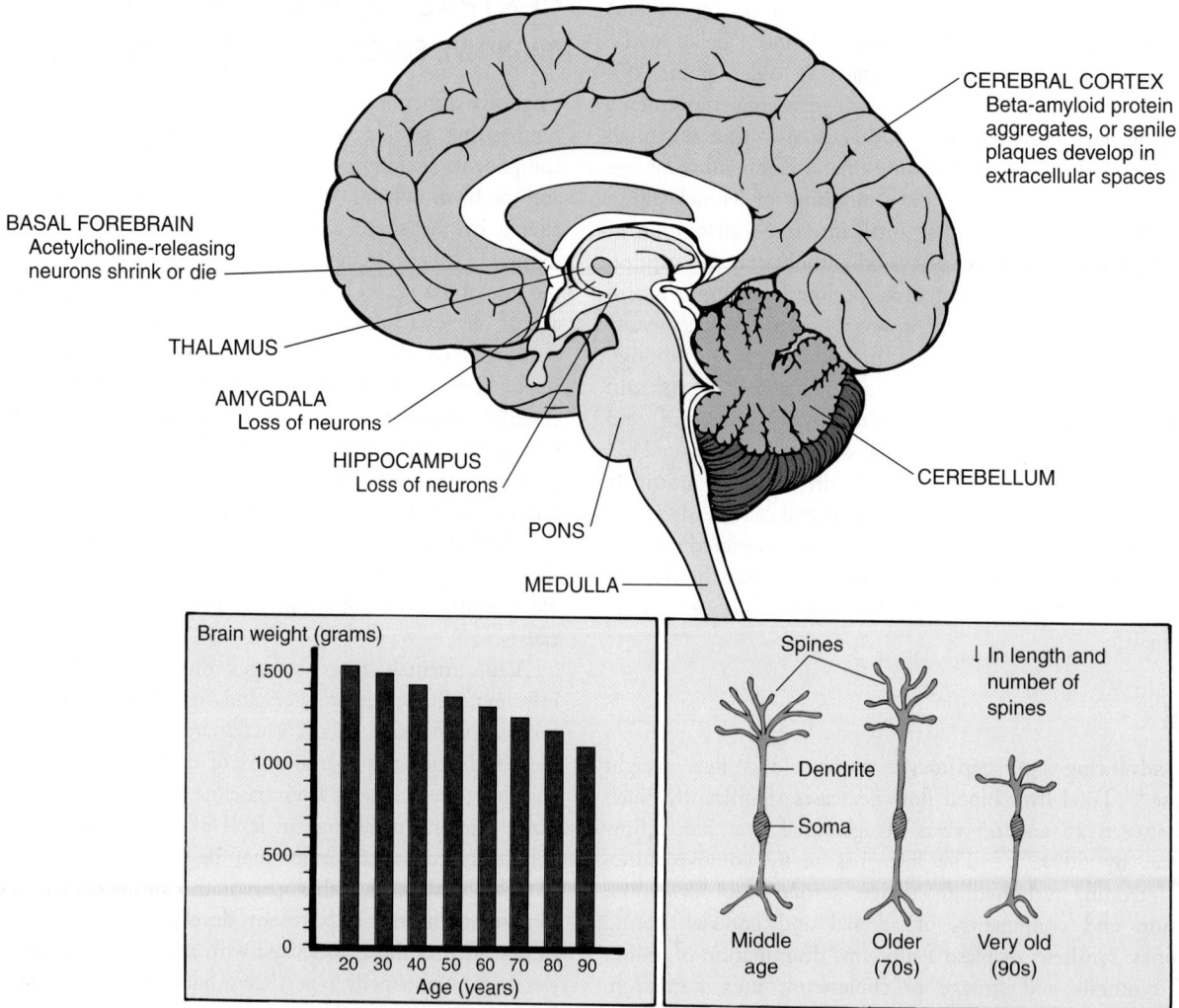

Figure 14-2 Summary of age-related changes in the brain. *(From Selkoe DJ:* Aging brain, aging mind, *Sci Am 267:134-142, 1992.)*

age, the length of the dendritic spines increases, but then it decreases after late old age (>90 years).[93,96] Shrinking of large neurons and degenerative changes occurring in the cell bodies and axons of certain acetylcholine-secreting neurons have been reported. These changes may explain alterations in the processing and receiving of information.[93]

With advancing age, lipofuscins, neuritic plaques, and neurofibrillary bodies appear within the cytoplasm of the neuron.[96] Lipofuscins, or age pigments, are granules containing a dark, fluorescent pigment. They are derived from lipid-rich membranes that have been partially disintegrated and oxidized. It is still not clear whether lipofuscin accumulation is harmful to the brain.[96] Neuritic, or senile, plaques are aggregates of the beta-amyloid protein, and they also accumulate in the brain of normal senescent persons. Neuritic plaques are found in the hippocampus, the cerebral cortex, and other brain regions.[95,96] Neurofibrillary tangles, which are bundles of helically wound protein filaments, occur in the hippocampus with advancing age in healthy persons.[97] However, they are present in larger numbers in persons with neuropathologic disorders such as Alzheimer's disease. It has been suggested that neurofibrillary tangles interfere with neuronal signaling.[93,96]

In the senescent brain, synaptogenesis (synaptic regeneration) still occurs after partial nerve degeneration.[99] After a nerve fiber is damaged, neighboring undamaged neurons often sprout new fibers and form new connections. However, synaptogenesis occurs at a slower rate in the older brain.[99]

NEUROTRANSMITTER SYNTHESIS

Advancing age is associated with changes in neurotransmitter function. Altered neurotransmitter function can result from changes in the available precursors for neurotransmitter synthesis, changes in the neurotransmitter receptor, or changes in the activity of the enzymes that synthesize and degrade the neurotransmitter. Various methods are used to examine changes in neurotransmitter function, including measurement of neurotransmitter levels, neurotransmitter turnover, and receptor number and binding. Changes in neurotransmitter systems in the aging brain are equivocal and are more than likely a result of the different methods used to study the neurotransmitter systems.[100] For example, in some studies, neurotransmitters have been quantified by measuring (1) the concentration of the neurotransmitters, (2) the breakdown or activation products, and (3) the activity of the enzyme responsible for the synthesis or breakdown of the neurotransmitters. Gottstein and Held[101] suggested that age-related changes in neurotransmitter levels might cause a "desynchronization" in neurotransmission, thereby affecting many neurologic functions. Acetylcholine (ACh), dopamine (DA), serotonin (5–HT), glutamate, and γ-aminobutyric acid (GABA) all decrease with increasing age.

In addition to age-related neurotransmitter dysfunction, certain disorders frequently encountered in the older adult, such as Alzheimer's disease, Parkinson's disease, multiple sclerosis, depression, and delirium, may further contribute to neurologic dysfunction associated with neurotransmitters.[102] Similarly, many medications (e.g., histamine blockers, benzodiazepines,

anticholinergics, antiarrhythmics, antimicrobials, antiemetics) administered in critical care directly affect neurotransmitter function and contribute to the incidence of delirium.[103,104]

CEREBRAL METABOLISM AND BLOOD FLOW

Cerebral blood flow (CBF) decreases with advancing age. This decrease parallels the decrease in brain weight and is most likely caused by the reduction in neuron number and metabolic needs of the cerebral tissue.[92,101] Cerebral blood flow is also influenced by age-related changes in blood pressure, barometric response to positional change, and the severity of cerebrovascular disease.[105]

IMMUNE SYSTEM

Several changes in immune function render the older adult more susceptible to infections.[106-111] Infections in the geriatric population are associated with higher rates of mortality.[111] Common infections in the older adult are associated with bacterial pneumonia, urinary tract infection, intraabdominal infections, gram-negative bacteremia, and decubitus ulcers.[111] The reasons for the increased susceptibility are multifactorial and include changes in cell-mediated and humoral-mediated immunity; breakdown in physical barriers, such as the skin and oral mucosa; and changes in nutrition.

CELL-MEDIATED AND HUMORAL-MEDIATED IMMUNITY

Immune system function depends on many cell types with distinct functions. T cells are the primary effector of cell-mediated immunity, whereas bone marrow–derived B cells produce antibodies that are the effector cells of humoral-mediated immunity.[106,108,110] With aging, cell-mediated immunity declines. Even though the total number of T cells remains unchanged with advancing age, T-cell function decreases.[108,110] For example, there is a decrease in T-cell production of interleukin 2 (IL-2) and in differentiation of T cells into effector cells. IL-2 is essential for activation of B cells, which eventually differentiate into antibody-secreting cells. Subsets of T cells mature into cytotoxic cells, whereas other T cells activate B cells and stimulate B-cell proliferation. Changes in B-lymphocyte function are not as well understood, even though with age the ability of B cells to produce antibodies to new antigens declines.[106,108] Although there is no evidence that age-associated changes directly affect phagocytosis and chemotaxis or the bactericidal action of neutrophils, compromised immune-mediated responses have been identified in areas with reduced blood supply such as the skin.[106]

Older patients are not necessarily more likely to contract an infectious illness, but the ability of the aging bone marrow to increase neutrophil production in response to infection may be impaired and older individuals may be less able to eradicate infection quickly. Elderly patients with major infections often have normal white blood cell counts, but the differential count usually shows a large proportion of immature forms.[72]

ADDITIONAL RISK FACTORS

Multiple concurrent chronic illnesses produce systemic stressors that ultimately diminish immune functioning. The critical care nurse must be aware that an exacerbation of preexisting illness such as diabetes or emphysema may manifest before infection is suspected. Introducing bacteria through invasive devices such as central lines or chest tubes may threaten an already suppressed immune system. Nutritional deficiencies, particularly protein malnutrition, are a common problem among older adults. Inadequate protein intake can develop from prolonged anorexia and cognitive impairment. Protein malnutrition is associated with a shrinkage of lymphoid tissue, which then diminishes T-cell functioning and cell-mediated immunity.[109]

Inadequate emptying of urine because of bed rest, obstruction, or side effects from anticholinergic medications can result in stagnation of urine and recurrent urinary tract infections. Long-term placement of urinary catheters is a significant source of bacturia. However, treatment with antibiotic therapy is not indicated unless the patient becomes symptomatic with anorexia or cognitive impairment or has a history of a chronic illness, such as diabetes or chronic obstructive pulmonary disease.[106,111,112]

CHANGES IN PHARMACOKINETICS AND PHARMACODYNAMICS

The many benefits of modern advancements in pharmacologic therapy are frequently counterbalanced by adverse drug effects, medication interactions, and therapeutic failure.[107] Adverse drug effects and medication interactions are related to pharmacokinetics and pharmacodynamics. There are many age-related changes in drug pharmacokinetics, which is the manner in which the body absorbs, distributes, metabolizes, and excretes a drug.[90,91,107] The aging process is associated with changes in gastric acid secretion, which can alter the ionization or solubility of a drug and hence its absorption[90,91] (Table 14-4).

Drug distribution depends on body composition and on the physiochemical properties of the drug. With advancing age, fat content increases, lean body mass decreases, and total body water decreases, which can alter the drug disposition.[91] For example, because of the increase in the ratio of body fat content to body weight, lipophilic drugs have a greater volume of distribution per body weight in older adults compared with younger adults. Other age-related factors[90,113] affecting drug disposition are listed in Table 14-4.

The senescent liver and kidneys are less able to metabolize and excrete a drug, which also affects clinical outcomes. For example, the rate of absorption, time to peak plasma concentration, and clearance of loop diuretics is reduced in older adults, which may necessitate high dosing regimens in order to facilitate diuresis.[114,115] This poses an increased risk of metabolic acidosis, since the higher diuretic dose increases competition for the organic acid transport pathway at the proximal tubule. Using the example of diuretics, bioavailability between agents may also be variable. For instance, bumetanide has a fairly consistent bioavailability in advanced age, whereas that of furosemide varies from 20% to 80%.[115]

Similarly, other drugs associated with management of common disorders seen in critically ill patients—such as digoxin, angiotensin II–converting enzyme (ACE) inhibitors, and angiotensin II receptor blockers (ARBs)[115,116]—have delayed excretion, increased serum concentration, and more prolonged duration of action because their excretion parallels GFR, which decreases

TABLE 14-4 Age-Related Changes in Pharmacokinetics

Pharmacokinetic Parameter	Definition	Age-Related Changes
Absorption	Receptor-coupled or diffusional uptake of drug into tissue	Decreased absorptive surface area of small intestine Decreased splanchnic blood flow Increased gastric acid pH Decreased gastrointestinal motility
Distribution	Theoretic space (tissue) or body compartment into which free form of drug distributes	Decreased lean body mass and total body water Increased total body fat Decreased serum albumin level Increased α_1-acid glycoprotein
Metabolism	Chemical change in drug that renders it active or inactive	Decreased liver mass Decreased activity of microsomal drug-metabolizing enzyme system Decreased total liver blood flow
Excretion	Removal of drug through an eliminating organ, often the kidney; some drugs are excreted in bile or feces, in saliva, or through the lungs	Decreased renal blood flow and glomerular filtration rate Decreased distal renal tubular secretory function

Data from Gilman AG et al, editors: *Goodman and Gilman's the pharmacological basis of therapeutics,* ed 8, London, 1990, Pergamon Press; Vestal RE, Cusack BJ: Pharmacology and aging. In Schneider EL, Rowe JW, editors: *Handbook of the biology of aging,* San Diego, 1990, Academic Press.

with age.[110] Table 14-4 describes age-related changes in drug pharmacokinetics.

Age-related changes in pharmacodynamics have also been reported. Pharmacodynamics refers to the pharmacologic or physiologic response to a drug that occurs after the drug interacts with its receptor on the plasma membrane. The chronotropic and inotropic effects of β-adrenergic agonists reportedly decrease in older adults.[117,118] There also are reports that age produces no change in heparin-stimulated increases in partial thromboplastin time, whereas the effects of warfarin (Coumadin) are very susceptible to medication interactions.

The Critical Care Safety Study found that 61% of adverse events in the ICU were associated with medications. The average age of patients observed in these areas was greater than 60 years. Medications groups most often associated with errors were cardiovascular drugs (24%), anticoagulants (20%), and antiinfective agents (13%).[119] The Beers Criteria is a list of medications that have more risk than benefit when given to the elderly (www.dcri.duke.edu/ccge/curtis/beers.html).[120]

The use of multiple medications in the presence of multiple comorbidities has been associated with an increase in adverse drug reactions. Although this is not always avoidable, it is important to avoid choosing an agent for its side effect profile (e.g., diphenhydramine for sedative effects) and to monitor the effects of the chosen agent. A major cause of therapeutic failure is the underuse or inappropriate use of drug therapy that is indicated for the treatment of a particular problem. It is not uncommon for delirium that is not associated with a withdrawal syndrome to be treated with benzodiazepines in critical care. However, this frequently makes agitation worse, once the sedative effects are gone, in comparison with a low-dose antipsychotic agent.[103,104,121]

PHYSICAL EXAMINATION AND DIAGNOSTIC PROCEDURES

The various physiologic changes that occur with aging warrant special physical examination techniques.[122] The clinician must distinguish between changes in health caused by physiologic or pathologic processes, and the nurse must ensure that the physical examination is conducted under optimal conditions. When beginning a physical examination, the clinician should consider the ability of the gerontologic patient to cooperate and to hear, as well as his or her activity level. The patient's comfort and energy levels must be considered. Before beginning an examination, the nurse must ensure that the room's noise and temperature levels and the patient's position in the bed are optimal and comfortable.[123]

HEAD AND NECK

Normal funduscopic findings include a diminished pupillary response to penlight, a decrease in near and peripheral vision, and a loss of visual acuity to dim light. These changes result from an increase in opacity of the lens and a decrease in ciliary movement.[124,125] It is not uncommon to find irises that are pale blue or light gray, which stems from a decrease in melanocyte production.[124,125] Around the periphery of the iris, fat deposits may also be found, which are referred to as arcus senilis. The eyes may appear sunken or recessed because of a loss of subcutaneous tissue. These clinical manifestations may also be signs of dehydration; however, in older adults, these may be normal findings. The pupils may appear small, which can be unrelated to changes in neurologic status or medication administration. The pupil at 60 years is one third of the size of a pupil at 20 years.[125] Patients may complain of dry, itching eyes, which result from a decrease in lacrimal activity.[125]

Although healthy older adults usually do not have any remarkable deficit in taste, smell is significantly diminished.[126] However, taste is likely to be markedly affected in the patient with metabolic imbalance who is receiving multiple medications.

Loss of dentition is not a normal process of aging. It indicates poor nutrition or poor oral hygiene. Older adults commonly experience gradual hearing loss.[127] On physical examination, the older adult may have a reduced ability to distinguish low- and high-pitched sounds and may have difficulty in understanding high-pitched and rushed speech. The hearing loss is related to atrophy of the auditory nerve and the organ of Corti.[127]

INTEGUMENTARY AND MUSCULOSKELETAL SYSTEMS

The loss of elastic and connective tissue causes the skin to wrinkle; skin wrinkles and sagging may be found over many areas of the body. The appearance and number of skin wrinkles also depend greatly on environmental agents and exposure to ultraviolet rays.[125] The underlying structures such as veins and muscles are more visible because of the transparency of the skin. Because of the loss of skin turgor, especially in the hands, the nurse assesses for dehydration by pinching the skin tissue over the sternum or forehead. Table 14-5 summarizes age-related changes in the skin and their associated nursing interventions.

The nurse may find multiple ecchymotic areas because of decreased protective subcutaneous tissue layers, increased capillary fragility, and flattening of the capillary bed, which predispose older adults to developing ecchymoses.[128-131] In conjunction with frequent aspirin use, these physiologic factors result in an increased bleeding tendency and the appearance of ecchymotic areas. However, areas of ecchymosis may indicate elder abuse.

Changes that occur in the musculoskeletal system are a decrease in lean body mass; a compression of the spinal column, which results from thinning of the cartilage between vertebrae; and a decrease in the mobility of skeletal joints.[132,133] Despite the ubiquitous finding of reduced joint mobility, no exact physiologic process gives rise to the altered mobility. It is possible that the reduced synovial fluid production that occurs with aging causes changes in function. This may produce some changes in range of motion.

Bone demineralization afflicts men and women as they age, but it occurs four times more often in women than in men. Bone demineralization refers to an increase in osteoplast and

TABLE 14-5 Age-Related Changes in the Integumentary System

Skin Problem	Underlying Mechanisms	Nursing Interventions
Delayed wound healing	↓ Vascular supply to dermis ↓ Connective tissue layer ↓ Subcutaneous tissue layer Impaired inflammatory response ↓ New connective tissue proliferation	Use nonrestrictive dressings Weigh patient daily Support nutritional needs
Thermoregulation	↓ Subcutaneous tissue layer ↓ Number of capillary arterioles supplying skin ↓ Number of eccrine (sweat glands)	Monitor room temperature
Pressure ulcers	↓ Flattening of capillary bed ↓ Thinning of epidermis	Reposition patient every 2 hr Use pressure-relieving devices
IV infiltrations	↓ Connective tissue layer Vascular fragility	Monitor peripheral IV site hourly Discontinue IV administration at first sign of infiltration
Diminished skin turgor	↓ Connective tissue layer ↓ Eccrine and sebaceous gland activity	Bathe patient with tepid water Avoid use of deodorant soap

osteoclast activity, which decreases calcium absorption into the bone.[133] Mineral loss (calcium and phosphorus) with a decrease in bone mass is referred to as *osteoporosis*.[133] Osteoporosis produces bones that are more "porous" or fragile. With extensive bone demineralization, an elderly patient may sustain multiple fractures. There is an accelerated incidence of osteoporosis in women, which occurs after the onset of menopause. A decrease in estrogen is implicated in this process, because estrogen replacement may arrest the osteoporosis process (although it does not reverse it). The exact mechanism whereby estrogen affects bone mass is unknown. Evidence indicates that estrogen stimulates intestinal absorption of calcium, and the loss of estrogen action after menopause may in part be related to postmenopausal osteoporosis.[133] Decreased intake of dietary calcium, immobility, excess glucocorticoid secretion, and smoking all contribute to the development of osteoporosis. The nurse should be alert for physical signs of deformities associated with osteoporosis, such as kyphosis or scoliosis, which may place limitations on physical mobility or lead to gait instability.

RESPIRATORY AND CARDIOVASCULAR SYSTEMS

Many of the physiologic changes that occur with aging and the mechanisms underlying them were addressed earlier in this chapter. The physical correlates to these changes are described in this section. The aging thorax has a greater anterior-posterior diameter than in a younger adult, and there is some degree of kyphosis. On initial auscultation, bibasilar crackles may be heard; however, they should clear after several deep breaths and coughing. Bibasilar crackles that do not clear with deep inspirations are suggestive of pathology. The cough reflex also is diminished, which predisposes the elderly patient to aspiration. No changes are observed with palpation, but the nurse needs to assess for areas of tenderness, which could be the result of old fractures. Increased resonance with percussion is observed. Changes in tests of pulmonary function are listed in Tables 14-2 and 14-3.

There are relatively few modifications in the assessment of cardiovascular function and age-related physical findings in the older adult. The resting heart rate decreases and systolic blood pressure increases with age. Manifestations of left ventricular hypertrophy and aortic sclerosis may include a prominent cardiac apex impulse, a prominent S_4 sound at the cardiac apex, a single S_2 sound (with expiration), and a short, early-peaking systolic murmur.[79]

GASTROINTESTINAL AND RENAL SYSTEMS

On physical examination of the nonobese older adult, the abdominal organs are more easily palpated because of a decrease in subcutaneous tissue. Despite a change in gastrointestinal motility, bowel sounds are normoactive. There are no remarkable physical assessment considerations with the hepatic-biliary and renal systems and no age-related change in liver function tests. Blood urea nitrogen (BUN) and serum creatinine levels can be normal or decreased in older adults (Box 14-1).

The GFR decreases with age. In the hospital, the GFR is estimated from the CrCl, usually by collecting a 24-hour urine sample to measure creatinine excretion. Endogenous creatinine is a metabolic byproduct of muscle metabolism that is excreted by the kidney and is not reabsorbed. With advancing age, muscle mass decreases, thereby reducing the renal load of serum concentration of creatinine. In the geriatric patient, neither the creatinine excreted nor the plasma creatinine level may reflect the change in GFR. In older adults, the Cockcroft-Gault equation often is used to assess CrCl and GFR (in milliliters per minute), because it incorporates the serum creatinine concentration, body weight (in kilograms), age (in years), and gender as variables.[73] The Cockcroft-Gault equation for males is

$$CrCl = (140 - Age)/72 \times Serum\ creatinine \times Weight$$

For females, this calculated value is multiplied by 0.85.

Box 14-1 lists the effects of aging on other laboratory tests that may or may not have clinical significance.[107,134]

BOX 14-1   EFFECTS OF AGING ON VARIOUS LABORATORY VALUES

VALUES THAT DO NOT CHANGE WITH AGE

- Hemoglobin, hematocrit
- Platelet count
- White blood cell count with differential
- Serum electrolytes
- Coagulation profile
- Liver function tests
- Thyroid function tests
- NC or ↓ Blood urea nitrogen
- NC or ↓ Creatinine

VALUES THAT CHANGE WITH AGE BUT HAVE LITTLE CLINICAL SIGNIFICANCE

- ↓ Calcium
- ↑ Uric acid

VALUES THAT CHANGE WITH AGE AND HAVE CLINICAL SIGNIFICANCE

- ↓ Erythrocyte sedimentation rate
- ↓ Arterial oxygen pressure
- ↑ Blood glucose
- ↓ or ↑ Serum lipid profile
- ↓ Albumin

NC, no change; ↓ decreased; ↑ increased.
From Duthie EH, Abbasi AA: Laboratory testing: current recommendations for older adults, *Geriatrics* 46:41, 1991.

CENTRAL NERVOUS SYSTEM

Physical examination of the central nervous system begins with a review of the older patient's mental status. The nurse assesses the patient's level of consciousness, ability to communicate and follow commands, and short- and long-term memory. In the critical care unit, parameters may be altered by hypoxia, electrolyte imbalances, or various medications. The practitioner may observe that the patient occasionally forgets minor details. The slow, gradual decline in some cognitive functions, as evidenced by forgetfulness, is considered normal.[135,136] However, forgetting important information such as a name, address, and marital status is not part of the normal aging process. Some older adults have problems with short-term memory but their long-term memory is intact. Older adults are commonly labeled "demented" or "confused." These cognitive syndromes have different causes and are not a normal part of aging. Foreman and colleagues[137] have reviewed impaired cognition in the older adult patient. Hearing dysfunction associated with aging affects spoken communication, and careful attention should be paid in assessing cognition to ensure that answers are in response to the questions posed.

The neurologic examination for the geriatric patient always includes an assessment of muscle strength, reflexes, sensation, and cranial nerves.[138] There may be some changes in fine and gross motor skills. Handgrip strength declines with age and may correlate with a decreased ability to perform fine motor activity (e.g., tying a shoelace). Age diminishes the geriatric patient's vibratory sense, primarily in the lower extremities. Reflexes are slowed as a result of neuronal loss.[138] Neurologic deficits may ultimately alter the patient's ability to perform self-care. Changes in older adults' cognitive function may alter their ability to follow instructions and interpret patient-teaching instructions regarding their care in the critical care unit. The critical care nurse evaluates the patient's gait if the patient is ambulatory.

IMMUNE SYSTEM

Infections in the older adult initially may appear as an acute onset of mental status changes, anorexia, urinary incontinence, falls, or generalized weakness.[111,139] These may be signs of a urinary tract infection or pneumonia, two common infections in older adults. Because the response of the immune system is attenuated, signs such as fever and chills initially may be absent.

Summary

The older adult requires more intense observation and consideration in the critical care unit, because his or her system has become less adaptable to stress and illness. Table 14-6 summarizes the major changes in the various systems, along with clinical considerations.[1,79,140] As shown in Figure 14-3, many physiologic changes occur with advancing age, and each change may render a particular system less adaptable to stress. Changes in one system may affect another system in the presence of disease. The inability to adapt poses a significant risk for functional decline after discharge. Older adults at greatest risk include those with poor nutritional status or cognitive dysfunction and those who required assistance with at least two activities of daily living before admission.[141]

The critical care nurse must be aware of socioeconomic factors that confront older adult patients and lifestyle adjustments such as the death of a spouse or friend. Changes in Medicare payment for hospitalization and medication have also placed a financial burden on such patients. To provide the best care and prevent iatrogenic complications, the critical care nurse must consider all physiologic and psychological factors that affect the older adult patient.

Cardiovascular System

- Aorta and other arteries become stiff and less pliable, leading to increased workload on the heart to perfuse tissue.
- Systolic and diastolic pressures increase, along with an increase in systemic vascular resistance and a decrease in cardiac output.
- There is a loss of capacity in the myocardium and arterial system and decreased ability to respond and recover from periods of physiologic and psychological stress.

TABLE 14-6 Summary of Age-Related Physiologic Changes and Related Clinical Considerations

Age-Related Effect	Clinical Considerations
Cardiovascular System	
↓ Inotropic and chronotropic response of myocardium to catecholamine stimulation	The increase in cardiac output during stress or exercise is achieved by an increase in diastolic filling (increased dependence on Starling's law of the heart)
↑ Myocardial collagen content	Leads to a decrease in the compliance of the ventricle (higher filling pressures are needed to maintain stroke volume)
↓ Baroreceptor sensitivity	↑ Tendency for orthostatic hypotension after prolonged bed rest or if patient is taking antihypertensive medication or has systolic hypertension
Prolonged rate of relaxation	May predispose the elderly patient to hemodynamic derangements in the presence of tachydysrhythmias, hypertension, or ischemic heart disease
↓ Compliance of blood vessels	↑ Peripheral vascular resistance and blood pressure
Respiratory System	
↓ Strength of the respiratory muscles, recoil of lungs, chest wall compliance, and efficiency and number of cilia in airways	↑ Susceptibility to aspiration, atelectasis, and pulmonary infection Patient may require more frequent deep breathing, coughing, and position change
↓ Pao_2 level	↓ Ventilatory response to hypoxia and hypercapnia ↑ Sensitivity to narcotics
Renal System	
↓ Glomerular filtration rate	Careful observation of patient when administering aminoglycosides, antibiotics, and contrast dyes
↓ Ability to concentrate and conserve water	May predispose patient to development of dehydration and hypernatremia, especially if patient is fluid-restricted and insensible losses are high (e.g., during mechanical ventilation or fever)
↓ Ability to excrete salt and water loads, as well as urea, ammonia, and drugs	Observe for clinical manifestations of fluid overload and drug reactions
↓ Response to an acid load	After an acid load (i.e., metabolic acidosis), the elderly patient may be in a state of uncompensated metabolic acidosis for a longer period
Liver	
↓ Total liver blood flow	Adverse drug reactions, especially with polypharmacy
Gastrointestinal System	
Diminished ability to swallow	May predispose elderly patient to aspiration pneumonia Assess for proper fit of dentures and ability to chew Flex head forward 45 degrees Develop awareness for complaints of food or medications "sticking in throat"
Impaired esophageal motility	Assess for complaints of heartburn or epigastric discomfort Avoid prolonged supine position
Delayed emptying of liquids	Examine abdomen for distention Investigate complaints of anorexia
↓ Stool weight and transit time	Obtain thorough bowel history and note routine use of laxatives Increase intake of dietary fiber and assess for fecal incontinence and impaction
Neurologic System	
↑ Cranial dead space	Elderly persons may sustain a significant amount of hemorrhage before symptoms are apparent
↓ Number of neurons and dendrites and length of dendrite spines	Delayed or impaired processing of sensory and motor information
Delay in the rate of synaptogenesis Changes in neurotransmitter turnover	May cause desynchronization of neurotransmission

Modified from Rebenson-Piano M: The physiologic changes that occur with aging, *Crit Care Q* 12:1-14, 1989.

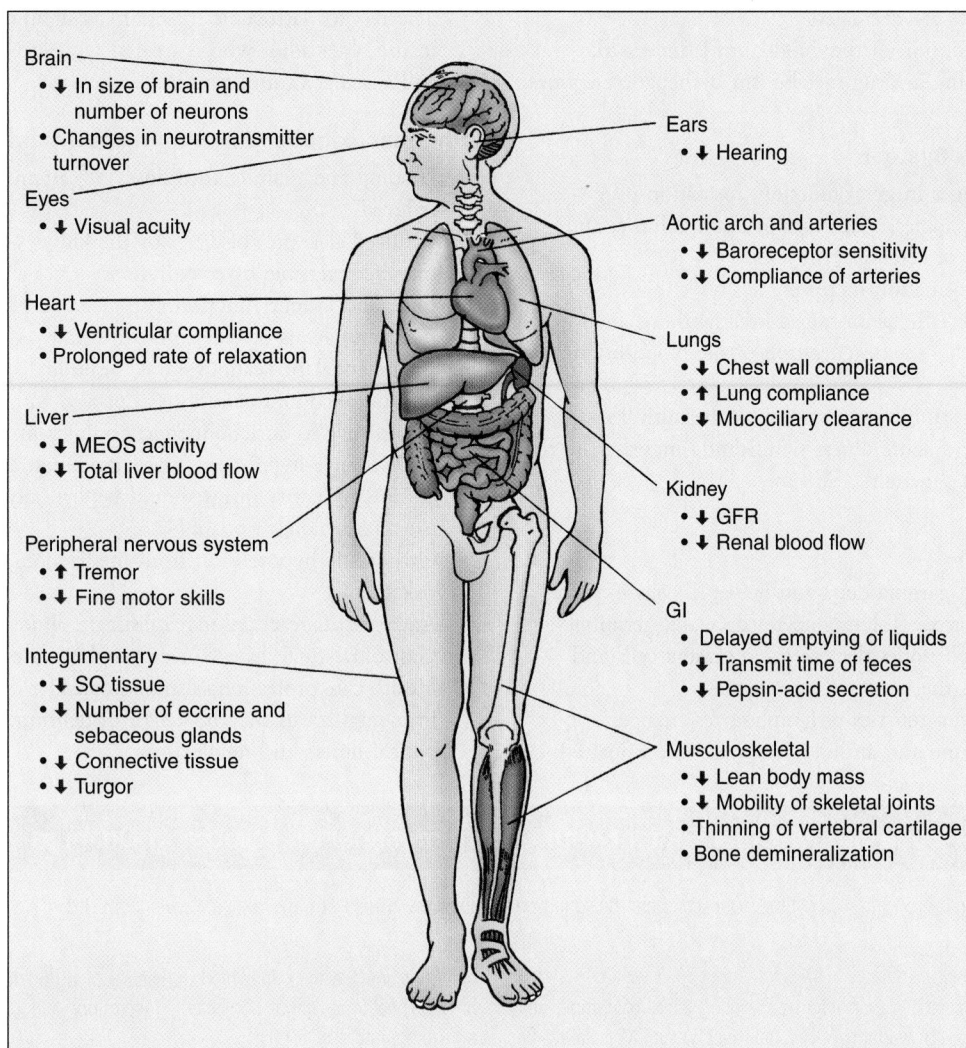

Figure 14-3 Summary of the physiologic changes that occur in all systems and that the critical care nurse must consider in caring for the elderly patient in the critical care unit. GFR, glomerular filtration rate; GI, gastrointestinal; MEOS, microsomal enzyme oxidative system; SQ, subcutaneous.

- Decreased myocardial efficiency results in less relaxation during diastole.
- The alteration in baroreceptor function leads to changes in compensatory responses.

Pulmonary System

- Lung tissue stiffens.
- Diffusion of gases is impaired by 8% per year after age 65 years.
- There is a decrease in vital capacity and maximal breathing capacity.
- Increased weakness of diaphragm and abdominal and accessory muscles leads to decreased ability to inhale and exhale.
- Decreased respiratory reserve may cause rapid decompensation and require longer periods of mechanical ventilation than in younger patients.

Renal System

- Decreased renal blood flow leads to a decrease in glomerular filtration and decreased renal tubule function.
- There is decreased elimination of physiologic substances (i.e., BUN and creatinine).
- Creatinine clearance, rather than the serum creatinine level, provides a more accurate indication of renal function.
- The older adult is predisposed to developing metabolic acidosis, volume depletion, and hyperchloremia.

Gastrointestinal System

- Gastric emptying, splenic blood flow, and gastrointestinal motility are decreased; gastrointestinal pH and thinning or reduction of the absorptive surface of the gut are increased.
- *H. pylori* infection and medication effects increase the risk for gastrointestinal bleeding.

- Absorption rates are decreased.
- Bacterial colonization of the duodenum is increased.
- There is a decline in drug metabolism by hepatic enzymes.

Central Nervous System

- There are changes in gyral function, formation of neurofibrillary tangles, a decrease in brain volume, and increase in size of cerebral ventricles.
- Senile plaque formation increases.
- There are changes in neurotransmitter synthesis and function, and there is degeneration of the blood-brain barrier.
- Environmental stimuli associated with the critical care environment and acute illness significantly increase the risk for cognitive decline and delirium.

Immune System

- The number of gamma/delta and helper T cells increases, suppressor/cytotoxic T lymphocytes decrease, germinal centers of lymph nodes decrease, and plasma cells and lymphocytes in the bone marrow increase.
- Cell surface characteristics of lymphocytes change.
- Humoral immune and antibody responses are impaired.

- The risk for iatrogenic infections is significantly increased in the older adult who is treated with indwelling catheters and vascular cannulation.

Pharmacokinetics and Pharmacodynamics

- Loading and maintenance doses of certain drugs should be reduced.
- Reduced clearance of drugs by the kidneys from dehydration may be reversible by rehydration.
- Liver and kidney function tests need to be repeated at regular intervals or when new drugs are added.
- Nonessential medications should be limited, and patients should be monitored for toxic effects associated with new medications.
- Drugs such as anticholinergics, opioids or narcotic analgesics, sedative-hypnotics, benzodiazepines, and nonsteroidal antiinflammatory drugs should be critically evaluated before use and avoided if possible.
- Orthostatic hypotension from medications may increase the risk of falls.
- Adverse drug reactions may mimic the abnormal signs of aging.
- Gastrointestinal disturbances may be caused by medications.
- Health care professionals should consider that subtle changes in mental status may be a sign of delirium from the critical illness and medications.

Case Study: Older Patient with Gastrointestinal Bleeding and Delirium

evolve Answers to the Case Study Questions can be found on the Evolve web site at http://evolve.elsevier.com/Urden/.

Brief Patient History

Mr. Smith is a 75-year-old man who has a long history of chronic atrial fibrillation treated with warfarin. Over the past week, Mr. Smith has experienced intermittent epigastric pain and black stools. He is now dizzy and weak.

Clinical Assessment

Mr. Smith is admitted to the intensive care unit from the emergency department. He recently began taking ciprofloxacin for a urinary tract infection. He also has been taking an aspirin each day because he heard it was "good for you." He recently began taking over-the-counter ibuprofen for his stomach pain and general aches. He does not have a history of cognitive impairment and otherwise appears in good health. However, during the assessment, you notice that he is inattentive at times, seems to doze on and off when unstimulated, and is confused about person and place episodically. This acute change in mental status evidenced by fluctuating symptoms, inattention, and a change in level of consciousness suggests the presence of delirium.

Diagnostic Procedures

Mr. Smith's admission laboratory work reveals a hemoglobin level of 7 g/dL and an international normalized ratio (INR) of 7. His baseline vital

signs include the following: blood pressure of 80/60 mm Hg, heart rate of 150 beats/min (atrial fibrillation), respiratory rate of 30 breaths/min, and temperature of 99.3° F.

Medical Diagnosis

Mr. Smith is diagnosed with gastrointestinal bleeding and delirium.

Questions

1. What major outcomes do you expect to achieve for this patient?
2. What problems or risks must be managed to achieve these outcomes?
3. What interventions must be initiated to monitor, prevent, manage, or eliminate the problems and risks identified?
4. What interventions should be initiated to promote optimal functioning, safety, and well-being of the patient?
5. What possible learning needs do you anticipate for this patient?
6. What cultural and age-related factors may have a bearing on the patient's plan of care?

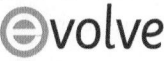 Be sure to check out the bonus material, including free self-assessment exercises, on the Evolve web site at http://evolve.elsevier.com/Urden/.

References

1. Marik PE: Management of the critically ill geriatric patient, *Crit Care Med* 34:S176, 2006.

2. *Profile of Older Americans: 2007*, Administration on Aging, U.S. Department of Health and Human Services. Retrieved on February 12, 2009. www.aoa.gov/prof/Statistics/profile/2007/2007profile.pdf.

3. Resnick NM, Dosa D: Geriatric medicine. In Kasper D et al, editors: *Harrison's principles of internal medicine*, ed 16, New York, 2005, McGraw-Hill.

4. Levine BS, Craven RF: Physiologic adaptations with aging. In Woods SL et al, editors: *Cardiac nursing*, ed 5, Philadelphia, 2005, Lippincott Williams & Wilkins.

5. Polanczyk C et al: Impact of age on perioperative complications and length of stay in patients undergoing noncardiac surgery, *Ann Intern Med* 134:637, 2001.

6. Eghbali M et al: Collagen accumulation in heart ventricles as a function of growth and aging, *Cardiovasc Res* 23:723, 1989.

7. Wegelius O, von Knorring J: The hydroxyproline and hexosamine content in human myocardium at different ages, *Acta Med Scand Suppl* 412:233, 1964.

8. Francis GS et al: Pathophysiology of heart failure. In Fuster V et al, editors: *Hurst's the heart*, ed 12, New York, 2008, McGraw-Hill.

9. Eaton L: Cardiovascular function. In Lueckenotte AG, editor: *Gerontologic nursing*, ed 2, St. Louis, 2000, Mosby.

10. Nadelmann J et al: Prevalence, incidence and prognosis of recognized and unrecognized myocardial infarction in persons aged 75 years or older: The Bronx Aging Study, *Am J Cardiol* 66:533, 1990.

11. Mukerji V et al: The clinical description of angina pectoris in the elderly, *Am Heart J* 117:705, 1989.

12. Lakatta EG et al: Aging and cardiovascular disease in the elderly. In Fuster V et al, editors: *Hurst's the heart*, ed 12, New York, 2008, McGraw-Hill.

13. Alexander, KP et al: Acute coronary care in the elderly, part II: ST-segment-elevation myocardial infarction. A scientific statement for healthcare professionals from the American Heart Association Council on Clinical Cardiology, in collaboration with the Society of Geriatric Cardiology. *Circulation* 115:2570, 2007.

14. Gerstenblith G et al: Echocardiographic assessment of normal adult aging population, *Circulation* 56:273, 1977.

15. Seifer CM, Kenny RA: Aging and geriatric heart disease. In Crawford MH et al, editors: *Cardiology*, ed 2, St. Louis, 2004, Mosby.

16. Lakatta EG et al: Prolonged contraction duration in the aged myocardium, *J Clin Invest* 55:61, 1975.

17. Cinelli P et al: Effects of age on mean heart rate variability, *Aging* 10:146, 1987.

18. Ribera JM et al: Cardiac rate and hyperkinetic rhythm disorders in healthy elderly subjects: evaluation by ambulatory electrocardiographic monitoring, *Gerontology* 35:158, 1989.

19. Jose AD: Effect of combined sympathetic and parasympathetic blockage on heart rate and cardiac function in man, *Am J Cardiol* 18:476, 1966.

20. Rodeheffer RJ et al: Exercise cardiac output is maintained with advancing age in human subjects: cardiac dilation and increased stroke volume compensate for a diminished heart rate, *Circulation* 69:203, 1984.

21. Aronow WS: Effects of aging on the heart. In Tallis RC, Fillit HM, editors: *Brocklehurst's textbook of geriatric medicine and gerontology*, ed 6, London, 2003, Churchill Livingstone.

22. Bonow RO et al: Effects of aging on asynchronous left ventricular regional function and global ventricular filling in normal human subjects, *J Am Coll Cardiol* 11:50, 1988.

23. Miller TR et al: Left ventricular diastolic filling and its association with age, *Am J Cardiol* 58:531, 1986.

24. Davidson WR, Fee WC: Influence of aging on pulmonary hemodynamics in a population free of coronary artery disease, *Am J Cardiol* 65:1454, 1990.

25. Bachman S et al: Effect of aging on the electrocardiogram, *Am J Cardiol* 48:513, 1981.

26. Horwitz LN, Lynch RA: Managing geriatric arrhythmias: I. General considerations, *Geriatrics* 46:31, 1991.

27. Carom AJ et al: The rhythm of the heart in active elderly subjects, *Am Heart J* 99:598, 1980.

28. Fleg JL, Kennedy HL: Cardiac arrhythmias in 9 healthy elderly population: detection by a 24–hour ambulatory electrocardiography, *Chest* 81:638, 1982.

29. Aronow WS: Cardia arrhythmias. In Tallis RC, Fillit HM, editors: *Brocklehurst's textbook of geriatric medicine and gerontology*, ed 6, London, 2003, Churchill Livingstone.

30. McNamara RL et al: Management of atrial fibrillation: review of the evidence for the role of pharmacologic therapy, electrical cardioversion, and echocardiography. *Ann Intern Med* 139:1018, 2003.

31. Fang MC et al: Age and the risk of warfarin-associated hemorrhage: the anticoagulation and risk factors in atrial fibrillation study. *J Am Geriatr Soc* 54:1231, 2006.

32. Bristow MR et al: Cardiac-resynchronization therapy with or without an implantable defibrillator in advanced chronic heart failure, *N Engl J Med* 350:2140, 2004.

33. Docherty JR: Cardiovascular responses in aging: a review, *Pharmacol Rev* 42:103, 1990.

34. Yin FCP et al: Age-associated decrease in ventricular response to haemodynamic stress during beta-adrenergic blockade, *Br Heart J* 40:1349, 1978.

35. Elliott HL et al: Effects of age in the responsiveness of vascular alpha-adrenoreceptors in man, *J Cardiovasc Pharmacol* 4:388, 1982.

36. Strogatz DS et al: Correlates of postural hypotension in a community sample of elderly blacks and whites, *J Am Geriatr Soc* 39:562, 1991.

37. Applegate WB et al: Prevalence of postural hypotension at baseline in the Systolic Hypertension in the Elderly Program (SHEP) cohort, *J Am Geriatr Soc* 39:1057, 1991.

38. Smith JJ et al: The effect of age on hemodynamic response to graded postural stress in normal men, *J Gerontol* 42: 406, 1987.

39. Dambrink JHA, Wieling W: Circulatory response to postural change in healthy male subjects in relation to age, *Clin Sci* 72:335, 1987.

40. Yin FCP et al: Role of aortic input impedance in the decreased cardiovascular response to exercise in aging dogs, *J Clin Invest* 68:28, 1981.

41. Potter JF: Hypertension. In Tallis RC, Fillit HM, editors: *Brocklehurst's textbook of geriatric medicine and gerontology*, ed 6, London, 2003, Churchill Livingstone.

42. Schoenberger JA: Epidemiology of systolic and diastolic systemic blood pressure elevation in the elderly, *Am J Cardiol* 57:45c, 1986.

43. Lawn RM: Lipoprotein(a) in heart disease, *Sci Am* 266:54, 1992.

44. Rowe JW: Clinical consequences of age-related impairments in vascular compliance, *Am J Cardiol* 60:68G, 1987.

45. Kreisberg RA, Kasim S: Cholesterol metabolism and aging, *Am J Med* 82:54, 1987.

46. Davis CE et al: Lipoprotein-cholesterol distributions in selected North American populations: The Lipid Research Clinics Program Prevalence Study, *Circulation* 2:302, 1980.

47. Hall JE, Coleman TG, Guyton AC: The renin-angiotensin system: normal physiology and changes in older hypertensives, *J Am Geriatr Soc* 37:801, 1989.

48. Crane MG, Harris JJ: Effect of aging on renin activity and aldosterone excretion, *J Lab Clin Med* 87:947, 1976.

49. Webster JR, Kadah H: Unique aspects of respiratory disease in the aged, *Geriatrics* 46:31, 1991.

50. Connolly MJ: Age-related changes in the respiratory system. In Tallis RC, Fillit HM, editors: *Brocklehurst's textbook of geriatric medicine and gerontology*, ed 6, London, 2003, Churchill Livingstone.

51. Connolly MJ: Asthma and chronic obstructive pulmonary disease. In Tallis RC, Fillit HM, editors: *Brocklehurst's textbook of geriatric medicine and gerontology*, ed 6, London, 2003, Churchill Livingstone.

52. Thurlbeck WM: Growth, aging and adaptation. In Murray JF, Nadel JA, editors: *Textbook of respiratory medicine*, Philadelphia, 1988, Saunders.

53. Levitzky MG: Effects of aging on the respiratory system, *Physiologist* 27:102, 1984.

54. Mittman C et al: Relationship between chest wall and pulmonary compliance and age, *J Appl Physiol* 20:1211, 1965.

55. Rizzato G, Marazzine L: Thoracoabdominal mechanisms in elderly men, *J Appl Physiol* 28:457, 1970.

56. Gutmann E, Hanzlikova V: Fast and slow motor units in aging, *Gerontology* 22:280, 1976.

57. Pontoppidan HH, Beecher HK: Progressive loss of protective reflexes in the airway with advance of age, *JAMA* 1974:2209, 1960.

58. Belman MJ, Gaesser GA: Ventilatory muscle training in the elderly, *J Appl Physiol* 64:899, 1988.

59. Knudson RJ et al: Changes in the normal maximal expiratory flow-volume curve with growth and aging, *Am Rev Respir Dis* 127:725, 1983.

60. Turner JM et al: Elasticity of human lungs in relation to age, *J Appl Physiol* 25:664, 1968.

61. Pierce JA, Hocott JB: Studies on the collagen and elastin content of the human lung, *J Clin Invest* 39:8, 1960.

62. Pierce JA, Ebert RV: Fibrous network of the lung and its change with age, *Thorax* 20:469, 1965.

63. Semmens M: The pulmonary artery in the normal aged lung, *Br J Dis Chest* 64:65, 1970.

64. Sorbini CA et al: Arterial oxygen tension in relation to age in healthy subjects, *Respiration* 25:3, 1968.

65. LeBlanc P et al: Effects of age and body position on "airway closure" in man, *J Appl Physiol* 28:448, 1970.

66. Holland J et al: Regional distribution of pulmonary ventilation and perfusion in elderly subjects, *J Clin Invest* 47:81, 1968.

67. Knudson RJ et al: Effect of aging alone on mechanical properties of the normal adult human lung, *J Appl Physiol* 43:1054, 1977.

68. Knudson RJ et al: The maximal expiratory flow-volume curve: normal standards, variability, and effects of age, *Am Rev Respir Dis* 113:587, 1976.

69. Medbo A, Melbye H: Lung function testing in the elderly: can we still use FEV$_1$/FVC <70% as a criterion of COPD? *Respir Med* 101:1097, 2007.

70. Wahba WH: Influence of aging on lung function: clinical significance of changes from age twenty, *Anesth Analg* 62:764, 1983.

71. Weder AB: The renally compromised older hypertensive: therapeutic considerations, *Geriatrics* 46:36, 1991.

72. Rosenthal RA, Kavic SM: Assessment and management of the geriatric patient, *Cri Care Med* 32:S92, 2004.

73. Gilbert BR, Vaughan ED: Pathophysiology of the aging kidney, *Clin Geriatr Med* 6(1):12, 1990.

74. Kasiske BL: Relationship between vascular disease and age-associated changes in the human kidney, *Kidney Int* 31:1153, 1987.

75. Anderson S, Brenner BM: Effects of aging on the renal glomerulus, *Am J Med* 80:435, 1986.

76. Clark JA, Coopersmith CM: Intestinal crosstalk: a new paradigm for understanding the gut as the "motor" of critical illness, *Shock* 28:384, 2007.

77. Tepper RE, Katz S: Geriatric gastroenterology: overview. In Tallis RC, Fillit HM, editors: *Brocklehurst's textbook of geriatric medicine and gerontology*, ed 6, London, 2003, Churchill Livingstone.

78. Greenwald DA, Brandt LJ: The upper gastrointestinal tract. In Tallis RC, Fillit HM, editors: *Brocklehurst's textbook of geriatric medicine and gerontology*, ed 6, London, 2003, Churchill Livingstone.

79. Fletcher K: Optimizing reserve in hospitalized elderly, *Crit Care Nurs Clin North Am* 19:285, 2007.

80. Thomson AB, Keelan M: The aging gut, *Can J Physiol Pharmacol* 64:30, 1986.

81. Bansal SK et al: Upper gastrointestinal hemorrhage in the elderly: a record of 92 patients in a joint geriatric/surgical unit, *Age Ageing* 16:279, 1987.

82. Moore JG et al: Effect of age on gastric emptying of liquid-solid meals in man, *Dig Dis Sci* 28(4):340, 1983.

83. Schuster MM: Disorders of the aging GI system, *Hosp Pract* 11:95, 1976.

84. Curran J: Overview of geriatric nutrition, *Dysphagia* 5:72, 1990.

85. Hogenauer & Hammer H: Maldigestion and malabsorption. In Feldman M, Friedman LS, Brandt LJ, editors: *Slesinger and Fordtran's Gastrointestinal and Liver Disease: Pathophysiology, diagnosis, management*, ed 8, Philadelphia, 2006, Saunders.

86. Sato TG et al: Age changes in the human liver of the different races, *Gerontology* 16:368, 1970.

87. Bach B et al: Disposition of antipyrine and phenytoin correlated with age and liver volume in man, *Clin Pharmacokinet* 6:389, 1981.

88. James OFW: The liver. In Tallis RC, Fillit HM, editors: *Brocklehurst's textbook of geriatric medicine and gerontology* ed 6, London, 2003, Churchill Livingstone.

89. Schmucker DL, Wang RK: Age-related changes in liver drug metabolism: structure versus function, *Proc Soc Exp Biol Med* 165:178, 1980.

90. Guay DRP et al: The pharmacology of aging. In Tallis RC, Fillit HM, editors: *Brocklehurst's textbook of geriatric medicine and gerontology*, ed 6, London, 2003, Churchill Livingstone.

91. Yuen GJ: Altered pharmacokinetics in the elderly, *Clin Geriatric Med* 6:257, 1990.

92. Stuart-Hamilton IA: Normal cognitive aging. In Tallis RC, Fillit HM, editors: *Brocklehurst's textbook of geriatric medicine and gerontology*, ed 6, London, 2003, Churchill Livingstone.

93. Quinn J, Kaye J: The neurology of aging, *Neurologist* 7:98, 2001.

94. Wilcock GK: Alzheimer's disease. In Tallis RC, Fillit HM, editors: *Brocklehurst's textbook of geriatric medicine and gerontology*, ed 6, London, 2003, Churchill Livingstone.

95. Rockwood K, Erkinjuntti T: Vascular dementia. In Tallis RC, Fillit HM, editors: *Brocklehurst's textbook of geriatric medicine and gerontology*, ed 6, London, 2003, Churchill Livingstone.

96. Arriagada P et al: Neurofibrillary tangles but not senile plaques parallel duration and severity of Alzheimer's disease, *Neurology* 42:631, 1992.

97. Selkoe DJ: Aging brain, aging mind, *Sci Am* 267:134, 1992.

98. Morris JC, McManus DQ: The neurology of aging: normal versus pathologic change, *Geriatrics* 46:47, 1991.

99. Lytle LD, Altar A: Diet, central nervous system, and aging, *Fed Proc* 38:2017, 1979.

100. Cotman CW: Synaptic plasticity, neurotropic factors and transplantation in the aged brain. In Schneider EL, Rowe JW, editors: *Handbook of the biology of aging*, San Diego, 1990, Academic Press.

101. Gottstein U, Held K: Effects of aging on cerebral circulation and metabolism in man, *Acta Neurol Scand Suppl* 72:54-55, 1979.

102. Meara J: Parkinsonism and other movement disorders. In Tallis RC, Fillit HM, editors: *Brocklehurst's textbook of geriatric medicine and gerontology*, ed 6, London, 2003, Churchill Livingstone.

103. Pompei P: Delirium. In Tallis RC, Fillit HM, editors: *Brocklehurst's textbook of geriatric medicine and gerontology*, ed 6, London, 2003, Churchill Livingstone.

104. Litton KA: Delirium in the critical care patient: what the professional staff needs to know, *Crit Care Nurs Q* 26:208, 2003.

105. Potter JF: Hypertension. In Tallis RC, Fillit HM, editors: *Brocklehurst's textbook of geriatric medicine and gerontology*, ed 6, London, 2003, Churchill Livingstone.

106. Gravenstein S et al: Clinical immunology of aging. In Tallis RC, Fillit HM, editors: *Brocklehurst's textbook of geriatric medicine and gerontology*, ed 6, London, 2003, Churchill Livingstone.

107. Hanlon JT et al: Geriatric pharmacotherapy. In Tallis RC, Fillit HM, editors: *Brocklehurst's textbook of geriatric medicine and gerontology*, ed 6, London, 2003, Churchill Livingstone.

108. Miller RA: Immune system. In Masoro EJ, editor: *Handbook of physiology: aging*, New York, 1995, Oxford University Press.

109. Terpenning MS, Bradley SF: Why aging leads to increased susceptibility to infection, *Geriatrics* 46:77, 1991.

110. Miller RA: The aging immune system: primer and prospectus, *Science* 273:70, 1996.

111. Moran D: Infections in the elderly, *Topics Emerg Med* 25:174, 2003.

112. President's Commission for the Study of Ethical Problems in Medicine and Biomedical and Behavioral Research: *Deciding to forgo life-sustaining treatment: a report on the ethical, medical and legal issues on treatment decisions*, Washington, DC, 1993, U.S. Government County Office.

113. Schwertz DW, Bushmann MT: Pharmacogeriatrics, *Crit Care Q* 12:26, 1989.

114. Gilman AG et al, editors: *Goodman and Gilman's the pharmacological basis of therapeutics*, ed 8, London, 1990, Pergamon.

115. Gillespie ND, Struthers AD: Chronic cardiac failure. In Tallis RC, Fillit HM, editors: *Brocklehurst's textbook of geriatric medicine and gerontology*, ed 6, London, 2003, Churchill Livingstone.

116. The SCOPE Study Group: The Study on Cognition and Prognosis in the Elderly (SCOPE): principal results of a randomized double-blind intervention trial, *J Hypertens* 21:875, 2003.

117. Bertel O et al: Decreased beta-adrenoreceptor responsiveness as related to age, blood pressure and plasma catecholamines in patients with essential hypertension, *Hypertension* 2:130, 1980.

118. Kendall MJ et al: Responsiveness to beta-adrenergic receptor stimulation: the effects of age are cardioselective, *Br J Clin Pharmacol* 14:821, 1982.

119. Rothschild JM et al: The critical care safety study: the incidence and nature of adverse events and serious errors in intensive care, *Crit Care Med* 33:1694, 2005.

120. Fick DM, Cooper JW, Wade WE, et al: Updating the Beers criteria for potentially inappropriate medication use in older adults: results of a US consensus panel of experts, *Arch Intern Med* 163:2716, 2003.

121. Balas MC et al: Delirium doulas: an innovative approach to enhance care for critically ill older adults, *Crit Care Nurse* 24:36, 2004.

122. Fields SD: History-taking in the elderly: obtaining useful information, *Geriatrics* 46(8):26, 1991.

123. Geokas MC: The aging process, *Ann Intern Med* 113:455, 1990.

124. Mobbs CV: Neurobiology of aging. In Tallis RC, Fillit HM, editors: *Brocklehurst's textbook of geriatric medicine and gerontology*, ed 6, London, 2003, Churchill Livingstone.

125. Brodie SE: Aging and disorders of the eye. In Tallis RC, Fillit HM, editors: *Brocklehurst's textbook of geriatric medicine and gerontology*, ed 6, London, 2003, Churchill Livingstone.

126. Blandford G: Eating disorders. In Tallis RC, Fillit HM, editors: *Brocklehurst's textbook of geriatric medicine and gerontology*, ed 6, London, 2003, Churchill Livingstone.

127. Weinstein BE: Disorders of hearing. In Tallis RC, Fillit HM, editors: *Brocklehurst's textbook of geriatric medicine and gerontology*, ed 6, London, 2003, Churchill Livingstone.

128. Brooke RC, Griffiths CE: Aging of the skin. In Tallis RC, Fillit HM, editors: *Brocklehurst's textbook of geriatric medicine and gerontology*, ed 6, London, 2003, Churchill Livingstone.

129. Pittman J: Effect of aging on wound healing current concepts, *J WOCN* 34:412, 2007.

130. Kelly L, Mobily PR: Iatrogenesis in the elderly, *J Gerontol Nurs* 17(9):24, 1991.

131. Shenefelt PD, Fenske NA: Aging and the skin: recognizing and managing common disorders, *Geriatrics* 45(10):57, 1990.

132. Francis RM: Metabolic bone disease. In Tallis RC, Fillit HM, editors: *Brocklehurst's textbook of geriatric medicine and gerontology*, ed 6, London, 2003, Churchill Livingstone.

133. Tobias JH, Sharif M: Bone and joint aging. In Tallis RC, Fillit HM, editors: *Brocklehurst's textbook of geriatric medicine and gerontology*, ed 6, London, 2003, Churchill Livingstone.

134. Edwards N, Baird C: Interpreting laboratory values in older adults, *Medsurg Nurs* 14:220, 2005.

135. Quinn J, Kaye J: The neurology of aging, *The Neurologist* 7:98, 2001.

136. Howieson DB et al: Natural history of cognitive decline in the old, *Neurology* 60:1489, 2003.

137. Foreman MD et al: Impaired cognition in the critically ill elderly patient: clinical implications, *Crit Care Q* 12:61, 1989.

138. Boss BJ: Normal aging in the nervous system: implications for SCI nurses, *SCI Nurs* 8(2):42, 1991.

139. Henshke PJ: Infections in the elderly, *Med J Aust* 158:830, 1993.

140. Piano MR: The physiologic changes that occur with aging, *Crit Care Q* 12:1, 1989.

141. Covinsky KE et al: Loss of independence in activities of daily living in older adults hospitalized with medical illnesses: increased vulnerability with age, *J Am Geriatr Soc* 51:451, 2003.

Perianesthesia Management

$\mathcal{M}$any advances in anesthetic agents and monitoring have resulted in more precise and safer delivery of anesthetic agents. However, caring for the critically ill patient who is emerging from anesthesia requires diligent monitoring of the patient's physical and psychological status to prevent potential complications that may occur as a result of the anesthetic agents or techniques. To provide safe and competent patient care, the critical care nurse needs to be aware of anesthetic agents and techniques and the physiologic and psychological responses of patients who are subjected to anesthesia.[1,2]

SELECTION OF ANESTHESIA

The complex structure of the anesthetic agents, combined with potential drug interactions and the patient's physical condition, can make it difficult to predict exactly how a patient will respond when emerging from anesthesia. An understanding of general principles prepares the nurse for the most commonly expected outcomes.[2,3] The American Society of Anesthesiologists physical status classification is a widely accepted method of preoperative patient evaluation. It serves as a guide to communicate clinical conditions and predict risks for anesthesia (Box 15-1). Preoperative evaluation allows the anesthesiologist to modify care for patients at high risk for surgery.[4]

The type of anesthesia used for surgery may be local, regional, or general. Local and regional anesthetics eliminate the sensation of pain to a specific part of the body without loss of protective reflexes or consciousness. Many patients also receive intravenous sedation with benzodiazepines to relieve anxiety, provide amnesia, and promote relaxation. Local anesthesia with sedation is commonly referred to as *conscious* or *procedural* sedation. Depending on the amount of sedation given and the patient' response, the level of consciousness can range from light to deep. Further information on sedation is provided in Chapter 9. Regional anesthesia is achieved through the use of nerve blocks or spinal or epidural catheters. Spinal anesthesia involves injecting the lumbar subarachnoid space with local anesthetics. Epidural anesthesia involves injecting the epidural space with local anesthetics or opioids, or both. Spinal and epidural anesthesia cause sensory and motor anesthesia. The advantages of epidural over spinal anesthesia are a decreased incidence of spinal headache and increased ability to provide postoperative pain management. General anesthesia is a controlled state of unconsciousness: the patient is not arousable, there is partial or complete loss of protective reflexes, and the airway needs to be continuously monitored and maintained. The preferred method of maintaining the patient's airway during general anesthesia is with an endotracheal tube.[3-6]

Several factors influence the choice of anesthetic agent and the mode of delivery, including age and physical status of the patient, the type of surgery, the skills of the anesthesia care provider and surgeon, and the patient's wishes.

GENERAL ANESTHESIA

The objectives of general anesthesia are analgesia, amnesia/hypnosis, blocking of reflexes, and skeletal muscle relaxation. There are four distinct phases or stages of anesthesia.

Stage I, commonly called the *stage of analgesia,* begins with the initiation of an anesthetic agent and ends with the loss of consciousness. This stage has been described as the lightest level of anesthesia and represents mild sensory and mental depression. Patients can open their eyes on command, breathe normally, and maintain protective reflexes. The patient's pain threshold is not appreciably lowered during this stage.[2,3,5] Stage II, also called the *stage of delirium,* begins with the loss of consciousness and ends with the onset of a regular pattern of breathing and the disappearance of the eyelid reflex. It is characterized by excitement, which can include uncontrolled movement and potentially dangerous responses to noxious stimuli. Other responses include vomiting, laryngospasm, tachycardia, and even cardiac arrest. If vomiting occurs, the patient is at risk for aspiration because of the loss of protective reflexes that is associated with this stage of anesthesia. With the use of newer and faster-acting anesthetic agents, this stage is passed through rapidly, decreasing the risk of complications. The use of propofol, etomidate, or short-acting barbiturates during the induction of anesthesia also facilitates rapid transition through stage II.[2,3,5]

Stage III is the *stage of surgical anesthesia.* It lasts from the onset of a regular pattern of breathing to the cessation of breathing. This is the goal for anesthesia, because the response to surgical incision is absent. Patients experience a depression in all elements of nervous system function (i.e., sensory depression, loss of recall, reflex depression, and some skeletal muscle relaxation). Each anesthetic agent affects the patient's clinical signs differently; therefore, monitoring the effects of anesthesia depends on the specific properties of each agent.[2,3,5]

BOX 15-1   AMERICAN SOCIETY OF ANESTHESIOLOGISTS' PHYSICAL STATUS CLASSIFICATION

- Category 1: Normal, healthy patient
- Category 2: Patient with mild systemic disease
- Category 3: Patient with severe systemic disease (e.g., hypertension, diabetes)
- Category 4: Patient with severe systemic disease that is a threat to life
- Category 5: Patient with high morbidity
- Category 6: Brain death

Stage IV is considered the *stage of overdose* and occurs when the patient receives too much anesthesia. In this stage, the patient shows signs of circulatory failure, and full cardiovascular and pulmonary support must be provided.[2,3,5]

During general anesthesia, the goal is to keep the patient in stage III. If the patient is not given enough anesthesia, he or she may experience recall or awareness during surgery (see Patient Safety Alert: Preventing and Managing the Impact of Anesthesia Awareness). If the patient is given too much anesthesia, stress on the patient and recovery time increase. The level of anesthesia is monitored by continual assessment of the patient's clinical presentation. Changes in breathing pattern and decreased to absent eye movement, muscle tone, and lacrimation are some of the indicators of the depth of anesthesia. External monitoring devices used to assess levels of anesthesia include lower esophageal contractility, heart rate variability, surface electromyogram, spontaneous electroencephalographic activity monitors, and evoked potentials.[6-9]

Patient Safety Alert

Preventing and Managing the Impact of Anesthesia Awareness

Anesthesia awareness, also called unintended intraoperative awareness, occurs under general anesthesia when a patient becomes cognizant of some or all events during a procedure and has direct recall of those events. Because of the routine use of neuromuscular blocking agents (paralytics) during general anesthesia, the patient is often unable to communicate with the surgical team when this occurs.

The frequency of anesthesia awareness has been found in multiple studies to range between 0.1% and 0.2% of all patients undergoing general anesthesia.[1-3] General anesthesia is administered to 21 million patients annually in the United States, so 20,000 to 40,000 cases of anesthesia awareness occur each year. Patients experiencing awareness report auditory recollections (48%), sensations of not being able to breathe (48%), and pain (28%).[1] More than 50% experience mental distress after surgery, including an indeterminate number with posttraumatic stress syndrome.[2,3] Some patients describe these occurrences as their "worst hospital experience," and some determine to never again undergo surgery.

The incidence of awareness is reported to be greater in patients for whom the dose of general anesthetic must be smaller and carefully titrated to decrease significant side effects, such as a patient who is hemodynamically unstable. Procedures typically identified as falling into this category are some cardiac, obstetric, and major trauma cases.[4] Factors contributing to the risk of anesthesia awareness include the increasing use of intravenous delivery of anesthesia, as opposed to inhalation, and the premature lightening of anesthesia at the end of procedures to facilitate operating room turnover.

Monitoring of patients under general anesthesia to prevent anesthesia awareness can be challenging. Despite a variety of available monitoring methods, awareness is difficult to recognize while it is occurring. Typical indicators of physiologic and motor response, such as high blood pressure, fast heart rate, movement, and hemodynamic changes, are often masked by the use of paralytic agents to achieve necessary muscle relaxation during the procedure, as well as the concurrent administration of other drugs necessary to the patient's management, such as beta-blockers or calcium channel blockers.

To overcome the limitations of current methods to detect anesthesia awareness, new methods are being developed that are less affected by the drugs typically used during general anesthesia. These devices measure brain activity rather than physiologic responses. These electroencephalography devices (also called level-of-consciousness, sedation-level, or anesthesia-depth monitors) include the Bispectral Index (BIS), spectral edge frequency (SEF), and median frequency (MF) monitors. These devices may have a role in preventing and detecting anesthesia awareness in patients with the highest risk, thereby ameliorating the impact of anesthesia awareness. A body of evidence has not yet accumulated to precisely define the role of these devices in detecting and preventing anesthesia awareness; The Joint Commission expects additional studies on these subjects to emerge. In its review of the BIS monitor, the U.S. Food and Drug Administration determined that "Use of BIS monitoring to help guide anesthetic administration may be associated with the reduction of the incidence of awareness with recall in adults during general anesthesia and sedation."

The anesthesia professional must often balance the psychological risks of anesthesia awareness against the physiologic risks of excessive anesthesia for many critical medical conditions. The Joint Commission has asked the American Society of Anesthesiologists (ASA) and the American Association of Nurse Anesthetists (AANA) to address the adequacy of current monitoring practices regarding anesthesia levels, including those practices that involve little or no technologic support.

Reducing the Risk of Anesthesia Awareness

The ASA and the AANA provide guidelines for administering and monitoring anesthesia. Specific recommendations for the prevention of awareness were addressed in the February 2000 issue of *Anesthesiology*[4]:

- Consider premedication with amnesic drugs (e.g., benzodiazepines, scopolamine), particularly when light anesthesia is anticipated.
- Administer more than a "sleep dose" of induction agents if they will be followed immediately by tracheal intubation. Avoid muscle paralysis unless absolutely necessary and, even then, avoid total paralysis (by using only the amount clinically required).

Continued

Patient Safety Alert—*cont'd*

- Conduct periodic maintenance of the anesthesia machine and its vaporizers, and meticulously check the machine and its ventilator before administering anesthesia.
- Be alert to patients taking beta-blockers, calcium channel blockers, or other drugs that can mask physiologic responses to inadequate anesthesia.

Managing the Impact of Anesthesia Awareness

Anesthesia awareness cannot always be prevented. Health care practitioners must be prepared to acknowledge and manage the occurrence of anesthesia awareness with compassion and diligence. The following practices are suggested when patients report awareness[4]:

- Interview the patient after the procedure, taking a detailed account of his or her experience and including it in the patient's chart.
- Apologize to the patient if anesthesia awareness occurred.
- Assure the patient of the credibility of his or her account, and sympathize with the patient's suffering.
- Explain what happened and its reasons (e.g., the necessity to administer light anesthesia in the presence of significant cardiovascular instability).
- Offer the patient psychological or psychiatric support, including referral to a psychiatrist or psychologist.
- Notify the patient's surgeon, nurse, and other key personnel about the incident and the subsequent interview with the patient.

Surgical team members should also be educated about anesthesia awareness and its managament.

Joint Commission Recommendations

Anesthesia awareness is underrecognized and undertreated in health care organizations. The Joint Commission recommends that health care organizations performing procedures under general anesthesia take the following steps to help prevent and manage anesthesia awareness:

1. Develop and implement an anesthesia awareness policy that addresses the following:
   - Education of clinical staff about anesthesia awareness and how to manage patients who have experienced awareness.
   - Identification of patients at proportionately higher risk for an awareness experience and discussion with such patients, before surgery, of the potential for anesthesia awareness.
   - The effective application of available anesthesia monitoring techniques, including timely maintenance of anesthesia equipment.
   - Appropriate postoperative follow-up of all patients who have undergone general anesthesia, including children.
   - The identification, management, and, if appropriate, referral of patients who have experienced awareness.
2. Ensure access to necessary counseling or other support for patients who are experiencing posttraumatic stress syndrome or other mental distress.

References

1. Sebel PS et al: The incidence of awareness during anesthesia: a multicenter United States study, *Anesth Analg* 99: 833-839, 2004.
2. Lennmarken C, Sandin R: Neuromonitoring for awareness during surgery, *Lancet* 363:1747-1748, 2004.
3. Osterman JE et al: Awareness under anesthesia and the development of post-traumatic stress disorder, *Gen Hosp Psychiatry* 23:198-204, 2001.
4. Ghoneim MM: Awareness during anesthesia, *Anesthesiology* 92(2):597-602, 2000.

Bibliography

Ekman A et al: Reduction in the incidence of awareness using BIS monitoring, *Acta Anaesthesiol Scand* 48:20-26, 2004.

Liska JM: *Silenced screams: surviving anesthetic awareness during surgery—a true-life account*, Park Ridge, IL, 2002, AANA Publishing, Council for Public Interest in Anesthesia.

Myles et al: Bispectral index monitoring to prevent awareness during anaesthesia: the B-Aware randomised controlled trial, *Lancet* 363:1757-1763, 2004.

Modified from the Joint Commission: Sentinel Event Alert, Issue 32, October 6, 2004. Available at www.jointcommission.org/SentinelEvents/SentinelEventAlert/sea_32.htm (accessed January 2009).

BOX 15-2   IDEAL CHARACTERISTICS OF ANESTHETIC AGENTS AND ADJUNCTS

- Rapid onset of action
- Controllable duration of action
- Identifiable levels of depth
- Technically easy to administer
- No untoward effects on vital signs
- No toxic metabolites
- Predictable elimination
- High specificity of action
- High margin of safety
- Useful with all ages
- Cost-effective
- Rapid emergence

ANESTHETIC AGENTS

Usually, two or more anesthetic agents are used in combination to achieve the desired level of anesthesia. To anticipate the patient's response, it is important for the nurse to have knowledge of the anesthetic agents that are used and their usual physiologic effects.

The ideal characteristics of anesthetic agents and adjuncts are listed in Box 15-2.[2]

INHALATION AGENTS

Inhalation agents are used for induction and maintenance of anesthesia or, in combination with other anesthetic agents, to maintain stage III anesthesia. They can be classified as volatile or gaseous. Volatile agents are further classified as halogenated hydrocarbons or ethers, are liquid at room temperature, and

TABLE 15-1 Pharmacologic Management: Inhalation Anesthetics

DRUG	CHARACTERISTICS	EFFECTS	CONSIDERATIONS
Nitrous oxide	Light anesthetic; carrier for other inhalation agents; always given with oxygen	Anesthetic and analgesic; little pulmonary, cardiac, or CNS effects; increases intracranial pressure; amnesia	Eliminated by ventilation; nausea and vomiting; diffusion hypoxia; mild myocardial depression
Isoflurane (Forane)	Pungent, ether-like odor; low potential for toxicity; successful ambulatory agent	Higher cardiovascular stability; potentiates muscle relaxants	Mild depression of spontaneous ventilation; postoperative shivering; fewer dysrhythmias noted
Desflurane (Suprane)	Strong, pungent odor; rapid onset; requires warmed vaporizer for administration	Minimal metabolism; respiratory depression; cardiovascular depression; no lingering analgesia	Observe for breath holding; coughing and laryngospasm; needs immediate analgesia
Sevoflurane (Ultane)	None irritating to airway; choice for pediatric anesthetic	Minimal airway irritation; rapid elimination; great precision and control over anesthetic depth	May trigger malignant hypothermia; observe for breath holding

CNS, central nervous system; SVR, systemic vascular resistance.

have a boiling point of 20° C. Gaseous agents are gases at room temperature. Inhaled anesthetics are delivered through the respiratory tract and are absorbed into the circulation through the alveoli. The effects of inhalation agents depend on alveolar ventilation, the ventilation-perfusion ratio, coadministered gases, gas flow, and the physicochemical properties of the gas. Their exact mechanism of action is unknown, but all cause central nervous system (CNS) depression and a state of unconsciousness that is deep enough to allow surgery. Table 15-1 lists the inhalation anesthetics presently used and their chief characteristics, effects, and nursing implications.[10]

INTRAVENOUS ANESTHETICS

Because inhalation anesthetics can produce adverse effects such as vasodilation, hypotension, dysrhythmias, and myocardial depression, other medications and methods of delivery have been sought to provide general anesthesia. Intravenous anesthetics are commonly used in the perioperative period. Intravenous anesthetics are grouped by their primary pharmacologic action as nonopioid or opioid intravenous agents. The nonopioid agents are further divided into the barbiturates, nonbarbiturates, and tranquilizers. These drugs can be administered by intermittent intravenous push dosing to induce anesthesia or by continuous intravenous drip to maintain anesthesia.[2,11]

Nonopioid Intravenous Anesthetics. The nonopioid drugs appear to interact with γ-aminobutyric acid (GABA) in the brain. GABA is an inhibitory neurotransmitter. Activation of the GABA receptors inhibits the postsynaptic neurons and results in a loss of consciousness. Barbiturates bind to GABA postsynaptic receptors, inhibiting neuronal activity and causing a loss of consciousness. Tranquilizers such as benzodiazepines potentiate the action of GABA, leading to inhibition of neuronal activity. Nonbarbiturate induction agents, such as etomidate, antagonize the muscarinic receptors in the

CNS and work as opioid agonists, resulting in a hypnotic state and loss of consciousness.[2,11] Table 15-2 presents the nonopioid intravenous anesthetics and their effects and nursing considerations.

Benzodiazepine Antagonists. Flumazenil (Romazicon) antagonizes or reverses the sedative, amnesic, anxiolytic, and muscle-relaxant effects of benzodiazepines. However, flumazenil does not reverse benzodiazepine-induced respiratory or cardiac depression. Flumazenil is specific for the benzodiazepine receptors and does not reverse the effects of barbiturates or opiates. It should be used with great caution in patients who have a history of seizures or chronic benzodiazepine use, because it can precipitate seizures. The incidence of postoperative nausea and vomiting is also increased with its use. Because flumazenil has a shorter duration of action than most of the benzodiazepines, the risk of resedation can occur after the initial dose starts to wear off, especially when high doses of benzodiazepines are administered. The patient must be monitored for resedation and other residual effects. If the patient develops signs of resedation, flumazenil is repeated at 20-minute intervals. Flumazenil has proved to be a valuable asset in the care of the patient who has received an excessive dose of a benzodiazepine such as midazolam or lorazepam. Consequently, flumazenil is very useful intraoperatively, postoperatively, and in the intensive care unit.[2,11,12]

Opioid Intravenous Anesthetics. Intravenous opioid anesthetics play an important role in clinical anesthesia. These drugs enhance the effectiveness of inhalation agents by providing the analgesic portion of the anesthetic process. Intravenous opioids blunt the sympathetic response to painful stimuli during anesthesia. The use of opioids allows for reduction in the concentration of the inhalation agent to be administered, resulting in a safer process. Opioids bind to specific receptors and produce a morphine-like or opioid agonist effect. Opioids are used to manage acute and chronic pain and are administered for general anesthesia, sedation, and pain relief during regional anesthesia;

TABLE 15-2   Pharmacologic Management: Nonopioid Intravenous Anesthetics

DRUG	CHARACTERISTICS	EFFECTS	CONSIDERATIONS
Barbiturates			
Thiopental (Pentothal)	Good patient acceptance; quick onset; very brief duration; no analgesia	CNS depression; spontaneous ventilation arrested; loss of laryngeal reflexes; causes histamine release (vasodilation, hypotension, and flushing)	IV administration painful; may cause myoclonus and hiccoughs; increased risk of aspiration
Methohexital (Brevital)	Similar to thiopental but twice as potent; used in pediatric patients; no analgesia; hepatic metabolism	Similar to thiopental; lowers seizure threshold (epileptiform)	Similar to thiopental; burns when given IV
Nonbarbiturates			
Etomidate (Amidate)	Agent of choice in patients with cardiovascular disease	Heart rate and cardiac output remain constant; minimal negative inotropic effects; suppression of adrenal function	May cause nausea and vomiting; burns when given IV; may cause myoclonus and hiccoughs
Propofol (Diprivan)	No analgesic effect; avoid in patients with coronary stenosis, ischemia, or hypovolemia; antiemetic properties; hepatic metabolism	Patient wakes up clearly and quickly, myocardial depressant; may decrease blood pressure 20%-25%	Rapid emergence may hasten pain awareness; low incidence of postoperative side effects; pain on administration
Dissociative Anesthetic			
Ketamine (Ketalar)	Profound analgesia and anesthesia; provides amnesia; may be used alone, may be given IV, IM, or PO	Produces cardiovascular and respiratory stimulation; may increase blood pressure and heart rate 10%-50%; increases intracranial pressure	Monitor for and prevent emergent reactions; titrate pain medications
Butyrophenones			
Haloperidol (Haldol)	Limited use in anesthesia because of long duration; antipsychotic; antiemetic	—	High incidence of extrapyramidal reactions
Droperidol (Inapsine)	Major tranquilizer; works with CNS as dopamine antagonist; hepatic metabolism; used in low doses for antiemetic prophylaxis	Prevents and treats nausea and vomiting; neuroleptic, causing amnesia or indifference to surroundings; adrenergic blocker, causing extrapyramidal muscle movements, hypotension, and peripheral vasodilation	Postanesthetic dysphoria (internalized overwhelming fear); effects last longer than those of narcotics (rare in low doses); prolongs QT interval.
Benzodiazepines			
Diazepam (Valium)	Rapid onset; long half-life; potent amnesic; effective anxiolysis; renal excretion	—	Titrate pain medications; monitor vital signs for respiratory depression
Midazolam (Versed)	Rapid onset; short duration; potent amnesic; effective anxiolysis; hepatic metabolism	—	Lower dose in elderly, debilitated, COPD, and liver disease patients; titrate pain medications; monitor vital signs
Lorazepam (Ativan)	Slow onset of action; long duration; anticonvulsant action; renal excretion	Pronounced sedation; minimal cardiovascular effects	Poor IV compatibility; titrate pain medications; monitor vital signs and for respiratory depression; watch for orthostatic hypotension

CNS, central nervous system; COPD, chronic obstructive pulmonary disease; IM, intramuscular; IV, intravenous.

TABLE 15-3 Pharmacologic Management: Opioid Adjunctive Agents*

CLINICAL USES	IMPLICATIONS	CONSIDERATIONS
Preoperative sedation	Monitor for hypotension	Keep naloxone (Narcan) available
Induction of anesthesia	Monitor for bradycardia	Keep resuscitation equipment available
Maintenance of anesthesia	Monitor for respiratory depression	Respiratory depressant effect may outlast analgesia
Postoperative pain management	May cause nausea and vomiting	

*Agents include alfentanil (Alfenta), fentanyl (Sublimaze), ketorolac (Toradol), morphine, and sufentanil (Sufenta).

they are important in all phases of the perioperative experience.[2,11] Table 15-3 presents a summary of clinical uses and nursing implications for the most frequently used opioids.

Opioid Antagonists. Opioid antagonists are used to reverse the effects of opioids, particularly respiratory depression. The drug of choice in perianesthesia care is naloxone (Narcan). Naloxone competes with and displaces the opioid on the receptor site; it therefore reverses respiratory depressant and analgesic effects of opioids. Naloxone is titrated to the patient's response. The onset of action is 1 to 2 minutes and the duration of action is 1 to 4 hours. If adequate reversal has not been achieved after 3 to 5 minutes, naloxone administration is repeated until reversal is complete.[12,13] If long-acting opioids are used, the patient must be monitored for respiratory insufficiency, because the depressant effects of the opioids may return. Often, a low-dose, continuous intravenous drip of naloxone proves effective. Close monitoring of vital signs is critical. One adverse effect to watch for when excessive doses of naloxone are given is an increase in blood pressure, which may occur in response to pain. In addition, tachycardia, nausea, vomiting, or diaphoresis may occur if the reversal is too rapid. Naloxone must be used with caution in patients with cardiac irritability and in patients who are physically dependent on opioids, because reversal may precipitate an acute withdrawal syndrome.[12,13]

NEUROMUSCULAR BLOCKING AGENTS

Neuromuscular blocking agents (NMBAs), or muscle relaxants, interrupt the transmission of impulses from the nerve to the muscle, causing a decrease in muscle activity. Decreasing muscle activity allows the surgeon to operate in a quiet field and decreases the need for deep anesthesia. These drugs have contributed greatly to clinical anesthesia. However, the use of NMBAs is not limited to the operating room; they are used to facilitate endotracheal intubation, to terminate laryngospasm, to eliminate chest wall rigidity that may occur after the rapid injection of potent opioids, and to facilitate mechanical

ventilation by producing total paralysis of the respiratory muscles. NMBAs cause paralysis of the respiratory muscles, and the patient receiving these agents requires support of ventilation with a handheld bag-valve-mask or a mechanical ventilator. NMBAs do not have analgesic, amnesic, anxiolytic, or sedative effects. The paralyzed patient is not able to communicate his or her needs; NMBAs must be used in combination with other medications to prevent pain and provide sedation.[3,14,15]

Skeletal muscle contraction occurs when acetylcholine is released from the motor neuron and binds to receptor sites on the muscle fiber (i.e., neuromuscular junction), resulting in depolarization. Skeletal muscle relaxation occurs when the release of acetylcholine ceases and any residual acetylcholine is destroyed by the enzyme acetylcholinesterase, resulting in repolarization. NMBAs interfere with the relationship between acetylcholine and the receptor. There are two general categories of skeletal muscle relaxants: nondepolarizing and depolarizing.[14-16]

Depolarizing agents compete with acetylcholine at the neuromuscular junction, causing the muscle to depolarize and inhibiting repolarization. The muscle stays in a prolonged depolarized state, and movement is inhibited. The principal depolarizing skeletal muscle agent is succinylcholine (Anectine). After succinylcholine attaches to the receptor, a brief period of depolarization occurs, which is manifested by transient muscular fasciculations. Succinylcholine has a rapid onset, 30 to 60 seconds, and a short duration of action, 5 to 10 minutes. It is frequently used to facilitate intubation. The actions of succinylcholine cannot be pharmacologically reversed.[2,5,14,17]

Nondepolarizing NMBAs usually are longer-acting agents than depolarizing agents. Nondepolarizing agents do not cause muscle contraction or depolarization. They compete with and block the uptake of acetylcholine at the muscle receptor site and prevent repolarization. Sustained muscle relaxation occurs, and voluntary control of skeletal muscle contraction is weakened or lost.[2,5,14,16]

Table 15-4 presents a pharmacologic overview of the commonly used skeletal muscle relaxants. A number of factors can potentiate the effects of nondepolarizing NMBAs or antagonize them; these factors are listed in Box 15-3.[15,16]

Neuromuscular Blocking Agent Antagonists. The pharmacologic actions of nondepolarizing NMBAs can be reversed by anticholinesterase drugs such as neostigmine (Prostigmin). These drugs increase the amount of acetylcholine available at the receptor sites by preventing its destruction by acetylcholinesterase. This promotes more effective competition of acetylcholine with the nondepolarizing skeletal muscle relaxant that is occupying the receptor sites. Because of the increased availability and mobilization of the acetylcholine, the concentration gradient favors acetylcholine and the removal of the nondepolarizing agent from the receptors, resulting in the return of normal skeletal muscle depolarization and contraction.[15] These drugs also produce undesired side effects by increasing the level of acetylcholine at receptor sites in the heart, the lungs, the eyes, and gastrointestinal tract, which can lead to bradycardia, bronchospasm, miosis, and increased peristalsis and secretion. To prevent or minimize these effects, anticholinergic agents such as atropine

TABLE 15-4 Pharmacologic Management: Neuromuscular Blocking Agents*

	IMPLICATIONS	
CHARACTERISTICS	DEPOLARIZING	NONDEPOLARIZING
Compete with acetylcholine at the myoneural junction Shorter-acting agents are most appropriate for anesthesia Provide surgical relaxation Facilitate intubation Assist in ventilatory support	Reversible only with time Use cautiously in patients with neuromuscular disease, such as myasthenia gravis or muscular dystrophy Adverse effects include bradycardia, tachycardia, ventricular dysrhythmias, asystole, hypertension, hyperkalemia Increases intraocular, intracranial, and intragastric pressure Precipitates muscle fasciculations and pain Prolongs respiratory depression Histamine release causes hypotension Use cautiously in patients with head injury, cerebral edema, trauma, burns, electrolyte imbalances, and renal or hepatic disease Be alert for manifestations of malignant hyperthermia	Reversible with time and anticholinesterase Use cautiously in patients with hepatic or renal disease, obesity, asthma, or chronic obstructive pulmonary disease Adverse effects include tachycardia, hypertension, hypotension, bronchospasms, and flushing

*Long-acting agents include doxacurium (Nuromax), gallamine (Flaxedil), pancuronium (Pavulon), and pipecuronium (Arduan); intermediate-acting agents include atracurium (Tracrium) and vecuronium (Norcuron); short-acting agents include rocuronium (Zemuron), and succinylcholine (Anectine), which is a depolarizing agent.

BOX 15-3   FACTORS INFLUENCING NEUROMUSCULAR BLOCKADE

POTENTIATING FACTORS
- Hypocalcemia
- Hypokalemia
- Hyponatremia
- Hypermagnesemia
- Acidosis
- Hypothermia
- Antibiotics (gentamicin; tobramycin; amikacin; kanamycin; neomycin; polymyxin A, B, and E; clindamycin; tetracyclines; piperacillin; streptomycin)
- Antidysrhythmics (procainamide, lidocaine, quinidine)
- β-Adrenergic blockers
- Calcium channel blockers
- Diuretics (furosemide, thiazides)
- Droperidol
- Inhalation agents
- Cyclosporine
- Lithium
- Dantrolene
- Etomidate
- Hepatic failure
- Renal failure
- Neuromuscular diseases

ANTAGONIZING FACTORS
- Phenytoin
- Carbamazepine
- Aminophylline
- Theophylline
- Sympathomimetic agents
- Corticosteroids
- Azathioprine

or glycopyrrolate (Robinul) are given with the reversal agent.[2,4,5,10] Table 15-5 outlines the common NMBA reversal agents used in anesthesia and their nursing implications.

PERIANESTHESIA ASSESSMENT AND CARE

The goal of management in the immediate postoperative period is the recognition and immediate treatment of any problems, to eliminate or lessen complications that may occur. This requires the collaborative effort of the nurse, the anesthesiologist, and the surgeon. Physical assessment of the postanesthesia patient begins immediately on admission to the unit. The nurse admitting the patient receives a report from the anesthesia care provider. The nurse should get information related to the patient's general condition, the operation performed, the type of anesthesia administered, estimated blood loss, total intake and output during surgery, and any problems or complications encountered in the operating room (see Patient Safety Alert: Hand-off Communication).[2]

Assessment of the cardiopulmonary system is the immediate priority. The patient's airway is assessed to ensure that it is patent, and the patient's breathing pattern is evaluated to ensure that it is unlabored. The patient's blood pressure, pulse, rate of respiration, and oxygen saturation level are checked and recorded. All dressings and drains are quickly inspected for gross bleeding. After these initial observations have been made, it is essential to systematically assess the patient's total condition.[2,6,18]

RESPIRATORY FUNCTION

Because patients have experienced some interference with their respiratory system, postanesthesia maintenance of adequate gas exchange is a crucial aspect of care in the immediate postoperative period. Oxygen administration may be used in the immediate postoperative phase. Any change in respiratory function must be detected early so that appropriate measures can be taken to ensure adequate oxygenation and ventilation. Respiratory function is evaluated by using physical assessment skills: inspection, palpation, percussion, and auscultation. Several preexisting conditions can increase the probability that ventilatory support will be needed in the postoperative period. These include preexisting lung disease, thoracic or upper abdominal surgery, history of smoking, recent opioid administration, and low oxygen saturation before surgery.[2,4,6]

Patient Safety Alert

Hand-off Communication

National Patient Safety Goal (NPSG).02.05.01
The [organization] implements a standardized approach to hand-off communications, including an opportunity to ask and respond to questions.

Rationale for NPSG.02.05.01
Health care has numerous types of [patient] hand-offs, including, but not limited to, nursing shift changes; physician transfer of complete responsibility for a [patient]; physician transfer of on-call responsibility; acceptance of temporary responsibility for staff leaving the unit for a short time; anesthesiologist report to postanesthesia recovery room nurse; nursing and physician hand-off from the emergency department to inpatient units, different hospitals, nursing homes, and home health care; and critical laboratory and radiology results sent to physician offices. The primary objective of a hand-off is to provide accurate information about a [patient]'s care, treatment, and services; current condition; and any recent or anticipated changes. The information communicated during a hand-off must be accurate in order to meet [patient] safety goals.

Elements of Performance for NPSG.02.05.01
1. The hospital's process for effective hand-off communication includes the following: interactive communication that allows for the opportunity for questioning between the giver and receiver of patient information.
2. The hospital's process for effective hand-off communication includes the following: up-to-date information regarding the patient's condition, care, treatment, medications, services, and any recent or anticipated changes.
3. The hospital's process for effective hand-off communication includes the following: a method to verify the received information, including repeat-back or read-back techniques.
4. The hospital's process for effective hand-off communication includes the following: an opportunity for the receiver of the hand-off information to review relevant patient historical data, which may include previous care, treatment, and services.
5. Interruptions during hand-offs are limited to minimize the possibility that information fails to be conveyed or is forgotten.

From The Joint Commission. Accreditation Program: Critical Access Hospital, 2009 National Patient Safety Goals, p. 7. Available at www.jointcommission.org (accessed January 2009).

Pulse oximetry, a noninvasive technique, measures oxygen saturation of functional hemoglobin. Pulse oximetry can be used to identify hypoxemia, and it should be used on all postoperative patients. If the patient is intubated and being mechanically ventilated, capnography can be used to assess the adequacy of ventilation. Arterial blood gas measurements can be used to definitively confirm abnormal pulse oximetry or capnography values. Normal pulse oximetry values are 97% to 99%; however, preanesthetic baseline values must be noted. Some patients normally have lower saturation values on room air for a variety of reasons, and attempting to maintain higher oxygen saturation levels may result in prolonged oxygen therapy.[20]

Routine oxygen administration in the postanesthesia recovery period can be accomplished with the use of nasal cannula (prongs) or a facemask. Surgery and anesthesia often interrupt the normal functioning of the nose, so humidification or nebulization with oxygen delivery may be needed. Humidifiers convert water from the liquid to the gaseous state, whereas nebulizers produce tiny water particles. This is especially helpful at higher flow rates.[21]

Some patients recovering from anesthesia require mechanical ventilation. Various modes, such as positive end-expiratory pressure (PEEP), continuous positive airway pressure (CPAP), and synchronized intermittent mandatory ventilation (SIMV), are used to improve the respiratory status of the patient.[21]

Stir-Up Regimen. A significant aspect of perianesthesia nursing management is the stir-up regimen. The regimen is aimed at the prevention of complications, primarily atelectasis and venous stasis. The stir-up regimen consists of five major activities—deep-breathing exercises, coughing, positioning, mobilization, and pain management.[22]

Deep-Breathing Exercises. The major factor contributing to postoperative pulmonary complications is low lung volumes resulting from a shallow, monotonous, sighless breathing pattern caused by general anesthesia, opioids, and pain. The patient must be stimulated to take three or four deep breaths every 5 to 10 minutes. Full lung expansion is important, and every effort must be made to enhance the patient's ability to accomplish it.

The sustained maximal inspiration (SMI) maneuver is a method to enhance the lung volumes of postoperative patients. The SMI maneuver consists of having the patient inhale as close to lung capacity as possible and, at the peak of inspiration, hold that volume for 3 to 5 seconds before exhaling it. This maneuver is more effective than simple deep breathing in preventing reduced lung volumes in the immediate postanesthesia periods. If the patient's vital capacity is inadequate or if anesthesia respiratory depression is prolonged, deep breathing and the SMI maneuver may be augmented with a manual resuscitation bag connected to an oxygen source or with an intermittent positive-pressure breathing apparatus.

Incentive spirometry has become increasingly popular and is used to assist with preventing and treating atelectasis, promoting normal lung expansion, and improving oxygenation. Incentive spirometry devices allow patients visual feedback and observation of inspiratory volume. Instruction and practice before surgery provide patients with the opportunity to master the device and establish their baseline levels before anesthetic and surgical interventions.[22]

TABLE 15-5 Pharmacologic Management: NMBA Reversal Agents

DRUG	CHARACTERISTICS	EFFECTS	CONSIDERATIONS
Neostigmine (Prostigmin)	Binds with cholinesterase and inactivates it Preserves endogenous anticholinesterase	Antidote for nondepolarizing NMBAs Prevents postoperative distention and urinary retention Muscarinic effects cause bradycardia, broncho-constriction, peripheral vasodilation, and coronary vasoconstriction	Does not cross blood-brain barrier Lasts 30-90 min May be given with atropine and glycopyrrolate to decrease muscarinic effects Use cautiously in patients with asthma or coronary disease
Pyridostigmine (Regonol)	Analogue of neostigmine with fewer adverse effects Only 20% as potent as neostigmine Rapid onset of action (5-15 min)	Antidote for nondepolarizing NMBAs Muscarinic effects less severe than those of neostigmine	Longer half-life Lasts 120 min May be given with atropine and glycopyrrolate Use cautiously in patients with asthma, peptic ulcer, epilepsy, or pregnancy
Edrophonium (Tensilon)	Cholinergic Short-acting anticholinesterase	Parasympathetic effects: GI: Salivation, dysphasia, nausea, vomiting, increased peristalsis CV: bradycardia, cardiac dysrhythmias, hypotension RESP: Increased pharyngeal and tracheobronchial secretions EENT: Lacrimation, miosis, diplopia	Must be given with atropine Very rapid onset but brief duration of action Use cautiously in presence of asthma, peptic ulcer, or bradycardia
Atropine	Anticholinergic Antimuscarinic Chronotropic stimulator in event of bradycardia	Preanesthetic medication to prevent or reduce respiratory tract secretions Restoration of cardiac rate during anesthesia Antidote for cholinesterase inhibitors Causes decreased sweating and predisposition to heat prostration	Crosses blood-brain barrier Ensures adequate hydration Provides temperature control to prevent hyperpyrexia
Glycopyrrolate (Robinul)	Similar to atropine Longer duration	Less incidence of dysrhythmias Slow increase in heart rate Protection against peripheral muscarinic effects of neostigmine and pyridostigmine	Does not cross blood-brain barrier Contraindicated in presence of glaucoma, peptic ulcer, or COPD

COPD, chronic obstructive pulmonary disease; CV, cardiovascular; EENT, eyes, ears, nose, and throat; GI, gastrointestinal; NMBA, neuromuscular blocking agent; RESP, respiratory.

Coughing. The patient must be instructed to cough and to perform SMI maneuvers. The best way to clear the air passages of obstructive secretions is with a purposeful cough. For the patient recovering from anesthesia, the cascade cough is the most effective coughing maneuver. Instruct the patient to take a rapid, deep inhalation. This will increase the volume of air in the lungs and dilate the airways, allowing air to pass behind the retained secretions. On exhalation, have the patient perform multiple coughs. With each cough the length of the airways increases, enhancing the effectiveness of the cough. Coughing should be done only by patients with secretions, because it can promote atelectasis.[22]

Coughing is most effective with the patient sitting upright. Splinting of incisions and adequate analgesia facilitate coughing. If the patient is unable to sit upright, place the patient in a side-lying position with hips and knees flexed, or in a semi-Fowler's position with the head and arms supported with pillows and the knees flexed. This positioning decreases abdominal tension and allows maximal movement of the diaphragm, improving the effectiveness of the cough.

Between cascade cough maneuvers, the patient is encouraged to inhale and close the glottis. This dilates the airways, increases intrathoracic pressure, and compresses the smaller airways, pushing the secretions toward the larger airways where they can be expectorated in succeeding cough maneuvers.

When a large amount of secretions accumulates in the patient's lungs and cannot be handled effectively by coughing, suctioning must be instituted. Suctioning is not without complications and should be done only when necessary and not routinely.[22]

Positioning. Patients recovering from anesthesia are maintained in a semiprone, side-lying position if possible. The semiprone position promotes maintenance of a patent airway, prevents aspiration, and permits optimal ventilation of the lower lung lobes. Frequent repositioning of patients (at least every hour) from side to side is essential for the prevention of atelectasis and venous stasis. Patients are encouraged to turn and change positions as soon as possible.

Mobilization. To prevent venous stasis, patients must be encouraged to move their legs and arms rhythmically, flexing and extending their extremities. Mobilization and flexion of the muscles aids venous return, improves cardiac output

(CO), and prevents venous stasis and the formation of deep vein thrombosis.[22]

Pain Management. Adequate pain control is a major consideration in the recovering patient (Box 15-4). Without it, it is difficult to implement the first four interventions of the stir-up regimen. Poorly controlled pain can have serious consequences in terms of hemodynamic responses to catecholamines and physical limitations on respiratory function. On the other hand, the medications used to control pain may in themselves have deleterious effects on hemodynamic and respiratory function. Opioids depress the cough reflex, ciliary activity, and the respiratory center in the brain and should not be used

---

BOX 15-4   ASPAN POSITION STATEMENT ON PAIN MANAGEMENT

The American Society of PeriAnesthesia Nurses (ASPAN) has the responsibility for defining the practice of perianesthesia nursing. An integral part of this responsibility involves identifying the educational requirements and competencies essential to perianesthesia nursing practice and the educational needs of the patients and family regarding pain assessment and management.

ASPAN sets forth this position statement to promote the optimal level of ractice and to present a consistent standard of care that documents sound clinical judgment in the management of postoperative pain.

BACKGROUND

ASPAN has defined a standard for pain management (Standard XI) with the intent of providing guidelines that represent what is believed to be an optimal level of practice. To assist members in achieving this standard, ASPAN published pain management competency material in the Competency Based Orientation and Credentialing Program. In response to continued concerns from perianesthesia nurses, ASPAN's Standards and Guidelines Committee conducted a review of the literature to identify current issues related to pain assessment and management. The following issues were identified:

1. As many as 50% of postoperative patients in hospitals and outpatient surgical centers are undermedicated and suffer unrelieved pain.[1-4]
2. The practice of undermedicating for pain occurs regardless of the patient's age.[5,6]
3. Frequently the patient's self-report of pain is not taken into consideration when choosing the dosage of medication to give for pain relief.[7,8]
4. Inadequate pain management affects postoperative recovery and behaviors associated with that recovery.[5,6,9]
5. A prevalent cause of ineffective pain management is the professional's lack of knowledge related to pain physiology, medications, and protocols.[4,10]
6. There is still an overriding concern that the use of opioids in the treatment of acute postoperative pain control will contribute to psychological dependence.[11]
7. Patient and family education addressing postsurgical pain management remains inconsistent.[12]
8. Pain management should begin preoperatively with patient and family education addressing use of a pain scale and methods of postoperative pain control.

9. The Agency for Health Care Policy and Research (AHCPR) suggests that practitioners are too rigid when managing acute postoperative pain and should set goals to reduce its incidence and severity. Guidelines have been published by this agency for acute pain management.[13]

POSITION

It is therefore the position of ASPAN that a collaborative plan should be developed between the anesthesia department and the perianesthesia nurses to address pain management within the perianesthesia setting. The following points of action should be addressed:

1. The goal should be to relieve as much pain as possible to allow for activity, relaxation, prevention of complications, and promotion of optimal health and healing.
2. Areas of education in pain management for health care professionals should include the following:
   a. Physiology of pain management.
   b. Assessment techniques
   c. Methods of intervention (pharmacologic and nonpharmacologic)
   d. Management of side effects and complications related to each intervention
   e. Evaluation of successful management
   f. Ethical considerations
   g. Age and cultural considerations
   h. Patient and family education issues
3. Whenever possible, the patient's plan of care for pain management should begin during the preoperative interview.
4. The patient's self-report of pain is the best measurement tool to use when assessing pain.
5. The use of reliable and valid pain scales should be a standard part of the pain assessment.
6. Measurement of outcomes should reflect timely, appropriate interventions and achievement of desired effects.

EXPECTED OUTCOMES

Perianesthesia nurses need to familiarize themselves with this position statement and inform and educate peers, nurse managers, hospital administrators, and physicians.

Anesthesiologists and perianesthesia nurses need to collaborate in the development of a multidisciplinary plan of care (e.g., protocol, critical pathway, care map) to provide safe, appropriate, and effective pain management.

Continued

BOX 15-4   ASPAN POSITION STATEMENT ON PAIN MANAGEMENT—*cont'd*

ASPAN, as the voice of perianesthesia nursing practice, must externalize this information by sharing this position statement with regulatory agencies and professional organizations that interface with perianesthesia nursing areas.

APPROVAL OF STATEMENT

This statement was recommended by a vote of the ASPAN Board of Directors on April 16, 1999, and approved by a vote of the ASPAN Representative Assembly on April 18, 1999, in Honolulu, Hawaii.

References

1. Most patients face pain, often unrelieved, after surgery, *Am J Nurs* 96(3):68, 1996.
2. Campese C: Development and implementation of a pain management program, *AORN J* 64:931-940, 1996.
3. Bormann D, Hansen K: Improving pain management through staff education, *Nurs Manage* 28(7):55-57, 1997.
4. Thornborough J: Developing a pain management protocol in the PACU, *Surg Nurse* 20(5):23-27, 1998.
5. Fortin J et al: The postoperative pain experience: a description based on the McGill Pain Questionnaire, *Clin Nurs Res* 1(3):292-304, 1992.
6. Pasero C, McCaffrey M: Managing postoperative pain in the elderly, *Am J Nurs* 96(10):38-46, 1996.
7. Reid D et al: Postoperative pain, *Can Nurse* 88(7):55, 1992.
8. Malek C, Olivieri R: Pain management: documenting the decision-making process, *Nurs Case Manage* 1(2):64-76, 1996.
9. Getker-Black S et al: Preoperative self-efficacy and postoperative behaviors, *Appl Nurs Res* 5(3):134-139, 1992.
10. Carr E: Overcoming barriers of effective pain control, *Prof Nurse* 12:412-416, 1997.
11. Aiher J et al: Children win with improved pain management, *Can Nurse* 88(1):19-21, 1992.
12. Jones S, Villalobos J: Incorporating clinical research findings into practice, *J Nurs Staff Dev* 12(1):46, 1996.
13. Agency for Health Care Policy and Research: *Acute pain management in infants, children, and adolescents: operative and medical procedures*, Rockville, MD, 1992, U.S. Department of Health and Human Services.

Bibliography

American Nurses Association: *Code for nurses with interpretative statements*, Washington, DC, 1995, ANA.

American Society of PeriAnesthesia Nurses: *Competency-based orientation and credentialing program*, Cherry Hill, NJ, 1997, ASPAN.

Bishop A, Scudder J: *Nursing ethics: therapeutic caring presence*, Boston, 1996, Jones & Bartlett.

Heiser R et al: The use of music during the immediate postoperative recovery period, *AORN J* 65:777-778, 781–785, 1997.

Miaskowski C et al: Interdisciplinary guidelines for the management of acute pain: implications for quality improvement, *J Nursing Care Qual* 7:1-6, 1992.

Schwartz-Barcott C et al: Client-nurse interaction: testing for its impact in preoperative instruction, *Int J Nurs Stud* 31:23-35, 1994.

Surgical patient's no. 1 fear: pain, *Today's Surg Nurse* 18:7, 1996.

Wong D: Video Presentation. Pain Assessment in Children and Infants.

Information from the American Society of PeriAnesthesia Nurses, 10 Melrose Avenue, Suite 110, Cherry Hill, NJ 080037-3696; (877) 737-9696; fax: (856) 616-9601; e-mail: aspan@aspan.org; 1997-2001.

indiscriminately. However, if the patient refuses to deep breathe, cough, or move because of pain, he or she is at risk for postoperative respiratory and embolic complications.

Pain accelerates the cardiovascular system by activating the sympathetic nervous system and the adrenal system. Normally, this causes an increase in heart rate and blood pressure. However, anesthesia and some cardiac medications can blunt the sympathetic response; asking the patient his or her pain level is the most valid method of assessing pain levels (see Chapter 9). It has been suggested that pain, especially at upper abdominal and thoracic sites, decreases or eliminates the normal sighing (yawning) mechanism. The absence of an appropriate sigh leads to reduced lung volumes and, ultimately, to atelectasis and pneumonia. Appropriate pain relief in these patients reduces the postoperative incidence of atelectasis and pneumonia.[23]

After the assessment has been made and it has been determined that the patient is experiencing acute postoperative pain, certain interventions are suggested. If the patient has received an inhalation anesthetic, such as isoflurane, and demonstrates manifestations of acute pain, relief is instituted early in the postanesthetic period. Similarly, patients undergoing a nitrous oxide–opioid technique are medicated early in the immediate postoperative period, particularly if the intraoperative opioids were of short duration. If medications such as sufentanil and morphine were used intraoperatively, opioids must be administered with caution to avoid respiratory depression as a result of the synergistic action of the intraoperative and postoperative opioid agonists. Because of the synergistic effects of the medications, it may be necessary to decrease the amount of opioids administered during the first 24 hours after administration of anesthesia, but this decision must always be based on the patient's report of pain and clinical status.[10,23-26]

CARDIOVASCULAR FUNCTION

Evaluation of the cardiovascular system involves assessment of the heart, circulating blood, and the arteriovenous system. These three basic components control CO. Because tissue perfusion depends on a satisfactory CO, most of the assessment is aimed at evaluating this component.[27]

In most patients, the nurse uses physical assessment skills to evaluate cardiovascular function. The patient's overall condition is observed, especially skin color and turgor. Peripheral cyanosis, edema, jugular venous distention, shortness of breath, and many other findings may be indicative of cardiovascular problems. All operative sites are checked for blood loss, and the amount of blood lost during surgery and the patient's most recent hemoglobin level are noted.[2,6,19]

The patient's blood pressure must be assessed and correlated to the preoperative assessment, intraoperative course, and anesthetic course. The major component of systolic pressure is stroke volume, and the major component of diastolic pressure is systemic vascular resistance (SVR). Changes in the patient's systolic or diastolic pressure or narrowing of the pulse pressure may indicate cardiovascular comprominse.[19] Peripheral pulses are assessed bilaterally. The rate, character, and any irregularities are documented and reported to the physician if clinically indicated.[19] Electrocardiographic (ECG) monitoring is also essential in the immediate postoperative recovery period. Dysrhythmias of any type may occur at any time and in any patient during the postoperative period.[2,6,19]

Two components of CO are heart rate and stroke volume. If CO is compromised, one of the first compensatory responses is an increase in heart rate, followed by peripheral vasoconstriction. Medications such as beta-blockers and angiotensin-converting enzyme inhibitors, as well as anesthetic agents, can impair the patient's ability to initiate that response. The nurse must be aware of the patient's preoperative medications and the impact they may have in the initial phase of recovery. Hemodynamic monitoring is commonly used with higher-acuity patients in the postanesthesia recovery period. Hemodynamic monitoring is usually accomplished by a pulmonary artery catheter and intraarterial blood pressure monitoring.

CENTRAL NERVOUS SYSTEM FUNCTION

Assessment of the CNS in the immediate postanesthesia period typically involves only gross evaluation of behavior, level of consciousness, intellectual performance, and emotional status. Anesthetic agents are usually reversed before the patient leaves the operating room, and the nurse should anticipate that the patient will be responsive. However, even if anesthesia is not reversed, most patients can respond within 90 minutes from time of admission to the unit. A more detailed assessment of the CNS is necessary for patients who have undergone CNS surgery.[2]

Occasionally, a patient becomes agitated and thrashes about; this behavior is referred to as *emergence delirium*. It occurs more often in adolescents and young adults than in patients of other age groups. Emergence delirium also tends to occur more commonly in patients who have undergone intraabdominal or intrathoracic procedures.[2,28]

THERMAL BALANCE

Measurement of the patient's body temperature in the immediate postanesthesia recovery period is particularly important. Factors influencing the body temperature include type of anesthesia, preoperative medication, age of patient, site and temperature of intravenous fluids, body surface exposure, temperature of irrigation solutions, temperature of the ambient air, and vasoconstriction (from blood loss or anesthetic agents). Hypothermia (temperature <36° C) and hyperthermia (temperature >38° C) are associated with physiologic alterations that may interfere with recovery.[29]

The body maintains its temperature in a narrow range, between 36° C and 38° C. This is accomplished by a balance of heat production and heat loss that is controlled by the thermoregulation mechanisms in the CNS. These mechanisms receive input from various thermoreceptors located in the skin, nose, oral cavity, thoracic viscera, and spinal cord. They then send sensory information in hierarchic order to the spinal cord, the reticular formation, and the primary control center in the hypothalamic region of the brain.[29]

The central temperature controls maintain body temperature through physiologic and behavioral responses. The physiologic thermoregulatory responses consist of sweating, shivering, and alterations in peripheral vasomotor tone. These responses fine-control the regulatory process of body temperature; heat is conserved by vasoconstriction and lost by vasodilation and sweating. The physiologic responses also can lower the metabolic rate to decrease heat production or increase muscle tone and shivering to increase heat production. Behavioral thermoregulation is accomplished by subjective feelings of discomfort or comfort. For example, in a hot environment a person seeks air conditioning, and in a cold environment a person seeks heat. Behavioral thermoregulation is a stronger response mechanism, but it cannot fine-tune body temperature as the physiologic responses can.[29]

FLUID AND ELECTROLYTE BALANCE

Evaluation of a patient's fluid and electrolyte status involves total body assessment. Imbalances readily occur in the postoperative patient because of a number of factors, including restriction of food and fluids preoperatively, fluid loss during surgery, and stress. The normal body response to stress, surgery, trauma, and anesthesia is to release the antidiuretic hormone responsible for the retention of water and sodium. Postanesthesia patients often have abnormal avenues of fluid loss after surgery.

Each patient must be evaluated to determine his or her baseline requirements and the fluid needed to replace abnormal losses. Most patients in the immediate postanesthesia recovery period receive intravenous fluids. It is important to know what fluids, if any, are to follow and whether the infusion is to be discontinued. All intravenous sites are checked regularly for signs of extravasation, phlebitis, and infection.

Oral intake is prohibited after anesthesia until the patient regains laryngeal and pharyngeal reflexes. These reflexes are demonstrated by the patient's ability to gag and swallow effectively. The management of postoperative nausea and vomiting remains critical.

Normal output in the average adult results from urinary output and insensible losses, including evaporation of water from the skin and exhalation during respiration. A lower-than-normal urinary output can be expected in the immediate postanesthesia recovery period as a result of the body's normal reaction to stress. External losses from vomiting, nasogastric tubes, T-tubes, and wound drainage are assessed and monitored. Accurate measurement and recording of all intake and output is vital in the assessment of the patient's fluid and electrolyte status.[30]

In the surgical patient, intravenous access to the circulatory system is necessary for the administration of anesthesia, resuscitation drugs, blood and blood products, and fluid and electrolyte solutions. Postoperative parenteral fluid requirements vary with the patient's preoperative status and with the surgical procedure. Disease processes, tissue injuries, and operative procedures greatly influence the physiology of fluids and electrolytes in the body.

In deciding the type of fluid to use in the postanesthesia recovery period, the clinician can differentiate between crystalloids and colloids, between maintenance and replacement fluids, and among fluids of differing tonicity. Because of the large variety of fluid solutions, some general guidelines are recommended in clinical practice. Crystalloids are typically used as maintenance fluids to compensate for insensible fluid losses and as replacement fluids to correct body fluid deficits (i.e., treatment of specific fluid and electrolyte disturbances). Maintenance fluid requirements are calculated according to body weight and are used to replace insensible losses from the lungs, skin, urine, and feces. Adults typically require 1.5 to 2 mL/kg/hour. When crystalloids are used to replace blood loss, the replacement factor is 5 mL of crystalloid for each 1 mL of blood loss. Isotonic solutions, 0.9% normal saline, or lactated Ringer's solution, are usually administered in the immediate postoperative period. Colloids typically are used for fluid replacement associated with severe hypotension or shock resuscitation. In general, they do not leave the intravascular space and therefore require lower infusion volumes to achieve volume replacement.[30]

The goal of fluid therapy in the immediate postanesthesia recovery period is the restoration of blood volume and tissue perfusion. Recovery after surgery is a dynamic process, and fluid reassessment is conducted periodically. Fluid challenges may be necessary in the hypovolemic patient or in the patient with clinical manifestations of hypoperfusion. The decision of whether to use crystalloids or colloids for fluid resuscitation is complex, controversial, and often determined by physician preference. Either can meet the replacement needs of the patient and achieve the desired outcome when administered appropriately. As with any therapeutic intervention, complications can occur with fluid administration, and the patient should be monitored closely.

Blood and blood components are reserved for specific patient situations. Red blood cells are indicated to increase oxygen-carrying capacity in patients with anemia. Platelets are used to treat bleeding associated with deficiencies in platelet number or function. Fresh-frozen plasma is transfused to increase clotting factor levels in patients with demonstrated deficiencies. A good understanding of the fluid types available, a systematic approach to evaluating fluid depletion, and awareness of the indications for blood component therapy allow the nurse to make appropriate decisions when implementing fluid therapy in the immediate postanesthesia period.[2]

PSYCHOSOCIAL STATUS

Assessment of the patient's psychosocial and emotional well-being is an important component of perianesthesia care. As with any other assessment, this must be made in the context of the whole patient. Almost all patients experience a degree of anxiety about anesthesia and the surgical procedure and a fear of postoperative pain. The physical manifestations include increased heart rate and blood pressure; pale, cool skin; increased respiratory rate; increased muscle tone; restlessness; agitation; and dilated pupils.[31]

OTHER POSTANESTHESIA CARE UNIT NURSING CONSIDERATIONS

In the postanesthesia care unit (PACU), assessment and nursing care are based on the complexity and acuity of the patient's condition.[32] Concerns are growing regarding the use of the PACU as an overflow unit for critically ill patients. Issues surrounding these concerns are competencies of staff; adequacy of equipment, medications, supplies, and technology; and appropriate nurse staffing.[33] Refer to Box 15-5 for guidelines for the overflow of critical care patients into the PACU.[34]

GENERAL COMFORT MANAGEMENT[†]

General comfort and safety measures are important parts of postanesthesia care. For safety, at least two nurses (one of whom is a registered nurse) must always be present whenever patients are recovering. An unconscious patient must never be left alone, and side rails must be raised on the bed whenever direct care is not being provided. The wheels of the bed must be locked to prevent sliding when care is being rendered.

General physical measures such as cleanliness must not be overlooked in the postanesthesia recovery period. Comfort measures are important to the total well-being of postanesthesia patients but are often forgotten in the hustle of caring for them. As soon as the patient is settled into the unit and has been assessed, all excess skin preparations and electrodes are removed; in addition to providing comfort, washing off excess skin preparations gives the nurse an excellent opportunity to further assess the patient's general condition. A back rub at this time may prevent later complaints of discomfort from positioning for long periods in the operating room. This is also a good time to change the patient's position, assist with range-of-motion exercises, and encourage deep breathing. Frequent position changes help prevent atelectasis, promote circulation, and prevent pressure sores from developing on the skin surfaces.

Oral care is comforting to the patient who has had no oral intake and has been medicated with an anticholinergic or glycopyrrolate to reduce secretions. When patients are fully conscious and their laryngeal reflexes have returned, they may rinse their mouth with mouthwash and water. Ice chips and small sips of water or juice may be offered to patients who can tolerate fluids. A non–petroleum-based ointment is applied to the lips after oral care to prevent drying and consequent cracking.

Patients often complain of being cold when returning from the operating suite. This is a result of the effects of anesthesia and premedications and the cool atmosphere of the operating suite. The normothermic patient may shiver or complain of feeling cold, so warm blankets may provide psychological comfort. Blankets of any type must not, however, obscure the intravenous lines, arterial lines, or other monitoring apparatus from the direct view of the attending nurse. The patient's temperature must be monitored closely to avoid overheating.

[†]From: O'Brien D: Patient education and care of the perianesthesia patient. In Drain CB, Odom-Forren, J editors: *Perianesthesia nursing: a critical care approach*, ed 5, Philadelphia, 2008, Saunders.

BOX 15-5   A JOINT POSITION STATEMENT ON ICU OVERFLOW PATIENTS

ISSUE

A phase I postanesthesia care unit (PACU) is a critical care area providing postanesthesia nursing care for patients immediately after operative and invasive procedures, before discharge to the phase II ambulatory setting, the inpatient surgical unit, and the intensive care unit.

Perianesthesia nurses have identified concerns regarding the increasing use of the phase I PACU for the care of surgical and nonsurgical intensive care unit (ICU) patients when ICU beds are not available in the facility.

PURPOSE

As professional societies involved in the provision of care for operative and invasive procedures and critically ill patients, the American Society of PeriAnesthesia Nurses (ASPAN), the American Association of Critical-Care Nurses (AACN), and the American Society of Anesthesiologists (ASA) collaborated to develop criteria for the purposes of maintaining quality care in the PACU, ensuring quality care for the ICU patient, and promoting the safe practice of perianesthesia nursing and critical care nursing.

ASPAN exists to promote quality and cost-effective care for patients, their families, and the community through public and professional education, research, and standards of practice. ASPAN has the responsibility for defining the practice of perianesthesia nursing. An integral part of this responsibility involves identifying the educational requirements and competencies essential to perianesthesia practice and recommending acceptable staffing requirements for the perianesthesia environment.

AACN was established to provide the highest quality resources to maximize nurses' contributions to care for critically ill patients and their families. AACN provides and inspires leadership to develop standards and guidelines that establish work and care environments that are respectful, healing, and humane.

ASA was established to raise and maintain the standard of the medical practice of anesthesiology and improve the care of the patient during anesthesia and recovery, and ASA is involved in the provision of critical care medicine in the ICU.

BACKGROUND

In response to concerns expressed by perianesthesia nurses around the country, the ASPAN Standards and Guidelines Committee conducted a review of current literature and perianesthesia nursing practice to identify issues related to the care of critically ill surgical and nonsurgical patients in phase I PACUs during times when all other ICU beds are full. The review identified the following trends:

1. Staffing requirements identified for phase I PACUs may be exceeded during times when PACUs are being utilized for ICU overflow patients.[1]
2. The phase I PACU nurse may be required to provide care to a surgical or nonsurgical ICU patient despite a lack of proper training and the required valid care competencies.[1]
3. Phase I PACUs may be unable to receive patients normally admitted from the operating room when staff are caring for ICU overflow patients.[1]
4. Because the need to send ICU overflow patients to the phase I PACU does not occur regularly, the PACU and hospital management may not be properly prepared to deal with the admission and discharge of phase I PACU and ICU patients.[1]

STATEMENT

When it is necessary to admit ICU overflow patients or to prolong the stay of the surgical ICU patient in the phase I PACU, ASPAN, AACN, and ASA recommend that the following criteria be met:

1. The primary responsibility for the phase I PACU is to provide the optimal standard of care to the postanesthesia patient and to effectively maintain the flow of the surgery schedule.
2. Appropriate staffing requirements should be met to maintain safe, competent nursing care of the postanesthesia patient and the ICU patient.[2] Staffing criteria for the ICU patient should be consistent with ICU guidelines and based on individual patient acuity and needs.[3]
3. Phase I PACUs are by their nature critical care units, and PACU staff should meet the competencies required for the care of the critically ill patient. These competencies include, but are not limited to, ventilator management, hemodynamic monitoring, and medication administration, as appropriate to the patient population.
4. Management should develop and implement a comprehensive resource utilization plan with ongoing assessment that supports the staffing needs for PACU and ICU patients when the need for overflow admission arises.[3]
5. Management should have a multidisciplinary plan to address appropriate utilization of ICU beds. Admission and discharge criteria should be used to evaluate the necessity for critical care and to determine the priority for admissions.[3]

EXPECTED ACTIONS

ASPAN, AACN, and the ASA committees (Anesthesia Care Team, Critical Care Medicine, and Trauma Medicine) recognize the complexity of caring for patients in a dynamic health care environment where reduced availability of resources and expanding roles for the registered nurse have an impact on patient care. We encourage all members to actively pursue the education and development of competencies required for the care of the critically ill patient in the perianesthesia environment. We also encourage members to actively identify strategies for collaboration and problem solving to address complex staffing issues.

This information and position is to be shared with all individuals, organizations, and institutions involved in the care of the critically ill patient in the perianesthesia environment.

References

1. Johannes MS: A new dimension of the PACU: the dilemma of the ICU overflow patient, *J Post Anesth Nurs* 9:297-300, 1994.
2. American Society of PeriAnesthesia Nurses: *Resource 3: Patient classification/ recommended staffing guidelines in the standards of perianesthesia nursing practice*, Thorofare, NJ, 1998, pp 27-28, ASPAN.
3. Medina J: *Staffing blueprint: constructing your staffing solutions*, Alisa Viejo, CA, 1999, American Association of Critical-Care Nurses.

Information from the American Society of PeriAnesthesia Nurses: American Association of Critical-Care Nurses; American Society of Anesthesiologists: Anesthesia Care Team Committee; Committee on Critical Care Medicine and Trauma Medicine; June 2000.

In addition to the physical comfort measures, psychological comfort should be provided. Reorientation, especially to time and place, is important to the postanesthesia patient, as is constant reassurance that the surgery has been completed and that all went well. The nurse's presence at the bedside or gentle touch may also be comforting to the patient.[22]

MANAGEMENT OF POSTANESTHESIA PROBLEMS AND EMERGENCIES

In the immediate postoperative period, significant physiologic changes occur as the patient emerges from the effects of anesthesia. Factors that influence the development of problems are listed in Box 15-6.[35]

RESPIRATORY PROBLEMS AND EMERGENCIES

Respiratory problems occur with some regularity in the postanesthesia period. All general anesthetic agents and opioid analgesic drugs have respiratory depressant effects. Acute pain also impairs the ability to breathe deeply. Most respiratory problems are related to upper airway obstruction, although other problems can occur, including acute respiratory failure, aspiration, pulmonary edema, and respiratory arrest.[8]

Airway Obstruction. Slack nasal or oropharyngeal muscles, rigid neck muscles, or secretions in the upper respiratory tract can cause obstruction of the airway. Soft tissue obstruction occurs when the pharynx is blocked and air cannot flow in and out. The most common cause of soft tissue obstruction is the tongue. Clinical manifestations of an airway obstruction include snoring, stridor, flaring of the nostrils, retractions at the intercostal spaces and the suprasternal notch, abnormal use of accessory muscles, asynchronous movements of the chest and abdomen, increased pulse rate, decreased oxygen saturation level, and decreased breath sounds.

Management of an airway obstruction begins with immediate recognition. Stimulation may be all that is necessary to relieve the obstruction and obtain a patent airway. With the nonreactive patient, the head tilt–chin lift maneuver or elevation of the mandible at its angles (jaw thrust) can be used to displace the tongue and open the airway. If patency of the airway cannot be achieved

---

> ## BOX 15-6   FACTORS INFLUENCING THE DEVELOPMENT OF POSTOPERATIVE PROBLEMS
>
> - Intraoperative complications
> - Type of anesthetic technique
> - Preoperative condition of patient
> - Length and type of surgery
> - Urgency of surgery
> - Poorly controlled pain
> - Other drugs administered intraoperatively
> - Changes in fluid status and electrolyte balance
> - Alterations in body temperature

---

by either of these methods, an oropharyngeal or nasopharyngeal airway is inserted. A nasopharyngeal airway is usually better tolerated, although it can occasionally cause nasal bleeding. Oropharyngeal airways should be used only for an unconscious patients, because they can cause gagging, vomiting, and laryngospasm in the awake patient. The patient can also be turned on his or her side to a lateral position, which facilitate displacement of the tongue and drainage of secretions. If the obstruction is still unrelieved, positive-pressure mask ventilation, intubation, tracheotomy, or cricothyrotomy may be required.[3,4,35,36]

Laryngeal Edema. Laryngeal edema is defined as swelling of the laryngeal tissue. This edema can cause various degrees of airway obstruction. Manifestations include stridor, retraction, hoarseness, and a crouplike cough. Apprehension and restlessness may be present in the awake patient.

Management consists of placing the patient in the upright position; using cool, humidified oxygen; and administering nebulized racemic epinephrine. If the laryngeal edema is a result of an allergic reaction, the reaction must be managed with epinephrine, bronchodilators, and antihistamines. Reintubation is performed only if the patient's symptoms cannot be controlled by an inhalation treatment within 30 minutes, if hypercarbia persists, or if the patient appears to be in respiratory distress. If reintubation is done, the endotracheal tube must be at least one size smaller than the previous tube used, and an air leak must be present around the cuff.[36,37]

Laryngospasm. Laryngospasm is caused by reflex contractions of the pharyngeal muscles, which results in spasms of the vocal cords and the inability of the patient to take a breath. The spasms may result in partial or complete airway obstruction. Involvement of the intrinsic laryngeal muscles causes a reflex closure of the glottis, which results in an incomplete obstruction. Involvement of the extrinsic muscles causes a reflex closure of the larynx, which results in a complete airway obstruction. Signs and symptoms of laryngospasm include dyspnea, hypoxia, hypoventilation, absence of breath sounds, and hypercarbia. Crowing sounds may be heard if the spasm is incomplete. The chest does not expand normally, and a rocking motion of the chest wall that stimulates abdominal breathing may be present. The patient panics if awake.

Several factors can help identify the patient at risk for a laryngospasm. Preoperatively, risks include a history of asthma, chronic obstructive pulmonary disease (COPD), or smoking. Intraoperatively, risks include the use of an endotracheal tube, anesthetic agents, "light" anesthesia, multiple attempts at intubation, and surgical airway manipulation. After surgery, risks include coughing, "bucking" on the endotracheal tube, repeated suctioning, and excessive secretions in the nasopharyngeal area. Laryngospasm may also be precipitated by irritants and foreign bodies.

Laryngospasm is an emergency that requires an immediate response; otherwise, the patient may rapidly deteriorate. Management is initiated by removing the stimulus, along with any irritants such as secretions, blood, or an artificial airway that is too long. The patient's head must be hyperextended and positive-pressure mask ventilation instituted on 100% oxygen. The anesthesiologist is notified immediately. If complete obstruction is unrelieved by positive-pressure ventilations, a small dose of succinylcholine (10 to 20 mg) may be needed to relax the vocal cords to allow for ventilation. Positive-pressure mask ventilation is continued until full muscle function has resumed. Endotracheal intubation is required if the laryngospasm persists or if refractory hypoxemia develops, even though it may cause further irritation of the airways. Medications that may be used in the treatment of laryngospasm include lidocaine, steroids, and atropine.

After the spasm, the patient continues to receive supplemental oxygen until stable. It is also important at that time for the nurse to reassure the patient that the spasm has resolved. The patient's feelings of being unable to breathe during laryngospasm are intense, and emotional support from the nurse is imperative.[5,37,38]

Bronchospasm. Bronchospasm is a lower airway obstruction that is characterized by spasmodic contractions of the bronchial tubes. Bronchial airway constriction is a result of an increase in smooth muscle tone in the airways, and bronchospasms develop when the smooth muscles constrict and obstruct the airway. Inflammation has also been recognized as a fundamental component of bronchospasms.

Bronchiolar constriction may be centrally generated, as in asthma, or it may be a local response to airway irritation. Manifestations include wheezing; noisy, shallow respirations; chest retractions; and use of accessory muscles. The patient can exhibit shortness of breath, coughing, and a prolonged expiratory phase of respiration. Hypertension and tachycardia may be present. The patient's level of consciousness may range from lethargy to extreme anxiety.

Patients who smoke and those with chronic bronchitis have essentially irritable airways that react to stimulation. A preoperative history of asthma, a recent upper respiratory infection, severe emphysema, pulmonary fibrosis, and radiation pneumonitis are indicators of a greater risk of bronchospasm. Stimuli that may produce a bronchospasm postoperatively include secretions, vomitus, and blood. Patients who have had laryngoscopy, bronchoscopy, or other surgical stimulation are also at increased risk of bronchospasm. Some drugs are also thought to predispose the patient to bronchoconstriction resulting from cholinomimetic stimulation; these drugs include physostigmine, neostigmine, edrophonium, and barbiturates. Other histamine-releasing drugs, such as tubocurarine, morphine, metocurine, and atracurium, may potentially foster bronchospasm.

Bronchospasm is treated initially by removal of any possible irritants or drugs. The first line of therapy consists of inhaled bronchodilators. These inhalants cause fewer cardiovascular side effects than systemically administered drugs. Common inhalant medications used are isoetharine, metaproterenol, albuterol, and beclomethasone. Systemic bronchodilators and antiinflammatory agents may also be required at times. Epinephrine or isoproterenol is occasionally needed as a continuous infusion. Intravenous methylprednisolone manages the inflammatory aspect of bronchospasm. Cholinergics have been given by nebulizer to decrease secretions.[37,38]

Noncardiogenic Pulmonary Edema. Pulmonary edema may be defined simply as increased total lung water. Fluid can accumulate in the interstitial spaces or in the alveoli as the result of cardiogenic or pulmonary capillary processes. Noncardiogenic pulmonary edema in the postanesthesia recovery period can result from pulmonary aspiration, blood transfusion reaction, allergic drug reaction, upper airway obstruction, or sepsis. The most common causative factor seems to be an upper airway obstruction, usually laryngospasm. Often, a short episode of airway obstruction occurred in the operating room. Noncardiogenic pulmonary edema has also been reported after the administration of naloxone to patients who have received general anesthesia. Reversal of the analgesics causes a rise in the level of adrenal catecholamines, which can lead to pulmonary hypertension and probably increased pulmonary vascular permeability.

During laryngospasm, the patient is inhaling against a closed glottis. This generates an increase in negative intrathoracic pressure. A tremendous subatmospheric transpulmonary pressure gradient is created that causes transudation, or leakage of fluid, from the pulmonary capillaries into the interstitium.

Management consists of maintenance of an unobstructed airway and supplemental oxygen to correct hypoxemia. Those patients who cannot maintain adequate oxygenation with a mask may require the use of CPAP or even mechanical ventilation with PEEP. The use of PEEP or CPAP improves hypoxemia by restoring the functional residual capacity. Vigorous pulmonary toilet and the use of hemodynamic monitoring may be required if the patient's blood pressure is labile and fluid balance is difficult to maintain. Morphine can be titrated to relieve anxiety. Corticosteroid therapy can be used to decrease laryngeal edema and stabilize the pulmonary membrane. Noncardiogenic pulmonary edema occurs rapidly and requires early assessment and immediate intervention.[39,40]

Aspiration. Aspiration can be defined as the passage of regurgitated gastric contents or other foreign materials into the trachea and down to the smaller air units. It can occur during the period of reduced protective airway reflexes. The most common and most severe form of aspiration is the aspiration of gastric contents. The gastric acid in gastric contents damages the alveolar and capillary endothelial cells. Fluid rich with protein leaks into the interstitium and alveoli. This results in atelectasis and consolidation. Pulmonary compliance and functional residual capacity are decreased, and airway resistance and intrapulmonary shunting are increased, with hypoxemia resulting.

If aspiration is suspected, management begins with lowering the patient's head, if possible. The patient is positioned to the side or the head is turned to the side to permit gravity to pull secretions from the trachea. Management centers on promoting tissue oxygenation by maintaining arterial oxygenation by means of CPAP and supplemental oxygen. Positive-pressure ventilation by mask can be applied if the patient is awake and can protect his or her airway or by an endotracheal tube if the patient cannot tolerate the mask or requires higher levels of airway pressure.[37,38]

Hypoxemia. Administration of oxygen by facemask or nasal cannula to recovering patients may be needed to prevent hypoxemia in the postoperative patient. Respiratory depressant effects of residual agents may result in a shallow breathing pattern with an increased ratio of dead space to tidal volume. This is even more evident in patients after upper abdominal surgery, and the reduction in the effective ventilation can have serious effects on oxygenation.[35]

The most common cause of hypoxemia is ventilation-perfusion mismatching. Atelectasis often occurs as a result of bronchial obstruction by secretions or blood. Reduction in functional residual capacity (FRC) is caused by the effects of anesthesia and, in the case of upper abdominal surgery, by the surgical procedure. When FRC falls below closing capacity, dependent alveoli occlude, leading to increased mismatching. Impairment of hypoxic pulmonary vasoconstriction by inhalation agents and some vasoactive drugs potentiates this effect.[37]

Hypoventilation. Central respiratory depression is caused by all anesthetic agents. This may lead to significant hypoventilation and hypercarbia. Impaired respiratory muscle function, particularly after upper abdominal surgery, may contribute to the problem of carbon dioxide elimination. Incomplete reversal of neuromuscular blockade must also be considered. Other contributory factors may include tight dressings and body casts, obesity, and gastric dilation. Increased carbon dioxide production may occur as a result of shivering or sepsis. This leads to hypercarbia in patients who are unable to increase ventilation enough to compensate.

Hypercarbia resulting from postoperative hypoventilation may cause hypertension and tachycardia, increasing the risk of myocardial ischemia in susceptible individuals. Hypoventilation, by itself or in combination with the other factors previously discussed, can cause hypoxemia. Very high levels of carbon dioxide may have sedative effects. Evaluation of suspected hypoventilation requires measurement of arterial blood gases.

Careful titration of opioid antagonists, such as naloxone, may be effective in improving ventilation without compromising pain relief. Planning ahead to provide adequate postoperative pain relief is essential for maintaining ventilation, particularly in patients undergoing abdominal or thoracic procedures. Placing obese patients in a head-up position and relieving the effects of tight dressings and casts can also be important. Hypoventilation that cannot be improved sufficiently by noninvasive means requires intubation and mechanical ventilation until the patient can maintain adequate ventilation.[8,38]

CARDIOVASCULAR PROBLEMS AND EMERGENCIES

In the immediate postoperative period, cardiovascular complications causing an alteration in CO can occur. These include anesthetic effects on cardiac function, myocardial dysfunction, dysrhythmias, hypertension, and hypotension. These conditions may occur individually or in combination.[6,37,41]

Effects of Anesthesia on Cardiac Function. In the immediate postoperative period, the residual effects of anesthetic agents and their adjuncts must be considered in the evaluation of a patient who has cardiac dysfunction. Volatile anesthetic agents such as sevoflurane and isoflurane can cause a dose-related reduction in myocardial function. The actions of these agents may be observed for several hours after the conclusion

of surgery.[2,4] Nitrous oxide is an inhalation agent that demonstrates insignificant cardiac depression. However, the combined action of opioids given during emergence from nitrous oxide can result in marked cardiovascular depression.[2]

Therapy directed toward mitigating the myocardial depressant effects of inhalation anesthetic agents primarily focuses on increasing preload. Elevation of the legs and a crystalloid fluid bolus are commonly sufficient treatment, but ephedrine or other positive inotropic agents may be needed.[10]

Individually, most opioids and benzodiazepines only moderately depress cardiac function. Opioids reduce the sympathetic response and enhance vagal and parasympathetic tone. This results in vasodilation and a decrease in SVR. Benzodiazepines also cause vasodilation and a decrease in the SVR. Used in combination, these medications can have a significant effect on the cardiovascular system. Specifically, the overall reaction may include a lowered SVR, heart rate, ventricular contractility, catecholamine level, baroreceptor reflex, CO, and blood pressure. Aggressive administration of crystalloid solutions may be required to counteract these effects. High-dose opioids combined with vecuronium produce a negative inotropic and chronotropic effect. Patients may require short-term vascular support until these medications dissipate.[13,37]

Barbiturates depress the activity of the vasomotor center, causing peripheral vasodilation and hypotension. These actions are dose related and are more marked in the presence of underlying cardiovascular disease. Ketamine has a direct myocardial depressant effect that is usually counterbalanced by its indirect effect on the autonomic nervous system to increase heart rate and blood pressure. In patients who are unable to mount a sympathetic response to stress, ketamine causes a net decrease in CO. Propofol causes a dose-dependent decrease in blood pressure primarily because of a decrease in SVR. This must be considered when caring for patients who are hypovolemic or have minimal cardiac reserves.[38,42]

Local anesthetic agents can cause cardiovascular toxicity if inadvertently injected into the systemic circulation or if an excessive dosage of the agent is used. Decreased myocardial contractility, reduced SVR, and diminished CO have resulted from these agents. Cardiovascular compromise appears to occur in a dose-related fashion. Management of the cardiovascular complications associated with local anesthetic agents includes measures to increase preload, namely elevation of legs and fluid administration. In refractory cases, ephedrine may also be needed.[2,4,37]

Myocardial Dysfunction. During the immediate postoperative period, the causes of myocardial depression include pathologic processes and aberrant physiologic states, in addition to anesthetic side effects. These processes may occur alone or in combination and may be particularly hazardous in the presence of underlying cardiac disease.

Myocardial ischemia results from an imbalance of oxygen supply and demand. Commonly, ischemia results from a decrease in myocardial blood flow caused by atherosclerosis, vasospasm, or hypotension. In the postoperative period, the stress of surgery and the actions of certain anesthetic agents can increase myocardial ischemia.[37,41]

Dysrhythmias. In the immediate postanesthetic period, patients are predisposed to a variety of cardiac dysrhythmias. The most common dysrhythmias are sinus tachycardia, sinus bradycardia, premature ventricular contractions, supraventricular tachydysrhythmias, and ventricular tachycardia. A variety causes can result in dysrhythmias including circulatory instability, preexisting heart disease, an increase in vagal tone, drugs, pain, electrolytic disturbances, and hypoxemia.[18]

Accurate interpretation and identification of the dysrhythmia are essential, because therapeutic intervention is based on diagnosis. Appropriate skin preparation and lead placement are extremely important to ensure a clear, readable tracing that is free from artifact. Additional 12-lead electrocardiographic capabilities should be used if an interpretation cannot be made from tracings obtained with bedside monitoring.

The hemodynamic effects of the dysrhythmia also should be thoroughly assessed. The clinical presentation of the dysrhythmia determines the severity of underlying cardiac disease and the type of treatment. Tachydysrhythmias shorten diastolic filling time and interfere with coronary artery perfusion. These two effects, coupled with an increase in myocardial oxygen consumption, may produce cardiac decompensation. Bradycardia can produce a clinically significant decrease in CO if stroke volume is limited by underlying cardiac disease or if the venous return is reduced. The cause of the rhythm disturbance should be considered.[42]

General anesthesia lowers the dysrhythmia threshold of the myocardium. Inhalation agents sensitize the myocardium to catecholamines and depress sinoatrial (SA) and atrioventricular (AV) nodal function. Junctional rhythms and premature ventricular contractions are the most common dysrhythmias. Ketamine produces sympathetic stimulation, resulting in tachycardia and hypertension. Succinylcholine stimulates the cholinergic receptors, enhancing vagal tone, and it can produce sinus bradycardia or junctional escape rhythms. Opioids may cause bradycardia because of direct stimulation of the vagus nerve.

Endogenous catecholamine levels in postoperative patients are elevated because of the pain and stress of surgery. Increased catecholamine levels increase sinus and AV node rates, as well as atrial and ventricular irritability. The direct result is tachydysrhythmias and atrial or ventricular premature contractions.[37,41,42]

Postoperative Hypertension. Hypertension is not an unusual occurrence in the immediate postoperative period. The diagnosis of hypertension must be considered in the context of an elevated blood pressure in relation to the patient's preoperative and intraoperative blood pressure range. Most commonly, postoperative hypertension is related to fluid overload, heightened sympathetic nervous system activity, or preexisting hypertension. Postoperative hypertension, even as a transient episode, can have significant cardiovascular and intracranial consequences, so aggressive diagnosis and treatment are indicated.

Increased sympathetic tone in the immediate postoperative period may result from the stress of surgery, postoperative pain, anxiety or restlessness during emergence from anesthesia, bladder or bowel distention, or hypothermia. Stimulation of the autonomic nervous system can occur because of hypoxia or hypercarbia. These factors can occur alone or in combination.

Pain is one of the most common sources of increased sympathetic tone. Administering adequate amounts of analgesics, repositioning the patient for comfort, providing reassurance, and limiting environmental stimuli can contribute to alleviating postoperative pain and to lowering blood pressure. Hypothermia and shivering also contribute to postoperative hypertension and are easily treated with warm blankets, active warming devices, and warm intravenous fluids. Bladder distention contributes to postoperative hypertension and must be alleviated. Placement of a urinary catheter may be needed. Hypoxia and hypercarbia must also be treated.

Pharmacologic treatment of postoperative hypertension includes the use of vasodilators, adrenergic inhibitors, and calcium channel blockers. The use of these agents is necessary when hypertension persists despite conservative measures previously mentioned.[8,41]

Postoperative Hypotension. Maintenance of blood pressure depends on adequate preload, myocardial contractility, and afterload. The most common cause of hypotension is intravascular volume depletion caused by inadequate replacement of blood loss, third space fluid loss, insensible loss, and urinary output. Pulmonary embolism may also reduce preload by blocking flow of blood to the left side of the heart. Reduced myocardial contractility may be a result of the effects of anesthetic drugs, myocardial ischemia, or dysrhythmias. Reduced afterload in the form of low SVR may occur as a result of sepsis, hyperthermia, sympathectomy, or large arteriovenous shunts, as seen in chronic liver failure.

Prolonged hypotension can lead to serious ischemic organ damage. Prompt treatment is essential. If the underlying cause is not immediately apparent, the first treatment is an attempt to increase preload by elevating the patient's legs and infusing fluids. Examination of the ECG monitor for dysrhythmias or evidence of ischemia may help guide therapy. The lungs are examined for evidence of pulmonary edema or tension pneumothorax. Vasopressors may be administered to maintain perfusion while additional monitoring modalities are evaluated and established. Insertion of a central venous catheter allows measurement of right ventricular filling pressure and may be used to guide fluid administration in patients with normal myocardial function. In the presence of left ventricular dysfunction or when the cause remains unclear, a pulmonary artery catheter may be inserted to guide therapy through evaluation of left-sided filling pressure, CO, and SVR. The use of additional fluids, inotropic agents, or vasoconstrictor or vasodilator drugs is determined by these measurements.[8,37]

THERMOREGULATORY PROBLEMS AND EMERGENCIES

Patients recovering from anesthesia usually experience some form of thermoregulatory imbalance (i.e., a core body temperature that is outside the normothermic range of 36° C to 38° C). Hypothermia and hyperthermia can occur in the postoperative patient. Management of these alterations is important, because they are associated with other physiologic alterations that may interfere with recovery.

Hypothermia. Hypothermia is a common occurrence intraoperatively and postoperatively, because the conditions associated with surgery and anesthesia typically inhibit the body's heat-generating mechanisms and favor its heat-loss mechanisms.[43] Hypothermia occurs when systemic heat loss lowers core body temperature below 36° C. Causes include wound and skin exposure, respiratory gas exchange, fluid and blood administration, use of mechanical warming or cooling devices, chemical reactions, alterations in body temperature regulation, and disease states. Clinical manifestations of hypothermia include bluish tint to the skin (peripheral cyanosis), shivering and an increase in metabolic rate (early sign), dysrhythmias, and a decrease in metabolic rate (late sign), oxygen consumption, muscle tone, heart rate, and level of consciousness.[29]

Hypothermia has several adverse effects, including discomfort, vasoconstriction, and shivering. It depresses the myocardium and increases susceptibility to ventricular dysrhythmias. Significant hypothermia slows metabolic processes, leading to reduced drug biotransformation and impaired renal transport. This may prolong drug effects and delay emergence.[29,43]

Shivering. Shivering may be a result of the compensatory response to hypothermia or the effects of anesthetic agents, and it can produce an increase in the metabolic rate. Under these conditions, increased oxygen consumption and greater carbon dioxide production can increase the ventilatory requirements. If these requirements are not met, the $PaCO_2$ increases and the PaO_2 can decrease, especially if any significant intrapulmonary shunting coexists. The demand for blood flow by the diaphragm can increase sharply, requiring CO and myocardial workload to increase and causing an increase in myocardial oxygen consumption. This can result in myocardial ischemia, particularly in elderly patients and patients with coronary artery disease.[29,43]

Vasoconstriction, a particularly deleterious consequence of postoperative hypothermia, may be responsible for unexplained hypertension in the postanesthesia period. Because vasoconstriction can increase SVR and myocardial workload, the potential for myocardial ischemia exists. Vasoconstriction can mask hypovolemia, and sudden reductions in blood pressure can occur as the patient warms and vasodilates.[44] Delayed drug clearance as a consequence of hypothermia is particularly significant in elderly patients who may already have impaired drug-clearing mechanisms and a decreased metabolic rate. For example, the maximal rate of renal excretion of a drug can decline by 10% for every 0.6° C drop in body temperature. Elderly hypothermic patients are more likely to have residual paralysis because of muscle relaxants that are difficult to reverse pharmacologically.[45]

Management of the hypothermic patient is directed toward the restoration of normothermia. Rewarming prevents the thermoregulatory responses to cold, such as shivering. Management depends on the degree of temperature loss. If the patient's body temperature is between 36° C and 37° C, the patient can simply be covered with warmed blankets, and heat lamps can be used to keep the patient adequately warm. If the patient's body temperature is less than 36° C, rapid rewarming is required to decrease the possible complications of hypothermia and the postanesthesia recovery time. Convective warming devices provide a safe and effective means of rewarming the patient. In patients with a normal metabolic rate, a setting of "low" or "medium" increases the mean body temperature by about 1° C

per hour. A "high" setting increases the mean body temperature by about 1.5° C per hour.[2,4] Other methods of rewarming are thermal mattresses, fluid and blood warming, and environmental warming. Supplemental oxygen must be administered to meet the increased metabolic demand in shivering patients. Patients who are shivering may respond to a small dose of meperidine (Demerol).[44]

Hyperthermia. By definition, hyperthermia occurs at any core body temperature above normal. Severe, clinically significant hyperthermia results when core temperature exceeds 40° C. Although it is not as common perioperatively as hypothermia, hyperthermia is nevertheless a serious complication of surgery. Postoperative temperature elevations may be caused by accidental overwarming of the patient during surgery, infection, sepsis, or transfusion reactions. Because an elevated temperature increases oxygen demand and, subsequently, the ventilatory and cardiac workload, a hyperthermia patient with poor cardiac reserve suffers serious consequences.[46]

Postoperative fever must be distinguished from other hyperthermic syndromes. A fundamental difference exists between fever and specific hyperthermic states. In non–fever-related hyperthermic states, body temperature rises above normal despite the body's heat-dissipating mechanisms (e.g., vasodilation, sweating). Excessive heat gain from internal or external factors exceeds the body's cooling capabilities, with a consequent rise in body temperature.[2,4]

In contrast, fever results from a resetting to a higher temperature from the normal set point. Until the body reaches its new set point temperature, heat-generating mechanisms (i.e., vasoconstriction and shivering) are activated. After the new set point temperature is reached, there is an equilibrium between heat generation and heat loss. Unlike hyperthermia, with fever there is no physiologic activity to bring body temperature back to normal. Factors that can contribute to raising core body temperature and fever during the perioperative period are listed in Box 15-7.[2,43]

Primary therapy for hyperthermia includes cooling and decreasing thermogenesis. Cooling by evaporative or direct

---

BOX 15-7 FACTORS INFLUENCING TEMPERATURE AND FEVER

CAUSES OF ELEVATED CORE TEMPERATURE
- Blood transfusion
- Drug-induced fever
- Overuse of techniques to prevent hypothermia
- Hypothalamic injury
- Malignant hyperthermia
- Warm environment
- Use of anticholinergics
- Endocrine disorders
- Neurogenic hyperthermia

CAUSES OF POSTOPERATIVE FEVER
- Atelectasis
- Wound infection
- Abscess formation
- Fat emboli after bone trauma
- Drug reactions
- Malignancy
- Silent aspiration
- Dehydration
- Blood transfusion reaction
- Central nervous system damage
- Urinary tract infections
- Phlebitis, deep vein thrombosis
- Pulmonary emboli

external methods has proved effective. This includes ice packs, a cool environment, and cooling blankets. Gastric and bladder lavage have also proved effective. Although physical cooling is an appropriate therapy for other hyperthermias, attempts to cool a febrile patient may be resisted by the thermoregulatory system. Consequently, the first course of action is to restore normothermia with the use of antipyretic drugs. Antipyretics are useful because they have the ability to prevent prostaglandin synthesis in the hypothalamus. Measures to manage the febrile patient include using antipyretics (as indicated), providing a sponge bath with tepid water, keeping the environment cool, using a cooling blanket for sustained fever, and monitoring fluid and electrolyte balance as fluid needs increase during fever. The possibility of malignant hyperthermia (MH) must always be considered.[46]

Malignant Hyperthermia. Malignant hyperthermia is a genetically determined condition. MH is precipitated by certain general inhalation anesthetics, depolarizing skeletal muscle relaxants, local anesthetics, and stress. The incidence of MH ranges from 1 in 15,000 in children to 1 in 50,000 in adults. The onset of MH usually occurs during induction of anesthesia has been reported up to 72 hours after introduction of the triggering agent. Because successful management of MH depends on early assessment and prompt intervention, the nurse must be knowledgeable about the pathophysiology and treatment of this syndrome.[46,47]

Identification before anesthesia of patients who may be susceptible to MH is of major therapeutic importance. Patient history or genealogy going back two generations may be positive. Physical examination may reveal myopathies such as cryptorchidism, pectus carinatum, kyphosis, lordosis, ptosis, or hypoplastic mandible. Electromyographic changes are seen in fewer than half of MH-susceptible patients.[2,4,47]

The most definitive test for detecting MH susceptibility is a biopsy of skeletal muscle. Samples are obtained from the quadriceps muscles and are subjected to isometric contractor testing. The skeletal muscle of the MH-susceptible patient has an increased isometric tension when exposed to caffeine or halothane.[47]

When a susceptible patient is exposed to a triggering agent for MH, such as isoflurane, the clinical features are produced by an excess of calcium ions in the myoplasm. With an elevated calcium ion concentration in the myoplasm, skeletal muscle contraction is intense and prolonged, leading to a hypermetabolic state of acid and heat production. More specifically, heat is produced by the accelerated and continued synthesis and use of adenosine triphosphate (ATP) during glycolysis. The metabolic byproduct of glycolysis, lactic acid, is transported to the liver and then back to the metabolically active muscle, where the cycle repeats. Respiratory acidosis and metabolic acidosis develop because of this hypermetabolic state, and symptoms such as tachycardia, tachypnea, ventricular dysrhythmias, and unstable blood pressure appear. Because of intense vasoconstriction, the skin is mottled and cyanotic.[47] Box 15-8 lists the clinical manifestation of MH.

Elevated body temperature can actually be a late sign of MH. For this reason, the nurse must not prolong the assessment of the patient on the assumption that the patient's temperature must be significantly elevated before intervention is attempted. After the patient's temperature begins to rise, it may increase at a rate of 0.5° C every 15 minutes and may approach levels as high as 46° C.[2]

Muscle rigidity occurs in about 75% of the patients who experience MH. This is especially true in MH-susceptible patients after the administration of succinylcholine. Muscle rigidity may be so severe that the nurse cannot open the patient's mouth to insert an airway. The onset of skeletal muscle rigidity after the administration of succinylcholine could be a sign of impending development of MH.[46,47]

Various environmental and pharmacologic agents can stimulate an acute episode of MH (Box 15-9). Fatigue, emotional

---

BOX 15-8 SIGNS AND SYMPTOMS OF MALIGNANT HYPERTHERMIA

- Hypoxemia
- Metabolic acidosis
- Respiratory acidosis
- Hyperkalemia
- Myoglobinuria
- Elevated creatine phosphokinase
- Tachycardia
- Tachypnea
- Ventricular dysrhythmias
- Cyanosis
- Skin mottling
- Fever—hot, flushed skin
- Rigidity
- Profuse sweating
- Unstable blood pressure

Modified from Drain CB, Odom-Forren J: *Perianesthesia nursing: a critical care approach,* ed 5, Philadelphia, 2008, WB Saunders.

BOX 15-9 ENVIRONMENTAL AND PHARMACOLOGIC TRIGGERS OF MALIGNANT HYPERTHERMIA

ENVIRONMENTAL STIMULI
- Extensive skeletal muscle injury
- Emotional crisis
- Very hot and humid weather
- Strenuous and prolonged exercise

PHARMACOLOGIC AGENTS
- Halothane
- Enflurane
- Isoflurane (?)
- Succinylcholine
- *d*-Tubocurarine
- Gallamine (?)
- Amide local anesthetics—lidocaine, mepivacaine, bupivacaine, etidocaine
- Caffeine

From Drain CB, Odom-Forren J: *Perianesthesia nursing: a critical care approach,* ed 5, Philadelphia, 2008, WB Saunders.

upset, or very hot and humid weather can trigger a waking febrile episode. The anesthetic agents that may trigger MH seem to affect the sarcoplasmic reticulum. Because of their widespread use, volatile anesthetic agents (e.g., isoflurane) and succinylcholine are the most common triggering agents. In MH-susceptible patients and in patients who have had an episode of MH in the operating room, all possible triggering agents must be stringently avoided. As another precaution, because emotional upsets trigger MH, nurses must provide a stress-free environment for the MH-susceptible patient.[46,47]

The cornerstone of successful management of MH is early detection. If the patient develops acute MH, all inhalation anesthetics are stopped, the patient is hyperventilated with 100% oxygen, sodium bicarbonate (1 to 2 mg/kg) is administered, and dantrolene is given. To administer dantrolene, it must be diluted with sterile water. Cooling measures, such as administering cold intravenous fluids, packing the patient in ice, and irrigating body cavities (e.g., stomach, bladder) with cold fluids, are initiated. Accurate intake and output records are essential because large amounts of fluids and diuretics are given. Laboratory tests, such as complete blood cell counts (CBC) and coagulation studies, are closely scrutinized for signs of bleeding or the onset of disseminated intravascular clotting. Ongoing ECG and temperature monitoring are also essential. It is recommended that all emergency drugs be available on a special cart in the operating room or in the PACU.[46,47]

NEUROLOGIC PROBLEMS AND EMERGENCIES

Almost all patients exhibit some level of arousal within 90 minutes after anesthesia is completed. Although many factors are known to prolong anesthetic effects, most reports of delayed arousal and emergence delirium are anecdotal.

Delayed Arousal. Delayed awakening after general anesthesia is a common and often easily explained problem. It can usually be attributed to prolonged action of anesthetic drugs, metabolic causes, or neurologic injury. In most cases, prolonged sedation is the result of residual general anesthetic. Hypoventilation resulting from a high concentration of inhaled anesthetic limits exhalation of the agent and prolongs its retention. Opioids used as adjunct therapy may contribute to hypercarbia and sedation as well. Hypothermia, advanced age, hepatic dysfunction, and renal disease may contribute to prolonged recovery from anesthetics by heightening sensitivity or delaying elimination, or both. The use of premedication may also prolong recovery, especially if opioids or benzodiazepines, particularly lorazepam, are used.[48]

In addition to experiencing a slowing elimination of potent inhalation anesthetic, the hypoventilating patient may develop hypoxia and hypercapnia. The hypercapnia may cause significant narcosis and may potentiate the depressive effects of the anesthetics. In the diabetic patient, the administration of chlorpropamide or excessive insulin preoperatively may cause postoperative hypoglycemia, unconsciousness, or even coma.[49]

Severe electrolyte disturbances are most commonly seen after excessive water absorption during transurethral prostate surgery. The subsequent dilution hyponatremia may manifest as sedation, coma, or hemiparesis. Dilution hyponatremia may also be seen

after the inappropriate release of antidiuretic hormone. Hypocalcemia after parathyroid surgery may result in delayed awakening. High magnesium levels after prolonged administration of magnesium sulfate to the eclamptic or preeclamptic patient may also result in prolonged postoperative sedation and in muscle weakness after cesarean section under general anesthesia.[30]

Neurologic injury and subsequent unconsciousness may be the result of an unsuspected cerebral vascular accident. Intracranial hemorrhage may result from hypertensive responses to anesthetic agents or surgical manipulations, especially in the patient receiving anticoagulant therapy. Paradoxic air emboli may cross a patent foramen ovale in the presence of a right-to-left shunt. Direct emboli from cardiac valves, intracardiac thrombi, and atherosclerotic vessels may also be a threat. Fat emboli can occur after massive long-bone or tissue damage and may not appear until during or after surgical manipulation or reduction of the fracture. Deliberate, induced hypotension in normal patients is not usually associated with neurologic damage. However, uncontrolled intraoperative hypotension may result in ischemia, especially in the patient with hypertension or carotid occlusive disease.[48]

The successful management of delayed arousal depends on careful consideration of the differential diagnosis. A thorough review of the patient's preoperative medical condition and the intraoperative course (surgical and anesthetic) usually points to a cause. If the cause of the sedation is not immediately obvious, the first consideration must be assessing the patient's oxygenation and ensuring adequate gas exchange. Pulse oximetry, end-tidal carbon dioxide measurement, and arterial blood gas analysis can give an estimate of any ventilatory depression and rule out ongoing hypoxia and hypercarbia factors.[48,50]

If the cause is thought to be residual inhalation anesthetic, maintenance of adequate ventilation should be sufficient treatment. If mass spectrophotometry is available, it can provide an estimate of exhaled anesthetic concentrations and confirm the diagnosis. Residual opioids can be reversed by naloxone, and anticholinergic CNS depression can be reversed by physostigmine. The benzodiazepine antagonist flumazenil has been shown to directly antagonize the CNS sedative and amnesic effects of the benzodiazepines.[2]

Body temperature is determined, and warming is instituted if hypothermia exists. Serum electrolytes and magnesium and calcium levels are checked if ion disturbance is suspected. Blood for a serum glucose assay may also be drawn, but the simple fingerstick glucose determination is faster and accurate enough to exclude hypoglycemia from consideration if the result is normal. Other laboratory tests may be useful if hepatic or renal disease is being considered. Unless perioperative events point specifically to it, neurologic injury is usually a diagnosis of exclusion. If other causes of prolonged arousal have been excluded, a thorough neurologic consultation is obtained.[48]

Emergence Delirium. Most patients emerge from general anesthesia in a calm, tranquil manner. Some patients, however, emerge in a state of excitement, a condition characterized by restlessness, disorientation, crying, moaning, or irrational talking. In the extreme form of excitement, which is referred to as *emergence delirium,* the patient screams, shouts, and thrashes about wildly. This condition is seen most frequently after tonsillectomy, thyroid surgery, circumcision, hysterectomy, and perineal and abdominal wall procedures.[37,50]

Hypoxia with resulting air hunger and hypercarbia may appear as restlessness, disorientation, slurred speech, and agitation. Hyponatremia, hypochloremia, and acid-base changes can all be seen during the immediate postoperative period and can be the cause of mental confusion. Pain is a common cause of restlessness and is frequently seen postoperatively. Urinary bladder and gastric distention, which can cause considerable discomfort, are easily overlooked.[37,50]

Drug reactions are commonly implicated as the cause of postoperative agitation. Such reactions are less common than they once were, because the use of offending drugs is less prevalent. The most frequently implicated drugs are the anticholinergics, most notably scopolamine and atropine. They have been shown to have CNS-toxic effects that can include psychotic behavior, delirium, and motor disturbance. Ketamine is also associated with a high incidence of unpleasant agitation. Neuroleptic drugs such as droperidol, especially in high doses, may be associated with development of dyskinesia and involuntary muscle activity and with postoperative confusion.[48]

The patient's state of apprehension or anxiety can have a marked effect on emergence agitation; it is especially notable in apprehensive patients and, conversely, in those who are seemingly unconcerned about forthcoming major surgery. Factors such as fear of disfigurement (e.g., caused by cancer surgery) and feelings of suffocation also increase the likelihood of emergence excitement. Young patients tend to have an increased incidence of postoperative excitation, as do patients undergoing emergency procedures. Several psychiatric factors have been shown to increase the incidence of postoperative delirium, including a history of alcoholism, insomnia, depression, or debility.[37,50]

If emergence delirium occurs, the patient's status is thoroughly evaluated. Management includes determining a cause, initiating specific therapy, and protecting patients from injuring themselves. When the nurse encounters a restless, confused postoperative patient, the first measure is to ensure that the agitation is not the result of hypoxia. Presuming pain to be the cause of agitation in a hypoxic patient and treating the excitement with opioids or sedatives can have disastrous consequences. Hypoxia must be quickly excluded from the differential diagnosis by pulse oximetry or arterial blood gas determination, or both.[2,3,6,49]

Hyponatremia may be suspected in the confused patient after prostate surgery, especially if the surgery was prolonged. A serum electrolyte determination can confirm the diagnosis. The treatment usually consists of fluid restriction and, rarely, hypertonic saline administration. Severe acid-base disturbances can be diagnosed and therapy directed by arterial blood gas determination. If pain appears to be the diagnosis after exclusion of hypoxia, intravenous opioids may be administered in small increments. The CNS effects of the anticholinergics are usually dramatically reversed by the administration of physostigmine. The incidence of hallucinations with ketamine may be decreased by benzodiazepine or droperidol administration. Gastric distention may be relieved by nasogastric aspiration, and urinary bladder distention is easily treated with catheterization.[2,4,6]

When dealing with perioperative anxiety, the best treatment is prevention. Some patients need reassurance that they will not experience intraoperative awareness and will receive pain medication, if needed, on awakening.[6,7,51]

Occasionally, the nurse is faced with a restless postoperative patient who does not seem to be getting relief from opioid administration. Small intravenous doses of a short-acting benzodiazepine such as midazolam may be warranted. The anxiolytics are administered in reduced doses, because their respiratory depressant effects are cumulative with those of existing opioids, sedatives, and residual general anesthetics. If overt psychotic behavior is apparent despite adequate treatment, psychiatric consultation should be obtained.[50]

The patient's respiratory function and airway patency are checked first, because restlessness is a well-known manifestation of hypoxia. Other causes of emergence delirium include a full bladder, cramped or sore muscles and joints from prolonged abnormal positioning on the operating table, pain, incomplete reversal of NMBAs, withdrawal from alcohol and other drugs, acid-base disturbances, and electrolyte abnormalities. The restless patient requires constant, careful observation. Gentle physical restraint may be required to prevent injury. Several nurses or other personnel may be needed. If hypoxia, pain, and a full bladder are ruled out, a change in positioning may have a quieting effect.[2]

NAUSEA AND VOMITING

Nausea and vomiting, although usually not life-threatening, are probably the most unpleasant and lasting memories many patients have of their anesthesia. Although the incidence has decreased in recent years, nausea and vomiting still result in significant postoperative morbidity and patient discomfort. Nausea is described as a subjective, unpleasant mental experience that usually leads to vomiting. Retching is the rhythmic muscular activity that usually precedes vomiting. Vomiting is defined as the forceful expulsion of gastrointestinal contents through the mouth.[52]

Decidedly unpleasant, vomiting can also be dangerous. The physical exertion may increase postoperative bleeding and disrupt delicate suture lines. Tearing or rupture of the esophagus is probably rare but must be a concern in patients with a history of esophageal pathology. Aspiration of emesis is a life-threatening complication in a patient whose airway-protective reflexes are blunted by residual anesthetic or sedative drugs or damaged by surgical activity. If the vomiting is protracted, dangerous hypokalemia, hypochloremia, hyponatremia, and dehydration may develop. Nausea and vomiting are also the leading causes of unexpected hospitalization after surgery.[52,53]

Many medications are associated with nausea and vomiting, but postoperative nausea and vomiting is not isolated to a specific type of anesthetic agent. The use of nitrous oxide is said to cause nausea and vomiting by gastric distention, sympathetic stimulation, and changes in middle ear pressure. Adjunct drugs given preoperatively or in conjunction with the inhalation anesthetic may themselves be suspected of contributing to the high rate of emetic sequelae. The opioids, when given as premedications, may contribute to nausea and vomiting. Some of the newer general anesthetics have resulted in less nausea and vomiting than their predecessors. When administered alone or in conjunction with the opioids, the anticholinergics can act as potent antiemetics.[54]

Muscle relaxants are thought not to influence postoperative vomiting. However, the reversal of muscle relaxants may contribute to postoperative vomiting. Neostigmine has potent muscarinic effects; it may increase intestinal peristalsis and may even trigger spasm.[15,16]

Spinal anesthesia has long been known to trigger a substantial incidence of nausea and vomiting. During spinal anesthesia, a systolic blood pressure lower than 80 mm Hg results in a significant incidence of emesis. The administration of 100% oxygen to these patients has substantially decreased the development of emesis.[55]

Gastric distention and irritation cause nausea and vomiting by direct stimulation of the vomiting center. The stomach may become distended during anesthesia by manual insufflation by mask induction. Swallowing of air or blood may also result in significant stomach irritation. Acute appendicitis or bowel obstruction is notoriously associated with preoperative and postoperative emesis.

The site of the surgery may also influence the development of postoperative nausea and vomiting. Gastrointestinal procedures have a high frequency of postoperative emesis. Laparoscopic, ophthalmic, and otologic procedures have a high incidence. The duration of the procedure may affect the frequency. Pain triggers nausea and vomiting in many patients.[54]

Patients with a history of motion sickness are most likely to experience postoperative emetic sequelae with each subsequent anesthesia. Some patients experience nausea after fasting, even before the administration of any drugs. Many patients develop nausea on their first movement and therefore may have emesis during transport.[22,53] Female gender also has been associated with higher incidence of postoperative emesis. The incidence of nausea and vomiting tends to decrease with advancing age.[54]

Other circumstances may act to increase the likelihood of postoperative emesis in any given patient. Patients with a full stomach from a recent meal or swallowed blood are more likely to vomit on induction of or emergence from anesthesia. Alcohol intoxication or illicit drug use may increase the frequency of emesis. Vigorous nasopharyngeal or oropharyngeal suctioning can elicit a strong gag reflex and trigger vomiting. In neurosurgical patients, especially those with closed head injury, increased intracranial pressure may trigger nausea and vomiting.[56]

The most effective treatment of postoperative nausea and vomiting is prevention. Several maneuvers merit mention as being fairly simple to perform and effective in their usefulness. Avoidance of gastric insufflation is paramount. Swallowing of blood should be prevented during oral, pharyngeal, or nasal surgery. If distention is suspected, it should be decompressed intraoperatively.[2,4,45] A nasogastric tube is placed to empty fluid and gases from the stomach, but its presence may trigger gagging and subsequent vomiting. An oral airway may elicit the same response in a partially conscious patient and is removed at the first signs of gagging to prevent vomiting and subsequent aspiration.[56]

Many drugs have been shown to possess antiemetic qualities, and prophylactic antiemetics and combination medications

have been shown to be effective is decreasing or preventing postoperative nausea and vomiting. Available antiemetics include anticholinergics, phenothiazines, antihistamines, butyrophenones, and antidopaminergics. Complementary therapies, including acupuncture and aromatherapy with peppermint oil, have also been shown to be effective in relieving symptoms.[57]

It is important to remember the supportive care of the nauseated and vomiting patient. If vomiting is severe, electrolyte replacement must be considered. Prolonged vomiting may result in hypovolemia. Intravenous fluids may need to be increased to compensate for fluid losses. Opioids must never be withheld from the nauseated patient complaining of pain, because pain itself may be the cause of the vomiting.[56,58]

Summary

Selection of Anesthesia

- The type of anesthesia used for surgery may be local, regional, or general.
- Local and regional anesthetics eliminate the sensation of pain to a specific part of the body without loss of protective reflexes or consciousness.
- General anesthesia is a controlled state of unconsciousness; the patient is not arousable, there is partial or complete loss of protective reflexes, and the airway needs to be continuously monitored and maintained.

Perianesthesia Assessment and Care

- Caring for the critically ill patient who is emerging from anesthesia requires monitoring of the patient's physical and psychological status to prevent potential complications that may occur as a result of anesthesia or surgical procedures.
- Knowledge of the preoperative history is important in evaluating and managing postoperative care.
- Communication and hand-off among the anesthesia care provider, the operating room nurse, and the registered nurse caring for the patient in the immediate postoperative period is important for continuity and safe patient care.
- The goal of patient management in the immediate postoperative period is recognition and immediate treatment of any problems to eliminate or lessen complications.
- Assessment of the cardiopulmonary system is the immediate priority.
- The stir-up regimen is probably the most important aspect of perianesthesia nursing management and consists of five major activities: deep-breathing exercises, coughing, positioning, mobilization, and pain management.

Management of Postanesthesia Problems and Emergencies

- The most frequent complications include respiratory compromise, hypovolemia, hypothermia, and cardiac dysrhythmias.
- The most common adverse reaction is postoperative nausea and vomiting.

- The most lethal complication is malignant hyperthermia.
- Respiratory issues include upper airway obstruction, laryngeal edema, laryngospasm, bronchospasm, acute respiratory failure, aspiration, pulmonary edema, and respiratory arrest.

- Pain management is a priority; inadequate pain control can interfere with respiratory function and adequate ventilation, affect hemodynamic status, and have a prolonged psychological impact.

Case Study: Patient with Complex Perianesthesia Management

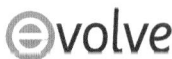 Answers to the Case Study Questions can be found on the Evolve web site at http://evolve.elsevier.com/Urden/.

Brief Patient History

Ms. C is a 60-year-old, bilingual Hispanic woman. She has a history of colon cancer with metastasis, and she has been taking the equivalent of 400 mg of morphine each day for the past 2 weeks in order to effectively manage her pain. Ms. C is a recovering alcoholic and opioid addict but has been "clean" for 6 years. Other significant medical history includes hypertension, which has been controlled for the past 2 years with Lisinopril 10 mg daily. She has undergone a colon resection with general anesthesia (combination of inhalation and intravenous opioid and nonopioid agents), which took several hours to complete. Her vital signs were stable throughout the surgical procedure. Ms. C received a total of 20 mg of morphine during the 4 hours she was in the perianesthesia unit.

Clinical Assessment

Ms. C is admitted to the surgical intensive care unit from the perianesthesia unit because of difficulty in controlling her hypertension. She is somnolent but arousable to painful stimuli; however, she states in Spanish that she is having abdominal pain. Ms. C's skin is warm and dry; her breaths are being taken through her nose, but respirations are slow and shallow.

Diagnostic Procedures

Ms. C's baseline vital signs are: blood pressure (BP), 190/92; heart rate (HR), 120 (sinus tachycardia); respiratory rate (RR), 14; temperature (T), 97.8° F; chest x-ray, right lower lobe atelectasis; hemoglobin, 9; hematocrit, 27; pulse oximetry O_2 saturation, 80% on 100% O_2 via non-rebreather mask; end-tidal CO_2, 70 mm Hg. Ms. C reports that her pain is an 8 out of 10. Riker Sedation-Agitation Scale is 2.

Medical Diagnosis

Ms. C is diagnosed with respiratory depression and hypoxemia secondary to opioid analgesia.

Questions

1. What major outcomes do you expect to achieve for this patient?
2. What problems or risks must be managed to achieve these outcomes?
3. What interventions must be initiated to monitor, prevent, manage, or eliminate the problems and risks identified above?
4. What interventions should be initiated to promote optimal functioning, safety, and well-being of the patient?
5. What possible learning needs would you anticipate for this patient?
6. What cultural and age-related factors might have a bearing on the patient's plan of care?

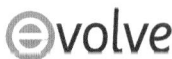 Be sure to check out the bonus material, including free self-assessment exercises, on the Evolve web site at http://evolve.elsevier.com/Urden/.

References

1. Krenzischek DA et al: Patient safety: perianesthesia nursing's essential role in safe practice, *J Perianesth Nurs* 22:385, 2007.
2. Drain CB, Odom-Forren J: *Perianesthesia nursing: a critical care approach*, ed 5, Philadelphia, 2008, Saunders.
3. Barone CP et al: Postanesthetic care in the critical care unit, *Crit Care Nurse* 24(1):38, 2004.
4. Fleisher LA: Risk of anesthesia. In Miller R, ed: *Anesthesia*, ed 6, Philadelphia, 2005, Churchill Livingstone.
5. Wilson M: Giving postanesthesia care in the critical care unit, *Dimen Crit Care Nurs* 19:38, 2000.
6. Wadlund DL: Prevention, recognition, and management of nursing complications in the intraoperative and postoperative surgical patient, *Nurs Clin North Am* 41:151, 2006.
7. Sandlin D: Anesthesia awareness, *J Perianesth Nurs* 21:135, 2006.
8. Geisz-Everson M, Wren KR: Awareness under anesthesia, *J Perianesth Nurs* 22:85, 2007.
9. Leslie K et al: Patients' knowledge of attitudes towards awareness and depth of anaesthesia monitoring, *Anaesth Intensive Care* 31:63, 2003.
10. Goldman L et al: *Cecil's textbook of medicine*, ed 23, St Louis, 2007, Saunders.
11. Hodgson BB, Kizior RJ: *Saunders nursing drug handbook 2008*, ed 15, St Louis, 2008, Saunders.
12. Gahart BL, Nazareno AR: *2005 intravenous medications*, ed 21, St Louis, 2005, Elsevier.
13. Mokhlesi B, Corbridge T: Toxicology in the critically ill patient, *Clin Chest Med* 24:689, 2003.
14. Kirby RR et al: *Clinical anesthesia practice*, ed 2, Philadelphia, 2001, Saunders.
15. Katz RL: Muscle relaxants: clinical considerations, *Semin Anesth* 14:1, 1995.
16. Katz RL: Muscle relaxants: new drugs and special situations, *Semin Anesth* 14:245, 1995.
17. Sloan TB: Anesthetics and the brain, *Anesthesiol Clin North Am* 20:265, 2002.
18. Stoelting RK, Miller RD: *Basics of anesthesia*, ed 5, New York, 2005, Churchill Livingstone.
19. American Society of PeriAnesthesia Nurses et al: *Perianesthesia nursing core curriculum: preoperative, phase I and phase II PACU nursing*, Philadelphia, 2004, Saunders.
20. Schutz, SL: Oxygen saturation monitoring by pulse oximetry. In McHale DJ, Carlson KK: *AACN procedure manual for critical care*, ed 5, Philadelphia, 2005, Saunders.

21. Watson C: Respiratory complications associated with anesthesia, *Anesthesiol Clin North Am* 20:275, 2002.

22. O'Brien D: Patient education and care of the perianesthesia patient. In Drain CB, Odom-Forren, J editors: *Perianesthesia nursing: a critical care approach*, ed 5, Philadelphia, 2008, Saunders.

23. Dunwoody CJ et al: Assessment, physiological monitoring, and consequences of inadequately treated acute pain, *Pain Manage Nurs* 9(1 suppl):S11, 2008.

24. Auburn D et al: Relationships between measurement of pain using visual analog score and morphine requirements during postoperative period, *Anesthesiology* 8:1415, 2003.

25. Golembiewski JA: Morphine and hydromorphone for postoperative analgesia: focus on safety, *J Perianesth Nurs* 18:120, 2003.

26. Polomano, RC et al: Perspective on pain management in the 21st century, *Pain Manage Nurs* 9(1 suppl):S3, 2008.

27. Blank T, Less DL: Cardiac physiology. In Miller R, editor: *Anesthesia*, ed 6, New York, 2004, Churchill Livingstone.

28. Lepousé C et al: Emergence delirium in adults in the post-anaesthesia care unit, *Br J Anaesth* 96:747, 2006.

29. AORN Recommended Practices Committee: Recommended practice for the prevention of unplanned perioperative hypothermia, *AORN J* 85:972, 2007.

30. Kaye AD, Kucere IJ: Intravascular fluid and electrolyte physiology. In Miller R, editor: *Anesthesia*, ed 6, New York, 2005, Churchill-Livingstone.

31. Rosen S et al: Calm or not calm: the question of anxiety in the perianesthesia patient, *J Perianesth Nurs* 23:237, 2008.

32. Kiekkas P et al: Nursing activities and use of time in the postanesthesia care unit, *J Perianesth Nurs* 20:311, 2005.

33. American Association of Critical-Care Nurses: Criteria for overflow patient care in PACUs, *AACN News* 17(8):16, 2000.

34. Mamaril M: The official ASPAN position: ICU overflow patients in the PACU, *J Perianesth Nurs* 16:274, 2001.

35. Litwack K: *Post anesthesia care nursing*, ed 2, St Louis, 1995, Mosby.

36. Wright SM: Assessment and management of the airway. In Drain CB, Odom-Forren J, editors: *Perianesthesia nursing: a critical care approach*, ed 5, Philadelphia, 2008, Saunders.

37. O'Brien D: Postanesthesia care complications. In Drain CB, Odom-Forren J, editors: *Perianesthesia nursing: a critical care approach*, ed 5, Philadelphia, 2008, Saunders.

38. Odom JL: Airway emergencies in the post anesthesia care unit, *Nurs Clin North Am* 28:483, 1993.

39. Ward D: Avoiding ventilatory emergencies, *Semin Anesth* 15(2):183, 1996.

40. van Vugt R et al: Negative pressure pulmonary oedema, *Eur J Anaesthesiol* 24:1057, 2007.

41. Weitz HH: Perioperative cardiac complications, *Med Clin North Am* 85:1151, 2001.

42. Sloan SB, Weitz HH: Postoperative arrhythmias and conduction disorders, *Med Clin North Am* 85:1171, 2001.

43. Kurz A: Thermal care in the perioperative period, *Best Pract Res Clin Anaesthesiol* 22:39, 2008.

44. De Witte J, Sessler DI: Perioperative shivering: physiology and pharmacology, *Anesthesiology* 96:467, 2002.

45. Hildebrand F et al: Pathophysiologic changes and effects of hypothermia on outcome in elective surgery and trauma patients, *Am J Surg* 187:363, 2004.

46. McHenry CR et al: Recognition, management, and prevention of specific operating room catastrophies, *J Am Coll Surg* 198:810, 2004.

47. Hommertzheim R, Steinke EE: Malignant hyperthermia: the perioperative nurse's role, *AORN J* 83:151, 2006.

48. Delinger K: Prolonged emergence and failure to regain consciousness. In Gravenstein N, Kirby R, editors: *Complications in anesthesiology*, ed 2, Philadelphia, 1996, Lippincott.

49. Benumof JL: *Airway management: principles and practice*, St Louis, 1996, Mosby.

50. O'Brien D: Acute postoperative delirium: definitions, incidence, recognition, and interventions, *J Perianesth Nurs* 17:384, 2002.

51. Klock A, Roxzen MF: Anesthesiologist's role as perioperative physician, *Anesth Analg* 83(4):67, 1996.

52. Mazze R, Wharton RS: Fluid and electrolyte problems. In Gravenstein N, Kirby R, editors: *Complications in anesthesiology*, ed 2, Philadelphia, 1996, JB Lippincott.

53. Gan TJ et al: Consensus guidelines for managing postoperative nausea and vomiting, *Anesth Analg* 97:62, 2003.

54. Habib AS, Gan TJ: Evidence-based management of postoperative nausea and vomiting: a review, *Can J Anaesth* 51:326, 2004.

55. Wilhelm SM et al: Prevention of postoperative nausea and vomiting, *Ann Pharmacother* 41:68, 2007.

56. Odom-Forren J et al: Evidence-based interventions for post discharge nausea and vomiting: a review of the literature, *J Perianesth Nurs* 21(6):411, 2006.

57. Mamaril ME et al: Prevention and management of postoperative nausea and vomiting: a look at complementary techniques, *J Perianesth Nurs* 21:404, 2006.

58. Grove TM: Management of problems in the post anesthesia care unit. I. General considerations, pain, neurological problems, nausea, and vomiting, *Curr Rev Post Anesth Care Nurs* 18:1, 1996.

Chapter

16

Cardiovascular Anatomy and Physiology

ANATOMY

Discussion of the anatomy of the heart and blood vessels in this text begins on a macroscopic level with a description of the major structures and then progresses to the cellular and molecular levels for each structure.

MACROSCOPIC STRUCTURE

Structures of the Heart. The heart is situated in the anterior thoracic cavity, just behind the sternum (Fig. 16-1). Several important structures are located behind the heart, including the esophagus, the aorta, the vena cava, and the vertebral column. The position of the heart within the chest cavity is such that the chambers normally described as "right" and "left" are really anterior and posterior.[1,2] The right ventricle constitutes the majority of the anterior surface (closest to the chest wall) and also the inferior surface (directly above the diaphragm). The left ventricle makes up the anterolateral (front and side) and posterior surfaces. The base of the heart is superior (atrial and great vessel level), and the tip (apex) is inferior (ventricular level), above the diaphragm. The base of the heart includes not only the superior portion of the heart itself but also the roots of the aorta, vena cava, and pulmonary vessels.

The increasing use of thoracic computed tomography in critical care has highlighted the anatomic inaccuracy of the terms right and left ventricle, because these terms do not relate to the position of the heart in the chest when described in standard anatomic position (i.e., upright and facing the observer).[1,2] However, there is no impetus to change the traditional nomenclature.

Size and Weight of the Heart. The average human heart is about the size of the clenched fist of that individual. In the adult, this averages 12 cm in length and 8 to 9 cm in breadth at the broadest part. In adult men, the weight of the normal heart averages 310 g, and that of women averages 255 g. There are no significant differences in ventricular wall thickness between men and women. Body weight is a better predictor of healthy heart weight than is body surface area or height. Pathologic conditions such as hypertension increase the weight of the heart muscle because of ventricular hypertrophy.[3]

Layers of the Heart. There are four distinct layers of the heart: the pericardium, the epicardium, the myocardium, and the endocardium.

Pericardium. The heart and the origins of the great vessels are surrounded by a triple-layered sac called the *pericardium.* Ligaments anchor the outer pericardium to the diaphragm and great vessels so that the heart is maintained in a fixed position within the thoracic cavity.[4] The pericardium also provides a physical barrier to infection. The outermost *fiberous pericardium* is a thick envelope that is tough and inelastic.[4] Inside the fibrous layer is an inner, serous sac that can be divided into two layers, known as parietal and visceral. The *parietal pericardium* forms an inner, serous lining that adheres to the tough, outer pericardium.[4] The *visceral pericardium* (also known as the *epicardium*) is flexible, adheres directly to the heart, and folds with the surface contours of the heart.[4] The space between these two layers normally contains a very small amount of pericardial fluid (approximately 20 to 25 mL) that is secreted, reabsorbed, and serves as a lubricant between the layers.[4] The fibrous, outer pericardial sac is noncompliant and unable to adapt to rapid increases in cardiac size or the amount of fluid in the sac.[5] For example, blood can collect in this sac abnormally, as occurs in cardiac tamponade, or serum can collect in it, as in pericardial effusion. If the fluid collection in the sac impinges on ventricular filling, ventricular ejection, or coronary artery perfusion, a clinical emergency may exist that necessitates removal of the excess pericardial fluid to restore normal cardiac function.

Epicardial Fat. In adults, a layer of adipose tissue is typically present beneath the visceral pericardium and may surround the heart. This epicardial fat accumulates along the routes of the major coronary arteries and veins. Autopsy data indicate that epicardial fat increases until age 20 to 40 years, but thereafter, the quantity does not depend on age.[6] Epicardial fat covers 80% of the surface of the heart and constitutes about 20% of the total weight of the heart, with the largest quantity positioned over the right ventricle.[4,6] If a person is overweight or obese with a large quantity of visceral and subcutaneous adipose tissue, there is usually more epicardial fat present.[7] Because obesity is endemic in modern society, epicardial fat is receiving more attention.[6] Epicardial fat is hypothesized to increase the risk of coronary artery disease (CAD), because it contains smaller adipocytes than other fat deposits, has a different fatty acid composition, and has a higher protein content. This composition facilitates the infiltration of free fatty acids and

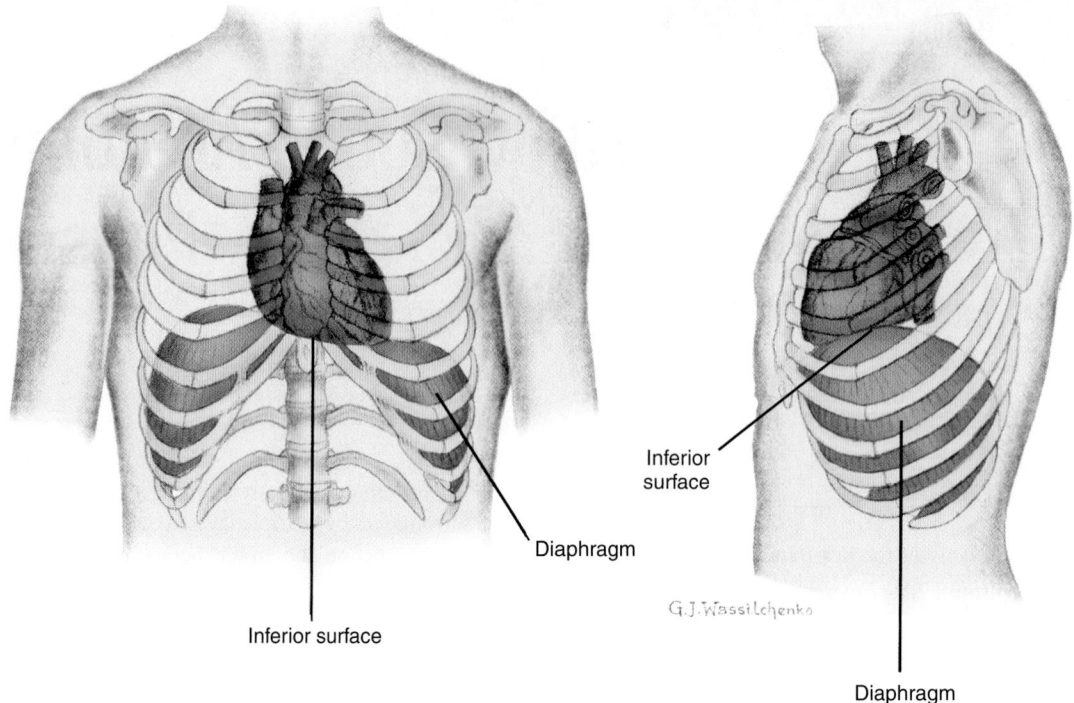

Figure 16-1 Anatomic location of the heart within the thoracic cavity.

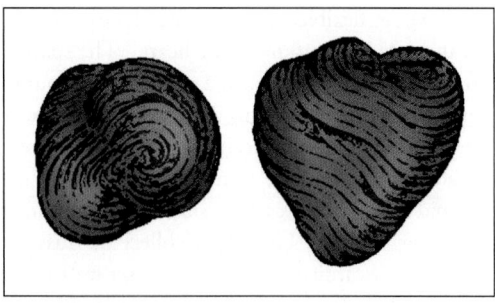

Figure 16-2 Macroscopic structure of the spiral musculature of the ventricular walls.

adipokines into coronary arteries.[6,7] The fibrous, outer pericardium does not contain any fat deposits.[4]

Epicardium. The epicardium is tightly adhered to the heart and base of the great vessels as described earlier. The coronary arteries lie on the top of the visceral epicardium.[8]

Myocardium. The next layer of the heart is the myocardium, a thick, muscular layer. This layer includes all of the atrial and ventricular muscle fibers necessary for contraction. The fibers of the myocardium do not have the same thickness throughout the ventricular walls. The left ventricle is much thicker than the right ventricle or the atria. The fibers are organized so that the force of contraction is most efficient in ejecting blood toward the outflow tracts in a wringing motion from the apex toward the base[9] (Fig. 16-2). The myocardium is the muscle that is damaged by a "heart attack" or transmural myocardial infarction (MI).

Endocardium. The innermost layer is the endocardium, which is a thin layer of endothelium and connective tissue lining the inside of the heart. This layer is continuous with the endothelial of the great vessels to provide a continuous closed system. Disruption in the endothelium as a result of surgery, trauma, or congenital abnormality can predispose the endocardium to infection. This infective endocarditis is a devastating disease that, if left untreated, can lead to massive valve damage or sepsis and death.

Cardiac Chambers. The human heart has four chambers: the left and right atria and the left and right ventricles. The atria are thin-walled and normally low-pressure chambers. They function to receive blood from the vena cava and pulmonary arteries and to pump blood into their respective ventricles. Atrial contraction, also known as atrial kick, contributes approximately 20% of blood flow to ventricular filling; the other 80% occurs passively during diastole. The ventricles are the primary pumping chambers of the heart. The healthy left ventricle is about 10 to 13 mm thick, and the interior chamber appears round in cross section.[10] The healthy right ventricle is approximately 3 mm thick, appears to have a triangular shape when viewed from the side, and has a crescent shape when viewed in cross section[2] (Fig. 16-3). The right ventricle pumps blood into the low-pressured pulmonary circulation, which has a normal mean pressure of approximately 15 mm Hg. The left ventricle must generate tremendous force to eject blood into the aorta (normal mean pressure of approximately 100 mm Hg). Because of left ventricular wall thickness and the large force it must generate, the left ventricle is considered to be the major pump of the heart. When the left ventricular muscle is damaged from cardiomyopathy or infarction, the effective pumping pressure is diminished, leading to increased left atrial pressure, pulmonary vasculature congestion, and ultimately, systemic venous congestion.

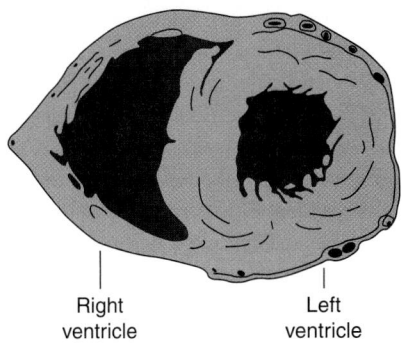

Figure 16-3 A transverse section of the ventricles of the adult heart. The right ventricle forms the greater part of the anterior surface of the heart, and the wall of the left ventricle is three times as thick as the wall of the right ventricle. *(From Quaal S: Comprehensive intraaortic balloon pumping, ed 2, St. Louis, 1993, Mosby.)*

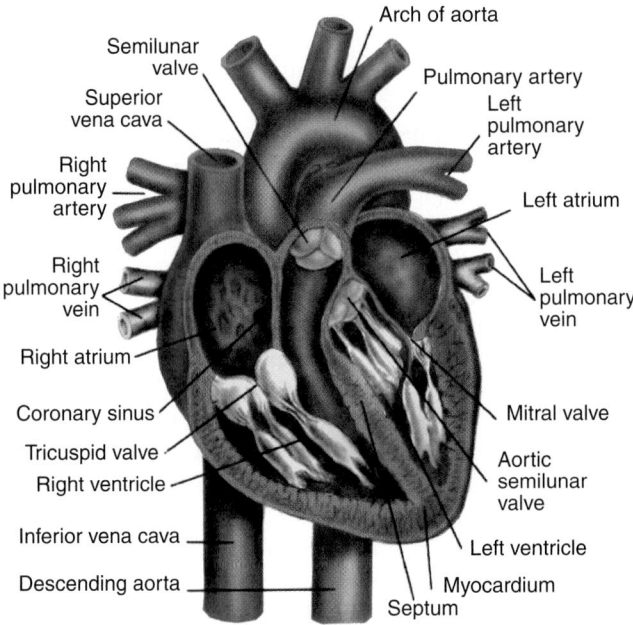

Figure 16-4 Cross-sectional view of the heart. Notice the position of the four cardiac valves. *(From Thompson JM et al: Mosby's clinical nursing, ed 5, St. Louis, 2002, Mosby.)*

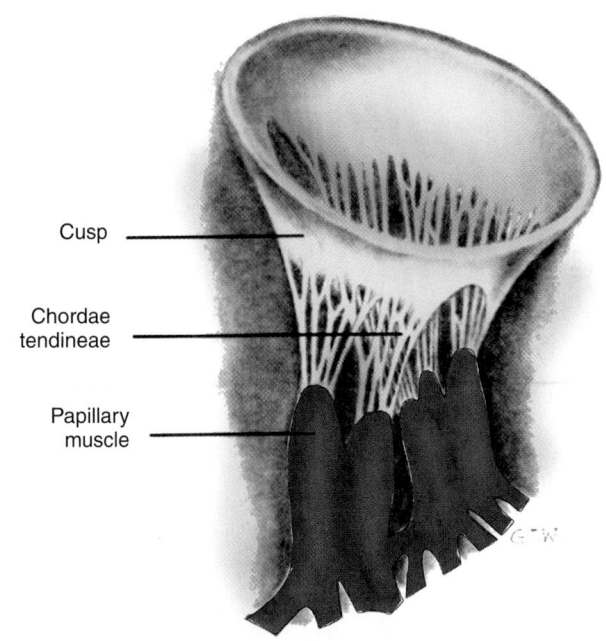

Figure 16-5 The mitral valve and the relationship of the cusps, chordae tendineae, and the papillary muscles.

during ventricular systole (contraction). The *chordae tendineae* and *papillary muscles*, which attach to the tricuspid and mitral valves, give the valves stability and prevents valve leaflet eversion during systole (Fig. 16-5). Papillary muscles arise from the ventricular myocardium and derive their blood supply from the coronary arteries. Each papillary muscle gives rise to approximately 4 to 10 main chordae tendineae, which divide into finer and finer cords as they approach and attach to the valve leaflets.[11] The chordae tendineae are fibrous, avascular structures covered by a thin layer of endocardium. A dysfunction of the chordae tendineae or of a papillary muscle can cause incomplete closure of an AV valve, which results in backflow of blood into the atrium and produces a murmur. For example, after an acute MI, the papillary muscles may be at risk for rupture as a result of inadequate blood supply from the coronary circulation.[12] If a papillary muscle in the left ventricle ruptures, the mitral valve leaflets do not close completely. Clinically, this causes acute mitral regurgitation and an audible murmur that can be auscultated with a stethoscope.

Semilunar Valves. The semilunar valves are the pulmonic and aortic valves. Each valve has three cuplike leaflets (Fig. 16-6). These valves separate the ventricles from their respective outflow arteries (Table 16-1). During ventricular systole (contraction), the semilunar valves open, allowing blood to flow out of the ventricles. As systole ends and the pressure in the outflow arteries exceeds that of the ventricles, the semilunar valves close, preventing blood regurgitation back into the ventricles. In most individuals, the aortic valve has three leaflets. In about 1% of the population, it is bicuspid (a two-leaflet valve), which increases susceptibility to aortic valve failure over time.[13,14] Aortic valve dysfunction, from any cause, not only affects the valve leaflets but also pathologically alters the shape of the left ventricle.

Cardiac Valves. Cardiac valves are composed of flexible, fibrous tissue. A normal valve has the translucent appearance of a rose petal. The valve structure allows blood to flow in only one direction. The opening and closing of the valves depends on the relative pressure gradients on either side of the valve. The four cardiac valves lie in an oblique plane of collagen described as the *fibrous skeleton.* Four adjacent rings of connective tissue contain and support the cardiac valves (Fig. 16-4).

Atrioventricular Valves. The two atrioventricular (AV) valves are named for their location between the atria and the ventricles. These are the tricuspid valve on the right and the mitral valve on the left. The mitral valve is described as having two leaflets, although the "leaflets" are a continuous, noninterrupted structure.[11] The AV valves are open during ventricular diastole (filling) and prevent backflow of blood into the atria

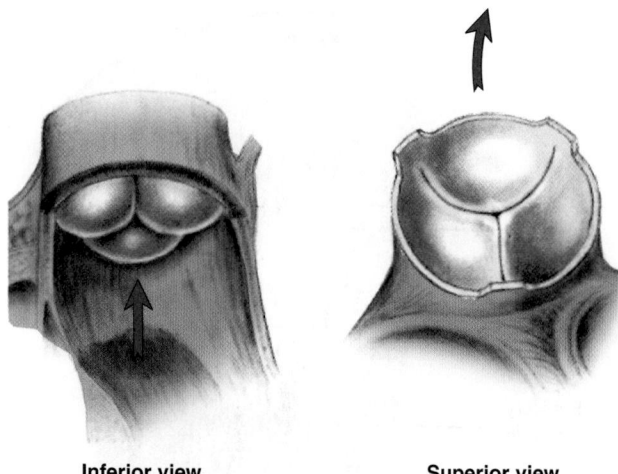

Inferior view   **Superior view**

Figure 16-6 The aortic valve and its cuplike leaflets.

TABLE 16-1 Cardiac Valves and Their Locations

Valve	Type	Situated Between
Tricuspid	Atrioventricular	Right atrium and right ventricle
Pulmonic	Semilunar	Right ventricle and pulmonary artery
Mitral	Atrioventricular	Left atrium and left ventricle
Aortic	Semilunar	Left ventricle and aorta

TABLE 16-2 Intrinsic Pacemaker Rates of Cardiac Conduction Tissue

Location	Rate (beats/min)
Sinoatrial (SA) node	60-100
Atrioventricular (AV) node	40-60
Purkinje fibers	15-40

The Conduction System. To analyze electrical activity within the heart, it is helpful to understand the three main areas of impulse propagation and conduction: the sinoatrial (SA) node, the AV node, and the conduction fibers within the ventricle, specifically the bundle of His, the bundle branches, and the Purkinje fibers.

The Sinoatrial Node. The SA node is considered the natural pacemaker of the heart because it has the highest degree of automaticity, producing the fastest intrinsic heart rate (Table 16-2). The node is a spindle-shaped structure located near the entrance of the superior vena cava, on the posterior aspect of the right atrium. Some normal variability in the position and shape of the node exists. The SA node is supplied from the right coronary system in 66% of people and from the left coronary system in 34%.[15] The SA node contains two types of cells, the specialized pacemaker cells found in the node center and the border zone cells. Both cell types have inherent pacemaker

properties (they automatically depolarize 60 to 100 times per minute). The cells in the nodal center are responsible for the pace-making of the heart, whereas the intrinsic depolarization capability of the fibers in the border zone is depressed by surrounding atrial tissue.

Once the center nodal cells depolarize, the impulse is conducted through the nodal border zone toward the atrium. Atrial depolarization occurs cell to cell and through three specialized conduction pathways that exit the SA node (Fig. 16-7A). These *internodal pathways* are directed to the AV node.[16,17] An intraatrial conduction pathway, known as *Bachmann's bundle,* travels from the right to the left atrium.[18,19]

The Atrioventricular Node. The AV node is located posteriorly on the right side of the interatrial septum, on the floor of the right atrium. The AV node receives its blood supply from the first posterior septal branch of the right (90%) or left (10%) coronary artery.[20] Because the atria and ventricles are separated by nonconductive tissue, electrical impulses initiated in the atria are conducted to the ventricles only via the AV node.[21,22] The AV node performs four essential functions to support cardiac conduction:

1. The AV node delays the conduction impulse from the atria (0.8 to 1.2 seconds) to provide time for the ventricles to fill during diastole.
2. The AV node controls the number of impulses that are transmitted from the atria to the ventricles. This prevents rapid irregular atrial heart rhythms from destabilizing the ventricular rhythm.
3. The AV node acts as a backup pacemaker if the faster SA node fails. Normally, the intrinsic AV nodal rate is slower than the SA nodal rate (see Table 16-2). When an impulse from the SA node arrives at the AV node, the AV nodal tissue becomes depolarized and the AV nodal pacemaker timing is reset (see Fig. 16-7B). This prevents the AV node from initiating its own pacemaker impulse that would compete with the SA node.
4. The AV node can conduct retrograde (backward) impulses through the node. If the SA and AV pacemaker cells fail to fire, an electrical impulse may be initiated in the ventricles and conducted backward via the AV node. Retrograde conduction time is usually longer than antegrade (forward) conduction.

Bundle of His, Bundle Branches, and Purkinje Fibers. Electrical impulses are conducted in the ventricles through the bundle of His, the bundle branches, and the Purkinje fibers (see Fig. 16-7C). These structures run through the subendocardium, down the right side of the interventricular septum. About 12 mm from the AV node, the bundle of His divides into the right and left bundle branches. The right bundle branch continues down the right side of the interventricular septum toward the right apex. The left bundle branch is thicker than the right and takes off from the bundle of His at almost a right angle. It traverses the septum to the subendocardial surface of the left interventricular wall, where it divides into a thin, anterior branch and a thick, posterior branch. Functionally, when one of the left branches is blocked, it is referred to as a *hemiblock.* All of the bundle branches are subject to conduction defects

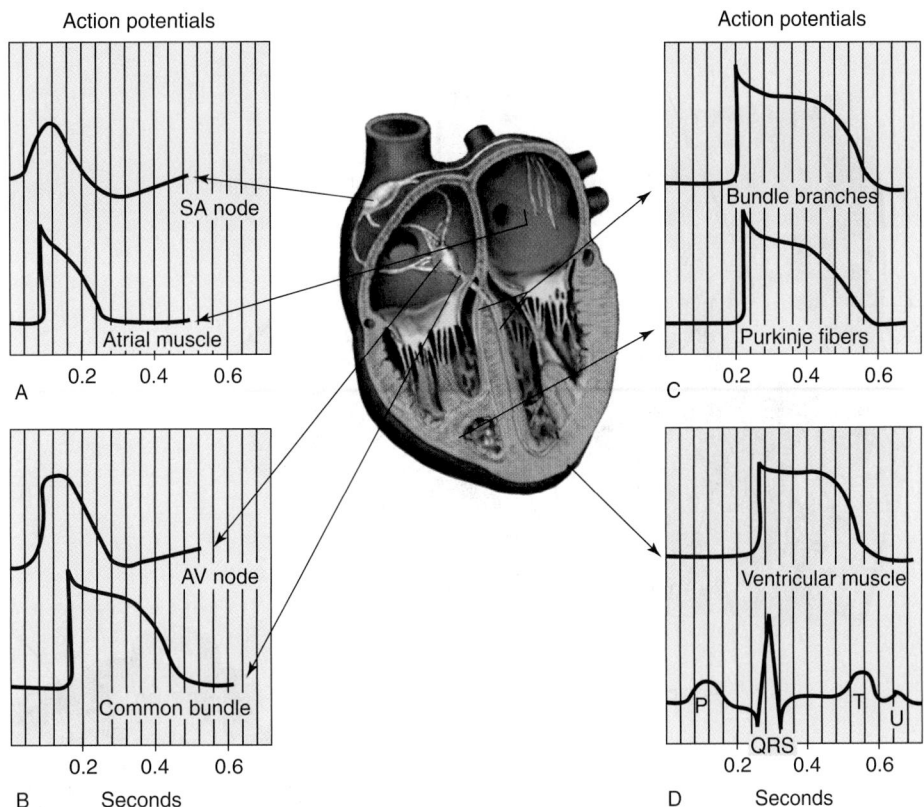

Figure 16-7 Heart with normal conduction pathways and transmembrane action potentials of sinoatrial (SA) node and atrial muscle *(A)*; atrioventricular (AV) node and common bundle *(B)*; bundle branches *(C)*; and ventricular muscle *(D)*. *(From Thompson JM et al: Mosby's clinical nursing, ed 5, St. Louis, 2002, Mosby.)*

(bundle branch blocks) that give rise to characteristic changes in the 12-lead electrocardiogram (ECG).

The right bundle branch and the two divisions of the left bundle branch eventually divide into the Purkinje fibers. These divide many times, terminating in the subendocardial surface of both ventricles. The Purkinje fibers have the fastest conduction velocity of all heart tissue. Ventricular muscle depolarization follows (see Fig. 16-7D).

Coronary Blood Supply. The coronary circulation consists of those vessels that supply the heart structures with oxygenated blood (coronary arteries) and then return the blood to the general circulation (coronary veins). The right and left coronary arteries arise at the base of the aorta, immediately above the aortic valve (Fig. 16-8). They then traverse the outside of the heart, above the epicardium, in the natural grooves (sulci) between the chambers. To perfuse the thick heart muscle, branches from these main arteries arise at acute angles, penetrating the muscular wall and eventually feeding the endocardium (Fig. 16-9).

The right coronary artery (RCA) serves the right atrium and the right ventricle in most people. In more than half of the population (66%), the sinus node artery, which supplies the SA node, arises from the RCA.[15] The AV node is supplied via the RCA in most of the population. The term *dominant coronary artery* is used to describe the artery that supplies the posterior part of heart. In 70% of the population, the RCA is dominant, supplying the posterior cardiac wall.

The left coronary artery is a short but important artery that divides into two large arteries, the left anterior descending

(LAD) and the circumflex (Cx). These vessels serve the left atrium and most of the left ventricle (Fig. 16-10). The SA node is supplied from the left coronary arterial system in 34% of people.[15]

The coronary arteries are end-arteries, meaning that they supply a discrete area of myocardium and have limited collateral circulation. End-arteries are also susceptible to obstruction by atherosclerotic plaque or thrombus that can result in loss of blood flow to the myocardial muscle normally supplied by that artery. This can be fatal, depending on the location of the obstruction. Blockage of coronary arterial blood flow, especially in the left main coronary artery, usually results in death from massive infarction of the left ventricle. If the blocked artery supplies a smaller section of myocardium, the result may be an MI but not death.

Several clinical situations merit a brief discussion here. During ventricular contraction, no blood flows to the cardiac tissues because of the contracted state of the cardiac muscle and resulting occlusion of arteries within the musculature. Coronary artery circulation is highest during early diastole, after the aortic valve has closed. During an episode of tachycardia, diastolic time is greatly diminished; hence coronary perfusion time is lessened. This offers an explanation for compromised coronary blood flow and fall in blood pressure during times of rapid heart rate.

Coronary Veins. The cardiac (coronary) veins, carrying deoxygenated blood are adjacent to the paths of the coronary arteries with one significant difference. The coronary veins ultimately join together to become the *coronary sinus* (the largest

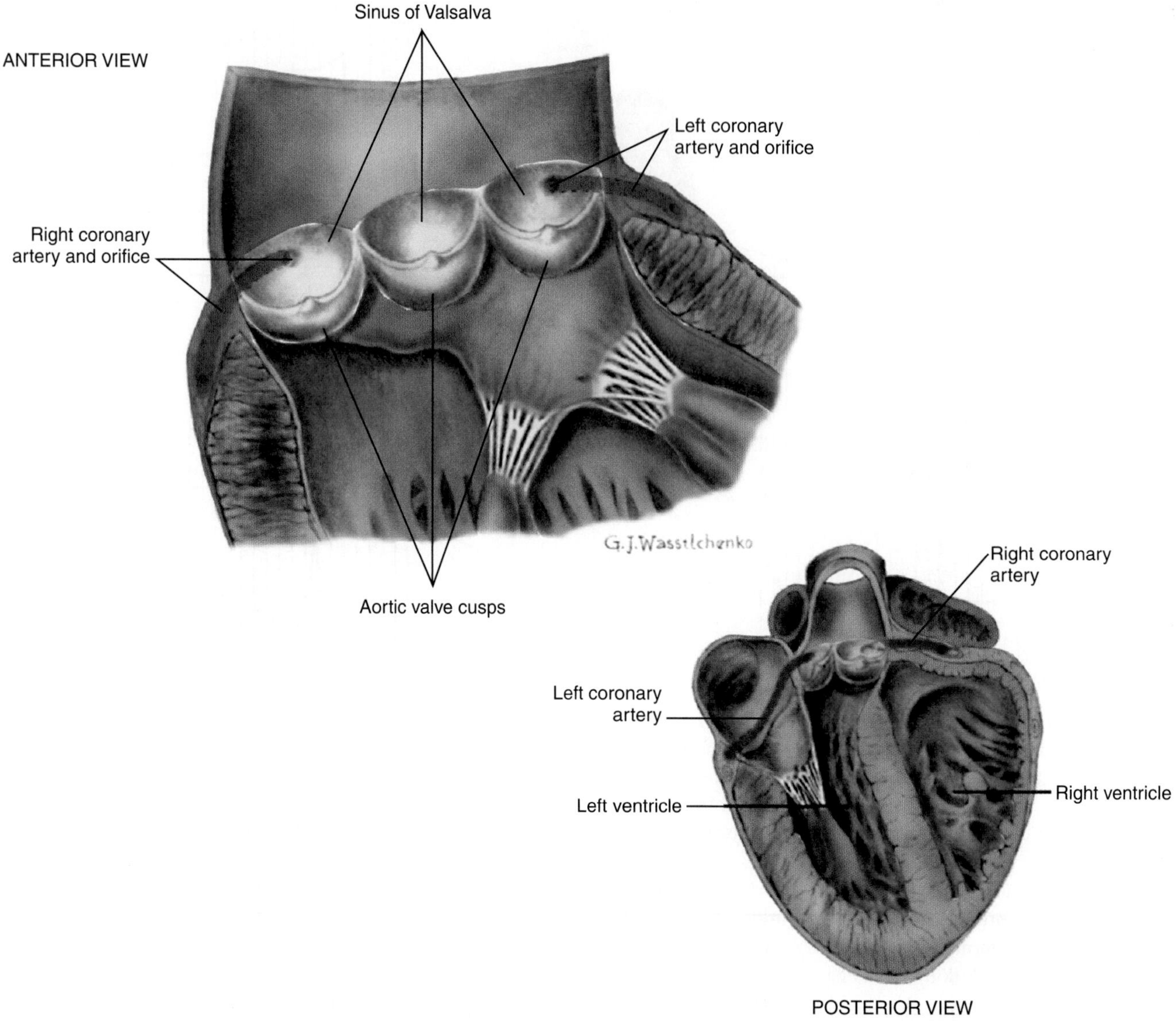

ANTERIOR VIEW

Sinus of Valsalva

Left coronary
artery and orifice

Right coronary
artery and orifice

Aortic valve cusps

G.J.Wasstlchenko

Right coronary
artery

Left coronary
artery

Left ventricle

Right ventricle

POSTERIOR VIEW

Figure 16-8 Proximity of the right and left coronary arteries to the aortic valve and the sinus of Valsalva.

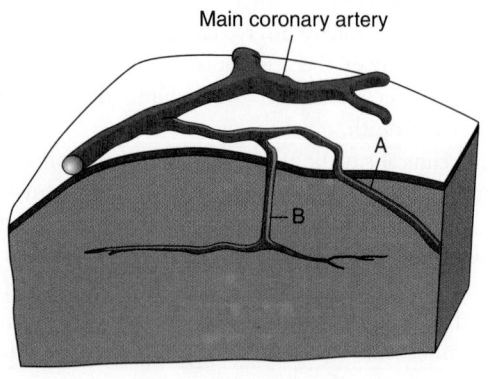

Main coronary artery

Figure 16-9 Intramyocardial distribution of coronary arteries. *A,* Epicardial arteries rise at acute angles from main coronary vessels to supply the epicardial surface of the heart. *B,* Smaller vessels branch at oblique angles from main coronary vessels that penetrate deeper into the myocardium and endocardium (intramural arteries). *(Redrawn from Quaal S: Comprehensive intraaortic balloon pumping, ed 2, St. Louis, 1993, Mosby.)*

cardiac vein), which primarily empties into the back of the right atrium. The coronary venous blood then mixes with the systemic venous blood in the right atrium.[23]

Physiologic Cardiac Shunts. A shunt occurs when there is mixing of deoxygenated blood (usually venous blood with reduced oxygen content) with arterial oxygenated blood. In the heart, there is a specific situation in which this is a normal physiologic process. The *thebesian veins* are small vessels that connect capillary beds directly with the cardiac chambers via irregular endothelium-lined sinuses within the myocardium. The thebesian veins add a small quantity of deoxygenated blood to the oxygenated blood in the left ventricle.

An example of an abnormal, or pathologic, intracardiac shunt is an opening in the ventricular septum, between the left and right sides of the heart. In the ventricle this septal opening, called a *ventricular septal defect* (VSD), allows mixing of blood from both ventricles. The clinical impact depends on the size of the intracardiac shunt. A VSD is a congenital opening

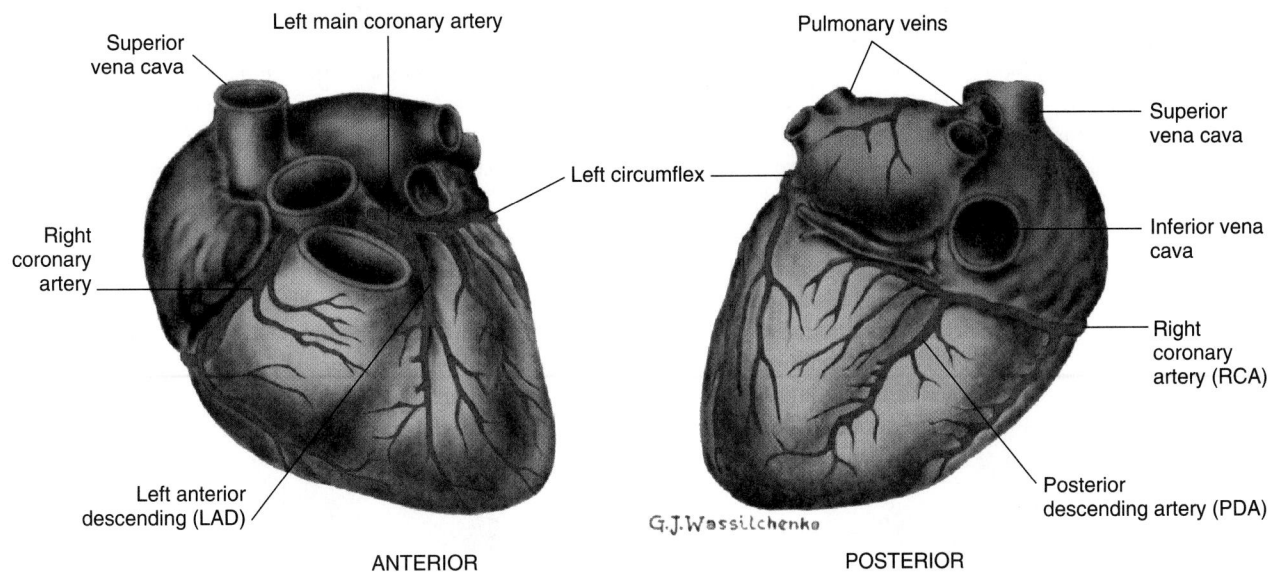

Figure 16-10 Anterior and posterior views of the coronary artery circulation and major vessels.

between the ventricles; a ventricular septal rupture (VSR) can occur as a complication of a large anterior-wall MI, as described in Chapter 19.

MAJOR CARDIAC VESSELS

Aorta. The aorta is the largest artery in the body. It carries oxygenated blood from the left ventricle to the rest of the body. The aorta is separated from the left ventricle by the aortic valve. Just above the aortic valve are two small openings that represent the origins of the right and left coronary arterial systems (see Fig. 16-8). These opening are known by several names, including the *coronary ostia* and the *sinus of Valsalva.*

Pulmonary Artery. The pulmonary artery carries deoxygenated blood from the right ventricle to the pulmonary arterioles. The pulmonary artery is separated from the right ventricle by the pulmonic valve. The main pulmonary artery divides into a right and a left branch, directing blood to the right and the left lung vasculature. The pulmonary artery is the only artery in the body that carries deoxygenated blood.

Pulmonary Veins. The four pulmonary veins return oxygenated blood from the lungs to the left atrium. These are the only veins in the body that carry oxygenated blood. The veins drain into the back wall of the left atrium (see Fig. 16-10). There are no valves to inhibit the flow of blood into the left atrium. Blood flow is accomplished by simple hydrostatic pressure gradients. The pressure must be lower in the left atrium than in the pulmonary circulation for flow to occur in a forward direction. Tissue from the left atrium may grow into the pulmonary vein orifices. This opportunistic tissue is a frequent cause of atrial fibrillation.[24]

The Systemic Circulation. If the task of the heart is to generate enough pressure to pump the blood, it is the function of the vascular structures to act as conduits to carry vital oxygen and nutrients to each cell and also to carry away waste products. The ability to exchange those nutrients and waste products at

the cellular level is of primary importance. The vascular system acts not only as a conducting system for the blood but also as a control mechanism for the pressure in the heart and vessels. It is the complex interplay between heart and blood vessels that maintains adequate pressure and velocity within this system for optimal functioning.

The Arterial System. Arteries are constructed of three layers (Fig. 16-11). The *adventitia,* the outermost layer, is composed largely of a connective tissue coat to provide strength and shape to the vessel. The *media,* or muscular middle layer, is made up of smooth muscle and elastic tissue. The muscular layer changes the lumen diameter when necessary. The innermost layer, or *intima,* consists of a thin lining of endothelium and a small amount of elastic tissue. The smooth endothelial lining decreases resistance to blood flow and minimizes opportunity for platelet aggregation.

The intimal and the adventitial layers remain relatively constant in the vascular system, whereas the elastin and smooth muscle in the media vary in proportion, depending on the size and type of the vessel. The aorta contains the greatest amount of elastic tissue. This is necessary because of the sudden shifts in pressure created by the left ventricle. The arterioles, or smaller arteries, and precapillary sphincters have more smooth muscle than do the larger arteries and aorta, because they function to change the luminal diameter when regulating blood pressure and blood flow to the tissues (Fig. 16-12).

Blood Flow and Blood Pressure. The pulsatile nature of arterial flow is caused by intermittent cardiac ejection and the stretch of the ascending aorta. The pressure wave initiated by left ventricular ejection (Fig. 16-13) travels considerably faster than does the blood itself. When an examiner palpates a pulse, it is the propagation of the pressure wave that is perceived.

In the normal arterial system, the blood flow is described as laminar, or streamlined, because the fluid moves in one direction. However, there are differences in the linear velocities within a blood vessel. The layer of blood immediately adjacent to the vessel wall moves relatively slowly because of the friction created as it comes in contact with the motionless vessel wall. In contrast, the more central blood in the lumen travels more rapidly (Fig. 16-14).

Clinical implications include conditions in which the vessel wall has an abnormality such as a small clot or plaque deposit. This disruption in the streamlined flow can set up eddy currents that may predispose the area to platelet aggregation and atherosclerosis.

Blood pressure measurement has several components. The *systolic blood pressure* (SBP) represents the ventricular volume ejection and the response of the arterial system to that ejection. The *diastolic blood pressure* (DBP) value indicates the ventricular resting state of the arterial system. The *pulse pressure* is the difference between the SBP and the DBP. The *mean arterial pressure* (MAP) is the mean value of the area under the blood pressure curve (Fig. 16-15). Blood pressure may be measured several ways. Direct measurement is accomplished by means

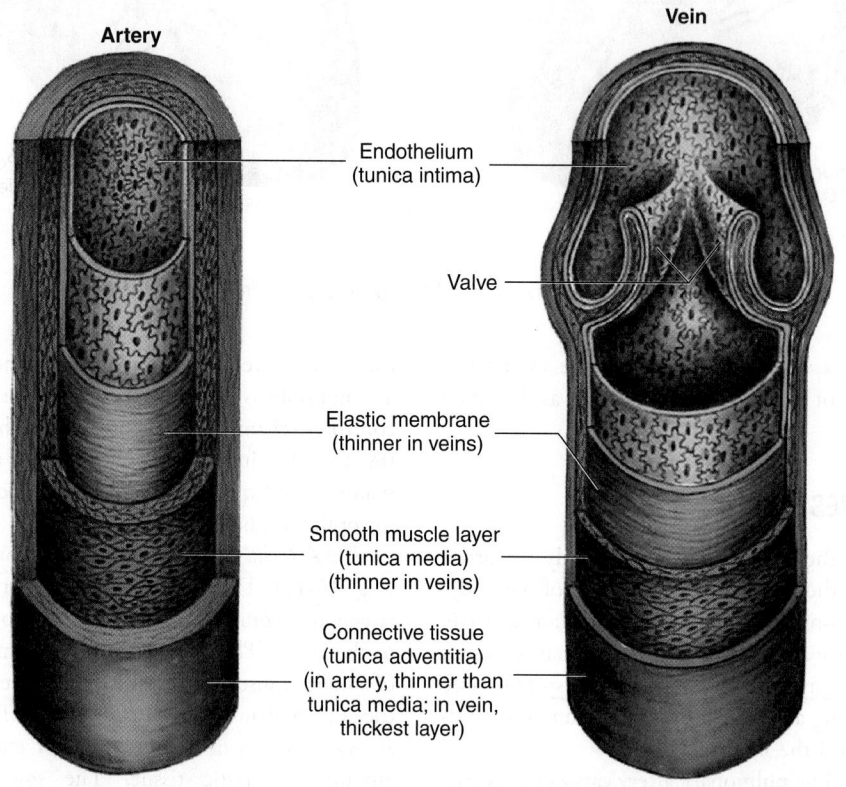

Figure 16-11 Cross section of an artery and vein showing the three layers: tunica intima, tunica media, and tunica adventitia. Notice the difference in wall thickness between the artery and the vein and the lack of valves within the artery. *(From Thompson JM et al: Mosby's clinical nursing, ed 5, St. Louis, 2002, Mosby.)*

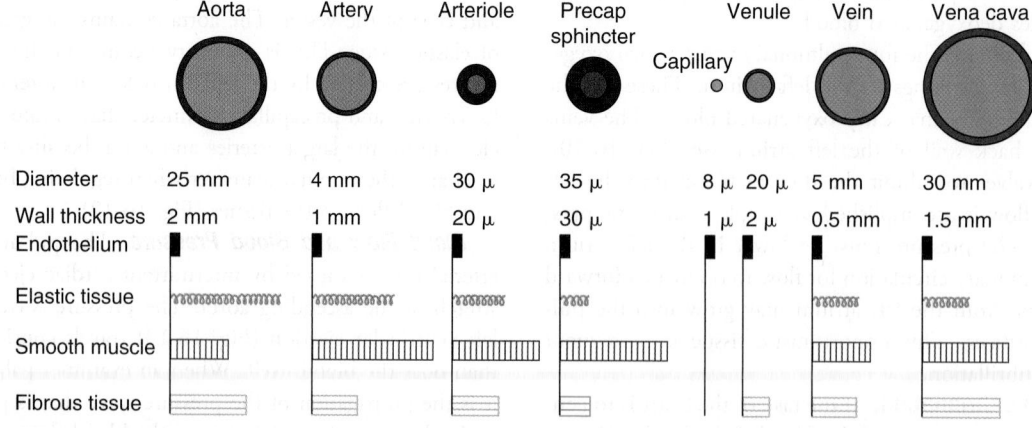

Figure 16-12 Internal diameter, wall thickness, and relative amounts of the principal components of the vessel circulatory system. Cross sections of the vessels are not drawn to scale because of the huge range from aorta to vena cava to capillaries. *(From Berne RM, Levy MN: Cardiovascular physiology, ed 8, St. Louis, 2001, Mosby.)*

of a catheter inserted into an artery. The blood pressure is measured in millimeters of mercury (mm Hg). The most common indirect method is by means of a stethoscope and sphygmomanometer (Fig. 16-16). Figure 16-17 graphically summarizes blood pressures in various portions of the systemic circulatory system.

Vascular resistance is a reflection of arteriolar tone. The large amount of smooth muscle in the arterioles allows for relaxation or contraction of these vessels, which causes changes in the resistance and redistribution of blood flow. Resistance is the opposition to flow caused by the blood vessels. Most changes in resistance are caused by alterations in the tone of the arterial vessel walls, especially in the arterioles. The purpose of this mechanism is to maintain a constant blood pressure in the arterial system. The clinician can never assume that blood flow and blood pressure are identical. For example, poor blood flow to the tissues because of vasoconstricted peripheral arterioles causes the blood to back up and increases the blood pressure. A higher

blood pressure is a compensatory mechanism but does not necessarily mean that there is adequate tissue perfusion.

It is also possible to calculate the resistance within the systemic vascular system, described by the phrase *systemic vascular resistance* (SVR). In the pulmonary circulation, it is termed *pulmonary vascular resistance* (PVR). These derived values are based on calculations from other hemodynamic parameters, as described in Chapters 18 and Appendix B.

The Microcirculation. The *microcirculation* consists of arterioles, arterial capillaries, venous capillaries, and venules (Fig. 16-18). Oxygen, nutrients, hormones, and waste products are exchanged between the bloodstream and adjacent cells. The microcirculation has a vital role in the regulation of oxygen supply and demand at the tissue level.[25] The density and anatomy of the microcirculation vary and depend on the metabolic needs of each tissue or organ.[25]

Precapillary sphincters are small cuffs of smooth muscle that control blood flow at the junction of the arterioles and the capillaries. The precapillary sphincters allow selective blood flow into capillary beds, depending on their contractile state, and are innervated by the sympathetic nervous system (SNS) and epinephrine released by the adrenal glands.

As the blood reaches the capillary level, the pulsatile nature of arterial flow is dampened (see Fig. 16-17). Even though the diameter of a capillary is less than that of an arteriole, the pressure and flow velocity in the capillary bed is low as a result of the large cross-sectional area of the branching capillary bed (see Fig. 16-18). The capillary consists of a single cell layer of endothelium and is devoid of muscle or elastin (see Fig. 16-12). This arrangement allows solutes to diffuse in and out of the capillaries unimpeded by mechanical barriers. Capillaries normally retain large structures, such as red blood cells, but are highly permeable to smaller solutes, such as electrolytes.

The Venous System. As the blood leaves the capillary system, it passes through the venules and into the veins. Venules and veins contain elastic tissue, smooth muscle, and fibrous tissue (see Fig. 16-12). The veins, however, contain a greater percentage of smooth muscle and fibrous tissue, to accommodate the large venous volume and demand for reserve capacity. The majority of circulating blood is contained in the venous system. Veins are referred to as *capacitance vessels* (Fig. 16-19). Approximately 75% of the total blood volume is found in the veins.[26] This enables the body to tap into a large reserve during times of need. For example, when a person changes from a supine to a

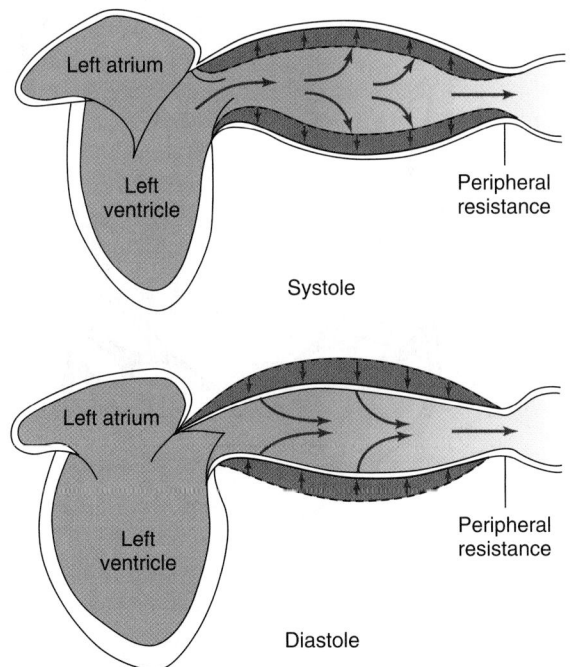

Figure 16-13 Elastic and recoil properties of the aorta. *(From Berne RM, Levy MN: Cardiovascular physiology, ed 8, St. Louis, 2001, Mosby.)*

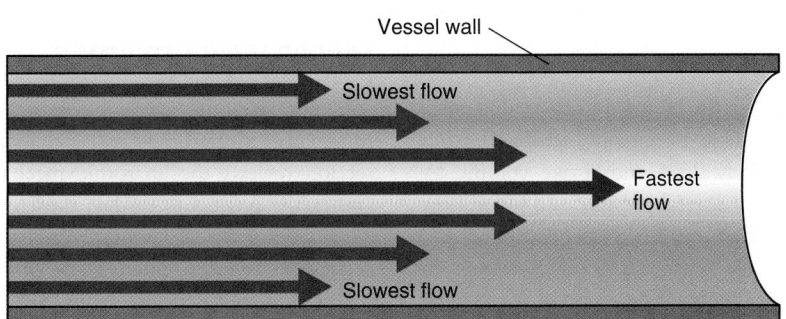

Figure 16-14 Laminar flow in an artery.

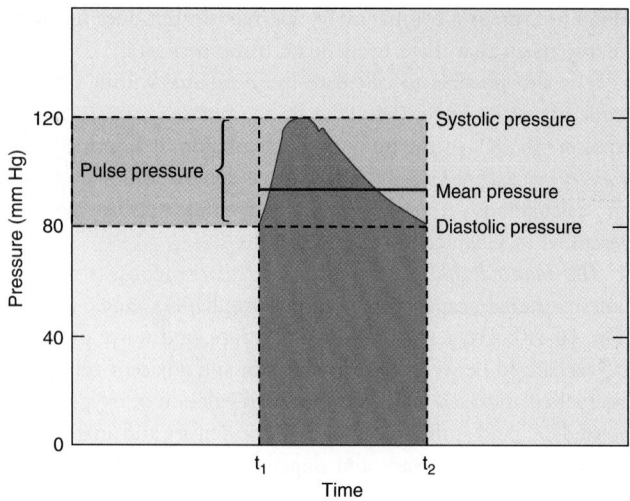

Figure 16-15 Arterial systolic, diastolic, pulse, and mean pressures. *(From Berne RM, Levy MN: Cardiovascular physiology, ed 8, St. Louis, 2001, Mosby.)*

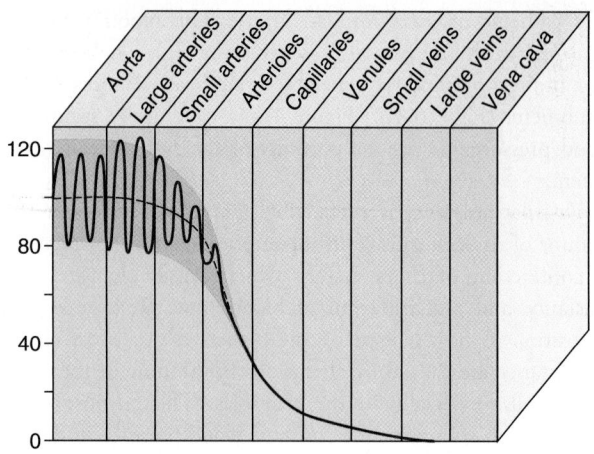

Figure 16-17 Blood pressures in various portions of the systemic circulatory system.

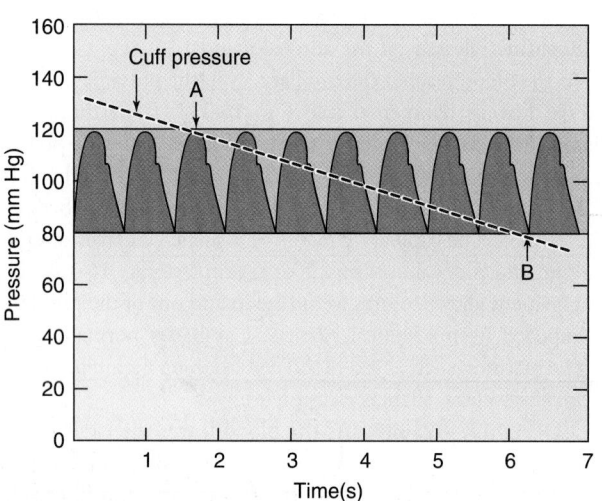

Figure 16-16 Principles of blood pressure measurement with a sphygmomanometer. The oblique line represents pressure in the inflatable bag in the cuff. At cuff pressures greater than the systolic pressure (*to the left of* A), no blood progresses beyond the cuff, and no sounds can be detected below the cuff with the stethoscope. At cuff pressures between the systolic and diastolic levels (*between* A *and* B), spurts of blood traverse the arteries under the cuff and produce Korotkoff sounds. At cuff pressures lower than the diastolic pressure (*to the right of* B), arterial flow past the region of the cuff is continuous, and no sounds are audible. *(From Berne RM, Levy MN: Cardiovascular physiology, ed 8, St. Louis, 2001, Mosby.)*

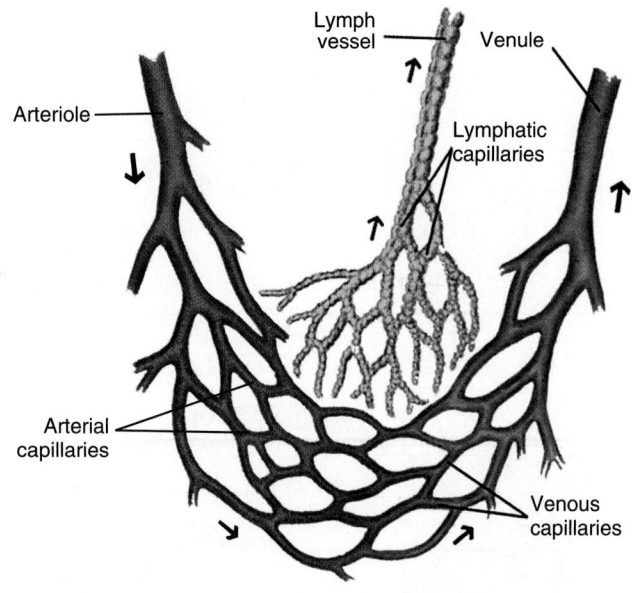

Figure 16-18 Microcirculation. Notice the branching nature and large cross-sectional area of the capillary bed. *(From Thompson JM et al: Mosby's clinical nursing, ed 5, St. Louis, 2002, Mosby.)*

during position changes, especially from supine to standing. Before helping the patient to stand, the nurse must allow him or her to "dangle" (sit on the side of the bed) to check for adequate venous reserves.

MICROSCOPIC STRUCTURE

To appreciate the unique pumping ability of the heart, the nurse must understand cardiac cell structure and function. This section reviews the anatomic mechanisms responsible for the contractile process in cardiac muscle cells.

Cardiac Fibers. Cardiac muscle fibers are typically found in a latticework arrangement. The fiber cells (myofibrils) divide, rejoin, and then separate again, but they retain distinct cellular walls and possess a single nucleus. Individual cardiac muscle cells are known as *myocytes*. The myocytes are connected by

sitting position, approximately 7 to 10 mL blood per kilogram of body weight pools in the legs. Potentially, cardiac output could decrease by approximately 20% and stroke volume by 20% to 50%. However, normal arterial pressure and blood flow are maintained by a combination of reflex vasoconstriction and redistribution of blood from the venous capacitance vessels. In humans, these capacitance reservoirs are greatest in the spleen, liver, and intestines. Patients with decreased blood reserves, who are dehydrated or hypovolemic, require special caution

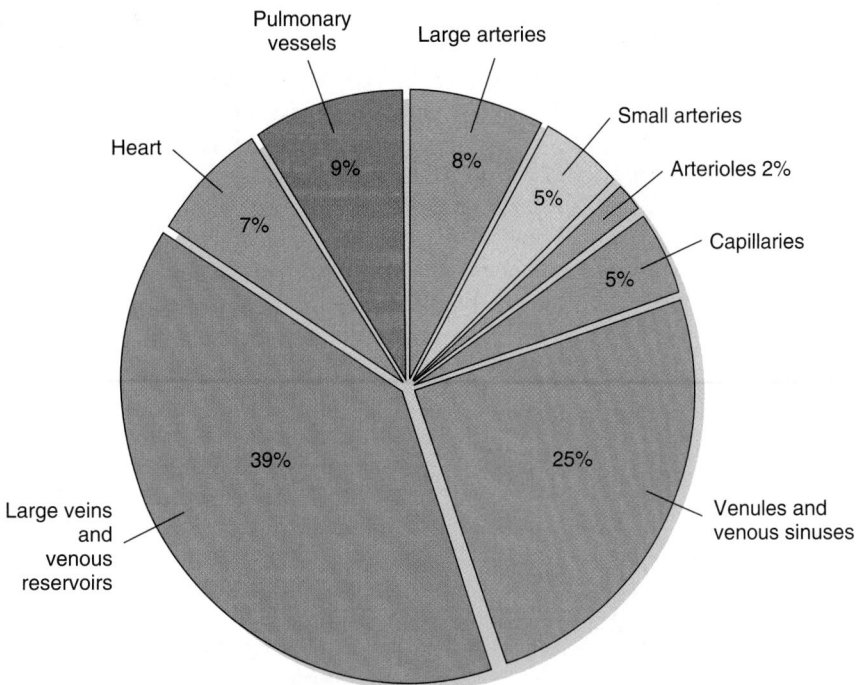

Figure 16-19 Percentage of the total blood volume in each portion of the circulation system.

specialized junctional complexes called *intercalated disks* that assist in the propogation of deolarization. Myocardial muscle cells differ greatly from skeletal muscle, where the cells are fused together to form a continuous fiber with many nuclei.

In general, cardiac myofibrils run on a longitudinal axis, and the fibers appear striped, or striated. When viewed under an electron microscope, these striations are seen to be the contractile proteins (Fig. 16-20). The areas separating each myocardial cell from its neighbor, called *intercalated disks* are continuous with the *sarcolemma*, or cell membrane. The point at which a longitudinal branch of one cell meets the branch of another is called a tight junction (or gap junction) that are contained within the intercalated discs. These junctions offer much less impedance to electrical flow than does the sarcolemma, so depolarization occurs from one cell to another with relative ease. The cardiac muscle is a functional syncytium: depolarization initiated in any cardiac cell quickly spreads to all of the heart.

Cardiac Cells. Each cardiac cell contains many intracellular proteins that contribute to contraction. Two important contractile proteins are *actin* and *myosin*. These proteins abound in the cell in organized longitudinal arrangements. When visualized by electron microscopy, the myosin filaments appear thick, whereas the actin filaments, which are almost twice as prevalent, appear thin. The actin filaments are connected to a *Z-line* (also known as z disk, or z band) on one end, leaving the other end free to interact with the myosin cross-bridges.[27] In the resting muscle cell, the actin and myosin partially overlap. Myosin has three distinct regions, the head, the hinge and the tail. The ends of the myosin filament that overlap with actin have tiny projections named *myosin heads* that contain a binding site for actin (Fig. 16-21). In order for contraction to occur, the myosin heads must interact with actin to form cross-bridges (see Fig. 16-21).

The sarcomere is the functional unit of cardiac contraction and is defined as the region between two Z-lines. In a normal resting state, the sarcomere is about 2.0 to 2.2 mm long (Fig. 16-22). The myosin filaments are situated in the middle of the sarcomere and are attached to the Z-line of the sarcomere by the protein *titan*. Each sarcomere consists of a central *A-band* (thick filaments) and two halves of the *I-band* (thin filaments), as shown in Figure 16-22C. The I-bands from two adjacent sarcomeres meet at the Z-line. The central portion of the A-band is the *M-line*, which does not contain actin. Figure 16-22C shows the position of titin, the thin filaments and the thick filaments in the sarcomere. The thin filament is composed of helical chains of actin globular proteins that coil around a long filament of tropomyosin, and three regulatory *troponin* proteins: Tn-T, Tn-C, and Tn-I. The troponin complex is attached to actin at regularly spaced intervals. Troponin proteins regulate the cross-bridge cycling between actin and myosin.

Another extremely important intracellular structure necessary for successful contraction is the *sarcoplasmic reticulum*. Calcium ions are stored in the in the sarcoplasmic reticulum and released for use after depolarization (Fig. 16-22A). Deep invaginations into the sarcomere are called *transverse tubules*, or *T tubules*. The T tubules are essentially an extension of the cell membrane (sarcolema); they conduct depolarization to structures deep within the cytoplasm, such as the sarcoplasmic reticulum. The T tubules connect to the sarcomeres at the Z-line, as shown in Figure 16-22B. The Z-line is composed of interconnecting proteins such as *desmin* and *alpha-actinin* that link actin to the Z-line. The cardiac cells abound with mitochondria, which contain respiratory enzymes necessary for oxidative phosphorylation (Fig. 16-20). This enables the cell to keep up with the tremendous energy requirements of repetitive contraction.

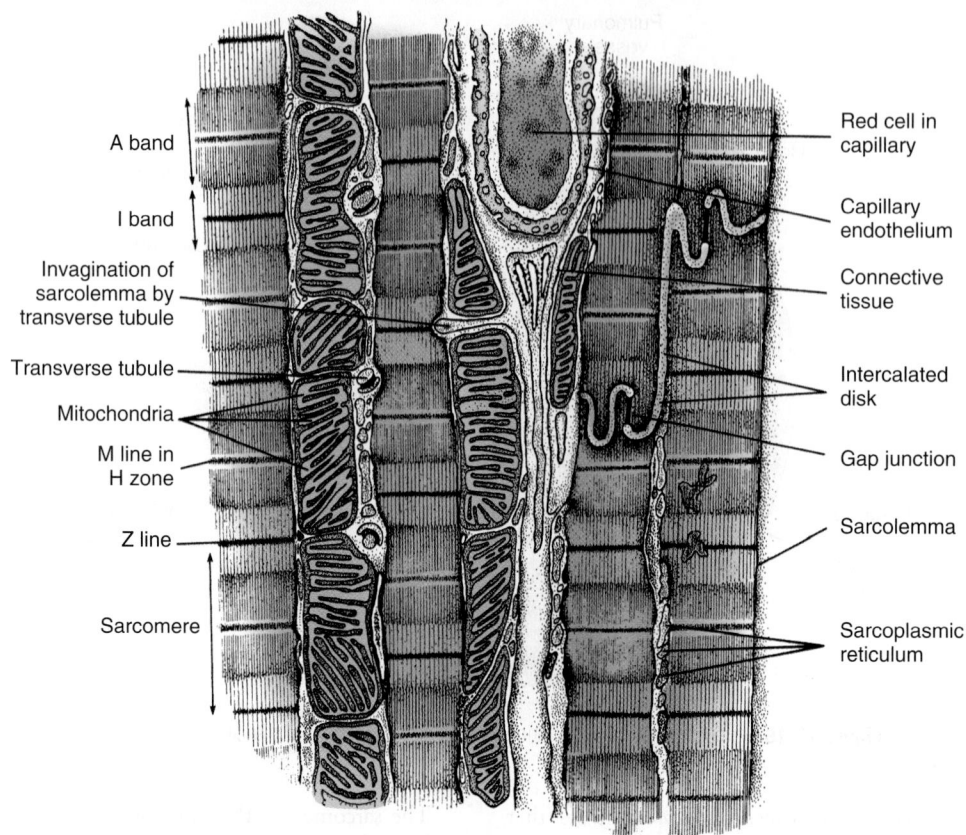

Figure 16-20 Diagram of an electron micrograph of cardiac muscle showing the large numbers of mitochondria, the intercalated disks with tight junctions, the transverse tubules, and the longitudinal tubules (also known as the *sarcoplasmic reticulum*) (approximately ×30,000). *(From Berne RM, Levy MN: Cardiovascular physiology, ed 8, St. Louis, 2001, Mosby.)*

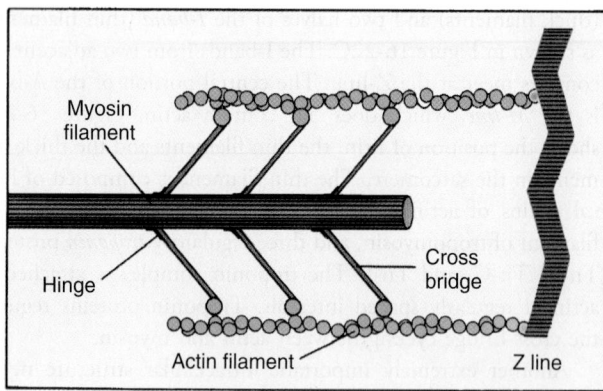
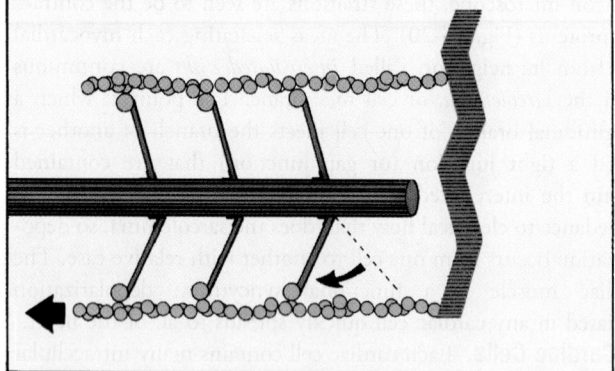

Figure 16-21 Actin and myosin filaments and cross-bridges responsible for cell contraction.

When cardiac cells are damaged by trauma or ischemia, the myocardial cells release protein biomarkers such as troponin that when measured by laboratory analysis, can help determine the extent of injury (see Chapter 18).

PHYSIOLOGY

The electrical and mechanical properties of cardiac tissue have fascinated scientists for more than 100 years. These properties include excitability, conductivity, automaticity, rhythmicity, contractility, and refractoriness. The following section relates these concepts specifically to cardiac cells (Table 16-3).

ELECTRICAL ACTIVITY

Transmembrane Potentials. Electrical potentials across cell membranes are present in essentially all cells of the body. Some cells, such as nerve and muscle cells, are specialized for conduction of electrical impulses along their membranes. This electrical potential, or transmembrane potential, refers to the relative electrical difference between the interior of a cell and

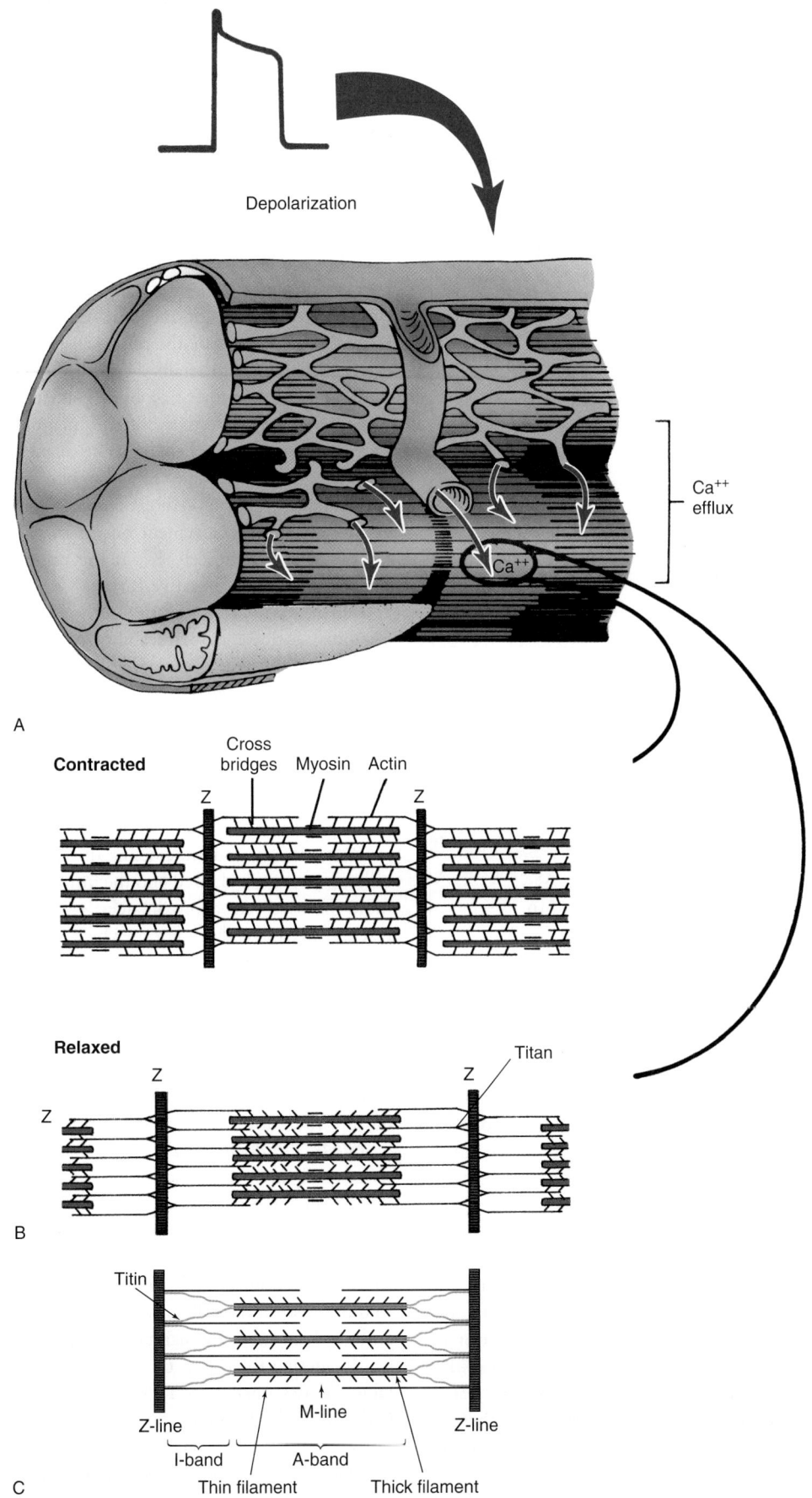

Figure 16-22 *A,* Depolarization of a myocardial cell causes release of calcium from the sarcoplasmic reticulum and the transverse tubules. *B,* Calcium release allows for the cross-bridges on the myosin filaments to attach to the actin filaments to effect cell contraction. *C,* The sarcomere lies between two Z-lines. The sarcomere is composed of a central A-band which contains thick filaments, and two halves of the I-band that contain thin filaments. The center of the A-band is the M-line. Titin spans from the Z-line to the M-line. *(A and* B *from Quaal S: Comprehensive intraaortic balloon pumping, ed 2, St. Louis, 1993, Mosby;* C *from Shiels HA, White E: Commentary: The Frank-Starling mechanism in vertebrate cardiac myocytes,* J Exp Biol *211:2005-2013, 2008.)*

TABLE 16-3 Terms Related to Cardiac Tissue Function

Term	Definition
Excitability	Ability of a cell or tissue to depolarize in response to a given stimulus
Conductivity	Ability of cardiac cells to transmit a stimulus from cell to cell
Automaticity	Ability of certain cells to spontaneously depolarize ("pacemaker potential")
Rhythmicity	Automaticity generated at a regular rate
Contractility	Ability of the cardiac myofibrils to shorten in length in response to an electrical stimulus (depolarization)
Refractoriness	State of a cell or tissue during repolarization, when the cell or tissue cannot depolarize regardless of the intensity of the stimulus or requires a much greater stimulus than is normally required

TABLE 16-4 Approximate Concentrations of Potassium, Sodium, and Calcium Ions in a Resting Myocardial Cell

Ion	Extracellular Concentration (mEq/L)	Intracellular Concentration (mEq/L)
K^+	4	135
Na^+	145	10
Ca^{2+}	2	0.1

that of the fluid surrounding the cell. *Ionic channels* are pores in cell membranes that allow for passage of specific ions at specific times or in response to specific signals. Transmembrane potentials and ionic channels are extremely important in myocardial cells because they form the basis for electrical impulse conduction and muscular contraction. Knowledge of the normal structure and function of cardiac ion channels is increasingly important as a basis for understanding the genesis of lethal cardiac dysrhythmias and for development of cardiac drugs designed to treat these channelopathies.

Resting Membrane Potential. In a myocardial cell at rest, the normal resting membrane potential (RMP) is approximately −80 to −90 millivolts (mV). This means that the interior of the cell is relatively negative compared with the exterior medium. The relative negativity of the cell interior is created by an uneven distribution of positively and negatively charged ions. When the cell is at rest, more positively charged ions are outside the cell than are inside the cell.

When the cell is at rest, the intracellular potassium ion (K^+) concentration is very high, and the intracellular sodium ion (Na^+) level is low. Conversely, the extracellular K^+ concentration is relatively low, compared with a high concentration of Na^+ (Table 16-4). Calcium (Ca^{2+}) has a much higher

concentration outside than inside the cell when the cell is at rest. These large differences in individual ion concentrations create chemical gradients. A *chemical gradient* describes the tendency of an ion to move from an area of higher solute concentration to an area of lower concentration. However, an *electrical gradient* is also present, which causes the positively charged ions to move to an area of relative negativity. For example, the chemical gradient of K^+ forces it to move out of the cell, because the intracellular K^+ concentration is so much higher than that of the outside medium. However, as a result of the relative negativity inside the cell (−80 to −90 mV), the electrical gradient works to retain the positively charged K^+ ion. An important factor influencing both gradients is membrane permeability, or the selectivity of the membrane to ionic movements. Even at rest, there is some slight movement of ions across the cell membrane. For example, the cell membrane is approximately 50 times more permeable to K^+ than it is to Na^+. Because K^+ movement out of the cell results in greater negativity inside the cell, K^+ is the principal ion responsible for maintaining the negative RMP.

Phases of the Action Potential. In a myocardial cell, when a sudden increase in permeability of the membrane to Na^+ occurs, a rapid sequence of events follows that lasts a fraction of a second. This sequence of events is termed *depolarization*. The graphic representation of depolarization and repolarization is termed the action potential (AP) (Fig. 16-23). The ionic currents cause changes in electrical potentials that are known as *AP phases 0, 1, 2, 3,* and *4*. These phases give the AP a characteristic shape (Table 16-5; see Fig. 16-7).

Phase 0. The sodium crossing the cell membrane causes the cell to become depolarized and the interior of the cell to become more positive. At approximately −65 mV, the membrane reaches threshold, the point at which the inward Na^+ current overcomes the efflux of K^+. This is accomplished by means of the fast Na^+ channels. With the fast Na^+ channels open, the inward rush of Na^+ is extremely rapid and briefly causes the inside of the cell to become slightly more positive than the outside of the cell. This series of events is graphically described as phase 0 of the AP and is reflected in the overshoot of the AP, during which the charge is 20 to 30 mV.

Phase 1 and Phase 2. When the rapid influx of Na^+ is terminated, a brief period of partial repolarization occurs as the AP slope returns toward zero (phase 1 of the AP). The plateau that follows is described as phase 2. During this phase, another set of channels, the slow Na^+ and Ca^{2+} channels, open to allow the influx of Ca^{2+} and Na^+. During phase 2, K^+ tends to diffuse out of the cell, balancing the slow inward flux of Na^+ and Ca^{2+} and thereby maintaining the plateau of the AP. The Ca^{2+} entering the cell at this phase causes cardiac contraction, which is described later in this chapter. The inward flux of Ca^{2+} during this phase can be influenced by many factors. For example, calcium channel–blocking drugs, such as verapamil and diltiazem, inhibit the inward Ca^{2+} current into pacemaker tissue, especially the AV node. For this reason, this class of drugs are used therapeutically to slow the rate of atrial tachydysrhythmias and protect the ventricle from excessive atrial impulses, as described in the section on cardiac drugs in Chapter 20.

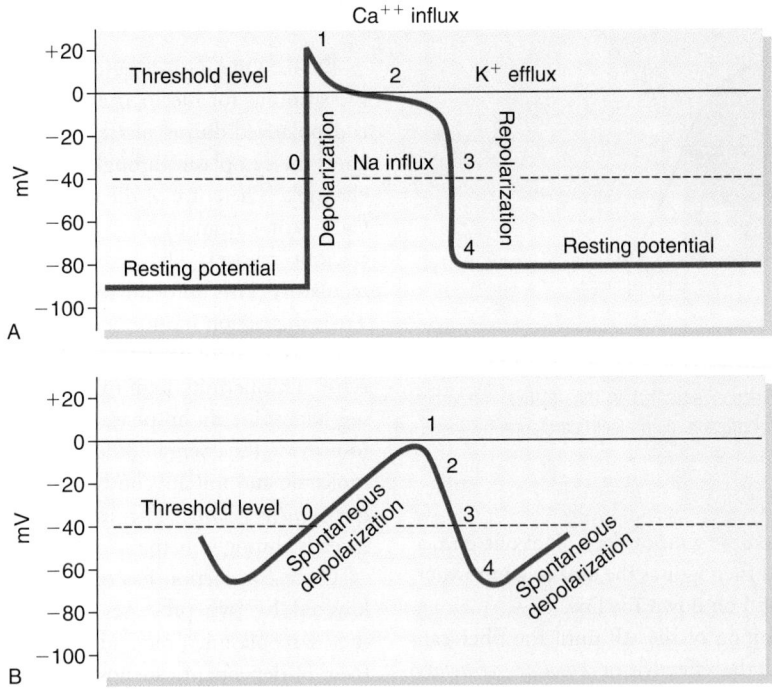

Figure 16-23 Cardiac action potentials. *A,* Action potential phases 0 to 4 of a nonpacemaker cell. *B,* Action potential of a pacemaker cell. *(From Thompson JM et al: Mosby's clinical nursing, ed 5, St. Louis, 2002, Mosby.)*

TABLE 16-5 Phases 0 through 4 of a Cardiac Cell Action Potential

Phase	Description	Ionic Movement	Mechanisms
0	Upstroke	Na^+ into cell	Fast Na^+ channels open
1	Overshoot	—	Fast Na^+ channels close
2	Plateau	Na^+ and Ca^{2+} into cell, K^+ out	Multiple channels (Ca^{2+}, Na^+, K^+) open to maintain membrane voltage
3	Repolarization	K^+ out of cell	Ca^{2+} and Na^+ channels close; K^+ channel remains open
4	Resting membrane potential	Na^+ out, K^+ in	Na^+/K^+ pump

Phase 3. The repolarization phase is described as phase 3, and it depends on two processes. The first is the inactivation of the slow channels, which prevents further influx of Ca^{2+} and Na^+. The other is the continued efflux of K^+ out of the cell. Both processes cause the intracellular environment to become more negative, thereby reestablishing the RMP. On the AP, phase 3 is seen as a gradual descent during which the interior of the cell becomes more negative relative to the outside.

Phase 4. In phase 4, the AP returns to an RMP of −80 to −90 mV. The excess Na^+ that entered the cell during depolarization is removed from the cell in exchange for K^+ by means of the Na^+/K^+ pump. This mechanism returns the intracellular concentrations of Na^+ and K^+ to the levels present before depolarization and is essential for normal ionic balance and preparation for the next depolarization (see Table 16-5).

Fiber Conduction and Excitability. Different parts of the conduction system require different electrical currents and create individual transmembrane APs, as shown in Figure 16-7. Ionic shifts within the endocardium, myocardium, and epicardium are not uniform, although the clinical significance of this finding is not clear. Propagation of an AP along a cardiac fiber occurs as a result of ionic shifts (discussed earlier). As a local section of the cell becomes depolarized, reaches threshold, and completely depolarizes, it affects the adjacent area of the cell and initiates depolarization in that area. The AP propagates down the fiber in a wavelike fashion (Fig. 16-24). This is somewhat analogous

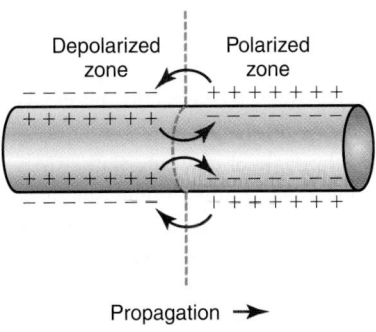

Figure 16-24 Schematic representation of the propagation of an action potential along a cell membrane.

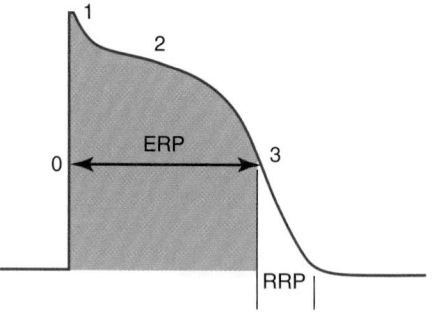

Figure 16-25 The two parts of the refractory period. The effective (absolute) refractory period (ERP) extends from phase 0 to approximately −50 mV in phase 3. The remainder of the action potential is the relative refractory period (RRP). *(From Conover MB:* Understanding electrocardiography, *ed 8, St. Louis, 2002, Mosby.)*

to a trail of gunpowder. When the gunpowder is lit at one end, a small area ignites, burns, and then ignites the area of gunpowder immediately adjacent to it and on down the line.

The time from the beginning of the AP until the fiber can accept another AP is called the effective or *absolute refractory period.* During this period, the cell cannot be depolarized regardless of the amount or intensity of the stimulus. This period lasts from the beginning of depolarization until the interior of the cell has repolarized to approximately −50 mV during phase 3. Immediately after the absolute refractory period is the *relative refractory period.* At this time, the cell is not fully repolarized but could depolarize with a strong enough stimulus (Fig. 16-25). This period lasts from approximately −50 mV during phase 3 until the cell returns to RMP (phase 4); at that point, the cell is fully repolarized and is again ready to respond to the next stimulus. The concept of relative versus absolute refractory periods is useful for understanding the genesis of ventricular dysrhythmias (see Chapter 18). In brief, a cell cannot be stimulated to depolarize until it has at least partially recovered from the previous impulse. This means that an ectopic impulse cannot be propagated during the absolute refractory period.

Pacemaker Cell versus Nonpacemaker Cell Action Potentials. The AP is representative of the depolarization of nonpacemaker myocardial cells. The AP generated by a Purkinje fiber is similar to that of a ventricular myocardial cell except that phase 2 is usually more prolonged in the Purkinje fiber. Atrial myocardial cells exhibit a shortened plateau (phase 2) when compared with ventricular cells. The pacemaker cells of the SA node have an AP that is very different from that of a myocardial cell or a Purkinje cell. In the SA node, the RMP is not as negative, approximately −65 mV. Rather than having an RMP that remains constant, the pacemaker cells slowly depolarize at a steady rate until threshold is reached (see Fig. 16-23B). The lack of a steady-state RMP is largely the result of a continual Na$^+$ influx through the slow channels. This mechanism explains how the cells can spontaneously depolarize (automaticity). It also provides the basis for understanding alterations in the pacemaker cells. The frequency of pacemaker cell discharge may be altered by changing the rate of depolarization or by raising or lowering the cellular RMP.

MECHANICAL ACTIVITY

Excitation-Contraction Coupling. The electrical activity is the stimulus for mechanical contraction. As the myocardial cell is depolarized during phase 2 of the AP, extracellular Ca^{2+} ions enter the cytoplasm through the cell membrane via special Ca^{2+} channels. The entry of the Ca^{2+} ions is the trigger for release of Ca^{2+} stores from the sarcoplasmic reticulum (calcium-induced calcium release). The cytoplasmic Ca^{2+} then binds with the regulatory Tn-C protein to induce a conformational change in Tn-I; this action induces a conformational change in Tn-T that moves the tropomyosin away from the myosin-binding site on actin. This permits actin to interact with myosin, thereby releasing adensoine diphosphate (ADP) and an inorganic phosphate to provide the energy needed for myosin to slide along the actin molecule and initiate contraction. This mechanism is known as *cross-bridge cycling.* The result is myocardial contraction that spreads throughout the myocardium.

Once contraction has occurred, intracellular Ca^{2+} levels are lowered by two processes. Most Ca^{2+} is taken backup into the sarcoplasmic reticulum via a Ca^{2+} and magnesium (Mg^{2+})-dependent, adenosine triphosphate (ATP)–based process. In addition, the Na$^+$/Ca^{2+} exchange system located in the sarcolema moves Ca^{2+} outside the cell. This decreases the concentration of Ca^{2+} in the cytoplasm, leading to muscular relaxation.

THE CARDIAC CYCLE

The term *cardiac cycle* refers to one complete mechanical cycle of the heartbeat, beginning with ventricular contraction and ending with ventricular relaxation.

Atrial Systole. The atria fill by passive filling from the vena cave (right atrium) and the pulmonary veins (left atrium). During diastole the mitral and tricuspid vales are open, allowing for passive filling into the ventricles. Following electrical depolarization of the atria (the p wave), atrial contraction (atrial systole) is initiated causing additional blood to enter the ventricular chamber. This is also referred to as *atrial kick.* The next action is that the mitral and tricuspid valves will close.

Isovolumic Contraction. Ventricular depolarization from the QRS electrical stimulus depolarizes the septum and papillary muscles first. The ventricles then begin to tense, starting with the inner endocardium and traversing the myocardium toward the outer epicardium. This increases the pressure within the ventricular chambers. This is known as *isovolumic contraction,* because, even though the ventricular muscle is contracting, the volume of blood within the ventricles does not change. In Figure 16-26 this is seen as a rapid rise in left ventricular pressure.

Ventricular Systole. Ventricular systole represents the ventricular ejection portion of the cardiac cycle. As the ventricular tension increases, the intraventricular pressures exceed the pressure in the aorta and pulmonary arteries, causing the aortic and pulmonic valves to open. The amount of blood ejected from the ventricles with each beat is called the *stroke volume* (SV). In a healthy heart, more than half of the total ventricular blood

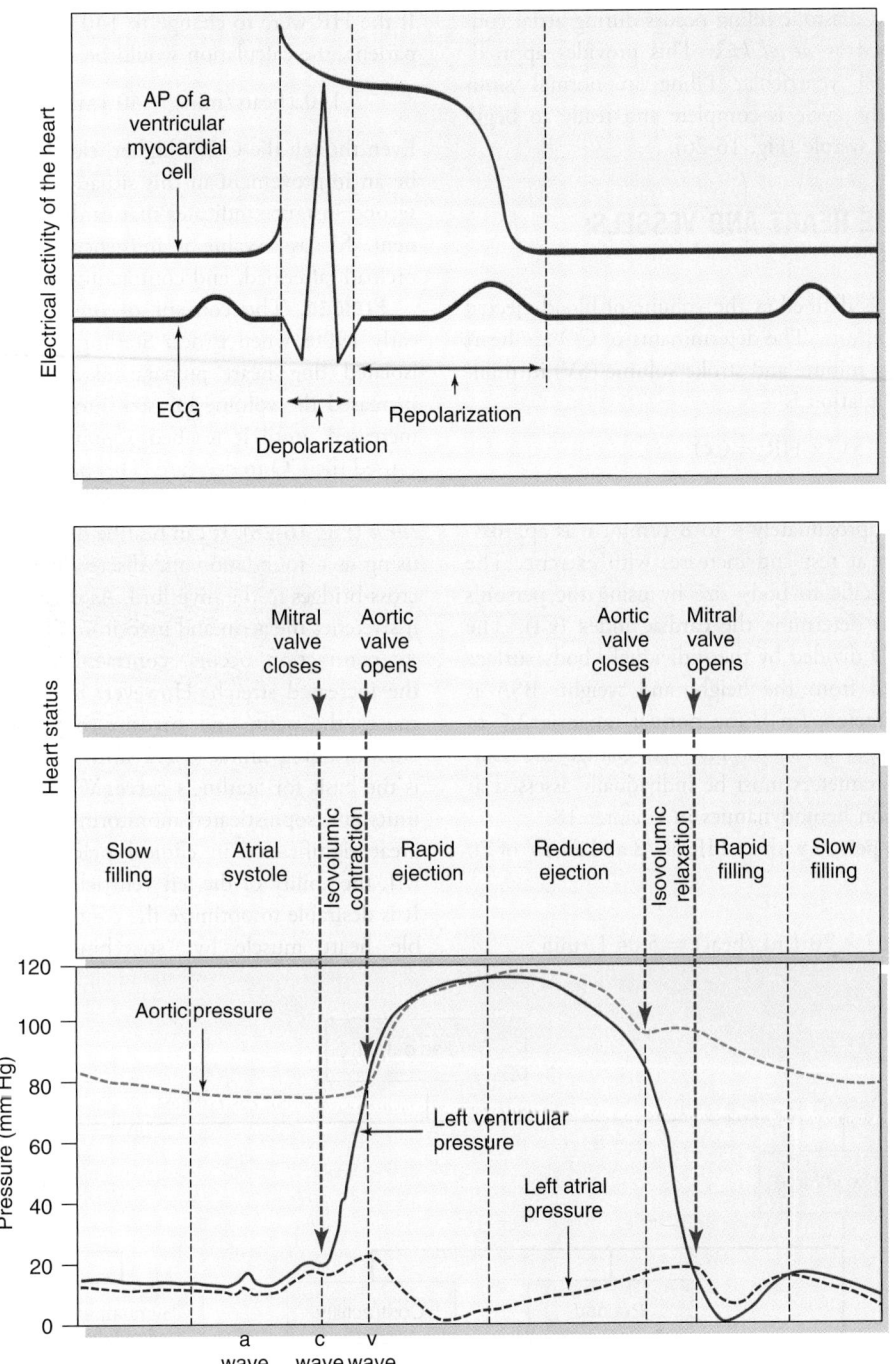

Figure 16-26 The cardiac cycle.

volume is ejected; the blood that remains in the ventricles is the *residual* or *end-systolic* volume.

The ejection fraction (EF) is the ratio of the SV ejected from the left ventricle per beat to the volume of blood remaining in the left ventricle at the end of diastole (left ventricular end-diastolic volume, or LVEDV). EF is expressed as a percentage, and a normal value is 50% or greater. An EF of less than 35% indicates poor ventricular function (as in cardiomyopathy), poor ventricular filling, obstruction to outflow (as in some valve stenosis conditions), or a combination of these conditions.

Isovolumic Relaxation. The next phase is *isovolumic relaxation*, which occurs between the closure of the semilunar (aortic and pulmonic) valves and the opening of the AV (mitral and tricuspid) valves. All four valves are closed, and pressure within the ventricular chamber falls to below atrial pressure without any change in intraventricular volume. At this point the mitral and tricuspid vales open.

Ventricular Diastole. Once the AV valves open, the majority of ventricular filling occurs. The next phase is a reduced ventricular filling period where blood flows passively from the periphery and pulmonary vasculature into the ventricles. The last part of ventricular diastolic filling occurs during atrial contraction, also described as *atrial kick*. This provides approximately 20% of total ventricular filling in normal sinus rhythm. With this, the cycle is complete and ready to begin once again with atrial systole (Fig. 16-26).

INTERPLAY OF THE HEART AND VESSELS: CARDIAC OUTPUT

Cardiac output (CO) is defined as the volume of blood ejected from the heart in 1 minute. The determinants of CO are heart rate (HR) in beats per minute and stroke volume (SV) in milliliters per beat. The equation is

$$SV \times HR = CO$$

CO is usually expressed in liters per minute. The normal CO in the human adult is approximately 4 to 8 L/min; it is approximately 4 to 6 L/min at rest and increases with exercise. The CO can be made specific to body size by using the person's height and weight to determine the cardiac index (CI). The CI is equal to the CO divided by the individual's body surface area (BSA) calculated from the height and weight. BSA is expressed in square meters (m^2), the normal range is 2.5 to 4.5 $L/min/m^2$. Changes in SV or HR can change the CO. However, all three parameters must be individually assessed as described in the section hemodynamics in Chapter 18.

For example, for a person with an HR of 72 and an SV of 70 ml, the CI would be

$$72 \text{ (beats/min)} \times 70 \text{ (mL/beat)} = 5.04 \text{ L/min}$$

If the HR were to change to 140 and the SV to 40 mL in this patient, the calculation would be

$$140 \text{ (beats/min)} \times 40 \text{ (mL/beat)} = 5.6 \text{ L/min}$$

Even though the CO is higher, clearly the faster HR would not be an improvement in this situation. The decreased SV in the second instance indicates that cardiac decompensation is imminent. SV as a value is influenced by three primary factors: preload, afterload, and contractility (Fig. 16-27).

Preload. The concept of preload was introduced in the early 1900s when Ernest Starling described his findings in an isolated dog heart preparation. Starling found that, as he increased the volume infused into a denervated heart, the CO increased, until it reached a point at which further infusion caused the CO to decrease. This has become known as *Starling's law of the heart,* and it is graphically described as the *Starling curve* (Fig. 16-28). It can best be described on a molecular basis, using as a foundation the discussion of the actin and myosin cross-bridges in the myofibril. As the diastolic volume increases, it stretches the actin and myosin molecules in their resting state. As contraction occurs, contractility increases as a result of the increased stretch. However, if the stretch is excessive and causes the actin and myosin to be stretched beyond their cross-bridging limits (>2.2 mm), contractility decreases. This is the basis for Starling's curve. With the advent of critical care units and sophisticated monitoring, this principle has acquired great significance in clinical practice. For example, after an MI, the ability of the left ventricle to pump may be impaired. It is desirable to optimize the contractility of the remaining viable heart muscle by "stretching" it with added volume.

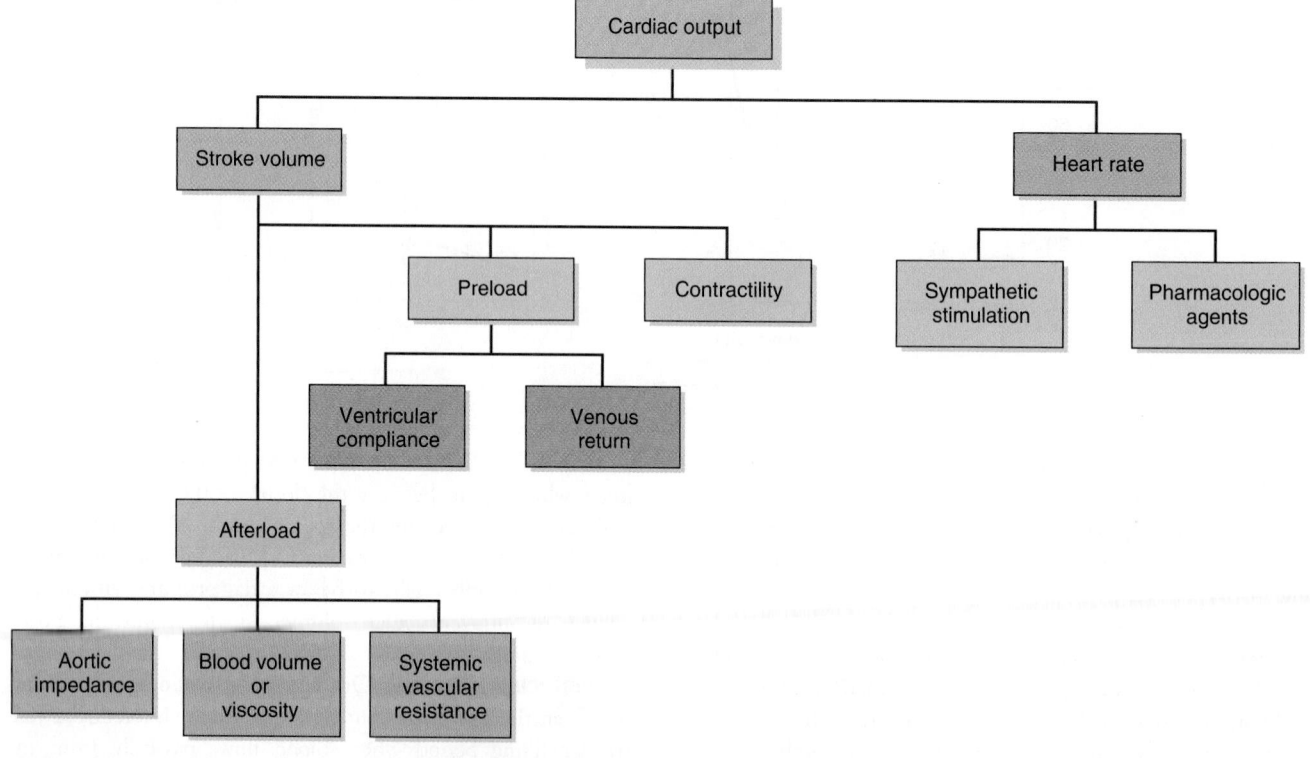

Figure 16-27 Determinants of cardiac output.

However, if the intravascular volume exceeds the stretch limit, CO diminishes.

Preload, then, is the volume of blood in the left ventricle at the end of diastole. The pressure created by this volume is described as the *left ventricular end-diastolic pressure* (LVEDP). Factors affecting LV preload include venous return to the heart, total blood volume, and atrial kick. Factors affecting the compliance (ability to stretch) of the ventricles are the stiffness and the thickness of the muscular wall. For example, the hypovolemic patient has too little preload, whereas the patient with heart failure has too much preload. One way to measure preload is through the pulmonary artery occlusion pressure (PAOP). This value was previously known as the pulmonary arterial wedge pressure (PAWP) or the pulmonary capillary wedge pressure (PCWP). Clinical application of the PAOP is discussed in Chapter 18.

Afterload. Afterload can be defined as the ventricular wall tension or stress during systolic ejection. It is commonly described by the term *systemic vascular resistance (SVR)* or, less frequently, *peripheral vascular resistance.* An increase in afterload usually means an increase in the work of the heart. Afterload is increased by factors that oppose ejection. Examples of increased afterload include aortic impedance (high diastolic aortic pressure, aortic stenosis), septal hypertrophy (obstruction in the outflow tract), vasoconstriction (increased SVR), and hypertension. Therapeutic management to decrease afterload is aimed at decreasing the work of the heart through the use of vasodilators to decrease the myocardial oxygen demand.

An increase in afterload evokes autoregulation, in which the ventricle adapts to changes in filling pressure without a continued increase in resting fiber length. For example, when the SVR increases abruptly during vasoconstriction, ventricular diastolic pressure rises temporarily until the ventricle reaches a new equilibrium level of pressure.

Contractility. Contractility refers to the heart's contractile force. Also known as *inotropy* (*ino* ["strength"] and *tropy* ["enhancing"]), it can be positive (i.e., stronger contraction) or negative (i.e., weaker contraction). Contractility can be increased by Starling's mechanism. It also is altered by the SNS and by pharmacologic agents that mimic the SNS (i.e., sympathomimetics) (see Fig. 16-27).

REGULATION OF THE HEARTBEAT

Nervous Control. The autonomic nervous system (ANS) is composed of two competing neurologic systems of control. The parasympathetic nervous system (PNS) and the SNS operate to create a balance and homeostasis between relaxation and *fight-or-flight* readiness. They affect cardiovascular function by slowing the HR during periods of calm and increasing it in response to sympathetic stimulation. Table 16-6 summarizes the effects of these divisions of the ANS on the heart.

Parasympathetic fibers are concentrated near the SA and AV conduction tissue and in the atria. Specifically, this involves the right and left vagus nerves (Fig. 16-29). Stimulation of the vagus nerve produces bradycardia as a result of hyperpolarization of phase 4 of the AP, which causes the slope to take longer to reach threshold. Sympathetic tone also concomitantly decreases.

Sympathetic nerve fibers are subepicardial and follow the path of the major coronary arteries.[28] When stimulated, sympathetic fibers directly alter ventricular function and increase the HR and contractility.

Intrinsic Regulation. Supplementing the nervous control of the heart are several reflexes that serve as feedback mechanisms to the brain. These reflexes work to maintain even blood flow, oxygenation, and perfusion.

Baroreceptors. The *baroreceptors,* or pressure sensors, are located in the aortic arch and the carotid sinuses. They are more sensitive to wall changes (wall stretch) in these areas than to the absolute pressure. As the receptors sense a change in wall conformation, usually as a result of a change in pressure, the ANS is activated to raise the HR (in the case of decreased pressure) or lower it (in response to increased pressure). For example, a decrease in blood pressure alters the baroreceptor input to the vasomotor center in the medulla (brainstem), causing a reflex tachycardia. The baroreflex also initiates changes in venous tone to alter CO according to need. Venoconstriction increases blood return to the heart and augments SV.

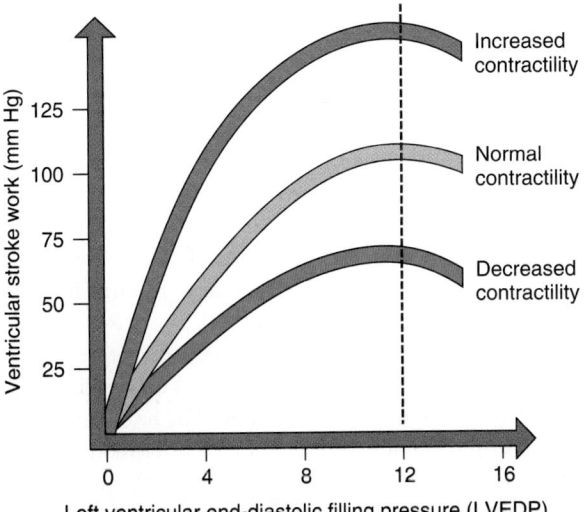

Figure 16-28 Starling curve. As the left ventricular end-diastolic pressure (LVEDP) increases, so does ventricular stroke work or contractility. When left ventricular filling pressure exceeds a maximal point, contractility and cardiac output diminish.

TABLE 16-6	Summary of the Effects of the Parasympathetic and Sympathetic Nervous Systems on the Heart	
Function	**Parasympathetic**	**Sympathetic**
Automaticity	Decrease	Increase
Contractility	Decrease	Increase
Conduction velocity	Decrease	Increase
Chronotropy (rate)	Decrease	Increase

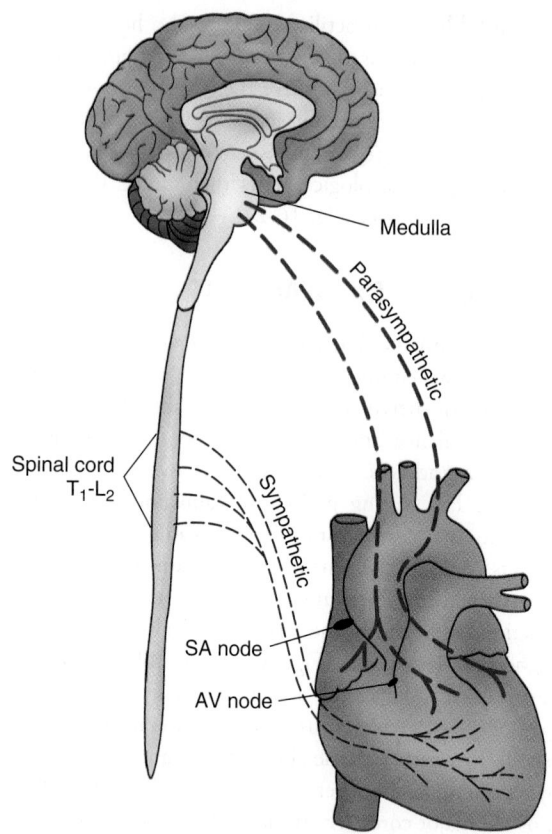

Figure 16-29 Autonomic nervous system innervation of nodal tissue and myocardium by parasympathetic vagus nerve fibers and sympathetic chains. *(Modified from Quaal S: Comprehensive intraaortic balloon pumping, ed 2, St. Louis, 1993, Mosby.)*

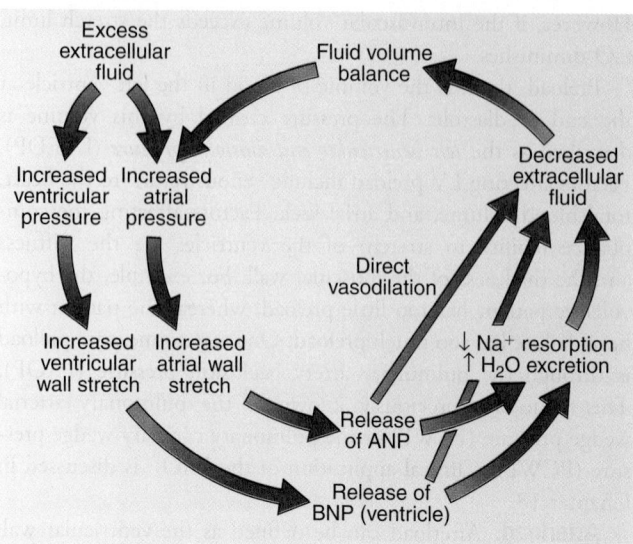

Figure 16-30 The release of atrial peptide (ANP) from the atrium and brain natriuretic peptide (BNP) from the ventricle in response to volume overload.

Chemoreceptors. The arterial *chemoreceptors,* or *carotid and aortic bodies,* are located in the carotid arteries and at the bifurcation of the aortic arch.[29] They possess a rich capillary blood supply and extensive innervation of the peripheral nervous system. Their primary function is to maintain homeostasis during hypoxemia.[29] The chemoreceptors signal changes in oxygen tension (PaO_2 <80 mm Hg), or a carbon dioxide tension ($PaCO_2$) of greater than 40 mm Hg, but not to changes in acid-base (pH). Changes in the pH level are detected by central chemoreceptors in the brainstem (medulla oblongata). Information about changes in these paramenters is communicated to the SNS via the brainstem causing altering the heart rate. Stimulation of the carotid or aortic chemoreceptors normally causes an increase in respiratory rate and depth.

Right Atrial Receptors. The *Bainbridge reflex* is attributed to receptors in the right atrium. When the pressure in the right atrium rises sufficiently to stimulate these stretch receptors, it causes a reflex tachycardia. The purpose of this reflex is possibly to protect the right side of the heart from an overload state and to quickly equalize filling pressures of the right and left sides of the heart.

Natriuretic Peptides. Another cardiac control mechanism involves the natriuretic peptide system (Fig. 16-30).[30] The heart secretes two major natriuretic peptides. The atrial myocardium secretes *atrial natriuretic peptide* (ANP) in response to atrial stretch, and the ventricular myocardium secretes *brain*

natriuretic peptide (BNP) if there is stretch of the ventricular chamber.[30] Both peptides cause vasodilatation, increase natriuresis (Na^+ and water loss via the kidneys), and inhibit the SNS and the renin-angiotensin-aldosterone system (RAAS).[30] Clinically, BNP levels are measured to confirm the diagnosis of acute heart failure.[31] A recombinant form of human BNP, nesiritide (Natrecor), is used therapeutically to mimic the clinical effects of BNP and treat symptoms of heart failure.[31]

Renin-Angiotensin-Aldosterone System. The RAAS system is activated by low blood pressure or intravascular volume depletion. The juxtaglomerular cells of the kidney, located near the afferent arteriole, are activated by low renal blood flow. As shown in Table 16-7, this stimulates release of the hormone renin. Renin converts the protein angiotensinogen to angiotensin I. When angiotensin I passes through the pulmonary vascular bed, it is activated by angiotensin-converting enzyme (ACE) to become angiotensin II. Angiotensin II is a powerful agent with two principal actions. It activates peripheral vascular receptors to vasoconstrict the systemic arterial system and increase blood pressure, and it activates the release of aldosterone from the adrenal glands. Aldosterone works at the distal convoluted tubule in the kidney to retain sodium and, consequently, water. Many drugs are used to manipulate the RAAS system to manage symptoms of heart failure (see " Heart Failure" in Chapter 19 and "Cardiac Drugs" in Chapter 20).

Respiratory Influences. Other influences involve the respiratory cycle and its effect on HR and SV. Normally, the HR varies slightly with the respiratory cycle. The heart usually accelerates on inspiration and decelerates with exhalation (see "Sinus Dysrhythmia" in Chapter 18). Left ventricular SV decreases during normal inspiration. Possible reasons include normal fluctuations in sympathetic and vagal tone during respiration or any of the following alterations: decreased intrathoracic pressure contributing to increased venous return; the Bainbridge reflex; activation of stretch receptors in the lungs; interactions between the respiratory and cardiac centers in the medulla; increased

TABLE 16-7 Interplay between the Renin-Angiotensin-Aldosterone and Antidiuretic Hormone Systems To Maintain Fluid Balance

Hormone	Effect*
Renin ↓	Reduction in vascular volume or low arterial blood pressure stimulates renin release from juxtaglomerular cells near kidney.
Angiotensinogen ↓	Angiotensinogen is produced in liver.
Angiotensin I ↓	Lungs release ACE to convert angiotensin I to angiotensin II.
Angiotensin II ↓	Angiotensin II activates peripheral vascular receptors to increase SVR and raise arterial blood pressure. Angiotensin II release also stimulates adrenal glands to release aldosterone. ADH is released from the posterior pituitary when angiotensin II causes constriction of the renal arterioles and when the hypothalamus detects intracellular dehydration.
Aldosterone	Aldosterone acts on the kidney distal tubules to retain sodium; when salt is retained, so is water.

*Overall effect is to increase intravascular volume and raise blood pressure.
ACE, angiotensin-converting enzyme; ADH, antidiuretic hormone; SVR, systemic vascular resistance.

capacity of the pulmonary vessels during lung inflation; decreased left ventricular compliance resulting from increased right ventricular return; increased impedance to left ventricular outflow related to the pleural pressure changes; or neural reflex mechanisms that are independent of mechanical influences.

CONTROL OF PERIPHERAL CIRCULATION

Intrinsic Control. Intrinsic, or local, control of the arterial peripheral circulation is most influential at the arteriolar level. The arterioles are the major resistance vessels because of the amount of smooth muscle in the vessel walls (see Fig. 16-12). The arteriole has the potential for increasing or decreasing its lumen substantially. Several local factors influence this balance, including pharmacologic stimuli from locally released catecholamines, histamine, acetylcholine, serotonin, angiotensin, adenosine, and prostaglandins. These agents can be induced by a variety of mechanisms, such as tissue injury, hypoxemia, or hormones. Other factors that influence circulation locally are temperature and carbon dioxide.

Extrinsic Control. Extrinsic control is mediated by two major mechanisms: the ANS and the peripheral vascular reflexes.

The ANS exerts dual antagonistic control over most organ systems via the sympathetic (constriction) and parasympathetic (dilation) nerve fibers. Stimulation of the vasomotor center in the medulla causes increased mean arterial pressure and HR by enhancing sympathetic outflow and possibly inhibiting parasympathetic outflow. The sympathetic outflow targets the resistance arterioles, causing vasoconstriction. Inhibition of these areas produces the opposite effect—vasodilation. Sympathetic fibers causing vasoconstriction supply the arteries, arterioles, and veins.

The capacitance vessels (veins) contain up to 75% of the blood volume.[25,26] Increases in venous tone (venoconstriction) increase the volume of blood returning to the right side of the heart and augment SV. The most richly innervated venous beds are those in the splanchnic (spleen) and cutaneous (skin)

TABLE 16-8 Regions in the Medulla That Affect Cardiovascular Activity

Region	Activity
Dorsal lateral medulla (pressor region)	Vasoconstriction Cardiac acceleration Enhanced contractility
Ventromedial medulla (depressor region)	Direct spinal inhibition Inhibition of the pressor region

circulations.[26] The venous and arterial vascular systems are interdependent; they dilate and constrict in unison.[26] One does not act without the other. Table 16-8 summarizes the sympathetic receptors, including location and effects of stimulation

Control of peripheral circulation is a combination of intrinsic and extrinsic mechanisms. Additional influences include emotions, temperature, and humoral substances. For example, when red blood cells are exposed to hypoxia at the tissue level, they release the vasodilators nitric oxide and adenosine triphosphate, to increase oxygen delivery.[25]

Summary

- Knowledge of normal cardiovascular anatomy and physiology is vital for a complete understanding of the changes that occur in cardiac disease states.
- The major anatomic structures of the heart include the pericardium, myocardium, endocardium, coronary arteries, coronary veins, atria, ventricles, heart valves, and electrical conduction system.
- The electrical conduction system, the mechanical events of the cardiac cycle, the autonomic nervous system, and the preload volume in the veins act synergistically to ensure optimal cardiac output and hemodynamic stability in a state of health.

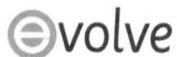 Be sure to check out the bonus material, including free self-assessment exercises, on the Evolve web site at http://evolve.elsevier.com/Urden/.

References

1. Anderson RH et al: Cardiac anatomy revisited, *J Anat* 205(3):159-177, 2004.
2. Haddad F et al: Right ventricular function in cardiovascular disease. Part I. Anatomy, physiology, aging, and functional assessment of the right ventricle, *Circulation* 117(11):1436-1448, 2008.
3. Frey N et al: Hypertrophy of the heart: a new therapeutic target? *Circulation* 109(13):1580-1589, 2004.
4. D'Avila A et al: Pericardial anatomy for the interventional electrophysiologist, *J Cardiovasc Electrophysiol* 14(4):422-430, 2003.
5. Goldstein JA: Cardiac tamponade, constrictive pericarditis, and restrictive cardiomyopathy, *Curr Probl Cardiol* 29(9):503-567, 2004.
6. Rabkin SW: Epicardial fat: properties, function and relationship to obesity, *Obes Rev* 8(3):253-261, 2007.
7. Sacks HS, Fain JN: Human epicardial adipose tissue: a review, *Am Heart J* 153(6):907-917, 2007.
8. Olivey HE et al: Coronary vessel development the epicardium delivers, *Trends Cardiovasc Med* 14(6):247-251, 2004.
9. Anderson RH et al: The anatomical arrangement of the myocardial cells making up the ventricular mass, *Eur J Cardiothorac Surg* 28(4):517-525, 2005.
10. Partridge JB, Anderson RH: Left ventricular anatomy: its nomenclature, segmentation, and planes of imaging, *Clin Anat* 22(1):77-84, 2009.
11. Muresian H: The clinical anatomy of the mitral valve, *Clin Anat* 22(1):85-98, 2009.
12. Segal BL: Valvular heart disease, part 2: Mitral valve disease in older adults, *Geriatrics* 58(10):26-31, 2003.
13. Robicsek F et al: The congenitally bicuspid aortic valve: how does it function? Why does it fail? *Ann Thorac Surg* 77(1):177-185, 2004.
14. Tzemos N et al: Outcomes in adults with bicuspid aortic valves, *JAMA* 300 (11):1317-1325, 2008.
15. Berdajs D et al: The clinical anatomy of the sinus node artery, *Ann Thorac Surg* 76(3):732-735, 2003.
16. James TN: The internodal pathways of the human heart, *Prog Cardiovasc Dis* 43(6):495-535, 2001.
17. Bharati S: Anatomy of the atrioventricular conduction system, *Circulation* 103(12):E63-E64, 2001.
18. Anderson RH, Cook AC: The structure and components of the atrial chambers, *Europace* 9(suppl 6):vi 3-vi9, 2007.
19. Platonov PG: Interatrial conduction in the mechanisms of atrial fibrillation: from anatomy to cardiac signals and new treatment modalities, *Europace* 9(suppl 6):vi10-vi16, 2007.
20. Pejković B et al: Anatomical aspects of the arterial blood supply to the sinoatrial and atrioventricular nodes of the human heart, *J Int Med Res* 36(4):691-698, 2008.
21. James TN: Structure and function of the sinus node, AV node and His bundle of the human heart. Part I. Structure, *Prog Cardiovasc Dis* 45 (3):235-267, 2002.
22. James TN: Structure and function of the sinus node, AV node and his bundle of the human heart. Part II. Function, *Prog Cardiovasc Dis* 45(4):327-360, 2003.
23. von Ludinghausen M: The venous drainage of the human myocardium, *Adv Anat Embryol Cell Biol* 168:I-VIII, 1-104, 2003.
24. Perez-Lugones A et al: Evidence of specialized conduction cells in human pulmonary veins of patients with atrial fibrillation, *J Cardiovasc Electrophysiol* 14(8):803-809, 2003.
25. den Uil CA et al: The microcirculation in health and critical disease, *Prog Cardiovasc Dis* 51(2):161-170, 2008.
26. Peters J et al: The importance of the peripheral circulation in critical illnesses, *Intensive Care Med* 27(9):1446-1458, 2001.
27. Pyle WG, Solaro RJ: At the crossroads of myocardial signaling: the role of Z-discs in intracellular signaling and cardiac function, *Circ Res* 94(3):296-305, 2004.
28. Zipes DP: Heart-brain interactions in cardiac arrhythmias: role of the autonomic nervous system, *Cleve Clin J Med* 275(suppl 2):S94-S96, 2008.
29. Prabhakar NR, Peng YJ: Peripheral chemoreceptors in health and disease, *J Appl Physiol* 96(1):359-366, 2004.
30. Suttner SW, Boldt J: Natriuretic peptide system: physiology and clinical utility, *Curr Opin Crit Care* 10(5):336-341, 2004.
31. Maisel A: Circulating natriuretic peptide levels in acute heart failure, *Rev Cardiovasc Med* 8(suppl 5):S13-S21, 2007.

Cardiovascular Clinical Assessment

*P*hysical assessment of the cardiovascular patient is a skill that must not be lost amid the technology of the critical care setting. Data collected from a thorough, thoughtful history and examination contribute to both the nursing and the medical decisions for therapeutic interventions.

HISTORY

The patient history is important because it provides data that contribute to the cardiovascular diagnosis and treatment plan. For a patient in acute distress, the history is curtailed to just a few questions about the patient's chief complaint, the precipitating events, and current medications (see Data Collection: Cardiovascular History). For a patient without obvious distress, the history focuses on the following four areas:

1. Review of the patient's present illness.
2. Overview of the patient's general cardiovascular status, including previous cardiac diagnostic studies, interventional procedures, cardiac surgeries, and current medications (i.e., cardiac, noncardiac, and over-the-counter drugs).
3. Examination of the patient's general health status, including family history of coronary artery disease (CAD), hypertension, diabetes, peripheral arterial disease, or stroke.
4. Survey of the patient's lifestyle, including risk factors for CAD.

One of the unique challenges in cardiovascular assessment is identifying when "chest pain" is of cardiac origin and when it is not. The following safety information should always be considered:

- If there is any evidence of CAD or risk of heart disease, assume that the chest pain is caused by myocardial ischemia until proven otherwise.
- Questions to elicit the nature of the chest pain cover five basic areas: quality, location, duration of pain, factors that provoke the pain, and factors that relieve the pain. Questions that may help elicit this information are listed in Table 17-1.
- There may be little correlation between the severity of chest discomfort and the gravity of its cause. This is a result of the subjective nature of pain and the unique

presentation of ischemic disease in women, elderly patients, and individuals with diabetes.
- Subjective descriptors vary greatly among individuals. Not all patients use the word "pain"; some may describe "pressure," "heaviness," "discomfort," or "indigestion."
- There is not always a correlation between the location of chest discomfort and its source because of *referred pain*. For example, in patients with gastroesophageal reflux disease (GERD), esophageal spasm can cause visceral substernal chest pain that radiates to the left arm and jaw, described by patients as "heartburn."[1,2]
- Other nonpainful symptoms that may signal cardiac dysfunction are dyspnea, palpitations, cough, fatigue, edema, ischemic leg pain, nocturia, syncope, and cyanosis.

In a meta-analysis of the evaluation of stable, intermittent chest pain, a patient's description of chest pain was found to be the most important predictor of underlying coronary disease.[3] In the evaluation of acute chest pain, the 12-lead electrocardiogram was the most useful bedside predictor for a diagnosis of ST-elevation myocardial infarction (STEMI).[3]

PHYSICAL EXAMINATION

A comprehensive physical assessment is fundamental to the achievement of an accurate diagnosis. The nurse who has developed the skills of inspection, palpation, and auscultation can be confident when assessing patients with cardiovascular disease. Percussion is not employed when assessing the cardiovascular system.

INSPECTION

Face. The face is observed for the color of the skin (i.e., cyanotic, pale, or jaundiced) and for apprehensive or painful expressions. The skin, lips, tongue, and mucous membranes are inspected for pallor or cyanosis. *Central cyanosis* is a bluish discoloration of the tongue and sublingual area. Multiracial studies indicate that the tongue is the most sensitive site for observation of central cyanosis, which must be recognized and treated as a medical emergency. Pulse oximetry, arterial blood gas analysis, and treatment with 100% oxygen must be instituted immediately.

Data Collection

Cardiovascular History

COMMON CARDIOVASCULAR SYMPTOMS
- Chest pains
- Palpitations
- Dyspnea
- Cough, hemoptysis
- Nausea
- Nocturia
- Edema
- Dizziness, syncope, visual changes
- Claudication, extremity pain or paresthesias
- Fatigue

PATIENT PROFILE
- Baseline cognitive functioning
- Health habits
  - Use of tea and coffee; over-the-counter drug use; smoking; exercise; sleep; dietary habits
  - Use of illegal recreational drugs (e.g., cocaine)
  - Use of alcohol (occasional, daily)
- Lifestyle pattern and responsibilities
- Working, relaxing, coping, cultural habits
- Social support systems
- Recent life changes within the past 12 months
- Emotional state
- Evidence of psychologic stress, anger, anxiety, depression
- Perception of illness and its meaning for the future

RISK FACTORS
- Male / Female,
- Age, cultural identity
- Family history of premature CAD (65 years or younger)
- Smoking history
- Hypertension
- Hyperlipidemia
- Sedentary lifestyle
- Diabetes mellitus
- Obesity
- Kidney failure

FAMILY HISTORY
- CAD at age 65 years or younger
- Myocardial infarction or early death of unknown origin
- Hypertension
- Stroke
- Diabetes mellitus
- Lipid disorders
- Collagen vascular disease

CARDIAC STUDIES OR INTERVENTIONS DONE IN THE PAST
- Cardiac catheterization
- Electrophysiology study
- Cardiac ultrasound (echocardiogram)
- 12-Lead electroencephalogram
- Exercise electrocardiography test (stress test)
- Myocardial imaging with radiographic isotopes (e.g., thallium, dipyridamole [Persantine], dobutamine)
- Thrombolytic therapy
- Percutaneous transluminal coronary angioplasty
- Atherectomy
- Stent placement
- Valvuloplasty

MEDICAL HISTORY
Childhood
- Murmurs, cyanosis, streptococcal infections, rheumatic fever
Adult
- Diseases and abnormalities
  - Heart failure (right or left sided), CAD, heart valve disease, mitral valve prolapse, myocardial infarction, peripheral vascular disease, diabetes mellitus, hypertension, hyperlipidemia, dysrhythmias, murmurs, endocarditis, visual defects, recent weight changes, psychiatric illnesses, thrombophlebitis, deep vein thrombosis, systemic or pulmonary emboli
- Surgical history
  - Cardiovascular: coronary artery bypass grafting, valvular placement, peripheral vascular bypasses or repairs, pacemaker, defibrillator implants (ICDs)
  - Other body systems: neurologic, gastrointestinal, musculoskeletal, pulmonary, renal, immunologic, hematologic
- Allergies, especially to emergency medications (lidocaine, morphine), radiographic contrast agents, or iodine (shellfish)
- Recent dental work or infection

CURRENT MEDICATION USAGE
- ACE inhibitors
- Anticoagulants
- Antidysrhythmics
- Antihypertensives
- Antiplatelet agents
- Angiotensin receptor blockers
- Beta-blockers
- Calcium channel blockers
- Cholesterol-lowering agents
- Digitalis
- Diuretics
- Nitrates
- Hormone replacement therapy
- Oral contraceptives
- Potassium, calcium
- Nonprescription medications/herbal remedies

ACE, angiotensin-converting enzyme; CAD, coronary artery disease; ICDs, implantable cardioverter defibrillators.

TABLE 17-1 Clarifying Chest Pain Symptoms by Asking Specific Questions

Determine	Typical Question
Location, radiation	Where is it? Does it move or stay in one place?
Quality	What's it like?
Quantity	How severe is it? How frequent? How long does it last?
Chronology	When did it begin? How has it progressed? What are you doing when it occurs? What do you do to get rid of it?
Associated findings	Do you feel any other symptoms at the same time?
Treatment sought and effect	Have you seen a physician in the past for this same problem? What was the treatment?
Personal perception	What do you think this is from? Why do you think it happened now?

Thorax. The anterior thorax and posterior thorax are inspected for skeletal deformities that may displace the heart and cause cardiac compromise. The skin on the chest wall and abdomen is inspected for scars, bruises, wounds, and bulges associated with pacemaker or defibrillator implants. Respiratory rate, pattern, and effort are also observed and recorded.

Abdomen. The abdomen is assessed for signs of distention or ascites that may be associated with right-sided heart failure. Abdominal adiposity is a known risk factor for CAD.

Nail Beds and Cyanosis. The nail beds are inspected for signs of discoloration or cyanosis. *Clubbing* in the nail bed is a sign associated with long-standing central cyanotic heart disease or pulmonary disease with hypoxemia.[4] Clubbing describes a nail that has lost the normal angle between the finger and the nail root; the nail becomes wide and convex. The terminal phalanx of the finger also becomes bulbous and swollen, sometimes described as *drumstick fingers*.[5] Clubbing is rare and is a sign of severe central cyanosis (Fig. 17-1). Platelet-derived vascular endothelial growth factor is thought to play a key role in the development of clubbing.[6]

Peripheral cyanosis, a bluish discoloration of the nail bed, is more commonly seen. Peripheral cyanosis results from a reduction in the quantity of oxygen in the peripheral extremities from arterial disease or decreased cardiac output (CO). Clubbing never occurs as a result of peripheral cyanosis.

Lower Extremities. The legs are inspected for signs of peripheral arterial or venous vascular disease. The visible signs of arterial vascular disease include pale, shiny legs with sparse hair growth. Venous disease creates an edematous limb with deep red rubor, brown discoloration, and, frequently, leg ulceration. A comparison of arterial and venous disease is presented in Table 17-2.

Clubbing of Nail Beds

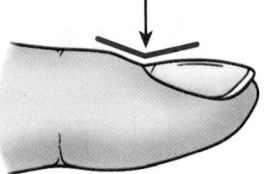

Normal nail shows a slight angle between root of nail bed and finger.

Normal Finger and Nail Bed

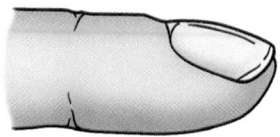

Early clubbing shows loss of angle at root of nail bed. Finger tip is of normal size.

Early Clubbing

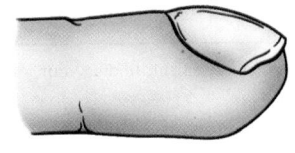

Moderate clubbing shows bulging of angle at root of nail bed. Distal finger/toe is enlarged.

Moderate Clubbing

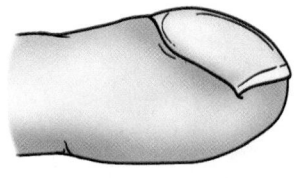

Advanced clubbing shows bulging and widening of nail bed. Distal finger/toe is bulbous.

Advanced Clubbing

Figure 17-1 Clubbing of the nail beds.

Posture. Body posture can indicate the amount of effort it takes to breathe. For example, sitting upright to breathe may be necessary for the patient with acute heart failure, and leaning forward may be the least painful position for the patient with pericarditis.

Weight. The weight in proportion to height is assessed to determine whether the patient is obese or cachectic.

Mentation. The patient is observed for signs of confusion or lethargy that may indicate hypotension, low CO, or hypoxemia.

Jugular Veins. The jugular veins of the neck are inspected for a noninvasive estimate of intravascular volume and pressure. The external jugular veins are observed for *jugular vein distention* (JVD) (Fig. 17-2 and Box 17-1). JVD is caused by an elevated central venous pressure (CVP).[7] This occurs with fluid volume overload and right ventricular dysfunction, which elevates right atrial pressure.[8] The right internal jugular vein can be used for measurement of CVP in centimeters of water (Fig. 17-3 and Box 17-2).[9-11]

Abdominojugular Reflux. The abdominojugular reflux sign can assist with the diagnosis of right ventricular failure.

TABLE 17-2   Inspection and Palpation of Extremities: Comparison of Arterial and Venous Disease

Characteristic	Arterial Disease	Venous Disease
Hair loss	Present	Absent
Skin texture	Thin, shiny, dry	Flaking, stasis, dermatitis, mottled
Ulceration	Located at pressure points; painful, pale, dry with little drainage; well-demarcated with eschar or dried; surrounded by fibrous tissue; granulation tissue scant and pale	Usually at the ankle; painless, pink, moist with large amount of drainage; irregular, dry, and scaly; surrounded by dermatitis; granulation tissue healthy
Skin color	Elevational pallor, dependent rubor	Brown patches, rubor, mottled cyanotic color when dependent
Nails	Thick, brittle	Normal
Varicose veins	Absent	Present
Temperature	Cool	Warm
Capillary refill	Greater than 3 seconds	Less than 3 seconds
Edema	None or mild, usually unilateral	Usually present foot to calf, unilateral or bilateral
Pulses	Weak or absent (0 to 1+)	Normal, strong, and symmetric

Modified from Krenzer ME: Peripheral vascular assessment: finding your way through arteries and veins, *AACN Clin Issues* 6(4):631, 1995.

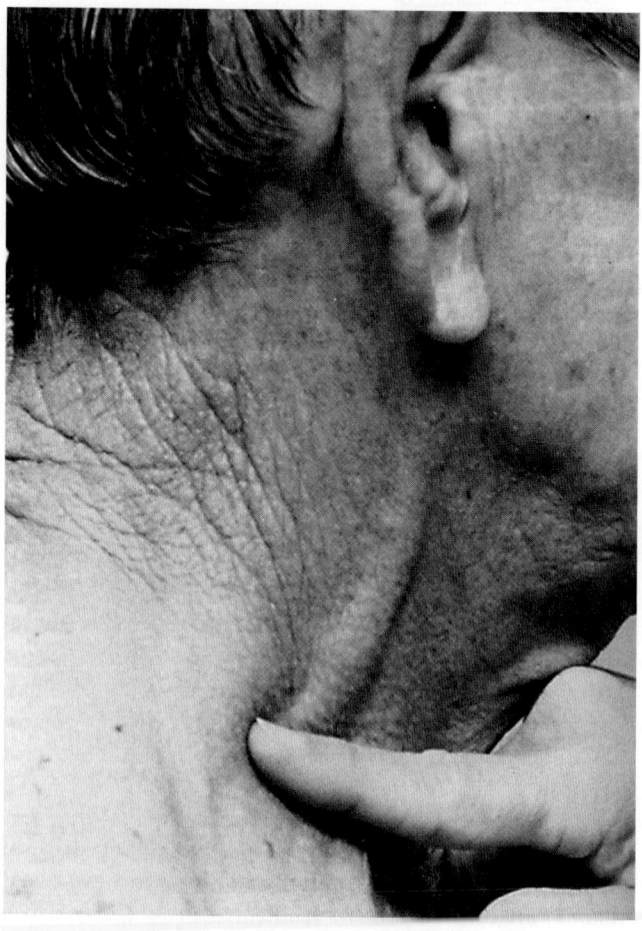

Figure 17-2 Assessment of jugular vein distention (JVD). Applying light finger pressure over the sternocleidomastoid muscle, parallel to the clavicle, helps identify the external jugular vein by occluding flow and distending it. The finger pressure is released, and the patient is observed for true distention. If the patient's trunk is elevated to 30 degrees or more, JVD should not be present.

BOX 17-1   PROCEDURE FOR ASSESSING JUGULAR VEIN DISTENTION

1. Patient reclines at a 30- to 45-degree angle.
2. The examiner stands on the patient's right side and turns the patient's head slightly toward the left.
3. If the jugular vein is not visible, light finger pressure is applied across the sternocleidomastoid muscle just above and parallel to the clavicle. This pressure fills the external jugular vein by obstructing flow (see Fig. 17-2).
4. After the location of the vein has been identified, the pressure is released, and the presence of jugular vein distention (JVD) is assessed.
5. Because inhalation decreases venous pressure, JVD should be assessed at end-exhalation.
6. Any fullness in the vein extending more than 3 cm above the sternal angle is evidence of increased venous pressure. Generally, the higher the sitting angle of the patient when JVD is visualized, the higher the central venous pressure.
7. Documentation: JVD is reported by including the angle of the head of the bed at the time JVD was evaluated (e.g., "presence of JVD with the head of the bed elevated to 45 degrees").

This noninvasive test is used in conjunction with measurement of JVD. The procedure for assessing abdominojugular reflux is described in Box 17-3. A positive abdominojugular reflux sign is an increase in the jugular venous pressure (CVP equivalent) of greater than 3 cm sustained for at least 15 seconds.[12]

Thoracic Reference Points. The thoracic cage is divided with imaginary vertical lines (sternal, midclavicular, axillary, vertebral, and scapular), and the intercostal spaces are divided with horizontal lines to serve as reference points in locating or

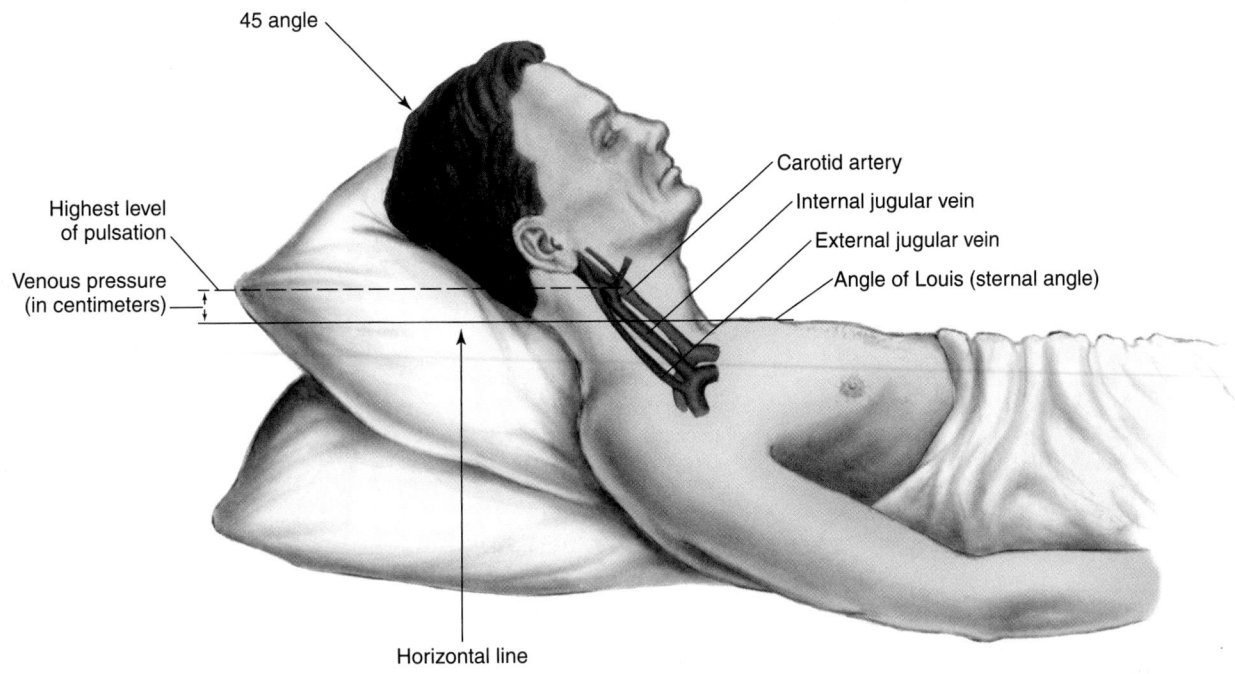

Figure 17-3 Position of internal and external jugular veins. Pulsation in the internal jugular vein can be used to estimate central venous pressure. (*Modified from Thompson JM et al:* Mosby's clinical nursing, *ed 5, St Louis, 2002, Mosby.*)

BOX 17-2	**PROCEDURE FOR ASSESSING CENTRAL VENOUS PRESSURE**

1. The patient reclines in the bed. The highest point of pulsation in the internal jugular vein is observed during exhalation.
2. The vertical distance between this pulsation (top of the fluid level) and the sternal angle is estimated or measured in centimeters.
3. This number is then added to 5 cm for an estimation of CVP. The 5 cm is the approximate distance of the sternal angle above the level of the right atrium (see Fig. 17-3).
4. Documentation: The degree of elevation of the patient is included in the report (e.g., "CVP estimated at 13 cm, using internal jugular vein pulsation, with the head of the bed elevated 45 degrees").

BOX 17-3	**PROCEDURE FOR ASSESSING ABDOMINOJUGULAR REFLUX**

1. Ask the patient to relax and breathe normally through an open mouth.
2. Measure the jugular vein distention (JVD) in the patient's right internal jugular vein, following the procedure described in Box 17-1.
3. Apply firm pressure of approximately 20 to 35 mm Hg to the patient's midabdomen for 15 to 30 seconds, and remeasure the JVD during the compression.
4. Measure the right JVD a third time after the compression is released.
5. Ask the patient not to tense or hold the breath during the test. (Doing so increases venous return to the heart and may produce a falsely positive result.)
6. A positive abdominojugular reflux (AJR) is identified when abdominal compression causes a sustained JVD increase of 4 cm or more. This sign is indicative of right-sided heart failure.
7. A normal AJR is reported if there is no rise in JVD, a transient (<10 seconds) rise in JVD, or a rise in JVD less than or equal to 3 cm sustained throughout compression.

---

describing cardiac findings (Fig. 17-4). The ribs are numbered from 1 (the first rib below the clavicle) to 12. The intercostal space below each rib is numbered the same as the rib that lies above it. The second rib is the easiest to locate, because it is attached to the sternum at the angle of Louis. This angle (also called the *sternal angle*) is the bony ridge on the sternum that lies approximately 2 inches below the sternal notch (see Fig. 17-4A). After the second rib has been located, it can be used as a reference point to count off the other ribs and intercostal spaces.

Apical Impulse. The anterior thorax is inspected for the *apical impulse,* sometimes referred to as the *point of maximal impulse* (PMI). The apical impulse occurs as the left ventricle contracts during systole and rotates forward, causing the left ventricular apex of the heart to hit the chest wall. The apical impulse is a quick, localized, outward movement normally located just lateral to the left midclavicular line at the fifth

intercostal space in the adult patient (Fig. 17-5). The apical impulse is the only normal pulsation visualized on the chest wall. In the patient without cardiac disease, PMI may not be noticeable (see Fig. 17-5).

PALPATION

Palpation is a technique that uses the sense of touch in the tips of the fingers and the palm of the hand.

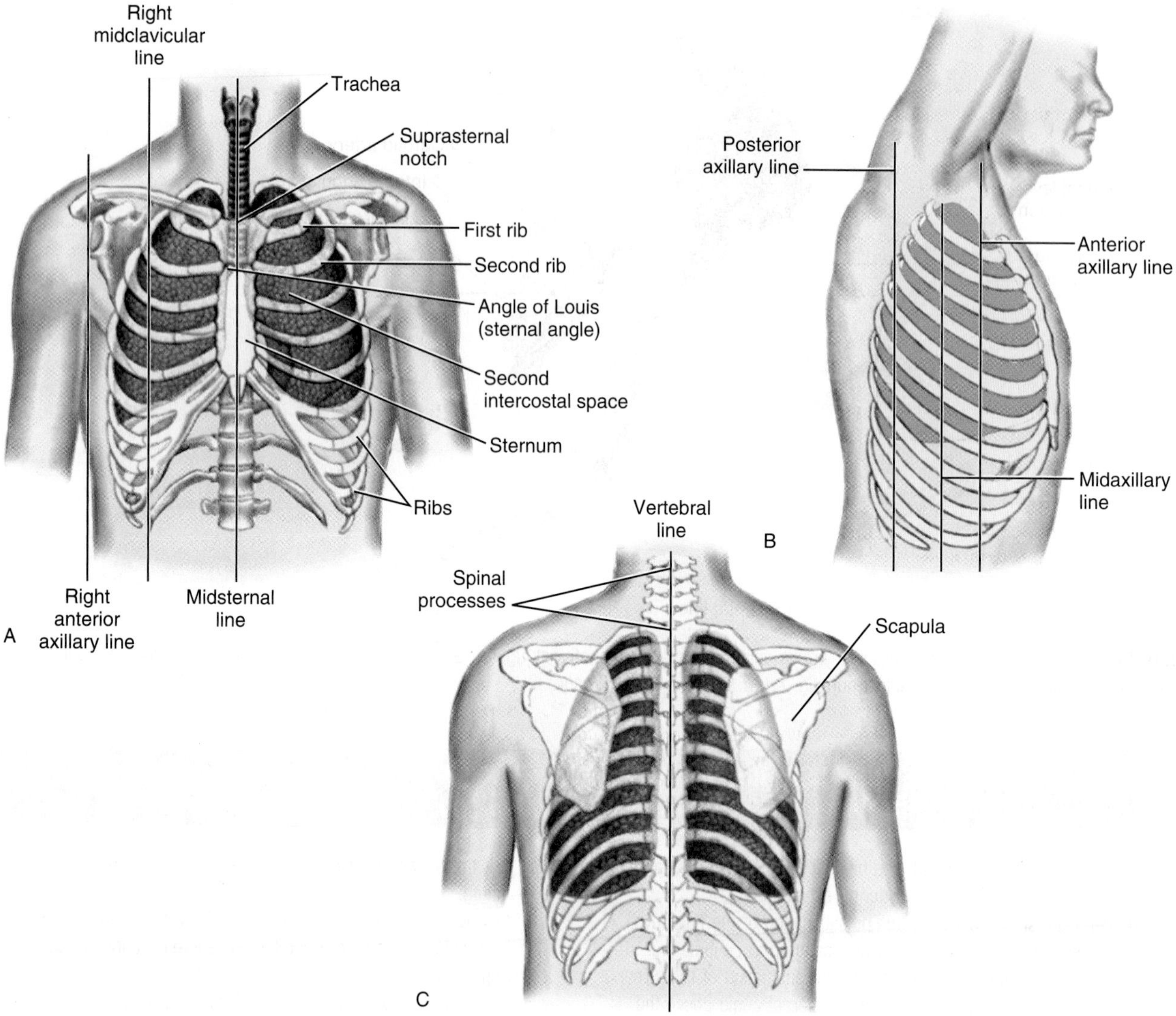

Right
midclavicular
line

Trachea

Suprasternal
notch

First rib

Second rib

Angle of Louis
(sternal angle)

Second
intercostal space

Sternum

Ribs

Right
anterior
axillary line

Midsternal
line

A

Posterior
axillary line

Anterior
axillary line

Midaxillary
line

B

Vertebral
line

Spinal
processes

Scapula

C

Figure 17-4 Thoracic landmarks. *A,* Anterior thorax. *B,* Right lateral thorax. *C,* Posterior thorax.

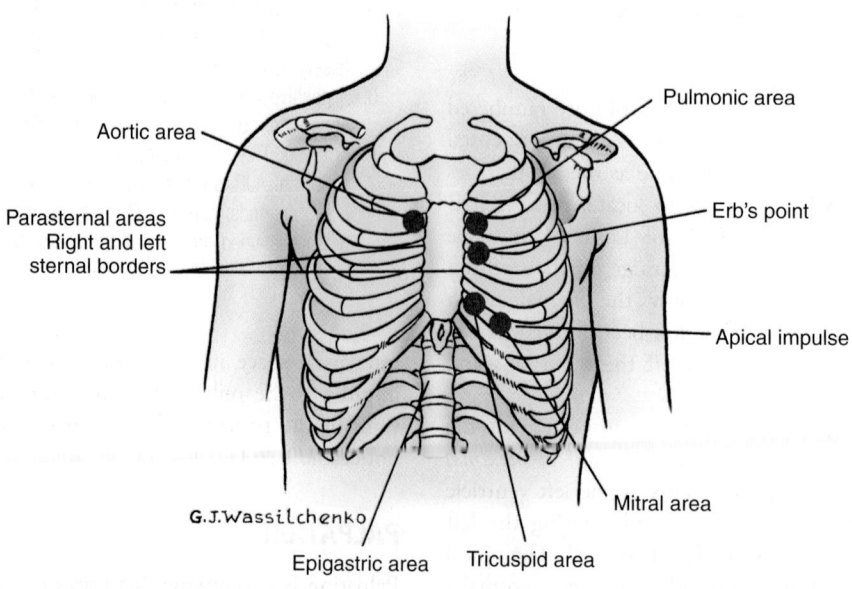

Aortic area

Pulmonic area

Parasternal areas
Right and left
sternal borders

Erb's point

Apical impulse

G.J.Wassilchenko

Mitral area

Epigastric area   Tricuspid area

Figure 17-5 Thoracic palpation and auscultation points.

Arterial Pulses. Seven pairs of bilateral arterial pulses are palpated. The examination incorporates bilateral assessment of the carotid, brachial, radial, ulnar, popliteal, dorsalis pedis, and posterior tibial arteries. The pulses are palpated separately and compared bilaterally to check for consistency. Pulse volume is graded on a scale of 0 to 3+ (Box 17-4). The abdominal aortic pulse can also be palpated.

Carotid Pulses. The carotid arteries are assessed at the medial midneck region. If blood flow through the carotid arteries is compromised by atherosclerotic plaque, firm palpation could cause total occlusion. The touch is light, and only one carotid artery at a time is gently palpated.

Brachial, Ulnar, and Radial Pulses. The brachial pulse is assessed by gently palpating the inner aspect of the slightly bent elbow with the fingers. The radial pulse is palpated in the medial area of the wrist (thumb side). The ulnar artery is palpated at the opposite side of the wrist (little finger side). The radial and ulnar arterial pulses must be assessed before an arterial line is inserted; this test, known as the *Allen test,* is described in Box 17-5.

Femoral Pulses. The femoral arteries are palpated by pressing deeply into the groin beneath the inguinal ligament, approximately midway between the anterior superior iliac spine and the symphysis pubis.

Popliteal Pulses. The popliteal pulse is palpated behind the knee. The leg is very slightly bent, and the clinician's two hands gently cup the patient's knee with the thumbs on top of the kneecap. The pulse is palpated by the fingertips, behind the knee.

Dorsalis Pedis and Posterior Tibial Pulses. The pulses of the lower leg and foot are assessed to determine flow to the limb and to assess adequacy of CO to the extremities. The dorsalis pedis pulse is located on the upper aspect of the foot. The posterior tibial pulse is located behind the medial malleolus (inner ankle bone) of the lower leg.

Descending Aorta Pulse. When the patient is lying in a supine position, the abdominal aortic pulsation is located in the epigastric area and can be felt as a forward movement when firm fingertip pressure is applied above the umbilicus. If prominent or diffuse, the pulsation may indicate an abdominal aneurysm.

A diminished or absent pulse may indicate low CO, arterial stenosis, or occlusion proximal to the site of the examination. An abnormally strong or bounding pulse suggests the presence of an aneurysm or an occlusion distal to the examination site. If a distal pulse cannot be palpated using light finger pressure, a Doppler ultrasound stethoscope can increase diagnostic accuracy.[13] It is important to mark the location of the audible signal with an indelible ink marker pen for future evaluation of pulse quality.

Capillary Refill. Capillary refill assessment is a maneuver that uses the patient's nail beds to evaluate arterial circulation to the extremity and overall perfusion. The nail bed is compressed to produce blanching, after which release of the pressure should result in a return of blood flow and baseline nail color in less than 2 seconds.[14] The severity of arterial insufficiency is directly proportional to the amount of time required to reestablish flow and color.

Edema. Edema is fluid accumulation in the extravascular spaces of the body. The dependent tissues within the legs and sacrum are particularly susceptible. The nurse should observe whether the edema is dependent, unilateral or bilateral, pitting or nonpitting. The amount of edema is quantified by measuring the circumference of the limb or by pressing the skin of the feet, ankles, and shins against the underlying bone. Edema is a symptom associated with several diseases, and further diagnostic evaluation is required to determine the cause. Although no universal scale for pitting edema exists, typical scales use a 0 to 4+ system (Table 17-3).

BOX 17-4   PULSE PALPATION SCALE

0	Not palpable
1+	Faintly palpable (weak and thready)
2+	Palpable (normal pulse)
3+	Bounding (hyperdynamic pulse)

BOX 17-5   PROCEDURE FOR ASSESSMENT OF ARTERIAL BLOOD SUPPLY TO THE HAND: THE ALLEN TEST

Before a radial artery is punctured or cannulated, the Allen test is performed to assess blood flow to the hand and ensure that it is adequate.

ALLEN TEST BY VISUAL INSPECTION

1. If the patient is alert and cooperative, he or she is asked to repeatedly make a tight fist to squeeze the blood out of the hand.
2. The radial artery is compressed with firm thumb pressure by the examiner.
3. The patient is requested to open the hand, palm side up, while the radial artery is still occluded.
4. Pressure is released, and the time it takes for the color to return to the hand is noted.
    If the ulnar artery is patent, the color will return within 3 seconds. The patient may describe a tingling in the palm as blood flow returns. Delayed color return (a "failed" Allen test) implies that the ulnar artery is

inadequate; the radial artery is the only source of blood flow to the hand and must not be punctured or cannulated.

ALLEN TEST WITH PULSE OXIMETRY

1. If the patient is unable to cooperate to make a fist, an alternative approach is to use a pulse oximeter that displays a pulse waveform.
2. Place the pulse oximeter on the middle finger and establish an adequate pulse amplitude display on the monitor.
3. Simultaneously compress the radial and ulnar arteries until the waveform clearly decreases or vanishes.
4. Release pressure off the ulnar artery only. If the ulnar artery is patent, the pulse amplitude recovers its normal appearance.
5. Repeat the procedure with the radial artery.
6. Only if there is adequate blood supply to the hand can arterial catheterization of the radial artery be accomplished safely.

TABLE 17-3   Pitting Edema Scale

Scale	Edema	INDENTATION DEPTH English Units	INDENTATION DEPTH Metric Units	Time to Baseline
0	None	0	0	
1+	Trace	0-0.25 inch	<6.5 mm	Rapid
2+	Mild	0.25-0.5 inch	6.5-12.5 mm	10-15 sec
3+	Moderate	0.5-1 inch	12.5 mm-2.5 cm	1-2 min
4+	Severe	>1 inch	>2.5 cm	2-5 min

AUSCULTATION

Blood Pressure Measurement. Blood pressure measurement is an essential component of every complete physical examination. Hypertension is diagnosed as a systolic blood pressure (SBP) of 140 mm Hg or higher, or a diastolic blood pressure (DBP) of 90 mm Hg or above.[15] Prehypertension is defined an SBP in the range of 120 to 139 mm Hg in association with a DBP between 80 to 89 mm Hg.[15,16] The incidence of hypertension in the United States has increased dramatically as a result of an aging population and an increasing prevalence of obesity. During the period from 1999 to 2000, 65 million adults in the United States were hypertensive, compared with 50 million in 1988 through 1994—an increase of 30%.[17] Risk of hypertension increases with older age. More than 90% of people who have a normal blood pressure at 55 years of age eventually develop hypertension, according to findings from the Framingham Heart Study.[16]

In the critical care setting, systemic blood pressure can be measured directly or indirectly. Arterial monitoring devices (see Chapter 18) that directly measure arterial pressure by means of an invasive technique requiring placement of an arterial catheter are considered the gold standard.[18] Correct use of a stethoscope and sphygmomanometer or electronic measuring devices can produce indirect blood pressure values that closely reflect direct measurements (within 1 to 3 mm Hg). The following discussion reviews the essential elements of noninvasive blood pressure monitoring.

Noninvasive Blood Pressure Monitoring. The most common peripheral locations for blood pressure monitoring are the bilateral brachial arteries. The pressure is measured in both arms to rule out subclavian arterial stenosis. Normally, the difference in pressure between the arms is only 5 to 10 mm Hg. A finding of more than 15 mm Hg difference between the bilateral arm pressures suggests arterial obstruction on the side with the lower pressure.[19] Asymmetry is documented so that all subsequent measurements can be made on the arm with the higher pressure.

Correct positioning of the extremity being measured is essential. As long as the arm or leg is at the level of the heart, the blood pressure can be measured in any position. Falsely elevated readings are obtained if the arm is lower than the heart, and falsely low pressures are measured if the arm is higher than the heart.[18]

Orthostatic Hypotension. When a healthy person stands, 10% to 15% of the blood volume is pooled in the legs; this reduces venous return to the right side of the heart, which decreases CO and lowers arterial blood pressure.[20] The fall in blood pressure activates baroreceptors; the subsequent reflex increase in sympathetic outflow and parasympathetic inhibition leads to peripheral vasoconstriction, with increased heart rate and contractility.[20] Postural (orthostatic) hypotension occurs when the SBP or BP drops 10 to 20 mm Hg after a change from the supine to the upright posture.[20,21] It is usually accompanied by complaints of dizziness, lightheadedness, or syncope. If a patient experiences these symptoms, it is important to complete a full set of postural vital signs before increasing the patient's activity level (Box 17-6). Orthostatic hypotension can have many causes. The three most common causes of orthostatic vital sign changes (i.e., drop in blood pressure and rise in heart rate) observed in critical care are

1. Intravascular volume depletion or fluid loss caused by bleeding, excessive diuresis, or fever
2. Inadequate vascular vasoconstrictor mechanisms to constrict the arterial bed, which can occur in elderly patients after prolonged immobility[21] or as a result of spinal cord injury
3. Autonomic insufficiency caused by administration of pharmacologic agents such as beta-blockers, angiotensin-converting enzyme (ACE) inhibitors, and calcium channel blockers

Blood Pressure Cuff Size. Correct size and placement of the inflatable bladder (inside the nondistensible cuff) are crucial to obtaining an accurate blood pressure measurement.[18] The bladder width should be 40% of the circumference of the limb (arm or leg) to be measured.[18] The length of the bladder should be long enough to encircle at least 80% of the width of the limb in adults.[18] Cuffs that are too small can give falsely high readings, and cuffs that are too large can give falsely low readings. It is also important that the meniscus of the mercury be at eye level when the blood pressure is measured.[18] Box 17-7 lists the key points to observe when obtaining standard blood pressure readings.

Korotkoff Sounds. Obtaining systemic blood pressure readings involves auscultation of *Korotkoff sounds,* the sounds created by turbulence of blood flow within a vessel caused by constriction of the blood pressure cuff. The pressure in the cuff is inflated above the normal systolic pressure. As the pressure in

BOX 17-6 MEASUREMENT OF POSTURAL (ORTHOSTATIC) VITAL SIGNS

GUIDELINES

1. Record blood pressure (BP) and heart rate (HR) in each position.
2. Do not remove cuff between measurements.
3. Record all associated signs and symptoms.
4. Clearly document patient position.

Lying

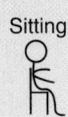
Sitting

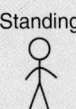
Standing

TECHNIQUE

1. Keep patient as flat as possible for 10 minutes before the initial assessment.
2. Patient supine: Obtain initial BP and HR measurements.

3. Patient sitting with legs hanging: Measure immediately and after 2 minutes.
4. Patient standing: Measure immediately and after 2 minutes. If BP and HR are stable but orthostasis is suspected, BP and HR can be repeated every 2 minutes. Note that this is rarely practical for the critically ill patient.

RESULTS

Normal Changes
HR increases by 5 to 20 beats/min (transiently).
Systolic BP drops 10 mm Hg.
Diastolic BP drops 5 mm Hg.

Positive Orthostasis
Drop in systolic BP by more than 20 mm Hg.
Drop in diastolic BP by more than 10 mm Hg within 3 minutes.

BOX 17-7 OBTAINING ACCURATE BLOOD PRESSURE READINGS

- Compare right and left measurements.
- Position the extremity at the level of the heart.
- Document the position of the patient.
- Ensure proper cuff size.
- Measure readings at eye level at top of meniscus.

---

the cuff is reduced, the Korotkoff sounds change in quality and intensity. These sounds are divided into five stages.[18] The SBP is the highest point at which initial tapping occurs. DBP is equated with the complete disappearance of Korotkoff sounds. There is often a muffling of diastolic sounds before they completely disappear. Because complete disappearance of the Korotkoff sounds corresponds more closely to intraarterial catheter measurement, this is the value that should be recorded.[18]

Auscultatory Gap. In elderly patients with systolic hypertension, the presence of an *auscultatory gap* is not uncommon. It is important to inflate the cuff to greater than the patient's normal systolic pressure to avoid this gap and a subsequent underestimation of SBP.[18] Use of an initial palpation estimate of the SBP taken before auscultation with a stethoscope is one recommended method to accurately determine the upper SBP.[18]

Automated Blood Pressure Devices. Electronic automated devices are frequently used for measuring blood pressure and have replaced the mercury sphygmomanometer in many places. The mercury used in the sphygmomanometer is a nondegradable environmental pollutant that is difficult to dispose of safely. For this reason, mercury sphygmomanometers have been phased out of use in many hospitals.[18]

In readings from automated devices, the systolic number is accurate, but the diastolic value is often calculated from the SBP and the mean arterial pressure (MAP) and therefore may not be accurate.[18] Devices placed on the arm or leg are considered accurate (as long as the cuff size is correct) for systolic measurement and trending of blood pressure. There is considerable controversy about automated devices applied to the wrist or finger, and this method should not be used to monitor blood pressure in any critically ill or cardiac patient.[18]

Automatic blood pressure cuff placement should be rotated frequently to avoid excessive irritation to the extremity, especially when the automatic cuff is set to cycle more frequently than every 15 minutes.

Pulse Pressure. *Pulse pressure* describes the difference between the systolic and diastolic values. The normal pulse pressure is 40 mm Hg (i.e., the difference between an SBP of 120 mm Hg and a DBP of 80 mm Hg). In the critically ill patient, a low blood pressure is frequently associated with a narrow pulse pressure. For example, a patient with a blood pressure of 90/72 mm Hg has a pulse pressure of 18 mm Hg. The narrowed pulse pressure is a temporary compensatory mechanism caused by arterial vasoconstriction resulting from volume depletion or heart failure. The narrow pulse pressure ensures that the MAP (78 mm Hg in this example) remains in a therapeutic range to provide adequate organ perfusion.

In contrast, a hypotensive septic patient who exhibits vasodilation will have a wide pulse pressure and inadequate organ perfusion. If the blood pressure is 90/36 mm Hg, the pulse pressure is 54 mm Hg, and the MAP calculates to an inadequate 54 mm Hg. In both of these examples, the SBP is the same (90 mm Hg); the difference in pulse pressure is a function of intravascular volume and vascular tone.

Pulsus Paradoxus. In normal physiology, the strength of the pulse fluctuates throughout the respiratory cycle. When the "pulse" is measured using the SBP, the pressure is observed to decrease slightly during inspiration and to rise slightly during respiratory exhalation. The normal difference is 2 to 4 mm Hg.[8] In some clinical conditions, such as cardiac tamponade, the blood pressure decline is abnormally large during inspiration. In general, an inspiratory decline of SBP greater than 10 mm Hg is considered diagnostic of *pulsus paradoxus*.[22-24] The traditional

MEASUREMENT WITH A SPHYGMOMANOMETER

1. The patient should be lying supine in a comfortable position.
2. The breathing pattern should be of normal depth and rate to avoid excessive respiratory interference.
3. Blood pressure is measured following standard procedures (see Boxes 17-6 and 17-7). The sphygmomanometer cuff is inflated to a pressure greater than the systolic blood pressure (SBP), and Korotkoff sounds are auscultated over the brachial artery while the cuff is deflated at rate of approximately 2 to 3 mm Hg per heartbeat.
4. The peak SBP during expiration (i.e., the pressure at which Korotkoff sounds are heard only during expiration) should be identified and then reconfirmed.
5. The cuff is then deflated slowly to establish the SBP at which Korotkoff sounds become audible during both inspiration and expiration.
6. If the auscultated difference between these two SBP values exceeds 10 mm Hg during quiet respiration, a paradoxical pulse is present.

MEASUREMENT BY WAVEFORM ANALYSIS

1. A pulse oximetry sensor with a visible pulse waveform can be used as an additional measurement device.
2. In the critical care unit, an arterial waveform from an indwelling arterial catheter (if present) can be used to measure the difference in SBP between expiration and inspiration.

First Heart Sound (S_1)
- High-pitched
- Loudest in mitral area (apex)

Split S_1
- Normal split less than 20 msec
- Split heard best in tricuspid area
- Important to differentiate between split S_1 and S_4
- Occurs immediately before carotid upstroke

Second Heart Sound (S_2)
- High-pitched
- Loudest in aortic area (base)

Split S_2
- Normal split less than 30 msec
- Split heard best in pulmonic area
- ↑ Split with inhalation
- ↓ Split with exhalation

↑, increased; ↓, decreased.

technique for measuring pulsus paradoxus using a sphygmomanometer and a blood pressure cuff[18] and pulse oximetry[22-24] is described in Box 17-8.[18] If the patient is hypotensive, pulsus paradoxus is more accurately assessed in the critical care unit by monitoring a pulse oximetry waveform or an indwelling arterial catheter waveform.[22-24]

Pulsus Alternans. *Pulsus alternans* describes a regular pattern of pulse amplitude changes that alternate between stronger and weaker beats. This finding is suggestive of end-stage left ventricular heart failure.

Vascular Bruits. The carotid and femoral arteries are auscultated for bruits. A bruit, a high-pitched "sh-sh" sound, is an extracardiac vascular sound that vacillates in volume with systole and diastole. An abnormal bruit is produced as blood flows through a partially occluded vessel. Auscultation of a bruit can expedite the diagnosis of suspected arterial obstruction.

Normal Heart Sounds. Auscultation of the heart is the most challenging part of the cardiac physical examination, and, in an era of increasing technologic demands, it is daunting to new clinicians.[25] To summarize the advice given by most experts, the examiner must do the following:

1. Auscultate systematically across the precordium.[26]
2. Visualize the cardiac anatomy under each point of auscultation, expecting to hear the physiologically associated sounds.[26]
3. Memorize the cardiac cycle to enhance the ability to hear abnormal sounds.[26]
4. Practice, practice, practice.[27]

First and Second Heart Sounds. Normal heart sounds are referred to as the *first heart sound* (S_1) and the *second heart sound* (S_2). S_1 is the sound associated with mitral and tricuspid valve closure and is heard most clearly in the mitral and tricuspid areas. S_2 (aortic and pulmonic closure) can be heard best at the second intercostal space to the right and left of the sternum (see Fig. 17-5). Both sounds are high-pitched and heard best with the diaphragm of the stethoscope (Box 17-9). Each sound is loudest in an auscultation area located downstream from the actual valvular component of the sound, as shown in Figure 17-6.

Physiologic Splitting of S_1 and S_2. Each normal heart sound has two components (right and left). Mitral valve closure and tricuspid valve closure are both responsible for S_1, and aortic valve and pulmonic valve closure are responsible for S_2. All the components of the split sounds are high-pitched and best heard with the diaphragm of the stethoscope (Fig. 17-7). Normally, sounds emitted from the left side are louder than those from the right, because left ventricular contraction occurs milliseconds before that of the right ventricle. Physiologic splitting is accentuated by inspiration and usually disappears on expiration. This splitting is most easily detected on inspiration because there is an increased blood return to the right side of the heart and a decreased amount of blood return to the left side of the heart. As a result, pulmonic valve closure is delayed because of the extra time needed for the increased blood volume to pass through the pulmonic valve, and aortic valve closure is early because of the relatively smaller amount of blood ejected from the left ventricle. The resulting heart sound is a split S_2 (the closure of each valve is audible, because there is more time between left and right contractions) (see Fig. 17-7).

Pathologic Splitting of S_1 and S_2. A variety of abnormalities can alter the intensity and timing of split heart sounds. For example, during auscultation in the pulmonic area, a pathologic split is audible with a stethoscope if the pulmonic valve closure occurs after the aortic valve closure. Pathologic splitting of S_1 and S_2 is associated with specific cardiovascular conditions such as pulmonary hypertension, pulmonic stenosis, and right ventricular failure and with electrical conduction disturbances such as right bundle branch block and premature ventricular contractions.

Aortic
Pulmonic
Tricuspid
Mitral
G.J.Wassilchenko

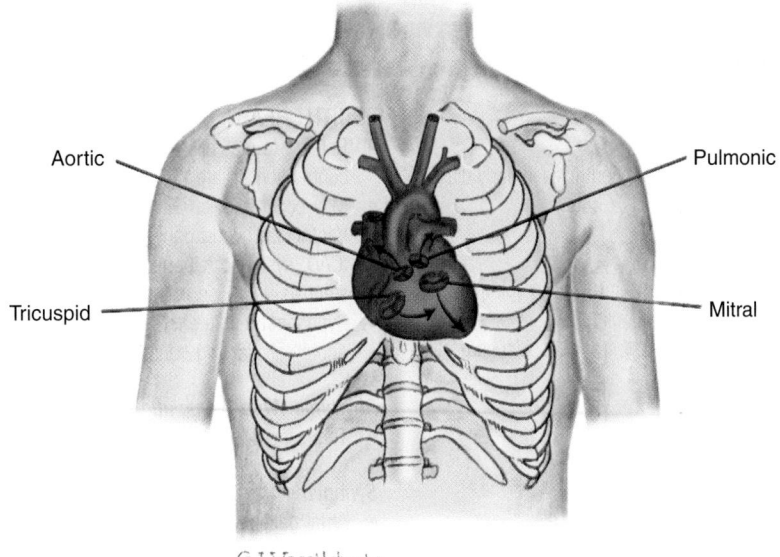

Figure 17-6 Transmission of heart sounds to the thorax and their relationship to the anatomic position of the heart valves.

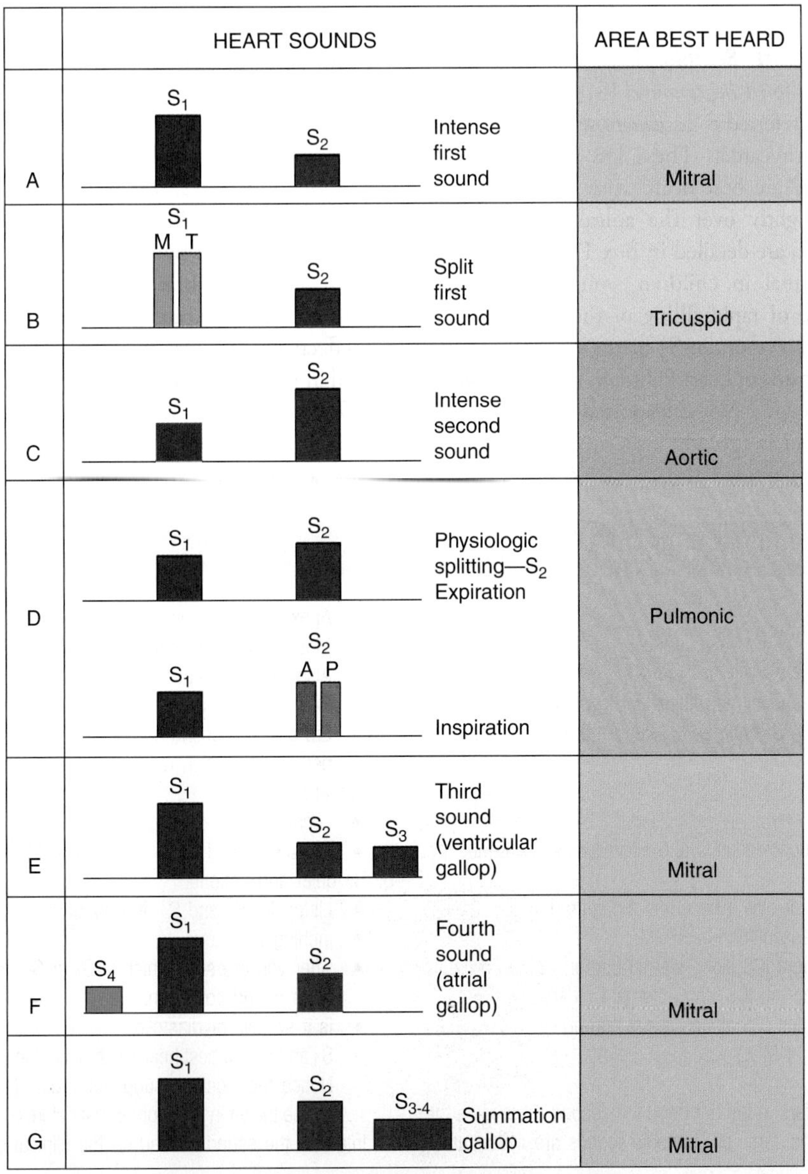

HEART SOUNDS
AREA BEST HEARD
A
S_1
S_2
Intense first sound
Mitral
B
S_1
M T
S_2
Split first sound
Tricuspid
C
S_1
S_2
Intense second sound
Aortic
D
S_1
S_2
Physiologic splitting—S_2 Expiration
S_1
S_2
A P
Inspiration
Pulmonic
E
S_1
S_2
S_3
Third sound (ventricular gallop)
Mitral
F
S_4
S_1
S_2
Fourth sound (atrial gallop)
Mitral
G
S_1
S_2
$S_{3\text{-}4}$
Summation gallop
Mitral

Figure 17-7 Characteristics of normal and abnormal heart sounds and the auscultatory area where each is best heard.

BOX 17-10 CHARACTERISTICS OF THE THIRD AND FOURTH HEART SOUNDS

THIRD HEART SOUND (S_3)

Physiologic Causes
- Related to diastolic motion and rapid filling of ventricles in early diastole
- Can be normal in children and young adults (<40 yr)

Pathologic Causes
- Ventricular dysfunction with an increase in end-systolic volume (MI, heart failure, valvular disease, systemic or pulmonary hypertension)
- Hyperdynamic states (anemia, thyrotoxicosis, mitral or tricuspid regurgitation)

Rhythmic Word Association
- Kentucky: S_1, S_2, S_3

Synonyms
- Ventricular gallop
- Protodiastolic gallop

FOURTH HEART SOUND (S_4)
- Related to diastolic motion and ventricular dilation with atrial contraction in late diastole
- May occur with or without cardiac decompensation
- Ventricular hypertrophy with a decrease in ventricular compliance (CAD, systemic hypertension, cardiomyopathy, aortic or pulmonary stenosis, increase in intensity with acute MI or angina)
- Hyperkinetic states (anemia, thyrotoxicosis, arteriovenous fistula)
- Acute valvular regurgitation

Rhythmic Word Association
- Tennessee: S_4, S_1, S_2

Synonyms
- Atrial gallop
- Presystolic gallop

CAD, coronary artery disease; MI, myocardial infarction.

Abnormal Heart Sounds

Third and Fourth Heart Sounds. The abnormal heart sounds are known as the *third heart sound* (S_3) and the *fourth heart sound* (S_4); they are referred to as *gallops* when auscultated during an episode of tachycardia. These low-pitched sounds occur during diastole and are best heard with the bell of the stethoscope positioned lightly over the apical impulse. The characteristics of S_3 and S_4 are detailed in Box 17-10. The presence of S_3 may be normal in children, young adults, and pregnant women because of rapid filling of the ventricle in a young, healthy heart.[28] However, an S_3 in the presence of cardiac symptoms is an indicator of heart failure in a noncompliant ventricle with fluid overload.[29] Not unexpectedly, the development of an S_3 heart sound is strongly associated with elevated levels of brain natriuretic peptide (BNP).[29,30]

Auscultation of an S_4 also leads the examiner to suspect heart failure and decreased ventricular compliance. An S_4, also referred to as an atrial gallop, occurs at the end of diastole (just before S_1), when the ventricle is full. It is associated with atrial contraction, also called atrial kick.

Heart Murmurs. *Heart valve murmurs* are prolonged extra sounds that occur during systole or diastole. Murmurs are produced by turbulent flood flow through the chambers of the heart, which results in vibrations that occur during systole or diastole. Most murmurs are caused by structural cardiac changes. The steps to effectively and accurately auscultate for cardiac murmurs are listed in Box 17-11. Murmurs are characterized by specific criteria:

Timing: place in the cardiac cycle (systole/diastole)

Location: where it is auscultated on the chest wall (mitral/aortic area)

BOX 17-11 TECHNIQUE OF AUSCULTATION OF HEART SOUNDS AND MURMURS

1. Stethoscope
   - Diaphragm
     Larger surface area
     Brings out higher frequency and filters out low frequency
     Use for listening to S_1/S_2 (split S_1/S_2), loud murmurs, pericardial friction rubs
   - Bell
     Smaller surface area
     Filters out high-frequency sounds and accentuates low-frequency sounds
     Rest lightly on area (or else it becomes a diaphragm)
2. Location: heart sounds auscultated at APTM
   A: aortic area (second right ICS along sternal border)
   P: pulmonic area (second left ICS along sternal border)
   T: tricuspid area (fourth left ICS along sternal border)
   M: mitral area (fifth ICS at MCL)
3. "Know your bases"
   - Base of the heart refers to the right and left second ICS beside the sternum S_2 where the aortic or pulmonic sounds are auscultated

   - Apex or left ventricular area refers to the fifth ICS along the MCL
     Most commonly referred to as the PMI
     Also referred to as the mitral area
     S_1 and mitral sounds are loudest here
   - Erb's point: second aortic area (third left ICS along sternal border); pericardial friction rubs are heard best here
4. Palpation
   - Location
   - Palpate carotid pulse (or watch ECG to identify S_1 and S_2)
5. Be quiet and patient!
   - Listen for S_1 and S_2 first, ignoring all other sounds.
   - Inching technique
   - After you are sure which is S_1 or S_2, try to determine when the other sound comes in,
   - Is it systolic or diastolic?
   - S_3 and S_4 are best heard with patient in left lateral decubitus position. Notice the location (suggests origin of sound). Notice the timing (S_4 comes just before S_1, and S_3 comes just after S_2).
6. Interpret the sounds based on the clinical condition.

ECG, electrocardiogram; ICS, intercostal space; MCL, midclavicular line; PMI, point of maximal impulse.

Radiation: how far the sound spreads across chest wall

Quality: whether the murmur is blowing, grating, or harsh

Pitch: whether the tone is high or low

Intensity: the loudness is graded on a scale of 1 through 6; the higher the number, the louder the murmur (Box 17-12).

The four most common valvular murmurs auscultated in adults are briefly discussed in the following paragraphs. For more information on valvular anatomy, refer to Chapter 16.

Mitral Stenosis. Mitral stenosis describes a narrowing of the mitral valve orifice. This produces a low-pitched murmur, which varies in intensity and harshness depending on the degree of valvular stenosis. It occurs during diastole, is auscultated at the mitral area (fifth intercostal space, midclavicular line), and does not radiate. As the mitral stenosis progresses, left atrial enlargement occurs, often leading to atrial fibrillation and the development of left atrial thrombi.[31] The increased left atrial pressure also creates pulmonary congestion, breathlessness, moist cough, and symptoms of right-sided heart failure.

Mitral Regurgitation. Mitral regurgitation is described as acute or chronic. Causes of acute mitral regurgitation include rupture of a papillary muscle after an acute myocardial infarction and rupture of one or more chordae tendineae. As a result, when the ventricle contracts during systole, a jet of blood is sent retrograde to the left atrium, causing a sudden increase in left atrial pressure, acute pulmonary edema, and low CO and leading to cardiogenic shock. Chronic mitral regurgitation is most often seen in the elderly as the valve structures sag and stretch over time. The murmur of mitral regurgitation is auscultated in the mitral area and occurs during systole. It is high-pitched and blowing, although the pitch and intensity vary depending on the degree of regurgitation.[31] As mitral regurgitation progresses, it radiates more widely, sometimes to under the left arm.

Aortic Stenosis. Aortic stenosis describes a narrowing of the aortic valve orifice. As a result, the left ventricle faces increasing difficulty in ejecting blood to the aorta. The ventricle responds by increasing intraventricular pressure and adding muscle mass (left ventricular hypertrophy), but over time, due to the pressure load and the stenotic aortic valve, the left ventricle will fail and lose contractile force. The decreased blood volume entering the aorta during systole means that the coronary arteries do not fill efficiently, and chest pain is a common symptom of aortic stenosis. This chest pain can be difficult to differentiate from angina caused by CAD, especially in the older adult.[32] Other symptoms include dizziness, syncope, and breathlessness caused by left-sided heart failure. After symptoms occur, the clinical course is poor unless the aortic valve is replaced. Two years after onset of aortic stenosis symptoms, survival is poor without aortic valve replacement.[32] The murmur of aortic stenosis occurs during systole. It is auscultated at the aortic area (second intercostal space, right sternal border). Aortic stenosis produces a low-pitched murmur that does not radiate, although the tone of the murmur varies depending on the degree of valvular obstruction. Because there is not a strong correlation between the loudness of the murmur, clinical symptoms, and the severity of the stenosis, it is advisable to perform an echocardiogram to visualize the valve after an aortic stenosis murmur is detected.[33]

Aortic Insufficiency. Aortic regurgitation, also commonly known as aortic insufficiency, describes an incompetent aortic valve. It is often described in layperson's terms as a "leaking valve." After the left ventricle has ejected blood into the aorta, the valve normally closes, maintains a tight seal, and prevents blood from moving back into the left ventricle. If the valve cusps do not maintain this seal, the sound of blood flowing back into the left ventricle during diastole is heard as a decrescendo high-pitched, blowing murmur.[34] This early diastolic murmur is initially audible at the aortic area (second intercostal space, right sternal border), but as the aortic regurgitation progresses, it can be auscultated along the length of the left sternal border.[32] As with all valvular murmurs, the pitch and intensity vary with the degree of regurgitation. Box 17-13 provides expected abnormal findings at each of the key auscultatory areas; Table 17-4 compares the features of the most common valvular murmurs.

Innocent Murmurs. In children, adolescents, and healthy young adults, systolic "high-flow" murmurs are common and are a result of vigorous ventricular contraction. These nonpathologic murmurs are termed *innocent murmurs*. They are always systolic, have a low to medium pitch (heard best with the bell of the stethoscope), and are grade 1 to 2 intensity with a blowing quality. They are often heard best in the tricuspid area and do not radiate (Box 17-14).

Murmurs Associated With Myocardial Infarction. At the bedside, the nurse is often the first person to auscultate a new murmur. The holosystolic or pansystolic murmurs that can occur acutely as a complication of myocardial infarction are good examples.

BOX 17-12 GRADING OF CARDIAC MURMURS

Grade	Description
1	Very faint; may be heard only in a quiet environment
2	Quiet but clearly audible
3	Moderately loud
4	Loud; may be associated with a palpable thrill
5	Very loud; thrill easily palpable
6	Very loud; may be heard with stethoscope off the chest Thrill palpable and visible

---

BOX 17-13 AUSCULTATION OF THE CARDIAC VALVES

AORTIC AREA
- S_2 loud
- Aortic systolic murmur

PULMONIC AREA
- S_2 loud and split with inhalation
- Pulmonic valve murmurs

ERB'S POINT
- S_2 split with inhalation
- Aortic diastolic murmur
- Pericardial friction rub

TRICUSPID AREA
- S_1 split
- Right ventricular S_3 and S_4
- Tricuspid valve murmurs
- Murmur of ventricular septal defect

MITRAL AREA
- S_1 loud
- Left ventricular S_3 and S_4
- Mitral valve murmurs

TABLE 17-4 Characteristics of Some Murmurs

Defects	Timing in the Cardiac Cycle	Pitch, Intensity, Quality	Location, Radiation
Systolic Murmurs			
Mitral regurgitation	S_1 — S_2	High Harsh Blowing	Mitral area May radiate to axilla
Tricuspid regurgitation	S_1 — S_2	High Often faint, but varies Blowing	Tricuspid RLSB, apex, LLSB, epigastric areas Little radiation
Ventricular septal defect	S_1 — S_2	High Loud Blowing	Left sternal border
Aortic stenosis	S_1 — S_2	Chhhh hh Medium Rough, harsh	Aortic area to suprasternal notch, right side of neck, apex
Pulmonary stenosis	S_1 — S_2	Low to medium Loud Harsh, grinding	Pulmonic area No radiation
Diastolic Murmurs			
Mitral stenosis	S_2 — Atrial kick — S_1	Low Quiet to loud with thrill Rough rumble	Mitral area Usually no radiation
Tricuspid stenosis	S_2 — Atrial kick — S_1	Medium Quiet; louder with inspiration Rumble	Tricuspid area or epigastrium Little radiation
Aortic regurgitation	S_2 — S_1	High Faint to medium Blowing	Aortic area to LLSB and aorta Erb's point
Pulmonic regurgitation	S_2 — S_1	Medium Faint Blowing	Pulmonic area No radiation

Atrial kick, atrial contraction; LLSB, left lower sternal border; RLSB, right lower sternal border.

> ### BOX 17-14   DESCRIPTION OF INNOCENT MURMURS
>
> - Always systolic
> - Soft, short (grade 1 or 2, low pitched)
> - Modified by change in position
> - Normal S_2
> - Most common at left sternal border

Papillary Muscle Rupture. The auscultation of a new, high-pitched, holosystolic, blowing murmur at the cardiac apex heralds mitral valve regurgitation resulting from papillary muscle dysfunction. This murmur may be soft (grade 1 or 2) and may occur only during ischemic episodes when the papillary muscle contractility is impaired, but its presence is associated with persistent pain, ventricular failure, and higher mortality. If the murmur is loud (grade 5 or 6), harsh, and radiating in all directions from the apex, the papillary muscle or chordae tendineae may have ruptured. The clinical auscultation of a new murmur should be confirmed by transthoracic or transesophageal echocardiography (TEE).[35] Papillary muscle rupture is an emergency situation requiring immediate medical and surgical intervention.

Ventricular Septal Rupture. Ventricular septal rupture is a rare emergency situation that can occur after an acute myocardial infarction. Ventricular septal rupture describes a new opening in the septum between the two ventricles. It creates a harsh, holosystolic murmur that is loudest (by auscultation) along the left sternal border. The clinical picture associated with acute ventricular septal rupture is that of acute ventricular failure and cardiogenic shock. Immediate diagnosis and treatment are necessary to prevent death.

Cardiac Rubs

Pericardial Friction Rub. A *pericardial friction rub* is a sound that can occur within 2 to 7 days after a myocardial infarction. The friction rub results from pericardial inflammation *(pericarditis)*. Classically, a pericardia friction rub is a grating or scratching sound that is both systolic and diastolic, corresponding with cardiac motion within the pericardial sac. It is often associated with chest pain, which can be aggravated by deep inspiration, coughing, swallowing, and changing position. It is important to differentiate pericarditis from acute myocardial ischemia, and the detection of a pericardial friction rub through auscultation can assist in this differentiation, leading to effective diagnosis and treatment.

Summary

- An accurate history from the patient, or from a family member or significant other who knows the individual's current state of health, is essential. Signs and symptoms experienced by the patient offer clues as to the underlying causes of the cardiac condition. If the patient exhibits obvious signs of acute distress (shortness of breath, pink-frothy sputum, hypotension, tachycardia, pallor, sweating), or complains of chest pain or pressure, the questions are brief and focused in order to identify the immediate problem.
- Inspection is used to identify whether the patient is anxious or relaxed. Inspection is also employed to identify serious conditions such as cyanosis, clubbing of the fingernails, or significant peripheral edema.
- Palpation of the major pulses is a routine part of the cardiovascular physical exam. Normally pulses are equal bilaterally., and loss of a pulse on one side may indicate the presence of atherosclerotic arterial vascular disease.
- Auscultation of heart sounds and murmurs is a skill that takes time and practice to master. When performed skillfully, the auscultation can reveal much about cardiac function and blood flow.

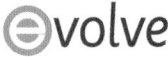 Be sure to check out the bonus material, including free self-assessment exercises, on the Evolve web site at http://evolve.elsevier.com/Urden/.

References

1. Ang D et al: Mechanisms of heartburn, *Nat Clin Pract Gastroenterol Hepatol* 5(7):383-392 2008.
2. Faybush EM, Fass R: Gastroesophageal reflux disease in noncardiac chest pain, *Gastroenterol Clin North Am* 33(1):41-54, 2004.
3. Chun AA, McGee SR: Bedside diagnosis of coronary artery disease: a systematic review, *Am J Med* 117(5):334-343, 2004.
4. Marrie TJ, Brown N: Clubbing of the digits, *Am J Med* 120(11):940-941, 2007.
5. Spicknall KE et al: Clubbing: an update on diagnosis, differential diagnosis, pathophysiology, and clinical relevance, *J Am Acad Dermatol* 52(6): 1020-1028, 2005.
6. Martinez-Lavin M: Exploring the cause of the most ancient clinical sign of medicine: finger clubbing, *Semin Arthritis Rheum* 36(6):380-385, 2007.
7. Vinayak AG et al: Usefulness of the external jugular vein examination in detecting abnormal central venous pressure in critically ill patients, *Arch Intern Med* 166(19):2132-2137, 2006.
8. Brennan JM et al: A comparison by medicine residents of physical examination versus hand-carried ultrasound for estimation of right atrial pressure, *Am J Cardiol* 99(11):1614-1616, 2007.
9. Drazner MH et al: Prognostic importance of elevated jugular venous pressure and a third heart sound in patients with heart failure, *N Engl J Med* 345(8):574-581, 2001.
10. Drazner MH et al: Third heart sound and elevated jugular venous pressure as markers of the subsequent development of heart failure in patients with asymptomatic left ventricular dysfunction, *Am J Med* 114(6):431-437, 2003.
11. Sinisalo J et al: Simplifying the estimation of jugular venous pressure, *Am J Cardiol* 100(12):1779-1781, 2007.
12. Wiese J: The abdominojugular reflux sign, *Am J Med* 109(1):59-61, 2000.

13. Khan NA et al: Does the clinical examination predict lower extremity peripheral arterial disease? *JAMA* 295(5):536-546, 2006.

14. Lewin J, Maconochie I: Capillary refill time in adults, *Emerg Med J* 25(6):325-326, 2008.

15. Chobanian AV et al: Seventh report of the Joint National Committee on Prevention, Detection, Evaluation, and Treatment of High Blood Pressure, *Hypertension* 42(6):1206-1252, 2003.

16. Chobanian AV: Prehypertension revisited, *Hypertension* 48(5):812-814, 2006.

17. Fields LE et al: The burden of adult hypertension in the United States 1999 to 2000: a rising tide, *Hypertension* 44(4):398-404, 2004.

18. Perloff D et al: *Human blood pressure determination by sphygmomanometry*, ed 6, Dallas, TX, 2001, American Heart Association.

19. Shadman R et al: Subclavian artery stenosis: prevalence, risk factors, and association with cardiovascular diseases, *J Am Coll Cardiol* 44(3):618-623, 2004.

20. Naschitz JE, Rosner I: Orthostatic hypotension: framework of the syndrome, *Postgrad Med J* 83(983):568-574, 2007.

21. Marcus GM et al: Relationship between accurate auscultation of a clinically useful third heart sound and level of experience, *Arch Intern Med* 166(6):617-622, 2006.

22. Swami A, Spodick DH: Pulsus paradoxus in cardiac tamponade: a pathophysiologic continuum, *Clin Cardiol* 26(5):215-217, 2003.

23. Stone MK et al: Respiratory changes in the pulse-oximetry waveform associated with pericardial tamponade, *Clin Cardiol* 29(9):411-414, 2006.

24. Wu LA, Nishimura RA: Images in clinical medicine: pulsus paradoxus, *N Engl J Med* 349(7):666, 2003.

25. Treadway K: Heart sounds, *N Engl J Med* 354(11):1112-1113, 2006.

26. Chizner MA: Cardiac auscultation: rediscovering the lost art, *Curr Probl Cardiol* 33(7):326-408, 2008.

27. Barrett MJ et al: Mastering cardiac murmurs: the power of repetition, *Chest* 126(2):470-475, 2004.

28. Mehta NJ, Khan IA: Third heart sound: genesis and clinical importance, *Int J Cardiol* 97(2):183-186, 2004.

29. Shah SJ et al: Physiology of the third heart sound: novel insights from tissue Doppler imaging, *J Am Soc Echocardiogr* 21(4):394-400, 2008.

30. Marcus GM et al: Usefulness of the third heart sound in predicting an elevated level of B-type natriuretic peptide, *Am J Cardiol* 93(10):1312-1313, 2004.

31. Segal BL: Valvular heart disease, part 2: mitral valve disease in older adults, *Geriatrics* 58(10):26-31, 2005.

32. Segal BL: Valvular heart disease, part 1: diagnosis and surgical management of aortic valve disease in older adults, *Geriatrics* 58(9):31-35, 2003.

33. Attenhofer Jost CH et al: Echocardiography in the evaluation of systolic murmurs of unknown cause, *Am J Med* 108(8):614-620, 2000.

34. Heidenreich PA et al: A systolic murmur is a common presentation of aortic regurgitation detected by echocardiography, *Clin Cardiol* 27(9):502-506, 2004.

35. Czarnecki A et al: Acute severe mitral regurgitation: consideration of papillary muscle architecture, *Cardiovasc Ultrasound* 6:5, 2008.

Cardiovascular
Diagnostic Procedures

CARDIOVASCULAR ASSESSMENT AND MONITORING

BEDSIDE HEMODYNAMIC MONITORING

Hemodynamic monitoring is at a critical juncture. The technology that launched invasive hemodynamic monitoring is more than 30 years old, and the search to find viable replacement monitoring technologies that are minimal or noninvasive is intense. This has created a new challenge in critical care. Although the use of invasive therapies is declining, they are still employed for hemodynamically unstable patients. Critical care nurses must be knowledgeable about traditional hemodynamic monitoring methods and be able to apply established physiologic principles in new situations. As the technology evolves, the critical care nurse will apply the same physiologic principles to the new methods to ensure safety and optimal outcomes for each patient. This discussion of hemodynamic monitoring describes established and emerging technologies.

Equipment. A traditional hemodynamic monitoring system has four component parts as shown in Figure 18-1 and described in the following list:

1. An invasive catheter and high-pressure tubing connect the patient to the transducer.
2. The transducer receives the physiologic signal from the catheter and tubing and converts it into electrical energy.
3. The flush system maintains patency of the fluid-filled system and catheter.
4. The bedside monitor contains the amplifier with recorder, which increases the volume of the electrical signal and displays it on an oscilloscope and on a digital scale in millimeters of mercury (mm Hg).

Although many different types of invasive catheters can be inserted to monitor hemodynamic pressures, all such catheters are connected to similar equipment (see Fig. 18-1). Even so, there remains considerable variation in the way different hospitals configure their hemodynamic systems. The basic setup consists of the following:

- A bag of 0.9% sodium chloride (normal saline) is used as a flush solution. In some hospitals heparin is added as an anticoagulant. A pressure infusion cuff covers the bag of flush solution and is inflated to 300 mm Hg.
- The system contains intravenous tubing, three-way stopcocks, and an in-line flow device attached for continuous

fluid infusion and manual flush. High-pressure tubing must be used to connect the invasive catheter to the transducer to prevent damping (flattening) of the waveform.
- A pressure transducer is used. Modern transducers are disposable, use a silicon chip, and are highly accurate.

Heparin. The use of the anticoagulant heparin added to the normal saline (NS) flush setup to maintain catheter patency remains controversial. A systematic review of the literature showed that a heparinized flush solution is associated with a longer duration of catheter patency.[1] Other units do not use heparin because of concern about development of the autoimmune condition known as heparin-induced thrombocytopenia (HIT). This is sometimes described as a "heparin allergy" and, when present, is associated with a dramatic drop in platelet count, and thrombus formation. Some trials have not found platelet counts or catheter duration to be influenced by heparin.[2,3] If heparin is used in the flush infusion, monitoring the trend in the platelet count is recommended.[4]

The flush solutions and tubing are usually changed every 72-96 hours. There is variety; some hospitals change flush solutions every 24 hours. For this reason, it is essential to be familiar with the specific written procedures that concern hemodynamic monitoring equipment in each critical care unit.

Calibration of Equipment. To ensure accuracy of hemodynamic pressure readings, two baseline measurements are necessary:

1. Calibration of the system to atmospheric pressure, also known as *zeroing the transducer*
2. Determination of the phlebostatic axis for transducer height placement, also called *leveling the transducer*[5]

Zeroing the Transducer. To calibrate the equipment to atmospheric pressure, referred to as zeroing the transducer, the three-way stopcock nearest to the transducer is turned simultaneously to open the transducer to air (atmospheric pressure) and to close it to the patient and the flush system. The monitor is adjusted so that "0" is displayed, which equals atmospheric pressure. Atmospheric pressure is not zero; it is 760 mm Hg at sea level. Using zero to represent current atmospheric pressure provides a convenient baseline for hemodynamic measurement purposes.

Some monitors also require calibration of the upper scale limit while the system remains open to air. At the end of the calibration procedure, the stopcock is returned to the closed position

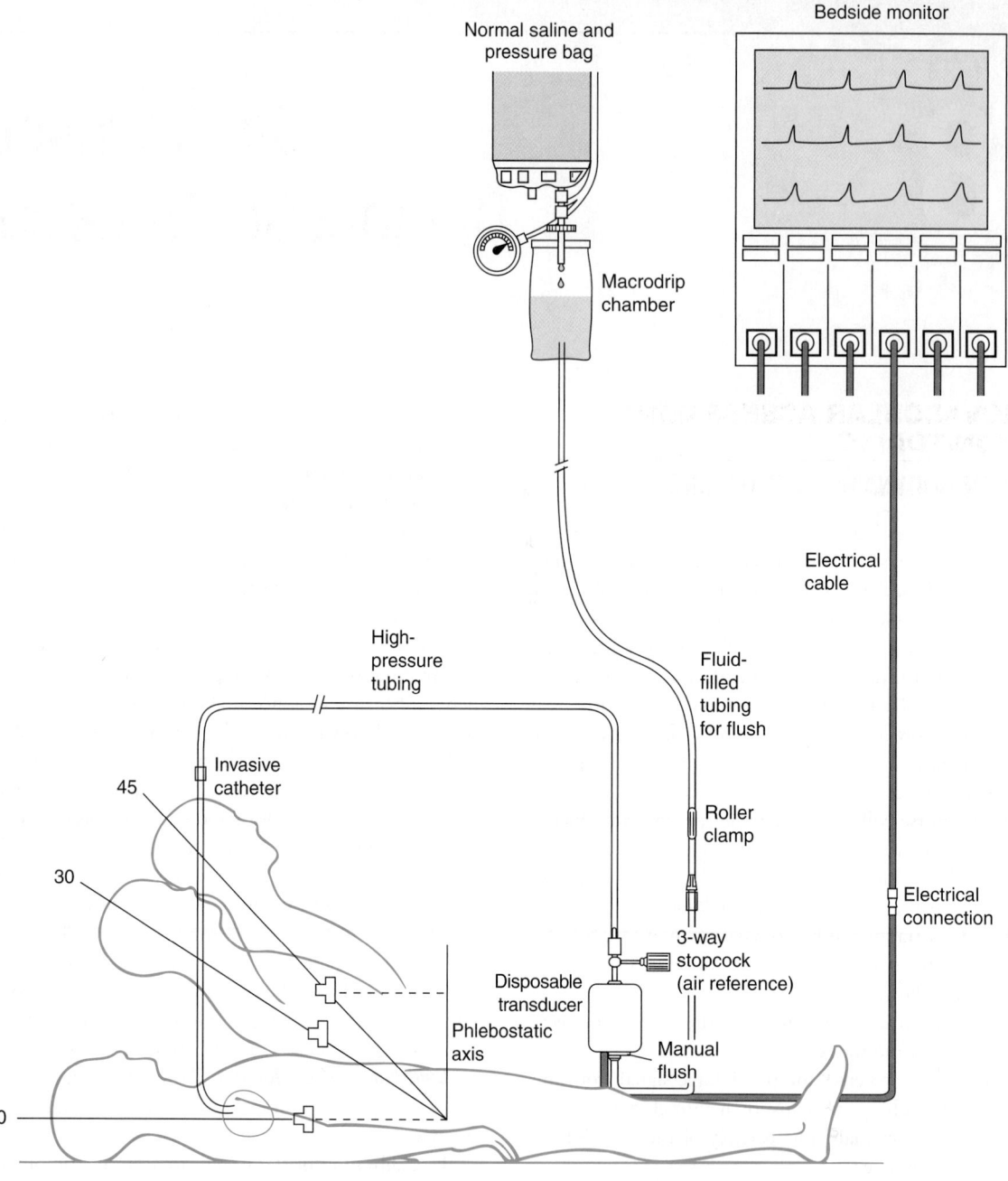

Normal saline and
pressure bag

Bedside monitor

Macrodrip
chamber

High-
pressure
tubing

Electrical
cable

Fluid-
filled
tubing
for flush

Invasive
catheter

45

Roller
clamp

30

Electrical
connection

3-way
stopcock
(air reference)

Disposable
transducer

Phlebostatic
axis

Manual
flush

0

Patient with invasive catheter

Figure 18-1 The four parts of a hemodynamic monitoring include an invasive catheter attached to high-pressure tubing to connect to the transducer; a transducer; a flush system, including a manual flush; and a bedside monitor.

and a closed cap is placed over the open port. At this point, the patient's waveform and hemodynamic pressures are displayed.

Disposable transducers are very accurate, and after they are calibrated to atmospheric pressure, drift from the zero baseline is minimal. Although in theory this means that repeated calibration is unnecessary, clinical protocols in most units require the nurse to calibrate the transducer at the beginning of each shift for quality assurance.

Phlebostatic Axis. The phlebostatic axis is a physical reference point on the chest that is used as a baseline for consistent

transducer height placement. To obtain the axis, a theoretic line is drawn from the fourth intercostal space, where it joins the sternum to a midaxillary line on the side of the chest. The midaxillary line is one half of the anteroposterior depth of the lateral chest wall.[5] This point approximates the level of the atria, as shown in Figure 18-1. It is used as the reference mark for central venous pressure (CVP) and pulmonary artery catheter transducers. The level of the transducer "air reference stopcock" approximates the position of the tip of an invasive hemodynamic monitoring catheter within the chest.

NIC

Invasive Hemodynamic Monitoring

Definition

Measurement and interpretation of invasive hemodynamic parameters to determine cardiovascular function and regulate therapy as appropriate

Activities

Assist with insertion and removal of invasive hemodynamic lines.

Assist with Allen test for evaluation of collateral ulnar circulation before radial artery cannulation, if appropriate.

Assist with chest x-ray examination after insertion of pulmonary artery catheter.

Zero and calibrate equipment every 4 to 12 hours, as appropriate, with transducer at the level of the right atrium.

Monitor blood pressure (systolic, diastolic, and mean), central venous/right atrial pressure, pulmonary artery pressure (systolic, diastolic, and mean), and pulmonary artery occlusion pressure.

Monitor hemodynamic waveforms for changes in cardiovascular function.

Compare hemodynamic parameters with other clinical signs and symptoms.

Use closed-system cardiac output setup.

Obtain cardiac output by administering cardiac output injectate within 4 seconds, and average three injections that are within less than 1 L of each other.

Monitor pulmonary artery and systemic arterial waveforms; if damping occurs, check tubing for kinks or air bubbles, check connections, aspirate clot from tip of catheter, gently flush system, or assist with repositioning of catheter.

Document pulmonary artery and systemic arterial waveforms.

Monitor peripheral perfusion distal to catheter insertion site every 4 hours or as appropriate.

Monitor for dyspnea, fatigue, tachypnea, and orthopnea.

Monitor for forward progression of pulmonary catheter resulting in spontaneous wedge, and notify physician if it occurs.

Refrain from inflating balloon more frequently than every 1 to 2 hours, or as appropriate.

Monitor for balloon rupture (e.g., assess for resistance when inflating balloon and allow balloon to passively deflate after obtaining pulmonary artery occlusion pressure).

Prevent air emboli (e.g., remove air bubbles from tubing; if balloon rupture is suspected, refrain from attempts to reinflate balloon and clamp balloon port).

Maintain sterility of ports.

Maintain closed-pressure system to ports, as appropriate.

Perform sterile dressing changes and site care, as appropriate.

Inspect insertion site for signs of bleeding or infection.

Change IV solution and tubing every 24 to 72 hours, based on protocol.

Monitor laboratory results to detect possible catheter-induced infection.

Administer fluid and/or volume expanders to maintain hemodynamic parameters within specified range.

Administer pharmacologic agents to maintain hemodynamic parameters within specified range.

Instruct patient and family on therapeutic use of hemodynamic monitoring catheters.

Instruct patient on activity restriction while catheters remain in place.

From Bulechek GM et al: *Nursing interventions classification (NIC)*, ed 5, 2008, St Louis, Mosby.

Leveling the Transducer. Leveling the transducer is different from zeroing. This process aligns the transducer with the level of the left atrium. The purpose is to line up the *air-fluid interface* with the left atrium to correct for changes in *hydrostatic pressure* in blood vessels above and below the level of the heart.[5]

A carpenter's level or laser-light level can be used to ensure that the transducer is parallel with the phlebostatic axis reference point. When there is a change in the patient's position, the transducer must be leveled again to ensure accurate hemodynamic pressure measurements are obtained.[5] Errors in measurement can occur if the transducer is placed below the phlebostatic axis because the fluid in the system weighs on the transducer, creating additional hydrostatic pressure, and produces a falsely high reading. For every inch the transducer is below the tip of the catheter, the fluid pressure in the system increases the measurement by 1.87 mm Hg. For example, if the transducer is positioned 6 inches below the tip of the catheter, this falsely elevates the displayed pressure by 11 mm Hg.

If the transducer is placed above this atrial level, gravity and lack of fluid pressure will give an erroneously low reading. For every inch the transducer is positioned above the catheter tip, the measurement is 1.87 mm Hg less than the true value. If several clinicians are taking measurements, the reference point can be marked on the side of the patient's chest to ensure accurate measurements.[5] The Nursing Interventions Classification (NIC) feature on Invasive Hemodynamic Monitoring summarizes other nursing activities associated with hemodynamic monitoring.

Patient Position. Position of the hemodynamically monitored patient would not be an issue if critical care patients only lay flat in the bed. However, lying flat is not always a comfortable position, especially if the patient is alert or if the head of the bed needs to be elevated to decrease the work of breathing.

Head of Bed Position. Nurse researchers have determined that the CVP, pulmonary artery pressure (PAP), and pulmonary artery occlusion pressure (PAOP, also called *pulmonary artery wedge pressure* [PAWP]) can be reliably measured at head-of-bed positions from 0 (flat) to 60 degrees if the patient is lying on his or her back (supine).[5] If the patient is normovolemic and hemodynamically stable, raising the head of the bed usually does not affect hemodynamic pressure measurements. If the patient is so hemodynamically unstable or hypovolemic that raising the head of the bed negatively affects intravascular volume distribution, the first priority is to correct the hemodynamic instability and leave the patient in a supine position. In summary, most patients do not need the head of the bed to be lowered to 0 degrees to obtain accurate CVP, PAP, or PAOP readings.

Lateral Position. The landmarks for leveling the transducer are different if the patient is turned to the side. Researchers have evaluated hemodynamic pressure measurement readings with the patients in the 30- and 90-degree lateral positions with the head of the bed flat, and they found the measurements to be reliable.[5] In the 30-degree angle position, the landmark to use for leveling the transducer is one half of the distance from the surface of the bed to the left sternal border.[5] In the 90-degree right-lateral position, the transducer fluid-air interface was positioned at the fourth ICS at the midsternum. In the 90 degree left-lateral position, the transducer was positioned at the left parasternal border (beside the sternum).[5] It is important to know that measurements can be recorded in nonsupine positions, because critically ill patients must be turned to prevent development of pressure ulcers and other complications of immobility.

INTRAARTERIAL BLOOD PRESSURE MONITORING

Indications. Intraarterial blood pressure monitoring is indicated for any major medical or surgical condition that compromises cardiac output (CO), tissue perfusion, or fluid volume status. The system is designed for continuous measurement of three blood pressure parameters: systole, diastole, and mean arterial blood pressure (MAP). The direct arterial access is helpful in the management of patients with acute respiratory failure who require frequent arterial blood gas measurements.

Catheters. The size of the catheter used is proportionate to the diameter of the cannulated artery. In small arteries—such as the radial and dorsalis pedis—a 20-gauge, 3.8-cm to 5.1-cm, nontapered catheter is used most often. If the larger femoral or axillary arteries are used, a 19- or 20-gauge, 16-cm catheter is used.

The catheter insertion is usually percutaneous, although the technique varies with vessel size. Catheters are most often inserted in the smaller arteries, using a "catheter-over-needle" unit in which the needle is used as a temporary guide for catheter placement. With this method, after the unit has been inserted into the artery, the needle is withdrawn, leaving the supple plastic catheter in place. Insertion of a catheter into a larger artery typically uses the Seldinger technique, which involves the following steps:

1. Entry into the artery using a needle
2. Passage of a supple guidewire through the needle into the artery
3. Removal of the needle
4. Passage of the catheter over the guidewire
5. Removal of the guidewire, leaving the catheter in the artery

Insertion and Allen Test. Several major peripheral arteries are suitable for receiving a catheter and for long-term hemodynamic monitoring. The most frequently used site is the radial artery. The femoral artery is a larger vessel that is also frequently cannulated. Other smaller arterials such as the dorsalis-pedis, axillary, or brachial arteries are avoided if possible, and only used when other arterial access is unavailable.

The major advantage of the radial artery is the supply of collateral circulation to the hand provided by the ulnar artery

through the palmar arch in most of the population. Before radial artery cannulation, collateral circulation must be assessed by using Doppler flow or by the Allen test according to institutional protocol.[6-8] In the Allen test the radial and ulnar arteries are compressed simultaneously. The patient is asked to clench and unclench the hand until it blanches. One of the arteries is then released, and the hand should immediately flush from that side. The same procedure is repeated for the remaining artery.

Nursing Management. Intraarterial blood pressure monitoring is designed for continuous assessment of arterial perfusion to the major organ systems of the body. MAP is the clinical parameter most often used to assess perfusion, because MAP represents perfusion pressure throughout the cardiac cycle. Because one third of the cardiac cycle is spent in systole and two thirds in diastole, the MAP calculation must reflect the greater amount of time spent in diastole. This MAP formula can be calculated by hand or with a calculator, where diastole times 2 plus systole is divided by 3 as shown in the formula below:

$$\frac{(\text{Diastole} \times 2) + (\text{Systole} \times 1)}{3} = \text{MAP}$$

A blood pressure of 120/60 mm Hg produces a MAP of 80 mm Hg. However, the bedside hemodynamic monitor may show a slightly different digital number because most computers calculate the area under the curve of the arterial line tracing (Table 18-1). The MAP represents an estimate of organ perfusion pressure.[9]

Perfusion Pressure. A MAP greater than 60 mm Hg is necessary to perfuse the coronary arteries A higher MAP may be required to perfuse the brain and the kidneys. A MAP between 70 and 90 mm Hg is ideal for the cardiac patient to decrease left ventricular (LV) workload. After a carotid endarterectomy or neurosurgery, a MAP of 90 to 110 mm Hg may be more appropriate to increase cerebral perfusion pressure. Systolic and diastolic pressures are monitored in conjunction with the MAP as a further guide to the accuracy of perfusion. If CO decreases, the body compensates by constricting peripheral vessels to maintain the blood pressure. In this situation, the MAP may remain constant but the pulse pressure (difference between systolic and diastolic pressures) narrows. The following examples explain this point:

Mr. A: BP, 90/70 mm Hg; MAP, 76 mm Hg

Mr. B: BP, 150/40 mm Hg; MAP, 76 mm Hg

Both patients have a perfusion pressure of 76 mm Hg, but they are clinically very different. Mr. A is peripherally vasoconstricted, as is demonstrated by the narrow pulse pressure (90/70 mm Hg). His skin is cool to touch, and he has weak peripheral pulses. Mr. B has a wide pulse pressure (150/40 mm Hg), warm skin, and normally palpable peripheral pulses. Nursing assessment of the patient with an arterial line includes comparison of clinical findings with arterial line readings, including perfusion pressure and MAP.

Pulse Pressure. A clinical example of hemodynamic nursing assessment can be seen in patient JW 1 day after

TABLE 18-1 Hemodynamic Pressures and Calculated Hemodynamic Values

Hemodynamic Pressure	Definition and Explanation	Normal Range
Mean arterial pressure (MAP)	Average perfusion pressure created by arterial blood pressure during the cardiac cycle. The normal cardiac cycle is one third systole and two thirds diastole. These three components are divided by 3 to obtain the average perfusion pressure for the whole cardiac cycle.	70-100 mm Hg
Central venous pressure (CVP)	Pressure created by volume in the right side of the heart. When the tricuspid valve is open, the CVP reflects filling pressures in the right ventricle. Clinically, the CVP is often used as a guide to overall fluid balance.	2-5 mm Hg 3-8 cm water (H_2O)
Left atrial pressure (LAP)	Pressure created by the volume in the left side of the heart. When the mitral valve is open, the LAP reflects filling pressures in the left ventricle. Clinically, the LAP is used after cardiac surgery to determine how well the left ventricle is ejecting its volume. In general, the higher the LAP, the lower the ejection fraction from the left ventricle.	5-12 mm Hg
Pulmonary artery pressure (PAP) PA systolic (PAS) PA diastolic (PAD) PAP mean (PAP_M)	Pulsatile pressure in the pulmonary artery measured by an indwelling catheter.	PAS 20-30 mm Hg PAD 5-10 mm Hg PAP_M 10-15 mm Hg
Pulmonary artery occlusion pressure (PAOP)*	Pressure created by the volume in the left side of the heart. When the mitral valve is open, the PAOP reflects filling pressures in the pulmonary vasculature, and pressures in the left side of the heart are transmitted back to the catheter "wedged" into a small pulmonary arteriole.	5-12 mm Hg
Cardiac output (CO)	Amount of blood pumped out by a ventricle. Clinically, it can be measured using the thermodilution CO method, which calculates CO in liters per minute (L/min).	4-6 L/min (at rest)
Cardiac index (CI)	CO divided by the body surface area (BSA), with tailoring of CO to individual body size. A BSA conversion chart is necessary to calculate CI, which is considered more accurate than CO because it is individualized to height and weight. CI is measured in liters per minute per square meter of BSA (L/min/m²).	2.2-4.0 L/min/m²
Stroke volume (SV)	Amount of blood ejected by the ventricle with each heartbeat the SV. Hemodynamic monitoring systems calculate SV by dividing cardiac output (CO in L/min) by the heart rate (HR) and then multiplying the answer by 1000 to change liters to milliliters (mL).	60-70 mL
Stroke volume index (SI)	SV indexed to the BSA.	40-50 mL/m²
Systemic vascular resistance (SVR)	Mean pressure difference across the systemic vascular bed divided by blood flow. Clinically, SVR represents the resistance against which the left ventricle must pump to eject its volume. This resistance is created by the systemic arteries and arterioles. As SVR increases, CO falls. SVR is measured in Wood units or dyn·sec·cm^{-5}. If the number of Wood units is multiplied by 80, the value is converted to dyn·sec·cm^{-5}.	10-18 Wood units or 800-1400 dyn·sec·cm^{-5}
Systemic vascular resistance index (SVRI)	SVR indexed to BSA.	2000-2400 dyn·sec·cm^{-5}
Pulmonary vascular resistance (PVR)	Mean pressure difference across pulmonary vascular bed divided by blood flow. Clinically, PVR represents the resistance against which the right ventricle must pump to eject its volume. This resistance is created by the pulmonary arteries and arterioles. As PVR increases, the output from the right ventricle decreases. PVR is measured in Wood units or dyn·sec·cm^{-5}. PVR is normally one sixth of SVR.	1.2-3.0 Wood units or 100-250 dyn·sec·cm^{-5}

*Pulmonary artery occlusion pressure (PAOP) was formerly called pulmonary capillary wedge pressure (PCW or PCWP) or pulmonary arterial wedge pressure (PAWP).

Continued

TABLE 18-1 Hemodynamic Pressures and Calculated Hemodynamic Values—*cont'd*

Hemodynamic Pressure	Definition and Explanation	Normal Range
Pulmonary vascular resistance index (PVRI)	PVR indexed to BSA.	225-315 dyn·sec·cm^{-5}/m^2
Left cardiac work index (LCWI)	Amount of work the left ventricle does *each minute* when ejecting blood. The hemodynamic formula represents pressure generated (MAP) multiplied by volume pumped (CO). A conversion factor is used to change mm Hg to kilogram-meter (kg-m). LCWI is always represented as an indexed volume (BSA chart). LCWI increases or decreases because of changes in pressure (MAP) or volume pumped (CO).	3.4-4.2 kg-m/m^2
Left ventricular stroke work index (LVSWI)	Amount of work the left ventricle performs with *each heartbeat*. The hemodynamic formula represents pressure generated (MAP) multiplied by volume pumped (SV). A conversion factor is used to change mL/mm Hg to gram-meter (g-m). LVSWI is always represented as an indexed volume. LVSWI increases or decreases because of changes in the pressure (MAP) or volume pumped (SV).	50-62 g-m/m^2
Right cardiac work index (RCWI)	Amount of work the right ventricle performs *each minute* when ejecting blood. The hemodynamic formula represents pressure generated (PAP mean) multiplied by volume pumped (CO). A conversion factor is used to change mm Hg to kilogram-meter (kg-m). RCWI is always represented as an indexed value (BSA chart). Similar to LCWI, the RCWI increases or decreases because of changes in the pressure (PAP mean) or volume pumped (CO).	0.54-0.66 kg-m/m^2
Right ventricular stroke work index (RVSWI)	Amount of work the right ventricle does *each heartbeat*. The hemodynamic formula represents pressure generated (PAP mean) multiplied by volume pumped (SV). A conversion factor is used to change mm Hg to gram-meter (g-m). RVSWI is always represented as an indexed value (BSA chart). Similar to LVSWI, the RVSWI increases or decreases because of changes in the pressure (PAP mean) or volume pumped (SV).	7.9-9.7 g-m/m^2

coronary artery bypass grafting (CABG). JW recently was been weaned from dopamine (Intropin) and sodium nitroprusside (Nipride) and received a diuretic (20 mg of furosemide [Lasix] given intravenously). He voided 800 mL of urine by means of the urinary catheter during the past 2 hours. JW's MAP remains at 80 mm Hg, but his pulse pressure has narrowed by 30 mm Hg from 120/60 to 100/70 mm Hg. His heart rate has increased from 90 to 110 beats per minute. This clinical situation is not uncommon after furosemide administration, but the narrowed pulse pressure and increased heart rate may indicate hypovolemia. The nurse caring for JW will monitor the trend of the MAP. If the MAP begins to decrease and JW shows signs of a low CO, his physician will be notified. In most nonemergency situations, following the trend of the arterial pressure is more valuable than an isolated measurement.

Cuff Blood Pressure. If the arterial line becomes unreliable or dislodged, a cuff pressure can be used as a reserve system. In the normovolemic patient, little difference exists between the cuff blood pressure and arterial pressure. When the arterial catheter is functioning accurately, it is considered the gold standard.[10]

Slight pressure differences are to be expected between the cuff and the arterial catheter because the invasive catheter measures flow within the artery, whereas the arm cuff (sphygmomanometer and stethoscope) measures pressure from the outside. In the normovolemic patient, differences of 5 to 10 mm Hg do not affect clinical management. If the patient has a low CO or is in shock, the cuff pressure is unreliable because of peripheral vasoconstriction, and an arterial line is inserted. If there is any doubt about the accuracy of the arterial waveform or pressure reading, a cuff blood pressure reading is always taken.

Arterial Pressure Waveform Interpretation. As the aortic valve opens, blood is ejected from the left ventricle and is recorded as an increase of pressure in the arterial system. The highest point recorded is called *systole*. After peak ejection (systole), the force decreases, and the pressure drops. A notch (dicrotic notch) may be visible on the downstroke of this arterial waveform, representing closure of the aortic valve. The *dicrotic notch* signifies the beginning of diastole. The remainder of the downstroke represents diastolic runoff of blood flow into the arterial tree. The lowest point recorded is called *diastole*. A normal arterial pressure tracing is shown in Figure 18-2. Notice that electrical stimulation (QRS) is always first and that the arterial pressure tracing follows the initiating QRS.

Decreased Arterial Perfusion. Specific problems with heart rhythm can translate into poor arterial perfusion if CO

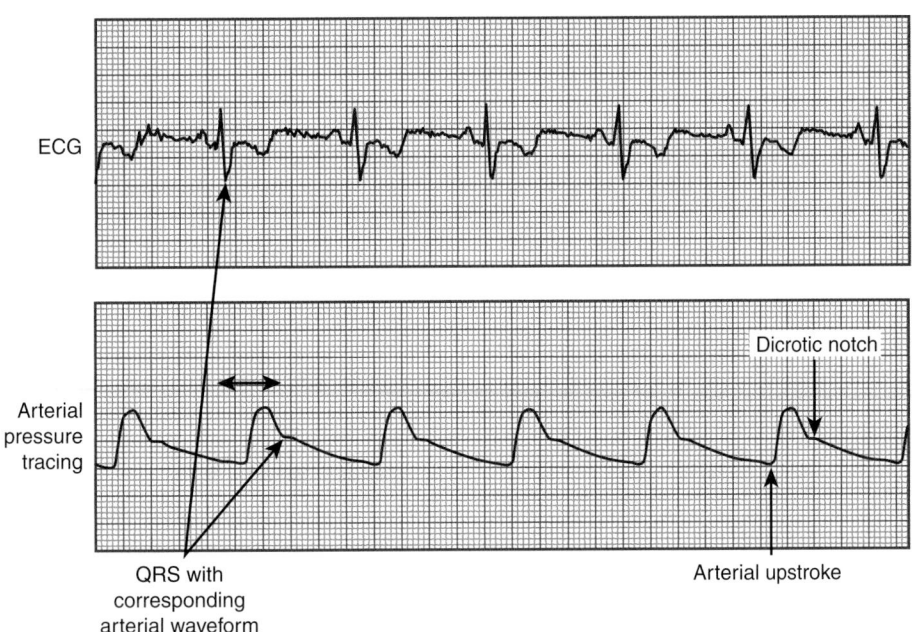

Figure 18-2 Simultaneous ECG and normal arterial pressure tracing.

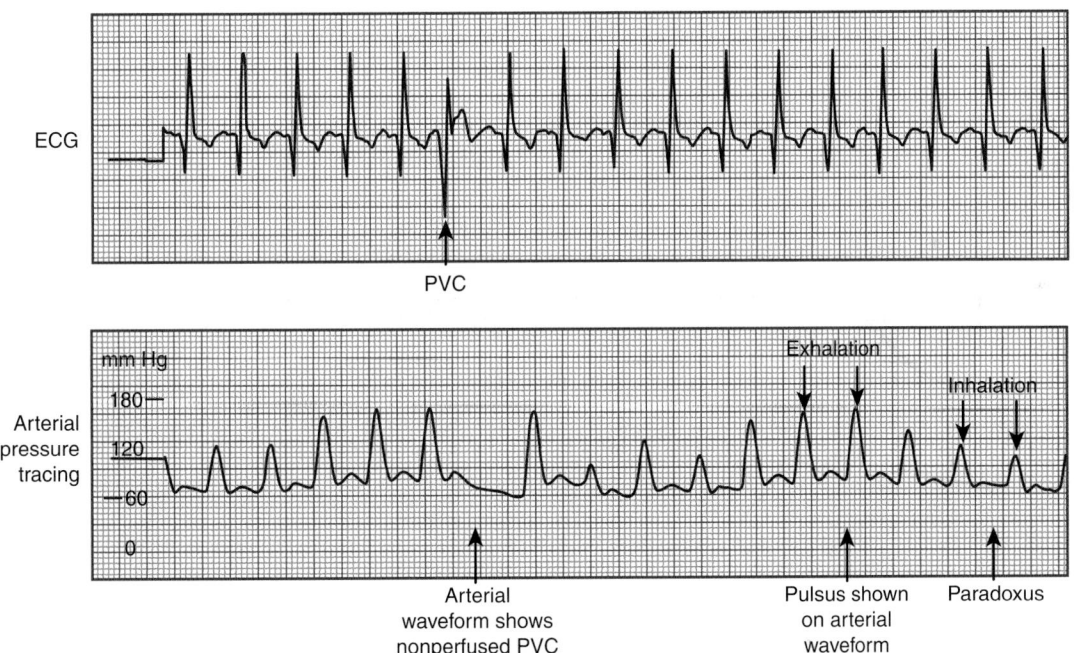

Figure 18-3 Simultaneous ECG and arterial pressure tracings show a normal arterial waveform with a nonperfused premature ventricular contraction (PVC). The arterial waveform also shows evidence of pulsus paradoxus in a patient who is mechanically ventilated.

decreases. Poor perfusion may be seen as a single, nonperfused beat after a premature ventricular contraction (PVC) (Fig. 18-3) or as multiple, nonperfused beats (Fig. 18-4). In ventricular bigeminy, every second beat is poorly perfused (Fig. 18-5). A disorganized atrial baseline resulting from atrial fibrillation creates a variable arterial pulse because of the differences in stroke volume between each beat (Fig. 18-6). All of these examples illustrate that when two beats are close together, the left ventricle does not have time to fill adequately, and the second beat is inadequately perfused or is not perfused at all.

Pulse Deficit. A pulse deficit occurs when the apical heart rate and the peripheral pulse are not equal. In the critical care unit, this can be seen on the bedside monitor. Normally, there is one arterial upstroke for each QRS, and if there are more QRS complexes than arterial upstrokes, a pulse deficit is present, as shown in Figures 18-3 and 18-6. To identify a pulse deficit in an unmonitored patient, a stethoscope is placed over the apex of the heart. The heartbeat can be heard, but it cannot be felt as a radial pulse. To determine whether a pulse deficit is significant, it is necessary to evaluate the clinical impact on the patient and whether any change in MAP or pulse pressure has occurred. Generally, the more nonperfused beats, the more serious the problem.

Pulsus Paradoxus. Pulsus paradoxus is a decrease of more than 10 mm Hg in the arterial waveform that occurs during inhalation (inspiration). It is caused by a fall in CO as a result

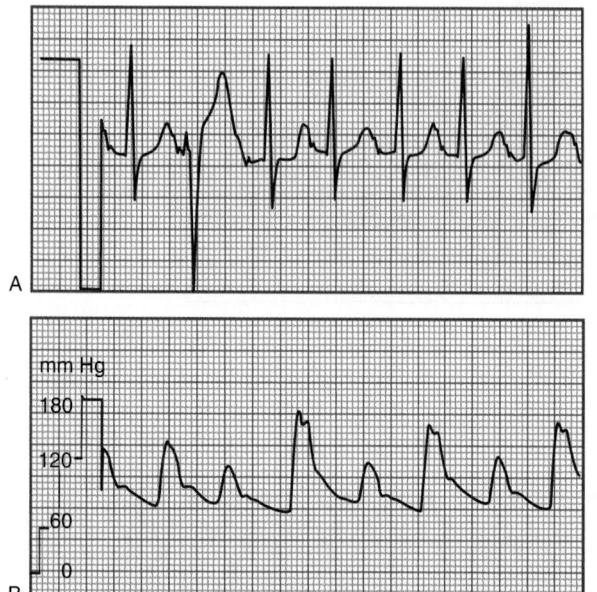

Figure 18-4 Simultaneous ECG *(A)* and arterial pressure *(B)* tracings show pulsus alternans. A nonperfused premature ventricular contraction (PVC) is also present.

of increased negative intrathoracic pressure during inhalation. As pressure within the thorax falls, blood pools in the large veins of the lungs and thorax, and stroke volume is decreased. The procedure for identification of pulsus paradoxus is discussed in Chapter 17 (see Box 17-8).

In certain clinical conditions, the pulsus paradoxus is obvious and can be clearly seen on an arterial waveform. It can be used as a clinical diagnostic test in a patient with cardiac tamponade, pericardial effusion, or constrictive pericarditis. Pulsus paradoxus commonly occurs in hypovolemic surgical patients who are mechanically ventilated with large tidal volumes (see Fig. 18-3).

Pulsus Alternans. In pulsus alternans, every other arterial pulsation is weak. This sometimes occurs in individuals with advanced left ventricular failure.

Damped Waveform. If the arterial monitor shows a low blood pressure, it is the responsibility of the nurse to determine whether it is a patient problem or a problem with the equipment, as described in Table 18-2. A low arterial blood pressure waveform is shown in Figure 18-7. In this case, the digital readout correlated well with the patient's cuff pressure, confirming that the patient was hypotensive. This arterial waveform is more rounded, without a dicrotic notch, compared with the normal waveform in Figure 18-2. A damped (flattened) arterial waveform is shown in Figure 18-8. In this case, the patient's cuff pressure was significantly higher than the digital readout, representing a problem with equipment. A damped waveform occurs when communication from the artery to the transducer is interrupted and produces false values on the monitor and oscilloscope. Damping is caused by a fibrin "sleeve" that partially occludes the tip of the catheter, by kinks in the catheter or

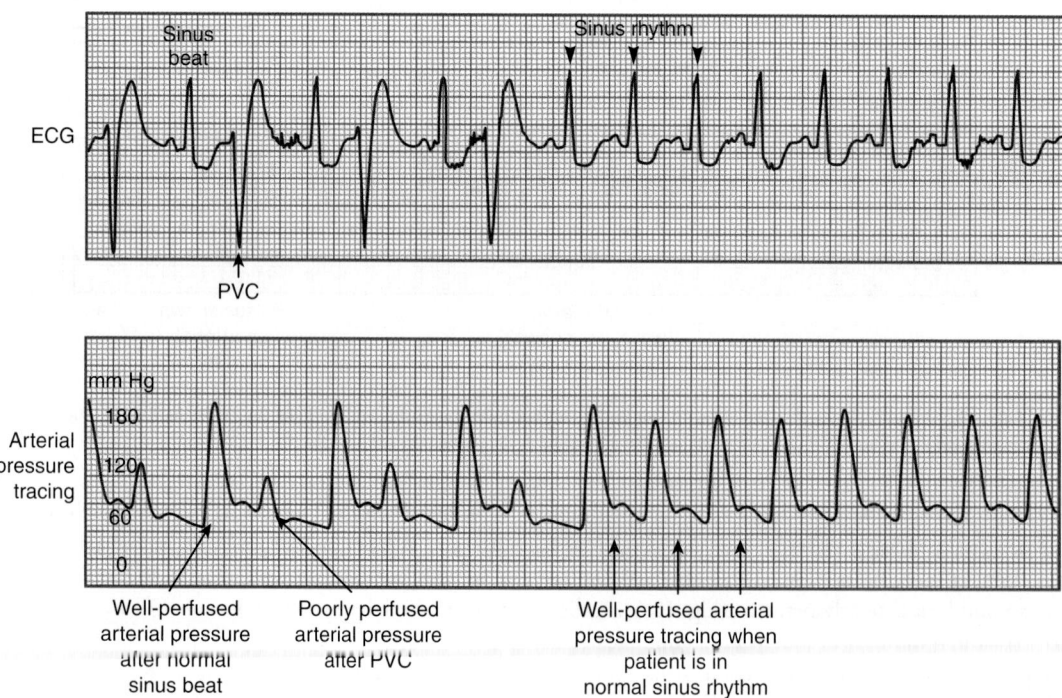

Figure 18-5 Simultaneous ECG and arterial pressure tracings show ventricular bigeminy in which every other ventricular beat is poorly perfused on the arterial pressure waveform in the first part of the tracing. In the second half of the tracing, there is a well-perfused arterial pressure tracing as the patient converts to normal sinus rhythm.

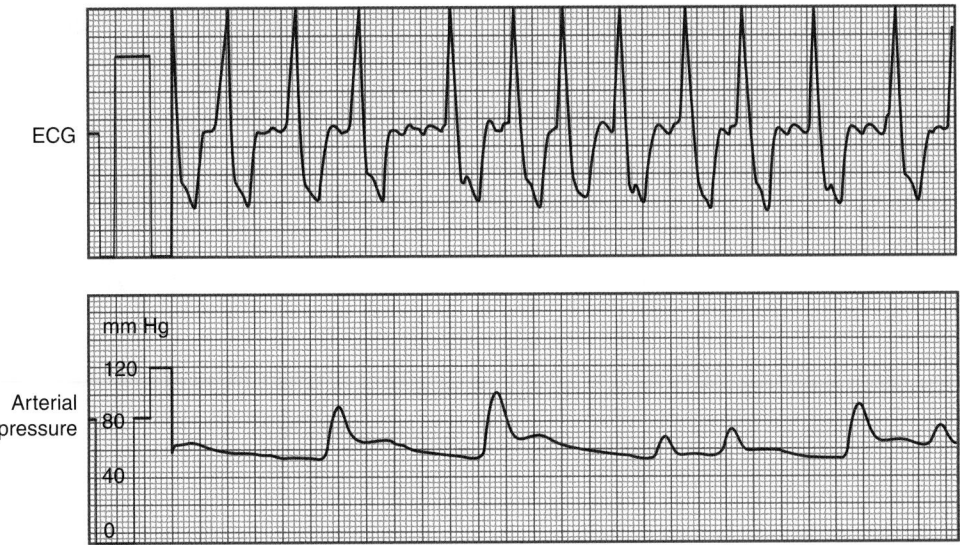

ECG

Arterial
pressure

mm Hg
120
80
40
0

Figure 18-6 Simultaneous ECG and arterial pressure tracings show atrial fibrillation, which results in irregular atrial pulsations. They create differences in beat-to-beat ventricular upstroke volume, resulting in diminished or absent ventricular output, as seen on the arterial waveform.

TABLE 18-2 Nursing Measures to Ensure Patient Safety and to Troubleshoot Problems with Hemodynamic Monitoring Equipment

Problem	Prevention	Rationale	Troubleshooting
Overdamping of waveform	Provide continuous infusion of solution containing heparin through an in-line flush device (1 unit of heparin for each 1 mL of flush solution).	Ensure that recorded pressures and waveform are accurate because a damped waveform gives inaccurate readings.	Before insertion, completely flush the line and/or catheter. In a line attached to a patient, back flush through the system to clear bubbles from tubing or transducer.
Underdamping ("overshoot" or "fling")	Use short lengths of noncompliant tubing. Use fast-flush square wave test to demonstrate optimal system damping. Verify arterial waveform accuracy with the cuff blood pressure.	If the monitoring system is underdamped, the systolic and diastolic values will be overestimated by the waveform and the digital values. False high systolic values may lead to clinical decisions based on erroneous data.	Perform the fast-flush square wave test to verify optimal damping of the monitoring system.
Clot formation at end of the catheter	Provide continuous infusion of solution containing heparin through an in-line flush device (1 unit of heparin for each 1 mL of flush solution).	Any foreign object placed in the body can cause local activation of the patient's coagulation system as a normal defense mechanism. The clots that are formed may be dangerous if they break off and travel to other parts of the body.	If a clot in the catheter is suspected because of a damped waveform or resistance to forward flush of the system, gently aspirate the line using a small syringe inserted into the proximal stopcock. Flush the line again after the clot is removed, and inspect the waveform. It should return to a normal pattern.
Hemorrhage	Use luer-lock (screw) connections in line setup. Close and cap stopcocks when not in use. Ensure that the catheter is sutured or securely taped in position.	A loose connection or open stopcock creates a low-pressure sump effect, causing blood to back into the line and into the open air. If a catheter is accidentally removed, the vessel can bleed profusely, especially with an arterial line or if the patient has abnormal coagulation factors (resulting from heparin in the line) or has hypertension.	After a blood leak is recognized, tighten all connections, flush the line, and estimate blood loss. If the catheter has been inadvertently removed, put pressure on the cannulation site. When bleeding has stopped, apply a sterile dressing, estimate blood loss, and inform the physician. If the patient is restless, an armboard may protect lines inserted in the arm.

Continued

TABLE 18-2 Nursing Measures to Ensure Patient Safety and to Troubleshoot Problems with Hemodynamic Monitoring Equipment—*cont'd*

Problem	Prevention	Rationale	Troubleshooting
Air emboli	Ensure that all air bubbles are purged from a new line setup before attachment to an indwelling catheter. Ensure that the drip chamber from the bag of flush solution is more than one-half full before using the in-line, fast-flush system. Some sources recommend removing all air from the bag of flush solution before assembling the system.	Air can be introduced at several times, including when central venous pressure (CVP) tubing comes apart, when a new line setup is attached, or when a new CVP or pulmonary artery (PA) line is inserted. During insertion of a CVP or PA line, the patient may be asked to hold his or her breath at specific times to prevent drawing air into the chest during inhalation. The in-line, fast-flush devices are designed to permit clearing of blood from the line after withdrawal of blood samples. If the chamber of the intravenous tubing is too low or empty, the rapid flow of fluid will create turbulence and cause flushing of air bubbles into the system and into the bloodstream.	Because it is impossible to get the air back after it has been introduced into the bloodstream, prevention is the best cure. If air bubbles occur, they must be vented through the in line stopcocks and the drip chamber must be filled. The left atrial pressure (LAP) line setup is the only system that includes an air filter specifically to prevent air emboli.
Normal waveform with *low* digital pressure	Ensure that the system is calibrated to atmospheric pressure. Ensure that the transducer is placed at the level of the phlebostatic axis.	To provide a 0 baseline relative to atmospheric pressure. If the transducer has been placed *higher* than the phlebostatic level, gravity and the lack of hydrostatic pressure will produce a false *low* reading.	Recalibrate the equipment if transducer drift has occurred. Reposition the transducer at the level of the phlebostatic axis. Misplacement can occur if the patient moves from the bed to the chair or if the bed is placed in a Trendelenburg position.
Normal wave form with *high* digital pressure	Ensure that the system is calibrated to atmospheric pressure. Ensure that the transducer is placed at the level of the phlebostatic axis.	To provide a 0 baseline relative to atmospheric pressure. If the transducer has been placed *lower* than the phlebostatic level, the weight of hydrostatic pressure on the transducer will produce a false *high* reading.	Recalibrate the equipment if transducer drift has occurred. Reposition the transducer at the level of the phlebostatic axis. This situation can occur if the head of the bed was raised and the transducer was not repositioned. Some centers require attachment of the transducer to the patient's chest to avoid this problem.
Loss of waveform	Always have the hemodynamic waveform monitored so that changes or loss can be quickly noted.	The catheter may be kinked, or a stopcock may be turned off.	Check the line setup to ensure that all stopcocks are turned in the correct position and that the tubing is not kinked. Sometimes, the catheter migrates against a vessel wall, and having the patient change position restores the waveform.

tubing, or by air bubbles in the system. Troubleshooting techniques (see Table 18-2) are used to find the origin of the problem and to remove the cause of damping.

Underdamped Waveform. Another cause of distortion of the arterial waveform is underdamping, often called *overshoot* or *fling*. Underdamping is recognized by a narrow, upward systolic peak that produces a falsely high systolic reading compared with the patient's cuff blood pressure as shown in Figure 18-9. The overshoot is caused by an increase in dynamic response or increased oscillations within the system.

Fast-Flush Square Waveform Test. The monitoring system's dynamic response can be verified for accuracy at the

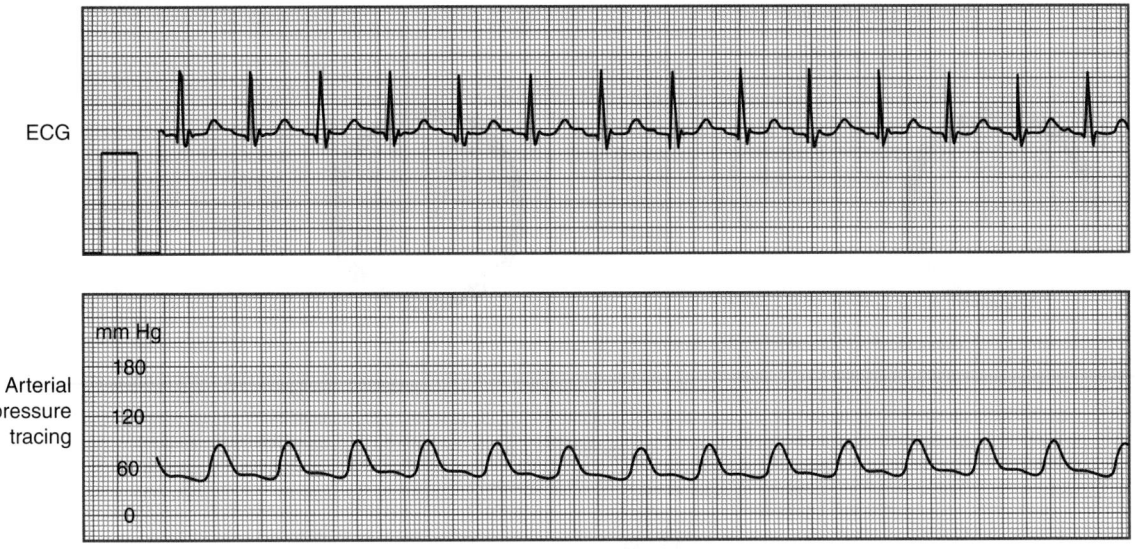

Figure 18-7 Simultaneous ECG and arterial pressure tracings show a low arterial pressure waveform.

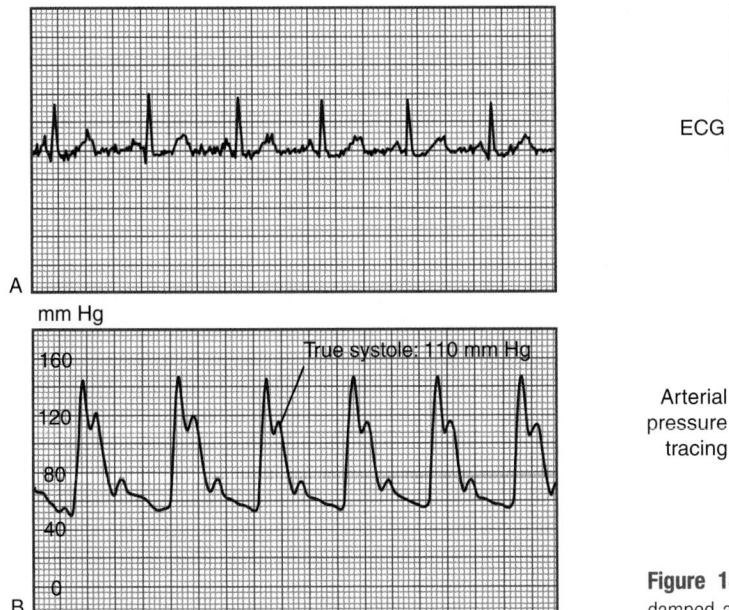

Figure 18-8 Simultaneous ECG *(A)* and arterial pressure *(B)* tracings show the overshoot, or fling, caused by a heightened dynamic response in the monitoring system. The monitor recorded an arterial line blood pressure of 141/51 mm Hg. The patient's true blood pressure with a cuff was 110/54 mm Hg. The 110 mm Hg cuff systolic pressure is consistent with the arterial line tracing without "overshoot."

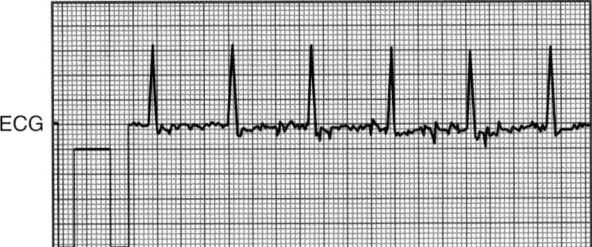

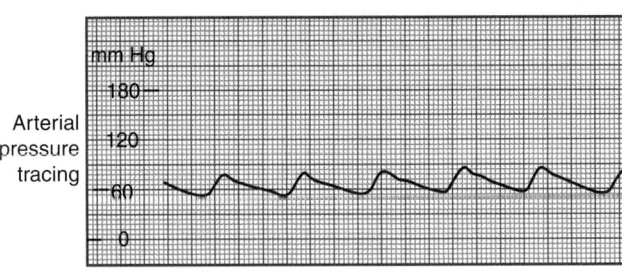

Figure 18-9 Simultaneous ECG and arterial pressure tracings show a damped arterial pressure waveform.

bedside by the *fast-flush square waveform test,* also called the *dynamic frequency response test.*[5] The nurse performs this test to ensure that the patient pressures and waveform shown on the bedside monitor are accurate.[5] The test makes use of the manual flush system on the transducer. Normally, the flush device allows only 3 mL of fluid/hr. With the normal waveform displayed, the manual fast-flush procedure is used to generate a rapid increase in pressure, which is displayed on the monitor oscilloscope. As shown in Figure 18-10, the normal dynamic response waveform shows a square pattern with one or two oscillations before the return of the arterial waveform. If the system is overdamped, a sloped (rather than square) pattern is seen. If the system is underdamped, additional oscillations—or vibrations—are seen on the fast-flush square wave test. This test can be performed with any hemodynamic monitoring system. If air bubbles, clots, or kinks are in the system, the waveform becomes damped, or flattened, and this is reflected in the square waveform result.

This is an easy test to perform, and it should be incorporated into nursing care procedures at the bedside when the hemodynamic system is first set up, at least once per shift, after opening the system for any reason, and when there is concern about the accuracy of the waveform.[5] If the pressure waveform is distorted or the digital display is inaccurate, the troubleshooting methods described in Table 18-2 can be implemented. The nurse caring

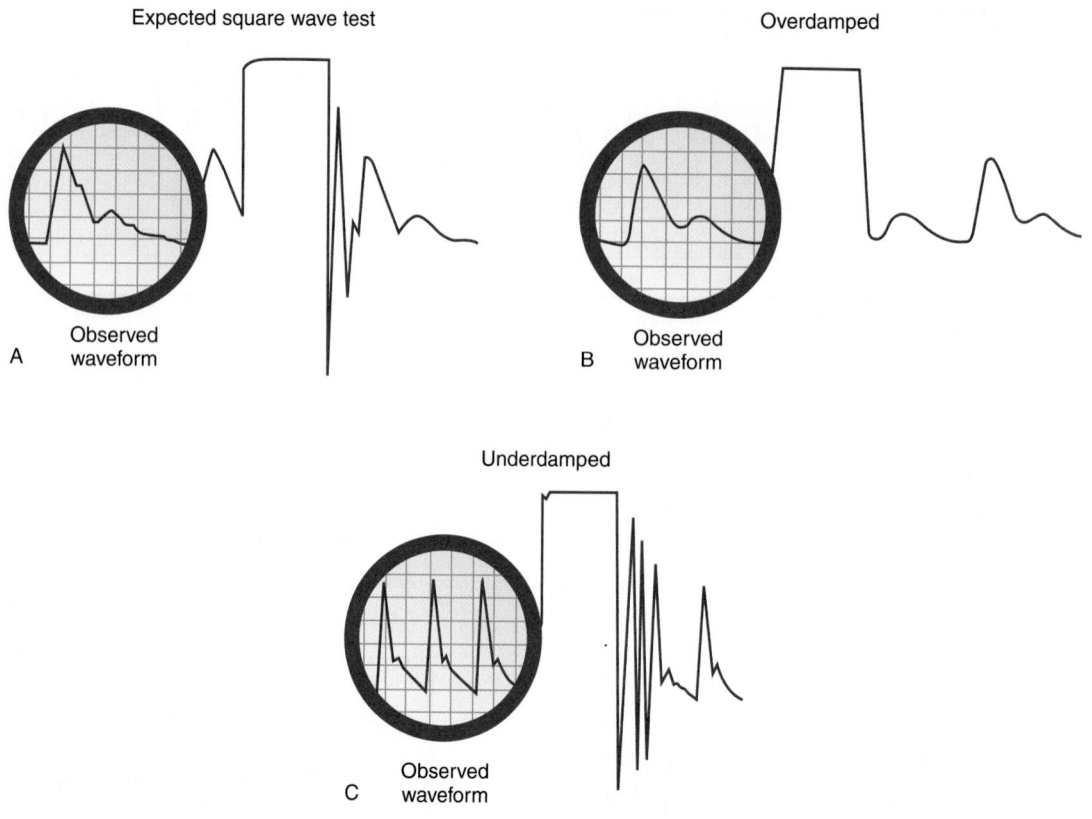

Figure 18-10 Square wave test. *A,* Expected square wave test result. *B,* Overdamped. *C,* Underdamped. *(From Darovic GO:* Hemodynamic monitoring: invasive and noninvasive clinical application, *ed 3, Philadelphia, 2002, WB Saunders.)*

◼ Patient Safety Alert

Clinical Alarm Systems

Clinical Alarm System Effectiveness
1. Implement regular preventive maintenance and testing of alarm systems.
2. Ensure that alarms are activated with appropriate settings and are sufficiently audible with respect to distances and competing noise within the unit.

Clinical Alarm Safety
Alarm Identification
1. Audible and visual indication should be present for any condition that poses a risk to the patient. Indicators should be visible from at least 10 feet (3 m).
2. Cause of the alarm must be easily identifiable by the health care practitioner.
3. Life-threatening conditions should be clearly differentiated from noncritical alarm situations.

4. High-priority alarms should override low-priority alarms.
5. Alarm must be sufficiently loud or distinctive to be heard over the environmental noise of a busy critical care unit.
6. It should never be possible to turn the volume control to "off."

Disabling and Silencing Alarms
1. Alarm silence must have visual indicator to clearly show it is disabled.
2. Critical alarms should not be permanently overridden (turned "off").
3. New, life-threatening alarm conditions should override a silenced alarm.

Power
Battery units should initiate an alarm before a unit stops working effectively.

Alarm Limits
1. Alarm limits can be adjusted to meet the clinical needs of a patient. The system should default to standard settings between patients.
2. Alarm limits should preferably be displayed on the monitor.

Data from www.jointcommission.org/ and Critical alarms and patient safety. ECRI's guide to developing effective alarm strategies and responding to JCAHO's alarm-safety goal, *Health Devices* 31(11):397-412, 2002.

---

for the patient with an arterial line must be able to assess whether a low MAP or narrowed perfusion pressure represents decreased arterial perfusion or equipment malfunction. Assessment of the arterial waveform on the oscilloscope, in combination with clinical assessment, and use of the square waveform test will yield the answer.

Alarms. All critically ill patients must have the hemodynamic monitoring alarms on and adjusted to sound an audible alarm if the patient should experience a change in blood pressure, heart rate, respiratory rate, or other significant monitored variable. The key issues concerning monitor alarms are presented in the Patient Safety Alert feature on Clinical Alarm Systems.

CENTRAL VENOUS PRESSURE MONITORING

Indications. CVP monitoring is indicated whenever a patient has significant alteration in fluid volume (see Table 18-1). The CVP can be used as a guide in fluid volume replacement in hypovolemia and to assess the impact of diuresis after diuretic administration in the case of fluid overload. When a major intravenous line is required for volume replacement, a central venous catheter (CVC) is a good choice because large volumes of fluid can easily be delivered.

Central Venous Catheters. A range of CVC options are available as single-, double-, triple- and quad-lumen infusion catheters, depending on the specific needs of the patient. CVCs are made from a variety of materials ranging from polyurethane to silicone; most are soft and flexible. Some catheters incorporate an antimicrobial coating to reduce the risk of bloodstream infections.

Insertion. The large veins of the upper thorax— subclavian (SC) and internal jugular (IJ)—are most commonly used for percutaneous CVC line insertion. The femoral vein in the groin is used when the thoracic veins are not accessible. All three major sites have advantages and disadvantages.

Internal Jugular Vein. The IJ vein is the most frequently used access site for CVC insertion. Compared with the other thoracic veins, it is the easiest to canalize. If the IJ vein is not available, the external jugular (EJ) vein may be accessed, although blood flow is significantly higher in the IJ vein, making it the preferred site. Another advantage of the IJ vein is that the risk of creating an iatrogenic pneumothorax is small. Disadvantages to the IJ vein are patient discomfort from the indwelling catheter when moving the head or neck and contamination of the IJ vein site from oral or tracheal secretions, especially if the patient is intubated or has a tracheostomy. This may be the reason why catheter-related infections are higher in the IJ than the SC position for indwelling catheters left in place for more than 4 days.[11,12]

Subclavian Vein. If the anticipated CVC dwelling time is prolonged more than 5 days, the SC site is preferred. The SC position has the lowest infection rate and produces the least patient discomfort from the catheter. The disadvantages are that the SC vein is more difficult to access and carries a higher risk of iatrogenic pneumothorax or hemothorax, although the risk varies greatly, depending on the experience and skill of the physician inserting the catheter.

Femoral Vein. The femoral vein is considered the easiest cannulation site because there are no curves in the insertion route. The large diameter of the femoral vein carries a high blood flow that is advantageous for specialized procedures such as continuous renal replacement therapy (CRRT) or plasmapheresis. Disadvantages are that the patient cannot bend at the hip, because this interrupts blood flow through the catheter and may lead to thrombus formation; risk of retroperitoneal bleed; and a higher rate of nosocomial infections, probably due to site location near the groin area.[11]

During insertion of a catheter in the SC or IJ vein, the patient may be placed in a Trendelenburg position. Placing the head in a dependent position causes the IJ veins in the neck to become more prominent, facilitating line placement. To minimize the risk of air embolus during the procedure, the patient may be asked to "take a deep breath and hold it" any time the needle or catheter is open to air. The tip of the catheter is designed to remain in the vena cava and should not migrate into the right atrium. If the IJ or SC veins are not available, the femoral veins can be used for CVC access. The femoral veins are farther away from the heart; for accurate CVP measurements, the tip of the catheter must be advanced into the inferior vena cava near the right atrium. Because many patients are awake and alert when a CVC is inserted, a brief explanation about the procedure can minimize patient anxiety and result in cooperation during the insertion. This cooperation is important, because CVC insertion is a sterile procedure and because the supine or Trendelenburg position may not be comfortable for many patients. The electrocardiogram (ECG) should be monitored during CVC insertion because of the associated risk of dysrhythmias.

All central catheters are designed for placement by percutaneous injection after skin preparation and administration of a local anesthetic. A prepackaged CVC kit typically is used for the procedure. The standard CVC kit contains sterile towels, chlorhexidine and alcohol for skin preparation, a needle introducer, a syringe, guidewire, and a catheter. The Seldinger technique, in which the vein is located by using a "seeking" needle and syringe, is the preferred method of placement. A guidewire is passed through the needle, the needle is removed, and the catheter is passed over the guidewire. After the catheter is correctly placed in the vena cava, the guidewire is removed. A sterile intravenous tubing and solution is attached, and the catheter is sutured in place.

An important development in central venous catheter management is adherence to the Centers for Disease Control (CDC) and Institute for Healthcare Improvement (IHI) bundle approach to prevent blood stream infections. The CVC bundle places a strong emphasis upon infection control during insertion to protect the patient. The IHI recommends meticulous hand hygiene, 2% chlorhexidine gluconate in 70% isopropyl patient skin preparation, full-barrier precautions for each CVC insertion, and optimal catheter site selection. In many hospitals the nurse is authorized to stop the procedure if these insertion infection control guidelines are not followed. A daily review to determine whether the catheter is still required is recommended to ensure CVCs are removed promptly when no longer needed.

After thoracic CVC placement, a chest radiograph is obtained to verify placement and the absence of an iatrogenic hemothorax or pneumothorax, especially if the SC vein was accessed. The use of Doppler ultrasound guidance to find the vein and guide insertion may reduce the incidence of iatrogenic complications.[11] In the rare case when it is not possible to insert a CVC percutaneously, a surgical cutdown may be performed.

Central Venous Catheter Complications. The CVC is an essential tool in care of the critically ill patient, but it is associated with some risks, and it is the responsibility of all clinicians to be informed about these hazards and to follow hospital procedures to avoid iatrogenic complications. CVC complications include air embolus, catheter-associated thrombus formation, and infection.

Air Embolus. The risk of air embolus, although uncommon, is always present for the patient with a central venous line in place. Air can enter during insertion[13] through a disconnected or broken catheter by means of an open stopcock,[14] or air can enter along the path of a removed CVC.[15] This is more likely if the patient is in an upright position, because air can be pulled into the venous system with the increase in negative intrathoracic pressure during inhalation. If a large volume of air is infused rapidly, it may become trapped in the right ventricular outflow tract, stopping blood flow from the right side of the heart to the lungs. Based on animal studies, this volume is approximately 4 mL/kg.[16] If the air embolus is large, the patient will experience respiratory distress and cardiovascular collapse. An auscultatory clinical sign specifically associated with a large venous air embolism is *mill wheel murmur*.[13-15] A mill wheel murmur is a loud, churning sound heard over the middle chest, caused by the obstruction to right ventricular outflow. Treatment involves administering 100% oxygen and placing the patient on the left side with the head downward (left lateral Trendelenburg position).[14] This position displaces the air from the right ventricular outflow tract to the apex of the heart, where the air may be aspirated by catheter intervention or gradually absorbed by the bloodstream as the patient remains in the left lateral Trendelenburg position. Precautions to prevent an air embolism in a CVP line include using only screw (Luer-Lock) connections, avoiding long loops of intravenous tubing, and using closed-top screw caps on the three-way stopcock.

Thrombus Formation. Clot formation (thrombus) at the CVC site is unfortunately common. Ultrasound studies have found asymptomatic thrombus formation to be in the range of 33% to 67% when the catheter is in place for more than 7 days.[11] Symptomatic thrombi are reported in 0% to 5% of those cases.[11,12] Thrombus formation is not uniform; it may involve development of a *fibrin sleeve* around the catheter, or the thrombus may be attached directly to the vessel wall. Other factors that promote clot formation include rupture of vascular endothelium, interruption of laminar blood flow, and physical presence of the catheter, all of which activate the coagulation cascade. The risk of thrombus formation is higher if insertion was difficult or there were multiple needlesticks.[11] Gradual thrombus formation may lead to "sudden" CVC occlusion. Usually, the CVC becomes more difficult to withdraw blood from, or the CVP waveform becomes intermittently damped over a period of hours or even 1 to 2 days and is reported as "needing frequent flushes" to remain patent. This situation is caused by the continued lengthening of a fibrin sleeve that extends along the catheter length from the insertion site past the catheter tip.[11,12] Some catheters are heparin coated to reduce the risk of thrombus formation, although the risk of HIT, reported to be 0.4% with indwelling CVC, does not make this a benign option.[12] Sometimes, CVC complications are additive; for example, the risk of catheter-related infection is increased in the presence of thrombi. The thrombus likely serves as a culture medium for bacterial growth.[12]

Infection. Infection related to the use of CVCs is a major problem. Risk factors for catheter-related infections include extremes of age, impaired host defense mechanisms, severe illness, malnutrition, and presence of other invasive lines. It is estimated that more than 50,000 infections related to CVC use occur annually in the United States, with associated mortality rates between 10% and 20%.[12]

The incidence of infection strongly correlates with the length of time the CVC has been inserted.[17] Catheters that are in place less than 3 days rarely lead to infection, providing standard insertion and management procedures are followed. If the CVC remains between 3 and 7 days, the infection rate is 3% to 5%. Catheters remaining in one site more than 7 days have an infection rate of 5% to 10%.[12]

CVC-related infection is identified at the catheter insertion site or as a bloodstream infection (septicemia). Systemic manifestations of infection can be present without inflammation at the catheter site. To determine whether a suspect catheter is contaminated, after removal the tip may be placed in a sterile container and cultured. No decrease in infections was found when catheters were routinely changed to prevent infectious, and this practice is no longer recommended.[18] A "suspect" CVC changed over guidewire risks a higher rate of infection.[17,18] Prevention is the best defense against complications resulting from infections. Most infections are transmitted from the skin, and infection prevention begins prior to insertion of the CVC. Insertion guidelines state that the physician must use effective hand-washing procedures, clean the insertion site with 2% chlorhexidine gluconate in 70% isopropyl, use sterile technique during catheter insertion, and maintain maximal sterile barrier precautions (see the Patient Safety Alert feature on Guidelines for Prevention and Management of Central Venous Catheter Infections).[18]

All clinicians must use good hand-washing technique and follow aseptic procedures during site care and any time the CVC system is entered to withdraw blood, give medications, or change tubing.[18,19] The infusion of high-dextrose solutions such as total parental nutrition (TPN) may be associated with an increased risk of infection. Methods to lower TPN-related complications include use of a single-lumen CVC that is not accessed for other medications or laboratory samples.

Incidence of infection is higher with use of occlusive dressings that do not allow removal of moisture. Transparent, breathable dressings that allow removal of skin moisture are recommended. Site dressings that have antimicrobial properties are being used to lower infection rates. Improvements in catheter design may also help to reduce central line infection. Some catheters are impregnated with an antimicrobial substance[18] or have a silver-impregnated, tissue-barrier cuff attached to the catheter. These catheters are designed to lower the rate of CVC infection.

Nursing Management. In the critically ill patient, the CVC is used to monitor CVP and waveform. The CVP catheter is used to measure the filling pressures of the right side of the heart. During diastole, when the tricuspid valve is open and blood is flowing from the right atrium to the right ventricle, the CVP accurately reflects right ventricular end-diastolic pressure (RVEDP). The normal CVP is 2 to 5 mm Hg (3 to 8 cm H_2O).

Patient Safety Alert

Guidelines for Prevention and Management of Central Venous Catheter Infections

1. Use effective hand washing.
2. Educate and train health care providers who insert and maintain central venous catheters (CVCs) to follow infection-control guidelines. Empower nurses to stop the insertion procedure if the infection control guidelines are not being followed.
3. Use maximal sterile barrier precautions during CVC insertion.
4. Use 2% chlorhexidine in 70% isopropyl alcohol for skin antisepsis prior to insertion.
5. Select optimal catheter site, avoid the femoral venous site in adults when possible.
6. Avoid routine replacement of CVCs as a strategy to prevent infection.
7. Daily assessment as to whether the CVC is still required. If not needed, promptly pull the catheter.
8. Insert antiseptic- or antibiotic-impregnated, short-term CVCs if the rate of infection is high despite adherence to other strategies (e.g. education or training, maximal sterile barrier precautions, 2% chlorhexidine skin preparation).
9. Confirm clinical suspicion of infection by taking cultures of blood and catheter samples.
10. Initially, treat intravascular catheter infection with intravenous (IV) antimicrobial therapy, considering severity of patient's acute illness, underlying disease, and potential pathogens. After the catheter-related pathogen is documented, narrow the focus of antimicrobial therapy to treat specific organisms.
11. Remove the CVC if infected.

Data from O'Grady NP et al: Guidelines for the prevention of intravascular catheter-related infections, Am J Infect Control 30(8):476-489, 2002; Boyce JM, Pittet D: Guideline for Hand Hygiene in Health-Care Settings. Recommendations of the Healthcare Infection Control Practices Advisory Committee and the HIPAC/SHEA/APIC/IDSA Hand Hygiene Task Force, Am J Infect Control 30(8):S1-S46, 2002. Institute for Healthcare Improvement (IHI) Implement the Central Line Bundle; www.ihi.org/IHI/Topics/CriticalCare/IntensiveCare/Changes/Implementthe CentralLineBundle.htm (accessed April 2009).

Low Central Venous Pressure. A low CVP often occurs in the hypovolemic patient and suggests that insufficient blood volume is in the ventricle at end-diastole to produce an adequate stroke volume. To maintain normal CO, the heart rate (HR) must increase. This HR increase produces the tachycardia often observed in hypovolemic states and increases myocardial oxygen demand.

The CVP is used in combination with the MAP and other clinical parameters to assess hemodynamic stability. In the hypovolemic patient, the CVP falls before a significant fall in MAP occurs, because peripheral vasoconstriction keeps the MAP normal. The CVP is an excellent early-warning system for the patient who is bleeding, vasodilating, receiving diuretics, or being rewarmed after cardiac surgery.

High Central Venous Pressure. An elevated CVP occurs in cases of fluid overload. To circulate the excess blood volume,

the heart must greatly increase its contractile force to move the large volume of blood. This increases the cardiac workload and increases myocardial oxygen consumption. The critical care nurse follows the trend of the CVP measurements to determine subsequent interventions for optimal fluid volume management.

Central Venous Pressure Limitations. The CVP is not a reliable indicator of left ventricular dysfunction. LV dysfunction, which can occur after an acute myocardial infarction (MI), increases filling pressures on the left side of the heart. The CVP, because it measures RVEDP, remains normal until the increase in pressure from the left side of the heart is reflected back through the pulmonary vasculature to the right ventricle. In this situation, a pulmonary artery catheter that measures pressures on the left side of the heart is the monitoring method of choice. More information on PAP monitoring is provided later in this chapter.

Water versus Mercury Central Venous Pressure. CVP values are measured in millimeters of mercury (mm Hg) if bedside hardwire monitoring is used. If a patient is admitted from a medical-surgical unit with a water manometer CVP and clinicians want to know the relationship between the two values, it involves a straightforward calculation based on the following standard relationship: 1 mm Hg (mercury pressure) is equivalent to 1.36 cm H_2O (water pressure). Although the numeric value in cm H_2O will be higher, the values are clinically equivalent for the specific patient. To convert water manometer pressure to mercury pressure, the water-pressure value is divided by 1.36 ($H_2O \div 1.36$). To convert mercury pressure to water pressure, the mercury value is multiplied by 1.36 (mm Hg $\times$ 1.36).

Removal. Removal of the CVC usually is a nursing responsibility. Complications are infrequent, and the ones to anticipate are bleeding and air embolus. Recommended techniques to avoid air embolus during CVC removal include removing the catheter when the patient is supine in bed (not in a chair) and placing the patient flat or in reverse Trendelenburg position if the patient's clinical condition permits this maneuver.[93] Patients with heart failure, pulmonary disease, and neurologic conditions with raised intracranial pressure (ICP) should not be placed flat. If the patient is alert and able to cooperate, he or she is asked to take a deep breath to raise intrathoracic pressure during removal.[20] After removal, to decrease the risk of air entering by a "track," an occlusive dressing is applied to the site.[20] If bleeding at the site occurs after removal, firm pressure is applied. If a patient has prolonged coagulation times, fresh-frozen plasma or platelets may be prescribed before CVC removal.

Patient Position. To achieve accurate CVP measurements, the phlebostatic axis is used as a reference point on the body, and the transducer or water manometer zero must be level with this point. If the phlebostatic axis is used and the transducer or water manometer is correctly aligned, any head-of-bed position of up to 60 degrees may be used for CVP accurate readings for most patients.[5] Elevating the head of the bed is especially helpful for the patient with respiratory or cardiac problems who cannot tolerate a flat position.

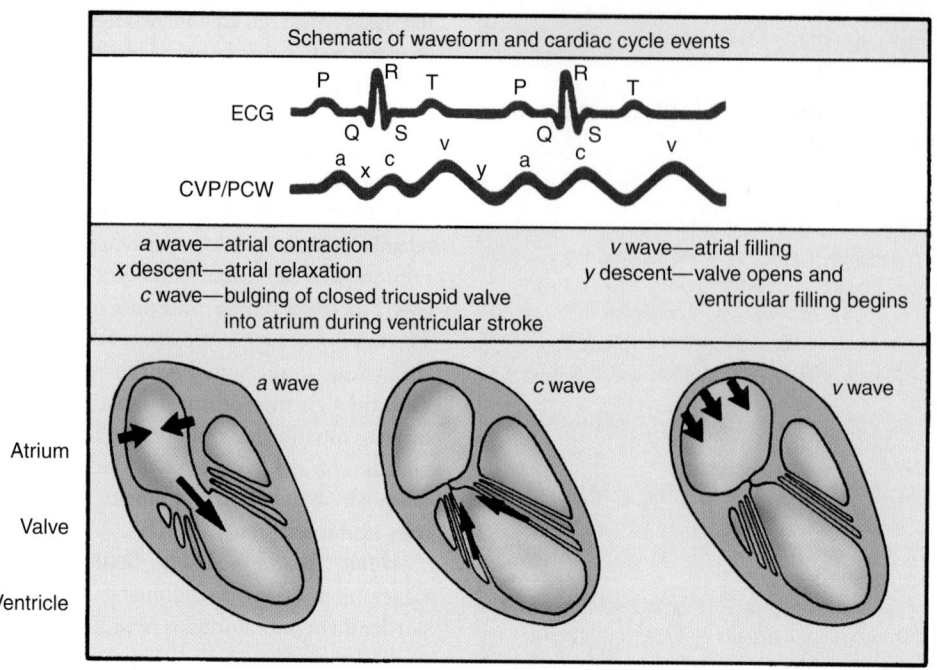

Figure 18-11 Cardiac events that produce the CVP waveform with *a*, *c*, and *v* waves. The *a* wave represents atrial contraction. The *x* descent represents atrial relaxation. The *c* wave represents the bulging of the closed tricuspid valve into the right atrium during ventricular systole. The *v* wave represents atrial filling. The *y* descent represents opening of the tricuspid valve and filling of the ventricle.

Central Venous Pressure Waveform Interpretation. The normal right atrial (CVP) waveform has three positive deflections—*a*, *c*, and *v* waves—that correspond to specific atrial events in the cardiac cycle (Fig. 18-11). The *a* wave reflects atrial contraction and follows the P wave seen on the ECG. The downslope of this wave is called the *x* descent and represents atrial relaxation. The *c* wave reflects the bulging of the closed tricuspid valve into the right atrium during ventricular contraction; this wave is small and not always visible, but corresponds to the QRS-T interval on the ECG. The *v* wave represents atrial filling and increased pressure against the closed tricuspid valve in early diastole. The downslope of the *v* wave is named the *y* descent and represents the fall in pressure as the tricuspid valve opens and blood flows from the right atrium to the right ventricle.

Cannon Waves. Dysrhythmias can change the pattern of the CVP waveform. In a junctional rhythm or after a PVC, the atria are depolarized after the ventricles if retrograde conduction to the atria occurs. This may be seen as a retrograde P wave on the ECG and as a large combined *ac* or *cannon wave* on the CVP waveform (Fig. 18-12). These cannon waves can be easily detected as large pulses in the jugular veins. Other pathologic conditions, such as advanced right ventricular failure or tricuspid valve insufficiency, allow regurgitant backflow of blood from the right ventricle to the right atrium during ventricular contraction, producing large *v* waves on the right atrial waveform. In atrial fibrillation, the CVP waveform has no recognizable pattern because of the disorganization of the atria.

Specialized Catheters. A CVC that incorporates a fiberoptic sensor to continuously measure central venous oxygen saturation (ScvO₂) can be used as a traditional CVC and additionally used to follow the trend of venous oxygen saturation.[21] The physiology underlying use of this fiberoptic technology is discussed later in sections on monitoring mixed venous oxygen saturation (S$\bar{\text{v}}$O₂) and ScvO₂.

LEFT ATRIAL PRESSURE MONITORING

Indications. Left atrial pressure (LAP) monitoring is used in rare cases after major cardiac surgery. Until the advent of the pulmonary artery catheter in the 1970s, LAP monitoring was used to assess hemodynamics on the left side of the heart. It is no longer used for routine monitoring, but it is a clinical choice on rare occasions in the postoperative management of the cardiac surgery patient who has significant pulmonary hypertension. In this situation, accurate LAPs may be difficult to obtain with a pulmonary artery catheter.

Insertion. The LAP catheter is inserted into the left atrium during open heart surgery. The single-lumen catheter exits through the chest wall and is attached to a hemodynamic monitoring setup that contains an in-line air filter.

Nursing Management. Placement of the LAP catheter directly into the left atrium places the patient at risk for air or tissue emboli. Nursing care is planned to reduce these equipment-related risks. To reduce the risk of air emboli, an in-line air filter is added to the flush system that contains heparin. If the waveform becomes damped, noninvasive methods of troubleshooting—such as repositioning the patient—are performed. The catheter is not manually flushed, because to do so may increase the risk of emboli resulting from clot formation at the tip of the catheter. Pericardial tamponade is a potential complication of LAP catheter removal. Mediastinal chest tubes

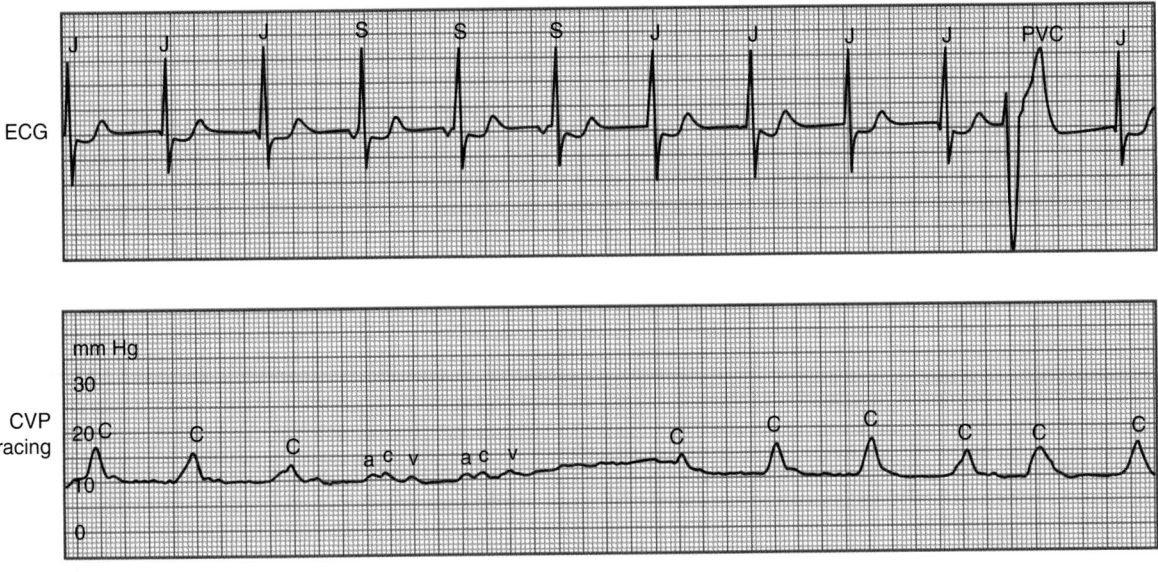

Figure 18-12 Simultaneous electrocardiographic and central venous pressure (CVP) tracings. The CVP waveform shows large cannon waves (*c* waves) corresponding to the junctional beats or premature ventricular contractions *(bottom strip)*. As the patient converts to sinus rhythm, the CVP waveform has a normal configuration. ac, normal right atrial pressure tracing; c, cannon waves on CVP tracing; J, junctional rhythm followed by cannon waves on CVP waveform; PVC, premature ventricular contraction followed by cannon wave on CVP; S, sinus rhythm followed by normal CVP tracing with *a*, *c*, and *v* waves.

are left in position until after the catheter is removed. Because of these risks, the LAP catheter is rarely left in place for more than 48 hours.

Left Atrial Pressure Waveform Interpretation. The LAP waveform consists of two positive deflections, the *a* and *v* waves. The *a* wave represents atrial contraction, and the *v* wave represents filling of the left atrium against a closed mitral valve. Normal LAP pressure ranges from 5 to 12 mm Hg and is elevated with mitral valve disease or severe heart failure on the left side.

Direct monitoring of the LAP waveform is a component of cardiac catheterization when a catheter may be passed from the right atrial to the left atrium in a *transseptal* or *transatrial* approach. Use of an LAP implantable monitor has been studied in patients with heart failure.[22]

PULMONARY ARTERY PRESSURE MONITORING

The pulmonary artery (PA) catheter is the most invasive of the critical care monitoring catheters. It is also known as a *right heart catheter* or *Swan-Ganz catheter* (named after the catheter's inventors). The practice of routinely using PA catheters has been called into question and is highly controversial. Several randomized, controlled trials of critically ill patients have not demonstrated a benefit to use of the PA catheter. A randomized, controlled trial of 676 critical care patients with acute respiratory distress syndrome (ARDS) in France reported no difference in mortality rates for patients when treatment was guided by PA catheter and for patients without this information.[23] A randomized, controlled trial of 1000 patients with acute lung injury in the United States found no difference in mortality rates for patients when treatment was guided by a PA catheter

and those for whom diagnostic information was obtained from a CVP.[24]

The impact of PA catheterization on mortality rates for patients with acute heart failure has also been examined. A randomized, controlled trial of 433 patients with acute heart failure in the United States reported no difference in mortality based on whether fluid volume management was guided by PA catheter insertion or not.[25] Similar results were reported from a British multicenter trial enrolling more than 1000 critical care patients; there were no differences in mortality or in length of stay.[26,27] No survival benefit was found in a randomized, controlled trial enrolling older high-risk surgical patients who required critical care monitoring when treatment was guided by PA catheter diagnostics or not.[28] Systematic reviews and meta-analysis of studies of PA catheter use have reached similar conclusions—that insertion of a PA catheter is neutral, it neither conferred a benefit nor increased risk to the patient. There was no increase in mortality or increase in the number of days in the critical care unit or the hospital.[29,30]

These findings have raised concerns about routine use of PA catheters for critically ill patients. The PA catheter is invasive. It previously seemed intuitive that the diagnostic information provided would confer a survival advantage over less invasive methods, but research has shown this is not the case. In 2000, the number of PA catheters used in the United States was reported as 1.5 million annually; 30% were used in cardiac surgery units, 30% in cardiac catheterization laboratories and coronary care units, 25% in high-risk surgery and trauma units, and 15% in medical intensive care units.[31] As a result of studies that document the failure of the PA catheter to lower mortality, the use of PA catheters has declined considerably. A study of PA catheterization between 1993 and 2004 reported a decline of 65% in PA catheter use in critically ill patients.[32]

Clinicians who do not frequently work with PA catheters are less knowledgeable about waveform analysis and interpretation of data. With the decline in PA catheterization, this issue has become even more important. As a response to this concern, several professional organizations, including the American Association of Critical-Care Nurses (AACN), the Society of Critical Care Medicine (SCCM), and the American College of Chest Physicians (ACCP), endorse the Internet-based Pulmonary Artery Catheter Education Project (PACEP). This Web site (www.pacepp.org) is free and is designed to provide education about PA catheters to improve the quality of hemodynamic monitoring practices.

The PA catheter is subsequently described in the context that its use has become much less frequent in critical care units, although right heart catheterization is still used as a diagnostic tool in the cardiac catheterization laboratory. Although the PA catheter has not been associated with increased harm, the lack of benefit means it will play a less important role in patient care management in the future. In some critical care units, the PA catheter may be reserved for patients who are refractory to conventional treatment,[33] but in many settings, it will be replaced by less invasive technologies such as echocardiography.

Indications. The thermodilution PA catheter is used for diagnosis and evaluation of heart disease, shock states, ARDS, and medical conditions that compromise CO or fluid volume status. The PA catheter can be used to evaluate patient response to treatment, as described in Table 18-3. The PA catheter can simultaneously assess pulmonary artery systolic and diastolic pressures, pulmonary artery mean pressure, and PAOP (wedge pressure). The PA catheter is used to measure CO, determine mixed-venous oxygen saturation, and calculate additional hemodynamic parameters.

Cardiac Output Determinants. Cardiac output (CO) is the product of heart rate (HR) multiplied by stroke volume (SV). Stroke volume is the volume of blood ejected by the heart during each beat (reported in milliliters).

$$HR \times SV = CO$$

The normal adult stroke volume is 60 to 70 mL. The clinical factors that contribute to the heart's stroke volume are preload, afterload, and contractility (Fig. 18-13). These three factors may be monitored using the PA catheter. Another contributor to CO is heart rate, which is usually recorded from the ECG leads.

Oxygen Supply and Demand. When the peripheral tissues need more oxygen (e.g., during exercise or fever), the normal, healthy heart can augment heart rate and stroke volume and greatly increase CO. In the critically ill patient, when the tissues require more oxygen, these normal mechanisms are often non-functional, and it is the critical care nurse who assesses the need for and then optimizes hemodynamic function. The following discussion is intended to provide a basic understanding of the

clinical factors that determine CO and the role of the critical care nurse in caring for the patient with an alteration in any of these factors.

Preload. Clinicians commonly describe the hemodynamic numbers related to preload as *filling pressures*. These values refer to the pressures resulting from the volumes in the atria and ventricles. These pressure numbers include pulmonary artery diastolic pressure (PADP) and PAOP (or wedge pressure), which measure preload in the left side of the heart, and CVP, which measures preload in the right side of the heart.

Preload is the *volume* in the ventricle at end-diastole. Because diastole is the filling stage of the cardiac cycle, the volume in the ventricle at end-diastole represents the presystolic volume available for ejection for that cardiac cycle. It is not possible to measure left ventricular volume directly in the critical care unit. However, the presence of blood within the ventricle creates pressures that can be measured by the PA catheter and transducer and can be displayed on the bedside monitor.

Measurement of Preload. When the PA catheter is correctly positioned with the tip in one of the large branches of the pulmonary artery, the only valve between the PA catheter tip and the left ventricle is the mitral valve. During diastole, when the mitral valve is open, no obstruction exists between the tip of the PA catheter and the left ventricle (Fig. 18-14). The left ventricular preload volume creates left ventricular end-diastolic pressure (LVEDP). This is measured clinically by the PAOP. The PAOP and PADP are the values most often referred to in this chapter, because they are the values most often used in clinical practice. Normal LAP or PAOP is 5 to 12 mm Hg.

Frank-Starling Law of the Heart. Clinically the PAOP has significance because a change in left ventricular volume (preload) is reflected by a change in the measured PAOP (wedge pressure). Change in preload relies on the *Frank-Starling law of the heart*. This concept states that the force of ventricular ejection is directly related to two elements:

1. Volume in the ventricle at end-diastole (preload)
2. Amount of myocardial stretch placed on the ventricle as a result

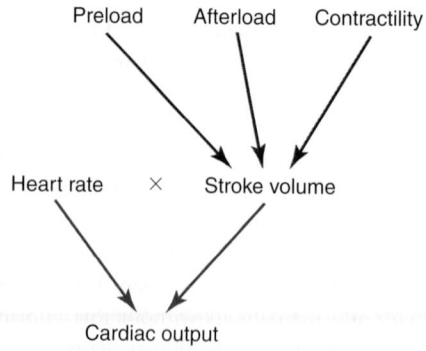

Figure 18-13 Preload, afterload, and contractility contribute to the heart's stroke volume. Stroke volume × Heart rate = Cardiac output.

TABLE 18-3 Pulmonary Artery Catheters: Selected Indications for Use and Response to Treatment

Diagnostic Indications*	Possible Cause	Associated Clinical Findings	Hemodynamic Profile†	Treatment and Expected Response
Hypovolemic shock	Trauma Surgery Bleeding Burns Excessive diuresis	Cardiovascular: sinus tachycardia, ↓ BP (SBP <90 mm Hg), weak peripheral pulses Pulmonary: lungs clear Renal: ↓ urinary output Skin: normal skin temperature, no edema Neurologic: variable	Low CO Low CI (2.2 L/min/m²) High SVR (>1600 dyn·sec·cm⁻⁵) Low PAP Low PAOP	Treatment: Fluid challenge Expected hemodynamic response: ↓ HR ↑ BP ↑ PAP ↑ PAOP ↑ CVP ↑ CO/CI ↓ SVR
Septic shock	Sepsis	Cardiovascular: sinus tachycardia, ↓ BP (SBP <90 mm Hg), bounding peripheral pulses Pulmonary: lungs may be clear or congested, depending on the origin of the sepsis Renal: ↓ urinary output Skin: warm and flushed Neurologic: variable	High CO (>8 L/min) High CI Low SVR (<600 dyn·sec·cm⁻⁵) Low PAP Low PAOP Low CVP	Treatment: IV fluid to maintain hemodynamic function Fluid challenge Peripheral vasoconstricting agent (alpha) to ↑ SVR Antibiotics and laboratory cultures to find site of infection Consider rhAPC Expected hemodynamic response: ↓ HR ↑ BP ↑ PAP ↑ PAOP ↑ CVP ↑ CO and CI ↑ SVR S̄v̄O₂ = 70%
Multisystem failure shock	Multiple organ dysfunction syndrome (MODS)	Cardiovascular: normal sinus rhythm or sinus tachycardia, ↓ BP, weak peripheral pulses Pulmonary: lungs may be clear or congested, depending on the site of sepsis; acidosis based on arterial blood gas values, may require mechanical ventilation Renal: ↓ urinary output, may have ↑ BUN and ↑ creatinine levels Skin: cool and mottled	Low CO Low CI (<2.2 L/min/m²) High SVR (>1600 dyn·sec·cm⁻⁵) High or low PAP High or low PAOP High or low CVP	Treatment: Vasodilators to ↓ SVR, Antibiotics Support of body system as necessary (e.g., mechanical ventilation, hemodialysis)

*Patients undergoing major vascular or cardiac surgery may also have a pulmonary catheter in situ to follow the trend of the cardiac output and cardiac index, systemic vascular resistance and pulmonary vascular resistance, and fluid status during the first 24 hours after surgery.

†See Table 18-1 for definitions and Appendix B for normal values of hemodynamic parameters listed in this table.

1BP, blood pressure; BUN, blood urea nitrogen; CI, cardiac index; CO, cardiac output; CVP, central venous pressure; CWI, cardiac work index; HR, heart rate; IABP, intraaortic balloon pump; IV, intravenous; PAOP, pulmonary artery occlusion pressure; PAP, pulmonary artery pressure; PVR, pulmonary vascular resistance; rhAPC, recombinant human activated protein C; SPB, systolic blood pressure; SVI, stroke volume index; S̄v̄O₂, mixed venous oxygen saturation; SVR, systemic vascular resistance; VSWI, ventricular stroke work index; ↓, decrease or decreased; ↑, increase or increased.

Continued

TABLE 18-3 Pulmonary Artery Catheters: Selected Indications for Use and Response to Treatment—*cont'd*

Diagnostic Indications	Possible Cause	Associated Clinical Findings	Hemodynamic Profile[†]	Treatment and Expected Response
		Neurologic: variable, depending on fluid status and drugs used in treatment		Expected hemodynamic response: ↓ HR ↑ BP Normalized PAP, PAOP, CVP ↓ SVR ↓ PVR ↑ CO and CI
Cardiogenic shock	Left ventricular pump failure caused by acute myocardial infarction or severe mitral or aortic valve disease	Cardiovascular: sinus tachycardia, possibly dysrhythmias, systolic BP <90 mm Hg, S_3 or S_4, weak peripheral pulses Pulmonary: lungs may have crackles or pulmonary edema Renal: ↓ urinary output Skin: cool, pale, and moist	Low CO Low CI (<2.2 L/min/m^2) High SVR (>1600 dyn·sec·cm−5) High PAP High PAOP (>15 mm Hg) High CVP Low SVI Low left CWI Low left VSWI	Treatment: Inotropic drugs to ↑ left ventricular contractility Vasodilators or IABP to ↓ afterload Diuretics to ↓ preload Optimization of heart rate and control of dysrhythmias Expected hemodynamic response: ↓ HR ↑ BP ↓ PAP ↓ PAOP ↓ CVP ↓ SVR ↑ CO and CI ↑ SVI ↑ Left CWI ↑ Left VSWI
Acute respiratory distress syndrome (ARDS) or noncardiogenic pulmonary edema	Trauma Sepsis Shock Inhaled toxins (smoke, chemicals, 100% oxygen) Aspiration of gastric contents Metabolic disorders	Neurologic: may have ↓ mentation caused by low BP and CO Cardiovascular: sinus tachycardia, high or low BP, normal peripheral pulses Pulmonary: poor oxygenation and pulmonary edema, ↑ respiratory rate, or need for mechanical ventilation Renal: ↑ or ↓ urinary output Skin: normal temperature Neurologic: anxiety or confusion associated with respiratory distress and poor oxygenation	Normal CO Normal CI Normal SVR Normal PAOP High PAP High PVR (>250 dyn·sec·cm^{-5}) Low right CWI Low right VSWI	Treatment: Eliminate cause of ARDS Support pulmonary function as necessary Expected hemodynamic response: ↓ HR Normal BP ↓ PAP ↓ PVR ↑ Right CWI ↑ Right VSWI Normal CO and CI Normal SVR

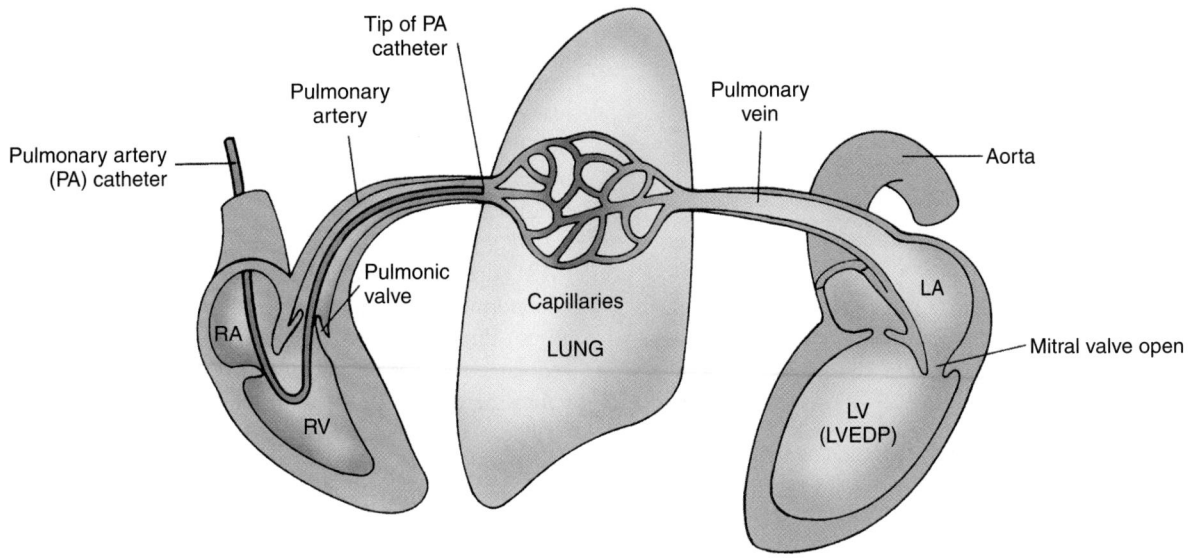

Figure 18-14 Relationship of the pulmonary artery occlusion pressure (PAOP) (i.e., wedge pressure) to the left ventricular end-diastolic pressure (LVEDP) (i.e., preload). In most clinical situations, the PAOP accurately reflects the LVEDP. During diastole, when the mitral valve is open, there are no other valves or other obstructions between the tip of the catheter and the left ventricle (LV). The pressure exerted by the volume in the LV is reflected through the left atrium (LA), through the pulmonary veins, and to the pulmonary capillaries. PA, pulmonary artery; RA, right atrium; RV, right ventricle.

If the volume in the left ventricle is low, CO is also suboptimal. If intravenous fluids (volume) are infused, CO increases as LV volume and myocardial fiber stretch increase. This is true up to a point. Past this point, more fluid volume overdistends the ventricle and stretches the myocardial fibers so much that CO decreases. This scenario is seen clinically in the setting of acute heart failure with pulmonary edema. The increased volume in the overdistended left ventricle raises pressure in the left ventricle, left atrium, and pulmonary veins (that drain into the left atrium), and it ultimately raises pulmonary capillary pressures measured as an increased wedge pressure (PAOP). The impact of preload on CO is represented in Figures 18-15 and 18-16, using the Frank-Starling curve as a model.

Ejection Fraction. The relationship of preload to the CO is complex because not all of the preload volume is ejected with every heartbeat. The percentage of preload volume ejected from the left ventricle per beat is measured during cardiac catheterization and is described as the ejection fraction (EF). A normal ejection fraction in a healthy heart is 70%. In clinical practice, most cardiologists will accept an EF value of greater than 50% as normal. The volume ejected from the left ventricle with each beat is known as the stroke volume, which can be calculated at the bedside by dividing the CO by the heart rate per minute (SV = CO ÷ HR).

Cardiac Dysfunction. A significant relationship exists between LVEDP and cardiac muscle dysfunction. As a general rule, the higher the pressure inside the left ventricle, the greater the degree of cardiac dysfunction. The pressure rises at end-diastole (end of filling) because the compromised ventricle cannot eject all of the preload blood volume. In a patient with heart failure, the preload volume may be 100 mL. However, the stroke volume ejected may be only 30 mL. The ejection fraction in this patient is 30% (normal EF is greater than 50%). The remaining

preload volume (70 mL in this example) significantly elevates left ventricular pressures. When the mitral valve opens at the beginning of diastole, the pressure in the left atrium needs to be slightly higher than pressures in the left ventricle to allow filling. The 70 mL remaining in the ventricle produces high LV diastolic pressures. This elevates the left atrial filling pressure and consequently elevates the PAOP (wedge pressure). In this example, the left ventricle is overstretched by excessive preload, and cardiac output therefore is below normal. A plan of care for

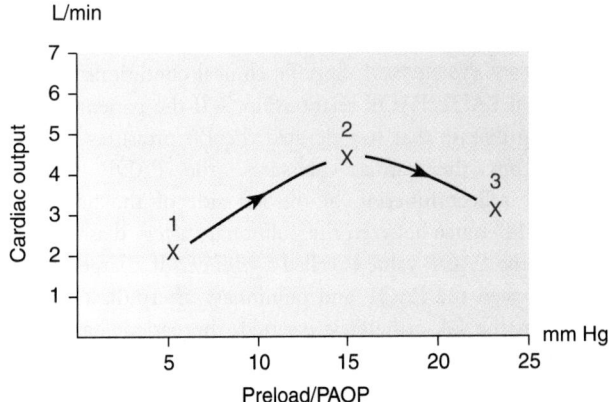

Figure 18-15 Impact of preload on cardiac output. *1,* Poor cardiac output (CO) with low preload as a result of hypovolemia. *2,* Hypovolemia is corrected after the administration of 2 L of intravenous fluid. The preload volume in the ventricle is increased, and pulmonary artery occlusion pressure (PAOP) has risen. Because of the increased fiber stretch from the increase in preload, CO also has risen. *3,* After the infusion of an additional 2 L of intravenous solution, the myocardial fibers are overdistended, preload (PAOP) has increased, and CO has fallen as the volume in the left ventricle rises.

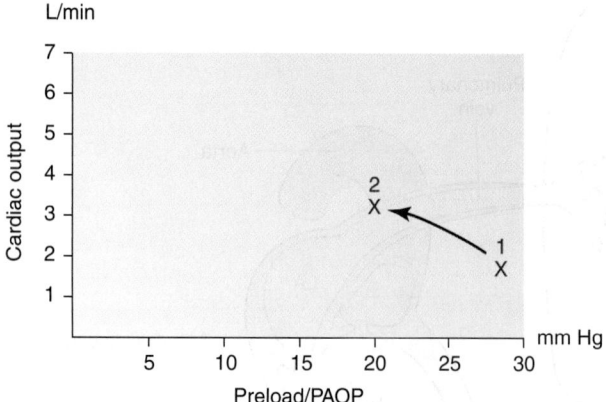

Figure 18-16 Impact of preload and venodilation on cardiac output (CO). *1,* After an acute anterior wall myocardial infarction that has created significant left ventricular dysfunction, this patient has left ventricle (LV) pump failure with low CO and elevated filling pressures (i.e., pulmonary artery occlusion pressure [PAOP]). One of the clinical problems faced by this patient is too much preload. *2,* After administration of diuretics to reduce volume and nitroglycerin to dilate the venous system, preload is reduced and CO rises.

this patient includes decreasing LV preload through (1) restriction of intravenous and oral fluids, (2) venodilation, and (3) diuresis. The myocardial dysfunction will lead to heart failure symptoms that are discussed further in Chapter 19.

Pulmonary Artery Diastolic Pressure and Pulmonary Artery Occlusion Pressure Relationship. LVEDP can be estimated by indirect measures using the PA catheter. The most accurate is the PAOP method. The second method involves measuring PADP during diastole when the normal PADP is equal to or 1 to 3 mm Hg higher than the mean PAOP and LVEDP. It is physiologically impossible for the PAOP to be higher than the PADP. The clinician must recalibrate and troubleshoot the monitoring system if this appears to occur (see Table 18-2).

Pulmonary Hypertension. Specific clinical conditions can alter the normal PADP/PAOP relationship.[34] If the patient has vascular lung disease that has elevated the PA pressures independently from the cardiac pressures, the PADP will not accurately reflect function of the left side of the heart. The numeric difference between the pulmonary artery diastolic pressure and the PAOP value is called a *gradient.* If a large gradient exists between the PAOP and pulmonary artery diastolic pressure when the PA catheter is inserted, the patient has pulmonary hypertension (Table 18-4, illustration C). Pulmonary hypertension is further discussed in Chapter 19.

Heart Failure. In failure of the left side of the heart, the PAOP and PADP are elevated and approximately equal (see Table 18-4, illustration B). The heart failure may cause secondary pulmonary hypertension. Over time, the damage to the lung vasculature occurs because of exposure to high LV pressure.

Mitral Stenosis. Pathology of the mitral valve—stenosis or regurgitation—alters the accuracy of PAOP and PADP as parameters of left ventricular function. In mitral valve stenosis, LAP and PAOP are increased and cause pulmonary congestion;

however, these elevated values do not reflect the LVEDP because a stenotic mitral valve decreases normal blood flow from the left atrium to the left ventricle, decreasing left ventricular preload and consequently lowering LVEDP. A nonstenotic mitral valve is essential for accurate readings because a narrowed mitral valve increases LAP, PAOP, and PADP in the presence of a normal LVEDP.

Mitral Regurgitation. In patients with mitral regurgitation (MR), the mean PAOP reading is artificially elevated because of abnormal backflow of blood from the left ventricle to the left atrium during systole. This PAOP reading is distinguished by very large *v* waves on the PAOP (wedge) tracing and may not reflect the true LVEDP (see Table 18-4, illustration F).

The *v* waves can be dramatic in some patients. However, the size of the *v* wave is related to the amount of MR and to the compliance of the left atrium. If the MR is chronic and the left atrium is compliant, *v* waves may be small. In the setting of acute MR after infarction of a papillary muscle, the noncompliant atrium contributes to the development of large *v* waves. Reading the PAOP tracing in the presence of MR is difficult. If the *v* waves are large (acute MR), they cannot be used to estimate LV preload. If the *v* wave is small (chronic MR), the mean PAOP or LAP can still estimate LV preload (LVEDP). Echocardiography also is used to confirm the presence of MR.[35]

Afterload. *Afterload* is defined as the pressure the ventricle generates to overcome the resistance to ejection created by the arteries and arterioles. It is a calculated measurement derived from information obtained from the PA catheter. As a response to increased afterload, ventricular wall tension rises. After a decrease in afterload, wall tension is lowered. The technical name for afterload is *systemic vascular resistance.*

Systemic Vascular Resistance. Resistance to ejection from the left side of the heart is estimated by calculating the systemic vascular resistance (SVR). The formula, normally calculated by the bedside computer, is as follows:

$$SVR = \frac{MAP - CVP}{CO} \times 80$$

The normal value is 800 to 1200 dyn·sec·cm^{-5}. To index this value to the patient's body surface area, the cardiac index (CI) is placed in the formula in the same position as the CO. The critical care nurse frequently manipulates prescribed vasoactive drugs to therapeutically alter afterload. In general, the lower the SVR, the higher the CO.

Pulmonary Vascular Resistance. Resistance to ejection from the right side of the heart is estimated by calculating the pulmonary vascular resistance (PVR). The PVR value is normally one sixth of the SVR. Normal PVR is 100 to 250 dyn·sec·cm^{-5}. The formula to calculate PVR is listed in Appendix B. In acute lung injury and in ARDS, the PVR rises above normal, and traditionally, a PA catheter was used to monitor vasodilator therapy and fluid management. However, because research trials have not shown a survival benefit to patients with ARDS and acute lung injury who received invasive PA monitoring compared with CVP monitoring, the PA catheter is less likely to be used.[23,24]

TABLE 18-4 **Clinical Interpretation of Pulmonary Artery Waveforms**

PA Pressure	Clinical Interpretation	Waveform Interpretation*
Pulmonary artery systolic (PAS) pressure	PAS pressure reflects the systolic pressure in the pulmonary vasculature. Waveform **A** is a normal waveform. The elevated values in pulmonary hypertension may be caused by idiopathic sources, some congenital heart defects, or lung disease.	**A** — Normal
Pulmonary artery diastolic (PAD) pressure	In the patient with healthy lung vasculature, PAD pressure reflects left ventricular end-diastolic pressure (LVEDP), as shown in waveform **B**. Even if the patient experiences heart failure, the pulmonary artery occlusion pressure (PAOP) and PAD increase together.	**B** — PAD/PAOP Correlation in a Patient With Normal Lungs
	In the presence of acute respiratory distress syndrome or pulmonary hypertension, PAD pressure is not an accurate reflection of PAOP, as shown in waveform **C**.	**C** — Poor PAD/PAOP Correlation in a Patient With Pulmonary Hypertension
Mean pulmonary artery pressure (PAP mean or PAP$_M$)	PAP mean pressure is used in the calculation of pulmonary vascular resistance (PVR) and pulmonary vascular resistance index (PVRI), as described in Table 18-1. High mean pressures can reflect cardiac or pulmonary disease. Low mean pressures reflect hypovolemia. Waveform **D** shows PAP mean placement.	**D** — Placement of PAP Mean Value
Pulmonary artery occlusion pressure (PAOP) or pulmonary artery wedge pressure (PAWP)	In the healthy patient, PAOP reflects blood in the left ventricle at end-diastole (LVEDP). The normal PAOP waveform is a left atrial waveform, as shown in waveform **E**. If a patient has mitral valve regurgitation, the *v* waves are larger than normal, increasing PAOP and possibly not reflecting true LVEDP, as shown in waveform **F**. PAOP is elevated in many cardiac disease states in which left ventricular function is compromised. PAOP is low in hypovolemic states.	**E** — Normal PAOP Tracing With *a* and *v* Waves **F** — PAOP Tracing With Elevated *v* Waves Caused by Mitral Valve Regurgitation

*Pressures on the *y* axis are given in millimeters of mercury (mm Hg).

Afterload Reduction. Pharmacologic manipulation of afterload to improve cardiac performance is commonly used with the critically ill patient. Many drugs with different modes of action are available. Drugs that vasodilate the arterial system and reduce SVR when given as a continuous infusion include sodium nitroprusside (Nipride) and high-dose nitroglycerin (NTG).[36] Other vasodilators commonly used include intravenous hydralazine and oral angiotensin-converting enzyme

(ACE) inhibiting drugs. Vasodilation of the pulmonary arterial vasculature is achieved by several medications, including dobutamine at less than 5 mcg/kg/min and prostaglandin infusions.[34]

If the SVR is extremely low (e.g., less than 500 dyn·sec·cm^{-5}), as may occur in sepsis, the CO will be elevated, and MAP will be low. In this situation, volume and vasopressors are infused to increase MAP and the SVR. After adequate volume resuscitation, the Surviving Sepsis Campaign guidelines recommend centrally administered dopamine, which increases MAP by affecting CO, or norepinephrine (Levophed), which increases MAP by vasoconstriction of the peripheral vasculature to increase SVR.[37] Frequent assessment of the peripheral circulation is required when drugs that increase SVR are used, because excessive vasoconstriction can negatively affect tissue perfusion.

One case can serve as an example. Mr. T had a large anterior wall MI 2 days earlier. As a result, he has symptoms of acute heart failure, an elevated SVR of 1840 dyn·sec·cm^{-5}, and a low CO of 2.8 L/min. In a heart with decreased contractility after an acute MI, an afterload measurement above the normal range lowers CO. To optimize Mr. T's cardiac function, systemic vasodilators (afterload-reducing drugs) are infused to lower the SVR into the normal range. After the administration of sodium nitroprusside (1 to 4 mcg/kg/min), Mr. T's SVR decreased to 970 dyn·sec·cm^{-5}, and his CO increased to 4.1 L/min. In this situation, decreasing the SVR to ejection greatly increased the amount of blood ejected from the left ventricle.

For a person with a normal heart without cardiac dysfunction, an elevated SVR may have minimal impact on CO. In summary, the importance of afterload on CO is related to the functional quality of the myocardium. Whether the heart muscle is globally damaged (cardiomyopathy) or regionally damaged (MI), small changes in SVR can produce significant changes in CO.

Contractility. Many factors have an impact on contractility, including preload volume as measured by PAOP, afterload (SVR), myocardial oxygenation, electrolyte balance, positive and negative inotropic drugs, and the amount of functional myocardium available to contribute to contraction. These factors can have a positive inotropic effect, enhancing contractility, or a negative inotropic effect, decreasing contractility. Significant factors related to contractility that can be measured by the PA catheter include preload filling pressures, afterload, and CO. Additional contractility numbers can be calculated and are displayed in the hemodynamic profile on the bedside monitor. These include left and right ventricular stroke work index values (LVSWI and RVSWI). These values estimate the force of cardiac contraction (see Table 18-1).

Preload has an impact on contractility by means of Starling's mechanism. As volume in the ventricle rises, contractility increases. If the ventricle is overdistended with volume, contractility falls (see Figs. 18-15 and 18-16). Afterload alters contractility by changes in resistance to ventricular ejection. If afterload is high, contractility is decreased. If afterload is low, contractility

is augmented. Hypoxemia acts as a negative inotrope. The myocardium must have oxygen available to the cells to contract efficiently.

Optimizing Contractility. Intravenous drugs such as dopamine, dobutamine, and milrinone are prescribed for their positive inotropic effect. The nurse considers the impact of these pharmacologic agents on contractility when following the trend of the patient's hemodynamic profile. No single hemodynamic number reflects contractility. However, if left ventricular contractility is increased in response to treatment, this effect is frequently reflected by changes in PAOP (wedge pressure) and by an increase in CO and LVSWI.

Pulmonary Artery Catheters. The traditional PA catheter, invented by Swan and Ganz, has four lumens for measurement of right atrial pressure (RAP) or CVP, PA pressures, PAOP, and CO (Fig. 18-17A). Multifunction catheters may have additional lumens, which can be used for intravenous infusion (Fig. 18-17B) and to measure continuous mixed venous oxygen saturation ($S\bar{v}O_2$), right ventricular volume, and continuous CO (Fig. 18-17C). Other PA catheters include transvenous pacing electrodes to pace the heart if needed.

The PA flow directed catheter is 110 cm long. The most commonly used size is 7.5 or 8.0 Fr, although 5.0 and 7.0 Fr sizes are available. Each of the four lumens exits into the heart or pulmonary artery at a different point, graduated along the catheter length (see Fig. 18-17A).

Right Atrial Lumen. The proximal lumen is situated in the right atrium and is used for intravenous infusion, CVP measurement, withdrawal of venous blood samples, and injection of fluid for CO determinations. This port is often described as the *right atrial port,* also called the *CVP port.*

Pulmonary Artery Lumen. The distal PA lumen is located at the tip of the PA catheter and is situated in the pulmonary artery. It is used to record pulmonary artery pressures and can be used for withdrawal of blood samples to measure mixed venous blood gases (e.g., $S\bar{v}O_2$).

Balloon Lumen. The third lumen opens into a balloon at the end of the catheter that can be inflated with 0.8 mL (7 Fr) to 1.5 mL (7.5 Fr) of air. The balloon is inflated during catheter insertion after the catheter reaches the right atrium to assist in forward flow of the catheter and to minimize right ventricular ectopy from the catheter tip. The balloon is also inflated to obtain the PAOP measurements when the PA catheter is correctly positioned in the pulmonary artery.

Thermistor Lumen. The fourth lumen is a thermistor (temperature sensor) used to measure changes in blood temperature. It is located 4 cm from the catheter tip and is used to measure thermodilution CO. The connector end of the lumen is attached directly to the CO computer.

Additional Features. If continuous $S\bar{v}O_2$ is measured, the catheter has an additional fiberoptic lumen that exits at the tip of the catheter (see Fig. 18-17C). If cardiac pacing is used, two PA catheter methods are available. One type of catheter has three atrial (A) and two ventricular (V) pacing electrodes attached to the catheter so that when it is properly positioned, the patient can be connected to a pacemaker and be AV paced.

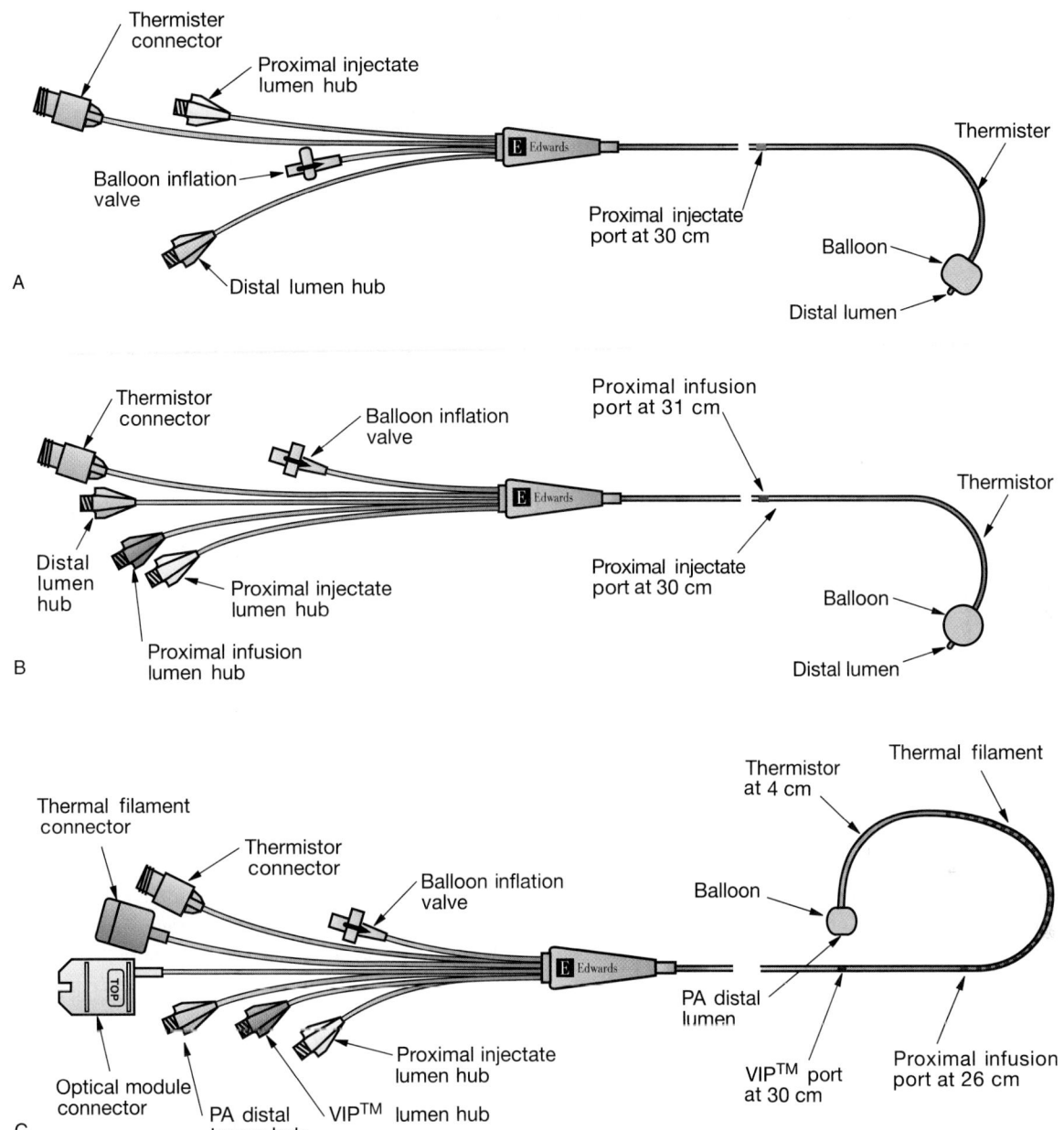

Figure 18-17 Types of pulmonary artery catheters. *A,* Four-lumen catheter. *B,* Five-lumen catheter that includes an additional venous infusion port (VIP) into the right atrium. *C,* Seven-lumen catheter that includes a VIP port and two additional lumens for continuous cardiac output (CCO) and a thermal filament and for continuous mixed venous oxygen saturation (S$\bar{\text{v}}$o$_2$) monitoring (i.e., optical module connector). An additional option is to combine the use of the CCO filament and the thermistor response time to calculate continuous end-diastolic volume (CEDV). *(©2001 Edwards Lifesciences LLC. All rights reserved. Reprinted with permission of Edwards Lifesciences, Swan-Ganz is a trademark of Edwards Lifesciences Corporation, registered in the US Patent and Trademark Office.)*

The other catheter method uses a specific transvenous pacing wire that is passed through an additional catheter lumen and exits into the right ventricle if ventricular pacing is required. A right ventricular volumetric PA catheter is available that measures stroke volume in the right ventricle.

Insertion. If a PA catheter is to be inserted into a patient who is awake, some brief explanations about the procedure are helpful to ensure that the patient understands what is going to happen. The initial insertion techniques used for placement of a PA catheter are similar to those described for CVC insertion. Because the PA catheter is positioned within the heart chambers and pulmonary artery on the right side of the heart, catheter passage is monitored using fluoroscopy or waveform analysis on the bedside monitor (Fig. 18-18).

Before inserting the catheter into the vein, the physician—using sterile technique—tests the balloon for inflation and flushes the catheter with normal saline solution to remove any air.

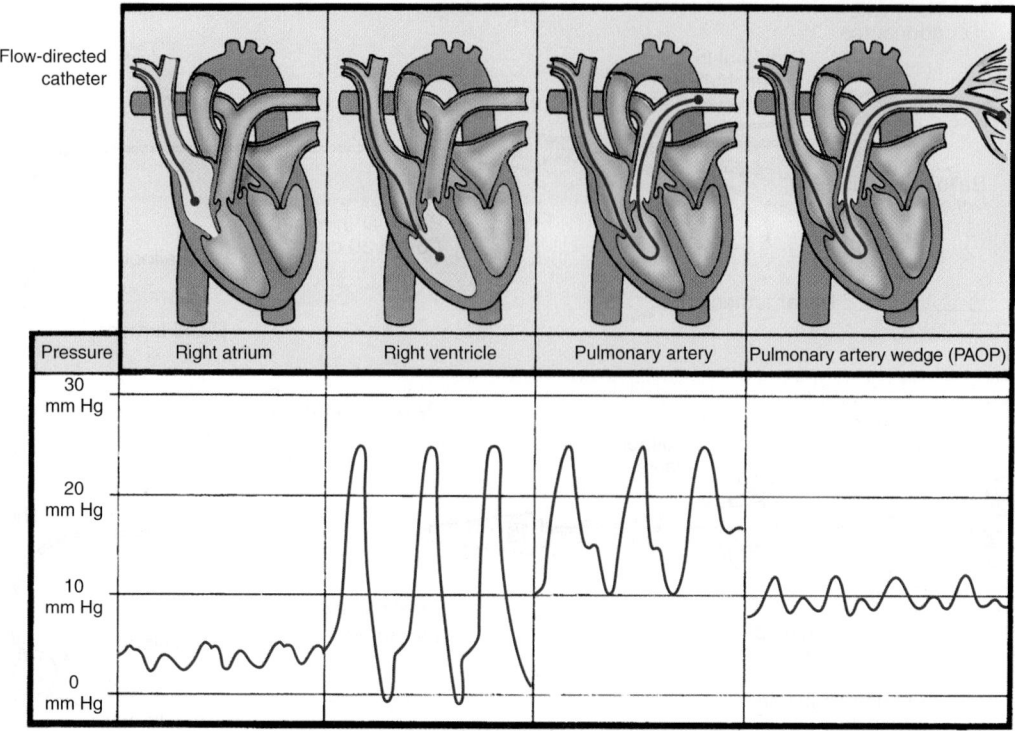

Figure 18-18 Pulmonary artery (PA) catheter insertion with corresponding waveforms.

The PA catheter is then attached to the bedside hemodynamic line setup and monitor so that the waveforms can be visualized while the catheter is advanced through the right side of the heart (see Fig. 18-18). A larger introducer sheath (8.5 Fr)—which has the tip positioned in the vena cava and has an additional intravenous side-port lumen—is often used to cannulate the vein first.[38] This introducer sheath is known by several different names in clinical practice, including *sheath, cordis, introducer,* or *side port.* This introducer sheath remains in place, and the supple PA catheter is threaded through it into the vena cava and into the right side of the heart.

Pulmonary Artery Waveform Interpretation. Each chamber of the heart has a distinctive waveform with recognizable characteristics. It is the responsibility of the critical care nurse to recognize each waveform displayed on the bedside monitor when the catheter enters the corresponding chamber during insertion and during routine monitoring.[38]

Right Atrial Waveform. As the PA catheter is advanced into the right atrium during insertion, a right atrial waveform must be visible on the monitor, with recognizable *a, c,* and *v* waves (see Fig. 18-18). The normal mean pressure in the right atrium is 2 to 5 mm Hg. Before passage through the tricuspid valve, the balloon at the tip of the catheter is inflated for two reasons. First, it cushions the pointed tip of the PA catheter so that if the tip comes into contact with the right ventricular wall, it will cause less myocardial irritability and, consequently, fewer ventricular dysrhythmias. Second, inflation of the balloon assists the catheter to float with the flow of blood from the right ventricle into the pulmonary artery. It is because of these features and the balloon that PA catheters are described as *flow-directional catheters.*

Right Ventricular Waveform. The right ventricular waveform is distinctly pulsatile, with distinct systolic and diastolic pressures. Normal right ventricular pressures are 20 to 30 mm Hg systolic and 0 to 5 mm Hg diastolic. Even with the balloon inflated, it is not uncommon for some ventricular ectopy to occur during passage through the right ventricle. All patients who have a PA catheter inserted must have simultaneous ECG monitoring, with defibrillator and emergency resuscitation equipment nearby.

Pulmonary Artery Waveform. As the catheter enters the pulmonary artery, the waveform again changes. The diastolic pressure rises. Normal PA pressures range from 20 to 30 mm Hg systolic over 10 mm Hg diastolic. A dicrotic notch, visible on the downslope of the waveform, represents closure of the pulmonic valve.

Pulmonary Artery Occlusion Waveform (Wedge). While the balloon remains inflated, the catheter is advanced into the wedge position. This maneuver produces the PAOP. The waveform decreases in size and is nonpulsatile, reflecting a normal left atrial tracing with a and v wave deflections. This is known as a *wedge tracing,* because the balloon is "wedged" into a small pulmonary vessel, but it is technically described as the PAOP (see Fig. 18-18). The balloon occludes the pulmonary vessel so that the PA catheter tip and lumen are exposed only to LAP and is protected from the pulsatile influence of the pulmonary artery. When the balloon is deflated, the catheter should spontaneously float back into the PA. When the balloon is reinflated, the wedge tracing should be visible. The normal PAOP ranges from 5 to 12 mm Hg.

After insertion, the introducer is sutured to the skin, the catheter, which lies within the introducer, is secured with tape or with a specialized catheter securement device. A chest radiograph is taken to verify placement. If the catheter is advanced too far into the pulmonary bed, the patient is at risk for pulmonary infarction. If the PA catheter is not sufficiently advanced into the pulmonary artery, it will not be useful for PAOP readings. However, in many critical care units, if the patient's PADP and PAOP values approximate (within 0 to 3 mm Hg), the PADP is reliably used to follow the trend of LV filling pressure (preload). This prevents possible trauma from frequent balloon inflation; in such a situation, the PA catheter is consciously pulled back into a nonwedging position in the pulmonary artery.

After insertion of the catheter, the chest radiograph or fluoroscopy is used to verify the PA catheter position to make sure that it is not looped or knotted in the right ventricle and to rule out pneumothorax or hemorrhagic complications. A thin plastic cuff can be placed on the outside of the catheter when it is inserted to maintain sterility of the part of the PA catheter that exits from the patient. If the PA catheter is not in the desired position or if it migrates out of position, it can be repositioned. The plastic cuff is designed to keep the external catheter sterile for a short period after insertion.

Medical Management. Controversy exists in the medical community over the use of PA catheters and rates of use have declined in response to lack of benefit demonstrated in clinical trials.[23-30] Medical goals of hemodynamic monitoring include assessment of adequacy of perfusion in stable patients, early detection of decreased perfusion, titration of therapy to meet specific therapeutic outcomes, and differentiation of different organ system dysfunctions. Practice guidelines are available for physicians who routinely work with PA catheters.[39]

Nursing Management. The more knowledgeable the critical care nurse can become about use of the PA catheter, the more accurate and effective the nursing management interventions will be.[5,40] Factors that affect PA measurement are the head-of-bed position and lateral body position relative to transducer height placement, respiratory variation, and use of positive end-expiratory pressure (PEEP).

Patient Position. The patient does not need to be flat for accurate pressure readings to be obtained. In the supine position, when the transducer is placed at the level of the phlebostatic axis, a head-of-bed position from flat up to 60 degrees is appropriate for most patients.[5] It is important to know that PADP and PAOP measurements in the lateral position may be significantly different from those taken when the patient is lying supine. If there is concern about the validity of pressure readings in a particular patient, it is more reliable to take measurements with the patient on his or her back, with the head of bed elevated from flat to 60 degrees as tolerated. After a patient changes position, a stabilization period of 5 minutes is recommended before taking pressure readings if the patient has a healthy heart (normal left ventricle), and a stabilization period of 15 minutes is recommended if the patient has LV dysfunction.[41]

Respiratory Variation. All PADP and PAOP (wedge) tracings are subject to respiratory interference, especially when the patient is on a positive-pressure, volume-cycled ventilator.[5,38] During the positive-pressure inhalation phase, the increase in intrathoracic pressure may "push up" the pulmonary artery tracing, producing an artificially high reading (Fig. 18-19A). During inhalation with spontaneous breaths, negative intrathoracic pressure "pulls down" the waveform, producing an erroneously low measurement (see Fig. 18-19B). To minimize the impact of respiratory variation, the PADP is read at end-expiration, which is the most stable point in the respiratory cycle when intrapleural pressures are close to zero.[38] If the digital number fluctuates with respiration, a printed readout on paper can be obtained to verify true PADP. In some clinical settings, ECG signals or airway pressure and flow are recorded simultaneously with the PADP/PAOP tracing to identify end-expiration.[5]

Positive End-Expiratory Pressure. Some clinical diagnoses, such as ARDS, require the use of high levels of PEEP set with the ventilator to treat refractory hypoxemia. If a PEEP of greater than 10 cm H_2O is used, PAOP (wedge) and pulmonary artery pressures will be artificially elevated, and CO may be negatively affected.[42,43] Because of this impact of PEEP, in the past, patients in some critical care units were taken off the ventilator to record pulmonary artery pressure measurements. It has since been shown that this practice closes alveoli, decreases the patient's oxygenation level, and may result in persistent hypoxemia.

Because patients remain on PEEP for treatment, they remain on it during measurement of pulmonary artery pressures. In this situation, the trend of pulmonary artery readings is more important than one individual measurement. The most important factor is not one individual measurement or the absolute number obtained; it is instead the trend of the measurements being used as a basis for clinical interventions to support and improve cardiopulmonary function in the critically ill.

Avoiding Complications. Potential cardiac complications include ventricular dysrhythmias, endocarditis, valvular damage, cardiac rupture, and cardiac tamponade. Potential pulmonary complications include rupture of a pulmonary artery, pulmonary artery thrombosis, embolism or hemorrhage, and infarction of a segment of lung. The PA catheter tracing is continuously monitored to ensure that the catheter does not migrate forward into a spontaneous wedge or PAOP position. A segment of lung can suffer infarction if the wedged catheter occludes an arteriole for a prolonged period. If the catheter is spontaneously wedged, the critical care nurse can gently pull the catheter back out of the wedge position if the institutional policy allows.[44]

Infection is always a risk with a PA catheter. The risks are similar to those discussed in the section on CVCs (see the Patient Safety Alert feature on Guidelines for Prevention and Management of Central Venous Catheter Infections).

Pulmonary Artery Catheter Removal. PA catheters can be safely removed from the patient by critical care nurses competent in this procedure.[5,44,45] Removal is not usually associated with major complications. The most common incidents are PVCs in about 2% of patients as the catheter is pulled through the right ventricle.[5,45,46]

Cardiac Output. The PA catheter measures CO using an intermittent (bolus) or a continuous CO method.

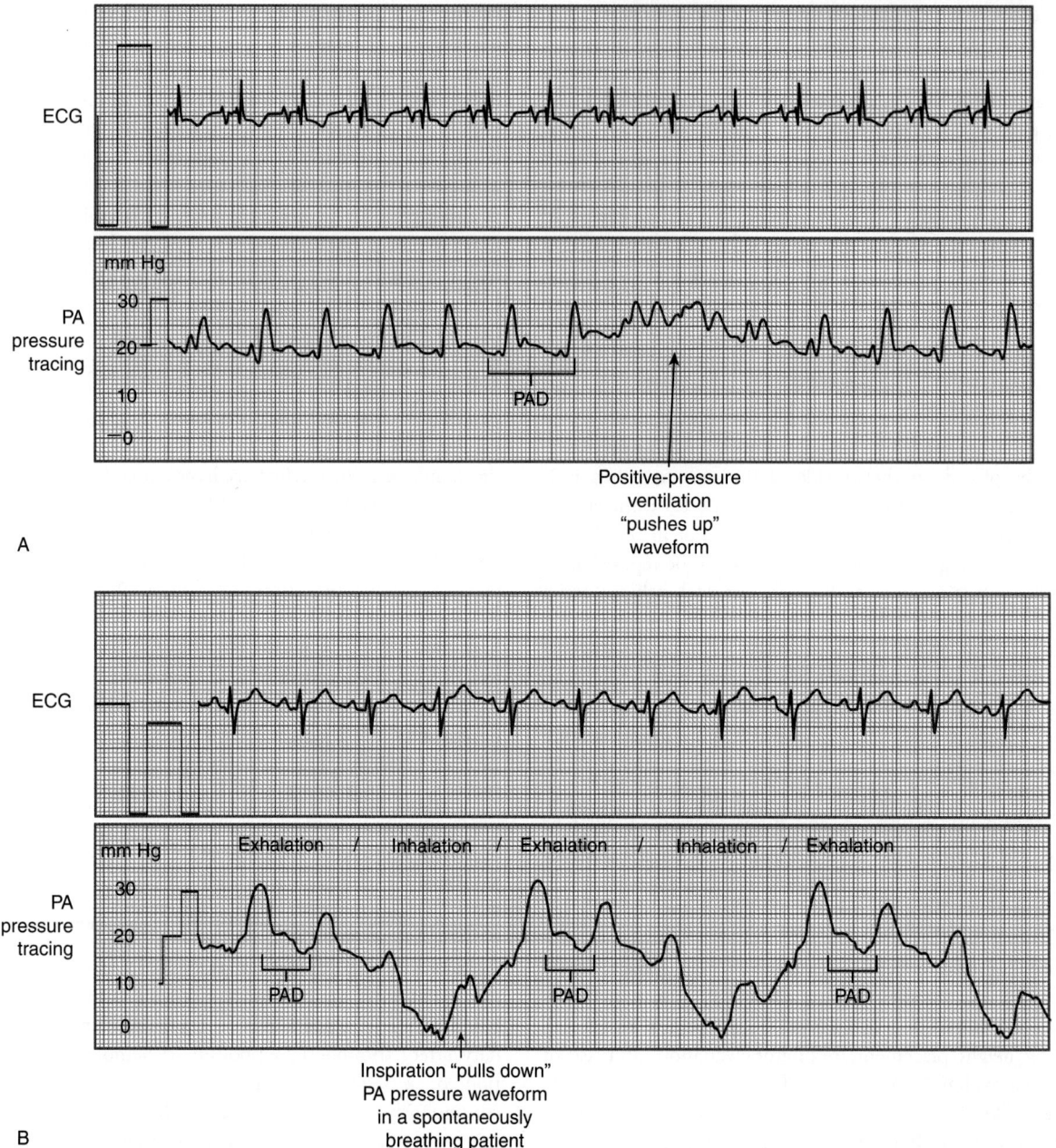

Figure 18-19 Pulmonary artery (PA) waveforms that demonstrate the impact of ventilation on PA pressure readings. For accuracy, PA pressures are read at the end of exhalation. *A,* In positive-pressure ventilation, the increase in intrathoracic pressure during inhalation "pushes up" the PA pressure waveform, creating a falsely high reading. *B,* In spontaneous breathing, the decrease in intrathoracic pressure during normal inhalation "pulls down" the PA waveform, creating a falsely low reading.

Thermodilution Cardiac Output Bolus Method. The bolus thermodilution method is performed at the bedside and results in CO calculated in liters per minute. Three CO values that are within a 10% mean range are obtained at one time and are averaged to calculate CO. A known amount (5 mL) of iced or, more typically, 10 mL of room-temperature normal saline solution is injected into the proximal lumen of the PA catheter. The injectate exits into the right atrium and travels with the flow of blood past the thermistor (temperature sensor) located at the distal end of the catheter in the pulmonary artery. The injectate can be delivered by hand injection using individual

syringes of saline. Frequently, a closed in-line system attached to a 500-mL bag of normal saline is used as a reservoir to deliver the individual injections.[47]

Sometimes, the right atrial (proximal) port is clotted and not usable. If another right atrial port is available, it can be substituted. However, if a usable port is not available, to ensure accurate CO data, a new pulmonary artery catheter is inserted.

Cardiac Output Curve. The thermodilution CO method uses the indicator-dilution method, in which a known temperature is the indicator. It is based on the principle that the change in temperature over time is inversely proportional to

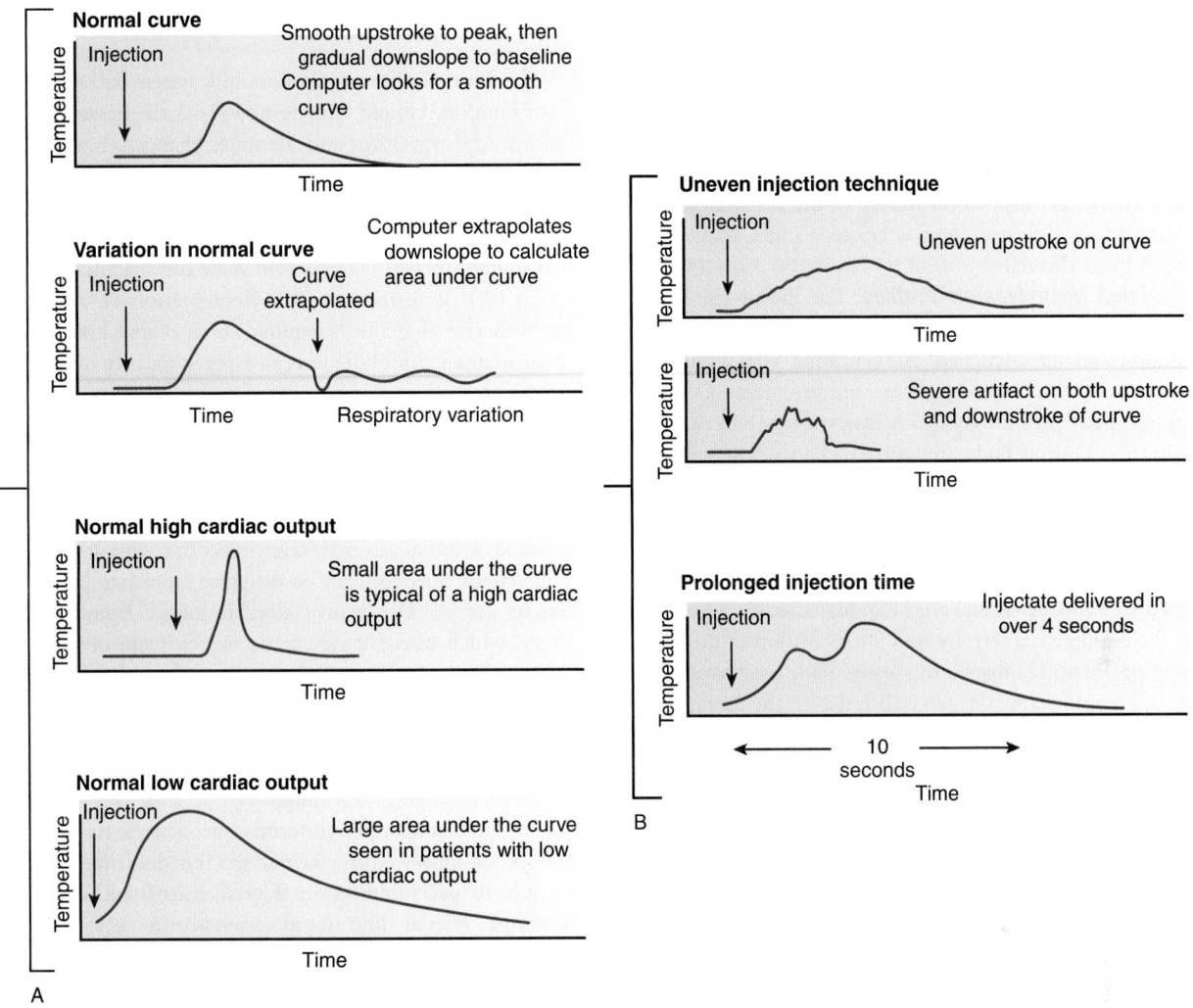

Figure 18-20 *A,* Variations in the normal cardiac thermodilution bolus output curve. *B,* Abnormal cardiac output curves produce an erroneous cardiac output value.

blood flow. Blood flow can be diagrammatically represented as a CO curve on which temperature is plotted against time (Fig. 18-20A). Most hemodynamic monitors display this CO curve, which must then be interpreted to determine whether the CO injection is valid. The normal curve has a smooth upstroke, with a rounded peak and a gradually tapering downslope. If the curve has an uneven pattern, it may indicate faulty injection technique, and the CO measurement must be repeated. Patient movement or coughing also alters the CO measurement (see Fig. 18-20B).

Injectate Temperature. If the CO is within the normal range, it is equally accurate whether iced or room temperature injectate is used. However, if the COs are extremely high or very low, iced injectate may be more accurate. To ensure accurate readings, the difference between injectate temperature and body temperature must be at least 10° C, and the injectate must be delivered within 4 seconds, with minimal handling of the syringe to prevent warming of the solution. This is particularly important if iced injectate is used. With all delivery systems, the injectate is delivered at the same point in the respiratory cycle, usually end-exhalation.

Patient Position and Cardiac Output. In the normovolemic, stable patient, reliable CO measurements can be obtained in a supine position (patient lying on his or her back) with the head of the bed elevated up to 45 degrees. If the patient is hypovolemic or unstable, leaving the head of the bed in a flat position or only slightly elevated is the most clinically appropriate choice. CO measurements performed when the patient is turned to the side are not considered as accurate as those performed with the patient in the supine position.

Clinical Conditions That Alter Cardiac Output. Two clinical conditions produce errors in the thermodilution CO measurement: tricuspid valve regurgitation and ventricular septal rupture. If the patient has tricuspid valve regurgitation, the expected flow of blood from the right atrium to the pulmonary artery is disrupted by backflow from the right ventricle to the right atrium. This creates a lower CO measurement than the patient's actual output. If the person has an intracardiac left-to-right shunt, as occurs after ventricular septal rupture, the thermodilution CO measures the large pulmonary volume and records a higher CO than the patient's true systemic output.

Continuous Invasive Cardiac Output Measurement. The bolus thermodilution method is reliable but performed intermittently. Continuous CO monitoring using a PA catheter is also frequently used in clinical practice. One method employs a thermal filament on the PA catheter to emit small energy signals (the indicator) into the bloodstream. These signals are then detected by the thermistor near the tip of the PA catheter. The equivalent of an indicator curve is created, and a CO value is calculated from this data.

Calculated Hemodynamic Profiles. For the patient with a thermodilution PA catheter in place, additional hemodynamic information can be calculated using routine vital signs, CO, and body surface area (BSA). These measurements are calculated using specific formulas that are indexed to a patient's body size using the DuBois body area surface chart or the computer program associated with the current generation of hemodynamic monitors.

The calculated values used in the hemodynamic profiles are described in Table 18-1. Clinical use of these profiles is described in two case studies. In Hemodynamic Profile 1 (Box 18-1), the example is a step-by-step interpretation of the hemodynamic profile to familiarize the reader with use of calculated values. In Hemodynamic Profile 2 (Box 18-2), the example uses only values indexed to body weight and illustrates the impact of treatment on these values over time.

Noninvasive and Minimally Invasive Measurement of Cardiac Output. As a result of the perceived risks associated with use of the pulmonary artery thermodilution catheter, combined with studies that have not shown improved outcomes with routine monitoring, there is tremendous interest in finding less invasive methods of CO measurement. All of these evolving techniques are less invasive that the PA catheter, one is *noninvasive* and others are described as *minimally invasive* and involve vascular catheters or esophageal probes as described in Table 18-5. All have been compared with the thermodilution CO method.

Noninvasive Cardiac Output Measurement. Thoracic bioimpedance cardiography is a noninvasive method of continuous CO measurement. Impedance cardiography works by emitting a low-voltage, high-frequency, alternating electrical current through the thorax by means of skin electrodes. The sensing electrodes detect changes in electrical impedance within the thorax. Because blood flow through the thoracic aorta causes shifts in impedance, this information can be used to calculate stroke volume and continuous CO. This is the least invasive method of monitoring continuous CO.

Minimally Invasive Cardiac Output Measurement. Several technologies offer different levels of minimal invasiveness for continuous CO monitoring (see Table 18-5). Pulse contour waveform analysis is the least invasive of this group. It allows stroke volume or CO to be derived from the arterial waveform. These technologies require the patient to have a functional venous catheter and arterial catheter in place. A significant advantage to the pulse contour waveform method is that the patient does not have to be intubated or sedated to tolerate the monitoring system. Three commercial systems that use pulse contour

waveform technology have undergone trials in critically ill patients.

The lithium dilution cardiac output system (LiDCO, LiDCO Ltd., London, United Kingdom) assesses the power of the arterial pressure waveform and identifies changes in arterial power to reflect changes in stroke volume. To obtain an accurate baseline measure of stroke volume, a subtherapeutic dose of lithium is injected into the venous line and measured at the arterial sensor for calibration. The values obtained are comparable to thermodilution CO measurements.[48,49] Recalibration of the system to establish a new baseline is required about every 8 hours according to the manufacturer but closer to every 4 hours to maintain accurate CO according to researchers who have used this system.[48,50]

The pulse contour cardiac output system (Pulsion Medical Systems, Munich, Germany) obtains a continuous CO measurement by analyzing the systolic component of the systolic arterial waveform. Three calibrations using cold saline are required at initial setup (venous injections with arterial sensor). The venous injection can be delivered from jugular or femoral venous access. The transit time is longer from the femoral artery, which causes a systematic overestimate of the CO, but once recognized, this can be accounted for by following the trend of measurements.[51] The manufacturer recommends recalibration every 8 hours, but researchers reported that recalibration was required every 4 to 6 hours or even hourly to maintain accurate CO readings.[48,52,53]

The Vigileo Monitor (Edwards Lifesciences, Irvine, CA) uses pulse contour waveform technology but does not require calibration. A specialized sensor (Flotrac sensor) added to the conventional arterial line setup assesses arterial pressure at a frequency of 100 Hz to characterize the arterial pulse waveform. This information is combined with patient variables (age, sex, weight) in a proprietary algorithm to estimate stroke volume and CO.[48,54] The validation studies show conflicting results; some researchers reported that the system was not able to maintain accurate CO readings, and others found it tracked hemodynamic changes accurately in response to vasopressors.[48,54]

The esophagus is used as the monitoring site for patients who are deeply sedated or are under general anesthesia in the operating room. The esophageal Doppler and transesophageal echocardiography (TEE) are considered less invasive that a PA catheter. Insertion of the esophageal Doppler is reported to be similar to insertion of a gastric tube, although the probe is relatively inflexible and stiff.[55,56] The probe is inserted 35 to 40 cm from the teeth. The tip of the probe rests near T5-T6 on the vertebral column, where the esophagus typically is parallel with the descending aorta.[56] There are at least two types of esophageal Doppler monitors available, with proprietary differences in the methods of CO measurement. When the probe is correctly placed, this method has a high degree of accuracy for CO measurement.[56] Both methods depend on correct placement and on the skill of the operator. TEE is discussed further under "Transesophageal Echocardiography."

A third technology involves partial carbon dioxide (CO_2) rebreathing and uses a modified Fick principle for CO applied to CO_2. The NICO system involves the addition of an extra

BOX 18-1 HEMODYNAMIC PROFILE 1

ADMISSION

Mr. SR has a medical history of cardiomyopathy and chronic obstructive pulmonary disease (COPD). He is admitted to a coronary care unit because of an exacerbation of his biventricular heart failure. He has been complaining about anginal pain and shortness of breath. His nursing diagnoses are Decreased Cardiac Output and Impaired Gas Exchange.

Height	163 cm	PAD	27 mm Hg	PVR	322 dyn·sec·cm^{-5}
Weight	79 kg	PAP$_M$	36 mm Hg	PVRI	612 dyn·sec·cm^{-5}/m^2
Body surface area (BSA)	1.9 m^2	PAOP	26 mm Hg	LCW	2.1 kg-m
		CVP	24 mm Hg	LCWI	1.1 kg-m/m^2
HR	104 beats/min	CO	2.48 L/min	LVSW	2.4 g-m
ABP		CI	1.31 L/min/m^2	LVSWI	10.7 g-m/m^2
Systolic	88 mm Hg	SV	23.8 mL	RCW	1.21 kg-m
Diastolic	51 mm Hg	SI	12.5 mL/m^2	RCWI	0.64 kg-m/m^2
MAP	63 mm Hg	SVR	1257 dyn·sec·cm^{-5}	RVSW	11.7 g-m
PAS	55 mm Hg	SVRI	2388 dyn·sec·cm^{-5}/m^2	RVSWI	6.2 g-m/m^2

ANALYSIS OF THE HEMODYNAMIC PROFILE*

Profile	Analysis
HR (heart rate)	Heart rate of 104 beats/min is above normal limits (normal, 60-100 beats/min).
ABP (arterial blood pressure)	Narrow pulse pressure of 88/51 mm Hg with a low mean arterial pressure (MAP) of 63 mm Hg (normal MAP, 65-90 mm Hg).
Pulmonary artery pressure	Pulmonary artery pressures are elevated (55/27 mm Hg), consistent with diagnosis of cardiomyopathy, failure of left side of heart, and COPD (normal PAP, 25/10 mm Hg).
PAOP (pulmonary artery occlusion pressure)	Elevated PAOP (26 mm Hg), consistent with diagnosis of cardiomyopathy and failure of left side of heart (normal PAOP, 5-12 mm Hg).
CVP (central venous pressure)	Elevated CVP (24 mm Hg), consistent with diagnosis of cardiomyopathy, failure of right side of heart, and COPD (normal CVP, 4-6 mm Hg).
CO (cardiac output) and CI (cardiac index)	Poor CO and CI (CO, 2.48 L/min; CI, 1.31 L/min/m^2). Both values are below normal (normal CO, 4-6 L/min; normal CI, 2.2-4 L/min/m^2).
SV (stroke volume) and SI (stroke volume index)	SV and SI are low (SV, 23.8 mL; SI, 12.5 mL/m^2). These results would be anticipated from the low cardiac output (normal SV, 60-70 mL; normal SI, 40-50 mL/min/m^2).
SVR (systemic vascular resistance) and SVRI (systemic vascular resistance index)	SVR and SVRI are at the upper normal range (SVR, 1257 dyn·sec·cm^{-5}; SVRI, 2388 dyn·sec·cm^{-5}/m^2). These values are not contributing to the low cardiac output at this time (normal SVR, 800-1400 dyn·sec·cm^{-5}; normal SVRI, 2000-2400 dyn·sec·cm^{-5}/m^2).
PVR (pulmonary vascular resistance) and PVRI (pulmonary vascular resistance index)	PVR and PVRI are elevated (PVR, 322 dyn·sec·cm^{-5}; PVRI 612 dyn·sec·cm^{-5}/m^2). High pulmonary vascular resistance may be contributing to the low cardiac output (normal PVR, 100-250 dyn·sec·cm^{-5}; normal PVRI, 225-315 dyn·sec·cm^{-5}/m^2).
LCWI (left cardiac work index) and LVSWI (left ventricular stroke work index)	Both LCWI and LVSWI are below normal (LCWI, 1.1 kg-m/m^2; LVSWI, 10.7 g-m/m^2), indicating that left ventricular myocardial damage may be present. This is consistent with Mr. SR's diagnosis of cardiomyopathy (normal LCWI, 3.4-4.2 kg-m/m^2; normal LVSWI, 50-62 g-m/m^2).
RCWI (right cardiac work index) and RVSWI (right ventricular stroke work index)	RCWI is normal, but RVSWI is below normal (RCWI, 0.64 kg-m/m^2; RVSWI, 6.2 g-m/m^2), indicating that right ventricular myocardial damage may be present. This is consistent with Mr. SR's diagnosis of cardiomyopathy and history of COPD (normal RCWI, 0.54-0.66 kg-m/m^2, normal RVSWI, 7.9-9.7, g-m/m^2).
Nursing impression	The hemodynamic data confirm the nursing clinical diagnosis of poor CO. The goal is to improve CO within the limits of Mr. SR's myocardial dysfunction and COPD. As CO improves and PA pressures decrease, the patient will have less pulmonary congestion, which will improve alveolar gas exchange.

*Formulas and normal values for the hemodynamics values are given in Table 18-1 and in Appendix B.

---

circuit (tubing loop) to the ventilator tubing, and it can be used only with intubated, mechanically ventilated patients. A sensor that uses infrared light absorption measures CO_2, and a second sensor measures airflow in the circuit tubing to collect data during a breathing cycle. CO_2 production is calculated as the product of minute ventilation and CO_2 concentration. Arterial CO_2 content is derived from end-tidal CO_2 and the CO_2 dissociation curve. The differences in these values are then used to calculate the CO.[52] The validation studies have produced inconsistent results for the accuracy of the derived CO; this might have resulted from intrapulmonary shunt in the critically ill. This system also requires frequent calibration.

BOX 18-2   HEMODYNAMIC PROFILE 2

1. ADMISSION

Mrs. JL has been admitted to the critical care unit with pulmonary edema. She has a history of anterior wall myocardial infarction and severe chronic obstructive pulmonary disease (COPD).

Height	159 cm	MAP	106 mm Hg	SI	9.9 mL/m^2
Weight	45.8 kg	PAS	53 mm Hg	SVRI	5351 dyn·sec·cm^{-5}/m^2
Body surface area (BSA)	1.40 m^2	PAD	27 mm Hg	PVRI	1046 dyn·sec·cm^{-5}/m^2
		PAP$_M$	44 mm Hg	LCWI	1.9 kg-m/m^2
HR	131 beats/min	PAOP	27 mm Hg	LVSWI	14.3 g-m/m^2
ABP		CVP	19 mm Hg	RCW	0.78 kg-m/m^2
Systolic	160 mm Hg	CO	1.82 L/min	RCWI	5.9 g-m/m^2
Diastolic	80 mm Hg	CI	1.3 L/min/m^2		

Analysis of the Hemodynamic Profile*

In the above hemodynamic profile, notice the fast heart rate; high MAP; high PA and CVP filling pressures; low CI, SI, LVSWI, and RVSWI; and high SVRI and PVRI. These values are consistent with a diagnosis of failure of the left side of the heart, causing pulmonary edema, which may lead to cardiogenic shock. Treatment is focused on increasing the cardiac index by lowering SVRI and PVRI and using IV sodium nitroprusside and intravenous (IV) nitroglycerin in continuous infusion.

2. THREE HOURS LATER

Height	159 cm	MAP	83 mm Hg	SI	16.5 mL/m^2
Weight	45.8 kg	PAS	41 mm Hg	SVRI	3088 dyn·sec·cm^{-5}/m^2
Body surface area (BSA)	1.40 m^2	PAD	26 mm Hg	PVRI	300 dyn·sec·cm^{-5}/m^2
		PAP$_M$	33 mm Hg	LCWI	2.1 kg-m/m^2
HR	113 beats/min	PAOP	26 mm Hg	LVSWI	18.6 g-m/m^2
ABP		CVP	11 mm Hg	RCWI	0.84 kg-m/m^2
Systolic	104 mm Hg	CO	2.61 L/min	RVSWI	7.4 g-m/m^2
Diastolic	69 mm Hg	CI	1.86 L/min/m^2		

Analysis of Hemodynamic Profile 2

Results 3 hours after sodium nitroprusside administration showed improving hemodynamics, demonstrated as normal MAP and lower intracardiac filling pressures (PA and CVP). However, CI and SI remain low; and SVRI is above normal. Mrs. JL remains in severe left ventricular failure because of her low CI.

3. THE NEXT DAY

Height	159 cm	MAP	77 mm Hg	SI	22.5 mL/m^2
Weight	45.8 kg	PAS	31 mm Hg	SVRI	2423 dyn·sec·cm^{-5}/m^2
Body surface area (BSA)	1.40 m^2	PAD	15 mm Hg	PVRI	273 dyn·sec·cm^{-5}/m^2
		PAP$_M$	23 mm Hg	LCWI	2.4 kg-m/m^2
HR	104 beats/min	PAOP	15 mm Hg	LVSWI	22.9 g-m/m^2
ABP		CVP	4 mm Hg	RCWI	0.74 kg-m/m^2
Systolic	111 mm Hg	CO	3.28 L/min	RVSWI	7.1 g-m/m^2
Diastolic	60 mm Hg	CI	2.34 L/min/m^2		

Analysis of Hemodynamic Profile 3

The next day, Mrs. JL's hemodynamics have improved with continued use of sodium nitroprusside and nitroglycerin. The CI value is in the low-normal range, and SVRI and PVRI values are in the high-normal range. LVSWI remains low, reflecting the patient's compromised left ventricle from a prior anterior wall myocardial infarction.

---

*See Box 18-1 for explanation of abbreviations and Table 18-1 and Appendix B for an explanation of hemodynamic values.

These emerging technologies are likely to improve over time. The impetus for improvement is the push toward less invasive methods to replace the PA catheter. The different technologies have very different advantages and disadvantages, and more innovations are certainly on the horizon.

CONTINUOUS MONITORING OF VENOUS OXYGEN SATURATION

Indications. Continuous monitoring of venous oxygen saturation is indicated for the critically ill patient who has the potential to develop an imbalance between oxygen supply and

TABLE 18-5 Cardiac Output Measurement

Device Name	Probe Placement	Method	Cardiac Output Calculation	Clinical Issues
Noninvasive Methods				
Bioimpedance	External electrodes placed on the neck and chest	Thoracic electric bioimpedance	1. A small alternating current is applied across the chest by skin electrodes. 2. Pulsatile changes in thoracic blood volume result in changes in electrical impedance. The rate of change of impedance during systole is measured and used to calculate CO.	Noninvasive Less accurate with low body temperature
Minimally Invasive Methods				
Pulse Contour Waveform Methods				
LiDCO (LiDCO Ltd., Cambridge, United Kingdom)	Requires a venous access catheter (central or peripheral) and an arterial catheter with a lithium-monitoring sensor attached	Pulse contour waveform analysis method (calibrated)	Independent calibration with a lithium dilution technique is initially required: 1. A small, subtherapeutic dose of isotonic lithium chloride is injected through the venous catheter. 2. The lithium is detected at the arterial sensor (femoral artery), where a fixed flow pump ensures constant flow. 3. A concentration-time curve is produced for lithium before recirculation. 4. CO is calculated based on the lithium dose given and the measurement of area under the curve.	Easy to set up, uses conventional venous and arterial catheters; can measure extravascular lung water for patients in pulmonary edema. CO measurement is affected by artifact on arterial waveform and by irregular and damped arterial waveforms; can be used in conscious and in unresponsive patients. Requires calibration at least every 8 hours to maintain accuracy; cannot be used in patients on lithium therapy because this interferes with the calibration.
PiCCO (Pulsion Medical Systems, Munich, Germany)	Requires a central venous access catheter and uses a specialized arterial thermistor-tipped catheter in the femoral artery	Pulse contour waveform analysis method that uses transpulmonary thermodilution	1. A set volume of cold saline is injected through the central venous catheter. The arterial thermistor-tipped catheter detects the blood temperature change. 2. Continuous CO measurements are achieved by analyzing the systolic component of the arterial waveform.	CO measurement is affected by artifact on arterial waveform and irregular arterial waveforms. Three calibrations are required initially, and frequent recalibration is required to maintain accuracy.

Continued

TABLE 18-5 Cardiac Output Measurement—*cont'd*

Device Name	Probe Placement	Method	Cardiac Output Calculation	Clinical Issues
Vigileo (Edward Lifesciences, Irvine, CA)	Requires a functional arterial catheter	Pulse contour waveform analysis method (does not require calibration)	1. Calculates CO by use of the arterial pressure waveform analysis in conjunction with patient data (age, sex, height, weight). 2. Uses an internal proprietary algorithm based on the principle that pulse pressure (difference between systolic and diastolic pressure) is proportional to stroke volume and inversely proportional to aortic compliance. 3. Aortic pressure is sampled at 100 Hz and is updated every 20 seconds.	Does not require external calibration but requires zeroing of the transducer Lack of calibration procedures is controversial.
Esophageal Probe Methods				
Esophageal Doppler	Ultrasound probe placed in the lower esophagus	Stroke volume is calculated by measurement of the aortic blood velocity in the descending thoracic aorta (by continuous wave Doppler) plus calculation of the cross-sectional area of the aorta; these values are used to calculate the CO.	1. Measurement of the aorta cross-sectional area, measured using M-mode ultrasound, and multiplying this value by blood velocity to calculate flow or CO. 2. The value of total CO is derived from a nomogram using aortic blood velocity, height, weight, and age.	Useful in the operating room or with deeply sedated patients. Probe is stiff, and placement is not well tolerated by conscious patients.
Transesophageal echocardiography (TEE)	Ultrasound probe placed in the esophagus	Probe placement allows imaging of the left ventricular outflow tract. Stroke volume is measured by Doppler.	1. The left ventricular (LV) outflow tract area is measured; this value is squared and multiplied by the velocity time interval of blood flow and heart rate. 2. LV stroke volume can be measured, as can heart rate to use the SV × HR = CO formula.	Useful in the operating room or with deeply sedated patients Probe is stiff, and placement is not well tolerated by conscious patients. Requires skill to accurately position probe to visualize the LV outflow tract.
Partial CO_2 Rebreathing Method				
NICO$_2$ (Philips, Respironics)	Addition of a partial CO_2 rebreathing circuit to ventilator	Partial CO_2 rebreathing method	CO measurement is based on changes in respiratory CO_2 concentration obtained from a short period of rebreathing. CO_2 elimination is calculated by sensors that measure flow, airway pressure, and CO_2 concentration. These variables are used in the Fick partial rebreathing formula to calculate CO.	Can be used only in intubated and ventilated patients. Specialized additional tubing setup on ventilator Cannot be used in patients who cannot tolerate hypercapnia (elevated CO_2) CO measurement is altered by intra-pulmonary shunt.

CO, cardiac output; CO_2, carbon dioxide; HR, heart rate; LV, left ventricle SV, stroke volume.

metabolic tissue demand. This includes patients in severe sepsis or shock, those after high-risk cardiac surgery, and patients with severe respiratory compromise, such as ARDS.

Continuous venous oxygen monitoring permits a calculation of the balance achieved between arterial oxygen supply (SaO_2) and oxygen demand at the tissue level by sampling desaturated venous blood from the pulmonary artery catheter distal tip. This sample is called *mixed venous oxygen saturation* ($S\bar{v}O_2$) because it is a mixture of all of the venous blood drained from many body tissues. The same fiberoptic technology has been used in combination with a fiberoptic triple-lumen CVC. In this situation, the venous blood is sampled from the superior vena cava, just above the right atrium, and the central venous oxygen saturation ($ScvO_2$) is measured.

Under normal conditions, the cardiopulmonary system achieves a balance between oxygen supply and demand. Four factors contribute to this balance:

1. Cardiac output (CO)
2. Hemoglobin (Hgb)
3. Arterial oxygen saturation (SaO_2)
4. Tissue oxygen metabolism ($\dot{V}O_2$)

Three of these factors (CO, Hgb, and SaO_2) contribute to the supply of oxygen to the tissues. Tissue metabolism ($\dot{V}O_2$) determines oxygen consumption or the quantity of oxygen extracted at tissue level that creates the demand for oxygen. The relationships of these factors are illustrated in Fig. 18-21.

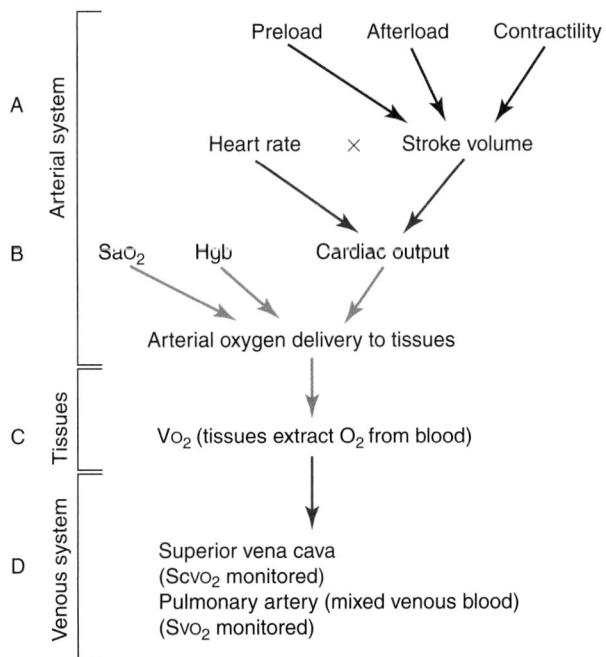

Figure 18-21 Several factors contribute to the mixed venous oxygen saturation ($S\bar{v}O_2$) value. *A,* Cardiac output (CO) is determined by heart rate (central venous oxygen saturation [$ScvO_2$] HR) × stroke volume (SV). *B,* The oxygen saturation (SaO_2), hemoglobin (Hgb) level, and CO contribute to arterial oxygen delivery at the tissue level. *C,* Tissues extract and use the oxygen carried in the blood. This process of cellular oxygen consumption is $\dot{V}O_2$. *D,* Blood returns to the superior vena cava (recorded as $ScvO_2$) and then to the pulmonary artery, where the mixed venous blood is recorded as $S\bar{v}O_2$.

In addition to measurement of venous oxygen saturation, it is possible to calculate the quantity of oxygen (in mL/min) that is provided to the tissues by the cardiopulmonary system and to assess the amount of oxygen consumed by the body tissues. These calculations rely on principles of oxygen transport physiology and are the basis for calculation of $S\bar{v}O_2$. These formulas are explained in greater detail in Table 18-6 and are listed in Appendix B.

Catheters. The type of catheter used to measure venous oxygen saturation is defined by where the fiberoptic tip is located, either at the tip of a CVC or on the distal tip of a PA catheter.

$S\bar{v}O_2$ Catheter. The pulmonary arterial $S\bar{v}O_2$ catheter has the traditional four lumens plus a lumen containing two or three optical fibers. The fiberoptics are attached to an optical module that is connected to a small bedside computer. The optical module transmits a narrow band of light down one optical fiber. This light is reflected off the hemoglobin in the blood and returns to the optical module through the receiving fiberoptic. The $S\bar{v}O_2$ signal is recorded on a continuous display.

$ScvO_2$ Catheter. The central venous $ScvO_2$ technology is incorporated into a multilumen CVC. The fiberoptic catheter tip is positioned in a central vein, such as the superior vena cava. The technology used to measure the venous saturation is identical in both types of catheters, and the same continuous display module is used for both catheters.

The $ScvO_2$ catheter has been successfully used to guide hemodynamic fluid resuscitation in septic patients.[57] The relationship between the values obtained from the traditional PA ($S\bar{v}O_2$) catheter and the central venous ($ScvO_2$) catheter are very similar, although the $ScvO_2$ values are slightly higher. The trend of parallel measurements (up or down as patient condition changes) is in the same direction in about 90% of cases.

$S\bar{v}O_2$ or $ScvO_2$ Calibration. The catheter is calibrated before insertion into the patient through a standardized color reference system, which is part of the catheter package. Insertion technique and sites are identical to those used for placement of conventional PA or CVC catheters. Waveform analysis or venous saturation measurement, or both, can be used for accurate placement. After the catheter is inserted, recalibration is unnecessary unless the catheter becomes disconnected from the optical module.

To recalibrate the fiberoptic module to verify accuracy when the catheter is already inserted in a patient, a mixed venous blood sample ($S\bar{v}O_2$) or central venous sample ($ScvO_2$) must be withdrawn from the appropriate catheter tip and sent to the laboratory for oxygen saturation analysis. In many critical care units, this is a standard daily procedure to ensure that readings used to guide patient care remain accurate.[58]

Nursing Management. $S\bar{v}O_2$ monitoring provides a continuous assessment of the balance of oxygen supply and demand for an individual patient. Nursing assessment includes evaluation of the $S\bar{v}O_2$ or $ScvO_2$ value and evaluation of the four factors (SaO_2, CO, Hgb, and $\dot{V}O_2$) that maintain the oxygen supply-demand balance.

Normal $S\bar{v}O_2$ Values. Normal $S\bar{v}O_2$ is approximately 75% in the healthy individual (range, 60% to 80%). In critically ill

TABLE 18-6 Calculations of Oxygen Transport Physiology

Name	Formula	Normal Value	Explanation
Arterial oxygen saturation (SaO_2)	$\dfrac{HgbO_2}{Hgb + HgbO_2} \times 100$	>96%	SaO_2 is determined by the amount of oxygen bound to hemoglobin (oxyhemoglobin [$HgbO_2$,]) divided by the total hemoglobin ($Hgb + HgbO_2$). Normally, 96% of oxygen is bound to hemoglobin (Hgb).
Blood oxygen content CaO_2 (arterial) CvO_2 (venous)	(O_2 dissolved) + (O_2 saturation) ($Po_2 \times 0.003$) + ($1.34 \times Hgb \times So_2$)	19-20 mL/dL 12-15 mL/dL	Blood oxygen (O_2) content is the amount of oxygen dissolved in 100 mL (1 dL) of blood. It can be calculated for arterial blood (CaO_2) and for venous blood (CvO_2). Measured in units of mL/dL, it is the combination of dissolved O_2 (PaO_2) and O_2 saturation (SaO_2).
Blood oxygen transport (i.e., oxygen delivery)	$CO \times CaO_2 \times 10$ (arterial) $CO \times CvO_2 \times 10$ (venous)	1000 mL/min 750 mL/min	Oxygen transport represents the amount (mL) of oxygen transported to or from the tissues each minute (mL/min). Arterial O_2 transport is a measure of the O_2 delivered to the tissues. Venous O_2 transport reflects the venous return to the right side of the heart. Oxygen transport is calculated by multiplying the cardiac output (CO) by the oxygen content (CaO_2 or CvO_2) and by the number 10. The difference between normal arterial and normal venous O_2 return represents oxygen consumption by the tissues.
Tissue oxygen consumption ($\dot{V}o_2$)	Arterial O_2 transport minus venous O_2 transport ($CO \times CaO_2 \times 10$) − ($CO \times CvO_2 \times 10$)	250 mL/min	Oxygen consumption is the amount of oxygen consumed by the tissues in 1 minute. To calculate $\dot{V}o_2$, the arterial oxygen transport and venous oxygen transport values (calculated in mL/min) must be known. The difference is $\dot{V}o_2$.
Arterial-venous oxygen difference (a-v O_2 difference)	Arterial O_2 content minus venous O_2 content $CaO_2 - CvO_2$	3.0-5.5 mL/dL	The a-v O_2 difference is the difference between the arterial oxygen content (CaO_2) and the venous oxygen content (CvO_2). Because CaO_2 and CvO_2 are measured in mL/dL, the a-v O_2 difference is also measured in mL/dL.
Mixed venous oxygen saturation ($S\bar{v}O_2$)	Arterial O_2 transport minus tissue O_2 consumption equals venous O_2 return ($CO \times CaO_2 \times 10$) − $\dot{V}o_2$	60%-80%	$S\bar{v}O_2$ is the venous oxygen return that is bound (saturated) to hemoglobin. Saturation is measured as a percentage (%). The $S\bar{v}O_2$ value is a function of the amount of oxygen delivered to the tissues minus the amount of oxygen consumed by the tissues ($\dot{V}o_2$) and is measured in mL/min. The higher the amount (mL) of oxygen in the venous return, the greater the hemoglobin saturation.

patients, an $S\bar{v}O_2$ value between 60% and 80% is evidence of adequate balance between oxygen supply and demand.

Normal $Scvo_2$ Values. The normal values for the $Scvo_2$ catheter are slightly higher,[21] because the reading is taken before the blood enters the right heart chambers, where the *cardiac sinus* (vein) delivers venous blood drained from the myocardium into the right atrium. The heavily desaturated myocardial blood decreases the oxygen saturation slightly. For this reason, $S\bar{v}O_2$ values are always slightly lower than $Scvo_2$ readings in the same patient.[21]

One clinical rule of thumb is to subtract 30 from the arterial oxygen saturation, and the resulting value should represent an acceptable mixed venous oxygen saturation. For example,

$$SaO_2 \text{ is } 100\% - 30\% = 70\% \ S\bar{v}O_2$$

$$SaO_2 \text{ is } 95\% - 30\% = 65\% \ S\bar{v}O_2$$

If the $S\bar{v}O_2$ or $Scvo_2$ value changes by more than 10% and this change is maintained for more than 10 minutes, the clinician must determine which of the four factors is affecting $S\bar{v}O_2$.[58]

$S\bar{v}O_2$ or $Scvo_2$ and Arterial Oxygen Saturation. A change in $S\bar{v}O_2$ or $Scvo_2$ may be caused by a change in arterial oxygen oxygen saturation (SaO_2). If the SaO_2 is increased because supplemental oxygen is being administered, the $S\bar{v}O_2$ also will increase. If the oxygen supply is disrupted and SaO_2 is decreased, $S\bar{v}O_2$ will decrease. The $S\bar{v}O_2$ can be decreased by

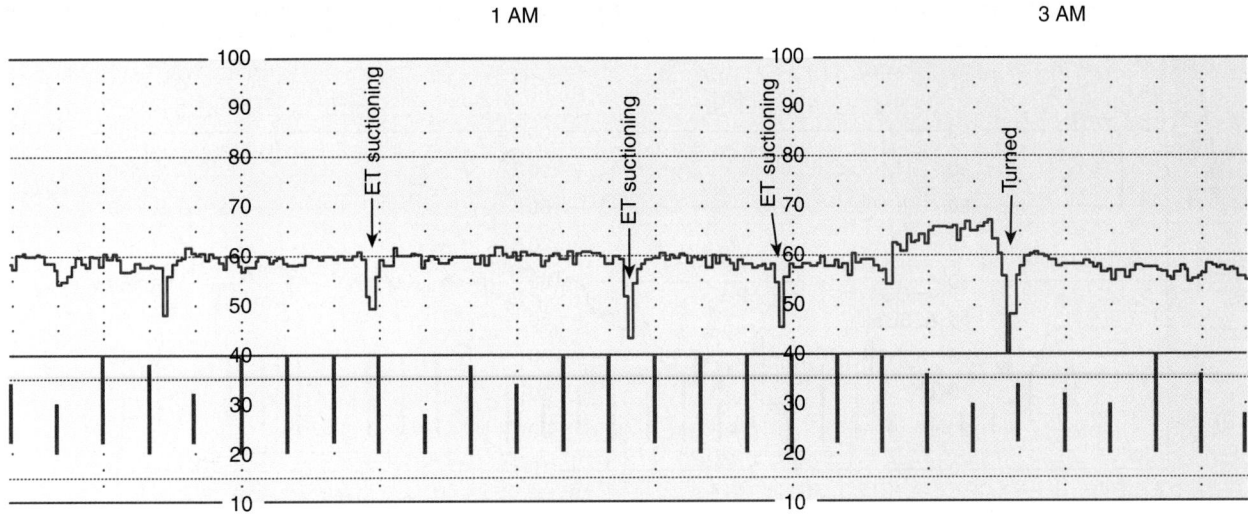

Figure 18-22 The $S\bar{v}O_2$ value decreases during endotracheal (ET) suctioning. The ET suction decreases the oxygen saturation (SaO_2) level. The baseline $S\bar{v}O_2$ value is low (60%) because the patient has acute respiratory distress syndrome (ARDS) and is hypoxemic.

any action or disease that reduces oxygen supply, including ARDS, endotracheal suctioning, removing a patient from the ventilator, or removing supplementary oxygen. Figure 18-22 demonstrates a drop in $S\bar{v}O_2$ during suctioning in a patient with ARDS. Transient decreases in $S\bar{v}O_2$ or $ScvO_2$ related to a nursing action such as endotracheal suctioning are not usually a cause for concern. Some patients may be slow to resaturate up to the presuction level of $S\bar{v}O_2$ or $ScvO_2$. In this case, an appropriate nursing intervention is to wait until the venous oxygen saturation has again returned to baseline before initiating other nursing activities.

$S\bar{v}O_2$ or $ScvO_2$ and Cardiac Output. A change in $S\bar{v}O_2$ or $ScvO_2$ may be caused by an alteration in CO. Four hemodynamic factors affect CO: preload, afterload, contractility, and heart rate (see Fig. 18-21). Changes in one or more of these individual factors affects CO. Figure 18-23 shows an improvement in a patient's $S\bar{v}O_2$ concentration from 70% to 80% after volume administration that increased preload (point A). Later, this patient's CO fell abruptly during a short run of ventricular tachycardia (VT) (point B). Any major loss of heart rate causes a decrease in CO. Alterations in contractility, preload, and afterload (SVR) also have the potential to alter CO.

Because CO is an important component of the continuous $S\bar{v}O_2$ value, several researchers have investigated whether $S\bar{v}O_2$ could be substituted for thermodilution CO as a monitoring tool. Studies of adult patients after cardiac surgery and acute MI indicate that a sustained change in the $S\bar{v}O_2$ value does not automatically mean there has been a change in CO. No consistent or reliable correlation was found between $S\bar{v}O_2$ and CO in these clinical studies. Instead, a change in $S\bar{v}O_2$ indicates a need to check a CO at the bedside to determine the cause of the change in venous oxygen saturation. The $S\bar{v}O_2$ measurement is very sensitive and serves as an early warning for changes in patient condition, whether or not the change is the result of an alteration in CO. Monitoring $S\bar{v}O_2$ is an additional level of hemodynamic monitoring but does not replace thermodilution CO.

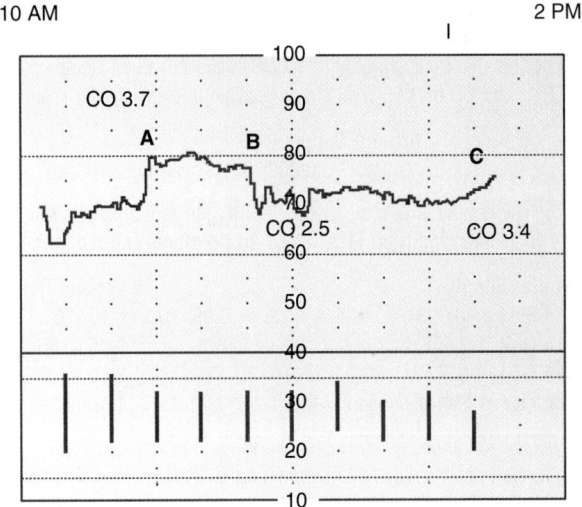

Figure 18-23 Impact of changes in cardiac output (CO) on $S\bar{v}O_2$ values. *Point A:* Just before point A, $S\bar{v}O_2$ readings are low because CO and pulmonary artery pressures were low as a result of excessive diuresis. Infusion of 500 mL of colloid solution and 1000 mL of lactated Ringer's solution crystalloid increased the $S\bar{v}O_2$ level and improved the CO, which rose to 3.7 L/min. *Point B:* A short run of ventricular tachycardia caused the CO to fall abruptly to 2.5 L/min and decreased the $S\bar{v}O_2$ value. *Point C:* The beginning of an upward trend in $S\bar{v}O_2$ is related to administration of fluids and to improvement in CO and in filling pressures. CO is now 3.4 L/min. The graph represents a 4-hour printout; the space between each dotted line represents 20 minutes.

This principle is clearly illustrated in the $S\bar{v}O_2$ Hemodynamic Profile 3 (Box 18-3), in which an increase in $S\bar{v}O_2$ is not associated with a significant rise in CO. The rationale and explanation for this finding is also discussed in the section on assessment of oxygen consumption.

$S\bar{v}O_2$ or $ScvO_2$ and Hemoglobin. Hemoglobin is the transport mechanism for oxygen in the blood. If the hemoglobin level falls as a result of bleeding or red cell destruction, the body maintains

BOX 18-3 HEMODYNAMIC PROFILE 3

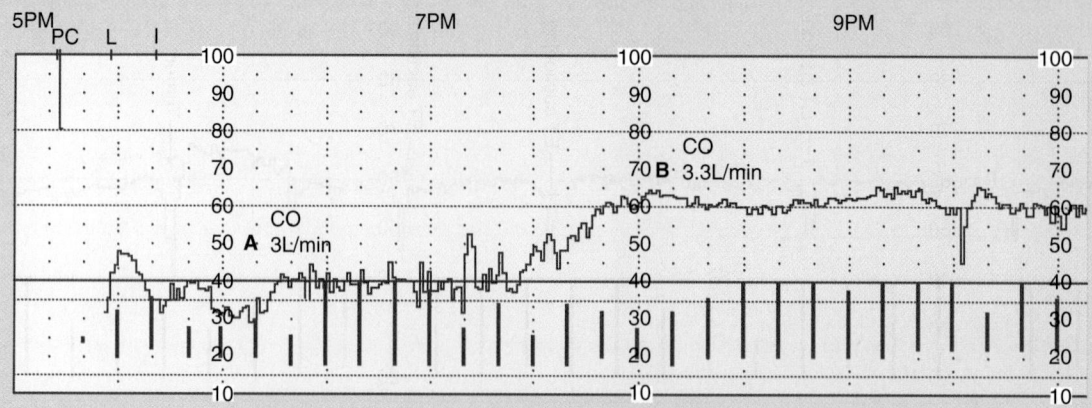

Mr. EH has just been admitted to the cardiovascular critical care unit after open heart surgery. At *point A* in the figure, he has an extremely low mixed venous oxygen saturation ($S\bar{v}o_2$) value of 40%. An $S\bar{v}o_2$ value below 40% indicates that the oxygen supply is not adequate to meet the demands of the body tissues, resulting in metabolic acidosis. To determine the reason for the low $S\bar{v}o_2$ level, values must be known for the hemoglobin (Hgb) level, the arterial oxygen saturation (Sao_2), the cardiac output (CO), and the tissue oxygen consumption ($\dot{V}o_2$). EH'S Hgb value is 11.6 g/dL (normal male Hgb, 13.5-18.0 g/dL), which is acceptable after major surgery; the Sao_2 is 99.6% (normal, 97%), which is high because this patient started receiving mechanical ventilation with 70% oxygen immediately after surgery; and the CO is low at 3.15 L/min (normal, 4-6 L/min). EH is receiving dopamine (5 mcg/kg/min) for his low CO. He is shivering and cold because his body temperature is only 35.2° C after the surgery. Using the values of Hgb of 11.6 g/dL, Sao_2 of 99.6%, and CO of 3.15 L/min, it is possible to calculate the tissue oxygen consumption ($\dot{V}o_2$) for EH.

Arterial Supply	Venous Return
CO ($Pao_2 \times 0.003$) + ($1.34 \times$ Hgb $\times Sao_2$) 10	$-$ CO ($Pvo_2 \times 0.0031$) + ($1.34 \times$ Hgb $\times S\bar{v}o_2$) 10 $= \dot{V}o_2$

To calculate arterial oxygen supply, the oxygen in the venous return, $\dot{V}o_2$, and the difference between the arterial (a) and venous (v) oxygen content (a-v O_2 difference), insert EH's values (**in boldface**) into the previous formula.

Arterial Supply	Venous Return	$\dot{V}o_2$	a-v O_2 Difference
3.15 (**354** $\times 0.003$) + ($1.34 \times$ **11.6** $\times$ **0.99**) 10 $-$	**3.15** (**20** $\times 0.003$) + ($1.34 \times$ **11.6** $\times$ **0.38**) 10		
3.15 (1.0) + 15.3) 10	**3.15** (0.06 + 5.90) 10		
3.15 (16.3) 10	**3.15** (5.90) 10		
505 mL/min (see illustration at top)	183 mL/min	$= 322$ mL/min	10.4 mL/dL

At *point A* in the preceding illustration, the arterial oxygen supply to the tissues is 505 mL/min (normal, 1000 mL/min), whereas the oxygen returned in the venous blood is only 183 mL/min (normal, 750 mL/min). EH's $\dot{V}o_2$ is elevated at 322 mL/min (normal, 250 mL/min). The clinical goals for this patient would be to (1) increase the CO and (2) use sedation or muscle relaxants to decrease oxygen consumption by controlling the shivering. The difference between the oxygen content in the arterial (a) and the venous (v) blood (a-v o_2 difference) is very large at 10.4 mL/dL (normal, 3.5-5.0 mL/dL). These calculated values confirm the nursing diagnosis of Ineffective Tissue Perfusion with a decreased cardiac output.

Two hours later, at *point B* (see illustration), EH's $S\bar{v}o_2$ has improved to a low-normal value of 60%. Additional inotropic drugs have been administered. At this time the Hgb is 10.8 g/dL, Sao_2 is 99.6%, and CO remains low at 3.3 L/min. The improvement in $S\bar{v}o_2$ has not been caused by a dramatic increase in CO. When EH's oxygen consumption is calculated at *point B*, it becomes evident that the decrease in physical activity after sedation with morphine to reduce shivering has improved the $S\bar{v}o_2$. EH's values are emphasized in bold.

Arterial Supply	Venous Return
CO ($Pao_2 \times 0.003$) + ($1.34 \times$ Hgb $\times Sao_2$) 10	$-$ CO ($Pvo_2 \times 0.003$) + ($1.34 \times$ Hgb $\times S\bar{v}o_2$) 10 $= \dot{V}o_2$

Arterial Supply	Venous Return	$\dot{V}o_2$	a-v O_2 Difference
3.3 (**266** $\times 0.003$) + ($1.34 \times$ **10.8** $\times$ **0.99**) 10 $-$	**3.3** (**28** $\times 0.003$) + ($1.34 \times$ **10.8** $\times$ **0.60**) 10		
3.3 (0.82 + 14.32) 10	**3.3** (0.86 + 8.6) 10		
3.3 (15.1) 1	**3.3** (9.4) 10		
498 mL/min	300 mL/min	$= 198$ mL/min	5.7 mL/dL

At *point B* in the illustration, EH's arterial oxygen supply is still low at 498 mL/min, and the oxygen in his mixed venous blood return remains low at 300 mL/min. $\dot{V}o_2$ is now lower than normal (typical after sedation) at 198 mL/min. At this time, the a-v O_2 difference is almost within the normal limits at 5.7 mL/dL. These findings are confirmed by the low-normal $S\bar{v}o_2$ value of 60% at *point B*. This case study illustrates the point that tissue oxygen consumption (O_2 demand) can be as important as cardiac output (CO) and oxygenation (O_2 supply) in determining mixed venous oxygen saturation ($S\bar{v}o_2$) in the patient with a compromised cardiovascular system.

See Table 18-6 for an explanation of abbreviations and Box 18-1 and Appendix B for explanation of hemodynamic values.

oxygen transport by increasing CO and using oxygen reserves in the venous blood return. The body can compensate efficiently for anemia. In the healthy person, the hemoglobin concentration must be extremely low before $S\bar{V}O_2$ decreases. However, in an anemic patient with a compromised cardiovascular system who cannot adequately increase CO, $S\bar{V}O_2$, or $ScvO_2$ declines as venous oxygen reserves are depleted by the body.

$S\bar{V}O_2$ or $ScvO_2$ and Oxygen Consumption. Oxygen consumption ($\dot{V}O_2$) describes the amount of oxygen the body tissues consume for normal function in 1 minute. If the body's metabolic demands increase because of exercise or increased metabolic rate, the body increases CO to augment oxygen supply and uses reserve oxygen in the venous system. Normal oxygen delivery to the tissues is 1000 mL (1 L) of oxygen per minute. At rest, a person may consume one fourth of the available oxygen, or 250 mL of oxygen per minute. This leaves a venous oxygen reserve of 750 mL of oxygen per minute (see Table 18-6). For the normal individual, the combination of increased CO and use of considerable venous oxygen reserve provides adequate compensation for increased metabolic needs. However, for the critically ill patient with cardiac or respiratory dysfunction, an increase in activity leading to increased oxygen consumption may overwhelm the cardiopulmonary system and oxygen reserves.

In the critically ill patient, nursing procedures can increase $\dot{V}O_2$ by 10% to 36% (Table 18-7). The critical care nurse can observe the effect of increased $\dot{V}O_2$ during routine nursing care and under conditions that increase metabolic rate. Activities such as turning, giving a backrub, or getting a patient out of bed are often accompanied by a sudden, temporary decrease in the patient's continuous $S\bar{V}O_2$ or $ScvO_2$ reading. After the physical activity is finished, most patients resaturate up to their preactivity venous saturation level within a few minutes. In critically ill patients, it may take up to 5 minutes for resaturation (increase in $S\bar{V}O_2$ or $ScvO_2$) to occur. In this situation, the appropriate nursing action is to observe the patient clinically in conjunction with monitoring $S\bar{V}O_2$ or $ScvO_2$ and to postpone additional maneuvers until the venous saturation has returned to baseline.

Many clinical conditions that dramatically increase $\dot{V}O_2$ consumption are often seen in critical care units. Conditions such as sepsis, multiple organ dysfunction syndrome (MODS), burns, head injury, and shivering can more than double the normal oxygen tissue requirements (see Table 18-7). Such dramatic increases in $\dot{V}O_2$ translate into a low $S\bar{V}O_2$ or $ScvO_2$ value, even if the CO is normal. This situation is demonstrated in Hemodynamic Profile 3, in which intense shivering resulted in increased tissue oxygen consumption and a low initial $S\bar{V}O_2$ value (point A); after sedation, the $S\bar{V}O_2$ value increased due to the normalization of tissue oxygen requirements (point B).

Normal $S\bar{V}O_2$ or $ScvO_2$. If $S\bar{V}O_2$ or $ScvO_2$ is within the normal range of 60% to 80% and the patient is not clinically compromised, the nurse can assume that oxygen supply and demand are balanced for that individual. The situation becomes out of balance when a decrease in oxygen delivery (SaO_2) occurs because of changes in CO or hemoglobin concentration, or an increase in oxygen demand (increased $\dot{V}O_2$) occurs.

Low $S\bar{V}O_2$ or $ScvO_2$. If $S\bar{V}O_2$ or $ScvO_2$ falls below 60% and is sustained, the clinician must assume that oxygen supply is not equal to demand (Table 18-8). It is helpful to assess the cause of decreased $S\bar{V}O_2$ or $ScvO_2$ in a logical sequence that reflects knowledge of the meaning of the venous saturation value. The following is one such assessment sequence:

TABLE 18-7 Alterations in Oxygen Consumption

Condition or Activity	% Increase Over Resting $\dot{V}O_2$	% Decrease Under Resting $\dot{V}O_2$
Clinical Conditions That Increase $\dot{V}O_2$		
Fever	10% (for each 1° C above normal)	
Skeletal injuries	10%-30%	
Work of breathing	40%	
Severe infection	60%	
Shivering	50%-100%	
Burns	100%	
Routine postoperative procedures	7%	
Nasal intubation	25%-40%	
Endotracheal tube suctioning	27%	
Chest trauma	60%	
Multiple organ dysfunction syndrome	20%-80%	
Sepsis	50%-100%	
Head injury, with patient sedated	89%	
Head injury, with patient not sedated	138%	
Critical illness in emergency department	60%	

Continued

TABLE 18-7 Alterations in Oxygen Consumption—*cont'd*

Condition or Activity	% Increase Over Resting $\dot{V}O_2$	% Decrease Under Resting $\dot{V}O_2$
Nursing Activities That Increase $\dot{V}O_2$		
Dressing change	10%	
Electrocardiogram	16%	
Agitation	18%	
Physical examination	20%	
Visitor	22%	
Bath	23%	
Chest x-ray examination	25%	
Position change	31%	
Chest physiotherapy	35%	
Weighing on sling scale	36%	
Conditions That Decrease $\dot{V}O_2$		
Anesthesia		25%
Anesthesia in burned patients		50%

Modified from White KM et al: The physiologic basis for continuous mixed venous oxygen saturation monitoring, *Heart Lung* 19(5 Pt 2):548-551, 1990.
$\dot{V}O_2$, oxygen consumption.

TABLE 18-8 Measurements of Mixed Venous Oxygen Saturation

$S\bar{v}O_2$ Measurement	Physiologic Basis for Changes in $S\bar{v}O_2$/$Scvo_2$	Clinical Diagnosis and Rationale
High $S\bar{v}O_2$ (80%-95%)	Increased oxygen supply Decreased oxygen demand	Patient receiving more oxygen than required by clinical condition Anesthesia, which causes sedation and decreased muscle movement Hypothermia, which lowers metabolic demand (e.g., during cardiopulmonary bypass) Sepsis caused by decreased ability of tissues to use oxygen at a cellular level False high-positive result because the pulmonary artery catheter is wedged in a pulmonary arteriole ($S\bar{v}O_2$ only)

Normal $S\bar{v}O_2$/$Scvo_2$ (60% to 80%)
Low $S\bar{v}O_2$/ $Scvo_2$ (<60%)
	Normal oxygen supply and metabolic demand
	Decreased oxygen supply caused by:
	  Low hemoglobin (Hgb)
	  Low arterial saturation (Sao_2)
	  Low cardiac output (CO)
	  Increased oxygen consumption ($\dot{V}O_2$)
		Balanced oxygen supply and demand
		Anemia or bleeding with compromised cardiopulmonary system
		Hypoxemia resulting from decreased oxygen supply or lung disease
		Cardiogenic shock caused by left ventricular pump failure
		Metabolic demand exceeds oxygen supply in conditions that increase muscle movement and increase metabolic rate, including physiologic states such as shivering, seizures, and hyperthermia and nursing interventions such as being weighed on a bed scale and turning

$Scvo_2$, central venous oxygen saturation; $S\bar{v}O_2$, mixed venous oxygen saturation.

1. Clinically assess the patient.
2. Assess whether the decreased $S\bar{v}O_2$ or $Scvo_2$ is caused by low oxygen supply. Verify the effectiveness of the ventilator or oxygen mask, or check arterial oxygen saturation (Sao_2) from arterial blood gas values.
3. Assess cardiac function by performing a CO measurement.
4. Assess the hemoglobin value by checking recent laboratory results or by withdrawing a blood sample for laboratory analysis.
5. Assess whether the decreased $S\bar{v}O_2$ or $Scvo_2$ is the result of a recent patient movement or nursing action that may have temporarily increased $\dot{V}O_2$.

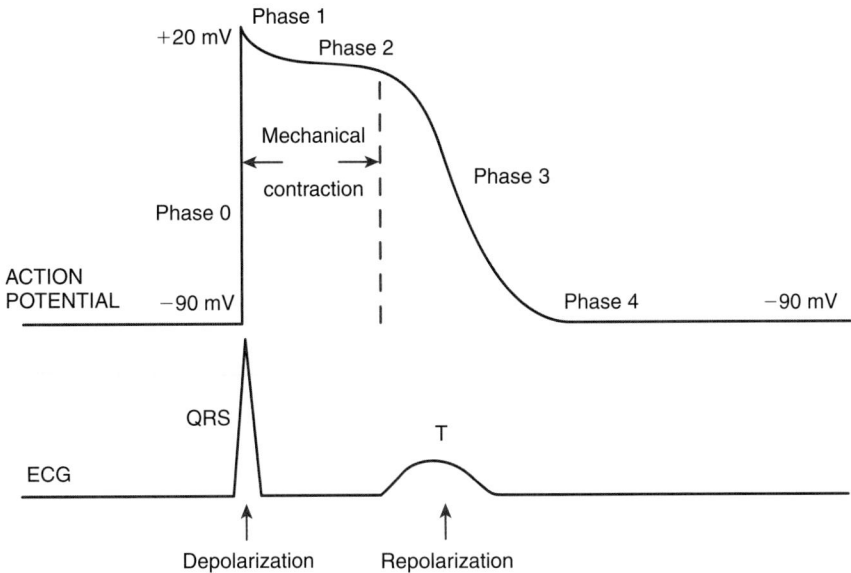

Figure 18-24 Correlation of the action potential of a ventricular myocardial cell with the electrical events recorded on the surface ECG. Notice that the ECG pattern is "silent" during phase 2 of the action potential. Mechanical contraction is occurring, but no significant electrical activity is present.

The concept of target values is helpful when designing protocols for hemodynamic monitoring. Target values for venous oximetry are an $S\bar{v}O_2$ of 70% or above and a $ScvO_2$ of 65% or above. The concept is that patients with values below these targets are at greater risk for organ hypoperfusion and increased mortality. This was seen in a study of intraoperative and postoperative surgical patients, in whom an $ScvO_2$ below 65% was associated with increased mortality.[59] However, cardiac surgery patients who were below the $ScvO_2$ 65% target did not have lower mortality rates.[60] Based on studies of patients with sepsis, the Surviving Sepsis Campaign guidelines recommend that $ScvO_2$ be maintained above 70% for septic patients.[37,57] This represents a clinically useful target to aim for even as research is ongoing to find the $ScvO_2$ value for optimal survival.

If $S\bar{v}O_2$ or $ScvO_2$ falls below 40%, and is maintained at this low value, the imbalance of oxygen supply and demand will not be adequate to meet tissue needs at the cellular level. At some point, the cells change from an aerobic to anaerobic mode of metabolism, which results in the production of lactic acid and is representative of a shock state in which cellular injury or cell death may result. At this point, every attempt must be made to determine the cause of the low $S\bar{v}O_2$ or $ScvO_2$ and to correct the oxygen supply-demand imbalance. To avoid the risk of lactic acidosis, it is helpful to watch the trend of the $S\bar{v}O_2$ or $ScvO_2$ and to intervene early with a goal of returning the venous oxygen saturation to 70%.[37]

High $S\bar{v}O_2$. In certain clinical conditions, $S\bar{v}O_2$ or $ScvO_2$ may increase to an above-normal level (>80%). This occurs during times of low oxygen demand (decreased $\dot{V}O_2$), such as during anesthesia or hypothermia. In some cases of septic shock, the tissue cells cannot use the oxygen supplied to them, and the oxygen is not extracted from the blood at the tissue level. In this situation, the venous oxygen reserve remains elevated, and the $S\bar{v}O_2$ or $ScvO_2$ value is higher than normal (see Table 18-8). If the

$S\bar{v}O_2$ PA catheter drifts into a wedged position, the $S\bar{v}O_2$ increases because the fiberoptic tip of the catheter comes into contact with newly oxygenated blood.

ELECTROCARDIOGRAPHY

Electrocardiography is a complex and important subject. Detailed evaluation of an ECG can provide a wealth of cardiac diagnostic information and often provides the basis on which other, definitive diagnostic tests are selected. The following sections discuss the many clinical factors that the critical care nurse considers when using ECG monitoring, specific dysrhythmias commonly encountered in clinical practice, and the skills needed for 12-lead ECG analysis. The intent is to provide a sound basis for understanding the value of the many clinical applications of electrocardiography.

Basic Principles of Electrocardiography. The ECG records electrical changes in heart muscle caused by an action potential. It does not record the mechanical contraction, which usually follows electrical depolarization immediately. A brief discussion of the cardiac action potential is included to reinforce the concept that the electrical changes occurring during electrical stimulation of the myocardial cell produce the deflections seen on the ECG tracing (Fig. 18-24).

Phase 0. During phase 0 (depolarization), the electrical potential changes rapidly from a baseline of −90 mV to +20 mV and stabilizes at about 0 mV. Because this is a significant electrical change, it appears as a wave on the ECG as the QRS.

Phases 1 and 2. During phases 1 and 2, an electrical plateau is created, and during this plateau, mechanical contraction occurs. Because there is no significant electrical change, nothing is shown on the ECG.

Phase 3. During phase 3 (repolarization), the electrical potential again changes, this time a little more slowly, from

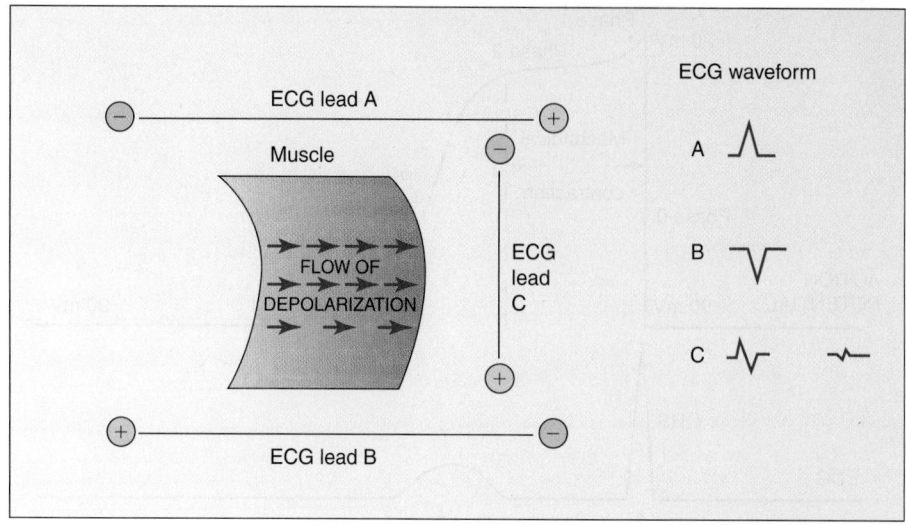

Figure 18-25 Effect of lead position on the ECG tracing. *A,* Flow of depolarization toward the positive electrode results in a positive deflection on the ECG. *B,* Flow of depolarization away from the positive electrode results in a negative deflection on the ECG. *C,* Flow of depolarization perpendicular to the positive electrode results in a biphasic or nearly isoelectric deflection on the ECG. This basic principle applies to the P wave and the QRS complex.

0 mV back to −90 mV. This is another major electrical event, and it is reflected on the ECG as a T wave.

Phase 4. During phase 4 (resting period), the chemical balance is restored by the sodium pump, but because positively charged ions are exchanged on a one-for-one basis, no electrical activity is generated, and no visible change occurs on the ECG tracing. For more information on the cardiac action potential, see "Phases of the Action Potential" in Chapter 16.

Electrocardiographic Leads. All electrocardiographs use a system of one or more leads. The basic 3-lead system consists of three bipolar electrodes that are applied to the chest wall and labeled right arm (RA), left arm (LA), and left leg (LL). The term *bipolar* means that each created ECG lead has a positive and a negative pole. One lead also acts as a ground. The function of the ground electrode is to prevent the display of background electrical interference on the ECG tracing. Leads do not transmit any electricity to the patient; they sense and record it.

The positive electrode on the skin acts as a camera. If the wave of depolarization travels toward the positive electrode, an upward stroke, or *positive deflection,* is written on the ECG paper (Fig. 18-25A). If the wave of depolarization travels away from the positive electrode, a downward line, or *negative deflection,* is recorded on the ECG (see Fig. 18-25B). When depolarization moves perpendicularly to the positive electrode, a biphasic complex occurs. Sometimes, the complex may even appear almost flat, or isoelectric, if the electrical forces traveling in opposite directions are equal and have the effect of canceling each other (see Fig. 18-25C). The size of the muscle mass being depolarized also has an effect, with the larger muscle mass (usually the left ventricle) having a greater influence on the tracing.

The wave of ventricular depolarization in the healthy heart travels from right to left and from head to toe. The appearance of the waveforms in different ECG leads depend on the location of the positive electrode.

12-Lead Electrocardiogram. The standard 12-lead ECG provides a picture of electrical activity in the heart using 10 different electrode positions to create 12 ECG images.[61-63] A standard 12-lead ECG contains six limb lead images and six chest (precordial) lead images, and the correct placement of these leads is vitally important to avoid misdiagnosis.[64] If a 12-lead ECG is being obtained, the limb electrodes are typically placed on the muscle of the limb avoiding bone, and the patient is asked to remain still. In the critical care unit, the electrodes are typically placed on the torso, near the origin of the limb, avoiding the clavicle bone (LA and RA) and the pelvis bone (LL and RL), as shown in Figure 18-26A. This arrangement is used because patients wear the electrodes for hours or days, and limb movement would distort the electrical baseline. Practically, this means that ECG waveforms on the bedside monitor will not be identical to those obtained by standard 12-lead ECG, for which the electrodes are placed directly on the extremities.[61]

Standard Limb Leads. The limb lead tracings are obtained by placing electrodes on all four extremities: left arm (LA), right arm (RA), Left leg (LL), and right leg (RL). Leads I, II, and III are *bipolar* limb leads that use limb lead electrodes paired as the positive and negative poles (see Fig. 18-26A). The electrodes are placed in a static position on the body, and the polarity is switched to achieve the desired view. This is done manually on the critical care bedside monitor or automatically by the electrocardiographic machine when a 12-lead ECG is obtained.

Lead I—positive electrode at LA and negative electrode at RA

Lead II—positive electrode at LL and negative electrode at LA

Lead III—positive electrode at LL and negative electrode at RA

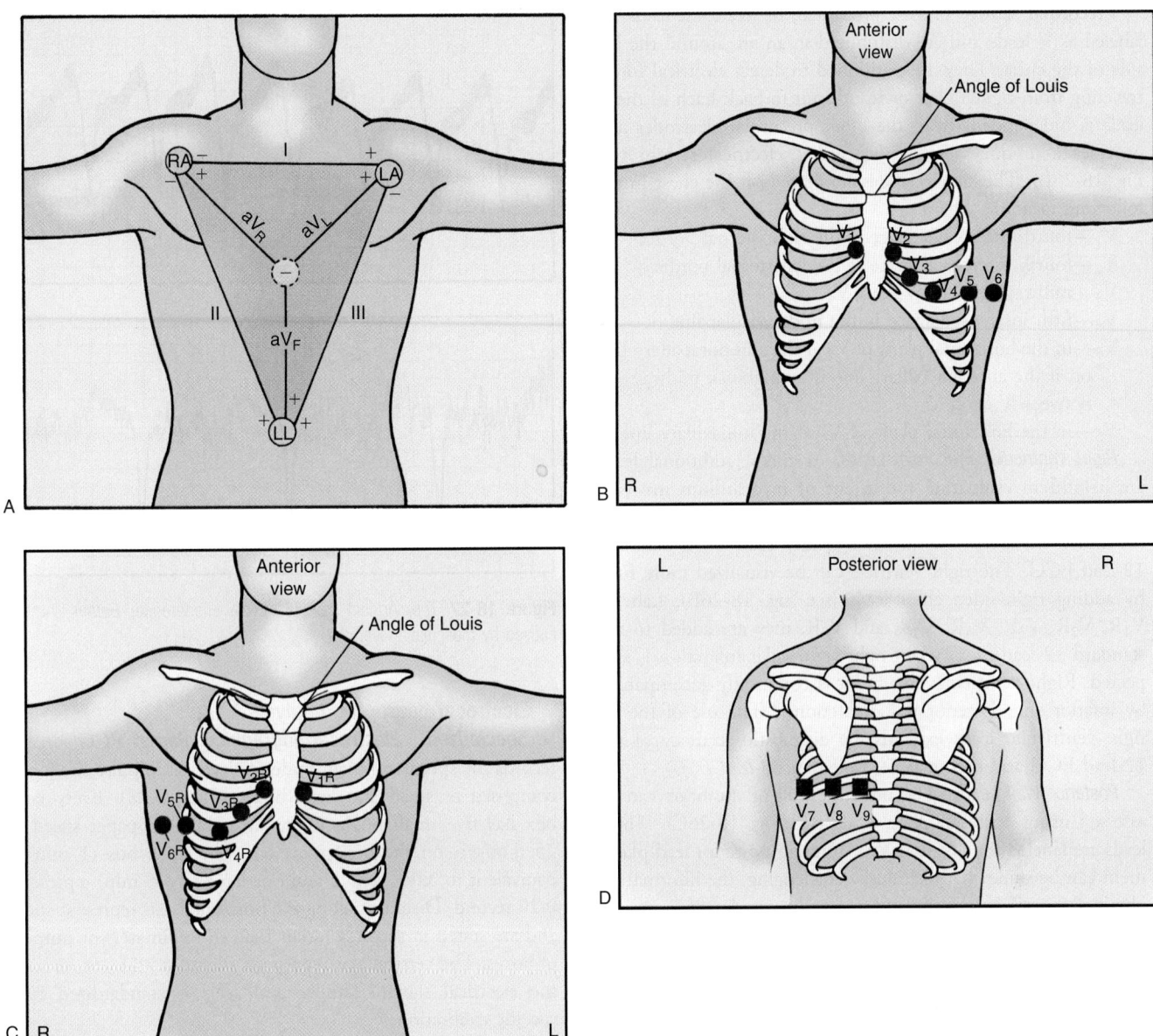

Figure 18-26 *A,* Standard limb leads. Leads are located on the extremities: right arm (RA), left arm (LA), and left leg (LL). The right leg electrode serves as a ground. Leads I, II, and III are bipolar, with each using a positive electrode and a negative electrode. Leads aVR, aVL, and aVF are augmented unipolar leads that use the calculated center of the heart as their negative electrode. *B,* Precordial leads. V_1 to V_6 are the six standard precordial leads and are placed as follows: V_1, fourth intercostal space, right sternal border; V_2, fourth intercostal space, left sternal border; V_3, equidistant between V_2 and V_4; V_4, fifth intercostal space, left midclavicular line; V_5, anterior axillary line, same horizontal level as V_4; V_6, midaxillary line, same horizontal level as V_4. *C,* The right precordial leads V_1R to V_6R are shown. They are not part of a standard 12-lead ECG but are used when a right ventricular infarction is suspected. Their placement is identical to V_3 to V_6, except that they are placed on the right side of the chest rather than on the left. *D,* Posterior precordial leads V_7, V_8, and V_9 are placed on the patient's left posterior chest at the same horizontal level as V_4 (fifth intercostal space). V_7 is on the posterior axillary line, V_8 is on the scapular line, and V_9 is on the spinal border. These leads may be added to the standard 12-lead ECG when a posterior wall infarction is suspected.

This configuration means that the three limb leads are linked in a circuit. The information obtained from the three limb leads is used to create a *central reference potential* that reflects the average potential of the RA, LA, and LL electrodes.[61] The central reference potential shown at the center of the electrode triangle in Figure 18-26A is used to calculate the augmented vector leads.

Augmented Vector Leads. The *augmented vector leads,* labeled aVR, aVL, and aVF, are created from the derived electrode pairs previously described. These augmented leads have only one positive electrode (see Fig. 18-26A), with the calculated central reference potential (center of triangle) acting as a negative electrode. Under these circumstances, the ECG tracing is ordinarily be very small, so the machine enhances, or *augments,* it. The term *vector* refers to directional force. The augmented vector leads are used in the interpretation of myocardial injury and infarction. The limb leads and the augmented vector leads are derived from the four limb electrodes. They provide the *frontal plane axis* of the 12-lead ECG.[61]

Precordial Leads. The six precordial, or left chest leads are labeled as V leads and are distributed in an arc around the left side of the chest. They are positioned to detect electrical forces traveling from right to left or from front to back Each of the V leads is independent from the other precordial electrodes and provides a unique view of the cardiac electrical system (see Fig. 18-26B). The six electrodes are placed on the chest in the following locations[61]:

V_1—fourth intercostal space at the right sternal border

V_2—fourth intercostal space at the left sternal border

V_3—midway between V_2 and V_4

V_4—fifth intercostal space in the midclavicular line

V_5—in the horizontal plane of V_4 at the anterior axillary line or, if the anterior axillary line is ambiguous, midway between V_4 and V_6

V_6—in the horizontal plane of V_4 at the midaxillary line

Right Ventricular Precordial Leads. At times, additional leads are helpful in evaluating the extent of myocardium involved in an acute MI. The right ventricle and the posterior wall of the heart are areas that are not clearly seen on a standard 12-lead ECG. The right ventricle can be visualized more fully by adding right-sided chest leads (see Fig. 18-26B). Labeled V_1R, V_2R, V_3R, V_4R, V_5R, and V_6R, they are added to the standard 12-lead ECG when right ventricular infarction is suspected. Right ventricular infarction is commonly accompanied by inferior and posterior wall infarction.[64] The use of the six right ventricular leads expands the diagnostic accuracy of the 12-lead ECG and is sometimes called an *18-lead ECG.*

Posterior Wall Leads. The posterior wall of the heart can be assessed using posterior chest leads (see Fig. 18-26C). These leads are labeled V_7, V_8, and V_9. Although posterior lead placement can be somewhat technically challenging, the information obtained is useful clinically and may influence decisions regarding clinical management. Approximately 4% of patients with an acute MI show evidence of isolated ST-segment elevation in the posterior leads (V_7, V_8, V_9).[65] The use of the posterior leads expands the diagnostic accuracy of the 12-lead ECG and can be described as a *15-lead ECG.*

Baseline Distortion. The tracing must have a flat baseline, which is that portion of the tracing between the various waveforms. Two forms of artifact can distort the baseline: 60-cycle interference and muscular movement. Sixty-cycle interference (Fig. 18-27A) results from leakage of electrical current somewhere within the system and appears as a generalized thickening of the baseline. It can usually be resolved by ensuring that all electrical equipment at the bedside is electrically grounded. Occasionally, it may be necessary to unplug one piece of equipment at a time until the offending device is found. Muscular movement (see Fig. 18-27B) is displayed as a coarse, erratic disturbance of the baseline. In most cases, asking the patient to lie quietly while the ECG is being run is sufficient. If movement is caused by shivering or seizure activity, it is best to wait until the activity subsides before obtaining the 12-lead ECG. When baseline tremor is caused by Parkinson's disease or another neuromuscular disorder, a resolution may not be possible. The artifact has an adverse effect on the accurate interpretation of the tracing, and may sometimes mimic lethal ventricular dysrhythmias.

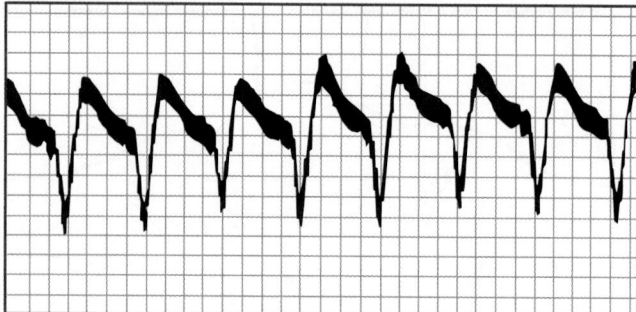

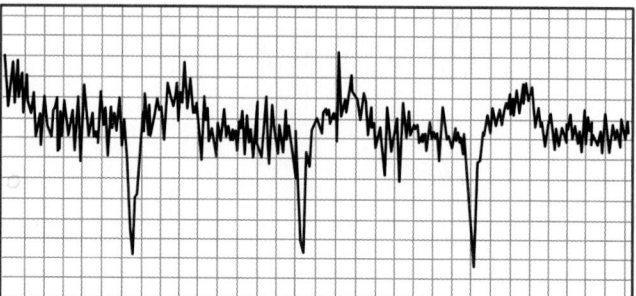

Figure 18-27 *Top,* Artifact from 60-cycle interference. *Bottom,* Artifact caused by muscular movement.

Electrocardiographic Analysis

Specialized Electrocardiographic Paper. ECG paper records the speed and magnitude of electrical impulses on a grid composed of small and large boxes (Fig. 18-28). Every large box has five small boxes in it. At a standard paper speed of 25 mm/sec, on the horizontal axis, one small box (1 mm) is equivalent to 0.04 second, and one large box (5 mm) represents 0.20 second. Distances along the horizontal axis represent speed and are stated in seconds rather than in millimeters or number of boxes. The vertical axis represents the magnitude, or force, of the electrical signal. The vertical scale is standardized to a specific calibration.

Calibration. At standard calibration, one small box equals 0.1 mm, and one large box equals 0.5 mm. It is important to look for the standardization mark, which is usually located at the beginning of the tracing (Fig. 18-29A). The mark indicates that in response to a standard electrical signal of 1 mV, the calibration signal rises two large boxes to make a calibration mark. ECGs are sometimes run at different calibrations. If at standard calibration some complexes are so tall they run off the paper, the tracing is repeated at one-half standard (see Fig. 18-29B), and the calibration mark rises only one large box. If all of the complexes on a standard tracing are very small, it may be repeated at double standard, with the calibration mark going up four large boxes (see Fig. 18-29C). In any case, the calibration must be clearly marked on the tracing, because some diagnostic conclusions are based on the magnitude of specific portions of the ECG complex.

Waveforms. The analysis of waveforms and intervals provide the basis for ECG interpretation (Fig. 18-30).

P Wave. The P wave represents atrial depolarization.

QRS Complex. The QRS complex represents ventricular depolarization, corresponding to phase 0 of the ventricular

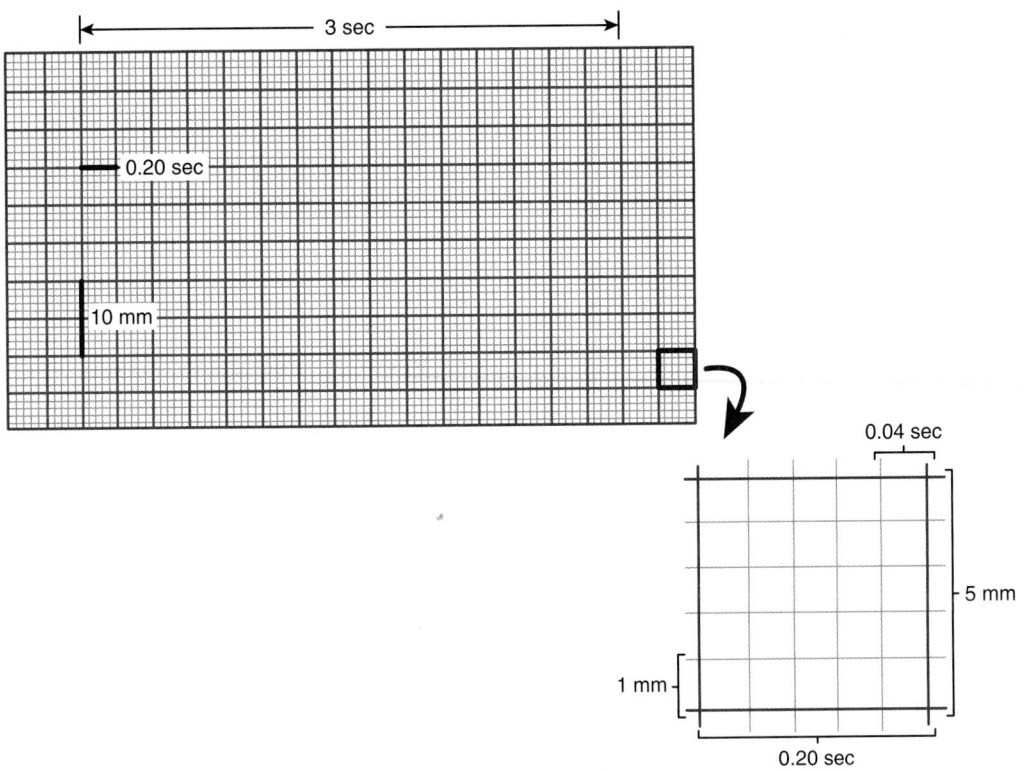

Figure 18-28 ECG graph paper. The horizontal axis represents time, and the vertical axis represents the magnitude of voltage. Horizontally, each small box is 0.04 second, and each large box is 0.20 second. Vertically, each large box is 5 mm. Markings are present every 3 seconds at the top of the paper for ease in calculating heart rate.

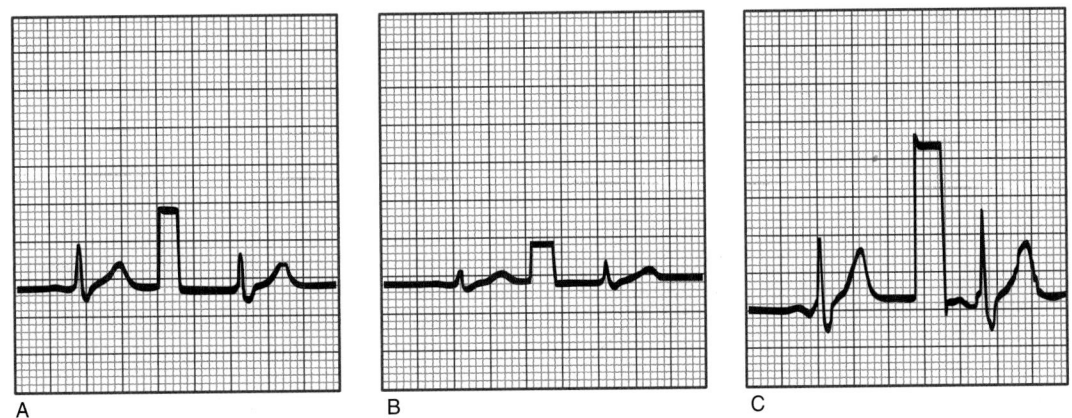

Figure 18-29 *A,* The machine is calibrated so that the normal standardization mark is 10 mm tall. *B,* Half standardization is used when QRS complexes are too tall to fit on the paper. *C,* Twice normal standardization is used when QRS complexes are too small to be adequately analyzed.

action potential. It is referred to as a *complex* because it consists of several different waves. The letter *Q* is used to describe an initial negative deflection; only if the first deflection from the baseline is negative will it be labeled a Q wave. The letter *R* applies to any positive deflection. If there are two positive deflections in one QRS complex, the second is labeled R′ ("R prime") and is commonly seen in lead V_1 in patients with right bundle branch block. The letter *S* refers to any subsequent negative deflections. Any combination of these deflections can occur and is collectively called the *QRS complex* (Fig. 18-31).

The QRS duration is normally less than 0.10 second (2.5 small boxes).

T Wave. The T wave represents ventricular repolarization, corresponding to phase 3 of the ventricular action potential. The onset of the QRS to approximately the midpoint or peak of the T wave represents an absolute refractory period, during which the heart muscle cannot respond to another stimulus no matter how strong that stimulus may be (Fig. 18-32). From the midpoint to the end of the T wave, the heart muscle is in the relative refractory period. The heart muscle has not yet fully

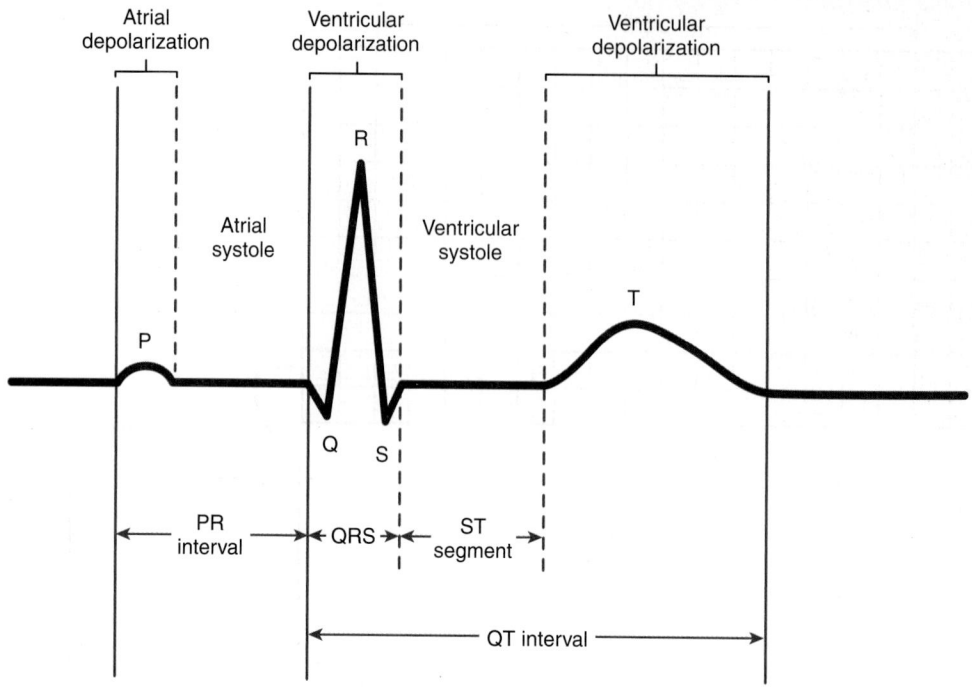

Figure 18-30 Normal ECG waveforms, intervals, and correlation with events of the cardiac cycle. The *P wave* represents atrial depolarization, followed immediately by atrial systole. The *QRS* represents ventricular depolarization, followed immediately by ventricular systole. The *ST segment* corresponds to phase 2 of the action potential, during which time the heart muscle is completely depolarized and contraction normally occurs. The *T wave* represents ventricular repolarization. The *PR interval,* measured from the beginning of the P wave to the beginning of the QRS, corresponds to atrial depolarization and impulse delay in the atrioventricular (AV) node. The *QT interval,* measured from the beginning of the QRS complex to the end of the T wave, represents the time from initial depolarization of the ventricles to the end of ventricular repolarization.

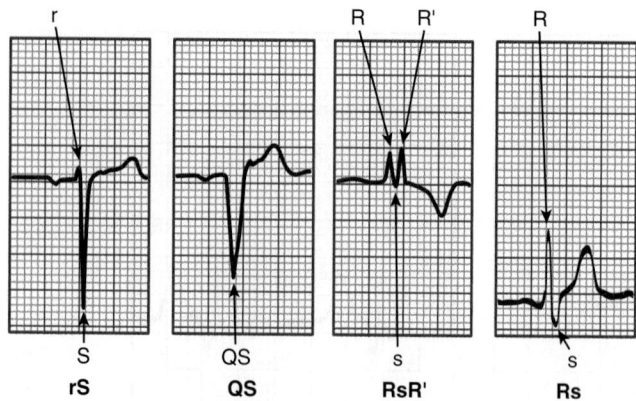

Figure 18-31 Examples of QRS complexes. Small deflections are labeled with lowercase letters, and uppercase letters are used for larger deflections. A second upward deflection is labeled R'.

recovered, but it can be depolarized again if a strong enough stimulus is received. This can be a particularly dangerous time for ventricular ectopy to occur, especially if any portion of the myocardium is ischemic, because the ischemic muscle takes even longer to fully repolarize. This sets the stage for the disorganized, self-perpetuating depolarizations of various sections of the myocardium known as *ventricular fibrillation* (VF).

Intervals Between Waveforms. The intervals between waveforms are evaluated (see Fig. 18-30).

PR Interval. The PR interval is measured from the beginning of the P wave to the beginning of the QRS complex. Normally,

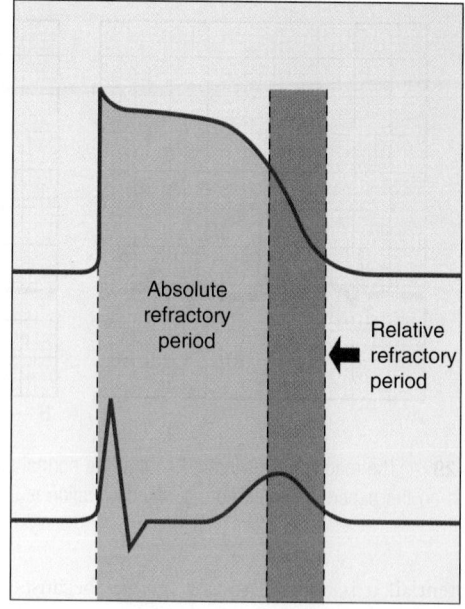

Figure 18-32 Absolute and relative refractory periods are correlated with the cardiac muscle's action potential and with an ECG tracing.

the PR interval is 0.12 to 0.20 second long and represents the time between sinus node discharge and the beginning of ventricular depolarization. Because most of this period results from delay of the impulse in the AV node, the PR interval is an indicator of AV nodal function.

In the electrophysiology laboratory and in some critical care units, these time values are described in milliseconds. There are 1000 milliseconds (msec) in 1 second. The normal PR interval value can also be written as 120 to 200 msec.

ST Segment. The ST segment is the portion of the wave that extends from the end of the QRS to the beginning of the T wave. Its duration is not measured. Instead, its shape and location are evaluated.[63] The ST segment is normally flat and at the same level as the isoelectric baseline. Any change from baseline is expressed in millimeters and may indicate myocardial ischemia (one small box equals 1 mm). ST-segment elevation (increase above baseline greater than 1 mm) is associated with acute myocardial injury, preinfarction, and pericarditis. ST-segment depression (decrease from baseline more than 1 mm) is associated with myocardial ischemia.[66] The ST segment must be monitored carefully in high-risk patients described later).[66]

QT Interval. The QT interval is measured from the beginning of the QRS complex to the end of the T wave and indicates the total time interval from the onset of depolarization to the completion of repolarization. There is no established bedside monitoring lead recommended for measuring the QT interval.[62] On the 12-lead ECG, the QT interval is usually the longest in precordial leads V$_3$ and V$_4$.[62] The important point is that each clinician measures the QT interval using the same ECG lead.[62] At normal heart rates, the QT interval is less than one half of the R-R interval when measured from one QRS complex to the next. However, the length of a QT interval depends on heart rate and must be adjusted according to the heart rate to be evaluated in a clinically meaningful way.

Because the QT interval shortens with faster heart rates and lengthen with slower heart rates, it is often written as a "corrected" value (QTc), meaning the QT value was mathematically corrected as if the heart rate were 60 beats/min.[67] This allows comparison of QTc across a range of heart rates. The corrected QT interval (QTc) is calculated by dividing the measured QT interval (in seconds) by the square root of the RR cycle length (see Fig. 18-3).[62,66] The normal QTc is less than 0.46 second (460 msec) in women and less than 0.45 second (450 msec) in men.[62] A prolonged QT interval is significant because it can predispose the patient to the development of polymorphic VT, known also as *torsades de pointes.* A long QT interval can be the result of a *congenital* chromosomal abnormality, or it can be *acquired* as a result of electrolyte imbalance or antidysrhythmic drug therapy.[68]

Quinidine is an antidysrhythmic drug commonly responsible for the acquired form of prolonged QT interval, although any class Ia drug (e.g., quinidine, procainamide, disopyramide) can lengthen the QT interval; class III drugs (e.g., amiodarone, ibutilide, sotalol) also can prolong the QT interval and initiate an episode of torsades de pointes.[68] When drugs associated with a high risk of torsades de pointes are started, it is important to record the QT and QTc interval and to continue to monitor the QT and QTc interval during treatment. Prolongation of the absolute QT interval beyond 0.5 second (500 msec) increases the risk of polymorphic VT.[68]

However, not all patients are at equal risk, and the reason some patients with a prolonged QT interval experience lethal

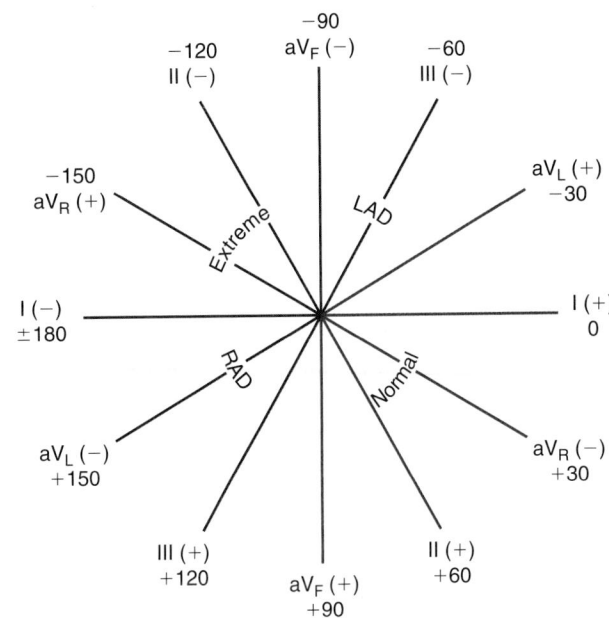

Figure 18-33 Hexaxial reference system. *LAD,* left-axis deviation; *RAD,* right-axis deviation.

ventricular dysrhythmias but others do not is not understood.[68] Researchers speculate that between 5% and 10% of patients with acquired long QT syndrome (drug induced) also carry a genetic predisposition for the syndrome.[68]

The risk of torsades de pointes is intensified in acquired and congenital long QT syndrome in the presence of hypokalemia or hypomagnesemia. Polymorphic VT occurs most frequently in the presence of a slow ventricular rate caused by heart block, a sinus pause, or sinus bradycardia.[68]

QT-interval monitoring is used as an indirect measure of ventricular repolarization.[62] It is often challenging on a bedside monitoring strip to determine precisely where the end of the QT interval occurs.[62,67]

Acute therapy is directed at increasing the heart rate, which will shorten the QT interval, stopping culprit medications and correcting electrolyte abnormalities. It may also include placement of a temporary pacemaker and intravenous magnesium, especially if serum levels of magnesium are low.

Ventricular Axis. Electrical impulses spread through cardiac muscle tissue in many directions at once when the ventricular muscle is depolarized. Using the 12-lead ECG, all of these individual forces can be averaged to describe the overall direction that current is traveling, which is called the *mean vector.* The mean vector can be plotted on a circular graph known as the *hexaxial reference system* (Fig. 18-33), and a degree can be assigned to it. This degree represents the ventricular axis.

Parameters for ventricular axis are not always listed in the same way in every hospital.[38] Normal axis may be listed as 0 to 90 degrees for a "quick look" or more accurately as −30 to +90 degrees. Right-axis deviation is present if the heart's electrical axis falls between +90 and +180 degrees. Right-axis deviation can be further delineated as moderate right-axis deviation when it is between +90 and +120 degrees, and marked right-axis deviation when it is between +120 and +180 degrees.

Left-axis deviation is present if the axis falls between −30 and −90 degrees. Moderate left-axis deviation describes an axis between −30 and −45 degrees. Marked left-axis deviation describes an axis between −45 and −90 degrees.

Figure 18-33 shows how to locate these points on the hexaxial reference wheel. If the axis plots in the upper left portion of the circle, also known as the *extreme quadrant* or *northwest quadrant*, it is called an *indeterminate axis*. This axis occurs rarely but can be seen when the wave of depolarization starts at the bottom of the ventricle—near the point of maximal impulse (PMI) or apex of the ventricle—and spreads upward toward the atria. Clinically, this can be seen in beats of ventricular origin, such as PVCs and some pacemaker-initiated beats.

Calculating the Ventricular Axis. The ventricular axis is calculated using the six limb leads (leads I, II, III, and aVR, aVL, aVF) in the three steps outlined below (ECG example in Fig. 18-34).

Step 1. Find the limb lead with the smallest QRS complex or the one that is the most *equiphasic* (equal portions above and below the baseline). In Figure 18-34, lead aVF is the smallest.

Step 2. Using the hexaxial reference system (see Fig. 18-33), locate the lead that is perpendicular to the one that had the smallest complex. For example, perpendicular to lead aVF is lead I, so the mean vector lies parallel with lead I.

Step 3. The third step is to determine whether the QRS complex is positive or negative in the lead parallel to the mean vector (in this case, lead I). If the QRS is positive, the mean vector is directed *toward* the positive electrode. If the QRS is negative, the mean vector is directed *away* from the positive electrode. In Figure 18-34, the QRS deflection in lead I is upright, or positive. The positive pole of lead I is at the right midpoint of the hexaxial reference system and corresponds to a numeric degree of zero, which is within the normal range (Box 18-4).

Cardiac Monitor Lead Analysis. During continuous cardiac monitoring, adhesive, pre-gelled electrodes are used to obtain an ECG tracing that is similar to one lead of a 12-lead ECG. At a minimum, this requires three electrodes. One of the electrodes acts as a positive pole, one as a negative pole, and one as a ground. In most critical care units, five electrodes are used. Five leads allow the clinician to monitor two leads simultaneously or to allow selection of several different leads at any time through a lead selector switch on the monitor. Typical placement of the five electrodes in a multilead system is right arm (RA), left arm (LA), left leg (LL), and right leg (RL), with one chest lead that usually is placed in the V_1 position, as illustrated in Figure 18-35.

The selection of an ECG monitoring lead is not a decision to be made casually or according to habit. The chosen monitoring lead should be directly related to the patient's clinical condition and recent clinical history.[62] If the patient has experienced ST-segment elevation associated with acute coronary syndrome, percutaneous catheter intervention (PCI), or recent cardiac

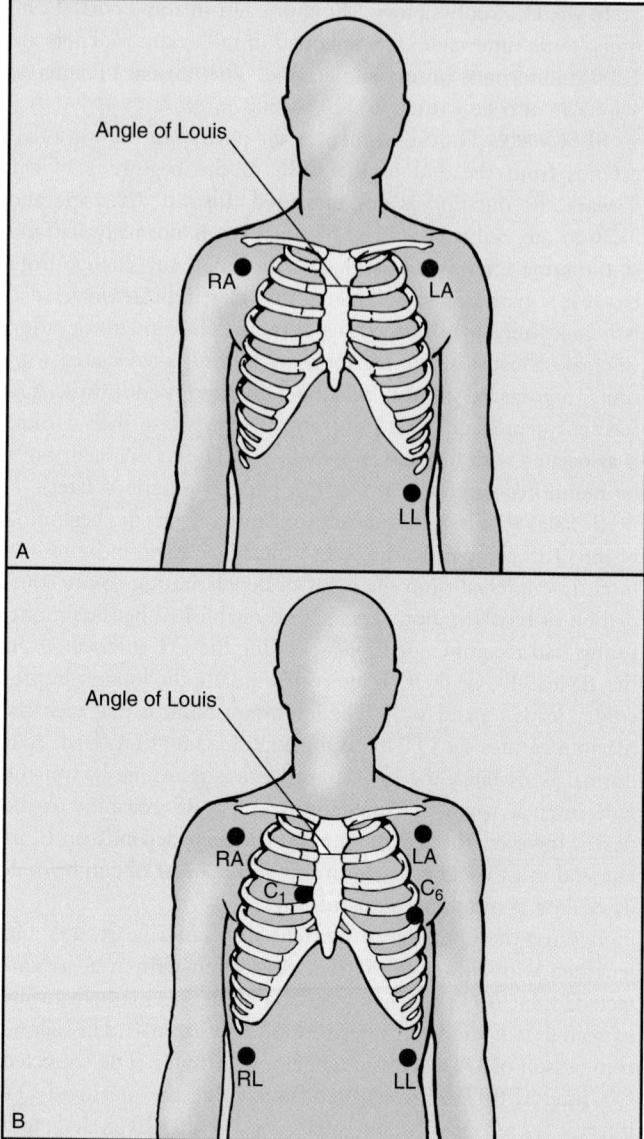

Figure 18-34 *A,* Three electrodes and lead-wire cables allow monitoring of three of the limb leads (I, II, and III) and can be rearranged to monitor MCL_1 and MCL_6. *B,* In the multilead monitoring system, five electrodes and lead-wire cables allow monitoring of any of the six standard limb leads (I, II, III, aVR, aVL, or aVF) and any one precordial lead (V_1 or V_6). C_1 indicates the proper position of the chest electrode for monitoring lead V_1, and C_6 indicates the proper position of the chest electrode for monitoring V_6. Color-coded cable attachments allow quick identification and accurate electrode placement.

BOX 18-4   STEPS IN DETERMINING THE AXIS

1. Find the most isoelectric limb lead.
2. Using the hexaxial reference system, find the lead that is perpendicular to the one identified in step 1.
3. Determine whether the QRS is positive or negative in the perpendicular lead.
4. Look at the corresponding positive or negative pole of the perpendicular lead on the hexaxial reference system.
5. The degree listed on the hexaxial reference system is the axis.

surgery, the leads that exhibited ST-segment elevation should used to guide selection of the optimal ECG monitoring leads.[62] Verify correct lead placement at the beginning of each shift.

Lead II. On a standard 12-lead ECG, lead II is formed by a positive electrode attached to the left leg, a negative electrode

attached to the right arm, and a ground electrode on the right leg. It is not practical to connect electrodes to the arms and legs during continuous monitoring, so the electrodes are placed on the torso near the origin of the limbs (Fig. 18-36). In the critical care unit, most patients have at least five electrodes placed, and the lead is selected by choosing a lead selector button on the monitor. If the monitored heart has a normal electrical axis, lead II displays a waveform that is predominantly upright, with a positive P wave and positive QRS waveform (see Fig. 18-36B). P waves are usually easy to identify in lead II, and it is recommended for monitoring of atrial dysrhythmias. However, it is difficult to identify right bundle branch block (RBBB) and left bundle branch block (LBBB) in this lead, because this is a vertical lead that does not clearly display horizontal interventricular conduction changes. Lead II is also nondiagnostic in differentiating VT from supraventricular tachycardia (SVT) with aberrant conduction. More information on differentiating VT from wide-complex SVT is provided later in this chapter.

Lead V₁. The V₁ electrode is placed at the fourth intercostal space to the right of the sternal border. Most of the electrical activity of the heart is directed toward the left ventricle and away from the V₁ electrode. For this reason, the normal QRS complex in lead V₁ is mostly negative (Fig. 18-37B). Any abnormal electrical activity directed toward the right ventricle, such as in RBBB, results in an upright QRS complex, often in an RSR' pattern.

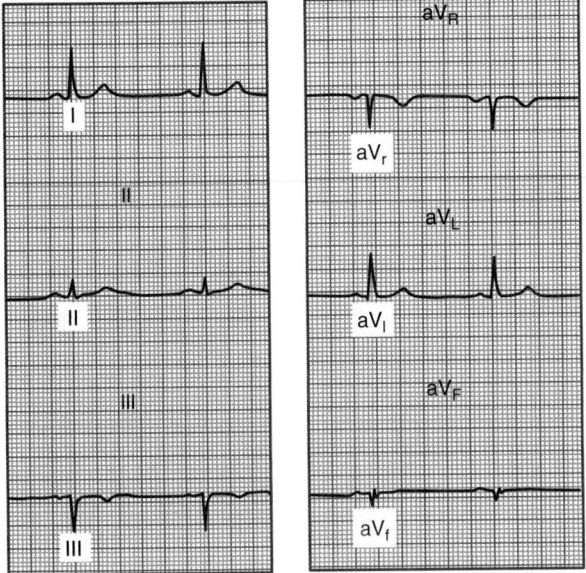

Figure 18-35 Limb leads of a normal ECG illustrate a normal axis of 0 degrees.

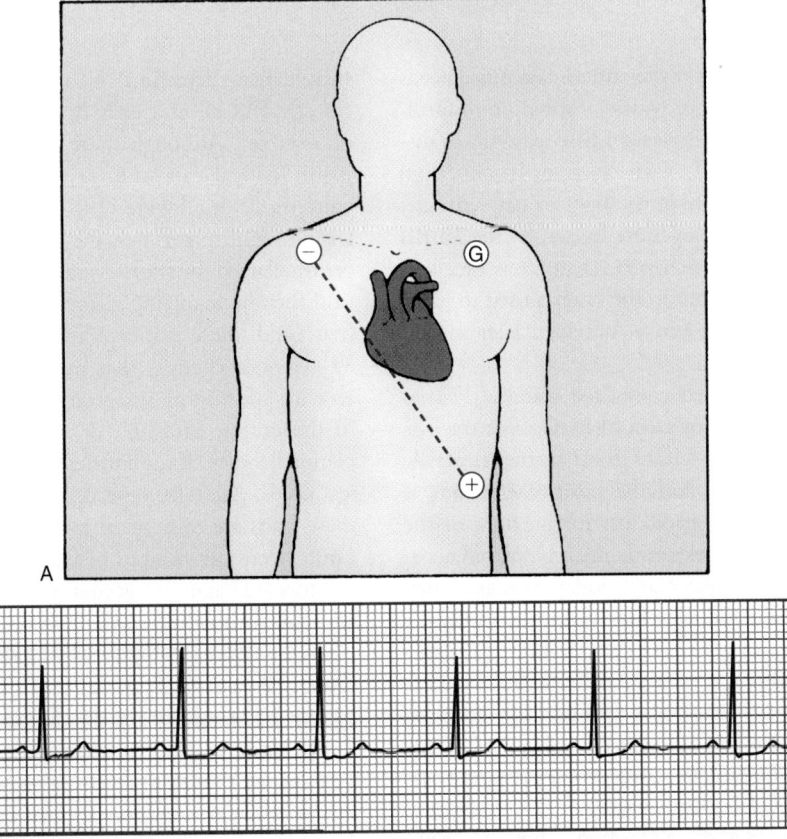

Figure 18-36 Monitoring lead II. *A,* Electrode placement. The negative electrode is placed below the right shoulder; the positive electrode is placed on the lower left torso (preferably below the rib cage); and the ground electrode is placed on the left shoulder. *B,* Typical ECG tracing in lead II.

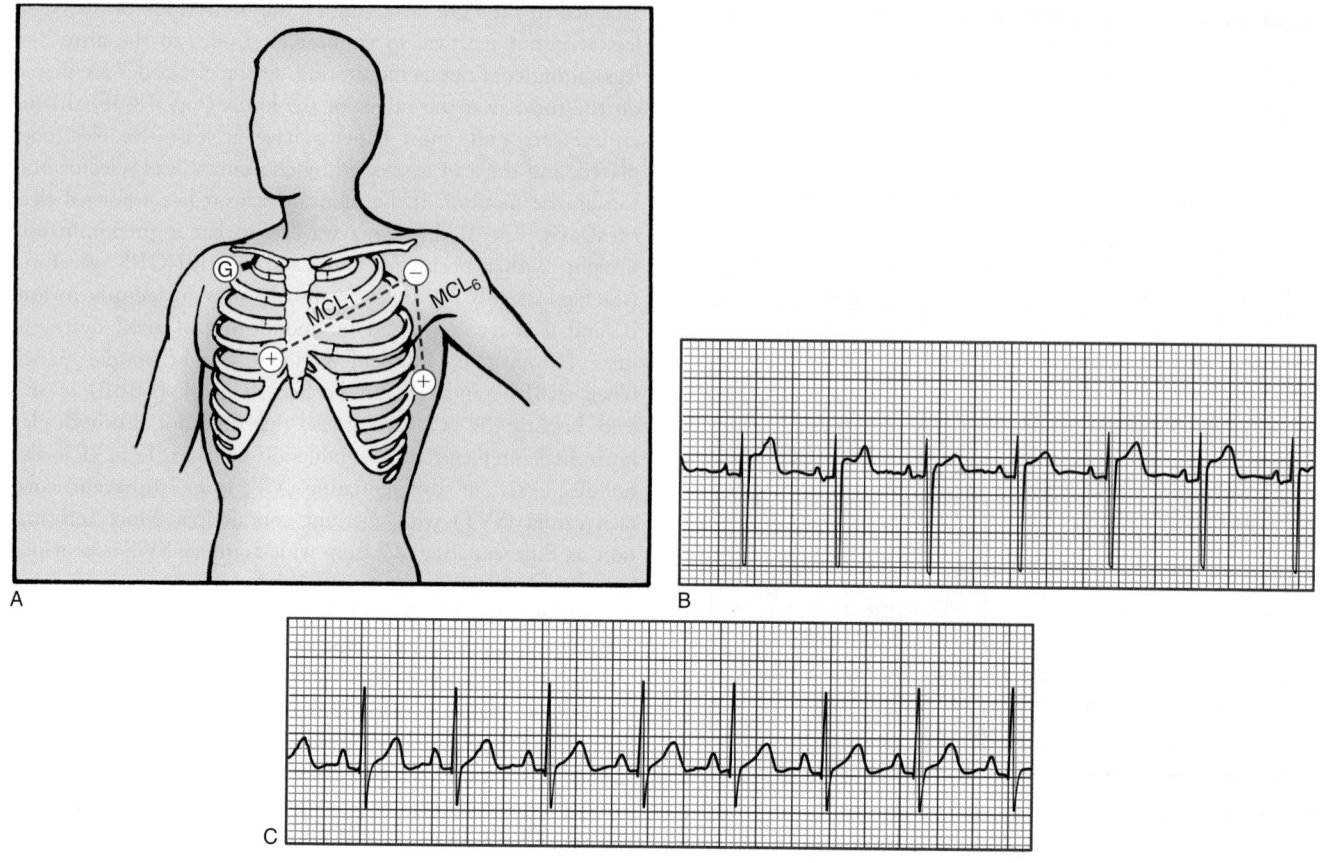

Figure 18-37 *A,* Monitoring lead placement for MCL$_1$ and MCL$_6$. *B,* Typical ECG tracing for MCL$_1$. *C,* Typical ECG tracing for MCL$_6$.

V$_1$ is the optimal lead to select if the critical care nurse needs to analyze ventricular ectopy. V$_1$ provides information to facilitate differentiation between RBBB versus LBBB pattern, or distinguish between VT and SVT with aberrant conduction; determine whether PVCs originate in the right or left ventricle, and clarify when ST-segment changes are caused by the RBBB and when they are the result of ischemia. Lead V$_1$ is excellent for this purpose. More information on the criteria used to identify these rhythms from the V$_1$ lead is provided later in this chapter.

MCL$_1$. MCL$_1$ means "modified chest lead using V$_1$." It is similar to a V$_1$ lead on a 5-lead or 12-lead ECG. The tracings are similar but not identical. In MCL$_1$ the negative electrode is placed on the right shoulder and the positive electrode is placed at the fourth intercostal space, just to the right of the sternum (see Fig. 18-37A). This electrode must be placed accurately. MCL$_1$ is an uncommon lead choice today. It is used only if monitoring with a 3-lead system (when V$_1$ is not available), which is a rare situation within any critical care unit. The normal QRS complex in lead MCL$_1$ has a mostly negative deflection (see Fig. 18-37B). In contrast, the normal QRS complex in lead MCL$_6$ has a mostly positive deflection because of the position of the MCL$_6$ lead placement on the left lateral mid-axillary chest wall (see Fig. 18-37C).

Electrocardiographic Lead Selection for Optimal Bedside Monitoring. In the early years of critical care nursing, the primary goals of cardiac monitoring were heart rate surveillance, detection of "warning" ventricular dysrhythmias (mostly PVCs), and early detection of lethal dysrhythmias (VF or asystole). Although these are still goals of ECG monitoring in the critical care unit, several more complex issues are now concerns. Not all wide QRS complex tachycardias are ventricular in origin; sometimes, they are supraventricular with aberrant ventricular conduction. Many patients are undergoing reperfusion therapy involving balloon angioplasty, stenting, or fibrinolysis, and these patients require continuous monitoring for ST-segment changes that may represent ischemia even in the absence of clinical symptoms. The nurse admitting a patient to the critical care unit or telemetry unit must make a well-planned choice of monitoring leads tailored to the patient's clinical needs. Accuracy of lead placement is extremely important if these leads are to be used for specialized diagnostic purposes.[66] Limb electrodes need to be placed close to where the limb joins the torso. Diagnostic accuracy is diminished if limb electrodes are moved too close to the heart.

Continuous Dysrhythmia Monitoring. Patients with serious cardiac diseases such as acute MI, heart failure, and cardiomyopathy are at risk for the development of bundle branch blocks, complex ectopy, and wide-complex tachycardias. These patients need to be monitored with a precordial lead that documents interventricular conduction changes. This is lead V$_1$.[69] Some 5-lead systems offer the clinician the choice of MCL$_1$ or V$_1$. The tracings in these two leads are not identical, and V$_1$ must be chosen over MCL$_1$ because it has a higher diagnostic accuracy.

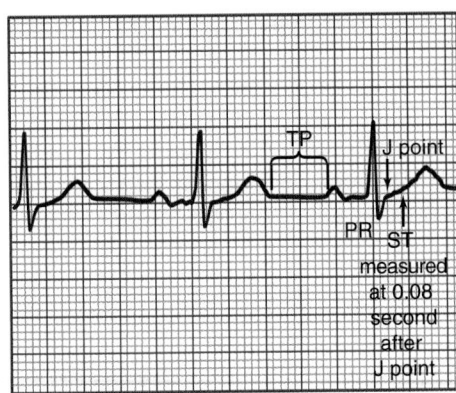

Figure 18-38 The TP interval is used as the reference point for the isoelectric line if the heart rate is slow enough for the TP interval to be clearly seen. If not, the PR interval can be used.

The six limb lead tracings also offer several monitoring choices that can be individualized to the clinical needs of the patient. Leads I and aVF are selected to detect a sudden change in ventricular axis. If ST-segment monitoring is required, the lead is selected according to the area of ischemia. If the ischemic area is not known, leads V_3 and III are recommended to detect ST-segment ischemia.[66] In inferior wall injury, leads II, III, and aVF are chosen; if lateral ischemia is present, lead I or aVL may be selected.

Continuous ST-Segment Monitoring. A key responsibility of the critical care nurse is monitoring for ECG changes that signify myocardial ischemia.[70] At the bedside, this takes the form of continuous ST-segment monitoring using the traditional bedside monitor and ECG electrodes. Increasingly, bedside monitoring systems incorporate ST-segment analysis to detect myocardial ischemia or injury. ST-segment changes may be accompanied by classic symptoms such as chest pain, or they may be "silent," without any clinical symptoms except ST-segment depression seen on the ECG monitor.[71]

The best way to choose a lead for monitoring the ST segment to detect ischemia is to look at the patient's 12-lead ECG during an episode of ischemia, if available. The standard 12-lead ECG obtained in an acute coronary syndrome before treatment or during a percutaneous coronary intervention (PCI) will reveal the leads that best demonstrate ischemia in that patient.[62,66] Under normal (nonischemic) conditions, the ST segment is at the same level as the TP segment, also known as the *isoelectric line* (Fig. 18-38).

Patients at risk for silent ischemia include anyone experiencing an acute coronary syndrome even if treated with thrombolytics, nitrates, or anticoagulation therapy. PCI patients are at risk for coronary artery repeat occlusion or spasm, reflected by ST-segment changes similar to those seen during PCI balloon inflation. Any patient admitted to the critical care unit with a history of prior MI, angina, diabetes, or kidney failure is a candidate for ST-segment monitoring.[62]

ST-segment deviation can have nonischemic causes and can create a false-positive alarm. Common culprits include hyperkalemia, pericarditis, hypokalemia, hypomagnesemia, hypothermia, ventricular aneurysm, hypothyroidism, pulmonary infarction,

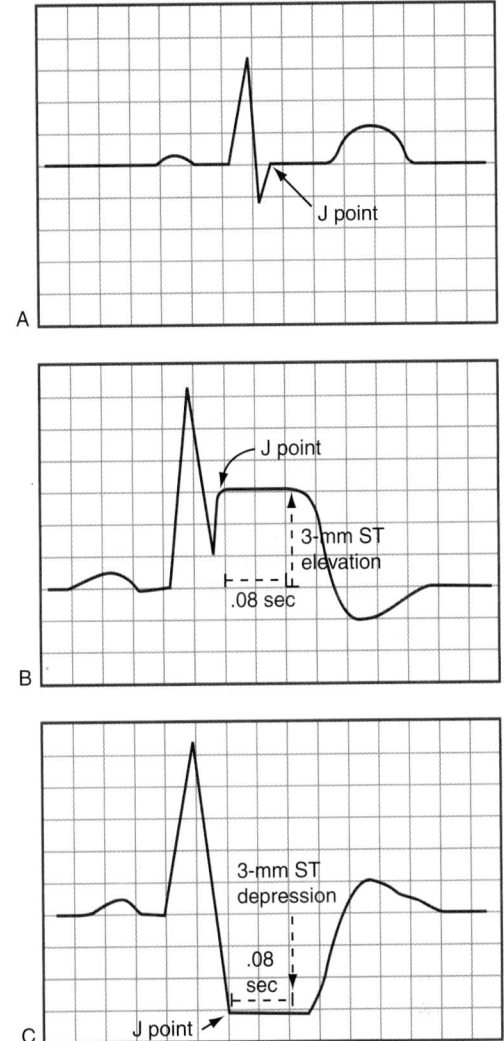

Figure 18-39 *A,* Normal position of the J point. *B,* A 3-mm ST-segment elevation. *C,* A 3-mm ST-segment depression. ST-segment changes are measured 60 to 80 msec (0.06 to 0.08 sec) after the J point.

and drugs such as quinidine and digitalis. Patients with subarachnoid hemorrhage (SAH) demonstrate ST-segment changes caused by excessive release of norepinephrine from the myocardial sympathetic nerves. The degree of myocardial necrosis and ST-segment elevation depends on the severity of neurologic injury.[72]

ST-segment deviation is measured as the number of millimeters of ST-segment vertical displacement from the isoelectric line or from the patient's baseline. The measurement position is typically selected 60 to 80 msec from the J point (Fig. 18-39). The J point is chosen to avoid monitoring the upstroke of the T wave.[67] On the bedside monitor, ST-segment elevation is displayed as a positive number, whereas ST-segment depression is indicated as a negative number (see Fig. 18-39). To be clinically significant, the ST segment must be displaced by at least 1 mm and last for at least 60 seconds.

When setting ST-segment alarm parameters, the patient's condition is always considered. The alarm may be set at 1 mm above and below the baseline ST-segment level in patients at high risk for ischemia. In stable, low-risk patients, the suggested setting is 2 mm above or below the isoelectric line.[62] The rationale for selection of wider ST-segment alarm parameters in more stable patients is that this may reduce the number of false ST-segment alarms.[62] This is important because stable patients tend to be more active, and when patients change position, it can alter the isoelectric baseline. If there are too many false ST-segment alarms, clinicians may be tempted to turn off or not pay attention to the alarm system. Poor electrode contact with the skin also is responsible for false ST-segment change alarms, emphasizing the need for adequate skin preparation before electrode placement.[62]

Some specific ECG patterns do not lend themselves to ST-segment monitoring, particularly rhythms that are associated with a wide QRS and distortion of the ST segment. This includes LBBB and RBBB, paced rhythms, and idioventricular rhythms. Other rhythms that make ST-segment monitoring problematic include erratic atrial fibrillation or atrial flutter that obscures the isoelectric baseline.[62] Agitated and restless patients make continuous ST-segment monitoring almost impossible.

Atrial Hypertrophy. Atrial chamber enlargement can be suspected from the 12-lead ECG because muscle size influences the ECG tracing, although the echocardiogram is considered the gold standard for diagnosis of cardiac chamber enlargement.[73] Atrial hypertrophy on the 12-lead ECG is identified by the size and shape of the P waves and is usually most obvious in lead II. Wide, m-shaped P waves are seen in *left atrial hypertrophy* and are called *P mitrale,* because left atrial hypertrophy is often caused by mitral stenosis (Fig. 18-40A). Tall, peaked P waves occur in *right atrial hypertrophy* and are referred to as *P pulmonale,* because this condition is often the result of chronic pulmonary disease (see Fig. 18-40B).

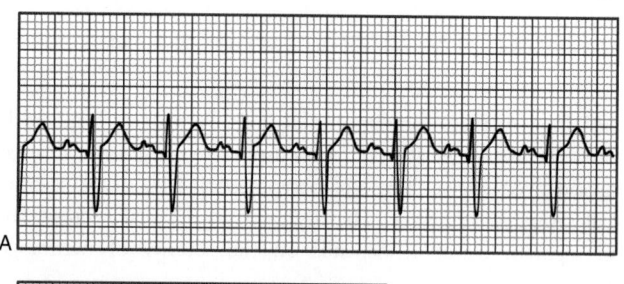

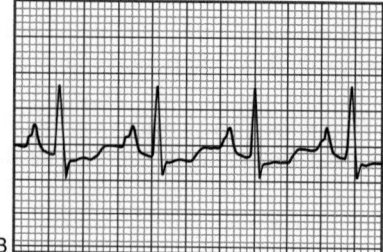

Figure 18-40 Atrial hypertrophy. *A,* In left atrial hypertrophy, the P wave is broad and notched and is sometimes called *P mitrale,* because it is often associated with mitral valve disease. *B,* In right atrial hypertrophy, the P wave is tall and peaked and is sometimes called *P pulmonale,* because it is often associated with pulmonary disease.

Ventricular Hypertrophy. Ventricular hypertrophy describes an increase in the size and muscle mass of one or both ventricles. Because a larger muscle is being depolarized, a greater amount of electrical activity is recorded on the ECG during depolarization. In ventricular hypertrophy, specific changes occur in the QRS complex. Upright QRS complexes become taller, and negative QRS complexes become even more negative. Often, the QRS becomes slightly wider, because it takes longer to depolarize a larger muscle. The QRS axis often shifts toward the enlarged ventricle, because a greater portion of the total electrical activity of the heart occurs there. A diagnosis of LV hypertrophy and LBBB on the 12-lead ECG is associated with increased cardiovascular mortality.[74,75] Although the 12-lead ECG can suggest hypertrophy, the echocardiogram is the most reliable diagnostic device, because it can visualize ventricular wall thickness and motion.[76]

Ischemia and Infarction. *Ischemia* occurs when the delivery of oxygen to the tissues is insufficient to meet metabolic demand. Cardiac ischemia in an unstable form occurs because of a sudden decrease in supply, such as when the artery is blocked by a thrombus or when coronary artery spasm occurs.[65,77] Stable angina can occur when a stenotic coronary artery is unable to adapt to sudden increase in demand created by exercise. Ischemia is by nature a transient process. The balance of supply versus demand is restored, and the muscle tissue recovers, or the imbalance becomes so great that the tissue can no longer survive, and it infarcts and becomes necrotic. Many nursing and medical interventions are directed toward saving as much ischemic tissue as possible.

Infarction refers to the death and disintegration of muscle cells and their eventual replacement by scar tissue. After infarction has occurred, the process cannot be reversed.[77]

Electrocardiographic Changes Indicating Ischemia and Infarction. Ischemia and infarction cause changes in the way cardiac muscle cells respond to electrical stimuli. These changes can usually be seen in a 12-lead ECG tracing.[78]

ST-segment elevation is seen when the positive electrode lies directly over an area of transmural (full-wall thickness) injury (Fig. 18-41A). This represents a preinfarction state, and interventions to unblock the occluded coronary artery must be initiated to prevent death of myocardium. ST-segment elevation is a precursor to an ST-elevation myocardial infarction (STEMI).[77]

Not every myocardial infarction is heralded by ST-segment elevation. When the patient has an MI without ST-segment elevation, it is described as a non–ST-elevation myocardial infarction (NSTEMI), but the diagnosis can be considerably more challenging without the signature ST-segment changes seen on the ECG.[65]

ST-segment depression occurs when the reduction of blood flow is limited to the endocardium and some normal muscle tissue remains between the ischemic area and the positive electrode (see Fig. 18-41B). ST-segment depression is seen because the positive electrode is separated from the ischemic area by normal tissue. T waves most commonly flatten or become inverted.

Infarction involves necrosis (death) of muscle cells with eventual formation of scar tissue. These cells can no longer be depolarized when an impulse reaches them. If the infarction involves the epicardial (outer) layer of the heart muscle or the entire thickness of the heart wall (transmural lesion), the QRS complex changes. Abnormal Q waves typically develop in the leads overlying the affected area. Occasionally, the entire QRS complex becomes smaller without development of Q waves.

Non–Q-wave Infarction. Not every acute MI results in a pathologic Q wave on the 12-lead ECG.[77] When the typical ECG changes are not present, the diagnosis depends on symptomatic clinical presentation, specific cardiac biomarkers (e.g., cTnI, cTnT, CK-MB), and non-ECG diagnostic tests such as cardiac catheterization.

Infarct Location by 12-Lead Electrocardiogram. The location of the infarction can be roughly determined by noting the specific leads in which the ST-segment and T-wave changes are seen on the 12-lead ECG. Table 18-9 summarizes of the anticipated 12-lead ECG changes.

Right ventricular infarction and posterior wall infarction are particularly difficult to identify on a standard 12-lead ECG, because none of the standard leads directly views these areas. A right ventricular infarction can be suspected and investigated in the setting of an acute inferior wall MI. To avoid missing this diagnosis, right-sided precordial leads (see Fig. 18-26B) can be placed, and a 12-lead ECG obtained for any patient with a suspected inferior right ventricular wall MI.[64]

A posterior wall MI may be suspected in a patient with an acute inferior wall MI when there is ST-segment depression in leads V_1, V_2, and V_3 on the standard 12-lead ECG. Tall, upright R waves may also be present. Posterior wall involvement can be verified by adding posterior precordial leads V_7, V_8, and V_9 (see Fig. 18-26D).[79]

Infarct Electrocardiographic Progression. When blood flow in a coronary artery is suddenly occluded, the entire area of heart muscle normally perfused by that artery becomes ischemic. Collateral arterioles exist, which overlap and supply the perimeter of this area and may prevent necrosis of some of the affected tissue. At the center of the ischemic area, collateral blood flow is minimal or does not exist at all. Within a few hours, this tissue begins to die. On the ECG tracing, this process is illustrated as follows. Within minutes of the onset of infarction, ST-segment elevation occurs in the leads directly overlying the affected heart wall. This ST-segment elevation persists for a period of hours to 1 day, gradually becoming less severe. Within the first few hours, T waves may become tall and symmetric. They are known as hyperacute T waves, and they indicate acute ischemia. Meanwhile, usually within 4 to 24 hours from the onset of the infarction, abnormal Q waves begin to develop in the affected leads, and T waves begin to invert. Sometimes, instead of Q waves developing, the R waves become smaller. This still indicates necrosis of muscle tissue. The ST segments become isoelectric again in a few days, and the T wave becomes symmetric and deeply inverted in the affected leads.

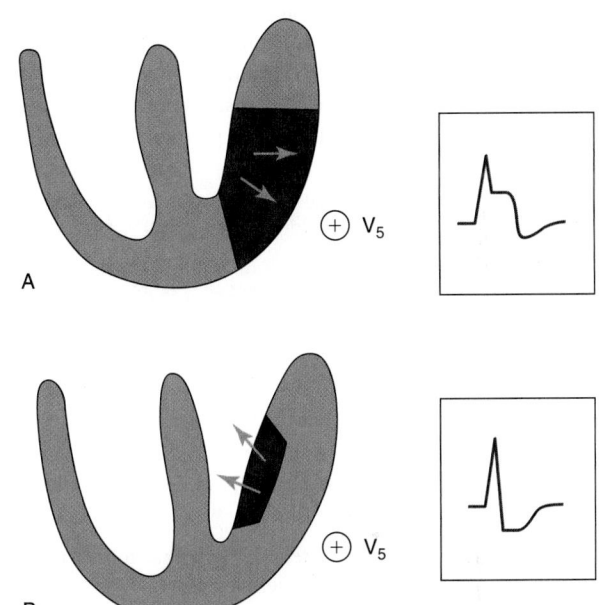

Figure 18-41 A, Acute transmural ischemia. The electrical forces *(arrows)* responsible for the ST segment are directed outward through the entire thickness of the heart muscle wall, causing ST-segment elevation in leads directly over the ischemic area. *B,* Acute subendocardial ischemia. The electrical forces responsible for the ST segment are deviated toward the inner layer of the heart, resulting in ST depression in leads directly over that area of the heart muscle wall.

TABLE 18-9 Electrocardiographic Changes during Myocardial Infarction

Location of Infarction	Artery Involved	Leads Involved	ECG Changes*
Anterior wall	LAD	V_{3-4}	Q waves, ST ↑, T ↓
Inferior wall	RCA or LCx	II, III, aVF	Q waves, ST ↑, T ↓
Ventricular septum	LAD	V_{1-2}	Q waves, ST ↑, T ↓
Lateral wall	LCx	V_{5-6}, I, aVL	Q waves, ST ↑, T ↓
Posterior wall	RCA or LCx	V_{1-3} (ant*); V_{7-9} (post†)	Tall, upright R; ST ↓; Upright T with ST ↑ V_{7-9}
Right ventricle	Proximal RCA	V_4R (right‡)	ST ↑

*See Figure 18-7B for ECG lead placement.
†See Figure 18-7D for ECG lead placement.
‡See Figure 18-7C for ECG lead placement.
ant, anterior; ECG, electrocardiographic; LCx, left circumflex artery; LAD, left anterior descending artery; post, posterior; right, right precordium; Q waves, pathologic Q waves; RCA, right coronary artery; ↑, elevated; ↓ depressed.

Occasionally, these T-wave changes never resolve. However, the T waves usually return to normal within several months. The Q waves may persist for the remainder of the patient's life, or they may get smaller over time and, in some individuals, disappear altogether. Table 18-10 summarizes the timing of these changes.

Intraventricular Ventricular Conduction Defects. Intraventricular conduction defects are the result of an abnormal pathway of conduction through the ventricles. Normally, conduction spreads from the AV node to the bundle of His and from there down the right and left bundle branches. The right bundle branch is long and thin and terminates in a mass of Purkinje fibers, which spread the wave of depolarization to the surrounding right ventricular muscle. After only a short distance, the left bundle branch divides into the left anterior fascicle, the left posterior fascicle, and the left septal fibers (Fig. 18-42). Each of these fascicles causes depolarization of separate areas of the left ventricle. If any part of the conduction

system fails, the muscle cells in that area will still depolarize, but not as quickly. Depolarization must then spread from cell to cell, a slower process than activation through specialized conduction pathways.

On the ECG, intraventricular conduction defects cause a widening of the QRS because of the slower spread of depolarization. The affected muscle tissue begins the slower cell-to-cell depolarization just as the other areas in the ventricle are almost finished. This later depolarization is then tacked onto the end of the normal QRS, making it prolonged and altering its shape.

Any part of the conduction system can be affected. The term *bundle branch block* refers to complete interruption of conduction through the right bundle or the entire left bundle branch. In complete RBBB or LBBB, the QRS is always 0.12 second (120 msec) or longer in duration. When only one fascicle of the left bundle branch is blocked, it is called a *hemiblock,* and the QRS duration is within normal limits, although it may be more prolonged than before the conduction disturbance occurred.

Right and Left Bundle Branch Blocks. The chest leads are the most useful in identifying complete RBBB and LBBB. V_1 and V_6 are the best leads from which to identify forces traveling in a horizontal direction, because they are located on the right and left sides of the heart, respectively. Figure 18-43A shows the normal sequence of ventricular activation and the usual shape of the QRS complex in V_1 and V_6.

Right Bundle Branch Block. In complete RBBB (see Fig. 18-43B), the right ventricle is not activated through the rapid conduction system. Instead, it must be activated slowly, from one cell to the next. Electrical forces, which are not counterbalanced by opposing forces on the left, travel toward the right at the end of the ventricular activation. The septum is depolarized first in a normal manner from left to right. Next, the wave of

TABLE 18-10	Timing of Electrocardiographic Changes
Time Frame	**Change**
Immediate	ST-segment elevation in leads over the area of infarction
Within a few hours	Giant, upright T waves
Several hours	ST segment normalizes; T waves invert symmetrically
Several hours to days	Q waves or reduced R waves; voltage may remain low permanently

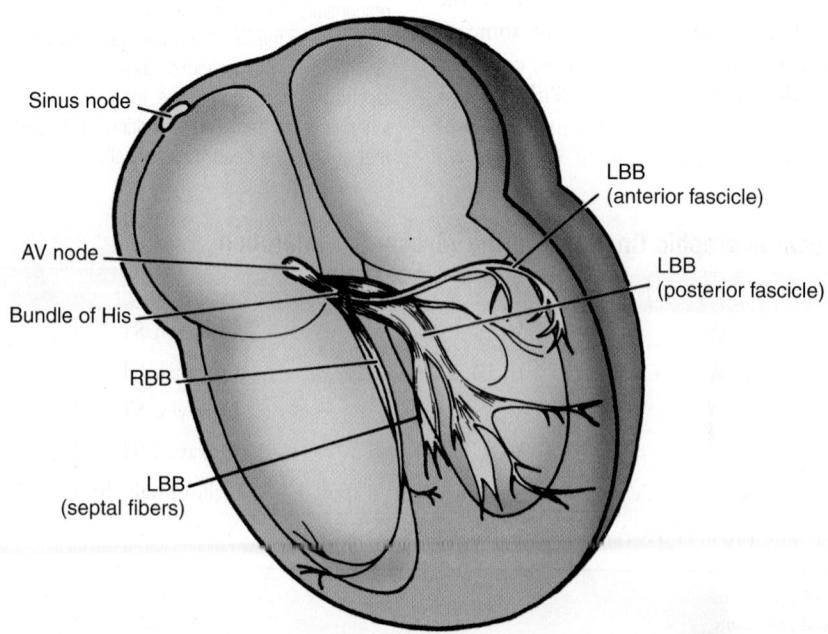

Figure 18-42 Cardiac conduction system. AV, atrioventricular; LBB, left bundle branch; RBB, right bundle branch. *(Modified from Conover MB:* Understanding electrocardiography, *ed 7, St Louis, 1996, Mosby.)*

depolarization spreads through the left ventricle and is recorded in lead V_1 as a tiny negative deflection. The final portion of the QRS complex is wide and upright, indicating final electrical forces traveling toward the right. This represents right ventricular depolarization that occurs after left ventricular depolarization is almost complete. In V_1, this QRS complex represents a classic pattern that is labeled rsR'; the ST segment representing repolarization is also abnormal and makes recognition of ST-segment changes related to ischemia impossible to detect by ECG monitoring.[80]

In lead V_6, the positive electrode is on the left side of the chest, and the waveforms are reversed. The final forces of the QRS complex are negative because they are traveling toward the right and away from the positive electrode of V_6. The final negative deflection in V_6 is smaller than the final upright deflection in lead V_1, because the positive electrode in V_6 is at a greater distance from the right ventricle.

Left Bundle Branch Block. In complete LBBB (see Fig. 18-43C), the conduction through the left ventricle must spread from cell to cell. Because a portion of the common left bundle normally initiates depolarization of the septum, the septum is depolarized in an abnormal direction, from right to left. In lead V_1, this is recorded as an initial negative deflection. Next, the right ventricle is depolarized, which is identified as a small upright notch in the QRS complex as the forces travel briefly toward the positive electrode of V_1. Sometimes, this notch is absent. The sequence of events has not changed, but the left ventricle is already beginning to be depolarized cell to cell and may offset the rightward forces of right ventricular depolarization. The final forces travel toward the left as the left ventricle is being depolarized. The left ventricle is a very large muscle mass, and these final electrical forces are large and wide. In lead V_1, the final deflection is a deep, negative deflection (S wave), whereas in lead V_6, these final forces inscribe a tall, upright deflection (R wave).

Presence of an LBBB makes diagnosis of an acute anterior wall MI extremely difficult because the change in repolarization masks ST-segment elevation.[81] Perhaps related to this difficulty in interpreting injury, patients with acute coronary syndrome in the presence of LBBB and associated LV hypertrophy have higher mortality rates than patients with acute coronary syndrome alone.[75] LBBB is a frequent finding in patients with dilated cardiomyopathy.[74]

Bundle branch blocks can easily be diagnosed at the bedside if the patient is being monitored with leads V_1 and V_6, respectively. A bundle branch block exists when the P wave is followed by a QRS complex that is wider than 0.12 second (120 msec); the presence of the P wave indicates that the complex did not originate from the ventricles.[81] To determine which bundle branch is blocked, the examiner looks at the last part of the QRS just before it returns to the baseline in leads V_1 and V_6. If upright in V_1 and negative in V_6, an RBBB exists. If negative in V_1 and upright in V_6, an LBBB is present.

Hemiblocks. Hemiblocks involve conduction failure of only part of the left bundle branch. In left anterior fascicular block, also called *left anterior hemiblock*, left ventricular depolarization begins in the left posterior fascicle and spreads anteriorly

through Purkinje fibers distal to the block. The QRS is only slightly prolonged, up to 0.02 second longer than the patient's previous QRS. However, the axis changes dramatically and becomes more negative than −30 degrees (left-axis deviation). Other causes of left-axis deviation must be ruled out before a clinical diagnosis of left anterior hemiblock can be made (Boxes 18-5 and 18-6). In left posterior fascicular block, also called *left posterior hemiblock*, the anterior portion of the left ventricle is depolarized first. Conduction then spreads slowly to the right, inferiorly and posteriorly. The QRS is slightly prolonged, although within normal limits. The axis then swings entirely the other direction and becomes greater than +90 degrees

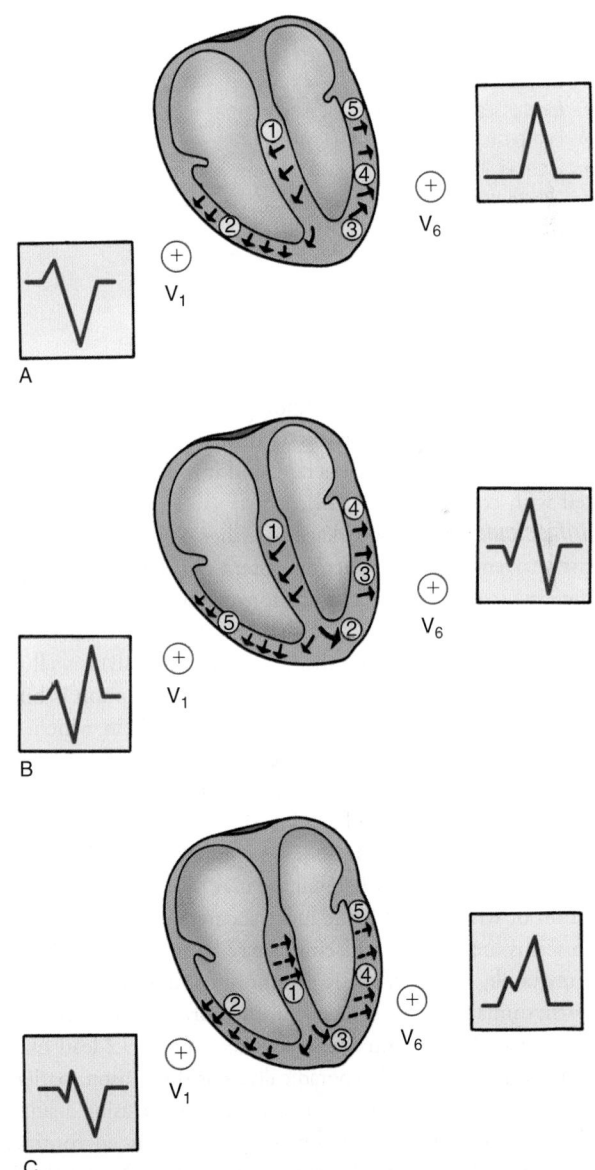

Figure 18-43 *A,* Sequence of ventricular depolarization and resulting QRS complex, as seen in leads V_1 and V_6. *B,* Sequence of ventricular depolarization for a right bundle branch block and resulting QRS complex, as seen in leads V_1 and V_6. *C,* Sequence of ventricular depolarization for a left bundle branch block and resulting QRS complex, as seen in leads V_1 and V_6.

BOX 18-5 **CAUSES OF LEFT-AXIS DEVIATION**

- Normal variation
- Mechanical shifts: exhalation; high diaphragm caused by pregnancy, ascites, or abdominal tumor
- Left anterior hemiblock
- Left ventricular hypertrophy
- Wolff-Parkinson-White syndrome
- Hyperkalemia
- Cardiomyopathy

BOX 18-6 **CAUSES OF RIGHT-AXIS DEVIATION**

- Normal variation
- Mechanical shifts: inhalation, emphysema
- Left posterior hemiblock
- Right ventricular hypertrophy
- Lateral wall myocardial infarction
- Right bundle branch block
- Dextrocardia

(right-axis deviation). Anterior hemiblock (causes left-axis deviation) is a relatively frequent finding in patients with arterial hypertension or cardiomyopathy (see Box 18-6).[82] In contrast, isolated posterior hemiblock is rare, and it is almost always associated with concomitant RBBB. [82]

Bifascicular Block. Blockage of either of the two branches of the left ventricular conduction system plus RBBB constitutes a *bifascicular block.* Any combination of these conduction disturbances can occur and can evolve into complete heart block. Normally, bifascicular block (hemiblock plus RBBB) is well tolerated, and no intervention is necessary. The exception is bifascicular block that develops during an acute MI, in which the evolving infarct may warrant placement of a temporary pacemaker prophylactically in case conduction tissue ischemia progresses to complete heart block.

Dysrhythmia Interpretation. In clinical practice, the terms *dysrhythmia* and *arrhythmia* often are used interchangeably. The question of which word is the more accurate is often discussed. Both terms are correct, and either may be used in practice. In this textbook, dysrhythmia is the more commonly used term. A dysrhythmia is any disturbance in the normal cardiac conduction pathway. Dysrhythmias can be detected on a 12-lead ECG, but they often occur only sporadically. For this reason, patients in a critical care unit are monitored continuously using a single- or dual-lead system, and rhythm strips are recorded routinely and any time the patient's heart rhythm changes. Dysrhythmias occur frequently in cardiac and noncardiac critically ill patients.[83,84] A systematic approach to assess a rhythm disturbance is an indispensable skill. Steps to accurately interpret a rhythm strip are introduced first, followed by specific criteria to evaluate common dysrhythmias encountered in clinical practice.

Heart Rate Determination. The first thing to assess when evaluating a rhythm strip is the ventricular rate. Regardless of the dysrhythmia involved, the ventricular rate holds the key to whether the patient can tolerate the dysrhythmia (i.e., maintain adequate blood pressure, CO, and mentation). If the ventricular rate is consistently greater than 200 or less than 30, emergency measures must be started to correct the rate. A detailed analysis of the underlying rhythm disturbance can proceed later, when the immediate crisis is over. The three methods for calculating rate (Fig. 18-44A) follow:

1. Number of R-R intervals in 6 seconds times 10 (ECG paper is usually marked at the top in 3-second increments, making a 6-second interval easy to identify)
2. Number of large boxes between QRS complexes divided into 300
3. Number of small boxes between QRS complexes divided into 1500

In the healthy heart, the atrial rate and the ventricular rate are the same. However, in many dysrhythmias, the atrial and ventricular rates are different, and both must be calculated. To find the atrial rate, the PP interval, instead of the R-R interval, is used in one of the three methods listed for determining rate.

The choice of method for calculating the heart rate depends on the regularity of the rhythm. If the rhythm is irregular, the first method (R-R intervals in 6 seconds × 10) is the only method that can be used (see Fig. 18-44B). If the rhythm is regular, it is more accurate to use the second or third method. The second method can be easier to use when two consecutive R waves fall exactly on dark lines, and it provides a rapid estimate of rate. The third method is recommended when both R waves do not fall exactly on dark lines.

Rhythm Determination. The term *rhythm* refers to the regularity with which the P waves or R waves occur. Calipers assist in determining rhythm. One point of the calipers is placed on the beginning of one R wave, and the other point is placed on the next R wave. Leaving the calipers "set" at this interval, each succeeding R-R interval is checked to be sure it is the same width as the first one measured.

In describing the rhythm, three terms are used. If the rhythm is *regular,* the R-R intervals are the same ± 10%. For example, if there are 20 small boxes in an R-R interval, an R wave could be off by two small boxes, but the rhythm would still be considered regular. If the rhythm is *regularly irregular,* the R-R intervals are not the same, but some sort of pattern is involved, which could be grouping, rhythmic speeding up and slowing down, or any other consistent pattern (Fig. 18-45A). If the rhythm is *irregularly irregular,* the R-R intervals are not the same, and no pattern can be found (see Fig. 18-45B).

P-Wave Evaluation. The P wave is analyzed by answering the following questions. First, is the P wave present or absent? Second, is it related to the QRS? It is hoped that one P wave will be in front of every QRS. Sometimes, two, three, or four P waves may be in front of every QRS. If this pattern is consistent, the P wave and QRS are still related, although not on a 1:1 basis.

PR-Interval Evaluation. The duration of the PR interval, which normally is 0.12 to 0.20 second (120 to 200 msec), is

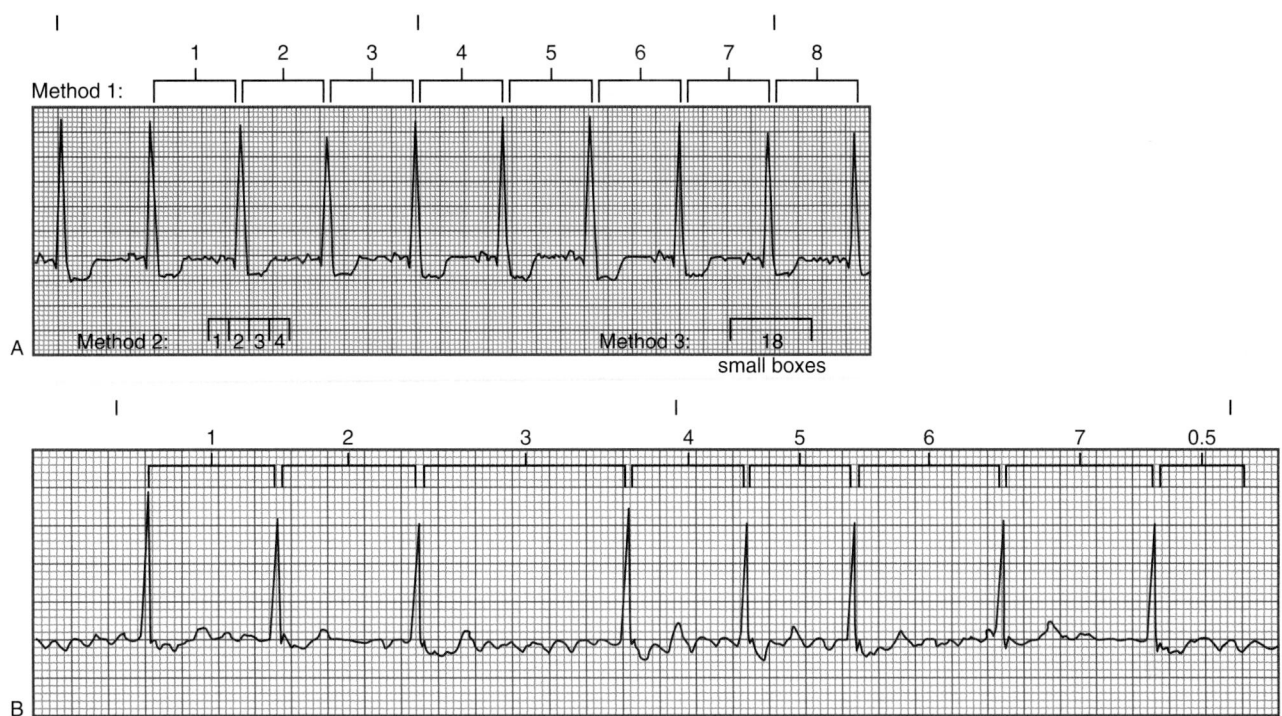

Figure 18-44 *A*, Calculation of the heart rate if the rhythm is regular. Method 1: number of R-R intervals in 6 seconds multiplied by 10 (e.g., 8 × 10 = 80/min). Method 2: number of large boxes between QRS complexes divided into 300 (e.g., 300 ÷ 4 = 75/min). Method 3: number of small boxes between QRS complexes divided into 1500 (e.g., 1500 ÷ 18 = 84/min). *B*, Rate calculation if the rhythm is irregular. Only method 1 can be used (e.g., 7.5 intervals × 10 = 75/min).

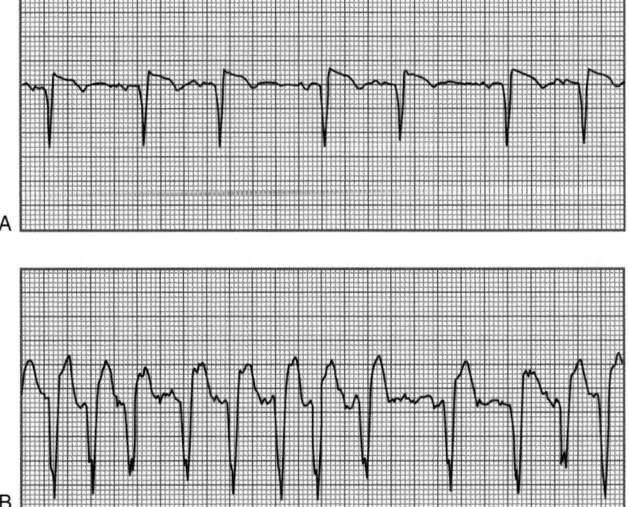

Figure 18-45 *A*, Regularly irregular rhythm is irregular but has a consistent pattern in that every other beat is premature. *B*, Irregularly irregular rhythm is irregular with no consistent pattern.

measured first. This is measured from the start of a visible P wave to the beginning of the next QRS (Fig. 18-46). All PR intervals on the strip are verified to be sure they have the same duration as the original interval.

QRS Complex Evaluation. The entire ECG strip must be evaluated to ascertain that the QRS complexes are consistently the same shape and width. The normal QRS duration is 0.06

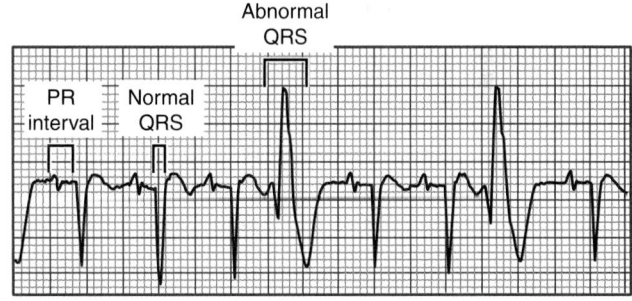

Figure 18-46 PR interval measurement, from the beginning of the P wave to the beginning of the QRS complex. The PR interval on this tracing is 0.20 second; the QRS duration illustrates normal and abnormal intervals. The narrow QRS complexes measure 0.08 second, which is normal. The wide QRS complexes measure 0.20 second and are caused by ventricular ectopy.

to 0.10 second (60 to 100 msec). If more than one QRS shape is on the strip, each QRS must be measured. The QRS is measured from where it leaves the baseline to where it returns to the baseline (see Fig. 18-46).

QT Evaluation. The length of the QT varies with the heart rate. The QT interval is shorter when the heart rate is faster. A QT interval corrected for heart rate (QTc) that is longer than 0.50 second (500 msec) is of concern, as discussed earlier under "QT Interval."

Sinus Rhythms. The cardiac cycle begins when an impulse originates in the sinus node. As the wave of depolarization spreads through the atria, a P wave is inscribed on the ECG.

The impulse is delayed briefly in the AV node, which corresponds to the PR interval on the ECG. After leaving the AV node, the wave of depolarization spreads rapidly through the bundle of His and the bundle branches and causes ventricular depolarization, which is recorded as a QRS complex by the ECG. Contraction immediately follows depolarization. Contraction is terminated by repolarization, which is demonstrated as a T wave on the ECG.

Normal Sinus Rhythm. If all of the events described for sinus rhythms occur in their normal sequence with normal rates and intervals, the patient is in normal sinus rhythm. The following are the criteria for normal sinus rhythm:

Rate. The intrinsic rate of the sinus node is 60 to 100 beats/min. *Intrinsic rate* is the normal rate at which a pacemaker site in the heart depolarizes automatically with no outside influences, such as drugs, fever, or exercise. In normal sinus rhythm, the rate must be whatever is normal for the sinus node (60 to 100 beats/min).

Rhythm. The rhythm must be regular ± 10%.

P wave. P waves must be present, and only one must precede every QRS complex.

PR interval. The PR interval represents delay in the AV node. In normal sinus rhythm, the PR interval is 0.12 to 0.20 second.

QRS. Size and shape do not matter in this complex, because it depends on lead placement and gain adjustments on the monitor. However, all QRS complexes must look alike. If conduction through the ventricles is normal, the QRS duration is 0.06 to 0.10 second. Figure 18-47 is an example of normal sinus rhythm in V1.

Sinus Bradycardia. Sinus bradycardia meets all of the criteria for normal sinus rhythm except that the rate is less than 60 beats/min (Table 18-11). It is normally seen in well-trained athletes at rest or in many other individuals during sleep. Other conditions in which sinus bradycardia occurs include vagal stimulation, increased intracranial pressure, drug therapy with digoxin or beta-blockers, and ischemia of the sinus node caused by an acute MI. Sinus bradycardia usually is not treated unless the patient displays symptoms of hypoperfusion, such as hypotension, dizziness, chest pain, or changes in level of consciousness.

Sinus Tachycardia. Sinus tachycardia meets all the criteria for normal sinus rhythm except that the rate is greater than 100 beats/min (see Table 18-11). Rates may be as high as

180 to 200 beats/min in healthy, young adults during strenuous exercise. However, in the critical care setting, bed rest is prescribed for most patients. It is wise to be skeptical of any "sinus tachycardia" with a rate greater than 150 and to search for a triggering focus other than the sinus node. For example, atrial flutter waves may be difficult to see at first glance because of baseline distortion caused by the high ventricular rate (Fig. 18-48).

Sinus tachycardia can be caused by a wide variety of factors, such as exercise, emotion, pain, fever, hemorrhage, shock, heart failure, and thyrotoxicosis.[85] Illegal stimulant drugs such as cocaine, "ecstasy," and amphetamines can raise the resting heart rate significantly.[85] Many drugs used in critical care can also cause sinus tachycardia; common culprits are aminophylline, dopamine, hydralazine, atropine, and catecholamines such as epinephrine. Tachycardia is detrimental to anyone with ischemic heart disease because it decreases the time for ventricular

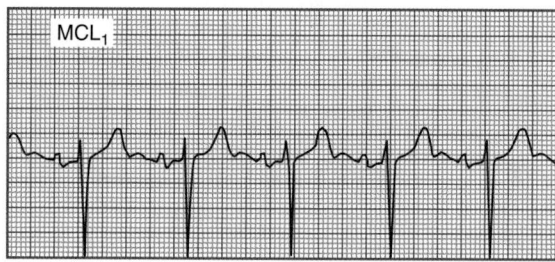

Figure 18-47 Normal sinus rhythm. The rate is 70, and the rhythm is regular. One P wave is present before each QRS complex. The PR interval is 0.18 second and does not vary throughout the strip. The QRS duration is 0.08 second. All evaluation criteria are within normal limits.

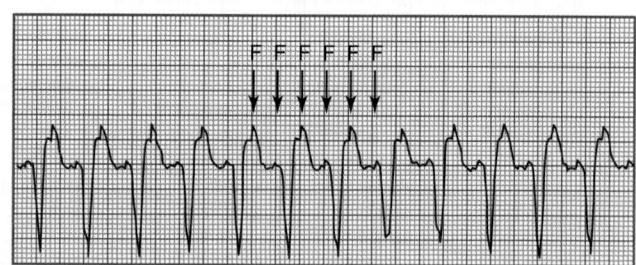

Figure 18-48 Although the tracing may be confused with sinus tachycardia, it is atrial flutter with 2:1 conduction. Notice how difficult it is to see the extra flutter waves (F) that are hidden in the QRS complexes.

TABLE 18-11 **Sinus Rhythms**

Parameters	Normal Sinus Rhythm	Sinus Bradycardia	Sinus Tachycardia	Sinus Dysrhythmia
Rate	60-100/min	<60/min	>100/min	Variable
Rhythm	Regular	Regular	Regular	Irregular; respiratory variation
P wave	Present, with one per QRS	Present, with one per QRS	Present, with one per QRS	Present, with one per QRS
PR interval	0.12-0.20 sec and constant	0.12-0.20 sec and constant	0.12-0.20 sec and constant	0.12-0.20 sec and constant
QRS	0.06-0.10 sec	0.06-0.10 sec	0.06-0.10 sec	0.06-0.10 sec

filling, decreases stroke volume, and compromises CO. Tachycardia increases heart work and myocardial oxygen demand while decreasing oxygen supply by decreasing coronary artery filling time.

If the cause of the tachycardia can be determined, such as fever or pain, it is treated rather than trying to treat the heart rate directly. Several drugs are available to decrease the heart rate if needed. Calcium channel blockers and beta-blockers are widely used for this purpose. However, a word of caution is warranted. CO is determined by heart rate and stroke volume. If an injured heart can no longer maintain an adequate stroke volume, heart rate can be increased to maintain CO and supply an adequate blood flow to vital body tissues. If a drug is administered to force the sinus node to slow, severe and relatively immediate heart failure can result. The sinus node is controlled by many neural and humoral influences in the body, and the rate is set to try to meet the perceived demands; a close examination of the reason for the tachycardia is mandatory before treatment decisions are made.

Sinus Dysrhythmia. Sinus dysrhythmia, commonly called *sinus arrhythmia* in clinical practice, meets all of the criteria for normal sinus rhythm except that the rhythm is irregular (see Table 18-11). This irregularity coincides with the respiratory pattern; heart rate increases with inhalation and decreases with exhalation[86] (Fig. 18-49). Sinus dysrhythmia often occurs in children and young adults, and the incidence decreases with age. No treatment is required. To avoid being misled by other rhythm disturbances, the examiner must look at all P waves closely to verify that they are all the same shape and that the PR intervals are all constant.

Atrial Dysrhythmias. Atrial dysrhythmias originate from an ectopic focus in the atria, somewhere other than the sinus node. The ectopic impulse occurs prematurely, before the normal sinus impulse occurs. The premature atrial depolarization may initiate a normal QRS complex, an abnormal or aberrant complex, or an SVT. Huge advances have been made in the understanding of the pathogenesis and management of atrial dysrhythmias.

Premature Atrial Contractions. Premature atrial contractions (PACs) are isolated, early beats from an ectopic focus in the atria. The underlying rhythm is usually sinus. The regular sinus rhythm is interrupted by an early, abnormally shaped atrial P wave. The early atrial wave usually looks different from the sinus P wave and may be inverted. The PR interval may be longer, shorter, or the same as the PR interval of a sinus impulse. The QRS that follows the ectopic atrial P wave can vary in shape depending on the degree of refractoriness of the AV node.

Normal, narrow QRS. If the atrial impulse arrives in the AV node after the AV node is fully repolarized, the impulse is conducted to the ventricles as a normal QRS. If the ventricles are also fully repolarized, conduction through the bundle branches is expected and a normal QRS is recorded on the ECG (Fig. 18-50A).

Wide QRS. Occasionally, the early ectopic P wave can be conducted through the AV node, but part of the conduction pathway through the ventricular bundle branches is blocked. Because the right bundle branch normally has the longest refractory period, it is usually the right bundle branch that is still blocked when the early impulse arrives. This produces a QRS that is wider than 0.12 second (120 msec) or wider than three small boxes on the ECG paper, with a shape consistent with RBBB (see Fig. 18-50B). Conduction through the ventricles that is different from normal is referred to as *aberrant*. Consequently, these early, abnormally conducted PACs are described as *aberrantly conducted PACs*.

Pause with no QRS. Sometimes, the ectopic P wave arrives so early that the AV node is still in its absolute refractory period. In this case, the wave of depolarization does not move past the AV node and no QRS follows. All that is seen on the ECG is an early, abnormal P wave followed by a pause until the next sinus P wave occurs (see Fig. 18-50C). This is called a *nonconducted PAC*. Usually, these P waves are so early that they are superimposed on the T wave of the previous beat, making them difficult to find. The pause that follows is still clearly seen. Whenever an unexpected pause occurs in a rhythm, the T wave preceding the pause must be examined very carefully and compared with other T waves on the same strip to locate distortions that may reveal a hidden early P wave.

PACs can occur in individuals with normal hearts. PACs are accentuated by emotional upheaval, nicotine, caffeine, and digitalis. Mitral valve prolapse is associated with an increased frequency of atrial dysrhythmias. Heart failure can cause PACs because of increased pressure within the atria. As atrial pressure begins to rise, the atrial walls are stretched, causing irritability of atrial cells and the occurrence of PACs.

Supraventricular Tachycardia. The term *supraventricular tachycardia* (SVT) is used clinically to describe a varied group

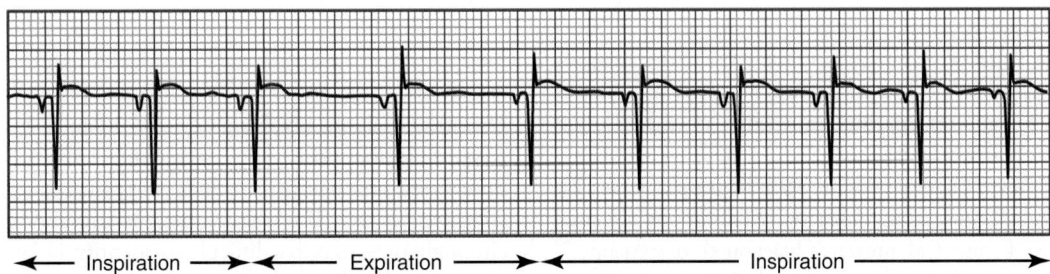

Figure 18-49 Sinus dysrhythmia. Notice the increased heart rate during inspiration and decreased heart rate during expiration.

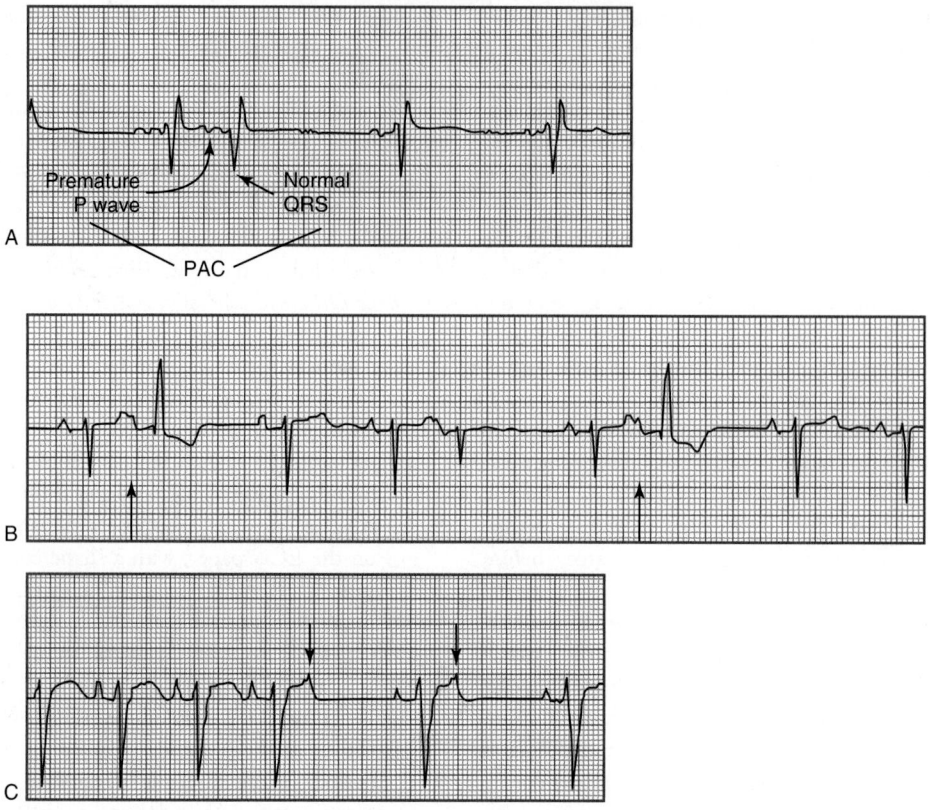

Figure 18-50 Premature atrial contractions (PACs). *A,* Normally conducted PAC. The early P wave is indicated by the *arrow,* and the QRS that follows has a normal shape and duration. *B,* Nonconducted (blocked) PACs. The early P waves are indicated by *arrows.* Notice how they distort the T waves, making them appear peaked compared with the normal T waves seen after the third and fourth QRS complexes. *C,* Right bundle branch block aberration after a PAC.

of dysrhythmias that originate above the AV node. SVT is not a specific term; it includes sinus tachycardia, atrial tachycardia, multifocal atrial tachycardia, atrial flutter, atrial fibrillation, and junctional tachycardia. Each of these entities has a distinct pathophysiology, specific therapy, and expected outcome. SVT may also be described as a *narrow-complex tachycardia,* defined as a QRS that is less than 0.12 second (120 milliseconds).[85] After the specific dysrhythmia is identified, it usually is referred to by a specific name, such as atrial fibrillation with a rapid ventricular response.[87] The term SVT is used to describe a rapid, sustained atrial or junctional tachycardia when the exact mechanism is unknown. Women are affected by episodic SVT at about twice the rate of men.[85]

In an acute situation, a rapid dysrhythmia may be difficult to identify precisely. SVT can cause hemodynamic instability. It is important to differentiate VT from SVT; the focus then can be directed toward rate control until the acute situation is resolved and hemodynamic stability is restored. At that point, a more careful analysis is needed to determine the specific dysrhythmia responsible for the SVT. The differentiation of wide-complex SVT from VT requires specific knowledge of the relevant ECG criteria (discussed later).

SVT is not always benign. About 15% of people with SVT experience syncope (lose consciousness). Medications are used to limit the SVT rate and prevent "blackouts" or syncope.[85] SVT that is persistent for weeks or months may lead to a tachycardia-mediated cardiomyopathy.[85] A baseline 12-lead ECG is helpful, and when possible, a 12-lead ECG should be obtained during the palpitations.[85]

Supraventricular Tachycardia with Aberrant Conduction. If the QRS in SVT is wider than 0.12 second, it is important to differentiate between SVT with aberrant conduction and VT (discussed later). SVT with aberrant conduction includes SVT with a bundle branch block[87] and SVT that uses an anomalous congenital additional fiber (accessory pathway), such as Wolff-Parkinson-White syndrome.[85,88] Patients with SVT with aberrant conduction are frequently misdiagnosed, and evaluation by a specialist is highly recommended.[85]

Paroxysmal Supraventricular Tachycardia. *Paroxysmal* means starting and stopping abruptly. *Paroxysmal supraventricular tachycardia* (PSVT) refers to the sudden interruption of sinus rhythm by an atrial ectopic focus that fires repetitively at a rate of 150 to 250 beats/min and eventually stops as suddenly as it began (Fig. 18-51).

The rhythm of PSVT is perfectly regular because the reentry loop has a specific length; each circuit through the loop requires exactly the same amount of time to complete. Reentry within the atria itself or involving the AV node is the mechanism responsible for most SVTs, including PSVT. Other common underlying mechanisms include abnormal automaticity and triggered activity. P waves are present and abnormally shaped, although they may be difficult to identify because they often blend in with the previous T wave because of the rapid rate. It is most helpful if the beginning of the PSVT run is captured

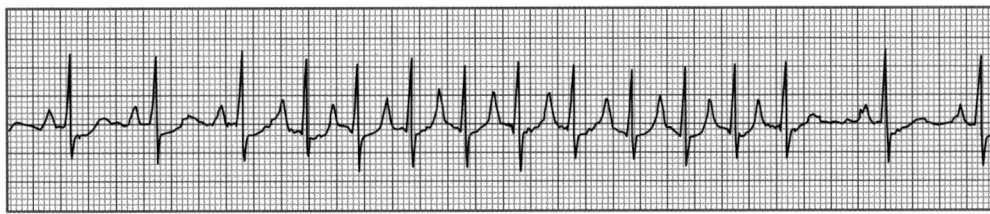

Figure 18-51 Paroxysmal supraventricular tachycardia (PSVT). Notice that the atrial rate during tachycardia is 158 beats/min. The run starts and stops abruptly.

TABLE 18-12 Atrial Dysrhythmias

Parameter	Paroxysmal Supraventricular Tachycardia	Multifocal Atrial Tachycardia	Atrial Flutter	Atrial Fibrillation
Rate				
Atrial	150-250/min	100-160/min	250-350/min	>350/min (unable to count it)
Ventricular	Same or less	Same	250-350/min, one half or less	100-180/min (uncontrolled); <100/min (controlled)
Rhythm	Regular	Irregular	Atrial: regular; ventricular: may or may not be regular	Irregularly irregular
P wave	Present; abnormally shaped	Present; three or more different shapes	F waves	Fibrillatory baseline
PR interval	May be normal or prolonged	Variable	Conduction ratio: flutter waves per QRS	Absent
QRS	0.06-0.10 sec	0.06-0.10 sec	0.06-0.10 sec	0.06-0.10 sec

and recorded on ECG paper, because the early, abnormal P wave is often easiest to identify in front of the first beat of the run. The PR interval should be the same for each cycle in the run, but it will probably be different from the PR interval of the patient's own normal sinus rhythm. As with PACs, the QRS complex is usually normal, because after the impulse passes through the AV node, conduction through the ventricles follows the usual pathway (Table 18-12). However, in PSVT (as discussed for SVT), aberrant conduction, often in the form of LBBB or RBBB, can occur with a wide QRS complex (>0.12 second); this creates difficulty in differentiating relatively benign PSVT from its more serious counterpart, VT.

Sometimes, because of refractoriness in the AV node, not all of the ectopic P waves are conducted to the ventricles. Usually, at least every other P wave conducts a QRS, described as a 2:1 ratio, but occasionally, the conduction relation may drop to three P waves for every QRS (3:1 ratio).

PSVT has essentially the same causal factors as PACs. PSVT has greater clinical significance, because it may be sustained for long periods and because it occurs at such a rapid rate. As stressed in the discussion of sinus tachycardia, rapid rates decrease ventricular filling time, increase myocardial oxygen consumption, and decrease oxygen supply. Heart failure, angina, or even MI can result. PSVT usually responds rapidly to medical management, which initially includes the use of vagal maneuvers. Vagal maneuvers used in critical care include the following[85]:

Valsalva maneuver. The patient is asked to "bear down," as if going to the bathroom.

Carotid sinus massage. It is performed on only one side of the neck over the carotid artery by a physician on a patient with a monitored ECG and avoided on older patients who may have atherosclerotic disease of the carotid arteries.

If vagal maneuvers are unsuccessful at terminating the PSVT, the next step usually is the use of intravenous drugs if the patient is hemodynamically stable.[85] The intravenous drug of choice to briefly block conduction through the AV node is adenosine (Adenocard). In PSVT, adenosine alone is often sufficient to restore normal sinus rhythm, but if not, it will unmask the ectopic P waves and confirm or provide strong clues to diagnose the SVT.[85] The usual dose is 6 mg given intravenously by rapid push, followed by a normal saline bolus. If this does not create a temporary AV block or restore sinus rhythm, a 12-mg intravenous dose is administered. Potential dysrhythmic side effects of adenosine include a 1% to 15% chance of initiating atrial fibrillation.[85] Adenosine is contraindicated in patients with severe asthma.[85]

Other intravenous drugs that may be used to slow the rate in PSVT are amiodarone (Cordarone), a class III antidysrhythmic with a rapid onset and a short half-life.[85] Alternatively, diltiazem, a class IV calcium channel blocker in the nondihydropyridine group, can be used. The action of these drugs is to slow conduction through the AV node.[85] If intravenous drugs do not convert the PSVT or sustained SVT or if the patient becomes hemodynamically unstable, the next step is electrical cardioversion.[85]

Multifocal Atrial Tachycardia. Multifocal atrial tachycardia (MAT), sometimes referred to as *chaotic atrial tachycardia,* occurs when there are numerous irritable atrial foci that intermittently fire and generate an impulse (Fig. 18-52). The atrial rate is greater than 100 beats/min but usually does not exceed 160 beats/min. The distinguishing feature on the ECG is that there are at least three different P-wave shapes, indicating at least three different irritable foci that can generate three different atrial rates.[85] MAT is always irregular and is frequently misdiagnosed and confused with atrial fibrillation.[85] MAT is most commonly seen in older patients with chronic obstructive pulmonary disease (COPD). COPD causes chronic pulmonary hypertension, which causes chronically elevated right atrial and right ventricular pressures. The abnormally high right atrial pressure causes stretching of the right atrial muscle cells and chronic irritability. Because the underlying cause cannot be resolved, this dysrhythmia is refractory to any treatment. There is no role for electrical cardioversion, antidysrhythmic drugs, or catheter ablation. Therapy is directed at limiting the effect of the COPD and correcting any electrolyte abnormalities.[85]

Atrial Flutter. Atrial flutter is recognized on the ECG by the *sawtooth* atrial pattern. These sawtooth-shaped atrial wavelets are not P waves; they are more appropriately called F waves (atrial flutter waves), as shown in Figure 18-53. Fortunately, the AV node does not allow conduction of all these impulses to the ventricles.

Pathogenesis of Atrial Flutter. Atrial flutter can be started by any isolated atrial impulse, but to be maintained, the atrial flutter requires a *reentry circular pathway* around macroscopic structures in the atria. Typically, these structures are in the right atrium and involve the vena cava and the tricuspid valve in an area known as the *cavotricuspid isthmus.* The *reentry loop* typically circles counterclockwise around the tricuspid valve[85] and can circle the inferior vena cava (IVC) or the IVC and the tricuspid valve. To maintain a viable, self-perpetuating reentry pathway, the loop must avoid the sinoatrial node and be large enough to always meet tissue that is ready to be depolarized (accept a new electrical stimulus). The atrial reentry rate in atrial flutter is typically between 250 to 350 beats/min, producing the classic sawtooth or flutter wave pattern.[85] The atrial

flutter wavelet always appears regular, because the circuit is always the same length and requires exactly the same amount of time to complete the reentry loop.

Atrial and Ventricular Rates in Atrial Flutter. When evaluating the rate of atrial flutter, it is important to calculate both atrial and ventricular rates. The ventricular rhythm is regular if the same number of flutter waves occurs between each QRS complex—in other words, if the degree of block at the AV node remains constant. Sometimes, the refractoriness in the AV node changes from beat to beat, resulting in an irregular ventricular response. When describing atrial flutter, the term *PR interval* no longer applies; instead, a conduction ratio, such as 3:1 or 4:1 (ratio of atrial waves to QRS complexes) is used. In normal sinus rhythm, measuring the PR interval allows evaluation of the speed of conduction through the AV node; in atrial flutter, the number of flutter waves that bombard the AV node before one is allowed to pass through to the ventricles is a measure of AV nodal conduction. After the impulse has passed the AV node, conduction through the ventricles is unaltered. The QRS duration remains normal or at least the same as it was in normal sinus rhythm (see Table 18-12).

The major factor underlying atrial flutter symptoms is the ventricular response rate. If the atrial rate is 300 beats/min and the AV conduction ratio is 4:1, the ventricular response rate is 75 beats/min and should be well tolerated. However, if the atrial rate is 300 beats/min but the AV conduction ratio is 2:1, the corresponding ventricular rate of 150 beats/min may cause angina, acute heart failure, or other signs of cardiac decompensation. An atrial rate of 250 beats/min with a 1:1 AV conduction ratio yields a ventricular response rate of 250 beats/min; the patient will be extremely symptomatic, and emergency measures are needed to decrease the ventricular rate.

Sometimes, it is difficult to identify the flutter waves, especially if the conduction ratio is 2:1. Vagal maneuvers or adenosine can be useful diagnostic tools to allow better visualization of the flutter waves (see Fig. 18-53A). Vagal maneuvers or intravenous adenosine cannot terminate atrial flutter but do create a temporary AV block to permit visualization of the atrial waveform and thereby facilitate accurate diagnosis, as seen in Figure 18-53B.

Atrial Flutter Management. Pharmacologic cardioversion using ibutilide (Corvert) is effective at converting hemodynamically stable atrial flutter to sinus rhythm in 38% to 76% of patients.[85] The reasons for the variance in conversion in clinical studies is unknown, but it was not related to the length of time the patients had been in atrial flutter. For patients who responded to the ibutilide, the average conversion time after

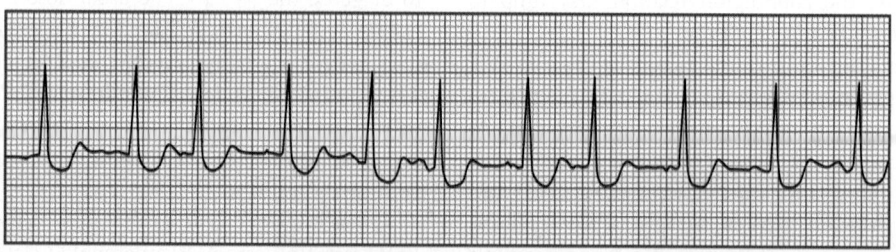

Figure 18-52 Multifocal atrial tachycardia (MAT). Notice that there are several differently shaped P waves and that the PR intervals vary.

infusion was 30 minutes.[85] One of the complications of ibutilide is polymorphic tachycardia—also known as *torsades de pointes*—but in studies of patients with atrial flutter, the rate of torsades de pointes was less than 3%.[85]

Antidysrhythmic drugs are prescribed in two ways to treat atrial flutter: to convert the rhythm to normal sinus rhythm (NSR) and to slow conduction through the AV node. Of the specific drugs that may convert stable atrial flutter to sinus rhythm, the most effective is ibutilide (discussed previously); other, less effective agents include flecainide, propafenone, sotalol, procainamide, and amiodarone.[85] Other AV node–blocking medications are used to control the ventricular rate in atrial flutter but are ineffective at terminating the dysrhythmia. These drugs include the calcium channel blockers, β-blockers, and digoxin. Amiodarone shares both properties. It can slow conduction through the AV node and convert the atrial dysrhythmia. These drugs are effective as a mechanism to control the ventricular rate before electrical cardioversion.[85]

Nonpharmacologic interventions to convert atrial flutter to sinus rhythm are the most effective; they include electrical cardioversion and atrial overdrive pacing. The conversation rate with DC cardioversion is between 95% and 100%.[85] If atrial flutter has been present for more than 48 hours, up to one third of patients will have thrombi in the atria, and anticoagulation is mandated before pharmacologic or electrical cardioversion. The risk of systemic emboli after cardioversion ranges from 2% to 7%.[85] Overdrive atrial pacing is often favored to convert atrial flutter after cardiac surgery. Epicardial wires that are placed at the time of surgery are connected to an external pacemaker. The overall success rate of atrial overdrive pacing is 83% (range, 55% to 100%).[85]

For about 60% of patients, sudden onset of atrial flutter is associated with an acute disease process such as acute MI or exacerbation of pulmonary disease, or it follows cardiac or pulmonary surgery.[85] In this scenario, after the acute disease is managed, the atrial flutter usually responds quickly to standard therapy, and long-term drug management is not required. If at any time the patient with atrial flutter becomes hemodynamically unstable, electrical cardioversion is the recommended emergency intervention.[85]

For patients with atrial flutter unrelated to an acute disease process, permanent termination of the atrial flutter circuit can be achieved by *radiofrequency ablation* (RFA). RFA is a catheter procedure used to create a line of conduction block across one of more sections of the reentry pathway. The most frequent location for RFA is a narrow band of tissue between the inferior vena cava and the tricuspid annulus known as the *cavotricuspid isthmus*.[85] Chapter 20 contains additional information on antidysrhythmic drugs.

Atrial Fibrillation. Atrial fibrillation is the most frequently encountered dysrhythmia in the developed world (Fig. 18-54). It affects an estimated 2.3 million individuals in the United States and 4.5 million people in the European Union. In the United States, the estimated annual cost to treat atrial fibrillation is about $3,000 per patient per year.[89] When first detected, atrial fibrillation may be described as *paroxysmal* (self-terminating) or *persistent* (not self-terminating); when all attempts at conversion to sinus rhythm have failed, it is described as *permanent* (Fig. 18-55).

Atrial fibrillation may be classified under the broad category of SVT, because the heart rate is rapid and many patients have symptoms of hypotension and breathlessness during paroxysmal atrial fibrillation when uncontrolled by medication. Nonsinus uncoordinated atrial electrical activation leads to a rapid deterioration in atrial mechanical function. The ECG tracing in atrial fibrillation is notable for an uneven atrial baseline that lacks clearly defined P waves and instead shows rapid oscillations or fibrillatory wavelets that vary in size, shape, and frequency.[89] The atrial fibrillatory waves are particularly easy to identify in the inferior ECG leads II, III, and AVF.

The ventricular response to atrial fibrillation is influenced by several factors: the efficiency of the AV node; autonomic nervous system activity—the level of sympathetic and parasympathetic (vagus nerve) tone; presence of medications that increase or slow conduction through the AV node–bundle branch conduction system; and various underlying heart conditions such as heart failure.[89,90] Atrial fibrillation displays irregular R-to-R intervals (different timing intervals between the QRS complexes) that do not show any logical pattern. The ability of the AV node and bundle branches to conduct or block the fibrillatory atrial impulses is key to the appearance of the QRS

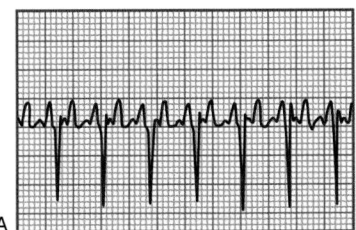

A

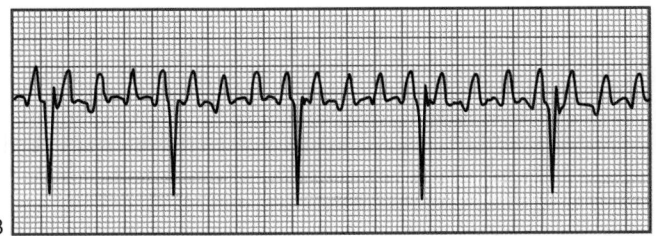

B

Figure 18-53 *A,* Initial strip shows atrial flutter with 2:1 conduction through the atrioventricular (AV) node. *B,* During carotid sinus massage, the AV conduction rate is decreased, more clearly revealing the flutter waves.

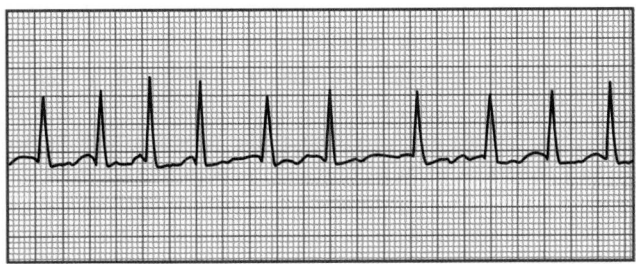

Figure 18-54 Atrial fibrillation. Notice the irregularly irregular ventricular rhythm.

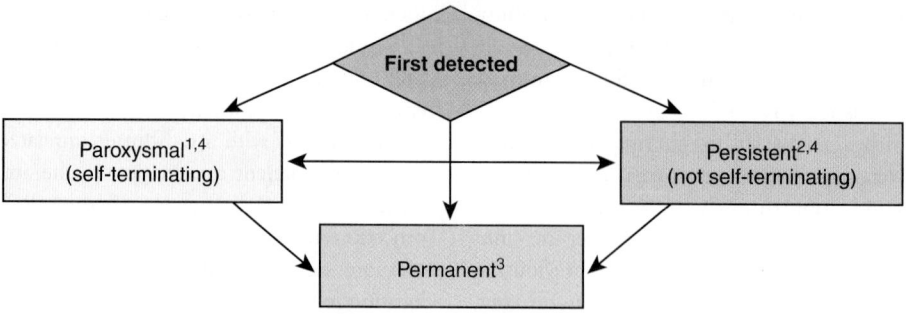

^{1}Episodes that generally last less than or equal to 7 days (most less than 24 h);
^{2}usually more than 6 days;
^{3}cardioversion failed or not attempted; and
^{4}both paroxysmal and persistent AF may be recurrent.

Figure 18-55 Patterns of new-onset atrial fibrillation. *(From Fuster V et al: ACC/AHA/ESC 2006 Guidelines for the Management of Patients with Atrial Fibrillation: a report of the American College of Cardiology/American Heart Association Task Force on Practice Guidelines and the European Society of Cardiology Committee for Practice Guidelines (Writing Committee to Revise the 2001 Guidelines for the Management of Patients With Atrial Fibrillation): developed in collaboration with the European Heart Rhythm Association and the Heart Rhythm Society, Circulation 114[7]:e257-e354, 2006.)*

on the surface ECG. In atrial fibrillation, the QRS complex shape is usually narrow and normal in appearance as long as the pathway through the ventricles is intact after the impulse leaves the AV node. The AV node acts as a filter to protect the ventricles from the hundreds of atrial impulses that occur each minute, although the AV node does not receive all of these atrial impulses. When the atrial muscle tissue immediately surrounding the AV node is in a refractory state, impulses generated in other areas of the atria cannot reach the AV node, which helps to explain the wide variation in R-R intervals during atrial fibrillation (see Table 18-12).

Pathogenesis of Atrial Fibrillation. The pathogenesis of atrial fibrillation has traditionally been ascribed to random electrical foci firing in the atria. Research using high-density atrial mapping, high-speed video recordings, and ECG analysis has uncovered distinct spatial organization within the atria.[89] Atrial fibrillation involves several reentry circuits within the atria, and in some cases, they originate at specific anatomic sites. The four pulmonary veins that drain into the left atrium are a trigger site for early atrial foci to initiate and propagate reentry circuits to maintain atrial fibrillation.[89] The earliest atrial ectopic foci have been electrically mapped 2 to 4 cm within the pulmonary veins.[91] The affected pulmonary veins contain thin myocardial sleeves that project into the pulmonary veins from the left atrium. This ectopic tissue resembles discontinuous fingerlike projections about 5 mm thick that extend as far as 4.5 cm into one or more pulmonary veins. The tissue ultimately becomes part of the venous wall. The spread of atrial fibrillation to the rest of the atria is thought to occur through multiple reentry *wavelets* that are maintained in perpetual motion by a "mother rotor," or dominant reentry circuit, that functions at a higher frequency, drives the atrial fibrillation, and originates from the ectopic pulmonary vein tissue.[91]

When a single focus can be identified, it is possible to encircle that area and isolate that site using RFA. There are several different RFA designs used to isolate foci that originate in the four pulmonary veins: encircling all four veins together or isolating

individual pulmonary veins or in pairs.[92] This catheter procedure is successfully used in many cardiac electrophysiology centers.

The atria demonstrate other pathologic changes in atrial fibrillation, typically atrial fibrosis and loss of atrial muscle mass.[89] Atrial fibrosis may precede the development of atrial fibrillation, and the ongoing fibrosis is hypothesized to contribute to persistent atrial fibrillation.[89] It is probable that there are several different types of atrial fibrillation involving different mechanisms. As electrophysiologic mapping techniques become more advanced, the mystery surrounding the origins of atrial fibrillation will become less cloudy. Although atrial fibrillation may look disorganized on the ECG baseline tracing, an electrical pattern exists within the atria. Knowledge of this pattern will ultimately lead to treatments that can help cure or control atrial fibrillation.

Types of Atrial Fibrillation. Atrial fibrillation is described by several additional labels that are associated with different clinical outcomes:

1. *Paroxysmal atrial fibrillation.* Atrial fibrillation that starts and stops abruptly is called *paroxysmal atrial fibrillation,* and it is often described as self-limiting (see Fig. 18-55).[89] The patient can often feel the palpitations and may describe it in many different ways, such as "like a bird fluttering in my chest." Sometimes, when the heart rate is really fast, it is not possible to identify the rhythm as atrial fibrillation and it may initially be labeled as an SVT. It is always helpful to catch the start or ending point of any SVT on an ECG rhythm strip so that the initial stimulus can be identified. A printed rhythm strip also permits a more precise analysis of the dysrhythmia after the patient's clinical condition has been stabilized. In the critical care unit, it is important to document occurrence of paroxysmal atrial fibrillation by placing an ECG rhythm strip in the medical record and noting any associated clinical symptoms. The goal of treatment is to convert the atrial fibrillation back to a sinus rhythm as soon as possible. Electrical or pharmacologic

cardioversion is most effective when the atrial fibrillation has been present for less than 24 hours.[89]

2. *Recurrent atrial fibrillation.* When a patient has two or more episodes of paroxysmal atrial fibrillation, it is described as *recurrent.* There is often a period during which patients may go in and out of atrial fibrillation, before the electrical atrial remodeling is complete and atrial fibrillation becomes the dominant and persistent rhythm.[89]

3. *Persistent atrial fibrillation.* When atrial fibrillation is sustained beyond 7 days or there are multiple bouts of paroxysmal atrial fibrillation, it is called *persistent* (see Fig. 18-55).[89] Research studies and clinical experience demonstrate that the longer a person remains in atrial fibrillation, the greater the degree of atrial electrical remodeling, and the more difficult it becomes to convert the atria back to sinus rhythm. Even after electrical cardioversion, when the ECG may show sinus rhythm, the mechanical function of the atria may take up to a week to return to normal.[91]

4. *Permanent atrial fibrillation.* When atrial fibrillation has lasted for more than 1 year it is described as *permanent.* Typically, attempts to electrically or pharmacologically convert the atrial fibrillation back to sinus rhythm have failed before atrial fibrillation is described as permanent (see Fig. 18-55).[89]

5. *Lone atrial fibrillation.* The expression *lone atrial fibrillation* is used to describe individuals younger than 60 years who have atrial fibrillation without structural heart disease. Approximately 30% to 45% of cases of paroxysmal atrial fibrillation, and 20% to 25% of cases of persistent atrial fibrillation occur in younger patients without demonstrable underlying heart disease.[89]

6. *Atrial fibrillation associated with underlying structural heart disease.* Some cardiac conditions are associated with atrial fibrillation, particularly hypertension, especially with associated left ventricular hypertrophy, heart failure, valvular heart disease, acute MI, myocarditis, and pericarditis.[89] In developed countries, rheumatic heart disease, which was prevalent at the beginning of the 20th century, now plays a minor role. When the atrial tissue of patients in persistent atrial fibrillation is examined histologically (tissue analysis), the atria show structural abnormalities beyond the changes known to be caused by the underlying heart condition. These changes are called *electrical atrial remodeling.* The longer the person remains in atrial fibrillation, the less likely is a return to sinus rhythm.[89]

7. *Atrial fibrillation associated with other conditions.* Noncardiac conditions associated with an increased incidence of atrial fibrillation are diabetes, pulmonary embolism, pneumonia, and thyrotoxicosis. After the acute condition is treated, the atrial fibrillation should resolve and not recur. Hyperthyroidism is a correctable cause of atrial fibrillation that can be effectively reversed in most cases by correcting the thyrotoxic condition. If not recognized and treated, excess thyroid hormone makes rate control difficult, increases risk of a thromboembolic event, and causes higher rates of morbidity and mortality.

8. *Vagal mediated atrial fibrillation.* This is a condition in which the autonomic nervous system triggers atrial fibrillation due to heightened vagal tone in susceptible individuals.[89] Vagally mediated atrial fibrillation is characterized by episodes occurring at rest or during sleep, usually in younger patients.[93]

9. *Silent atrial fibrillation.* In the critical care unit, all patients have ECG monitoring so detection of atrial fibrillation is not difficult. Clinical trial registries report between 10% and 50% of enrolled patients had clinically silent atrial fibrillation; this means that the atrial fibrillation was asymptomatic or minimally symptomatic and that the patient was unaware of the dysrhythmia.[94] Among patients with implantable recording pacemakers or defibrillators, the silent atrial fibrillation rate is 50% to 60%.[95] The presence of silent atrial fibrillation is of concern because atrial fibrillation causes a deterioration in atrial mechanical function, formation of atrial emboli, and increased risk of stroke, and it is harder to convert to sinus rhythm the longer it is present.

10. *Cardiac surgery postoperative atrial fibrillation.* Atrial fibrillation occurs in approximately 30% of patients after CABG.[96] If the CABG is combined with a mitral value replacement (MVR), the incidence of atrial fibrillation rises to 63.6%; if the CABG is combined with aortic valve replacement (AVR), the incidence of atrial fibrillation is 48.8%.[97] Most atrial fibrillation develops on the second to third postoperative day and affects patients with or without a history of atrial fibrillation.[97,98] Postoperative atrial fibrillation after cardiac surgery is associated with significant hemodynamic instability, increased length of hospital stay, decreased long-term survival, and increase in the risk of embolic stroke.[97,98] Beta-blockers are recommended as prophylaxis to reduce the incidence of atrial fibrillation after cardiac surgery.[99] Patients who undergo minimally invasive cardiac surgery may experience a lower incidence of atrial fibrillation compared with patients who have traditional cardiac surgery procedures.[98]

11. *Atrial electrogram after cardiac surgery.* Atrial and ventricular epicardial temporary pacemaker wires are frequently inserted during cardiac surgery in case postoperative pacing support is required during the postoperative course.[100] The atrial pacing wire or wires are placed on the right ventricle and exit the chest to the lower right side of the sternum.[98] If the atrial pacing lead is connected to an ECG monitoring lead, the atrial tracing is clearly visible and much larger than normal because the recording comes directly from the right atrium. The atrial electrogram (AEG) procedure is not frequently performed but is useful when it is not possible to differentiate whether a patient in SVT has P waves, flutter waves, or atrial fibrillation on the standard surface ECG.[98,100]

Atrial Fibrillation Risk Factors. As more research has focused on the cause of atrial fibrillation, a clearer picture of incidence and risk factors has emerged. Atrial fibrillation is present in 0.4% to 1% in the general population, but the incidence rises to more than 8% among those older than 80 years.[89] The median age of patients with atrial fibrillation is about 75 years.[89] Atrial fibrillation is the most common cardiac dysrhythmia in the United States and responsible for about one third of dysrhythmia related hospital admissions.[89] The risk of developing atrial fibrillation is higher for people with a history of hypertension, heart failure, obesity or MI.[89]

Atrial Fibrillation Management. There continues to be debate about the most effective treatment approach for atrial fibrillation, as shown in the algorithm to treat new-onset atrial fibrillation (Fig. 18-56). In the past, the gold standard was to convert the patient out of the atrial fibrillation back to sinus rhythm. However, for many older patients, staying out of atrial fibrillation is an unattainable goal. The major issues focus is on *rhythm* versus *rate* control. All patients with atrial fibrillation require anticoagulation to prevent thrombotic embolism and stroke.

Rhythm Control. For the hospitalized patient with *new-onset* atrial fibrillation with unstable hemodynamics, the focus is generally on rhythm control (conversion to sinus rhythm) using antidysrhythmic drugs or electrical cardioversion. Emergency drugs used to convert atrial fibrillation to sinus rhythm, also known as a chemical cardioversion, include amiodarone and ibutilide. Antidysrhythmic drugs used long-term to maintain the patient in sinus rhythm include amiodarone, disopyramide, flecainide, moricizine, procainamide, propafenone, quinidine, sotalol, and dofetilide or a combination of these medications as needed.[101] Even with drug therapy, recurrence of atrial fibrillation is likely.[101] Electrical cardioversion may be successful in converting the atria to sinus rhythm if attempted within a few days or weeks of the onset of atrial fibrillation. Its success is less likely if the atrial fibrillation has existed for a long time.[89] Without continued antidysrhythmic drug therapy, about 75% of cardioverted patients will be in atrial fibrillation at one year.[102]

Rate Control. The most frequently prescribed drugs used to control the ventricular rate in atrial fibrillation include calcium channel blockers, beta-blockers, and digoxin. These drugs work to slow conduction through the AV node. They have no impact on the fibrillating atria. In the past, it was assumed that rate control was an inferior strategy, because the patient stayed in atrial fibrillation, lost "atrial kick," and was presumed to have an increased risk of embolic stroke. Two multicenter trials have altered that perception: the *A*trial *F*ibrillation *F*ollow-up: *I*nvestigation of *R*hythm *M*anagement (AFFIRM) and the *RA*te Control vs. *E*lectrical Cardioversion for Persistent Atrial Fibrillation (RACE).[101] These two trials found similar morbidity, mortality, and quality of life in patients treated long term with rhythm conversion or rate control.[101] For long-term management of atrial fibrillation, rate control is the recommended approach, and therapeutic anticoagulation to prevent embolic stroke is

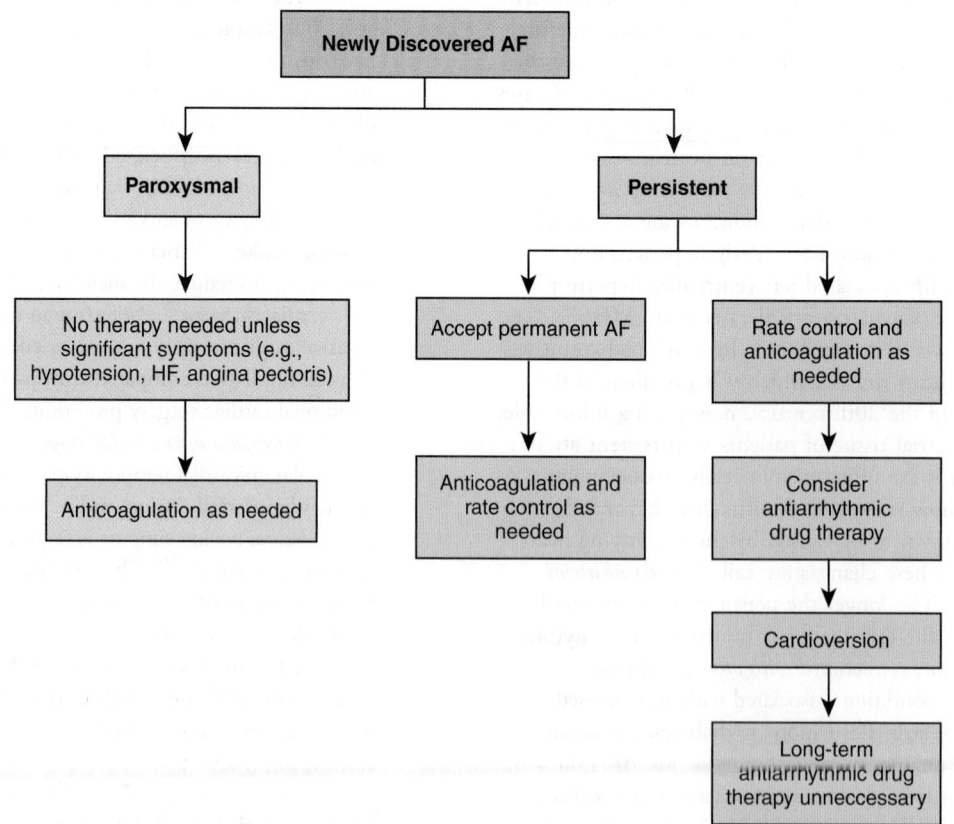

Figure 18-56 Management of new-onset atrial fibrillation. *(From Fuster V et al: ACC/AHA/ESC 2006 Guidelines for the Management of Patients with Atrial Fibrillation: a report of the American College of Cardiology/American Heart Association Task Force on Practice Guidelines and the European Society of Cardiology Committee for Practice Guidelines (Writing Committee to Revise the 2001 Guidelines for the Management of Patients With Atrial Fibrillation): developed in collaboration with the European Heart Rhythm Association and the Heart Rhythm Society, Circulation 114[7]:e257-e354, 2006.)*

mandatory.[103] Antidysrhythmic medications used to manage atrial fibrillation are listed in Chapter 20 (Table 20-16).

Anticoagulation in Atrial Fibrillation. Electrical and chemical (drug-induced) forms of cardioversion entail the threat of precipitating emboli into the systemic circulation. During atrial fibrillation, the atria do not contract, and blood may pool and promote clots that attach to the atrial walls (mural thrombi). If cardioversion is successful and normal sinus rhythm is restored, the atria again contract forcibly and, if thrombus formation has occurred, may send clots traveling through the pulmonary or systemic circulation. The atrial fibrillation antithrombotic recommendations subsequently described apply equally to patients with atrial flutter.[103]

To prevent embolic stroke, it is important to pay attention to the *48-hour rule.* Patients who have been in atrial fibrillation for 48 hours or longer (how long may not be known) must be adequately anticoagulated with an oral vitamin K antagonist (warfarin) to achieve a target international normalized ration (INR) of 2.5 (range, 2.0 to 3.0) for at least 3 weeks before elective cardioversion.[103] After successful cardioversion, patients should be anticoagulated for 4 weeks.[103]

TEE is helpful in identifying the presence or absence of thrombi in the fibrillating atria and is recommended as a screening tool before elective cardioversion.[103] It is especially helpful for patients in atrial fibrillation for less than 48 hours who, in the absence of atrial thrombi, may undergo cardioversion without anticoagulation.[103] TEE is described in more detail under "Transesophageal Echocardiography."

Patients who experience episodes of rapid atrial fibrillation for only a few hours or days at a time and then convert back to sinus rhythm spontaneously (paroxysmal atrial fibrillation) are also at risk for embolic stroke. Independent risk factors for stroke with atrial fibrillation include prior stroke or transient ischemic attack (TIA), hypertension, diabetes, and advancing age.[104] History of a prior stroke or TIA identifies patients at greatest risk.[104]

Nonpharmacologic Procedures to Treat Atrial Fibrillation. Several catheter interventions to treat atrial fibrillation are being explored, including atrial pacing, catheter isolation of the pulmonary veins, and combination catheter-surgical procedures. Atrial pacing is not indicated as a treatment for atrial fibrillation, although research into this procedure continues.[105]

The Cox-Maze III procedure (typically called the MAZE procedure) is an open heart surgical operation designed to permanently cure atrial fibrillation. It is suitable for only a tiny fraction of the individuals who have atrial fibrillation, usually those who have *lone atrial fibrillation* without other structural heart disease. For carefully selected patients, this surgery is successful more than 90% of cases. The cut-and-sew maze procedure has been replaced by interventions that use catheter-based radiofrequency energy sources to create lines of conduction block (scar) around the pulmonary veins with minimal risk for bleeding.[106] Alternative surgical approaches are under investigation, including minimally invasive epicardial "beating heart" techniques. Percutaneous catheter-based ablation procedures are listed as second-line therapy after medical therapy for atrial fibrillation.[89] As the technology advances, this may become a more widely available option.[107,108]

Junctional Dysrhythmias. Only certain areas of the AV node have the property of automaticity. The entire area around the AV node is collectively called the *junction;* impulses generated there are called *junctional.* After an ectopic impulse arises in the junction, it spreads in two directions at once. One wave of depolarization spreads upward into the atria and depolarizes them, causing the recording of a P wave on the ECG. This is called *retrograde (backward) conduction,* and the P wave is inverted when viewed in lead II. At the same time, another wave of depolarization spreads downward into the ventricles through the normal conduction pathway, producing a normal QRS complex. This is called *antegrade (forward) conduction.*

Depending on timing, the P wave (1) may be seen in front of the QRS, with a short PR interval of less than 0.12 second, (2) may be obscured entirely by the QRS, or (3) may immediately follow the QRS.

Premature Junctional Contraction. If only a single ectopic impulse originates in the junction, it is simply called a *premature junctional contraction.* On the ECG, the rhythm is regular from the sinus node, except for one early QRS complex of normal shape and duration. The P wave can be entirely absent. If a P wave can be found, it very closely precedes or follows the QRS. In lead II, the P wave appears inverted (having a negative deflection), because the atria are being depolarized from the AV node upward, which is the opposite direction from the wave of depolarization that occurs when triggered by the sinus node. If the P wave appears before the QRS, the PR interval is less than 0.12 second. Premature junctional contractions have virtually the same clinical significance as do PACs. However, if the patient is receiving digoxin, digitalis toxicity may be suspected. Although digoxin slows conduction through the AV node, it also increases automaticity in the junction.

Junctional Escape Rhythm. Sometimes, the junction becomes the dominant pacemaker of the heart (Table 18-13). Normally, the intrinsic rate of the junction is 40 to 60 beats/min. The intrinsic rate of the sinus node is 60 to 100 beats/min. Under normal conditions, the junction never has a chance to escape and depolarize the heart because it is overridden by the sinus node. However, if the sinus node fails, the junctional impulses can depolarize completely and pace the heart. This is called a *junctional escape rhythm,* and it is a protective mechanism

TABLE 18-13 Junctional Rhythms

Parameter	Junctional Escape Rhythm	Accelerated Junctional Rhythm	Junctional Tachycardia
Rate	40-60/min	60-100/min	>100/min
Rhythm	Regular	Regular	Regular
P waves	May be present or absent; inverted in lead II	May be present or absent; inverted in lead II	May be present or absent; inverted in lead II
PR interval	<0.12 sec	<0.12 sec	<0.12 sec
QRS	0.06-0.10 sec	0.06-0.10 sec	0.06-0.10 sec

to prevent asystole in the event of sinus node failure. Generally, a junctional escape rhythm (Fig. 18-57) is well tolerated hemodynamically, although efforts must be directed toward restoring sinus rhythm. Sometimes, a pacemaker is inserted as a protective measure because of concern that the AV junction may also fail.

Junctional Tachycardia and Accelerated Junctional Rhythm.

A junctional rhythm can also occur at a faster rate (see Table 18-13). As with sinus rhythm, the term *tachycardia* is reserved for rates greater than 100 beats/min; junctional tachycardia is a junctional rhythm, usually regular, at a rate greater than 100 beats/min. What if the junctional rate is greater than 60 beats/min and less than 100 beats/min (faster than the intrinsic rate of the junction but not fast enough to be considered a tachycardia)? The phrase *accelerated junctional rhythm* applies to this situation.[73] Accelerated junctional rhythm is usually well tolerated by the patient, mainly because the heart rate is within a reasonable range. Junctional tachycardia may not be tolerated as well, depending on the rate and the patient's underlying cardiac reserve. Digitalis toxicity is strongly suspected, because digoxin enhances automaticity of the AV node. For digitalis toxicity, the optimal strategy is to measure the digoxin serum level and to withhold digoxin until the dysrhythmia resolves.

Ventricular Dysrhythmias.

Ventricular dysrhythmias result from an ectopic focus in any portion of the ventricular myocardium. The usual conduction pathway through the ventricles is not used, and the wave of depolarization must spread from cell to cell. As a result, the QRS complex is prolonged and is always greater than 0.12 second. It is the width of the QRS, not the height that is important in the diagnosis of ventricular ectopy.

Premature Ventricular Contractions.

A single ectopic impulse originating in the ventricles is called a *premature ventricular contraction* (PVC). Some PVCs are very small in height but remain wider than 0.12 second. If in doubt, a different lead is evaluated. The shape of the QRS depends on the location of the ectopic focus. If the ectopic focus is in the right ventricle, the impulse spreads from right to left, and the QRS resembles an LBBB pattern, because the left ventricle is the last to be depolarized. In V_1, this is a wide, negative QRS (Fig. 18-58A). If the ectopic focus is in the left ventricular free wall, the wave of depolarization spreads from left to right (see Fig. 18-58B).

Because the ectopic focus may be any cell in the ventricle, the QRS can take an unlimited number of shapes or patterns. If all of the ventricular ectopic beats look the same in a particular lead, they are called *unifocal*, which means that they probably all result from the same irritable focus (Fig. 18-59A). Conversely, if the ventricular ectopics are of various shapes in the same lead, they are called *multifocal* (see Fig. 18-59B). Multifocal ventricular ectopics are more serious than unifocal ventricular ectopics, because they indicate a greater area of irritable myocardial tissue and are more likely to deteriorate into VT or fibrillation. In general, ventricular dysrhythmias have more serious implications than do atrial or junctional dysrhythmias and occur only rarely in healthy individuals.

A PVC originates in a ventricular cell that has become abnormally permeable to sodium, usually as a result of damage of one kind or another. Because of this new permeability to sodium, the cell reaches depolarization threshold before an impulse is received from the sinus node. After the depolarization threshold is reached, the cell automatically depolarizes,

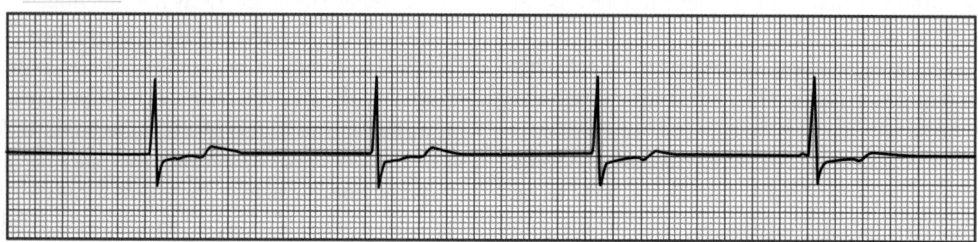

Figure 18-57 Junctional escape rhythm. The ventricular rate is 38. P waves are absent, and the QRS has a normal width.

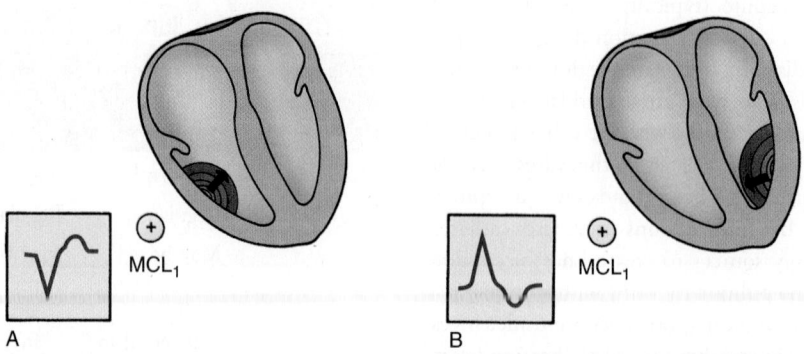

Figure 18-58 *A,* Right ventricular premature ventricular contraction (PVC). The spread of depolarization is from right to left, away from the positive electrode in lead V_1 (MCL$_1$), resulting in a wide, negative QRS complex. *B,* Left ventricular PVC. The spread of depolarization is from left to right, toward the positive electrode in lead V_1 (MCL$_1$). The QRS complex is wide and upright.

beginning total ventricular depolarization. Ordinarily, the ventricular impulse does not conduct back through the AV node; the sinus node is not disturbed and continues to depolarize the atria, resulting in a normal P wave. Conduction from the sinus node will not proceed into the ventricles if they are in a refractory state. The next sinus beat, assuming there is no further ventricular ectopy, conducts normally through the AV node and into the ventricles.

Compensatory Pause. If the interval from the last normal QRS preceding the PVC to the next one is exactly equal to two complete cardiac cycles (Fig. 18-60A), a compensatory pause is present. Because it does not usually occur in PACs or

premature junctional contractions, when present, it is somewhat diagnostic of ventricular ectopy. If the normal sinus P wave that occurs immediately after the PVC finds the ventricles sufficiently recovered to accept another impulse, a normal QRS results and the PVC is sandwiched between two normal beats (see Fig. 18-60B). This PVC is referred to as *interpolated,* meaning *between.* Interpolated PVCs usually occur when the PVC is very early or the normal sinus rate is relatively slow.

Occasionally, the ventricular impulse spreads backward across the AV node to depolarize the atria. When this occurs, the sinus node is reset and no full compensatory pause occurs.

Describing Ventricular Ectopy. PVCs can develop concurrently with any supraventricular dysrhythmia. It is not sufficient to describe a patient's rhythm as "frequent PVCs" or even "frequent unifocal PVCs." The underlying rhythm must always be described first, such as "sinus bradycardia with frequent unifocal PVCs" or "atrial fibrillation with occasional multifocal PVCs." Timing of PVCs can also be described. When a PVC follows each normal beat, *ventricular bigeminy* is present (Fig. 18-61). If a PVC follows every two normal beats, it is called *ventricular trigeminy.*

In individuals with underlying heart disease, PVCs or episodes of self-terminating VT are potentially malignant. Nonsustained VT is defined as three or more consecutive premature ventricular beats at a rate faster than 110 beats/min lasting less than 30 seconds.

Premature Ventricular Contraction Timing. The timing of PVCs can be important, especially if myocardial ischemia is present. The relative refractory period, represented on the ECG by the last half of the T wave, is a particularly vulnerable time for ectopy to occur because repolarization is not complete. Repolarization is even more delayed in ischemic tissue, so that various portions of the ventricular muscle are not repolarized simultaneously. If a PVC occurs at this critical point when only a part

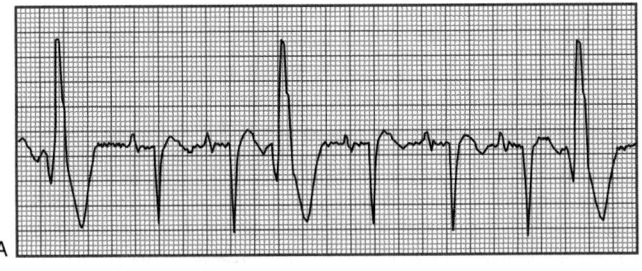

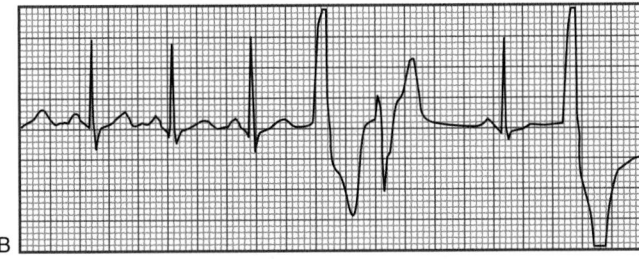

Figure 18-59 *A,* Unifocal premature ventricular contractions (PVCs). *B,* Multifocal PVCs.

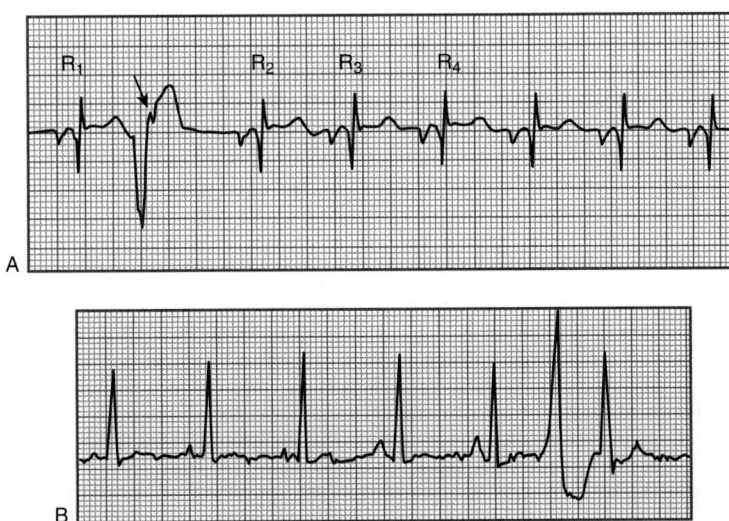

Figure 18-60 *A,* Premature ventricular contraction (PVC) with a fully compensatory pause. The interval between the two sinus beats that surround the PVC (R_1 and R_2) is exactly two times the normal interval between sinus beats (R_3 and R_4). The fully compensatory pause occurs because the sinus node continues to pace despite the PVC. Notice the sinus P wave *(arrow)* hidden in the ST segment of the PVC. This P wave did not conduct through to the ventricles because they had just been depolarized and were still in the absolute refractory period. *B,* Interpolated PVC. The PVC falls between two normal QRS complexes without disturbing the rhythm. Notice that the R-R interval between sinus beats remains the same.

of the muscle is repolarized, individual segments of muscle can depolarize separately from each other, resulting in VF. This is called the *R-on-T phenomenon* (Fig. 18-62).

Two consecutive PVCs are described as a *couplet*, and three consecutive PVCs are called a *triplet* or a *three-beat run of ventricular tachycardia*. More than three consecutive PVCs are considered VT, but it is still useful to state how many beats of VT occurred if the run was short, lasting fewer than 20 beats.

Causes of Premature Ventricular Contractions. PVCs can result from many causes. They have been known to occur, although rarely, in healthy individuals with no evidence of heart disease. The critical care nurse has an important role in identifying factors that may be causing or at least contributing to PVCs. Acute ischemia is the most dangerous cause of ventricular ectopy. Ischemia causes cell membrane permeability to change, giving rise to early depolarization and the initiation of ectopic impulses. Ventricular ectopy that occurs during an acute ischemic event may require treatment with intravenous amiodarone or other antidysrhythmic drugs.

Metabolic abnormalities are common causes of PVCs. Hypokalemia, hypoxemia, and acidosis predispose the cell membrane to instability and may cause ventricular ectopy. Treatment is directed toward identifying the metabolic disturbance and correcting it. Arterial blood gas values and serum potassium and magnesium levels are obtained if no recent results are available. The ability of oxygen and potassium values to change very rapidly in a critically ill patient must not be underestimated. If PVCs develop during suctioning of an intubated patient, a few additional breaths of 100% oxygen usually are sufficient to restore adequate oxygenation and to eliminate the ventricular ectopy.

Any form of heart disease can lead to ventricular ectopy. Patients with cardiomyopathy or ventricular aneurysms can have chronic, severe ventricular ectopy, which may prove to be refractory to any antidysrhythmic agent. Invasive procedures, such as insertion of a pulmonary artery catheter or cardiac catheterization, can cause PVCs by mechanically irritating the ventricular muscle. In these situations, the ectopy usually resolves with removal or advancement of the catheter.

Certain drugs can cause ventricular ectopy. Digitalis toxicity is often accompanied by PVCs, which are somewhat resistant to conventional antidysrhythmic therapy. Some class I antidysrhythmic drugs can cause more serious dysrhythmias than those they were intended to treat. This is called a *prodysrhythmic effect* (also described as a *proarrhythmic effect*), and it can sometimes be fatal.[109] These drugs prolong the QT interval by lengthening the ventricular refractory period. This is a therapeutic effect, but when the QT prolongation becomes excessive, a characteristic form of polymorphic VT called *torsades de pointes* develops (Fig. 18-63). In this dysrhythmia, the VT is very rapid, and the QRS complexes appear to twist in a spiral pattern around the baseline. Clinically, torsades de pointes is poorly tolerated because of the extremely rapid rate. If not terminated, death will result. Sometimes, torsades de pointes stops spontaneously, although the patient may experience a syncopal episode or seizure at the time of the dysrhythmia.

Premature Ventricular Contraction Management. Not all ventricular ectopy requires treatment. In individuals without significant

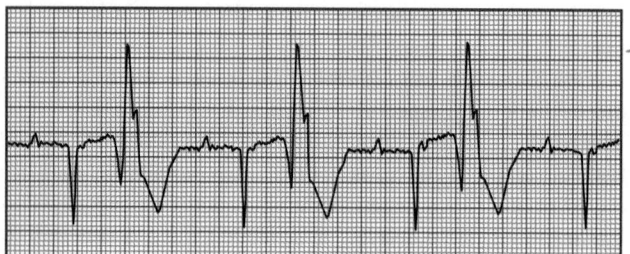

Figure 18-61 Ventricular bigeminy.

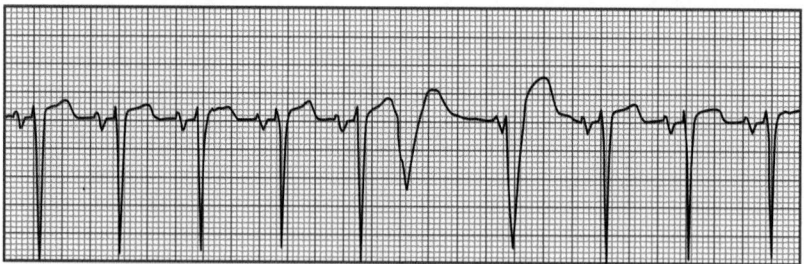

Figure 18-62 R-on-T phenomenon.

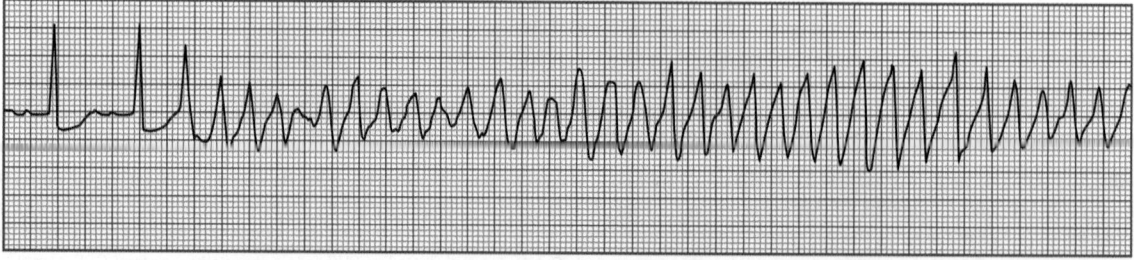

Figure 18-63 Torsades de pointes.

underlying heart disease, PVCs do not represent an increased risk for sudden death and are considered benign. If the patient complains of palpitations, therapy initially includes reassurance and elimination of such factors as caffeine or alcohol ingestion, emotional stress, and sympathomimetic drugs that increase ventricular irritability. If symptoms continue, mild tranquilizers can be administered or beta-blockers can be given to reduce the response to sympathetic stimulation. Antidysrhythmic drugs such as amiodarone or beta-blockers are used during an acute MI when the damaged myocardium increases the risk of isolated PVCs becoming VT. In contrast, if the patient with PVCs has a healthy heart, antidysrhythmic drugs are used as a last resort because of the risk of prodysrhythmia (the drugs increase the incidence of VT). Chapter 20 provides further information on antidysrhythmic drugs.

Idioventricular Rhythms. Sometimes, an ectopic focus in the ventricle can become the dominant pacemaker of the heart (Table 18-14). If the sinus node and the AV junction fail, the ventricles depolarize at their own intrinsic rate of 20 to 40 times per minute. This is called an *idioventricular rhythm* and is protective in nature. Rather than trying to abolish the ventricular beats, the aim of treatment is to increase the effective heart rate and reestablish a higher pacing site, such as the sinus node or the AV junction. Usually, a temporary pacemaker is used to increase heart rate until the underlying problems that caused failure of the other pacing sites can be resolved.

An *accelerated idioventricular rhythm* (AIVR) occurs when a ventricular focus assumes control of the heart at a rate greater than its intrinsic rate of 40 beats/min but less than 100 beats/min (Fig. 18-64). Although relatively benign in and of itself, this rhythm must be closely observed for any increase in rate, and the patient must be observed for hemodynamic deterioration. Usually, it is not treated pharmacologically if well tolerated with a stable blood pressure, although a transvenous temporary pacemaker should be inserted electively as a precaution against sudden hemodynamic deterioration. Intravenous lidocaine must never be administered to a patient with an idioventricular rhythm, because it suppresses the ventricular pacemaker and converts the rhythm to asystole.

Ventricular Tachycardia. Ventricular tachycardia (VT) is caused by a ventricular pacing site firing at a rate of 100 times or more per minute, usually maintained by a reentry mechanism within the ventricular tissue (Fig. 18-65). The complexes are wide, and the rhythm may be slightly irregular, often accelerating as the tachycardia continues (see Table 18-14). In most cases, the sinus node is not affected and it continues to depolarize the atria on schedule. P waves can sometimes be seen on the ECG tracing. They are not related to the QRS and may even appear to conduct a normal impulse to the ventricles if their timing is just right.

If the sinus impulse and the ventricular ectopic impulse meet in the middle of the ventricles, a fusion beat results.[110] Fusion beats are narrower than ventricular beats and look like a cross between the patient's sinus QRS and the ventricular ectopic QRS (Fig. 18-66). When present, P waves and fusion beats are helpful in verifying the diagnosis of VT as opposed to SVT. Differentiation between VT and SVT was discussed earlier.

More than 90% of VT occurs in the presence of structural cardiac disease, such as myocardial ischemia, congenital heart disease, valvular dysfunction, and cardiomyopathy. Other triggers include drug toxicity, electrolyte disturbances, and as an adverse reaction to certain antidysrhythmic drugs (prodysrhythmia).[109]

TABLE 18-14 Ventricular Rhythms

Parameter	Idioventricular Rhythm	Accelerated Idioventricular Rhythm	Ventricular Tachycardia	Ventricular Fibrillation
Rate	20-40/min	40-100/min	>100/min	None
Rhythm	Usually regular	Usually regular	Usually regular	Irregular
P waves	Absent or retrograde	Absent or retrograde	Absent or retrograde	None
PR interval	None	None	None	None
QRS	>0.12 sec	>0.12 sec	>0.12 sec	Fibrillatory waves

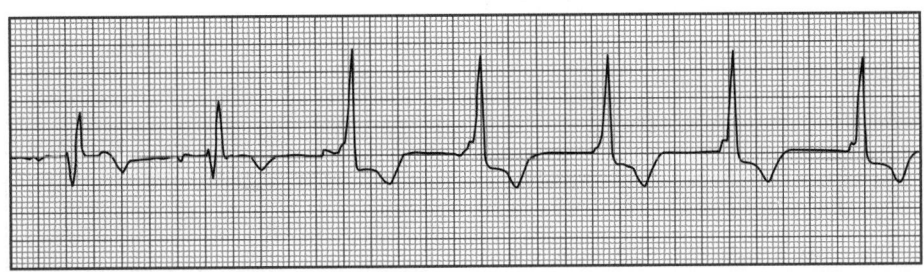

Figure 18-64 Accelerated idioventricular rhythm (AIVR). The QRS duration is 0.14 second, and the ventricular rate is 65.

VT is a serious dysrhythmia and must be treated quickly. The rapid ventricular rate makes this dysrhythmia poorly tolerated. The loss of the proper timing of atrial contraction, which would add volume to the ventricles just before contraction and enhance the force of contraction, is lost, greatly reducing CO. The decrease in CO may cause the patient to lose consciousness. If not terminated quickly, VT is likely to degenerate into VF and death.

How VT is clinically managed depends on whether the patient is stable or unstable, as well as whether a pulse and adequate blood pressure are present. Pulseless VT is a life-threatening condition. The patient will lose consciousness and will need immediate cardiopulmonary resuscitation and defibrillation as described in the American Heart Association (AHA) protocols for advanced cardiac life support (ACLS).

Patients with stable or wide-complex "slow VT" who have a heart rate below 150 beats/min, palpable pulse, and stable blood pressure may be treated pharmacologically with amiodarone, beta-blockers, lidocaine, procainamide, or overdrive pacing as described in the ACLS protocols.

After the acute episode is over, patients who have already experienced sustained VT or cardiac arrest continue to be at risk for sudden cardiac death. An extensive clinical evaluation of these patients is warranted, including cardiac catheterization and electrophysiologic testing with programmed ventricular stimulation. Therapy is aimed at preventing a recurrence of sustained VT or VF. It may include treating the underlying cause, administering antidysrhythmic drugs, performing ablation of the reentrant pathway within the ventricle, or inserting an implantable cardioverter defibrillator (ICD).

ICDs can be programmed to deliver several bursts of overdrive pacing to terminate stable VT before cardioversion. This has the advantage of being more comfortable for the patient, since it prevents the discomfort of an internal shock if the

overdrive pacing is successful. Most patients with an ICD are also managed with antidysrhythmic drugs. Antitachycardia (overdrive) pacing is an effective treatment if combined with defibrillation backup. It is risky without defibrillator support, since one of the complications of antitachycardiac pacing is acceleration of the VT toward a faster, pulseless VT, polymorphic VT, or even VF. Chapter 20 provides more information on implantable cardioverter defibrillators.

Ventricular Fibrillation. VF is the result of chaotic electrical activity in the ventricles from repetitive, small areas of reentry or a series of rapid discharges from various foci within the ventricular myocardium. This causes the ventricles to be unable to contract completely and effectively. The ventricles merely quiver, and no forward flow of blood occurs. Without forward flow, no palpable pulse or audible apical heart tones are present. Clinically, VF is indistinguishable from asystole (absence of electrical activity). On the ECG, VF appears as a continuous, undulating pattern without clear P, QRS, or T waves (Fig. 18-67). When VF occurs in the setting of an acute ischemic event and is accompanied by a significant amount of myocardial damage, the survival rate is poor. Resuscitation is often unsuccessful; recurrence rates are high for those who are resuscitated. VF is seen on the ECG as large, erratic undulations of the baseline (coarse VF) or as a mild tremor (fine VF). In VF, the patient does not have a pulse, no blood is being pumped forward, and defibrillation is the only definitive therapy. Coarse VF is more likely to be successfully defibrillated. Antidysrhythmic drugs such as intravenous amiodarone are administered if initial attempts at defibrillation fail. As with any cardiac arrest situation, supportive measures such as cardiopulmonary resuscitation (CPR), intubation, and correction of metabolic abnormalities are performed concurrently with definitive therapy.

Differential Diagnosis of a Wide QRS-Complex Tachycardia. Wide-complex tachycardias are typically caused by one of four mechanisms[111]:

1. VT
2. SVT with aberrancy due to conduction slowing in the bundle branch system
3. SVT with antegrade conduction over an accessory pathway
4. Ventricular paced rhythm

The challenge is to recognize the atypical wide-complex tachycardia. Tachycardias that are triggered by an ectopic atrial or junctional focus have a *supraventricular* origin, meaning that they come from an irritable site above the ventricles.[85] Typical SVT has a narrow QRS complex (less than 0.12 second),

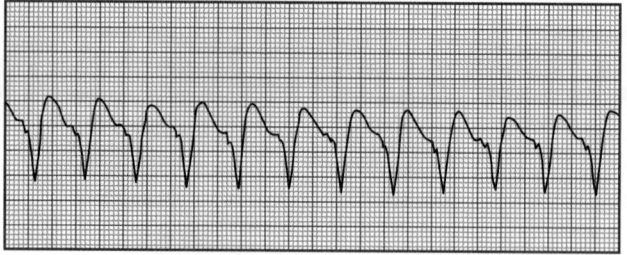

Figure 18-65 Ventricular tachycardia.

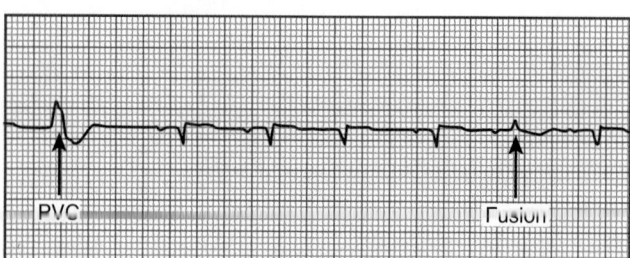

Figure 18-66 Ventricular fusion beat *(arrows).* The QRS duration is only 0.08 second, and the shape represents the normal QRS and the previous PVC.

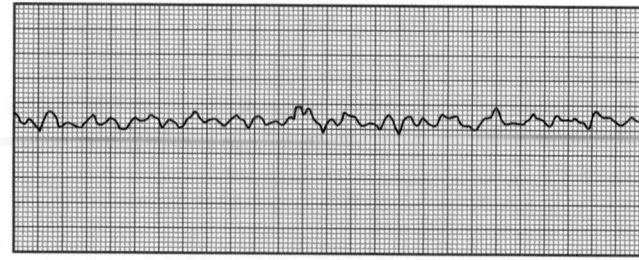

Figure 18-67 Ventricular fibrillation.

because the electrical impulse enters the ventricle through the AV node and still follows the normal conduction pathway by means of the bundle branches through the ventricles. VT always has a wide QRS complex (longer than 0.12 second), because the impulse begins somewhere within the ventricles and must spread slowly—cell to cell—without the benefit of the usual conduction system. It is easy to distinguish between typical SVT and VT by QRS width alone. Unfortunately, not all SVTs result in a narrow QRS complex. An SVT presents with a wide QRS complex in three situations:

1. The patient may already have a RBBB or LBBB, resulting in a wide QRS even during sinus rhythm. Understandably, if the patient develops an atrial or junctional tachycardia, the bundle branch block remains unchanged, and the QRS complex is still wide.[87]

2. A supraventricular impulse may arrive in the ventricles so early that only part of the conduction system is repolarized. One of the bundle branches is still refractory, causing the wave of depolarization to spread abnormally (aberrantly) through the ventricles and resulting in a wide QRS complex.

3. Occasionally, an anatomic variant occurs in which the patient has a small strip of muscle tissue connecting the atria with the ventricles and bypassing the AV node. This is called an *accessory pathway,* or *bypass tract,* the most common of which occurs in Wolff-Parkinson-White syndrome. This does not pose a hemodynamic problem in normal sinus rhythm, although it sometimes causes subtle ECG changes that allow it to be detected.[88] However, when rapid atrial dysrhythmias occur, they can be conducted directly to a portion of the ventricular myocardium without normal AV delay. Depolarization through the ventricles then proceeds from cell to cell rather than through the normal pathway of the conduction system, resulting in a wide QRS-complex tachycardia that closely resembles VT.

Significance of Ventricular Tachycardia and Supraventricular Tachycardia. Standard treatment for VT includes administration of intravenous amiodarone. In contrast, SVT is treated with a variety of drugs that work by blocking the AV node conduction pathway—diltiazem, verapamil, amiodarone, or digoxin. A problem occurs if the SVT has occurred as a result of the presence of an accessory pathway and the narrow complex tachycardia is treated with verapamil or other drugs that block the AV node but do not block the Wolff-Parkinson-White accessory pathway. The consequences can be acute, severe hypotension or loss of consciousness requiring immediate cardioversion. For this reason, it is important to be sure of the cause of the tachycardia in individuals who are relatively hemodynamically stable before treatment is initiated.

Regardless of the site of origin, a rapid wide QRS-complex tachycardia may not be well tolerated, mainly because of the fast heart rate that prevents adequate ventricular filling during diastole, as well as increasing myocardial oxygen demand while decreasing time available for coronary artery filling. Hemodynamic deterioration is evidenced by syncope, severe hypotension, or ischemic symptoms. In this case, emergency external cardioversion needs to be performed regardless of whether the tachycardia is of ventricular or supraventricular origin. Correct diagnosis of a wide QRS-complex tachycardia may have an impact on the long-term management of a patient as well. If atrial flutter or fibrillation is determined to be the underlying mechanism, long-term treatment probably includes amiodarone or a beta-blocker to reduce the heart rate response when these dysrhythmias occur. If VT is determined to be the underlying mechanism in a patient without a history of ventricular dysrhythmias, a careful search for the cause (e.g., hypoxemia, electrolyte imbalance, excess sympathetic stimulation, ischemia) is warranted. Depending on the clinical situation, the patient may require long-term antidysrhythmic therapy. If there is a history of VT or sudden cardiac death and the patient is already on antidysrhythmic therapy, a recurrent episode of VT indicates that the current treatment regimen is not effective and the therapy needs to be changed.

Clinical Differentiation of Ventricular Tachycardia from Supraventricular Tachycardia. Contrary to popular belief, hemodynamic stability or instability does not help to differentiate between VT and SVT with a wide QRS complex. In theory, an SVT is better tolerated, especially if atrial contraction is still occurring before each ventricular contraction (AV synchrony). However, clinically this is often variable. VT may be well tolerated, especially if the rate is less than 150 beats/min. Some patients can be in sustained VT for hours without significant hemodynamic compromise. Conversely, because AV synchrony is lost in atrial fibrillation or atrial flutter, and the ventricular response rate may be very rapid; ventricular filling and CO can be severely compromised.

Careful physical examination can be of value in determining the source of the tachycardia. The jugular venous pulse can be assessed for the presence of cannon *a* waves. When the atria contract at the same time as ventricular systole, the AV valves are closed and the blood in the atria is forced to regurgitate into the venous system. This is seen as a very large pulsation in the jugular vein. If it occurs sporadically (not with every beat), it is a sign of AV dissociation, or independent beating of the atria and ventricles. Heart sounds provide another diagnostic clue. Variation of the intensity of the first heart sound (S_1) from beat to beat favors VT, because this is also indicative of AV dissociation.

By far the most reliable means of diagnosing a wide QRS-complex tachycardia is through careful analysis of the ECG. Heart rate and rhythm are evaluated first, although they are not the only diagnostic indicators.

The QRS width is measured in more than one lead, because the lead with the widest QRS complex is the most reliable indicator of true QRS duration. (It is assumed that some portion of the QRS complex is isoelectric in leads where the QRS appears to be narrow.) QRS widths of less than 0.14 second favor SVT with aberrant conduction, whereas widths of greater than 0.14 second in an RBBB pattern or of greater than 0.16 second in an LBBB pattern favor VT.

The tracing is examined closely for the presence of P waves. If P waves can be identified and they do not correlate on a 1:1 basis with the QRS complexes, AV dissociation exists and strongly suggests VT.

Although P waves may be found in any lead, they are most likely to be visible in V_1 or lead II. When the sinus node remains in control of the atria and a ventricular ectopic focus is in control of the ventricles, it is likely that at some point the timing will be coordinated and, by chance, the sinus impulse will get to conduct through the AV node and begin to depolarize the ventricles just as the ventricular ectopic focus fires. The resulting QRS complex is a *fusion beat* (see Fig. 18-66), which looks like a blend of the patient's normal QRS and the wide QRS complex of the ventricular dysrhythmia. Fusion beats also strongly suggest VT.

Another helpful diagnostic criterion for VT is a QRS axis in the northwest quadrant of −90 degrees to −180 degrees (Fig. 18-68). An axis in this quadrant means that the wave of depolarization is directed upward and to the right, exactly the opposite of normal ventricular depolarization. Even when ventricular conduction is abnormal, as in bundle branch blocks, ventricular depolarization begins at the level of the AV junction and spreads downward toward the apex, although conduction disturbances direct the current flow more to the right or left than normal. Although not all VTs have an axis in the northwest quadrant, about one fourth of them do, and when present, an axis in the northwest quadrant confirms the diagnosis of VT. Figure 18-69 shows how this abnormal axis can be identified from a 5-lead ECG bedside monitor by observing the shape of the QRS in leads I and aVF.

The shape of the QRS complex in the right precordial lead V_1 or MCL_1 and the left precordial lead V_6 or MCL_6 can be diagnostic of VT or SVT with aberrant conduction.[69] Figure 18-69 summarizes these QRS patterns. If the QRS complex is entirely positive from V_1 through V_6 or entirely negative, the diagnosis is VT. This phenomenon is known as *precordial concordance.*

Nursing Management. Proper electrode placement and appropriate lead selection have already been discussed but cannot be overemphasized. In addition to correct lead placement and selection, every effort must be made to record the wide QRS complex tachycardia on a standard 12-lead ECG. Certainly,

emergency treatment must not be delayed if the patient is hemodynamically unstable, but documenting the dysrhythmia by recording a "stat" 12-lead ECG must be given a high priority if time permits. VT and SVT are often nonsustained, and waiting for a physician's order or the arrival of a technician to perform the test could result in failure to document the dysrhythmia at all, leaving the cause and subsequent therapy a mystery.

Atrioventricular Conduction Disturbance. Normally, the sinoatrial node triggers electrical depolarization in the heart. From there, the impulse travels through three internodal tracts in the right atrium to the AV node. The left atrium is depolarized by a conduction fiber known as *Bachman's bundle* that connects the right and left atria. The electrical impulse is briefly delayed in the AV node to allow the atria to contract and the mitral and tricuspid valves to close before the impulse is conducted to the bundle of His, the bundle branches, and the Purkinje fibers.

On the ECG, the ability of the AV node to conduct is evaluated by measuring the PR interval and the relationship of P waves to QRS complexes (Table 18-15). The normal PR interval, measured from the beginning of the P wave to the beginning of the QRS complex, ranges from 0.12 to 0.20 second.

First-Degree Atrioventricular Block. When all atrial impulses are conducted to the ventricles but the PR interval is greater than 0.20 second, a condition known as *first-degree AV block* exists (Fig. 18-70). First-degree AV block can be chronic or acute, and it may be caused by a multitude of conditions. Long-standing first-degree block may occur related to fibrosis and sclerosis of the conduction system, lack of blood supply to the conduction system due to coronary artery disease (CAD), valvular heart disease, myocarditis, and various cardiomyopathies. First-degree heart block that develops acutely is of much greater concern. Causes include drug toxicity related to digoxin, beta-blockers or amiodarone administration, acute myocardial ischemia or infarction, hyperkalemia, edema after valvular heart surgery, and increased vagal tone.[112,113] First-degree AV block represents slowed conduction through the

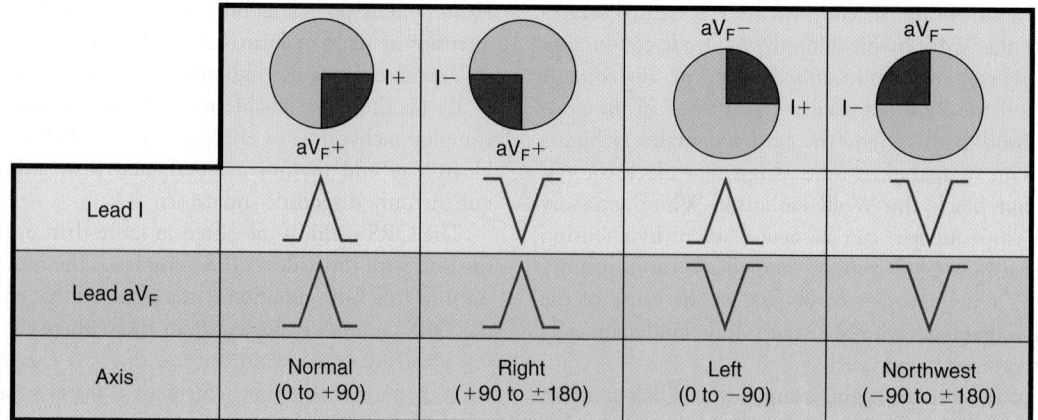

Figure 18-68 Determination of QRS axis quadrant by noting predominant QRS polarity in leads I and aVF. *Normal axis:* If QRS during tachycardia is primarily positive in both I and aVF, the axis falls within the normal quadrant from 0 to 90 degrees. *Right axis deviation:* If the QRS complex is primarily negative in I and positive in aVF, right axis deviation is present. *Left axis deviation:* If the QRS complex is predominantly positive in I and negative in aVF, left axis deviation is present. *Indeterminate axis:* If QRS is primarily negative in both I and aVF, a markedly abnormal "indeterminate," or "northwest," axis is present that is diagnostic of ventricular tachycardia. *(From Drew B: Bedside electrocardiographic monitoring: state of the art for the 1990s,* Heart Lung *20[6]:610-623, 1991.)*

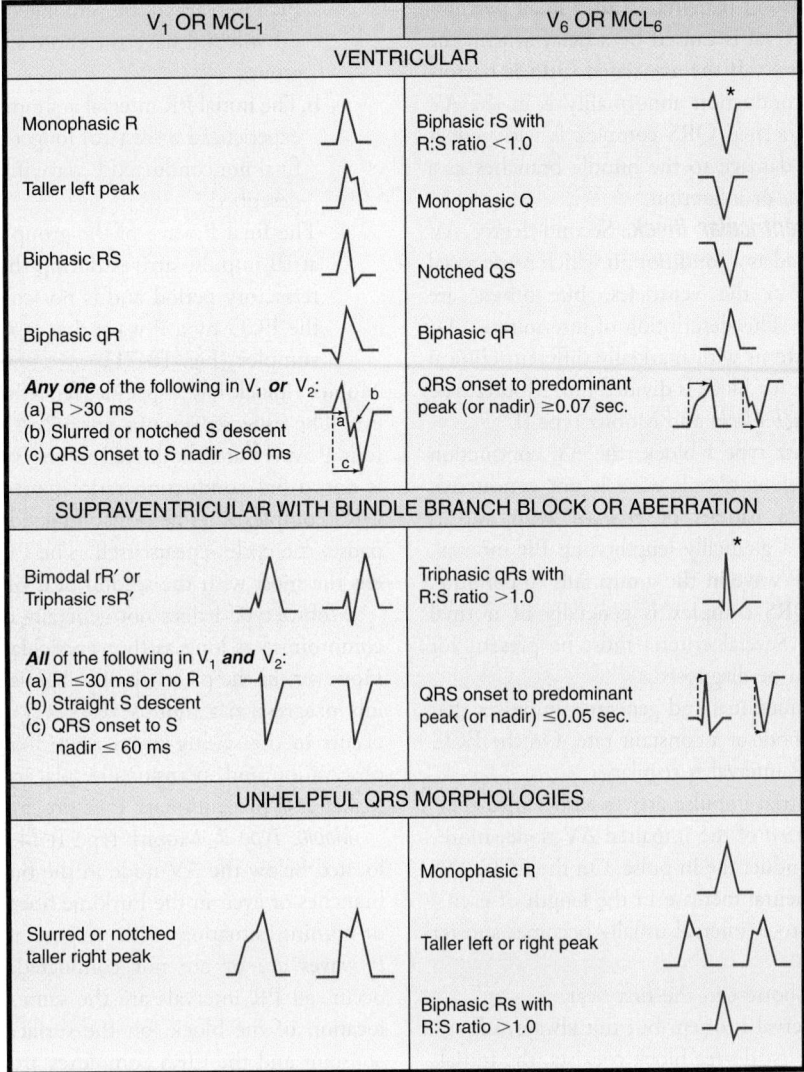

Figure 18-69 Summary of morphologic clues in V₁ or MCL₁ *(left column)* and in V₆ or MCL₆ *(right column)* that are valuable in distinguishing supraventricular tachycardia with bundle branch block or aberration from ventricular tachycardia. If wide-complex tachycardia with taller right peak pattern (i.e., unhelpful morphology) develops in a patient monitored with a single MCL₁ lead, the nurse changes leads to determine whether the wide complex falls into one of the diagnostic patterns in V₆ (MCL₆). *(From Drew B: Bedside electrocardiographic monitoring: state of the art for the 1990s,* Heart Lung *20[6]:610-623, 1991.)*

TABLE 18-15 Atrioventricular Block

Parameter	First Degree	Second-Degree Mobitz I (Wenckebach)	Second-Degree Mobitz II	Third Degree (Complete)
PR interval	>0.20 sec and constant	Increases with each consecutively conducted P wave	Constant	Varies randomly
P waves	1 P wave for each QRS	Intermittently not conducted, yielding more P waves than QRS complexes	Intermittently not conducted, yielding more P waves than QRS complexes	P waves independent and not related to QRS complexes
QRS	0.06-0.10 sec	0.06-0.10 sec	May be normal, but usually coexists with bundle branch block (>0.12 sec)	0.06-0.10 sec if junctional escape pacemaker activates the ventricles; >0.12 sec if ventricular escape pacemaker activates the ventricles

AV node in more than 90% of patients.[113] In a small percentage, the prolonged PR interval is caused by a delay within the atrial conduction pathways.[113] If the associated QRS is narrow it is likely that the only conduction abnormality is in the AV node. However, if the associated QRS complex is widened, it is likely that there is also damage to the bundle branches as a result of sclerosis, ischemia, or infarction.[113]

Second-Degree Atrioventricular Block. Second-degree AV block can be broadly defined as a condition in which some atrial impulses are conducted to the ventricles, but others are "blocked" at the AV node. This description of intermittent AV conduction covers two patterns with markedly different clinical significance: second-degree AV block is divided into Mobitz type I (also known as *Wenckebach block*) and Mobitz type II.

Mobitz Type I. In Mobitz type I block, the AV conduction times progressively lengthen until a P wave is not conducted. This typically occurs in a pattern of *grouped beats* and is observed on the ECG by a gradually lengthening PR interval, until ultimately the final P wave in the group fails to conduct. In Mobitz type I, the QRS complex is generally of normal width and appearance.[113] Several criteria must be present for Mobitz I (Wenckebach) to be diagnosed:

1. The sinus node is functional and generates impulses that conduct to the AV node at a constant rate. On the ECG the measured P-to-P interval is regular.

2. As each successive atrial impulse arrives earlier into the *relative refractory period* of the impaired AV node, more time is needed to conduct the impulse. On the ECG, this is seen as an incremental increase in the length of each PR interval. The R-to-R interval usually becomes shorter with each beat.

3. The PR interval is shortest in the first beat.
   a. The initial PR interval is often, but not always, of normal length. If first-degree block coexists, the initial PR interval will be prolonged, but this initial PR interval will still have the shortest measured interval of the group.
   b. The initial PR interval is shorter because the AV node has experienced a "rest" or longer recovery time due to the final nonconducted P wave in the group, as subsequently described.

4. The final P wave of the group is not conducted. The atrial impulse arrives during the AV node's absolute refractory period and is not conducted. This is seen on the ECG by a P wave that is *not* followed by a QRS complex (Fig. 18-71).

Mobitz I block has a specific, repeating pattern that catches the eye. The expected groups are 3:2, 4:3, or 5:4. For example, if four P waves are conducted to the ventricles and the fifth one is not, a 5:4 conduction ratio is present (five P waves to four QRS complexes). The nonconducted P ends a *group*. After the pause, the cycle repeats itself. The PR interval typically lengthens the most with the second beat of the cycle.[113]

Mobitz type I does not generally cause major hemodynamic compromise as long as the ventricular heart rate is maintained. However, in the presence of ischemia and infarction it can rapidly progress to a more severe level of block. If Mobitz type I occurs in the setting of an acute inferior wall infarction, close observation and, occasionally, placement of a temporary pacemaker as a precautionary measure are warranted.

Mobitz Type II. Mobitz type II block is always anatomically located below the AV node in the bundle of His in the bundle branches or even in the Purkinje fibers.[113] This results in an all-or-nothing situation with respect to AV conduction. Sinus P waves are or are not conducted. When conduction does occur, all PR intervals are the same. Because of the anatomic location of the block, on the surface ECG the PR interval is constant and the QRS complexes are wide (Fig. 18-72).

Mobitz II block is more ominous clinically than Mobitz I and often progresses to complete AV block. If the block involves the Purkinje fibers, an escape rhythm may not develop.[114] For this reason, it is important to prepare for *transcutaneous cardiac pacing* (TCP) by bringing the TCP device (often combined with a defibrillator) to the bedside as a precaution. TCP refers to external pacing from outside the chest wall. When pacing is required, two large pacing electrodes are placed on the chest. There is always a diagram on the machine showing where to place the pads on the chest. Consider the possibility that the patient will need a temporary transvenous pacemaker inserted and possibly require a permanent pacemaker before hospital discharge.

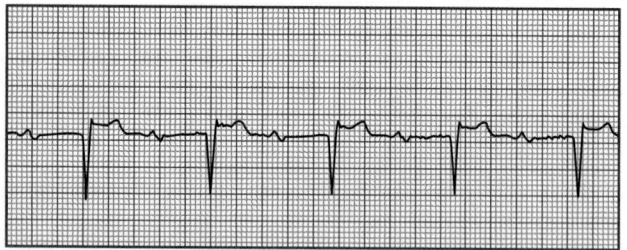

Figure 18-70 First-degree atrioventricular (AV) block. The PR interval is prolonged to 0.44 second.

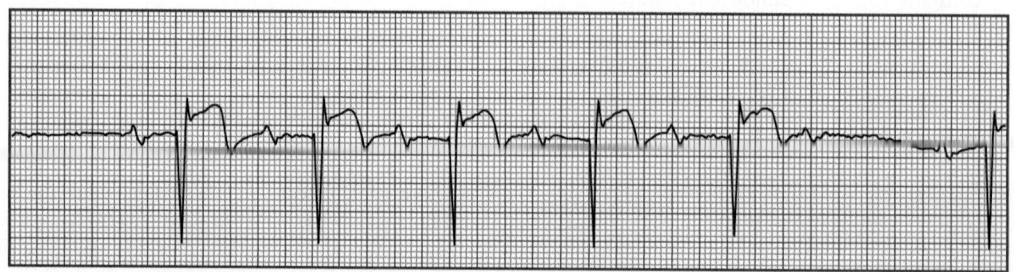

Figure 18-71 Mobitz type I (Wenckebach) second-degree atrioventricular (AV) block. Notice that the PR intervals gradually increase from 0.36 to 0.46 second until a P wave is not conducted to the ventricles.

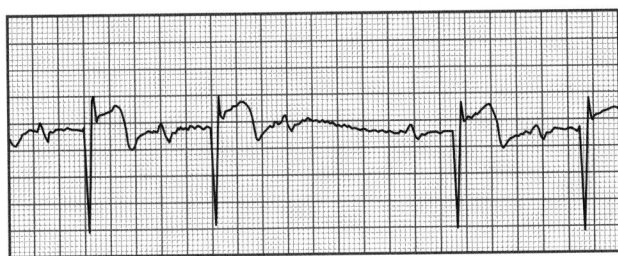

Figure 18-72 Mobitz type II second-degree atrioventricular (AV) block. Notice that the PR intervals remain constant.

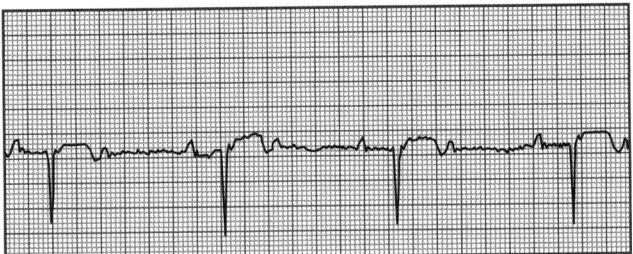

Figure 18-73 A 2:1 atrioventricular (AV) block. Because no two consecutive P waves are conducted, it is not possible to determine with certainty whether this is a Mobitz I or Mobitz II second-degree AV block.

2:1 Conduction. Occasionally, only every other P wave is conducted through the AV node (Fig. 18-73). This pattern may indicate Mobitz type I or Mobitz type II, because consecutive conduction of P waves—which reveal a lengthening or constant PR—does not occur. In Mobitz I, the conduction ratios may have decreased from 4:3 to 3:2 to 2:1, but the site and type of block have not changed. The change in conduction ratio may be caused by an increase in atrial rate, or it may change spontaneously.

In 2:1 conduction, it is impossible to be certain whether the block is Mobitz type I or type II from the surface ECG. If it occurs along with other Mobitz I ratios, it is probably still Mobitz I. If it is an isolated occurrence with no other strips for comparison, the QRS width and the PR interval offer valuable clues to the site of the block. In Mobitz I, the QRS is usually normal and the PR interval is usually prolonged. In Mobitz II, the QRS is usually wide and the PR interval is usually normal. During an acute inferior MI, Mobitz type I AV block with 2:1 conduction is much more common than is type II.

Third-Degree Atrioventricular Block. Third-degree, or complete, AV block is a condition in which no atrial impulses can conduct from the atria to the ventricles. This is also described by the terms *complete heart block* or *AV dissociation* to indicate that the atria and the ventricles are controlled by different pacemakers.[110] The block can be located at the level of the AV node or below the node within the bundle of His or the bundle branches. It can be caused by infraction, digitalis toxicity, or age-related degeneration of the conduction system in older patients.[115] It is hoped that a junctional focus or ventricular focus will depolarize spontaneously at its intrinsic rate of 20 to 40 beats/min and that ventricular contraction will continue. If not, asystole occurs; there is no pulse, and death will result if pacemaker support is not immediate.

On the ECG, P waves are present and usually occur at regular intervals. If a junctional focus is pacing the heart, normal QRS complexes are present but occur at a rate and timing interval totally independent of the P waves. The PR intervals vary widely, because the P wave and QRS are not related to each other. If a ventricular focus is pacing the heart, the QRS complex is wide and unrelated to the P waves (Fig. 18-74).

Management of Atrioventricular Block. Clinically, the consequences of AV block range from benign to life threatening. First-degree AV block is seldom of immediate concern but bears close observation for progression of the conduction disturbance. Second-degree Mobitz I (Wenckebach) is usually benign as long as the patient is not bradycardic. If hemodynamic compromise is present or deemed likely, a temporary pacemaker can be inserted prophylactically. Second-degree Mobitz II is more serious and often precedes complete AV block. Use of a temporary pacemaker is recommended, but its insertion can be elective if the patient remains hemodynamically stable. Complete heart block causes AV dissociation and is associated with a low CO that requires use of a pacemaker. In complete heart block, the patient may exhibit cannon waves as the dissociated atria contact against closed AV valves and create a "wave" on the atrial pressure waveform. An example of this phenomenon is shown in Figure 18-12. If the patient is hemodynamically unstable, external TCP can be used to maintain an adequate ventricular rate until a transvenous or permanent pacemaker can be inserted.

LABORATORY ASSESSMENT

Laboratory assessment of cardiovascular status is obtained through studies of blood serum. Accurate interpretation of these laboratory studies, along with the clinical picture, enables the critical care team to diagnose, treat, and assess the response to therapeutic interventions.

Laboratory studies of blood serum are performed to assess the following:

1. Electrolyte levels that can alter cardiac muscle contraction
2. Cardiac biomarkers that reflect myocardial cellular integrity or infarction
3. Hematologic status to evaluate risk of anemia and infection
4. Coagulation times
5. Serum lipid levels
6. Status of other organ systems that can secondarily affect cardiac function

ELECTROLYTES

Potassium. During depolarization and repolarization of nerve and muscle fiber, potassium and sodium exchange occurs intracellularly and extracellularly. The potassium gradient across the cell membrane determines conduction velocity and helps confine pacing activity to the sinus node. Excess or deficiency of potassium can alter myocardial muscle function. Normal serum potassium levels are 3.5 to 4.5 mEq/L.

Hyperkalemia. Elevated serum potassium, called *hyperkalemia,* can be caused by a variety of conditions that include excess potassium administration, extensive skeletal muscle destruction

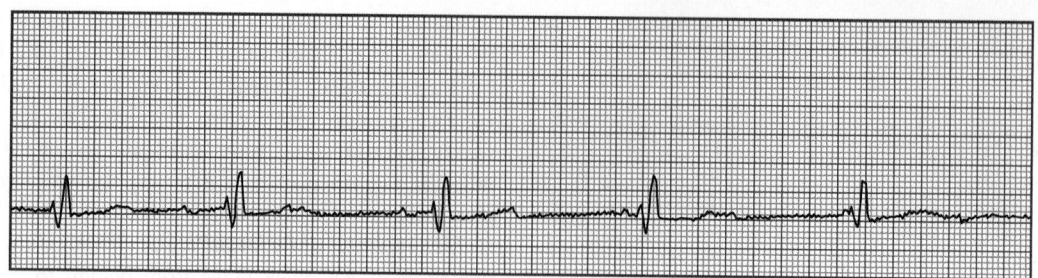

Figure 18-74 Third-degree (complete) heart block.

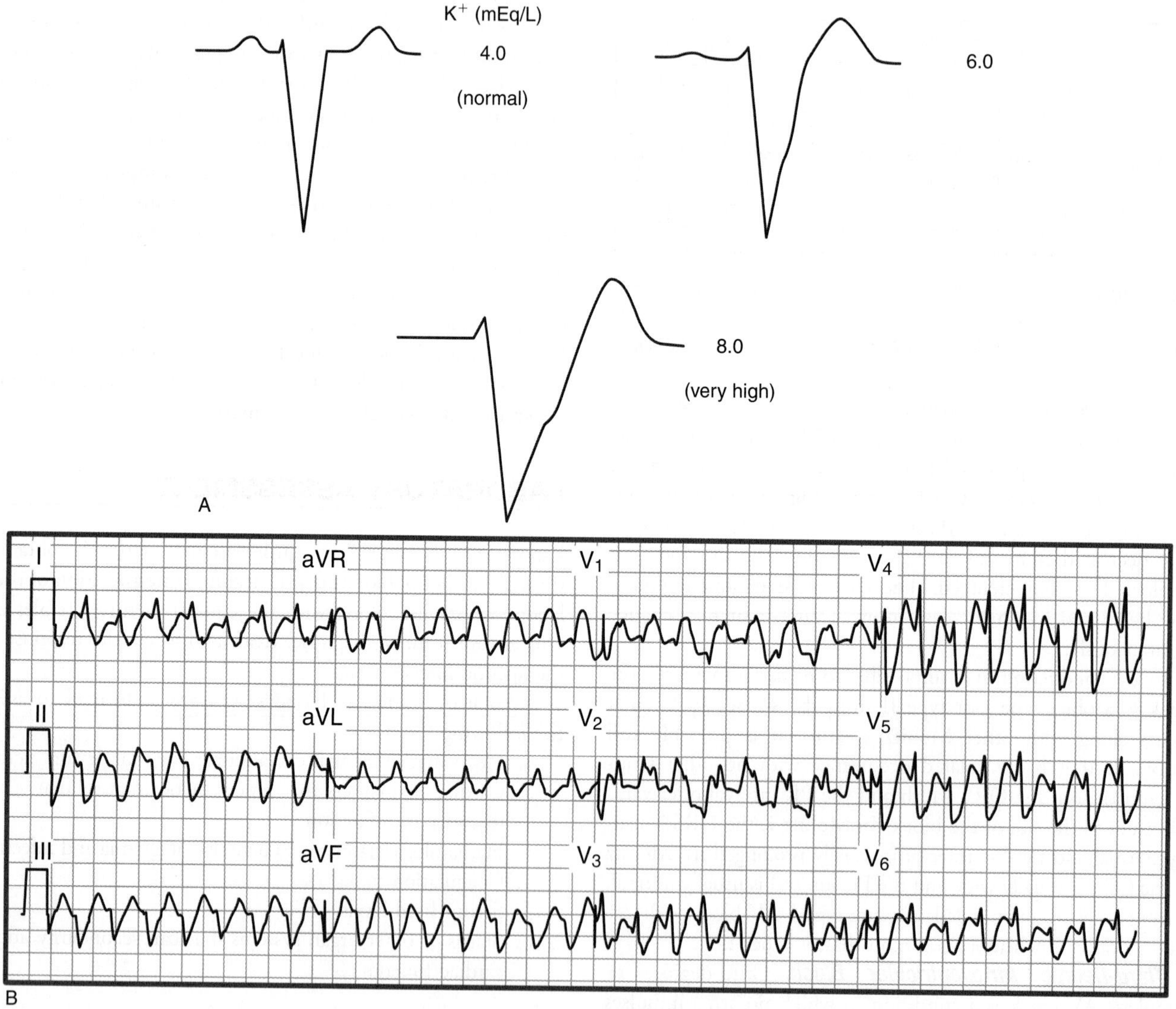

K⁺ (mEq/L)

4.0
(normal)

6.0

8.0
(very high)

A

B

Figure 18-75 Effects of hyperkalemia on the ECG. *A,* Stages in hyperkalemia from normal potassium levels to plasma levels of 8 mEq/L. At approximately 6 mEq/L, the P wave flattens, the QRS broadens, and the ST segment disappears, with the S wave flowing into the tall, tented T wave. *B,* A 12-lead ECG of a patient with a serum potassium level of 9.1 mEq/L.

(rhabdomyolysis), tumor lysis syndrome, kidney failure, and some drugs. Drugs that may induce hyperkalemia include potassium-sparing diuretics, angiotensin-converting enzyme (ACE) inhibitor drugs and angiotensin receptor blocker (ARB) drugs. Hyperkalemia elicits significant changes in the ECG because it decreases AV conduction velocity, slows ventricular depolarization, and accelerates repolarization.[116] As the serum levels of potassium rise above normal (>4.5 mEq/L), evidence

is clearly visible on the ECG (Fig. 18-75A). Tall, narrow peaked T waves are usually, although not uniquely, associated with early hyperkalemia and are followed by prolongation of the PR interval, loss of the P wave, widening of the QRS complex, heart block, and asystole.[116] Severely elevated serum potassium (>8 mEq/L) causes a wide QRS tachycardia, as shown in the 12-lead ECG in Figure 18-75B. If not corrected, severe hyperkalemia can lead to VF or cardiac standstill.

Hypokalemia

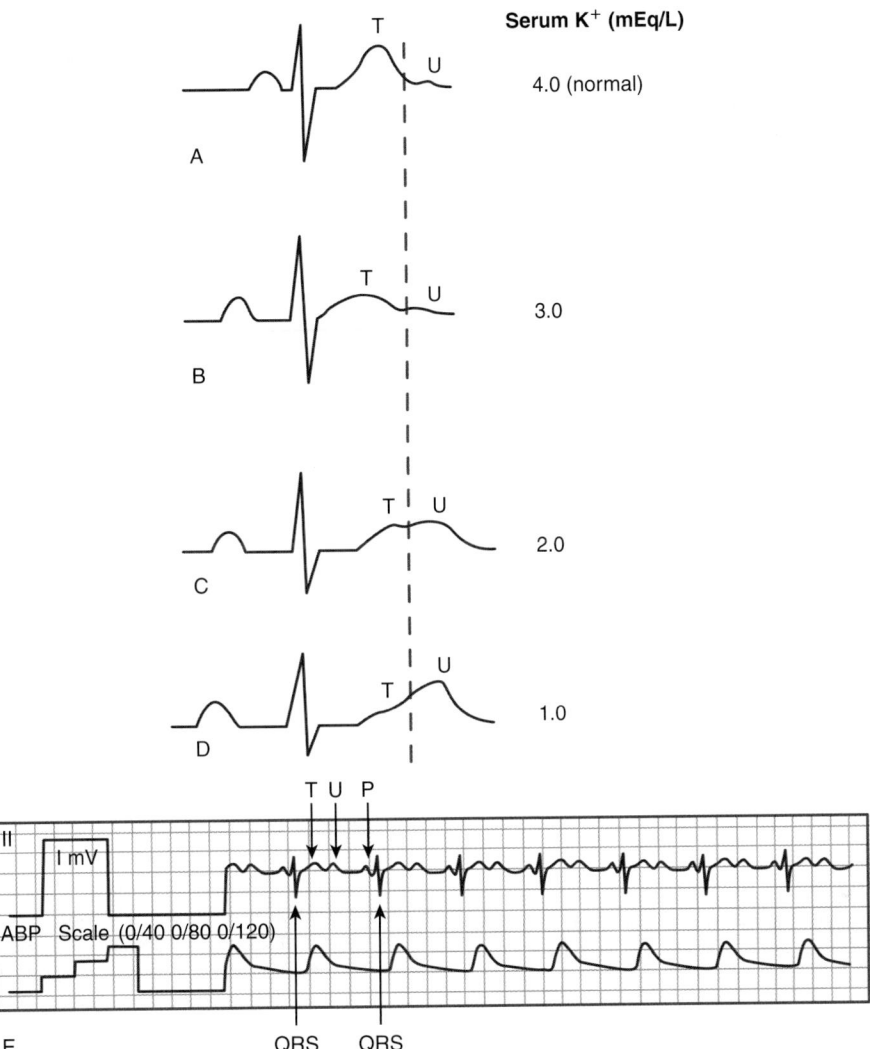

Figure 18-76 Effects of hypokalemia on the ECG. *A,* At a normal serum concentration of 3.5 to 4.5 mEq/L, the amplitude of the T wave is appreciably greater than that of the U wave. *B,* By the time the serum potassium level has dropped to 3 mEq/L, the amplitudes of the T and U waves are approaching each other. *C* and *D,* With a further drop in the level of potassium, the U wave begins to tower over and fuse with the T wave. *E,* ECG tracing from a patient with a serum potassium of 2.6 mEq/L shows a prominent U wave.

This life-threatening condition can be acutely managed with an intravenous insulin or glucose infusion that drives the potassium inside the cell and temporarily out of the serum. Potassium is permanently removed from the serum by cation-exchange resin products, such as Kayexalate, placed into the gastrointestinal tract or removed directly from the blood by hemodialysis. Coexisting low serum sodium, calcium, or pH levels potentiate the cardiac effects of hyperkalemia.

Hypokalemia. A low serum potassium (K^+) level, called *hypokalemia* (<3.5 mEq/L), is commonly caused by gastrointestinal losses, diuretic therapy with insufficient replacement, or chronic steroid therapy. Hypokalemia is also reflected by changes on the ECG (Fig. 18-76). The earliest ECG change is often PVCs, which can deteriorate into VT or VF without appropriate potassium replacement.

Hypokalemia impairs myocardial conduction and prolongs ventricular repolarization. This can be seen by a prominent U wave (a positive deflection after the T wave on the ECG). The U wave is not totally unique to hypokalemia, but its presence is a signal for the clinician to check the serum potassium level. In the critical care unit, where patients are receiving diuretics or have nasogastric tubes to suction, the serum potassium level is checked frequently by the critical care nurse and replaced intravenously to normal levels to prevent dysrhythmias. Great care must be taken when replacing potassium intravenously to ensure it is diluted sufficiently and administered slowly to prevent accidental overdose.[117] Potassium is considered a high-alert medication, and additional safety procedures are recommended for this drug (see the Patient Safety Alert feature on Medication Administration). If concomitant hypomagnesemia exists, successful replenishment of potassium deficit cannot be accomplished until the hypomagnesemia is reversed. Box 18-7 provides the electrolyte values that affect cardiac contractility.

Calcium. Calcium (Ca^{2+}) is an important cation in the body. Calcium metabolism is controlled by many factors, including normal parathyroid hormone (PTH) function, calcitonin, and vitamin D acting on target organs such as the kidney, bone, and gastrointestinal tract.[118] Calcium is an important mediator of many cardiovascular functions because of its effect on vascular tone, myocardial contractility, and cardiac excitability.[118]

Serum calcium values are recorded in three possible ways, depending on the hospital laboratory: milliequivalents per liter (mEq/L), milligrams per deciliter (mg/dL), or millimols per liter (mmol/L).

In the bloodstream, 55% of calcium is bound to protein (primarily albumin) and found in complexes with anions such as chloride and phosphate. As such, it is not physiologically available to the body.[118] The remaining 45% of calcium is biologically active and is called the *ionized calcium*.[118] The normal values for total and ionized serum calcium levels are listed in Box 18-7. The normal serum concentration of ionized calcium

---

Patient Safety Alert

Medication Administration

1. Accurate patient identification
   - Use at least two patient identifiers (not the patient's room number) when taking blood samples or administering medications or blood products. Examples include the patient name, date of birth, or hospital record number.
2. Effective communication among caregivers
   - Hospitals should have (or implement) a process for taking verbal or telephone orders that requires a verification "read back" of the complete order by the person receiving the order.
   - Because thousands of brand name and generic drugs are available, there is always the potential for error. Similar drug names, written or spoken, account for approximately 15% of all medication error reports to the U.S. Pharmacopeia (USP) Medication Errors Reporting Program.
   - In March 2001, the USP released "Use Caution, Avoid Confusion," an updated list highlighting hundreds of confusing drug name sets and identifying more than 750 unique drug names that have been reported to the Medication Errors Reporting Program. A poster and a laminated, quick-reference card are available for health care professionals free of charge from the USP by contacting USP's Practitioner and Product Experience department at 800-487-7776, or the list may be accessed from USP's website at www.usp.org/reporting/review/.
   - An organizational method to decrease the number of medication errors is the use of *computerized physician order entry* (CPOE), as advocated by the Leapfrog group (www.leapfroggroup.org).
   - Standardize the abbreviations, acronyms, and symbols used throughout the organization, including a list of abbreviations, acronyms, and symbols not to use.
   - Examples of problematic abbreviations include "U" for units and "μg" for micrograms. When handwritten, a capital U can be mistaken for a zero (0); in numerous case reports, an insulin dosage written in U was interpreted as 0. Using the abbreviation "μg" instead of "mcg" for micrograms is also problematic; when handwritten, the Greek letter μ can look like an "m."
   - Use of trailing zeros (e.g., 2.0 versus 2) and use a leading decimal point without a leading zero (e.g., .2 instead of 0.2) are dangerous prescription-writing practices. Misinterpretation has caused 10 fold dosing errors.
   - Information on similar medication issues is available on the Web pages (www.jointcommission.org) of The Joint Commission,

formerly called the Joint Commission for the Accreditation of Healthcare Organizations (JCAHO).
3. High-alert medication safety
   - Remove concentrated electrolytes (including but not limited to potassium chloride, potassium phosphate, and hypertonic sodium chloride) from patient care units.
   - Standardize and limit the number of drug concentrations available in the organization.
   - In the first 2 years after enacting a *sentinel event reporting mechanism*, the most common category was medication errors, and the most frequently implicated drug was potassium chloride (KCl). The Joint Commission reviewed 10 incidents of patient death resulting from misadministration of KCl. Eight were the result of direct infusion of concentrated KCl. In six of the eight cases, the KCl was mistaken for another medication, primarily because of similarities in packaging and labeling. Most often, KCl was mistaken for sodium chloride, heparin, or furosemide (Lasix).
   - The Joint Commission suggests that health care organizations *not* make concentrated KCl available outside the pharmacy unless appropriate, specific safeguards are in place.
4. Infusion pump safety
   - Ensure free-flow protection on all general-use and patient-controlled analgesia (PCA) intravenous (IV) infusion pumps used in the organization.
   - Infusion pumps that do not provide protection from the free flow of IV fluid or medication into the patient are hazardous. USP reported six cases in which a patient died because an IV pump did not provide protection from free flow of the IV solution. (October 1991 to November 1999: four additional cases resulted in near-death.)
   - *Free flow* occurs when IV solution flows freely under the force of gravity without being controlled by the infusion pump. Free flow typically occurs after the administration set is temporarily removed from the pump to transfer a patient to another area, change a patient's gown, or place a patient on a radiography table. Clinicians can greatly reduce this risk by using administration sets with set-based anti–free-flow mechanisms that prevent gravity free flow by closing off the IV tubing to prohibit flow when the administration set is removed from the pump.

The information in this feature can be accessed on the Web pages of the following three safety organizations:

www.jointcommission.org

www.usp.org

www.leapfroggroup.org

is maintained within very narrow limits; changes in ionized calcium level are responsible for the clinical effects of hypercalcemia and hypocalcemia. If a patient has an extremely low total serum calcium (<7.0 mg/dL), it is highly likely that the ionized calcium will also be low.[119] However, the only accurate way to determine the level of ionized calcium—described as physiologically active, unbound, or free—is to measure the ionized serum value with a laboratory assay. The mathematically calculated values that extrapolate from total calcium and serum albumin levels have been shown to be inaccurate.[120]

Hypercalcemia. Hypercalcemia is defined as increased amounts of ionized calcium (>4.8 mg/dL or 1.30 mmol/L) or increased amounts of total serum calcium (>10.5 mg/dL or 2.60 mmol/L). Serum calcium levels are increased by bone tumors; primary hyperparathyroidism caused by elevated PTH levels; excessive intake of supplemental calcium and vitamin D, usually in oral antacids; hypomagnesemia; and as a complication of kidney failure from decreased renal excretion of calcium.[120] Hypercalcemia affects many organs, causes smooth muscle relaxation, and can lead to neurologic changes such as lethargy, confusion, and even coma.[120] Elevated serum calcium has the cardiovascular effect of strengthening contractility and

shortening ventricular repolarization, demonstrated on the ECG by a shortened QTc interval.[120] Rhythm disturbances may include bradycardia; first-, second-, and third-degree heart block; and bundle branch block. Hypercalcemia can potentiate the effects of digitalis, precipitate digitalis toxicity, and cause hypertension.[118]

Management of hypercalcemia involves promotion of renal excretion of calcium by diuretics and high-volume intravenous normal saline at 200 to 300 mL/hr if tolerated by the cardiac, pulmonary, and renal systems. Patients who cannot tolerate this clinical regimen should be hemodialyzed using a low-calcium dialysate.[121]

Hypocalcemia. *Hypocalcemia* is defined as an ionized calcium level below normal (<4 mg/dL or <1.05 mmol/L) or a low total serum calcium level. Hypocalcemia (measured by ionized calcium) is a common finding and is reported to occur in 26% to 88% of critically ill patients, depending on the admitting diagnosis.[122] The more severe the patient's illness, the greater the risk of developing hypocalcemia.[122] Transfusions of blood from the blood bank lower serum calcium levels because the citrate used as an anticoagulant in banked blood binds to the calcium. This is called *citrate chelation.* If citrate is used during hemodialysis or plasmapheresis, it will have the same calcium-binding (chelating) effect.[122] Phosphate also binds to calcium and can lower the serum calcium level.[122] Metabolic alkalosis often coexists with hypocalcemia.[122] The cardiovascular effects of hypocalcemia include decreased myocardial contractility, decreased CO, and hypotension. Rhythm disturbances with severe hypocalcemia are variable, ranging from bradycardia to VT and asystole. When the ionized calcium is low, the ECG may show a prolonged QTc interval (Fig. 18-77). This predisposes a patient to the life-threatening ventricular dysrhythmia called *torsades de pointes.*

Management of hypocalcemia, especially when the ionized calcium is low, involves infusion of intravenous calcium chloride or IV calcium gluconate.[122,123]

- Calcium chloride provides 27 mg of elemental calcium/mL.
- Calcium gluconate provides 9 mg of elemental calcium/mL.

Magnesium. Magnesium (Mg^{2+}) is essential for many enzyme, protein, lipid, and carbohydrate functions in the body and is critical for the production and use of energy. The body

BOX 18-7 CHEMISTRY VALUES THAT AFFECT CARDIAC CONTRACTILITY AND CONDUCTION

Electrolyte	NORMAL RANGES*		
	mEq/L	mg/dL	mmol/L
Potassium (K^+)	3.5-4.5		3.50-4.50
Ionized calcium (Ca)		4.0-5.0	1.00-1.30
Total calcium (Ca^{2+})		8.5-10.5	2.00-2.60
Magnesium (Mg^{2+})	1.5-2.0	1.8-2.4	0.70-1.10

*Laboratory values may be reported as mEq/L, mg/dL, or mmol/L. Each measurement parameter used produces a different value. Some electrolytes are reported with more than one reference value. Different clinical laboratories use different reference values, and the cited reference values may vary slightly between hospital laboratories.

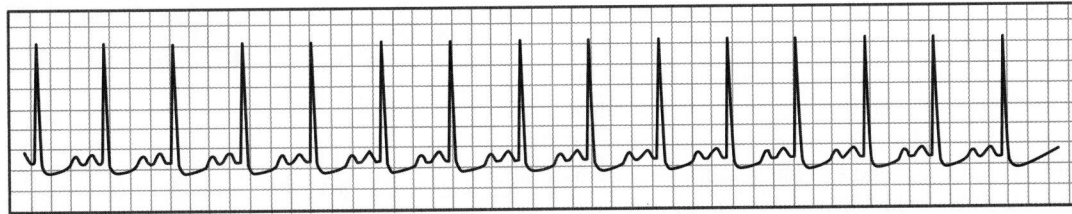

Figure 18-77 Abnormal QT prolongation in a hypocalcemic patient. The patient is a 50-year-old woman admitted to the critical care unit with a diagnosis of alcoholic liver disease and malnourishment. Total calcium concentration is 5.1 mg/dL, and the albumin level is 1.3 mg/dL. The QT interval (0.55 second) is markedly prolonged for the heart rate (100 beats/min). The QT interval varies with the heart rate and can be corrected (QT_c) as if the heart rate were 60 beats/min using the formula $\sqrt{QT/RR} = QT_c$. The QT_c should be 0.44 second or less. The QT_c in the ECG tracing shown is 0.55 second. Hypocalcemia lengthens ventricular repolarization. A quick method for assessing the QT interval is to remember that it is usually less than half of the R-R interval. If it is more than one half of the R-R interval, it is prolonged. *(From Yucha CB, Toto KH: Calcium and phosphorus derangements.* Crit Care Nurs Clin North Am *6[4]:747-766, 1994.)*

stores most magnesium in bone (53%), muscle (27%), and soft tissues (19%); only a tiny proportion resides within the bloodstream—red blood cells contain 0.5%, and serum contains 0.3%.[124] As with other electrolytes, the ionized portion of the serum magnesium is the biologically active component that is available for biochemical processes. Serum magnesium is 67% ionized, 19% protein bound, and 14% complexed.[124] The serum magnesium is what is normally measured in a routine blood test. Serum magnesium can be reported in units of mEq/L, mg/dL, or mmol/L, depending on the laboratory running the analysis. The normal serum range is from 1.5 to 2 mEq/L, 1.8 to 2.4 mg/dL, or 0.7 to 1.1 mmol/L. These represent the same serum level of magnesium despite different measurement guidelines used in the report. It is important to anticipate that normal reference values will vary between hospital laboratories.

Hypermagnesemia. The incidence of hypermagnesemia is rare in comparison with hypomagnesemia. It results from kidney failure, tumor lysis syndrome, or iatrogenic overtreatment.

Hypomagnesemia. A total serum magnesium concentration below 1.5 mEq/L defines *hypomagnesemia*. It is commonly associated with other electrolyte imbalances, most notably alterations in potassium, calcium, and phosphorus. Low serum magnesium levels can result from many causes. Hypomagnesemia is caused by insufficient intake in the diet or in total parental nutrition (TPN) and is associated with chronic alcohol abuse. In the critical care unit, aggressive diuresis with loop diuretics will lower serum potassium and magnesium levels.[124] Diarrhea can be a significant cause of magnesium loss because lower gastrointestinal fluids contain up to 15 mEq/L magnesium; vomiting or gastric suction causes less depletion because the upper gastrointestinal fluids contain about 1 mEq/L.[124] Another cause of magnesium depletion is rapid administration of citrated blood products, which causes the citrate to bind to the magnesium, a condition known as *citrate chelation*. In patients with chronic hypomagnesemia, the serum levels are replenished from the bone stores.[124]

Hypokalemia and hypocalcemia are likely to be unresponsive to replacement therapy until the hypomagnesemia is corrected.[118,124] Expected cardiac-related changes with hypomagnesemia include hypertension and vasospasm, including coronary artery spasm. Some studies have linked magnesium depletion to sudden cardiac death, to an increased incidence of acute MI, and to the occurrence of ventricular dysrhythmias.[124]

In hypomagnesemia, the ECG changes are similar to those seen with hypokalemia[124] and hypocalcemia: prolonged PR and QTc intervals, presence of U waves, T-wave flattening, and a widened QRS complex. Cardiac dysrhythmias may be supraventricular or ventricular and include torsades de pointes. Dysrhythmias associated with hypomagnesemia may not respond to the usual antidysrhythmic drugs, but they often respond well to magnesium infusions. The treatment of choice for torsades de pointes is intravenous magnesium sulfate. The dose of magnesium is adjusted based upon the severity of the clinical situation as described in the American Heart Association (AHA) guidelines.[125] In cardiac arrest with hypomagnesemia or torsades de pointes 1 to 2 g magnesium in 10 mls D5W is administered IV over 5 to 20 minutes. In torsades de pointes without cardiac arrest (the patient has a pulse), magnesium is administered more slowly. An initial bolus of 1 to 2 g magnesium in 50 to 100 ml D5W is infused IV over 5 to 60 minutes. This is followed by 0.5 to 1.0 g magnesium per hour to control breakthrough episodes of torsades de pointes.[125] It is important to evaluate kidney function when administering magnesium to avoid precipitating hypermagnesium states.

CARDIAC BIOMARKER STUDIES

Cardiac Biomarkers. Cardiac biomarkers, previously described by the term *cardiac enzymes,* are proteins that are released from severely damaged myocardial tissue cells.[65,77] When myocardial cells are damaged, they release detectable proteins into the bloodstream so that a rise in biomarkers can be correlated with myocardial cellular damage. The biomarkers that are routinely measured include cardiac *troponin I* (cTnI), cardiac *troponin T* (cTnT), and *CK-MB*. Table 18-16 summarizes the cardiac biomarkers related to myocardial injury and infarction.[126] Unfortunately, in many hospitals, the laboratory turnaround time for results of cardiac biomarkers is between 60 and 90 minutes, which limits the usefulness of the biomarkers in the emergency room when the patient is first admitted with symptoms of acute coronary syndrome.[126] If point-of-care testing at the bedside is used, the results are available more quickly and may be more helpful in the clinical decision-making process.[126]

Creatine Kinase-MB. The creatine kinase (CK) muscle/brain (MB) biomarker (CK-MB) is released as a result of myocardial damage, and serum levels rise 4 to 8 hours after MI, peak at 15 to 24 hours, and remain elevated for 2 to 3 days (see Table 18-16). Serial samples are drawn routinely every at 6- or 8-hour intervals, and three samples are usually sufficient to support or rule out the diagnosis of MI. CK-MB is never an isolated test; it is always performed in conjunction with cardiac troponin levels.

TABLE 18-16 Serum Biomarkers after Acute Myocardial Infarction

Serum Biomarker	Time to Initial Elevation (hours)*	Peak Elevation[†] (hours)*	Return to Baseline (days)*
Cardiac troponin I (cTnI)	3-12	24	5-10
Cardiac troponin T (cTnT)	3-12	12-48	5-14
CK-MB[‡]	3-12	24	2-3

*Time periods represent average reported values.
[†]Does not include patients who have had reperfusion therapy.
[‡]The creatine kinase (CK) enzyme consists of two subunits, the brain type (B) and the muscle type (M).

Troponin T and Troponin I. The *troponins* are biomarkers for myocardial damage found in cardiac muscle. cTnI and cTnT are more sensitive markers of myocardial damage than CK-MB, and as a result, more patients with myocardial damage are now being dectected.[65] Several different methods of laboratory assay are available, which means that normal serum levels will vary between different clinical settings, although cardiac serum cTnI and cTnT levels are low in the absence of myocardial muscle damage.[126]

The initial elevation of cTnI, cTnT, and CK-MB occurs 3 to 6 hours after the acute myocardial damage. This means that if an individual comes to the emergency department as soon as chest pain is experienced, the biomarkers will not have risen. For this reason, it is clinical practice to diagnose an acute MI by 12-lead ECG and clinical symptoms without waiting for elevation of cardiac biomarkers.

Because cTnI is found only in cardiac muscle, it is a highly specific biomarker for myocardial damage, considerably more specific than CK-MB. As a consequence, patients with a positive cTnI result and a negative CK-MB result usually rule in an acute MI.[127] A negative cTnI result that remains negative many hours after an episode of chest pain is a strong indicator that the patient is not experiencing an acute MI. Even with a negative cTnI result, symptoms of chest pain still indicate that the patient should have a comprehensive cardiac evaluation to determine if there is underlying CAD present that may later lead to complications.

Cardiac Biomarkers and Reperfusion. Management of STEMI includes opening the coronary artery obstructed by a thrombus and reperfusing the injured area as rapidly as possible.[77] Individuals who have recent onset of chest pain (within 12 hours) are candidates for reperfusion therapies, including fibrinolytic agents ("clot busters"), cardiac catheterization with PCIs such as balloon angioplasty, atherectomy, or stent placement. If successful, these interventions may totally abort the MI or limit the amount of cardiac muscle damage, resulting in an early rise and fall of the cardiac biomarkers as illustrated in Figure 19-12 of Chapter 19.[77] After reperfusion, the serum troponin levels rise dramatically and peak early. Cardiac biomarker samples are drawn at admission, before administration of thrombolytic therapy or PCI, and then at 6- or 8-hour intervals for 18 to 24 hours to detect any biomarker rise and assess the return of effective myocardial reperfusion.

Natriuretic Peptide Biomarkers in Heart Failure. Natriuretic peptides are biomarkers that provide additional information with which to accurately evaluate the breathless patient. It can be difficult to identify whether a dyspneic patient has a primary pulmonary problem or is exhibiting symptoms of acute heart failure with pulmonary edema. Cardiac natriuretic peptides are used to help make the correct diagnosis. In decompensated heart failure, the myocytes in the volume-distended heart release atrial natriuretic peptide (ANP) from the atria and brain natriuretic peptide (BNP) from the ventricles. Three laboratory assays are commercially available to measure BNP: a point-of-care test, a laboratory test for BNP, and a different laboratory test to measure the amino-terminal fragment of pro-BNP (NT-pro-BNP).[128] BNP has a half-life of about 20 minutes, whereas pro-BNP has a longer half-life of 1 to 2 hours.[129] The choice of test is generally dependent on what is available in the hospital.[129]

The greater the ventricular wall stress, the higher the BNP level rises. The BNP value is combined with the physical examination, the 12-lead ECG, and a chest radiograph to increase the accuracy of heart failure diagnosis (Fig. 18-78).[129] A patient with a BNP level below 100 pg/mL is unlikely to be in heart failure, and a patient with a BNP level above 400 pg/dL is almost definitely in heart failure. BNP is an excellent test to rule out acute heart failure.[128] The challenge lies in interpreting the results of patients with a BNP level between 100 and 400 pg/mL, sometimes described as the *gray zone*.[129] This highlights the importance of using a spectrum of clinical and diagnostic tests. As the symptoms of heart failure are successfully treated, the BNP level usually decreases toward the normal range.

Natriuretic peptides are also released from the endothelium and from the kidney, and they can alter the measured BNP levels. Renal filtration is one of the mechanisms by which BNP is cleared from the bloodstream. BNP levels are higher in patients with kidney failure, especially if the glomerular

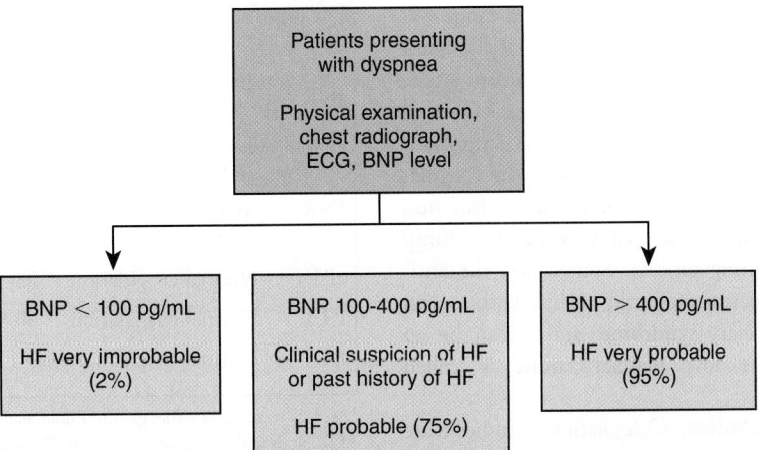

Figure 18-78 The B-type natriuretic peptide (BNP) algorithm in the diagnosis of heart failure.

filtration rate (GFR) is below 60 mL/min/1.7 m^2 due to renal natriuretic peptides.[128,129] BNP levels can also be elevated in high-CO septic shock, possibly because of endothelial natriuretic peptide release or myocardial damage.[128]

BNP levels are lower than expected in obese patients with heart failure, possibly because natriuretic peptide receptors in adipose tissue degrade BNP more rapidly.[129] Conditions such as mitral stenosis that cause pulmonary edema but protect the left ventricle are associated with lower BNP levels than expected from the clinical picture. Even with these caveats, the BNP remains an extremely useful addition in the diagnosis of heart failure.

HEMATOLOGIC STUDIES

Hematologic laboratory studies that are routinely ordered for the management of patients with altered cardiovascular status are red blood cell (RBC) or erythrocyte level, hemoglobin level, hematocrit level, and white blood cell (WBC) or leukocyte level.

Red Blood Cells. The normal amount of RBCs in a person varies with age, gender, environmental temperature, altitude, and exercise. Men produce 4.5 to 6 million RBCs/mm^3, whereas the normal level for women is 4 to 5.5 million/mm^3. *Anemia* is the clinical condition that occurs when not enough red blood cells are available to carry oxygen to the tissues. *Polycythemia* is the condition that occurs when excess RBCs are produced.

Hemoglobin. Hemoglobin levels normally range from 14 to 18 g/dL in men and from 12 to 16 g/dL in women.

Hematocrit. The hematocrit is the volume percentage of RBCs in whole blood. The value is 40% to 54% for men and 38% to 48% for women.

White Blood Cells. Most inflammatory processes that produce necrotic tissue within the heart muscle, such as rheumatic fever, endocarditis, and MI, increase the WBC level. WBCs are also known as leukocytes, and a WBC test may be called a serum leukocyte count. The normal WBC level for both genders is 5000 to 10,000 cells/mm^3. The WBC level also increases in response to infection.

Platelets. The normal platelet count is 150,000 to 400,000 cells/mm^3. Less commonly, the normal platelet count range will be written as 150 to 400 × 10^9/L. Normally, the platelet count is the only laboratory value that is reported. Unfortunately, there is no routine test available for critical care patients that can evaluate platelet functionality. Platelets are important because they are the first cells to be activated when the coagulation system is stimulated. Many drugs inhibit platelet function and make the platelets "slippery" so that they do not clump together to activate the clotting process. Sometimes, the antiplatelet action of a drug is its intended role, such as with aspirin used to prevent acute coronary syndrome, and it can be an unintended side effect. A low platelet count is called *thrombocytopenia*.

Blood Coagulation Studies. Coagulation studies are ordered to determine blood-clotting effectiveness. Anticoagulants—most notably heparin, direct thrombin inhibitors,

warfarin, and platelet inhibitory agents—are administered daily in critical care units for many clinical reasons. It is essential to understand the laboratory tests that are used to monitor the effectiveness of therapeutic anticoagulation.

Prothrombin Time. Most coagulation study results are reported as the length of time in seconds it takes for blood to form a clot in the laboratory test tube. The *prothrombin time* (PT) is no longer directly used to determine the therapeutic dosage of warfarin (Coumadin) necessary to achieve anticoagulation. The PT is not standardized between laboratories so the result of this test is always reported as a standardized *international normalized ratio* (INR).[130]

International Normalized Ratio. The INR was developed by the World Health Organization (WHO) in 1982 to standardize PT results among clinical laboratories worldwide. Table 18-17 shows target INR ranges for different cardiovascular conditions that require anticoagulation. It is recommended that the INR be used to guide anticoagulation therapy with warfarin rather than the PT, especially if the PT results are analyzed at more than one laboratory.

When a patient is first started on warfarin, it is important to know that it can take 72 hours or more to achieve a therapeutic level of anticoagulation. This is because the half-life of prothrombin is between 60 and 72 hours.[130] This delay in anticoagulation effectiveness also occurs if a patient is being converted from heparin anticoagulation—monitored by *activated partial thromboplastin* time (aPTT)—to warfarin anticoagulation (monitored by INR). To ensure a safe transition, a delay of 4 to 5 days must be anticipated in order to obtain two therapeutic INR values 24 hours apart before the heparin is discontinued.[130]

Activated Partial Thromboplastin Time. The aPTT is used to measure the effectiveness of intravenous or subcutaneous ultrafractionated heparin (UFH) administration. Coagulation

TABLE 18-17 Normal and Therapeutic Coagulation Values

Test	Clinical Condition	Normal Value	Therapeutic Anticoagulant Target Value
INR	Normal coagulation	<1.0	
INR	Atrial fibrillation		2.0-3.0
INR	Treatment of DVT/PE		2.0-3.0
INR	Mechanical heart valves		2.5-3.5
aPTT	Normal coagulation	28-38 sec	1.5-2.5 × normal
PTT	Normal coagulation	60-90 sec	1.5-2.0 × normal
ACT*	Normal coagulation	0-120 sec	150-300 sec

*ACT is normal, but therapeutic values may vary with type of activator used. ACT, activated coagulation time; aPPT, activated partial thromboplastin time; DVT, deep vein thrombosis; INR, international normalized ratio; PE, pulmonary embolism; PTT, partial thromboplastin time.

monitoring is required with UHF, although not with subcutaneous low-molecular-weight heparin, because of lower levels of plasma protein binding. In cases of over-anticoagulation with heparin, the antidote is protamine sulfate.

Activated Coagulation Time. An additional test of heparin effect is the *activated coagulation time* (ACT). The ACT can be performed outside of the laboratory setting in areas such as the cardiac catheterization laboratory, the operating room, or specialized critical care units. Normal and therapeutic values for all of these coagulation studies are shown in Table 18-17.

SERUM LIPID STUDIES

Four primary blood lipid levels are important in evaluating an individual's risk of developing or having progression of CAD: total cholesterol; low-density lipoprotein cholesterol (LDL-C); triglycerides; and high-density lipoprotein cholesterol (HDL-C). When levels of cholesterol low-density lipoproteins (LDLs) and triglycerides are elevated or the level of high-density lipoproteins (HDLs) is low, the patient is considered at risk for developing or having progression of CAD and is offered intensive interventions in diet therapy, exercise prescription, and drug therapy.[131]

Total Cholesterol. Cholesterol is a fatlike substance (lipid) that is present in cell membranes, is produced by the liver, and is a precursor of bile acids and steroid hormones. The cholesterol level in the blood is determined partly by genetics and partly by acquired factors such as diet, calorie balance, and level of physical activity. Cholesterol in excess amounts (>200 mg/dL) in the serum forces the progression of atherosclerosis (atherogenesis). Table 18-18 lists the desirable lipid levels to lower the risk of CAD and to reduce morbidity and mortality in patients with established CAD.

Low-Density Lipoproteins. About 60% to 70% of the total serum cholesterol is carried in the bloodstream, complexed as LDL-C. The LDL-C and total serum cholesterol levels are directly correlated with risk for CAD, and high levels of each are significant predictors of future acute MI in persons with established coronary artery atherosclerosis. LDL-C is the major atherogenic lipoprotein and is the primary target for cholesterol-lowering efforts.[131,132] Guidelines recommend maintaining an LDL-C level below 130 mg/dL for the patient with no history of atherosclerotic disease. A patient with known CAD but who is not high risk should aim for an LDL-C level below 100 mg/dL. The recommended target LDL-C level for high-risk patients with CAD has been lowered to 70 mg/dL.[132]

Very-Low-Density Lipoproteins and Triglycerides. The very-low-density lipoproteins (VLDLs) contain 10% to 15% of the total serum cholesterol along with most of the triglycerides in fasting serum. Elevated triglyceride levels are often associated with reduced HDL-C levels.[131]

High-Density Lipoproteins. HDLs are particles that carry 20% to 30% of the total serum cholesterol. A low HDL-C level (below 35 mg/dL) is another independent, significant risk factor for CAD. Several studies also support the finding that HDL-C helps protect against atherogenesis, and a level greater than 50 mg/dL may act as a shield against the risk of CAD.[131,132]

DIAGNOSTIC PROCEDURES

CARDIAC CATHETERIZATION AND CORONARY ARTERIOGRAPHY

Cardiac catheterization and coronary arteriography are routine diagnostic procedures for patients with known or suspected heart disease. Clinical indications for cardiac catheterization include myocardial ischemia, unstable angina, evolving MI, heart failure with a history that suggests CAD or cardiac valvular disease, and congenital heart disease. Cardiac catheterization is used to confirm physical findings and to provide a baseline for medical or surgical therapy.

Left-Heart Cardiac Catheterization. During catheterization of the left side of the heart, hemodynamic pressure measurements are taken in the aortic root, the left ventricle, and the left atrium. Radiopaque contrast (dye) is used to visualize the left ventricle (ventriculogram). This information is also used to calculated the LV ejection fraction. The coronary arteries are visualized and contrast dye is injected directly into each arterial system. The general term for vessel imaging is *angiogram* (veins and arteries), but the more specific term used to describe the visualization of the coronary arteries is *arteriogram.*

Right-Heart Cardiac Catheterization. Catheterization of the right side of the heart is performed using a thermodilution PA catheter. Information obtained includes hemodynamic pressure measurements in the right atrium, the right ventricle, the pulmonary artery, and the pulmonary artery occlusion wedge position, as well as the measurement of CO, calculated hemodynamic values, and oxygen saturations and an angiogram of the right-heart chambers using radiopaque contrast.

TABLE 18-18 **Desirable Lipid Levels**	
Lipid	**Desirable Level**
Total cholesterol	<200 mg/dL
	<130 mg/dL without CAD
LDL-C	<100 mg/dL with CAD but not considered high risk
	<70 mg/dL with CAD and considered at high risk for future coronary events
Triglycerides	<150 mg/dL
HDL-C	>40 mg/dL (male)
	>50 mg/dL (female)

Data from the Executive Summary of the Third Report of the National Cholesterol Education Program (NCEP) Expert Panel on Detection, Evaluation, and Treatment of High Blood Cholesterol in Adults (Adult Treatment Panel III), *JAMA* 285(19):2486-2497, 2001; Grundy SM et al: Implications of recent clinical trials for the national Cholesterol Education Program (NCEP) Adult Treatment Panel III (ATP III) Guidelines, *Circulation* 110:227-239, 1993.
CAD, coronary artery disease; HDL-C, high-density lipoprotein cholesterol; LDL-C, low-density lipoprotein cholesterol.

Procedure. Before the catheterization, the patient meets with the cardiologist to discuss the purpose, benefit, and risks of the study. For many patients, cardiac catheterization is the first major invasive procedure after a diagnosis of possible cardiac disease. The patient is often very anxious and has many questions. It is important that nursing and medical staff fully answer patients' questions about the catheterization experience.

The morning of the procedure the patient fasts except for ingesting prescribed cardiac medications. Light premedication is given before the patient goes to the catheterization laboratory. If there is a history of allergy, an antihistamine or corticosteroid may be administered to prevent an anaphylactic reaction to the radiopaque contrast. Throughout the cardiac catheterization, the patient remains awake and alert. He or she is positioned on a hard table with a C-shaped camera arm overhead or to the side. This arm can be moved to view the heart from several different angles.

Cardiac catheterization catheters, available in a variety of designs and sizes, are placed in the femoral vein and artery after the patient receives a local anesthetic. The choice of catheters is based on the cardiologist's experience and the diagnostic study required. The femoral artery is used to catheterize the left side of the heart, including the coronary arteries. The femoral vein is frequently used as the access vessel to pass catheters to the right side of the heart. During the study, the patient receives heparin systemically to reduce the risk of emboli. Many patients also receive nitroglycerin to control chest pain, particularly when the coronary arteries are full of contrast material during the coronary arteriographic procedure. At this time, the patient may also experience bradycardia or hypotension. To move the contrast dye more quickly and minimize the vagal effect on heart rate and blood pressure, the patient may be asked to cough. If the bradycardia persists, atropine or, occasionally, a transvenous pacemaker may be used. If hypotension continues, intravenous fluids are administered as a bolus. At the end of the study, the femoral catheters are removed from the vessels. After the catheterization, when the patient is stable, the cardiologist meets with the patient and family to discuss the findings and plan of care.

Nursing Management

Femoral Artery Site Care. After the diagnostic catheters (and the sheaths through which they are inserted) are removed from the femoral artery and vein, pressure is applied to the femoral vessels until bleeding has stopped. After catheterization, the patient remains flat for up to 6 hours (varies by institutional protocol and catheter size) to allow the femoral arterial puncture site to form a stable clot. Most bleeding occurs within the first 2 to 3 hours after the procedure. During this time, the groin site is checked frequently for evidence of bleeding or hematoma. Three methods may be used to control bleeding at the femoral arterial puncture site after catheter or sheath removal. The most basic method is manual pressure, in which a clinician holds pressure directly on the vein or artery until bleeding stops. The second method uses external mechanical compression over the site (C-clamp or Femstop). The third method is for the cardiologist to use an *arteriotomy closure device* at the end of the catheterization procedure. One closure device is designed to suture the artery closed as the sheath is removed; another option

is placement of a collagen plug into the track of the sheath insertion site. All of these methods are effective. After routine diagnostic cardiac catheterization procedures, there is no difference in the rate of femoral arterial site complications for the different methods. The patient is asked to lie still and not to bend at the hip. It usually takes about 40 minutes for a stable clot to form, but it can take longer in some patients, including those with a large body surface area.

Sometimes, when the patient needs to void urine, the movement can dislodge the clot. If the patient cannot void in the supine position, a urinary catheter is usually inserted for women and a condom catheter is used for men.

Peripheral Pulses. The peripheral pulses located distal to the arterial access site are monitored closely by the critical care nurse. If the femoral artery has been used, pedal and posterior tibial pulses are assessed. If an alternative access site such as the radial artery is used, the radial pulse is assessed. Pulses are assessed every 15 minutes for the first hour after the catheterization and every 30 minutes to 1 hour thereafter. The affected limb is assessed for changes in color, temperature, pain, or paresthesia to detect early evidence of acute arterial occlusion.

Rehydration. The patient is encouraged to drink large amounts of clear liquids, and the intravenous fluid rate is increased to 100 mL/hr. Fluid is given for rehydration because the radiopaque contrast acts as an osmotic diuretic. This is also used to prevent *contrast-induced nephropathy* or damage to the kidney from the contrast dye used to visualize the heart structures. Patients who have elevated blood urea nitrogen (BUN) or creatinine levels before catheterization are at risk for acute renal failure from the dye. For these patients, the quantity of contrast material is consciously limited, and fluid boluses are given to preserve kidney function.

Angina. The patient is assessed for chest pain after the procedure. Usually, sublingual nitroglycerin is sufficient to relieve the pain, discomfort, or pressure. Not all patients describe their angina as "pain," and many other descriptors may be used. Patients are encouraged to use the 0-to-10 pain scale to quantify the angina. A 12-lead ECG must be obtained immediately to identify the coronary arteries involved, and the cardiologist is notified. If the chest pain persists, this may indicate that a clot has formed in a coronary artery, and the patient may need to return to the cardiac catheterization laboratory for an interventional cardiology procedure. More information about PCI is provided under "Catheter Interventions for Coronary Artery Disease" in Chapter 20.

Dysrhythmias. Dysrhythmias are always a concern after an invasive cardiovascular diagnostic procedure. They result from the underlying cardiac disease and the low potassium levels that can occur after excessive diuresis.

Patient Education. Because of the invasive nature of cardiac catheterization, many patients express considerable anxiety. Relevant information concerns the sensory details of the procedure, such as lying flat and motionless on a hard table for many hours and sometimes experiencing a feeling of warmth when the dye is injected. Pain is uncommon because opiate analgesics and sedative medications are always provided. Information about possible outcomes—positive and negative—and possible complications must be provided to the patient. Postcatheterization requirements such as lying still and drinking large quantities of fluids are explained. The basic information can be provided using written material and videotapes, but it is vital to individualize the content and answer any specific concerns or questions. Patients are also asked to report any other unusual symptoms, such as chest pain or nausea.

ELECTROPHYSIOLOGY STUDY

Indications. The electrophysiology study (EPS) is an invasive diagnostic tool used to record intracardiac electrical activity. A person may have an EPS performed because of a history of a syncopal episode (loss of consciousness); rapid, wide-complex tachycardia; or other cardiac electrical problems not diagnosed by the noninvasive diagnostic studies such as the 12-lead ECG, treadmill stress test, signal-averaged ECG, or Holter monitoring. The EPS is performed in a specially equipped cardiac catheterization laboratory.

Before the electrophysiology study, written and verbal education is given to the patient and family to increase their sense of security and to decrease stress and anxiety. All antidysrhythmic medications are discontinued several days before the study so that any ventricular dysrhythmias may be readily induced during the EPS. Anticoagulants, especially warfarin, are also stopped before EPS. Premedication is administered before the study to induce a relaxed state, and during the procedure, the patient is conscious but receives sedative agents (midazolam) at regular intervals. The patient fasts 6 hours before the EPS and during the procedure lies supine on a hard table with a C-shaped or U-shaped camera arm to the side or overhead to verify the position of the EPS catheters in the heart.

Electrophysiology equipment for stimulation of dysrhythmias and monitoring is usually positioned nearby. A peripheral intravenous access line and surface ECG leads are placed, and electrophysiology catheters are inserted into the femoral vein and advanced to the right side of the heart under fluoroscopy. These catheters, similar to pacing catheters, are placed at specific anatomic sites within the heart to record the earliest electrical activity. The catheter placements are demonstrated in Figure 18-79, with catheter tip positions shown at the following locations:

1. High right atrium (HRA) near to the sinoatrial (SA) node
2. AV node
3. Coronary sinus (CS) behind the left atrial/ventricular border
4. His bundle (HB) near the tricuspid valve
5. Right ventricle (RV) near the apex

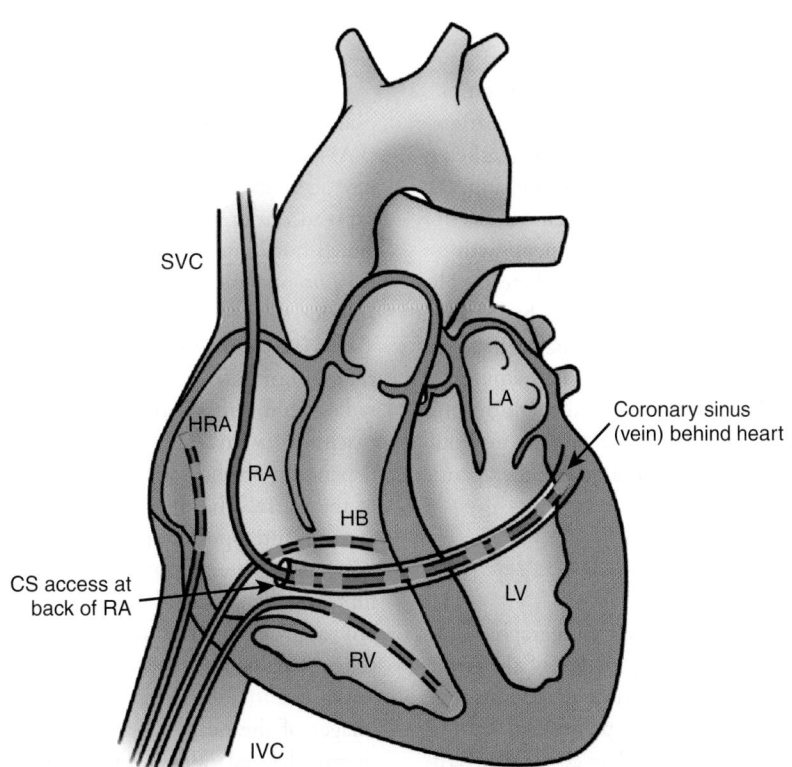

Placement of catheters in the heart in an electrophysiology study.

CS indicates coronary sinus: HB, His bundle; HRA, high right atrium; IVC, inferior vena cava; RV, right ventricle; SVC, superior vena cava.

Figure 18-79 Catheter placement within the heart during an electrophysiology study (EPS). LA, left atrium; LV, left ventricle; RA, right atrium.

During EPS, *programmed electrical stimulation* is used to trigger the dysrhythmia. This technique delivers pulses of two to four early paced beats by means of a specific catheter to the selected area of myocardium. During the EPS, the electrophysiologist looks for a site of early electrical activation that stimulates the myocardium before the sinoatrial node. The goal of EPS is to discover the origin of dysrhythmias that cannot be evaluated from the surface ECG alone.

Atrial Measurements. Typical measurements during EPS include sinus node recovery time (SNRT) and sinoatrial conduction time (SACT) plus atrial pacing to measure the atrial and AV node refractory periods. Coronary sinus pacing is used to induce left atrial tachydysrhythmias.[133] Atrial pacing usually is performed after the ventricular study to reduce the risk of putting the patient into atrial fibrillation or flutter because of retrograde conduction up the His bundle and AV node.[133]

Ventricular Measurements. Programmed electrical stimulation is used to induce the ventricular dysrhythmia, especially in patients who have experienced sustained or nonsustained VT, or survived a sudden cardiac death episode. To measure the retrograde V-to-A interval and stimulate the myocardium, the right ventricular catheter is selected to rapidly pace the right ventricle; the catheter then is moved to the right ventricular outflow tract (near the pulmonary valve), and the pacing stimulation is repeated. This protocol produces VT in 92% of patients with a known history of VT or VF.[133]

After the dysrhythmia is induced and diagnosed, it can be converted to normal sinus rhythm by 10 to 15 paced beats delivered at a rate faster than the VT or by cardioversion and defibrillation plus intravenous antidysrhythmic medications. At the end of the study, all of the electrophysiology catheters are removed before the patient returns to the nursing unit.

Implantable Cardioverter Defibrillators. When an electrophysiology follow-up study is required for a patient with an ICD, the device can substitute for the EP catheters. The ICD has sensing leads, pace termination, backup bradycardia pacing, and cardioversion and defibrillation capabilities. The EPS can be performed by the external ICD programmer in the EPS laboratory. The ICD generator and leads perform programmed electrical stimulation in a manner similar to a full EPS. Chapter 20 provides more information on the therapeutic uses of ICDs.

CHEST RADIOGRAPHY

Basic Principles and Technique. Chest radiography is the oldest noninvasive method for visualizing images of the heart, and it remains a frequently used and valuable diagnostic tool. Information about cardiac anatomy and physiology can be obtained with ease and safety at a relatively low cost. In the critical care unit, the nurse may be the first person to view the chest radiograph of an acutely ill patient. Critical care nurses also have an important role in ensuring the quality of the film through proper positioning and instruction of the patient. For these reasons, it is crucial to understand the basics of chest x-ray techniques and interpretation as they apply to the cardiovascular and pulmonary systems.

TABLE 18-19	Intrathoracic Structure X-Ray Densities	
Metal or Bone (White)	**Fluid (Gray)**	**Air (Black)**
Ribs, clavicle, sternum, spine	Blood	Lung
Calcium deposits	Heart	
Surgical wires or clips	Veins	
Prosthetic valves	Arteries	
Pacemaker wires	Edema	

Tissue Densities. As x-rays travel through the chest from the emitting tube to the film plate, they are absorbed to various degrees by the tissues through which they pass (Table 18-19). Very dense tissue, such as bone, absorbs almost all the x-rays, leaving the film unexposed, or white. The heart, the aorta, and the pulmonary vessels and the blood they contain are moderately dense structures, appearing as gray areas on the x-ray film. These vascular structures are surrounded by air-filled lung that allows the greatest penetration of x-rays, resulting in fully exposed (black) areas on the film. Thoracic structures can be studied best by examining their borders. Two structures with the same density, when located next to each other, have no visible border. If a structure is located next to a contrasting density (e.g., vascular structures next to an air-filled lung), even subtle changes in size and shape can be seen.

Standard Views. In most institutions, a standard radiographic examination of the heart and lungs consists of posterior-anterior (PA) and left lateral films. The standard film is taken in the radiology department with the patient in an upright position; the film exposed during a deep, sustained inhalation; and the x-ray tube aimed horizontally 6 feet from the film. This is referred to as a *PA film* because the beam traverses the patient from posterior to anterior.

Portable Chest Radiography. Because most patients in critical care units are too ill to go to the radiology department, chest radiographs are routinely obtained by using portable x-ray machines, with the patient sitting upright or lying supine, depending on the patient's clinical condition and the judgment of the nurse. The film plate is placed behind the patient's back and an anteroposterior (AP) projection is used, in which the x-ray beam enters from the front of the chest.[134] For the supine film, with the patient lying flat on the bed, the x-ray tube can be only approximately 36 inches from the patient's chest because of ceiling height and x-ray equipment construction. This results in a lower quality film from a diagnostic standpoint, because the images of the heart and great vessels are magnified and not as sharply defined. Whenever possible, the upright (AP) film is preferred to the supine (flat) one, because it provides a more accurate image, it shows more of the lung since the diaphragm is lower, and the thoracic structures appear sharper and less magnified.

Nursing Interventions to Produce an Optimal Chest Radiograph. The critical care nurse can have a big impact on the quality of the x-ray film. Several key elements must be considered[135]:

- The radiograph is taken when the patient has taken a deep breath (inspiration). During exhalation, the lungs are less full of air, which can make the lung tissue appear cloudy as if there is additional lung water. The heart also appears larger during exhalation. This could lead to an erroneous diagnosis of heart failure. Alert patients are encouraged to take in a deep breath and hold it while the exposure is obtained. For patients receiving mechanical ventilatory support, the exposure must be timed to coincide with maximal inhalation.
- It is important to remove extrinsic tubing and other movable objects from the patient's thorax to permit optimal visualization of the chest. Hands or arms should not be across the chest while the radiograph is obtained.
- The patient should sit upright in bed if the clinical condition allows for this position. Upright x-ray views have a sharper focus because the distance from the patient to the x-ray tube is closer to the standard 72 inches (6 feet).
- The nurse should ensure that the patient is straight in the bed rather than turned or twisted; this permits clearer visualization of the major thoracic structures.

Indications. There is considerable debate over the optimal frequency of the routine chest radiograph in the critical care unit.[136] The American College of Radiology (ACR) expert panel made these recommendations for portable x-ray machines used in the critical care unit[134]:

1. Daily chest radiograph are recommended for patients with acute cardiopulmonary problems and those receiving mechanical ventilation.
2. Patients who require cardiac monitoring but are otherwise stable need only an admission x-ray film.
3. A chest radiograph is obtained when a new thoracic device is placed or there is a specific question about the patient's cardiopulmonary status that the radiograph could address.

Chest Radiograph Analysis: Lines and Tubes. Evaluation of a chest film is a systematic process. All thoracic invasive tubes and lines must be located and identified. Major thoracic structures, including the lungs, pleural space, mediastinum, diaphragm, and vascular structures, are assessed and compared with previous films, if available. Variations from previous films can alert the clinician to possible complications and provide information about the patient's hemodynamic status.

Central Venous Catheter. CVCs are seen on the chest film as moderately radiopaque tubes extending centrally from a subclavian (SC), internal jugular (IJ), or femoral vein insertion site. The ideal location of the catheter tip is within the superior vena cava (SVC) so that it is close, but not inside, the right atrium. CVC misplacement during insertion ranges from 1% to 15% of cases.[134] The expertise of the clinician inserting the catheter and variations in patient anatomy are some of the reasons for the wide range of complications. The risk of pneumothorax is 5.6%.[134] A chest radiograph is required after CVC insertion using the IJ or SC vein.

Pulmonary Artery Catheter. A chest radiograph is required after insertion of a PA catheter, also known as a Swan-Ganz catheter. The primary clinical reason for the chest radiograph is to determine the position of the tip of the PA catheter. To wedge correctly, the noninflated catheter tip must lie within 2 cm of the hilar point of the lung and not extend beyond the proximal interlobar arteries.[134] The most serious potential complication is rupture of the pulmonary artery. This complication is rare but has a mortality rate of more than 70% when it does occur.[134]

Endotracheal Tube. A chest radiograph is always requested after endotracheal intubation, because physical examination is not sufficiently sensitive to determine endotracheal tube (ETT) malposition. Although clinical physical assessment can recognize a misplaced ETT in 2% to 5% of cases, suboptimal positioning is identified in 20% to 25% of cases by chest radiographs.[134]

Enteric Tube. Malposition of enteral feeding tubes occurs in 1% of cases and occurs more frequently with small-bore feeding tubes.[134] Because the consequences of delivering enteral nutrition into a nonenteric space are so severe for the patient, a chest radiograph is required after placement and before beginning tube feeds.

Chest Tube. Chest tubes contain a radiopaque line that makes them clearly visible on the chest radiograph. Chest tubes are located within the pleural or mediastinal space. Pulmonary chest tubes are placed to treat pneumothorax or hemothorax. Most pneumothoraces in the critical care unit are iatrogenic (e.g., ventilator barotrauma) or traumatic (e.g., complication of CVC placement), or they occur after cardiothoracic surgery.[137] One or two mediastinal drainage tubes are commonly inserted during cardiac surgery. One may be positioned superiorly to drain the anterior mediastinum, and the other is directed inferiorly to drain the left posterolateral pericardial space.

Intraaortic Balloon Catheter. An intraaortic balloon pump (IABP) provides mechanical support for the failing heart. The catheter that is evaluated on the chest radiograph is a 26- to 28-mm inflatable balloon that surrounds a catheter inserted into the descending aorta, usually percutaneously through the femoral artery. A chest radiograph must be obtained immediately after insertion to evaluate the position of the IABP catheter.[137] The distal tip of the IABP catheter contains a small radiopaque marker that is helpful in determining its position on the chest film. The tip of the IABP catheter must lie below the origin of the left subclavian artery in the descending thoracic aorta (just below the aortic arch). Even when inserted properly, there is a risk of aortic dissection. Aortic dissection is a life-threatening complication. It can be seen on the chest radiograph as a loss of sharpness of the borders of the descending thoracic aorta.

Pacemaker or Implantable Defibrillator. A *pacemaker* and ICD are cardiovascular devices that can be visualized on a chest film. There is considerable variety in the range of pacing electrodes that are encountered in critical care patients. If the pacemaker is permanently implanted, the entire system is seen on the chest film. If it is only a temporary pacemaker, the pulse generator is external to the body and is not seen on the chest radiograph. The pacing electrodes are radiopaque and look like white wires extending transvenously into the right side of the heart. Pacing wires sutured on the epicardium during cardiac surgery are visible on the right atrium and/or right ventricle.

TABLE 18-20 Cardiovascular Devices

Device	Function	Position
Pulmonary artery catheter	Measures pulmonary artery occlusion pressure and right heart pressures	Tip in right or left pulmonary artery
Central venous catheter	Central venous pressure measurement, venous access	Superior vena cava
Left atrium catheter	Left atrial pressure	Left atrium
Mediastinal chest tubes	Mediastinal fluid evacuation	Anterior mediastinum, posterior pericardium
Pacemaker leads	Cardiac pacing	Over right heart
Intraaortic balloon catheter	Assists left ventricular function	Tip just below top of aortic arch

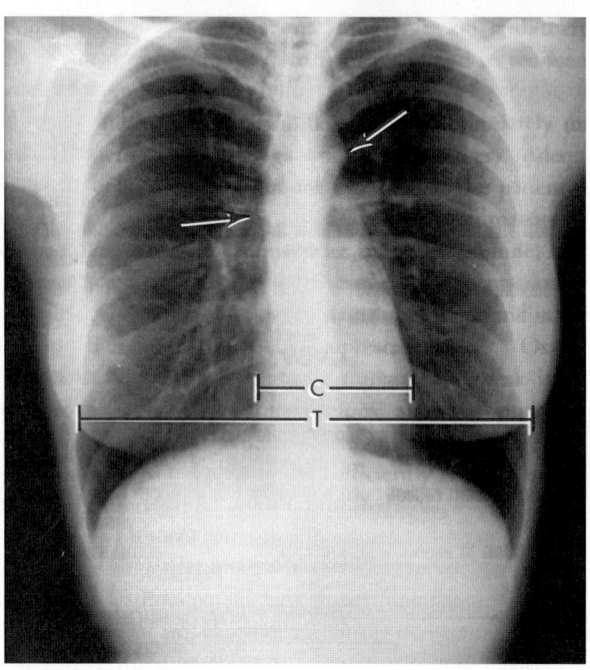

Figure 18-80 Determining the cardiothoracic ratio is a technique for estimating heart size on a posteroanterior chest radiograph. Normally, the cardiac diameter is 50% or less of the thoracic diameter when measured during full inhalation. The width of the vascular pedicle *(arrows)* is a more accurate indicator of systemic blood volume. C, maximal cardiac diameter; T, maximal thoracic diameter measured to the inside of the ribs.

Patients with a history of heart failure may have an additional pacing wire inserted into the coronary sinus (vein) to pace the left ventricle in addition to a right ventricular wire (biventricular pacing). Table 18-20 summarizes the most common cardiovascular devices and their correct position as seen on the chest radiograph.

Chest Radiograph Analysis: Cardiac and Pulmonary Factors. A wealth of physiologic data can be gleaned from a chest radiograph. To be valid, this information must be interpreted in the context of a thorough physical examination and clinical knowledge of the patient's condition.

Cardiac Heart Size. Comparison of the cardiothoracic (CT) ratio (Fig. 18-80) can be used to assess heart size. The normal heart size is less than one third of the diameter of the chest viewed on the radiograph. Patients with chronic heart failure have cardiomegaly (enlarged heart).

Pulmonary Edema. Pulmonary edema is a common finding in the critically ill. The "wet lungs" appear on the chest radiograph as white, dense, cloudy areas. Pulmonary edema shows up very clearly on the chest radiograph, although in the absence of a clinical history the radiograph is not sufficient to determine if the pulmonary edema is from a cardiac or a pulmonary cause.[134] If the pulmonary edema is caused by heart failure, sometimes described as *hydrostatic pulmonary edema,* the fluid may be in a "bat-wing" distribution, with the white areas concentrated in the hilar region (origin of the major pulmonary vessels). However, as the heart failure progresses, the quantity of fluid in the alveolar spaces increases, and the white, fluffy appearance is seen throughout the lung.

If the pulmonary edema is caused by ARDS, also known as *noncardiogenic pulmonary edema* or *permeability edema,* the distribution of fluid is randomly distributed. It may be described as diffuse bilateral infiltrates.[137]

Pneumonia. Hospital-acquired pneumonia (HAP) is a serious iatrogenic complication that may be detected on a chest radiograph. For the mechanically ventilated patient, the risk is increased because the normal oropharyngeal defenses are bypassed by intubation. This leaves the patient vulnerable for development of *ventilator-associated pneumonia* (VAP), a complication with a reported incidence of between 12% to 29% of cases and a mortality of up to 50%.[134] On the chest radiograph, any appearance of a new or progressive opacity (dense, white area) is a cause for concern and should be clinically investigated. More comprehensive information on pneumonia is provided in Chapter 24.

Pneumothorax. Pneumothorax, or air within the pleural cavity, is diagnosed by chest radiography. Normally, the pleura are not visible because they are adjacent to the chest wall. As the pneumothorax increases in size, the nurse can see the edge of the pleura as the trapped air separates it from the chest wall. The "pneumo" (air) appears black within the pleura. There are no lung markings in the pleural area, and the collapsed lung appears increasingly dense (gray or white). The biggest risk is development of a *tension pneumothorax* that will shift the mediastinal structures. This is also visible on a chest radiograph.

DIGITAL RADIOGRAPHY

Digital radiography systems are being widely implemented in hospitals.[134] In a digital radiograph, the image is divided into discrete elements (pixels) that are assigned a specific value and stored for later display on a computer screen or by means of a laser printer. Pixel sizes vary; the smaller the pixel, the better the resolution. Digital systems have many advantages. No film development is necessary, so the image can be displayed rapidly on a computer screen in the clinical area. The image can be expanded or compressed. This system also lends itself to computer-assisted diagnosis, which involves computer analysis of the image to detect and quantify pathologic findings. If a baseline film has been digitally recorded, the baseline film can be "subtracted" from the current film, highlighting any areas of change, such as increased heart size or new pulmonary infiltrates.

AMBULATORY ELECTROCARDIOGRAPHIC TESTS

Before coming to the critical care unit, a patient might have had other ECG tests to determine the degree of cardiovascular disease. *Ambulatory electrocardiography* is a technique that records the ECG of patients while they perform their usual activities. It is designed to document abnormal cardiac rhythms that occur at random or that are induced by specific circumstances such as emotional stress or physical activity. Clinical indications include palpitations, dizziness, syncope, and pacemaker evaluation. Two types of recording systems are available: *continuous* and *intermittent.* Many intermittent systems have a short memory loop that permits capture of recent symptoms.

Continuous Electrocardiographic Recording Systems. *Holter monitors* are the most widely used continuous recording systems. The patient wears skin electrodes and carries a small box that contains a digital or analog recorder. The monitor is carried by a shoulder strap or clipped to a belt or pocket for 24 hours and then is returned to the hospital or clinic for reading. This is a totally noninvasive procedure with no adverse effects. All Holter monitors record at least two leads to minimize inaccurate interpretation caused by artifact.

Electrocardiographic Monitoring Leads. Usually, five electrodes are placed. Two of them are positive electrodes, corresponding approximately to the V_1 and V_5 positions on a standard 12-lead ECG. Two negative electrodes and one ground also are placed. Occasionally, additional electrodes are used to improve diagnostic capabilities. For example, a separate lead can be used to detect pacemaker spikes if the patient is being monitored for pacemaker dysfunction. The skin electrodes are disposable, pre-gelled, and self-adhering. They should be kept dry—not because of any electrical danger but to prevent their falling off before the recording is completed.

Patient Education. If clear directions are provided to the patient, it will make a big difference to the quality of the final recording. The ambulatory monitor saves all of the ECG tracings for 24 hours. The final recording can display the time that an event occurred. Most also have an event marker, which the patient can press to indicate the onset of symptoms or another event that may be important. The patient is asked to keep a diary of activities, symptoms, and any medications that are taken.

Continuous recording systems are the most thorough form of ambulatory electrocardiography because they record every heartbeat for 24 hours. They do not require the active participation of the patient (although a detailed patient log is helpful) and therefore do not miss asymptomatic ECG changes or dysrhythmias that may be accompanied by a loss of consciousness. When dysrhythmias occur that correlate with symptoms or symptoms occur in the absence of dysrhythmias, one of the primary goals of Holter monitoring has been achieved. Unfortunately, most patients do not have typical symptoms daily. If no significant dysrhythmias or symptoms occur during the 24-hour monitoring period, the test is unhelpful. The only activities that are restricted while wearing a Holter monitor are those that would get the chest electrodes or monitor wet, eliminating swimming and taking a shower or tub bath. Sponge baths are permitted as long as the chest electrodes are avoided.

Intermittent Electrocardiographic Recording Systems. A portable monitor that does not record the ECG continuously can also be used to diagnose dysrhythmias. These may also be described as *event monitors.* The patient wears electrodes, but the device is not constantly recording. The patient is instructed to press a button when experiencing symptoms to initiate the recording manually in real time. The big advantage of the intermittent recording system is the ability to leave the recorder in place up to 96 hours, as well as the ability to trigger recording when the symptoms occur.

External Loop Recorders. The external loop recorder records continuously but only keeps the most recent 4 minutes of ECG activity on the memory loop. The memory loop in the device means the patient can press a button and intermittently record a specific event such as heart palpitations during or after the event has occurred. At a later time, the recorder is returned to the hospital or clinic for interpretation of the ECG. The recorder is small and can be clipped to a belt and worn for up to a month.

Implantable Electrocardiographic Recording Systems. For patients whose symptoms are not diagnosed with the traditional methods or who require longer periods of follow-up to diagnose syncope or intermittent dysrhythmias, a small, continuous *implantable loop recorder* may be inserted under the skin of the upper chest.[74] The recorder is about 2 inches by 1 inch by 1 inch. Insertion takes about 20 minutes under local anesthetic. It is especially useful if prior short-term ambulatory ECG recordings have failed to reveal an underlying problem. The inserted loop recorder continuously monitors the ECG rhythm for up to 14 months. After a syncopal episode (loss of consciousness), the patient or a family member places a small, hand-held activator on the chest wall over the loop recorder to capture the most recent ECG data. The stored ECG is subsequently analyzed to determine whether the syncopal episode was caused by a dysrhythmia. At this point, after a diagnosis is made, the implantable loop recorder can be safely removed.

Transtelephonic Electrocardiographic Systems. Transtelephonic monitors are intermittent monitoring systems that are not attached to the patient all the time. These monitors consist of a small box, about 4 inches by 2 inches, with four metal electrodes on the bottom. The box is issued to the patient for a specific time, often 1 month, and the patient carries the box at all times. Whenever symptoms are experienced, the patient places the recording box in the center of the chest and places the four metal electrodes in firm contact with the skin.

An alternative method is to use two arm bracelets containing metal electrodes rather than direct chest placement. A button is depressed to activate the recording, which lasts 1 to 2 minutes. The recording is stored until it is convenient for the patient to make a telephone call to send in the recording to a central analysis facility. At that time, the patient's telephone is placed over a transmitter on the box, and the recording is transmitted to the analysis facility, where it is printed out and analyzed as a readable ECG tracing.

Internet Remote Monitoring.
The transtelephonic system has been used for many years to remotely follow the function of ICDs or pacemakers. Newer technology options mean that patients who have recent-model ICDs or permanent pacemakers implanted can have their device monitored by an Internet-based, remote monitoring service. The patient dials a prearranged phone number to send the information to a protected site. The information is then downloaded by the dysrhythmia nurse or electrophysiologist to a secure Internet web page in the clinical setting. The clinician can view all the programmable details plus any dysrhythmic events or malfunction of the ICD or the pacemaker. The quantity and quality of information transmitted is superior to that transmitted with older transtelephonic systems. The patient does not need to have a computer available because the information is transmitted using a small portable monitor and any standard telephone line.

Patient Education.
A well-informed patient can greatly enhance the quality of the recording. Many patients' symptoms do not occur every day and may be missed during a random 24-hour recording. Often, symptoms tend to occur in association with specific activities. The patient is encouraged to be as active as possible. Keeping an accurate diary of activities is important, because it allows correlation of an identified dysrhythmia with a specific event.

Stress Tests: Exercise with Electrocardiographic Monitoring.
Exercise ECG, more commonly known as a stress test, consists of the recording of an ECG tracing during a period of *physiologic stress* on the heart muscle and its blood supply to uncover and diagnose ischemia, which is not apparent at rest. Physiologic stress is created by asking the patient to walk on a treadmill or to ride a stationary bicycle.

Physiology of Exercise on the Cardiovascular System.
Exercise places unique demands on the cardiovascular system. Systemic oxygen consumption increases markedly, requiring the heart to increase CO to meet these demands. Myocardial contractility increases, resulting in greater stroke volume and systolic blood pressure. Heart rate is increased as a result of circulating catecholamines. Normally, as heart rate and stroke volume rise, CO is increased dramatically, and the tissue needs for oxygen are met. This enhanced myocardial performance is not without a penalty. Even at rest, the heart muscle extracts 70% of the oxygen available in the circulating blood. When the myocardial demand for oxygen increases during exercise, coronary blood flow must increase to maintain an adequate oxygen supply. In people with CAD, coronary blood flow cannot increase sufficiently to meet the high metabolic needs of the myocardium during exercise, and ischemia results.

Stress Test Protocols.
Most exercise tests in the United States are performed using a treadmill on which the speed and slope can be varied or using a stationary bicycle. A number of protocols have been developed using a treadmill. Two popular ones are the *Bruce protocol,* in which the grade and speed are varied every 3 minutes, and the *Balke protocol,* in which speed remains constant and grade is gradually increased every minute. Regardless of the protocol used, the ECG is monitored continuously. Blood pressure is also measured and recorded every minute.

Heart Rate Criteria in Treadmill Stress Test.
The treadmill test is terminated when a desirable level, based on the patient's maximal stress test heart rate, is reached. The maximal predicted heart rate is estimated using the formula:

$$220 - \text{Patient's age}$$

Increasing the heart rate to 85% to 90% of the predicted maximum is preferred, and in most patients, this level of exercise is sufficient to unmask any significant CAD. The diagnostic value of the test is based on the maximal heart rate achieved, *not* on the length of time that the patient remains on the treadmill. A well-trained athlete may be able to stay on the treadmill for 15 minutes, whereas an older or sedentary person may tolerate it for only 3 to 5 minutes; however, if 85% of the predicted maximal heart rate is achieved, both tests are equally diagnostic. A person who is taking beta-blockers may not be able to reach his or her age-adjusted targeted heart rate because of the bradycardiac effect of this class of drugs.

The test workload also is described in metabolic equivalents (METs) of oxygen consumption.[138] The definition of 1 MET is 3.5 mL of oxygen per kilogram per minute at rest for a 70 kg, 40-year-old man. The stress test result may be described as "poor exercise tolerance" (3 to 4 METS) or "good exercise tolerance" (10 to 11 METS).

Clinical Reasons to Stop the Treadmill Test.
The test may be aborted before maximal heart rate is reached if symptoms occur. Reasons to halt the test include the development of moderate to severe angina (chest pain), signs of pallor or poor perfusion, and the patient asking to stop the test.[138] Other signs that can alert the nurse to stop the test include ST-segment elevation equal to or greater than 1.0 mm (one small box); ST depression equal to or greater than 2.0 mm (2 small boxes); cardiac dysrhythmias or a marked shift in ventricular axis; and increased symptoms, such as breathlessness or fatigue and a fall in blood pressure of 10 mm Hg or more from baseline.[138] Blood pressure is expected to rise during exercise, but a systolic blood pressure greater than 250 mm Hg or a diastolic blood pressure greater than 115 mm Hg is considered high enough to stop the test.[138]

Treadmill Tests after Myocardial Infarction.
A low-level stress test is sometimes performed before discharge from the hospital on patients who have had an acute MI. In this case, the heart rate is raised to only 120 or 130 beats per minute. ST-segment depression or elevation that occurs during the predischarge low-level stress test is a reliable indicator of additional myocardium at risk. However, exercise-induced angina or

abnormal blood pressure responses to exercise often do not appear during a low-level stress test, so a "normal" predischarge stress test must be followed later by a test closer to maximal level.

Nursing Management. During the exercise test, the patient is encouraged to continue as long as possible. However, the test is stopped if the patient requests because of symptoms such as fatigue, shortness of breath, leg cramps, significant ECG changes, blood pressure changes, or development of angina. After the exercise test is completed, the patient is assisted into a supine position. The ECG, the pulse rate, and blood pressure are monitored for at least 10 more minutes to detect dysrhythmias or signs of ischemia. The patient is instructed to rest for the next 30 to 60 minutes after release from the exercise laboratory. Hot showers should be avoided for 3 to 4 hours to prevent development of orthostatic hypotension. It is essential that nurses who monitor patients during this test are experienced and knowledgeable about all aspects of stress testing and emergency protocols. Emergency medications and a defibrillator must be available in the test area.

Patient Education. Many patients are anxious about undergoing exercise testing, and the anxiety is often multifactorial. Patients without known heart disease may be afraid that they will "fail" the test, find they have heart disease, and perhaps need open heart surgery. If the patient generally follows a sedentary lifestyle, anxiety may be caused by the fear of "collapsing" on the treadmill or spending several days recovering from exhaustion. Some are afraid that they will be forced to go beyond their endurance. Often, low-level exercise testing is performed before discharge on patients who have been hospitalized for an acute MI. These patients may be afraid that the strain on their heart is too great or that they will die during the test. Effective patient education can do much to allay these fears. In addition to describing the procedure itself, the nurse instructs the patient to fast for 3 hours before the test, refrain from smoking for at least 2 hours before the test, and wear comfortable shoes and loose-fitting clothes. Reassurance that the heart will be monitored closely during the test is also important.

SIGNAL-AVERAGED ELECTROCARDIOGRAM

The *signal-averaged electrocardiogram* (SAECG) is used to identify late potentials within the QRS complex. These low-amplitude waveforms cannot be detected on a standard surface ECG but can be recorded as an SAECG. Late potentials indicate slow conduction within the ventricular myocardium that can be a substrate for ventricular dysrhythmias and put the individual at risk for sudden cardiac death.[139]

SAECG is a noninvasive test. The patient lies in a supine position and is asked to keep muscle movement to a minimum. Cardiac electrode leads are applied to the anterior and posterior chest walls, and the leads are connected to a signal-averaged ECG computer. This computer produces a high-resolution, high-magnification ECG signal. This "noise-free" ECG is then analyzed for QRS duration and for the presence, duration, and measurement of late myopotentials. After computer

analysis, the SAECG is described as negative (normal) or positive (abnormal). A positive SAECG in combination with other specific indicators is a predictor of increased risk for sudden cardiac death.

Many patients with a positive SAECG (abnormal) produce a normal SAECG when placed on antidysrhythmic medications. The SAECG is not analyzed in isolation. It is used in conjunction with other cardiac diagnostic tests, including the EPS. It is a helpful adjunct to the EPS but does not replace it.

ECHOCARDIOGRAPHY

Echocardiography uses *waves of ultrasound* to obtain and display images of cardiac structures. Normal human hearing occurs at a sound frequency of 20 to 20,000 cycles per second (Hz). Ultrasound uses sound frequencies greater than 20,000 Hz. When used to image cardiac structures, the best results are achieved using 1.5 to 10 MHz. Usually, 2.25 MHz is used with adults to allow optimal depth penetration, whereas 3 to 5 MHz is used in pediatric patients to provide a clearer image of the smaller structures.

Ultrasound is reflected best at interfaces between tissues that have different densities. In the heart these are the blood, cardiac valves, myocardium, and pericardium. Because all these structures differ in density, their borders can be seen on the echocardiogram.

Echocardiography is used to detect cardiac abnormalities such as mitral valve stenosis and regurgitation, prolapse of mitral valve leaflets, aortic stenosis and insufficiency, hypertrophic cardiomyopathy, atrial septal defect, thoracic aortic dissection, cardiac tamponade, and pericardial effusion.[76] Echocardiography is quickly becoming a first-line hemodynamic assessment tool in the critical care unit.[140]

Transthoracic Echocardiography. When transthoracic echocardiography (TTE) is performed, the patient is in a supine, a left lateral, or a semirecumbent position. The position used depends on the patient's clinical condition and on which structures are to be examined. A transducer is placed on the skin, with lubricant between the transducer and the skin to improve contact and reduce artifact. The active element in the transducer is a piezoelectric crystal. *Piezoelectric* refers to the ability to transform electrical energy into mechanical energy (in this case, sound energy). The transducer emits ultrasound waves and receives a signal from the reflected sound waves. Periods of sound transmission alternate with periods of sound reception.

Ultrasonic waves do not travel through air very well, and they cannot penetrate very dense structures, such as bone. In adults, the transducer is usually placed in the third or fourth intercostal space to the left of the sternum, because at that point the pericardium is in direct contact with the chest wall and the ultrasonic waves are not obstructed by air or bone. Other positions are sometimes used if the standard location does not provide adequate visualization of the cardiac structures. In the critical care unit, the echocardiograph machine is usually brought to the bedside. The lighting in the room can be dimmed to improve the visual clarity of the images displayed on the screen.

The nursing care consists of monitoring the patient during the procedure, which is usually performed by an echocardiography technician. TTE is completely noninvasive; the nurse explains this and the purpose of the test to the patient and family. The procedure is not uncomfortable, but it may be tiresome for certain patients because of the length of the procedure, which is usually 30 to 60 minutes.

Motion-Mode Echocardiography. In motion-mode (M-mode) TTE, a thin beam of ultrasound is directed through the heart (Fig. 18-81A). Each interface is represented by a dot, and when recorded over time (like an ECG tracing), each dot becomes a line on an oscilloscope. A strip-chart recording can be made of this tracing as the heart beats. Heart motion is recorded over time, and a typical M-mode echo is shown in Figure 18-81B. M-mode echocardiograms are particularly useful in detecting small pericardial effusions and cardiac tamponade.

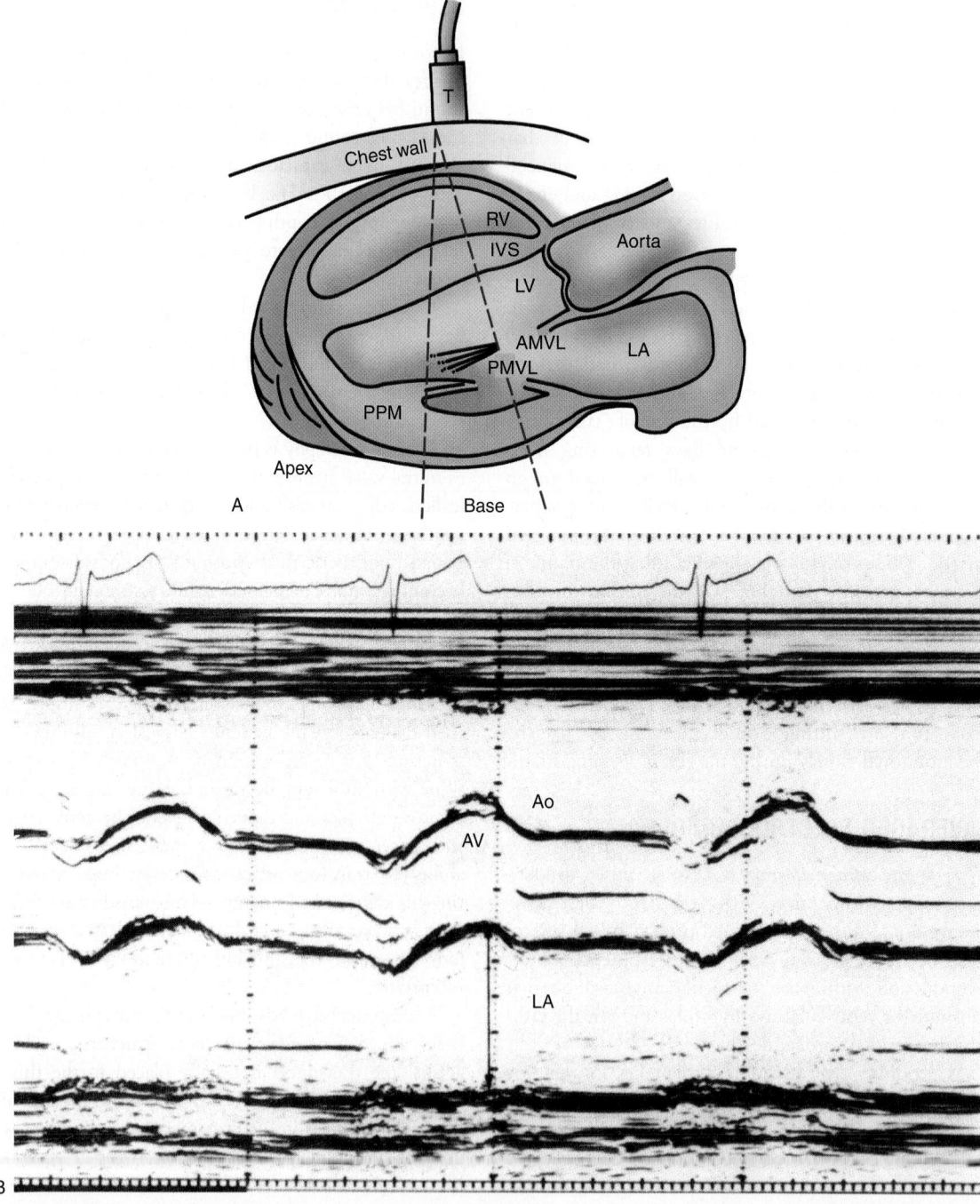

Figure 18-81 *A,* Schematic representation of cardiac structures traversed by two echobeams. *B,* Normal, M-mode echocardiogram at the level of the aorta, aortic valve leaflets, and left atrium. AMVL, anterior mitral valve leaflet; Ao, aorta; AV, aortic valve; IVS, interventricular septum; LA, left atrium; LV, left ventricle; PMVL, posterior mitral valve leaflet; PPM, posterior papillary muscle; RV, right ventricle; T, transducer. *(B from Kinney M et al: Andreoli's comprehensive cardiac care, ed 8, St Louis, 1995, Mosby.)*

Two-Dimensional and Three-Dimensional Echocardiograms. The two-dimensional (2-D) echocardiogram uses crystals in the transducer to create a cross-sectional imaging plane. Sections of the heart are then viewed from a number of different angles (Fig. 18-82). The picture is displayed on an oscilloscope, and digital photographs are taken to serve as a permanent record. The 2-D echocardiogram images a whole "slice" of the heart at once and is used for direct measurement of LV volumes and wall mass.[76] The 2-D slice also permits visualization of the cardiac structures in relation to each other and readily identifies valvular dysfunction and wall motion abnormalities after MI.[141]

A more recent innovation is the three-dimensional (3-D) echocardiogram. It produces a more realistic image of structures such as the mitral valve.[142]

Phonocardiogram. Phonocardiography is combined with echocardiography to evaluate valvular dysfunction. *Phono* (sound), *cardio* (heart), and *gram* (recording) provide a graphic display of the sounds that occur in the heart and great vessels. The transducer is placed on the chest wall to record heart sounds that correspond to auscultation with a traditional stethoscope. Chapter 17 provides more information on heart sounds.

Color-Flow Doppler Echocardiography. Doppler echocardiography provides a special kind of echocardiogram that assesses blood flow. It uses a pulsed or continuous wave of ultrasound that records frequency shifts of reflected sound waves, showing velocity and direction of blood flow relative to the transducer. Doppler signals are usually displayed in color. Known as *color-flow mapping* or *imaging,* this technique analyzes Doppler signals from multiple intracardiac sites simultaneously. The Doppler tracing for each site is displayed in a color-coded format superimposed on a real-time 2-D echocardiographic image. Flow toward the transducer is displayed in one color, whereas flow away from the transducer is displayed in a contrasting color. The brightness of the color varies to signify different flow velocities.

Doppler echocardiography is especially useful in individuals with valvular heart disease. The blood flow associated with regurgitation and stenosis can be detected, and estimates can be made of the severity of the disease. Doppler can accurately estimate right ventricular systolic pressure.[76] When several valves are involved, the Doppler technique can clarify the extent of damage to the individual valves. Other uses for Doppler echocardiography include evaluation of congenital shunts, measurement of volume flow and CO, and assessment of new structural abnormalities after acute MI.[141] By measuring flow velocity in the right ventricular outflow tract, mean pulmonary artery pressure can be estimated.

Transesophageal Echocardiography. TEE is a technique in which the transducer (single-plane, biplane, or multiplane device) is mounted on a flexible shaft similar to an endoscope and advanced into the esophagus, from where cardiac structures can be clearly visualized. The multiplane transducer has a single array of crystals that can be rotated in a 180-degree arc, requiring less manipulation of the probe within the esophagus. Because of the close anatomic relationship between the heart and the esophagus, TEE produces high-quality images of intracardiac structures and the thoracic aorta without the interference of the chest wall, bone, or air-filled lung.

The insertion procedure is similar to an upper gastrointestinal endoscopy. The patient is asked to fast for a minimum of 6 hours before the TEE to prevent nausea and vomiting. For an elective TEE, medication is usually given to inhibit salivary secretions, reducing the risk of aspiration. Analgesic and sedative agents are administered to reduce fear and anxiety and to provide retrograde amnesia. Routine antibiotic prophylaxis against bacteremia and endocarditis is not necessary, although it is considered for high-risk patients such as those with prosthetic valves, previous endocarditis, or very poor dentition. The pharyngeal region is anesthetized with 2% viscous lidocaine (Xylocaine) and 10% lidocaine spray to lessen the gag reflex and prevent retching and laryngospasm. The patient is usually placed in the left lateral decubitus position, although the supine position can be used in the critical care setting if necessary. A soft bite block is inserted between the teeth to prevent

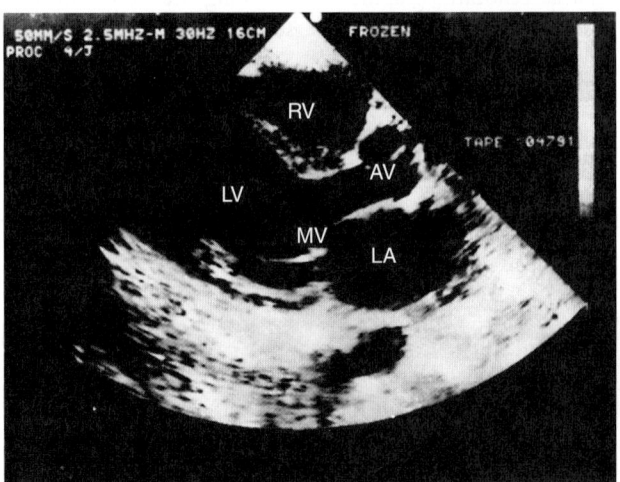

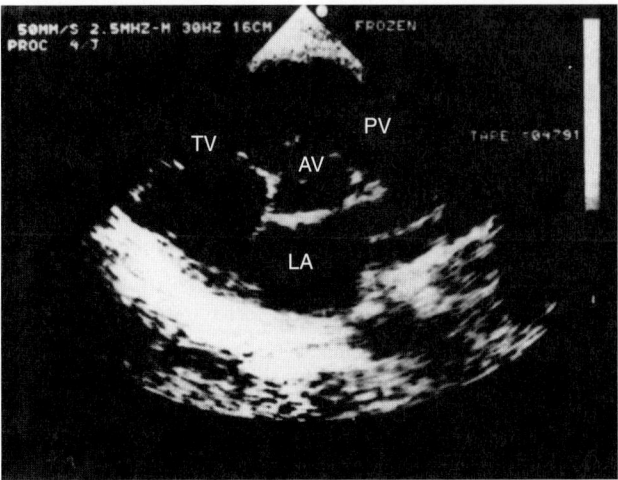

Figure 18-82 Two-dimensional echocardiogram. Notice that several sections of the heart can be viewed at one time and that it is easier to see the relationships of the chambers. *LA,* left atrium; *LV,* left ventricle; *MV,* mitral valve; *PV,* pulmonary vein *RV,* right ventricle; *TV,* tricuspid valve. *(From Kinney M et al: Andreoli's comprehensive cardiac care, ed 8, St Louis, 1995, Mosby.)*

damage to the echoscope. As the echoscope is inserted, the patient is asked to swallow. The echoscope is advanced to 25 cm from the mouth, and imaging is begun (Fig. 18-83). TEE is also used intraoperatively during cardiac surgery for valve repair and replacement.[76] The images obtained by TEE are superior to transthoracic views in a variety of ways. The entire thoracic aorta can be visualized clearly. Both atrial chambers are clearly seen with TEE, and the left atrial appendage is particularly well visualized, making TEE the procedure of choice for detection of left atrial thrombus. Diagnosis and quantification of atrial septal defects is possible with this method, and the addition of Doppler capabilities allows assessment of atrial shunting. TEE is useful in evaluating patients with valvular disorders, including infective endocarditis to visualize vegetations on the valve leaflets.[76]

Manipulation of the TEE probe within the esophagus can cause a vasovagal response, producing bradycardia and hypotension. The most serious risk of the procedure is esophageal bleeding. Individuals with liver cirrhosis or esophageal varices and patients on a heparin drip are also at risk for esophageal bleeding. TEE must always be performed under ECG and blood pressure monitoring, and if esophageal entry is difficult, it cannot be forced. In some hospitals, TEE can represent 5% to 10% of all echocardiographic studies. To remain competent at performing TEE safely, trained physicians must perform 10 to 25 TEE examinations per year to maintain the cognitive and technical skills necessary to maintain competence.[143] During

TEE, the patient's vital signs are closely monitored. Emergency resuscitation equipment must be present in case of a severe vasovagal episode (e.g., bradycardia, hypotension). Suction equipment must be at the bedside in the event that the patient vomits or has difficulty handling oral secretions.

Stress Echocardiography. Stress echocardiography is often used in the outpatient setting to identify stable angina. It provides a very accurate picture of the ischemic impact of CAD on the myocardium.[143,144] Stress echocardiography can diagnose regional (ischemia) and global (cardiomyopathy) abnormalities.[143,144] It may also be used after MI to evaluate the impact of necrosis on viable wall tissue. Physiologic stress from increased exercise creates an imbalance between myocardial oxygen supply and demand. This causes ischemia and eventually results in wall-motion abnormalities, which are detectable with an echocardiogram. Stress can be applied to the heart by physical and pharmacologic means.[143,144] One of two methods of physical exertion usually are employed; the patient can exercise on a treadmill or a stationary bicycle. The protocols used for physical echocardiographic stress testing are very similar to those used in the ECG stress test setting previously described (Table 18-21).

Dobutamine Stress Test. Pharmacologic stress is most frequently incited with a dobutamine infusion beginning at 5 mcg/kg/min and increasing as needed to 40 or 50 mcg/kg/min to achieve 85% of maximal heart rate.[144,145] Dobutamine causes myocardial ischemia through a dramatic increase in

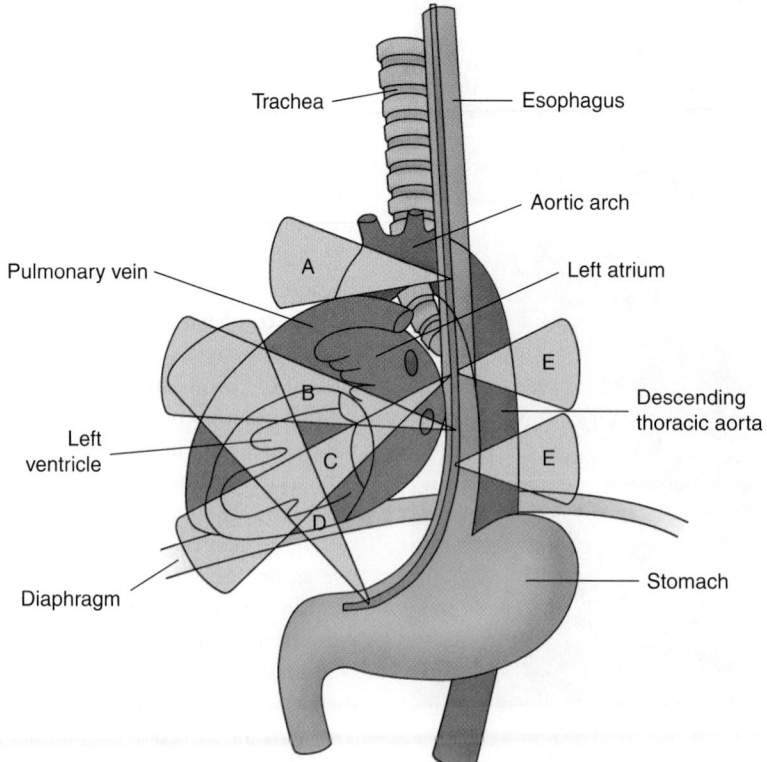

Figure 18-83 Diagram of common scan planes during a transesophageal echocardiogram (TEE) with a two-dimensional view. *A,* Horizontal scan plane of the aortic arch and distal portion of aorta. *B,* Basal, short-axis (transverse), long-axis (sagittal), and short-axis views of both atria. *C,* Four-chamber and left atrioventricular long-axis views. A sagittal scan plane can image a cross section of the left ventricle. *D,* Transgastric, short-axis view of the left and right ventricles. *E,* Transverse and sagittal scan sections of the descending aorta.

myocardial oxygen demand by an increase in heart rate, contractility, and systemic blood pressure. Potential side effects include hypotension, hypertension, dysrhythmias, nausea, headache, anxiety, and tremor. Atropine is also administered if the dobutamine infusion alone does not cause an adequate increase in heart rate.[145] Because of the potential risks of dobutamine stress echocardiography, it is recommended that qualified physicians be engaged in at least 100 studies a year to maintain competence.[143] Other vasodilating drugs used in pharmacologic stress tests are dipyridamole and adenosine.[145]

Intravascular Ultrasound. Intravascular ultrasound (IVUS) is used as an adjunct diagnostic technique during coronary angiography or during a coronary PCI. A miniature, flexible ultrasound catheter that incorporates a high-frequency transducer (20 to 40 MHz) provides high-resolution images of the coronary arterial wall. This technology is not an alternative to angiography but is used as a complementary diagnostic technique. IVUS permits an anatomic view of the interior of the coronary artery. The cardiologist can visualize the exact location of atherosclerotic plaque or see if a coronary stent has deployed (expanded) correctly against the vessel wall.[146]

Intracardiac Ultrasound. The use of intracardiac ultrasound is increasing. Flexible ultrasound catheters can be directed into the atria and ventricles. Diagnostic uses include direct visualization of intracardiac structures, replacement for TEE during interventional or selected surgical procedures, and views of the atrial or ventricular septum during a repair procedure.

Hand-Carried Ultrasound Devices. Portable ultrasound, or handheld ultrasound, is used in many critical care units and emergency departments. Portable ultrasound is designed to increase the accuracy of the bedside physical examination.[142]

TABLE 18-21 Stress Testing Methods

Test Parameters	Stress Electrocardiography	Stress Echocardiography	Stress Radionuclide Imaging
Exercise stress test	3-, 5-, or 12-lead ECG leads are attached to the chest and limbs to monitor the ECG *during* the exercise protocol.	The patient exercises according to protocol. Echocardiogram is recorded immediately *after* exercise.	The radiopharmaceutical (thallium 201 or technetium 99m) is injected before exercise. The patient exercises according to the protocol. The heart is scanned *after* exercise to view uptake of the radiotracer.
Pharmacologic stress test	Patient is at rest. IV drugs stimulate heart rate and contractility: Dosage starts with dobutamine at 5 mcg/kg/min and is increased as needed to increase the heart rate. ECG pattern is monitored during the drug infusions. Other drugs include adenosine and dipyridamole.	Patient is at rest. IV drugs stimulate heart rate and contractility: Dosage starts with dobutamine at 5 mcg/kg/min and is increased as needed to increase the heart rate. Echocardiogram is recorded during and after the drug infusions. Other drugs include adenosine and dipyridamole.	Patient is at rest. IV drugs simulate exercise: Dosage starts with dobutamine 5 mcg/kg/min and is increased as needed to increase the heart rate. Radionuclide image is scanned during and after pharmacologic stress. Other drugs include adenosine and dipyridamole.
Clinical indications	Used to rule out CAD Not as helpful if patient has a distorted ECG pattern at baseline due to LBBB, RBBB or internal ventricular pacemaker because ST-segment changes are obscured	Useful for patients with LBBB, RBBB, and implanted pacemaker, because the wall motion is visualized directly	Helpful for patients with LBBB, RBBB and implanted pacemaker It is useful before CABG to determine if bypass graft will supply blood to an ischemic area. There is no benefit in grafting an artery to an infarcted area.
Clinical outcome of a positive test result	Chest pain develops. ST-segment ECG pattern changes.	Chest pain develops. Wall motion abnormalities are visualized.	Areas of the heart that do not take up radiotracer are called *cold spots*. A cold spot is ischemic or infarcted tissue. A follow-up scan later the same day (or the next day with some radiotracers) shows whether the cold spot has filled in; if yes, the area is ischemic; if it remains cold, the area is infarcted.

CABG, coronary artery bypass graft; CAD, coronary artery disease; ECG, electrocardiographic; IV, intravenous; LBBB, left bundle branch block; RBBB, right bundle branch block.

MAGNETIC RESONANCE IMAGING

Magnetic resonance imaging (MRI) is a noninvasive imaging technique that can obtain specific biochemical information from body tissue without the use of ionizing radiation. The procedure does not present any known hazard to living cells. In many respects, the image created is superior to radiography and ultrasonography, because bone does not interfere with MRI.

Indications. Cardiac MRI can provide information about tissue integrity, cardiac wall-motion abnormalities, aneurysms, ejection fraction, CO, patency of proximal coronary arteries, and flow rates through coronary artery bypass grafts.[147,148] MRI is useful in diagnosing complications of MI, such as pericarditis or pericardial effusion, valvular dysfunction, ventricular septal rupture, aneurysm, and intracardiac thrombus.

Blood that is actively flowing does not emit a magnetic resonance signal; it provides a natural dark contrast material in the lumen of proximal coronary arteries. As a result, abnormalities of lumen size such as narrowing—which may provide evidence of obstruction—can be visualized.

How Magnetic Resonance Imaging Works. The physics behind MRI scanning is complex, but the basic concept is simple. Certain atoms within molecules act as tiny bar magnets with north and south poles. The nuclei spin around this axis like a spinning top. Under normal conditions, these small atomic magnets are arranged at random. If a patient is placed within a strong magnetic field, many of the nuclei line up in the same direction as the magnetic force. When a radiofrequency wave is sent, some of the nuclei absorb this energy, causing them to fall out of alignment and wobble like a gyroscope that is winding down. This wobbling out of alignment is called *resonance.* The process of returning to alignment with the magnetic field after the radiofrequency signal is turned off is called *relaxation.* These energy changes can be detected and recorded by the scanner.

Each type of atom has its own unique resonance and relaxation pattern. The easiest one to record is the hydrogen ion, although other atoms such as phosphorus, sodium, and carbon are being studied. Because there are two hydrogen ions per molecule of water, MRI is especially sensitive to changes in tissue water content. Myocardial ischemic injury results in predictable increases in regional myocardial water content, allowing differentiation between normal and ischemic tissue. Infarction leading to myocardial scarring results in tissue with a decreased water content, which can be identified on a magnetic resonance scan as an area of decreased signal intensity.

MRI works well for structures that have little or no motion, such as the brain. Cardiac applications have been limited because of the constant motion of the heart. In an attempt to overcome this limitation, various gating or slicing techniques have been used to time the images at exact phases of the cardiac cycle. The gating can be timed from the R wave of the ECG or from the arterial pulse tracing. Either method is satisfactory as long as the patient is in normal sinus rhythm. With any irregularity of the rhythm, the gating technique becomes much less helpful.

Metal Objects. MRI is a safe procedure. The main hazard is related to the presence of metal substances in the environment.

Because the magnetism used is approximately 40,000 times stronger than the magnetic field of the earth, metal objects such as intravenous line poles, infusion pumps, or oxygen tanks can become projectiles if they come close enough to the magnet's pull. No metal objects are permitted in the area of the MRI scanner. The patient must be asked about the presence of any metallic implants (pacemaker) or other metal (residual bullet or shrapnel) that may be moved by the magnetic force during the scan. Aneurysm clips are composed of ferromagnetic materials and can experience significant torque when exposed to the magnetic field. Box 18-8 lists some guidelines about which implants are safe and which are not. Another consideration is that exposure to the strong magnetic field may cause a cardiac pacemaker or ICD to turn off or switch modes.

Challenges with Magnetic Resonance Imaging. MRI has significant limitations that affect patients in the critical care setting. One of the challenges is that patients must leave the unit and be transported to the nuclear medicine laboratory for MRI. Standard ventilators, monitoring equipment, and infusion pumps cannot be used because these machines contain metal parts. Special ventilators with nonmagnetic accessories are available, as well as non-metal ECG, pulse oximetry sensors, and infusion pumps.

The narrow size of the magnet bore (tube or tunnel) requires the patient to lie flat and motionless for up to 7 minutes at a time. The close quarters inside the magnet bore tend to provoke claustrophobia in anyone already predisposed to it, and sedation may be required. The patient who is claustrophobic needs considerable reassurance and education before lying supine and motionless inside the MRI tube. A recent innovation is the use of open MRI scanners. The MRI tube is open at both ends so that the patient's head is not enclosed while the body is scanned.

CARDIAC RADIONUCLIDE IMAGING STUDIES

Several types of radionuclide imaging tests are available. As with diagnostic ECG and echocardiography, many of the radionuclide tests can be performed at rest and during exercise.

Purpose of Radionuclide Scans. The purpose of a radionuclide scan is to determine whether there is a perfusion defect in cardiac muscle. A scan is indicated for the person with chest pain and known or suspected CAD. The radionuclide scan is especially helpful for the person who has a coexisting LBBB or a permanent pacemaker where the QRS shape is distorted. Both situations make interpretation of acute angina challenging to interpret accurately on the 12-lead ECG. This has opened a window of opportunity for radionuclide imaging, in which the myocardial ability to receive blood flow is visualized directly.[149]

A radionuclide scan adds to the information that has been gained from a cardiac catheterization study and a 12-lead ECG. Coronary artery anatomy and patency is important because regional myocardial blood supply is always from a specific coronary artery and any blockage of an artery can lead to a discrete myocardial perfusion defect, meaning that the blood supply to this area is decreased (ischemic) or absent (infarcted). Although coronary arteriography defines the anatomy of the coronary arteries, it does not show whether the arteries perfuse the cardiac muscle.

Radionuclide Isotopes. The radioisotopes used in cardiac diagnostic imaging are very different from those used in oncology for tumor ablation. Diagnostic isotopes have a short half-life (minutes to hours) and are used in very small amounts to minimize radioactivity risk. Patients do not need to be isolated, and no specific precautions are required for blood, urine, stool, or other body fluids.

Thallium 201. Thallium 201 (^{201}Tl) is a low-energy radioactive isotope. It is an analogue of potassium and acts like potassium when injected into the bloodstream. Because thallium is similar to potassium, it is absorbed from the bloodstream by cardiac muscle cells as part of the sodium-potassium adenosine triphosphatase (ATPase) pump. Thallium uptake depends on two factors: the patency of the coronary arteries and the amount of healthy myocardium with a functional sodium-potassium ATPase pump. Areas of infarcted myocardium (dead tissue) do not take up thallium. After thallium has been injected, a specialized scintillation camera and associated computer system are used to scan the myocardium.

Technetium 99m. Technetium 99m (^{99m}Tc) is also used frequently. It is often attached to other tracer substances for diagnostic imaging (^{99m}Tc-sestamibi or ^{99m}Tc-tetrofosmin).[149] These substances are often described as *radiopharmaceuticals*.[149] ^{99m}Tc tracers are highly suited to imaging myocardium during ACS because the tracers do not redistribute over time (they remain in myocardium), allowing a second scan to be performed many hours later if needed.[149] In clinical practice, this is seldom practical, and use of radiopharmaceuticals in emergency situations is rare outside of research studies.[149] These tests are widely used when the patient's hemodynamic and cardiac condition is stable.

Stress Test Radionuclide Scan. This test takes place in a specialized nuclear medicine department. The walls of the testing space are normally lined with lead to prevent any radioactivity dispersal to other areas. A patent intravenous line is required. A radioisotope flow agent (^{201}Tl or ^{99m}Tc) is injected into the bloodstream before exercise to permit identification of perfused versus nonperfused (cold) areas. After the physical activity, a specialized perfusion-scanning camera is used to scan the heart. As with the other cardiac stress tests, the options to increase the heart rate and myocardial blood flow are physical exercise by the patient or infusion of a drug to achieve the same effect (see Table 18-21).

Exercise Radionuclide Scan Procedure. Before the *exercise radionuclide scan,* the procedure is fully explained to the patient, including a description of the equipment (ECG monitoring equipment, cardiovascular exercise treadmill or stationary bicycle, and an Anger gamma scintillation camera). The patient is usually fasting, because the scan involves vigorous exercise. Vasodilating medications that may alter the uptake of the radioisotope (nitrates, theophylline, and related drugs) are held (not taken by the patient) before any baseline study. Other medications that will not affect the outcome of the study can be taken as usual. A patent intravenous line is inserted before the test. In the laboratory, the patient is asked to exercise vigorously for 1 minute or more or until angina or fatigue develops. At this point, the isotope is injected into the bloodstream. After the

injection, the patient is asked to exercise vigorously for another minute to stress the heart and circulate the radioisotope. As soon as possible after exercise (within 10 minutes), the patient is asked to lie on the examination table for the first perfusion scan by the scintillation camera. The camera examines the heart from three angles—anterior, left anterior oblique, and left lateral oblique—to increase accuracy. On the camera screen, the heart image looks like a circle with a hole (doughnut shape). The myocardium appears, but the fluid-filled center does not.

Pharmacologic Radionuclide Scan Procedure. A patient who cannot tolerate a radionuclide-exercise stress test can undergo a pharmacologic radionuclide test at rest. The test can be performed with ^{201}Tl or ^{99m}Tc. In the absence of physical exercise, a dobutamine infusion is used to increase coronary artery and myocardial blood flow.[149] Maximal contractility is achieved with dobutamine at about 10 mcg/kg/min for normal hearts, the goal is to drive the heart rate to the 85% maximal heart rate predicted for that individual; if needed, atropine is added to achieve the desired heart rate.[150] After the first scan, the patient is removed from the scanner and the heart rate is allowed to return to baseline. After about 5 to 10 minutes, the patient is asked to return to the scanner to ensure the LV wall motion has also returned to baseline.[150] Other vasodilating medications that may be used for this study include adenosine and dipryidamole.[149] The choice of agent is dependent on the preference of the physician conducting the study.

Radionuclide Test Results. If no perfusion defect is seen, the test is complete for that patient. If a perfusion defect (dark area) is observed in the myocardium, the patient is asked to return for a repeat scan 2 to 4 hours later or the next day, depending on the radioisotope tracer that was used. If a perfusion defect is present 4 hours later, the area is infarcted. This is sometimes described as a *cold spot* or as a *fixed lesion*. If the perfusion defect has taken up the radioisotope since the first test (redistribution), the area is ischemic. An ischemic defect is amenable to reperfusion therapy such as CABG or a catheter-based procedure to open a coronary artery.

Summary

- Hemodynamic monitoring is one of the major reasons patients are admitted to the critical care unit.
- Accurate interpretation of hemodynamic parameters is an indispensable skill the critical care nurse must acquire to deliver safe patient care.
- Accurate ECG lead placement and interpretation of ECG rhythms in the context of a clinical diagnosis yields relevant information that contributes to optimal patient outcomes.
- Interpretation of the chest radiograph is used to noninvasively locate catheters, tubes, and implantable devices and to detect complications such as pulmonary edema, pneumonia, and pneumothorax.
- Echocardiography is frequently used in the critical care unit for rapid assessment of change in cardiac function; use will increase as this technology becomes smaller and more portable.

References

1. Halm MA: Flushing hemodynamic catheters: what does the science tell us? *Am J Crit Care* 17(1):73-76, 2008.
2. Del Cotillo M et al: Heparinized solution vs. saline solution in the maintenance of arterial catheters: a double blind randomized clinical trial, *Intensive Care Med* 34(2):339-343, 2008.
3. Hall KF et al: Effect of heparin in arterial line flushing solutions on platelet count: a randomised double-blind study, *Crit Care Resusc* 8(4):294-296, 2006.
4. Warkentin TE et al: Treatment and prevention of heparin-induced thrombocytopenia: American College of Chest Physicians Evidence-Based Clinical Practice Guidelines (8th edition), *Chest* 133(6 suppl):340S-380S, 2008.
5. American Association of Critical-Care Nurses (AACN): Pulmonary Artery Pressure Monitoring: AACN Practice Alert, 2004. Available at www.aacn.org (accessed February 2009).
6. Kohonen M et al: Is the Allen test reliable enough? *Eur J Cardiothorac Surg* 32(6):902-905, 2007.
7. Barone JE, Madlinger RV: Should an Allen test be performed before radial artery cannulation? *J Trauma* 61(2):468-470, 2006.
8. Agrifoglio M et al: The Allen test is not adequate enough for the screening of hand circulation, *Eur J Cardiothorac Surg* 33(4):754, 2008.
9. Hadian M, Pinsky MR: Functional hemodynamic monitoring, *Curr Opin Crit Care* 13(3):318-323, 2007.
10. Perloff D et al: *Human blood pressure determination by sphygmomanometry*, ed 6, Dallas, TX 2001, American Heart Association.
11. Polderman KH, Girbes AJ: Central venous catheter use. Part 1. Mechanical complications, *Intensive Care Med* 28(1):1-17, 2002.
12. Polderman KH, Girbes AR: Central venous catheter use. Part 2. Infectious complications, *Intensive Care Med* 28(1):18-28, 2002.
13. Maddukuri P et al: Echocardiographic diagnosis of air embolism associated with central venous catheter placement: case report and review of the literature, *Echocardiography* 23(4):315-318, 2006.
14. Collyer TC et al: Severe air embolism resulting from a perforated cap on a high-flow three-way stopcock connected to a central venous catheter, *Eur J Anaesthesiol* 24(5):474-475, 2007.
15. Deceuninck O et al: Images in cardiovascular medicine. Massive air embolism after central venous catheter removal, *Circulation* 116(19):e516-e518, 2007.
16. Wang AZ et al: The differences between venous air embolism and fat embolism in routine intraoperative monitoring methods, transesophageal echocardiography, and fatal volume in pigs, *J Trauma* 65(2):416-423, 2008.
17. Garnacho-Montero J et al: Risk factors and prognosis of catheter-related bloodstream infection in critically ill patients: a multicenter study, *Intensive Care Med* 34(12):2185-2193, 2008.
18. O'Grady NP et al: Guidelines for the prevention of intravascular catheter-related infections, *Infect Control Hosp Epidemiol* 23(12):759-769, 2002.
19. Boyce JM, Pittet D: Guideline for hand hygiene in health-care settings. Recommendations of the Healthcare Infection Control Practices Advisory Committee and the HIPAC/SHEA/APIC/IDSA Hand Hygiene Task Force, *Am J Infect Control* 30(8):S1-S46, 2002.
20. Dumont CP: Procedures nurses use to remove central venous catheters and complications they observe: a pilot study, *Am J Crit Care* 10(3):151-155, 2001.
21. Marx G, Reinhart K: Venous oximetry, *Curr Opin Crit Care* 12(3):263-268, 2006.
22. Ritzema J et al: Direct left atrial pressure monitoring in ambulatory heart failure patients: initial experience with a new permanent implantable device, *Circulation* 116(25):2952-2959, 2007.
23. Richard C et al: Early use of the pulmonary artery catheter and outcomes in patients with shock and acute respiratory distress syndrome: a randomized controlled trial, *JAMA* 290(20):2713-20, 2003.
24. Wheeler AP et al: Pulmonary-artery versus central venous catheter to guide treatment of acute lung injury, *N Engl J Med* 354(21):2213-2224, 2006.
25. Binanay C et al: Evaluation study of congestive heart failure and pulmonary artery catheterization effectiveness: the ESCAPE trial, *JAMA* 294(13):1625-1633, 2005.
26. Harvey S, Singer M: Managing critically ill patients with a pulmonary artery catheter, *Br J Hosp Med (Lond)* 67(8):421-426, 2006.
27. Harvey SE et al: Post hoc insights from PAC-Man—the U.K. pulmonary artery catheter trial, *Crit Care Med* 36(6):1714-1721, 2008.
28. Sandham JD et al: A randomized, controlled trial of the use of pulmonary-artery catheters in high-risk surgical patients, *N Engl J Med* 348(1):5-14, 2003.
29. Harvey S et al: Pulmonary artery catheters for adult patients in intensive care, *Cochrane Database Syst Rev* (3):CD003408, 2006.
30. Shah MR et al: Impact of the pulmonary artery catheter in critically ill patients: meta-analysis of randomized clinical trials, *JAMA* 294(13):1664-1670, 2005.
31. Bernard GR et al: Pulmonary artery catheterization and clinical outcomes: National Heart, Lung, and Blood Institute and Food and Drug Administration Workshop Report. Consensus statement, *JAMA* 283(19):2568-2572, 2000.
32. Wiener RS, Welch HG: Trends in the use of the pulmonary artery catheter in the United States, 1993-2004, *JAMA* 298(4):423-429 2007.
33. Cotter G et al: Hemodynamic monitoring in acute heart failure, *Crit Care Med* 36(1 suppl):S40-S43, 2008.
34. Zamanian RT et al: Management strategies for patients with pulmonary hypertension in the intensive care unit, *Crit Care Med* 35(9):2037-2050, 2007.
35. Marangelli V et al: Images in cardiovascular medicine. Three-dimensional imaging in rupture of papillary muscle after acute myocardial infarction, *Circulation* 111(23):e385-e387, 2005.
36. Coons JC, Seidl E: Cardiovascular pharmacotherapy update for the intensive care unit, *Crit Care Nurs Q* 30(1):44-57, 2007.
37. Dellinger RP et al: Surviving Sepsis Campaign: international guidelines for management of severe sepsis and septic shock: 2008, *Crit Care Med* 36(1):296-327, 2008.
38. Summerhill EM, Baram M: Principles of pulmonary artery catheterization in the critically ill, *Lung* 183(3):209-219, 2005.
39. Practice guidelines for pulmonary artery catheterization: an updated report by the American Society of Anesthesiologists Task Force on Pulmonary Artery Catheterization, *Anesthesiology* 99(4):988-1014, 2003.
40. Wiener B et al: Guideline development and education to insure accurate and consistent pulmonary artery wedge pressure measurement by nurses in intensive care units, *Dimens Crit Care Nurs* 26(6):263-268, 2007.
41. Bridges EJ: Pulmonary artery pressure monitoring: when, how, and what else to use, *AACN Adv Crit Care* 17(3):286-303, 2006.
42. Pinsky MR: Hemodynamic evaluation and monitoring in the ICU, *Chest* 132(6):2020-2029, 2007.
43. Frazier SK, Skinner GJ: Pulmonary artery catheters: state of the controversy, *J Cardiovasc Nurs* 23(2):113-121, 2008.
44. Antle DE: Ensuring competency in nurse repositioning of the pulmonary artery catheter, *Dimens Crit Care Nurs* 19(2):44-51, 2000.
45. Oztekin DS et al: Comparison of complications and procedural activities of pulmonary artery catheter removal by critical care nurses versus medical doctors, *Nurs Crit Care* 13(2):105-115, 2008.

46. Baldwin IC, Heland M: Incidence of cardiac dysrhythmias in patients during pulmonary artery catheter removal after cardiac surgery, *Heart Lung* 29(3):155-160, 2000.

47. Gawlinski A: Measuring cardiac output: intermittent bolus thermodilution method, *Crit Care Nurse* 20(2):118-120, 122-124, 2000.

48. Morgan P et al: Minimally invasive cardiac output monitoring, *Curr Opin Crit Care* 14(3):322-326, 2008.

49. Costa MG et al: Continuous and intermittent cardiac output measurement in hyperdynamic conditions: pulmonary artery catheter vs. lithium dilution technique, *Intensive Care Med* 34(2):257-263, 2008.

50. Cecconi M et al: A prospective study to evaluate the accuracy of pulse power analysis to monitor cardiac output in critically ill patients, *BMC Anesthesiol* 8:3, 2008.

51. Schmidt S et al: Effect of the venous catheter site on transpulmonary thermodilution measurement variables, *Crit Care Med* 35(3):783-786, 2007.

52. Hofer CK et al: What technique should I use to measure cardiac output? *Curr Opin Crit Care* 13(3):308-317, 2007.

53. Hamzaoui O et al: Effects of changes in vascular tone on the agreement between pulse contour and transpulmonary thermodilution cardiac output measurements within an up to 6-hour calibration-free period, *Crit Care Med* 36(2):434-440, 2008.

54. Button D et al: Clinical evaluation of the FloTrac/Vigileo system and two established continuous cardiac output monitoring devices in patients undergoing cardiac surgery, *Br J Anaesth* 99(3):329-336, 2007.

55. Prentice D, Sona C: Esophageal Doppler monitoring for hemodynamic assessment, *Crit Care Nurs Clin North Am* 18(2):189-193, 2006.

56. Turner MA: Doppler-based hemodynamic monitoring: a minimally invasive alternative, *AACN Clin Issues* 14(2):220-231, 2003.

57. Rivers E et al: Early goal-directed therapy in the treatment of severe sepsis and septic shock, *N Engl J Med* 345(19):1368-1377, 2001.

58. Jesurum J: Protocols for practice—SVO₂ monitoring, *Critical Care Nurse* 24(4):73-76, 2004.

59. Collaborative Study Group on Perioperative ScvO2 Monitoring: Multicentre study on peri- and postoperative central venous oxygen saturation in high-risk surgical patients, *Crit Care* 10(6):R158, 2006.

60. Ospina-Tascón GA et al: What type of monitoring has been shown to improve outcomes in acutely ill patients? *Intensive Care Med* 34(5):800-820, 2008.

61. Kligfield P et al: Recommendations for the standardization and interpretation of the electrocardiogram. Part I. The electrocardiogram and its technology: a scientific statement from the American Heart Association Electrocardiography and Arrhythmias Committee, Council on Clinical Cardiology; the American College of Cardiology Foundation; and the Heart Rhythm Society: endorsed by the International Society for Computerized Electrocardiology, *Circulation* 115(10):1306-1324, 2007.

62. Drew BJ et al: Practice standards for electrocardiographic monitoring in hospital settings: an American Heart Association scientific statement from the Councils on Cardiovascular Nursing, Clinical Cardiology, and Cardiovascular Disease in the Young: endorsed by the International Society of Computerized Electrocardiology and the American Association of Critical-Care Nurses, *Circulation* 110(17):2721-2746, 2004.

63. Drew BJ, Funk M: Practice standards for ECG monitoring in hospital settings: executive summary and guide for implementation, *Crit Care Nurs Clin North Am* 18(2):157-168, 2006.

64. Drew BJ: Pulling it all together: case studies on ECG monitoring, *AACN Adv Crit Care* 18(3):305-317, 2007.

65. Anderson JL et al: ACC/AHA 2007 guidelines for the management of patients with unstable angina/non ST-elevation myocardial infarction: a report of the American College of Cardiology/American Heart Association Task Force on Practice Guidelines (Writing Committee to Revise the 2002 Guidelines for the Management of Patients with Unstable Angina/Non ST-Elevation Myocardial Infarction): developed in collaboration with the American College of Emergency Physicians, the Society for Cardiovascular Angiography and Interventions, and the Society of Thoracic Surgeons: endorsed by the American Association of Cardiovascular and Pulmonary Rehabilitation and the Society for Academic Emergency Medicine, *Circulation* 116(7):e148-e304, 2007.

66. ST-Segment Monitoring, *Crit Care Nurse* 28(4):70-72, 2008.

67. Sommargren CE, Drew BJ: Preventing torsades de pointes by careful cardiac monitoring in hospital settings, *AACN Adv Crit Care* 18(3):285-293, 2007.

68. Roden DM: Drug-induced prolongation of the QT interval, *N Engl J Med* 350(10):1013-1022, 2004.

69. Jacobson C: Tools for teaching arrhythmias: wide QRS beats and rhythms—part II. QRS morphology clues, *AACN Adv Crit Care* 18(1):91-96, 2007.

70. Leeper B: Continuous ST-segment monitoring, *AACN Clin Issues* 14(2):145-154, 2003.

71. Pelter MM et al: Transient myocardial ischemia is an independent predictor of adverse in-hospital outcomes in patients with acute coronary syndromes treated in the telemetry unit, *Heart Lung* 32(2):71-78, 2003.

72. Tung P et al: Predictors of neurocardiogenic injury after subarachnoid hemorrhage, *Stroke* 35(2):548-551, 2004.

73. Pelter MM, Carey MG: P wave alterations, *Am J Crit Care* 16(2):187-188, 2007.

74. El-Menyar AA, Abdou SM: Impact of left bundle branch block and activation pattern on the heart, *Expert Rev Cardiovasc Ther* 6(6):843-857, 2008.

75. Pope JH et al: The impact of electrocardiographic left ventricular hypertrophy and bundle branch block on the triage and outcome of ED patients with a suspected acute coronary syndrome: a multicenter study, *Am J Emerg Med* 22(3):156-163, 2004.

76. Cheitlin MD et al: ACC/AHA/ASE 2003 guideline update for the clinical application of echocardiography: summary article: a report of the American College of Cardiology/American Heart Association Task Force on Practice Guidelines (ACC/AHA/ASE Committee to Update the 1997 Guidelines for the Clinical Application of Echocardiography), *Circulation* 108(9):1146-1162, 2003.

77. Antman EM et al: ACC/AHA guidelines for the management of patients with ST-elevation myocardial infarction—executive summary: a report of the American College of Cardiology/American Heart Association Task Force on Practice Guidelines (Writing Committee to Revise the 1999 Guidelines for the Management of Patients With Acute Myocardial Infarction), *Circulation* 110:588, 2004.

78. Birnbaum Y, Drew BJ: The electrocardiogram in ST elevation acute myocardial infarction: correlation with coronary anatomy and prognosis, *Postgrad Med J* 79(935):490-504, 2003.

79. Hinkle C, Stegall G: The possibility of obtaining 15- and 18-lead ECGs on all patients with myocardial infarction, *Crit Care Nurse* 20(2):125-126, 2000.

80. Pelter MM, Adams MG: ST segment changes in right bundle branch block, *Am J Crit Care* 14(4):341-342, 2005.

81. Pelter MM, Adams MG: Wide QRS duration, *Am J Crit Care* 13(4):355-356, 2004.

82. Elizari MV et al: Hemiblocks revisited, *Circulation* 115(9):1154-1163, 2007.

83. Goodman S et al: Supraventricular arrhythmias in intensive care unit patients: short and long-term consequences, *Anesth Analg* 104(4):880-886, 2007.

84. Annane D et al: Incidence and prognosis of sustained arrhythmias in critically ill patients, *Am J Respir Crit Care Med* 178(1):20-25, 2008.

85. Blomstrom-Lundqvist C et al: ACC/AHA/ESC guidelines for the management of patients with supraventricular arrhythmias—executive summary. a report of the American College of Cardiology/American Heart Association Task Force on Practice Guidelines and the European Society of Cardiology Committee for Practice Guidelines (Writing Committee to Develop Guidelines for the Management of Patients with Supraventricular Arrhythmias) developed in collaboration with NASPE-Heart Rhythm Society, *J Am Coll Cardiol* 42(8):1493-1531, 2003.

86. Yasuma F, Hayano J: Respiratory sinus arrhythmia: why does the heartbeat synchronize with respiratory rhythm? *Chest* 125(2):683-690, 2004.

87. Carey MG, Pelter MM: Rapid ventricular response, *Am J Crit Care* 17(1):83-84, 2008.

88. Pelter MM, Carey MG: Abnormal conduction, *Am J Crit Care* 17(2):173-174, 2008.

89. Fuster V et al: ACC/AHA/ESC 2006 Guidelines for the Management of Patients with Atrial Fibrillation: a report of the American College of Cardiology/American Heart Association Task Force on Practice Guidelines and the European Society of Cardiology Committee for Practice Guidelines (Writing Committee to Revise the 2001 Guidelines for the Management of Patients With Atrial Fibrillation): developed in collaboration with the European Heart Rhythm Association and the Heart Rhythm Society, *Circulation* 114(7):e257-e354, 2006.

90. Aronow WS: Etiology, pathophysiology, and treatment of atrial fibrillation. Part 1, *Cardiol Rev* 16(4):181-188, 2008.

91. Everett TH, Olgin JE: Basic mechanisms of atrial fibrillation, *Cardiol Clin* 22(1):9-20, 2004.

92. Calkins H et al: HRS/EHRA/ECAS expert consensus statement on catheter and surgical ablation of atrial fibrillation: recommendations for personnel, policy, procedures and follow-up. A report of the Heart Rhythm Society (HRS) Task Force on Catheter and Surgical Ablation of Atrial Fibrillation developed in partnership with the European Heart Rhythm Association (EHRA) and the European Cardiac Arrhythmia Society (ECAS); in collaboration with the American College of Cardiology (ACC), American Heart Association (AHA), and the Society of Thoracic Surgeons (STS). Endorsed and approved by the governing bodies of the American College of Cardiology, the American Heart Association, the European Cardiac Arrhythmia Society, the European Heart Rhythm Association, the Society of Thoracic Surgeons, and the Heart Rhythm Society, *Europace* 9(6):335-379, 2007.

93. Nemirovsky D et al: The electrical substrate of vagal atrial fibrillation as assessed by the signal-averaged electrocardiogram of the P wave, *Pacing Clin Electrophysiol* 31(3):308-313, 2008.

94. Crystal E, Connolly SJ: Atrial fibrillation: guiding lessons from epidemiology, *Cardiol Clin* 22(1):1-8, 2004.

95. Savelieva I, Camm J: Update on atrial fibrillation: part I, *Clin Cardiol* 31(2):55-62, 2008.

96. Eagle KA et al: American College of Cardiology; American Heart Association: ACC/AHA 2004 guideline update for coronary artery bypass graft surgery: a report of the American College of Cardiology/American Heart Association Task Force on Practice Guidelines (Committee to Update the 1999 Guidelines for Coronary Artery Bypass Graft Surgery), *Circulation* 110(14):e340-e437, 2004.

97. Kern LS: Postoperative atrial fibrillation: new directions in prevention and treatment, *J Cardiovasc Nurs* 19(2):103-115, 2004.

98. Kern LS et al: ECG monitoring after cardiac surgery: postoperative atrial fibrillation and the atrial electrogram, *AACN Adv Crit Care* 18(3):294-304, 2007.

99. Bradley D et al: Pharmacologic prophylaxis: American College of Chest Physicians guidelines for the prevention and management of postoperative atrial fibrillation after cardiac surgery, *Chest* 128(2 suppl):39S-47S, 2005.

100. Miller JN, Drew BJ: Atrial electrograms after cardiac surgery: survey of clinical practice, *Am J Crit Care* 16(4):350-356, 2007.

101. Kellen JC: Implications for nursing care of patients with atrial fibrillation: lessons learned from the AFFIRM and RACE studies, *J Cardiovasc Nurs* 19(2):128-137, 2004.

102. Weiss EM, Buescher T: Atrial fibrillation: treatment options and caveats, *AACN Clinical Issues* 15(3):362-376, 2004.

103. Singer DE et al: Antithrombotic therapy in atrial fibrillation: American College of Chest Physicians Evidence-Based Clinical Practice Guidelines (8th edition), *Chest* 133(6 suppl):546S-592S, 2008.

104. Stroke Risk in Atrial Fibrillation Working Group: Independent predictors of stroke in patients with atrial fibrillation: a systematic review, *Neurology* 69(6):546-554, 2007.

105. Knight BP et al: Role of permanent pacing to prevent atrial fibrillation: science advisory from the American Heart Association Council on Clinical Cardiology (Subcommittee on Electrocardiography and Arrhythmias) and the Quality of Care and Outcomes Research Interdisciplinary Working Group, in collaboration with the Heart Rhythm Society, *Circulation* 111(2):240-243, 2005.

106. Gillinov AM, Saltman AE: Surgical approaches for atrial fibrillation, *Med Clin North Am* 92(1):203-215, 2008.

107. Noheria A et al: Catheter ablation vs antiarrhythmic drug therapy for atrial fibrillation: a systematic review, *Arch Intern Med* 168(6):581-586, 2008.

108. Yamada T, Kay GN: Evidence-based approach to ablating atrial fibrillation, *Curr Cardiol Rep* 9(5):366-370, 2007.

109. Roden DM: Proarrhythmia as a pharmacogenomic entity: a critical review and formulation of a unifying hypothesis, *Cardiovasc Res* 67(3):419-425, 2005.

110. Jacobson C: Tools for teaching arrhythmias: wide QRS beats and rhythms. Part I. P waves, fusion, and capture beats, *AACN Adv Crit Care* 17(4):462-465, 2006.

111. Goldberger ZD et al: Approach to the diagnosis and initial management of the stable adult patient with a wide complex tachycardia, *Am J Cardiol* 101(10):1456-1466, 2008.

112. Berdajs D et al: Incidence and pathophysiology of atrioventricular block following mitral valve replacement and ring annuloplasty, *Eur J Cardiothorac Surg* 34(1):55-61, 2008.

113. Paul S: Understanding advanced concepts in atrioventricular block, *Crit Care Nurse* 21(1):56-66, 2001.

114. Adams-Hamoda MG, Pelter MM: Heart blocks, *Am J Crit Care* 12(1):77-78, 2003.

115. Pelter MM, Carey MG: Slow escape rhythms, *Am J Crit Care* 16(4):405-406, 2007.

116. Freeman K et al: Effects of presentation and electrocardiogram on time to treatment of hyperkalemia, *Acad Emerg Med* 15(3):239-249, 2008.

117. Sladdin C, Lee G: Safely treating hypokalaemia in high dependency cardiac surgical patients, *Nurs Crit Care* 11(6):267-272, 2006.

118. Ariyan CE, Sosa JA: Assessment and management of patients with abnormal calcium, *Crit Care Med* 32(4 suppl):S146-S154, 2004.

119. Dickerson RN et al: Low serum total calcium concentration as a marker of low serum ionized calcium concentration in critically ill patients receiving specialized nutrition support, *Nutr Clin Pract* 22(3):323-328, 2007.

120. Dickerson RN et al: Accuracy of methods to estimate ionized and "corrected" serum calcium concentrations in critically ill multiple trauma patients receiving specialized nutrition support, *JPEN J Parenter Enteral Nutr* 28(3):133-141, 2004.

121. Ma G et al: Electrocardiographic manifestations: digitalis toxicity, *J Emerg Med* 20(2):145-152, 2001.

122. Zivin JR et al: Hypocalcemia: a pervasive metabolic abnormality in the critically ill, *Am J Kidney Dis* 37(4):689-698, 2001.

123. Dickerson RN et al: Dose-dependent characteristics of intravenous calcium therapy for hypocalcemic critically ill trauma patients receiving specialized nutritional support, *Nutrition* 23(1):9-15, 2007.

124. Noronha JL, Matuschak GM: Magnesium in critical illness: metabolism, assessment, and treatment, *Intensive Care Med* 28(6):667-679, 2002.

125. 2005 American Heart Association guidelines for cardiopulmonary resuscitation and emergency cardiovascular care. *Circulation*; 112(24 suppl): IV1-196, 2005.

126. Novis DA et al: Biochemical markers of myocardial injury test turnaround time: a College of American Pathologists Q-Probes study of 7020 troponin and 4368 creatine kinase-MB determinations in 159 institutions, *Arch Pathol Lab Med* 128(2):158-164, 2004.

127. Lin JC et al: Rates of positive cardiac troponin I and creatine kinase MB mass among patients hospitalized for suspected acute coronary syndromes, *Clin Chem* 50(2):333-338, 2004.

128. Correa de Sa DD, Chen HH: The role of natriuretic peptides in heart failure, *Curr Cardiol Rep* 10(3):182-189, 2008.

129. Maisel A: Circulating natriuretic peptide levels in acute heart failure, *Rev Cardiovasc Med* 8(suppl 5):S13-S21, 2007.

130. Ansell J et al: Pharmacology and management of the vitamin K antagonists: American College of Chest Physicians Evidence-Based Clinical Practice Guidelines (8th edition), *Chest* 133(6 suppl):160S-198S, 2008.

131. Grundy SM et al: Implications of recent clinical trials for the National Cholesterol Education Program Adult Treatment Panel III guidelines, *Circulation* 110(2):227-239, 2004.

132. Grundy SM et al: Diagnosis and management of the metabolic syndrome: an American Heart Association/National Heart, Lung, and Blood Institute Scientific Statement, *Circulation* 112(17):2735-2752, 2005.

133. Attin M: Electrophysiology study: a comprehensive review, *Am J Crit Care* 10(4):260-273, 2001.

134. Trotman-Dickenson B: Radiology in the intensive care unit (part 1), *J Intensive Care Med* 18(4):198-210, 2003.

135. American College of Radiology (ACR): ACR practice guideline for the performance of pediatric and adult chest radiography, 2004. Available at www.acr.org (accessed February 2009).

136. Clec'h C et al: Are daily routine chest radiographs useful in critically ill, mechanically ventilated patients? A randomized study, *Intensive Care Med* 34(2):264-270, 2008.

137. Trotman-Dickenson B: Radiology in the intensive care unit (part 2), *J Intensive Care Med* 18(5):239-252, 2003.

138. Gibbons RJ et al: ACC/AHA 2002 guideline update for exercise testing: summary article: a report of the American College of Cardiology/American Heart Association Task Force on Practice Guidelines (Committee to Update the 1997 Exercise Testing Guidelines), *Circulation* 106(14): 1883-1892, 2002.

139. Marcus FI et al: Evaluation of the normal values for signal-averaged electrocardiogram, *J Cardiovasc Electrophysiol* 18(2):231-233, 2007.

140. Vieillard-Baron A et al: Echocardiography in the intensive care unit: from evolution to revolution?, *Intensive Care Med* 34(2):243-249, 2008.

141. Gueret P et al: Echocardiographic assessment of the incidence of mechanical complications during the early phase of myocardial infarction in the reperfusion era: a French multicentre prospective registry, *Arch Cardiovasc Dis* 101(1):41-47, 2008.

142. Mor-Avi V et al: Three-dimensional adult echocardiography: where the hidden dimension helps, *Curr Cardiol Rep* 10(3):218-225, 2008.

143. Quiñones MA et al: ACC/AHA clinical competence statement on echocardiography: a report of the American College of Cardiology/American Heart Association/American College of Physicians-American Society of Internal Medicine Task Force on clinical competence, *J Am Soc Echocardiogr* 16(4):379-402, 2003.

144. Douglas PS et al: ACCF/ASE/ACEP/AHA/ASNC/SCAI/SCCT/SCMR 2008 appropriateness criteria for stress echocardiography: a report of the American College of Cardiology Foundation Appropriateness Criteria Task Force, American Society of Echocardiography, American College of Emergency Physicians, American Heart Association, American Society of Nuclear Cardiology, Society for Cardiovascular Angiography and Interventions, Society of Cardiovascular Computed Tomography, and Society for Cardiovascular Magnetic Resonance: endorsed by the Heart Rhythm Society and the Society of Critical Care Medicine, *Circulation* 117(11): 1478-1497, 2008.

145. Picano E et al: The diagnostic accuracy of pharmacological stress echocardiography for the assessment of coronary artery disease: a meta-analysis, *Cardiovasc Ultrasound* 6:30, 2008.

146. McKay CR, Shavelle DM: Intravascular ultrasound in the coronary arteries, *Semin Vasc Surg* 19(3):132-138, 2006.

147. Constantine G et al: Role of MRI in clinical cardiology, *Lancet* 363 (9427):2162-2171, 2004.

148. Shan K et al: Role of cardiac magnetic resonance imaging in the assessment of myocardial viability, *Circulation* 109(11):1328-1334, 2004.

149. Klocke FJ et al: ACC/AHA/ASNC guidelines for the clinical use of cardiac radionuclide imaging–executive summary: a report of the American College of Cardiology/American Heart Association Task Force on Practice Guidelines (ACC/AHA/ASNC Committee to Revise the 1995 Guidelines for the Clinical Use of Cardiac Radionuclide Imaging), *J Am Coll Cardiol* 42(7):1318-1333, 2003.

150. Rerkpattanapipat P, Hundley WG: Dobutamine stress magnetic resonance imaging, *Echocardiography* 24(3):309-315, 2007.

Cardiovascular Disorders

Cardiovascular disease remains the leading cause of mortality in the United States. The estimated direct and indirect national cost in 2008 is $448.5 billion.[1] Cardiovascular diseases are the leading cause of death for women and men. There are almost 80 million adults in the United States living with cardiovascular disease. Cardiovascular disease accounts for one of every 2.8 deaths in the United States.[1] In terms of disability, the number of disability-adjusted life-years (DALYs) attributable to cardiovascular disease on a global basis is projected to double by the year 2020.[1] An understanding of the pathology of cardiovascular disease processes and clinical management allows the critical care nurse to accurately anticipate and plan interventions. This chapter focuses on cardiac disorders commonly seen in the critical care environment.

CORONARY ARTERY DISEASE

DESCRIPTION AND ETIOLOGY

The biggest contributor to cardiovascular-related morbidity and mortality is *coronary artery disease* (CAD). *Atherosclerosis* is a progressive disease that affects arteries throughout the body. In the heart, atherosclerotic changes are clinically known as CAD. This disease process is also known by the term *coronary heart disease* (CHD) because other heart structures ultimately become involved in the disease process. The atherosclerotic vascular changes that lead to CAD may begin in childhood.[2] Research and epidemiologic data collected during the past 50 years have demonstrated a strong association between specific risk factors and the development of CAD.[1] These risk factors are further delineated as nonmodifiable and modifiable coronary risk factors (Box 19-1).

RISK FACTORS FOR CORONARY ARTERY DISEASE

Age, Gender, and Race. The severe effects of CAD occur as a person ages. In general, CAD symptoms are seen in middle and old age.[1] Traditionally, CAD has been regarded as a male disease, but it is increasingly obvious that in modern society it affects both genders.[1] The average age for a person having a first heart attack is 65.8 years for men and 70.4 years for women.[1] Men typically develop external manifestations of the disease about 5 to 10 years earlier than women. Starting at age 75 years, the prevalence of cardiovascular disease is higher among women than men.[2,3] CAD rates for postmenopausal women are two to three times higher than those for premenopausal women of the same age.[1] People of color and multiracial populations of both genders have higher CAD mortality rates than do white populations of similar socioeconomic status.[1]

Family History. A positive family history is one in which a close blood relative has had a myocardial infarction (MI) or stroke before the age of 60. This family history suggests a genetic or lifestyle predisposition to the development of CAD. Individuals with a family history had a 50% greater risk of having an acute MI in the INTERHEART study.[4] This was a large, international, standardized case-control study of similar cohorts in 52 countries that was designed to examine the importance of risk factors for CAD on a worldwide basis.[4]

Hyperlipidemia. Hyperlipidemia is a leading factor responsible for severe atherosclerosis and the development of CAD. Determining total serum cholesterol and triglyceride levels is a helpful start in the evaluation process.[3,5] A lipid panel blood test can measure the following values:

- High-density lipoprotein (HDL) cholesterol
- Low-density lipoprotein (LDL) cholesterol
- Very-low-density lipoprotein (VLDL) cholesterol
- Triglycerides

Treatment of hyperlipidemia has advanced beyond the concept of lowering total cholesterol to treatment of specific lipoprotein abnormalities.[3,6-8] The target levels for specific serum lipids are listed in Table 19-1.

Total Cholesterol. The total cholesterol is the sum of the HDL, LDL, and VLDL cholesterol in the bloodstream. It is used as a starting point for lipid testing. A total cholesterol level higher than 200 mg/dL is an indication to investigate the lipid profile and other risk factors for CAD. More than 105 million American adults have a total blood cholesterol level at or above 200 mg/dL.[1]

High-Density Lipoprotein Cholesterol. HDL cholesterol is frequently described as the "good cholesterol" because higher serum levels exert a protective effect against acute atherosclerotic events. All the reasons are not completely understood, but one recognized physiologic effect is the ability of HDL to promote the efflux of cholesterol from cells. This process may minimize the accumulation of foam cells in the artery wall and decrease the risk of developing atherosclerosis.[9] High HDL

BOX 19-1   CORONARY ARTERY DISEASE RISK FACTORS

NONMODIFIABLE RISK FACTORS
- Age
- Gender
- Family history
- Race

MODIFIABLE RISK FACTORS
- Elevated serum lipids
- Hypertension
- Cigarette smoking
- Prediabetes or diabetes mellitus
- Diet high in saturated fat, cholesterol, and calories
- Elevated homocysteine level
- Metabolic syndrome
- Obesity
- Physical inactivity
- Postmenopause (modification is controversial)

TABLE 19-1   Lipid Guidelines and Risk for Coronary Artery Disease

Lipid	Target Value* (mg/dL)
Total cholesterol	<200
HDL cholesterol	
Men	>40
Women	>50
LDL cholesterol	
Very high risk	<70
High risk	<100
Low risk	<130
VLDL cholesterol	<30
Triglycerides	<150

*Values outside the target range increase the risk for coronary artery disease.
HDL, high-density lipoprotein; LDL, low-density lipoprotein; VLDL, very-low-density lipoprotein.

cholesterol levels confer antiinflammatory and antioxidant benefits on the arterial wall.[9] In contrast, a low HDL cholesterol level is an independent risk factor for the development of CAD and other atherosclerotic conditions. HDL cholesterol is generally higher in women, and levels can be raised by physical exercise and by stopping smoking. In patients with low HDL cholesterol levels, when lifestyle changes are ineffective, the HDL level can be raised by drugs such as extended-release nicotinic acid (niacin) and fibrates. In 2005, 17% of the adult U.S. population had HDL cholesterol levels below 40 mg/dL.[1]

Low-Density Lipoprotein Cholesterol. LDL cholesterol is usually described as the "bad cholesterol" because high levels are associated with an increased risk of acute coronary syndrome, stroke, and peripheral arterial disease (PAD). High

LDL levels initiate the atherosclerotic process by infiltrating the vessel wall and binding to the matrix of cells beneath the endothelium.[9] LDL cholesterol also exerts an inflammatory effect on the arterial vessel wall.[9] A high LDL cholesterol level is initially managed by nonpharmacologic lifestyle changes such as weight loss, smoking cessation, low-fat diet, physical exercise, and attainment of a normal body size as measured by the body mass index (BMI). If lifestyle changes are insufficient to reduce the LDL cholesterol level in the bloodstream, the drug category of choice is a *statin*. Numerous research studies have conclusively demonstrated that lowering the LDL cholesterol with statins for primary or secondary prevention is highly effective in lowering mortality due to CAD.[1,3] Therapy should be tailored to treat the individual cardiovascular risk profile. The target LDL cholesterol is determined according to the individual's risk profile as described in Table 19-1. Patients at highest risk are advised to maintain LDL cholesterol below 70 mg/dL; those at high risk, a level below 100 mg/dL; and those at low risk, LDL below 130 mg/dL. Controversy exists about whether the tiered LDL goals in the current guidelines are sufficiently low to prevent coronary atherosclerosis developing in persons without CAD. Some cardiologists advocate a reduction of the LDL goal to 50 to 70 mg/dL range for everyone, not just those with a known cardiovascular disease.[10] In 2005, 33% of the adult U.S. population had LDL cholesterol levels of 130 mg/dL or higher.[1]

Very-Low-Density Lipoprotein Cholesterol. VLDL cholesterol is not usually measured, although a normal value is about 30 mg/dL.[6] The value can be estimated by subtracting the sum of the HDL and LDL from the total cholesterol. When triglyceride levels are elevated, the VLDL cholesterol level also is high.

Triglycerides. Triglycerides are serum lipids that constitute an additional atherogenic risk factor. Triglycerides are carried by VLDL cholesterol in the bloodstream.[7] An optimal triglyceride level is below 150 mg/dL, and the more elevated the triglyceride serum level, the higher the risk of developing CAD. A value between 150 and 199 mg/dL is borderline high; a value between 200 and 500 mg/dL is high; and a value above 500 mg/dL signals a high risk of atherogenic complications and a strong risk for the presence or development of type 2 diabetes.

Lipoprotein(a). LDL cholesterol can be further analyzed by the category of lipid particles that make up the total LDL value. Researchers have investigated the function of several lipid particles to determine their role in the development of premature atherosclerotic CAD. One particle that has been extensively studied is *lipoprotein(a),* which is abbreviated Lp(a) and described verbally as "LP little a." Lp(a) is manufactured in the liver and circulates in the bloodstream bound to a large glycoprotein called *apolipoprotein(a),* abbreviated as apo(a).[11] The Lp(a)-apo(a) lipid particle concentration is elevated in the presence of inflammation, and it stimulates atheroma and clot formation in inflamed arteries.[11] This effect is thought to occur because the apo(a) is structurally similar to plasminogen, a protein essential for clot formation.

Lp(a) levels are 90% genetically determined. Elevated Lp(a) plasma levels constitute the most frequently encountered genetic lipid disorder in families with premature CAD.[11] Testing for Lp(a) is reserved for high-risk patient populations such as those with a strong family history of premature atherosclerotic disease and for patients with premature CAD who do not exhibit the expected cardiac risk factors. Reduction of Lp(a) levels to below 30 mg/dL is the therapeutic goal. This usually is achieved by ingesting high doses (3 to 4 g/day) of extended-release nicotinic acid (niacin). The Lp(a) level is not reduced by statins, drugs that traditionally lower LDL levels, or by physical exercise, a low-fat diet, weight loss, or tight control of blood glucose levels.[11] Lifestyle changes are recommended, and research is ongoing, but a cure is not yet discernible.

High-Fat Diet. A diet rich in saturated fats leads to elevated cholesterol levels in the blood. The first line of treatment to lower elevated serum cholesterol is a low-fat, high-fiber diet and increased physical exercise.[7,8] If these measures are not effective, lipid-lowering drugs are indicated.[1] This approach sounds simple, but less than one half of the people who qualify for lipid reduction therapy are taking their medications; only one third of treated patients reach their LDL target; and one half of patients prescribed a lipid-lowering drug stop taking it 6 months after starting it.[1] Although the drugs are very helpful for some, they are not a panacea for everyone.

Obesity. Obesity is a disease of modern times. Global estimates are more than 1 billion overweight adults, and at least 300 million of these people are obese. Obesity is often associated with a sedentary lifestyle. A high risk of coronary heart disease is among the well-established adverse health effects associated with excess weight. Hypertension, hypercholesterolemia, and diabetes are among the clinical conditions that are important mediators of this association.[12] In the United States in 2001, 122 million adults were overweight or obese.[13] In 2005, 66% of the U.S. population were overweight, and 31.4% were obese.[1] Obesity is defined using the BMI.

The BMI is a mathematic formula used to assess body weight relative to height. BMI is used to evaluate the threat of excess pounds as a risk factor for CAD and permits comparisons of people of different gender, age, height, and body type.[1] BMI is calculated as the weight in kilograms divided by the square of the height in meters (kg/m^2). The BMI calculation in metric and English units (pounds, inches) is shown in Box 19-2. A normal BMI is between 18.5 and 25 kg/m^2. A BMI between 25 and 30 kg/m^2 indicates the person is overweight. A BMI greater than 30 kg/m^2 is the definition of obesity.[1]

The distribution pattern of fat on the body is a CAD risk factor. The more weight carried in the abdominal area, producing a large waist, the greater the risk of CAD. Excess abdominal adiposity (apple body shape) indicates additional fat around the abdominal organs compared with individuals who have a smaller waist and larger hips (pear body shape). A waist size greater than 40 inches in men and 35 inches in women increases their risk for CAD. Physical exercise assists with weight reduction, lowers the risk for CAD, and decreases the risk of developing type 2 diabetes.

Physical Inactivity. Regular vigorous physical activity using large muscle groups promotes physiologic adaptation to aerobic exercise that can prevent the development of CAD and reduce symptoms in patients with established

---

BOX 19-2 HOW TO CALCULATE AND INTERPRET BODY MASS INDEX

USE A CALCULATOR TO DETERMINE THE BODY MASS INDEX (BMI)

Metric Units: Divide body weight in kilograms by height in meters; divide the result by height in meters:

$$BMI = (Weight_{kg}/Height_m) \div Height_m$$

Example: A person weighs 100 kg and is 1.90 m tall:

$$BMI = 100/1.90 \div 1.90 = 27.7$$

Pounds/Inches: Divide body weight in pounds by height in inches, divide that result by height in inches, and multiply by 703:

$$BMI = (Weight_{lb}/Height_{in}) \div Height_{in} \times 703$$

Example: A person weighs 222 pounds and is 6 feet 3 inches (75 inches) tall:

$$BMI = 222/75 \div 75 \times 703 = 27.7$$

HOW TO INTERPRET THE BMI RESULT

BMI (kg/m^2)	Weight Status
<18.5	Underweight
18.5-24.9	Normal weight
25-29.5	Overweight
>30	Obese

---

cardiovascular disease.[14] Exercise also reduces the incidence of many other diseases, including type 2 diabetes, osteoporosis, obesity, depression, and cancers of the colon and breast.[14] Many research trials have demonstrated the positive effects of physical activity on the other major cardiac risk factors.[14] Exercise alters the lipid profile by decreasing LDL cholesterol and triglyceride levels and increasing HDL cholesterol levels.[14] Exercise reduces insulin resistance at the cellular level, lowering the risk for developing type 2 diabetes, especially if combined with a weight-loss program.[14] Epidemiologic studies indicate that physical athletics as a young person do not confer protection in later years. A sedentary lifestyle has negative effects, regardless of age, gender, BMI, smoking status, presence or absence of hypertension, or abnormal lipoprotein profile. Lifelong physical activity is necessary to prevent atherosclerotic CAD and stroke.[14] The prevalence of adults not engaging in physical activity in the United States in 2006 was 30.9%.[1] In affluent countries, only one third of the population exercises moderately for the recommended 30 minutes, five times per week.

Hypertension. Normal blood pressure is described as a systolic blood pressure (SBP) below 120 mm Hg and a diastolic blood pressure (DBP) below 80 mm Hg. *Hypertension* is defined as an SBP greater than 140 mm Hg or DBP higher than 90 mm Hg. *Controlled hypertension* describes a situation in which administration of antihypertensive medications maintains the patient's blood pressure within the normal range.

Hypertension is a cardiac risk factor because the high SBP damages the arterial endothelium, leading to vascular inflammation that encourages formation of plaque. Hypertension is a complex, multifactorial disease process. Hypertension is divided into stages for the purposes of treatment, as shown in Table 19-2.

Prehypertension is an SBP of 120 to 139 mm Hg or DBP above 85 mm Hg.[1,13] In the United States, one in five adults

TABLE 19-2 Blood Pressure Guidelines and Risk for Coronary Artery Disease

Category	Systolic BP* (mm Hg)	Diastolic BP* (mm Hg)
Normal (optimal)*	<120	<80
Prehypertension	120-139	80-89
Stage 1 hypertension	140-159	90-99
Stage 2 hypertension	≥160	≥100

*Values greater than normal increase the risk for CAD and heart failure.
BP, blood pressure; CAD, coronary artery disease.

is prehypertensive. *Hypertension* is diagnosed when the blood pressure is above 140/90 mm Hg. Hypertension affects another one in four adults in the United States. After the blood pressure is above 140/80 mm Hg, hypertension is described as stage 1 or stage 2 (see Table 19-2).

Hypertension is often described as the "silent killer," because 30% of those affected are unaware they have seriously elevated blood pressure.[1] In the United States, one person in three has hypertension. Of those who know that they are hypertensive, 34% are on medication and have their blood pressure controlled; 25% are on medication but do not have their blood pressure under control; and 11% are hypertensive but are not taking any medication.[1] A higher percentage of men than women have hypertension until age 45, but from the ages of 45 to 54 years, the percentage of men and women with hypertension is similar.[1] It is essential that patients understand that sustained elevation of blood pressure leads inexorably toward atherosclerosis, heart failure, kidney failure, stroke, and heart attack.[13] So widespread is hypertension in industrialized societies that even a normotensive person at age 55 has a 90% lifetime risk of developing hypertension. This implies that even normotensive persons should adopt interventions to maintain a normal blood pressure.[13] The estimated direct and indirect cost of hypertension in the United States for 2008 is $69.4 billion.[1]

According to recent guidelines, the goal of treatment for the hypertensive person without other risk factors is to achieve a blood pressure below 140/80 mm Hg. For the hypertensive person who already has diabetes or kidney disease, the target blood pressure is below 130/80 mm Hg. A normal blood pressure is below 120/80 mm Hg.[13]

Lifestyle interventions that can normalize blood pressure include physical exercise, a low-salt diet, limiting alcohol intake, and achieving normal body weight. Most patients are started on a diuretic, and if this is insufficient, they may be placed on an angiotensin-converting enzyme inhibitor (ACEI), angiotensin receptor blocker (ARB), beta-blocker, or calcium channel blocker. Most patients require at least two medications, each from different drug classifications, to normalize their blood pressure.[13] Hypertensive emergencies with acute organ damage are discussed in the last section of this chapter.

Cigarette Smoking.
The greater the number of cigarettes smoked per day, the greater the risk of developing CAD, acute MI, and stroke.[1,14,16] In the United States, the prevalence of

smoking has always been lower among women than men.[1] Cigarette smoking unfavorably alters serum lipid levels, decreases the HDL cholesterol level, and increases LDL cholesterol and triglyceride levels. In the United States, smoking remains common, representing 20.9% of the adult population. Smoking increases the risk of coronary heart disease at all levels, including less than 5 cigarettes per day.[1] Smokers are two to four times more likely to develop CAD than nonsmokers.[1] Passive, secondhand smoke exposure also increases cardiovascular risk, and 34.7% of nonsmoking adults are exposed to environmental tobacco smoke at home or at work.[1,15-17]

Within 1 year of giving up cigarettes, an ex-smoker's risk of developing CAD decreases by 50%. With 15 smoke-free years, a person's risk falls to almost that of a lifetime nonsmoker.[1] Nicotine is addictive, and giving up smoking is difficult. People need tremendous support to be able to "kick the habit." The good news is that many do quit, and since 1965, smoking in the United States has declined by more than 40% among adults.[1] Chapter 25 provides patient education guidelines on how to stop smoking.

Diabetes Mellitus.
Individuals with diabetes mellitus (types 1 and 2) have a higher incidence of coronary heart disease than the general population. Data from the Framingham Heart Study indicates a doubling in the incidence of diabetes over the past 30 years and most dramatically during the 1990s.[1] Elevated blood glucose level is a known risk factor for development of vascular inflammation associated with atherosclerosis. The normoglycemia range is 70 to 110 mg/dL. It is recommended that patients in critical care have blood glucose levels maintained close to the normal range,[18] while avoiding hypoglycemic episodes.

A fasting blood glucose concentration between 110 and 125 mg/dL represents a prediabetic state and is a risk factor for the development of diabetes and CAD (Table 19-3). The upper limit for a normal fasting plasma glucose level is 126 mg/dL. Patients with diabetes have an increased risk of developing CAD and have worse clinical outcomes after acute coronary syndrome events.[19] In a multinational study of patients who were seen at hospitals with symptoms of acute coronary syndrome, almost one in four had a known history of diabetes.[20] More detailed information on type 2 diabetes and the use of insulin and oral medications to control blood glucose levels and combat insulin resistance is included in Chapters 36 and 37.

Chronic Kidney Disease.
Chronic kidney disease is considered a risk equivalent for CAD.[2,3,21] This means patients with chronic kidney disease have as much risk of experiencing a coronary event as if they already had CAD.[2,3,22] The risk of death for the patient with acute MI rises as the serum creatinine level increases.[22] In one study, the in-hospital mortality rates for patients with an acute MI were 2% for patients with normal kidney function, 6% for those with mild kidney failure, 14% for those with moderate kidney failure, 21% for those with severe kidney failure, and 30% for patients with end-stage kidney disease.[22]

Metabolic Syndrome.
Metabolic syndrome refers to the clustering of risk factors associated with cardiovascular disease and type 2 diabetes.[1] The age-adjusted prevalence of metabolic

TABLE 19-3   Fasting Blood Glucose and Risk for Coronary Artery Disease

Blood Glucose Level	Fasting Plasma Glucose Level* (mg/dL)
Normal	70-100
Prediabetic	100-125
Diabetic	126 or higher

*Values greater than normal increase the risk for CAD and kidney failure.
CAD, coronary artery disease.

TABLE 19-4   Blood Homocysteine Levels and Risk for Coronary Artery Disease

Category	Homocysteine Plasma Level* (mmol/L)
Normal homocysteine	5-15
Moderate risk	16-30
Intermediate risk	30-100
High risk	>100

Modified from Reeder SJ et al: Homocysteine: the latest risk factor for heart disease, *Dimens Crit Care Nurs* 19(1):22-28, 2000.
*Values greater than normal increase the risk for coronary artery disease.

syndrome in 2006 for adults in the United States was 23.9%.[1] The following are risk factors[23]:

1. Waist circumference greater than 40 inches (102 cm) in men and greater than 35 inches (88 cm) in women
2. Serum triglyceride level greater than 150 mg/dL ($\geq$1.7 mmol/L)
3. High-density lipoprotein (HDL) cholesterol level less than 40 mg/dL ($\leq$1.04 mmol/L) in men; less than 50 mg/dL ($\leq$1.29 mmol/L) in women
4. Blood pressure 130/85 mm Hg or higher, which is diagnostic for prehypertension or hypertension
5. Fasting glucose level is 100 to 110 mg/dL, which is diagnostic for prediabetes. A fasting blood glucose level greater than 126 mg/dL is diagnostic for diabetes.

It is perhaps obvious that individuals with the signs of metabolic syndrome are at increased risk for CAD; even so, it is surprising to what degree this holds true. In the Framingham epidemiologic study, presence of the factors associated with metabolic syndrome predicted 25% of all new-onset CAD and almost 50% of new-onset diabetes.[23]

Women and Heart Disease: Premenopause and Postmenopause. Serious CAD symptoms occur approximately 5 years later in women than in men.[24] The average age for the first acute MI in men is 65.8 years and in women is 70.4 years.[1] Incidence of CAD is two to three times higher among postmenopausal women than women who are premenopausal.[1] In the past, it seemed logical to prescribe *hormone replacement therapy* (HRT) to treat the symptoms of menopause. However, well-designed research trials discovered an increase in cardiovascular events in the first year of HRT (estrogen plus progestin), although cardiac events declined after the first year.[24,25] Subsequent studies have confirmed this result.[24] In 2004, the estrogen-only HRT trial was stopped by the National Institutes of Health (NIH) because of an increased risk of stroke among the women taking estrogen. For these reasons, HRT is no longer recommended for prevention of atherosclerotic cardiovascular disease.[26] Data from the Framingham Heart Study indicate the lifetime risk for cardiovascular disease is more than one in two for women at age 40.[1]

Cardiovascular disease kills more than one-half million women annually in the United States. To emphasize the magnitude of the problem, this represents more deaths than the next seven fatal diseases for women combined.[27] Mortality rates for women after an acute MI are higher than for men: 38% and

25%, respectively. Risk factors more strongly associated with acute MI in women compared to men include hypertension, diabetes mellitus, alcohol intake and physical inactivity.[25] Many reasons contribute to women having higher mortality from acute MI, including waiting longer to seek medical care, having smaller coronary arteries, being older when symptoms occur, and experiencing very different symptoms from those of men of the same age.[28] The 2007 evidence-based guidelines for cardiovascular disease prevention in women recommended a scheme for a general approach to the female patient that classifies her as high risk, at risk, or at optimal risk.[27] In 2007, 50% of women surveyed by the American Heart Association (AHA) recognized that heart disease was the leading cause of death among women. Risk factors more strongly associated with MI in women compared with men include hypertension, diabetes mellitus, alcohol intake, and physical inactivity.[27]

Hyperhomocysteinemia. Homocysteine plays an essential part in protein metabolism. It is a derivative of methionine, an amino acid found in dietary protein. Homocysteine is metabolized in the body by two metabolic pathways; one pathway requires folate and vitamin B_6, and the other depends on vitamin B_{12}.[29] A person missing these vitamins is unable to metabolize homocysteine. *Hyperhomocysteinemia,* or elevated levels of homocysteine in the bloodstream, is acquired or occurs as a genetic error of metabolism.[29] High levels are of concern because of the association with atherosclerotic CAD, stroke, and peripheral arterial disease. An optimal level of plasma homocysteine is thought to be between 5 and 15 mmol/L.[29,30] Between 5% and 7% of the population may have mild homocystinemia. Plasma levels associated with hyperhomocysteinemia are shown in Table 19-4.[29] High plasma homocysteine levels are associated with adverse cardiovascular events. Elevated homocysteine levels may be reduced by consumption of a varied diet with B vitamins. Typical nutritional sources of vitamin B_6, B_{12}, and folic acid which provides folate, are shown in Table 19-5. Individuals at high risk may need to take daily multiple vitamin supplements containing vitamins B_6, B_{12}, and folic acid.[30]

Vascular Inflammation. The link between vascular inflammation and atherosclerotic disease is well established.[31] However, measurement of this link has been more controversial.[31] Many researchers think the development of atherosclerotic

TABLE 19-5 Food Sources of Vitamin B₆, Vitamin B₁₂, and Folic Acid

Vitamin	RDA	Sources
B₆	2 mg	Chicken, fish, liver, pork, kidney, eggs, unmilled rice, soybeans, and whole-wheat foods
B₁₂	6 mcg	Peanuts, walnuts, and animal products
Folic acid	400 mcg	Citrus fruits, tomatoes, vegetables, and grain products

From Reeder SJ et al: Homocysteine: the latest risk factor for heart disease, *Dimens Crit Care Nurs* 19(1):22-28, 2000.
RDA, recommended dietary allowance.

TABLE 19-6 C-Reactive Protein and Risk for Coronary Artery Disease

Category	hs-CRP Level* (mg/L)
Low risk (normal)	<1
Moderate risk	1-3
High risk	>3

Data from Pearson TA et al: Markers of inflammation and cardiovascular disease, application to clinical and public health practice: a statement for healthcare professionals from the Centers for Disease Control and Prevention and the American Heart Association, *Circulation* 107(3):499-511, 2003.
*Values above 1 mg/dL increase the risk for CAD, but test results are not valid in the presence of infection or other inflammatory condition. Normal values may vary slightly between clinical laboratories; however, values below 1 mg/dL are usually considered normal. A test result greater than 10 mg/L suggests a noncoronary source of inflammation or infection.
CAD, coronary artery disease; hs-CRP, high-sensitivity C-reactive protein.

plaque occurs in response to inflammation. Noxious inflammatory agents circulate in the bloodstream and stimulate chemical mediators that directly modify the arterial wall (see "Pathophysiology of Coronary Artery Disease"). The initial inflammatory stimuli include increased blood glucose, elevated blood lipids, nicotine, and hypertension. However, other clinical conditions, such as connective tissue disorders and systemic infection, also produce an inflammatory state, and it is not clear what the impact of inflammation produced by these stimuli is on the vessels.[31] Research to identify prognostic inflammatory markers is ongoing.

C-Reactive Protein. The inflammatory marker most frequently cited is *C-reactive protein* (CRP). It is measured as high-sensitivity C-reactive protein (hs-CRP).[31] The higher the hs-CRP value, the greater the risk of a coronary event, especially if all other potential causes of systemic inflammation such as infection can be ruled out. Value ranges for hs-CRP are shown in Table 19-6. If other systemic inflammatory conditions such as bronchitis or a urinary tract infection are present, the hs-CRP test loses all predictive value.[31] CRP and other inflammatory markers are used to estimate the probability of future acute coronary events.[31,32] During acute coronary syndrome events, there is widespread activation of neutrophils in the cardiac circulation (measured from the coronary sinus), which suggests that inflammation is not limited to one unstable plaque.[33] Debate continues about whether CRP is simply a marker of vascular inflammation or also contributes to the proinflammatory state.[9]

Multifactorial Risk. The major risk factors for developing CAD have been extensively documented in large epidemiologic studies: smoking, family history, adverse lipid profile, and elevated blood pressure. Certain medical conditions are considered risk equivalents of CAD. A *risk equivalent* means the person has the same risk of having an acute MI as if they had coronary heart disease already. Two noncardiac medical conditions are considered risk equivalents for CAD: diabetes mellitus and chronic kidney disease. PAD and cerebral vascular disease are atherosclerotic conditions that are also considered CAD risk equivalents.

CAD has multifactorial causation; the greater the number of risk factors, the greater the risk of developing CAD.[1,3,23,34] The best time for an individual to make lifestyle changes is before symptoms of CAD occur. Patients with two or more risk factors or with one or more of the CAD risk-equivalent diseases have the greatest potential to benefit from risk factor reduction and lifestyle change.[3]

Primary versus Secondary Prevention of Coronary Artery Disease. If a person has symptoms of CAD or has previously had an acute coronary syndrome event, the goal of any lifestyle change or medication is called *secondary prevention*, or preventing another heart attack. If an individual matches the risk profile described previously but does *not* have symptoms of CAD or has *not* had an acute MI, the treatment plan is described as *primary prevention*. The constellation of cardiac risk factors is well established and can predict development of CAD for most populations in the developed industrial world.

PATHOPHYSIOLOGY OF CORONARY ARTERY DISEASE

Coronary heart disease is a progressive atherosclerotic disorder of the coronary arteries that results in narrowing or complete occlusion. *Atherosclerosis* affects the medium-size arteries that perfuse the heart and other major organs. Normal arterial walls are composed of three layers: the *intima* (inner lining), the *media* (middle muscular layer), and the *adventitia* (outer coat).

Development of Atherosclerosis. Atherosclerosis is a chronic inflammatory disorder that is characterized by an accumulation of macrophages and T lymphocytes in the arterial intimal wall. A high LDL cholesterol concentration is one of the triggers of vascular inflammation. The inflammation injures the wall, allowing the LDL cholesterol to move into the vessel wall below the endothelial surface.[9] Blood monocytes adhere to endothelial cells and migrate into the vessel wall. Within the artery wall, some monocytes differentiate into macrophages that unite with and then internalize LDL cholesterol. The *foam cells* that result are the marker cells of atherosclerosis.[9]

Elevated LDL cholesterol levels promote low-level endothelial inflammation that allows lipoproteins to infiltrate the intimal vessel wall. After it has infiltrated under the endothelium, LDL cholesterol tends to stay within the vessel wall rather than return to the circulation.[9] This contrasts with the actions of HDL cholesterol, which enters the vessel wall, helps efflux cholesterol from cells, and then returns to the circulation.[9] The actions of HDL cholesterol may help minimize the number of foam cells in the artery wall.[9]

Atherosclerotic Plaque Rupture. When a mature atherosclerotic plaque develops, it is not uniform in composition. It has a lipid liquid center filled with procoagulant factors. A connective tissue *fibrous cap* covers the top of the fluid lipid center.[31-33] The abrupt rupture of this cap allows procoagulant lipids to flood

into the vessel lumen and rapidly form a coronary thrombosis, as shown in Table 19-7. As the enlarging clot blocks blood flow through the coronary artery, a "heart attack" will occur unless there is adequate collateral circulation from other coronary vessels. Symptoms and suggested cardiac interventions at appropriate stages in development of CAD are listed in Table 19-7.

Plaques that are likely to rupture are saturated with macrophages and other inflammatory cells. These *vulnerable plaques* are usually not obstructive and are situated at bends or branch points in the arterial tree.[3] It is not known what factors cause the fibrous

TABLE 19-7 Timeline of Atherogenesis Development Depicted by Longitudinal Section of an Artery

Atherogenesis or Thrombogenesis	Associated Symptoms	Cardiac Intervention
A. Normal artery, normal vessel wall	No symptoms	Primary prevention of CAD recommended: consume a low-fat diet, take regular physical exercise, avoid smoking, and achieve normal BMI
B. Lipids in bloodstream	No symptoms	
C. Extracellular lipid accumulates in the intima of the artery (atheroma).	No symptoms	
D. Lipid accumulation evolves to become a fatty-fibrous (atherosclerotic) lesion. Some lesions contain a lipid interior covered by a fibrous cap.	Chest pain with exercise that is relieved by rest or NTG (stable angina) or possibly no symptoms until the lesion fills more than 75% of the vessel lumen	PCI if stable angina is present and CAD is diagnosed by cardiac catheterization.
E. Rupture of the cap allows lipid in the center to be released into the bloodstream, stimulating clot formation (thrombogenesis).	Chest pain not relieved by rest or NTG (ACS—unstable angina)	Call 911 for immediate transport to a hospital, preferably one with experience treating ACS
F. Fresh clot blocks the vessel; spasm of the artery may occur near the thrombus.	Chest pain unrelieved by rest or NTG—severity, location of angina, and associated symptoms vary greatly among individuals (ACS—acute MI)	Emergency intervention to open the artery: fibrinolytic or catheter-based procedure (PCI)
G. Vessel is open, but the atherosclerotic lesion remains.	No symptoms	Secondary prevention of CAD to prevent repeat MI; beta-blockers to prevent arrhythmias; ACE-1 drugs to prevent ventricular remodeling and heart failure; elective PCI

Illustration modified from Antman EM et al: ACC/AHA guidelines for the management of patients with ST-elevation myocardial infarction—executive summary, *Circulation* 110:588-636, 2004.
ACE-1, angiotensin-converting enzyme 1; ACS, acute coronary syndrome; BMI, body mass index; CAD, coronary artery disease; MI, myocardial infarction; NTG, nitroglycerin; PCI, percutaneous coronary intervention.

cap to rupture or erode. As deep fissures in the cap expose the procoagulant factors to the blood plasma, an unstoppable cycle is put into motion. When platelets in the bloodstream are exposed to collagen, necrotic debris, von Willebrand factor, and thromboxane, a clot is formed that can occlude the coronary artery. Highly fibrotic plaques do not rupture. The type of atherosclerotic plaque that is prone to rupture has a weak fibrous cap and a large amount of liquid cholesterol within the core (see Table 19-7).[33]

Plaque Regression. A reduction in blood cholesterol decreases atherosclerotic plaque size by decreasing the amount of liquid cholesterol within the plaque core.[7] Lowering cholesterol levels does not change the dimensions of the fibrous or calcified portions of the plaque. However, lower cholesterol levels reduce vascular inflammation and make vulnerable plaque less likely to rupture.

If diet is not effective in lowering blood cholesterol, lipid-lowering drugs are prescribed to lower the LDL cholesterol level below 100 mg/dL for patients at risk for CAD and to aim for an LDL level below 70 mg/dL for individuals with the highest-risk profile.[7] Drugs, diet, and exercise are used to lower the triglyceride levels to less than 150 mg/dL, and to raise HDL cholesterol levels above 40 mg/dL for men and above 50 mg/dL for women.[3,7,8,34]

ACUTE CORONARY SYNDROMES

The term *acute coronary syndrome* (ACS) is used to describe the array of clinical presentations of CAD that range from unstable angina to acute MI (see Table 19-7).[1,3,5] The general public and media describe an acute MI as a "heart attack." The following section discusses stable manifestations of CAD (stable angina) and acute manifestations described as an acute coronary syndrome (unstable angina and acute MI).

Angina. *Angina pectoris*, or chest pain, caused by myocardial ischemia is not a separate disease, but rather a symptom of CAD. It is caused by a blockage or spasm of a coronary artery, leading to diminished myocardial blood supply. The lack of oxygen causes myocardial ischemia, which is felt as chest discomfort, pressure or pain. Angina may occur anywhere in the chest, neck, arms, or back, but the most commonly described location is pain or pressure behind the sternum. The pain often radiates to the left arm but can also radiate down both arms and to the back, the shoulder, the jaw, or the neck (Fig. 19-1). Angina symptoms are not the same for all individuals, many patients may describe pressure or discomfort rather than pain and presenting symptoms can be highly individualized, as described in Box 19-3. Patients and families must be taught that angina does not always present in the dramatic heart attack scenario seen on television and in movies, in which the person clutches the throat or chest and exhibits extreme distress.[3]

Women and Angina. Many women experience a variety of different symptoms before an acute MI and during the acute event, as shown in Box 19-4.[35] The recognition and publicity about the fact that many women do not experience "crushing chest pain" is important if women's symptoms are not to be trivialized by clinicians.[36] It is important that all patients are made aware of *angina symptom equivalents,* such as unexpected shortness of breath, breaking out in a cold sweat, or sudden fatigue, nausea, or lightheadedness.[3] More women die every year in the United States of cardiovascular disease than men, a fact that is largely unknown.[27]

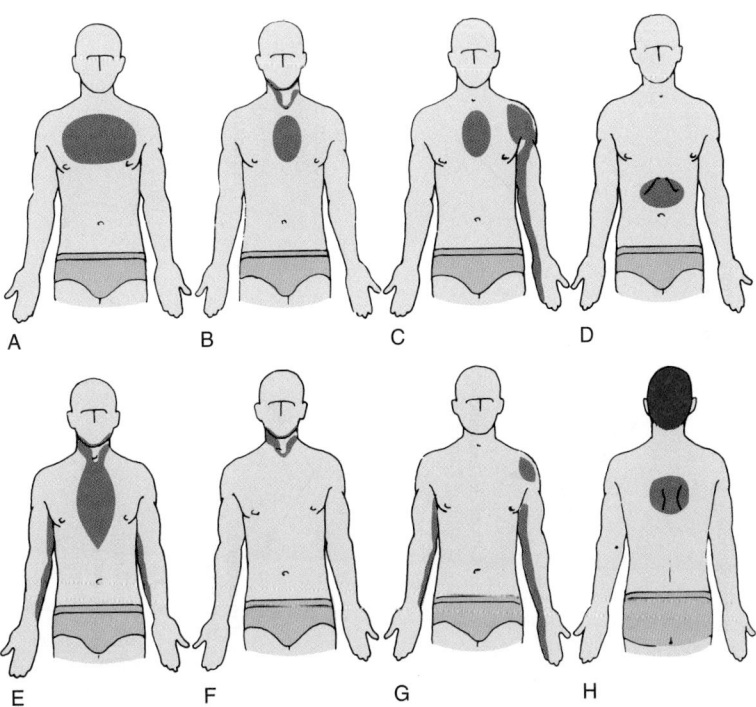

Figure 19-1 Common sites for anginal pain. *A,* Upper part of chest. *B,* Beneath sternum, radiating to neck and jaw. *C,* Beneath sternum, radiating down left arm. *D,* Epigastric. *E,* Epigastric, radiating to neck, jaw, and arms. *F,* Neck and jaw. *G,* Left shoulder. *H,* Intrascapular.

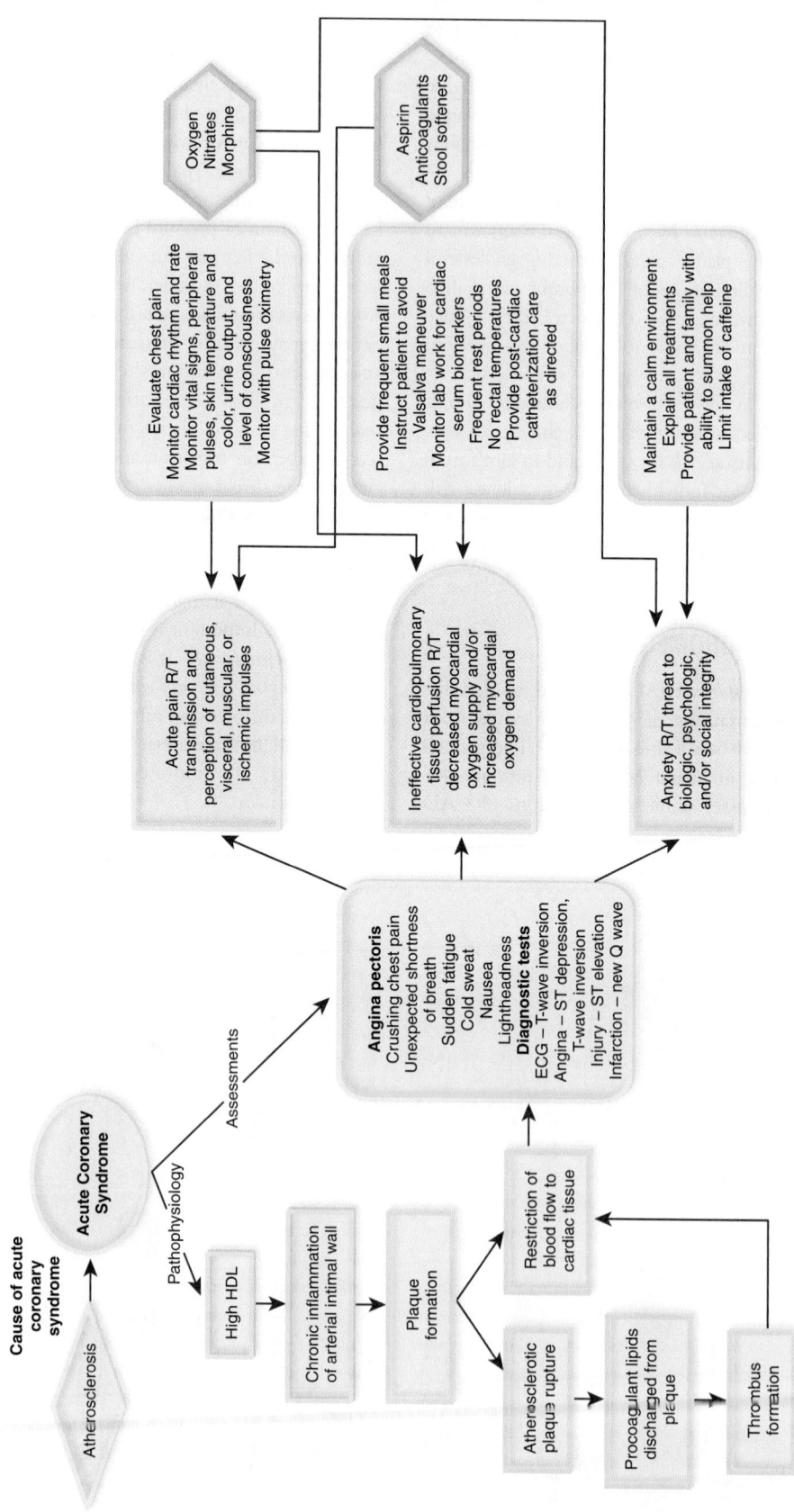

BOX 19-3   CHARACTERISTICS OF ANGINA PECTORIS

LOCATION
- Beneath sternum, radiating to neck and jaw
- Upper chest
- Beneath sternum, radiating down left arm
- Epigastric
- Epigastric, radiating to neck, jaw, and arms
- Neck and jaw
- Left shoulder, inner aspect of both arms
- Intrascapular

DURATION
- Less than 5 minutes
- Less than 5 minutes (stable)
- Longer than 5 minutes or worsening symptoms without relief from rest or sublingual nitroglycerin indicates preinfarction symptoms (unstable)

QUALITY
- Sensation of pressure or heavy weight on the chest
- Feeling of tightness, like a vise
- Visceral quality (deep, heavy, squeezing, aching)
- Burning sensation

- Shortness of breath, with feeling of suffocation
- Most severe pain ever experienced

RADIATION
- Medial aspect of left arm
- Jaw
- Left shoulder
- Right arm

PRECIPITATING FACTORS
- Exertion/exercise
- Cold weather
- Exercising after a large, heavy meal
- Walking against the wind
- Emotional upset
- Fright, anger
- Coitus

MEDICATION RELIEF
- Usually within 45 seconds to 5 minutes after sublingual nitroglycerin administration

BOX 19-4   CARDIOVASCULAR SYMPTOMS EXPERIENCED BY WOMEN BEFORE ACUTE MYOCARDIAL INFARCTION

Symptoms 1 Month before Acute MI	Symptoms during Acute MI
• Unusual fatigue (71%)	• Shortness of breath (58%)
• Sleep disturbance (48%)	• Weakness (55%)
• Shortness of breath (42%)	• Unusual fatigue (43%)
• Indigestion (39%)	• Cold sweat (39%)
• Anxiety (36%)	• Dizziness (39%)
• Heart racing (27%)	• Nausea (36%)
• Arms weak/heavy (25%)	• Arm heaviness or weakness (35%)
• Changes in thinking or memory (24%)	• Ache in arms (32%)
• Vision change (23%)	• Heat or flushing (32%)
• Loss of appetite (22%)	• Indigestion (31%)
• Hands or arms tingling (22%)	• Pain centered high in chest (31%)
• Difficulty breathing at night (19%)	• Heart racing (23%)

From McSweeney JC et al: Women's early warning symptoms of acute myocardial infarction, *Circulation* 108(21):2619-2623, 2003.
MI, myocardial infarction.

Stable Angina. *Stable angina* is predictable and caused by similar precipitating factors each time; typically, it is exercise induced. Patients become used to the pattern of this type of angina and may describe it as "my usual chest pain." Pain control should be achieved within 5 minutes by rest and by taking sublingual nitroglycerin. Stable angina is the result of fixed lesions (blockages) of more than 75% of the coronary artery lumen. Ischemia and chest pain occur when myocardial demand from exertion exceeds the fixed blood oxygen supply.[6] Additional information on CAD and stable angina is provided in the Evidence-Based Practice: Collaborative feature on Coronary Artery Disease and Stable Angina.

Unstable Angina. *Unstable angina* is defined as a change in a previously established stable pattern of angina. It is part of the continuum of ACS. Unstable angina usually is more intense than stable angina, may awaken the person from sleep, or may necessitate more than nitrates for pain relief. A change in the level or frequency of symptoms requires immediate medical evaluation. Severe angina that persists for more than 5 minutes, is worsening in intensity, and is not relieved by one nitroglycerin tablet is a medical emergency, and the patient or a family member must call 911 immediately.[3] The 911 (Emergency Medical Services [EMS]) system is available to 90% of the population of the United States.[3] In one study, patients with an acute MI who used 911 and were transported to the hospital by ambulance had significantly faster receipt of initial reperfusion therapies.[37] Family and friends are discouraged from driving a person experiencing unstable angina to the hospital and instead are encouraged to call 911. Patients should be instructed never to drive themselves but to contact the EMS by calling 911.

Unstable angina is an indication of atherosclerotic plaque instability. It can signal atherosclerotic plaque rupture and thrombus formation that can lead to MI. The patient who comes to the emergency department with recent onset of unstable angina but who has nonspecific or nonelevated ST-segment changes on the 12-lead electrocardiogram (ECG) may be admitted to the critical care unit to rule out MI. If the symptoms are typical of an MI, it is important to treat the patient according to the latest published guidelines, because not all patients who experience an MI have ST-segment elevation on the 12-lead ECG.[5]

Evidence-Based Practice: Collaborative

Coronary Artery Disease and Stable Angina

Summary of Evidence-Based Recommendations for Management of Coronary Artery Disease and Stable Angina

Strong evidence exists that the following lifestyle interventions help to prevent CAD:

- Diet
  Diet: low in salt and high in fiber, fruit, vegetables, and grains
  All dietary fat less than 30% of total calories; saturated fat less than 7%
  Multivitamin if homocysteine level is elevated
  Limit sugary foods.
  Limit calories if overweight.
  Omega-3 fatty acids included in diet
- Exercise
  Start by walking more often and increase physical exercise from there. Refer to cardiac rehabilitation program.
- Obesity
  Achieve healthy body weight.
- Addiction
  Stop cigarette smoking. Avoid exposure to environmental (second-hand) tobacco smoke at home and at work.
  Limit alcohol intake.

Strong evidence exists that the following diagnostic procedures help the patient with angina:

- When a patient presents with chest pain, quickly obtaining a detailed history of symptoms, focused physical examination, and risk factor assessment can help determine whether the probability of CAD is low, intermediate, or high.
- Initial laboratory tests include hemoglobin, fasting blood glucose, lipid panel.
- Obtain a baseline 12-lead ECG at rest, even if chest pain is not present.
- Obtain a 12-lead ECG during an episode of chest pain.
- Obtain a chest radiograph if symptoms of heart failure are present.
- Obtain an exercise 12-lead ECG if the condition is stable and symptoms suggest CAD or if the condition is stable with complete LBBB or RBBB that makes the ECG difficult to interpret for ischemia.
- Obtain cardiac echocardiography for patients with a systolic murmur suggestive of aortic stenosis.
- Use cardiac echocardiography to determine extent of LV hypertrophy or dysfunction.
- Stress cardiac echocardiography is recommended for patients with greater than 1 mm of ST-segment depression at rest (stress may be by physical exercise or by pharmacologic stimulation).
- Coronary angiography (typically as part of a cardiac catheterization procedure) is recommended for patients at high risk for adverse coronary events.

Initial Pharmacologic and Lifestyle Treatment Recommendations

- The goal of treatment is to eliminate chest pain.
- The 10 most important elements of CAD and stable angina management can be remembered using the A to E mnemonic:

A—Aspirin and antianginal drugs: Prescribe daily, low-dose (75 to 325 mg) aspirin; oral nitrates; and sublingual nitroglycerin for episodes of angina.

B—Beta-blockers and blood pressure: Use ACEI and beta-blockers to decrease blood pressure to less than 140/90 mm Hg if no other CAD risk factors are present and to less than 130/80 mm Hg if diabetes or kidney disease are present.

C—Cholesterol and cigarettes: Obtain a fasting lipid profile. Recommend diet or lipid reduction drug therapy (statin) to lower LDL-C to less than 100 mg/dL (<70 mg/dL if achievable), increase HDL-C to more than 40 mg/dL for men or more than 50 mg/dL for women, and reduce triglycerides to less than 150 mg/dL. Recommend adding plant stanols or sterols (2 g/day) or viscous fiber (>10 g/day), or both, to the diet to further lower LDL-C; add dietary omega-3 fatty acids in the form of fish or capsule (1 g/day). Always ask about tobacco use; strongly recommend smoking cessation; encourage nicotine replacement therapy (nicotine patches or gum) as needed.

D—Diet and diabetes: Prescribe a low-fat, calorie-appropriate diet and provide nutritional consultation as needed to achieve a fasting blood glucose level of 70 to 100 mg/dL and HbA$_{1c}$ of less than 7%.

E—Education and exercise: Provide education about risk factor modification and the CAD disease process; recommend daily exercise for 30 to 60 minutes (ideal) or at least seven times each week (minimum of 5 days per week). Achieve a BMI between 18.5 and 24.9 kg/m^2 and waist less than 40 inches for men or less than 35 inches for women. Treat depression if present. HRT is not recommended as a treatment for symptoms of coronary heart disease. Influenza vaccination is recommended.

Interventional and Surgical Recommendations for Stable High-Risk Patients

Patients are risk stratified according to their symptoms and the results of cardiac diagnostic tests.

- Percutaneous catheter interventions (PCI)
  Angioplasty, atherectomy, stent
  PCI is more frequently performed than open heart surgery for relief of anginal symptoms.
- Coronary artery bypass surgery (CABG)
  For patients with left main occlusion or multivessel disease
  For patients with two-vessel disease who have significant proximal LAD stenosis and an LV ejection fraction less than 50%

References

Gibbons RJ et al: ACC/AHA 2002 guideline update for the management of patients with chronic stable angina—summary article, *Circulation* 107(1):149-158, 2003.

Fraker TD et al: 2007 Chronic angina focused update of the ACC/AHA 2002 guidelines for the management of patients with chronic stable angina, *J Am Coll Cardio,* 50(23):2264-2274, 2007.

Mosca L et al: Evidence-based guidelines for cardiovascular disease prevention in women, *Circulation* 109(5):672-693, 2004.

ACEI, angiotensin-converting enzyme inhibitors; BMI, body mass index; CAD, coronary artery disease; ECG, electrocardiogram; HbA$_{1c}$, glycosylated hemoglobin; HDL-C, high-density lipoprotein cholesterol; HRT, hormone replacement therapy; LAD, left anterior descending coronary artery; LBBB, left bundle branch block; LDL-C, low-density lipoprotein cholesterol; LV, left ventricle; RBBB, right bundle branch block.

Variant Angina. *Variant angina*, or Prinzmetal's angina, is caused by spasm of a coronary artery.[38] Spasm can occur with or without atherosclerotic lesions. Variant angina commonly occurs when the individual is at rest, and it is often cyclic, occurring at the same time every day. It usually is associated with ST-segment elevation. Smoking, alcohol use, and illegal stimulant drug use (cocaine) may precipitate spasm. A definitive diagnosis of variant angina is made during a cardiac catheterization study. To force the artery to spasm, 50 mcg of ergonovine is intravenously administered every 5 minutes, until a maximum dose of 400 mcg has been administered or the signs and symptoms of coronary artery spasm appear. Signs of spasm include ST-segment elevation and chest pain. Nitroglycerin can rapidly reverse the effects of ergonovine.[38] Coronary artery spasm can occur with or without CAD. The prognosis is excellent when there is no significant coronary artery stenosis. Coronary artery spasm is treated with nitroglycerin or calcium channel blockers to vasodilate the coronary arteries.

Silent Ischemia. *Silent ischemia* describes a situation in which objective evidence of ischemia is observed on an ECG monitor but the person does not complain of anginal symptoms. Silent ischemia can occur in many clinical situations, as described in Box 19-5. One third of patients who are having a heart attack do not report chest pain as a symptom.[3] Diabetic patients are at particular risk for silent ischemia. Many patients who have had type 2 diabetes for more than 10 years have developed *autonomic neuropathy*, which decreases their ability to experience chest pain. Diabetic patients may misinterpret angina-equivalent symptoms such as nausea, vomiting, and diaphoresis as signaling a disruption in glucose control rather than a sign of myocardial ischemia.[3]

MEDICAL MANAGEMENT

Accurate assessment of chest pain symptoms is essential if unstable angina is to be recognized and treated effectively. Factors to consider when assessing chest pain are listed in Box 19-6. An important reason to ask questions about the chest pain is to differentiate between stable and unstable angina. The change from stable to unstable angina is potentially life threatening for the patient. If the ST segments are elevated or there is a newly documented left bundle branch block on the 12-lead ECG, the patient will be treated for acute MI.[3] However, if these classic ECG signs are missing and the chest pain continues, the current pharmacologic treatments of choice are aspirin, vasodilation by nitroglycerin, intravenous antiplatelet agents such as the glycoprotein (GP) IIb/IIIa inhibitors, and intravenous unfractionated

heparin (UFH).[5] Low-molecular-weight heparin (LMWH) combined with fibrinolysis is an alternative to heparin fibrinolysis for patients younger than 75 years with a serum creatinine level below 2.5 mg/dL for men and below 2 mg/dL for women.[3]

Another option is to transport the patient directly to the cardiac catheterization laboratory for direct visualization of the coronary arteries by the cardiologist. Recanalization of the coronary arteries is recommended, provided the institution performs more than 200 procedures annually or the individual physician performs more than 75 interventional procedures annually.[3,5]

NURSING MANAGEMENT

Nursing management of the patient with CAD and angina incorporates a variety of nursing diagnoses (see the Nursing Diagnosis feature on Coronary Artery Disease and Angina). Nursing interventions focus on early identification of myocardial ischemia, control of chest pain, recognition of complications, maintenance of a calm environment, and patient and family education.

BOX 19-6   FACTORS TO CONSIDER WHEN ASSESSING CHEST PAIN

- Onset: Was it sudden or gradual?
- Duration: Did pain last seconds or minutes? How soon after onset did the patient call for help?
- Precipitating factors: Was the patient up and moving around?
- Location: Was pain substernal? Was it located in same area as previous pain?
- Radiation: Did pain radiate to the jaw, neck, arm, or shoulder?
- Quality: Was pain similar to previous anginal pain? Less painful or more painful?
- Intensity: On a scale of 1 to 10, where would the patient rate the pain?
- Relieving factors: What made the pain better—changing position, nitroglycerin, oxygen, the presence of the nurse?
- Aggravating factors: Did things such as the environment, telephone calls, or waiting for help worsen the pain?
- Associated symptoms: Was the pain accompanied by nausea, vomiting, diaphoresis, or dyspnea?
- Emotional response: Was there an emotional response that intensified the pain—anxiety, fear, anger?

Nursing Diagnoses

Coronary Artery Disease and Angina

- Acute Pain related to transmission and perception of cutaneous, visceral, muscular, or ischemic impulses
- Ineffective Cardiopulmonary Tissue Perfusion related to decreased myocardial oxygen supply or increased myocardial oxygen demand, or both
- Activity Intolerance related to cardiopulmonary dysfunction
- Powerlessness related to lack of control over current situation
- Anxiety related to threat to biologic, psychologic, or social integrity
- Deficient Knowledge: Discharge Regimen related to lack of previous exposure to information (see the Patient Education feature on Coronary Artery Disease and Angina)

BOX 19-5   CLINICAL CHARACTERISTICS OF SILENT ISCHEMIA

- Objective electrocardiographic (ECG) evidence of myocardial ischemia without any chest pain or symptoms
- No anginal symptoms after a previous myocardial infarction (MI), but objective ECG evidence of myocardial ischemia continues
- Symptoms of angina with some episodes of ischemia and no symptoms with other ischemic events; patient may or may not have had a previous MI

Recognizing Myocardial Ischemia. Complaints of chest discomfort (angina) must be evaluated quickly, because angina is an indicator of myocardial ischemia (see Box 19-6). The patient is asked to rate the intensity of the chest discomfort on a scale of 0 to 10. Pain levels must be assessed with sensitivity to differences in cultural manifestations of pain. The words *chest pain* are not to be used exclusively, because some patients describe their angina as "pressure" or "heaviness." It is important to document the characteristics of the pain and the patient's heart rate and rhythm, blood pressure, respirations, temperature, skin color, peripheral pulses, urine output, mentation, and overall tissue perfusion. A 12-lead ECG is used to identify the area of ischemic myocardium. The major concern is that the chest pain may represent preinfarction angina, and early identification is essential so that the patient can be immediately treated. Treatment may include transfer to the cardiac catheterization laboratory for a coronary arteriogram and opening of a blocked artery. If the hospital does not have a cardiac catheterization laboratory, GP IIb/IIIa receptor blockers may be infused to prevent the evolution of the acute MI before transfer.[3,5]

Relieving Chest Pain. In the critical care unit, control of angina is achieved by a combination of supplemental oxygen, nitrates, analgesia, and surveillance of the angina and of the effects of pharmacologic therapy.

Oxygen: All patients with acute ischemic pain are administered supplemental oxygen to increase myocardial oxygenation. Use of pulse oximetry is recommended to guide therapy and maintain oxygen saturation above 90%.[3] Patients who develop symptoms of acute heart failure may require emergency intubation and mechanical ventilation to correct significant hypoxemia.[3,5]

Nitrates: A combination of intravenous and sublingual nitroglycerin is used to vasodilate the coronary arteries and decrease pain. After nitrate administration, the critical care nurse closely observes the patient for relief of chest pain, for return of the ST segment to baseline, and for the potential development of unwanted side effects such as hypotension and headache. Administration of a nitrate is avoided if the SBP is below 90 mm Hg. Drug interactions with nitrates are another potential cause for concern. The phosphodiesterase inhibitor medication sidenafil (Viagra) is prescribed for several conditions including pulmonary hypertension and erectile dysfunction. Sidenafil and nitrates in combination may contribute to a precipitous fall in blood pressure.[3,5]

Analgesia: Morphine (2 to 4 mg given intravenously) is the analgesic opiate of choice for preinfarction angina. It relieves pain and decreases fear and anxiety. After administration, the critical care nurse assesses the patient for pain relief and the development of unwanted side effects such as hypotension and respiratory depression.[3,5]

Aspirin: Chewing an oral non–enteric-coated aspirin (162 to 325 mg) at the beginning of chest pain has been shown to reduce mortality. The nonenteric formulation is preferred because it increases absorption in the mouth when chewed, not swallowed.[3,5]

Maintaining a Calm Environment. Patients admitted to a critical care unit with unstable angina experience extreme anxiety and fear of death. The critical care nurse is faced with the challenge of ensuring that the elements of a calm environment that can alleviate the patient's fear and anxiety are maintained, while being ready at all times to respond to an acute emergency, such as a cardiac arrest, or to assist with emergency intubation or insertion of hemodynamic monitoring catheters. Additional aspects of acute cardiac care are listed in the Nursing Interventions Classification feature on Cardiac Care: Acute.

NIC

Cardiac Care: Acute

Definition
Limitation of complications for a patient recently experiencing an episode of an imbalance between myocardial oxygen supply and demand resulting in impaired cardiac function

Activities
Evaluate chest pain (e.g., intensity, location, radiation, duration, precipitating and alleviating factors).
Provide immediate and continuous means to summon nurse, and let the patient and family know that calls will be answered immediately.
Monitor cardiac rhythm and rate.
Auscultate heart sounds.
Recognize the frustration and fright caused by inability to communicate and exposure to strange machinery and environment.
Auscultate lungs for crackles or other adventitious sounds.
Monitor neurologic status.
Monitor intake/output, urine output, and daily weight.
Select best ECG lead for continuous monitoring.
Obtain 12-lead ECG.
Determine cardiac serum biomarkers, CK-MB, or troponins T or I.

Monitor kidney function (e.g., blood urea nitrogen, serum creatinine).
Monitor liver function (e.g., ALT, AST, LDH).
Monitor laboratory values for electrolytes, which may increase the risk of dysrhythmias (e.g., serum potassium, magnesium).
Obtain chest radiograph.
Monitor trends in blood pressure and hemodynamic parameters, if available (e.g., central venous pressure, pulmonary artery occlusion [wedge] pressure).
Provide small, frequent meals.
Limit intake of caffeine, sodium, cholesterol, and foods high in fat.
Monitor the effectiveness of oxygen therapy.
Monitor determinants of oxygen delivery (e.g., Pao2, hemoglobin level, cardiac output).
Maintain an environment conducive to rest and healing.
Instruct the patient to avoid activities that result in the Valsalva maneuver (e.g., straining during bowel movement).
Administer medications that will prevent episodes of the Valsalva maneuver (e.g., stool softeners, antiemetics).
Refrain from taking rectal temperatures.
Prevent peripheral thrombus formation (e.g., if patient is immobile, turn every 2 hours and administer low-dose anticoagulants).
Administer medications to relieve or prevent pain and ischemia, as needed.
Monitor effectiveness of medication.

Modified from Bulechek GM et al: *Nursing interventions classification (NIC),* ed 5, St Louis, 2008, Mosby.

PATIENT EDUCATION

In the critical care unit, the patient's ability to retain educational information is severely affected by stress and pain. Patient education topics that should be discussed when the clinical condition has stabilized are listed in the Patient Education feature on Coronary Artery Disease and Angina. It is essential to teach avoidance of the Valsalva maneuver, which is defined as forced expiration against a closed glottis. This can be explained to the patient as "bearing down" when going to the bathroom or breath-holding when repositioning in bed. The Valsalva maneuver causes an increase in intrathoracic pressure that decreases venous return to the right side of the heart and is associated with low blood pressure and symptomatic bradycardia.

After the anginal pain is controlled, longer-term patient and family education can begin. Points to cover include risk factor modification, signs and symptoms of angina, when to call the physician, medications, and dealing with emotions and stress. However, because the acute hospital length of stay for uncomplicated angina is usually less than 3 days, referral to a cardiac rehabilitation program for a controlled exercise program and risk factor modification after discharge may be the most helpful teaching intervention a critical care nurse can provide. Clinical practice guidelines for the management of CAD and stable angina are listed in the Evidence-Based Practice: Collaborative feature on Coronary Artery Disease and Stable Angina.

Patient Education

Coronary Artery Disease and Angina

- Angina: Describe signs and symptoms such as pain, pressure, and heaviness in chest, arms, or jaw.
- Preinfarction or unstable angina: Any chest pain that is not relieved within 5 min by a sublingual nitroglycerin (NTG) tablet provides a reason to call 911 (emergency services).
- Use of the 0 to 10 pain scale: Notify critical care nurse or emergency personnel of any changes in pain intensity.
- Use of sublingual NTG for angina: Pain intensity should decrease on the pain scale after NTG administration. At home, NTG must be kept in a dark, air-tight container, or it loses its potency. To ensure potency, the NTG supply must be replaced about every 6 months. Active NTG has a slight burning sensation when placed under the tongue.
- Avoidance of the Valsalva maneuver
- Risk factor modification tailored to the patient's individual risk factor profile:
  - Decrease fat intake to 30% of total calories a day.
  - Stop smoking.
  - Reduce salt intake.
  - Control hypertension.
  - Treat diabetes and control blood glucose levels, if patient is diabetic.
  - Increase physical activity; achieve ideal body weight.
- Reference to cardiac rehabilitation program
- Medication teaching: indications, side effects
- Follow-up care after discharge
- Symptoms to report to a health care professional
- Discussion of how to handle emotional stress and anger

MYOCARDIAL INFARCTION

DESCRIPTION AND ETIOLOGY

Myocardial infarction (MI) is the term used to describe irreversible myocardial necrosis (cell death) that results from an abrupt decrease or total cessation of coronary blood flow to a specific area of the myocardium.[1] In the hospital, this is often referred to as an *acute MI*, indicating the sudden onset and the life-threatening nature of the event. Increasingly, an acute MI is described in relation to whether there was ST-segment elevation on the diagnostic 12-lead ECG. It may be labeled an acute *non–ST-segment elevation MI* (NSTEMI)[5] or an acute *ST-segment elevation MI* (STEMI).[3]

Three mechanisms can block the coronary artery and are responsible for the acute reduction in oxygen delivery to the myocardium:

1. Plaque rupture
2. New coronary artery thrombosis
3. Coronary artery spasm close to the ruptured plaque

Myocardial tissue can best be salvaged within the first 2 hours (120 minutes) after the onset of anginal symptoms, as illustrated in Fig. 19-2.[3] The earlier the myocardium is revascularized, the better the survival.[5] Unfortunately, many persons do not seek treatment until the acute phase has passed.[3]

PATHOPHYSIOLOGY

Ischemia. The outer region of the infarcted myocardial area is the *zone of ischemia,* as illustrated in Fig. 19-3. It is composed of viable cells. Priority interventions are targeted to save this viable muscle. Repolarization in this zone is temporarily impaired but eventually will be restored to normal. Repolarization of the cells in this area manifests as T-wave inversion (Fig. 19-4B).

Injury. The infarcted zone is surrounded by injured but still potentially viable tissue in an area known as the *zone of injury* (see Fig. 19-3). Cells in this area do not fully repolarize because of the deficient blood supply. This is recorded on the ECG as elevation of the ST segment (see Fig. 19-4C).

Infarction. The area of dead muscle (necrosis) in the myocardium is known as the *zone of infarction* (see Fig. 19-3). On the ECG, evidence of this zone is seen by new pathologic Q waves, which reflect a lack of depolarization from the cardiac surface involved in the MI (see Fig. 19-4D). As healing takes place, the cells in this area are replaced by scar tissue.

Transmural Myocardial Infarction or Q-Wave Myocardial Infarction. MIs are classified according to the location on the myocardial surface and the muscle layers affected. Not all infarctions cause necrosis in all layers, as shown in Figure 19-5. A transmural MI involves all three cardiac layers—the *endocardium,* the *myocardium,* and the *epicardium.* A transmural (full-thickness) MI usually provokes significant ECG changes (see Fig. 19-4). This is also described as a *Q-wave MI.* Not every acute MI produces a recognizable series of Q waves on the 12-lead ECG. Some patients who had a demonstrated Q wave on a 12-lead ECG as a result of an acute MI lose

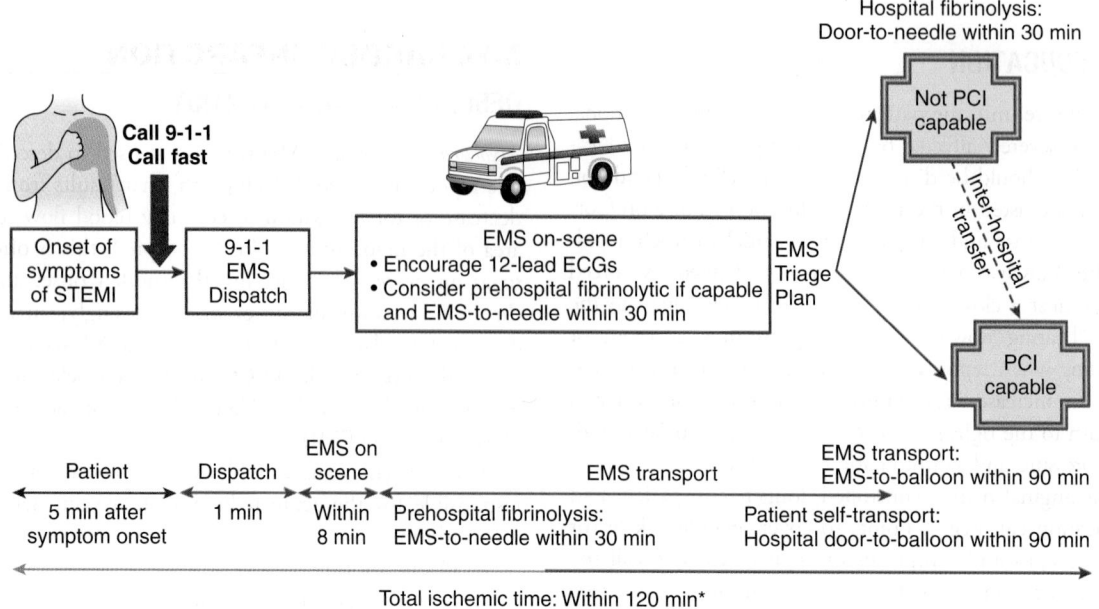

Figure 19-2 Evaluation of prehospital chest pain and ACS and treatment options. *(From the American Heart Association, 2004.)*

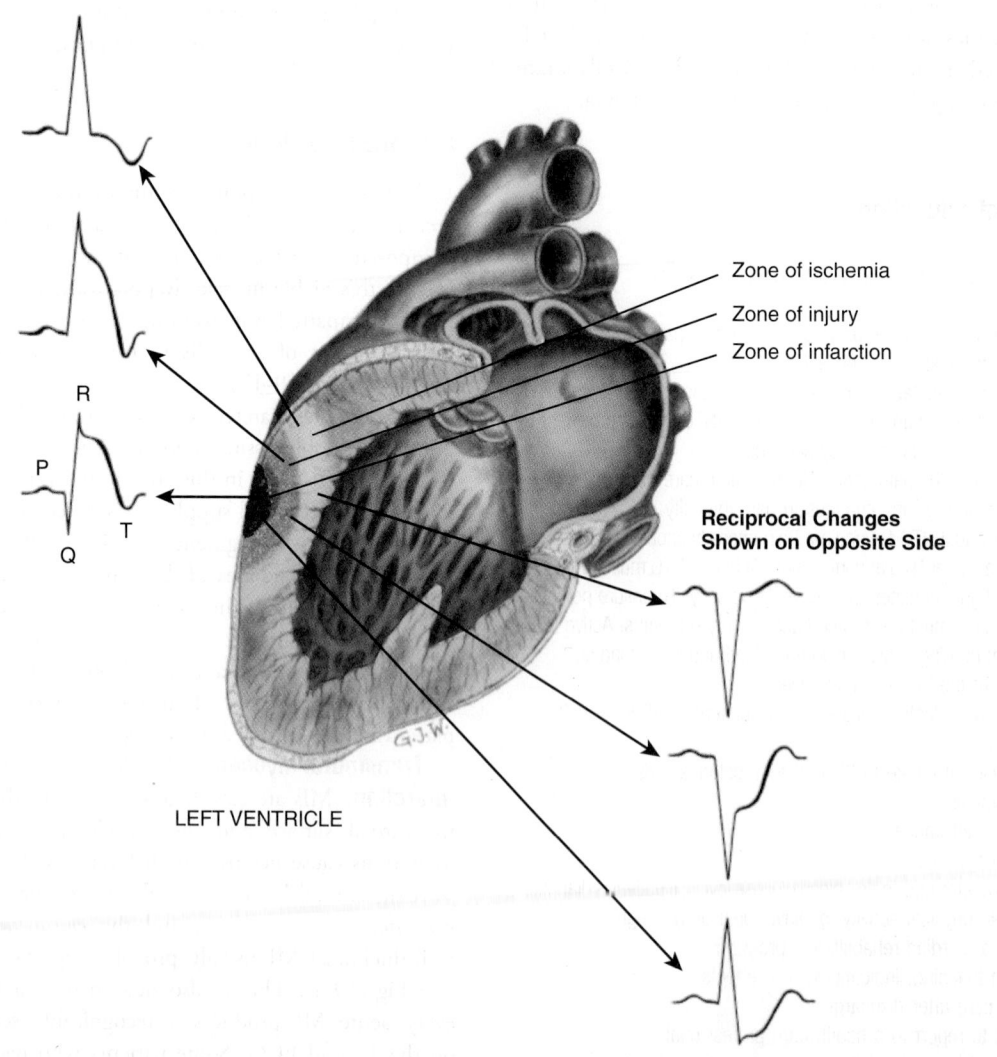

Figure 19-3 Zone of ischemia, zone of injury, and zone of infarction are shown through ECG waveforms and reciprocal waveforms corresponding to each zone.

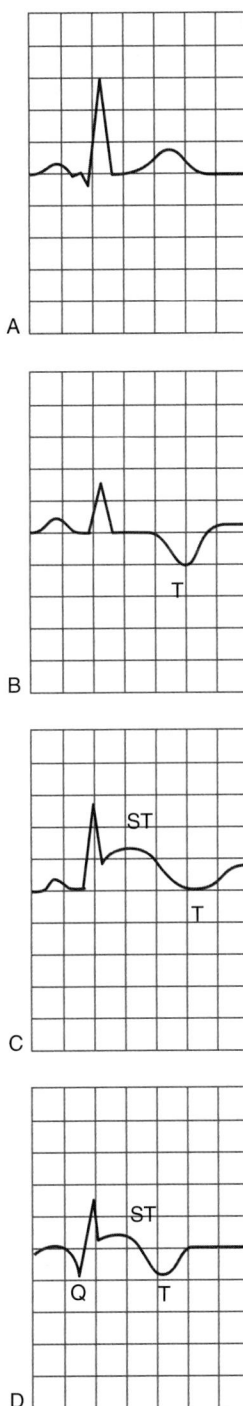

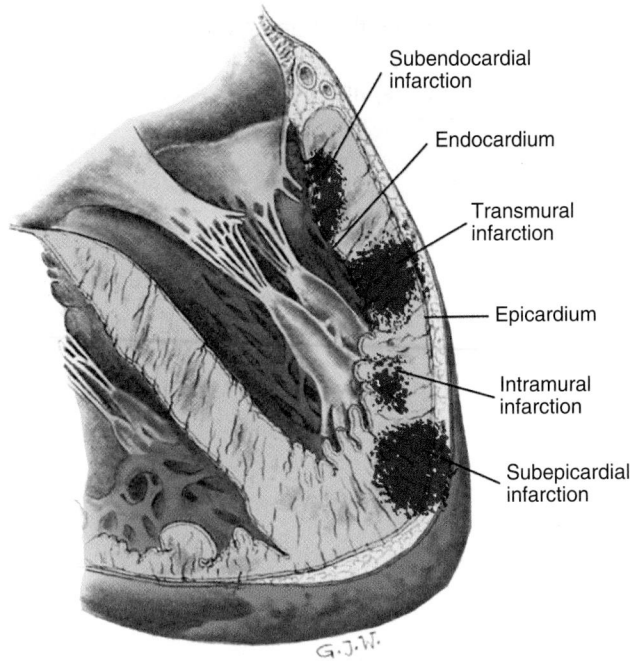

Figure 19-5 Location of infarctions in myocardium.

Figure 19-4 ECG changes indicative of ischemia, injury, and infarction (necrosis) of the myocardium. *A,* Normal ECG. *B,* Ischemia indicated by inversion of the T wave. *C,* Ischemia and current of injury indicated by T-wave inversion and ST-segment elevation. The ST segment may be elevated above or depressed below the baseline, depending on whether the tracing is from a lead facing toward or away from the infarcted area and depending on whether epicardial or endocardial injury occurs. Epicardial injury causes ST-segment elevation in leads facing the epicardium. *D,* Ischemia, injury, and myocardial necrosis. The Q wave indicates necrosis of the myocardium.

the Q wave months or years later. The reasons for this are unknown, but it may represent the development of collateral circulation.

12-Lead Electrocardiographic Changes. The ECG changes produced by a transmural infarction demonstrate alteration in myocardial depolarization (QRS complex) and repolarization (ST segment). The changes in repolarization are seen by the presence of new Q waves. These new, pathologic Q waves are deeper and wider than tiny Q waves found on the normal 12-lead ECG.[3]

Myocardial Infarction Location. The location of infarction is determined by correlating the ECG leads with Q waves and the ST-segment T-wave abnormalities (Table 19-8). Infarction most commonly affects the left ventricle and the interventricular septum; however, the right ventricle can be infracted, and many patients who sustain an inferior MI have some right ventricular damage. The ECG manifestations that are used to diagnose an MI and pinpoint the area of damaged ventricle include inverted T waves, ST-segment elevation, and pathologic Q waves in specific lead groupings as described subsequently.

Anterior Wall Infarction. Anterior wall infarction results from occlusion of the proximal left anterior descending artery (see Table 19-8). ST-segment elevation is expected in leads V_1 through V_4 on the 12-lead ECG, as shown in Figure 19-6. If the left main coronary artery is occluded, the ECG manifestations will involve almost all of the precordial leads V_1 through V_6 and leads I and aVL (see Table 19-8). These specific groups

TABLE 19-8 Correlations among Ventricular Surfaces, Electrocardiographic Leads, and Coronary Arteries

Surface of Left Ventricle	Electrocardiographic Leads	Coronary Artery Usually Involved
Inferior	II, III, aVF	Right coronary artery
Lateral	V_5-V_6, I, aVL	Left circumflex
Anterior	V_2-V_4	Left anterior descending
Anterior lateral	V_1-V_6, I, aVL	Left main coronary artery
Septal	V_1-V_2	Left anterior descending
Posterior	V_1-V_2	Left circumflex or right coronary artery (reciprocal changes)
	V_7-V_9 (direct)	

I lateral	aVR	V_1 septal	V_4 anterior
II inferior	aVL lateral	V_2 septal	V_5 lateral
III inferior	aVF inferior	V_3 anterior	V_6 lateral

of ECG changes that help to locate the part of the heart that is infarcting are called *indicative changes*. A large anterior wall MI may be associated with left ventricular pump failure, cardiogenic shock, or death.[3]

Left Lateral Wall Infarction. Left lateral wall infarction occurs as a result of occlusion of the circumflex coronary artery. On a 12-lead ECG, new Q waves and ST-segment T-wave changes are seen in leads I, aVL, V_5, and V_6 (Fig. 19-7). In reality, few patients present with only lateral wall ECG changes, and some anterior wall leads (V_3 and V_4) may show evidence of injury or infarction.

Inferior Wall Infarction. Inferior wall infarction occurs with occlusion of the right coronary artery. This infarction manifests by ECG changes in leads II, III, and aV_F (Fig. 19-8). Conduction disturbances are expected with an inferior wall MI and are related to the anatomy of the coronary arterial supply. Because the right coronary artery perfuses the sinoatrial (SA) node in slightly more than half of the population and supplies the proximal bundle of His and atrioventricular (AV) node in more than 90% of individuals, heart block and other conduction disturbances should be anticipated. Inferior wall MI carries a mortality rate of about 6%. If the right ventricle is involved, the mortality rate increases to 25% to 30%.[3]

Right Ventricular Infarction. Infarction of the right ventricle occurs when there is a blockage in a proximal section of the

right coronary artery. This places all of the right ventricle and the inferior wall at risk. Right ventricular ischemia can be demonstrated in up to one half of inferior wall STEMIs, although only 10% to 15% show the hemodynamic abnormalities associated with classic infarction of the right ventricle.[3] If massive infarction occurs, the patient can suffer cardiogenic shock, which carries a mortality rate of more than 50% in this population.[39]

To detect a right ventricular infarction, specific ECG lead placement is used. Electrodes are placed over the right precordium (chest) in a mirror image of the conventional left-sided leads. It is important to write R on the 12-lead ECG (e.g., V_1R-V_6R) in front of all of the recorded right ventricular chest leads to ensure that the lead location is clear. The limb leads are not affected. Figure 18-7C in Chapter 18 shows the correct position of the right-sided precordial leads used to diagnose an acute right ventricular MI.[40] The ECG voltage is much lower in the V_1R-V_6R leads, and when detected, ST-segment elevation is usually seen in V_4R (Fig. 19-9). The right ventricle has a very thin wall, which means that ST-segment elevation is detected only in the right ventricular leads during the acute phase of the infarction.[3]

Posterior Wall Infarction. Infarction in the posterior wall can occur because of a blockage in the right coronary artery or in the circumflex artery. This occurs because both arteries supply this section of the heart, although the right coronary artery is generally the dominant vessel. A posterior wall MI is difficult to detect but may be identified by specific leads placed in the left scapular area or by very tall R waves in leads V_1 and V_2 (Fig. 19-10). Figure 18-7D in Chapter 18 shows the correct placement of the left posterior leads used to diagnose an acute posterior MI.

Non–ST-Segment Elevation Myocardial Infarction. The 12-lead ECG is a highly useful diagnostic tool. For many years, it was considered the gold standard when diagnosing an acute MI. However, the ST segment is not elevated in every acute MI. One reason for the lack of ST-segment elevation may be that the infarction and subsequent necrosis are not full-thickness lesions. Because some of the muscle in the area can still be depolarized, ST-segment elevation may not occur. This type of MI is also less likely to develop Q waves on a subsequent 12-lead ECG after the acute phase has passed. This situation is diagnostically known as an NSTEMI.[5] This condition has previously been described by several names, including nontransmural MI, non–Q-wave MI, and subendocardial MI. Because patients who sustain an NSTEMI do have CAD, it is important that they be treated aggressively to minimize the size of the infarcted area. Without the visual clue of the ST-segment elevation on the 12-lead ECG, the patients cannot receive immediate intravenous fibrinolytic agents, but they can be appropriately managed in an interventional catheterization laboratory and receive GP IIb/IIIa inhibitor therapy, as illustrated in the timeline in Figure 19-2. The 12-lead ECG plays a vital role in identifying the treatment plan for an ACS. ST-segment elevation is helpful when present, but it would be a mistake to believe the patient is not in danger of MI if the ST segment is not elevated

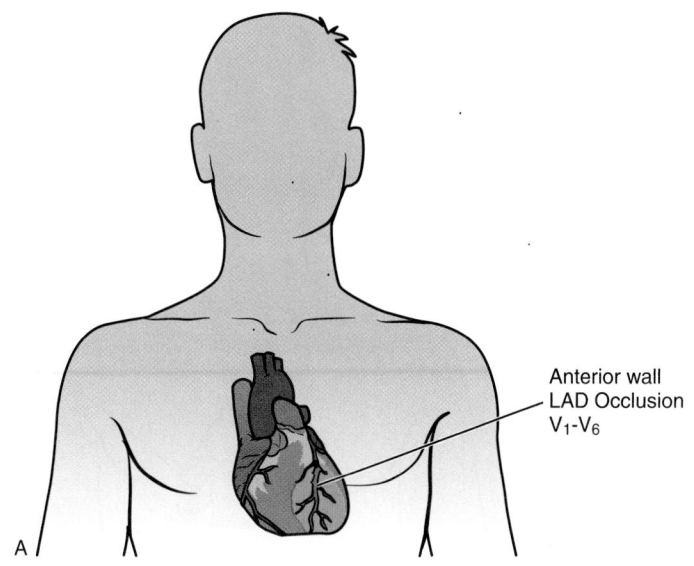

LIMB LEADS

PRECORDIAL LEADS

Lead I	AV$_R$	V$_1$	V$_4$
Lead II	AV$_L$	V$_2$	V$_5$
Lead III	AV$_F$	V$_3$	V$_6$

B

Example of an Acute Anterior Wall MI

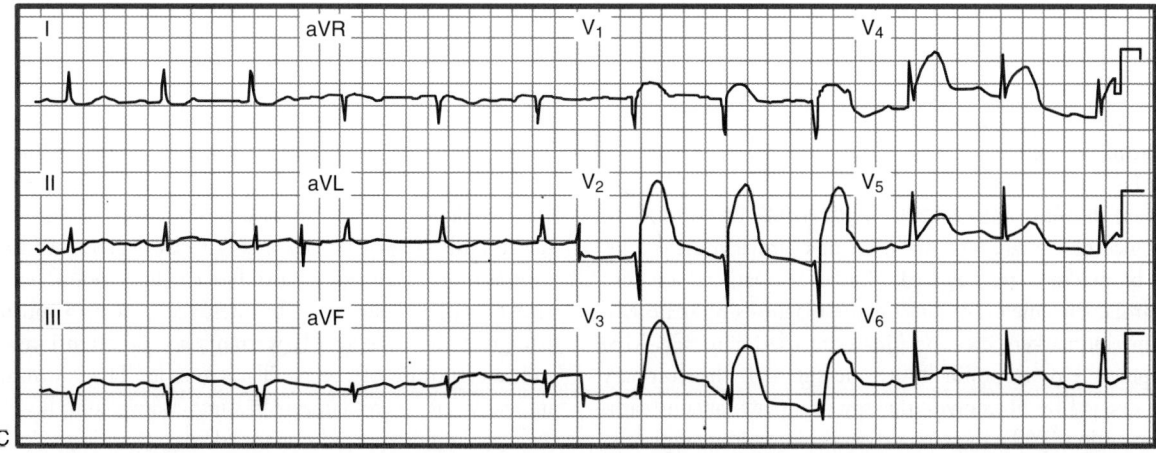

Figure 19-6 Changes seen on a 12-lead ECG with an anterior wall MI. *A,* Infarction location on the cardiac wall. *B,* ECG leads with expected ST-segment elevation. *C,* A 12-lead ECG from a patient experiencing left anterior wall MI. LAD, left anterior descending artery.

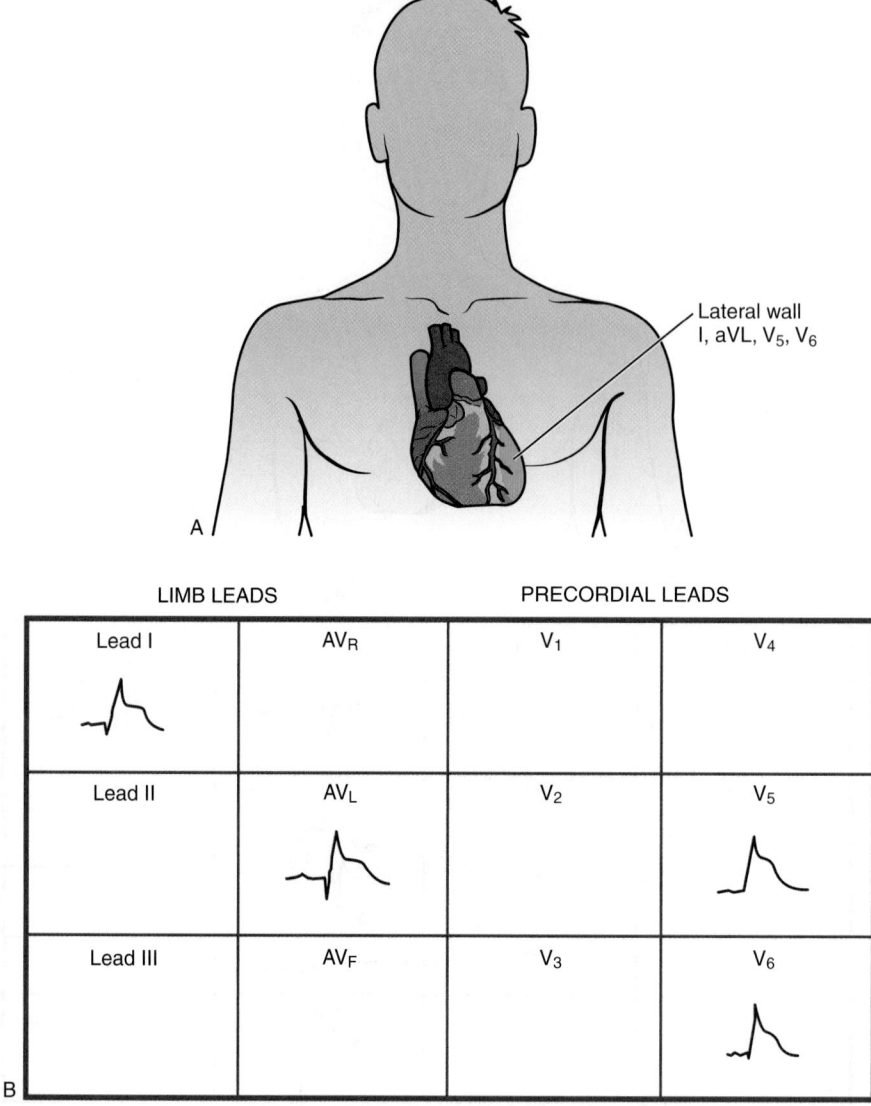

Figure 19-7 Changes seen on a 12-lead ECG with a lateral wall STEMI. *A,* Infarction location on the cardiac wall. *B,* ECG leads with expected ST-segment elevation.

(Fig. 19-11). In this case, the definitive diagnosis may be made in the cardiac catheterization laboratory or by elevation of specific cardiac biomarkers.

Cardiac Biomarkers during Myocardial Infarction. In the presence of damaged or necrosed myocardial muscle cells, cardiac biomarkers are released. These biomarkers are also called cardiac enzymes. To confirm the diagnosis of acute MI, the serum biomarkers creatine kinase-muscle/brain (CK-MB) and troponin I or troponin T are measured. If the coronary artery is opened by fibrinolytic therapy or a percutaneous catheter intervention (PCI), the biomarkers exhibit a more rapid rise and dramatic fall (Fig. 19-12). Information on biomarkers is also shown in Table 18-1 of Chapter 18.

Complications of Acute Myocardial Infarction. Many patients experience complications occurring early or late in the postinfarction course. These complications may result from

electrical dysfunction or from a cardiac contractility problem. The presence of a new murmur in a patient with an acute MI warrants special attention because it may indicate rupture of the papillary muscle. Electrical dysfunctions include bradycardia, bundle branch blocks, and various degrees of heart block. Pumping complications cause heart failure, pulmonary edema, and cardiogenic shock.[3] The presence of a new murmur in a patient with an acute MI warrants special attention as it may indicate rupture of the papillary muscle. The murmur can be indicative of severe damage and impending complications such as heart failure and pulmonary edema.

Sinus Bradycardia and Sinus Tachycardia. Sinus bradycardia (heart rate less than 60 beats/min) occurs in 30% to 40% of patients who sustain an acute MI.[2] It is more prevalent with an inferior wall infarction in the first hour after STEMI.[2] Symptomatic bradycardia with hypotension and low cardiac output

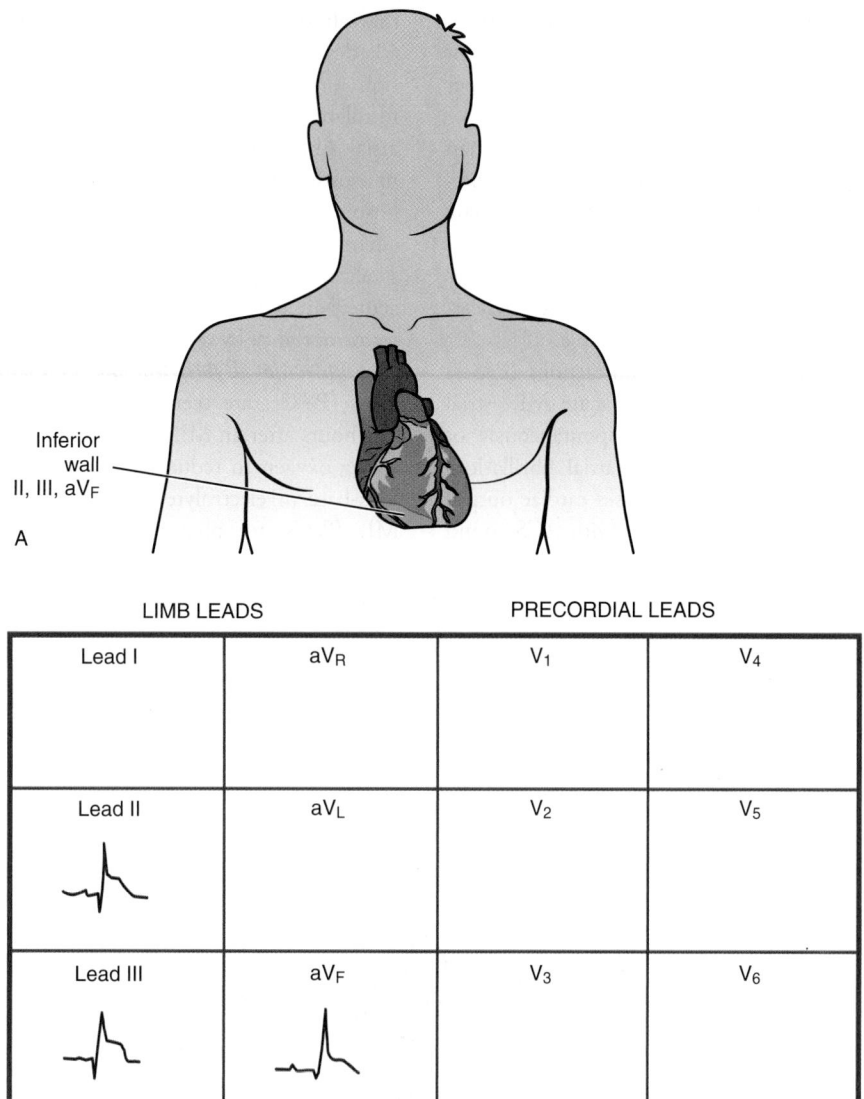

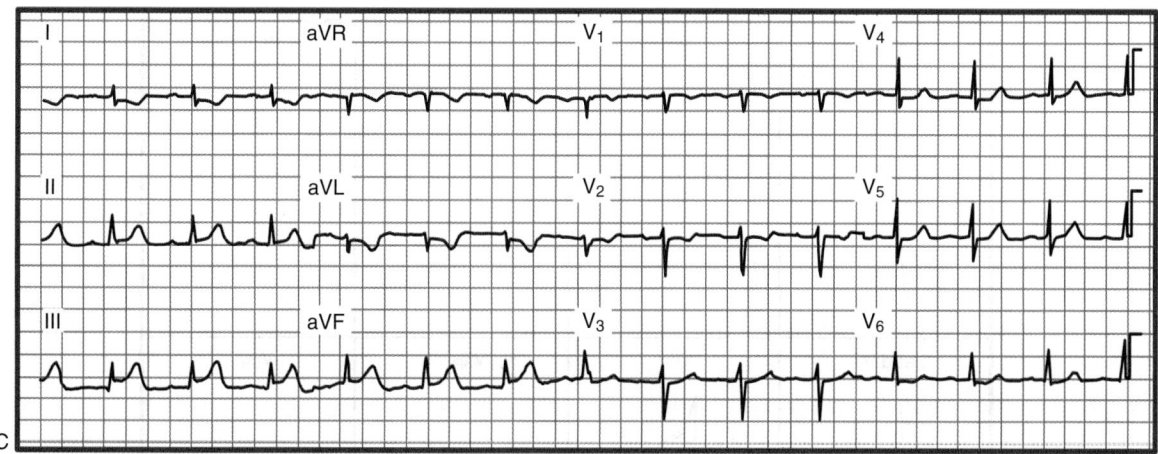

Figure 19-8 Changes seen on a 12-lead ECG with an inferior wall MI. *A,* Infarction location on cardiac wall. *B,* ECG leads with expected ST-segment elevation. *C,* A 12-lead ECG from a patient experiencing inferior wall MI.

is treated with atropine (0.5 to 1.0 mg by intravenous push), repeated every 3 to 5 minutes to a maximum dose of 0.03 mg/kg (e.g., 2 mg for a person who weighs 70 kg) per Advanced Cardiac Life Support (ACLS) Guidelines.

Sinus Tachycardia. Sinus tachycardia (heart rate more than 100 beats/min) most often occurs with an anterior wall MI. Anterior infarctions impair left ventricular pumping ability, thereby reducing the ejection fraction and the stroke volume. In an attempt to maintain cardiac output, the heart rate increases. Sinus tachycardia must be corrected, because it greatly increases myocardial oxygen consumption, leading to further ischemia.

Atrial Dysrhythmias. Premature atrial contractions (PACs) occur frequently in patients who sustain an acute MI. Atrial fibrillation is also common and may occur spontaneously or may be preceded by PACs. With onset of atrial fibrillation, the loss of organized atrial contraction decreases cardiac output by up to 20%. A global registry of patients with ACS found

that almost 8% have preexisting atrial fibrillation, and about 6% develop new-onset atrial fibrillation during their hospitalization for ACS.[41] Patients with new-onset or preexisting atrial fibrillation have higher morbidity rate than patients without atrial fibrillation during an ACS event. ACS patients with new-onset atrial fibrillation experience a greater number of in-hospital adverse events such as reinfarction, shock, pulmonary edema, bleeding, and stroke.[41] Atrial fibrillation during the hospitalization significantly affects risk of death in the setting of an acute MI; it increases in-hospital mortality by 20% and long-term mortality by 34%.[2]

Ventricular Dysrhythmias. Premature ventricular contractions (PVCs) are seen in almost all patients within the first few hours after an MI. They are initially controlled by administering oxygen to reduce myocardial hypoxia and by correcting acid-base or electrolyte imbalances. In the setting of an acute MI, PVCs are pharmacologically treated if they have the

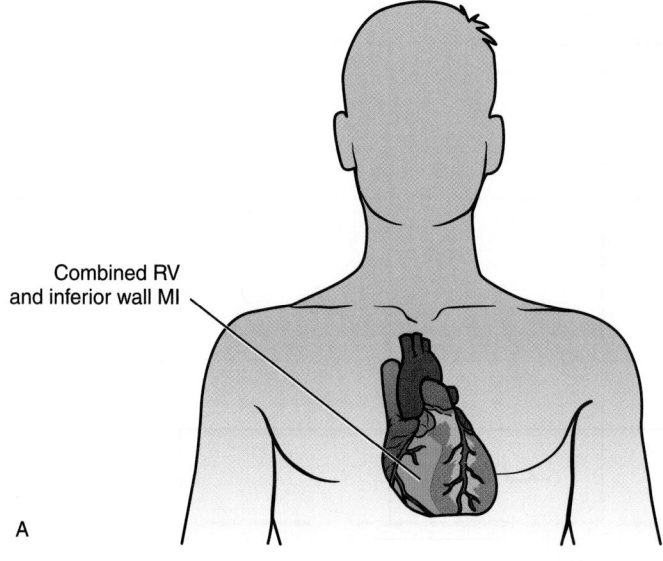

Figure 19-9 Changes seen on a 12-lead ECG with an inferior right ventricular (RV) STEMI. *A,* Picture of an RV wall myocardial infarction (MI). *B,* Acute inferior wall MI, with the right coronary artery (RCA) occluded.

(Continued)

following characteristics: frequent (>6/min), closely coupled (R-on-T phenomenon), multiform shapes, and occurrence in bursts of three or more, increasing the risk of sustained ventricular tachycardia (VT). Ventricular fibrillation (VF) is a life-threatening dysrhythmia associated with high mortality in acute MI. Beta-blockers often are prescribed after an acute MI to decrease mortality from ventricular dysrhythmias.[3]

Atrioventricular Heart Block during Myocardial Infarction. Heart block occurs in 6% to 14% of patients with STEMI, and those patients have increased mortality rates.[2] In STEMI, AV block most often occurs after an inferior wall infarction.

Because the right coronary artery supplies the AV node in 90% of the population, right coronary artery occlusion leads to ischemia and infarction of the AV node cells. The development of sudden heart block has become much less common because most patients receive fibrinolysis or undergo PCI to open the occluded vessel. In most cases, transcutaneous pacing is the primary intervention; transvenous pacemakers are used less frequently.[2]

Ventricular Aneurysm after Myocardial Infarction. A ventricular aneurysm (Fig. 19-13) is a noncontractile, thinned left ventricular wall that results from an acute transmural infarction.

Example of an Acute Inferior Wall and RV Wall MI. Shows ST elevation in leads II, III, AVF and reciprocal changes (ST depression) in anterior and lateral leads.

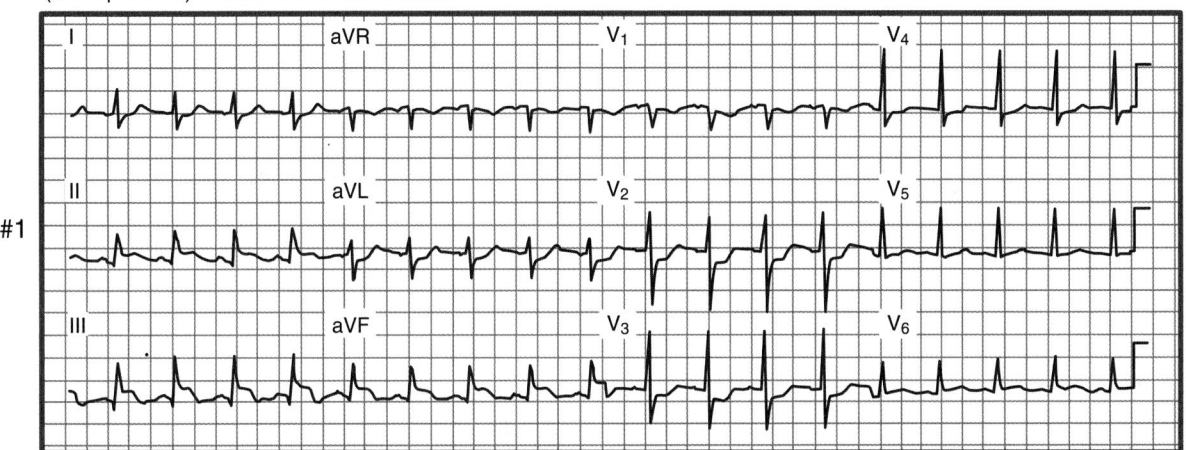

#1

Reciprocal changes seen in V_1, V_2, V_3, V_4, I, and aVL which provides a clue as to the extent of the MI.
Angiographic changes associated with an occlusion of the RCA.
These findings can range from:
- Proximal occlusion (near origin of RCA) which will produce both inferior MI, posterior MI and RV MI
- Middle RCA occlusion which will produce posterior and inferior MI
C - Distal RCA occlusion which will produce inferior wall MI

Example of an Acute RV MI in right precordial leads.

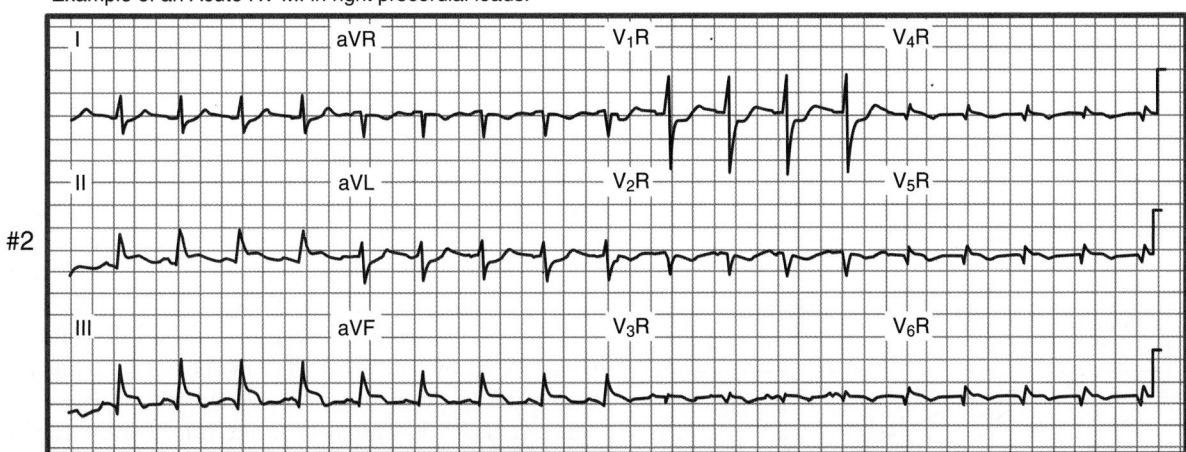

#2

ECG shows ST elevation in right precordial leads (V_3R to V_6R) indicating RV wall injury/infarct.
Note limb leads are identical in both ECGs.

D   **These two 12-lead ECGs are from the same patient with RV MI**

Figure 19-9, cont'd *C,* Example of an acute inferior RV wall MI with conventional 12-lead ECG. *D,* Example of an acute RV wall MI with a right-sided 12-lead ECG. Both 12-lead ECGs are taken from the same patient.

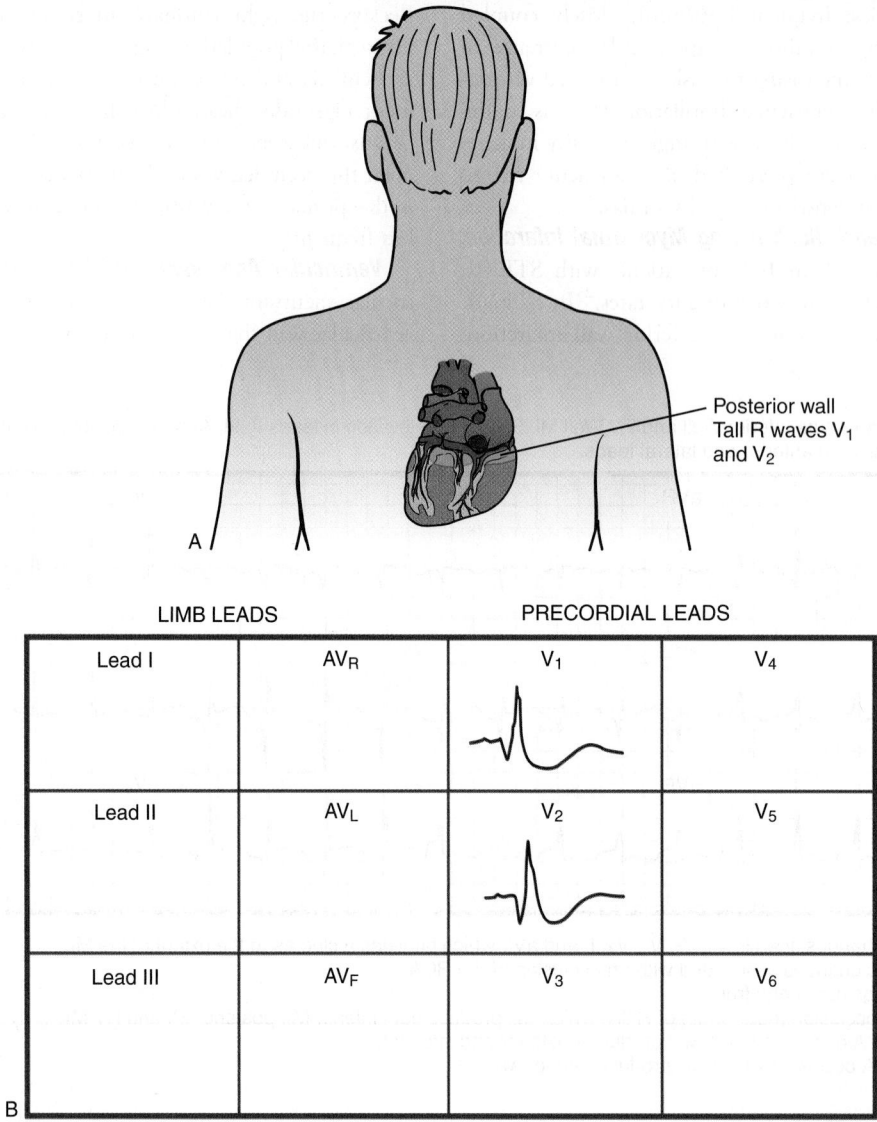

Posterior wall
Tall R waves V₁
and V₂

LIMB LEADS		PRECORDIAL LEADS	
Lead I	AV$_R$	V$_1$	V$_4$
Lead II	AV$_L$	V$_2$	V$_5$
Lead III	AV$_F$	V$_3$	V$_6$

Figure 19-10 Changes seen on a 12-lead ECG with STEMI. *A,* Infarction location on the cardiac wall. *B,* ECG leads with expected ST-segment elevation in the posterior wall STEMI.

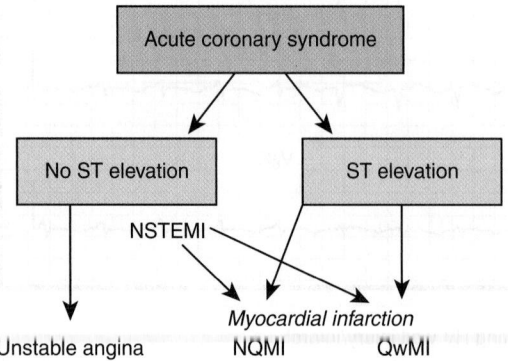

Figure 19-11 Acute coronary syndrome. *(Modified from Braunwald E et al: ACC/AHA guideline update for the management of patients with unstable angina and non-ST-segment elevation myocardial infarction—2002: summary article,* Circulation *106[14]:1893-1900, 2002.)*

It most often occurs in the setting of an acute left anterior descending artery occlusion with a wide area of infarcted myocardium.[2] The most effective prevention is early reperfusion of the myocardium, accomplished by opening the thrombosed coronary artery. In one study, the rate of ventricular aneurysm was reduced from 19% in untreated patients to 7% when the coronary artery was opened by fibrinolysis.[2] The most common complications of a ventricular aneurysm are acute heart failure, systemic emboli, angina, and VT. Treatment is directed toward management of these complications and surgical repair by left ventricular aneurysmectomy. The affected area may be described as *hypokinetic* (contracts poorly), *akinetic* (noncontractile scar tissue), or *dyskinetic* (scar tissue that moves in the opposite direction to the normal contractile myocardium). The prognosis depends on the size of the aneurysm, the level of overall left ventricular dysfunction, and the severity of coexisting CAD.

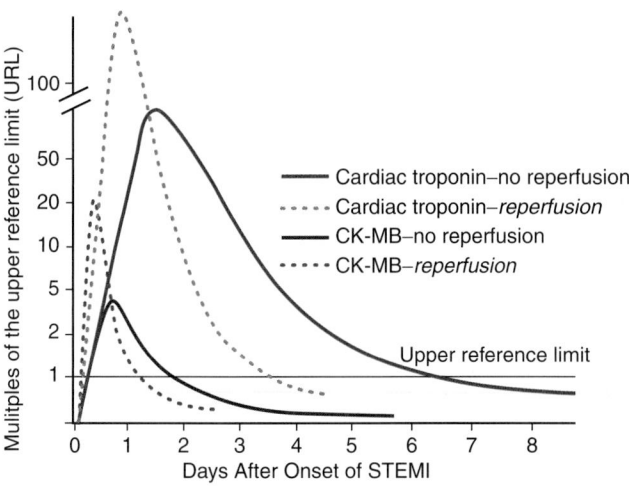

Figure 19-12 Cardiac biomarkers during MI. *(From Antman EM et al: ACC/ AHA guidelines for the management of patients with ST-elevation myocardial infarction—executive summary: a report of the American College of Cardiology/American Heart Association Task Force on Practice Guidelines [Writing Committee to Revise the 1999 Guidelines for the Management of Patients with Acute Myocardial Infarction], Circulation 110[9]:e82-292, 2004.)*

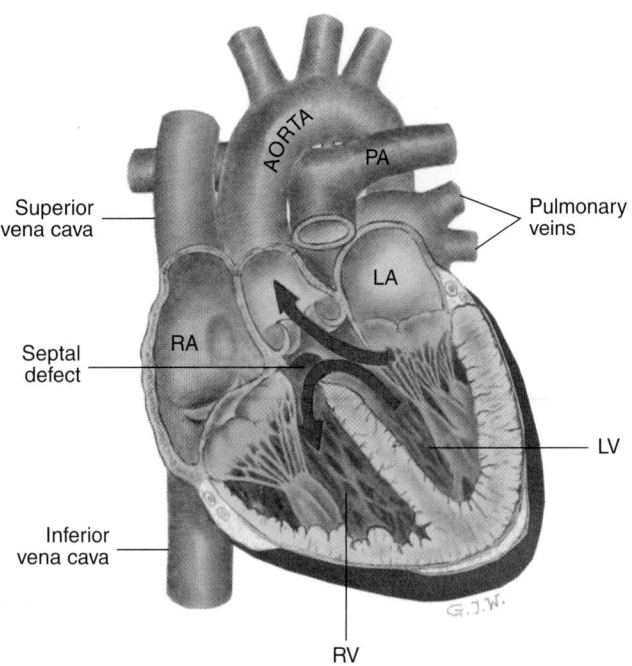

Figure 19-14 Ventricular septal rupture after acute myocardial infarction. LA, left atrium; LV, left ventricle; PA, pulmonary artery; RA, right atrium; RV, right ventricle.

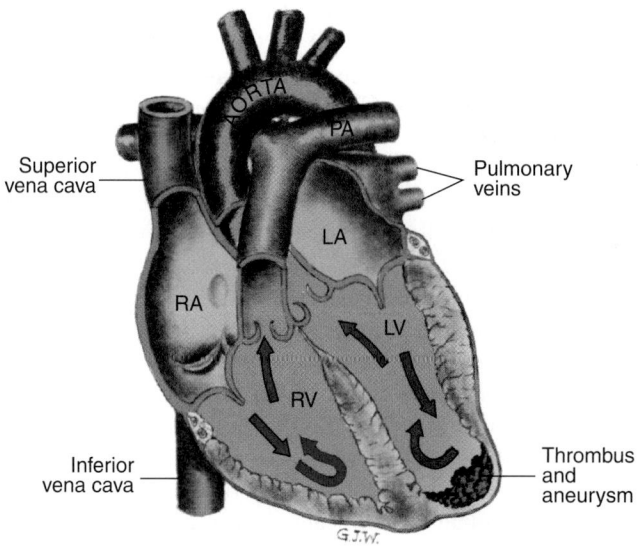

Figure 19-13 Ventricular aneurysm after acute myocardial infarction. LA, left atrium; LV, left ventricle; PA, pulmonary artery; RA, right atrium; RV, right ventricle.

Ventricular Septal Rupture after Myocardial Infarction.

Postinfarction rupture of the ventricular septal wall is a rare but potentially lethal complication of an acute anterior wall MI (Fig. 19-14). *Ventricular septal rupture,* also known as *acquired ventricular septal defect* (VSD), is an abnormal communication between the right and left ventricle. This complication occurs in less than 1% of all MIs, and the incidence has declined because most STEMI patients have the blocked coronary artery opened.[2] Nevertheless, rupture of the ventricular septum carries an extremely high mortality rate.[42] Mortality

rates between 35% and 73% are typical.[43,44] Most patients with septal rupture also have signs and symptoms of cardiogenic shock. Ventricular septal rupture manifests as severe chest pain, syncope, hypotension, and sudden hemodynamic deterioration caused by shunting of blood from the high-pressure left ventricle into the low-pressure right ventricle through the new septal opening. A holosystolic murmur (often accompanied by a thrill) can be auscultated and is best heard along the left sternal border. A diagnosis of postinfarction ventricular septal rupture can be made at the bedside with use of oxygen saturation assessment by means of a pulmonary artery catheter or by transesophageal echocardiography (TEE). Rupture of the septum is a medical and surgical emergency. The patient's condition is stabilized with vasodilators and an intraaortic balloon pump (IABP) to decrease afterload.[44] The goal of afterload reduction in this patient population is to decrease the amount of blood being shunted to the right side of the heart and consequently to increase the flow of blood to the systemic circulation. If the septal rupture is very small, and the patient's condition is sufficiently stable to wait for scar tissue to form before surgical repair, survival improves. Unfortunately, when the septal opening is large, the massive left to right shunt across the septum makes the chances of survival dismal with or without surgery.[43,44]

Papillary Muscle Rupture after Myocardial Infarction.

Papillary muscle rupture can occur when the infarct involves the area around one of the papillary muscles that support the mitral valve. Infarction of the papillary muscles results in ineffective mitral valve closure, and blood is forced back into the low-pressure left atrium during ventricular systole. The rupture may be partial or complete. Complete rupture is catastrophic

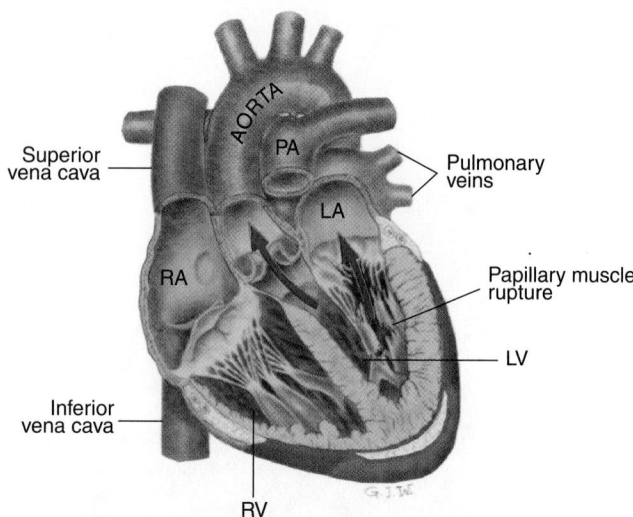

Figure 19-15 Papillary muscle rupture after acute myocardial infarction. LA, left atrium; LV, left ventricle; PA, pulmonary artery; RA, right atrium; RV, right ventricle.

and precipitates severe acute mitral regurgitation, cardiogenic shock, and high risk of death.

Partial rupture (Fig. 19-15) also results in mitral regurgitation, but the condition can be stabilized with aggressive medical management using the IABP and vasodilators. Urgent surgical intervention is required to replace the mitral valve.[45] As with other structural complications during acute MI, the incidence is decreased in patients who have their myocardium reperfused early.[2] Of the patients with acute MI who are admitted to the critical care unit in cardiogenic shock, 10% have papillary muscle rupture with acute mitral regurgitation. The mortality rate is 71% with medical treatment and 40% with surgical intervention to replace or repair the mitral valve.[2]

Cardiac Wall Rupture after Myocardial Infarction. Of the deaths that occur after MI, 1% to 6% can be attributed to cardiac rupture.[2] The incidence of cardiac wall rupture has two peak times. The first occurs within the first 24 hours and the second between the third and fifth postinfarction day when leukocyte scavenger cells are removing necrotic debris, thinning the myocardial wall.[2] The onset is sudden and usually catastrophic. Bleeding into the pericardial sac results in cardiac tamponade, cardiogenic shock, pulseless electrical activity (PEA), and death. Survival is rare. If rupture occurs in the hospital, emergency pericardiocentesis is required to relieve the tamponade until a surgical repair can be attempted. The best prevention is early reperfusion of the myocardium.[2]

Pericarditis after Myocardial Infarction. Pericarditis is inflammation of the pericardial sac. It can occur during a transmural MI or after an acute MI. Pericarditis may occur in 5% to 20% of transmural infarctions, but it is treated only if it is clinically significant.[46] The damaged epicardium becomes rough and inflamed and irritates the pericardium lying adjacent to it, precipitating pericarditis. Pain is the most common symptom of pericarditis, and a pericardial friction rub is the most common initial sign. The friction rub is best auscultated with a stethoscope at the sternal border and is described as a grating, scraping, or leathery scratching. Pericarditis frequently produces a pericardial effusion (fluid).[46] After the effusion occurs, the friction rub may disappear. On the 12-lead ECG, pericarditis may manifest as elevation of the ST segment in all of the typically upright leads.[47] Pericarditis is treated with nonsteroidal antiinflammatory drugs. Pericarditis that occurs as a late complication of acute MI is known as *Dressler's syndrome.*[46,48]

Heart Failure and Acute Myocardial Infarction. Almost 20% of patients with acute STEMI also have acute heart failure on admission to the hospital. These patients have often waited longer to come to the hospital and are older and more likely to be female. Compared with acute MI patients without heart failure, these patients have a higher risk of adverse in-hospital events and have longer lengths of stay and higher in-hospital mortality rates.[49] More detailed information about heart failure is presented later in this chapter.

MEDICAL MANAGEMENT

Quality outcomes research shows that compliance with the guidelines developed by the American College of Cardiology and the American Heart Association (ACC/AHA) decreases in-hospital mortality after acute MI.[50,51] Patients admitted to hospitals who adhere to the AHA/ACC guidelines for treatment of STEMI or NSTEMI have 8.3% in-hospital mortality rate, compared with a 15.3% mortality rate for patients managed at hospitals where the most recent guidelines are not fully used.[50,51] The guidelines are research based and are designed to improve the outcome of patients admitted to the hospital with an acute MI. Clinical guidelines address the issues of interventions to open the coronary artery, anticoagulation, prevention of dysrhythmias, tight glucose control, and prevention of ventricular remodeling after STEMI.[3]

Recanalization of the Coronary Artery. The essential immediate interventions are fibrinolytic therapy or PCI to open the occluded artery for the patient with an acute STEMI.[2] All clinical guidelines emphasize the need for patients with symptoms of ACS to be rapidly triaged and treated.[2]

Anticoagulation. In the acute phase after STEMI, heparin is administered in combination with fibrinolytic therapy to recanalize (open) the coronary artery.[2] For patients who will receive fibrinolytic therapy, an initial heparin bolus of 60 units/kg (maximum 4000 units) is given intravenously, followed by a continuous heparin drip at 12 units/kg/hr (maximum 1000 units/hour) to maintain an activated partial thromboplastin time (aPTT) between 50 and 70 seconds (1.5 to 2.0 times control). Alternatively, LMWH may be used at doses that provide full anticoagulation.[2]

It is also prudent to administer intravenous UFH or subcutaneous LMWH if the person is at risk for thrombus development.[2] For patients with known heparin induced thrombocytopenia (HIT), as an alternative to LMWH or UFH, a third class of antithrombotic drugs is available—direct antithrombotic agents (e.g., Hirudin, Bivalirudin, Argatroban, Fondaparinux)[52] Patients at risk for thrombotic emboli include those with an anterior wall infarction, atrial fibrillation, previous embolus, cardiomyopathy, or cardiogenic shock.

When the risk of systemic embolic complications remains high, especially in atrial fibrillation, the patient should be anti-coagulated with warfarin (Coumadin).[2]

Dysrhythmia Prevention. The antidysrhythmic with the best safety record after STEMI is amiodarone. The reduction in death related to decreased dysrhythmias after MI is 13%.[2] Beta-blockers are another class of antidysrhythmics that are recommended for all patients after STEMI. Beta-blockers prevent ventricular dysrhythmias, lower blood pressure, and prevent reinfarction, especially in patients with left ventricular dysfunction.[2]

Tight Glucose Control. Achievement of normal blood glucose levels during the acute phase and after MI improves survival.[2]

Prevention of Ventricular Remodeling. Many patients are at risk for development of heart failure after STEMI. Vasodilating drugs known as ACEIs or ARBs can stop or limit the ventricular remodeling that leads to heart failure. An ACEI is used, or if it is not tolerated, an ARB is indicated for all patients after STEMI.[2] Information about the clinical effects of heart failure is provided later in this chapter.

NURSING MANAGEMENT

Nursing management of the patient with an acute MI incorporates a variety of nursing diagnoses (see the Nursing Diagnoses feature on Myocardial Infarction). Nursing interventions focus on achieving a balance among myocardial oxygen supply and demand, preventing complications, and providing patient and family education.

Nursing Diagnoses

Myocardial Infarction

- Acute Pain related to transmission and perception of cutaneous, visceral, muscular, or ischemic impulses
- Decreased Cardiac Output related to alterations in preload
- Decreased Cardiac Output related to alterations in afterload
- Decreased Cardiac Output related to alterations in contractility
- Decreased Cardiac Output related to alterations in heart rate or rhythm
- Activity Intolerance related to cardiopulmonary dysfunction
- Ineffective Cardiopulmonary Tissue Perfusion related to decreased myocardial oxygen supply or increased myocardial oxygen demand, or both
- Disturbed Sleep Pattern related to fragmented sleep
- Anxiety related to threat to biologic, psychologic, or social integrity
- Ineffective Coping related to situational crisis and personal vulnerability
- Powerlessness related to lack of control over current situation or disease progression
- Deficient Knowledge: Discharge Regimen related to lack of previous exposure to information (see the Patient Education feature on Myocardial Infarction)

Balance of Myocardial Oxygen Supply and Demand. In the acute period, if severe heart muscle damage has occurred, myocardial oxygen supply is increased by the administration of supplemental oxygen to prevent tissue hypoxia. Many clinical signs manifest this imbalance (Box 19-7). Drugs play an increasingly important role in balancing supply and demand, and it is the critical care nurse who administers and monitors the effectiveness of these agents. For the patient with a low cardiac output, positive inotropic drugs such as dobutamine, dopamine, and milrinone are prescribed. These inotropic agents are used to increase cardiac contractility in the healthy areas of the heart (increasing oxygen supply), while avoiding damage to the recently infarcted areas. Myocardial oxygen supply can be further enhanced by the use of coronary artery vasodilators. Nitroglycerin is recommended for the first 48 hours to increase vasodilation and prevent myocardial ischemia.[2] Research evidence supports the administration of early beta-blockade therapy to decrease myocardial workload and to prevent dysrhythmias. Administration of beta-blockers reduces mortality by 14% in the first 7 days after an MI and by 23% in the long term.[2] However, if the patient is in cardiogenic shock, beta-blockers are withheld until the cardiac output has improved.[2] Other interventions to decrease cardiac work and myocardial oxygen consumption include bed rest with bedside commode privileges when the patient is clinically stable.

Prevention of Complications. A thorough grasp of the range of potential complications that can occur after STEMI is essential. Cardiac monitoring for early detection of ventricular dysrhythmias is ongoing. Assessment for signs of continued ischemic pain is important, because angina is a warning sign of myocardium at risk. In response to angina, a 12-lead ECG is obtained to determine if there is an extension of the infarct, nitroglycerin is administered, and the physician is notified immediately so that interventions may be initiated to limit the size of the MI. Heart failure is a serious complication after STEMI. When the patient's blood pressure is stable, treatment with ACEI is initiated. These vasodilators are used to prevent the left ventricular remodeling and dilation that occur in many patients after an acute MI. Hypotension is a potential complication of ACEI, especially with the first dose. It is an important nursing responsibility to monitor

---

BOX 19-7   CLINICAL MANIFESTATIONS OF ACUTE MYOCARDIAL INFARCTION

- Tachycardia with or without ectopy
- Bradycardia
- Normotension or hypotension
- Tachypnea
- Diminished heart sounds, especially S_1
- If left ventricular dysfunction present, may have S_3 and/or S_4
- Systolic murmur
- Pulmonary crackles
- Pulmonary edema

- Air hunger
- Orthopnea
- Frothy sputum
- Decreased cardiac output
- Decreased urine output
- Decreased peripheral pulses
- Slow capillary refill
- Restlessness
- Confusion
- Anxiety
- Agitation
- Denial
- Anger

blood pressure and patient symptoms after taking this medication. Surveillance to detect obvious and subtle signs of bleeding is also a priority because so many acute MI patients receive antiplatelet, anticoagulant, and fibrinolytic medications.[2]

In the first 24 hours, stable patients with acute MI may be given only a light diet, because their appetite is often poor. It is no longer considered necessary to restrict iced fluids or caffeine. While the patient is in bed, an upright position is preferred to foster better lung expansion. Deep breathing decreases the risk of atelectasis. An upright position also decreases venous return, lowers preload, and decreases cardiac work. The patient is taught to avoid increasing intraabdominal pressure (Valsalva maneuver). Stool softeners are given to the patient to lessen the risk of constipation from analgesics and bed rest and to decrease the risk of straining. The nurse controls the critical care unit environment by decreasing noise, diminishing sensory overload, and allowing adequate rest periods.

Depression after Myocardial Infarction. Depression is a phenomenon that occurs across a wide spectrum of human experience. The incidence of depression after an MI ranges from 17% to 27%. Key symptoms of depression mentioned frequently by cardiac patients are fatigue, change in appetite, and sleep disturbance. Depression is an independent risk factor for increased morbidity and mortality in those with coronary heart disease, and it is a treatable condition.

PATIENT EDUCATION

After the acute phase has passed, education for the patient and family focuses on risk factor reduction, manifestations of angina, when to call a physician or emergency services, medications, and resumption of physical and sexual activity (see the Patient Education feature on Myocardial Infarction). If possible, a referral is made to a cardiac rehabilitation program so that this education can be reinforced outside the acute care hospital environment.[53] Clinical practice guidelines for multidisciplinary care of the patient with an acute MI are listed in the Evidence-Based Practice: Collaborative feature on Acute Coronary Syndrome and Acute Myocardial Infarction.

Patient Education

Myocardial Infarction

- Pathophysiology of coronary artery disease, angina, and acute myocardial infarction
- Angina: Describe signs and symptoms, such as pain, pressure, or heaviness in chest, arms, or jaw.
- Use of the 0 to 10 pain scale: Notify critical care nurse or emergency personnel of any changes in chest pain intensity.
- Avoid the Valsalva maneuver.
- Risk factor modification tailored to the patient's individual risk factor profile:
  - Decrease daily fat intake to less than 30% of total calories.
  - Reduce total serum cholesterol to less than 200 mg/dL.
  - Reduce low-density lipoprotein (LDL) cholesterol to less than 70 mg/dL.
  - Stop smoking.
  - Reduce salt intake.
  - Control hypertension.
  - Control diabetes if patient is diabetic.
  - Increase physical activity.
  - Achieve ideal body weight if overweight.
- Reference to cardiac rehabilitation program
- Medication teaching: indications, side effects
- Follow-up care after discharge
- Symptoms to report to a health care professional
- Discussion of how to handle emotional stress and anger

Evidence-Based Practice: Collaborative

Acute Coronary Syndrome and Acute Myocardial Infarction (Non-STEMI and STEMI)

Prevention of Acute Coronary Syndrome
The term *ACS* is used to define the life-threatening consequences of CAD, notably unstable angina, non-STEMI, and STEMI:
- Unstable angina is a term that denotes chest pain that is not relieved by SL nitroglycerin or rest within 5 minutes.
- Non-STEMI is an acute MI *without* ST-segment elevation on the 12-lead ECG.
- STEMI is an acute MI *with* ST-segment elevation on the 12-lead ECG. All of the recommendations are class I, meaning that there is strong research evidence to support these recommendations.

Recommendations That Decrease the Risk of Developing Non-STEMI and STEMI
- Primary care providers should evaluate CAD risk factors for all patients every 3 to 5 years.
- The 10-year risk of ACS and acute MI should be assessed for all patients who have more than two major risk factors.

- An intensive risk factor modification program is recommended for patients with established CAD or high-risk equivalents such as diabetes or chronic kidney disease.

Recommendations That Patients Be Educated about Emergency ACS Symptoms
- A patient who has previously diagnosed CAD should take one SL nitroglycerin dose, and the patient (if alone) or a friend or relative should call 911 if chest pain or discomfort is unrelieved or worsening in 5 minutes.
- The same recommendation applies to a patient without known CAD. If pain is unrelieved with rest or worsening at 5 minutes, the patient (if alone) or a friend or relative should call 911.
- Patients with chest discomfort should be transported to the hospital by ambulance rather than be driven by a friend or relative.
- Family members should be advised to take a CPR course before an ACS emergency occurs. This will teach CPR skills, demonstrate use of an AED, and educate participants about the "chain of survival" concept.

Evidence-Based Practice: Collaborative—*cont'd*

Recommendations for Prehospital EMS-Paramedic First Responders
- First responders such as EMS-paramedics can provide early defibrillation and ACLS for patients in cardiac arrest.
- EMS personnel should administer 162 to 325 mg of nonenteric aspirin (chewed, not swallowed) to patients with chest pain and suspected STEMI.
- A prehospital fibrinolysis protocol is reasonable for patients with STEMI if there are physicians in the ambulance or if there is a well-organized EMS service with full-time paramedics plus 12-lead ECG transmission capability and online medical direction.
- Patients older than 75 years and those with cardiogenic shock should be transported to a hospital with the ability to provide fibrinolytics, emergency PCI, or emergency CABG. PCI or CABG, if needed, should be provided *within 18 hours* after the onset of cardiogenic shock.
- Patients with STEMI who have a contraindication to fibrinolytic therapy should be brought to a hospital capable of emergency PCI or CABG. At the scene, the door-to-departure time should be *less than 30 minutes*. PCI should be initiated *within 90 minutes* after initial medical contact.

Recommendations for Initial Emergency Clinical Management
- Hospitals should establish multidisciplinary teams to facilitate rapid triage of patients who present to the ED with chest pain.
- Use of written protocols is recommended to standardize care. An immediate cardiology consultation is advised if the patient's symptoms fall outside the written protocol.

STEMI
- Fibrinolytics for STEMI: Time from coming into contact with the health care system (paramedics or ED) to receiving fibrinolytics should be *less than 30 minutes*. A brief, focused neurologic examination to determine prior stroke or presence of cognitive defects is necessary before administration of fibrinolytics.
- PCI for STEMI: Time from coming into contact with the health care system (paramedics or ED) to balloon inflation PCI should be *less than 90 minutes*.

Non-STEMI
- If the level of risk for the patient with non-STEMI is not immediately apparent, a "chest pain unit" within the ED permits close surveillance by competent clinicians without immediate hospital admission.
- Glycoprotein IIb/IIIa inhibitors for non-STEMI, in addition to aspirin and heparin, are indicated if cardiac catheterization or PCI is planned.
- PCI may be indicated for non-STEMI.

Recommendations for Initial Emergency Physical Assessment
Vital Signs
- HR, BP, RR, temperature Spo_2, ECG monitor to detect presence of dysrhythmias

Physical Assessment
- Assess for warm or cool skin, color, capillary refill, peripheral pulses
- Auscultate heart for cardiac murmur or new S_3 or S_4
- Auscultate lungs for air entry plus crackles, wheezes
- Observe for breathlessness, frothy pink sputum (pulmonary edema)
- Ask patient, family, significant others for relevant history

Recommendations for Emergency Diagnostics
12-Lead ECG
- The 12-lead ECG should be shown to the ED physician within 10 minutes after the patient's arrival in the ED for all patients with chest discomfort or angina-equivalent symptoms.

- If the first ECG is normal but the patient continues to have symptoms of chest pain/discomfort, the 12-lead ECG should be repeated at 5- to 10-minute intervals, *or* continuous 12-lead ECG monitoring can be used.
- In patients with inferior wall infarction, RV infarction must be suspected and right-sided ECG leads recorded. V_4R is the diagnostic lead of choice to diagnose ST-segment elevation in the RV.

Laboratory Studies
- Laboratory tests should be performed as part of the general management of STEMI but should not delay the administration of reperfusion therapy.

Cardiac Biomarkers
- Measurement of cardiac-specific troponins is recommended for patients with coexistent skeletal muscle injury. Clinicians are advised not to wait for results of the biomarker assay before initiating reperfusion therapy. Point-of-care (handheld) biomarker assay results are permissible, but subsequent biomarker assays should be done by quantitative laboratory analysis.

Imaging Studies
- Portable chest radiograph: Obtaining the chest radiograph must not delay reperfusion therapy unless a major complication such as aortic dissection is suspected.
- Portable echocardiography (TTE or TEE) or MRI scan to distinguish aortic dissection from STEMI, for patients in whom the symptoms are not clear

Recommendations for Care
Prevent Hypoxia
- Supplemental oxygen administered to maintain Sao_2 greater than 90%

Coronary Vasodilation
- Nitroglycerin (0.04 mg SL every 5 minutes for three doses) is administered. If chest pain or discomfort is ongoing, start peripheral IV. Administer IV nitroglycerin for relief of chest pain, control of hypertension, or relief of pulmonary congestion.

Pain Control
- Morphine sulfate (2 to 4 mg IV) is administered; can increase to 2- to 8-mg IV increments at 5- to 15-minute intervals for STEMI pain control.

NSAIDS
- Discontinue NSAIDs (except for aspirin), both nonselective and COX-2 selective agents, at time of presentation with STEMI because of increased risk of mortality, reinfarction, hypertension, heart failure, and myocardial rupture associated with NSAID use.

Aspirin
- Aspirin 162 mg to be chewed for rapid buccal absorption

Beta-Blockers
- Oral beta-blocker therapy is administered to STEMI patients without contraindications to beta-blockade, irrespective of fibrinolytic or primary PCI reperfusion.
- Contraindications for beta-blockade with STEMI include signs of heart failure, low cardiac output, cardiogenic shock risk, heart block or prolonged PR interval (>0.24 second), and active asthma or reactive airway disease.
- While considering the options for reperfusion, beta-blockers are given if the patient has tachycardia or hypertension; otherwise, they are started as soon as possible after STEMI.

Angiotensin-Converting Enzymes Inhibitors
- Oral ACE inhibitors are indicated within the first 24 hours after STEMI

Recommendations for Emergency Interventions for STEMI
Fibrinolytic Drugs
- Fibrinolytic drugs are administered to STEMI patients with ST-segment elevation greater than 0.1 mV (1 mm or one small box) in two contiguous precordial (chest) leads *or* two adjacent limb leads, new LBBB or presumed new LBBB, and onset of symptoms less than 12 hours earlier.

Continued

Evidence-Based Practice: Collaborative—cont'd

- Before administration of fibrinolytic therapy, rule out neurologic contraindications.
- Rule out facial trauma, uncontrolled hypertension, or ischemic stroke within the last 3 months.
- If contraindications to fibrinolysis are present, PCI is the preferred method of reperfusion.

PCI

- Emergency diagnostic coronary angiography to identify blocked coronary artery before PCI
- Emergency PCI is recommended over fibrinolytic therapy if symptom onset was longer ago than 3 hours ago.
- Emergency PCI can be performed within 12 hours after symptom onset for patients with new LBBB or presumed new LBBB.
- Emergency PCI balloon inflation within 90 minutes after arrival at the hospital
- If cardiogenic shock develops less than 36 hours after MI, in patients younger than 75 years with ST-segment elevation, or in patients with new LBBB, "rescue PCI" is recommended within 18 hours after shock onset.

Cardiac Surgery

- Emergency CABG surgery is undertaken for specific indications in STEMI:

  Failed PCI with persistent pain or hemodynamic instability

  Recurrent ischemia refractory to medical therapy in patients with suitable anatomy who are not candidates for PCI

  Post-MI VSR or papillary muscle rupture, both of which frequently lead to cardiogenic shock

  Cardiogenic shock less than 36 hours after MI, in patients younger than 75 years with ST-segment elevation, or in patients with new LBBB who have multivessel or left main disease

  Recurrent ventricular dysrhythmias in patients with 50% or greater left main coronary artery lesion or triple-vessel disease or both

Recommendations for Secondary Prevention of Complications

Medications

- ACE inhibitors to prevent ventricular remodeling
- Beta-blockers to prevent ventricular dysrhythmias
- Diuretics if heart failure has developed
- Antihyperlipidemics if total cholesterol, LDL-C, or triglycerides are elevated

Recommendations for Management of Complications after STEMI

Cardiogenic Shock

- IABP for patients with hypotension (BP of 90 mm Hg or SBP of 30 mm Hg below baseline)

Ventricular Arrhythmias

- VF or pulseless VT is managed by standard ACLS criteria: unsynchronized biphasic shock of 200 joules, followed by 2 minutes (five cycles) of CPR; then another shock of 200 joules if patient has not converted, followed by 2 minutes of CPR. Vasopressors are given during CPR if intravenous or intraosseous access is available.
- Patients with hemodynamically significant VT more than 2 days after STEMI who have ongoing ventricular dysrhythmias are considered for implantation of an ICD.
- Patients with an EF between 30% and 40% at 1 month after STEMI should undergo an EPS, if they are inducible to VT/VF, an ICD is recommended to reduce risk of SCD.
- Patients with an EF of less than 30% at 1 month after STEMI are at high risk for SCD.

AV block

- Transvenous pacemaker (emergency) or permanent pacemaker (later elective) is inserted for symptomatic second- or third-degree AV block.
- All patients after STEMI who require permanent pacing should also be evaluated for ICD indications.

Provide Relevant Education

Medications

- Written and verbal instructions about medication dosages, administration, and side effects

Emergency Information

- Give patient and family information about calling 911 if pain/angina-equivalent symptoms persist or are worse after 5 minutes.
- Family members of high-risk patients are advised to take a CPR class and learn about AED.

Risk Factors

- Smoking cessation, hypertension control, weight control, normal blood glucose; low-fat diet; normal lipid panel
- Increase physical activity, no new HRT for women

Cardiac Rehabilitation

- Participation in a cardiac rehabilitation program will help the patient continue the process of risk factor and lifestyle modification.

References

Antman EM et al: ACC/AHA guidelines for the management of patients with ST-elevation myocardial infarction, *Circulation* 110:588-636, 2004.

Antman EM et al: 2007 focused update of the ACC/AHA 2004 guidelines for the management of patients with ST-elevation myocardial infarction, *Circulation* 117(2):296-329, 2008.

Braunwald E et al: ACC/AHA 2002 guideline update for the management of patients with unstable angina and non-ST-segment elevation myocardial infarction, *J Am Coll Cardiol* 40(7):1366-1374, 2002.

Anderson LJ et al: ACC/AHA 2007 guidelines for the management of patients with unstable angina and non–ST-segment elevation myocardial infarction, *J Am Coll Cardiol* 50(7):e1-e57, 2007.

ACE, angiotensin-converting enzyme; ACLS, advanced cardiac life support; ACS, acute coronary syndrome; AED, automated external defibrillator; AV, atrioventricular; BP, blood pressure, CABG, coronary artery bypass graft surgery; CAD, coronary artery disease; COX-2, cyclooxygenase 2; CPR, cardiopulmonary resuscitation; ECG, electrocardiogram; ED, emergency department; EF, ejection fraction; EMS, emergency medical services; EPS, electrophysiology study; HR, heart rate; HRT, hormone replacement therapy; IABP, intraaortic balloon pump; ICD, implantable cardioverter defibrillator; IV, intravenous; LBBB, left bundle branch block; LDL, low-density lipoprotein cholesterol; MI, myocardial infarction; MRI, magnetic resonance imaging; non-STEMI, non–ST-segment elevation myocardial infarction; NSAIDs, nonsteroidal antiinflammatory drugs; PCI, percutaneous coronary intervention; RR, respiratory rate; RV, right ventricle; Sao$_2$, arterial oxygen saturation; SCD, sudden cardiac death; SL, sublingual; Spo$_2$, oxygen saturation from external pulse-oximeter; STEMI, ST-segment elevation myocardial infarction; TEE, transesophageal echocardiogram; TTE, transthoracic echocardiogram; VF, ventricular fibrillation; VSR, ventricular septal rupture; VT, ventricular tachycardia.

SUDDEN CARDIAC DEATH

DESCRIPTION

Between 400,000 and 460,000 people die suddenly of cardiac causes each year.[1] This number represents 60% of all cardiac deaths.[1] These statistics represent deaths that occur outside the hospital with symptoms that last less than 1 hour or occur in a hospital emergency department.[54] Sudden cardiac death represents about 5% of the total annual mortality rate for all causes.[55]

When the onset of symptoms is rapid, the most likely mechanism of death is VT, which degenerates into VF. This syndrome is called *sudden cardiac death* (SCD). Despite aggressive cardiopulmonary resuscitation (CPR) initiated outside the hospital, few who sustain an out-of-hospital cardiac arrest survive to hospital discharge. Strategies that have been shown to improve resuscitation survival involve huge community-wide programs to teach laypersons CPR and how to use an automated external defibrillator (AED). With such a program in place and with accessible AED units and rapid EMS support, survival to hospital discharge has been shown to improve.[56]

ETIOLOGY

Most SCD incidents occur in patients with preexisting ventricular dysfunction resulting from cardiac disease. Specific SCD risk factors include extensive coronary atherosclerosis with or without a history of an acute MI; dilated or hypertrophic cardiomyopathy; valvular heart disease; autonomic nervous system abnormalities; electrical system abnormalities, such as AV block, Wolff-Parkinson-White (WPW) syndrome, prolonged QT syndrome, or Brugada syndrome; and taking medications that prolong the QT interval.[57-59] An ejection fraction less than 30% and a history of ventricular dysrhythmias are powerful predictors of SCD. Other risk factors are listed in Box 19-8. Unfortunately, many individuals are unaware of their risk, or there are other risk factors that have not yet been considered. In one longitudinal analysis, 48% of the SCD victims had not been previously diagnosed with cardiac disease.[54] Fifty percent of men and 64% of women who die suddenly of cardiovascular disease have no previous symptoms of the disease. Men account for 70% to 89% of SCD, an annual incidence that is three to four times higher for men than women.[1]

BOX 19-8 CAUSES OF SUDDEN CARDIAC DEATH

ACQUIRED SCD RISK

Most SCD patients are older adults and have a history of CAD, MI, and subsequent heart failure.

- Heart failure
  - Ejection fraction <30%
  - Heart structure is abnormal (systolic or diastolic ventricular dysfunction)
  - CAD and a history of MI that has produced scar tissue is the most common cause of VT/VF leading to SCD.
- Cardiomyopathy (dilated or ischemic)
  - Patients who are inducible for VT/VF in EPS are at highest risk.
  - Risk is decreased by implantation of an ICD and antidysrhythmic drug therapy.

GENETIC SCD RISK

Genetic cardiovascular disease accounts for 40% of SCD in young adults.

- Brugada syndrome
  - ECG signs: coved-type ST-segment elevation (>2 mm) in right precordial leads, although ECG variations also occur
  - Heart structure appears normal
  - High risk of VT or VF in otherwise young healthy adults
  - VT/VF often occurs at night, at rest
  - Represents 4% of all SCD; average age, 41 years
  - Represents up to 20% of genetic SCD patients
  - Hereditary: autosomal-dominant genetic transmission

- Five times more common in males
- Patients who are inducible in EPS are at increased risk
- Risk reduced by implantation of an ICD
- Wolff-Parkinson-White syndrome
  - Congenital accessory conduction pathway connects the atria and ventricles
  - Accessory pathway is *in addition* to the normal conduction system
  - Accessory pathway allows very rapid transmission of impulses leading to "preexcitation" of the ventricle that can degenerate into VT/VF, especially if atrial dysrhythmias are present
  - WPW syndrome is usually identified when patient is a teenager or young adult.
  - WPW syndrome is often recognized during exercise by palpitations or breathlessness.
  - It can be cured in many cases by radiofrequency ablation of the accessory pathway.
- Hypertrophic cardiomyopathy
  - There is a risk of VT/VF with exercise.
  - The HOCM form can be cured in many cases by alcohol ablation of the enlarged ventricular septum.
  - For other HCM patients, the risk is reduced by implantation of an ICD.
- Long QT syndrome
  - There is a risk of VT/VF with exercise.
  - The risk is reduced by implantation of an ICD.

CAD, coronary artery disease; *CV,* cardiovascular; ECG, electrocardiogram; EPS, electrophysiology study; HCM, hypertrophic cardiomyopathy; HOCM, hypertrophic subaortic obstructive cardiomyopathy; ICD, implantable cardioverter defibrillator; MI, myocardial infarction; SCD, sudden cardiac death; VF, ventricular fibrillation; VT, ventricular tachycardia; WPW, Wolff-Parkinson-White.

MEDICAL MANAGEMENT

Depending on the length of time the patient was unconscious as a result of the cardiac arrest, cognitive defects may be present because of the lack of cerebral blood flow and resultant hypoxia. The cardiac arrest may also have damaged the myocardium and other tissues. Therapy is tailored to the needs of the patient. For comatose patients at high risk for hypoxic brain injury after cardiac arrest, therapeutic hypothermia is initiated to preserve brain function. Survivors receive antidysrhythmic agents and have an implantable cardioverter defibrillator (ICD) unit inserted.[60-62] Prevention focuses on identification and treatment of high-risk cardiac patients (see "Implantable Cardioverter Defibrillator" and "Antidysrhythmic Drugs" in Chapter 20).

HEART FAILURE

DESCRIPTION AND ETIOLOGY

The number of patients with heart failure is increasing in the United States. More than 5 million Americans have a diagnosis of heart failure, and about 550,000 new cases are diagnosed each year.[1] This represents about 2.5% of the adult population.[1] More than 284,000 people die of heart failure each year.[1] Heart failure is primarily a disease of older persons. Approximately 6% to 10% of people older than 65 years have a diagnosis of heart failure; for patients who are hospitalized with this diagnosis, 80% are older than 80 years. The total inpatient and outpatient costs for heart failure exceed $38 billion annually, a sum that represents more than 5% of the total United States health care budget and increases significantly each year.[63]

PATHOPHYSIOLOGY

Heart failure is a response to cardiac dysfunction, a condition in which the heart cannot pump blood at a volume required to meet the body's needs. Any condition that impairs the ability of the ventricles to fill or eject blood can cause heart failure. CAD with resultant necrotic damage to the left ventricle is the underlying cause of heart failure in most patients. Other major conditions that lead to heart failure include valvular dysfunction, infection (myocarditis or endocarditis), cardiomyopathy, and uncontrolled hypertension.[63] Hypertension is the precursor of heart failure in women, whereas CAD, specifically MI, is the primary cause of heart failure in men.[64]

ASSESSMENT AND DIAGNOSIS

Heart failure is typically classified using the New York Heart Association (NYHA) criteria. Patients are assigned into four groups, I through IV, depending on the degree of symptoms and the amount of patient effort required to elicit symptoms (Table 19-9). Research-based clinical guidelines suggest adding a second level of classification that emphasizes the progressive nature of heart failure through stages identified by increasing symptom distress and intensified clinical interventions (Table 19-10).[63] Heart failure can manifest in many different

TABLE 19-9 New York Heart Association Functional Classification of Heart Failure

Class	Definition
I	Normal daily activity does not initiate symptoms.
II	Normal daily activities initiate onset of symptoms, but symptoms subside with rest.
III	Minimal activity initiates symptoms; patients are usually symptom free at rest.
IV	Any type of activity initiates symptoms, and symptoms are present at rest.

ways, depending on how far ventricular remodeling and dysfunction have advanced. Heart failure may be discovered because of a known clinical syndrome such as acute MI or because of decreased exercise tolerance, fluid retention, or admission to the critical care unit for an unrelated condition.[63] For patients with fluid retention, the most reliable clinical sign of fluid volume overload is jugular venous distention.[63] The procedure used to estimate jugular venous distention is described in Figure 17-2 and Box 17-1 of Chapter 17.

The first step in the diagnosis is to determine the underlying structural abnormality creating the ventricular dysfunction and symptoms. Various imaging tests are available to visualize cardiac anatomy, and laboratory tests are used to evaluate the impact of hormonal or electrolyte imbalance. The results of these tests permit the cardiology team to design a treatment plan to control symptoms and possibly correct the underlying cause. All patients do not have the same type of heart failure.

Left Ventricular Failure. Failure of the left ventricle is defined as a disturbance of the contractile function of the left ventricle, resulting in a low cardiac output state. This leads to vasoconstriction of the arterial bed that raises systemic vascular resistance (SVR), a condition also described as "high afterload," and creates congestion and edema in the pulmonary circulation and alveoli. Clinical manifestations include decreased peripheral perfusion with weak or diminished pulses; cool, pale extremities; and in later stages, peripheral cyanosis (Table 19-11). Over time, with progression of the disease state the fluid accumulation behind the dysfunctional left ventricle elevates pulmonary pressures, contributes to pulmonary congestion and edema, and produces dysfunction of the right ventricle, resulting in failure of the right side of the heart.

Right Ventricular Failure. Failure of the right side of the heart is defined as ineffective right ventricular contractile function. Pure failure of the right ventricle may result from an acute condition such as a pulmonary embolus or a right ventricular infarction, but it is most commonly caused by failure of the left side of the heart. The common manifestations of right ventricular failure are jugular venous distention, elevated central venous pressure (CVP), weakness, peripheral or sacral edema, hepatomegaly (enlarged liver), jaundice, and liver tenderness. Gastrointestinal symptoms include poor appetite, anorexia, nausea, and an uncomfortable feeling of fullness (see Table 19-11).

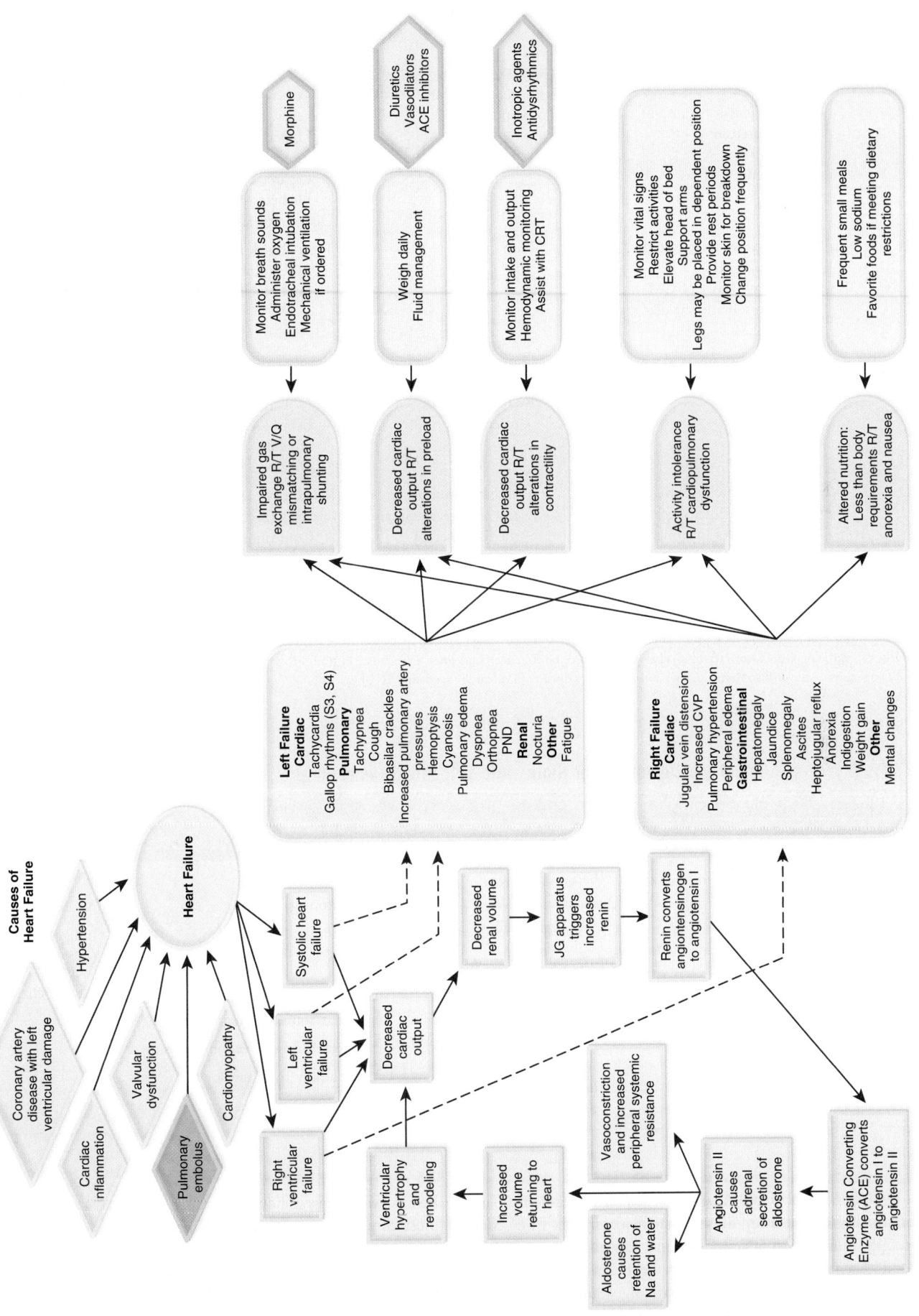

Causes of Heart Failure

Coronary artery disease with left ventricular damage

Hypertension

Cardiac inflammation

Valvular dysfunction

Pulmonary embolus

Cardiomyopathy

Heart Failure

Systolic heart failure

Left ventricular failure

Right ventricular failure

Decreased cardiac output

Decreased renal volume

JG apparatus triggers increased renin

Renin converts angiontensinogen to angiotensin I

Angiotensin Converting Enzyme (ACE) converts angiotensin I to angiotensin II

Angiotensin II causes adrenal secretion of aldosterone

Vasoconstriction and increased peripheral systemic resistance

Aldosterone causes retention of Na and water

Increased volume returning to heart

Ventricular hypertrophy and remodeling

Left Failure
Cardiac
Tachycardia
Gallop rhythms (S3, S4)
Pulmonary
Tachypnea
Cough
Bibasilar crackles
Increased pulmonary artery pressures
Hemoptysis
Cyanosis
Pulmonary edema
Dyspnea
Orthopnea
PND
Renal
Nocturia
Other
Fatigue

Right Failure
Cardiac
Jugular vein distension
Increased CVP
Pulmonary hypertension
Peripheral edema
Gastrointestinal
Hepatomegaly
Jaundice
Splenomegaly
Ascites
Heptojugular reflux
Anorexia
Indigestion
Weight gain
Other
Mental changes

Impaired gas exchange R/T V/Q mismatching or intrapulmonary shunting

Decreased cardiac output R/T alterations in preload

Decreased cardiac output R/T alterations in contractility

Activity intolerance R/T cardiopulmonary dysfunction

Altered nutrition: Less than body requirements R/T anorexia and nausea

Monitor breath sounds
Administer oxygen
Endotracheal intubation
Mechanical ventilation if ordered

Weigh daily
Fluid management

Monitor intake and output
Hemodynamic monitoring
Assist with CRT

Monitor vital signs
Restrict activities
Elevate head of bed
Support arms
Legs may be placed in dependent position
Provide rest periods
Monitor skin for breakdown
Change position frequently

Frequent small meals
Low sodium
Favorite foods if meeting dietary restrictions

Morphine

Diuretics
Vasodilators
ACE inhibitors

Inotropic agents
Antidysrhythmics

TABLE 19-10 Progression of Heart Failure

Stage	Structural Heart Disorder	Symptoms	Management

A	No, but at risk because of
	   Hypertension
	   CAD
	   Diabetes mellitus
		None	Preventive treatment of known risk factors
			   Hypertension
			   Lipid disorders
			   Cigarette smoking
			   Diabetes mellitus
			Discourage alcohol and illicit drug use

B	Yes, but without symptoms
	   Previous MI
	   Family history of CM
	   Asymptomatic valvular disease
	     or CM
		None	Treat all risk factors. If indicated, use the following:
			   ACE inhibitors
			   Beta-blockers

C	Yes, with prior or current symptoms	Shortness of breath
		Fatigue
		Reduced exercise
		   tolerance
			Treat all risk factors and HF symptoms:
			   Diuretics
			   ACE inhibitors
			   Beta-blockers
			   Digitalis
			   Dietary salt restriction

D	Yes, with refractory HF symptoms
	   despite maximal specialized
	   interventions (pharmacologic,
	   medical, nursing)
	Recurrently hospitalized for HF
	   symptoms
		Marked symptoms at
		   rest despite maximal
		   medical therapy
			Refractory HF requires interventions from previous
			   stages (A–C), plus the following:
			   Continuous IV inotropic support
			   Mechanical assist devices
			   Heart transplantation
			   Hospice care

Modified from Hunt SA et al: ACC/AHA 2005 guideline update for the diagnosis and management of chronic heart failure in the adult: a report of the American College of Cardiology/American Heart Association Task Force on Practice Guidelines, *Circulation* 112(12):e154-e235, 2005.
ACE, angiotensin-converting enzyme; CAD, coronary artery disease; CM, cardiomyopathy; HF, heart failure; IV, intravenous; MI, myocardial infarction.

TABLE 19-11 Clinical Manifestations of Right- and Left-Sided Heart Failure

LEFT VENTRICULAR FAILURE		RIGHT VENTRICULAR FAILURE	
Signs	Symptoms	Signs	Symptoms
Tachypnea	Fatigue	Peripheral edema	Weakness
Tachycardia	Dyspnea	Hepatomegaly	Anorexia
Cough	Orthopnea	Splenomegaly	Indigestion
Bibasilar crackles	Paroxysmal nocturnal dyspnea	Hepatojugular reflux	Weight gain
Gallop rhythms (S_3 and S_4)	Nocturia	Ascites	Mental changes
Increased pulmonary artery pressures		Jugular venous distention	
Hemoptysis		Increased central venous pressure	
Cyanosis		Pulmonary hypertension	
Pulmonary edema			

Systolic Heart Failure. *Systolic dysfunction* describes an abnormality of the heart muscle that markedly decreases contractility during systole (ejection) and lessens the quantity of blood that can be pumped out of the heart. Patients with a diagnosis of systolic heart failure have signs and symptoms of heart failure combined with a below-normal ejection fraction.

Left ventricular systolic dysfunction is the classic picture that most clinicians consider when thinking about heart failure. In addition to the signs and symptoms of left heart failure (described earlier), the patient has a low ejection fraction. There is some debate about how low the ejection fraction has to be to qualify as systolic heart failure, but the value usually is below

50%[65]; some clinicians cite numbers below 45% or 40%.[66,67] Symptoms of systolic heart failure include dyspnea, exercise intolerance, and fluid volume overload.

CAD and its sequelae represent the underlying cause in two thirds of patients with systolic heart failure.[63] The remaining patients with systolic dysfunction have *nonischemic cardiomyopathy* (interchangeably described as *dilated cardiomyopathy*)[68] that results from an identifiable cause such as hypertension, thyroid disease, cardiac valvular disease, alcohol use, or myocarditis.[63] If the cause is unknown, systolic dysfunction is described as *idiopathic dilated cardiomyopathy*.[63] The incidence of systolic heart failure in the general population is 3%; it increases with age, and the condition is more common in men.[67] Clinical findings that are required to make a diagnosis of systolic heart failure include the following[63]:

- Signs and symptoms of heart failure
- Left ventricular systolic dysfunction with an ejection fraction below normal

In systolic heart failure, the ventricular chambers change their shape, a detrimental development known as *ventricular remodeling.* The negative impact on the cardiac cells is different from the dysfunction and loss of myocytes from myocardial ischemia and infarction. Ventricular remodeling is modulated by catecholamines and activation of neurohormonal compensatory mechanisms. The heart chamber walls ultimately become dilated, thinned, and poorly contractile.

Significant hemodynamic changes occur as systolic dysfunction progresses. In systolic heart failure, the left ventricular end-diastolic volume (LVEDV) is high, which raises the left ventricular end-diastolic pressure (LVEDP) compared with a normal heart. The increase in intracardiac volume and pressure causes a rise in left atrial and pulmonary venous pressures. This means that all blood flowing into the heart through the pulmonary vascular bed is exposed to increased hydrostatic pressure, which is necessary to fill the congested heart. The increase in pulmonary vascular pressure causes transudation of fluid from the pulmonary capillaries into the alveolar interstitium, and this fluid is ultimately forced through the walls of the alveoli, causing pulmonary edema. The pulmonary complications of heart failure are described in greater detail later. The elevated left heart pressures eventually raise pressures in the right side of the heart and lead to secondary right heart failure. Right heart pressures are elevated in almost 80% of patients with chronically elevated left heart pressures.[63]

Diastolic Heart Failure. *Diastolic dysfunction* describes an abnormality of the heart muscle that makes it unable to relax, stretch, or fill during diastole. The ejection fraction can be normal or abnormal (low), and the patient may be symptomatic or symptom free.[65,69] Between 20% and 40% of patients with heart failure are believed to have diastolic muscle dysfunction.[63] The principal causes are similar to systolic heart failure (described earlier): CAD, myocardial ischemia, atrial fibrillation, uncontrolled hypertension in 75% of cases, and left ventricular hypertrophy in about 40%.[69] Some conditions that are known to markedly alter diastolic function include hypertrophic cardiomyopathy, restrictive cardiomyopathy, and infiltrative diseases such as amyloidosis and neoplastic infiltrate.[63,68] The incidence of diastolic heart failure is highest among patients older than 75 years, and the condition disproportionately affects elderly women.[63] It is postulated that the process of aging negatively impacts diastolic function, imposing stiffness and fibrosis on the cardiac muscle and cardiovascular vessels.[63]

Clinical findings that are required to make a diagnosis of diastolic heart failure include the following[63,65,66]:

- Signs and symptoms of heart failure
- Normal or only mildly abnormal left ventricular systolic dysfunction
- Abnormal left ventricular relaxation, filling, diastolic distensibility or diastolic stiffness

Diastolic heart failure is caused by dysfunction during the diastolic phase of the cardiac cycle. In affected patients, the heart muscle takes longer to relax compared with a normal heart, the ventricular chamber does not distend to accept the fill volume, and the myocardium remains stiff throughout diastole.[69,70] Normally, diastole is the filling stage of the cardiac cycle when the ventricle relaxes completely. The abnormal hemodynamics of diastolic heart failure can be elicited by diagnostic tests such as cardiac catheterization and a stress echocardiogram (see Chapter 18).[69] An ejection fraction above the range of 40% to 50% is considered normal for this population.

In diastolic heart failure, the LVEDP is high, whereas the LVEDV is paradoxically low compared with normal hearts.[65] Another diagnostic clue is that many patients with diastolic heart failure have normal intracardiac pressures at rest, but during exercise, the LVEDP and pulmonary vascular pressures rise rapidly.[65] This occurs because the noncompliant, stiff ventricle cannot increase stroke volume during exercise; cardiac output remains low even though physical demand is high. Patients with diastolic heart failure often experience a sudden rise in blood pressure and sinus tachycardia during exercise; they are exercise intolerant and experience fatigue, dyspnea, pulmonary venous congestion, and even pulmonary edema.[65,66,69]

Systolic versus Diastolic Heart Failure. It turns out to be impossible to accurately determine whether a patient has systolic or diastolic heart failure from clinical assessment alone.[65] Both types of heart failure produce similar signs and symptoms. The level of symptoms and quality of life vary between individuals and between men and women, even when the ejection fraction and presumed cardiac dysfunction is the same.[71] This may occur because most symptoms come from the neurohormonal compensatory mechanisms (described later) rather than the cardiac output. An elevated B-type natriuretic peptide (BNP) level (>100 pg/mL) is very useful to diagnose heart failure in patients with fluid overload and shortness of breath.[72] The BNP value tends to be higher for patients with a diagnosis of systolic heart failure compared with diastolic heart failure, although the difference is not reliable enough to be used to differentiate the two types of heart failure in clinical practice.[72] The more severe the heart failure, the higher the BNP level. The primary use of the BNP test is to determine whether the patient has heart failure.

The definitive diagnosis of the type of heart failure is often made using Doppler echocardiography. An echocardiogram performed at rest and during exercise (stress echo) permits visualization of heart wall movement during systole and diastole. Calculation of the ejection fraction can be determined using Doppler echocardiography or during a cardiac catheterization. These diagnostic tests also show that some patients exhibit combined systolic and diastolic heart failure.[65]

The annual mortality rate for diastolic heart failure is 5% to 8%, markedly less than the 10% to 15% annual mortality for patients with systolic heart failure. To put this in perspective, age-matched controls without any heart failure have an annual mortality rate of just 1%.[1,65,69]

It is not possible to distinguish whether a patient has systolic or diastolic heart failure simply by looking at the medications they are prescribed. The same drugs are used to treat the two types of heart failure, although the underlying rationales may be different.[66] For example, beta-blockers are used in diastolic heart failure to slow the heart rate, to prolong diastole to give more time for ventricular filling, and to modify the ventricular response to exercise, especially for patients who have a preserved ejection fraction.[66] When beta-blockers are prescribed for treatment of systolic heart failure, the intent is to preserve long-term inotropic (contractile) function and prevent ventricular remodeling.[66] Diuretics are used to treat both types of heart failure, although a smaller dosage is generally needed in diastolic heart failure.[66] ACEIs and ARBs are also used to treat both types of heart failure. The medications used to treat heart failure are further discussed in Chapter 20 (see Table 20-20).

Acute versus Chronic Heart Failure. Acute or chronic heart failure is determined by the rapidity with which the syndrome develops, the presence and activation of compensatory mechanisms, and the presence or absence of fluid accumulation in the interstitial space (see Table 19-10). In clinical practice guidelines, the terms *acute* and *chronic* have replaced the older name of *congestive heart failure* (CHF), because not all heart failure involves pulmonary congestion.[63] However, the description of a patient by CHF remains commonly employed in clinical practice.

Acute heart failure has a sudden onset, with no compensatory mechanisms. The patient may experience acute pulmonary edema, low cardiac output, or even cardiogenic shock. Patients with chronic heart failure are hypervolemic, have sodium and water retention, and have structural heart chamber changes such as dilation or hypertrophy.[63]

Chronic heart failure is ongoing, with symptoms that may be made tolerable by medication, diet, and a reduced activity level. The deterioration into acute heart failure can be precipitated by the onset of dysrhythmias, acute ischemia, sudden illness, or cessation of medications. This may necessitate admission to a critical care unit. Hypertension is the primary precursor of heart failure in women, whereas coronary heart disease, specifically MI, is the primary cause of heart failure in men.

NEUROHORMONAL COMPENSATORY MECHANISMS IN HEART FAILURE

When the heart begins to fail and the cardiac output is no longer sufficient to meet the metabolic needs of the tissues, the body activates several major compensatory mechanisms: the sympathetic nervous system, the renin-angiotensin-aldosterone system (RAAS), and if hypertension is present, the development of ventricular hypertrophy (see Table 19-10). This process ultimately reshapes the ventricle in a process described as *ventricular remodeling*. These pathophysiologic processes and the pharmacologic measures taken to limit ventricular remodeling are described in this section.

The *sympathetic nervous system* compensates for low cardiac output by increasing heart rate and blood pressure. As a result, levels of circulating catecholamines are increased, resulting in peripheral vasoconstriction. In addition to raising blood pressure and heart rate, catecholamines cause shunting of blood from nonvital organs, such as the skin, to vital organs, such as the heart and brain. This mechanism, although initially helpful, may become a negative factor if elevation of heart rate increases myocardial oxygen demand while shortening the amount of time for diastolic filling and coronary artery perfusion.

Activation of RAAS in heart failure promotes fluid retention.[63,73] The RAAS is activated by low cardiac output that causes the hormone *renin* to be secreted by the kidneys. A physiologic chain of events is then set in motion that leads to volume overload. The renin acts on *angiotensinogen* in the bloodstream and converts it to *angiotensin I;* when angiotensin passes through the lung tissues, it is activated by *ACE,* an enzyme that converts the angiotensin I to *angiotensin II,* a powerful vasoconstrictor that increases SVR, raises blood pressure, and increases the workload of the left ventricle; the increased SVR further lowers cardiac output. The mineralocorticoid hormone *aldosterone* is released from the adrenal glands and stimulates sodium retention by means of the distal tubules of the kidney. In response to the low cardiac output, the renal arterioles constrict, decrease glomerular filtration, and increase reabsorption of sodium from the proximal and distal tubules. To break the RAAS cycle of fluid retention in heart failure, two types of drugs are prescribed to interrupt the steps. To inhibit the conversion of angiotensin I to angiotensin II, an ACEI is prescribed (see Table 20-18 in Chapter 20). These agents prevent arterial vasoconstriction, decrease blood pressure and SVR, and decrease the amount of ventricular remodeling that often occurs with heart failure. A drug that inhibits angiotensin II directly may be prescribed instead. The drugs in this category are ARBs.[74] Aldactone (spirolactone) is a drug from a different category that is also prescribed to break the RAAS cycle. Aldactone is a *mineralocorticoid receptor antagonist* that inhibits (blocks) the retention of sodium from the distal tubules of the kidney.[73,75] Figure 19-16 shows the mechanism of action by which these drugs act on the RAAS.

Ventricular hypertrophy is the final compensatory mechanism. It is also strongly associated with preexisting hypertension. Because myocardial hypertrophy increases the force of contraction, hypertrophy helps the ventricle overcome an increase in afterload. When this mechanism is no longer efficient for the ventricle, it will remodel by dilation.

Ventricular remodeling occurs as a result of the previously described mechanisms. The shape of the ventricle is changed, or is remodeled, to resemble a round bowl. A dilated ventricle has poor contractility and is enlarged without hypertrophy.

Organs involved   **Pathophysiology**   **Drug actions**

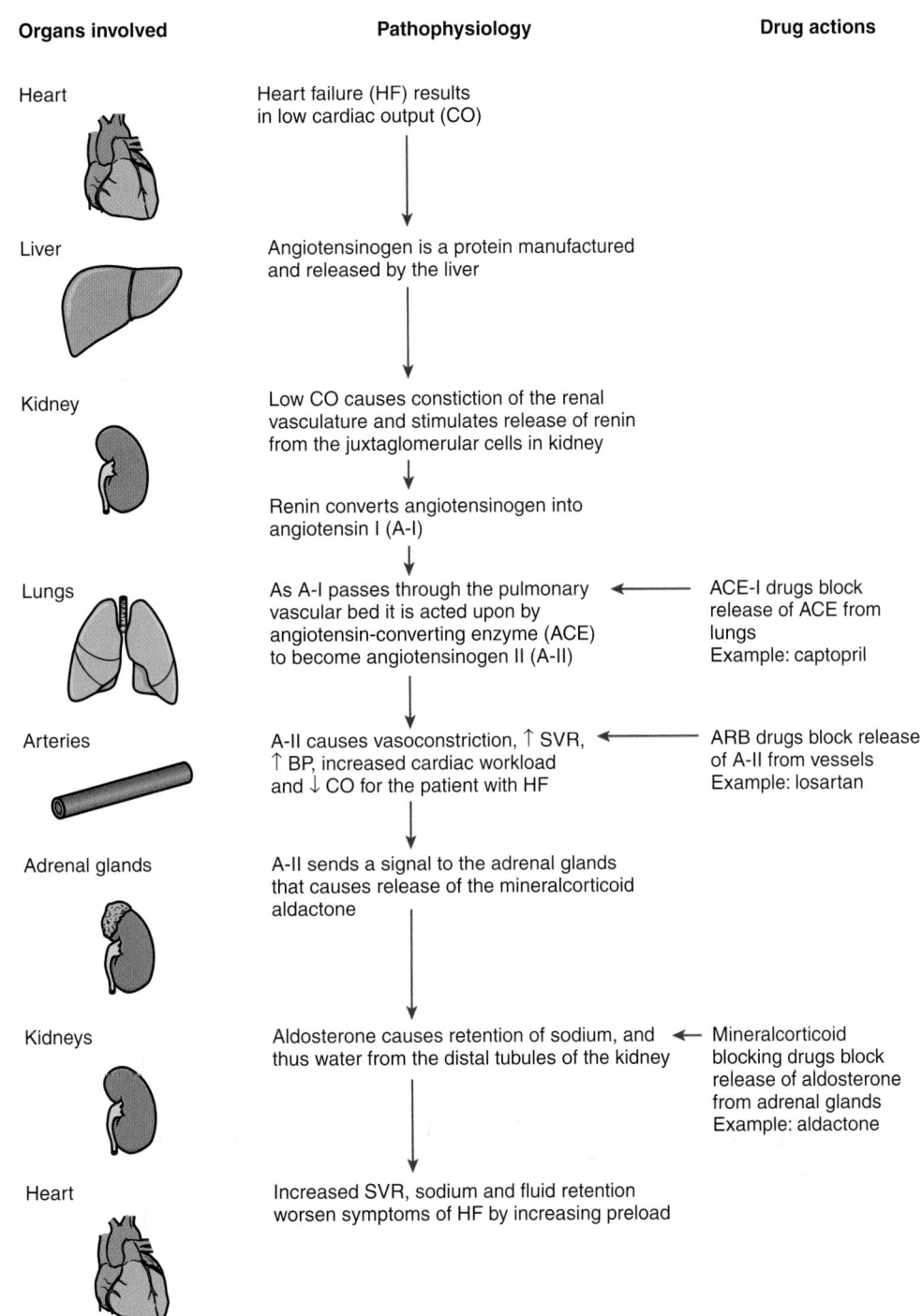

Heart — Heart failure (HF) results in low cardiac output (CO)

Liver — Angiotensinogen is a protein manufactured and released by the liver

Kidney — Low CO causes constiction of the renal vasculature and stimulates release of renin from the juxtaglomerular cells in kidney

Renin converts angiotensinogen into angiotensin I (A-I)

Lungs — As A-I passes through the pulmonary vascular bed it is acted upon by angiotensin-converting enzyme (ACE) to become angiotensinogen II (A-II) ← ACE-I drugs block release of ACE from lungs Example: captopril

Arteries — A-II causes vasoconstriction, ↑ SVR, ↑ BP, increased cardiac workload and ↓ CO for the patient with HF ← ARB drugs block release of A-II from vessels Example: losartan

Adrenal glands — A-II sends a signal to the adrenal glands that causes release of the mineralcorticoid aldactone

Kidneys — Aldosterone causes retention of sodium, and thus water from the distal tubules of the kidney ← Mineralcorticoid blocking drugs block release of aldosterone from adrenal glands Example: aldactone

Heart — Increased SVR, sodium and fluid retention worsen symptoms of HF by increasing preload

Figure 19-16 Renin-angiotensin-aldosterone system (RAAS), its role in heart failure, and drug actions.

Research trial evidence indicates that synergistic use of drugs from different categories—ACEI or ARB, Aldactone, plus beta-blockade—can halt or reduce the progression of heart failure remodeling.[74,76,77]

Pulmonary Complications of Heart Failure. The clinical manifestations of acute heart failure result from tissue hypoperfusion and organ congestion and are progressive. The severity of clinical manifestations progresses as heart failure worsens. Initially, manifestations appear only with exertion, but eventually, they also occur at rest.[63]

Shortness of Breath in Heart Failure. The patient experiences the feeling of shortness of breath first with exertion, but as heart failure worsens, symptoms are also present at rest. A diagnostic blood test is available to assist clinicians in differentiating whether a patient's shortness of breath is caused by cardiac failure or by pulmonary complications. BNP is released from the cardiac ventricles in response to increased wall tension. Heart failure increases left ventricular wall tension because of the excess preload in the ventricles. When the BNP blood level is greater than 100 pg/mL, the dyspnea is probably related to cardiac rather than pulmonary failure.[78,79] The more severe the heart failure, the higher the BNP test result.[80] If the patient has concomitant kidney disease, the BNP clinical diagnostic point to diagnose heart failure rises to greater than 200 pg/mL.[81] Breathlessness in heart failure is described by the following terms:

Dyspnea: the patient's sensation of shortness of breath, which from pulmonary vascular congestion and decreased lung compliance

Orthopnea: difficulty in breathing when lying flat because of an increase in venous return that occurs in the supine position

Paroxysmal nocturnal dyspnea: a severe form of orthopnea in which the patient awakens from sleep gasping for air

Cardiac asthma: dyspnea with wheezing, a nonproductive cough, and pulmonary crackles that progress to the gurgling sounds of pulmonary edema

Pulmonary Edema in Heart Failure. Pulmonary edema, or protein-laden fluid in the alveoli, inhibits gas exchange by impairing the diffusion pathway between the alveolus and the capillary. It is caused by increased left atrial and ventricular pressures and results in an excessive accumulation of serous or serosanguineous fluid in the interstitial spaces and alveoli of the lungs. The formation of pulmonary edema has two stages. The first stage is not as severe and is characterized by interstitial edema, engorgement of the perivascular and peribronchial spaces, and increased lymphatic flow (Fig. 19-17B). The later stage is characterized by alveolar edema resulting from fluid moving into the alveoli from the interstitium (see Fig. 19-17C). Eventually, blood plasma moves into the alveoli faster than the lymphatic system can clear it, interfering with diffusion of oxygen, depressing the arterial partial pressure of oxygen (PaO_2), and leading to tissue hypoxia (see Fig. 19-17D).

Heart failure patients in pulmonary edema are extremely breathless and anxious and have a sensation of suffocation. They expectorate pink, frothy liquid and feel as if they are drowning. They may sit bolt upright, gasp for breath, or thrash about. The respiratory rate is elevated, and accessory muscles of ventilation are used, with nasal flaring and bulging neck muscles. Respirations are characterized by loud inspiratory and expiratory gurgling sounds. Diaphoresis is profuse, and the skin is cold, ashen, and sometimes cyanotic, reflecting low cardiac output, increased sympathetic stimulation, peripheral vasoconstriction, and desaturation of arterial blood.

Arterial Blood Gases in Pulmonary Edema. Arterial blood gas values are variable. In the early stage of pulmonary edema, respiratory alkalosis may be present because of hyperventilation, which eliminates carbon dioxide. As the pulmonary edema progresses and gas exchange becomes impaired, acidosis (pH <7.35) and hypoxemia ensue. A chest radiograph usually confirms an enlarged cardiac silhouette, pulmonary venous congestion, and interstitial edema.

Cardiogenic versus Noncardiogenic Pulmonary Edema. In the critical care unit, when a patient develops pulmonary edema, it is often a challenge to determine whether the cause is cardiac, known as *cardiogenic pulmonary edema,* or the origin is pulmonary or systemic in origin. The latter is referred to as *noncardiogenic pulmonary edema* or, more commonly, *acute respiratory distress syndrome* (ARDS). Options to determine the cause of the pulmonary edema include use of the serum BNP level[81] or insertion of a pulmonary artery catheter. The pulmonary artery catheter is used to determine the patient's "wedge" pressure. It is essential to understand the different causes because the treatment of each form of pulmonary edema is

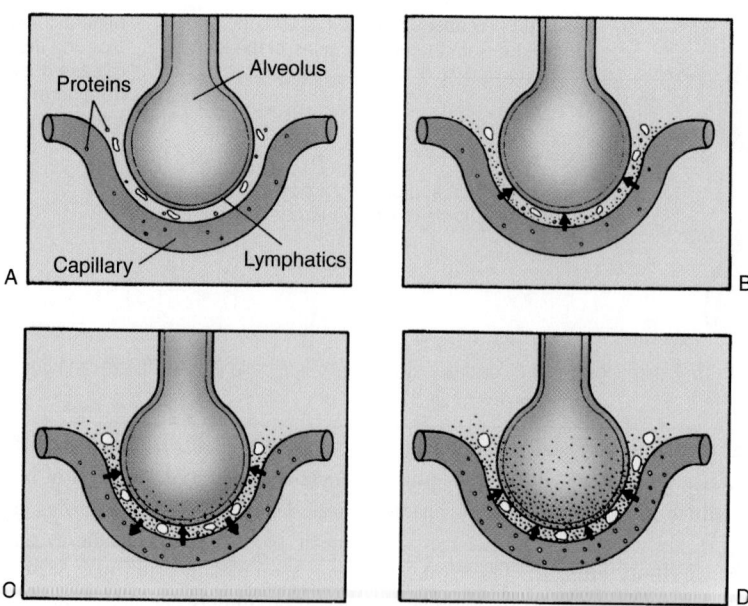

Figure 19-17 As pulmonary edema progresses, it inhibits oxygen and carbon dioxide exchange at the alveolar capillary interface. *A,* Normal relationship. *B,* Increased pulmonary capillary hydrostatic pressure causes fluid to move from the vascular space into the pulmonary interstitial space. *C,* Lymphatic flow increases in an attempt to pull fluid back into the vascular or lymphatic space. *D,* Failure of lymphatic flow and worsening of left-sided heart failure results in further movement of fluid into the interstitial space and the alveoli.

specific. Chapter 24 provides more information on the management of ARDS.

Dysrhythmias and Heart Failure. A ventricular ejection fraction below 30% and the presence of NYHA class III or IV heart failure are strongly associated with ventricular dysrhythmias and an increased risk for death.[82,83] Because sustained VT or VF initiates sudden cardiac death, high-risk patients with severe heart failure are prescribed antidysrhythmic drugs and have an ICD inserted.[83-85]

Many patients with heart failure also have atrial fibrillation. Digoxin is frequently prescribed for atrial fibrillation to control ventricular heart rate. Digoxin does not prolong life but makes patients feel less symptomatic. Digoxin may also work synergistically with specific beta-blockers (e.g., carvedilol) and make the symptoms more tolerable for patients with severe heart failure.[83,86]

MEDICAL MANAGEMENT

The goals of the medical management of heart failure are to relieve heart failure symptoms, enhance cardiac performance, and correct known precipitating causes of acute heart failure.

Relief of Symptoms and Enhancement of Cardiac Performance. In the acute phase of advanced heart failure, the patient may have a pulmonary artery catheter in place so that left ventricular function can be followed closely. Control of symptoms involves management of fluid overload and improvement of cardiac output by decreasing SVR and increasing contractility. Diuretics are administered to decrease preload and to eliminate excess fluid from the body.[75] If pulmonary edema develops, additional diuretics are used. Morphine is given to facilitate peripheral dilation and decrease anxiety. Afterload is decreased by vasodilators, such as sodium nitroprusside (Nipride) and nitroglycerin. Nitrates are used to decrease preload and vasodilate the coronary arteries if CAD is an underlying cause of the acute heart failure. For some patients, an IABP is temporarily required.[87] Contractility is initially increased by continuous infusion of positive inotropic drugs (dopamine) or by combination inodilators such as dobutamine or milrinone. Nesiritide (Natrecor) or intravenous BNP is indicated for the relief of patients with acutely decompensated heart failure who have dyspnea at rest. Nesiritide lowers pulmonary artery pressures and wedge pressure, which decreases symptoms of dyspnea.[88,89]

After the acute heart failure is controlled, the patient is weaned off intravenous medications, which are gradually replaced by oral agents. Before the transition out of the critical care unit, the heart failure patient will receive ACEIs to inhibit left ventricular chamber remodeling and slow left ventricular dilation.[63,73,76] If the patient does not tolerate ACEIs, ARBs may be substituted.[74] Low dosage beta-blockers such as carvedilol may also be prescribed, although strict surveillance is required to anticipate and avoid untoward negative inotropic effects.[83,90] Digoxin may be added to the regimen, especially if the person has concomitant atrial fibrillation.[86] Nonpharmacologic interventions that are increasingly used include *cardiac resynchronization therapy* (CRT).[91] CRT is biventricular pacing

where the right and left ventricles each have a pacing lead in contact with the myocardium. The right ventricular lead is inside the right ventricle, and the left ventricular lead is positioned into a left wall tributary of the coronary sinus vein.[91-93] In newer permanent pacemaker models, the right and left ventricular leads are paced to synchronize the ventricles and improve heart failure symptoms.

Correction of Precipitating Causes. After symptoms of heart failure are controlled, diagnostic studies such as cardiac catheterization, echocardiography, and thallium scanning are undertaken to uncover the cause of the heart failure and tailor long-term management to treat the cause. Some structural problems such as valvular disease may be amenable to surgical correction.

Palliative Care for End-Stage Heart Failure. In 2004, a consensus statement on palliative and supportive care in advanced heart failure was published.[94] Because heart failure is a progressive disease, some patients will not recover.[63] At some point, many NYHA class IV heart failure patients will become candidates for palliative care.[94] The primary aim of palliative care is symptom management. Symptom management strategies are deployed to emphasize relief of suffering. Fundamental to all symptom management strategies for heart failure is the optimization of medications according to current guidelines. The most common symptoms of advanced heart failure are dyspnea, pain, and fatigue.[94]

NURSING MANAGEMENT

Nursing management of the patient with heart failure incorporates a variety of nursing diagnoses (see the Nursing Diagnoses feature on Acute Heart Failure). Nursing management interventions are designed to achieve optimal cardiopulmonary function, promote comfort and emotional support, monitor the effectiveness of pharmacologic therapy, ensure nutritional intake is sufficient, and provide patient and family education.

Nursing Diagnoses

Acute Heart Failure

- Impaired Gas Exchange related to ventilation/perfusion mismatch or intrapulmonary shunting
- Decreased Cardiac Output related to alterations in preload
- Decreased Cardiac Output related to alterations in contractility
- Decreased Cardiac Output related to alterations in heart rate or rhythm
- Activity Intolerance related to cardiopulmonary dysfunction
- Anxiety related to threat to biologic, psychologic, or social integrity
- Ineffective Coping related to situational crisis and personal vulnerability
- Disturbed Sleep Pattern related to circadian desynchronization
- Deficient Knowledge: Discharge Regimen related to lack of previous exposure to information (see the Patient Education feature on Acute Heart Failure)

Optimizing Cardiopulmonary Function. The patient's ECG is evaluated for any dysrhythmias that may be present or may develop as a result of drug toxicity or electrolyte imbalance. Patients with heart failure are prone to digoxin toxicity because of decreased renal perfusion and to electrolyte imbalances. Breath sounds are auscultated frequently to determine the adequacy of respiratory effort and to assess for onset or worsening of pulmonary congestion. Oxygen through a nasal cannula is administered to relieve dyspnea. Diuretics or vasodilators are used to decrease excessive preload and afterload.[75,88] If the patient is not hypotensive, morphine may be administered to decrease hyperventilation and anxiety. If the patient's ventilatory status worsens, the nurse must be prepared for endotracheal intubation and mechanical ventilation. Obtaining daily weights is important until the weight stabilizes at a "dry" weight. Generally, the daily weight is used in fluid management and a weekly weight is optimally used for tracking body weight (e.g., muscle, fat).

Promoting Comfort and Emotional Support. During periods of breathlessness, activity must be restricted. Bed rest usually is prescribed for the patient, who is positioned with the head of the bed elevated to allow for maximal lung expansion. The arms can be supported on pillows so that no undue stress is placed on the shoulder muscles. The legs may be placed in a dependent position to encourage venous pooling, thereby decreasing venous return. Rest periods must be carefully planned and adhered to while independence within the patient's activity prescription is fostered. Vital signs are recorded before an activity is begun and after it is completed. Signs of activity intolerance, such as dyspnea, fatigue, sustained increase in pulse, and onset of dysrhythmias, are documented and reported to the physician. Activity is gradually increased according to the patient's tolerance. Skin breakdown is a risk because of the combination of bed rest, inadequate nutrition, peripheral edema, and decreased perfusion to the skin and subcutaneous tissue. Frequent position changes and mobilization can help to provide comfort and prevent this complication.

Monitoring the Effects of Pharmacologic Therapy. Patients experiencing acute heart failure require aggressive pharmacologic therapy.[83,89,95,96] The nurse must know the action, side effects, therapeutic levels, and toxic effects of the diuretics and venodilators used to decrease preload, the positive inotropic agents used to increase ventricular contractility, the vasodilators used to decrease afterload, and any antidysrhythmics used to control heart rate and prevent dysrhythmias. The patient's hemodynamic response to these agents is closely monitored. Fluid intake and output balances are tabulated daily or even hourly in the critical care unit.

Nutritional Intake. Patients experiencing heart failure often have decreased appetite and nausea, and small, frequent meals may be more appropriate than the standard three large meals. Food must be as tasty as possible; favorite foods and food from home may be incorporated into the diet as long as the foods are compatible with nutritional restrictions such as low levels of sodium to decrease the risk of fluid retention. Each patient must be assessed for nutritional imbalance individually. Some people with heart failure are well nourished, some are obese, and some are malnourished before they enter the hospital.

PATIENT EDUCATION

The nurse assesses the patient's and family's understanding of the pathophysiology and individual risk factor profile for heart failure.[97] Primary topics of education include the importance of a low-salt diet, daily weight, fluid restrictions, and written information about the multiple medications used to control the symptoms of heart failure (see the Patient Education feature on Acute Heart Failure).[63,98] Many patients with a diagnosis of heart failure also require education about lifestyle changes such as smoking cessation, weight loss, energy conservation, and how to incorporate exercise and sodium restriction into their daily life.[76,99,100] Achieving the optimal outcomes for the patient with heart failure requires contributions from a team of educated health care clinicians.[63,76,98,100] Collaborative multidisciplinary goals, developed from clinical practice guidelines for management of the patient with symptoms of heart failure, are listed in the Evidence-Based Practice: Collaborative feature on Heart Failure.

Patient Education

Acute Heart Failure

- Heart failure: pathophysiology of heart failure
- Fluid balance: low-salt diet to reduce fluid retention; intake and output measurement; signs of fluid overload, such as peripheral edema
- Daily weight: Increase or loss of 1 to 2 pounds in a few days is a sign of fluid gain or loss, not true weight gain or loss.
- Breathlessness: Increasing shortness of breath, wheezing, and sleeping upright on pillows are symptoms that must be monitored and reported to a health care professional.
- Activity: activity conservation with rest periods as heart failure progresses
- Medications: Medications are complex, and information must be given in writing and orally.
  - Preload: purpose of diuretics, increased urine output, and control of fluid volume
  - Afterload: purpose of vasodilators or angiotensin-converting enzyme (ACE) inhibitors in decreasing the workload of the heart
  - Heart rate: Purpose of digoxin is to control atrial fibrillation, a frequent dysrhythmia in heart failure.
  - Contractility: With the exception of digoxin, no oral contractility drugs are approved by the U.S. Food and Drug Administration (FDA).
  - Anticoagulation: Patients with distended atria and enlarged ventricles or with atrial fibrillation may be prescribed an anticoagulant such as warfarin (Coumadin); risks of bleeding, importance of correct dosages, prothrombin times, international normalized ratio (INR), and nutritional-pharmacologic interactions are emphasized.
- Follow-up care
- Symptoms to report to a health care professional

CARDIOMYOPATHY

DESCRIPTION AND ETIOLOGY

Cardiomyopathy is a disease of the heart muscle: *cardio* (heart), *myo* (muscle), and *pathy* (pathology). Cardiomyopathies are classified on the basis of structural abnormalities and, if known, genotype. The cardiomyopathic categories are hypertrophic, restrictive, and dilated, as illustrated in Figure 19-18.

Hypertrophic Obstructive Cardiomyopathy. Hypertrophic cardiomyopathy (HCM) is a genetically inherited disease that affects the myocardial sarcomere.[101,102] As HCM progresses, the left ventricle becomes stiff, noncompliant, and hypertrophied, sometimes in an asymmetric fashion.[101] HCM occurs in two forms. A well-known, but less frequent manifestation is a stiff, noncompliant myocardial muscle with left ventricular hypertrophy and bizarre cellular hypertrophy of the upper ventricular septum. This left ventricular septal hypertrophy obstructs outflow through the aortic valve, especially during exercise (see Fig. 19-18A). It also pulls the papillary muscle out of alignment, causing mitral regurgitation. This form of HCM was previously known as *idiopathic hypertrophic subaortic stenosis* (IHSS); however, because IHSS does not describe all patients with hypertrophied hearts, the more general term of HCM is now used.[101] Other patients with HCM have generalized left ventricular hypertrophy, but the septum is not more enlarged than the rest of the myocardium.[101] HCM causes significant diastolic dysfunction because the muscle-bound, stiff, noncompliant heart muscle cannot fill adequately during diastole.

Two advances in diagnostic medicine have propelled understanding of the differences between these two forms of HCM. Two-dimensional transthoracic echocardiography (TTE) is often useful as the first diagnostic test to identify HCM.[101] TTE enables visualization of the septal anatomy, septal movement, and ventricular wall thickness and motion. The second advance is diagnostic genetics. Genetic testing for HCM usually is performed at a center with expertise in this area.[101] HCM is inherited as an autosomal dominant trait, and the clinical expression is caused by mutations in any of one of 10 genes. Each different gene encodes different protein components of the myocardial sarcomere.[101] Genetic analysis is an area of ongoing research that will undoubtedly help clarify other aspects of this cardiomyopathy within the next decade.

Symptoms are similar to those seen with heart failure plus the symptoms of myocardial ischemia, supraventricular tachycardia (SVT), VT syncope, and stroke.[103] Symptoms usually are more intense with physical exercise, especially in the obstructive form of HCM, in which the aortic outflow tract is obstructed by the enlarged left ventricular septum. Because there is a known association between HCM and SCD, limitation of physical activity may be recommended. Causes of SCD are thought to stem from ventricular dysrhythmias and atrial fibrillation.[101] Episodes of paroxysmal atrial fibrillation occur in 20% to 25% of HCM patients.[101] The atrial dysrhythmias are related to increased age and atrial enlargement.[101] Pharmacologic management includes beta-blockers to decrease left ventricular workload, medications to control and prevent atrial and ventricular dysrhythmias, anticoagulation if atrial fibrillation or left ventricular thrombi are present, and drugs to manage heart failure. Interventional procedures include insertion of an ICD to decrease the risk of SCD, and percutaneous alcohol ablation of the intraventricular septum to decrease the size of the septal wall.[101,102] Surgical procedures such as septal myectomy and mitral valve replacement are options used less frequently than in the past.[101]

Evidence-Based Practice: Collaborative

Heart Failure

A collaborative heart failure management team provides an integrated approach to care to achieve clinical stability for the patient.

1. Ensure systematic assessment and management.
   - To achieve an absence of "congestion" and to stabilize patient's condition at the best "stage" possible when in hospital (see Tables 19-10 and 19-11)
   - To maintain the same stability once discharged home and to avoid hospital readmission
2. Counsel and educate patient and family after discharge from hospital. Patients and families should understand the following:
   - Heart failure disease process
   - Heart failure medications, dosages, medication schedule, drug side effects
   - Fluid balance related to salt-restriction diet (2 g/day of sodium), daily weight, diuretic regimen
   - When to call health care provider
   - Risk of additional complications: sudden cardiac death, progressive heart failure, need for other cardiac procedures (pacemaker, ICD, PCI) or cardiac surgery (bypass graft, valve replacement). Some patients may require a mechanical assist device or heart transplantation.
   - Purpose of "advance directive" for health care decisions

3. Promote patient compliance with treatment regimen.
   - Patient needs support from concerned companions and health care professionals.
   - Patient should remain physically active and involved with life.
4. Facilitate hospital discharge; implement outpatient models of health care delivery.
   - Close communication between inpatient and outpatient health care providers is essential.

References

Grady KL et al: Team management of patients with heart failure: a statement for healthcare professionals from the Cardiovascular Nursing Council of the American Heart Association, *Circulation* 102:2443-2456, 2000.

Hunt S et al: ACC/AHA guidelines for the evaluation and management of chronic heart failure in the adult: executive summary. A report of the American College of Cardiology/American Heart Association Task Force on Practice Guidelines (Committee to Revise the 1995 Guidelines for the Evaluation and Management of Heart Failure); developed in collaboration with the International Society for Heart and Lung Transplantation; endorsed by the Heart Failure Society of America, *Circulation* 104(24):2996-3007, 2001.

ICD, implantable cardioverter-defibrillator; PCI, percutaneous coronary intervention.

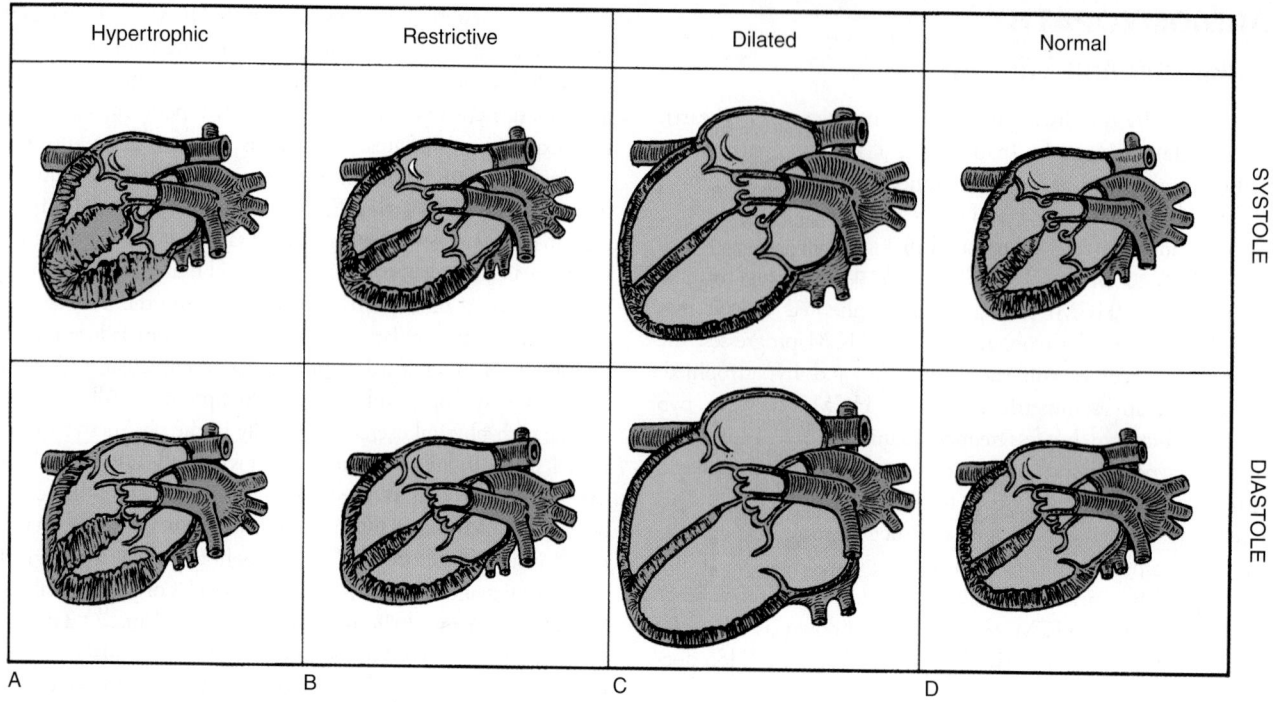

Figure 19-18 Types of cardiomyopathies and differences in ventricular diameter during systole and diastole compared with a normal heart. *A,* Hypertrophic. *B,* Restrictive. *C,* Dilated. *D,* Normal.

Dilated Cardiomyopathy. Dilated cardiomyopathy is characterized by gross dilation of both ventricles without muscle hypertrophy (see Fig. 19-18C). There are several distinct causes of dilated cardiomyopathy.

Ischemic Dilated Cardiomyopathy. Ischemic dilated cardiomyopathy results from repeated myocardial injury or infarction caused by the sequelae of CAD. It is the most common cause of dilated cardiomyopathy in the United States. The patient has signs and symptoms of systolic heart failure and a low ejection fraction.[67]

Familial Dilated Cardiomyopathy. When the cause of the dilated cardiomyopathy is unknown, it is called *idiopathic.* In some cases, the occurrence is linked to genetic inheritance. Scientific advances in molecular genetics permit detailed studies of families with a high incidence of dilated cardiomyopathy. It is thought that 10% to 50% of *familial idiopathic dilated cardiomyopathy* cases reflect genetic transmission.[104-106] In affected families, various genetic mutations occur in the gene that codes for the sarcomere contractile protein in the heart. The heritable trait can be expressed as an autosomal dominant or recessive inheritance pattern.[104-106] Preliminary research indicates that the genetic picture is highly individual for different family groups, even if the clinical picture appears similar.[104-106]

Other Causes of Dilated Cardiomyopathy. There are many other nonischemic, nongenetic known causes of dilated cardiomyopathy. Injury can be caused by valvular heart dysfunction that has placed extreme pressure or volume on the chambers, and viral or bacterial infections such as myocarditis can lead to inflammatory changes that permanently remodel the heart.[107] Other noncardiac causes include infiltration by systemic collagens as in amyloidosis or sarcoidosis.[108]

In dilated cardiomyopathy, the myocardial muscle fibers contract poorly, resulting in global left ventricular dysfunction, low cardiac output, atrial and ventricular dysrhythmias, blood pooling that leads to ventricular thrombi and embolic episodes, refractory heart failure, and premature death. The goals of the medical management of dilated cardiomyopathy are similar to those for systolic heart failure: improvement of pump function, removal of excess fluid, control of heart failure symptoms, anticipation and management of complications, and prevention of SCD.

Restrictive Cardiomyopathy. Restrictive cardiomyopathy is the least commonly encountered cardiomyopathy in industrialized societies (see Fig. 19-18B). As with the other cardiomyopathies, this form can be idiopathic or can have a known cause.[109,110] Restrictive cardiomyopathy results in ventricular wall rigidity as a consequence of myocardial fibrosis. The overall effect is the diastolic inhibition of ventricular filling. Diastolic heart failure, low cardiac output, dyspnea, orthopnea, and liver engorgement are the most common clinical manifestations of restrictive cardiomyopathy. Medical management includes beta-blockers to slow the heart rate and allow more time for ventricular filling, diuretics to remove excess fluid, and a low-sodium diet.

NURSING MANAGEMENT

Nursing management of the patient with cardiomyopathy incorporates a variety of nursing diagnoses related to the symptoms of heart failure. These nursing diagnoses are reviewed in the Nursing Diagnoses feature on Cardiomyopathy. Nursing interventions are individualized according to the type of cardiomyopathy and are focused on achievement of a stable fluid balance, monitoring the effects of pharmacologic therapy, safely increasing mobility, and providing patient and family education. As with heart failure, a collaborative team of compassionate, knowledgeable professionals is required to provide effective care and education for these challenging patients.[98]

Cardiomyopathy

- Decreased Cardiac Output related to alterations in preload
- Decreased Cardiac Output related to alterations in afterload
- Decreased Cardiac Output related to alterations in contractility
- Decreased Cardiac Output related to alterations in heart rate or rhythm
- Impaired Gas Exchange related to ventilation/perfusion mismatch or intrapulmonary shunting
- Activity Intolerance related to cardiopulmonary dysfunction
- Anxiety related to threat to biologic, psychologic, or social integrity
- Powerlessness related to lack of control over current situation or disease progression
- Deficient Knowledge: Discharge Regimen related to lack of previous exposure to information (see the Patient Education feature on Cardiomyopathy)

PATIENT EDUCATION

Education is tailored to the type of cardiomyopathy and to any associated conditions (see the Patient Education feature on Cardiomyopathy)

PULMONARY HYPERTENSION

DESCRIPTION AND ETIOLOGY

Pulmonary arterial hypertension (PAH) is a progressive, ultimately fatal disease of the pulmonary vasculature. PAH results from progressive narrowing of the small pulmonary arteries and arterioles resulting in increase in pulmonary vascular resistance. If untreated, PAH progresses to right ventricular failure and death.[111] It is a disease of the small pulmonary arteries that is characterized by vascular proliferation and remodeling.[112] It is discussed with the cardiovascular diseases that affect the arteries because it affects arterial vessels. PAH may arise as an isolated condition or be associated with other diseases.

World Health Organization Classification of Pulmonary Hypertension. The World Health Organization (WHO) classification of pulmonary hypertension, most recently updated in 2003 at the Third World Symposium of Pulmonary Hypertension, groups disorders according to similarities in pathophysiology and treatment (Table 19-12).[113] Some of the causes of PAH likely to be seen in a critical care unit are discussed in the following sections. Whatever the cause, the presence of PAH significantly increases morbidity and mortality of any underlying cardiac or pulmonary disease. PAH is a serious and frequently life-threatening condition that needs aggressive treatment.[111,114,115]

Functional Classification of Pulmonary Hypertension. A functional classification describes a grouping of physical symptoms that limit a patient's activity as a result of their disease condition. The AHA has used a functional classification for heart failure symptoms for many years (see Table 19-9). The NYHA heart failure classification was used for PAH symptoms,

Cardiomyopathy

Cardiomyopathy produces symptoms of heart failure; patient education covers many of the same issues discussed for heart failure.

- Cardiomyopathy: Explain pathophysiology of cardiomyopathy and heart failure.
- Fluid balance: low-salt diet to reduce fluid retention; intake and output measurement; signs of fluid overload, such as peripheral edema
- Daily weight: Increase or loss of 1 to 2 pounds in a few days is a sign of fluid gain or loss, not true weight gain or loss.
- Breathlessness: Increasing shortness of breath, wheezing, and sleeping upright on pillows are symptoms that must be monitored and reported to a health care professional.
- Activity: activity conservation with rest periods as heart failure progresses
- Medications: Medications are complex, and information must be given in writing and orally.
  - Preload: purpose of diuretics, increased urine output, and control of fluid volume
  - Afterload: purpose of vasodilators or angiotensin-converting enzyme (ACE) inhibitors in decreasing the workload of the heart
  - Heart rate: Purpose of digoxin is to control atrial fibrillation, a frequent dysrhythmia in heart failure; purpose of amiodarone is to control ventricular and atrial dysrhythmias, which are common in heart failure.
  - Contractility: With the exception of digoxin, no oral contractility drugs are approved by the U.S. Food and Drug Administration (FDA).
  - Decrease sympathetic response: Purpose of carvedilol (beta-blocker) is to lower cardiac response to adrenergic stimulation.
  - Anticoagulation: Patients with distended atria, enlarged ventricles, or atrial fibrillation may be prescribed anticoagulants (Coumadin) or aspirin, or both; risk of bleeding, importance of correct dosages, prothrombin times, international normalized ratio (INR), and nutritional-pharmacologic interactions are emphasized.
- Follow-up care
- Symptoms to report to a health care professional

until 2003, when a disease-specific functional classification was developed (Table 19-13).[114,115] The premise is the same as the NYHA classification, with the understanding that a higher number means the patient is more symptomatic, has greater limitation of activity, and risks higher mortality. The functional classification level strongly predicts mortality and is used to guide PAH therapy.[113,116,117]

Idiopathic Pulmonary Arterial Hypertension. If the cause of the PAH is unknown, it is called idiopathic pulmonary hypertension (IPAH) and is classified as WHO group I (see Table 19-12). IPAH is characterized by the following features (Fig. 19-19):

- Angioproliferative plexiform lesions of the endothelial cells
- Muscularization of precapillary arterioles
- Intimal endothelial cell proliferation and medial thickening due to vascular smooth muscle cell proliferation.

TABLE 19-12   WHO Classification of Pulmonary Hypertension

WHO Group I: Pulmonary Arterial Hypertension (PAH)

Idiopathic (IPAH)

Familial (FPAH)

Associated with other diseases (APAH): collagen vascular disease (e.g., scleroderma), congenital shunts between the systemic and pulmonary circulation, portal hypertension, human immunodeficiency virus (HIV) infection, drugs, toxins, or other diseases or disorders

Associated with venous or capillary disease

WHO Group II: Pulmonary Hypertension Associated with Left Heart Disease

Atrial or ventricular disease

Valvular disease (e.g., mitral stenosis)

WHO Group III: Pulmonary Hypertension Associated with Lung Diseases and/or Hypoxemia

Chronic obstructive pulmonary disease (COPD), interstitial lung disease (ILD)

Sleep-disordered breathing, alveolar hypoventilation

Chronic exposure to high altitude

Developmental lung abnormalities

WHO Group IV: Pulmonary Hypertension due to Chronic Thrombotic and/or Embolic Disease

Pulmonary embolism in the proximal or distal pulmonary arteries

Embolization of other matter, such as tumor cells or parasites

WHO Group V: Miscellaneous

WHO, World Health Organization.

TABLE 19-13   Functional Classification of Pulmonary Hypertension: WHO Classification

Category	Description
NYHA Functional Classification*	
Class 1	No symptoms with ordinary physical activity
Class 2	Symptoms with ordinary activity; slight limitation of activity
Class 3	Symptoms with less than ordinary activity; marked limitation of activity
Class 4	Symptoms with any activity or even at rest.
WHO Functional Assessment Classification	
Class I	Patients with PH but without resulting limitation of physical activity. Ordinary physical activity does not cause undue dyspnea or fatigue, chest pain, or near-syncope.
Class II	Patients with PH resulting in slight limitation of physical activity. They are comfortable at rest. Ordinary physical activity causes undue dyspnea or fatigue, chest pain, or near-syncope.
Class III	Patients with PH resulting in marked limitation of physical activity. They are comfortable at rest. Less than ordinary activity causes undue dyspnea or fatigue, chest pain, or near-syncope.
Class IV	Patients with PH with inability to carry out any physical activity without symptoms. These patients manifest signs of right-heart failure. Dyspnea and/or fatigue may even be present at rest. Discomfort is increased by any physical activity.

*Modified from New York Heart Association: *Diseases of the heart and blood vessels: nomenclature and criteria for diagnosis of the heart and great blood vessels,* ed 6, New York, Little, Brown, 1964.

NYHA, New York Health Association; PH, pulmonary hypertension; WHO, World Health Organization.

IPAH is rare, with an incidence of approximately 2 to 5 cases per million people per year. It has a female-to-male ratio of 1.7:1, and the mean age at diagnosis is 37 years.[118] PAH has an insidious onset, and diagnosis is difficult because of the nonspecific nature of the symptoms (e.g., dyspnea, fatigue). Frequently, by the time a firm diagnosis is made, the patient is highly symptomatic with anginal chest pain, near-syncope or syncope, and right ventricular heart failure.[118] Without treatment, PAH patients classified as NYHA class I or II survive an average of 5 years; class III patients survive 2.5 years, and class IV patients survive 6 months.[112]

Familial Pulmonary Arterial Hypertension.
Familial pulmonary arterial hypertension (FPAH) is a heritable condition that is classified in WHO group I (see Table 19-12). Several genes associated with FPAH have been confirmed, including *BMPR2* (bone morphogenic protein receptor II). Hereditary transmission of the *BMPR2* mutation leads to alteration of apoptosis that favors cellular proliferation.[118] In FPAH families, the children of patients have a 50% risk of inheriting the gene. However, not everyone who inherits the gene will exhibit the signs and symptoms of

disease, the reasons for which are not understood. Individuals who carry the *BMPR2* mutation gene have an estimated lifetime risk of 10% to 20% of developing the disease.[118]

Multiple genes and many environmental stimuli are thought to be involved in the pathogenesis of FPAH. This has led to the development of a multiple-hit hypothesis. This hypothesis predicts modifier genes and environmental stimuli influence primary gene abnormalities, such as the *BMPR2* mutation, to develop into clinically evident PAH.[111]

Associated Pulmonary Arterial Hypertension.
Pulmonary arterial hypertension can be related to risk factors or conditions such as associated pulmonary arterial hypertension (APAH). It is classified as a WHO group I disease (see Table 19-12). APAH includes a number of conditions associated with lesions in the small pulmonary muscular arterioles, such as collagen vascular disease, congenital systemic to pulmonary shunts, portal hypertension, human immunodeficiency virus (HIV) infection, and drug-related PAH. The risk of developing PAH increases with exposure to toxic drug or environmental stimuli. Drugs structurally derived

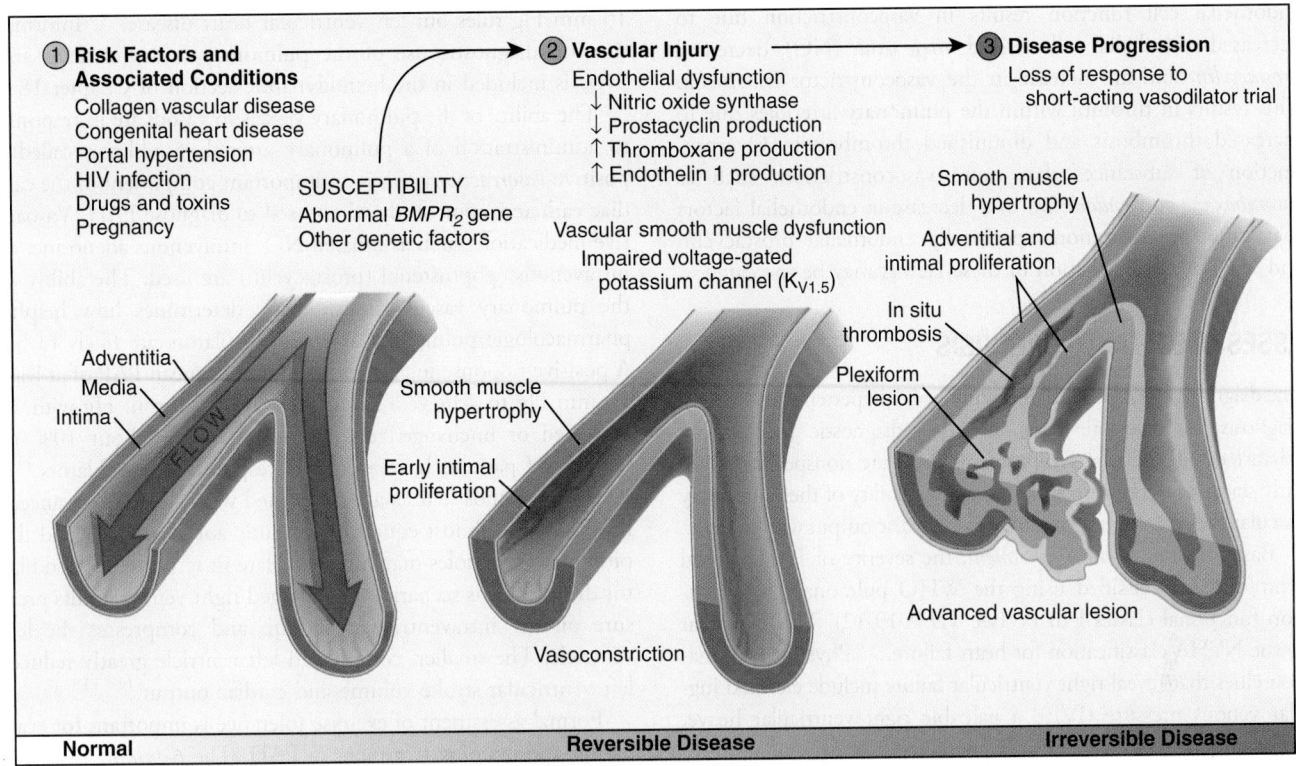

Figure 19-19 Pathogenesis of pulmonary arterial hypertension.

from amphetamine, especially the appetite suppressants *aminorex, fenfluramine,* and *dexfenfluramine,* have been associated with APAH. After studies connected these medications to PAH, they were all removed from the market.[118]

Pulmonary Venous Hypertension. Pulmonary hypertension that results from left heart disease is classified as a WHO group II condition (see Table 19-12). Pulmonary venous hypertension causes PAH by a different mechanism from those of other forms of pulmonary hypertension. It occurs as a result of elevated pressures in the left side of the heart that subsequently raise the pulmonary venous pressure. Patients with pulmonary venous hypertension have a history of CAD, acute MI, valvular disease, heart failure, or dilated cardiomyopathy. PAH develops initially as a passive process of back-pressure that produces upstream elevation in the pulmonary venous and ultimately pulmonary arterial pressure (PAP). Prolonged pressure elevation leads to an increase in pulmonary arteriolar resistance and persistent vascular changes.[118]

Pulmonary Hypertension Associated with Lung Disease or Hypoxemia. Chronic lung disease is often associated with hypoxemia and may entrain PAH. This group of disorders is classified as WHO group III (see Table 19-12). All patients with PAH feel short of breath with exercise, but patients with chronic obstructive pulmonary disease (COPD) or interstitial lung disease are breathless at rest. All patients with obstructive pulmonary disease have worse survival rates when pulmonary hypertension progresses.[118] Pulmonary function tests and sleep apnea studies are performed as part of the diagnostic workup for patients with PAH and lung disease.[119]

Chronic Thromboembolic Pulmonary Hypertension. PAH that results from chronic thromboembolic conditions, such as

chronic thromboembolic pulmonary hypertension (CTEPH), is classified as WHO group IV (see Table 19-12). PAH can happen acutely in response to a large pulmonary embolus that blocks flow to the pulmonary vascular bed. PAH can also occur after multiple microembolic thrombi that obstruct the smaller pulmonary arteries. If the risk of pulmonary emboli is recognized in the hypercoagulable patient, this condition is potentially preventable. The guidelines recommend that when PAH is diagnosed, a ventilation/perfusion scan (V/Q scan) be performed to determine the presence or absence of pulmonary emboli.[112]

Other Causes of Pulmonary Hypertension. Group V in the WHO classification (see Table 19-12) covers miscellaneous conditions, including sarcoidosis, histiocytosis X, lymphangiomatosis, and compression of pulmonary vessels (e.g., adenopathy, tumor, fibrosing mediastinitis).

PATHOPHYSIOLOGY

The pulmonary vascular bed is normally a high-flow, low-pressure, low-resistance system that easily adjusts to changes in cardiac output, oxygen demand, and exercise. In the presence of PAH, these characteristics are lost. Progressive and sustained elevation of pulmonary pressures with increased pulmonary vascular resistance leads to increased pressure on the right ventricle, increased right ventricular workload, right ventricular hypertrophy, heart failure, and death.

There are three major components in the pathogenesis of chronic PAH: endothelial dysfunction and vasoconstriction, vascular remodeling, and thrombosis. A fourth component is the development of plexiform lesions that irreversibly obliterate the pulmonary arterioles (see Fig. 19-19).[113] Impaired endothelial cell function results in vasoconstriction due to decreased endothelial cell–derived *nitric oxide* (NO), decreased *prostacyclin,* and an increase in the vasoconstrictor *endothelin.* This results in thrombi within the pulmonary arterioles due to increased thrombosis and diminished thrombolysis. Overproduction of substances that cause vasoconstriction, such as *thromboxane* and *endothelin,* or a decrease in endothelial factors that cause vasodilatation, specifically endothelial prostacyclin and NO, or a combination of these factors may be the catalyst.

ASSESSMENT AND DIAGNOSIS

The diagnosis of PAH is difficult. Pulmonary hypertension is often a diagnosis of exclusion when all other diagnostic theories are exhausted. The clinical symptoms of PAH are nonspecific in the early stages of the disease and reflect the inability of the pulmonary vascular bed to accommodate increased cardiac output with exercise.

Based on the *physical assessment,* the severity of PAH clinical symptoms are classified using the WHO pulmonary hypertension functional classes I to IV (see Table 19-12). This is similar to the NYHA classification for heart failure.[115] Physical examination clues that reveal right ventricular failure include elevated jugular venous pressure (JVP), a palpable right ventricular heave, hepatomegaly, ascites, and peripheral edema. Auscultation of heart sounds may reveals a prominent pulmonic component to the second heart sound, and a holosystolic blowing murmur from tricuspid regurgitation. Pulmonary edema suggests left ventricular dysfunction or a noncardiac cause such as ARDS.[117]

The *patient's signs and symptoms* early in PAH include fatigue and shortness of breath due to impaired oxygen transport and reduced cardiac output. Later symptoms include syncope from systemic hypotension as a result of low cardiac output and angina from the underfilled right and left ventricles. Patients may have intestinal edema, which can cause constipation, abdominal pain, malabsorption, and anorexia.[113]

Diagnostic tests that can assist with PAH diagnosis include the 12-lead ECG, the echocardiogram, and a right-sided cardiac catheterization. The most helpful noninvasive test is the echocardiogram. Echocardiography can estimate right atrial pressure and PAP, and it can determine the degree of right ventricular dysfunction.[117] Signs of significant disease include right ventricular dilation and hypertrophy; septal bowing into the left ventricle, creating a D-shaped left ventricle; right ventricular hypokinesis; tricuspid regurgitation; right atrial enlargement; and a dilated inferior vena cava.

The *12-lead ECG* is a noninvasive test that may show right axis deviation and right ventricular hypertrophy resulting from PAH. The 12-lead ECG is an adjunct test that can indicate the is strain on the right ventricle, but used alone, it cannot diagnose PAH.

The most helpful invasive diagnostic test is a *right-sided cardiac catheterization,* because it can provide verifiable numbers. To diagnose PAH, the mean PAP must be greater than 25 mm Hg at rest and above 30 mm Hg with exercise. Precise analysis of mixed venous oxygen saturation ($S\bar{v}O_2$) during insertion and passage of the pulmonary artery catheter through the cardiac chamber can allow diagnosis of intracardiac shunts. A pulmonary artery occlusion pressure (PAOP) less than 15 mm Hg rules out left ventricular heart disease.[117] Information on diagnostic use of the pulmonary artery catheter and $S\bar{v}O_2$ is included in the hemodynamic section of Chapter 18.

The ability of the pulmonary vessels to vasodilate in response to administration of a pulmonary arterial vasodilator, called a positive *vasoreactivity test,* is an important component of the cardiac catheterization study when used to diagnose PAH. Vasoactive medications such as inhaled NO, intravenous adenosine, or intravenous epoprostenol (prostacyclin) are used. The ability of the pulmonary vasculature to dilate determines how helpful pharmacologic pulmonary arterial vasodilators are likely to be. A positive response includes a reduction in mean PAP of at least 10 mm Hg to achieve a mean PAP below 40 mm Hg with an increased or unchanged cardiac output. Only about 10% to 20% PAH patients have a positive response to vasodilators.[113]

If the diagnostic tests are performed when PAH is advanced, the PAP may almost equal the systemic aortic pressure and the pulmonary arterioles may not vasodilate in response to vasodilator drugs. In this scenario, the enlarged right ventricle puts pressure on the intraventricular septum and compresses the left ventricle. The smaller, compressed left ventricle greatly reduces left ventricular stroke volume and cardiac output.[113,118]

Formal assessment of exercise tolerance is important for evaluation and ongoing treatment of PAH. The *6-minute walk distance* (6MWD) and a variety of treadmill exercise tests are used for this evaluation. In the 6MWD, the patient walks as far as possible for 6 minutes. The distance walked in 6 minutes has a strong association with mortality among patients with IPAH.[120] With serial measurements, the 6MWD test provides a benchmark to monitor disease severity, response to therapy, and progression of PAH.[111,112]

MEDICAL MANAGEMENT

Medical management focuses on early diagnosis, use of appropriate pharmacologic therapies, and prevention of complications. Goals of therapy include alleviation of symptoms, improvements in quality of life and survival. Improvements are measured by changes in functional class and exercise tolerance.[118] Because of the complexity of PAH medical management and the progressive nature of the disease process, the clinical practice guidelines recommend that patients be referred to a medical center that specializes in management of PAH patients.[119]

Medications. Most patients are maintained on a multidrug regimen that includes oral endothelin receptor antagonists, phosphodiesterase-5 (PDE-5) inhibitors, pulmonary vasodilators, prostacyclin derivatives, calcium channel blockers (early stage only), anticoagulants, diuretics, and oxygen. Figure 19-20 provides an example of how these drugs can be combined as part of a multidrug treatment regimen.[119]

Calcium channel blockers improve survival of PAH patients who demonstrate a significantly positive vasoreactivity test result during the right-sided cardiac catheterization (responders).[119] Long-acting calcium channel blockers include nifedipine, diltiazem, and amlodipine.[113] Most PAH patients are nonresponders and are more effectively managed with one of the newer drugs developed specifically to treat PAH (described later).[119]

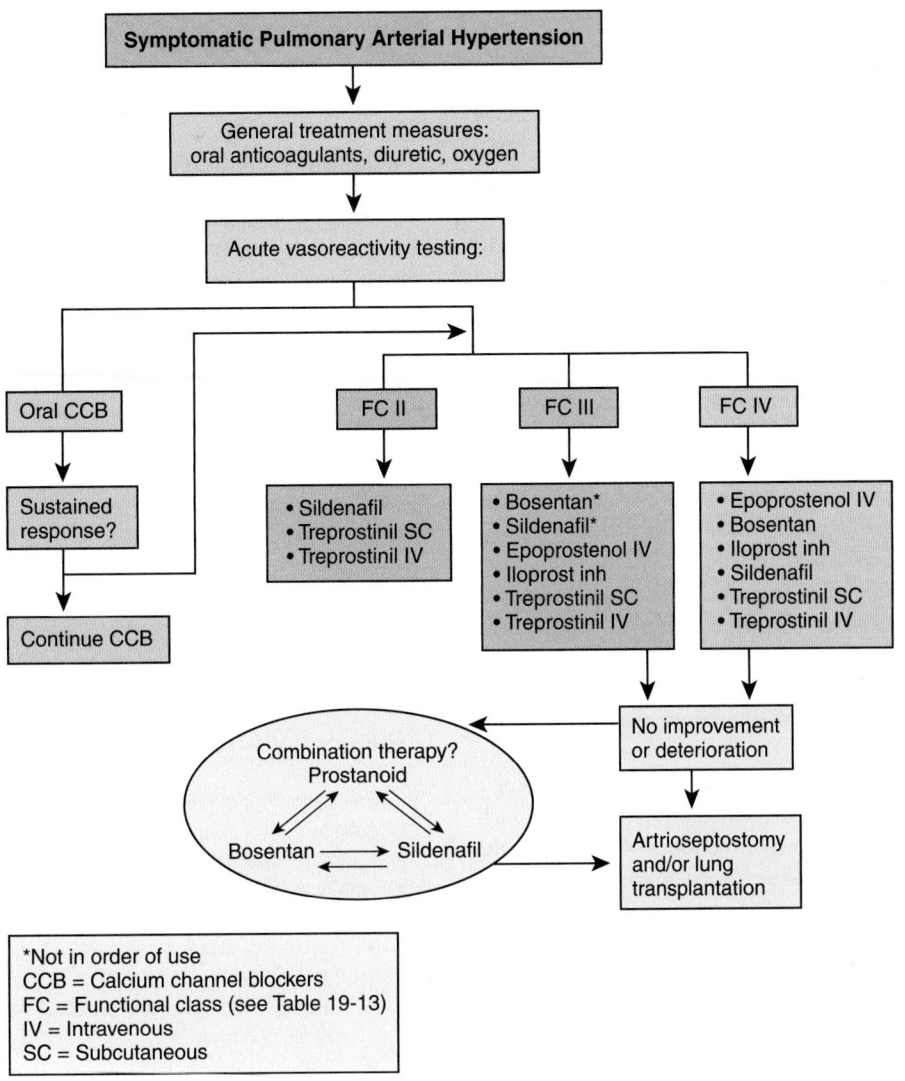

Figure 19-20 Combination drug therapy used to treat pulmonary arterial hypertension (PAH). *(Modified from Badesch DB et al: Medical therapy for pulmonary arterial hypertension: updated ACCP evidence-based clinical practice guidelines,* Chest *131[6]:1917-1928, 2007.)*

Endothelin receptor antagonists are used for treating PAH. Endothelin 1 is a potent vasoconstrictor and smooth muscle mitogen capable of inducing smooth muscle cell hypertrophy. There are two types of endothelin receptors. Endothelin A causes vasoconstriction and smooth muscle proliferation. Endothelin B causes vasodilatation and is involved in clearance of endothelin. *Bosentan* and *sitaxsentan* are oral endothelin receptor antagonists.[119] Bosentan is approved for WHO classes III and IV. In IPAH and scleroderma-related disorders, it improves symptoms, hemodynamics, and exercise capacity measured by 6MWD.[111,119] Sitaxsentan is useful in IPAH and PAH resulting from connective tissue and congenital heart disease. It improves exercise capacity and functional class.[113]

PDE-5 inhibitors are designed to inhibit the degradation of cyclic guanosine monophosphate (cGMP). These drugs promote pulmonary vasodilatation and decrease vascular smooth muscle cell proliferation. *Sildenafil* (Viagra) is a potent inhibitor of PDE-5; it is used for erectile dysfunction and is an effective treatment option for PAH.[111] Started as monotherapy, sildenafil is also used as part of a multidrug treatment regimen.[119]

NO is a potent vasodilator that dilates the pulmonary vasculature in ventilated lung units. It improves oxygenation and reduces PAP.[117] Inhaled NO is useful in critically ill mechanically ventilated patients, especially in combination with dobutamine or milrinone. Development of *methemoglobinemia*, NO_2 production, and rebound pulmonary hypertension with hemodynamic collapse after abrupt withdrawal limits NO use.

Prostacyclins are potent vasodilators affecting the pulmonary and systemic circulations, and they have antiproliferative and antiplatelet aggregatory effects.[119] Prostacyclin analogue drugs are known as *prostanoids.* There are three U.S. Food and Drug Administration (FDA) approved prostanoid drugs: epoprostenol (Flolan), treprostinil (Remodulin), and iloprost (Ventavis).[113,118-120]

Epoprostenol: In patients with advanced PAH and right ventricular failure, long-term therapy with intravenous epoprostenol can be life saving. Epoprostenol therapy is started in the hospital and continued long-term at home. Epoprostenol has a short elimination half-life of 3 to 6 minutes. Patients, who are critically ill and have functional class IV symptoms should be started on epoprostenol because it is the most rapidly effective therapy.[119] Epoprostenol provides a sustained survival benefit of 62.8% at 3 years, compared with 35.4% for historical controls.[113]

Treprostinil: A more recently approved prostanoid, treprostinil sodium is administered by a subcutaneous or intravenous infusion catheter and pump and has a half-life of 3 to 4 hours. Subcutaneous administration is safe and effective and avoids the risks of the indwelling catheter. However, it is associated with injection-site pain, which may not be tolerated. These prostacyclin analogues do not cure the PAH, but all vasodilate the pulmonary vascular bed, control symptoms, and prolong life in responsive patients.

Iloprost: Iloprost is an inhaled prostanoid administered with an ultrasonic nebulizer 6-12 times each day. Iloprost has a serum half-life of 20 to 25 minutes. Studies show it provides improved functional class, exercise capacity and pulmonary hemodynamics.[119] Recent studies on long term use and use as combination therapy with oral agents are demonstrating safety and efficacy.

Anticoagulation is an essential component of the pharmacologic management. Risk factors for venous thromboembolism, such as heart failure, right ventricular dysfunction, low stroke volume and decreased arterial pulse pressure, a sedentary lifestyle, and a thrombophilic predisposition are found in PAH. Warfarin (Coumadin) improves survival in IPAH and APAH. The usual target international normalized ratio (INR) of 2 to 3 is reduced to 1.5 to 2.5 when used with prostacyclin analogues.[113,120]

Diuretics are used to prevent right ventricular volume overload, edema, ascites, and malabsorption associated with bowel edema. Serum electrolytes and renal function are closely monitored.[118]

Supplemental oxygen (O_2) use is a key component of therapy for PAH.[119] Chronic hypoxemia from impaired cardiac output results in desaturation of mixed venous blood. It can also be related to right to left shunting through patent foramen ovale or heart defects.[120] Oxygen inhalation decreases PAPs and improves cardiac output. Hypoxia is a potent pulmonary vasoconstrictor. Oxygen saturation is preferably maintained above 90%.[117,118]

For patients who are refractory to pharmacologic management, a heart-lung transplant may be an option.[119,121] Detailed information on heart-lung transplantation is provided in Chapter 42.

NURSING MANAGEMENT

Nursing management of the patient with PAH incorporates a variety of nursing diagnoses related to the symptoms of breathlessness and right-sided heart failure. These nursing diagnoses are reviewed in the Nursing Diagnoses feature on Pulmonary Arterial Hypertension. Nursing interventions are individualized according to how advanced the symptoms of PAH are. Interventions focus on lowering PAPs, administration of pharmacologic therapy, monitoring of the effects and safety of all medications, treating pain that can occur at the site of injection (with epoprostenol or treprostinil), and providing patient and family education.

Nursing Diagnoses

Pulmonary Arterial Hypertension

- Impaired Gas Exchange related to ventilation/perfusion mismatch or intrapulmonary shunting
- Activity Intolerance related to cardiopulmonary dysfunction
- Decreased Cardiac Output related to alterations in afterload (pulmonary)
- Decreased Cardiac Output related to alterations in preload
- Decreased Cardiac Output related to alterations in contractility
- Decreased Cardiac Output related to alterations in heart rate or rhythm
- Disturbed Sleep Pattern related to sleep apnea
- Risk for Infection
- Anxiety related to biologic, psychologic, or social integrity
- Ineffective Coping related to situational crisis and personal vulnerability
- Deficient Knowledge: Discharge Regimen related to lack of previous exposure to information (see the Patient Education feature on Pulmonary Arterial Hypertension)

Patient Education

Pulmonary Arterial Hypertension

- Pathophysiology of pulmonary arterial hypertension and disease process
- Symptoms: dyspnea at rest or, more commonly, with exertion
- Activity conservation with scheduled rest periods
- Medications: purpose, side effects, special considerations
  - Epoprostenol (Flolan): intravenous (IV) by pump, half-life of 2 to 3 minutes
  - Treprostinil (Remodulin): IV or subcutaneous (SC) by pump, half-life of 3 hours
  - Bosentan (Tracleer): oral
  - Sildenafil (Viagra): oral
- Pain management at insertion site of IV or SC catheter
- Anticoagulation: purpose of international normalized ratio (INR); monitoring of skin, gums, urine, and stool for signs of bleeding; precautions to prevent bleeding when on anticoagulation (e.g., soft toothbrush, electric razor when shaving, avoid contact sports)
- Follow-up care after discharge
- Symptoms to report to a health professional

PATIENT EDUCATION

Before discharge from the hospital, the person with PAH needs to know the underlying reason for the disease process, if known. Provide all patients with a written medication list with the name and purpose of all their drugs. Specific education may be directed to management of a tunneled intravenous catheter or subcutaneous pump for administration and to infection control and sterile preparation of the prostacyclin analogue drug.[122] The name of the health care professional to contact for questions related to the PAH is also important (see the Patient Education feature Pulmonary Arterial Hypertension). A collaborative team of empathetic, educated professionals is essential to provide effective care for these challenging patients (see the Evidence-Based Practice: Collaborative feature on Pulmonary Arterial Hypertension).

Evidence-Based Practice: Collaborative

Pulmonary Arterial Hypertension

Recommendations for Early Detection and Screening for Pulmonary Arterial Hypertension

- Relatives of patients with familial pulmonary arterial hypertension (PAH) are recommended to undergo prenatal genetic testing before any pregnancy.
- Pregnancy is not recommended for female patients with PAH.
- If PAH is suspected, a 12-lead ECG is required as an early screening test to rule out other possible cardiac anomalies. The ECG is not diagnostic for PAH.
- If PAH is suspected, a chest radiograph can reveal features supportive of a PAH diagnosis.
- If PAH is suspected, Doppler echocardiography is recommended to noninvasively evaluate RV systolic pressures and to assess for anatomic abnormalities such as RA or RV enlargement, LV involvement, and intracardiac shunting.

Recommendations for Diagnostic Tests to Further Evaluate Pulmonary Arterial Hypertension

- In patients with unexplained PAH, testing for connective tissue disease and HIV infection is recommended.
- In patients with probable connective tissue PAH, a V/Q scan is recommended.
- Pulmonary function tests are recommended to rule out other causes of lung disease.
- Lung biopsy is not recommended. It carries a high risk and low diagnostic yield.
- Right-sided heart catheterization is recommended, as is acute vasoreactivity testing using a short-acting agent such as IV epoprostenol, IV adenosine, or inhaled NO.
- Serial assessments of functional class and endurance on a 6-minute walk are recommended.

Recommendations for General Management of Pulmonary Arterial Hypertension

- Anticoagulation with warfarin (Coumadin) should be considered.
- Diuretics as indicated.

- Supplemental oxygen should be used as necessary to maintain oxygen saturations higher than 90% at all times.
- Referral to a center that specializes in treatment of PAH is strongly recommended.

Recommendations for Medications to Treat Pulmonary Arterial Hypertension

- Most patients with PAH fail vasoreactivity testing, are not candidates for CCB drug trials, and should be considered for long-term therapy with a combination of the following drugs (see Fig. 19-20):
  Endothelin-receptor antagonists
    Bosentan (oral)
    Sitaxsentan (oral)
    Ambrisentan (oral)
  Phosphodiesterase inhibitors
    Sildenafil
  Prostanoids
    Epoprostenol (IV)
    Treprostinil (SC)
    Iloprost (inhaled)
- Patients with PAH in functional class IV are candidates for long-term treatment with IV epoprostenol.

References

Badesch DB et al: Medical therapy for pulmonary arterial hypertension: updated ACCP evidence-based clinical practice guidelines, *Chest* 131:1917-1928, 2007.

McGoon M et al: Screening, early detection, and diagnosis of pulmonary arterial hypertension: ACCP evidence-based clinical practice guidelines, *Chest* 126 (suppl 1):14S-34S, 2004.

McLaughlin V et al: ACCF/AHA 2009 Expert consensus document on pulmonary hypertension, *Circulation* 119:2250-2294, 2009.

CCB, calcium channel blocker; ECG, electrocardiogram; HIV, human immunodeficiency virus; IV, intravenous; LV, left ventricle; mPAP, mean pulmonary artery pressure; NO, nitrous oxide; PAH, pulmonary arterial hypertension; RA, right atrium; RV, right ventricle; SC, subcutaneous; V/Q, ventilation-perfusion.

ENDOCARDITIS

DESCRIPTION AND ETIOLOGY

Infective endocarditis (IE) is an infection on the endothelial surface of the heart, specifically thrombotic-fibrin vegetations on the cardiac valves. Although most commonly associated with valve leaflets, the chordae, chamber walls, paraprosthetic tissue, implanted shunts, conduits, and fistulas may also be affected.[123] The older term of bacterial endocarditis is no longer employed because nonbacterial organisms can be the infective source. The incidence of IE has not declined over the past 30 years, with 15,000 cases each year and a mortality rate of almost 40%.[124] IE is the fourth most common cause of life-threatening infectious syndromes (after urosepsis, pneumonia, and intraabdominal sepsis). The risk of acquiring IE is higher among patients with congenital heart disease, valvular heart disease, and prosthetic heart valves. Approximately 75% of patients have a preexisting structural abnormality of involved cardiac valve. Increasing incidence of invasive health care interventions such as implantable pacemakers and ICDs and an increase in elderly patients with degenerative valve disease increase the numbers at risk for IE.[124] Among intravenous drug abusers (IVDAs), the incidence of IE is 60 times that of age-matched controls.[125]

Development of IE depends on the following events:[126]

- Presence of a nonbacterial thrombotic lesion on a cardiac valve or endothelium
- Bacteremia (bacteria in bloodstream)
- Bacteria attaching to the nonbacterial thrombotic lesion
- Proliferation of bacteria on and within the lesion that may develop into a vegetation

Research suggests the source of the organism is less likely that previously thought to be related to a specific invasive procedure such as a urogenital procedure or dental work. Instead, IE results from the confluence of multiple daily bacteremic events in the presence of a susceptible cardiac lesion.[126]

PATHOPHYSIOLOGY

IE results from a bacterial or fungal organism in the bloodstream that successfully colonizes the cardiac endothelium. It is fatal if not treated. Bacterial organisms, typically streptococci, staphylococci, and enterococci, are the are the most common pathogens. An increase in multidrug-resistant organisms has led to increased numbers of patients, more serious complications, and higher mortality rates.[126,127] Sites where endocarditis vegetations occur correlate with aberrant intracardiac flow caused by valvular damage or septal defects. After vegetations have colonized, the bacteria multiply at a rapid rate inside a protective platelet-fibrin casing that sequesters the infection.[124]

ASSESSMENT AND DIAGNOSIS

Diagnosis must be made as soon as possible to initiate treatment and identify patients at high risk for complications. Diagnosis is guided by classic manifestations of bacteremia or fungemia, evidence of active valvulitis, peripheral emboli, and immunologic vascular phenomena.

Modified Duke Criteria. The 2005 AHA scientific statement on IE supports use of the modified Duke criteria for diagnosis, early identification, and treatment of IE. This system stratifies patients with suspected IE into three categories: definite cases, possible cases, and rejected cases (Table 19-14). A definite diagnosis of IE requires two major criteria, one major and three minor criteria, or five minor criteria. A possible diagnosis of IE requires one major criteria and one minor criteria or three minor criteria.[126,127]

Blood Cultures. Initial symptoms include fever, sometimes accompanied by rigor (shivering). Blood cultures are drawn during periods of elevated temperature to detect the infective organism. At least 10 mL of venous blood should be placed in each of the blood culture containers to ensure that the organism will be detected.[125] Culture-negative endocarditis occurs in up to one third of cases and usually is related to prior antibiotic use or infection by a *fastidious organism* that does not proliferate under conventional laboratory culture conditions.[123] White blood cell (WBC) counts are typically elevated, and the symptoms are identified in the Duke criteria (see Table 19-14).

Chest Radiograph. Cough and pleuritic chest pain are present in 40% to 60% of cases. The first noninvasive test is often a chest radiograph to detect nodular infiltrates, cardiomegaly, and enlarged pulmonary vessels.

Echocardiogram. The other essential noninvasive test is an echocardiogram of the heart valves to visualize vegetations. Transthoracic echocardiography (TTE) may be initially performed, but transesophageal echocardiography (TEE) is even more valuable because of the clarity of the heart valve images. TEE is more sensitive in detection of vegetation and abscesses.[127] Color-flow mapping is especially useful to visualize the severity a valvular regurgitation.[128]

TABLE 19-14 Modified Duke Criteria

Major Criteria*	Minor Criteria*
Blood culture positive for IE	Predisposition: persons with a heart condition or an injectable drug user
Evidence of endocardial involvement	Fever: temperature >38° C Vascular phenomena: major arterial emboli, septic pulmonary infarcts, mycotic aneurysm, intracranial hemorrhage, conjunctival hemorrhages and Janeway lesions
	Immunologic phenomena: glomerulonephritis, Osler's nodes, Roth's spots, and rheumatoid factor
	Microbial evidence: positive blood culture that does not meet any major criterion or serologic evidence of active infection with organism consistent with IE

Data from Baddour LM et al: Infective endocarditis: diagnosis, antimicrobial therapy, and management of complications. A statement for healthcare professionals from the Committee on Rheumatic Fever, Endocarditis, and Kawasaki Disease, Council on Cardiovascular Disease in the Young, and the Councils on Clinical Cardiology, Stroke, and Cardiovascular Surgery and Anesthesia, American Heart Association: endorsed by the Infectious Diseases Society of America, *Circulation* 111(23):e394-e434, 2005; Wilson W et al: Prevention of infective endocarditis: guidelines from the American Heart Association. A guideline from the American Heart Association Rheumatic Fever, Endocarditis, and Kawasaki Disease Committee, Council on Cardiovascular Disease in the Young, and the Council on Clinical Cardiology, Council on Cardiovascular Surgery and Anesthesia, and the Quality of Care and Outcomes Research Interdisciplinary Working Group, *Circulation* 116(15):1736-1754, 2007.
*A *definite* diagnosis of infective endocarditis (IE) requires two major criteria, or one major and three minor criteria, or five minor criteria. A *possible* diagnosis of IE requires one major criteria and one minor criteria or three minor criteria.

Complications. Heart failure is the most frequent complication of IE and the most frequent cause of death. Embolic complications are the second most common complication occurring in 22% to 50% of IE cases: 65% of the emboli occur in the central nervous system and can cause a stroke. Pulmonary embolism occurs in 66% to 75% of IVDA cases that involve vegetations on the tricuspid valve. Other organs affected by emboli include liver, spleen, kidney, abdominal mesenteric artery, and peripheral vessels. Septic emboli may be visible on the fingers and toes. Rate of emboli formation rapidly declines with appropriate intravenous antimicrobial administration.[127] Risk of death increases with the development of emboli and decreased arterial perfusion to vital organs. Clinical manifestations of endocarditis that may be discovered on physical examination are listed in Box 19-9.

MEDICAL MANAGEMENT

Treatment requires prolonged intravenous therapy with adequate doses of antimicrobial agents tailored to the specific IE microbe and patient circumstances. The antibiotic management of native valve endocarditis (NVE) is frequently different from treatment of prosthetic valve endocarditis (PVE) or IVDA

BOX 19-9 CLINICAL MANIFESTATIONS OF ENDOCARDITIS

- Fever
- Splenomegaly
- Hematuria
- Petechiae
- Cardiac murmurs
- Easy fatigability
- Osler nodes (small, raised, tender areas most commonly found in pads of fingers and toes)
- Splinter hemorrhages in nail beds
- Roth spots (round or oval spots consisting of coagulated fibrin; seen in the retina and lead to hemorrhage)

Nursing Diagnoses

Endocarditis

- Decreased Cardiac Output related to alterations in preload
- Decreased Cardiac Output related to alterations in afterload
- Decreased Cardiac Output related to alterations in contractility
- Decreased Cardiac Output related to alterations in heart rate or rhythm
- Activity Intolerance related to cardiopulmonary dysfunction
- Acute Pain related to transmission and perception of cutaneous, visceral, muscular, or ischemic impulses
- Risk for Infection related to invasive procedures
- Anxiety related to threat to biologic, psychologic, or social integrity
- Deficient Knowledge: Discharge Regimen related to lack of previous exposure to information (see the Patient Education feature on Endocarditis)

Patient Education

Endocarditis

- Pathophysiology of endocarditis
- Medications: importance of long-term intravenous antibiotics
- Temperature: daily temperature
- Infection control: prophylactic antibiotics related to dental work or other invasive procedures after current medical crisis is controlled
- Activity tolerance: Increase activity as tolerated and rest periods as needed.
- Heart failure: If symptoms of heart failure are present, education is given on fluid and sodium restriction, fluid balance, diuretic management, daily weight, and controlling breathlessness.
- Follow-up care after discharge
- Symptoms to report to a health care professional

endocarditis. Antibiotic treatment is prolonged, administered in high doses intravenously and may involve combination therapy.[127] Best outcomes are achieved if therapy is initiated before hemodynamic compromise.[125]

In many cases, antimicrobial drugs are not sufficient to cure the IE. Cardiac surgery to excise the damaged native or prosthetic valve is required for persistent vegetation, valve dysfunction, perivalvular extension, and aggressive fungal or antibiotic resistant bacteria. Usually, valve surgery is delayed until the patient is stable.[125] An increasing number of patients with uncomplicated IE are being discharged to home earlier than in the past and are continuing the intravenous antimicrobial therapy by means of a surgically or peripherally implanted long-term central venous catheter at home.[127]

NURSING MANAGEMENT

Nursing management of the patient with IE incorporates a variety of nursing diagnoses (see the Nursing Diagnoses feature on Endocarditis). Nursing interventions focus on timely antimicrobial administration to resolve the infection, prevent complications, provide pain medication, and individualize patient education.

Resolving the Infection. IE requires a long course of intravenous antibiotics, usually for 6 weeks. This is begun in the hospital and continued at home with an indwelling central catheter after the patient is in stable condition.[127] Nursing assessment includes monitoring for signs of worsening infection, such as persistent temperature elevation, malaise, weakness, easy fatigability, and night sweats, or new emboli on hands or feet (see the Patient Education feature on Endocarditis).

Preventing Complications. Between 20% and 60% of patients with IE experience complications.[124] The nursing assessment is attuned to the early detection of changes such as shortness of breath or chest pain with hemoptysis. As valvular dysfunction accelerates, acute heart failure develops. Cardiac assessment includes auscultation of heart sounds to detect the presence of or change in a cardiac murmur. This can be caused by worsening heart failure or by pulmonary emboli. Changes in level of consciousness, visual changes, or complaints of headache are always reported due to risk of emboli. Evaluation of liver and kidney function is essential to monitor the health of those organs due to embolic risk. With the complex and prolonged antibiotic therapy required for treating IE, adverse drug reactions constitute another important consideration.

PATIENT EDUCATION

The person with IE needs to know the manifestations of infection, how to take an oral temperature, and what medical procedures increase risk of a recurrence of IE. A written list of all medications must be supplied (see the Patient Education feature on Endocarditis). It is essential to reinforce the necessity of the patient providing other health care professionals such as the dentist or podiatrist with a comprehensive endocarditis history.[127,128] The known IVDA has a unique set of challenges to overcome.[129] Multidisciplinary support for the patient to meet the challenge of opiate withdrawal and psychological dependence is essential to prevent a relapse.[129] Many clinicians participate in the care of a patient with IE.

Evidence-Based Practice: Collaborative

Infective Endocarditis and Infective Endocarditis Prophylaxis

Diagnosis of Infective Endocarditis

The Modified Duke Criteria are recommended to guide diagnosis (see Table 19-14). Endocarditis prophylaxis is recommended for patients with

- Prosthetic heart valve with a history of infective endocarditis
- Valve repair
- Complex cyanotic congenital heart disease
- Congenital valve malformation such as bicuspid aortic valve
- HCM with latent or resting obstruction
- MVP with valvular regurgitation and/or thickened valve leaflets.

Special considerations apply for patients with prosthetic valve and IE:

- Patients with a risk for IE who have unexplained fever for more than 48 hours should have at least 2 sets of blood cultures obtained from different sites.
- Surgical valve replacement is indicated for patients with IE of a prosthetic valve who present in heart failure

Antimicrobial Therapy

Four features mark the antimicrobial therapy administered for IE:

1. It is prolonged.
2. It is bactericidal.
3. It is intravenous.
4. It is high dosage.

At least two sets of blood cultures are obtained every 24 to 48 hours until the bloodstream infection is cleared. IV antimicrobial therapy is continued after hospital discharge in the home setting.

Complications from Infective Endocarditis

- Emboli from infected heart valves occur in 22% to 50% of IE cases, and 65% of embolic events involve the central nervous system. The rate of embolic events drops significantly during and after 2 to 3 weeks of appropriate antimicrobial therapy.
- Acute heart failure has the greatest impact on overall prognosis.

Complications from Antibiotics

- Toxicity from the high doses of antibiotics may impair kidney function or vestibular function (balance).
- Diarrhea and colitis can be caused by a reaction to the antibiotic therapy or by overgrowth by *Clostridium difficile*.

Indications for Surgery

- Removal of infected device.
- Increase in size of valve vegetation despite appropriate antimicrobial therapy
- Mitral or aortic regurgitation with acute heart failure unresponsive to medical therapy
- One or more embolic events during the first 2 weeks of antimicrobial therapy.

References

Baddour LM et al: Infective endocarditis: diagnosis, antimicrobial therapy, and management of complications. A statement for healthcare professionals from the Committee on Rheumatic Fever, Endocarditis, and Kawasaki Disease, Council on Cardiovascular Disease in the Young, and the Councils on Clinical Cardiology, Stroke, and Cardiovascular Surgery and Anesthesia, American Heart Association; endorsed by the Infectious Diseases Society of America—executive summary, *Circulation* 111:3167-3184, 2005.

Bonow RO et al: ACC/AHA 2006 Guidelines for the management of patients with valvular heart disease: executive summary, *Circulation* 114:450-527, 2006.

Nishimura RA et al: ACC/AHA Practice guideline update on valvular heart disease: focused update on infective endocarditis, *Circulation* 118:887-896, 2006.

Wilson W et al: Prevention of infective endocarditis: guidelines from the American Heart Association. A guideline from the American Heart Association Rheumatic Fever, Endocarditis, and Kawasaki Disease Committee, Council on Cardiovascular Disease in the Young, and the Council on Clinical Cardiology, Council on Cardiovascular Surgery and Anesthesia, and the Quality of Care and Outcomes Research Interdisciplinary Working Group, *Circulation* 116(15):1736-1754, 2007.

HCM, hypertrophic cardiomyopathy; IE, infective endocarditis; MVP, mitral valve prolapse.

VALVULAR HEART DISEASE

DESCRIPTION AND ETIOLOGY

Valvular heart disease describes structural and functional abnormalities of single or multiple cardiac valves. The result is an alteration in blood flow across the valve. The two types of valvular lesions are stenotic and regurgitant. These are described with reference to the specific cardiac valves involved.

Usually, if a person is admitted to the critical care unit with valve disease, he or she is experiencing acute heart failure or is being admitted for cardiac surgical valvular replacement. In the past in the United States, most valvular lesions were rheumatic in origin, and damage was a direct result of group A β-hemolytic streptococcal pharyngitis. As a result of aggressive treatment of "strep throat," this has become a rare problem, and older patients now are more likely to be seen with symptoms of heart failure and degenerative valve changes. These changes may be described as myxomatous leaflet degeneration or annular calcification.[128,130]

PATHOPHYSIOLOGY

Mitral Valve Stenosis. Mitral valve stenosis describes a progressive narrowing of the mitral valve orifice. Primary cause is rheumatic carditis with rare occurrences related to congenital malformations. Mitral stenosis occurs in twice as many women as men.[130] Symptoms occur when the normal valve size is reduced to 2 cm^2 or less. Symptoms occur at rest when the valve area is reduced below 1 cm^2.[130] Narrowing is caused by aging valve tissue or by acute rheumatic valvulitis (Table 19-15A). The diffuse valve leaflets fibrose and fuse, reducing mobility and thickening the chordae tendineae. As a result, the mitral

TABLE 19-15 Valvular Dysfunction

	Pathophysiology	Clinical Manifestations	Physical Signs
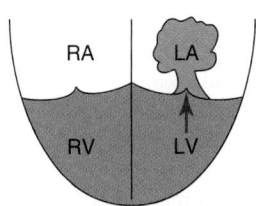 Mitral valve stenosis ⋮ indicates stenosis A	**Mitral Valve Stenosis** Left atrium must generate more pressure to propel blood beyond the lesion Rise in left atrial pressure and volume reflected retrograde into pulmonary vessels Right ventricular hypertrophy Right ventricular failure	Dyspnea on exertion Fatigue and weakness Pronounced respiratory symptoms (e.g., orthopnea, paroxysmal nocturnal dyspnea) Mild hemoptysis with bronchial capillary rupture Susceptibility to pulmonary infections	Chest radiograph: pulmonary congestion, redistribution of blood flow to upper lobes ECG: Atrial fibrillation and other atrial dysrhythmias Auscultation: diastolic murmur, accentuated S_1, opening snap Catheterization: elevated pressure gradient across valve; increased left atrial pressure, pulmonary artery wedge pressure, and pulmonary artery pressure; low cardiac output
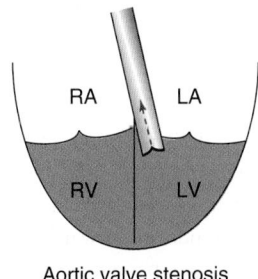 Mitral valve regurgitation indicates backward flow from a valve that is leaking or regurgitant B	**Mitral Valve Regurgitation** LV dilation and hypertrophy Left atrial dilation and hypertrophy	Weakness and fatigue Exertional dyspnea Palpitations Severe symptoms precipitated by LV failure, with consequent low output and pulmonary congestion	Chest radiograph: left atrial and LV enlargement, variable pulmonary congestion ECG: P mitrale, LV hypertrophy, atrial fibrillation Auscultation: murmur throughout systole Catheterization: opacification of left atrium during LV injection, *v* waves, increased left atrial and LV pressures Variable elevations of pulmonary pressures
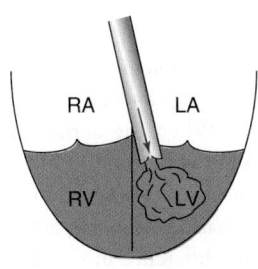 Aortic valve stenosis ⋮ indicates stenosis C	**Aortic Valve Stenosis** LV hypertrophy Progressive failure of ventricular emptying Pulmonary congestion Failure of right side of heart, with systemic venous congestion Sudden cardiac death	Exertional dyspnea Exercise intolerance Syncope Angina Heart failure (LV failure)	Chest radiograph: post-stenotic aortic dilation, calcification ECG: LV hypertrophy Auscultation: systolic ejection murmur Catheterization: significant pressure gradient, increased LV end-diastolic pressure
Aortic valve regurgitation indicates backward flow from a valve that is leaking or regurgitant D	**Aortic Valve Regurgitation** Increased volume load imposed on LV LV dilation and hypertrophy	Fatigue Dyspnea and exertion Palpitations	Chest radiograph: boot-shaped elongation of cardiac apex ECG: LV hypertrophy Auscultation: diastolic murmur Catheterization: opacification of LV during aortic injection Peripheral signs: hyperdynamic myocardial action and low peripheral resistance

Continued

TABLE 19-15 Valvular Dysfunction—*cont'd*

	Pathophysiology	Clinical Manifestations	Physical Signs

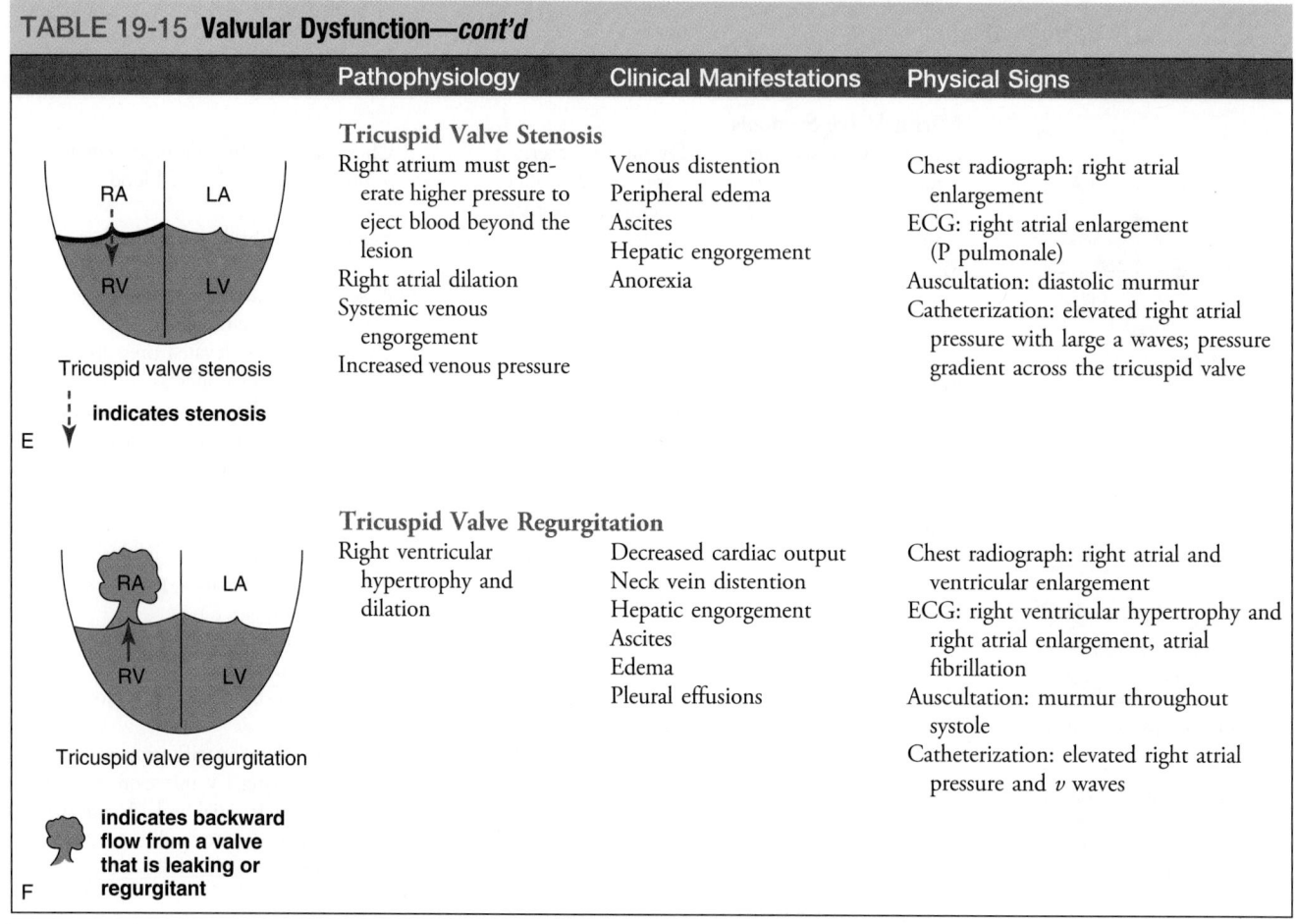

Tricuspid Valve Stenosis

E

Tricuspid valve stenosis

: indicates stenosis

	Pathophysiology	Clinical Manifestations	Physical Signs
	Right atrium must generate higher pressure to eject blood beyond the lesion Right atrial dilation Systemic venous engorgement Increased venous pressure	Venous distention Peripheral edema Ascites Hepatic engorgement Anorexia	Chest radiograph: right atrial enlargement ECG: right atrial enlargement (P pulmonale) Auscultation: diastolic murmur Catheterization: elevated right atrial pressure with large a waves; pressure gradient across the tricuspid valve

Tricuspid Valve Regurgitation

F

Tricuspid valve regurgitation

🍀 indicates backward flow from a valve that is leaking or regurgitant

	Right ventricular hypertrophy and dilation	Decreased cardiac output Neck vein distention Hepatic engorgement Ascites Edema Pleural effusions	Chest radiograph: right atrial and ventricular enlargement ECG: right ventricular hypertrophy and right atrial enlargement, atrial fibrillation Auscultation: murmur throughout systole Catheterization: elevated right atrial pressure and v waves

ECG, electrocardiogram; LV, left ventricular; P mitrale, m-shaped P waves that occur in left atrial hypertrophy and are often caused by mitral stenosis; P pulmonale, tall, peaked P waves that occur in right atrial hypertrophy and are often caused by chronic pulmonary disease.

valve can no longer open or close passively in response to left atrial and ventricular pressure changes. Blood flow across the valve is impeded. Mitral stenosis increases the risk of developing atrial fibrillation because of the high pressures in the left atrium that will stimulate left atrial remodeling and enlargement. Development of atrial fibrillation will significantly increase symptoms and may increase the need for surgical replacement of the valve.

Mitral Valve Regurgitation. Mitral valve regurgitation may result from rheumatic disease, aging of the valve, endocarditis, collagen vascular disease, or papillary muscle dysfunction[130] (see Table 19-15B). In mitral regurgitation, the valve annulus, leaflets, chordae tendineae, and papillary muscles may all be dysfunctional, or the dysfunction may be isolated to just one component of the valve. Mitral valve regurgitation results in retrograde flow of blood into the left atrium with each ventricular contraction. It is always described as chronic or acute because of the very different impact on the left-sided chambers.

With chronic mitral valve regurgitation, the left atrium has dilated to accommodate the additional regurgitant volume, whereas the left ventricle has hypertrophied (increased muscle) to maintain an adequate stroke volume and cardiac output. In contrast, acute mitral valve regurgitation is precipitated by chordae tendineae or papillary muscle rupture resulting from an acute MI or infectious endocarditis.[130] This is a medical emergency. The left atrium cannot accommodate the sudden increase in volume and pressure, and use of an IABP and inotropic drug support is often required to increase forward output and reduce pulmonary congestion. After the patient's condition has stabilized, surgical replacement or repair of the incompetent valve is performed.[130]

Aortic Valve Stenosis. Aortic valve stenosis describes a narrowing of the aortic valve area. It can result from aging, rheumatic valvulitis, or deterioration of a congenital bicuspid valve[130] (see Table 19-15C). The pathologic hallmarks are inflammation, fibrous valvular thickening, and tissue calcification resembling bone formation.[131] When the aortic valvular opening is reduced to less than 1.5 cm², the condition is classified as mild. Cardiac catheterization or Doppler echocardiography can identify a *gradient* of less than 25 mm Hg across the valve.[130] The gradient represents the difference in systolic pressure between the left ventricle and the aorta. A significant pressure difference is a diagnostic hallmark of valvular stenosis. If the valve orifice has narrowed to 1 cm² or less, the gradient will be greater than 40 mm Hg, and the diagnosis will be upgraded to severe aortic valve stenosis.[130] The impedance of left ventricular ejection into the aorta results in increased left ventricular systolic pressure, left ventricular hypertrophy, and eventually left ventricular dilation. When symptoms such as angina, dyspnea, syncope, and other indicators of heart failure develop, it is critical to intervene to prevent further damage to the left ventricle. Aortic valve replacement is usually indicated.

Aortic Valve Regurgitation. Aortic regurgitation, also known as aortic insufficiency, can occur as a result of rheumatic fever, systemic hypertension, Marfan syndrome, syphilis, rheumatoid arthritis, aging valve tissue, or discrete subaortic stenosis (see Table 19-15D). Aortic valve incompetence results in a reflux of blood back into the left ventricle during ventricular diastole. To accommodate this extra volume, the left ventricle initially dilates and then hypertrophies in an attempt to empty more completely and to meet the needs of the peripheral circulation. Aortic valve replacement is recommended for symptomatic patients with well-preserved or moderate left ventricular dysfunction.[130]

Tricuspid Valve Stenosis. Tricuspid valve stenosis is rarely an isolated lesion (see Table 19-15E). It often occurs in conjunction with mitral or aortic disease. Its origin most often is rheumatic fever or a complication of IVDA and resultant endocarditis.[130] Tricuspid valve stenosis increases the pressure work of the usually low-pressure right atrium, resulting in right atrial hypertrophy. The right atrium dilates in an attempt to accommodate the residual right atrial volume and the incoming venous return. As a result, systemic venous congestion occurs—the consequences of which include jugular venous congestion, liver failure, hepatomegaly, ascites, and peripheral edema.

Tricuspid Valve Regurgitation. Tricuspid valve regurgitation usually results from advanced failure of the left side of the heart that eventually affects the right side of the heart, severe pulmonary hypertension, or as a complication of IE. Other causes include carcinoid, rheumatoid arthritis, radiation therapy, trauma, and Marfan syndrome[130] (see Table 19-15F).

Pulmonic Valve Disease. Pulmonary valve disease is not a common disorder in adults. It is most often related to congenital anomalies and produces failure of the right side of the heart.

Mixed Valvular Lesions. Many persons have mixed valvular lesions as an element of stenosis and regurgitation. Mixed lesions can accentuate the severity of a condition. For example, when combined, aortic stenosis and aortic regurgitation increase left ventricular volume and pressure and thereby multiply the degree of left ventricular work.

MEDICAL MANAGEMENT

Management of valvular disorders includes pharmacologic therapy to control symptoms of heart failure and then cardiac surgical repair or replacement of the affected valve.[130,131] When surgery is not feasible, balloon dilation is a rare option selected for individuals too ill to undergo a major cardiac surgical procedure.[132]

NURSING MANAGEMENT

Nursing management of the patient with valvular disease incorporates a variety of nursing diagnoses (see the Nursing Diagnoses feature on Valvular Heart Disease). Nursing

---

Nursing Diagnoses

Valvular Heart Disease

- Decreased Cardiac Output related to alterations in preload
- Decreased Cardiac Output related to alterations in afterload
- Decreased Cardiac Output related to alterations in contractility
- Decreased Cardiac Output related to alterations in heart rate or rhythm
- Activity Intolerance related to cardiopulmonary dysfunction
- Deficient Knowledge: Discharge Regimen related to lack of previous exposure to information (see the Patient Education feature on Valvular Heart Disease)

---

management interventions focus on achievement of adequate cardiac output, maintenance of fluid balance, and patient and family education.

Cardiac Output. Low cardiac output is a common finding in patients with valvular heart disease. It can occur because of decreased forward flow through a stenotic valve, because of bidirectional flow across an incompetent valve, or because of associated heart failure. Vital signs and the effect of positive inotropic and afterload-reducing agents are assessed and documented. If the patient has hemodynamic catheters inserted, cardiac output and hemodynamic parameters are measured and evaluated. Patient care activities are carefully planned to provide adequate rest periods to prevent fatigue.

Fluid Balance. Fluid status is evaluated by auscultation of breath sounds for crackles, heart sounds for presence of an S_3, daily weights to trend a "sudden weight gain," and presence of peripheral edema. The appearance of pulmonary crackles or an S_3 heart sound confirms volume overload. The jugular vein is assessed for signs of increased distention. Diuretics and vasodilators are administered to counteract excess fluid retention. The patient is weighed daily, and fluid intake and output are monitored and recorded.

PATIENT EDUCATION

Education for the patient with acute or chronic heart failure caused by valvular dysfunction includes: (1) information related to diet, (2) fluid restrictions, (3) the actions and side effects of heart failure medications, (4) the need for prophylactic antibiotics before undergoing any invasive procedures such as dental work, and (5) when to call the health care provider to report a negative change in cardiac symptoms (see the Patient Education feature on Valvular Heart Disease). Many patients also require information about valvular heart surgery. Achieving the optimal outcomes for the patient with valve disease requires contributions from a team of educated health care clinicians. Collaborative multidisciplinary priorities are listed in the Evidence-Based Practice: Collaborative feature on Valvular Heart Disease. The heart valve replacement section in Chapter 20 provides more information on surgical management.

Patient Education

Valvular Heart Disease

- Pathophysiology of the valvular disease
- Infection control: prophylactic antibiotics related to dental work or other invasive procedures
- Heart failure: If symptoms of heart failure are present, education is provided on fluid and sodium restriction, fluid balance, diuretic management, daily weight, and controlling breathlessness.
- Surgery: If open heart surgery was performed, information about postsurgical recovery is provided.
- Medications: Medications may be complex, and information must be given in writing and orally.
- Preload: purpose of diuretics, increased urine output, and control of fluid volume
- Afterload: purpose of vasodilators or angiotensin-converting enzyme (ACE) inhibitors in decreasing the workload of the heart
- Heart rate: Purpose of digoxin is to control atrial fibrillation, a frequent dysrhythmia in heart failure.
- Contractility: With the exception of digoxin, no oral contractility drugs are approved by the U.S. Food and Drug Administration (FDA).
- Anticoagulation: Patients with distended atria, enlarged ventricles, atrial fibrillation, or mechanical valves may be prescribed anticoagulants (Coumadin); risks of bleeding, importance of correct dosages, prothrombin times, international normalized ratio (INR), and nutritional-pharmacologic interactions are emphasized.
- Follow-up care after discharge
- Symptoms to report to a health care professional

ATHEROSCLEROTIC DISEASES OF THE AORTA

DESCRIPTION

Two aortic conditions are described—aortic aneurysm and aortic dissection. Both disease states are the result of progressive atherosclerotic disease and systemic arterial hypertension.

Aortic Aneurysm. An aortic aneurysm is a localized dilation of the arterial wall that results in an alteration in vessel shape and blood flow. The first two parts of Figure 19-21 show the two types of vascular aneurysms. Aortic aneurysm is diagnosed most commonly in older adults. Abdominal aortic aneurysm is four times more common than is thoracic aneurysm.

Aortic Dissection. An aortic dissection occurs when a column of blood separates the vascular layers. This creates a false lumen, which communicates with the true lumen through a tear in the intima (see Fig. 19-21C).

ETIOLOGY

Ninety percent of patients with an aortic aneurysm have a history of systemic hypertension. Other causes of aortic aneurysm include the following:

- Atherosclerotic changes in the thoracic and abdominal aorta
- Blunt trauma
- Marfan syndrome
- Pregnancy
- Injury or dissection

Evidence-Based Practice: Collaborative

Valvular Heart Disease

Class I recommendations with strong evidence are provided.

Recommendations for Detection and Surveillance of Valvular Disease by Echocardiography
- Echocardiography is noninvasive and is used for all initial diagnosis and serial follow-up evaluations.

Recommendations for Aortic Stenosis
- Echocardiography is the primary diagnostic tool.
- Coronary arteriography is used before AVR if CAD is suspected.
- AVR recommended for symptomatic patients with severe AS; AVR can be combined with CABG surgery when CAD is present.

Recommendations for Aortic Regurgitation
- Echocardiography is the primary diagnostic tool.
- Cardiac catheterization is used if noninvasive tests are inconclusive.
- AVR is indicated for symptomatic patients with severe AR irrespective of LV systolic function.
- AVR is indicated for nonsymptomatic patients with severe AR with LV systolic dysfunction (ejection fraction < 0.5 [50%]); AVR can be combined with CABG surgery if CAD is present.

Recommendations for Mitral Stenosis
- Echocardiography is the primary diagnostic tool.

- Anticoagulation is indicated in MS patients with atrial fibrillation (paroxysmal, persistent, or permanent) and for MS patients in sinus rhythm with a prior embolic event or left atrial thrombus.
- Cardiac catheterization if noninvasive tests are inconclusive
- Mitral valve repair (preferable), or mitral valve replacement is indicated for symptomatic (NYHA functional class III or IV) moderate or severe MS if percutaneous mitral balloon valvotomy is contraindicated.

Recommendations for Mitral Regurgitation
- Echocardiography is the primary diagnostic tool.
- Cardiac catheterization if noninvasive tests are inconclusive or if additional hemodynamic measurements are required
- Mitral valve repair is the operation of choice over valve replacement in most patients with chronic MR.

See the Evidence-Based Practice feature on Infective Endocarditis for recommendations related to management of patients with valve disease and prosthetic valves.

References

Bonow RO et al: ACC/AHA 2006 guidelines for the management of patients with valvular heart disease: executive summary, *Circulation* 114:450-527, 2006.

Nishimura RA et al: ACC/AHA practice guideline update on valvular heart disease: focused update on infective endocarditis, *Circulation* 118:887-896, 2006.

AR, aortic regurgitation; *AS*, aortic stenosis; *AVR*, aortic valve replacement; *CABG*, coronary artery bypass graft; *CAD*, coronary valve disease; *IE*, infective endocarditis; *LV*, left ventricular; *MR*, mitral regurgitation; *MS*, mitral stenosis; *NYHA*, New York Heart Association.

ASSESSMENT AND DIAGNOSIS

An aortic aneurysm does not always produce symptoms. It may be detected during routine abdominal examination as a palpable, pulsatile mass located in the umbilical region of the abdomen to the left of the midline. A thoracic aneurysm may be identified on a routine chest radiograph. An aortic dissection is usually identified emergently by the onset of acute pain.

Aortic Aneurysm. An aneurysm less than 4 cm in diameter can be managed on an outpatient basis with frequent blood pressure monitoring and ultrasound testing to document any changes in the size of the aneurysm. The patient is encouraged to lose weight if obesity is a factor, quit smoking if a smoker, and have hypertension controlled to decrease hemodynamic stress on the site. An aortic aneurysm larger than 5 cm in diameter requires evaluation for surgical repair or placement of an aortic stent to eliminate the risk of rupture (see Chapter 20).

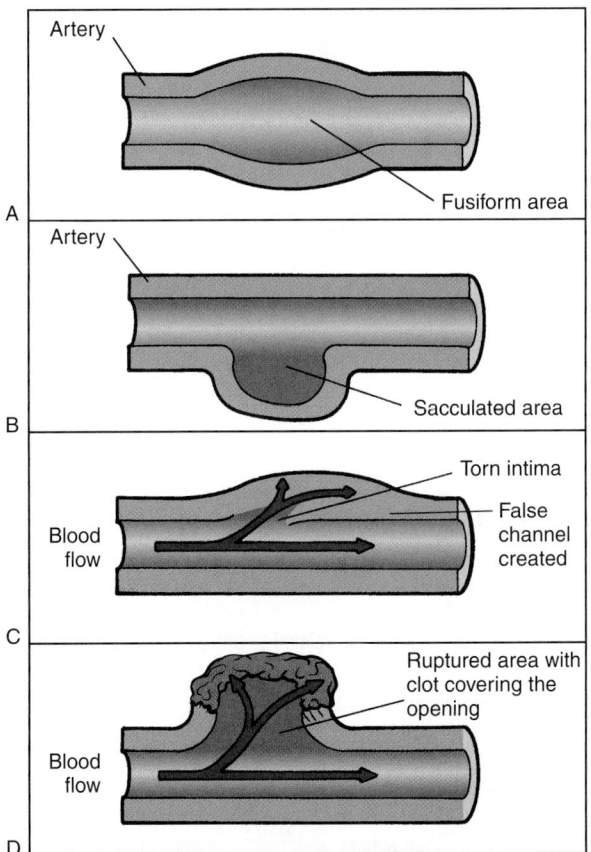

Figure 19-21 Four types of vascular injury. *A,* In the fusiform aneurysm, an entire segment of an artery is dilated, taking on a spindle or bulbous shape. Fusiform aneurysms occur most often in the abdominal aorta and result from atherosclerosis. *B,* A sacculated aneurysm involves only one side of an artery and usually is located in the ascending aorta. *C,* Dissection occurs because of a tear in the intima, resulting in the shunting of blood between the intima and media of a vessel. *D,* Pseudoaneurysm can result from arterial trauma, such as that caused by an arterial introducer sheath or intraaortic balloon catheter, when the arterial opening does not heal normally and is covered by a clot that may rupture at any time.

Aortic Dissection. Aortic dissections are classified according to the site of the tear. Two classification systems are used in clinical practice. These use the letters A and B or the numerals I, II, or III, as shown in Figure 19-22. The classic clinical presentation is the sudden onset of intense, severe, tearing pain, which may be localized initially in the chest, abdomen, or back. As the aortic tear (dissection) extends, pain radiates to the back or distally toward the lower extremities. Many patients have hypertension on initial presentation, and the focus is on control of blood pressure and early operation. Higher surgical mortality is found with patients who present with shock, hypotension, and signs of poor organ perfusion.[133]

The International Registry of Aortic Dissection (IRAD) records indicate that acute aortic dissection is more common in men (72%) than women (32%), but because women present at an older age and with greater delay, they have higher in-hospital mortality rates. The female mortality rate is twice that of an age-matched population of men.[134] Risk of aneurysm rupture and likelihood of poor outcome after rupture is greater with women[135] Morbidity and mortality associated with aortic dissection increase with advanced age.[133]

Cardiovascular warning signs may include severe hypertension, fleeting peripheral pulses, limb ischemia, or a new murmur indicative of aortic regurgitation. The most frequent acute neurologic changes include altered mental status and coma.[133,136] An ascending aortic dissection produces pain in the central chest or midscapular region of the back. A descending aortic dissection usually manifests by pain that radiates down the back, abdomen, or legs. The location of the dissection may be estimated according to the site of pain, although this does not eliminate the need for diagnostic procedures.

The two most helpful initial diagnostic tests are TTE and computed tomography (CT) because both permit rapid visualization of the thoracic structures. The chest radiograph is helpful only if the mediastinum is already widened. Diagnostic findings that identify high-risk patients include a widened mediastinum or an excessively dilated aorta. The definitive invasive diagnostic procedure is an aortogram (aortic angiogram with radiopaque contrast).

MEDICAL MANAGEMENT

Medical management of an aortic aneurysm depends on what symptoms are seen and hemodynamics. If the patient is stable, management is focused on controlling hypertension and educating the patient about the need for corrective surgery before the aneurysm is more than 5 cm wide. If the patient is seen with an acute aortic dissection, management involves immediate control of hypertension with intravenous drugs and control of pain with opiates. Progression of the dissection is evaluated by the patient's report of worsening or new pain. If the patient presents with hypotension or in cardiogenic shock, blood pressure support measures to maintain tissue perfusion are initiated. In such cases, emergency surgery may be performed. Surgery is usually required for dissections that involve the ascending aorta to prevent death from cardiac tamponade. This includes type A or type I and type II dissections (see Fig. 19-22). The surgical procedure

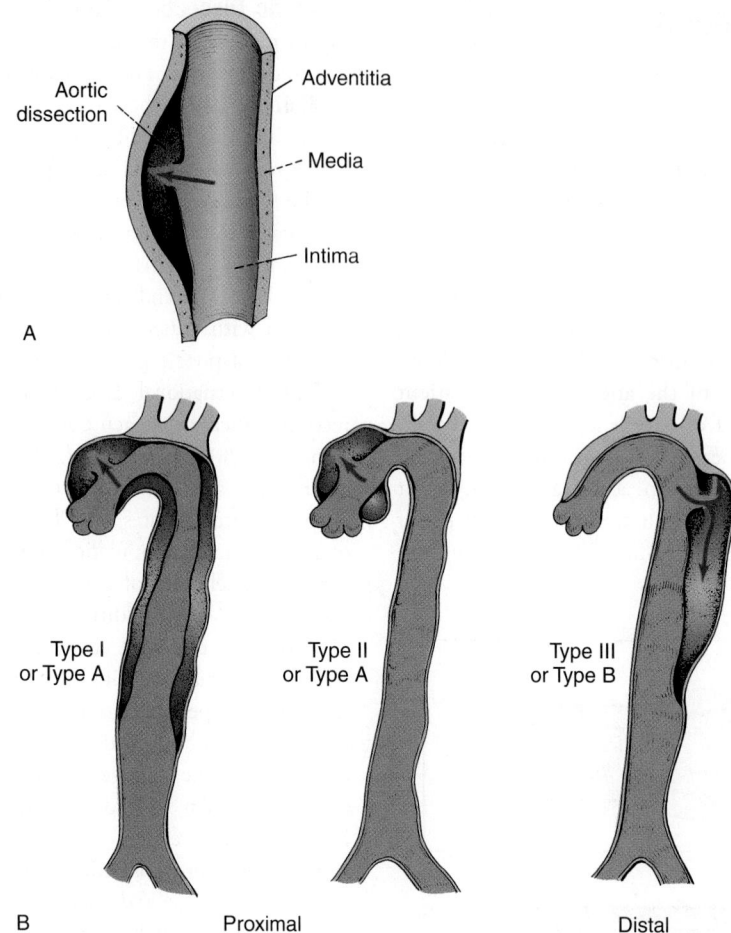

Figure 19-22 Aortic dissection. *A,* Separation of vascular layers. *B,* Classification of aortic dissection. *(Modified from Price SA, Wilson LM:* Pathophysiology: clinical concepts of disease processes, *ed 5, St Louis, 1997, Mosby.)*

includes resection of the affected area, followed by graft placement and restoration of blood flow to major branches of the aorta. Replacement of the aortic valve is performed if the dissection involves the valve. Dissections that involve the descending aorta (type B or type III) do not always require surgery.

NURSING MANAGEMENT

Nursing management of the patient with aortic aneurysm or aortic dissection incorporates a variety of nursing diagnoses (see the Nursing Diagnoses feature on Aortic Aneurysm and Aortic Dissection). Nursing interventions are directed toward control of hypertension, pain control, and education of the patient and family.

Hypertension Management. The cardiovascular status is assessed hourly, including monitoring blood pressure in both arms, checking peripheral pulses bilaterally, auscultating for an aortic murmur, and monitoring the ECG for ischemic changes or dysrhythmias. Patients usually require an arterial line and receive potent antihypertensive drugs such as labetalol, which combines beta-blocking activity to reduce cardiac output and lower blood pressure and peripheral alpha-blocking activity to vasodilate the arteries and decrease blood pressure.

Nursing Diagnoses

Aortic Aneurysm and Aortic Dissection

- Decreased Cardiac Output related to alterations in preload
- Acute Pain related to transmission and perception of cutaneous, visceral, muscular, or ischemic impulses
- Ineffective Peripheral Tissue Perfusion related to decreased peripheral blood flow
- Activity Intolerance related to cardiopulmonary dysfunction
- Ineffective Cardiopulmonary Tissue Perfusion related to decreased myocardial oxygen supply or increased myocardial oxygen demand, or both
- Risk for Infection related to invasive procedures
- Anxiety related to threat to biologic, psychologic, or social integrity
- Ineffective Renal Tissue Perfusion related to decreased renal blood flow
- Activity Intolerance related to cardiopulmonary dysfunction
- Deficient Knowledge: Discharge Regimen related to lack of previous exposure to information (see the Patient Education feature on Aortic Aneurysm and Aortic Dissection)

Pain Control. Acute pain is a classic sign of aortic dissection. Opiates and sedatives are administered to control pain, decrease anxiety, and increase comfort. Because these drugs can mask the pain of further dissection, they are administered judiciously. The patient's neurovascular status is assessed hourly. Documentation includes the presence and distribution of pain, pallor, paresthesia, paralysis, and movement of the limb.

PATIENT EDUCATION

In the acute period, education is limited to an explanation of the critical care environment and the importance of blood pressure control. If additional procedures such as aortography, CT, or surgery are to be performed, the critical care nurse assists with these explanations (see the Patient Education feature on Aortic Aneurysm and Aortic Dissection). Recommendations for prevention and treatment of atherosclerotic aortic aneurysm and dissection are listed in the Evidence-Based Practice: Collaborative feature on Aortic Aneurysm and Aortic Dissection.

Patient Education

Aortic Aneurysm and Aortic Dissection

- Pathophysiology of atherosclerotic aortic disease: aortic aneurysm or aortic dissection
- Hypertension control: Hypertension increases the risk of aneurysm rupture or aortic dissection.
- Pain control: use of 0 to 10 pain scale; information about availability of pain medications for acute pain
- Preprocedure teaching for aortic angiogram, CT scan, or transesophageal echocardiogram
- Preoperative teaching for aortic surgical repair
- Risk factor modification: After the acute episode, if the cause of the aortic aneurysm or aortic dissection is atherosclerosis, an individual risk factor profile is developed for each patient. Strategies to discuss include the following: decrease daily fat intake to less than 30% of total calories, achieve total blood cholesterol level of less than 200 mg/dL, stop smoking, reduce salt intake, control hypertension, treat diabetes if patient is diabetic, increase physical activity, achieve and maintain ideal body weight.
- Symptoms to report to a health care professional: pain, signs and symptoms of infection
- Follow-up care after discharge

Evidence-Based Practice: Collaborative

Aortic Aneurysm and Aortic Dissection

Recommendations for Prevention of Atherosclerotic Aortic Aneurysm and Dissection
- Hypertension is a major risk factor. There are no specific recommendations related to BP control and aortic disease. Reduction of BP to less than 130/80 mm Hg is consistent with recommendations for other atherosclerotic diseases (coronary and cerebrovascular).
- Cigarette smoking is a major risk factor for aortic disease. Smoking cessation is essential.
- Routine use of statins has been found to decrease the aneurysm rupture rate and may be effective in decreasing AAA growth rate.
- Aortic dissection also occurs as a complication of blunt chest trauma from high-speed motor vehicular trauma.

Recommendations for Treatment of Aortic Dissection
- Admission to the critical care unit for monitoring of heart rate and BP.
- Reduction of systolic BP using IV beta-blockers (Esmolol) or beta-blocker plus alpha-blocker combination (Labetalol). Beta-blockers are recommended because they reduce the force of blood ejected from the ventricle against the weakened aortic wall.
- If further systolic BP reduction is necessary, IV vasodilators (sodium nitroprusside) are added in addition to beta-blockers.
- Intubation and mechanical ventilation are recommended if there is profound hemodynamic instability.
- Pain relief (morphine sulfate) and sedation are recommended.
- Diagnosis of aortic dissection is made by clinical signs and location of the site of the tear and false lumen. CT is the most common diagnostic test in an emergency. MRI is often used for chronic stable dissections. TTE followed by TEE may also be used.
- Treatment recommendations depend on the classification of the dissection:

Type A (type I, type II) dissections that involve the aortic arch are repaired surgically to prevent aortic rupture or cardiac tamponade.

Type B (type III) dissections are recommended for medical treatment. Surgery or endovascular repair is recommended only in cases of persistent chest pain, aortic expansion, periaortic hematoma, or mediastinal hematoma.

- Type A aortic dissection is a high-risk diagnosis with an overall hospital mortality rate of 25%. Patients with type A dissections who are admitted to the hospital with hypotension have a higher risk of adverse events.

Recommendations for Treatment of Elective Abdominal Aortic Aneurysm
- Formation of AAA or dissection before the sixth decade of life is uncommon.
- Based on current evidence, a 5.5-cm aneurysm diameter is the best threshold for repair in the "average" male patient. Vascular surgery experts recommend that women have elective repair of aneurysm at 4.5 to 5.0 cm. Individual anatomy, patient age, and physical size must also be considered.
- Until the results of long-term randomized trials are available, the choice between endoluminal repair (stent) and open abdominal surgery depends on patient and physician preferences.

References

Erbel R et al: Diagnosis and management of aortic dissection, *Eur Heart J* 22(18): 1642-1681, 2001.

Brewster DC et al: Guidelines for the treatment of abdominal aortic aneurysms: report of a subcommittee of the Joint Council of the American Association for Vascular Surgery and Society for Vascular Surgery, *J Vasc Surg* 37(5):1106-1117, 2003.

Trimarchi S et al: Contemporary results of surgery in acute type A aortic dissection: the International Registry of Acute Aortic Dissection experience, *J Thorac Cardiovasc Surg* 129(1):112-122, 2005.

AAA, abdominal aortic aneurysm; BP, blood pressure; IV, intravenous; CT, computed tomography; MRI, magnetic resonance imaging; TTE, transthoracic echocardiography; TEE, transesophageal echocardiography.

PERIPHERAL ARTERIAL DISEASE

DESCRIPTION

Peripheral vascular disease (PVD) is divided into arterial and venous diseases of the peripheral vessels. Venous disease is a chronic condition that is managed on an outpatient basis and does not require admission to a critical care unit. In contrast, the arterial form of PVD (PAD) may require critical care admission for an acute thrombotic occlusion or after a vascular surgical procedure. PAD can occur in any peripheral artery. It is especially painful in the arteries that supply the lower extremities. The following descriptions relate to arterial PVD.

ETIOLOGY

Atherosclerosis is a common cause of chronic arterial occlusion in older adults. PAD affects less than 4% of people younger than 40 years but has an impact on almost 22% of those older than 70 years.[137] Risk factors are the same for PAD and CAD. Most patients diagnosed with PAD have at least one risk factor that predisposes them to development of CAD.[137] Diabetes, smoking, hypertension, hyperlipidemia, and male gender increase the risk of peripheral arterial occlusion.[137,138] As with CAD, the presence of kidney disease increases the incidence of concomitant PAD.[137,139,140]

PATHOPHYSIOLOGY

The most commonly affected vessels in the lower extremities are the superficial femoral artery and the popliteal artery in the legs, followed by the distal aorta and iliac arteries.

ASSESSMENT AND DIAGNOSIS

Ankle-Brachial Index. The ankle-brachial index (ABI) is a noninvasive test used to estimate the severity of arterial disease in the leg by comparing it to the measured arterial pressure in the arm. The SBP is measured on the arm and on the leg (just above the ankle). A cuff is used to occlude the pressure, and the SBP is measured at the posterior tibial pulse and the dorsalis pedis pulse locations.[137,139] The SBP can be palpated with the fingers or auscultated using a handheld 5- to 7-MHz Doppler device. To calculate the ABI, the arm SBP is divided into the ankle SBP number.[137,139] A normal ABI value is between 0.9 and 1.0, signifying that the peripheral arteries are normal. Patients with an ABI value between 0.71 and 0.9 have mild PAD; those with an ABI between 0.41 to 0.7 have moderate PAD; and an ABI less than 0.4 indicates severe PAD.[137,139] Generally, as the ABI value decreases, symptoms of peripheral ischemia increase.

Intermittent Claudication. Arterial occlusion obstructs blood flow to the distal extremity. The lack of blood flow produces ischemic muscle pain known as *intermittent claudication*. This cramping, aching pain while walking is often the first symptom of peripheral arterial occlusive disease. The pain is relieved by rest and may remain stable in occurrence and intensity for many years. Symptoms do not occur until more than 75% of the vessel lumen is occluded.

As with other atherosclerotic conditions, PAD is typically asymptomatic until the disease process is well advanced. Clinicians who rely on history of leg pain alone severely underestimate PAD in the early stages. Only about 10% of population with PAD has classic symptoms of intermittent claudication (leg pain associated with PAD). About 40% of patients with PAD are asymptomatic, and the remaining 50% have a variety of leg symptoms different from classic claudication.[141] The ABI can be used as a screening tool to detect the presence of PAD before symptoms occur.[137] Prevention measures can then be discussed with the patient.

Rest Pain. As PAD progresses, patients may develop pain at rest. Pain at rest threatens the viability of the limb and requires immediate catheter or surgical intervention to relieve the blockage and restore circulation to the extremity.

Acute Occlusion. The symptoms of acute occlusion from thrombosis are sudden onset of severe pain, loss of pulses, collapse of superficial veins, coldness, pallor, and impaired motor and sensory function. As with rest pain, acute occlusion requires immediate intervention to open the artery.

Atrophic Tissue Changes. Skin changes associated with PAD include thickening of the nails and drying of the skin. Hair loss is common on the lower leg, feet, and toes. Pallor and a temperature gradient may be present as a line of demarcation between areas that have adequate arterial perfusion and areas that are poorly perfused. Wasting of muscle or soft tissue may be seen. As the atherosclerotic arterial disease progresses, skin ulcerations and gangrene can occur.

MEDICAL MANAGEMENT

Medical therapy is geared toward controlling or eliminating risk factors, providing good foot care, and suggesting alterations in lifestyle to promote rest and pain relief. Pharmacologic management may include the use of anticoagulants, vasodilators, or antiplatelet agents. If these therapies do not produce positive results, the patient may be a candidate for percutaneous transluminal angioplasty (PTA), stent placement, or vascular bypass surgery. PTA or stent placement is effective if the lesion (blockage) is discrete and localized. However, if the arterial disease is diffuse, bypass surgery is usually performed. If gangrene (cell death) is present, limb or partial limb amputation is required.

NURSING MANAGEMENT

Nursing management of the patient with peripheral arterial insufficiency incorporates a variety of nursing diagnoses (see the Nursing Diagnoses feature on Peripheral Arterial Disease). Nurses assess the quality of the peripheral arterial pulses, intervene to maintain skin integrity and control pain, and educate the patient and family about PVD.

Arterial Pulses. Assessments of peripheral pulses, limb color, and temperature are critical in the evaluation of an ischemic limb. Arterial pulses are typically diminished, transiently present (intermittent vessel spasm), or absent distal to the site of occlusion. Diabetic patients have a much higher incidence of PVD (arterial and venous) than the general population. Most hospitals use a standard scale to improve documentation of pulses. If the pulse cannot be palpated, Doppler may be used to assess blood flow.

Nursing Diagnoses

Peripheral Arterial Disease

- Acute Pain related to transmission and perception of cutaneous, visceral, muscular, or ischemic impulses
- Ineffective Peripheral Tissue Perfusion related to decreased peripheral blood flow
- Activity Intolerance related to prolonged immobility or deconditioning
- Anxiety related to threat to biologic, psychologic, or social integrity
- Powerlessness related to lack of control over current situation or disease progression
- Deficient Knowledge: Discharge Regimen related to lack of previous exposure to information (see the Patient Education feature on Peripheral Arterial Disease)

Skin Integrity. Care is taken to protect the limb from injury and development of pressure ulcers. Healing is often impaired because of poor arterial blood flow or diabetes. Feet may be protected from injury by cotton or lamb's wool placed between the toes or by a bed cradle. However, for an acute ischemic limb, removal of the thrombus is the only treatment that can salvage ischemic tissue.

Pain Control. The term for pain during exercise in the presence of PAD is *intermittent claudication*. Leg pain that occurs after exercise, caused by increased muscle oxygen demand, can be effectively managed by stopping the exertion. However, pain at rest (without exercise) is a warning sign of an anoxic limb. The pain of an acute ischemic limb is extreme, and morphine is used for pain control. Ultimately, removal of the arterial obstruction is the only method to eliminate the pain.

PATIENT EDUCATION

Education topics include risk factor modification that emphasizes similar lifestyle changes to those recommended for patients with CAD, including smoking cessation, promoting exercise, maintenance of ideal body weight, inspection of the feet and legs, foot care, avoidance of foot trauma, and medications (see the Patient Education feature on Peripheral Arterial Disease). Many patients with PAD underestimate their risk of stroke or acute MI and do not understand that the risk factors for PAD are the same for all of the cardiovascular atherosclerotic diseases.[137] Walking is good exercise for increasing blood flow to the lower extremities and is highly recommended for the person with PAD.[141]

If a surgically implanted prosthetic bypass graft is in place, teaching must include information about IE precautions. If the patient is diabetic, education about diabetes management is included in the teaching plan. The Patient Education on Peripheral Arterial Disease feature lists the salient points to include when teaching patients and families about PAD. Symptoms of PAD are listed in the Evidence-Based Practice: Collaborative feature on Peripheral Arterial Disease.

Patient Education

Peripheral Arterial Disease

- Pathophysiology of peripheral arterial disease
- Daily inspection and care of feet and legs
- Avoidance of trauma to feet or legs
- Increase walking distance gradually
- Risk factor modification: After the acute episode, if the cause of the aortic aneurysm or aortic dissection is atherosclerosis, an individual risk factor profile is developed for each patient. Strategies to discuss include the following: decrease daily fat intake to less than 30% of total calories, achieve total blood cholesterol level of less than 200 mg/dL, stop smoking, reduce salt intake, control hypertension, control diabetes if patient is diabetic, increase physical activity, achieve and maintain ideal body weight.
- Preprocedure teaching about angiogram, percutaneous angioplasty, or stent placement in the lower extremities
- Risks and benefits of thrombolytic therapy for acute peripheral arterial occlusion
- Presurgery teaching for revascularization surgery
- Rehabilitation education if amputation is indicated
- Medications
- Antithrombotic therapy: usually, aspirin to decrease platelet adhesiveness
- Low-density lipoprotein cholesterol (LDL-C) lipid-lowering agents: 3-hydroxy-3-methylglutaryl coenzyme A (HMG CoA) reductase inhibitors
- Antihypertensive agents: antihypertensive medications and how to self-monitor blood pressure
- Symptoms to report to a health care professional: pain (chest or legs), leg or foot trauma
- Follow-up care after discharge

CAROTID ARTERY DISEASE

DESCRIPTION

The bifurcation of the carotid arteries is a common site of atherosclerotic plaque development (Fig. 19-23). Because these arterioles carry the blood supply to the brain, when they are obstructed, the presenting symptoms are neurologic. Carotid artery disease is a readily treatable obstruction to prevent a stroke. Blood supply to the brain is provided by two separate arterial systems: the vertebral arteries and the internal carotid arteries, branches of which anastomose to form the circle of Willis. Any abrupt interruption in circulation for 4 to 6 minutes can produce permanent brain damage. When circulation to an area is impaired gradually, collateral circulation is often able to develop and maintain an adequate supply of blood to that area of the brain. Abrupt interruption in blood supply leads to an area of brain tissue becoming ischemic and often permanently damaged.

ETIOLOGY

The most common cause of carotid artery disease in the United States is atherosclerosis.[140] Uncommon causes include fibromuscular dysplasia, irradiation, and arteritis. The risk factors for development of atherosclerotic carotid artery disease and stroke

Peripheral Arterial Disease

PAD affects 8 million men and women 40 years old or older in the United States. An international multidisciplinary group of clinicians has summarized evidence from clinical trials to begin the process of developing clinical guidelines.

Recommendations to Increase Awareness of PAD and Its Consequences

- Patients who are at highest risk of developing PAD are those who smoke cigarettes, have diabetes, and are older. In screening asymptomatic patients in high-risk groups, 30% to 50% of patients have PAD and do not know it.
- Other PAD risk factors include hypertension, hyperlipidemia, male sex, elevated C-reactive protein levels, elevated plasma fibrinogen levels, elevated blood glucose, prior MI, heart failure, and history of TIA or stroke.
- Patients with symptomatic PAD had a four to five times increased risk of stroke and a 20% to 60% increased risk of MI with a twofold to sixfold increased risk of death due to coronary heart disease compared with those without PAD.
- Many patients are not aware of the link between PAD and cardiac and cerebrovascular atherosclerotic disease.

Recommendations to Improve Identification of Patients with Symptomatic PAD

- Because PAD is asymptomatic in the early stages of the disease, the ABI is recommended as a screening tool in high-risk patients. See text for information on how to measure the ABI.

- If the diagnosis is not made until the patient complains of intermittent claudication (pain with walking), the disease is already at an advanced stage.

Recommendations to Treat Risk Factors Associated with PAD

- Smokers should stop smoking. This is not easy to do. Physician advice with frequent follow-up and pharmacologic therapy (nicotine replacement and bupropion) demonstrate 1-year success rates of 5%, 16%, and 30%, respectively.
- If the patient hyperlipidemic, achieve a normal lipid panel: reduce total serum cholesterol to less than 200 mg/dL and LDL-C to less than 70 mg/dL.
- Studies have not specifically examined the effect of controlling hypertension and diabetes on rates of PAD. However, extrapolating from the cardiac literature, researchers recommend reducing BP to less than 130/80 mm Hg and maintaining blood glucose within the normal range (70 to 110 mg/dL; $HbA_{1c} \leq 7\%$).
- Low-dose aspirin or another platelet-inhibitor drug is recommended.
- Exercise rehabilitation is recommended with promotion of daily walking. The goal is to increase the ability of the patient to walk longer distances without leg pain.

Reference

Hirsch et al: ACC/AHA 2005 practice guidelines for the management of patients with peripheral arterial disease, *Circulation* 113:e463-e654, 2006.

ABI, ankle brachial index; BP, blood pressure; HbA_{1c}, glycosylated hemoglobin; LDL-C, low-density lipoprotein cholesterol; PAD, peripheral arterial disease; MI, myocardial infarction; TIA, transient ischemic attack.

---

are similar to those for CAD and PAD. Patients with any of these conditions must be educated about the other disease processes. The modifiable risk factors include uncontrolled hypertension (SBP >160 mm Hg), atrial fibrillation, smoking, diabetes with uncontrolled blood glucose levels, and hyperlipidemia.[142] Women taking HRT after menopause also have an increased risk of stroke.[142] The incidence of carotid stenosis increases with age. Asymptomatic carotid artery stenosis with greater than 50% occlusion is present in 10% of men and 7% of women older than 50 years, and the risk of stroke doubles with each successive decade after age 55. The presence of coexisting CAD also increases incidence of stroke, with a relative risk of 1.73 for men and 1.55 for women.[142]

The major mechanisms by which atherosclerosis in the carotid arteries creates ischemic symptoms are embolization and thrombosis. Ulcerated carotid lesions with accumulated platelet and fibrin produce thrombi that travel along with cholesterol deposits to become emboli to the brain. Stenotic areas in the carotid arteries are prone to thrombosis because of sluggish flow across the lesions. Doppler studies can examine the carotid arteries noninvasively. If a stroke is suspected, an emergency CT scan of the head is the appropriate diagnostic test.[140]

Carotid artery disease can remain asymptomatic for many years. After emboli are dislodged, the manifestations of carotid artery disease are neurologic and include hemiparesis, dysphasia,

dysarthria, global aphasia, diplopia, vertigo, syncope, confusion, and monocular blindness. Neurologic symptoms that resolve completely within a short time are classified as transient ischemic attacks (TIAs). Symptoms that do not resolve are described as ischemic strokes.[143,144] If a patient has recently experienced a TIA, the risk of stroke is increased by more than 10% in the first 3 months, with the greatest risk in the first week.[142,144] Additional information on the neurologic management of the patient experiencing a stroke is provided in Chapter 28.

MEDICAL MANAGEMENT

Medical management is focused on lowering the atherosclerotic risk factors over which the patient has control. This includes regulation of hypertension, smoking cessation, seeking medical attention for treatable cardiac abnormalities such as atrial fibrillation, reducing weight, and reducing the cholesterol level to less than 200 mg/dL. Antithrombotic therapy (warfarin, aspirin, or other antiplatelet therapy) must be prescribed for patients with atrial fibrillation with a comprehensive individualized assessment of the relative risk of embolism versus the risk of bleeding complications.[142]

Asymptomatic patients who have carotid stenosis pose a quandary. In these patients the risk of stroke needs to be weighed against the risks of surgery—specifically, the increased risk of stroke during surgery. Current clinical guidelines suggest that patients with

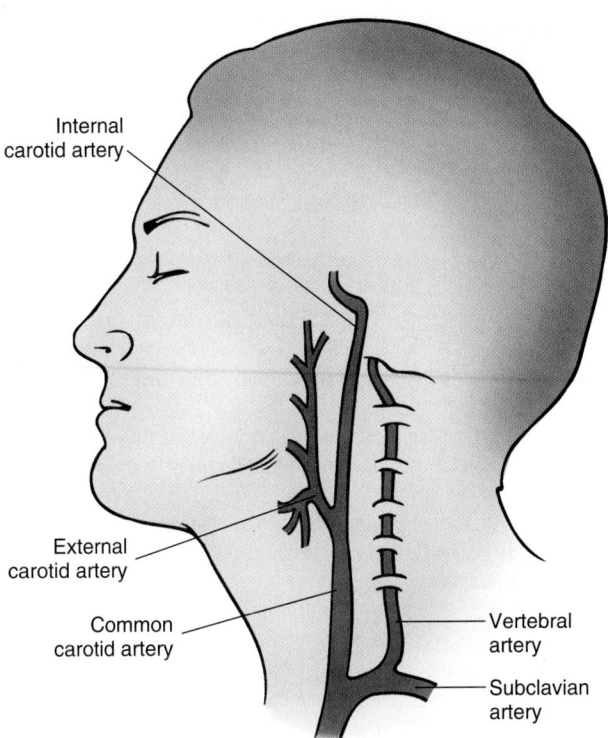

Figure 19-23 Common, internal, and external carotid arteries. Atherosclerotic plaque develops in the common carotid artery at the bifurcation into the internal and external carotid arteries. Plaque can develop in the common, internal, and external carotid arteries.

carotid stenosis greater than 60% will benefit from carotid surgical endarterectomy when performed by a surgeon with a history of less than 3% rates of operative morbidity and mortality.[142] The role of stent placement in the carotid artery is also under investigation.[145-148] Patients with carotid artery stenosis need to be informed about the risks involved with any procedure and their risk for future cerebrovascular events, such as stroke.

NURSING MANAGEMENT

Nursing management is focused on assessment of adequate cerebral perfusion represented by vital signs, respiratory pattern, level of consciousness, pupil reaction, pupil size, and possible cranial nerve deficits manifested by difficulty in swallowing, loss of gag reflex, changes in speech, and loss of facial symmetry. The National Institutes of Health (NIH) stroke scale is used to predict patient outcome on initial and ongoing assessment of TIA and stroke-related symptoms.[143] The nurse educates the patient and family about the causes of the current event and provides information on preventing further cerebrovascular events. Several nursing diagnoses are associated with management of the patient with carotid artery disease (see the Nursing Diagnoses feature on Carotid Artery Disease).

Neurologic Assessment. Neurologic assessment of the patient with carotid artery disease is divided into two parts: (1) level of consciousness, mental alertness, and cerebral perfusion and (2) cranial nerve function. A neurologic assessment is performed to make sure that the patient has not suffered a TIA or stroke. Questions to ascertain level of consciousness relate to

Nursing Diagnoses

Carotid Artery Disease

- Acute Pain related to transmission and perception of cutaneous, muscular, or ischemic impulses
- Ineffective Cerebral Tissue Perfusion related to vascular obstruction
- Anxiety related to threat to biologic, psychologic, or social integrity
- Deficient Knowledge: Discharge Regimen related to lack of previous exposure to information (see the Patient Education feature on Carotid Artery Disease)

time and place and reason for hospital admission. Mental alertness is assessed by the ability with which the patient responds to these and other questions. The person is asked to move all four limbs on command. To assess specific cranial nerves, the patient is asked to make a grimace, which should demonstrate bilateral facial symmetry; to stick out the tongue to ensure it is midline; and to swallow and speak, which should be done without difficulty (see "Cranial Nerves" in Chapter 26 and "Rapid Neurologic Examination" in Chapter 27.)

PATIENT EDUCATION

If a patient is admitted to a critical care unit who has known carotid artery disease and has not had a cerebrovascular event, preventive education is essential. It is important to discuss the mechanism of stroke in carotid artery disease. A stroke is most often caused by an embolic thrombus that has traveled in the bloodstream to a specific area of the brain. The thrombus may have originated in the atria during an episode of atrial fibrillation or in the carotid arteries. In the carotid arteries, a thrombus can develop across the narrowed carotid artery lumen, reducing flow and causing widespread cerebral hypoperfusion. Many patients who have atherosclerotic carotid artery disease also have CAD or PAD and are diabetic or hypertensive.[142] The major areas of patient education are listed in the Patient Education feature on Carotid Artery Disease. Recommendations for prevention of carotid artery disease are listed in the Evidence-Based Practice: Collaborative feature on Carotid Artery Disease.

Patient Education

Carotid Artery Disease

- Pathophysiology of atherosclerotic carotid artery disease
- Pathophysiology of embolic stroke (emboli from carotid artery)
- Warning signs of impending stroke
- Risk factor modification: After the acute episode, if the cause of the carotid artery disease is atherosclerosis, an individual risk factor profile is developed for each patient. Strategies to discuss include the following: decrease daily fat intake to less than 30% of total calories, achieve total blood cholesterol level of less than 200 mg/dL, stop smoking, reduce salt intake, control hypertension, control diabetes if patient is diabetic, increase physical activity, achieve and maintain ideal body weight
- Signs and symptoms to report to a health care professional
- Follow-up care after discharge

Evidence-Based Practice: Collaborative

Carotid Artery Disease

Recommendations for Prevention of Carotid Artery Disease

- Smokers should stop smoking and avoid exposure to environmental tobacco smoke (second-hand tobacco smoke). Smoking doubles the risk of stroke.
- Achieve a normal BP, preferably less than 120/80 mm Hg, for individuals at high risk of stroke. Oral antihypertensive drugs are prescribed if the target BP is not met with diet and exercise alone. Reduction of BP greatly reduces stroke incidence.
- Achieve and maintain normal weight. The target weight-to-height ratio is a BMI between 18.5 and 24.9 kg/m^2. A BMI above 25 kg/m^2 defines obesity. Obese patients are also identified as having a large waist circumference: more than 40 inches for men or more than 35 inches for women.
- Have serum lipids checked, and attain a normal lipid profile. Many patients are prescribed lipid-lowering drugs to achieve the following goals:
  Total cholesterol below 200 mg/dL
  LDL-C below 70 mg/dL if patient has CV disease risk factors (all patients with carotid arterial disease are likely to fall in this category), diabetes, or kidney disease
  Triglycerides below 150 mg/dL
- Normal fasting blood glucose level should be between 70 and 110 mg/dL. If the patient is diabetic, the HbA$_{1c}$ should be near normal or below 7%.
- A healthy diet should be instituted. Reduce saturated fat and add fruits and vegetables. Add omega-3 fatty acids as part of the treatment regimen to lower elevated triglycerides.
- Regular exercise is essential. The optimal goal is 30 to 60 minutes daily or at least three times weekly.

Recommended Medications

- Aspirin (50 to 325 orally each day) or other platelet-inhibitor medications are recommended. The combination of aspirin plus extended-

release dipyridamole and clopidogrel monotherapy are acceptable options for initial antiplatelet therapy.
- The statin class of drugs is recommended to aggressively lower lipid levels.
- Antihypertensive drugs are used to lower BP into normal range.

Recommendations Interventions for Carotid Artery Disease
Asymptomatic Patients

- Medical therapy without revascularization for low-grade carotid stenosis, defined as a carotid artery narrowed to less than 60% in asymptomatic patients
- Carotid endarterectomy and optimal medical therapy with carotid stenosis greater than 60% in asymptomatic patients with low-operative risk

Symptomatic Patients

- Medical therapy without revascularization for low-grade carotid stenosis, defined as a carotid artery narrowed to less than 50% in patients with symptoms
- Carotid endarterectomy and optimal medical therapy with carotid stenosis greater than 50% in patients with symptoms

References

Adams RJ et al: Update to the AHA/ASA recommendations for the prevention of stroke in patients with stroke and transient ischemic attack, *Stroke* 39 (5):1647-1652, 2008.

Hobson RW et al: Management of atherosclerotic carotid artery disease: clinical practice guidelines of the Society for Vascular Surgery, *J Vasc Surg* 48:480-486, 2008.

Sacco RL et al: Guidelines for prevention of stroke in patients with ischemic stroke or transient ischemic attack: a statement for healthcare professionals from the American Heart Association/American Stroke Association Council on Stroke; cosponsored by the Council on Cardiovascular Radiology and Intervention; the American Academy of Neurology affirms the value of this guideline, *Stroke* 37:577-617, 2006.

BP, blood pressure; BMI, body mass index; CAD, coronary artery disease; CV, cardiovascular; HbA$_{1c}$, glycosylated hemoglobin; LDL-C, low-density lipoprotein cholesterol.

VENOUS THROMBOEMBOLISM

DESCRIPTION

Venous thromboembolism (VTE) comprises two related conditions: deep vein thrombosis (DVT) and pulmonary embolism (PE). DVT describes a clot (thrombus) that forms in a large vein in the leg, pelvis, and less commonly, the arm. It is often accompanied by inflammation, pain, tenderness, and redness at the site of the thrombus. The concern is that the thrombus may migrate as a VTE through the venous circulation to the pulmonary vascular bed, causing a pulmonary embolism, development of pulmonary hypertension, or death.[149]

ETIOLOGY

At least 900,000 episodes of VTE leading to hospitalization and 300,000 related deaths occur in the United States annually.[150] Patients in the critical care unit face additional risks from invasive

procedures, immobility, and vascular inflammation. Other risk factors for VTE include increasing age, obesity, immobility, trauma, spinal cord injury, active cancer, major surgery, pregnancy, family history, and sepsis.[151] The VTE incidence is similar for men and women, unless a woman is taking HRT or a contraceptive pill, which increases her risk. Inherited coagulation disorders and hypercoagulability, also described as genetic thrombophilia, confer a propensity for clotting and increase the DVT risk profile in patients with this genetic inheritance.[151,152]

Three major predisposing factors are traditionally described as Virchow's triad: stasis of blood, endothelial injury, and hypercoagulability. Theories on the role of inflammation are adding to the risk profile of thrombosis generation.[152] Usually, two of these three conditions must be present for thrombosis to occur. Patients in critical care units generally have one or more risk factors that predispose them to the development of a venous thrombus. The hospitalized patient has more than a 100-fold increased incidence of acute VTE than someone in the community.[151] The incidence of DVT increases with age and markedly increases the patient's risk of fatal pulmonary embolism (see "Pulmonary Embolism" in Chapter 24).

ASSESSMENT AND DIAGNOSIS

Development of DVT may be insidious. Many patients with DVT are asymptomatic. Pain, if present, is described as an aching or throbbing sensation, which worsens with ambulation. A positive Homans sign, which is pain in the calf on dorsiflexion of the foot, heightens the suspicion of a DVT but is not considered a reliable marker. If DVT is present in the upper extremity, the entire arm swells. Other clinical manifestations include redness with swelling, increased skin temperature, dilation of superficial veins, and mottling and cyanosis caused by stagnant blood flow.

Venous Ultrasound and D-Dimer. When DVT is suspected, a noninvasive venous ultrasound test typically is used to evaluate vein patency.[153] If the thrombus is large and the vein is easy to visualize, the presence of a DVT can be confirmed by this method alone. However, when the results of the ultrasound are inconclusive, the addition of the D-dimer blood test increases diagnostic accuracy. The D-dimer test measures the presence of cross-linked fibrin derivatives in the serum. It is a sensitive marker of thrombosis but it lacks specificity. If the normal D-dimer serum value is elevated, it signifies the presence of clots, but the thrombi could be anywhere in the body. Ultrasound can help to localize the location of the DVT. Together, these two tests represent a useful and powerful diagnostic strategy.[152,153] When the D-dimer value is normal (not elevated), a DVT (or other thrombosis) can safely be ruled out.

Diagnosis of Pulmonary Embolism. If pulmonary embolism is suspected, CT of the thorax may be obtained. Contrast-enhanced CT-arteriography is faster and has greater sensitivity and specificity for detecting emboli in the pulmonary arteries.[153] A $\dot{V}/\dot{Q}$ scan is most likely to be diagnostic in the absence of disease, but it is less helpful in critically ill patients. A normal perfusion scan result effectively rules out acute pulmonary embolism.[152]

Current guidelines recommend evaluating the risk factors for each patient on an individual basis; maintaining a high index of suspicion and using thromboprophylaxis for at-risk patients; and if VTE is suspected, using clinical assessment, venous ultrasound, and the D-dimer assay to confirm or negate the presence of VTE.[149]

MEDICAL MANAGEMENT

Prevention of Venous Thromboembolism. Major therapeutic emphasis is placed on prophylaxis for critically ill patients at high risk for VTE.[95] Preventive measures include prophylactic anticoagulation with subcutaneous LMWH or UFH, increasing mobility, and use of sequential compression devices placed on the lower extremities.

Management of Diagnosed Venous Thromboembolism. The patient is confined to bed rest with elevation of the limb, and anticoagulation therapy is initiated. Analgesics are prescribed to reduce discomfort.

Anticoagulation. Anticoagulants are prescribed to reduce further clotting. The risks and benefits of therapeutic anticoagulation are discussed with the patient and family before therapy begins. In the acute phase, the VTE can be treated with intravenous heparin or subcutaneous LMWH. Subsequently, oral warfarin (Coumadin) may be used. Antiplatelet therapy with aspirin or other drugs is added to prevent VTE recurrence. Antiplatelet therapy alone does not provide protection against development of VTE.[149,154] None of the aforementioned antithrombotics dissolves the existing clot, but the drugs can prevent new thrombi from forming. Lytic therapy usually is reserved for massive pulmonary embolism. Patients receiving anticoagulation therapy require careful assessment for bleeding tendencies, including obtaining frequent bleeding studies—aPTT, INR, or prothrombin time (PT). Stool and urine are tested for presence of occult blood; gums are inspected for bleeding; and when endotracheal suctioning is required, it is important to be gentle and to assess for presence of blood in the aspirate. After the patient begins to ambulate, full-length, custom-fitted elastic stockings are ordered. Complaints or observation of dyspnea or chest pain must be quickly evaluated to assess the risk of pulmonary embolism. Medical management with anticoagulants is adequate for most patients; however, those at risk for pulmonary embolism (patients with cancer, bleeding disorders, or spinal cord injury) may require surgical intervention for protection. Possible procedures include venous embolectomy and insertion of an inferior vena cava filter.[152]

NURSING MANAGEMENT

The focus of nursing management is always to prevent the development of DVT. For the patient with DVT, the interventions include rest the affected extremity, prevention of complications that may result from VTE, and monitoring anticoagulant therapy. Several nursing diagnoses are used in the management of the patient with VTE (see the Nursing Diagnoses feature on Venous Thromboembolism).

Prevention of Thromboembolism. Normally, the simple action of walking helps return blood to the right side of the heart and prevents venous stasis that may lead to development of venous thrombi. For critically ill patients, immobility is often imposed because of the severity of the illness. After they become stable, most patients are assisted out of bed and helped to walk to restore the circulatory pump.

Nursing Diagnoses

Venous Thromboembolism

- Activity Intolerance related to prolonged immobility or deconditioning
- Acute Pain related to transmission and perception of cutaneous, visceral, muscular, or ischemic impulses
- Powerlessness related to lack of control over current situation or disease progression
- Anxiety related to threat to biologic, psychologic, or social integrity
- Deficient Knowledge: Discharge Regimen related to lack of previous exposure to information (see the Patient Education feature on Venous Thromboembolism)

Activity with Deep Vein Thrombosis. For the patient who has developed a DVT, physical activity is limited to prevent dislodgement of emboli. During the acute phase, self-care activities are limited, and bed rest is maintained. Range-of-motion exercises can be performed with any unaffected limb. The patient is instructed to avoid bending at the knees or hips because this impedes venous return. Antiembolism stockings that have been custom-fitted can be used. It is not clear when it is safe to resume normal activity, such as walking, after DVT. Usually, it is resumed after a Doppler study shows no evidence of DVT in the extremity and after symptoms have abated. Prevention strategies again become important, because the patient remains at risk for a recurrence. In general, early ambulation after surgery or other procedures and avoidance of bed rest are the most effective prevention strategies.

Risk of Pulmonary Embolism. The patient with a VTE is closely monitored for signs of pulmonary embolism and instructed to report immediately any chest pain, dyspnea, hemoptysis, or tachypnea. Risk factors for VTE are almost identical to those for pulmonary embolism. For patients who must remain immobile because of their clinical condition, external pneumatic compression devices, antiembolism stockings, and low-dose heparin are commonly used.[149,152,155]

Anticoagulation. Anticoagulant therapy is monitored by obtaining daily coagulation values—aPTT if the patient is receiving intravenous heparin and daily INR if the patient is receiving warfarin (Coumadin).[137] Although the American College of Clinical Pharmacology (ACCP) clinical practice guidelines limit routine coagulation monitoring recommendations for LMWH to anti-Xa levels in pregnant women only, this approach may be expanded to all patients in the future.[137] Signs of bleeding are monitored, and symptoms are treated promptly. For the critically ill patient, hemoglobin levels and hematocrit are monitored daily, and stools are assessed for occult blood. Avoidable mechanical trauma is minimized. The alert patient should be instructed to use a soft toothbrush and, if needed, an electric razor.

PATIENT EDUCATION

Patient education emphasizes VTE prevention for all patients who are immobile in the critical care unit for any length of time. This includes explanations about activity prophylaxis such as early ambulation after major surgery, external pneumatic compression boots, and low-dose heparin.

For patients who have a diagnosed DVT, education is focused on immobilization of the limb, avoidance of trauma to the limb, and elevation of the limb to decrease venous pooling and increase blood flow. If the patient is anticoagulated, the risks and benefits of this therapy are discussed, as well as the risk of VTE and pulmonary embolus. The patient is instructed to report any chest pain, shortness of breath, or respiratory distress (see the Patient Education feature on Venous Thromboembolism). A collaborative team of clinicians who are aware of current clinical recommendations is essential to provide effective care for all critical care patients at risk for VTE (see the Evidence-Based Practice: Collaborative feature on Venous Thromboembolism).

Patient Education

Venous Thromboembolism

- Pathophysiology of deep vein thrombosis
- Discuss risk of pulmonary embolus, need for antiembolism stockings or pneumatic compression devices on legs; avoid trauma to legs and report any chest pain, breathlessness, or increased respiratory rate.
- Medications: Anticoagulants (heparin or Coumadin) to prevent formation of new thrombus at the site; aspirin to decrease platelet aggregation

---

Evidence-Based Practice: Collaborative

Venous Thromboembolism

Summary of Evidence-Based Recommendations for VTE Prevention
Strong evidence exists for the following:
- For highest risk patients combine pharmacologic and mechanical prevention methods:
  - All patients admitted to the critical care unit must be assessed for risk of VTE.
  - Most critically ill patients will require thromboprophylaxis against VTE.
  - Aspirin *alone* should not be used for VTE prophylaxis for any patient group.
- Pharmacologic thromboprophylaxis with low dose UFH *or* LMWH (SQ) *or* fondaparinux
- Oral vitamin K agonists (warfarin) used to achieve a target INR of 2.5 (INR range, 2 to 3)

- Mechanical prophylaxis: graduated-compression stockings or intermittent pneumatic compression devices
- Some of the patients at highest risk for VTE include those undergoing open urologic surgery, gynecologic surgery, or total hip or knee procedures; all trauma patients with at least one risk factor; and medical patients with acute heart failure or acute respiratory failure. Others included in this group are immobile patients confined to bed who have at least one risk factor (e.g., age over 40 years, history of VTE).
- Rates of DVT in critical care patients not receiving prophylaxis range from 10% to 80%.

Reference

Geerts WH et al: Prevention of venous thromboembolism: American College of Chest Physicians Evidence-Based Clinical Practice Guidelines (8th edition), *Chest* 133 (6 suppl):381S-453S, 2008.

DVT, Deep vein thrombosis; *INR*, international normalized ratio; *IV*, intravenous; *LMWH*, low-molecular-weight heparin; *SQ*, subcutaneous; *VTE*, venous thromboembolism, *UFH* unfractionated heparin.

HYPERTENSIVE EMERGENCY

DESCRIPTION

Hypertensive emergency is relatively uncommon. It is seen in less than 1% of patients who are hypertensive, but when present, it is life threatening and demands early recognition and management to minimize morbidity and mortality. It was formerly known as hypertensive crisis or malignant hypertension. With the advent of so many categories of antihypertensive medications, this condition can be effectively managed in the critical care setting. Two forms of acute hypertension are recognized:

- *Hypertensive emergencies* pose a risk of end-organ damage and are life-threatening conditions. The target organ can be the heart (acute MI), the brain (stroke), or the kidney (renal failure).
- *Hypertensive urgencies* are characterized by a serious elevation in blood pressure but do not put the patient at risk for end-organ damage.[156,157]

ETIOLOGY

Hypertensive emergency may occur in patients with no history of the condition or can be precipitated by noncompliance with or inadequate drug therapy. In patients with no known history of hypertension, causes of hypertensive emergency include the following:

1. Acute renal failure
2. Acute central nervous system (CNS) events: hypertension that frequently accompanies subarachnoid hemorrhage (SAH), intracerebral hemorrhage, or a stroke
3. Acute aortic dissection: hypertension that frequently precedes dissection
4. Pregnancy-induced eclampsia: intense arterial vascular constriction, which raises blood pressure and decreases blood supply to the placenta
5. Pheochromocytoma: an adrenal tumor that produces epinephrine and norepinephrine and raises blood pressure as a result of the circulating catecholamines
6. Drug-induced hypertension: illegal drugs, particularly cocaine or amphetamines
7. Drug-food interactions: hypertensive response to tyramine-containing foods or beverages (beer or aged cheese) or during treatment with a monoamine oxidase inhibitor (MAOI), which is now rare because most patients are prescribed other antidepressant medications

PATHOPHYSIOLOGY

The exact trigger of a hypertensive crisis is often unknown. However, most patients suffer from known hypertension before the event, and the sudden rise in blood pressure is often related to the underlying disease process. Clinical manifestations of hypertensive emergency are listed in Table 19-16.

ASSESSMENT AND DIAGNOSIS

Hypertensive emergency can manifest as any of the following symptoms, depending on the target organ involved:

TABLE 19-16 Hypertensive Emergencies

Emergency	Possible Causes
Cardiovascular Compromise	
Chest pain	Unstable angina, myocardial infarction, aortic dissection
Acute heart failure	Myocardial infarction, severe hypertension
Hypertension after vascular surgery	Aortic aneurysmectomy, carotid endarterectomy, coronary artery bypass grafting
Central Nervous System Compromise	
Papilledema	Increased intracranial pressure—mass lesion Malignant hypertension—any cause
Headache, agitation, lethargy, confusion	Hypertensive encephalopathy—any cause, subarachnoid hemorrhage, stroke
Coma	Stroke, advanced hypertensive encephalopathy, trauma, tumor
Seizures	Advanced hypertensive encephalopathy, CNS tumor, eclampsia, stroke (less common)
Focal neurologic deficit	Stroke, CNS tumor, hypertensive encephalopathy
Acute renal failure	Malignant hypertension, vasculitis, scleroderma, glomerulonephritis
Catecholamine excess	Pheochromocytomas, MAOI in combination with certain drugs and foods; abrupt withdrawal of antihypertensive medications such as clonidine, guanabenz, or beta-blockers

CNS, central nervous system; MAOI, monoamine oxidase inhibitor.

1. CNS compromise, identified by headache, blurred vision, change in level of consciousness, or coma
2. Cardiovascular compromise, identified by the chest pain of an ACS or aortic dissection
3. Acute kidney failure, identified by a sudden absence of urine output
4. Catecholamine excess

Worsening of symptoms may indicate hypertensive encephalopathy. Diagnostic studies include blood pressure measurement in both arms and placement of an intraarterial line for close monitoring of blood pressure. A 12-lead ECG is taken to evaluate for evidence of acute MI or left ventricular hypertrophy.

MEDICAL MANAGEMENT

Hypertensive Emergencies. Hypertensive emergencies are defined as an acute blood pressure elevation greater than 180/120 mm Hg complicated by impending or progressive target organ dysfunction.[156,157] Hypertensive emergencies with the risk of end organ damage necessitate admission of the patient to the critical care unit, where intravenous antihypertensive therapy can be administered and blood pressure can be monitored continuously by means of an arterial line. Several intravenous medications in many different drug classes are available for acute reduction of blood pressure. Ideally, the drug should be targeted to the specific condition. Sodium nitroprusside is frequently the first drug used to lower blood pressure in hypertensive emergency. Sodium nitroprusside is useful because of its half-life of seconds. It is not suitable for long-tem use because of development of a metabolite that causes cyanide-like toxicity.[158,159] Short-acting beta-blockers that are effective are labetalol and esmolol. Beta-blockers are especially effective if aortic dissection is present. For patients with heart failure, the intravenous ACEI enalaprilat lowers blood pressure. For hypertensive patients with chest pain, the vasodilator nitroglycerin (NTG) is used. For patients with renal compromise, the dopamine receptor antagonist (DA₁) fenoldopam may be used to lower blood pressure and increase blood flow to the kidneys.[158,160] Hydralazine is the intravenous agent of choice in eclampsia because it does not cross the placental barrier. The calcium channel blocker nicardipine, and the combination alpha-beta blocker labetalol, are less likely to decrease cerebral blood flow, and have been used for patients with CNS compromise.[158,159] The alpha-blocker phentolamine is used for patients in pheochromocytoma crisis.[156-158] Sometimes, combinations of the aforementioned agents are more effective in hypertension control. The intravenous diuretic furosemide (Lasix) is useful for patients with fluid retention.[160]

Initial goals of therapy in hypertensive emergencies limit reducing mean arterial blood pressure by no more than 20% to 25% over a period of several minutes to several hours.[157,160] There is variability depending on the target organ that is affected. When the brain is the target organ, cerebral hypoperfusion can occur if blood pressure is lowered too rapidly. The guidelines for treating stroke do not recommend a rapid reduction of blood pressure. If the blood pressure is excessively high, the aim is to reduce by not more than 20% to 15% in the first 24 hours.[159] The blood pressure spontaneously decreases during the first 10 days after a stroke.[160] For the patient with CAD experiencing a hypertensive emergency, the need to maintain adequate DBP to allow for coronary artery filling is paramount.[156] If vasodilator therapy drops the diastolic pressure too far—when coronary artery filling occurs—myocardial ischemia may result.[160] The question of how much to decrease the blood pressure in a hypertensive emergency is not simply a matter of reading the number on the monitor from the patient's arterial line; it involves an assessment of the underlying pathology and an appreciation of the physiologic requirements of the affected target organ. The "Vasodilator Drugs" section in Chapter 20 provides more information on specific agents.

Hypertensive Urgencies. Hypertensive urgencies may not necessitate admission to a critical care unit, because organ damage is not evident and the patient may be treated with rapid-acting oral antihypertensive agents. There are many drug categories available including ACEIs, ARBs, calcium channel blockers, and beta-blockers. A loop diuretic (e.g., furosemide) often is prescribed in addition to the antihypertensive agents when the patient has fluid retention.

NURSING MANAGEMENT

The focus of nursing management for the patient with hypertensive crisis is to return the blood pressure to the desired range without introducing other complications as a result of the therapy. After the hypertension is controlled, the nurse identifies the factors that resulted in this life-threatening condition. Several nursing diagnoses are associated with hypertensive crisis (see the Nursing Diagnoses feature on Hypertensive Emergency).

During the acute phase, the patient is observed closely for clinical manifestations in other organ systems, including the neurologic, cardiac, and renal systems.[160] Neurologic compromise may be manifested by mental confusion, stupor, seizures, coma, or stroke. Cardiac compromise may be exhibited by aortic dissection, myocardial ischemia, or dysrhythmias. Acute renal failure may not be evident immediately, but urine output, BUN, and serum creatinine values are evaluated over several days to determine whether the kidneys were affected by the hypertensive episode. When short-acting intravenous antihypertensive agents are administered, the blood pressure is closely monitored. If potent antihypertensive drugs such as sodium nitroprusside or labetalol are being used, an arterial line must be inserted, and the drugs must be infused through an infusion pump.

PATIENT EDUCATION

Patient education during the acute phase of a hypertensive emergency is limited to an explanation of the need to control blood pressure and the purpose of the equipment used in the critical care unit. After the hypertensive crisis is resolved, the focus of education is on lifestyle changes to modify risk factors. Hypertension is emphasized as a risk factor for atherosclerotic arterial disease of the heart, brain, and peripheral arterial system. A more complete discussion of hypertension as a cardiovascular risk factor is provided at the beginning of this chapter. The major points to discuss with the patient are listed in the Patient Education feature on Hypertensive Emergency. Management of hypertensive emergencies and urgencies are listed in the Evidence-Based Practice: Collaborative feature on Hypertensive Emergencies.

Nursing Diagnoses

Hypertensive Emergency

- Ineffective Cerebral Tissue Perfusion related to vasospasm or hemorrhage
- Ineffective Cardiopulmonary Tissue Perfusion related to acute myocardial ischemia
- Anxiety related to threat to biologic, psychologic, or social integrity
- Deficient Knowledge: Discharge Regimen related to lack of previous exposure to information (see the Patient Education feature on Hypertensive Emergency)

Summary

- The number of patients with cardiovascular disease continues to grow.[161]
- Considerable research and clinical progress has clarified the diagnosis and management of many cardiac conditions.
- Atherosclerosis provides a common link among CAD, atherosclerotic aortic disease, PAD, and carotid artery disease. The risk factors and general management strategies for all of these diseases are the same.
- Acute myocardial infarction, aortic aneurysm, aortic dissection, and embolic stroke represent the acute manifestations of chronic disease progression.
- Heart failure is a consequence of damaged heart muscle that results form MI, cardiomyopathy, valve disease, or hypertension.
- Conditions such as PAH and valvular disease have diverse causes.
- Cardiac patients are vulnerable to complications such as VTE, IE, and hypertensive emergency.

Patient Education

Hypertensive Emergency

- Pathophysiology of hypertensive crisis
- Normal and abnormal blood pressure values
- Self-monitoring of blood pressure at home
- Connection between hypertension and other atherosclerotic diseases such as coronary artery disease, peripheral arterial disease (PAD), and cerebrovascular disease
- Warning signs of a "heart attack" or myocardial infarction
- Warning signs of a "brain attack" or stroke
- Warning signs of intermittent claudication or PAD
- Risk factors modification: After the acute episode, if the cause of the carotid artery disease is atherosclerosis, an individual risk factor profile is developed for each patient. Strategies to discuss include the following: decrease daily fat intake to less than 30% of total calories, achieve total blood cholesterol level of less than 200 mg/dL, stop smoking, reduce salt intake, control hypertension, control diabetes if patient is diabetic, increase physical activity, achieve and maintain ideal body weight.
- Medications: antihypertensive medications, rationale, and side effects
- Signs and symptoms to report to a health care professional
- Follow-up care after discharge

Evidence-Based Practice: Collaborative

Hypertensive Emergencies

Definition
Hypertensive emergency is defined as an acute BP elevation greater than 180/120 mm Hg complicated by impending or progressive target organ dysfunction.

Recommendations
- Early identification of hypertensive emergency in the emergency room and admission to an intensive care unit is recommended.
- Patients with hypertensive emergency should have continuous BP monitoring.
- IV drugs are used to reduce BP (not necessarily to normal) to prevent or limit target organ damage.
- Initial goal is to reduce BP by no more than 25%. For example, reduce SBP to 160 mm Hg and DBP to 100 to 110 mm Hg in the 2 to 6 hours after admission.
- Decreasing the BP gradually is recommended to avoid cerebral, coronary, and renal ischemia.
- Drugs that cause rapid falls in blood pressure are not recommended in the management of acute hypertensive emergency. For this reason, short-acting nifedipine is *not* endorsed (SL or IV).
- Further gradual reductions in BP can be achieved in the following 24 to 48 hours.

Special Situations: Hypertension and Acute Ischemic Stroke
- For patients admitted with an ischemic stroke, there is no clinical evidence to support rapid reduction in BP.
- For patients with SBP greater than 220 mm Hg or DBP between 120 and 140 mm Hg, BP should be lowered cautiously by 10% to 15% only.

- If the DBP is greater than 140 mm Hg, SNP is recommended to cautiously lower the SBP by about 10%.
- If the SBP is greater than 185 mm Hg or the DBP greater than 110 mm Hg, the use of thrombolytic therapy (tPA) is contraindicated within the first 3 hours after an acute ischemic stroke. The BP must be lowered before the administration of tPA.
- Careful monitoring of the patient for signs of neurologic deterioration related to the lower pressure is mandated in all situations.

Special Situation: Hypertension and Aortic Dissection
- Patients with aortic dissection should have their SBP lowered to less than 100 mm Hg if tolerated.

Ultimate Blood Pressure Target Goal
- The goal of therapy for all patients is a target BP of 140/90 mm Hg or lower before discharge from the hospital. Some patients will require oral medications to achieve this target.
- Target BP is 130/80 mm Hg or lower for patients with known hypertension, kidney failure, diabetes, or cardiovascular disease. Almost all patients with these conditions will require oral medications to achieve their target BP. Many patients require two or more oral drugs.

Reference
Chobanian AV et al: Seventh report of the Joint National Committee on Prevention, Detection, Evaluation, and Treatment of High Blood Pressure, *Hypertension* 42(6):1206-1252, 2003.

BP, Blood pressure; DBP, diastolic blood pressure; IV, intravenous; SBP, systolic blood pressure; SL, sublingual; SNP, sodium nitroprusside; tPA, tissue plasminogen activator.

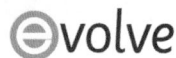 Be sure to check out the bonus material, including free self-assessment exercises, on the Evolve web site at http://evolve.elsevier.com/Urden/.

References

1. American Heart Association: *Heart disease and stroke statistics—2008 update*, Dallas, 2008, American Heart Association.

2. Antman EM et al: 2007 Focused update of the ACC/AHA 2004 guidelines for the management of patients with ST-Elevation Myocardial Infarction: a report of the American College of Cardiology/American Heart Association Task Force on Practice Guidelines; developed in collaboration with the Canadian Cardiovascular Society endorsed by the American Academy of Family Physicians: 2007 Writing Group to Review New Evidence and Update the ACC/AHA 2004 Guidelines for the Management of Patients with ST-Elevation Myocardial Infarction, writing on behalf of the 2004 Writing Committee, *Circulation* 117(2):296-3293, 2008.

3. Fraker TD et al: 2007 Chronic angina focused update of the ACC/AHA 2002 guidelines for the management of patients with chronic stable angina: a report of the American College of Cardiology/American Heart Association Task Force on Practice Guidelines Writing Group to develop the focused update of the 2002 guidelines for the management of patients with chronic stable angina, *J Am Coll Cardiol* 50(23):2264-2274, 2007.

4. Yusef S et al, INTERHEART Study Investigators: Effect of potentially modifiable risk factors associated with myocardial infarction in 52 countries (The INTERHEART Study): case-control study, *Lancet* 364 (9438):937-952, 2004.

5. Anderson LJ et al: ACC/AHA 2007 guidelines for the management of patients with unstable angina/non-ST-elevation myocardial infarction: a report of the American College of Cardiology/American Heart Association Task Force on Practice Guidelines (Writing Committee to Revise the 2002 Guidelines for the Management of Patients with Unstable Angina/Non-ST-Elevation Myocardial Infarction), *J Am Coll Cardiol* 50(7):1-57, 2007.

6. Gibbons RJ et al: ACC/AHA 2002 guideline update for the management of patients with chronic stable angina—summary article: a report of the American College of Cardiology/American Heart Association Task Force on Practice Guidelines (Committee on the Management of Patients with Chronic Stable Angina), *Circulation* 107(1):149-158, 2003.

7. Executive summary of the third report of the National Cholesterol Education Program (NCEP) Expert Panel on Detection, Evaluation, and Treatment of High Blood Cholesterol in Adults (Adult Treatment Panel III), *JAMA* 285(19):2486-2497, 2001.

8. Grundy SM et al: Implications of recent clinical trials for the National Cholesterol Education Program Adult Treatment Panel III guidelines, *Circulation* 110(2):227-239, 2004.

9. Barter PJ et al: Antiinflammatory properties of HDL, *Circ Res* 95(8):764-772, 2004.

10. O'Keefe JH Jr et al: Optimal low-density lipoprotein is 50 to 70 mg/dL: lower is better and physiologically normal, *J Am Coll Cardiol* 43(11):2142-2146, 2004.

11. Futterman LG, Lemberg L: Lp(a) lipoprotein: an independent risk factor for coronary heart disease after menopause, *Am J Crit Care* 10(1):63-67, 2001.

12. Jensen KM et al: Obesity, behavioral lifestyle factors, and risk of acute coronary events, *Circulation* 117;3062-3069, 2008.

13. Chobanian AV et al: Seventh report of the Joint National Committee on Prevention, Detection, Evaluation, and Treatment of High Blood Pressure, *Hypertension* 42(6):1206-1252, 2003.

14. Thompson PD et al: Exercise and physical activity in the prevention and treatment of atherosclerotic cardiovascular disease: a statement from the Council on Clinical Cardiology (Subcommittee on Exercise, Rehabilitation, and Prevention) and the Council on Nutrition, Physical Activity, and Metabolism (Subcommittee on Physical Activity), *Circulation* 107 (24):3109-3116, 2003.

15. Brook RD et al: Air pollution and cardiovascular disease: a statement for healthcare professionals from the Expert Panel on Population and Prevention Science of the American Heart Association, *Circulation* 109 (21):2655-2671, 2004.

16. Sargent RP et al: Reduced incidence of admissions for myocardial infarction associated with public smoking ban: before and after study, *BMJ* 328(7446):977-980, 2004.

17. Houterman S et al: Smoking, blood pressure and serum cholesterol-effects on 20-year mortality, *Epidemiology* 14(1):24-29, 2003.

18. Garber AJ et al: American College of Endocrinology position statement on inpatient diabetes and metabolic control, *Endocr Pract* 10(1):77-82, 2004.

19. McGuire DK et al: Association of diabetes mellitus and glycemic control strategies with clinical outcomes after acute coronary syndromes, *Am Heart J* 147(2):246-252, 2004.

20. Franklin K et al: Implications of diabetes in patients with acute coronary syndromes: the Global Registry of Acute Coronary Events, *Arch Intern Med* 164(13):1457-1463, 2004.

21. Sarnak MJ et al: Kidney disease as a risk factor for development of cardiovascular disease: a statement from the American Heart Association Councils on Kidney in Cardiovascular Disease, High Blood Pressure Research, Clinical Cardiology, and Epidemiology and Prevention, *Hypertension* 42(5):1050-10605, 2003.

22. Wright RS et al: Acute myocardial infarction and renal dysfunction: a high-risk combination, *Ann Intern Med* 137(7):563-570, 2002.

23. Grundy SM et al: Clinical management of metabolic syndrome: report of the American Heart Association/National Heart, Lung, and Blood Institute/American Diabetes Association conference on scientific issues related to management, *Circulation* 109(4):551-556, 2004.

24. Grady D et al: Cardiovascular disease outcomes during 6.8 years of hormone therapy: Heart and Estrogen/progestin Replacement Study follow-up (HERS II), *JAMA* 288(1):49-57, 2002.

25. Hulley S et al: Randomized trial of estrogen plus progestin for secondary prevention of coronary heart disease in postmenopausal women. Heart and Estrogen/progestin Replacement Study (HERS) Research Group, *JAMA* 280(7):605-613, 1998.

26. Anderson GL et al: Effects of conjugated equine estrogen in postmenopausal women with hysterectomy: the Women's Health Initiative randomized controlled trial, *JAMA* 291(14):1701-1712, 2004.

27. Mosca L et al: Evidence-based guidelines for cardiovascular disease prevention in women: 2007 update, *Circulation* 115:1481-1501, 2007.

28. Lefler LL, Bondy KN: Women's delay in seeking treatment with myocardial infarction: a meta synthesis, *J Cardiovasc Nurs* 19(4):251-268, 2004.

29. Reeder SJ et al: Homocysteine: the latest risk factor for heart disease, *Dimens Crit Care Nurs* 19(1):22-28, 2000.

30. Aronow WS: Homocysteine: the association with atherosclerotic vascular disease in older persons, *Geriatrics* 58(9):22-24, 27–28, 2003.

31. Pearson TA et al: Markers of inflammation and cardiovascular disease: application to clinical and public health practice: a statement for healthcare professionals from the Centers for Disease Control and Prevention and the American Heart Association, *Circulation* 107(3):499-511, 2003.

32. Speidl WS et al: High-sensitivity C-reactive protein in the prediction of coronary events in patients with premature coronary artery disease, *Am Heart J* 144(3):449-455, 2002.

33. Buffon A et al: Widespread coronary inflammation in unstable angina, *N Engl J Med* 347(1):5-12, 2002.

34. King SB 3rd et al: 2007 Focused update of the ACC/AHA/SCAI 2005 guideline update for percutaneous coronary intervention: a report of the American College of Cardiology/American Heart Association Task Force on Practice Guidelines, 2007 Writing Group to Review New Evidence and Update the ACC/AHA/SCAI 2005 Guideline Update for Percutaneous Coronary Intervention, writing on behalf of the 2005 Writing Committee, *J Am Coll Cardiol* 51(2):172-209, 2008.

35. McSweeney JC et al: Women's early warning symptoms of acute myocardial infarction, *Circulation* 108(21):2619-2623, 2003.

36. Bairey Merz N et al: Women's ischemic syndrome evaluation: current status and future research directions. Report of the National Heart, Lung and Blood Institute workshop, October 2-4, 2002: executive summary, *Circulation* 109(6):805-807, 2004.

37. Canto JG et al: Use of emergency medical services in acute myocardial infarction and subsequent quality of care: observations from the National Registry of Myocardial Infarction 2, *Circulation* 106(24):3018-3023, 2002.

38. Keller KB, Lemberg L: Prinzmetal's angina, *Am J Crit Care* 13(4):350-354, 2004.

39. Jacobs AK et al: Cardiogenic shock caused by right ventricular infarction: a report from the SHOCK registry, *J Am Coll Cardiol* 41(8):1273-1279, 2003.

40. Lanza M: Right ventricular myocardial infarction: when the power fails, *Dimens Crit Care Nurs* 21(4):122-126, 2002.

41. Mehta RH et al: Comparison of outcomes of patients with acute coronary syndromes with and without atrial fibrillation, *Am J Cardiol* 92(9):1031-1036, 2003.

42. Birnbaum Y et al: Ventricular septal rupture after acute myocardial infarction, *N Engl J Med* 347(18):1426-1432, 2002.

43. Crenshaw BS et al: Risk factors, angiographic patterns, and outcomes in patients with ventricular septal defect complicating acute myocardial infarction. GUSTO-I (Global Utilization of Streptokinase and TPA for Occluded Coronary Arteries) Trial Investigators, *Circulation* 101(1):27-32, 2000.

44. Deja MA et al: Post infarction ventricular septal defect: can we do better, *Eur J Cardiothorac Surg* 18(2):194-201, 2000.

45. Birnbaum Y et al: Mitral regurgitation following acute myocardial infarction, *Coron Artery Dis* 13(6):337-344, 2002.

46. Maisch B et al: Guidelines on the diagnosis and management of pericardial diseases executive summary: the Task Force on the Diagnosis and Management of Pericardial Diseases of the European Society of Cardiology, *Eur Heart J* 25(7):587-610, 2004.

47. Wang K et al: ST-segment elevation in conditions other than acute myocardial infarction, *N Engl J Med* 349(22):2128-2135, 2003.

48. Paelinck B, Dendale PA: Images in clinical medicine: cardiac tamponade in Dressler's syndrome, *N Engl J Med* 348(23):1-8, 2003.

49. Wu AH et al: Hospital outcomes in patients presenting with congestive heart failure complicating acute myocardial infarction: a report from the Second National Registry of Myocardial Infarction (NRMI-2), *J Am Coll Cardiol* 40(8):1389-1394, 2002.

50. Szekendi MK: Compliance with acute MI guidelines lowers inpatient mortality, *J Cardiovasc Nurs* 18(5):356-359, 2003.

51. Eagle KA et al: Adherence to evidence-based therapies after discharge for acute coronary syndromes: an ongoing prospective, observational study, *Am J Med* 117(2):73-81, 2004.

52. Moser KD, Riegal B: *Cardiac nursing: a companion to Braunwald's heart disease*, St Louis, 2008, WB Saunders.

53. Balady GJ et al: Core components of cardiac rehabilitation/secondary prevention programs: a statement for healthcare professionals from the American Heart Association and the American Association of Cardiovascular and Pulmonary Rehabilitation Writing Group, *Circulation* 102(9):1069-1073, 2000.

54. Fox CS et al: Temporal trends in coronary heart disease mortality and sudden cardiac death from 1950 to 1999: the Framingham Heart Study, *Circulation* 110(5):522-527, 2004.

55. Chugh SS et al: Current burden of sudden cardiac death: multiple source surveillance versus retrospective death-certificate based review in a large U.S. community, *J Am Coll Cardiol* 44(6):1268-1275, 2004.

56. Hallstrom AP et al: Public-access defibrillation and survival after out-of-hospital cardiac arrest, *N Engl J Med* 351(7):637-646, 2004.

57. Priori SG et al: Task Force on Sudden Cardiac Death of the European Society of Cardiology, *Eur Heart J* 22(16):1374-1450, 2001.

58. Antzelevitch C et al: Brugada syndrome: report of the second consensus conference; endorsed by the Heart Rhythm Society and the European Heart Rhythm Association, *Circulation* 111(5):659-670, 2005.

59. Goldberger JJ et al: American Heart Association/American College of Cardiology Foundation/Heart Rhythm Society scientific statement on noninvasive risk stratification techniques for identifying patients at risk for sudden cardiac death: a scientific statement from the American Heart Association Council on Clinical Cardiology Committee on Electrocardiography and Arrhythmias and Council on Epidemiology and Prevention, *J Am Coll Cardiol* 52(14):1179-1199, 2008.

60. Epstein AE et al: ACC/AHA/HRS 2008 guideline for device-based therapy of cardiac rhythm abnormalities: a report of the American College of Cardiology/American Heart Association Task Force on Practice Guidelines (Writing Committee to Revise the ACC/AHA/NASPE 2002 Guideline Update for Implantation of Cardiac Pacemakers and Antiarrhythmic Devices) developed in collaboration with American Association of Thoracic Surgery and the Society of Thoracic Surgeons, *J Am Coll Cardiol* 51(21):1-62, 2008.

61. Steinbeck G: Evolution of implantable cardioverter defibrillator indications: comparison of guidelines in the United States and Europe, *J Cardiovasc Electrophysiol* 13(suppl 1):S96-S99, 2002.

62. Epstein AE: An update on implantable cardioverter-defibrillator guidelines, *Curr Opin Cardiol* 19(1):23-25, 2004.

63. Hunt SA et al: ACC/AHA 2005 guideline update for the diagnosis and management of chronic heart failure in the adult: a report of the American College of Cardiology/American Heart Association Task Force on Practice Guidelines (Writing Committee to Update the 2001 Guidelines for the Evaluation and Management of Heart Failure) developed in collaboration with the American College of Chest Physicians and the International Society for Heart and Lung Transplantation; endorsed by the Heart Rhythm Society, *Circulation* 112:154-235, 2005.

64. Levy D et al: Long term trends in the incidence and survival with heart failure, *N Engl J Med* 347:1397-1402, 2002.

65. Zile MR, Brutsaert DL: New concepts in diastolic dysfunction and diastolic heart failure. Part I. Diagnosis, prognosis, and measurements of diastolic function, *Circulation* 105(11):1387-1393, 2002.

66. Zile MR, Brutsaert DL: New concepts in diastolic dysfunction and diastolic heart failure. Part II. Causal mechanisms and treatment, *Circulation* 105(12):1503-1508, 2002.

67. Henry LB: Left ventricular systolic dysfunction and ischemic cardiomyopathy, *Crit Care Nurs Q* 26(1):16-21, 2003.

68. Bolliger K, Sadar AM: Care and management of the patient with right heart failure secondary to diastolic dysfunction: an advanced practice perspective and case review, *Crit Care Nurs Q* 26(1):22-27, 2003.

69. Aurigemma GP, Gaasch WH: Clinical practice: diastolic heart failure, *N Engl J Med* 351(11):1097-1105, 2004.

70. Zile MR et al: Diastolic heart failure: abnormalities in active relaxation and passive stiffness of the left ventricle, *N Engl J Med* 350(19):1953-1959, 2004.

71. Riedinger MS et al: Quality of life in patients with heart failure: do gender differences exist? *Heart Lung* 30(2):105-116, 2001.

72. Maisel AS et al: Bedside B-type natriuretic peptide in the emergency diagnosis of heart failure with reduced or preserved ejection fraction. Results from the Breathing Not Properly (BNP) multinational study, *J Am Coll Cardiol* 41(11):2010-2017, 2003.

73. Thohan V et al: Aldosterone antagonism and congestive heart failure: a new look at an old therapy, *Curr Opin Cardiol* 19(4):301-308, 2004.

74. Patten RD, Soman P: Prevention and reversal of LV remodeling with neurohormonal inhibitors, *Curr Treat Options Cardiovasc Med* 6(4):313-325, 2004.

75. Paul S: Balancing diuretic therapy in heart failure: loop diuretics, thiazides, and aldosterone antagonists, *Congest Heart Fail* 8(6):307-312, 2002.

76. Paul S: Ventricular remodeling, *Crit Care Nurs Clin North Am* 15(4):407-411, 2003.

77. Dimopoulos K et al: Meta-analyses of mortality and morbidity effects of an angiotensin receptor blocker in patients with chronic heart failure already receiving an ACE inhibitor (alone or with a beta-blocker), *Int J Cardiol* 93(2-3):105-111, 2004.

78. McCullough PA, Sandberg KR: B type natriuretic peptide and renal disease, *Heart Fail Rev* 8(4):355-358, 2003.

79. Maisel AS et al: Impact of age, race, and sex on the ability of B-type natriuretic peptide to aid in the emergency diagnosis of heart failure: results from the Breathing Not Properly (BNP) multinational study, *Am Heart J* 147(6):1078-1084, 2004.

80. Maisel AS et al: Rapid measurement of B-type natriuretic peptide in the emergency diagnosis of heart failure, *N Engl J Med* 347(3):161-167, 2002.

81. McCullough PA et al: Uncovering heart failure in patients with a history of pulmonary disease: rationale for the early use of B-type natriuretic peptide in the emergency department, *Acad Emerg Med* 10(3):198-204, 2003.

82. Buxton AE et al: Relation of ejection fraction and inducible ventricular tachycardia to mode of death in patients with coronary artery disease: an analysis of patients enrolled in the multicenter unsustained tachycardia trial, *Circulation* 106(19):2466-2472, 2002.

83. Stroe AF, Gheorghiade M: Carvedilol: beta-blockade and beyond, *Rev Cardiovasc Med* 5(suppl 1):S18-S27, 2004.

84. Zhang J: Sudden cardiac death: implantable cardioverter defibrillators and pharmacological treatments, *Crit Care Nurs Q* 26(1):45-49, 2003.

85. Whang W et al: Heart failure and the risk of shocks in patients with implantable cardioverter defibrillators: results from the Triggers of Ventricular Arrhythmias (TOVA) study, *Circulation* 109(11):1386-1391, 2004.

86. Khand AU et al: Carvedilol alone or in combination with digoxin for the management of atrial fibrillation in patients with heart failure, *J Am Coll Cardiol* 42(11):1944-1951, 2003.

87. Chen EW et al: Relation between hospital intra-aortic balloon counterpulsation volume and mortality in acute myocardial infarction complicated by cardiogenic shock, *Circulation* 108(8):951-957, 2003.

88. Burger AJ et al: Effect of nesiritide (B-type natriuretic peptide) and dobutamine on ventricular arrhythmias in the treatment of patients with acutely decompensated congestive heart failure: the PRECEDENT study, *Am Heart J* 144(6):1102-1108, 2002.

89. Colbert K, Greene MH: Nesiritide (Natrecor): a new treatment for acutely decompensated congestive heart failure, *Crit Care Nurs Q* 26(1):40-44, 2003.

90. Abraham WT, Iyengar S: Practical considerations for switching beta-blockers in heart failure patients, *Rev Cardiovasc Med* 5(suppl 1): S36-S44, 2004.

91. Albert NM: Cardiac resynchronization therapy through biventricular pacing in patients with heart failure and ventricular dyssynchrony, *Crit Care Nurse* 23(suppl 3):2-13, 2003.

92. Abraham WT, Hayes DL: Cardiac resynchronization therapy for heart failure, *Circulation* 108(21):2596-2603, 2003.

93. Young JB et al: Combined cardiac resynchronization and implantable cardioversion defibrillation in advanced chronic heart failure: the MIRACLE ICD Trial, *JAMA* 289(20):2685-2694, 2003.

94. Goodlin SJ et al: Consensus statement: palliative and supportive care in advanced heart failure, *J Card Fail* 10(3):200-209, 2004.

95. Rudisill PT et al: The use of beta-blockers in the treatment of chronic heart failure, *Crit Care Nurs Clin North Am* 15(4):439-446, 2003.

96. Fonarow GC et al: Organized Program to Initiate Lifesaving Treatment in Hospitalized Patients with Heart Failure (OPTIMIZE-HF): rationale and design, *Am Heart J* 148(1):43-51, 2004.

97. Callahan HE: Families dealing with advanced heart failure: a challenge and an opportunity, *Crit Care Nurs Q* 26(3):230-243, 2003.

98. Grady KL et al: Team management of patients with heart failure: a statement for healthcare professionals from the Cardiovascular Nursing Council of the American Heart Association, *Circulation* 102(19):2443-2456, 2000.

99. Coviello JS, Nystrom KV: Obesity and heart failure, *J Cardiovasc Nurs* 18(5):360-366, 2003.

100. Sneed NV, Paul SC: Readiness for behavioral changes in patients with heart failure, *Am J Crit Care* 12(5):444-453, 2003.

101. Maron BJ et al: American College of Cardiology/European Society of Cardiology clinical expert consensus document on hypertrophic cardiomyopathy: a report of the American College of Cardiology Foundation Task Force on Clinical Expert Consensus Documents and the European Society of Cardiology Committee for Practice Guidelines, *J Am Coll Cardiol* 42(9):1687-1713, 2003.

102. Nishimura RA, Holmes DR Jr: Clinical practice: hypertrophic obstructive cardiomyopathy, *N Engl J Med* 350(13):1320-1327, 2004.

103. Elliott P, McKenna WJ: Hypertrophic cardiomyopathy, *Lancet* 363 (9424):1881-1891, 2004.

104. Kamisago M et al: Mutations in sarcomere protein genes as a cause of dilated cardiomyopathy, *N Engl J Med* 343(23):1688-1696, 2000.

105. Li D et al: Novel cardiac troponin T mutation as a cause of familial dilated cardiomyopathy, *Circulation* 104(18):2188-2193, 2001.

106. Murphy RT et al: Novel mutation in cardiac troponin I in recessive idiopathic dilated cardiomyopathy, *Lancet* 363(9406):371-372, 2004.

107. Noutsias M et al: Current insights into the pathogenesis, diagnosis and therapy of inflammatory cardiomyopathy, *Heart Fail Monit* 3(4): 127-135, 2003.

108. Syed J, Myers R: Sarcoid heart disease, *Can J Cardiol* 20(1):89-93, 2004.

109. Ammash NM et al: Clinical profile and outcome of idiopathic restrictive cardiomyopathy, *Circulation* 101(21):2490-2496, 2000.

110. Felker GM et al: Underlying causes and long-term survival in patients with initially unexplained cardiomyopathy, *N Engl J Med* 342 (15):1077-1084, 2000.

111. Gabbay E et al: Assessment and treatment of pulmonary arterial hypertension: an Australian perspective in 2006, *Intern Med J* 37(1):38-48, 2007.

112. McGoon M et al: Screening, early detection, and diagnosis of pulmonary arterial hypertension: ACCP evidence-based clinical practice guidelines, *Chest* 126(1 suppl):14S-34S, 2004.

113. Rubenfire M et al: Pulmonary hypertension in the critical care setting: classification, pathophysiology, diagnosis, and management, *Crit Care Clin* 23(4):801-834, 2007.

114. Rubin LJ: Diagnosis and management of pulmonary arterial hypertension: ACCP evidence-based clinical practice guidelines, *Chest* 126(1 suppl):7S-10S, 2004.

115. Rubin LJ: Diagnosis and management of pulmonary arterial hypertension: ACCP evidence-based clinical practice guidelines, *Chest* 126(1 suppl):4S-6S, 2004.

116. Gaine S: Pulmonary hypertension, *JAMA* 284(24):3160-3168, 2000.

117. Zamanian RT et al: Management strategies for patients with pulmonary hypertension in the intensive care unit, *Crit Care Med* 35(9):2037-2050, 2007.

118. McLaughlin VV, McGoon MD: Pulmonary arterial hypertension, *Circulation* 114(13):1417-1431, 2006.

119. Badesch DB et al: Medical therapy for pulmonary arterial hypertension: updated ACCP evidence-based clinical practice guidelines, *Chest* 131 (6):1917-1928, 2007.

120. Humbert M et al: Treatment of pulmonary arterial hypertension, *N Engl J Med* 351(14):1425-1436, 2004.

121. Doyle RL et al: Surgical treatments/interventions for pulmonary arterial hypertension: ACCP evidence-based clinical practice guidelines, *Chest* 126(1 suppl):63S-71S, 2004.

122. Doran AK et al: Guidelines for the prevention of central venous catheter-related blood stream infections with prostanoid therapy for pulmonary arterial hypertension, *Int J Clin Pract Suppl* 160:5-9, 2008.

123. Lester SJ, Wilansky S: Endocarditis and associated complications, *Crit Care Med* 35(8 suppl):S384-S391, 2007.

124. Bashore M et al: Update on infective endocarditis, *Curr Probl Cardiol* 31 (4):274-352, 2006.

125. Horstkotte D et al: Guidelines on prevention, diagnosis and treatment of infective endocarditis—executive summary: the Task Force on Infective Endocarditis of the European Society of Cardiology, *Eur Heart J* 25(3):267-276, 2004.

126. Wilson W et al: Prevention of infective endocarditis: guidelines from the American Heart Association. A guideline from the American Heart Association Rheumatic Fever, Endocarditis, and Kawasaki Disease Committee, Council on Cardiovascular Disease in the Young, and the Council on Clinical Cardiology, Council on Cardiovascular Surgery and Anesthesia, and the Quality of Care and Outcomes Research Interdisciplinary Working Group, *Circulation* 116(15):1736-1754, 2007.

127. Baddour LM et al: Infective endocarditis: diagnosis, antimicrobial therapy, and management of complications. A statement for healthcare professionals from the Committee on Rheumatic Fever, Endocarditis, and Kawasaki Disease, Council on Cardiovascular Disease in the Young, and the Councils on Clinical Cardiology, Stroke, and Cardiovascular Surgery and

Anesthesia, American Heart Association: endorsed by the Infectious Diseases Society of America, *Circulation* 111(23):e394-e434, 2005.

128. Nishimura RA et al: ACC/AHA 2008 guideline update on valvular heart disease: focused update on infective endocarditis. A report of the American College of Cardiology/American Heart Association Task Force on Practice Guidelines, *Circulation* 11(8):887-895, 2008.

129. Broyles LM, Korniewicz DM: The opiate-dependent patient with endocarditis: addressing pain and substance abuse withdrawal, *AACN Clin Issues* 13(3):432-451, 2002.

130. Bonow RO et al: ACC/AHA 2006 guidelines for the management of patients with valvular heart disease: a report of the American College of Cardiology/American Heart Association Task Force on Practice Guidelines (Writing Committee to Revise the 1988 Guidelines for the Management of Patients with Valvular Heart Disease) developed in collaboration with the Society of Cardiovascular Anesthesiologists; endorsed by the Society for Cardiovascular Angiography and Interventions and the Society of Thoracic Surgeons, *Circulation* 114(5):e84-e231, 2006.

131. Akat K et al: Aortic valve calcification: basic science to clinical practice, *Heart* 2008 Jul 16 (Epub ahead of print).

132. Rosengart TK et al: Percutaneous and minimally invasive valve procedures: a scientific statement from the American Heart Association Council on Cardiovascular Surgery and Anesthesia, Council on Clinical Cardiology, Function Genomics and Translation Biology Interdisciplinary Working Group, and Quality of Care and Outcomes Research Interdisciplinary Working Group, *Circulation* 117(13):1750-1767, 2008.

133. Trimarchi S et al: Role and results of surgery in acute type B aortic dissection: insights from the International Registry of Acute Aortic Dissection (IRAD), *Circulation* 114(1 suppl):I357-I364, 2006.

134. Golledge J, Powell JT: Medical management of abdominal aortic aneurysm, *Eur J Vasc Endovasc Surg* 34(3):267-273, 2007.

135. Norman PE, Powell JT: Abdominal aortic aneurysm: the prognosis in women is worse than in men, *Circulation* 115(22):2865-2869, 2007.

136. Tsai TT et al: Long-term survival in patients presenting with type A acute aortic dissection: insights from the International Registry of Acute Aortic Dissection (IRAD), *Circulation* 114(1 suppl):I350-I356, 2006.

137. Hirsch AT et al: ACC/AHA 2005 practice guidelines for the management of patients with peripheral arterial disease (lower extremity, renal, mesenteric, and abdominal aortic): a collaborative report from the American Association for Vascular Surgery/Society for Vascular Surgery, Society for Cardiovascular Angiography and Interventions, Society for Vascular Medicine and Biology, Society of Interventional Radiology, and the ACC/AHA Task Force on Practice Guidelines (Writing Committee to Develop Guidelines for the Management of Patients with Peripheral Arterial Disease). Endorsed by the American Association of Cardiovascular and Pulmonary Rehabilitation; National Heart, Lung, and Blood Institute; Society for Vascular Nursing; TransAtlantic Inter-Society Consensus; and Vascular Disease Foundation, *Circulation* 113(11):e463-e654, 2006.

138. Argacha JF et al: Acute effects of passive smoking on peripheral vascular function, *Hypertension* 51(6):1506-1511, 2008.

139. Menke A et al: Relation of borderline peripheral arterial disease to cardiovascular disease risk, *Am J Cardiol* 98(9):1226-1230, 2006.

140. Meschia JF et al: Diagnosis and invasive management of carotid atherosclerotic stenosis, *Mayo Clin Proc* 82(7):851-858, 2007.

141. Garg PK et al: Physical activity during daily life and mortality in patients with peripheral arterial disease, *Circulation* 114(3):242-248, 2006.

142. Goldstein LB et al: Primary prevention of ischemic stroke: a guideline from the American Heart Association/American Stroke Association Stroke Council: cosponsored by the Atherosclerotic Peripheral Vascular Disease Interdisciplinary Working Group; Cardiovascular Nursing Council; Clinical Cardiology Council; Nutrition, Physical Activity, and Metabolism Council; and the Quality of Care and Outcomes Research Interdisciplinary Working Group, *Circulation* 113(24):e873-e923, 2006.

143. Alexandrov AW: Methodologic challenges in the design and conduct of hyperacute stroke research, *AACN Adv Crit Care* 19(2):186-201, 2008.

144. Sacco RL et al: Guidelines for prevention of stroke in patients with ischemic stroke or transient ischemic attack: a statement for healthcare professionals from the American Heart Association/American Stroke Association Council on Stroke; co-sponsored by the Council on Cardiovascular Radiology and Intervention; the American Academy of Neurology affirms the value of this guideline, *Stroke* 37(2):577-617, 2006.

145. Gurm HS et al: Long-term results of carotid stenting versus endarterectomy in high-risk patients, *N Engl J Med* 358(15):1572-1579, 2008.

146. Hopkins LN et al: Carotid artery revascularization in high surgical risk patients with the NexStent and the Filterwire EX/EZ: 1-year results in the CABERNET trial, *Catheter Cardiovasc Interv* 71(7):950-960, 2008.

147. Iyer SS et al: Carotid artery revascularization in high-surgical-risk patients using the Carotid WALLSTENT and FilterWire EX/EZ: 1-year outcomes in the BEACH Pivotal Group, *J Am Coll Cardiol* 51(4):427-434, 2008.

148. Mas JL et al: Endarterectomy versus stenting in patients with symptomatic severe carotid stenosis, *N Engl J Med* 355(16):1660-1671, 2006.

149. Geerts WH et al: Prevention of venous thromboembolism: American College of Chest Physicians Evidence-Based Clinical Practice Guidelines (8th edition), *Chest* 133(6 suppl):381S-453S, 2008.

150. Wakefield TW et al: Mechanisms of venous thrombosis and resolution, *Arterioscler Thromb Vasc Biol* 28(3):387-391, 2008.

151. Heit JA: The epidemiology of venous thromboembolism in the community, *Arterioscler Thromb Vasc Biol* 28(3):370-372, 2008.

152. Tapson VF: Acute pulmonary embolism, *N Engl J Med* 358(10):1037-1052, 2008.

153. Moll S: A clinical perspective of venous thromboembolism, *Arterioscler Thromb Vasc Biol* 28(3):373-379, 2008.

154. Kearon C et al: Antithrombotic therapy for venous thromboembolic disease: American College of Chest Physicians Evidence-Based Clinical Practice Guidelines (8th edition), *Chest* 133(6 suppl):454S-545S, 2008.

155. Snow V et al: Management of venous thromboembolism: a clinical practice guideline from the American College of Physicians and the American Academy of Family Physicians, *Ann Fam Med* 5(1):74-80, 2007.

156. Elliott WJ: Clinical features in the management of selected hypertensive emergencies, *Prog Cardiovasc Dis* 48(5):316-325, 2006.

157. Varon J: Treatment of acute severe hypertension: current and newer agents, *Drugs* 68(3):283-297, 2008.

158. Feldstein C: Management of hypertensive crises, *Am J Ther* 14(2):135-139, 2007.

159. Marik PE, Varon J: Hypertensive crises: challenges and management, *Chest* 131(6):1949-1962, 2007.

160. Slama M, Modeliar SS: Hypertension in the intensive care unit, *Curr Opin Cardiol* 21(4):279-287, 2006.

161. Hirsh J et al: Parenteral anticoagulants: American College of Chest Physicians Evidence-Based Clinical Practice Guidelines (8th edition), *Chest* 133(6 suppl):141S-159S, 2008.

Cardiovascular Therapeutic Management

PACEMAKERS

Pacemakers are electronic devices that can be used to initiate the heartbeat when the heart's intrinsic electrical system cannot effectively generate a rate adequate to support cardiac output. Pacemakers may be used temporarily, either supportively or prophylactically, until the condition responsible for the rate or conduction disturbance resolves. They also may be used on a permanent basis if the patient's condition persists despite adequate therapy. The use of permanent pacemakers as a form of device-based therapy is gaining popularity.[1]

This section emphasizes temporary pacemakers, because the critical care nurse is responsible for preventing, assessing, and managing pacemaker malfunctions when these devices are used in the clinical setting. A brief discussion of permanent pacemakers is provided, and similarities between implanted and temporary pacemakers are presented where appropriate.

INDICATIONS FOR TEMPORARY PACING

The clinical indications for instituting temporary pacemaker therapy are similar regardless of the cause of the rhythm disturbance that necessitates the placement of a pacemaker (Box 20-1). The causes range from drug toxicities and electrolyte imbalances to sequelae related to acute myocardial infarction (MI) or cardiac surgery.

Therapeutic Indications. Dysrhythmias that are unresponsive to drug therapy and result in compromised hemodynamic status are a definite indication for pacemaker therapy. The goal of therapy in the case of bradydysrhythmia is to increase the ventricular rate and thereby enhance cardiac output. Alternately, overdrive pacing can be used to decrease the rate of a rapid supraventricular or ventricular rhythm. This rapid pacing of the heart (i.e., overdrive pacing) functions to prevent the breakthrough ectopy that can result from a slow rate or to interrupt an ectopic focus and allow the natural pacemaker to regain control. Temporary pacing may be used in the treatment of symptomatic bradycardia or progressive heart block that occurs as a result of myocardial ischemia or drug toxicity. After cardiac surgery, temporary pacing may be used to improve a transiently depressed, rate-dependent cardiac output. Conduction disturbances that occur after valvular surgery can be managed effectively with temporary pacing.

Diagnostic Indications. Several diagnostic uses for temporary pacing have evolved. Electrophysiology studies (EPS) are performed in cardiac catheterization laboratories equipped with specialized pacing equipment. During an EPS, special pacing electrodes are used to diagnose the patient's potential for dysrhythmias.[2] These electrodes are used to induce dysrhythmias in patients with recurrent symptomatic tachydysrhythmias. This allows the physician to closely evaluate the particular dysrhythmia and determine appropriate therapy. For those patients whose tachydysrhythmia is found to be refractory to conventional antidysrhythmic therapy, radiofrequency (RF) current catheter ablation of the responsible tissue can be done safely and effectively in the electrophysiology laboratory. After a mapping procedure has localized the site of dysrhythmia formation, short bursts of RF current are delivered through the catheter, destroying the offending tissue with heat. RF ablation is more effective than its predecessor, direct current (DC) ablation, because it delivers a more precise, localized ablation current that lowers the incidence of complications and does not require general anesthesia.[2] Ablation has been shown to be an effective treatment for patients with symptomatic supraventricular tachycardias that result from atrioventricular (AV) node reentry or accessory pathways, such as Wolff-Parkinson-White syndrome.[3]

The atrial electrogram (AEG) is simply an amplified recording of atrial activity that can be obtained through the use of an atrial pacing electrode or an esophageal pill electrode and a standard electrocardiogram (ECG) machine. It may be used after cardiac surgery to facilitate the diagnosis of supraventricular dysrhythmias in patients with temporary atrial epicardial wires already in place.[4]

THE PACEMAKER SYSTEM

A pacemaker system is a simple electrical circuit consisting of a pulse generator and a pacing lead (an insulated electrical wire) with one, two, or three electrodes.

Pacing Pulse Generator. The pulse generator is designed to generate an electrical current that travels through the pacing lead and exits through an electrode (exposed portion of the wire) that is in direct contact with the heart. This electrical current initiates a myocardial depolarization. The current then seeks to return by one of several pathways to the pulse generator to complete the circuit.

The power source for a temporary external pulse generator is a standard 9-volt alkaline battery inserted into the generator. Implanted permanent pacemaker batteries are usually long-lived lithium cells.

Pacing Lead Systems. The pacing lead used for temporary pacing may be bipolar or unipolar. In a bipolar system, two electrodes (positive and negative) are located within the heart, whereas in a unipolar system, only one electrode (negative) is in direct contact

with the myocardium. In both systems, the current flows from the negative terminal of the pulse generator, down the pacing lead to the negative electrode, and into the heart. The current is then picked up by the positive electrode (ground) and flows back up the lead to the positive terminal of the pulse generator.

The bipolar lead used in transvenous pacing has two electrodes on one catheter (Fig. 20-1). The distal, or negative, electrode is at the tip of the pacing lead and is in direct contact with the heart, usually inside the right atrium or ventricle. Approximately 1 cm from the negative electrode is a positive electrode. The negative electrode is attached to the negative terminal, and the positive electrode is attached to the positive terminal of the pulse generator, either directly or by means of a bridging cable (see Fig. 20-1B).

An epicardial lead system is often used for temporary pacing after cardiac surgery. The bipolar epicardial lead system has two separate insulated wires (one negative and one positive electrode) that are loosely secured with sutures to the cardiac chamber to be paced. Both leads are in contact with the myocardial tissue, so either wire may be used as the negative, or pacing, electrode. The remaining wire is then used as the positive, or ground, electrode.

BOX 20-1	**INDICATIONS FOR TEMPORARY PACING**

- Bradydysrhythmias
  - Sinus bradycardia and arrest
  - Sick sinus syndrome
  - Heart blocks
- Tachydysrhythmias
  - Supraventricular
  - Ventricular
- Permanent pacemaker failure
- Support of cardiac output after cardiac surgery
- Diagnostic studies
  - Electrophysiology studies (EPS)
  - Atrial electrograms (AEG)

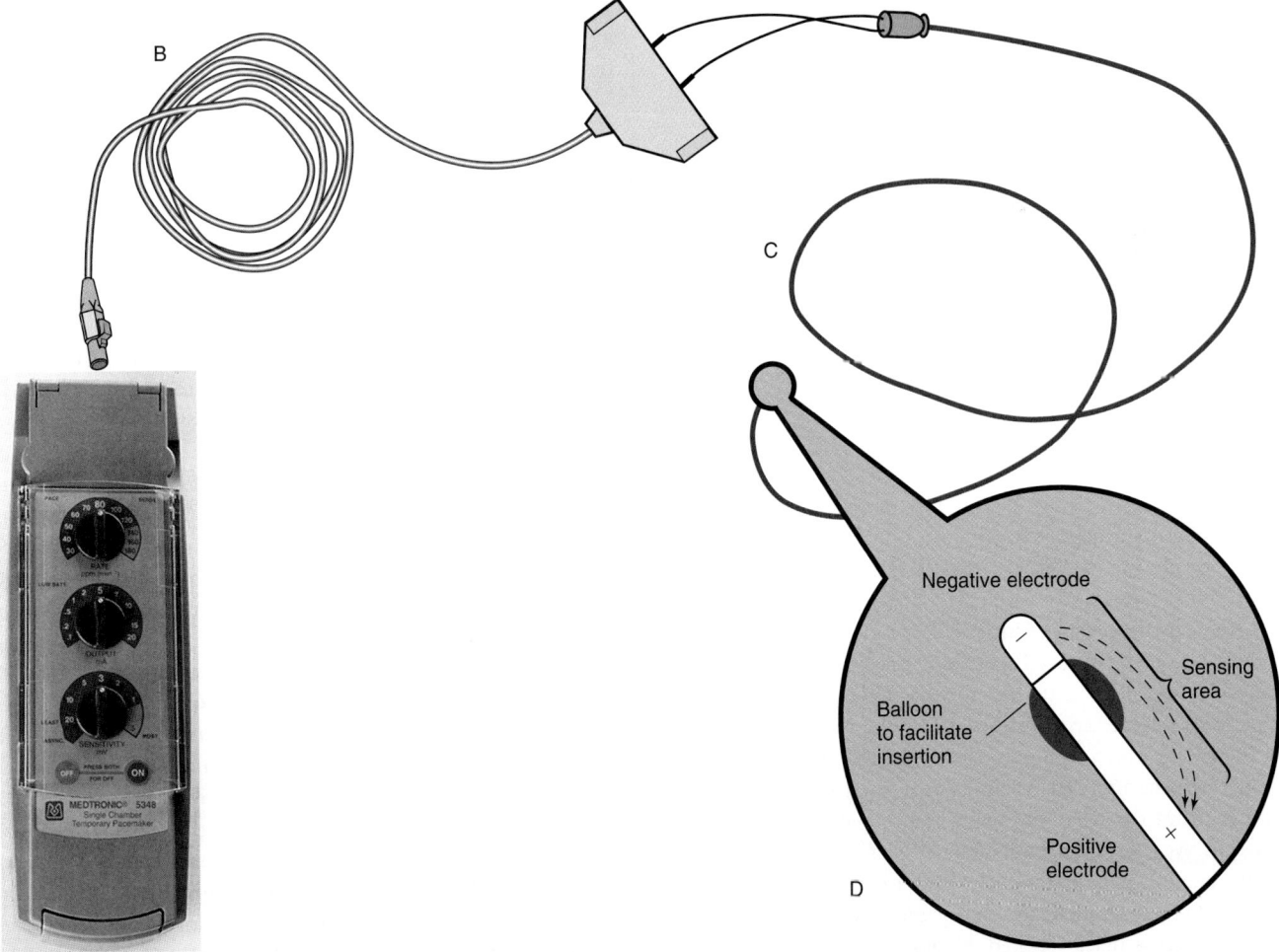

Figure 20-1 The components of a temporary bipolar transvenous catheter. *A,* Single-chamber temporary (external) pulse generator. *B,* Bridging cable. *C,* Pacing lead. *D,* Enlarged view of the pacing lead tip. (*A, Courtesy Medtronic Inc., Minneapolis, MN.*)

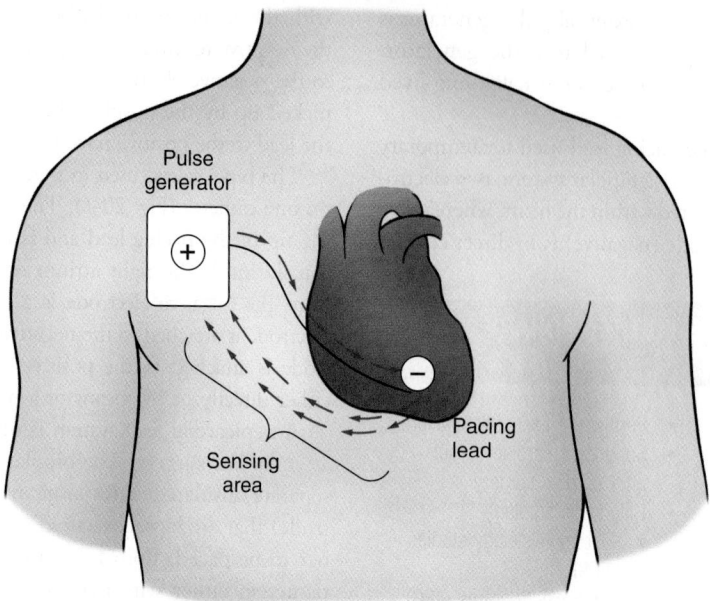

Figure 20-2 The components of a permanent unipolar transvenous pacing system.

BOX 20-2 ROUTES FOR TEMPORARY PACING

TRANSCUTANEOUS
Emergency pacing is achieved by depolarizing the heart through the chest by means of two large skin electrodes.

TRANSTHORACIC
A pacing wire is inserted emergently by threading it through a transthoracic needle into the right ventricle.

EPICARDIAL
Pacing electrodes are sewn to the epicardium during cardiac surgery.

TRANSVENOUS (ENDOCARDIAL)
The pacing electrode is advanced through a vein into the right atrium or right ventricle, or both.

A unipolar pacing system (epicardial or transvenous) has only one electrode (the negative electrode) making contact with the heart. For a permanent pacemaker, the positive electrode can be created by the metallic casing of the subcutaneously implanted pulse generator (Fig. 20-2), or as is the case with a unipolar epicardial lead system, the positive electrode can be formed by a piece of surgical steel wire sewn into the subcutaneous tissue of the chest or the metal portion of a surface ECG electrode.

Because the unipolar pacing system has a wide sensing area as a result of the relatively long distance between the negative and positive electrodes, it has better sensing capabilities than does a bipolar system. However, this feature makes the unipolar system more susceptible to sensing extraneous signals, such as the electrical artifacts created by normal muscle movements (i.e., myopotentials) or by external electromagnetic interference (EMI), which may result in inappropriate inhibition of the pacing stimulus. This problem is of more concern in permanent

pacing systems, in which the "can" of the pacemaker generator may be used as a part of the pacing circuit. Because the can is located near a large muscle mass, upper body movement can result in the inappropriate sensing of myopotentials.[5]

PACING ROUTES

Several routes are available for temporary cardiac pacing (Box 20-2). Permanent pacing usually is accomplished transvenously, although when a thoracotomy is otherwise indicated, as in cardiac surgery, the physician may elect to insert permanent epicardial pacing wires.

Transcutaneous cardiac pacing involves the use of two large skin electrodes, one placed anteriorly and the other posteriorly on the chest, connected to an external pulse generator. It is a rapid, noninvasive procedure that nurses can perform in the emergency setting and is recommended as a primary intervention in the advanced cardiac life support (ACLS) algorithm for the treatment of symptomatic bradycardia.[6] Improved technology related to stimulus delivery and the development of large electrode pads that help disperse the energy have helped reduce the pain associated with cutaneous nerve and muscle stimulation. Discomfort may still be an issue for some patients, particularly when higher energy levels are required to achieve capture. This route is typically used as a short-term therapy until the situation resolves or another route of pacing can be established.

The insertion of temporary epicardial pacing wires has become a routine procedure during most cardiac surgical cases. Ventricular and, in many cases, atrial pacing wires are loosely sewn to the epicardium. The terminal pins of these wires are pulled through the skin before the chest is closed. If both chambers have pacing wires attached, the atrial wires exit subcostally to the right of the sternum and the ventricular wires exit in the same region but to the left of the sternum. These wires can be removed several days after surgery by gentle traction at the skin surface with minimal risk of bleeding.[7]

Temporary transvenous endocardial pacing is accomplished by advancing a pacing electrode wire through a vein, often the subclavian or internal jugular vein, and into the right atrium or right ventricle (RV). Insertion can be facilitated through direct visualization with fluoroscopy or by the use of the standard ECG. In some cases, the pacing wire is inserted through a special pulmonary artery catheter by means of a port that exits in the right atrium or right ventricle.

FIVE-LETTER PACEMAKER CODES

In the 1960s, pacemaker terminology was limited to *fixed-rate* and *demand* pacing; *AV sequential* pacing was introduced in the early 1970s. Although these terms are still useful for understanding pacemaker function (Box 20-3), the continued expansion of functional capabilities of pulse generators has made it necessary to develop a more precise classification system. In 1974, the Inter-Society Commission for Heart Disease (ICHD) adopted a three-letter code for describing the various pacing modalities available. The code has since undergone several revisions, including the addition of two more letters representing programming characteristics and multisite pacing functions, to accommodate the development of newer devices that are rate responsive or that pace from more than one site within the atria and the ventricles. Table 20-1 describes the current five-letter code.[8] The original three-letter code remains adequate to describe temporary pacemaker function.

The original code is based on three categories, each represented by a letter. The first letter refers to the cardiac chamber that is paced. The second letter designates which chamber is sensed, and the third letter indicates the pacemaker's response to the sensed event. These three letters are used to describe the mode of pacing. For example, a VVI pacemaker paces the ventricle when the pacemaker fails to sense an intrinsic ventricular depolarization, but sensing of a spontaneous ventricular depolarization inhibits ventricular pacing. A VOO pacemaker paces the ventricle at a fixed rate and has no sensing capabilities. Table 20-2 provides a description of temporary pacing modes.

Physiologic pacing modes are those in which the normal physiologic, or sequential, relationship between atrial and ventricular stimulation and contraction is maintained. AV synchrony increases the volume in the ventricle before contraction and helps to improve cardiac output. This may be achieved with atrial pacing in patients who have an intact conduction system, one in which each atrial pacing stimulus depolarizes the atria and is then conducted through to the ventricles. When atrial-to-ventricular conduction is impaired (i.e., during heart block), AV synchrony may be maintained by dual-chamber pacing modes. The DDD mode is most common dual-chambered mode used.[5] In DDD pacing, atrial and ventricular leads are used for pacing and sensing. In response to sensed activity, the pacemaker inhibits the pacing stimulus; a sensed P wave in the atrium inhibits the atrial spike, and a sensed R wave in the ventricle inhibits the ventricular pacing spike. A sensed P wave may also be used to trigger a ventricular pacing stimulus if normal conduction through the AV node is impaired. Although the DDD mode is more complicated to program and interpret than earlier modes, it offers the most options for maintaining physiologic pacing.

PACEMAKER SETTINGS

The controls on all external temporary pulse generators are similar. Their functions must be thoroughly understood so that pacing can be initiated quickly in an emergency situation and troubleshooting can be facilitated if problems with the pacemaker arise.

The *rate control* (Fig. 20-3) regulates the number of impulses that can be delivered to the heart per minute. The rate setting

---

BOX 20-3 PACEMAKER TERMINOLOGY

FIXED-RATE (ASYNCHRONOUS)
Delivers a pacing stimulus at a set (fixed) rate regardless of the occurrence of spontaneous myocardial depolarization; occurs in nonsensing modes

DEMAND (SYNCHRONOUS)
Delivers a pacing stimulus only when the heart's intrinsic pacemaker fails to function at a predetermined rate; the pacing stimulus is either inhibited or triggered by the sensing of intrinsic activity

ATRIOVENTRICULAR SEQUENTIAL (DUAL-CHAMBER)
Delivers a pacing stimulus to both atrium and ventricle in physiologic sequence with sufficient atrioventricular delay to permit adequate ventricular filling

---

TABLE 20-1 NASPE/BPEG Generic Code

Position I: Chambers Paced	Position II: Chambers Sensed	Position III: Response to Sensing	Position IV: Rate Modulation	Position V: Multisite Pacing
0 = None	0 = None	0 = None	0 = None	0 = None
A = Atrium	A = Atrium	T = Triggered	R = Rate Modulation	A = Atrium
V = Ventricle	V = Ventricle	I = Inhibited		V = Ventricle
D = Dual (A + V)	D = Dual (A + V)	D = Dual (T + I)		D = Dual (A + V)

Modified from Bernstein AD et al: The Revised NASPE/BPEG generic pacemaker code for antibradycardia, adaptive-rate and multisite pacing, *PACE* 25:260-264, 2002.
BPEG, British Pacing and Electrophysiology Group; NASPE, North American Society of Pacing and Electrophysiology.

TABLE 20-2   Examples of Temporary Pacing Modes

Pacing Mode	Description
Asynchronous	
AOO	Atrial pacing, no sensing
VOO	Ventricular pacing, no sensing
DOO	Atrial and ventricular pacing, no sensing
Synchronous	
AAI	Atrial pacing, atrial sensing, inhibited response to sensed P waves
VVI	Ventricular pacing, ventricular sensing, inhibited response to sensed QRS complexes
DVI	Atrial and ventricular pacing, ventricular sensing; both atrial and ventricular pacing are inhibited if a spontaneous ventricular depolarization is sensed
Universal	
DDD	Both chambers are paced and sensed; inhibited response of the pacing stimuli to sensed events in their respective chambers; triggered response to sensed atrial activity to allow for rate-responsive ventricular pacing

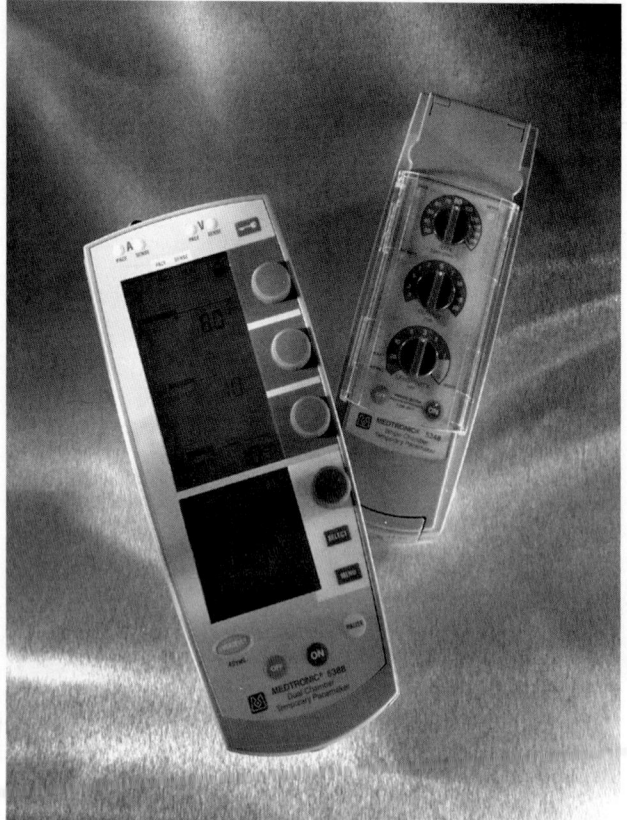

Figure 20-3 Temporary pulse generators (external). *A,* Dual-chamber pulse generator. *B,* Single-chamber pulse generator. *(Courtesy Medtronic Inc., Minneapolis, MN.)*

depends on the physiologic needs of the patient, but it usually is maintained between 60 and 80 beats/min. Pacing rates for overdrive suppression of tachydysrhythmias may greatly exceed these values. Some generators have special controls for overdrive pacing that allow for rates of up to 800 stimuli per minute. If the pacemaker is operating in a dual-chamber mode, the ventricular rate control also regulates the atrial rate.

The *output dial* regulates the amount of electrical current, measured in milliamperes (mA), that is delivered to the heart to initiate depolarization. The point at which depolarization occurs, called *threshold*, is indicated by a myocardial response to the pacing stimulus (i.e., capture). Threshold can be determined by gradually decreasing the output setting until 1:1 capture is lost. The output setting is then slowly increased until 1:1 capture is reestablished; this threshold to pace is less than 1 mA with a properly positioned pacing electrode. The output is set two to three times higher than threshold, because thresholds tend to fluctuate over time. Box 20-4 details the procedure for measuring pacing thresholds. Separate output controls for atrium and ventricle are used with a dual-chamber pulse generator.

The *sensitivity control* regulates the ability of the pacemaker to detect the heart's intrinsic electrical activity. Sensitivity is measured in millivolts (mV) and determines the size of the intracardiac signal that the generator will recognize. If the sensitivity is adjusted to its most sensitive setting—a setting of 0.5 to 1.0 mV—the pacemaker can respond even to low-amplitude electrical signals coming from the heart. Turning the sensitivity to its least sensitive setting (i.e., adjusting the dial to a setting of 20 mV or to the area labeled *async*) results in inability of the pacemaker to sense any intrinsic electrical activity and causes the pacemaker to function at a fixed rate. A sense indicator (often a light) on the pulse generator signals each time intrinsic cardiac electrical activity is sensed. A pulse generator may be designed to sense atrial activity or ventricular activity, or both. Box 20-5 describes the procedure for measuring sensitivity. The sensitivity is set at half of the value of the sensitivity threshold to ensure that all appropriate intrinsic cardiac signals are sensed. For example, if the measured sensitivity threshold is 3 mV, the generator is set at 1.5 mV. The pacemaker's sensing ability can be quickly evaluated by observing for a change in pacing rhythm in response to spontaneous depolarizations.

The *AV interval control* (available only on dual-chamber generators) regulates the time interval between the atrial and ventricular pacing stimuli. This interval is analogous to the PR interval that occurs in the intrinsic ECG. Proper adjustment of this interval to between 150 and 250 milliseconds (msec) preserves AV synchrony and permits maximal ventricular stroke volume and enhanced cardiac output.

Temporary DDD pacemakers have several other digital controls that are unique to this newer type of temporary pulse generator (see Fig. 20-3B). The *lower rate,* or *base rate,* determines the rate at which the generator will pace when intrinsic activity falls below the set rate of the pacemaker. The *upper rate* determines the fastest ventricular rate the pacemaker will deliver in response to sensed atrial activity. This setting is needed to protect the patient's heart from being paced in response to rapid atrial dysrhythmias. The *pulse width,* which can be adjusted

---

BOX 20-4	DETERMINING THE TEMPORARY PACEMAKER PACING THRESHOLD

1. Adjust the pacemaker rate setting so that patient is 100% paced. It may be necessary to increase the pacing rate to achieve this setting.
2. Gradually decrease the output (milliampere, mA) setting until 1:1 capture is lost. The pacing threshold is the point at which capture is lost.
3. Slowly increase the output setting until 1:1 capture is reestablished. With a properly positioned pacing electrode, the pacing threshold should be less than 1.0 mA.
4. Set the output setting two to three times higher than measured threshold, because thresholds tend to fluctuate over time.
5. If a dual-chamber pulse generator is being used, evaluate pacing thresholds for the atrial and ventricular leads separately.

BOX 20-5	DETERMINING THE TEMPORARY PACEMAKER SENSITIVITY THRESHOLD

- Set the sensitivity control to its most sensitive setting.
- Adjust the pulse generator rate to 10 beats/min less than the patient's intrinsic rate (the flash indicator should flash regularly).
- Reduce the generator output to the minimal value to eliminate the risk of competing with the intrinsic rhythm.
- Gradually increase the sensitivity value until the sense indicator stops flashing and the pace indicator starts flashing.
- Decrease sensitivity until the sense indicator begins to flash again; this is the sensitivity threshold.
- Adjust the sensitivity setting on the generator to half of the threshold value; restore the generator output and rate to their original values.

---

from 0.05 to 2 msec, controls the length of time that the pacing stimulus is delivered to the heart. There also is an *atrial refractory period,* programmable from 150 to 500 msec, which regulates the length of time, after a sensed or paced ventricular event, during which the pacemaker cannot respond to another atrial stimulus. An emergency button is also available on most models to allow for rapid initiation of asynchronous (DOO) pacing during an emergency.

On all temporary pacemakers, an on/off switch is provided with a safety feature that prevents the accidental termination of pacing. On new generators, there is also a locking feature to prevent unintended changes to the prescribed settings.

PACING ARTIFACTS

All patients with temporary pacemakers require continuous ECG monitoring. The pacing artifact is the spike that is seen on the ECG tracing as the pacing stimulus is delivered to the heart. A *P wave* is visible after the pacing artifact if the atrium is being paced (Fig. 20-4A). Similarly, a *QRS complex* follows a ventricular pacing artifact (see Fig. 20-4B). With dual-chamber pacing, a pacing artifact precedes both the P wave and the QRS complex (see Fig. 20-4C).

Not all paced beats look alike. For example, the artifact (spike) produced by a unipolar pacing electrode is larger than that produced by a bipolar lead (Fig. 20-5). The QRS complex of paced beats appears different, depending on the location of the pacing electrode. If the pacing electrode is positioned in the RV, a left bundle branch block (LBBB) pattern is displayed on the ECG. A right bundle branch block (RBBB) pattern is visible if the pacing stimulus originates from the left ventricle (LV).

PACEMAKER MALFUNCTIONS

Most pacemaker malfunctions can be categorized as abnormalities of pacing or of sensing. Problems with pacing can involve failure of the pacemaker to deliver the pacing stimulus, a pacing stimulus that fails to depolarize the heart, or an incorrect number of pacing stimuli per minute.

Pacing Abnormalities. Failure of the pacemaker to deliver the pacing stimulus results in disappearance of the pacing artifact, even if the patient's intrinsic rate is less than the set rate on the pacer (Fig. 20-6). This can occur intermittently or continuously and can be attributed to failure of the pulse generator or its battery, a loose connection between the various components of the pacemaker system, broken lead wires, or stimulus inhibition as a result of EMI. Tightening connections, replacing the batteries or the pulse generator itself, or removing the source of EMI may restore pacemaker function.

If the pacing stimulus fires but fails to initiate a myocardial depolarization, a pacing artifact will be present but will not be followed by the expected P wave or QRS complex, depending on the chamber being paced (Fig. 20-7). This *loss of capture* most often can be attributed to displacement of the pacing electrode or to an increase in threshold (electrical stimulus necessary to elicit a myocardial depolarization) as a result of drugs, metabolic disorders, electrolyte imbalances, or fibrosis or myocardial ischemia at the site of electrode placement. In many cases, increasing the output (mA) elicits capture. For transvenous leads, repositioning the patient onto the left side may improve lead contact and restore capture.

Pacing can occur at inappropriate rates. For example, impending battery failure in a permanent pacemaker can result in a gradual decrease in the paced rate, also referred to as *rate drift.* Inappropriate stimuli from a pacemaker may result in a pacemaker-mediated tachycardia. This usually is caused by sensing of inappropriate signals in a dual-chamber pacemaker that is in a trigger mode, such as DDD. The tachycardia can be terminated by placing a magnet over the generator to transiently suspend sensing.[1]

Sensing Abnormalities. Sensing abnormalities include both undersensing and oversensing.

Undersensing. *Undersensing* is the inability of the pacemaker to sense spontaneous myocardial depolarizations. Undersensing results in competition between paced complexes and the heart's intrinsic rhythm. This malfunction is manifested on the ECG by pacing artifacts that occur after or are unrelated to spontaneous complexes (Fig. 20-8). Undersensing can result

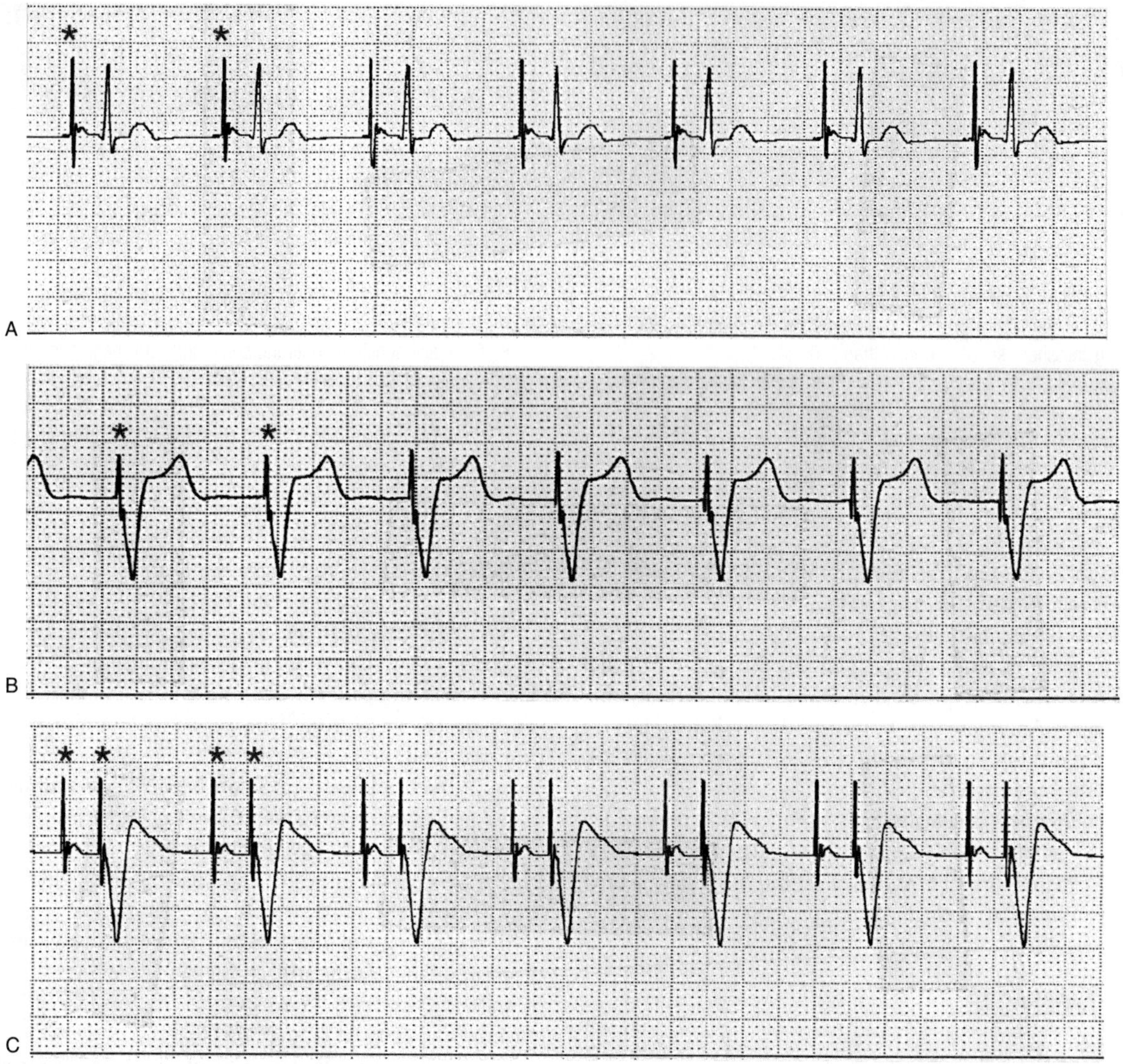

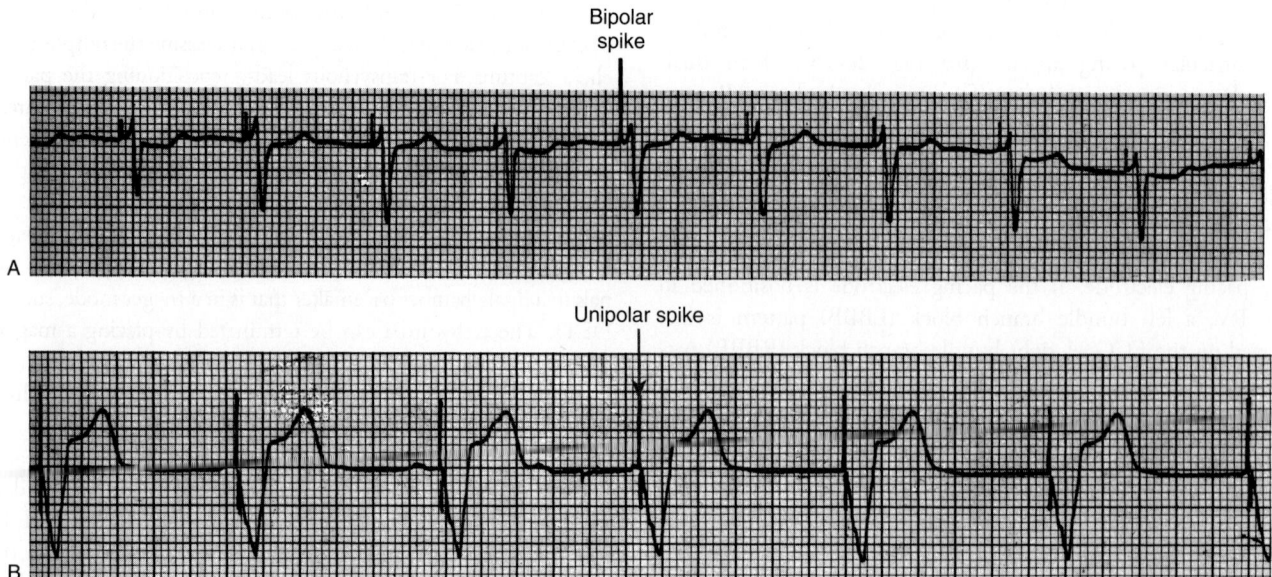

Figure 20-4 Pacing examples. *A,* Atrial pacing. *B,* Ventricular pacing. *C,* Dual-chamber pacing. Each *asterisk* represents a pacemaker impulse.

Figure 20-5 Bipolar and unipolar pacing. *A,* Bipolar pacing artifact. *B,* Unipolar pacing artifact. *(Modified from Conover MB:* Understanding electrocardiography, *ed 8, St Louis, 2003, Mosby.)*

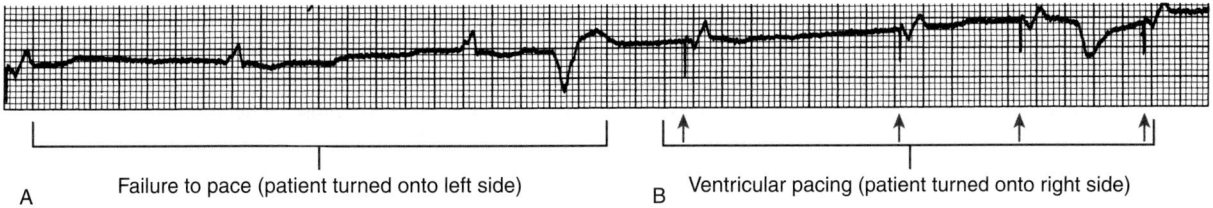

A   Failure to pace (patient turned onto left side)   B   Ventricular pacing (patient turned onto right side)

Figure 20-6 Pacemaker malfunction: failure to pace. *A,* Patient with a transvenous pacemaker is turned onto the left side. Immediately, there is a failure to pace (i.e., loss of pacer artifacts on the electrocardiogram). The patient's heart rate is extremely low without pacemaker support. *B,* The nurse turns the patient onto the right side, the transvenous electrode floats into contact with the right ventricular wall, and pacing is resumed. *(From Kesten KS, Norton CK: Pacemakers: patient care, troubleshooting, rhythm analysis, Baltimore, 1985, Resource Applications.)*

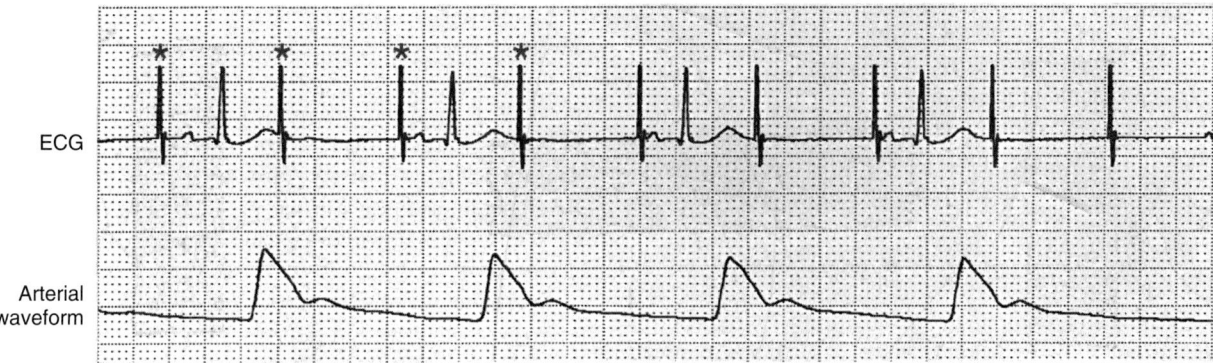

ECG

Arterial
waveform

Figure 20-7 Pacemaker malfunction: failure to capture. Atrial pacing and capture occur after pacer spikes 1, 3, 5, and 7. The remaining pacer spikes fail to capture the tissue, resulting in loss of the P wave, no conduction to the ventricles, and no arterial waveform. Each *asterisk* represents a pacemaker impulse.

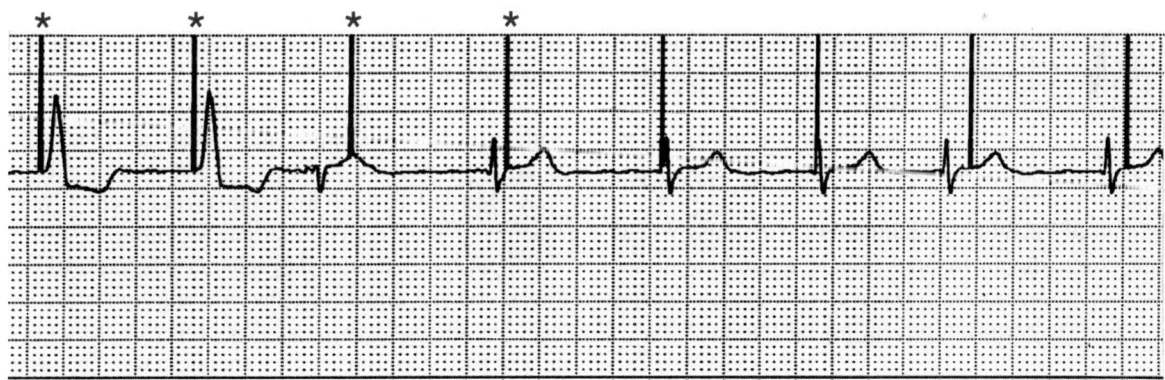

Figure 20-8 Pacemaker malfunction: undersensing. After the first two paced beats, a series of intrinsic beats occur; the pacemaker unit fails to sense these intrinsic QRS complexes. These spikes do not capture the ventricle because they occur during the refractory period of the cardiac cycle. Each *asterisk* represents a pacemaker impulse.

in the delivery of pacing stimuli into a relative refractory period of the cardiac depolarization cycle (see Fig. 18-13 in Chapter 18). A ventricular pacing stimulus delivered into the downslope of the T wave (R-on-T phenomenon) is a real danger with this type of pacer aberration, because it may precipitate a lethal dysrhythmia. The nurse must act quickly to determine the cause and initiate appropriate interventions. Often, the cause can be attributed to inadequate wave amplitude (height of the P or R wave). If this is the case, the situation can be promptly remedied by increasing the sensitivity by moving the sensitivity dial toward its lowest

setting. Other possible causes include inappropriate (asynchronous) mode selection, lead displacement or fracture, loose cable connections, and pulse generator failure.

Oversensing. Oversensing occurs as a result of inappropriate sensing of extraneous electrical signals that leads to unnecessary triggering or inhibition of stimulus output, depending on the pacer mode. The source of these electrical signals can range from tall peaked T waves to EMI in the critical care environment. Because most temporary pulse generators are programmed in demand modes, oversensing results in unexplained pauses in the ECG tracing as the extraneous signals are sensed and inhibit pacing. Often, moving the sensitivity dial toward 20 mV (less sensitive) stops the pauses. With permanent pacemakers, a magnet may be placed over the generator to restore pacing in an asynchronous mode until appropriate changes in the generator settings can be programmed.

MEDICAL MANAGEMENT

The physician determines the pacing route based on the patient's clinical situation. Transcutaneous pacing typically is used in emergent situations until a transvenous lead can be secured. If the patient is undergoing heart surgery, epicardial leads may be electively placed at the end of the operation. The physician places the transvenous or epicardial pacing lead or leads, repositioning them as needed to obtain adequate pacing and sensing thresholds. Decisions regarding lead placement may later limit the pacing modes available to the clinician. For example, to perform dual-chamber pacing, both atrial and ventricular leads must be placed. In an emergency, however, interventions are focused on establishing ventricular pacing, and atrial lead placement may not be feasible. After lead placement, the initial settings for output and sensitivity are determined, the pacing rate and mode are selected, and the patient's response to pacing is evaluated.

NURSING MANAGEMENT

Nursing responsibilities in the care of a patient with a temporary pacemaker are associated with several nursing diagnoses (see the Nursing Diagnoses feature on Temporary Pacemaker) and can be combined into four primary areas: assessment and prevention of pacemaker malfunction, protection against microshock, surveillance for complications such as infection, and patient education.

Prevention of Pacemaker Malfunction. Continuous ECG monitoring is essential to facilitate prompt recognition of and appropriate intervention for pacemaker malfunction. Proper care of the pacing system can prevent pacing abnormalities.

Nursing Diagnoses

Temporary Pacemaker

- Decreased Cardiac Output related to alterations in heart rate
- Ineffective Cardiopulmonary Tissue Perfusion related to acute myocardial ischemia
- Risk for Infection related to invasive monitoring devices
- Anxiety related to threat to biologic, psychological, or social integrity
- Disturbed Body Image related to functional dependence on life-sustaining technology
- Deficient Knowledge: Discharge Regimen related to lack of previous exposure to information (see the Patient Education feature on Temporary Pacemaker)

The temporary pacing lead and bridging cable must be properly secured to the body with tape to prevent accidental displacement of the electrode, which can result in failure to pace or sense. The external pulse generator can be secured to the patient's waist with a strap or placed in a telemetry bag for the mobile patient. If the patient is on a regimen of bed rest, the pulse generator can be suspended with twill tape from an IV pole mounted overhead on the ceiling. This prevents tension on the lead while the patient is moved (given adequate length of bridging cable) and alleviates the possibility of accidental dropping of the pulse generator.

The nurse inspects for loose connections between the leads and pulse generator on a regular basis. Replacement batteries and pulse generators must always be available on the unit. Although the battery has an anticipated life span of 1 month, it probably is sound practice to change the battery if the pacemaker has been operating continually for several days. Newer generators provide a low-battery signal 24 hours before complete loss of battery function occurs to prevent inadvertent interruptions in pacing. The pulse generator must always be labeled with the date on which the battery was replaced.

Microshock Protection. It is important to be aware of all sources of EMI within the critical care environment that may interfere with the pacemaker's function. Sources of EMI in the clinical area include electrocautery, defibrillation current, radiation therapy, magnetic resonance imaging devices, and transcutaneous electrical nerve stimulation (TENS) units.[9] In most cases, if EMI is suspected of precipitating pacemaker malfunction, conversion to the asynchronous mode (fixed rate) can maintain pacing until the cause of the EMI is removed.

Because the pacing electrode provides a direct, low-resistance path to the heart, the nurse takes special care while handling the external components of the pacing system, to avoid conducting stray electrical current from other equipment. Even a small amount of stray current transmitted through the pacing lead could precipitate a lethal dysrhythmia. The possibility of microshock can be minimized by wearing rubber gloves when handling the pacing wires and by proper insulation of terminal pins of pacing wires when they are not in use. The latter precaution can be accomplished by the use of caps provided by the manufacturer or by improvising with a plastic syringe or section of disposable rubber glove. The wires are taped securely to the patient's chest to prevent accidental electrode displacement. Additional safety measures include using a nonelectric or a properly grounded electric bed, keeping all electrical equipment away from the bed, and permitting the use of only rechargeable electric razors.

Infection Risk. Infection at the lead insertion site is a rare but serious complication associated with temporary pacemakers. The site is carefully inspected for purulent drainage, erythema, and edema, and the patient is observed for signs of systemic infection. Site care is performed according to the institution's policies and procedures. Although most infections remain localized, endocarditis can occur in patients with endocardial pacing leads. A less common complication associated with transvenous pacing is myocardial perforation, which can result in rhythmic hiccoughs or cardiac tamponade.

PATIENT EDUCATION

Patient teaching for the person with a temporary pacemaker emphasizes the prevention of complications (see the Patient Education feature on Temporary Pacemaker). The patient is instructed not to handle any exposed portion of the lead wire and to notify the nurse if the dressing over the insertion site becomes soiled, wet, or dislodged. The patient also is advised not to use any electrical devices brought in from home that could interfere with pacemaker functioning. Patients with temporary transvenous pacemakers need to be taught to restrict movement of the affected extremity to prevent lead displacement.

PERMANENT PACEMAKERS

More than 180,000 permanent pacemakers are implanted annually in the United States, and critical care nurses are likely to encounter these devices in their clinical practice.[10] These pacemakers were originally designed to provide an adequate ventricular rate in patients with symptomatic bradycardia. Today, the goal of pacemaker therapy is to simulate, as much as possible, normal physiologic cardiac depolarization and conduction. Sophisticated generators permit rate-responsive pacing, effecting responses to sensed atrial activity (DDD) or to a variety of physiologic sensors (body motion, QT interval, minute ventilation). For patients who do not have a functional sinus node that can increase their heart rate, rate-responsive pacemakers have been shown to improve exercise capacity and quality of life.[11] Table 20-3 describes the types of rate-responsive pacing generators in clinical use. The concept of physiologic pacing continues to evolve, because studies have indicated that pacing initiated from the RV apex—even in a dual-chamber mode—may promote heart failure in patients with permanent pacemakers.[1] This has prompted further research to identify alternative sites for pacing and modes that can maximize intrinsic AV conduction and minimize ventricular pacing.[11]

The patient who has undergone implantation of a permanent pacemaker has an anticipated length of hospital stay of 1 to 5 days. The longer length of stay is for patients with serious complications such as MI or shock.

Patient Education: Temporary Pacemaker

- Description of pacemaker therapy
- Care of the pacemaker system
  Minimize handling of leads or cables
  Notify nurse if dressing becomes wet or loose
- Activity restrictions (minimize upper-extremity movement with transvenous leads)
- Electrical safety precautions (no electric razors)
- Symptoms to report (dizziness)

Technologic advances in the computer industry have had a major impact on today's permanent pacemakers. Microprocessors have allowed for the development of increasingly smaller generators despite the incorporation of more complex features. Today's generators are smaller, more energy-efficient, and more reliable than previous models. An example of a modern pacemaker is shown in Fig. 20-9. A new trend in permanent pacemakers has been the use of these devices as a type of nonpharmacologic therapy for treatment of conditions such as heart failure and atrial fibrillation.

Cardiac Resynchronization Therapy. About one third of patients with severe heart failure have ventricular conduction delays (prolonged QRS duration or bundle branch block). These conduction delays have been shown to create a lack of synchrony

---

TABLE 20-3 **Permanent Pacemaker Rate-Response Pacing Modes**

Pulse Generator	Description
AAIR	AAI features plus rate-responsive pacing; used for patients with a symptomatic bradycardia who have a paceable atrium and intact atrioventricular conduction
VVIR	VVI features plus rate-responsive pacing; used for patients with an atrium that is unpaceable as a result of chronic atrial fibrillation or other atrial dysrhythmia
DDDR	DDD features plus rate-responsive pacing; used for patients with a symptomatic bradycardia in which the atrium is paceable but atrioventricular conduction is, or may become, unreliable

---

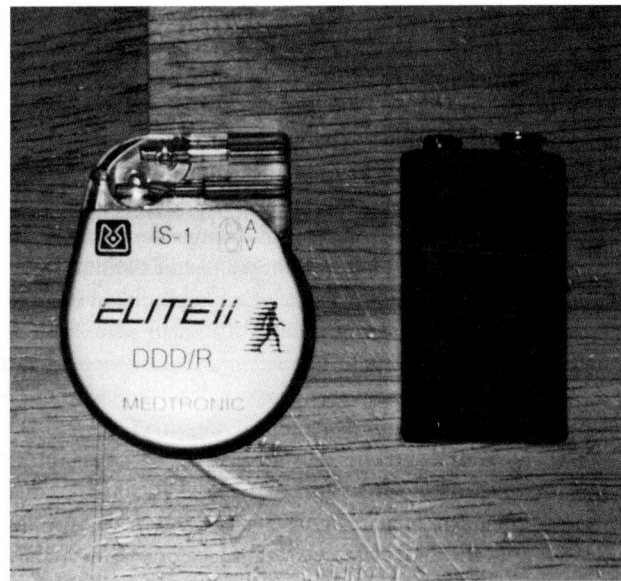

Figure 20-9 A permanent pacemaker (Medtronic Elite II) is placed next to a 9-volt battery for comparison of size. This dual-chamber generator is 7.5 mm thick and weighs only 26 g.

between the contractions of the LV and RV. The hemodynamic consequences of this dyssynchrony include impaired ventricular filling with decreased ejection fraction, cardiac output, and mean arterial pressure.[12] Cardiac resynchronization therapy (CRT) uses atrial pacing plus stimulation of both the LV and RV (biventricular pacing), in an attempt to optimize atrial and ventricular mechanical activity. The CRT device uses three pacing leads, one each in the right atrium and the RV and a specially designed transvenous lead that is inserted through the coronary sinus to pace the LV.[12] Because many patients with heart failure are also at risk for sudden cardiac death, biventricular pacing is available on some implantable cardioverter defibrillators (ICDs). A number of clinical trials have shown symptomatic and structural cardiac improvement with this new therapy.[13]

Atrial Arrhythmia Suppression. There is a growing incidence of atrial fibrillation, and atrial pacing has been proposed as a possible preventative therapy for this dysrhythmia in selected patients. Atrial pacing in patients with bradycardia has been shown to lower the recurrence of atrial fibrillation, especially compared with ventricular pacing.[14] Most pacemakers can be programmed to *mode switch* to a non–P wave tracking mode if rapid atrial rates are sensed.[1] Strategies for patients with paroxysmal atrial fibrillation, which include pacing both atriums (bi-atrial pacing) and transiently pacing the atrium at a rate higher than the patient's intrinsic sinus rate, require further study.[15]

Medical Management. Permanent pacemakers may be implanted with the patient under local anesthesia in the operating room or in the cardiac catheterization laboratory. Transvenous leads usually are inserted through the cephalic or subclavian vein and positioned in the right atrium or RV, or both, with fluoroscopic guidance. Satisfactory lead placement is determined by testing the stimulation and sensitivity thresholds with a pacing system analyzer. The leads are then attached to the generator, which is inserted into a surgically created pocket in the subcutaneous tissue below the clavicle.

Nursing Management. Nursing management for patients after permanent pacemaker implantation includes monitoring for complications related to insertion and for pacemaker malfunction. Postoperative complications are rare but include cardiac perforation and tamponade, pneumothorax, hematoma, lead displacement, and infection.[16]

Identification of permanent pacemaker malfunction is the same as that described previously for temporary pacemakers. To evaluate pacemaker function, the nurse must know at least the pacemaker's programmed mode of pacing and the lower rate setting. With permanent pacemakers, settings are adjusted noninvasively through a specialized programmer that uses pulsed magnetic fields or an RF signal. If a pacemaker problem is suspected, ECG strips are obtained, and the physician is notified so that the pacemaker settings can be reprogrammed as needed. If the patient experiences symptoms of decreased cardiac output, he or she may require support with temporary transcutaneous pacing until the problem is corrected.

Critical care nurses also may be involved in monitoring patients with permanent pacemakers after discharge. Some units are equipped with transtelephonic monitoring equipment that allows patients to transmit information over the telephone from a monitoring device in their home. Transmission of the patient's ECG can provide information to confirm proper pacemaker function (capture and sensing) and to determine battery status (rate). Newer technology that uses an Internet-based remote monitoring system for pacemaker follow-up may soon replace standard transtelephonic ECG evaluation.[17]

The foregoing discussion provides an introduction to the basic concepts of pacemaker therapy. However, the nurse who cares for patients with permanent or temporary pacemakers must be familiar with even the most sophisticated modes of pacemaker function. Only by keeping pace with current technology can the nurse accurately interpret pacer function and thereby safely and effectively care for patients with pacemakers.

IMPLANTABLE CARDIOVERTER DEFIBRILLATORS

An implantable cardioverter defibrillator (ICD) is an electronic device that is used in the treatment of tachydysrhythmias. The ICD is capable of identifying and terminating life-threatening ventricular dysrhythmias. Initially, an ICD was recommended only for patients who had survived an episode of cardiac arrest caused by ventricular fibrillation (VF) or ventricular tachycardia (VT). Later, a number of clinical trials compared ICD therapy for such secondary prevention of sudden cardiac death with antidysrhythmic drug therapy and found improved survival with the ICD.[1] As a result, ICD use was expanded to include primary prevention of sudden cardiac death in patients with coronary artery disease (CAD), previous MI, or LV dysfunction in whom VT or VF was inducible during EPS. Trials have shown improved survival with ICD implantation in high-risk patients (i.e., those with previous MI and an ejection fraction <35%) even without evidence of VT or VF on an EPS.[13] These results have further increased the number of patients who receive an ICD.

THE ICD SYSTEM

The ICD system contains (1) sensing electrodes to recognize the dysrhythmia and (2) defibrillation electrodes or patches that are in contact with the heart and can deliver a shock. These electrodes are connected to a generator that is surgically placed in the subcutaneous tissue of the upper left abdominal quadrant or the pectoral region (Fig. 20-10). The early-model generators could defibrillate or cardiovert only lethal dysrhythmias. The current generation of devices delivers a tiered therapy, with options for programmable antitachycardia pacing, bradycardia backup pacing, low-energy cardioversion, and high-energy defibrillation. With tiered therapy, antitachycardia pacing is used as the first line of treatment in some cases of VT. If the VT can be pace-terminated successfully, the patient will not receive a shock from the generator and may not even realize that the ICD terminated the dysrhythmia. If programmed bursts of pacing do not terminate the VT, the ICD will cardiovert the rhythm. If the dysrhythmia deteriorates into VF, the ICD is programmed to defibrillate at a higher energy. If the dysrhythmia terminates spontaneously, the device will not discharge. Occasionally, the

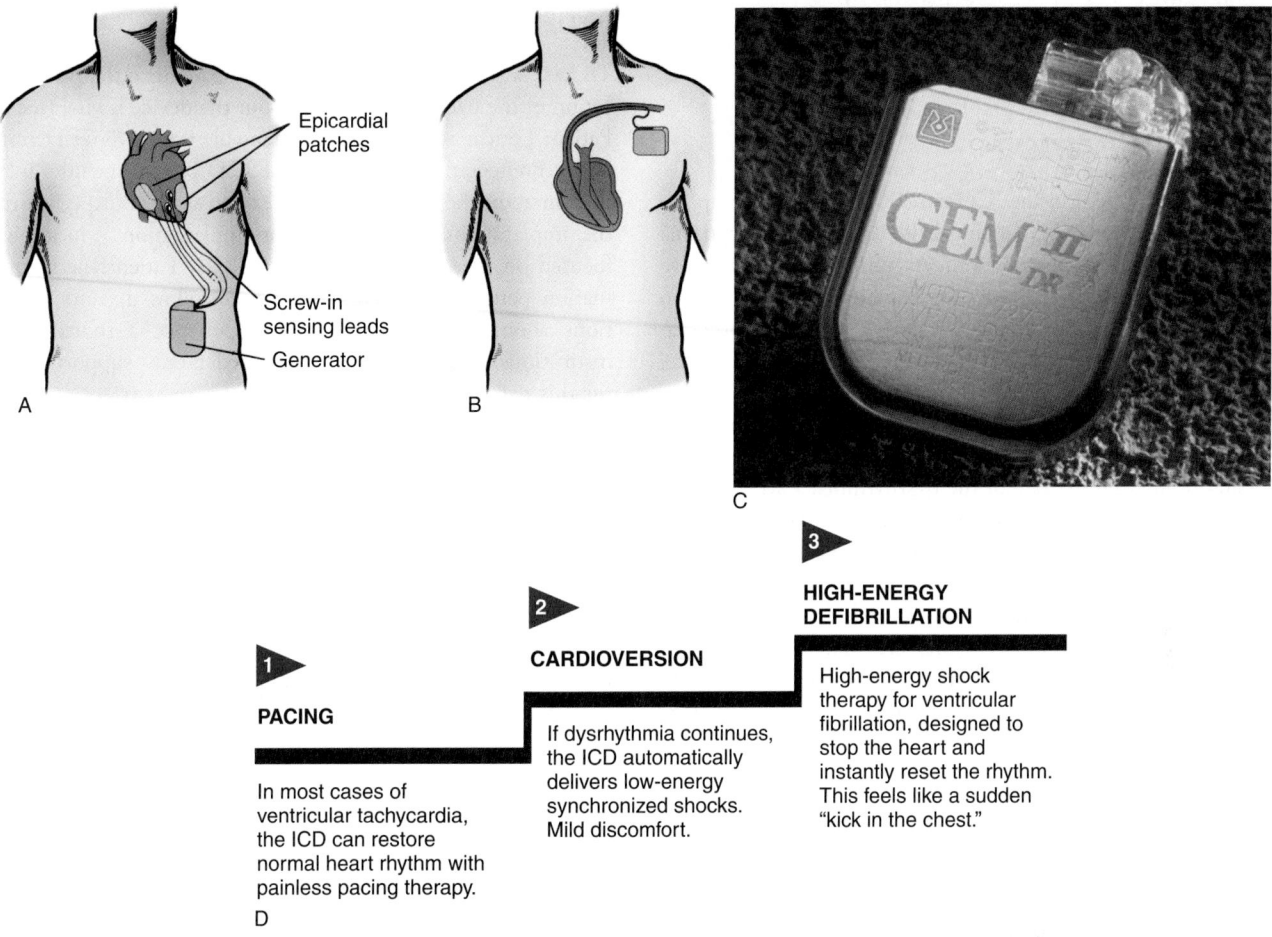

Figure 20-10 *A,* Placement of an implantable cardioverter defibrillator (ICD) and epicardial lead system. The generator is placed in a subcutaneous "pocket" in the left upper abdominal quadrant. The epicardial screw-in sensing leads monitor the heart rhythm and connect to the generator. If a life-threatening dysrhythmia is sensed, the generator can pace-terminate the dysrhythmia or deliver electrical cardioversion or defibrillation through the epicardial patches. With this system, the leads and patches must be placed during an open chest procedure (sternal surgery or thoracotomy). *B,* In the transvenous lead system, open chest surgery is not required. The pacing, cardioversion, and defibrillation functions are all contained in a lead (or leads) inserted into the right atrium and ventricle. New generators are small enough to place in the pectoral region. *C,* An example of a dual-chamber ICD (Medtronic Gem II DR) with tiered therapy and pacing capabilities. *D,* Tiered therapy is designed to use increasing levels of intensity to terminate ventricular dysrhythmias. *(Courtesy Medtronic Inc., Minneapolis, MN.)*

electrical rhythm may deteriorate to asystole or a slow idioventricular rhythm; in such cases, the bradycardia backup pacing function is activated.

Product development for ICDs has resulted in dual-chamber devices with leads in both atria and ventricles. The introduction of atrial leads allows for dual-chamber pacing to optimize hemodynamic performance and atrial sensing to more accurately discriminate between atrial and ventricular tachycardias and to decrease the incidence of inappropriate shocks. Implantable defibrillators with atrial capabilities may also be used to deliver therapies such as cardioversion or antitachycardia pacing to patients with atrial tachydysrhythmias, but their use may be limited because of the painful nature of the shocks.[18] ICDs may also incorporate triple-lead systems (leads in one atrium and both ventricles) to allow for CRT and defibrillation in one device. Other developments in ICD technology include improved diagnostic and telemetry functions, such as the ability to provide real-time electrograms obtained from the ICD electrodes or the ability to perform remote device interrogation by telephone or Internet.[19]

INSERTION OF ICD

The ICD has progressed in both programmable functions and insertion design. Initially, all ICDs were implanted surgically during open heart surgery, with electrode patches sewn directly onto the epicardium, or by means of a thoracotomy incision, with the electrode patches attached to the outside of the pericardium. Today's smaller generators, combined with the use of transvenous leads, obviate the need for major surgery. Transvenous electrode leads are inserted into the subclavian vein and advanced into the right side of the heart, where contact with the endocardium is achieved. To improve defibrillation efficacy, an additional subcutaneous patch may be placed with some models. The endocardial leads are used for sensing, pacing, cardioversion, and defibrillation. They are connected to the generator by tunneling through the subcutaneous tissue, and thoracotomy is avoided. The endocardial lead system offers several advantages: it is less invasive, requires shorter hospitalization, and is associated with significantly lower implantation mortality. Technical advances and the development of smaller ICDs have made it feasible to implant these devices in the pectoral position, similar to permanent pacemakers.

MEDICAL MANAGEMENT

Medical management in the ICD patient begins before implantation with a thorough evaluation of the patient's dysrhythmia and underlying cardiac function. A number of noninvasive studies are available to help identify patients at risk for sudden cardiac death, including signal-averaged ECG, echocardiography, baroreceptor sensitivity testing, and heart rate variability studies. Typically, patients identified as being at risk for sudden cardiac death undergo an EPS to determine the origin of the dysrhythmia and the effect of antidysrhythmic agents in suppressing or altering the rate of the dysrhythmia. Further assessment of cardiac status is made to determine whether additional interventions (e.g., cardiac surgery, angioplasty) are indicated to improve cardiac function. This part of the workup may include cardiac catheterization, stress testing, and echocardiography. Based on the evaluation, decisions are made regarding the implantation approach (e.g., thoracotomy at the time of surgery, nonthoracotomy) and the type of therapy required (e.g., antitachycardia pacing, cardioversion, defibrillation).

An electrophysiologist performs the initial programming of the device at the time of implantation. During implantation, defibrillation threshold measurements are obtained. This involves inducing the dysrhythmia and then evaluating the device's ability to terminate it. After it has been determined that the ICD functions appropriately, further follow-up is conducted on an outpatient basis to monitor the number of discharges and the battery life of the device.

NURSING MANAGEMENT

If the ICD system was implanted during open heart surgery, the postoperative nursing management is similar to that for any patient undergoing cardiac surgery. If an endocardial lead system is implanted, the nursing management is less intense and the hospital stay is shorter. The nursing diagnoses and management of the patient with an ICD are listed in the Nursing Diagnoses feature on Implantable Cardioverter Defibrillator. In the case of a ventricular dysrhythmia, it is important to know the type of ICD implanted, how the device functions, and whether it is activated (i.e., on). If the patient experiences a shockable rhythm, the nurse should be prepared to defibrillate in the event that the device fails. During external defibrillation, the paddles or patches should not be placed directly over the ICD generator. Standard paddle placement may need to be altered in patients with ICDs to achieve successful defibrillation.[6] Most patients continue to take some antidysrhythmic medications to decrease the number of shocks required and to slow the rate of the tachycardia. Complications associated with the permanent ICD include infection from the implanted system, broken leads, and sensing of supraventricular tachydysrhythmias resulting in unneeded discharges.

PATIENT EDUCATION

To facilitate a positive psychologic adjustment to the ICD, education of the patient and family about the device is vital (see the Patient Education feature on Implantable Cardioverter Defibrillator). Preoperative teaching for the ICD patient includes information about how the device works and what to expect during the implantation procedure. After implantation, education is focused on aspects of living with an ICD. Patients need information pertaining to scheduled device follow-up and instructions about what to do if they experience a shock. Many institutions also have successfully used family support groups for this patient population.

FIBRINOLYTIC THERAPY

Fibrinolytic therapy is an important clinical intervention for the patient experiencing acute ST-elevation myocardial infarction (STEMI). Before the introduction of fibrinolytic agents, medical management of acute MI was focused on decreasing myocardial oxygen demands to minimize myocardial necrosis and preserve ventricular function. Today, efforts to limit the size of the infarction are directed toward timely reperfusion of the

---

Nursing Diagnoses

Implantable Cardioverter Defibrillator

- Decreased Cardiac Output related to alterations in heart rate
- Ineffective Cardiopulmonary Tissue Perfusion related to acute myocardial ischemia
- Activity Intolerance related to cardiopulmonary dysfunction
- Acute Pain related to transmission and perception of cutaneous, visceral, muscular, or ischemic impulses
- Disturbed Body Image related to change in body structure, function, or appearance
- Compromised Family Coping related to critically ill family member
- Deficient Knowledge: Discharge Regimen related to lack of previous exposure to information (see the Patient Education feature on Implantable Cardioverter Defibrillator)

Patient Education: Implantable Cardioverter Defibrillator

- Pathophysiology of the underlying disease process, including sudden cardiac death and ventricular dysrhythmias
- Information regarding how the implantable cardioverter defibrillator is programmed to function
- Actions to take if a shock occurs
- Importance of continuing antidysrhythmic medications
- Activity limitations related to driving and avoiding strong magnetic fields
- Signs and symptoms of device failure
- Follow-up schedule with health care professional
- Cardiopulmonary resuscitation (CPR) training for family members

jeopardized myocardium through restoration of blood flow in the culprit vessel (the open artery theory). Two options are available for opening the artery—fibrinolytics and mechanical intervention. Although mechanical catheter-based intervention has been proven to be yield better outcomes when performed in a timely fashion, only 25% of U.S. hospitals are estimated to have this capability.[20] For this reason, fibrinolytic therapy continues to play a major role in the treatment of acute MI.

The use of fibrinolytic therapy is predicated on the theory that the significant event in acute coronary syndromes (e.g., unstable angina, acute MI) is the rupture of an atherosclerotic plaque with thrombus formation (Fig. 20-11). The thrombus, which is composed of aggregated platelets bound together with fibrin strands, occludes the coronary artery, depriving the myocardium of oxygen previously supplied by that artery. The administration of a fibrinolytic agent results in lysis of the acute thrombus, resulting in recanalization, or opening, of the obstructed coronary artery and restoration of blood flow to the affected tissue. After perfusion is restored, adjunctive measures are taken to prevent further clot formation and repeat occlusion.

ELIGIBILITY CRITERIA

Certain criteria have been developed, based on research findings, to determine the patient population that would most likely benefit from the administration of fibrinolytic therapy. Patients with recent onset of chest pain (<12 hours' duration) and persistent ST elevation (>0.1 mV in two or more contiguous leads) are considered candidates for fibrinolytic therapy.[21] Patients who present with bundle branch blocks that may obscure ST-segment analysis and a history suggesting an acute MI are also considered candidates for therapy (see "Myocardial Infarction" in Chapter 19). The goal of therapy is to administer fibrinolytic therapy within 30 minutes after presentation ("door to needle"), because early reperfusion yields the greatest benefit.[22]

Exclusion criteria are usually based on the increased risk of bleeding incurred from the use of fibrinolytics. Patients who have stable clots that might be disrupted by fibrinolytic therapy (recent surgery, trauma, or a cerebrovascular accident) usually are not considered candidates for fibrinolytic therapy. Other common criteria for the use of fibrinolytic therapy are presented in Box 20-6.

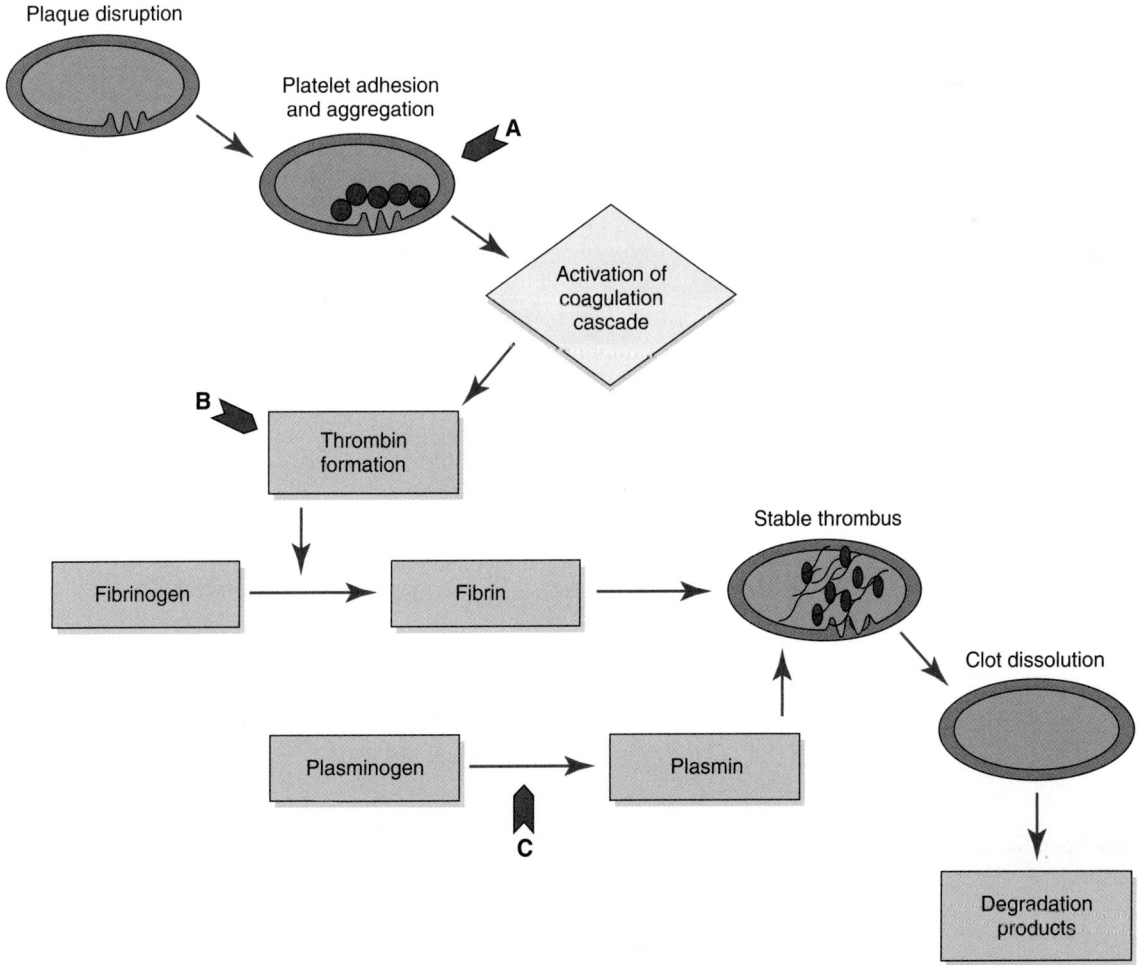

Figure 20-11 Thrombus formation and site of action of medications used in the treatment of acute myocardial infarction. *A,* Site of action of antiplatelet agents such as aspirin and glycoprotein IIb/IIIa inhibitors. *B,* Heparin bonds with antithrombin III and thrombin to create an inactive complex. *C,* Fibrinolytic agents convert plasminogen to plasmin, an enzyme responsible for degradation of fibrin clots.

Currently, fibrinolytic therapy is not indicated for patients with unstable angina or non–ST-elevation myocardial infarction (NSTEMIs). It is believed that these conditions result from plaque rupture with the formation of an only partially occlusive thrombus. Fibrinolysis breaks up the clot and releases thrombin, and this can paradoxically increase the material necessary for further thrombosis.[23] Instead, these patients are treated with antiplatelet agents (e.g., aspirin, clopidogrel, glycoprotein IIb/IIIa inhibitors) and antithrombin drugs (e.g., heparin).

FIBRINOLYTIC AGENTS

Four fibrinolytic agents are currently available for intravenous treatment of acute STEMI. All of these agents stimulate lysis of the clot by converting inactive plasminogen to plasmin, an enzyme responsible for degradation of fibrin (see Fig. 20-11). Streptokinase (SK) and urokinase were the first generation of fibrinolytic agents and had their primary effect on circulating plasminogen. Urokinase availability has been limited because

---

BOX 20-6 FIBRINOLYTIC THERAPY SELECTION CRITERIA

- No more than 12 hours from onset of chest pain (less if possible)
- ST-segment elevation on electrocardiogram or new-onset left bundle branch block
- Ischemic chest pain unresponsive to sublingual nitroglycerin
- No conditions that might cause a predisposition to hemorrhage

---

of manufacturing problems. Newer fibrinolytic agents (e.g., alteplase, reteplase, tenecteplase) have a greater effect on clot plasminogen than on circulating plasminogen and are therefore considered clot selective. A comparison of currently approved fibrinolytic agents is provided in Table 20-4. Because patients with an area of plaque disruption are still at risk for clot formation and reocclusion, fibrinolytic therapy is used in conjunction with anticoagulants and antiplatelet agents. Current guidelines recommend that heparin be administered for a minimum of 48 hours after fibrinolytic therapy. Low-molecular-weight heparin (LMWH) is considered an acceptable alternative in patients younger than 75 years who have adequate renal function. Antiplatelet therapy with clopidogrel is recommended for 14 days, and aspirin should be continued indefinitely.[24]

Streptokinase. SK is a fibrinolytic agent derived from β-hemolytic streptococci, which, when combined with plasminogen, catalyzes the conversion of plasminogen to plasmin, the enzyme responsible for clot dissolution in the body. SK can be administered intravenously or by an intracoronary approach, which necessitates cardiac catheterization. The efficacy of both routes has been established, although use of the intracoronary route is not considered practical, because the instrumentation required for this route would be similar to that required for a percutaneous intervention.[25]

The three major problems associated with the use of SK are its systemic lytic effects coupled with a long half-life, potential antigenic effects if readministered, and hypotension. Because the anticoagulant action of SK is systemic (non–clot specific) and prolonged (half-life of 20 to 25 minutes), bleeding is the

---

TABLE 20-4 Pharmacologic Management: Fibrinolytic Agents for Use in Acute Myocardial Infarction

DRUG	DOSAGE	ACTIONS	SPECIAL CONSIDERATIONS
Clot-Specific			
tPA (alteplase)	IV: 100 mg over 90 min with the first 15 mg given as a bolus	Binds to fibrin at the clot and promotes activation of plasminogen to plasmin	Short half-life, so heparin is usually given with the drug as a bolus and afterward as an infusion. Aspirin is begun with administration of the drug and continued daily.
rPA (reteplase)	IV: 10 units given as a bolus over 2 minutes, repeated in 30 min	Binds to fibrin at the clot and promotes activation of plasminogen to plasmin	Heparin is started with administration of the drug and continued for 24 hr. Aspirin is begun with administration of the drug and continued daily.
TNKase (tenecteplase)	IV: 30-50 mg based on body weight, given as a single bolus	Binds to fibrin at the clot and promotes activation of plasminogen to plasmin	Heparin is started with administration of the drug. Aspirin is begun with administration of the drug and continued daily.
Non–Clot-Specific			
SK (streptokinase)	IV: 1.5 million units given over 60 min	Catalyzes the conversion of plasminogen to plasmin, which causes lysis of fibrin; has systemic lytic effects	May cause allergic reactions and hypotension. Heparin may be administered IV or SQ. Aspirin is begun with administration of the drug and continued daily.

IV, intravenous; rPA, recombinant plasminogen activator; SQ, subcutaneous; tPA, tissue plasminogen activator.

most common complication. Patients require careful observation during the 12 hours immediately after administration (Box 20-7). Because SK is a bacterial protein, it can produce a variety of allergic reactions, including anaphylaxis, especially when administered to a patient who has received SK therapy previously or who has had a recent streptococcal infection. The nurse must be familiar with the possible allergic manifestations (Box 20-8) and understand that symptoms may develop several days after infusion, as a result of delayed antibody formation. Diphenhydramine (Benadryl) or steroids are often prescribed before SK administration to blunt this unwanted effect. Hypotension is sometimes associated with the rapid administration of SK. This fall in blood pressure usually responds to volume replacement but occasionally requires vasopressor support.

Tissue Plasminogen Activator. Marketed under the trade name Activase, tissue plasminogen activator (tPA) or alteplase is a naturally occurring enzyme (i.e., nonantigenic) that is clot specific and has a very short half-life (3 to 4 minutes). It converts plasminogen to plasmin after binding to the fibrin-containing clot. This clot-specific action results in an increased concentration and activity of plasmin at the site of the clot, where it is needed. It was hoped that this characteristic of tPA would prevent the induction of a systemic lytic state, such as occurs with SK therapy. However, studies comparing the adverse effects of SK and tPA showed a similar incidences of bleeding after administration.[21] tPA was approved specifically for intravenous administration. Several different dosing regimens have been proposed and tested in the clinical setting, but accelerated-dose tPA is considered most effective means of establishing early patency of the occluded vessel.[22]

Recombinant Plasminogen Activator. Recombinant plasminogen activator (rPA), or reteplase, is a variant of the natural human enzyme tPA. Reteplase is less fibrin selective and has a longer half-life than tPA, making it suitable for bolus administration rather than as a continuous infusion. This new-generation plasminogen activator is given as a double bolus and then followed with a heparin infusion. Unlike tPA, reteplase does not require weight-based dosing. Studies have shown that reteplase is as effective as tPA in the treatment of acute MI and is easier to administer.[22]

Tenecteplase. Tenecteplase (TNKase) is the newest of the fibrinolytic agents. It is a genetically engineered variant of alteplase with slower plasma clearance and better fibrin specificity. Studies have shown that TNKase is as effective as alteplase, with similar rates of bleeding complications between the two agents.[21] TNKase requires only a single bolus injection, which may help facilitate more rapid treatment both in and out of the hospital. Although the need for weight-based dosing is a potential disadvantage of the drug, tenecteplase is currently the most widely used thrombolytic agent in the United States.[25]

Outcomes of Fibrinolytic Therapy. The benefit of fibrinolytic therapy correlates with the degree of restoration of normal blood flow in the infarct-related artery. Coronary artery patency is defined by angiographic perfusion grades developed by the Thrombolysis in Myocardial Infarction (TIMI) study group in 1985 (Box 20-9).[26] Achievement of TIMI grade 3 flow is associated with the best long-term survival. Studies also indicate that rapid restoration of normal blood flow, within 90 minutes after treatment, results in improved LV function and reduced mortality. The three fibrin-specific fibrinolytics have been shown to achieve TIMI 3 flow in 54% to 63% of patients at 90 minutes.[25]

The area of fibrinolytic therapy continues to evolve, and drug dose ranges and regimens are subject to change when research findings are updated. Whereas fibrinolytic agents target the fibrin portion of the clot, other treatment strategies are focusing on the platelet portion of the clot (see Fig. 20-11). Clinical trials evaluating the combination of glycoprotein IIb/IIIa receptor antagonists with fibrinolytic agents (at half-dose) found outcomes equivalent to those of fibrinolytics alone, but with an increased risk for bleeding.[27] There was also speculation

---

BOX 20-7 SIGNS OF INADEQUATE HEMOSTASIS RELATED TO FIBRINOLYTIC THERAPY

- Bleeding or hematoma at puncture sites
- Hematuria, hematemesis, hemoptysis, melena, epistaxis
- Bruising or petechiae (pinpoint hemorrhages)
- Flank ecchymoses with complaints of low back pain (suggestive of retroperitoneal bleeding)
- Gingival bleeding
- Change in neurologic status (intracranial bleeding)
- Deterioration in vital signs, decreased hematocrit values (internal bleeding)

BOX 20-8 POSSIBLE ALLERGIC MANIFESTATIONS RELATED TO STREPTOKINASE THERAPY

- Anaphylaxis
- Urticaria
- Itching
- Nausea
- Flushing
- Fever
- Chills

BOX 20-9 FLOW IN THE INFARCT-RELATED ARTERY AS DESCRIBED IN THE THROMBOLYSIS IN MYOCARDIAL INFARCTION TRIAL

Perfusion Grades	Flow in the Infarct-Related Artery
TIMI 3	Normal or brisk flow through the coronary artery
TIMI 2	Partial flow, slower than in normal vessels
TIMI 1	Sluggish flow with incomplete distal filling
TIMI 0	No flow beyond the point of occlusion

Modified from The TIMI Study Group: The thrombolysis in myocardial infarction (TIMI) trial: phase I findings, *N Engl J Med* 312:932, 1985.
TIMI, Thrombolysis in Myocardial Infarction Trial

that a planned strategy for administering fibrinolytics or glyco-protein IIb/IIIa receptor antagonists, or both, to patients who must be transported to another facility for percutaneous intervention would improve outcomes. Although promising in theory, this facilitated approach to revascularization has not been shown to be beneficial and may increase the risk for bleeding complications in some patients.[28]

EVIDENCE OF REPERFUSION

Several phenomena may be observed after the reperfusion of an artery that has been completely occluded by a thrombus (Box 20-10). Recognition of these noninvasive markers of recanalization is essential for documenting the patient's response to fibrinolytic therapy.

Pain and Reperfusion Dysrhythmias. Initially, when there is reperfusion, ischemic chest pain ceases abruptly as blood flow is restored. Another reliable indicator of reperfusion is the appearance of various "reperfusion dysrhythmias." Premature ventricular contractions (PVCs), bradycardias, heart block, VT, and, rarely, VF may occur. The reason for the occurrence of these dysrhythmias remains unclear, but they are thought to be the result of restored flow to ischemic tissue. Reperfusion dysrhythmias are usually self-limiting or nonsustained, and aggressive antidysrhythmic therapy is not required. However, vigilant monitoring of the patient's ECG is essential, because a stable condition can deteriorate rapidly and the dysrhythmias may necessitate emergency treatment.

ST Segment. Another noninvasive marker of recanalization is rapid return to baseline of the elevated ST segments, which indicates restoration of blood flow to previously ischemic myocardial tissue. A monitoring lead should be chosen that clearly demonstrates ST elevation before initiation of therapy[29] (see "Continuous ST-Segment Monitoring" in Chapter 18).

Creatine Kinase. The serum concentration of creatine kinase (formerly known as creatine phosphokinase) rises rapidly and markedly after reperfusion of the ischemic myocardium. This phenomenon is called *washout,* because it is thought to result from the rapid readmission of creatine kinase—an enzyme released by damaged myocardial cells—into the circulation after restoration of blood flow to previously unperfused areas of the heart (see "Cardiac Biomarkers" in Chapter 18).

Residual Coronary Artery Stenosis. Fibrinolytic therapy has been determined to be a successful strategy for reopening occluded coronary arteries in the setting of acute MI. It limits infarct size, salvaging myocardium and significantly reducing morbidity and mortality associated with cardiogenic shock and

VF. However, residual coronary artery stenosis resulting from the atherosclerotic process remains, even after successful fibrinolysis. Subsequent prevention of reocclusion is critical to preserving myocardial function and preventing the risk of late complications. Fibrinolytic therapy is therefore recognized as an emergency procedure to restore patency until more definitive therapy can be initiated to effectively reduce the degree of stenosis (an interventional catheter procedure) or to bypass the offending occlusion (coronary artery bypass grafting [CABG]).

NURSING MANAGEMENT

Nursing management of the patient undergoing fibrinolytic therapy begins with identifying potential candidates. In many institutions, checklists are used to facilitate the rapid identification of patients who are candidates for fibrinolytics. The nurse prepares the patient for fibrinolytic therapy by starting intravenous lines and obtaining baseline laboratory values and vital signs. Throughout the administration of the fibrinolytic agent, assessment of the patient continues for clinical indicators of reperfusion and complications related to therapy. Several nursing diagnoses are linked to management of the patient receiving fibrinolytic therapy (see the Nursing Diagnoses feature on Fibrinolytic Therapy).

The most common complication related to thrombolysis is bleeding, from the fibrinolytic therapy itself and also because the patients routinely receive anticoagulation therapy for several days to minimize the possibility of rethrombosis. The nurse must continually monitor for clinical manifestations of bleeding (see Box 20-7). Mild gingival bleeding and oozing around venipuncture sites is common and not a cause of concern. Should serious bleeding occur, such as intracranial or internal bleeding, all fibrinolytic and heparin therapies are discontinued and volume expanders or coagulation factors, or both, are administered.

In addition to accurate assessment of the patient for evidence of bleeding, nursing management includes preventive measures to minimize the potential for bleeding. For example, patient handling is limited, injections are avoided if at all possible, and additional pressure is provided to ensure hemostasis at venipuncture and arterial puncture sites. Intravenous lines are placed before lytic therapy is administered, and a heparin lock may be used for obtaining laboratory specimens during treatment.

BOX 20-10 NONINVASIVE EVIDENCE OF REPERFUSION

- Cessation of chest pain
- Reperfusion dysrhythmias, primarily ventricular
- Return of elevated ST segments to baseline
- Early and marked peaking of creatine kinase concentration and troponins

---

Nursing Diagnoses

Fibrinolytic Therapy

- Ineffective Cardiopulmonary Tissue Perfusion related to acute myocardial ischemia
- Acute Pain related to transmission and perception of cutaneous, visceral, muscular, or ischemic impulses
- Anxiety related to threat of biologic, psychological, or social integrity
- Deficient Fluid Volume related to absolute loss
- Deficient Knowledge: Discharge regimen related to lack of previous exposure to information (see the Patient Education feature on Fibrinolytic Therapy)

PATIENT EDUCATION

Education for the patient receiving fibrinolytic therapy includes information regarding the actions of fibrinolytic agents, with emphasis on precautions to minimize bleeding (see the Patient Education feature on Fibrinolytic Therapy). For example, the patient is cautioned against vigorous tooth brushing and told to refrain from using straight-edge razors. Information is provided regarding ongoing risk factor management in the prevention of atherosclerotic CAD.

CATHETER INTERVENTIONS FOR CORONARY ARTERY DISEASE

During the past 3 decades, the use of catheter procedures to open coronary arteries blocked or narrowed by CAD has expanded dramatically. These procedures are grouped by the term *percutaneous coronary intervention* (PCI). Today, PCI includes PTCA, atherectomy, and stent implantation. Advances in device technology, along with more effective anticoagulant and antiplatelet regimens, have reduced complication rates and improved procedural outcomes.[30] Patients undergoing PCI based interventions have an anticipated hospital stay of 1 to 3 days.

Percutaneous transluminal coronary angioplasty (PTCA), frequently abbreviated to *balloon angioplasty* or simply *angioplasty*, was introduced in 1977 as an alternative to coronary surgical revascularization. PTCA avoids the risks involved with cardiac surgery (general anesthesia, sternotomy, extracorporeal circulation, and mechanical ventilation) and significantly decreases convalescence time. Disadvantages include acute complications related to the procedure itself, restenosis or renarrowing of the vessel after the procedure, and difficulty in accessing certain lesions. Research in this area has continued, and a growing number of interventional devices have been developed to address the limitations of conventional angioplasty.

INDICATIONS FOR CATHETER-BASED INTERVENTIONS

Indications for catheter-based interventions have been considerably broadened since the initial application of balloon angioplasty. Whereas only patients with single-vessel CAD were once considered for PTCA, patients with multivessel disease, even those who have previously undergone saphenous vein

Patient Education: Fibrinolytic Therapy

- Pathophysiology of atherosclerosis
- Risk factor management
- Description of fibrinolytic agent and how it works
- Measures to minimize bleeding and bruising associated with fibrinolytic therapy
- Recognition and actions to take for recurrent ischemic symptoms
- Information regarding prescribed medications (antiplatelet agents, anticoagulants)

grafting, internal mammary artery (IMA) grafting, or fibrinolytic therapy for acute MI, may now be candidates for catheter intervention. Previously seen as a rescue procedure to reduce a severe stenosis that persisted after fibrinolytic therapy, PCI has become preferred as the initial method of treatment for acute MI (primary PCI).[31]

Earlier restrictions regarding the characteristics and location of the atherosclerotic lesion have also changed with operator experience and improved technology. Distal, moderately calcified, and bifurcation stenoses are considered suitable for PCI. Left main coronary artery lesions, although considered high risk, have been successfully dilated under certain conditions. It is now possible to traverse and dilate a totally occluded vessel. Lesion morphology related to shape, size, location, and amount of calcification has been more clearly defined through clinical experience and is used to guide the selection of specific catheter-based interventions[32] (see "Coronary Artery Disease" in Chapter 19).

SURGICAL BACKUP

Initially, most institutions required that patients preparing to undergo PTCA be candidates for CABG. Complications such as intimal dissection with abrupt closure of the vessel could arise during the procedure, requiring the patient to undergo emergency CABG. Today, most dissections are effectively treated with stent placement, with less than 1% of patients requiring emergency bypass surgery. As a result, most institutions use an informal surgical backup plan, such as the first available operating room. Nevertheless, the availability of cardiac surgical services on site is still recommended. The one exception is in institutions that offer PCI only for treatment of acute STEMI. In this setting, an organized plan for emergent transfer to a surgical center may be used in lieu of on-site surgical access.[32]

PERCUTANEOUS TRANSLUMINAL CORONARY ANGIOPLASTY

PTCA involves the use of a balloon-tipped catheter that, when advanced through an atherosclerotic lesion (atheroma), can be inflated intermittently for the purpose of dilating the stenotic area and improving blood flow through it (Fig. 20-12). The high inflation pressure of the balloon stretches the vessel wall,

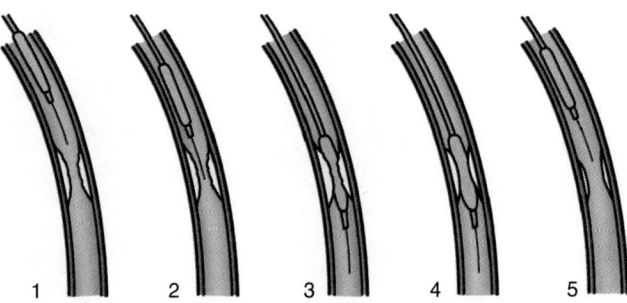

Figure 20-12 Percutaneous transluminal coronary angioplasty (PTCA) is used to open a stenotic vessel occluded by atherosclerosis.

fractures the plaque, and enlarges the vessel lumen. After balloon deflation, the vessel exhibits some degree of elastic recoil, resulting in a residual stenosis of approximately 30%.[33] A successful angioplasty procedure is one in which the stenosis is reduced to less than 50% of the vessel lumen diameter.[32]

LIMITATIONS

Although PTCA has relatively high success rates in initially opening occluded vessels, this technique by itself has major limitations, including the risk of acute vessel closure and a high frequency of restenosis. In the early application of angioplasty, acute closure occurred in up to 8% of patients as a result of dissection of the vessel wall and associated thrombus formation or vessel spasm. Restenosis occurred in more than one third of patients who underwent PTCA within the first 6 months and was diagnosed when patients experienced a recurrence of anginal symptoms.[34] Studies showed that restenosis was influenced by the final lumen diameter achieved by the procedure, the severity of elastic recoil of the vessel walls in response to the balloon inflation, and the amount of intimal hyperplasia that occurred as the vessel healed over the treated area. Patient characteristics such as a history of diabetes or unstable angina were also found to increase the risk of restenosis.[35]

After the limitations of angioplasty were recognized, devices were sought to more completely remove plaque and open the vessel at the time of the intervention. Coronary atherectomy and placement of endovascular prostheses (stents) are interventional technologies developed to address the problems of acute closure and restenosis associated with PTCA. Currently, PTCA is rarely used alone as an intervention, except to treat lesions in very small coronary arteries.[33] Nevertheless, balloon angioplasty remains an essential technique in PCI for dilating vessels and for deploying intracoronary stents.

ATHERECTOMY

Atherectomy is the excision and removal of the atherosclerotic plaque by cutting, shaving, or grinding. Specialized coronary catheters are used. Initially, atherectomy devices were used alone in an attempt to avoid the trauma to the vessel that was known to occur with balloon angioplasty and to more efficiently remove the atherosclerotic plaque, thereby decreasing the rate of restenosis. Later, as restenosis was also found to occur with these devices, balloon angioplasty was added as an adjunctive therapy to optimize the diameter of the vessel lumen and offset the intimal hyperplasia that occurred as a result of the procedure. Despite significant improvements in initial procedural success, atherectomy failed to significantly reduce the rate of restenosis.[36] In the current era of stenting, atherectomy devices are used in less than 5% of procedures.[33]

Two atherectomy devices are used in coronary intervention: directional coronary atherectomy (DCA) and rotational ablation (Rotablator). Both devices are approved by the U.S. Food and Drug Administration (FDA) for use in peripheral arteries. Because these devices use different mechanisms, they may offer special advantages for different types of lesions.

Directional Coronary Atherectomy. The DCA catheter consists of a rotating, cup-shaped blade within a windowed cylindrical chamber on one side and a low-inflation balloon on the other. The catheter is positioned within the lesion, and the balloon is inflated, forcing the atheromatous plaque into the chamber window. The cutting blade is then used to shave the protruding plaque, which is collected within the chamber. The ability to turn the catheter in various directions within the vessel led to the name of the device. A DCA catheter is pictured in Figure 20-13A. Because DCA extracts pieces of atheroma that can be studied microscopically (rather like a biopsy specimen), it has contributed significantly to our understanding

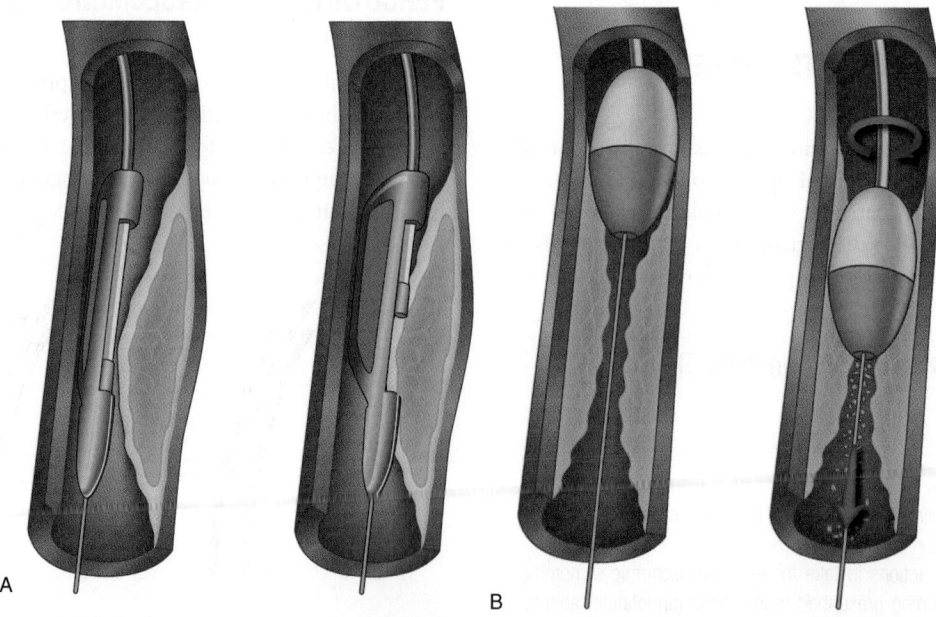

Figure 20-13 Atherectomy devices. *A,* Directional coronary atherectomy catheter. *B,* Rotational atherectomy catheter.

of both the pathogenesis of CAD and the restenosis process caused by intimal hyperplasia after catheter interventions. A randomized trial showed no clinical benefit for the use of DCA in combination with stenting, compared with stenting alone.[37] As a result, DCA is currently used only for noncalcified lesions that involve a bifurcation of a major side branch or in the ostium of the left anterior descending (LAD) artery.[30]

Rotablator. The Rotablator device has a high-speed, rotating, diamond-coated bur that drills through the plaque, creating tiny particles. (see Fig. 20-13B). The particulate matter is carried through the bloodstream and disposed of by the reticuloendothelial system. This atherectomy device is currently used to debulk heavily calcified lesions that cannot be dilated by angioplasty or prevent delivery of a coronary stent. Rotational atherectomy may also be used for chronic total occlusion and for calcified bifurcation lesions.[30]

CORONARY STENTS

A major development in the field of interventional cardiology has been the coronary stent prosthesis. A stent is a metal structure that is introduced into the coronary artery over a guidewire and expanded into the vessel wall at the site of the lesion. Bare metal stents were first used to treat acute or threatened vessel closure after failed PTCA.[34] The stent acted as a scaffold to tack dissection flaps against the vessel wall and provided mechanical support to minimize elastic recoil. Subsequent studies confirmed the clinical benefits of stents, which led to elective coronary stenting as a primary procedure. Stent implantation was initially limited to large vessels (>3 mm) with proximal, discrete lesions. Improvements in stent design and operator technique allow for their deployment in smaller vessels with diffuse disease, vessels with lesions at bifurcations, and vessels with thrombus. Multiple stents may be implanted sequentially within a vessel to fully cover the area of the lesion. Stents are currently the predominant form of PCI and are used in more than 90% of all interventional procedures.[10]

Numerous stents are available. They are composed of various types of metal (stainless steel, titanium, cobalt chromium) and come in a variety of configurations (e.g., mesh, coil). Most stents are balloon expandable Fig. 20-14.

Stent Thrombosis. Early use of stents was hampered by the high incidence of subacute stent thrombosis. Unlike the abrupt closure that often occurred in the first 24 hours after PTCA, stent thrombosis tended to occur during the first 2 to 14 days after stent placement.[33] To prevent acute thrombosis of the stent, intense anticoagulation was initially used during and after stent placement. Consequently, bleeding was a major complication in the early phases of stent placement. Clinical studies have since indicated that subacute stent thrombosis is caused by incomplete stent opening or deployment. High-pressure balloon inflations within the stent are used to fully open the stent, so reduced anticoagulation is sufficient to maintain stent patency. Dual antiplatelet therapy (aspirin and a thienopyridine) has been shown to be more important than anticoagulation in preventing stent thrombosis.[38] These agents are administered before the procedure and continued at

discharge.[39] More potent antiplatelet agents (glycoprotein IIb/IIIa inhibitors) have become available to reduce the formation of intracoronary thrombosis after PCI. Initially used only in patients with high risk for abrupt closure after PCI, these agents have been found to have benefit across the spectrum of interventional procedures, from PTCA to atherectomy to stenting.[39]

Abciximab (ReoPro) was the first of the glycoprotein IIb/IIIa inhibitors to be approved by the FDA as an adjunct to PTCA for the prevention of abrupt closure of arteries in high-risk patients. Later, two additional agents, eptifibatide (Integrilin) and tirofiban (Aggrastat), were approved. These drugs act on the glycoprotein IIb/IIIa receptors on the platelet membrane to inhibit the final phase of platelet aggregation and prevent platelets from binding with fibrinogen. Indications and dosing of these agents are provided in Table 20-5.

In-Stent Restenosis. Bare metal stents have been shown to decrease the incidence of restenosis when compared with balloon angioplasty, most likely as a result of achieving the largest possible lumen diameter at the time of the intervention.[30] Stents have not, however, proved to be a cure for restenosis as was once hoped. Restenosis within the stent is caused by intimal hyperplasia and can occur in a diffuse pattern throughout the stent, as discrete lesions within the body of the stent, or at the stent margins. The incidence of in-stent restenosis requiring intervention is approximately 20% within the first 6 months after implantation of a bare metal stent.[34] Factors that increase the risk of in-stent restenosis are listed in Box 20-11.

Drug-Eluting Stents. In an effort to minimize restenosis, drug-eluting stents (DES) were developed. These stents have polymer coatings impregnated with drugs that are released slowly into the endothelium at the site of stent placement to inhibit cellular proliferation. DES coated with sirolimus (an immunosuppressive drug used to prevent organ transplant rejection) and paclitaxel (an anticancer agent) have been approved by the FDA.[40] In initial trials, DES were found to decrease the 6-month restenosis rate to less than 10%, and they soon became the predominant stent, implanted in 90% of patients. Some trials demonstrated similar efficacy between bare metal stents and DES in long-term outcomes (stent thrombosis, MI, or death) and raised concerns regarding the possibility of late stent thrombosis (>1 year) in DES.[41,42] As a result, DES usage has decreased somewhat to between 60% and 70% of patients.[43] Because a DES delays endothelialization, dual antiplatelet therapy must be continued for a longer period to prevent stent thrombosis. A DES is also considerably more expensive than a bare metal stent. A comparison of bare metal stents and DES is provided in Table 20-6.

Procedure. PCI is performed in the cardiac catheterization laboratory under fluoroscopy. Patients typically receive antiplatelet therapy (clopidogrel and aspirin) before beginning the procedure. An introducer catheter, or sheath, is inserted percutaneously into the femoral artery. Alternatively, access to the arterial system can be obtained through the radial or brachial artery. In some cases, a venous sheath is inserted and used to perform a right heart catheterization or to insert a pacing catheter, or both. A catheter with pacing capabilities may be indicated if dilation of the right coronary artery or circumflex

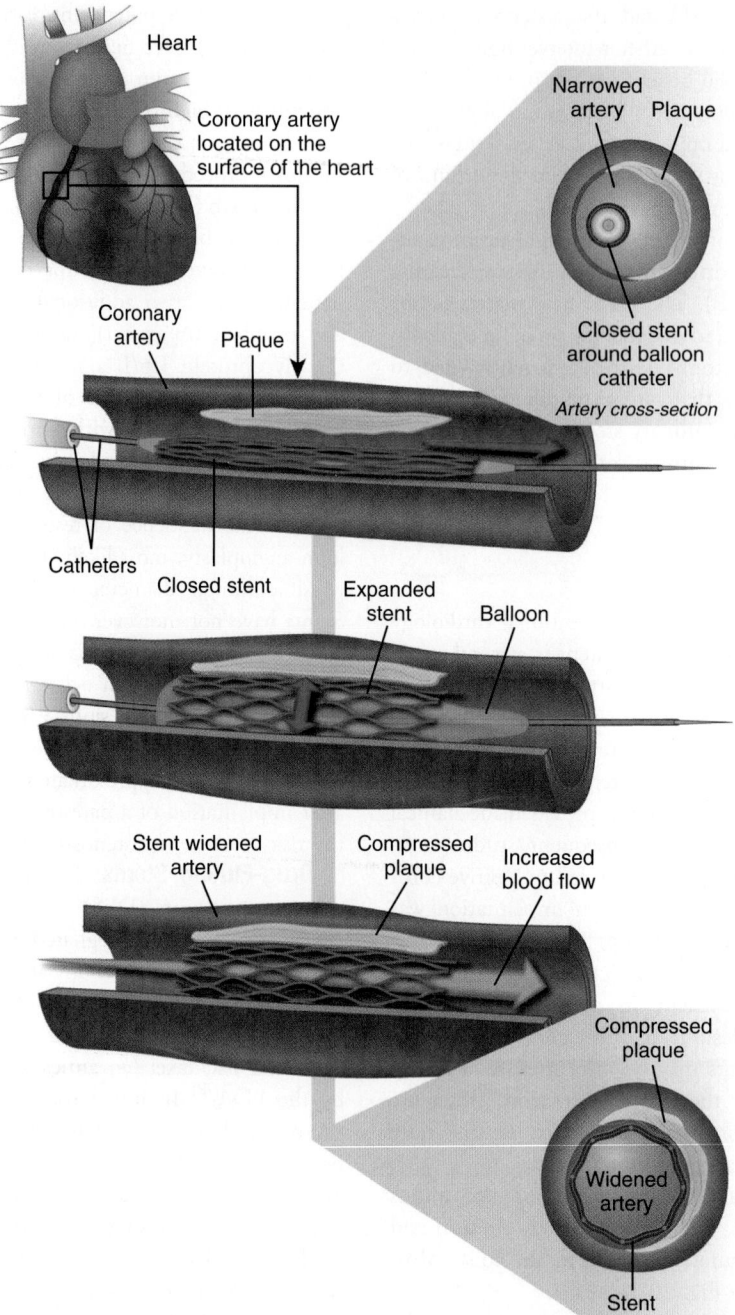

Figure 20-14 The intracoronary stent is a balloon-expandable stent.

artery is anticipated, because the blood supply to the conduction system of the heart may be interrupted, requiring emergency pacing. The patient is systemically anticoagulated to prevent clots from forming on or in any of the catheters. Unfractionated heparin is used most often, with dosing adjusted to achieve a target activated clotting time. Other anticoagulants may be used based on physician preference or if the patient cannot tolerate heparin. Newer anticoagulant agents are described in Table 20-7. A special guiding catheter, designed to engage the coronary ostia, is inserted through the arterial sheath and advanced in a retrograde manner through the aorta. Nitroglycerin or calcium channel blockers may be given at this time to prevent coronary artery spasm and to maximize coronary

vasodilation during the procedure. A guidewire is then advanced down the coronary artery and negotiated across the occluding atheroma. The balloon catheter is advanced over this guidewire and positioned across the lesion. The balloon is inflated and deflated repetitively (each inflation not to exceed 90 seconds) until evidence of dilation is demonstrated on an angiogram (Fig. 20-15). For lesions that do not respond well to angioplasty, additional plaque removal may be done with an atherectomy device.

In most procedures, vessel dilation is followed by deployment of an intracoronary stent. A stent is positioned at the target side, the stent is expanded, and the catheter is removed, leaving the stent in place. Intravascular ultrasound is used by

TABLE 20-5 Pharmacologic Management: Glycoprotein IIB/IIIA Inhibitors

DRUG	INDICATIONS AND DOSE	SPECIAL CONSIDERATIONS
Abciximab (ReoPro)	ACS: 0.25 mg/kg IVP, then 10 mcg/min until PCI PCI: 0.25 mg/kg IVP, then 0.125 mcg/kg/min × 12 hr	Used concomitantly with heparin and aspirin May affect platelet function for up to 48 hr after infusion
Eptifibatide (Integrilin)	ACS: IV bolus or 180 mcg/kg followed by an infusion of 2 mcg/kg/min for up to 72 hr; if the patient undergoes PCI, the dose is decreased to 0.5 mcg/kg/min and continued for 24 hr after the procedure, for a total of 96 hr PCI: 135 mcg/kg IVP, followed by an infusion of 0.5 mcg/kg/min × 24 hr	Concomitant heparin and aspirin may be administered Platelet function returns to baseline within 6-8 hr Contraindicated in patients with significant kidney dysfunction
Tirofiban (Aggrastat)	ACS (with or without PCI): 0.4 mcg/kg/min for 30 min, then continued at 0.1 mcg/kg/min for 48-108 hr after ACS or for patients undergoing PCI	Administered in combination with heparin for patients undergoing PCI Platelet function returns to baseline within 4-8 hr Dosage should be reduced in patients with severe kidney dysfunction

ACS, acute coronary syndrome; IV, intravenous; IVP, intravenous push; PCI, percutaneous coronary intervention.

BOX 20-11 RISK FACTORS FOR IN-STENT RESTENOSIS

PATIENT FACTORS
- Diabetes mellitus
- Acute or chronic renal failure

ANATOMIC FACTORS
- Longer lesions (>20 mm)
- Small vessel diameter (<3.0 mm)
- Complex, branched lesions

TABLE 20-6 Comparison of Bare Metal and Drug-Eluting Stents

Characteristics	Bare Metal Stent	Drug-Eluting Stent
Restenosis rate (at 6 months)	15-20%	5-10%
Cost	$800-1000 per stent	$2400-3000 per stent
Duration of dual antiplatelet therapy	2-4 wk	12 mo
Recommended lesion features	Short lesions <20 mm Large vessel diameter >3.0 mm	Longer lesions >20 mm Small vessel diameter <3.5 mm

some clinicians to evaluate the vessel lumen diameter after stent deployment to ensure optimal expansion.[38] Information obtained by ultrasonography provides a better estimate of residual plaque than that provided by angiography, because contrast material may surround the lattice-work of the stent, giving the appearance of a large lumen even when the stent is not fully open. The patient is transferred to the coronary care or angioplasty unit after the procedure for care and observation. Heparin or other anticoagulants are usually discontinued immediately after the procedure, to facilitate early sheath removal. Sheaths are removed within 2 to 4 hours after the procedure when the activated clotting time (ACT) returns to normal, or sooner if a vascular closure device is used. If glycoprotein IIb/IIIa inhibitors were initiated during the procedure, they are continued for 12 to 24 hours, depending on the agent used. Dual antiplatelet therapy with clopidogrel and aspirin is routinely prescribed at discharge. Recommendations for clopidogrel administration vary based on the type of stent used, typically 4 weeks for bare metal stents and 1 year for DES, whereas aspirin is continued indefinitely. Conventional medications for treatment of CAD, such as intravenous nitroglycerin and calcium channel blockers, may also be prescribed.

Acute Complications. The incidence of serious cardiac complications after PCI, including coronary spasm, coronary artery dissection, and acute coronary thrombosis, has decreased significantly with improvements in technology. Stents have proved efficacious in the repair of coronary dissections, decreasing the need for emergency bypass surgery. Acute thrombosis has decreased with the use of glycoprotein IIb/IIIa inhibitors. Other complications that can occur in the period immediately after PCI include bleeding and hematoma formation at the site of vascular cannulation, compromised blood flow to the involved extremity, retroperitoneal bleeding, contrast-induced renal failure, dysrhythmias, and vasovagal response (hypotension, bradycardia, and diaphoresis) during manipulation or removal of introducer sheaths.

Late Complications. Restenosis after PCI continues to be a problem, although rates are much lower with DES than with angioplasty alone. Patients at greatest risk are those with complex lesions, multivessel disease, or diabetes.[44] Treatment options for in-stent restenosis include balloon dilation, debulking with an atherectomy device, implantation of another DES or brachytherapy—the localized delivery of intracoronary radiation through

TABLE 20-7 Pharmacologic Management: Anticoagulants

CLASSIFICATION AND DRUGS	MECHANISM OF ACTION	INDICATIONS	SPECIAL CONSIDERATIONS
Heparin			
Heparin sodium	Enhances activity of antithrombin III, a natural anticoagulant	Prevention of clotting in patients with MI and those undergoing PCI or cardiac surgery	Effectiveness of treatment may be monitored by aPTT or ACT Response is variable because of binding with plasma proteins Effects may be reversed with protamine sulfate Risk of developing HIT
Low-Molecular-Weight Heparin			
Dalteparin (Fragmin) Enoxaparin (Lovenox)	Enhances activity of antithrombin III	Prophylaxis and treatment of thromboembolic complications after surgery Prevention of clots in patients with unstable angina and MI	More predictable response than heparin, because the drug is not largely bound to protein aPTT not particularly useful in monitoring treatment
Direct Thrombin Inhibitor			
Lepirudin (Refludan) Bivalirudin (Angiomax) Argatroban (Argatroban)	Directly inhibits thrombin	Prophylaxis and treatment of thrombosis in patients with HIT Prevention of clots in patients with unstable angina or PCI	aPTT may be monitored daily Dose should be adjusted for patients with renal insufficiency No reversal agent is available

ACT, activated clotting time; aPTT, activated partial thromboplastin time; HIT, heparin-induced thrombocytopenia; MI, myocardial infarction; PCI percutaneous coronary intervention.

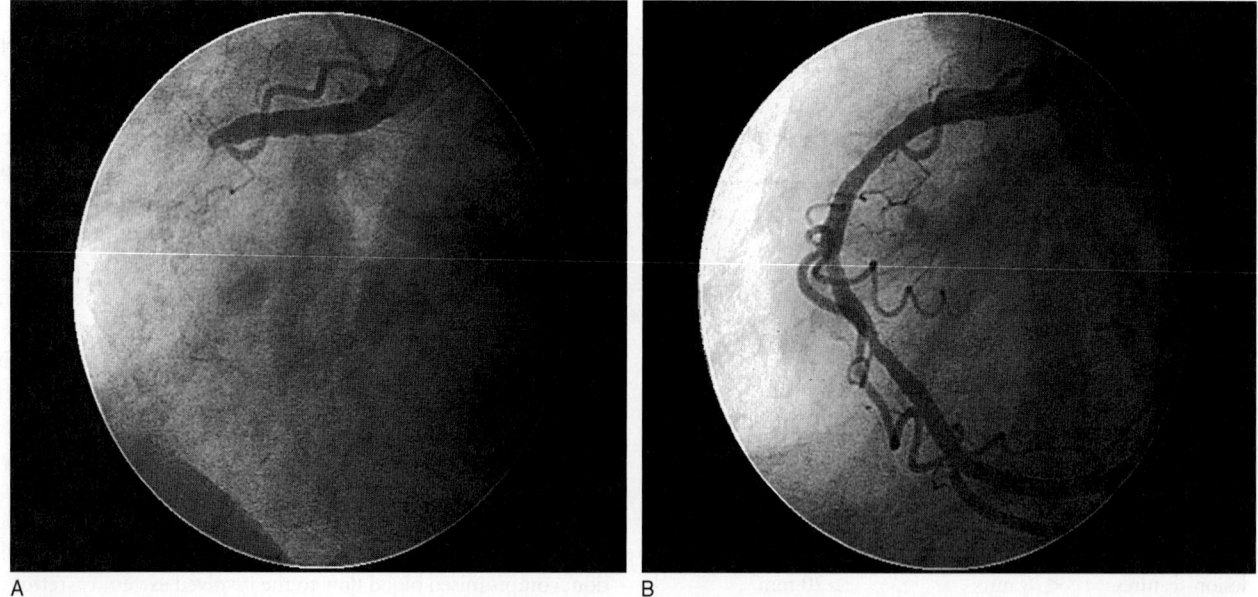

A   B

Figure 20-15 *A,* Coronary arteriogram of an acute proximal total occlusion of the right coronary artery (RCA). The patient had sudden onset of chest pain at home and was emergently admitted to the cardiac catheterization laboratory. *B,* The same vessel as in *A* after successful coronary atherectomy and intracoronary thrombolytic therapy to open the occluded artery. Symptoms of chest pain resolved after the procedure.

specialized catheters. Because healing within the stent is delayed, late thrombosis may occur in patients with DES. Late thrombosis, although rare, is associated with a 45% mortality rate. Premature discontinuation of antiplatelet therapy is the strongest predictor of late stent thrombosis, especially with DES.[34]

NURSING MANAGEMENT

Nursing management and nursing diagnoses after PCI focus on accurate assessment of the patient's condition and prompt intervention (see the Nursing Diagnoses feature on Percutaneous

Percutaneous Transluminal Coronary Angioplasty, Coronary Atherectomy, and Stenting

- Ineffective Cardiopulmonary Tissue Perfusion related to acute myocardial ischemia
- Ineffective Peripheral Tissue Perfusion related to decreased peripheral blood flow
- Activity Intolerance related to prolonged immobility or deconditioning
- Acute Pain related to transmission and perception of cutaneous, visceral, muscular, or ischemic impulses
- Anxiety related to threat to biologic, psychological, or social integrity
- Deficient Knowledge: Discharge Regimen related to lack of previous exposure to information (see the Patient Education feature on Percutaneous Transluminal Coronary Angioplasty, Coronary Atherectomy, and Stenting)

Transluminal Coronary Angioplasty, Coronary Atherectomy, and Stenting). The nurse at the bedside is in a unique position to continuously monitor for clinical manifestations of potential problems and to take quick and appropriate action to minimize the deleterious effects of complications related to the interventional catheter procedure.

Angina. It is essential that the nurse observe the patient for recurrent angina or ST elevation, which are clinical indicators of myocardial ischemia. Monitoring leads should be selected that will reflect ischemia in the vessels that were treated during the intervention. Angina during interventional cardiology procedures is an expected occurrence at the time of balloon inflation or manipulation within the coronary artery. Intraprocedural angina is caused by the temporary interruption of blood flow through the involved artery, which should subside with deflation or removal of the balloon or nitroglycerin administration, or both. Angina after a coronary interventional procedure may be caused by transient coronary vasospasm, or it may signal a more serious complication—acute thrombosis. In any case, the nurse must act quickly to assess for manifestations of myocardial ischemia and initiate clinical interventions as indicated. The physician usually orders intravenous nitroglycerin to be titrated to alleviate chest pain. Continued angina despite maximal vasodilator therapy usually rules out transient coronary vasospasm as the source of ischemic pain, and a return to the cardiac catheterization laboratory must be considered.

Renal Protection. Patients undergoing PCI are exposed to significant amounts of contrast dye, with its associated nephrotoxicity. Renal protective strategies may be implemented before the procedure, especially for patients with evidence of baseline renal impairment. This may include preprocedural hydration, infusion of sodium bicarbonate, and administration of N-acetylcysteine (Mucomyst).[45] After PCI, hydration is important to maintain adequate flow through the kidneys. Intravenous fluids are administered, and patients are encouraged to take oral fluids as tolerated.[46]

Femoral Site Care. While the sheath is in place or after its removal, bleeding or hematoma at the sheath insertion site may occur due to the effects of anticoagulation. The nurse observes the patient for bleeding or swelling at the puncture site and frequently assesses adequacy of circulation to the involved extremity. The nurse also assesses the patient for back pain, which can indicate retroperitoneal bleeding from the internal arterial puncture site. The patient is instructed to keep the involved leg straight and not to elevate the head of the bed any more than 30 degrees while the sheath is in place (to prevent dislodgment) and for several hours after its removal (to prevent bleeding), unless a vascular closure device is used. After sheath removal, direct pressure is applied to the puncture site for 15 to 30 minutes; a sandbag may be ordered if direct pressure is inadequate for hemostasis. For stent placement or atherectomy, which require a larger sheath size, a C-clamp or femoral compression device may be used to apply continuous pressure for 1 to 2 hours to ensure adequate hemostasis.

Patients usually are allowed to resume ambulation 6 to 8 hours after the procedure, depending on institutional protocol. Excessive bleeding or hematoma formation can become a serious problem if it results in hypotension or compromised blood flow to the involved extremity. Pulses are usually monitored every 15 minutes for the first 2 hours after the procedure and then every 1 to 2 hours until the sheaths are removed. After sheath removal, pulses are again monitored at 15-minute intervals for a brief period.

In the last decade, percutaneous vascular hemostatic devices have been introduced to address the problem of achieving adequate hemostasis at the femoral access site after sheath removal. Active closure devices utilize mechanical sutures, collagen plugs, or metal clips to close the vessel when the sheath is removed. Advantages of these devices include a reduced time to hemostasis of under than 5 minutes regardless of the patient's level of anticoagulation, earlier ambulation, and increased patient comfort.[47] Perclose has marketed a percutaneous vascular surgical device that is inserted into the femoral artery in the same position as a conventional introducer sheath. The device contains needles and sutures that are used to suture the artery closed after the interventional procedure (Fig. 20-16). Angioseal is a vascular hemostatic device that uses a collagen plug to seal the arterial puncture site. Gentle pressure is maintained over the puncture site for approximately 5 minutes, until hemostasis is achieved. The StarClose vascular closure device consists of a tiny circumferential nitinol (nickel and titanium) clip that is applied to surface of the vessel to close the femoral artery at the end of the procedure.

Reports of complications and increased cost have limited the use of active closure devices by some clinicians.[47,48] To avoid these complications, a number of products have been developed to enhance manual compression and shorten the time required to achieve hemostasis. Some of these devices rely on the delivery of prothrombotic materials by a patch, whereas others increase local pressure over the puncture site. These devices do not offer immediate closure, but may decrease the time to ambulation.[47] A comparison of vascular closure systems is provided in Table 20-8.

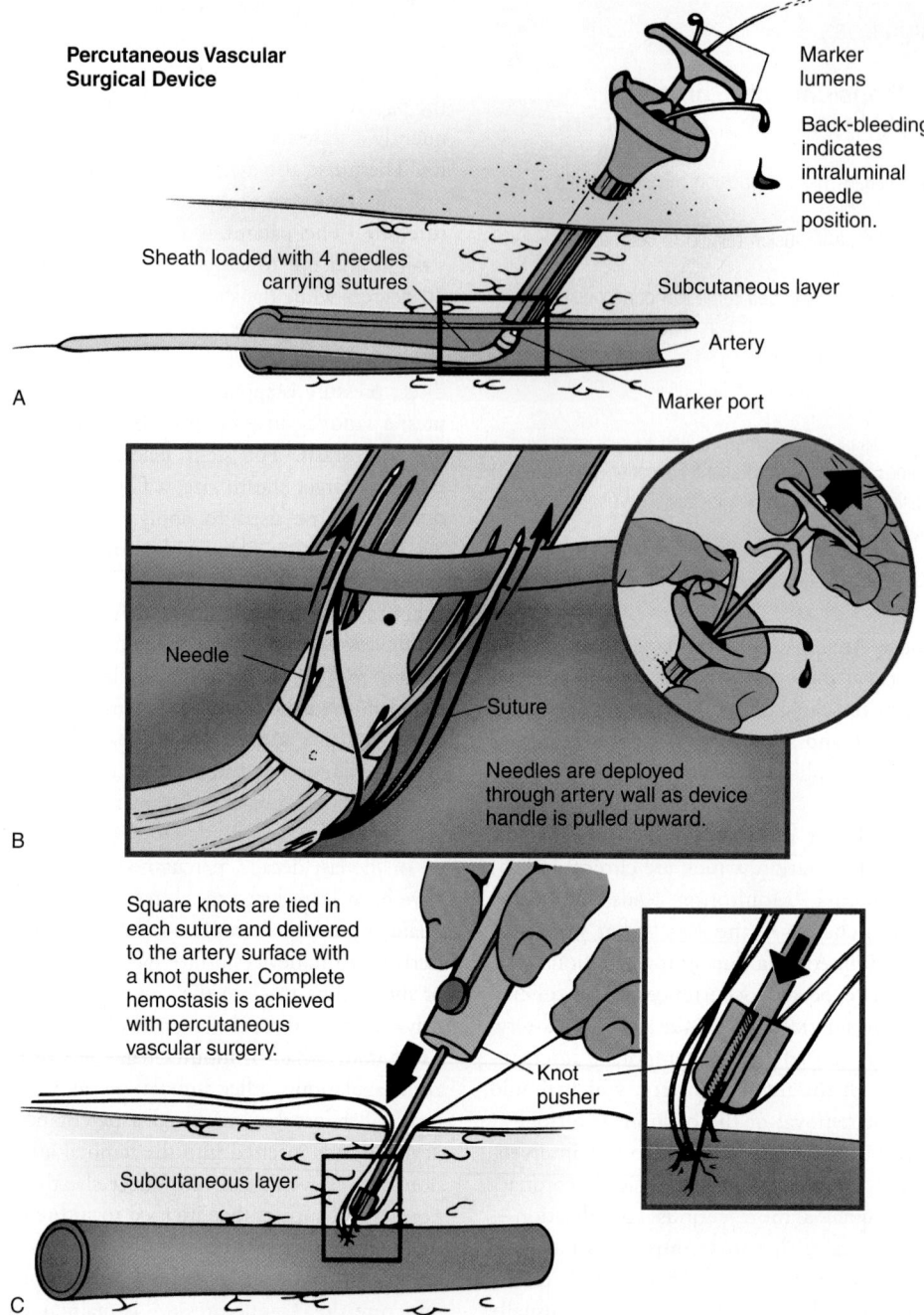

Percutaneous Vascular Surgical Device

Marker lumens

Back-bleeding indicates intraluminal needle position.

Sheath loaded with 4 needles carrying sutures

Subcutaneous layer

Artery

Marker port

A

Needle

Suture

Needles are deployed through artery wall as device handle is pulled upward.

B

Square knots are tied in each suture and delivered to the artery surface with a knot pusher. Complete hemostasis is achieved with percutaneous vascular surgery.

Knot pusher

Subcutaneous layer

C

Figure 20-16 Example of a percutaneous vascular surgical device used to close the femoral artery after catheter interventions for coronary artery disease. *A,* Insertion of the device into the femoral artery. *B,* After the interventional procedure, the device is removed by pulling upward to allow the needles in the device to close the artery. *C,* The sutured artery is secured with a knot pusher. *(Courtesy Perclose, Inc., Redwood City, CA.)*

PATIENT EDUCATION

In most cases, patients undergoing elective angioplasty, atherectomy, or stent procedures are hospitalized for approximately 24 hours. All patients require education about their medication regimen and about risk-factor modification (see the Patient Education feature on Percutaneous Transluminal Coronary Angioplasty, Coronary, Atherectomy, and Stenting). Because of the abbreviated hospital stay, the nurse often has time to do little more than identify the offending risk factors and initiate basic instruction. Patients are referred to local cardiac rehabilitation centers for more extensive teaching and follow-up to facilitate understanding and compliance with risk factor modification.

TABLE 20-8 Vascular Closure Devices

Technology and Examples	Description	Comments
Patch Chito-seal Closur P.A.D. D-Stat Syvek Patch	Patches that contain materials to promote clotting are applied directly to the puncture site, along with manual compression.	Less expensive than active closure devices. No foreign material is left in the patient.
Suture Perclose A.T. Proglide	Sutures deployed through the sheath are used to close the arteriotomy site.	Allows for immediate reaccess through the site if needed (see Fig. 20-16). Device failure may require surgical repair.
Plug or Sealant Angioseal Duett Mynx	Placement of a procoagulant sealant such as collagen or thrombin is used to close the artery. Angioseal also includes an intravascular suture to anchor the collagen plug in place. The Mynx system uses a balloon catheter to inject sealant into the puncture site tract.	Reaccess must be done 1 cm above the previous arterial access site to avoid dislodging the sealant. Extrusion of the sealant into the vessel may compromise the arterial lumen. Components are absorbed within 30-90 days, depending on the sealant used.
Clip or Staple EVS-Angiolink StarClose	Circumferential staples or clips are deployed at the site of the arteriotomy to close the vessel.	Extravascular clip does not compromise the artery lumen.

Patient Education: Percutaneous Transluminal Coronary Angioplasty, Coronary Atherectomy, and Stenting

- Pathophysiology of atherosclerosis
- Risk factor modification (diet, exercise, smoking cessation, weight loss)
- Information about prescribed medications (e.g., antiplatelet agents, nitrates, calcium channel blockers)
- Symptoms to report to the health care professional (chest pain, shortness of breath, bleeding)
- Follow-up appointments

Another point of instruction that must be addressed is the patient's knowledge deficit related to discharge medications. Patients are sent home on a regimen of antiplatelet drugs and drugs for secondary prevention, such as lipid-lowering agents and blood pressure medications. A nitrate such as isosorbide may be prescribed to promote vasodilation, or, if the patient has demonstrated evidence of a vasospastic component to the disease, calcium channel blockers may be used. It is essential that the patient clearly understand the rationale for therapy and the potential side effects of each drug. Patients also need to understand the importance of not discontinuing their antiplatelet therapy; deaths have been reported when patients discontinued this therapy before elective procedures.[49] It is important that patients be provided with written information and a number to call if problems occur.

BOX 20-12 INDICATIONS FOR BALLOON VALVULOPLASTY

AORTIC
- Nonsurgical candidate with incapacitating symptoms
- Patient with aortic stenosis who requires urgent noncardiac surgery
- Patient with severe heart failure or cardiogenic shock because of aortic stenosis whose condition needs to be stabilized until valve replacement is deemed safer
- Patient with poor left ventricular function, low cardiac output, and a small gradient across a stenotic aortic valve whose need for aortic valve replacement requires assessment

MITRAL
- As an alternative to open mitral commissurotomy

PERCUTANEOUS VALVE REPAIR

Percutaneous catheter technology has also been adapted to allow for nonsurgical interventions for stenotic cardiac valves. Percutaneous balloon valvotomy has become an accepted alternative to surgical approaches in patients with mitral or pulmonic valve stenosis. Aortic valvotomy has a limited role in adults, because restenosis and clinical deterioration occur within 6 to 12 months in most patients, and the procedure is associated with significant morbidity and mortality (Box 20-12).[50]

Balloon valvotomy is performed in the cardiac catheterization laboratory. The procedure is similar to a routine cardiac catheterization, including cannulation of the femoral artery and vein with percutaneous introducer sheaths. The balloon dilation catheter is then threaded over a guidewire across the stenotic valvular orifice. The valves may be approached retrograde through the aorta or antegrade across the interatrial septum. In the antegrade transseptal approach, the balloon catheter is passed across the interatrial septum, which results in the creation of a small atrial septal defect.[51] Subsequent inflations of the balloon increase the valve opening by separating fused commissures, cracking calcified leaflets, and stretching valve structures. Inflations are continued until the balloon "waist" disappears, which indicates full inflation. Regurgitant flow can result, particularly after mitral valvotomy, and may result in the need for emergent valve replacement if severe. The risks of balloon valvotomy are similar to those inherent in most catheterization procedures and include cardiac perforation, thromboembolic events, dysrhythmias, and vascular complications caused by the sheath. Postprocedural nursing management is similar to that for other percutaneous cardiac catheter procedures.

A number of additional percutaneous procedures for valve repair are being evaluated in clinical trials. Percutaneous aortic valve replacement has shown promising results as a possible treatment for aortic stenosis. This procedure involves the use of a valvuloplasty balloon catheter to deliver a stainless steel stent with an attached bovine valve within the native aortic valve. After the stent is in position, the balloon is inflated to deploy the stent-valve.[52] Investigational percutaneous treatments for mitral valve repair include correction of mitral regurgitation with a leaflet clip or an annular ring.[53]

CARDIAC SURGERY

Nursing management of the patient undergoing cardiac surgery is demanding but exciting work that requires the talents of an experienced team of critical care nurses. The following discussion introduces basic cardiac surgical techniques and principles of cardiopulmonary bypass and highlights the key points about postoperative care of the adult patient who requires valve replacement or coronary artery revascularization.

CORONARY ARTERY BYPASS SURGERY

Since its introduction more than 2 decades ago, CABG has proved to be safe and effective in relieving uncontrolled angina pectoris in most patients. With lifestyle changes, improved pharmacological therapy and improvements in PCI techniques, much debate has been generated regarding the efficacy of surgical therapy for CAD. Information on "Coronary Artery Disease" is presented in Chapter 19 and "Catheter Interventions for Coronary Artery Disease" are discussed earlier in this chapter.

The combined results of three major randomized trials support the view that CABG affords dramatic improvement of symptoms and quality of life. CABG is more effective than medical therapy (i.e. pharmacologic therapy and PCI) for improving survival in patients with left main coronary artery disease, triple-vessel disease, or double-vessel disease involving the LAD artery and for relief of exercise-induced ischemia or chronic ischemia leading to LV dysfunction. Medical therapy is recommended if the ischemia is prevented by antianginal drugs that are well tolerated by the patient.[54] Surgical revascularization has been shown to be more efficacious than stenting in patients with multivessel disease.[55] If arterial grafts are used, CABG has superior long-term patency rates, surpassing those of angioplasty or stents.[56] Bypass surgery may allow for more complete revascularization, because it can be used on vessels that are not amenable to treatment with a percutaneous approach, such as those with total occlusions or excessive tortuosity.

The anticipated length of stay for CABG ranges from 5 to 9 days. The longer length of stay is for patients who undergo cardiac catheterization and CABG surgery.

Myocardial revascularization involves the use of a conduit, or channel, designed to bypass an occluded coronary artery. The two most common conduits are the saphenous vein graft and the internal mammary artery (IMA) graft. Saphenous vein grafting involves the anastomosis of an excised portion of the saphenous vein proximal to the aorta and distal to the coronary artery below the obstruction (Fig. 20-17). Traditionally, the saphenous vein graft was obtained through an open incision, but endoscopic harvesting of this vessel is now possible. This minimally invasive technique of graft procurement decreases postoperative pain and reduces leg wound infection.[57]

The IMA, which usually remains attached to its origin at the subclavian artery, is swung down and anastomosed distal to the coronary artery (Fig. 20-18). Either the right IMA or the left IMA may be used as a conduit. Of note, emergency CABG may preclude the use of the IMA because of the extra time required to mobilize the artery and the inability to effect cardioplegia through this conduit. However, the current trend is to use arterial conduits such as the IMA whenever possible, because their long-term patency rates are superior to those of the saphenous vein graft.[58]

The right gastroepiploic artery (GEA) has also been introduced as an alternative conduit for CABG. The artery, which is a branch of the gastroduodenal artery, is pulled up to the pericardial cavity and anastomosed to a distal portion of the coronary artery (Fig. 20-19). Although it is a little smaller in diameter than the IMA, studies indicate that patency rates are excellent.[59] Because of its size and anatomic location, the gastroepiploic artery is well suited for bypassing the right coronary artery, the circumflex artery, or the posterior descending artery. However, the technical aspects of obtaining this conduit may limit its widespread use.

The potential benefit of long-term patency associated with arterial conduits has revived interest in the use of radial artery grafts. First introduced as a potential conduit for myocardial revascularization in the 1970s, radial artery grafts were

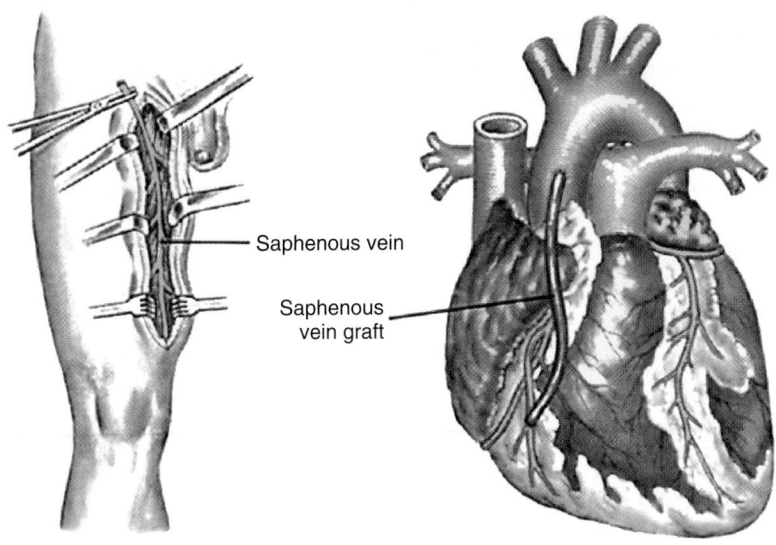

Saphenous vein

Saphenous
vein graft

Figure 20-17 Saphenous vein graft.

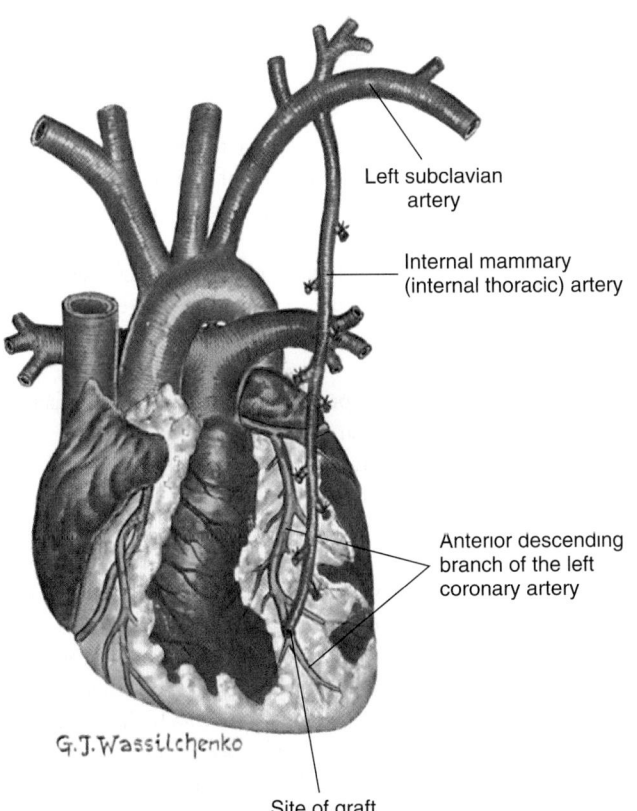

Left subclavian
artery

Internal mammary
(internal thoracic) artery

Anterior descending
branch of the left
coronary artery

G.J.Wassilchenko

Site of graft

Figure 20-18 Internal mammary artery graft.

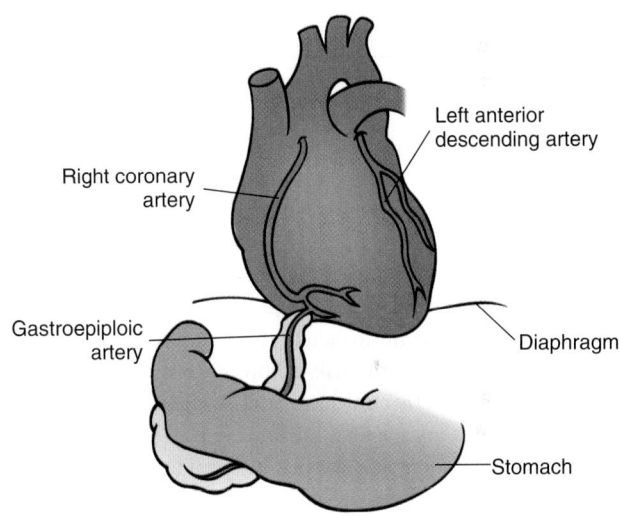

Left anterior
descending artery

Right coronary
artery

Gastroepiploic
artery

Diaphragm

Stomach

Figure 20-19 Gastroepiploic artery graft.

VALVULAR SURGERY

Valvular disease results in various hemodynamic dysfunctions that usually can be managed medically as long as the patient remains symptom-free. There is reluctance to intervene surgically early in the course of this disease because of the surgical risks and long-term complications associated with prosthetic valve replacement. These consequences, however, must be weighed against the possibility of irreversible deterioration in LV function that may develop during the compensated asymptomatic phase (see "Valvular Heart Disease" in Chapter 19).

Surgical therapy for aortic valve disease consists primarily of aortic valve replacement, although repairs may be done for selected regurgitant valves.[51] Three surgical procedures are available to treat mitral valve disease: commissurotomy, valve repair, and valve replacement. Commissurotomy is performed for mitral stenosis; the fused leaflets are incised, and calcium deposits are

abandoned because of a high incidence of early graft occlusion and vasospasm. Current early patency rates of 90% or better have been attributed to improved harvesting techniques and the use of postoperative calcium channel blockers to minimize vasospasm.[60] A comparison of conduits used for myocardial revascularization is provided in Table 20-9.

TABLE 20-9 Conduits Used for Coronary Artery Bypass Grafts

Type of Graft	Advantages	Disadvantages
Saphenous vein	Easily harvested Length allows for multiple grafts No anatomic limitations to graft sites	Long-term patency is not as good as that of arterial grafts Requires at least two anastomosis sites Associated with leg edema postoperatively
Internal mammary artery	Improved patency over venous grafts Requires only one anastomosis	Requires extensive dissection Not accessible for emergency bypass Associated with increased chest wall discomfort postoperatively Anatomic limitations to bypassing some areas of the heart
Gastroepiploic artery	Improved patency over venous grafts Requires only one anastomosis Associated with increased gastrointestinal complications postoperatively	Technically difficult to harvest Not accessible for emergency bypass Anatomic limitations to bypassing some areas of the heart
Radial artery	Improved patency over venous grafts Easily harvested	Requires adequate collateral flow to the hand through the ulnar artery May be associated with higher rates of vasospasm Requires two anastomosis sites

débrided to increase valve mobility. Repair of damaged leaflets may be accomplished with pericardial patches. In the setting of mitral regurgitation, valve repair may include reshaping of the leaflets and the use of a ring to reduce the size of the dilated mitral annulus, enhancing leaflet coaptation (annuloplasty). Although it is technically more demanding, valve repair is preferred over replacement to avoid the complications inherent with a prosthetic valve: the risk of thromboembolic events and the need for long-term anticoagulation.[61] If reconstruction of the mitral valve is not possible, it is replaced.

The patient undergoing valvular surgery has an anticipated length of hospital stay from 5 to 9 days. The longer length of stay is for patients who undergo cardiac catheterization in addition to valvular surgery. Prosthetic valves are designed with an orifice, through which blood flows, and an occluding structure that opens and closes. The two categories of prosthetic valves are mechanical valves and biologic valves, or tissue valves. *Mechanical valves* are made from combinations of metal alloys, Pyrolite carbon, Dacron, and Teflon and have rigid occluding devices (Fig. 20-20). Their construction renders them highly durable, but all patients with mechanical valves require anticoagulation to reduce the incidence of thromboembolism. *Biologic valves* are constructed from animal or human cardiac tissue and have flexible occluding mechanisms. Because of their low thrombogenicity, tissue valves offer the patient freedom from therapeutic anticoagulation. Their durability, however, is limited by their tendency toward early calcification. Box 20-13 provides a description of various valvular prostheses.

The first mechanical valve had a ball-in-cage design. The Starr-Edwards valve is the only example of this type of valve still in use today. Later valves used a tilting-disk mechanism to occlude blood flow. The Björk-Shiley tilting-disk valve was discontinued in the United States because of mechanical failure, but patients with this valve are still alive today. Most valves used today have a bi-leaflet design, the first of which was introduced by St. Jude Medical in 1977. One of the primary goals in mechanical valve research is to design a valve that can alleviate the causes of thrombosis: surface roughness, turbulent flow, and stagnation in valve pivots. Two of the newest valves on the market, the ATS and the On-X, offer several new improvements in this area.[62]

The choice of a valvular prosthesis depends on many factors. Because mechanical valves are more durable, for example, they may be preferred for a young person who is anticipated to have a relatively long life span ahead. Similarly, a bioprosthesis (tissue valve) may be chosen for an elderly patient; the valve has a reduced longevity, but this disadvantage is offset by the older patient's shorter life expectancy.[51] For patients with medical contraindications to anticoagulation and for those whose past compliance with drug therapy has been questionable, a tissue valve may be selected. Technical considerations, such as the size of the annulus (or the anatomic ring in which the valve sits), also can influence the choice of valve; for example, a bioprosthesis may be too big for a small aortic root.

CARDIOPULMONARY BYPASS

Cardiopulmonary bypass is a mechanical means of circulating and oxygenating a patient's blood while diverting most of the circulation from the heart and lungs during cardiac surgical procedures. The extracorporeal circuit consists of cannulas that drain off venous blood, an oxygenator that oxygenates the blood by one of several methods, and a pump head that pumps the arterialized blood back to the aorta through a single cannula. The patient is systemically heparinized before initiation of bypass to prevent clotting within the bypass circuit.

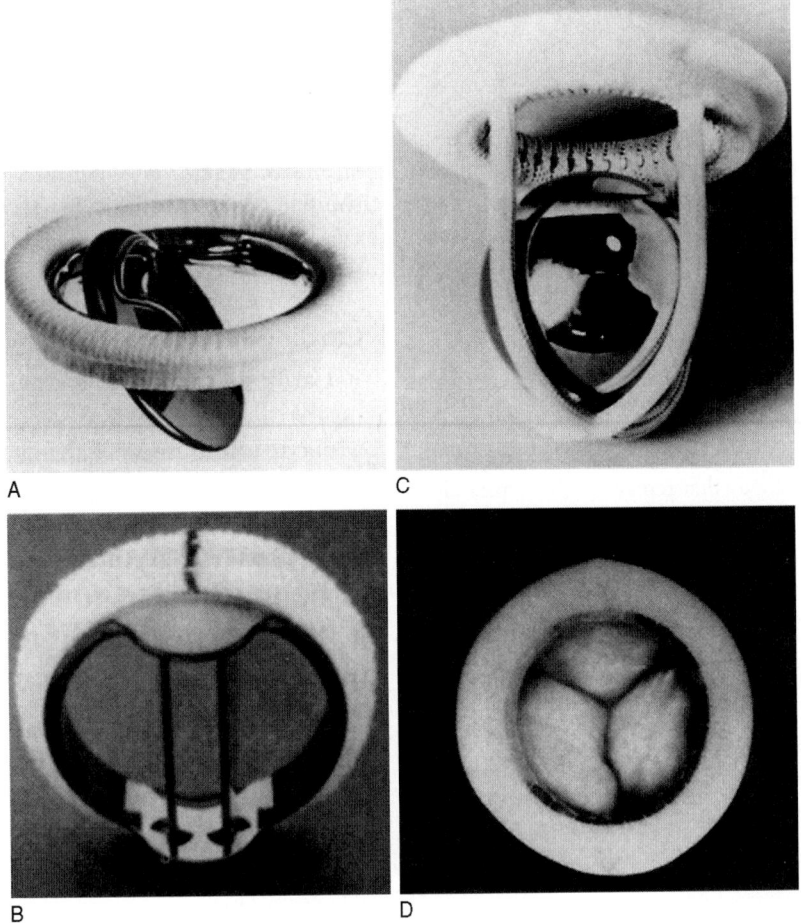

Figure 20-20 Prosthetic valves. *A,* The Björk-Shiley tilting-disk valve has a pyrolytic-carbon disk, Stellite cage, and Teflon cloth sewing ring. The valve opens to 60 degrees. *B,* The Starr-Edwards caged-ball valve model 6320, with a completely cloth-covered Stellite cage and a hollow Stellite ball, has a specific gravity approximating that of blood. *C,* The St. Jude Medical mechanical heart valve is a mechanical central-flow disk. *D,* In the Hancock II porcine aortic valve, the flexible Derlin stent and sewing ring are covered in Dacron cloth. *(A, B, and D from Eagle K et al, editors:* The practice of cardiology, *ed 2, Boston, 1989, Little, Brown; C, courtesy St Jude Medical, Inc., Copyright 1993, St. Paul, MN.)*

BOX 20-13   CLASSIFICATION OF PROSTHETIC CARDIAC VALVES

MECHANICAL VALVES
Caged-ball: a ball that moves freely within a three- or four-sided metallic cage mounted on a circular sewing ring
- Starr-Edwards

   Tilting-disk: a free-floating, lens-shaped disk mounted on a circular sewing ring
- Björk-Shiley (discontinued)
- Medtronic Hall
- Omniscience
- Monostrut

   Bi-leaflet: two semicircular leaflets, mounted on a circular sewing ring that opens centrally
- St. Jude Medical
- Duromedics

- CarboMedics
- On-X ATS

BIOLOGIC OR TISSUE VALVES (BIOPROSTHESES)
Porcine heterograft: a porcine aortic valve mounted on a semiflexible stent and preserved in glutaraldehyde
- Hancock
- Carpentier-Edwards
- Toronto Stentless (St. Jude)
- Free Style Stentless (Medtronic)

   Homograft: a human heart valve (aortic or pulmonic) harvested from a donated heart and cryopreserved; may or may not be mounted on a support ring

Systemic hypothermia during bypass can reduce tissue oxygen requirements to 50% of normal, which affords the major organs additional protection from ischemic injury. Lowering the body temperature to about 28° C (82.4° F) is accomplished through a heat exchanger incorporated into the pump. The blood is warmed to normal body temperature before bypass is discontinued.

The technique of hemodilution also is used to enhance tissue oxygenation by improving blood flow through the systemic and pulmonary microcirculation during bypass. *Hemodilution* refers to the dilution of the patient's own (autologous) blood with the isotonic crystalloid solution used to prime the pump. Capillary perfusion is enhanced by hemodilution, because the reduced viscosity (stickiness) of the blood decreases both resistance to flow through the capillaries and the possibility of microthrombi formation. At the completion of cardiopulmonary bypass, the large quantities of "pump blood" that remain in the bypass circuit can be collected and used for initial postoperative volume replacement.

In response to findings that the low cardiac output syndrome often seen postoperatively might be a result of intraoperative myocardial ischemia or necrosis, efforts have been directed toward providing additional protection to the myocardium during bypass. Rapidly stopping the heart in diastole by perfusing the coronary arteries with a cold potassium cardioplegic (heart-paralyzing) agent has been the method of choice for intraoperative myocardial protection. Continued research in this area has resulted in the emergence of blood as a vehicle for the cardioplegic components to enhance the supply of oxygen and nutrients to the arrested myocardial cells.[63] Warm (normothermic) cardioplegia may also be used and is believed by some to result in less ventricular dysfunction postoperatively.[64] Regardless of the type of cardioplegic solution used, it must be reinfused at regular intervals during bypass to keep the heart in an arrested state and to minimize myocardial oxygen requirements.

Numerous clinical sequelae can result from cardiopulmonary bypass (Table 20-10). Knowledge of these physiologic effects allows the nurse to anticipate problems and intervene effectively.

POSTOPERATIVE MANAGEMENT

Medical and nursing management of the postoperative cardiac surgery patient are often overlapping. The physician prescribes therapeutic interventions and identifies specific hemodynamic end points that are individualized for each patient. The nurse

---

TABLE 20-10 Physiologic Effects of Cardiopulmonary Bypass

Effects	Causes
Intravascular fluid deficit (hypotension)	Third-spacing Postoperative diuresis Sudden vasodilation (drugs, rewarming)
Third-spacing (weight gain, edema)	Decreased plasma protein concentration Increased capillary permeability
Myocardial depression (decreased cardiac output)	Hypothermia Increased systemic vascular resistance Prolonged cardiopulmonary bypass pump run Preexisting heart disease Inadequate myocardial protection
Coagulopathy (bleeding)	Systemic heparinization Mechanical trauma to platelets Depressed release of clotting factors from liver as a result of hypothermia
Pulmonary dysfunction (decreased lung mechanics and impaired gas exchange)	Decreased surfactant production Pulmonary microemboli Interstitial fluid accumulation in lungs
Hemolysis (hemoglobinuria)	Red blood cells damaged in pump circuit
Hyperglycemia (rise in serum glucose concentration)	Decreased insulin release Stimulation of glycogenolysis
Hypokalemia (low serum potassium concentration)	Intracellular shifts during bypass and postoperative diuresis
Hypomagnesemia (low serum magnesium concentration)	Postoperative diuresis resulting from hemodilution
Neurologic dysfunction (decreased level of consciousness, motor/sensory deficits)	Inadequate cerebral perfusion Microemboli to brain (air, plaque fragments, fat globules)
Hypertension (transient rise in blood pressure)	Catecholamine release and systemic hypothermia causing vasoconstriction

is then responsible for applying these therapies to maintain the patient's hemodynamic parameters within the desired range. For example, orders may be written to maintain the patient's blood pressure, filling pressures, cardiac output, and systemic vascular resistance (SVR) within a desired range, using a combination of volume, vasodilator, and inotropic infusions. In most institutions, standard protocols are used to facilitate the postoperative nursing diagnoses and management of cardiac surgical patients (see the Nursing Diagnoses feature on Open Heart Surgery).

Cardiovascular Support. Postoperative cardiovascular support often is indicated because of a low output state resulting from preexisting heart disease, a prolonged cardiopulmonary bypass pump run, inadequate myocardial protection, or some combination of these factors. Cardiac output can be maximized by adjustments in heart rate, preload, afterload, and contractility.

Heart Rate. In the presence of low cardiac output, the heart rate can be appropriately regulated by means of temporary pacing or drug therapy. Temporary epicardial pacing usually is instituted when the heart rate of the adult patient who has had cardiac surgery drops to less than 80 beats/min. In the case of tachycardia, intravenous beta-blockers (esmolol) or calcium channel blockers (diltiazem) may be used in the acute postoperative period to slow supraventricular rhythms with a ventricular response that exceeds 110 beats/min. Because ventricular ectopy can result from hypokalemia, serum potassium levels are maintained in the high-normal range (4.5 to 5 mEq/L) to provide some margin for error. Maintaining serum magnesium in a therapeutic range (2 mEq/L) has also been shown to reduce the incidence of dysrhythmias in the postoperative period.[65]

Nursing Diagnoses

Open Heart Surgery

- Decreased Cardiac Output related to alterations in preload
- Decreased Cardiac Output related to alterations in afterload
- Decreased Cardiac Output related to alterations in contractility
- Decreased Cardiac Output related to alterations in heart rate or rhythm
- Impaired Gas Exchange related to ventilation/perfusion mismatching or intrapulmonary shunting
- Ineffective Airway Clearance related to excessive secretions or abnormal viscosity of mucus
- Activity Intolerance related to cardiopulmonary dysfunction
- Deficient Fluid Volume related to absolute loss
- Risk for Infection related to invasive procedures
- Acute Pain related to transmission and perception of cutaneous, visceral, muscular, or ischemic impulses
- Anxiety related to threat to biologic, psychological, or social integrity
- Disturbed Sleep Pattern related to fragmented sleep
- Deficient Knowledge: Discharge Regimen related to lack of previous exposure to information (see the Patient Education feature on Open Heart Surgery)

Atrial fibrillation occurs in one third of patients after cardiac surgery, with a peak occurrence in the first 2 to 3 days after surgery. This rhythm may induce hemodynamic compromise, prolong hospitalization, and increase the patient's risk of stroke. Prophylactic administration of antidysrhythmic agents such as beta-blockers has been shown to decrease the incidence of atrial fibrillation and its clinical sequelae.[66]

Preload. In most patients, reduced preload is the cause of low postoperative cardiac output. If a pulmonary artery catheter has been inserted during surgery, monitoring of the pulmonary artery occlusion pressure (PAOP), also known as the *wedge pressure*, can provide a more convenient and accurate guide to LV preload than monitoring of central venous pressure (CVP) alone. To enhance preload, volume may be administered in the form of crystalloid, colloid, or packed red cells. It is not uncommon to achieve the greatest hemodynamic stability in cardiac surgery patients when filling pressures (PAOP or pulmonary artery diastolic pressure [PADP]) are in the range of 18 to 20 mm Hg (normally 5 to 12 mm Hg).

Afterload. Partly as a result of the peripheral vasoconstrictive effects of hypothermia, many patients who have had cardiac surgery demonstrate postoperative hypertension. Although it is transient, postoperative hypertension can precipitate or exacerbate bleeding from the mediastinal chest tubes. The high SVR (afterload) resulting from the intense vasoconstriction can increase LV workload. Vasodilator therapy with intravenous sodium nitroprusside or nitroglycerin often is used to reduce afterload, control hypertension, and improve cardiac output.

A significant percentage of patients experience hypotension after cardiopulmonary bypass, associated with peripheral vasodilation and a low SVR. This is believed to occur, in part, because of the systemic inflammatory response to cardiopulmonary bypass. Therapy for hypotension after cardiac surgery usually includes volume loading and vasopressors such as phenylephrine or vasopressin to tighten the peripheral vasculature and maintain an adequate mean arterial pressure.[67]

Contractility. If the adjustments in heart rate, preload, and afterload fail to produce significant improvement in cardiac output, contractility can be enhanced with positive inotropic support or intraaortic balloon pumping (IABP) to augment circulation (discussed later).

Temperature Regulation. Hypothermia can contribute to depressed myocardial contractility in the patient who has had cardiac surgery. Hypothermia may contribute to postoperative bleeding, because the functioning of clotting factors is depressed during hypothermia. After surgery, patients may be rewarmed with the use of warmed air or water blankets. To prevent subsequent excessive temperature elevations, care must be taken to remove the blankets promptly when the body temperature reaches 98.6° F (37° C).

Control of Bleeding. Postoperative bleeding from the mediastinal chest tubes can be caused by inadequate hemostasis, disruption of suture lines, or coagulopathy associated with cardiopulmonary bypass or hypothermia. Bleeding is more likely to occur with IMA grafts as a result of the extensive chest wall dissection required to free the IMA. If bleeding in excess of 150 mL/hr occurs early in the postoperative period, clotting factors (fresh-frozen plasma, fibrinogen, and platelets) and additional protamine (used to reverse the effects of heparin) may be administered, along with prompt blood replacement. Other medications used in the treatment of postoperative bleeding are described in Table 20-11.

Autotransfusion devices, which facilitate the collection and reinfusion of shed mediastinal blood, previously were used in some institutions. Routine autotransfusion of shed mediastinal blood is no longer recommended, because it may further exacerbate bleeding by activating the extrinsic clotting pathway and increase the risk of infection.[68] The use of positive end-expiratory pressure (PEEP) in conjunction with mechanical ventilation may be helpful in controlling excessive bleeding in some cases by increasing the intrathoracic pressure enough to effect tamponade of oozing mediastinal blood vessels.[68] Rewarming the patient reverses the depressed manufacture and release of clotting factors that results from hypothermia. However, persistent mediastinal bleeding—usually in excess of 500 mL in 1 hour or 300 mL/hr for 2 consecutive hours despite normalization of clotting studies—is an indication for re-exploration of the surgical site.

Chest Tube Patency.
Chest tube stripping to maintain patency of the tubes is controversial because of the high negative pressure generated by routine methods of stripping. It is believed to result in tissue damage that can contribute to bleeding. This risk must be carefully weighed against the real danger of cardiac tamponade if blood is not effectively drained from around the heart. Chest tube stripping often is advocated in instances of excessive postoperative bleeding. However, the technique of "milking" the chest tubes is advisable for routine postoperative care, because this technique generates less negative pressure and decreases the risk of bleeding.

Cardiac Tamponade.
Cardiac tamponade may occur after surgery if blood accumulates in the mediastinal space, impairing the heart's ability to pump. Signs of tamponade include elevated and equalized filling pressures (e.g., CVP, PADP, PAOP), decreased cardiac output, decreased blood pressure, jugular venous distention, pulsus paradoxus, muffled heart sounds, sudden cessation of chest tube drainage, and a widened cardiac silhouette on chest x-ray films. Interventions for tamponade may include emergency sternotomy in the intensive care unit or a return to the operating room for surgical evacuation of the clot.

Pulmonary Care.
Until recently, overnight intubation to facilitate lung expansion and optimize gas exchange was common for patients who had undergone cardiac surgery. Newer protocols that facilitate early extubation (within the first 4 to 8 hours) have been implemented in most institutions.[69] Early extubation requires a multidisciplinary approach that incorporates anesthesiologists, surgeons, nurses, and respiratory therapists. Potential candidates must be identified before surgery so that the anesthetic regimen can be modified to support early extubation. One approach is to use short-acting anesthetic agents such as propofol (Diprivan) at the end of the surgery and to minimize the use of opioids. Another option is to administer neostigmine and glycopyrrolate at the end of the surgery, to reverse the neuromuscular blockade used during the procedure.

After surgery, patients are evaluated for hemodynamic stability, adequate control of bleeding, and normothermia. After these criteria have been met, the patient is weaned off propofol or given neuromuscular reversal agents, and ventilator weaning can begin. If needed, opioids are given in small increments to manage pain and anxiety. Patients who exhibit hemodynamic instability or intraoperative complications or who have underlying pulmonary disease related to long-term valvular dysfunction may require longer periods of mechanical ventilation. After extubation, supplemental oxygen is administered, and patients are medicated for incisional pain to facilitate adequate coughing and deep breathing.

Neurologic Complications.
The transient neurologic dysfunction often seen in patients who have had cardiac surgery has been attributed to decreased cerebral perfusion, cerebral microemboli, and the systemic inflammatory response. It was once thought to be primarily caused by cardiopulmonary bypass, but newer evidence indicates that cognitive decline may be influenced more by patient-related factors such as the degree of preexisting cerebral vascular disease or diabetes.[70] Compounding these are environmental factors such as sensory deprivation and sensory overload associated with being in a critical care unit. The term *postcardiotomy delirium* has been used to describe this postoperative syndrome that initially may manifest as only a mild impairment of orientation but that may progress to agitation, hallucinations, and paranoid delusions. One study indicated that mild preoperative cognitive impairment might be a useful predictor of who is likely to develop postcardiotomy delirium.[71]

TABLE 20-11 Pharmacologic Management: Postoperative Bleeding		
DRUG	**DOSE**	**ACTION AND SIDE EFFECTS**
Amicaproic acid (Amicar)	Loading dose: 5 g over 1 hr, followed by continuous infusion of 1 g/hr for 8 hr or until bleeding is controlled	Inhibits conversion of plasminogen to plasmin to prevent fibrinolysis, helping to stabilize clots
Desmopressin acetate (DDAVP)	0.3 mg/kg IV over 20-30 min	Improves platelet function by increasing levels of factor VIII. Side effects include facial flushing, tachycardia, headache, and hypotension
Protamine sulfate	25-30 mg IV slowly over 10 min	Neutralizes the anticoagulant effect of heparin. Can cause hypotension, bradycardia, and allergic reactions

Treatment of delirium may require the use of medications such as benzodiazepines or haloperidol (Haldol). Environmental modifications such as noise reduction, restoring normal day/night lighting patterns, and placing familiar objects at the bedside may help to calm and reorient the patient. Liberalization of visitation policies to allow family members a prolonged presence at the bedside is also highly desirable. Nursing management is organized to maximize optimal sleep patterns whenever possible.

Infection. Postoperative fever is fairly common after cardiopulmonary bypass. However, persistent temperature elevation to greater than 101° F (38.3° C) must be investigated. Sternal wound infections and infective endocarditis are the most devastating infectious complications, but leg wound infection, pneumonia, and urinary tract infection also can occur. Infection rates are greater in diabetic patients. Studies have shown that maintaining the blood glucose concentration between 80 and 110 mg/dL in the perioperative period by means of a continuous insulin infusion may decrease the risk of infection in this population.[72]

Kidney Involvement. Hemolysis caused by trauma to the red blood cells in the extracorporeal circuit results in hemoglobinuria, which can damage kidney tubules. Small amounts of furosemide (Lasix) usually are given to promote urine flow if the urine output is low (<25 to 30 mL/hr) and tinged pink.

Guidelines for Coronary Artery Bypass Grafting. The American College of Cardiology and the American Heart Association have developed a set of clinical practice guidelines for care of the patient undergoing CABG.[54] These guidelines are designed to support clinical decision making with research evidence (see the Evidence-Based Practice feature on Coronary Artery Bypass Graft Surgery).

Evidence-Based Practice: Collaborative

Coronary Artery Bypass Graft Surgery

A summary is provided of evidence and evidence-based review recommendations for management of the coronary artery bypass graft (CABG) surgery patient.

Strong Evidence to Support CABG in the Following Circumstances
CABG for Stable and Unstable Angina
- Significant left main coronary artery stenosis.
- Left main equivalent stenosis: significant (≥70%) stenosis of the proximal left anterior descending (LAD) artery and proximal left circumflex artery.
- Three-vessel disease. Survival benefit is greater in patients with abnormal left ventricular function; such as left ventricular ejection fraction (LVEF) less than 0.50 (50%), or large areas of demonstrable myocardial ischemia.
- One- or two-vessel disease plus extensive ischemia and LVEF less than 0.50 (50%).
- Disabling or unstable angina despite maximal noninvasive therapy if surgery can be performed with acceptable risk. If the angina is not typical, objective evidence of ischemia should be obtained.
- Unstable angina or non–ST-elevation myocardial infarction (NSTEMI) if emergency percutaneous coronary intervention (PCI) revascularization is not optimal or possible, or ongoing ischemia is not responsive to maximal nonsurgical therapy.

CABG during ST-Elevation Myocardial Infarction
- Emergent or urgent CABG in patients with ST-elevation myocardial infarction (STEMI) should be undertaken in the following circumstances:
  1. Failed angioplasty with persistent pain or hemodynamic instability in patients with coronary anatomy suitable for surgery
  2. Persistent or recurrent ischemia refractory to medical therapy in patients with coronary anatomy suitable for surgery who have a significant area of myocardium at risk and who are not candidates for PCI
  3. At the time of surgical repair of postinfarction ventricular septal rupture or mitral valve insufficiency

4. Cardiogenic shock in patients younger than 75 years old with STEMI or left bundle-branch block or posterior myocardial infarction (MI) who develop shock within 36 hours after MI and are suitable candidates for revascularization that can be performed within 18 hours after shock, unless further support is futile because of the patient's wishes or because of contraindications or unsuitability for further invasive care

CABG Criteria for Life-Threatening Ventricular Dysrhythmias
- Life-threatening ventricular dysrhythmias in the presence of left main coronary artery stenosis greater than or equal to 50% or three-vessel coronary disease.

CABG Plus Valve Surgery Criteria
- Patients undergoing CABG who also have severe aortic stenosis should undergo aortic valve replacement (AVR). Severe aortic stenosis is measured by a mean gradient greater than or equal to 50 mm Hg or a Doppler velocity greater than or equal to 4 m/sec.

Reduction in Intraoperative Complications
- Significant atherosclerosis of the ascending aorta mandates a surgical approach that minimizes the possibility of arteriosclerotic emboli and stroke.
- Blood cardioplegia should be considered in patients undergoing cardiopulmonary bypass accompanying CABG surgery for acute MI or unstable angina.
- In every patient undergoing CABG, the left internal mammary artery should be given primary consideration for revascularization of the LAD artery.

Transmyocardial Revascularization
- Transmyocardial surgical laser revascularization, alone or in combination with CABG surgery, is reasonable in patients with angina refractory to medical therapy who are not candidates for PCI or surgical revascularization.

Reduction in Risk of Infection
- Preoperative antibiotic administration should be used in all patients to reduce the risk of postoperative infection.

Continued

Evidence-Based Practice: Collaborative—*cont'd*

- A deep sternal wound infection should be treated with aggressive surgical débridement and early revascularized muscle flap coverage, unless there are complicating circumstances.

Prevention of Postoperative Dysrhythmias

- Preoperative or early postoperative administration of beta-blockers in patients without contraindications should be used as the standard therapy to reduce the incidence and clinical sequelae of atrial fibrillation after CABG surgery.

Antiplatelet Therapy

- Aspirin is the drug of choice for prophylaxis against early saphenous vein graft closure.
- If clinical circumstances permit, clopidogrel should be withheld for 5 days before the performance of CABG surgery.

Pharmacologic Management of Hyperlipidemia

- All CABG surgery patients should receive statin therapy unless otherwise contraindicated.

Smoking Cessation Is Important

- All smokers should receive educational counseling and be offered smoking cessation therapy after CABG surgery.
- Pharmacologic therapy including nicotine replacement and bupropion (in selected patients) should be offered to patients indicating a willingness to quit.

Cardiac Rehabilitation Is Beneficial

- Cardiac rehabilitation should be offered to all eligible patients after CABG.

Moderate Evidence Exists to Support the Following

Assessment of Preoperative Risk

- Preoperative statistical risk models may be used to obtain objective estimates of cardiac surgical operative mortality.
- After MI that leads to clinically significant right ventricular dysfunction, it is reasonable to delay surgery for 4 weeks to allow recovery.

CABG Risk-Benefit Analysis for Stable and Unstable Angina

- CABG can be beneficial for patients who have proximal or nonproximal LAD stenosis with one- or two-vessel disease. The decision depends on extent of ischemia and LVEF (see section on *Strong Evidence*).

CABG during ST-Elevation Myocardial Infarction

- CABG may be performed as primary reperfusion in patients who have suitable anatomy, who are not candidates for or have had previous failed fibrinolysis or PCI, and who are not in the early hours (6 to 12 hours) of evolving STEMI. In patients who have had a STEMI or an NSTEMI, CABG mortality is elevated for the first 3 to 7 days after infarction, and the benefit of revascularization must be balanced against this increased risk. Beyond 7 days after infarction, the revascularization criteria described in the section on *Strong Evidence* are applicable.

CABG Plus Valve Surgery Criteria

- For patients with a preoperative diagnosis of clinically significant mitral regurgitation, concomitant mitral valve repair or replacement at the time of CABG is probably indicated.
- For patients undergoing CABG who have moderate aortic stenosis, concomitant AVR is probably indicated. Moderate aortic stenosis is measured by a mean transvalve gradient of 30 to 50 mm Hg or a Doppler velocity of 3 to 4 m/sec.
- Patients undergoing CABG who have mild aortic stenosis may be considered candidates for AVR if the risk of the combined procedure is acceptable. Mild aortic stenosis is measured by a mean gradient less than 30 mm Hg or a Doppler velocity less than 3 m/sec.

Reduction in Risk of Thrombus Formation

- After cardiac surgery, patients with atrial fibrillation that is recurrent or that persists longer than 24 hours should receive warfarin anticoagulation for 4 weeks.
- Long-term anticoagulation (3 to 6 months) is indicated for the patient with recent anteroapical infarct and persistent wall-motion abnormality after CABG surgery.
- Preoperative screening with echocardiography is considered for patients who have had a recent anterior MI to detect left ventricular thrombus; if thrombus is present, the timing or surgical approach may be altered.

Reduction in Risk of Carotid Disease and Stroke

- Carotid endarterectomy is probably indicated before CABG surgery or concomitant with CABG in patients who have a symptomatic carotid stenosis and in asymptomatic patients who have a unilateral or bilateral internal carotid stenosis of 80% or greater.
- Carotid screening is probably indicated in the following subsets of patients: age greater than 65 years, left main coronary artery stenosis, peripheral arterial disease, history of smoking, history of transient ischemic attack or stroke, carotid bruit on examination.

Cardiac Biomarker Elevation and Outcome

- Assessment of cardiac biomarkers in the first 24 hours after CABG may be considered. Patients with the highest elevations of creatine kinase-MB (>5 times the upper limit of normal) are at increased risk for subsequent adverse events.

Adjuncts to Myocardial Protection

- Use of prophylactic intraaortic balloon pump (IABP) support as an adjunct to myocardial protection is probably indicated in patients with evidence of ongoing myocardial ischemia or a subnormal cardiac index.

Reduction in Risk of Infection

- The risk for deep sternal wound infection is reduced by aggressive control of perioperative hyperglycemia with a continuous intravenous insulin infusion.

Prevention of Postoperative Dysrhythmias

- Preoperative administration of amiodarone reduces the incidence of postcardiotomy atrial fibrillation and is an appropriate prophylactic therapy for patients at high risk for postoperative atrial fibrillation who have contraindications to therapy with beta-blockers (see section on *Strong Evidence*).
- Digoxin and nondihydropyridine calcium channel blockers are useful for control of ventricular rate but at present have no indication for prophylactic use.
- Low-dose sotalol can be considered to reduce the incidence of atrial fibrillation after CABG in patients who are not candidates for traditional beta-blockers.

Reference

Eagel A et al: ACC/AHA 2004 guideline update for coronary artery bypass surgery: a report of the American College of Cardiology/American Heart Association Task Force on Practice Guidelines (Committee to Update the 1999 Guidelines for Coronary Artery Bypass Graft Surgery). *Circulation* 110(14):e340-e437, 2004.

PATIENT EDUCATION

Patient education includes information related to the surgical procedure, risk factor management, and prevention of atherosclerosis. Patients who have undergone valve surgery may also require information regarding the need for antibiotic prophylaxis before invasive procedures and specific instructions pertaining to their anticoagulation regimen (see the Patient Education feature on Open Heart Surgery).

TECHNICAL ADVANCES

Minimally Invasive Cardiac Surgery. Over the past decade, new techniques have been developed to address some of the problems associated with traditional cardiac surgery procedures. Many of these procedures can be accomplished without a median sternotomy, by means of a series of holes, or ports, in the chest and small thoracotomy incisions. CABG or valve surgery is then be performed using a thoracoscope for visualization and specially designed instruments.[73] As technology has improved, minimally invasive procedures have become an option for an expanding number of patients.[74] These procedures may be performed without cardiopulmonary bypass ("off-pump" or "beating heart") or with a less invasive, catheter-based system of cardiopulmonary bypass with access through the femoral artery and vein.[73]

In an effort to avoid the adverse effects of cardiopulmonary bypass, off-pump coronary artery bypass (OPCAB) is performed in approximately 20% to 30% of cases.[74] A variety of incisional approaches can be used. In minimally invasive direct coronary artery bypass graft (MIDCABG) surgery, a small left anterior thoracotomy incision is used to directly harvest the left IMA, which is then anastomosed to the LAD artery. Alternative approaches may use a segment of saphenous vein or radial artery, one end of which is attached to the left IMA and the other to accessible coronary arteries.[73] Some surgeons may opt for a standard median sternotomy approach to allow for bypassing of distal vessels. Several techniques are used to stabilize the operative area

during an OPCAB procedure. Immobilization devices that use compression or suction to create an immobile area have been developed to stabilize cardiac wall motion at the site of the anastomosis. Drugs that temporarily decrease the heart rate (e.g., esmolol, diltiazem) or cause transient cardiac asystole (e.g., adenosine) may also be used to further limit cardiac motion.[74]

Results from OPCAB surgery have been mixed. Some studies have demonstrated improvements in morbidity, including decreased transfusion requirements, shortened time on the ventilator, decreased length of stay, and a lower incidence of stroke and renal complications.[75] Others have shown no advantage over conventional surgery.[76,77] OPCAB may be most beneficial in patients with significant comorbid conditions and in those with contraindications to cardiopulmonary bypass.[78]

Minimally invasive procedures will continue to be refined with the use of robotic equipment in cardiac surgery, currently under clinical investigation at a small number of centers. Robotic-assisted surgery allows the surgeon to view a computer-enhanced image while manipulating instruments through small portholes using robotic arms. This provides increased surgical precision and the ability to perform conventional procedures with smaller incisions.[73]

Transmyocardial Revascularization. Transmyocardial revascularization (TMR) is a surgical technique for the treatment of severe CAD that is not amenable to traditional revascularization procedures.[79] In this procedure, a laser is used to create full-thickness channels in the ventricular wall to increase blood flow to ischemic areas. TMR may be performed alone or in conjunction with CABG in an effort to improve myocardial oxygenation, reduce angina, and improve the patient's functional status.

The surgical version of this procedure involves an anterolateral thoracotomy for exposure of the LV. The procedure is performed on a beating heart without the use of cardiopulmonary bypass in patients under general anesthesia. Approximately 20 to 40 channels are created in the myocardial wall with laser bursts timed to occur when the ventricle is full of blood. Bleeding is controlled with manual pressure at the laser site. After surgery, patients are monitored in the critical care unit to allow for detection and treatment of dysrhythmias, myocardial ischemia, and bleeding. Nitrates may be used to promote coronary perfusion, and antidysrhythmic agents may be prescribed to decrease ventricular irritability.[73] In clinical trials, TMR was strongly correlated with improvement in anginal symptoms and improved activity tolerance when compared with maximal medical therapy, although there was no change in mortality.[80] Initially, the benefit of this procedure was believed to be derived from the channels that allowed oxygenated blood from the LV to perfuse the myocardium. Later studies indicated that the channels close over time, and a more the likely mechanism is that the laser induces angiogenesis (growth of new vessels) to improve blood flow to the myocardium.[79] TMR has also been shown to be a useful adjunct to cardiac surgery for patients in whom complete surgical revascularization is not feasible.[81]

Surgical Treatment of Cardiac Dysrhythmias. The *maze procedure* is a surgical intervention for patients with atrial fibrillation that has not responded to medical therapy. A series of scars are made in the atrial tissue to create an electrical maze that disrupts the reentrant pathways and directs the sinus

---

Patient Education

Open Heart Surgery

- Pathophysiology of disease (coronary artery or valvular disease)
- Risk factor modification to prevent coronary artery disease (smoking cessation, regular exercise, weight loss)
- Postoperative incisional care
- Activity limitations (no lifting, pushing, or pulling of anything heavier than 10 pounds for 6 to 8 weeks; no driving for 6 to 8 weeks)
- Recommended exercise progression after surgery
- Recommended diet after surgery
- Information regarding prescribed medications (including prescribed pain medication)
- Anticipated mood changes after surgery
- Follow-up appointment for clinic or primary physician
- Additional information for valve patients
- Symptoms of endocarditis
- Antibiotic prophylaxis before invasive procedures
- Information regarding anticoagulant therapy and follow-up

impulse through the AV node. The procedure also includes surgical isolation of the pulmonary veins, which are thought to be responsible for initiation of atrial fibrillation, and removal of the left and right atrial appendages.[82] The goal of treatment is not only to prevent the recurrence of atrial tachydysrhythmias but to restore sinus rhythm and AV synchrony, if possible. If the sinus node is no longer functioning, a pacemaker may be implanted to restore an AV sequential rhythm. Initially, the scars were created with a "cut and sew" technique, but the development of specialized ablation catheters enabled the creation of lesion lines with other energy sources, such as RF current, microwave energy, or cryoablation.[83] Success rates for the surgical maze procedure have been promising, and modifications of the procedure have led to a less invasive thoracoscopic version of the procedure: the mini-maze.[82] The mini-maze is performed off pump using an RF clamp to ablate tissue and isolate the pulmonary veins. After either procedure, patients require monitoring for arrhythmias. Continued atrial fibrillation is common, because it takes months for the scar tissue to fully mature.[83]

Although future trends in the surgical management of cardiac disease are difficult to predict, the critical care nurse must continue to be prepared to meet the challenge of providing a high level of nursing management at the bedside. A solid knowledge base and keen assessment skills are prerequisites for the accurate anticipation of problems and prompt intervention necessary to stabilize the patient and prevent the occurrence of life-threatening complications.

MECHANICAL CIRCULATORY ASSIST DEVICES

Mechanical circulatory assist devices are used in the treatment of heart failure when conventional pharmacologic therapy has proved ineffective. The primary goals of mechanical assist devices are to decrease myocardial workload and maintain adequate perfusion to vital organs. If the acute heart failure is reversible, a short duration of ventricular assistance is used to allow the myocardium time to recover. If the condition is irreversible, a mechanical assist device may be used as a bridge to heart transplantation for qualified candidates or as a destination therapy for those who have no other surgical options.

INTRAAORTIC BALLOON PUMP

IABP is the most widely used temporary mechanical circulatory assist device for supporting failing circulation (Box 20-14). Its therapeutic effects are based on the hemodynamic principles of diastolic augmentation and afterload reduction.

The most commonly used intraaortic balloon (IAB) catheter consists of a single, sausage-shaped polyurethane balloon that is wrapped around the distal end of a vascular catheter and positioned in the descending thoracic aorta just distal to the takeoff of the left subclavian artery. The second generation of IAB catheters is more flexible and can be wrapped to a smaller diameter than their predecessors and therefore can be inserted into

---

BOX 20-14   INDICATIONS FOR USE OF THE INTRAAORTIC BALLOON PUMP

- Left ventricular failure after cardiac surgery
- Unstable angina refractory to medications
- Recurrent angina after acute myocardial infarction
- Complications of acute myocardial infarction
  Cardiogenic shock
  Papillary muscle dysfunction or rupture with mitral regurgitation
  Ventricular septal rupture
  Refractory ventricular dysrhythmias

---

the femoral artery percutaneously rather than surgically. When attached to a bedside pumping console and properly synchronized to the patient's cardiac cycle, the IAB inflates during diastole and deflates just before systole.

Initially, as the balloon is inflated in diastole concurrent with aortic valve closure, the blood in the aortic arch above the level of the balloon is displaced retrograde (backward) toward the aortic root, augmenting diastolic coronary arterial blood flow and increasing myocardial oxygen supply (Fig. 20-21A). The blood volume in the aorta below the level of the balloon is propelled forward toward the peripheral vascular system, which may enhance renal perfusion. Subsequently, the deflation of the balloon just before the opening of the aortic valve creates a potential space or vacuum in the aorta, toward which blood flows unimpeded during ventricular ejection (see Fig. 20-21B). This decreased resistance to LV ejection, or decreased afterload, facilitates ventricular emptying and reduces myocardial oxygen demands. The overall physiologic effect of IABP therapy is an improvement in the balance between myocardial oxygen supply and demand. Contraindications to IABP include aortic aneurysm, aortic valve insufficiency, and severe peripheral vascular disease.[84]

Medical Management. The IAB may be inserted in the operating room, the cardiac catheterization laboratory, or the critical care unit. The IAB catheter is usually inserted percutaneously through the femoral artery and advanced to the correct position in the descending thoracic aorta. The physician may insert the balloon through an introducer sheath or perform a sheathless insertion to minimize the degree of vessel occlusion created by the catheter. If percutaneous catheter placement is not feasible, the catheter may be placed through surgical cutdown or by a direct thoracic approach. After insertion, the balloon is attached to the console and filled with the prescribed volume of helium, and pumping is initiated. If the balloon fails to unwrap completely during filling, the physician may rapidly inflate and deflate the balloon manually, using a syringe.

Nursing Management. The management of the pumping console and its timing functions may be performed by the nurse caring for the patient or delegated to specially trained personnel on the unit. In either situation, several important nursing diagnoses and management responsibilities relate to the management of the patient receiving IABP therapy (see the Nursing Diagnoses feature on Intraaortic Balloon Pump).

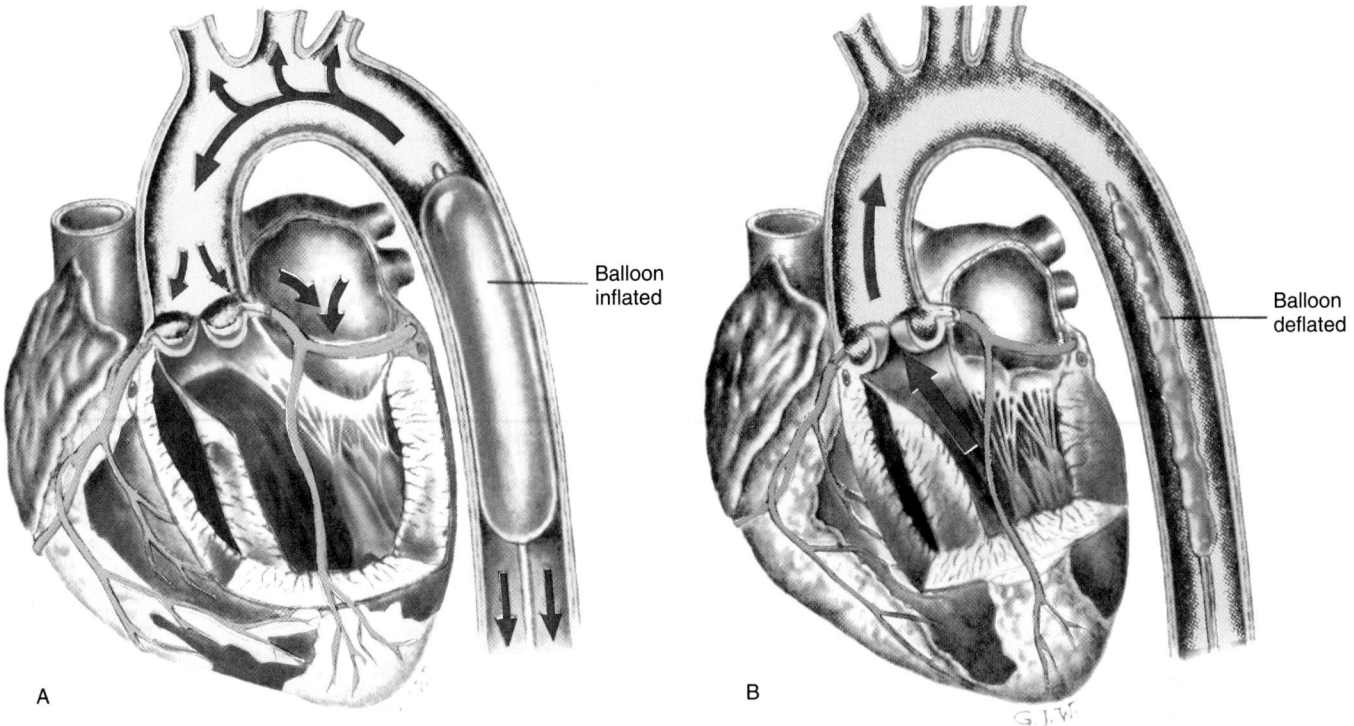

Figure 20-21 Mechanisms of action of the intraaortic balloon pump. *A,* Diastolic balloon inflation augments coronary blood flow. *B,* Systolic balloon deflation decreases afterload.

Nursing Diagnoses

Intraaortic Balloon Pump

- Decreased Cardiac Output related to alterations in preload
- Decreased Cardiac Output related to alterations in afterload
- Decreased Cardiac Output related to alterations in contractility
- Decreased Cardiac Output related to alterations in heart rate or rhythm
- Activity Intolerance related to cardiopulmonary dysfunction
- Ineffective Cardiopulmonary Tissue Perfusion related to acute myocardial ischemia
- Ineffective Peripheral Tissue Perfusion related to decreased peripheral blood flow
- Risk for Infection related to invasive procedures
- Disturbed Sleep Pattern related to circadian desynchronization
- Disturbed Body Image related to functional dependence on life-sustaining technology
- Deficient Knowledge: Discharge Regimen related to lack of previous exposure to information (see the Patient Education feature on Intraaortic Balloon Pump)

Dysrhythmias. The ECG and arterial pressure tracings are constantly monitored to verify the timing and effect of balloon counterpulsations (Fig. 20-22). For counterpulsation to occur, the pump must receive a trigger signal to identify the beginning of a new cardiac cycle. The trigger can be the R wave of the ECG, the upstroke of the arterial pressure waveform, or a pacemaker spike.[84] Dysrhythmias can adversely affect the timing of balloon inflation and deflation, so rhythm disturbances must be detected and treated promptly. Current IABPs have automatic timing features that use internal algorithms to adjust inflation and deflation in response to changes in the patient's heart rate or rhythm. New catheters are available that incorporate a fiber-optic sensor to enhance the quality of the arterial waveform obtained from the IAB catheter and improve timing. Mean arterial pressure is ideally maintained at approximately 80 mm Hg with adequate pumping.

Peripheral Ischemia. The most common complication of IABP support is lower extremity ischemia resulting from occlusion of the femoral artery by the catheter itself or by emboli caused by thrombus formation on the balloon.[85] Although ischemic complications have decreased with sheathless insertion techniques and the introduction of smaller balloon catheters (7.5 versus 9.5 Fr), evaluation of peripheral circulation remains an important nursing assessment.[86] The presence and quality of peripheral pulses distal to the catheter insertion site are assessed frequently, along with color, temperature, and capillary refill of the involved extremity. Doppler localization of peripheral pulses may be required if pulses are difficult to palpate on the cannulated extremity. Signs of diminished perfusion must be reported immediately. Anticoagulation (e.g., heparin infusion) may be prescribed to decrease the incidence of thrombosis. Other vascular complications associated with IABP include acute aortic dissection and the development of pseudoaneurysms at the catheter insertion site.

Balloon Perforation. Another potential complication of IABP therapy is balloon perforation. Perforation occurs because of repeated contact of the balloon membrane with calcified plaque in the aorta as the balloon inflates and deflates.

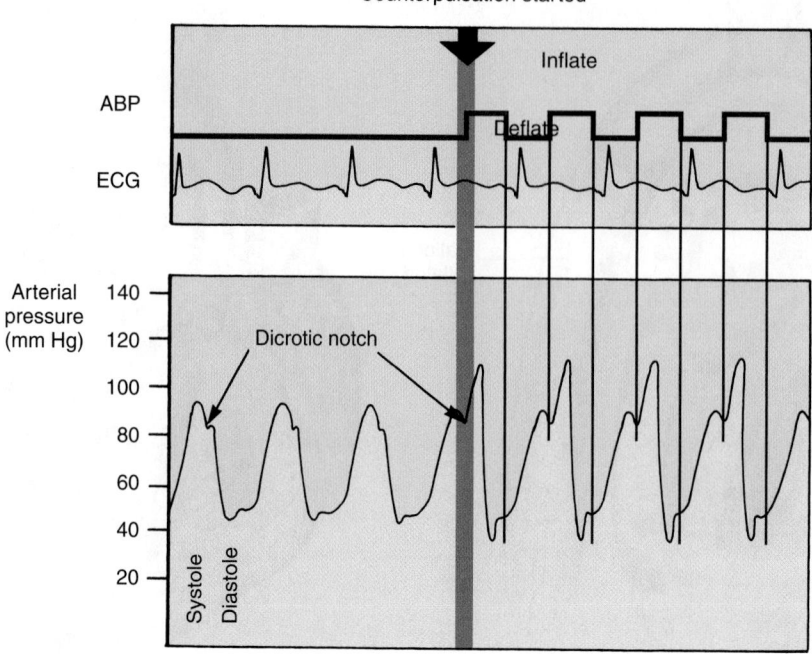

Figure 20-22 The timing and effect of balloon counterpulsations. Timing is adjusted by synchronizing balloon inflation with the dicrotic notch on the arterial waveform, resulting in an elevated diastolic pressure. Inflation is maintained throughout diastole to augment coronary perfusion. Deflation occurs just before the next systole, resulting in a reduced systolic pressure and decreased afterload. *(From Guzzetta CE, Dossey BM:* Cardiovascular nursing: holistic practice, *St. Louis, 1992, CV Mosby.)*

The patient is monitored for evidence of a balloon leak, such as a gas leak alarm from the pump console or the presence of blood in the IAB tubing. If a balloon leak is detected, pumping is stopped and the physician is immediately notified so that the balloon can be removed. If the balloon is not promptly removed or pumping is attempted after the perforation, the IAB may become entrapped as the blood hardens within the catheter, creating a mass. If this occurs, the balloon must be surgically removed.

Balloon Catheter Position. The balloon catheter must be maintained in proper position to optimize its effectiveness and minimize complications. The balloon may migrate proximally and occlude the left subclavian artery, or it may move distally, compromising renal circulation. Careful assessment of the left radial pulse and urinary output is essential. Measures to prevent accidental displacement of the balloon catheter include ensuring that the patient observes complete bed rest, with the head of the bed elevated no more than 30 degrees, and avoids any flexion of the involved hip.

Preventing Complications. Log rolling, in which the patient is moved from side to side every 2 hours, is used to maintain skin integrity and to prevent pulmonary atelectasis. Some institutional protocols call for implementation of continuous lateral rotation therapy to help facilitate pulmonary toilet in the patient with an IABP. Because thrombocytopenia may occur as a result of mechanical destruction of the platelets by the pumping action of the balloon, platelet counts are closely monitored and the patient is observed for evidence of bleeding. Because infection of the insertion site is a potential complication, the dressing is changed in accordance with the hospital policy for other invasive lines.

Patient Education

Intraaortic Balloon Pump

- Description of the intraaortic balloon pump (IABP) and how it works
- Activity restrictions (minimize leg movement)
- Symptoms to report to the health care professional (pain in the back, leg, or chest)

Psychological Needs. The psychological needs of the patient must be considered while on IABP therapy. Sleep deprivation is common and is related in part to the continuous nursing management requirements for the patient and the noise level in the unit, including the sounds made by the balloon pumping device. Anxiety related to fear of non-recovery and loss of control because of forced immobility is a common occurrence.

Weaning. Weaning from the IABP is considered after hemodynamic stability has been achieved with no, or only minimal, pharmacologic support. One weaning procedure consists of slowly decreasing the pumping frequency from every beat to every eighth beat, as tolerated. Another weaning method involves a gradual decrease in balloon volume.[87] To prevent thrombus formation on the balloon surface, the IABP must remain at a minimal pumping ratio (or volume) until its removal.

Patient Education. Patient education for the patient with an IAB is presented in the Patient Education feature on Intraaortic Balloon Pump. Many of the IABP manufacturers provide helpful educational booklets designed for patients and families.

TABLE 20-12 Ventricular Assist Devices

Type	Indications	Description
External		
Abiomed BVS 5000	Short-term univentricular or biventricular support	A two-chamber pump connected to the patient by tubing The pump contains bladders that fill by gravity and trigger ejection when they are full. They are mounted on an IV pole and positioned at a level relative to the patient. Systemic anticoagulation is required. Device may be changed noninvasively to the AB5000, an external pneumatic pump that allows for increased mobility in hospital or transport to another facility.
Thoratec PVAD	Short-term univentricular or biventricular support	A pneumatically driven pump that contains a plastic blood sac and two mechanical valves The device senses when the sac is full and triggers the ejection of blood. The pump is located on the patient's abdomen and connected to a large console, which limits mobility. Systemic anticoagulation is required.
Impella Recover LP 2.5	Short-term left ventricular support	A percutaneously inserted catheter with a miniaturized pump at the distal tip that provides continuous flow up to 2.5 L/min The catheter is placed retrograde across the aortic valve to pull blood from the left ventricle, which is returned to ascending aorta.
Tandem Heart	Short-term left ventricular support	A percutaneously inserted device that provides continuous flow up to 4 L/min Inflow is obtained from a catheter positioned in the left atrium (by a transseptal approach), and outflow is through the femoral artery. Device allows for transport to a center for long-term therapy.
Implantable		
Heartmate VE	Long-term left-ventricular support as bridge to transplantation or destination therapy	An electrically driven pump that is implanted in the abdomen and contains two porcine valves Textured surfaces allow patients to be maintained on aspirin. The pump is connected to a direct power source by a cable and may be operated by battery for 6-8 hr.
Heartmate II LVAS	Long-term ventricular support as a bridge to transplantation; under investigation for destination therapy	An electrically driven rotary pump that produces nonpulsatile flow Continuous flow is quiet, and minimal moving parts may lead to improved durability. Smaller size allows for implantation in patients with body surface area $<1.5 \ m^2$. Anticoagulation and antiplatelet therapy are required. Controller is powered by batteries or a standard electrical outlet.
Novacor LVAS	Long-term left-ventricular support as bridge to transplantation; under investigation for destination therapy	An electrically driven pulsatile pump implanted in the upper abdomen A percutaneous drive line connects to an external controller and can operate on battery for short periods (4 hr). Systemic anticoagulation is required.

VENTRICULAR ASSIST DEVICES

The ventricular assist device (VAD) is designed to support a failing natural heart with flow assistance. Diversion of varying amounts of systemic blood flow around a failing ventricle by means of a pump reduces cardiac workload while maintaining adequate perfusion to sustain end-organ function. VADs can be used to support a failing RV or LV, or both.[88]

VADs are currently indicated for three types of clinical applications. The first category of patients includes those who, despite aggressive medical therapy, continue to demonstrate persistent cardiac failure but who have the potential for regaining normal heart function if the heart is given time to rest. This category, called *bridge to recovery,* consists of patients who have acute post-surgical myocardial dysfunction, are in refractory cardiogenic shock after acute MI, or have acute viral myocarditis. The second category, called *bridge to transplantation,* includes those patients with decompensated chronic heart failure who need circulatory support until heart transplantation can be performed. The third category, called *destination therapy,* was recently approved by the FDA. These are patients with severe heart failure who are not candidates for heart transplantation and for whom the VAD may provide improved survival and quality of life.[89]

Several VADs have been approved by the FDA, and a number of other devices are in clinical trials.[90] All consist of a blood pump, cannula, and some type of power source. Some devices displace blood to create pulsatile flow, whereas others create continuous flow and are therefore pulseless.[89] Device selection is based on individual VAD capabilities and institutional preference (Table 20-12). External VADs are used primarily for short-term support, and smaller implantable VADS are used for long-term therapy. Percutaneous devices have become available to increase the ease of insertion in these very unstable patients. Percutaneous devices allow for short-term support until patients recover or receive a longer-term device.[990-92]

The left ventricular assist device (LVAD) is used most commonly because LV failure occurs more often than does RV failure. Use of biventricular support (bi-VAD) may be needed in the acute phase, because RV failure often follows LV failure. Outflow cannulas that divert blood from the heart to the LVAD for LV support are surgically placed in the left atrium or the LV apex, depending on the indication for the device. For example, if the patient is "pending recovery" of the natural heart, preservation of LV function mandates left atrial cannulation. The right atrium is cannulated for outflow for RV support. Inflow back to the heart from the pump is accomplished by cannulation of the aorta or femoral artery for the LVAD and or pulmonary artery for the right ventricular assist device (RVAD) (see Fig. 20-23 for cannula placement in bi-VAD configuration of the Abiomed pump). Flow rates between 1 and 6 L/min are used to maintain adequate cardiac output while decreasing ventricular workload.

Nursing Management. Nursing diagnoses and management for a patient with a VAD include monitoring for hemodynamic changes and for complications related to the device (see the Nursing Diagnoses feature on Ventricular Assist Device). The same interventions to optimize cardiac output by manipulation of heart rate, preload, afterload, and contractility that are

used for cardiac surgery patients apply to patients with a VAD. Adequate filling volumes are required to maintain pump flow. Afterload reduction may be needed to improve output from the unassisted ventricle when univentricular support is used. Complications common to all types of VADs include bleeding,

Nursing Diagnoses

Ventricular Assist Device

- Decreased Cardiac Output related to alterations in preload
- Decreased Cardiac Output related to alterations in afterload
- Decreased Cardiac Output related to alterations in contractility
- Decreased Cardiac Output related to alterations in heart rate or rhythm
- Activity Intolerance related to cardiopulmonary dysfunction
- Ineffective Cardiopulmonary Tissue Perfusion related to acute myocardial ischemia
- Ineffective Peripheral Tissue Perfusion related to decreased peripheral blood flow
- Risk for Infection related to invasive procedures
- Disturbed Sleep Pattern related to circadian desynchronization
- Disturbed Body Image related to functional dependence on life-sustaining technology
- Deficient Knowledge: Discharge Regimen related to lack of previous exposure to information (see the Patient Education feature on Ventricular Assist Device)

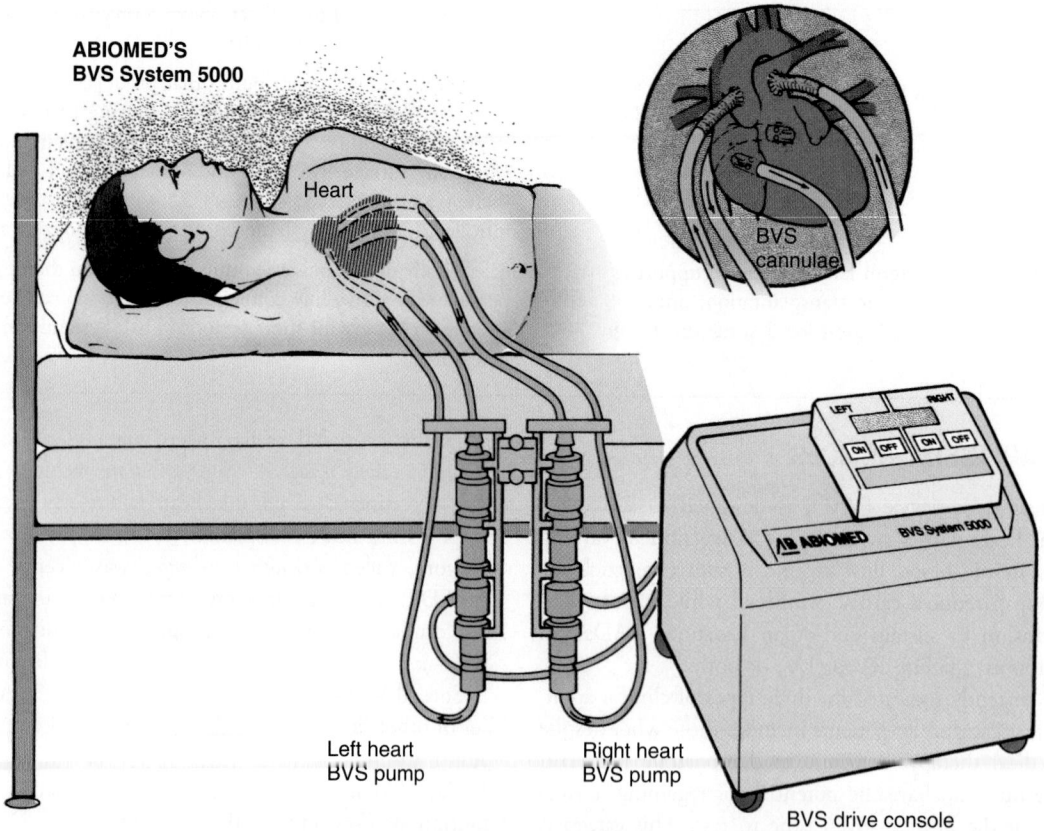

Figure 20-23 Diagram of a bi-ventricular support (BVS) system. *(Courtesy Abiomed, Inc., Danvers, MA.)*

infection, thromboembolism, and device failure, although complication rates vary among the different models.[89]

Device Failure. Because of the life-saving nature of this therapy, device failure is a life-threatening event. VAD designs vary considerably, and troubleshooting methods for device failure are unique to each device. The nurse must be aware of signs of device malfunction as well patient factors (volume status, dysrhythmias, RV failure) that may affect VAD function.

Anticoagulation. The requirement for anticoagulation varies with the type of VAD, the flow rate, and institutional protocol. If patients are anticoagulated with heparin, nurses are responsible for maintaining the ACT within a therapeutic range and monitoring for complications of bleeding. If bleeding occurs, additional coagulation studies, such as activated partial thromboplastin time (aPTT), prothrombin time (PT), international normalized ratio (INR), and fibrinogen and platelet counts, may be performed. Continued bleeding may necessitate withholding the heparin infusion and administering fresh-frozen plasma and platelets. If patients are not anticoagulated, the risk of thrombi obstructing a VAD cannula increases, as does the risk of an embolic event.

Infection. Patients with a VAD are at considerable risk for infection. The most common infection is pneumonia resulting from immobility and the need for ventilatory support. Other infectious risks are posed by the presence of invasive catheters and the surgically implanted VAD. Infection is prevented by the use of strict aseptic technique with all invasive tubing and dressing changes. Site care varies, depending on institutional protocols and the type of VAD that is used. Nurses monitor patients for infection by measuring temperatures, inspecting insertion sites and incisions, and obtaining daily leukocyte counts. If an infection is suspected, pan-cultures (blood, urine, and sputum) are taken to guide appropriate antibiotic therapy.

Weaning. Weaning is accomplished by gradually decreasing the flow rate to allow the patient's ventricle to contribute more to total blood flow. Controversy exists with regard to anticoagulation; however, during weaning of VAD flow rates to less than 2 L/min, ACTs are maintained between 160 and 400 seconds with heparin, depending on institutional protocols. This minimizes the potential for thrombus formation in the extracorporeal circuit during weaning but also increases the risk of bleeding and therefore necessitates close monitoring.

Patient Education. The rapid and acute nature of cardiogenic shock limits the nurse's ability to prepare patients and families for VAD insertion. Despite the critical nature of the illness, nurses explain the reason for the use of the VAD and provide information about the critical care environment and equipment (see the Patient Education feature on Ventricular Assist Device). Technologic advances and approval of devices for destination therapy are likely to increase the number of VAD patients discharged to home. These patients and their families require education related to care of the device and reinforcement on the components of heart failure management.

VASCULAR SURGERY

Vascular surgery may be used as a treatment for arterial occlusive disease or to correct structural abnormalities such as aneurysms. Because atherosclerosis is a diffuse disease that affects both the peripheral vessels and the coronary arteries, patients undergoing arterial vascular surgery are at high risk for perioperative cardiac events. The nursing care of patients after vascular surgery focuses not only on observations for surgical complications such as hematoma or reocclusion but also on prompt recognition and appropriate treatment of complications that may arise from the impact of the procedure on preexisting cardiac, pulmonary, or kidney disease.

CAROTID ENDARTERECTOMY

Carotid endarterectomy (CEA) may be beneficial in both symptomatic and asymptomatic patients with stenoses greater than 60% to 70%.[93] The procedure is performed through a neck incision that allows for visualization of the vessel. The plaque is removed, and the vessel is closed directly or with a patch composed of saphenous vein or a prosthetic material. A Jackson-Pratt drain may be placed at the end of the procedure to minimize hematoma formation. Complications after carotid endarterectomy include perioperative MI, cerebral ischemia or infarction, bleeding, and cranial nerve damage.

Postoperative Nursing Management. Patients require 12 to 24 hours of intensive nursing assessment in the period immediately after carotid endarterectomy. Complications are rare but may be life threatening and require rapid intervention. Serial assessments are performed, and the surgeon is promptly notified of significant changes in the patient's status.

Neurologic Assessment. Frequent neurologic assessments are performed as the patient awakens from anesthesia and then hourly for the first 12 hours. These assessments should include level of consciousness, orientation, pupil response, motor function, and evaluation of cranial nerve function (e.g., swallowing or gag reflexes, hoarseness, tongue movement, facial drooping). Compression, traction, or inadvertent severing can damage nerves that lie in or near the surgical field. The most common injuries are damage to the laryngeal and hypoglossal nerves. Most cranial nerve dysfunction resolves within a short time.[94]

Bleeding. Bleeding is assessed by observation of the dressing for drainage or swelling and measurement of output from the neck drain, if present. If hematoma formation occurs internally, it may impinge on the trachea, so the patient is also monitored for signs of a compromised airway. In addition to monitoring respiratory rate and oxygen saturation, the nurse assesses the patient for tracheal deviation and for symptoms of upper airway obstruction such as stridor or wheezing. A small venous hematoma may respond to manual pressure, but larger arterial hematomas that expand rapidly require emergent return to the operating room for reexploration and evacuation.

Cardiovascular Monitoring. Continuous ECG monitoring with ST-segment monitoring is used to detect myocardial ischemia after carotid endarterectomy. Bradycardia is common as a result of baroreceptor stimulation during the operative procedure but is usually hemodynamically tolerated as long as the patient's blood pressure is adequate. Manipulation of the carotid bulb during the surgery often results in hemodynamic instability in the immediate postoperative period. Usually, an arterial line is placed to allow for prompt detection and treatment of hypotension or hypertension. Adequate blood pressure control in the postoperative period is of paramount importance. Hypertension increases the risk of bleeding at the suture line and is typically treated with short-acting vasodilators such as sodium nitroprusside. A relative hypotension compared with the patient's baseline value results in inadequate cerebral perfusion and potential neurologic deficits, so vasopressors such as phenylephrine may be used to maintain an adequate blood pressure.

Carotid Stents. Although carotid endarterectomy has been the gold standard for treatment of patients with significant carotid artery stenosis, carotid stenting is increasingly being used as an alternative in patients considered to be at high surgical risk.[95] This procedure is performed with the use of local anesthesia and percutaneous cannulation similar to that used in coronary stenting. The use of embolic protection devices to trap and remove embolic particles generated during the procedure improves neurologic outcomes.[96] Typically, patients are monitored in a critical care unit overnight to allow for frequent neurologic assessments and treatment of hemodynamic instability.[97] Patients are also monitored for potential complications related to vascular access sheaths.

ABDOMINAL AORTIC ANEURYSM REPAIR

An abdominal aortic aneurysm (AAA) usually is repaired when the aneurysm is 5 cm or larger. The procedure is performed with the patient under general anesthesia and involves surgical access through a midline abdominal incision or a flank incision (retroperitoneal approach). Clamping of the aorta proximal and distal to the dilated area isolates the aneurysm. The aneurysmal portion of the aorta is replaced with a prosthetic graft, which is then enclosed within the aneurysmal sac.

Postoperative complications include myocardial ischemia or infarction, bleeding, acute renal failure, and distal embolization. Rarely, colon or spinal cord ischemia may occur because of interruption of blood flow during aortic cross-clamping or embolization. After the procedure, patients are monitored in the critical care unit for 24 to 48 hours, with a total length of hospital stay being 5 to 9 days.

Postoperative Management. Nursing assessment of vital signs along with assessment of peripheral perfusion is performed

frequently in the early postoperative period. Continuous ECG monitoring with ST-segment analysis is used to detect myocardial ischemia. An arterial line is placed to allow for prompt detection and treatment of hypotension or hypertension. Hypertension increases the risk of bleeding at the suture lines and is often treated with short-acting vasodilators such as sodium nitroprusside. Hypotension may result in compromised perfusion to organs or the extremities and is treated with volume replacement and vasopressors as needed. Hourly assessment of urine output is performed to evaluate kidney function. If urine output is less than 30 mL/hr, diuretics or low-dose dopamine may be used after correction of hypovolemia. The dressing is assessed for bleeding, and potential signs of internal hemorrhage from the graft site (hypotension, complaints of back pain) are further evaluated with serial hematocrit measurements. Patients without preoperative pulmonary conditions may be rapidly weaned from ventilatory support, with supplemental oxygen given as needed to maintain oxygen saturation in the normal range.

Endovascular Stent Grafts. The endoluminal placement of stent grafts is a newer, less invasive approach for repair of an AAA. In this procedure, a sutureless vascular graft is implanted into the abdominal aorta through a femoral arteriotomy (Fig. 20-24). The stent isolates the aneurysmal wall from intraluminal blood pressure to prevent further expansion or rupture of the aneurysm.[98] This procedure can be performed with the patient under epidural anesthesia, with minimal blood loss and a shorter length of stay. As a result, endovascular procedures may be attempted in patients who would otherwise be deemed inoperable due to comorbid conditions. Although the operative mortality and morbidity may be less with endovascular stents, randomized studies have shown no significant difference in long-term survival between open surgical and endovascular interventions in patients with AAA.[99,100] Reintervention is required more frequently with endovascular repair.[98]

PERIPHERAL VASCULAR PROCEDURES

Progression of peripheral arterial disease can lead to critical limb ischemia. This may initially manifest as intermittent claudication, but if left untreated, it can progress to rest pain, ulceration, or even gangrene. Initial treatment focuses on lifestyle modification, such as smoking cessation, adequate diabetic control, effective treatment of hypertension, and management of dyslipidemia. Pharmacologic interventions such as antiplatelet and antithrombotic agents may be used. If these nonoperative strategies fail, patients may be considered for surgical or interventional revascularization by means of surgical bypass, percutaneous transluminal angioplasty (PTA), or stent placement.[101]

Surgical Revascularization. *Arteriosclerosis obliterans* is a condition in which atherosclerosis produces progressive obstruction of medium-to-larger arteries. These lesions commonly occur at bifurcations of the abdominal aorta and the iliac, femoral, popliteal or tibial, and peroneal arteries. The surgical procedure is chosen based on the site of the vascular lesion or lesions and the patient's operative risk. For example, aortofemoral bypass grafting is the preferred operation for treatment of aortoiliac occlusive disease in low-risk patients, because it results in the highest patency rates. But axillobifemoral bypass

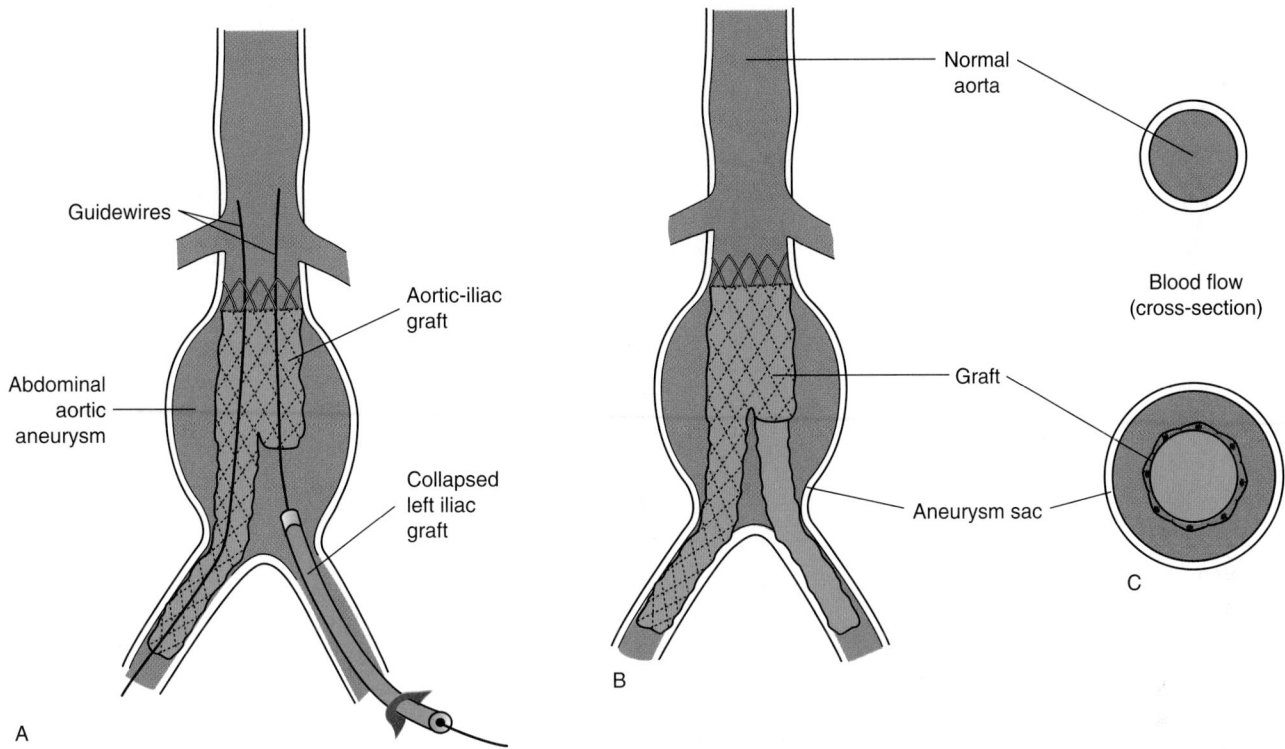

Figure 20-24 Placement of an endovascular aortic stent. *A,* With fluoroscopic guidance, the collapsed stent is inserted through an incision in the femoral or iliac artery over a guidewire. *B,* The positioned stent is opened with a balloon and anchored to the vessel by several small hooks. *C,* The stent isolates the aneurysmal wall from intraluminal blood pressure.

or unilateral femorofemoral bypass may be selected in higher-risk patients, because these procedures can be performed with regional anesthesia.[102] Types of peripheral vascular procedures are shown in Fig. 20-25.

Choice of Conduit. Conduits available for peripheral vascular bypass include vein grafts (reversed saphenous vein, arm vein, or human umbilical vein) and synthetic grafts made of polytetrafluoroethylene. As in CABG, the type of conduit used has an impact on the patency rate of the graft. Veins are the preferred conduit because of better patency rates (60% to 80% at 5 years) and lower potential for infection.[102]

Nursing Management. The primary focus of nursing care in the immediate postoperative period is assessment of the adequacy of perfusion to the limb supplied by the graft and identification of surgical complications. Pulse checks are performed frequently, and the surgeon is notified of any decrease in the strength of the Doppler signal. Because distal perfusion is compromised in this patient population, nursing measures to prevent skin breakdown (e.g., sheepskin, frequent repositioning, foot cradles) are implemented. If the graft was placed above the renal arteries, kidney function may be impaired as a result of interruption of renal blood flow during graft placement. Urine output is therefore assessed hourly and supported with fluids, diuretics, and low-dose dopamine as needed. ST-segment monitoring is performed to detect episodes of myocardial ischemia throughout the perioperative period.

Percutaneous Carotid Interventions. PTA can be performed to treat occlusion or narrowing in the peripheral vasculature by means of catheters similar to those used in PTCA. As

with coronary angioplasty, advances in catheter design and the development of intravascular stents have resulted in a dramatic increase in the number of percutaneous procedures performed. PTA was traditionally limited to the treatment of short, focal stenoses or occlusions but is now routinely used to treat more extensive diseased segments, as an emergency treatment to attempt limb salvage before surgical bypass, and as an alternative for patients who are poor surgical candidates. Intravascular stents may be used in combination with PTA, depending on lesion morphology and location. Complications of interventional vascular procedures include hematoma formation at the site of the arteriotomy, formation of a pseudoaneurysm, distal embolization, and thrombotic occlusion.

Acute occlusion of a peripheral artery may occur as a result of local thrombosis, emboli, trauma, or compression. Left untreated, the resultant ischemia may lead to amputation of the affected limb. Catheter-based interventions that may be used to recanalize acutely occluded arteries include intra-arterial infusions of fibrinolytic medications and the use of thrombectomy devices to fragment and remove the clot. If these interventions are unsuccessful, surgical revascularization may be performed.[103]

EFFECTS OF CARDIOVASCULAR DRUGS

Multiple medications are used in the treatment of critically ill cardiovascular patients. The critical care nurse is responsible for preparation and administration of these drugs and often is required to titrate the dose on the basis of the patient's hemodynamic response.

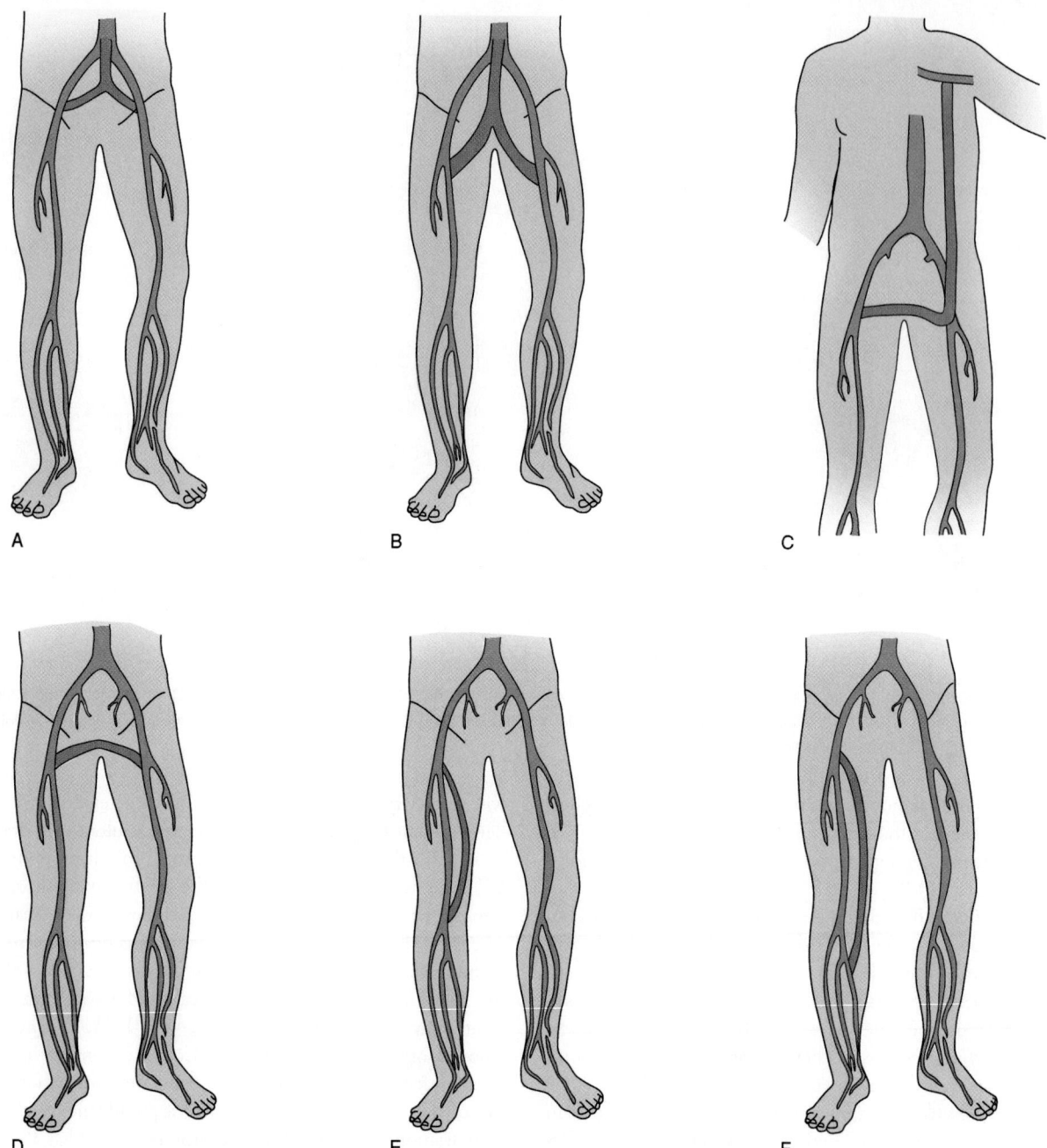

Figure 20-25 Peripheral arterial bypass procedures. *A*, Aortoiliac bypass. *B*, Aortobifemoral bypass. *C*, Axillobifemoral bypass. *D*, Femorofemoral bypass. *E*, Femoropopliteal bypass. *F*, Femorotibial bypass.

The medications used to treat cardiovascular disease are rapidly changing and expanding as more is learned about the pathophysiology of cardiac disease and as improved formulas are developed by pharmaceutical companies. The critical care nurse who has a general understanding of the mechanisms of action of the various drug classifications can readily apply this knowledge to new drugs within the same classification. The following discussion provides a concise review of drugs commonly administered to support cardiovascular function in the critical care setting. The emphasis is on intravenously administered medications that are used for the acute rather than the chronic management of cardiovascular conditions.

ANTIDYSRHYTHMIC DRUGS

Antidysrhythmic drugs comprise a diverse category of pharmacologic agents used to terminate or prevent an array of abnormal cardiac rhythms. These drugs commonly are classified according to their primary effect on the action potential of cardiac cells (Fig. 20-26). The classification scheme shown in Table 20-13 is the most commonly used system. Classification of newer agents is more difficult, because some of these agents have characteristics of more than one class and others have no characteristics of the current system.

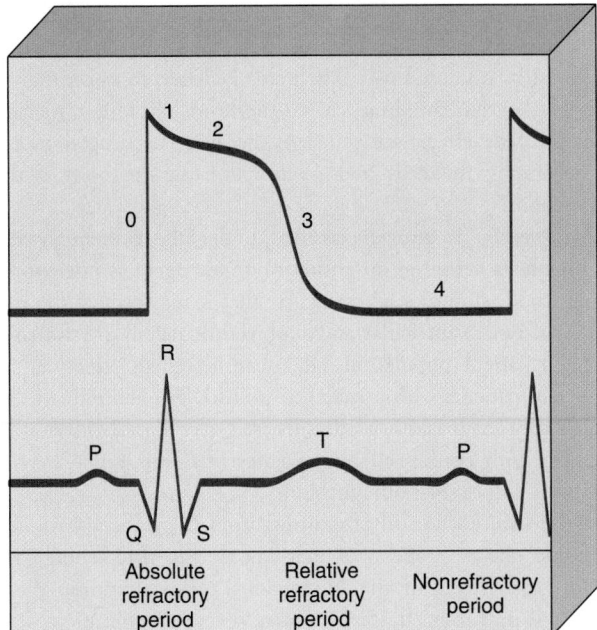

Figure 20-26 The phases of the cardiac action potential and their relationship to the heart's refractory periods. *Phase 0,* Depolarization with rapid influx of sodium. *Phase 1,* Rapid repolarization with rapid efflux of potassium ions and decreased sodium conductance. *Phase 2,* Plateau with slow influx of sodium and calcium ions. *Phase 3,* Repolarization with continued efflux of potassium ions. *Phase 4,* Resting phase with restoration of ionic balance by sodium and potassium pumps.

TABLE 20-13 Classification of Antidysrhythmic Agents

Class	Action	Drugs
I	Blocks sodium channels (stabilizes cell membrane)	
IA	Blocks sodium channels and delays repolarization, lengthening the duration of the action potential	Quinidine Procainamide Disopyramide
IB	Blocks sodium channels and accelerates repolarization, shortening the duration of the action potential	Lidocaine Mexiletine Tocainide
IC	Blocks sodium channels and slows conduction through the His-Purkinje system, prolonging the QRS duration	Flecainide Encainide Propafenone
II	Blocks β-receptors	Esmolol Metoprolol Propranolol
III	Slows repolarization and prolongs the duration of the action potential	Amiodarone Ibutilide Sotalol Dofetilide
IV	Blocks calcium channels	Diltiazem Verapamil

Class I Drugs. Class I agents are sodium channel blockers that decrease the influx of sodium ions through "fast" channels during phase 0 depolarization. This prolongs the absolute (effective) refractory period, thereby decreasing the risk of premature impulses from ectopic foci. These drugs also depress automaticity by slowing the rate of spontaneous depolarization of pacemaker cells during the resting phase (phase 4).

Class I drugs can be further subdivided into three groups according to their potency as sodium channel inhibitors and their effect on phase 3 repolarization. Class IA agents—*quinidine, procainamide,* and *disopyramide*—block both the fast sodium channels and phase 3 repolarization, thus prolonging the action potential duration. Clinically, this may result in measurable increases in the QRS duration and lengthening of the QT interval. All class IA agents may depress myocardial contractility, with disopyramide having the most potent negative inotropic effect. Drugs in class IB have only a moderate effect on sodium channels and accelerate phase 3 repolarization to shorten the action potential duration; *lidocaine, mexiletine,* and *tocainide* belong in this group. Class IC agents are the most potent sodium channel blockers and have little effect on repolarization. Class IC drugs increase the PR and QRS intervals. Included in this group are *encainide, flecainide,* and *propafenone.* The results of the Cardiac Arrhythmia Suppression Trial (CAST) indicated that treatment with encainide and flecainide may be associated with increased mortality, and the use of these agents in clinical practice has decreased.[104]

Class II Drugs. Class II drugs are β-adrenergic blockers (beta-blockers). They inhibit dysrhythmias mediated by the sympathetic nervous system by competing with endogenous catecholamines for available receptor sites. As a result, spontaneous depolarization during the resting phase (phase 4) is depressed, and AV conduction is slowed. Drugs in this class can be further subdivided into cardioselective agents (those that block only β1-receptors) and noncardioselective agents (those that block both β1- and β2-receptors). Knowledge of the effects of adrenergic-receptor stimulation allows for anticipation of both the therapeutic responses brought about by beta-blockade and the potential adverse effects of these agents (Table 20-14). For example, bronchospasm can be precipitated by noncardioselective beta-blockers in a patient with chronic obstructive

TABLE 20-14 Effects of Adrenergic Receptors

Receptor	Location	Response to Stimulation
Alpha (α)	Vessels of skin, muscles, kidneys, and intestines	Vasoconstriction of peripheral arterioles
Beta1 (β1)	Cardiac tissue	Increased heart rate Increased conduction Increased contractility
Beta2 (β2)	Vascular and bronchial smooth muscle	Vasodilation of peripheral arterioles Bronchodilation

pulmonary disease (COPD) caused by blockade of the effects of β_2-receptors in the lungs. Beta-blockers also are negative inotropes and must be used cautiously in patients with LV dysfunction. Although numerous beta-blockers are marketed, only *esmolol, metoprolol,* and *propranolol* are available as intravenous agents for the treatment of acute dysrhythmias. Of these, esmolol (Brevibloc) offers significant advantages for the critically ill patient because of its short half-life (approximately 9 minutes). It is used in the treatment of supraventricular tachycardias, such as atrial fibrillation and atrial flutter.

Class III Drugs. Class III agents include *amiodarone, dofetilide, ibutilide,* and *sotalol.* These agents markedly slow the rate of phase 3 repolarization, increasing the effective refractory period and the action potential duration. Although their effects on the action potential are similar, these drugs differ greatly in their mechanism of action and their side effects. At this time, sotalol is approved only for oral use. Intravenous amiodarone was originally approved for the treatment of serious ventricular dysrhythmias refractory to other medications. Because of its effectiveness, it is now used for both atrial and ventricular dysrhythmias.[105] Dofetilide (Tikosyn) is a new class III antidysrhythmic agent used for the conversion to and maintenance of normal sinus rhythm in patients with highly symptomatic atrial fibrillation or atrial flutter. Because dofetilide prolongs the refractoriness of both atrial and ventricular tissue, prolongation of the QT interval can occur and is associated with an increased risk of torsades de pointes.[106] Therapy with dofetilide is initiated in a hospital setting under close monitoring. Ibutilide (Covert) is a short-term antidysrhythmic agent used for the rapid conversion of acute atrial fibrillation or atrial flutter to sinus rhythm. The drug is administered as a 10-minute infusion in a carefully monitored clinical setting. The most serious side effect of ibutilide is its potential for inducing life-threatening dysrhythmias, especially torsades de pointes.[107]

Class IV Drugs. Class IV agents are calcium channel blockers that inhibit the influx of calcium through slow calcium channels during the plateau phase (phase 2). This effect occurs primarily in tissue in which slow calcium channels predominate, primarily the sinus and AV nodes and the atrial tissue. *Verapamil* was the first drug in this category available as an intravenous antidysrhythmic. It depresses sinus and AV node conduction and is effective in terminating supraventricular tachycardias caused by AV nodal reentry. *Diltiazem* (Cardizem) has become available in intravenous form and is thought to be as effective as verapamil in treating supraventricular dysrhythmias, with fewer hypotensive side effects. Because accessory pathways are not affected by calcium channel blockade, both of these agents must be avoided when treating atrial fibrillation in patients with Wolff-Parkinson-White syndrome.[105]

Unclassified Antidysrhythmics. *Adenosine* (Adenocard) is an antidysrhythmic agent that remains unclassified under the current system. Adenosine occurs endogenously in the body as a building block of adenosine triphosphate (ATP). Given in intravenous boluses, adenosine slows conduction through the AV node, causing transient AV block. It is used clinically to convert supraventricular tachycardias and to facilitate

differential diagnosis of rapid dysrhythmias. Because of its short half-life, the drug is administered intravenously as a rapid bolus, followed by a saline flush. The bolus is delivered as centrally as possible, so that the drug reaches the heart before it is metabolized.[105] Side effects are transient, because the drug is rapidly taken up by the cells and is cleared from the body within 10 seconds.

Magnesium is also unclassified under the present system. Although its action as an antidysrhythmic agent is not entirely understood, clinical studies suggest that it may reduce the incidence of both ventricular and supraventricular dysrhythmias in selected patient populations. It is considered the treatment of choice in patients with torsades de pointes. For acute treatment, 1 to 2 g of magnesium is administered over 1 to 2 minutes. In patients with confirmed hypomagnesemia, this bolus may be followed with a 24-hour infusion.[105]

Side Effects. Antidysrhythmic drugs carry the risk of serious side effects, some of which can be life threatening. The major side effects of the intravenous antidysrhythmic agents are listed in Table 20-15. The most severe complication is the potential for a prodysrhythmic effect. This may result in worsening of the underlying dysrhythmia, the occurrence of a new dysrhythmia, or the development of a bradydysrhythmia. For example, torsades de pointes is a prodysrhythmia caused by a number of drugs. Because the development of a prodysrhythmia is unpredictable, the nurse plays an important role in evaluating ECG changes, monitoring drug levels, and assessing patient symptoms. Antidysrhythmic agents may also alter the amount of energy required for defibrillation and pacing. For example, increases in the dose of an antidysrhythmic drug may increase the amount of output (mA) required to depolarize the myocardium.

Treatment of Atrial Fibrillation. More than 2 million people in the United States have atrial fibrillation, and extensive research has been done on the treatment of this disorder. The goals of pharmacologic therapy for atrial fibrillation include reestablishing and maintaining sinus rhythm, decreasing the rapid ventricular response during episodes of atrial fibrillation, and preventing the risk of thromboembolism. Table 20-16 reviews current drugs used in the treatment of atrial fibrillation. Results of some clinical trials suggest that rate control is equivalent to restoration of sinus rhythm in terms of mortality.[107,108]

INOTROPIC DRUGS

Critically ill patients with compromised cardiac function often require the use of medications to enhance myocardial contractility (positive inotropes). Clinically available inotropes include cardiac glycosides, sympathomimetics, and phosphodiesterase inhibitors. These agents increase myocardial contractility, resulting in improved cardiac output, more complete emptying of the ventricles, and decreased filling pressures.

Cardiac Glycosides. Cardiac glycosides include digitalis and its derivatives. Although these drugs have been used for centuries, their slow onset of action and risk of toxicity make them more appropriate for management of chronic heart

TABLE 20-15 Pharmacologic Management: Selected Antidysrhythmic Agents

DRUG AND SITE OF ACTION	INDICATIONS	DOSAGE	MAJOR SIDE EFFECTS
Sinus Node, Atria, or AV Node			
Adenosine	SVT, PSVT	6 mg IV rapid push; if unsuccessful, repeat with 12 mg over 1-2 sec; follow with IV fluid 10 mL flush (NS or D_5W)	Transient; flushing, dyspnea, hypotension
Digoxin	AFib, AF, PSVT	0.5-1 mg loading dose in divided doses; maintenance dose of 0.125-0.375 mg daily	Bradycardia, heart block Toxicity: CNS and GI symptoms
Diltiazem	SVT, AFib, AF	Bolus dose of 0.25 mg/kg IV over 2 min, followed by an infusion of 5-15 mg/hr	Bradycardia, hypotension, AV block
Esmolol	ST, SVT	Loading dose of 500 mcg/kg over 1 min, followed by an infusion of 50 mcg/kg/min for 4 min; repeat procedure every 5 min, increasing infusion by 25-50 mcg/kg/min to maximum of 200 mcg/kg/min	Hypotension, bradycardia, heart failure
Ibutilide	AFib, AF	0.010-0.025 mg/kg infused over 10 min (may repeat once) or 1 mg diluted in 50 mL infused over 10 min (may repeat once)	Minimal side effects except for rare polymorphic VT (torsades de pointes)
Propranolol	SVT	1-3 mg IV every 5 min, not to exceed 0.1 mg/kg	Bradycardia, heart block, heart failure
Verapamil	AF, PSVT	5-10 mg IV, may repeat in 15-30 min	Hypotension, bradycardia, heart failure
Ventricle			
Lidocaine	PVCs, VT, VF	1-1.5 mg/kg bolus, followed by continuous infusion of 1-4 mg/min	CNS toxicity, nausea, vomiting with repeated doses
Atria and Ventricle			
Amiodarone	VT/VT arrest	300 mg IV push; may repeat with 150 mg in 3-5 min (maximum dose, 2.2 g/24 hr)	Hypotension, abnormal liver function tests
	Stable VT, AFib, AF	150 mg IV over 10 min, followed by 360 mg over 6 hr (1 mg/min); maintenance infusion of 0.5 mg/min	
Procainamide	AF, SVT, PVCs, VT	Loading dose of 12-17 mg/kg at a rate of 20 mg/min, followed by infusion of 1-4 mg/min	Hypotension, GI effects Widening of QRS and QT lengthening

AF, atrial flutter; AFib, atrial fibrillation; AV, atrioventricular; CNS, central nervous system; D_5W, 5% dextrose in water; GI, gastrointestinal; IV, intravenous; NS, normal saline; PSVT, paroxysmal supraventricular tachycardia; PVCs, premature ventricular contractions; ST, sinus tachycardia; SVT, supraventricular tachycardia; VT, ventricular tachycardia; VF, ventricular fibrillation.

failure. Because digoxin also causes slowing of the sinus rate and a decrease in AV conduction, it may be administered intravenously in the acute care setting to control supraventricular dysrhythmias.

Sympathomimetic Agents. Sympathomimetic agents stimulate adrenergic receptors, thereby simulating the effects of sympathetic nerve stimulation. Included in this category are naturally occurring catecholamines (epinephrine, dopamine, and norepinephrine) and synthetic catecholamines (dobutamine and isoproterenol). The cardiovascular effects of these drugs, which vary according to their selectivity for specific receptor sites, are often dose dependent as well. Table 20-17 describes the cardiovascular effects of sympathomimetic drugs at various dosages.

Dopamine (Intropin) is one of the most widely used drugs in the critical care setting. It is a chemical precursor of norepinephrine, which, in addition to both α- and β-receptor stimulation, can activate dopaminergic receptors in the renal and mesenteric blood vessels. The actions of this drug are entirely dose related.[109] At low dosages of 1 to 2 mcg/kg/min, dopamine stimulates dopaminergic receptors, causing renal and mesenteric vasodilation. The resultant increase in renal perfusion increases urinary output. However, it is clear that this increase in urine output does not confer protection against the

TABLE 20-16 Pharmacologic Management: Atrial Fibrillation

TREATMENT GOAL	CLASSIFICATION AND DRUGS	SPECIAL CONSIDERATIONS

Conversion or maintenance of sinus rhythm	Class IA
	  Quinidine
	  Procainamide (Pronestyl)
	  Disopyramide (Norpace)
		Class IA drugs prolong QT intervals and may cause torsades de pointes. Rate control should be achieved before initiation of therapy.

	Class IC
	  Flecainide (Tambocor)
	  Propafenone (Rhythmol)
		Class IC drugs are prodysrhythmic in patients with CAD or previous MI and should be avoided in these patients.

	Class III
	  Amiodarone (Cordarone)
	  Dofetilide (Tikosyn)
	  Ibutilide (Corvert)
	  Sotalol (Betapace)
		Amiodarone and sotalol also have beta-blocking properties and may help with rate control. Treatment with dofetilide requires careful monitoring for prodysrhythmic effects. Ibutilide is an IV agent and is used for conversion only.

Control of ventricular rate	Beta-blockers
	  Esmolol (Brevibloc)
	  Metoprolol (Lopressor)
	  Propranolol (Inderal)
		IV esmolol may be used in acute settings to control ventricular rate. Oral agents are used for maintenance therapy. Beta-blockers provide good rate control during exercise.

	Calcium channel blockers
	  Diltiazem (Cardizem)
	  Verapamil (Isoptin)
		Intravenous calcium channel blockers may be used in emergency situations, followed by oral agents for maintenance therapy.

	Digitalis compounds Digoxin (Lanoxin)	Digoxin does not effectively control rate with exercise, so it may be used in combination with other drugs.

Prevention of thromboembolism	Anticoagulants
	  Heparin
	  Warfarin (Coumadin)
		Heparin may be used in emergency situations, before cardioversion. Warfarin is used long term, with monitoring to achieve an INR of 2.0-3.0.

	Antiplatelet agents Aspirin	Aspirin may be used in patients with contraindications to warfarin or in low-risk patients younger than 65 years.

CAD, coronary artery disease; INR, international normalized ratio; IV, intravenous; MI, myocardial infarction.

development of acute renal failure. Moderate dosages result in stimulation of β_1-receptors to increase myocardial contractility and improve cardiac output. At dosages greater than 10 mcg/kg/min, dopamine predominantly stimulates α-receptors, resulting in vasoconstriction that often negates both the β-adrenergic and the dopaminergic effects.

Dobutamine (Dobutrex) is a synthetic catecholamine with predominantly β_1-adrenergic effects. It also produces some β_2 stimulation, resulting in a mild vasodilation. Dobutamine is as effective as dopamine in increasing myocardial contractility and is useful in the treatment of heart failure, especially in hypotensive patients who cannot tolerate vasodilator therapy. The usual dosage range is 2.5 to 20 mcg/kg/min, titrated on the basis of hemodynamic parameters.

Epinephrine (Adrenalin) is produced by the adrenal gland as part of the body's response to stress. This agent has the ability to stimulate both α- and β-receptors, depending on the dose administered (see Table 20-17). At doses of 1 to 2 mg/min, epinephrine binds with β-receptors to increase heart rate, cardiac conduction, contractility, and vasodilation, thereby increasing cardiac output. As the dosage is increased, α-receptors are stimulated, resulting in increased vascular resistance and increased

blood pressure. At these doses, epinephrine's impact on cardiac output depends on the heart's ability to pump against the increased afterload. Epinephrine accelerates the sinus rate and may precipitate ventricular dysrhythmias in the ischemic heart. Other side effects include restlessness, angina, and headache.

Norepinephrine (Levophed) is similar to epinephrine in its ability to stimulate β- and α-receptors, but it lacks the β_2 effects of epinephrine. At low infusion rates, β_1-receptors are activated to produce increased contractility, augmenting cardiac output. At higher doses, the inotropic effects are limited by marked vasoconstriction mediated by α-receptors. Clinically, norepinephrine is used most often as a vasopressor to elevate blood pressure in shock states.

Isoproterenol (Isuprel) is a pure β-receptor stimulant with no α-adrenergic effects. It produces dramatic increases in heart rate, conduction, and contractility through β_1 stimulation and vasodilation through β_2 stimulation. Isoproterenol also produces vasodilation of the pulmonary arteries and bronchodilation. It greatly increases the automaticity of cardiac cells and frequently precipitates dysrhythmias, such as PVCs and even VT. These effects limit its usefulness in most patients and it is rarely used.

Phosphodiesterase Inhibitors. Phosphodiesterase inhibitors are inotropic agents that also are potent vasodilators

TABLE 20-17 Physiologic Effects of Sympathomimetic Agents

Drug	Dosage	RECEPTOR ACTIVATED*				CARDIOVASCULAR EFFECTS		
		Alpha	Beta$_1$	Beta$_2$	Dopa	CO	HR	SVR
Dobutamine	<5 mcg/kg/min	0	↑↑	↑	0	↑↑	↑	↓
	5-20 mcg/kg/min	0	↑↑↑	↑↑	0	↑↑↑	↑↑	↓↓
Dopamine	<3 mcg/kg/min	0	↑	↑	↑↑↑	0/↑	0/↑	0
	3-10 mcg/kg/min	↑↑	↑↑↑	↑	↑↑↑	↑↑↑	↑	↑
	11-20 mcg/kg/min	↑↑↑	↑↑↑	↑	↑↑	↑↑	↑↑	↑↑↑
Epinephrine	<2 mcg/min	0	↑	↑↑	0	0/↑	0/↑	↓
	2-8 mcg/min	↑↑	↑↑↑	↑↑	0	↑↑↑	↑↑	↑
	9-20 mcg/min	↑↑↑	↑↑↑	↑↑	0	↑↑	↑↑	↑↑↑
Isoproterenol	1-7 mcg/min	0	↑↑↑	↑↑↑	0	↑↑↑	↑↑↑	↓↓↓
Norepinephrine	<2 mcg/min	↑↑↑	↑↑	0	0	↑	0/↑	↑↑↑
	2-16 mcg/min	↑↑↑↑	↑↑	0	0	↓	↑	↑↑↑↑
Phenylephrine	10-100 mcg/min	↑↑↑↑	0	0	0	0	↓	↑↑↑

*See Table 20-14 for actions of receptors.

0, no effect; ↑, increased (number of arrows indicates degree of effect); ↓, decreased (number of arrows indicates degree of effect); CO, cardiac output; HR, heart rate; SVR, systemic vascular resistance.

(inodilators). Drugs in this classification inhibit the enzyme phosphodiesterase, resulting in increased levels of cyclic adenosine monophosphate (AMP) and intracellular calcium. Amrinone (Inocor) and milrinone (Primacor) were the first of these agents approved for use in the United States. Increases in cardiac output occur as a result of increased contractility (inotropic effects) and decreased afterload (vasodilative effects). Filling pressures tend to decrease, while the heart rate and blood pressure remain fairly constant. Amrinone may cause thrombocytopenia, so platelet counts are monitored and patients are observed for hemorrhagic complications. Milrinone is associated with a lower rate of thrombocytopenia but can induce ventricular dysrhythmias (PVCs, VT) in a significant number of patients.[110]

VASODILATOR DRUGS

Vasodilators are pharmacologic agents that improve cardiac performance by various degrees of arterial or venous dilation, or both. The goal of vasodilator therapy may be reduction of preload or of afterload, or both. Afterload reduction is accomplished by vasodilation of arterial vessels. This results in decreased resistance to LV ejection and may improve cardiac output without increasing myocardial oxygen demands. Reduction of preload is accomplished by dilation of venous vessels to increase capacitance. This results in decreased filling pressures for a failing heart. These drugs may be classified into four groups on the basis of mechanism of action (Table 20-18).

Direct Smooth Muscle Relaxants. Direct-acting vasodilators include sodium nitroprusside, nitroglycerin, and hydralazine. These drugs produce relaxation of vascular smooth muscle through the activation of nitric oxide, which results in decreased peripheral vascular resistance (PVR). Hypotension

may occur as a result of peripheral vasodilation, and headaches may be caused by cerebral vasodilation. Compensatory mechanisms can occur in response to the drop in blood pressure. These include baroreceptor activation that causes reflex tachycardia and activation of the renin-angiotensin-aldosterone system (RAAS) (see Fig. 19-16), with resultant sodium and water retention.

Sodium nitroprusside (Nipride) is a potent, rapidly acting venous and arterial vasodilator that is particularly suitable for rapid reduction of blood pressure in hypertensive emergencies and perioperatively. It also is effective for afterload reduction in the setting of severe heart failure. The drug is administered by continuous intravenous infusion, with the dosage titrated to maintain the desired blood pressure and SVR. Prolonged administration can result in thiocyanate toxicity, manifested by nausea, confusion, and tinnitus.[111]

Intravenous nitroglycerin (Tridil) causes both arterial and venous vasodilation, but its venous effect is more pronounced. It is used in the critical care setting for the treatment of acute heart failure, because it reduces cardiac filling pressures, relieves pulmonary congestion, and decreases cardiac workload and oxygen consumption. Nitroglycerin dilates the coronary arteries and is a useful adjunct in the treatment of unstable angina and acute MI. The initial dosage is 10 mcg/min, and the infusion is titrated upward to achieve the desired clinical effect: a reduction or elimination of chest pain, decreased PAOP (wedge pressure), or a decrease in blood pressure. Nitroglycerin is administered prophylactically to prevent coronary vasospasm after coronary angioplasty, atherectomy, stent insertion, or fibrinolytic therapy. The most common side effects of this drug are hypotension, flushing, and headache.[110]

Hydralazine (Apresoline) is a potent arterial vasodilator. It seldom is given as a continuous infusion; rather, it is

TABLE 20-18 Pharmacologic Management: Characteristics of Selected Vasodilators

CLASSIFICATION AND DRUGS	DOSAGE	PRELOAD	AFTERLOAD	SIDE EFFECTS
Direct Smooth Muscle Relaxants				
Sodium nitroprusside (Nipride)	0.25-6 mcg/kg/min IV infusion	Moderate	Strong	Hypotension, thiocyanate toxicity, reflex tachycardia
Nitroglycerin (Tridil)	5-300 mcg/min IV infusion	Strong	Mild	Headache, reflex tachycardia, hypotension
Calcium Channel Blockers				
Nicardipine (Cardene)	5 mg/hr IV, titrated to 15 mg/hr	None	Strong	Hypotension, headache, reflex tachycardia
Nifedipine (Procardia)	10-30 mg PO	None	Strong	Hypotension, headache, reflex tachycardia
Angiotensin-Converting Enzyme Inhibitors				
Captopril (Capoten)	6.25-100 mg PO every 8-12 hr	Moderate	Moderate	Hypotension, chronic cough, neutropenia
Enalapril (Vasotec)	0.625 mg IV over 5 min, then every 6 hr	Moderate	Moderate	Hypotension, elevation of liver enzymes
α-Adrenergic Blockers				
Labetalol (Normodyne)	20-80 mg IV bolus every 10 min, then 1-2 mg/min infusion	Moderate	Moderate	Orthostatic hypotension, bronchospasm, AV block
Phentolamine (Regitine)	1-5 mg IV slowly every 6 hours	Moderate	Moderate	Hypotension, tachycardia

AV, atrioventricular; IV, intravenous; PO, orally.

TABLE 20-19 Pharmacologic Management: Characteristics of Calcium Channel Blockers

DRUG	ACTIONS	DOSAGE	SPECIAL CONSIDERATIONS
Dihydropyridines			
Nicardipine (Cardene)	Short-term control of hypertension	5 mg/hr IV, titrated to 15 mg/hr	Hypotension, headache, nausea
Nifedipine (Procardia)	Hypertension	10-30 mg PO	Hypotension, headache, reflex tachycardia
Benzothiazepines			
Diltiazem (Cardizem)	SVT, AFib, AF, angina	Bolus dose of 0.25 mg/kg IV over 2 min, followed by an infusion of 5-15 mg/hr	Bradycardia, hypotension, atrioventricular block
Phenylalkylamines			
Verapamil (Calan, Isoptin)	AF, PSVT	5-10 mg IV, may repeat in 15-30 min	Hypotension, bradycardia, heart failure

AF, atrial flutter; AFib, atrial fibrillation; IV, intravenous; PO, by mouth; PSVT, paroxysmal supraventricular tachycardia; SVT, supraventricular tachycardia.

administered in slow intravenous doses of 5 to 10 mg every 4 to 8 hours. Occasionally, hydralazine is given as an intermediate drug during the transition between weaning of a continuous infusion and initiation of oral antihypertensive medications. The major side effect is reflex tachycardia mediated by the sympathetic nervous system. This may be diminished by the concomitant administration of beta-blockers.

Calcium Channel Blockers. Calcium channel blockers are a chemically diverse group of drugs with differing pharmacologic effects (Table 20-19).

Nifedipine (Procardia) and nicardipine (Cardene) are dihydropyridines. Drugs in this group of calcium channel blockers (with the suffix *pine*) are used primarily as arterial vasodilators. These agents reduce the influx of calcium in the arterial resistance vessels. Both coronary and peripheral arteries are affected. They are used in the critical care setting to treat hypertension. Nifedipine is available only in an oral form, but in the past it was prescribed sublingually during hypertensive emergencies. Reports of adverse events associated with sublingual nifedipine have prompted the FDA to strongly discourage sublingual use.[112] Nicardipine has become available as an intravenous calcium channel blocker, and it offers more accurate titration for effective control of hypertension. Side effects of nifedipine and nicardipine are related to vasodilation and include hypotension, reflex tachycardia, flushing, headache, and ankle edema.

Diltiazem (Cardizem) is from the benzothiazine group of calcium channel blockers. *Verapamil* (Calan, Isoptin) is part of the phenylalkylamine group. The different classifications account for the differing actions of these calcium channel blockers. These drugs dilate coronary arteries but have little effect on the peripheral vasculature. They are used in the treatment of angina, especially that which has a vasospastic component, and as antidysrhythmics in the treatment of supraventricular tachycardias.

Angiotensin-Converting Enzyme Inhibitors. Angiotensin-converting enzyme (ACE) inhibitors produce vasodilation by blocking the conversion of angiotensin I to angiotensin II. Because angiotensin is a potent vasoconstrictor, limiting its production decreases PVR. In contrast to the direct vasodilators and nifedipine, ACE inhibitors do not cause reflex tachycardia or induce sodium and water retention. However, these drugs may cause a profound fall in blood pressure, especially in patients who are volume-depleted. Blood pressure must be monitored carefully, especially at the initiation of therapy.

Captopril (Capoten) and *enalapril* (Vasotec) are used in patients with heart failure to decrease SVR (afterload) and PAOP (preload). Captopril is available only in an oral form, but it has a relatively rapid onset of action (approximately 1 hour). Enalapril is available in an intravenous form and may be used to decrease afterload in more emergent situations.

B-Type Natriuretic Peptide. *Nesiritide* (Natrecor) is a new vasodilator used in the treatment of acute heart failure. This agent is a recombinant form of human brain natriuretic peptide (BNP), the hormone released by cardiac cells in response to ventricular distention. The primary effects of nesiritide include decreased filling pressures (PAOP, CVP), reduced vascular resistance (SVR, PVR), and increased urine output. Compared with traditional vasodilator therapy for acute heart failure, nesiritide reportedly is as effective as the traditional agents and has fewer side effects (e.g., headache).[110] The recommended dose is an intravenous bolus of 2 mcg/kg, followed by a continuous infusion of 0.01 mcg/kg/min. The primary side effect is hypotension. If this occurs, nesiritide may need to be discontinued for a time and then restarted at a lower dose after the patient has stabilized.[110] Extensive analysis of clinical studies indicated that this drug may be associated with an increased risk of worsening kidney function and short-term mortality compared with traditional treatment of acute decompensated heart failure. As a result, an expert panel recommended that use of nesiritide be strictly limited to hospitalized patients with refractory heart failure until further study is completed.[113]

Alpha-Adrenergic Blockers. Peripheral adrenergic blockers block α-receptors in arteries and veins, resulting in vasodilation. Orthostatic hypotension is a common side effect and may result in syncope. Long-term therapy also may be complicated by fluid and water retention.

Labetalol (Normodyne), a combined peripheral alpha-blocker and cardioselective beta-blocker, is used in the treatment of acute stroke and hypertensive emergencies.[114] Because the blockade of β_1-receptors permits the decrease of blood pressure without the risk of reflexive tachycardia and increased cardiac output, this drug also is useful in the treatment of acute aortic dissection.[115]

Phentolamine (Regitine) is a nonselective peripheral alpha-blocker that deceases blood pressure through arterial vasodilation. The half-life is 19 minutes when given intravenously. It is administered slow IV push, 1 to 5 mg every 6 hours to reduce blood pressure.[111] This drug is used only in very specific circumstances. Phentolamine is the drug of choice in to control blood pressure and sweating caused by *pheochromocytoma*, an epinephrine (adrenalin)-secreting tumor that can arise from the adrenal medulla.[111]

Phentolamine also is used to treat the *extravasation of dopamine* or other vasopressors into peripheral tissues. If this occurs, 5 to 10 mg is diluted in 10 mL normal saline and administered intradermally into the infiltrated area as soon as possible following the extravasation.

Dopamine Receptor Agonists. Fenoldopam (Corlopam) is the first of a new class of vasodilators called *selective, specific dopamine (D_1) receptor agonists.*[111] The drug is a potent vasodilator that affects peripheral, renal, and mesenteric arteries. It is administered by continuous intravenous infusion beginning at 0.1 mcg/kg/min and titrated up to the desired blood pressure effect, with a maximum recommended dose of 0.5 mcg/kg/min. It can be administered as an alternative to sodium nitroprusside or other antihypertensives in the treatment of hypertensive emergencies. Fenoldopam can be used safely in patients with kidney dysfunction.[111]

Vasopressors. Vasopressors are sympathomimetic agents that mediate peripheral vasoconstriction through stimulation of α-receptors (see Table 20-14). This results in increased SVR and elevates blood pressure. Some of these drugs (epinephrine and norepinephrine) also have the ability to stimulate β-receptors. Vasopressors are not widely used in the treatment of critically ill cardiac patients, because the dramatic increase in afterload is taxing to a damaged heart. Occasionally, vasopressors may be used to maintain organ perfusion in shock states. For example, phenylephrine (Neo-Synephrine) or norepinephrine (Levophed) may be administered as a continuous intravenous infusion to maintain organ perfusion by increasing SVR in cases of severe sepsis or septic shock.

Vasopressin, also known as antidiuretic hormone (ADH), has become popular in the critical care setting for its vasoconstrictive effects. At higher doses, vasopressin directly stimulates V1 receptors in vascular smooth muscle, resulting in vasoconstriction of capillaries and small arterioles. A one-time dose of 40 units intravenously is recommended in the ACLS guidelines as first-line drug therapy for VF, pulseless VT asystole, or pulseless electrical activity (PEA).[116] Continuous infusions of 0.02 unit/min up to 0.1 unit/min have been used in the treatment of vasodilatory shock in patients with refractory hypotension after cardiopulmonary bypass.[65]

In septic shock vasopressin levels have been reported to be lower than anticipated for a shock state.[117] Vasopressin continuous infusion of 0.03 unit/min may be added to the norepinephrine infusion in refractory shock per the 2008 surviving sepsis guidelines.[117] Patients must be assessed for side effects such as heart failure caused by the antidiuretic effects, and monitored for increased risk of ischemia in the myocardium, spleen and periphery.[117] Vasopressin should be infused through a central line to avoid the risk of peripheral extravasation and resultant tissue necrosis. Placement of an arterial line in shock-states to monitor blood pressure and SVR is recommended.[117]

DRUG TREATMENT OF HEART FAILURE

Almost 5 million Americans have heart failure, making it a major chronic health issue.[118] The goals of treatment in heart failure include alleviating symptoms, slowing the progression of the disease, and improving survival. Findings from a number of randomly controlled clinical trials have resulted in guidelines for the pharmacologic treatment of heart failure.[119,120] More information about heart failure is available in Chapter 19. Table 20-20 reviews the drugs currently recommended for the treatment of heart failure.

TABLE 20-20 Pharmacologic Management: Heart Failure

CLASSIFICATION AND DRUG	MECHANISM OF ACTION	EFFECTS	SPECIAL CONSIDERATIONS
ACE Inhibitors			
Captopril (Capoten) Enalapril (Vasotec) Lisinopril (Prinivil)	Interferes with the renin-angiotensin-aldosterone system by preventing conversion of angiotensin I to angiotensin II	Decreases afterload Decreases preload Reverses ventricular remodeling	Agents appear equivalent in treatment of heart failure Monitor closely for hypotension when initiating therapy May be contraindicated in patients with renal insufficiency
Angiotensin Receptor Blockers			
Losartan (Cozaar) Valsartan (Diovan)	Interferes with the renin-angiotensin-aldosterone system by blocking the effect of angiotensin II at the angiotensin II receptor site	Decreases afterload Decreases preload Reverses ventricular remodeling	Reserved for patients who cannot tolerate ACE inhibitors due to side effects such as severe cough or angioedema
Beta-Blockers			
Metoprolol (Lopressor) Carvedilol (Coreg)	Counteracts the SNS response activated in heart failure by blocking receptor sites. Metoprolol is a cardioselective β-blocker, whereas carvedilol blocks α- and β-receptor sites.	Slows heart rate Prevents dysrhythmias Decreases blood pressure Reverses ventricular remodeling	Not initiated during decompensated stage of heart failure Use cautiously in patients with reactive airway disease, poorly controlled diabetes, bradydysrhythmias, or heart block Carvedilol dose is increased slowly, while monitoring for symptoms caused by vasodilation, such as dizziness or hypotension
Aldosterone Antagonists			
Spironolactone (Aldactone)	Counteracts the effects of aldosterone, which include sodium and water retention	Decreases preload Decreases myocardial hypertrophy	May increase serum potassium
Inotropes			
Digoxin (Lanoxin)	Affects the Na$^+$,K$^+$-ATPase pump in myocardial cells to increase the strength of contraction	Increases contractility Increases cardiac output Prevents atrial dysrhythmias	Risk of toxicity is increased with hypokalemia

ACE, Angiotensin-converting enzyme; Na$^+$/K$^+$-ATPase, sodium-potassium adenosine triphosphatase; SNS, sympathetic nervous system.

Case Study: Patient with a Cardiac Problem

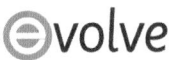 Answers to the Case Study Questions can be found on the Evolve web site at http://evolve.elsevier.com/Urden/.

Brief Patient History

Mrs. G is a 54-year-old African American woman who has been having intermittent indigestion for the past month. She has a history of hypertension and hyperlipidemia. She was admitted as an inpatient on a medical floor for management of her blood pressure and is scheduled to undergo endoscopy tomorrow. Mrs. G suddenly becomes diaphoretic and complains of nausea and epigastric pain.

Clinical Assessment

The rapid response team is called to evaluate Mrs. G. When the team arrives at her bedside, she continues to complain of pain which now radiates to her neck and back. She has some slight shortness of breath and is vomiting.

Diagnostic Procedures

The admission electrocardiogram (ECG) shows ST-segment elevation in II, III, and AVF.

Baseline vital signs include the following: blood pressure of 160/90 mm Hg, heart rate of 98 beats/min (sinus rhythm), respiratory rate of 18 breaths/min, temperature of 99° F, and O_2 saturation of 94%.

Medical Diagnosis

Mrs. G is diagnosed with an inferior myocardial infarction.

Questions

1. What major outcomes do you expect to achieve for this patient?
2. What problems or risks must be managed to achieve these outcomes?
3. What interventions must be initiated to monitor, prevent, manage, or eliminate the problems and risks identified?
4. What interventions should be initiated to promote optimal functioning, safety, and well-being of the patient?
5. What possible learning needs do you anticipate for this patient?
6. What cultural and age-related factors may have a bearing on the patient's plan of care?

Be sure to check out the bonus material, including free self-assessment exercises, on the Evolve web site at http://evolve.elsevier.com/Urden/.

References

1. Schoenfeld MH: Contemporary pacemaker and defibrillator device therapy: challenges confronting the general cardiologist, *Circulation* 115:638, 2007.
2. Tracy CM et al: ACC/AHA clinical competence statement on invasive electrophysiology studies, catheter ablation, and cardioversion, *Circulation* 114:1654, 2006.
3. Marine JE: Catheter ablation therapy for supraventricular arrhythmias, *JAMA* 298(23):2768, 2007.
4. Miller JN, Drew BJ: Atrial electrograms after cardiac surgery: survey of clinical practice, *Am J Crit Care* 16(4):350, 2007.
5. Stone KR, McPherson: Assessment and management of patients with pacemakers and implantable cardioverter defibrillators, *Crit Care Med* 32 (suppl):S155, 2004.
6. American Heart Association: ECC Guidelines. Part 5. Electrical therapies: automated external defibrillators, defibrillation, cardioversion and pacing, *Circulation* 112(8):IV-35, 2005.
7. Reade MC: Temporary epicardial pacing after cardiac surgery: a practical review. Part I. General considerations in the management of epicardial pacing, *Anaesthesia* 62:264, 2007.
8. Bernstein AD et al: The revised NASPE/BPEG generic pacemaker code for antibradycardia, adaptive-rate and multi-site pacing, *Pacing Clin Electrophysiol* 25:260, 2002.
9. Dyrda K, Khairy P: Implantable rhythm devices and electromagnetic interference: myth or reality? *Expert Rev Cardiovasc Ther* 6(6):823, 2008.
10. Rosamond W et al: Heart disease and stroke statistics—2008 update: a report from the American Heart Association Statistics Committee and Stroke Statistics Subcommittee, *Circulation* 117:e25, 2008.
11. Epstein AE et al: ACC/AHA/HRS 2008 guidelines for device-based therapy of cardiac rhythm abnormalities: executive summary, *Circulation* 117:2820, 2008.
12. Saul L: Cardiac resynchronization therapy, *Crit Care Nurse Q* 30(1):58, 2007.
13. Goldberger Z, Lampert R: Implantable cardioverter-defibrillators: expanding indications and technologies, *JAMA* 295(7):809, 2006.
14. Palazzo MO: Atrial fibrillation and the postoperative cardiac surgical patient, *Crit Care Nurs Clin North Am* 19:395, 2007.
15. Knight BP: Role of permanent pacing to prevent atrial fibrillation: science advisory from the American Heart Association Council on Clinical Cardiology and the Quality of Care and Outcomes Research Interdisciplinary Working Group in collaboration with the Heart Rhythm Society, *Circulation* 111:240, 2005.
16. Woodruff J, Prudente LA: Update on implantable pacemakers, *J Cardiovasc Nurs* 20(4):261, 2005.
17. Wilkoff BL: Pacemaker remote follow-up evaluation and review: results of the PREFER trial. Late-breaking clinical trials session. Presented at the Heart Rhythm Society 2008 Scientific Sessions, May 15, 2008, San Francisco, California.
18. Kadish A, Mandeep M: Heart failure devices: implantable cardioverter-defibrillators and bi-ventricular pacing therapy, *Circulation* 111:3327, 2005.
19. Angerstein RL et al: Enhancing care for cardiac resynchronization therapy patients: device diagnostics and clinical application, *J Cardiovas Nurs* 21 (5):397, 2006.
20. Faxon DP: Development of systems of care for ST-elevation myocardial infarction patients: current state of ST-elevation myocardial infarction care, *Circulation* 116(2):e29, 2007.
21. Antman EM et al: ACC/AHA guidelines for the management of patients with ST-elevation myocardial infarction, *J Am Coll Cardiol* 44:671, 2004.
22. Peacock WF et al: Reperfusion strategies in the emergency treatment of ST-elevation myocardial infarction, *Am J Emerg Med* 25:353, 2007.
23. Peterson ED et al: ACC/AHA 2007 guidelines for the management of patients with unstable angina/non–ST-elevation myocardial infarction, *Circulation* 116:e148, 2007.
24. Antman EM et al: 2007 Focused update of the ACC/AHA 2004 guidelines for the management of patients with ST-elevation myocardial infarction, *Circulation* 117:296, 2007.

25. Kiernan TJ, Gersh BJ: Thrombolysis in acute myocardial infarction: Current status, *Med Clin North Am* 91:617, 2007.

26. The TIMI Study Group: The Thrombolysis In Myocardial Infarction (TIMI) trial: phase I findings, *N Engl J Med* 312:932, 1985.

27. Gelfand EV, Cannon CP: Myocardial infarction: contemporary management strategies, *J Intern Med* 262:59, 2007.

28. Zimarino M et al: Facilitated PCI: rationale, current evidence, open questions and future directions, *J Cardiovasc Pharmacol* 51:3, 2008.

29. Drew BJ et al: Practice standards for electrocardiographic monitoring in hospital settings: an AHA scientific statement, *Circulation* 110:2721, 2004.

30. Sharma SK, Chen V: Coronary interventional devices: balloon, atherectomy, thrombectomy and distal protection devices, *Cardiol Clin* 24:201, 2006.

31. Singh KP, Harrington RA: Primary percutaneous intervention in acute myocardial infarction, *Med Clin North Am* 91:639, 2007.

32. King SB et al: ACCF/AHA/SCAI 2007 update of the clinical competence statement on cardiac interventional procedures, *Circulation* 116:98, 2007.

33. Pompa JJ, Baim DS, Resnic FS: Percutaneous coronary and valvular intervention. In Libby P et al, editors: *Braunwald's heart disease*, ed 8, Philadelphia, 2007, Saunders.

34. Newsome LT, Kutcher MA, Royser RL: Coronary artery stents. Part I. Evolution of percutaneous intervention, *Anesth Analges* 107:552, 2008.

35. Rajagopal V, Rockson SG: Coronary restenosis: a review of mechanisms and management, *Am J Med* 115:547, 2003.

36. Bittl JA et al: Meta-analysis of randomized trials of percutaneous transluminal coronary angioplasty versus atherectomy, cutting balloon atherotomy, or laser angioplasty, *J Am Coll Cardiol* 43:936, 2004.

37. Stankovic G et al: Comparison of directional coronary atherectomy and stenting verus stenting alone for the treatment of de novo and restenotic coronary artery narrowing, *Am J Cardiol* 93:953, 2004.

38. King SB et al: ACC/AHA/SCAI 2005 guideline update for percutaneous coronary intervention: a report of the ACC/AHA task force on practice guidelines, *Circulation* 117:261, 2008.

39. Levine GN et al: Newer pharmacotherapy in patients undergoing percutaneous interventions: a guide for pharmacists and other health professionals, *Pharmacotherapy* 26:1537, 2006.

40. Sims JM: Update on drug-eluting stents, *Dimens Crit Care Nurs* 26 (6):237, 2007.

41. Kastrati A et al: Analysis of 14 trial comparing sirolimus-eluting stents with bare-metal stents, *N Engl J Med* 356:1030, 2007.

42. Stone GW et al: Safety and efficacy of sirolimus-and paclitaxel-eluting stents, *N Engl J Med* 356:998, 2007.

43. King et al: 2007 focused update of the ACC/AHA/SCAI 2005 guideline update for percutaneous coronary intervention, *Circulation* 117:261, 2008.

44. Carmenzind E: Treatment of in-stent restenosis: back to the future? *N Engl J Med* 355:2149, 2006.

45. Wong EM et al: A review of the management of patients after percutaneous coronary intervention, *Int J Clin Pract* 60(5):582, 2006.

46. McCullough PA, Berman AD: Percutaneous coronary interventions in the high-risk renal patient: strategies for renal protection and vascular protection, *Cardiol Clin* 23:299, 2005.

47. Dauerman HL et al: Vascular closure devices: the second decade, *J Am Coll Card* 50(17):1617, 2007.

48. Jozic J et al: Timing and correlates of very early major adverse clinical events following percutaneous coronary intervention, *J Invasive Cardiol* 20(3):113, 2008.

49. Grines CL et al: Prevention of premature discontinuation of dual antiplatelet therapy in patients with coronary artery stents, *Circulation* 115:813, 2007.

50. Rosengart TK et al: Percutaneous and minimally invasive valve procedures: a scientific statement from the AHA Council on Cardiovascular Surgery and Anesthesia, Council on Clinical Cardiology, Functional Genomics and Translational Biology Interdisciplinary Working Group, and Quality of Care and Outcomes Research Interdisciplinary Working Group, *Circulation* 117:1750, 2008.

51. Bonow RO et al: ACC/AHA guidelines for the management of patients with valvular heart disease, *Circulation* 114:450, 2006.

52. Lauck S, et al: A new option for the treatment of aortic stenosis: percutaneous aortic valve replacement, *Crit Care Nurse* 28(3):40, 2008.

53. Mack MJ: Percutaneous treatment of mitral regurgitation: so near, yet so far, *J Thorac Cardiovasc Surg* 135:237, 2008.

54. Eagle KA et al: ACC/AHA 2004 guideline update for coronary artery bypass graft surgery: a report of the American College of Cardiology/American Heart Association Task Force on Practice Guidelines (Committee to Update the 1999 Guidelines for Coronary Artery Bypass Graft Surgery), *Circulation* 110(14):e340-e437, 2004.

55. Booth J et al: Randomized, controlled trial of coronary artery bypass surgery versus percutaneous coronary intervention in patients with multivessel coronary artery disease: six-year follow-up from the Stent or Surgery Trial (SoS), *Circulation* 118(4):381, 2008.

56. Bravata DM et al: Systematic review: The comparative effectiveness of percutaneous coronary interventions and coronary artery bypass graft surgery, *Ann Intern Med* 147:1, 2007.

57. Lai T et al: The transition from open endoscopic saphenous vein harvesting and its clinical impact, *Tex Heart Inst J* 33:316, 2006.

58. Desai ND, Fremes SE: Radial artery conduit for coronary revascularization: as good as the internal thoracic artery? *Curr Opin Cardiol* 22:534, 2007.

59. Tavilla G et al: Long-term follow-up of coronary artery bypass grafting in three-vessel disease using exclusively pedicled bilateral internal thoracic and right gastroepiploic arteries, *Ann Thorac Surg* 77(3):794, 2004.

60. Collins P et al: Radial artery versus saphenous vein patency randomized trial: five year angiographic follow-up, *Circulation* 117:2859, 2008.

61. Hill KM: Surgical repair of cardiac valves, *Crit Care Nurs Clin North Am* 19:353, 2007.

62. Gott VL et al: Mechanical heart valves: 50 years of evolution, *Ann Thorac Surg* 76:S2230, 2003.

63. Louagie YA et al: Continuous cold blood cardioplegia improves myocardial protection: a prospective randomized study, *Ann Thorac Surg* 77 (2):664, 2004.

64. Mallidi HR et al: The short-term and long-term effects of warm or tepid cardioplegia, *J Thorac Cardiovasc Surg* 125:711, 2003.

65. Katz EA: Pharmacological management of the postoperative cardiac surgical patient, *Crit Care Nurs Clin North Am* 19:487, 2007.

66. Mayson SE et al: The changing face of postoperative atrial fibrillation prevention: a review of current medical therapy, *Cardio Rev* 15:231, 2007.

67. Andre AC, DelRossi A: Hemodynamic management of patients in the first 24 hours after cardiac surgery, *Crit Care Med* 33:2082, 2005.

68. Ferraris VA et al: Perioperative blood transfusion and blood conservation in cardiac surgery: The Society of Thoracic Surgeons and The Society of Cardiovascular Anesthesiologists clinical practice guideline, *Ann Thorac Surg* 83:S27, 2007.

69. Martin CG, Turkelson SL: Nursing care of patient's undergoing coronary artery bypass grafting, *J Cardiovasc Nurs* 21:109, 2006.

70. Selnes OA: Etiology of cognitive changes after CABG surgery: more than just the pump? *Nature* 5(6):314, 2008.

71. Veliz-Reissmuller G et al: Pre-operative mild cognitive dysfunction predicts the risk for post-operative delirium after elective cardiac surgery, *Aging Clin Exp Res* 19:172, 2007.

72. Streeter NB: Considerations in prevention of surgical site infections following cardiac surgery, *J Cardiovasc Nurs* 21:E14, 2006.

73. Miga KC: Trends in cardiac surgery: exploring the past and looking into the future, *Crit Care Nurs Clin North Am* 19:343, 2007.

74. Schatzer MB et al: To pump or not to pump? *Crit Care Nurse Q* 30(1):67, 2007.

75. Puskas JD et al: Off-pump vs conventional coronary artery bypass grafting: early and 1-year graft patency, cost, and quality of life outcomes—a randomized trial, *JAMA* 291(15):1841, 2004.

76. Legare JF et al: Coronary bypass surgery performed off pump does not result in lower in-hospital morbidity than coronary artery bypass grafting on pump, *Circulation* 109:887, 2004.

77. Hravnak M et al: Short term complications and resource utilization in matched subjects after on-pump or off-pump primary isolated coronary artery bypass, *Am J Crit Care* 13:499, 2004.

78. Verma S et al: Off-pump coronary artery bypass surgery: fundamentals for the clinical cardiologist. *Circulation* 109:1206, 2004.

79. Horvath KA: Transmyocardial laser revascularization, *J Card Surg* 23:266, 2008.

80. Tasse J, Arora R: Transmyocardial revascularization: peril and potential, *J Cardiovasc Pharm Ther* 12:44, 2007.

81. Bridges CR et al: The Society of Thoracic Surgeons practice guidelines series: transmyocardial revascularization. *Ann Thorac Surg* 77:1494, 2004.

82. Schouchoff B: Surgical approaches for atrial fibrillation, *Crit Care Nurse Q* 30:233, 2007.

83. Kern LS et al: ECG monitoring after cardiac surgery: postoperative atrial fibrillation and the atrial electrogram, *AACN Adv Crit Care* 18:294, 2007.

84. Trost JC, Hillis DL: Intra-aortic balloon counterpulsation, *Am J Cardiol* 97:1391, 2006.

85. Erdogen HB et al: In which patients should sheathless IABP be used? An analysis of vascular complications in 1211 cases, *J Card Surg* 21(4):342, 2006.

86. Reid MB, Cottrell D: Nursing care of patients receiving intra-aortic balloon counterpulsation, *Crit Care Nurse* 25(5):40, 2005.

87. Lewis PA, Courtney M: Weaning intraaortic balloon counterpulsation: the evidence. *Br J Card Nurs* 1(8):385, 2006.

88. Shannon D et al: Mechanical circulatory support devices, *AACN Adv Crit Care* 17(4):368, 2006.

89. Richards NM, Stahl MA: Ventricular assist devices in the adult, *Crit Care Nurs Q* 30(2):104, 2007.

90. Boehmer JP, Popjes E: Cardiac failure: mechanical support strategies, *Crit Care Med* 34(9):S268, 2006.

91. Lee MS, Makkar RR: Percutaneous left ventricular support devices, *Cardiol Clin* 24:265, 2006.

92. Windecker S: Percutaneous left ventricular assist devices for treatment of patients with cardiogenic shock, *Curr Opin Crit Care* 13:521, 2007.

93. Hobson RW et al: Management of atherosclerotic carotid artery disease: clinical practice guidelines of the Society for Vascular Surgery, *J Vasc Surg* 48(2):480, 2008.

94. Kumar R, Chaturvedi S: Surgery insight: carotid endarterectomy—which patients to treat and when? *Nature* 4:621, 2007.

95. van der Vaart MG et al: Endarterectomy or carotid artery stenting: the quest continues, *Am J Surg* 195(2):259, 2008.

96. Lopez AC: New techniques in carotid stenting, *Nurs Practitioner* 33(4):43, 2008.

97. Gupta R, Horowitz M, Jovin TG: Hemodynamic instability after carotid artery angioplasty and stent placement: a review of the literature, *Neurosurg Focus* 18(1):e6, 2005.

98. Greenhalgh RM, Powell JT: Endovascular repair of abdominal aortic aneurysm, *Clin Ther* 358(5):494, 2008.

99. Blankensteijn J et al: Two-year outcomes after conventional or endovascular repair of abdominal aortic aneurysms, *N Engl J Med* 352, 2398, 2005.

100. Greenhalgh RM et al: Endovascular aneurysm repair versus open repair in patients with abdominal aortic aneurysm (EVAR trial 1): randomized controlled trial, *Lancet* 365, 2179, 2005.

101. Perera GB, Lyden SP: Current trends in lower extremity revascularization, *Surg Clin North Am* 87:1135, 2007.

102. Hirsch AT et al: ACC/AHA 2005 practice guidelines for the management of patients with peripheral arterial disease (lower extremity, renal, mesenteric, and abdominal aortic), *Circulation* 113:e463, 2006.

103. Sieggreen M: Recognize acute arterial occlusion, *Nursing 2007 Crit Care* 2(5):50, 2007.

104. Siddiqui A, Kowey PR: Sudden death secondary to cardiac arrhythmias: mechanisms and treatment strategies, *Curr Opin Cardiol* 21:517, 2006.

105. American Heart Association: ECC Guidelines. Part 7.4. Monitoring and medications, *Circulation* 112(8):IV-78, 2005.

106. Alexander E, Friedman L: Update on the clinical impact and issues surrounding dofetilide (Tikosyn) therapy, *AACN Adv Crit Care* 17:102, 2006.

107. Fuster V et al: ACC/AHA/ESC 2006 guidelines for the management of patients with atrial fibrillation: a report of the American College of Cardiology/American Heart Association Task Force on Practice Guidelines and the European Society of Cardiology Committee for Practice Guidelines, *Circulation* 114:257, 2006.

108. Steinberg JS et al: Analysis of cause-specific mortality in the Atrial Fibrillation Follow-up Investigation of Rhythm Management (AFFIRM) study. *Circulation* 109:1973, 2004.

109. Cooper BE: Review and update on inotropes and vasopressors, *AACN Adv Crit Care* 19:5, 2008.

110. Coons JC: Cardiovascular pharmacotherapy update for the intensive care unit, *Crit Care Nurse Q* 30:44, 2007.

111. Schulenburg M: Management of hypertensive emergencies: implications for the critical care nurse, *Crit Care Nurse Q* 30:86, 2007.

112. Monsoor AF, von Hagel-Keefer LA: The dangers of immediate release nifedipine in hypertensive emergencies, *Pharm Ther* 27:362, 2002.

113. Sacker-Bernstein JD et al: Short-term risk of death after treatment with nesiritide for decompensated heart failure, *JAMA* 293:1900, 2005.

114. Feldstein C: Management of hypertensive crisis, *Am J Ther* 14(2):135, 2007.

115. Jain AR et al. Treatment of hypertension in acute ischemic stroke, *Curr Treat Options Neurol* 11:20-25, 2009.

116. Hays AJ, Corso Y: Pharmacotherapy for a pulseless cardiac arrest, *AACN Adv Crit Care* 18:337, 2007.

117. Dellinger RP et al: Surviving sepsis campaign: International guidelines for management of severe sepsis and septic shock: 2008, *Crit Care Med* 36:296-327, 2008.

118. Schocken DD et al: Prevention of heart failure. A scientific statement from the American Heart Association Councils on Epidemiology and Prevention, Clinical Cardiology, Cardiovascular Nursing, and High Blood Pressure Research; Quality of Care and Outcomes Research Interdisciplinary Working Group, and Functional Genomics and Translational Biology Interdisciplinary Working Group. *Circulation* 117:2544-2565, 2008.

119. Hunt SH et al: ACC/AHA 2005 guideline update for the diagnosis and management of chronic heart failure in the adult, *Circulation* 112:e154, 2005.

120. Quinn B: Pharmacological treatment of heart failure, *Crit Care Nurs Q* 30:299, 2007.

Pulmonary Anatomy and Physiology

Chapter
21

The pulmonary system consists of the thorax, conducting airways, respiratory airways, and pulmonary blood and lymph supply. The primary functions of the pulmonary system are ventilation and respiration. *Ventilation* is the movement of air in and out of the lungs. *Respiration* is the process of gas exchange by means of movement of oxygen from the atmosphere into the bloodstream and movement of carbon dioxide from the bloodstream into the atmosphere. The anatomic structures that constitute the pulmonary system are intimately related to function, and structural abnormalities can readily translate into pulmonary disorders. An applicable knowledge of anatomy and physiology is imperative in caring for the patient with pulmonary dysfunction.

THORAX

The thorax contains the major organs of respiration. It consists of the thoracic cage, lungs, pleura, and muscles of ventilation. Together, these structures form the ventilatory pump, which performs the work of breathing.

THORACIC CAGE

The thoracic cage is a cone-shaped structure that is rigid but flexible. It must be somewhat rigid to protect the underlying structures, but it must be flexible to accommodate inhalation and exhalation. The cage consists of 12 thoracic vertebrae, each with a pair of ribs. Posteriorly, each rib is attached to its own vertebra, but anteriorly, attachment varies (Fig. 21-1). The first seven pairs of ribs are attached directly to the sternum. The 8th, 9th, and 10th pairs are attached by cartilage to the ribs above. Because the 11th and 12th ribs have no anterior attachment, they sometimes are referred to as *floating ribs*. The second rib is attached to the sternum at the angle of Louis, which is the raised ridge that can be felt just below the suprasternal notch.[1]

LUNGS

The lungs are cone-shaped organs that have a total volume of approximately 3.5 to 8.5 liters. The superior portion is known as the *apex*, and the inferior portion is known as the *base*. The

apical portion of each lung rises a few centimeters above the clavicle (see Fig. 21-1). Each lung is firmly attached to the thoracic cavity at the hilum and at the pulmonary ligament.[2]

Lobes and Segments. The lungs are divided into lobes and segments (Fig. 21-2), with the lobes being separated by pleural membrane–covered fissures. The right lung, which is larger and heavier than the left, is divided into upper, middle, and lower lobes. The left lung is divided into only an upper and a lower lobe.[2] A portion of the left lung, the lingula, corresponds anatomically with the right middle lobe. The horizontal fissure divides the right upper lobe from the right middle lobe. The oblique fissure divides the right upper and middle lobes from the lower lobe and the left upper lobe from the lower lobe. The lobes are divided into 18 segments, each of which has its own bronchus branching immediately off a lobar bronchus. Ten segments are located in the right lung and eight in the left lung.[1]

Mediastinum. The area between the two lungs, the mediastinum, contains the heart, great vessels, lymphatics, and the esophagus. A portion of the mediastinal area contains the root of the lungs, also known as the hilum, in which the visceral and parietal pleural membranes form a sheath around the main stem bronchi, the major blood vessels, and the nerves that enter and exit the lungs.[2]

PLEURA

The pleura is a thin membrane that lines the outside of the lungs and the inside of the chest wall. The visceral pleura adheres to the lungs, extending onto the hilar bronchi and into the major fissures. The parietal pleura lines the inner surface of the chest wall and mediastinum.[2] The two pleural surfaces are separated by an airtight space, which contains a thin layer of lubricating fluid. Pleural fluid allows the visceral and parietal pleural membranes to glide against each other during inhalation and exhalation.[1,3] The pleural space has the capacity to hold much more fluid than its normal volume of a few milliliters.[1]

Intrapleural Pressure. The pleural space has a pressure within it called the *intrapleural pressure*, which differs from the intrapulmonary (pressure within the lungs) and atmospheric pressures.[4] Under normal conditions, intrapleural pressure is less than intrapulmonary pressure and less than atmospheric

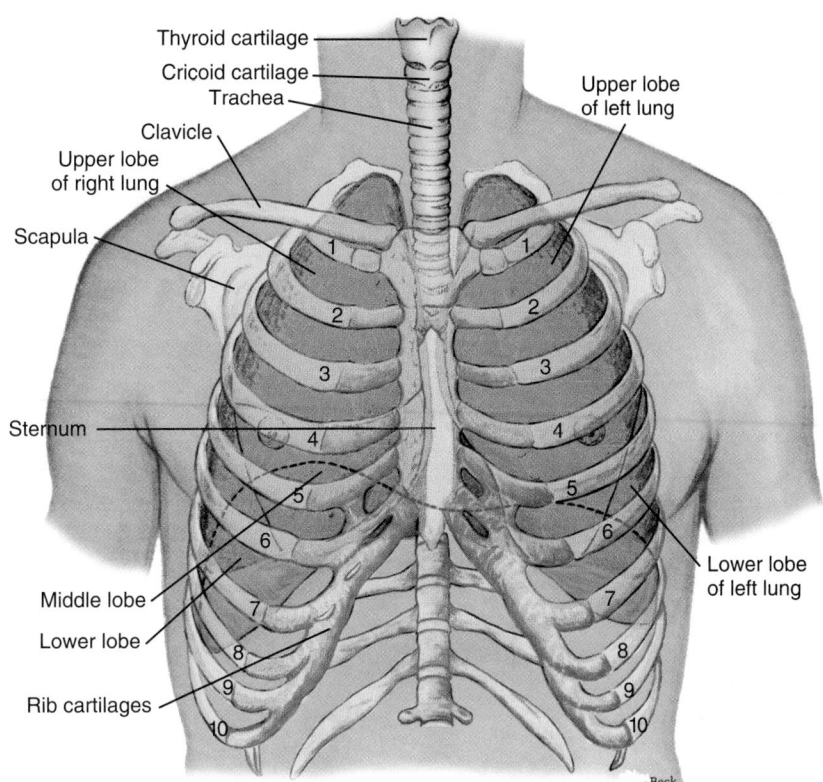

Figure 21-1 Ventilatory structures of the chest wall and lungs, showing the ribs *(numbered)* and lobes of the lungs. Each intercostal space takes the number of the rib above it. The *dotted line* indicates the location of the diaphragm at inhalation and exhalation. Notice the apex of each lung rising above the clavicle. *(From Thibodeau GA:* Anthony's textbook of anatomy and physiology, *ed 13, St Louis, 1990, Mosby.)*

pressure, with a normal range of −4 to −10 cm H_2O during exhalation and inhalation, respectively.[3] A deep inhalation can generate intrapleural pressures of −12 to −18 cm H_2O. This negative intrapleural pressure results from forces within the chest wall that exert pressure to pull the parietal pleura outward and away from the visceral pleura while the elastic fibers within the lungs exert pressure to pull the visceral pleura inward away from the parietal pleura. The constant pull of the two pleural membranes in opposite directions causes the pressure within the space to be subatmospheric.[4] The negative pressure in the pleural space keeps the lungs inflated (Box 21-1). If atmospheric pressure enters the pleural space, all or part of a lung will collapse, producing a pneumothorax.[1]

MUSCLES OF VENTILATION

The muscles of ventilation (Fig. 21-3) are governed by the regulatory activity of the central nervous system, which sends messages to the muscles to stimulate contraction and relaxation. This muscular activity controls inhalation and exhalation. Muscles that increase the size of the chest are called *muscles of inhalation;* those that decrease the size of the chest are called *muscles of exhalation.*[5]

Inhalation. The main muscle of inhalation is the diaphragm. The diaphragm is a dome-shaped, fibromuscular septum that separates the thoracic and abdominal cavities. It is connected to the sternum, ribs, and vertebrae. During normal, quiet breathing, the diaphragm does approximately 80% of

the work of breathing. On inhalation, the diaphragm contracts and flattens, pushes down on the viscera, and displaces the abdomen outward. Diaphragmatic contraction also lifts and expands the rib cage to some extent.[1,5,6]

The action of the diaphragm is governed by the medulla, which sends its impulses through the phrenic nerve. The phrenic nerve arises from the cervical plexus through the fourth cervical nerve, with secondary contributions by the third and fifth cervical nerves. For this reason and because the diaphragm does most of the work of inhalation, trauma involving levels C3 to C5 causes ventilatory dysfunction.[5]

Other muscles of inhalation include those that lift the rib cage. The most important of these are the external intercostal muscles, which elevate the ribs and expand the chest cage outward. The scalene, anterior serratus, and sternocleidomastoid muscles also participate to elevate the first two ribs and sternum.[1,5,6]

Exhalation. Exhalation in the healthy lung is a passive event requiring very little energy. Exhalation occurs when the diaphragm relaxes and moves back up toward the lungs. The intrinsic elastic recoil of the lungs assists with exhalation. Because exhalation is a passive act, there are no true muscles of exhalation other than the internal intercostal muscles, which assist the inward movement of the ribs. During exercise, however, exhalation becomes a more active event, requiring some participation of the accessory muscles of ventilation. Several muscles of the abdomen are thought to contribute to active exhalation.[4,5]

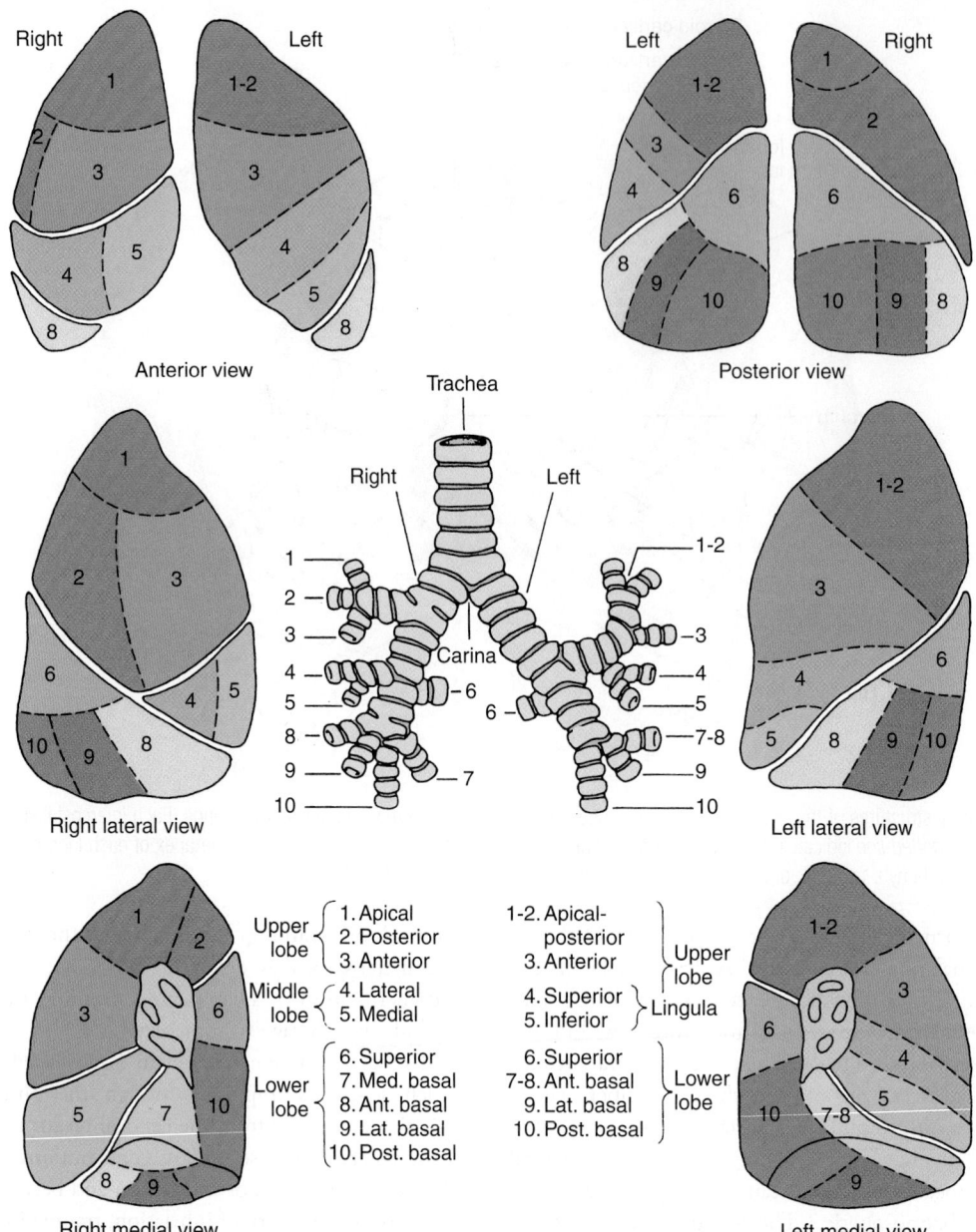

Figure 21-2 Lungs are divided into lobes and segments. Notice the differences between the right and left lungs. *(From Wilkins RL et al, editors: Egan's fundamentals of respiratory care, ed 9, St Louis, 2008, Mosby.)*

Accessory Muscles. The accessory muscles of ventilation usually are considered to be those that enhance chest expansion during exercise but that are not active during normal, quiet breathing. These muscles include the scalene, sternocleidomastoid, and other chest and back muscles, such as the trapezius and the pectoralis major.[1,5,6]

CONDUCTING AIRWAYS

The conducting airways consist of the upper airways, the trachea, and the bronchial tree (Fig. 21-4). The purposes of the conducting airways are to warm and humidify the inhaled air,

to act as a protective mechanism that prevents the entrance of foreign matter into the gas exchange areas, and to serve as a passageway for air entering and leaving the gas exchange regions of the lungs.[1-3]

UPPER AIRWAYS

The upper airways consist of the nasal and oral cavities, the pharynx, and the larynx (see Fig. 21-4). Their main contribution to ventilation is the conditioning of inspired air. *Conditioned air* is air that has been warmed, humidified, and cleansed of some irritants. Warming and humidifying, which are essential to prevent irritation of the lower airways, occur

The lungs stay inflated because the pressure surrounding them (intrapleural) is always less than the pressure within them (intrapulmonary).

WHY IS THE INTRAPLEURAL PRESSURE LESS THAN THE INTRAPULMONARY PRESSURE?

The intrapleural pressure is always (1) less then intrapulmonary pressure, (2) less than atmospheric pressure, and (3) considered negative because of the pull of the two pleural membranes in opposite directions. The parietal pleura is pulled outward by forces within the chest wall, whereas the visceral pleural is pulled inward by the force of the elastic fibers within the lungs.

WHY DO THE TWO PLEURAL MEMBRANES PULL IN OPPOSITE DIRECTIONS?

The parietal pleura, attached to the chest, is pulled outward because the elastic fibers within the intercostal muscles exert outward pressure on the ribs. These fibers are in a relaxed state when the rib cage is fully expanded, such as during a deep inhalation. The visceral pleura is attached to the lungs and is pulled inward because the elastic fibers within the lungs that are responsible for elastic recoil exert pressure to make the lungs smaller. Elastic fibers in the lung are in a relaxed position only when the lung is at its smallest configuration, as occurs with a pneumothorax. Because of the opposite pull of the chest wall and the lung and because the pleural membranes are attached to these structures, there is a constant pull of the two membranes in opposite directions. The subatmospheric pressure that results within the pleural space and the greater-than-atmospheric intrapulmonary pressure within the lungs allows the lungs to remain inflated. Anything that causes the pressure within the pleural space to rise to atmospheric pressure or above will cause the lung to collapse—a pneumothorax.

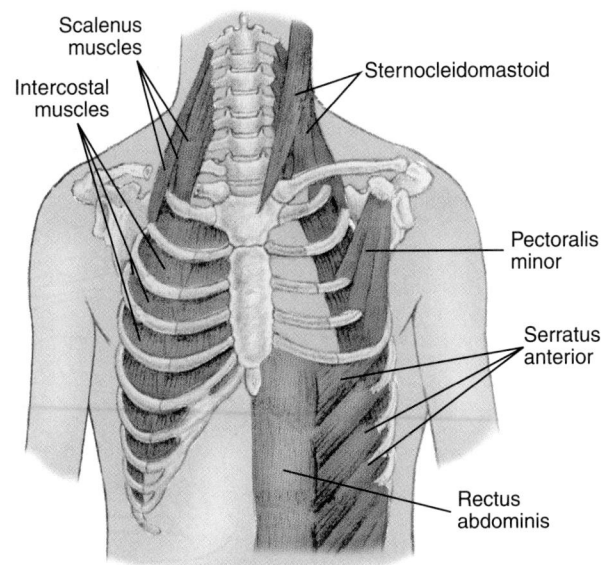

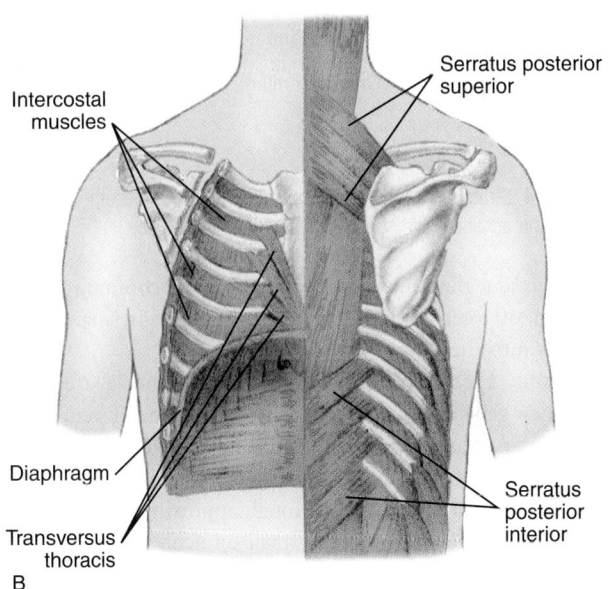

Figure 21-3 Muscles of ventilation. *A,* Anterior view. *B,* Posterior view.

mainly within the nose by means of a dense vascular network that lines the nasal passages. The air is cleansed by the coarse hairs that line the nasal passages and filter large inhaled particles.[1,3]

Epiglottis. The epiglottis is located in the upper airways. It protects the lower airways by closing the opening to the trachea during swallowing so that food passes into the esophagus and not the trachea. The epiglottis is a thin, leaf-shaped, elastic cartilage that is located directly posterior to the root of the tongue and attached to the thyroid cartilage (see Fig. 21-4). It opens widely during inhalation, permitting air to pass through the trachea into the lower airways.[1]

TRACHEA

The trachea is a hollow tube approximately 11 cm (4.5 inches) long and 2.5 cm (1 inch) in diameter (Fig. 21-5). It begins at the cricoid cartilage and ends at the bifurcation (major carina) from which the two main stem bronchi arise. The carina is positioned approximately at the level of the aortic arch, the fifth thoracic vertebra,[7] or just below the level of the angle of Louis.[1] The trachea consists of smooth muscle supported anteriorly by

16 to 20 C-shaped, cartilaginous rings. They prevent tracheal collapse during bronchoconstriction and strong coughing. The posterior wall of the trachea lies contiguous with the anterior wall of the esophagus. Having no cartilaginous support, this wall is composed only of muscle tissue, which is separated from the anterior esophageal wall by loose connective tissue (see Fig. 21-5, inset).[1]

BRONCHIAL TREE

The two main stem bronchi are structurally different (see Fig. 21-5). The left bronchus is slightly narrower than the right, and because of its position above the heart, the left bronchus angles directly toward the left lung at approximately 45 to 55 degrees from the midline. The right bronchus is wider and angles at 20 to 30 degrees from the midline. Because of this

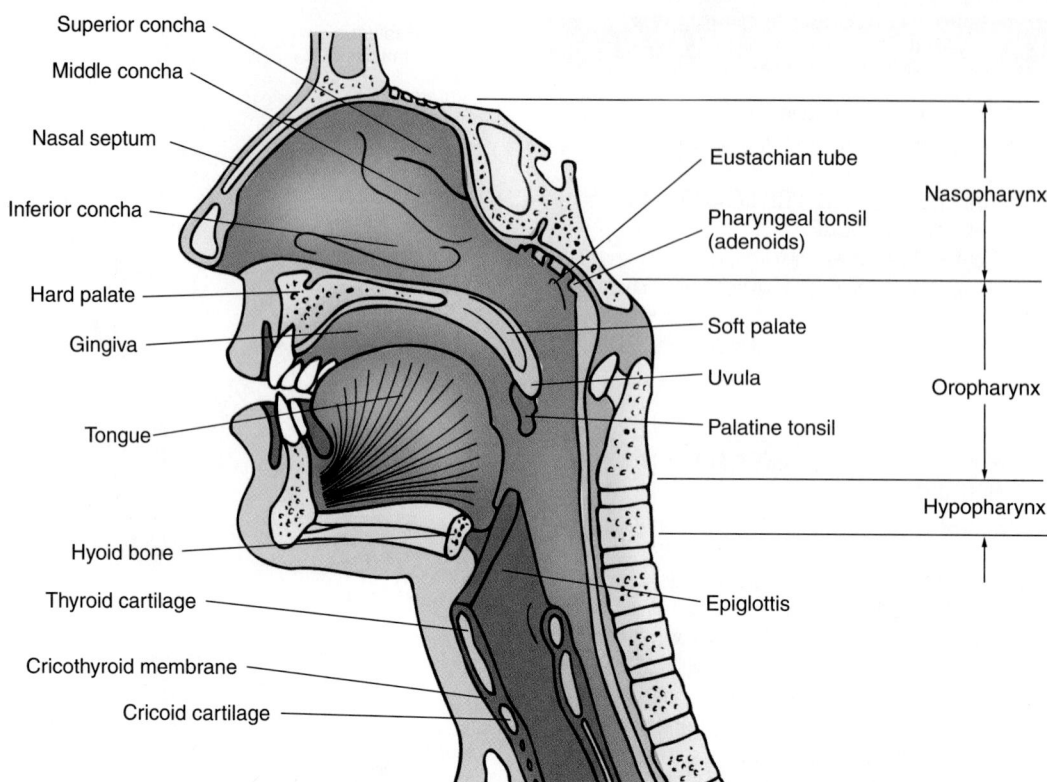

Figure 21-4 Structures of the upper airways. Notice the placement of the epiglottis. *(From Ellis PD, Billings DM: Cardiopulmonary resuscitation: procedures for basic and advanced life support, St Louis, 1980, Mosby.)*

angulation and the forces of gravity, the most common site of aspiration of foreign objects is through the right main stem bronchus into the lower lobe of the right lung.[2,3]

Bronchi. Each branching of the tracheobronchial tree produces a new generation of tubes (Fig. 21-6). The main stem bronchi are the first generation; the next branch, the five lobar bronchi, is the second generation. The third generation includes the 18 segmental bronchi. The fourth through approximately the ninth generations are referred to as the small bronchi, beginning with the subsegmental bronchi. In these bronchi, diameters decrease; however, because the number of bronchi increases with each generation, the total cross-sectional area increases with each generation. This great increase in the cross-sectional area of the lung is significant because it allows easy ventilation despite decreasing airway lumens.[1]

Bronchioles. The final subdivision of the conducting airways is the bronchioles. These tubes have a diameter less than 1 mm and have no connective tissue and cartilage within their walls. Their walls do, however, contain smooth muscle.[2] When smooth muscle constriction occurs, these airways may close completely because of the lack of structural support. The terminal bronchioles form the last branch of the conducting airways, after which the gas exchange areas of the lungs begin. There are more than 32,000 terminal bronchioles total.[1]

Defense System. The main defense system within the airways is the mucociliary escalator, or mucous blanket, a combination of mucus and cilia. The mucus, which floats atop the cilia (Fig. 21-7), traps foreign particles. Ciliary movement then propels the entire mucous blanket and any trapped particles

upward toward the pharynx at an average speed of 1 mm/min in the smaller bronchioles and 12 mm/min in the larger airways and trachea.[8] After the pharynx is reached, the mucus is swallowed or cleared. The submucous glands of the airways produce approximately 100 mL of mucus per day, with all but about 10 mL resorbed through the bronchial lining.[7] The mucociliary escalator is so efficient that almost no particles larger than 3 μm reach the alveoli.

The cough reflex is another protective mechanism in the lungs. Excessive amounts of foreign particles in the trachea and bronchi can initiate the cough reflex. Once initiated, the rapid expulsion of air carries away any foreign particles with it.[9]

RESPIRATORY AIRWAYS

The respiratory airways consist of the respiratory bronchioles and the alveoli. The respiratory airways also are known as the *terminal respiratory units*, or the *acini*. Gas exchange takes place in these areas of the lungs.

RESPIRATORY BRONCHIOLES

Each terminal bronchiole gives rise to two respiratory bronchioles, with each branching two to four more times.[2] The respiratory bronchioles form the transition zone of the lungs, acting as conducting airways and gas exchange units. While air is moving through them, alveolar outpouchings on their surfaces allow gas exchange to take place (see Fig. 21-6).[1]

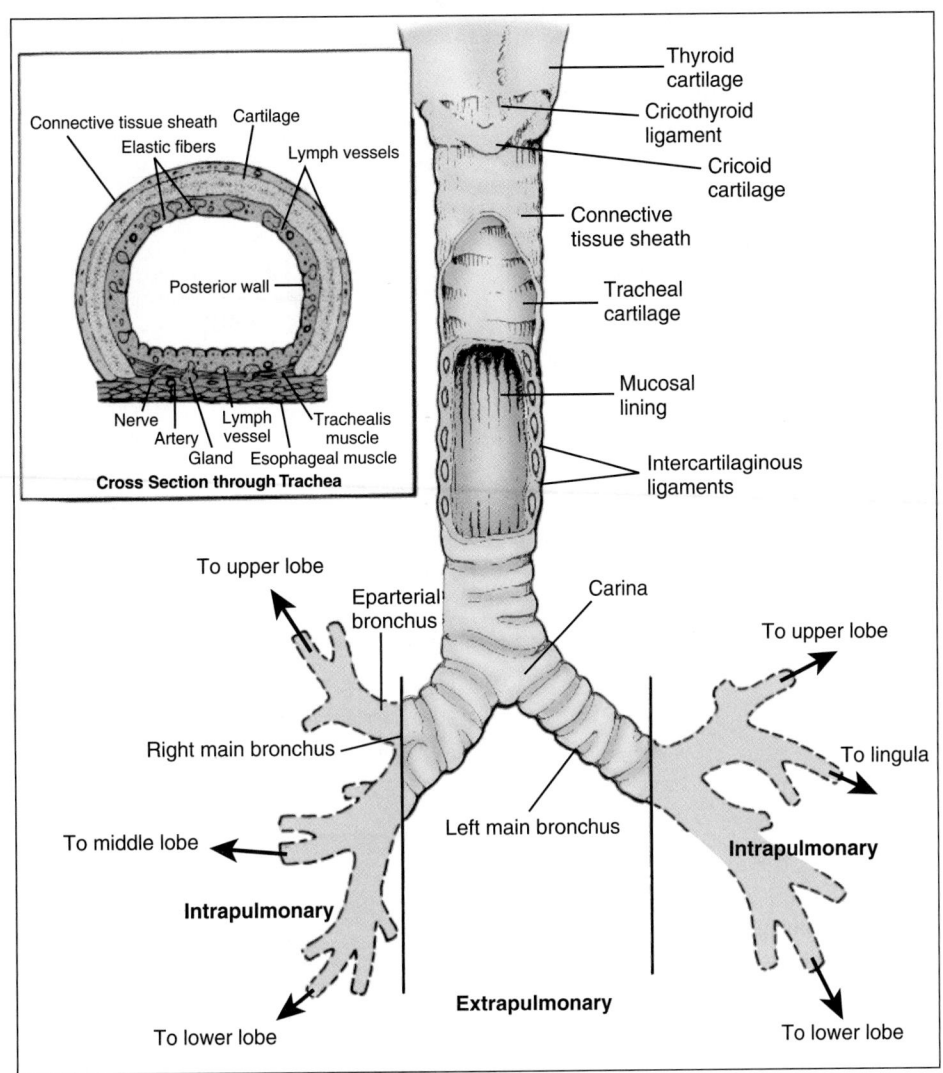

Figure 21-5 Anterior view of the trachea and primary bronchi and a cross section *(inset)* through a part of the trachea, including a C-shaped cartilaginous element. *(From Martin DE:* Respiratory anatomy and physiology, *St Louis, 1988, Mosby.)*

Labels (clockwise from top right): Thyroid cartilage; Cricothyroid ligament; Cricoid cartilage; Connective tissue sheath; Tracheal cartilage; Mucosal lining; Intercartilaginous ligaments; Carina; To upper lobe; To lingula; Intrapulmonary; To lower lobe; Left main bronchus; Extrapulmonary; To lower lobe; Intrapulmonary; To middle lobe; Right main bronchus; Eparterial bronchus; To upper lobe

Inset labels: Connective tissue sheath; Cartilage; Elastic fibers; Lymph vessels; Posterior wall; Nerve; Artery; Gland; Lymph vessel; Trachealis muscle; Esophageal muscle; **Cross Section through Trachea**

Conducting Airways				Respiratory Unit
Trachea	Segmental bronchi	Subsegmental bronchi (bronchioles)		Alveolar ducts
		Nonrespiratory	Respiratory	
Generations	8	16	24	26

Figure 21-6 Conducting and respiratory airways. Notice the escalating branching with increasing generations *(From Thompson JM et al:* Mosby's clinical nursing, *ed 5, St Louis, 2002, Mosby.)*

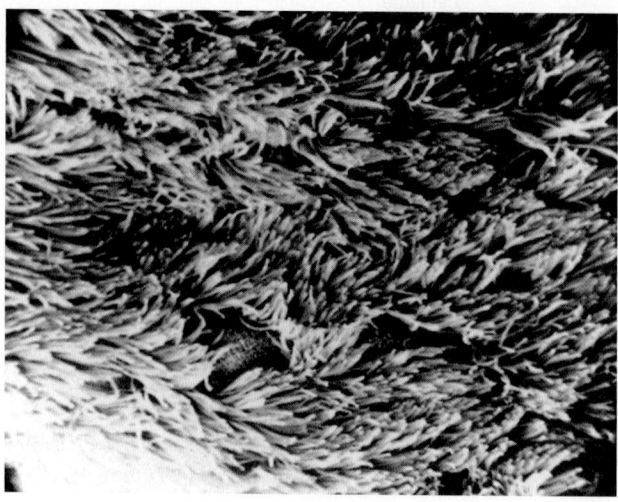

Figure 21-7 Scanning electron micrograph of the luminal surface and cilia of a bronchiole from a normal adult male (×2000). *(From Ebert RV, Terracio MJ: Observation of the secretion on the surface of the bronchioles with the scanning electron microscope, Am Rev Respir Dis 112:491, 1975.)*

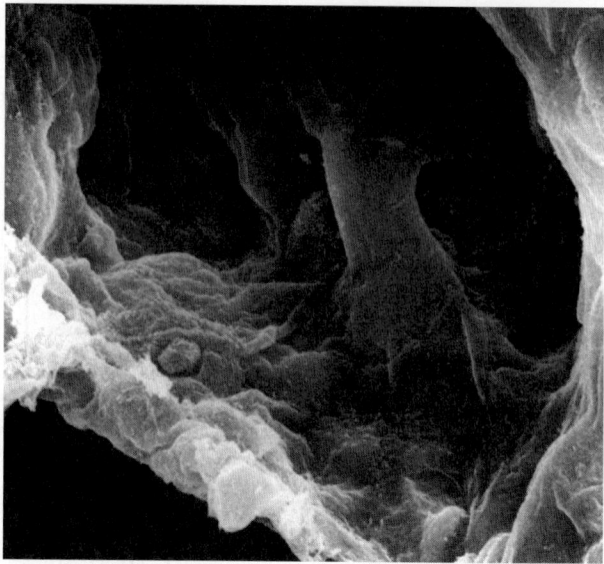

Figure 21-8 Detail of an alveolar surface composed chiefly of type I alveolar epithelial cells (scale: 1 cm of picture width = 3.46 μm). *(From Martin DE: Respiratory anatomy and physiology, St Louis, 1988, Mosby.)*

ALVEOLI

Each respiratory bronchiole gives rise to several alveolar ducts, which terminate in clusters of 10 to 16 alveoli (see Fig. 21-6). Each terminal respiratory unit contains approximately 100 alveolar ducts and 2000 alveoli.[2] The alveolus is the primary site of gas exchange and the end point in the respiratory tract. Approximately 300 million alveoli are in the two lungs. The alveoli are composed of several types of cells, including type I and II alveolar epithelial cells and alveolar macrophages.[1,3]

Type I Alveolar Epithelial Cells. Type I alveolar epithelial cells comprise approximately 90% of the total alveolar surface within the lungs (Fig. 21-8). They are the chief structural cells of the alveolar wall and play a major role in the maintenance of the gas-blood barrier and gas exchange. Type I cells are extremely susceptible to injury and become inflamed when exposed to inhaled toxins.[1,8]

Collateral Air Passages. A variety of collateral air passages are located within the lower regions of the lungs. Within the walls of the type I cells are the pores of Kohn (Fig. 21-9), which allow collateral movement of air between alveoli. The canals of Lambert are collateral air pathways that exist between the alveoli and the respiratory and terminal bronchioles.[8] They are of particular benefit when a respiratory bronchiole is blocked or collapsed, because they allow gas to pass into alveoli distal to the blockage. Collateral air passages are of significant benefit in any pathologic condition of the lung that results in obstruction of airflow into a portion of the lungs. However, these pores and canals also allow the movement of microorganisms through lung tissue.[1,2]

Type II Alveolar Epithelial Cells. Type II alveolar epithelial cells occur in much greater numbers than type I cells, but because of their minute size, they comprise a smaller portion of the total alveolar wall. After injury to the alveolar wall, type II cells rapidly divide to line the surface; later, they transform

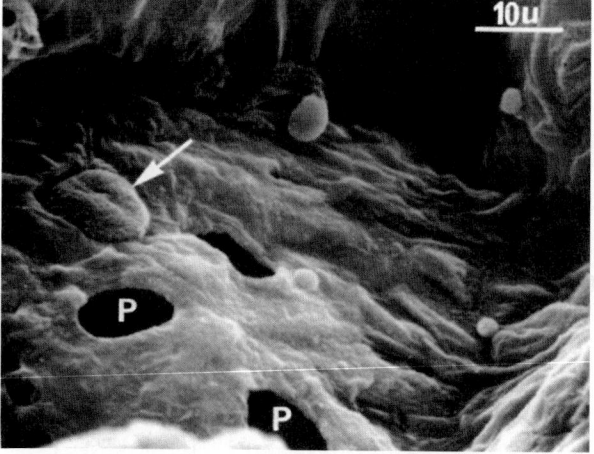

Figure 21-9 Scanning electron micrograph of the surface of a human alveolus shows the pores of Kohn (P) and a macrophage *(arrow)* (×1500). *(Courtesy M.S. Wang, MD.)*

into type I cells. The most important function of the type II cells is their ability to produce, store, and secrete pulmonary surfactant (Fig. 21-10).[1,3,8]

Surfactant. Surfactant is a phospholipid composed of fatty acids bound to lecithin. Like other surfactants, such as detergents and soaps, pulmonary surfactant functions to lower surface tension of the alveoli. Whereas with detergents and soaps this decrease in surface tension cleans clothes, within the lungs, it stabilizes the alveoli, increases lung compliance, and eases the work of breathing. When pulmonary disease disrupts the normal synthesis and storage of surfactant, the lungs become less compliant, and the work of breathing increases. Severe loss of surfactant results in alveolar instability and collapse and impairment of gas exchange.[10]

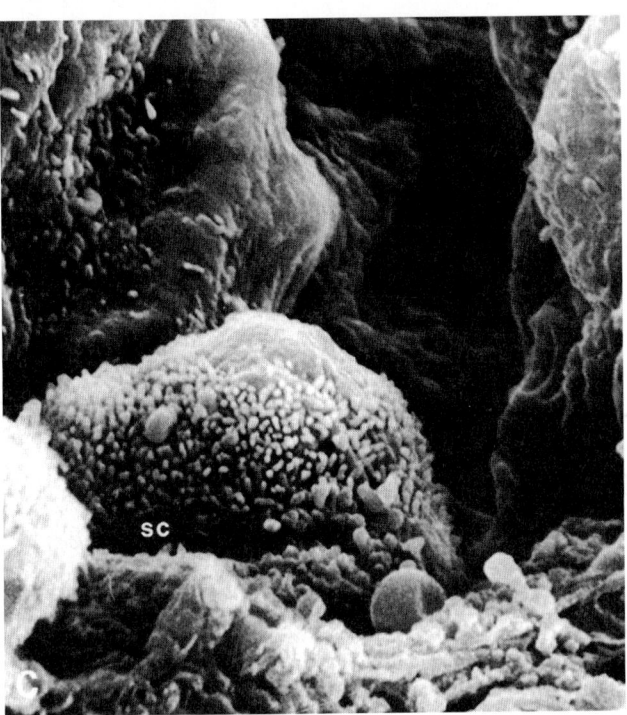

Figure 21-10 Type II alveolar epithelial cell. Notice the presence of brush microvilli on all except the bald top of the round luminal surface. Type II cells produce surfactant (scale: 1 cm of picture width = 0.85 μm.) *(From Martin DE:* Respiratory anatomy and physiology, *St Louis, 1988, Mosby.)*

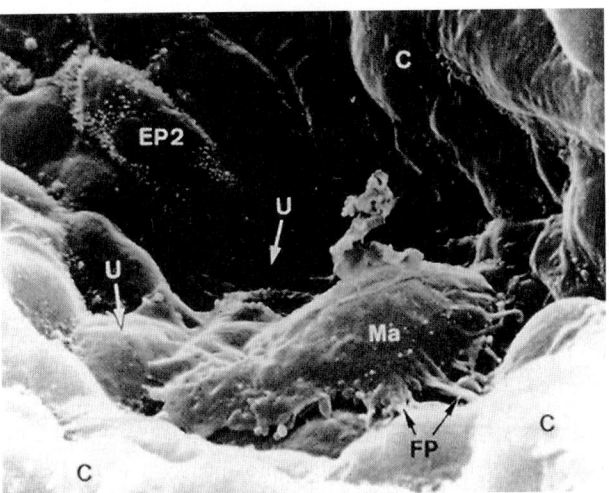

Figure 21-11 Scanning electron micrograph of a healthy human lung shows an alveolar macrophage (Ma) attached to the epithelium partly by filopodia (FP) and forming an undulating membrane (U) in the direction of forward movement to the left. Several capillaries (C) are evident, and a type II alveolar epithelial cell (EP2) can be seen in the background (original magnification ×3700.) *(From Gehr P et al: The normal human lung: ultrastructure and morphometric estimation of diffusion capacity,* Respir Physiol *32[2]:121, 1978.)*

Defense System. Alveolar macrophages are monocytes that originate in the bone marrow and are released into the bloodstream (Fig. 21-11).[1-3] On entering the pulmonary capillary circulation, they move through the capillary membrane wall into the interstitial space and through to the alveoli. In the alveoli, the monocytes transform into macrophages and assume a phagocytic role. They move from alveolus to alveolus through the pores of Kohn, keeping the alveoli clean and sterile through phagocytosis and microbial killing activity, which includes the secretion of hydrogen peroxide, lysozyme, and other substances that kill microorganisms.[2,3]

PULMONARY BLOOD AND LYMPH SUPPLY

Two vascular systems and one lymphatic system make up the pulmonary blood and lymph supply. The pulmonary circulation is the vascular system that forms the gas exchange network surrounding the alveoli. The bronchial circulation is the vascular system that perfuses the tracheobronchial tree.[1]

PULMONARY CIRCULATION

The pulmonary circulatory system begins at the pulmonary artery, which receives venous blood from the right side of the heart. The pulmonary artery then divides into left and right branches and continues to branch until it forms the capillaries that surround the alveoli (Fig. 21-12). After gas exchange takes

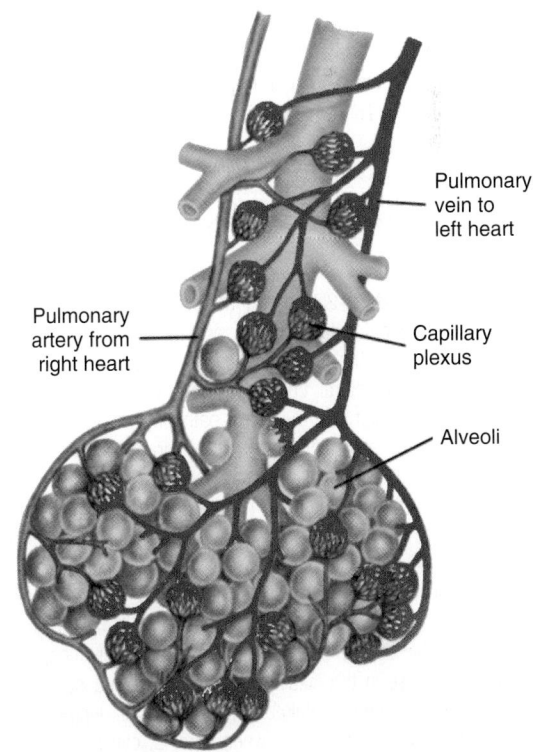

Figure 21-12 Terminal ventilation and perfusion units of the lung. Pulmonary arterial blood is venous *(dark gray),* and pulmonary venous blood is oxygenated *(blue). (From Thompson JM et al:* Mosby's clinical nursing, *ed 5, St Louis, 2002, Mosby.)*

place, the blood is returned to the left side of the heart through the pulmonary veins.[1,2]

Pulmonary Artery Pressures. The pulmonary circulation is by far the largest vascular bed within the body, and it is the only one that receives the entire cardiac output. Just as the systemic circulation has a systolic and a diastolic blood pressure, so does the pulmonary circulation. However, because of the relative lack of smooth muscle within the vessels of the pulmonary circulation, the pressures are vastly lower than within the systemic circulation.[1,3] Pulmonary artery systolic (PAS) pressure ranges from 15 to 30 mm Hg, pulmonary artery diastolic (PAD) pressure ranges from 4 to 12 mm Hg, and pulmonary artery mean (PAM) pressure ranges from 9 to 18 mm Hg.[11] Because of the low pulmonary artery pressures, right ventricular wall thickness needs to be only approximately one third of left ventricular wall thickness. However, just as hypertension can occur within the systemic circulation, it also can occur within the pulmonary circulation (Box 21-2).[12]

ALVEOLAR-CAPILLARY MEMBRANE

The vessels of the alveolar-capillary membrane form a network around each alveolus that is so dense it forms an almost continuous sheet of blood covering the alveoli.[2] The interior diameter of each capillary segment is just large enough to allow red blood cells to squeeze by in single file so that their cell membranes touch the capillary walls (Fig. 21-13).[4] In this way, oxygen and carbon dioxide need not pass through significant amounts of plasma when diffusing into and out of the alveoli, making a highly efficient vehicle for gas exchange. Each red blood cell spends approximately three fourths of a second in the alveolar-capillary network and is exposed to the alveolar gas of two or three alveoli.[1] In that short time, hemoglobin is brought

from its normal venous blood saturation level of 75% to its arterial saturation of more than 96%.[4] Hemoglobin levels have been shown to reach normal within only a 0.25-second exposure to alveolar gas; under conditions such as in tachycardia, in which the red blood cells spend less time within the pulmonary capillary network, normal oxygenation can still occur.[3]

Membrane Layers. The alveolar-capillary membrane is less than 0.5 μm thick[13] and is composed of several layers of cells: the alveolar epithelium, the alveolar basement membrane, the interstitial space, the capillary basement membrane, and the capillary endothelium (Fig. 21-14). Oxygen and carbon dioxide traverse easily across these layers, which present no barrier to diffusion because the membrane is very thin.[3]

BRONCHIAL CIRCULATION

The bronchial circulation, also known as the *systemic blood supply to the lungs*, is the system that perfuses the tracheobronchial tree, the visceral pleura, interstitial and connective tissue, some arteries and veins, lymph nodes, and the nerves within the thoracic cavity. The bronchial arteries that perfuse structures in the left side of the thorax branch off the aorta, and those that perfuse the right-sided structures branch from the intercostal, subclavian, or internal mammary artery. After perfusing the specific lung structures, most of the venous blood returns to the right side of the heart; however, some venous blood from the

---

BOX 21-2   PULMONARY HYPERTENSION

Pulmonary hypertension is defined as increased pressure (PAS >35 mm Hg and PAM >25 mm Hg at rest or >30 mm Hg with exertion) within the pulmonary arterial system. It occurs when the cross-sectional area of the pulmonary bed decreases as a result of vasoconstriction or structural changes in the vascular bed. These changes may be a result of a variety of pathophysiologic conditions, including impedance to pulmonary venous drainage (e.g., mitral stenosis); increased pulmonary blood flow (e.g., septal defect); impedance to flow through large pulmonary arteries (e.g., pulmonary embolus) or small pulmonary blood vessels (e.g., collagen vascular diseases); and impedance to flow from hypoxic vasoconstriction.

The pulmonary hypertension resulting from hypoxic vasoconstriction, although caused in part by vasospasm, is largely a result of alterations in the structure of the blood vessels of the pulmonary circulation, which results in an increase in the medial thickness and a reduction in the size of the vascular lumen. Pulmonary hypertension increases the afterload of the right ventricle and, when chronic, can result in right ventricular hypertrophy (cor pulmonale) and failure.

PAM, pulmonary artery mean pressure; PAS, pulmonary artery systolic pressure.

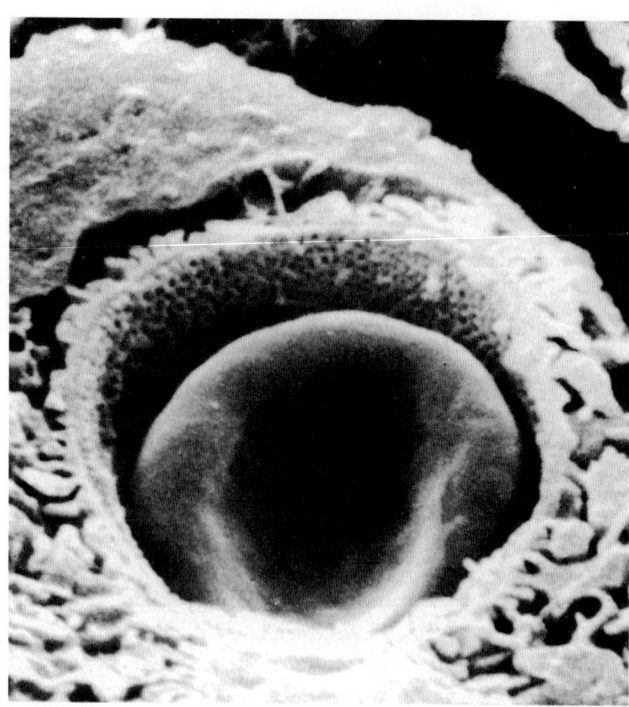

Figure 21-13 Scanning electron micrograph of a red blood cell in a capillary. Notice that the diameters of both are similar. In many instances, the red blood cells course through even smaller capillaries, often through capillaries that are one half of the diameter of the red blood cell. This is possible because the cells are pliable, mainly as a result of their biconcave disk shape. *(From Martin DE:* Respiratory anatomy and physiology, *St Louis, 1988, Mosby.)*

bronchial circulation returns directly into the pulmonary veins and the left atrium.[14]

Physiologic Shunting. The left atrium normally contains pure oxygenated blood, with a hemoglobin saturation level of 100%. The mixing of venous blood from the bronchial circulation with the oxygenated blood in the left atrium decreases the saturation of left atrial blood to a range between 96% and 99%. For this reason, while a person is breathing room air, the oxygen saturation of arterial blood is less than 100%. The dumping of venous blood into the left atrium is known as an *anatomic shunt.* The thebesian veins, which drain the right coronary circulation, are also responsible for the addition of venous blood to the left atrium. These two systems constitute the normal anatomic shunt, which comprises approximately 3% to 5% of the total cardiac output.[15]

LYMPHATIC CIRCULATION

The lungs are more richly supplied with lymphatic tissue than any other organ, perhaps because of their constant exposure to the external environment. The lymphatic vessels parallel much of the pulmonary vasculature and the tracheobronchial tree to the level of the terminal and respiratory bronchioles. Lymphatic vessels also are located within the connective tissue of lung parenchyma and within the pleural membranes. These vessels eventually drain into the primary lymph nodes located at the hila of the lungs. The lymphatic system in the lungs serves two purposes. As part of the immune system, it is responsible

for removing foreign particles and cell debris from the lungs and for producing antibody- and cell-mediated immune responses. It also is responsible for removing fluid from the lungs and for keeping the alveoli clear.[1-3]

VENTILATION

Air moves into and out of the lungs because of the difference between intrapulmonary pressure (pressure inside the lungs) and atmospheric pressure (Fig. 21-15). The movement of air into the lungs is known as *inhalation*, and the movement of air out of the lungs is known as *exhalation*. At the command of the central nervous system, the muscles of ventilation contract, the thorax and lungs expand, and intrapulmonary pressure falls. When the pressure falls below atmospheric pressure, air enters the lungs, and inhalation occurs. At the end of inhalation, the muscles of ventilation relax, the thorax contracts and the lungs are compressed, and intrapulmonary pressure rises. When the pressure rises above atmospheric pressure, air exits the lungs, and exhalation occurs.[4,16]

WORK OF BREATHING

The work of breathing is the amount of work that must be performed to overcome the elastic and resistive properties of the lungs. The elastic properties are determined by lung recoil,

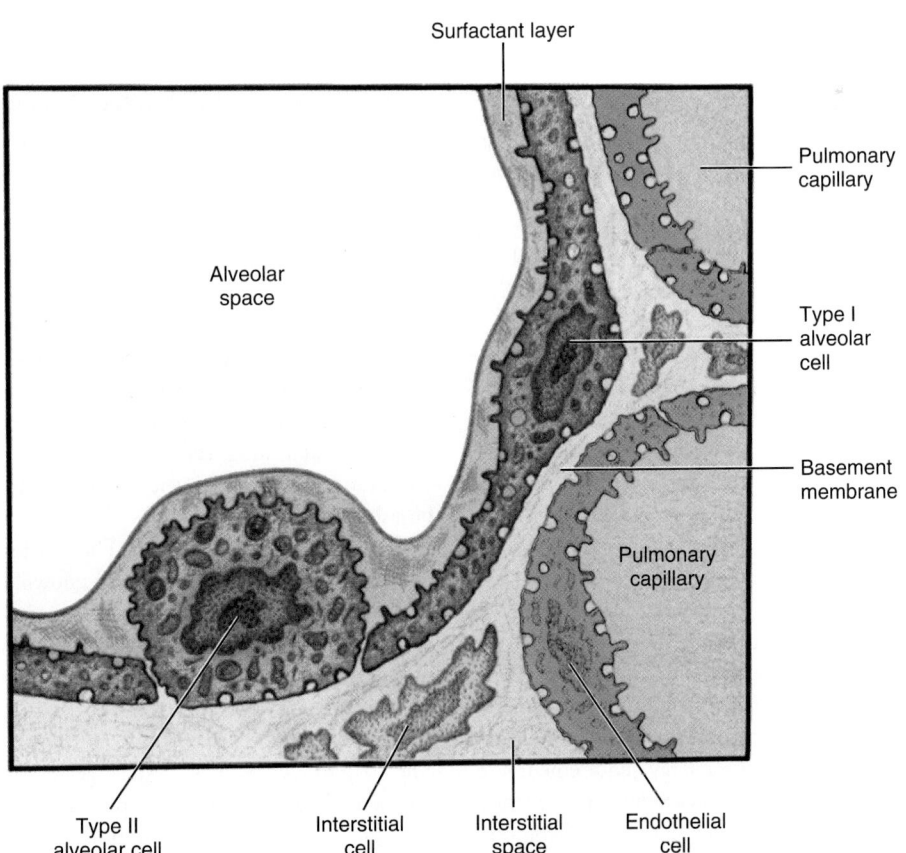

Surfactant layer

Pulmonary capillary

Alveolar space

Type I alveolar cell

Basement membrane

Pulmonary capillary

Type II alveolar cell

Interstitial cell

Interstitial space

Endothelial cell

Figure 21-14 Layers of the alveolar-capillary membrane. *(From Thompson JM et al: Mosby's clinical nursing, ed 5, St Louis, 2002, Mosby.)*

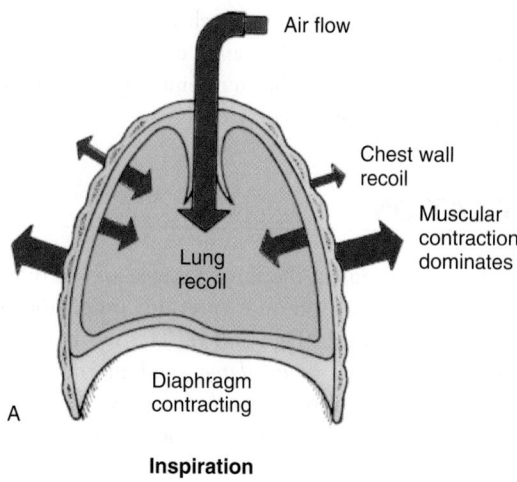

Inspiration

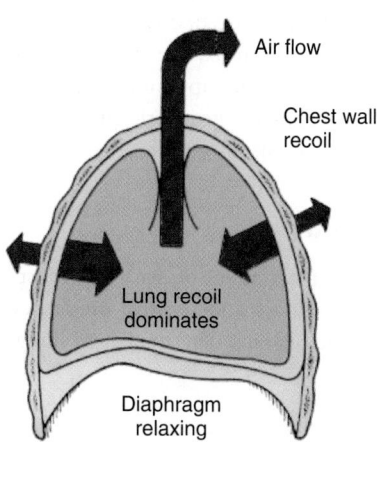

Expiration

Figure 21-15 The processes of inhalation and exhalation. *A,* During inhalation, the muscles of ventilation contract, the thorax and lungs expand, and air enters the lungs. *B,* During exhalation, the muscles of ventilation relax, the thorax and lungs are compressed, and air exits the lungs. *(Modified from McCance KL, Huether SE, editors:* Pathophysiology: the biologic basis for disease in adults and children, *ed 5, St Louis, 2006, Mosby.)*

chest wall recoil, and the surface tension of the alveoli. The resistive properties are determined by airway resistance.[1,16,17] Normally, the work of breathing occurs during inhalation, but even exhalation can be a strain when lung recoil, chest wall recoil, or airway resistance is abnormal.[4,16]

During normal, quiet ventilation, only 1% to 2% of basal oxygen consumption is required by the pulmonary system.[17] During heavy exercise, the amount of energy required by the pulmonary system can become progressively greater. The work of breathing can be a factor that limits exercise in the patient with pulmonary disease. Pathologic conditions of the pulmonary system can drastically change the energy requirement for ventilation. Pulmonary diseases that decrease lung compliance (e.g., atelectasis, pulmonary edema), decrease chest wall compliance (e.g., kyphoscoliosis), increase airway resistance (e.g., bronchitis, asthma), or decrease lung recoil (e.g., emphysema) can

---

BOX 21-3 HOW LUNG DISEASE CAN ALTER VENTILATION

Normal muscular action of the diaphragm, flexibility of the rib cage, elasticity of the lungs, and airway diameter are instrumental in allowing easy inhalation and exhalation. Any interference with these actions impairs normal ventilation. Pulmonary diseases can be categorized as obstructive or restrictive, depending on how the underlying cause affects normal ventilation.

Restrictive diseases limit lung or chest wall movement and include diffuse interstitial lung fibrosis, atelectasis, kyphoscoliosis, and severe chest wall pain. These conditions can be acute or chronic, and because they restrict lung or chest wall expansion, or both, patients have smaller tidal volumes but an increased ventilatory rate to maintain minute ventilation.

Obstructive diseases impede normal airflow. The classic examples are emphysema, in which airflow is decreased because of a decrease in lung recoil, and asthma, in which airflow is decreased because of diffuse airway narrowing. Emphysema results in lungs that inflate easily but, lacking the normal elastic recoil, do not compress to assist with exhalation. Patients with emphysema may have little difficulty inhaling but struggle to exhale.

---

increase the work of breathing so much that one third or more of the total body energy is used for ventilation (Box 21-3).[4,16]

PULMONARY VOLUMES AND CAPACITIES

Pulmonary ventilation can be described in terms of volumes and capacities (Fig. 21-16). Tidal volume (V_T) is the amount of air inhaled and exhaled with each breath. Inspiratory reserve volume (IRV) is the maximum amount of air that can be inhaled over and above the normal tidal volume. Expiratory reserve volume (ERV) is the maximum amount of air that can be exhaled beyond the normal tidal volume. The residual volume (RV) is the amount of air left in the lungs after a complete exhalation. Inspiratory capacity (IC) is the sum of the tidal volume and the inspiratory reserve. Functional residual capacity (FRC) is the sum of the expiratory reserve volume and the residual volume. Vital capacity (VC) is the sum of the inspiratory reserve volume, the tidal volume, and the expiratory reserve volume. Total lung capacity (TLC) is the sum of all four volumes and represents the maximal amount of air that can be inhaled.[3,16]

Physiologic Dead Space. The portion of total ventilation that participates in gas exchange is known as *alveolar ventilation.* The portion of ventilation that does not is known as *wasted ventilation.* The areas in the lungs that are ventilated but in which no gas exchange occurs are known as *dead space regions.* The conducting airways are referred to as *anatomic dead space* because they are ventilated but not perfused and therefore not able to participate in gas exchange. Some ventilation goes to unperfused alveoli. Without perfusion, gas exchange cannot take place, and the ventilation is wasted. These unperfused alveoli are known as *alveolar dead space.* Anatomic dead space plus alveolar dead space is called *physiologic dead space.*[3,15,16]

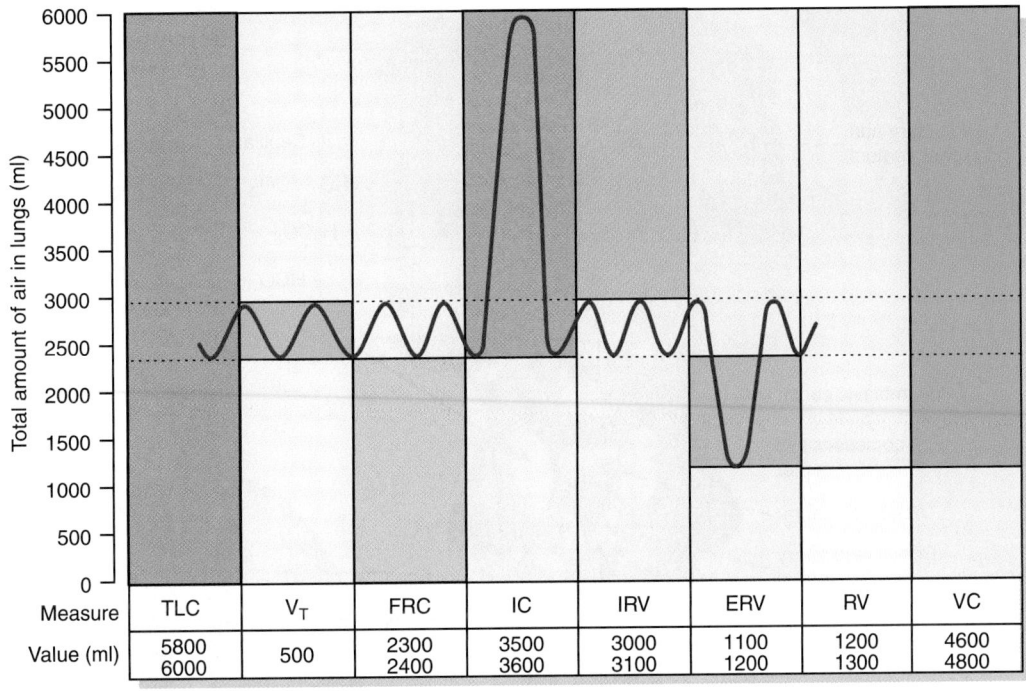

Figure 21-16 For lung volume measurements, all values are approximately 25% less in women. ERV, expiratory reserve volume; IC, inspiratory capacity; IRV, inspiratory reserve volume; FRC, functional residual capacity; TLC, total lung capacity; RV, residual volume; VC, vital capacity; V_T, tidal volume.

REGULATION OF VENTILATION

Regulation of ventilation by the brain is complex and not completely understood. Ventilation is regulated by a triad comprising a controller (located within the central nervous system), a group of effectors (muscles of ventilation), and a variety of sensors that include chemoreceptors (central and peripheral) and mechanoreceptors (located in chest wall and lungs). Efferent nerve fibers convey impulses from the controller to the effectors, whereas afferent nerve fibers carry impulses from some of the sensors to the controller (Fig. 21-17).[18]

Controller. The central nervous system houses what is known as the *controller of ventilation*. The controller is not located in one specific area; rather, it is in several areas that work together to provide coordinated ventilation. The brainstem regulates automatic ventilation, the cerebral cortex allows voluntary ventilation, and neurons housed in the spinal cord process information from the brain and from the peripheral receptors, allowing them to send final information to the muscles of ventilation.[18]

Brainstem. In the brainstem, the medulla oblongata and the pons are involved in ventilation. Four different groups of neurons are thought to participate in the regulation of inhalation and exhalation. The dorsal respiratory group, located in the medulla, is responsible for the basic rhythm of ventilation. Cells in this area are thought to automatically fire and trigger inhalation. The pneumotaxic center in the pons is responsible for limiting inhalation and triggering exhalation. This response also facilitates control of the rate and pattern of respiration. The ventral respiratory group, located in the medulla, is responsible for inspiration and expiration during periods of increased ventilation. The apneustic center in the lower pons is thought to

work with the pneumotaxic center to regulate the depth of inspiration.[18]

Cerebral Cortex. The cerebral cortex functions by allowing voluntary ventilation to override the automatic controls of the medulla and pons. Voluntary ventilatory control is most important during behavioral states such as crying, laughing, singing, and talking. During these states, voluntary control may override the automatic control, which responds chiefly to chemical stimuli and to changes in lung inflation.[3,18]

Effectors. The effectors of ventilation are the muscles of ventilation (see Fig. 21-3). In considering their function in the control of ventilation, the most important issue is that they function in a coordinated fashion. The central nervous system regulates this function.[18]

Sensors. The main sensors for the regulation of ventilation are the central and peripheral chemoreceptors (see Fig. 21-17). These chemoreceptors respond to changes in the chemical composition of the blood or other fluid around them. Other sensors that are found in the lung include the irritant receptors, stretch receptors, and the juxtacapillary (J) receptors.[3,18]

Central Chemoreceptors. The central chemoreceptors are located near the ventral surface of the medulla in the chemosensitive area (see Fig. 21-17). These chemoreceptors are surrounded by cerebral extracellular fluid and respond primarily to changes in the hydrogen ion concentration of that fluid. Ventilation increases when the hydrogen ion concentration rises and decreases when the hydrogen ion concentration falls. A rise in the partial pressure of carbon dioxide ($PaCO_2$) causes the movement of carbon dioxide across the blood-brain barrier into the cerebrospinal fluid, stimulating the movement of hydrogen ions into the brain's extracellular fluid. These hydrogen ions

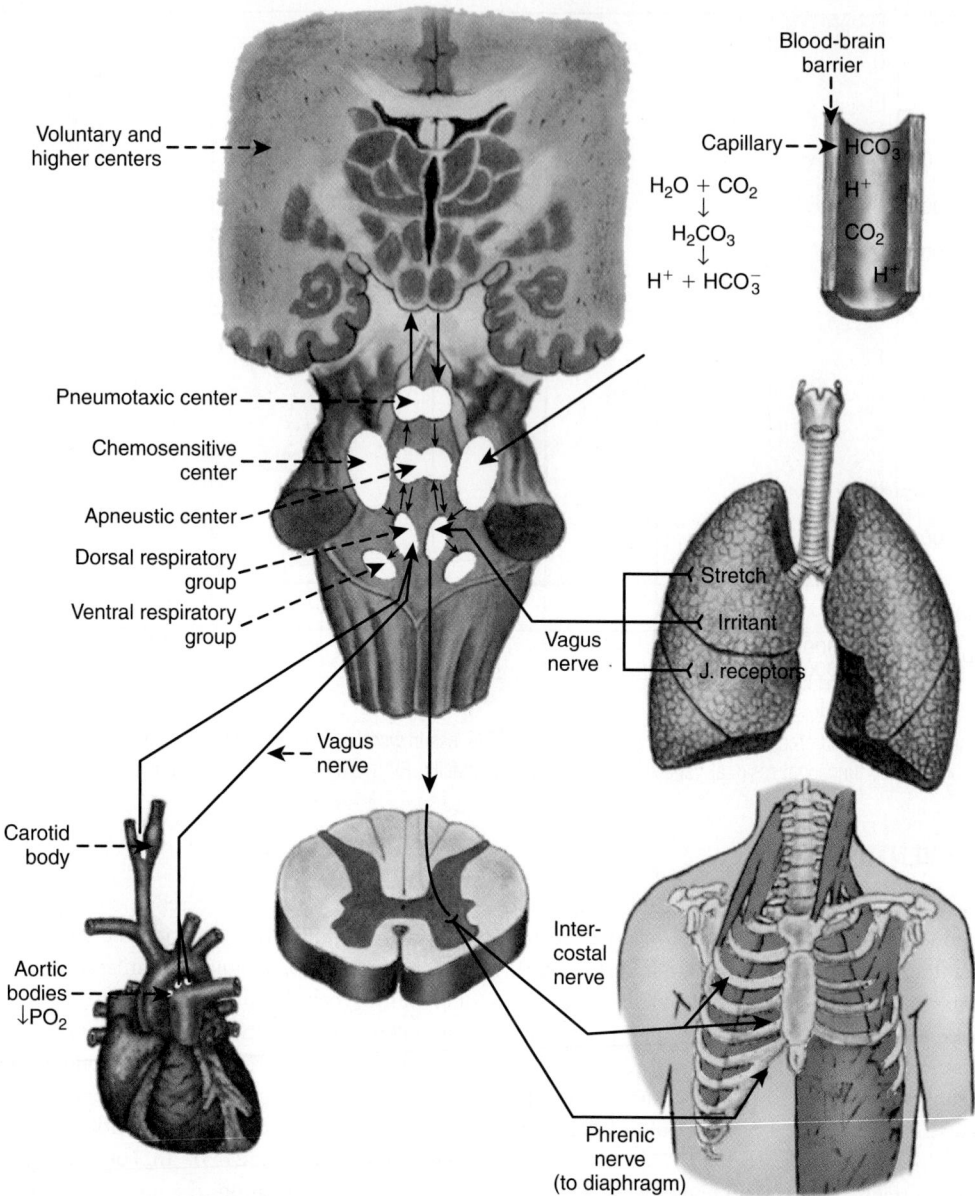

Figure 21-17 Respiratory control system. *(From McCance KL, Huether SE, editors:* Pathophysiology: the biologic basis for disease in adults and children, *ed 5, St Louis, 2006, Mosby.)*

then stimulate the chemoreceptors, and ventilation is increased. The increase in ventilation causes exhalation of excess carbon dioxide, the $PaCO_2$ falls, and ventilation returns to normal. Central chemoreceptors are not affected by changes in the partial pressure of oxygen (PaO_2).[18]

Peripheral Chemoreceptors. The peripheral chemoreceptors are located above and below the aortic arch and at the bifurcation of the common carotid arteries (see Fig. 21-17). The most important action of the peripheral chemoreceptors is their response to changes in the PaO_2, because they are the primary receptors that increase ventilation in response to arterial hypoxemia. Immediate hyperventilation, one of the principal compensatory mechanisms in response to hypoxemia, is governed by these chemoreceptors. The peripheral chemoreceptors also respond to changes in $PaCO_2$ and hydrogen ion concentration. An increase in either results in an increase in ventilation. Studies indicate that the peripheral chemoreceptors probably are more involved with short-term response to carbon dioxide, whereas the central chemoreceptors are responsible for the long-term response to carbon dioxide.[18]

Other Receptors. Irritant receptors lie between airway epithelial cells, and they stimulate bronchoconstriction and hyperpnea in response to inhaled irritants. Stretch receptors, which are located in the airways, are stimulated by changes in lung volume. They inhibit inhalation and are thought to protect the lung from overinflation (Hering-Breuer reflex). J receptors lie in the alveolar walls close to the capillaries. They are stimulated by engorgement of the pulmonary capillaries and an increase in the interstitial fluid volume. Stimulation of the J receptors is thought to cause rapid, shallow breathing.[19]

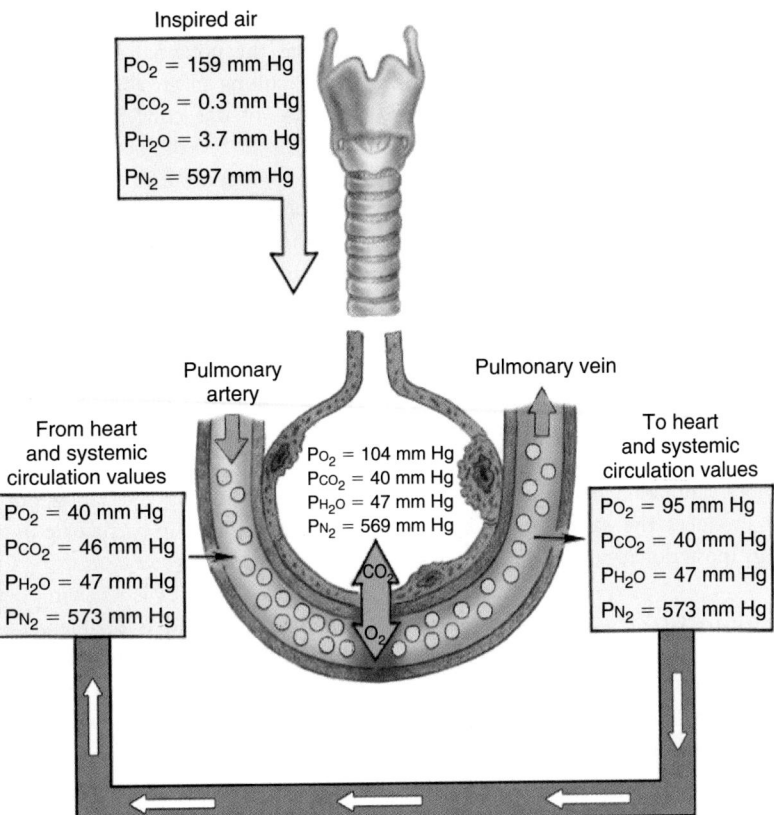

Inspired air

$P_{O_2} = 159$ mm Hg

$P_{CO_2} = 0.3$ mm Hg

$P_{H_2O} = 3.7$ mm Hg

$P_{N_2} = 597$ mm Hg

Pulmonary artery

Pulmonary vein

From heart and systemic circulation values

$P_{O_2} = 40$ mm Hg

$P_{CO_2} = 46$ mm Hg

$P_{H_2O} = 47$ mm Hg

$P_{N_2} = 573$ mm Hg

$P_{O_2} = 104$ mm Hg

$P_{CO_2} = 40$ mm Hg

$P_{H_2O} = 47$ mm Hg

$P_{N_2} = 569$ mm Hg

To heart and systemic circulation values

$P_{O_2} = 95$ mm Hg

$P_{CO_2} = 40$ mm Hg

$P_{H_2O} = 47$ mm Hg

$P_{N_2} = 573$ mm Hg

Figure 21-18 Process of respiration. *(From Thompson JM et al:* Mosby's clinical nursing, *ed 5, St Louis, 2002, Mosby.)*

RESPIRATION

Respiration refers to the movement of oxygen and carbon dioxide. Gas exchange that takes place at the lung level through the alveolar-capillary membrane is referred to as *external respiration*. The diffusion of gases in and out of the cells at the tissue level is referred to as *internal respiration*.[3]

DIFFUSION

Oxygen and carbon dioxide move throughout the body by diffusion. Diffusion moves molecules from an area of high concentration to an area of low concentration. The difference in the concentrations of the gases is referred to as the *driving pressure*. The greater the driving pressure of the gas through the membrane, the greater the rate of diffusion.[3] Within the lungs, diffusion occurs because of the difference in the driving pressure between the pulmonary capillaries and the alveoli. Oxygen is in high concentration within the alveoli and exerts a higher driving pressure as compared with the pulmonary capillaries; therefore, oxygen moves by diffusion from the alveoli into the pulmonary capillaries. Carbon dioxide is in higher concentration and has a higher driving pressure within the pulmonary capillaries compared with the alveoli; therefore, carbon dioxide diffuses out of the capillaries into the alveoli, where it is exhaled (Fig. 21-18). The driving pressure of oxygen is lower at higher altitudes because the effects of gravity on the gases

are lessened,[20] and it is higher when supplemental oxygen is administered.[21]

In addition to the driving pressure of gases, several other factors affect the rate of diffusion. They include the thickness of the alveolar-capillary membrane,[3] the surface area of the membrane,[22] and the diffusion coefficient of the gas.[21] An increase in the thickness of the alveolar-capillary membrane (e.g., pulmonary edema, fibrosis)[3] or a decrease in the surface area of the membrane (e.g., pneumonectomy, lobectomy, pulmonary embolus, emphysema)[22] decreases the rate of diffusion. The diffusion coefficient of each gas is determined by its solubility. The higher the diffusion coefficient, the faster the gas diffuses. Carbon dioxide has a much higher diffusion coefficient than oxygen, and carbon dioxide diffuses 20 times more rapidly than does oxygen.[21]

VENTILATION/PERFUSION RELATIONSHIPS

Ventilation ($\dot{V}$) and perfusion ($\dot{Q}$) should be equally matched at the alveolar capillary membrane level for optimal gas exchange to take place, but because of normal regional variations in the distribution of ventilation and perfusion, this is not the case. Normally, alveolar ventilation is approximately 4 L/min, and pulmonary capillary perfusion is approximately 5 L/min. The normal ventilation/perfusion ratio ($\dot{V}/\dot{Q}$) ratio is 4:5, or 0.8.[15,21]

DISTRIBUTION OF VENTILATION

The distribution of ventilation throughout the lungs is not even. This is the result of a variety of factors, including the configuration of the thorax and the effects of gravity on intrapleural pressure. The thorax allows more lung expansion at the base than at the apex, which permits more ventilation to the base and limits ventilation to the apex. Gravity also produces regional variations in intrapleural pressure. At rest, the negative intrapleural pressure at the apex is greater than at the base, and alveoli in the apexes are larger and have more air left in them at the end of expiration. Because the alveoli are larger, they are less compliant and more difficult to inflate. On inhalation, the alveoli at the base expand more because they have less pressure to overcome.[3,15,16] In the upright person, the base of the lung receives about four times more ventilation than the apex.[16] In the supine person, gravity produces the same effects in the dependent zones of the lungs (posterior regions).[3,15,16]

DISTRIBUTION OF PERFUSION

The distribution of perfusion through the lungs is related to gravity and intraalveolar pressures. Because of the effects of gravity, the pressure in the capillaries in the lungs is higher in the bases than in the apexes. This promotes preferential blood flow to the gravity-dependent areas of the lungs. Intraalveolar pressures also vary throughout the different regions of the lungs, with the highest pressure in the apexes and the lowest pressure in the bases. In some areas of the lungs, the intraalveolar pressure has the potential of exceeding capillary hydrostatic pressure, resulting in an absence of blood flow to these areas. On the basis of this concept, the lung can be divided into three zones. Zone 1 is the nondependent portion of the lung, which has the potential of no perfusion. Zone 2 is the middle portion of the lung, which receives various degrees of blood flow. Zone 3 is the gravity-dependent area of the lung, which receives a constant blood flow (Fig. 21-19).[3,15]

VENTILATION/PERFUSION MISMATCH

A variety of factors can affect the matching of ventilation to perfusion in the lungs, and their relationship can be considered as a continuum (Fig. 21-20). At one end of the continuum, the alveolus is receiving ventilation but is not receiving any perfusion and is unable to participate in gas exchange. This situation is referred to as *alveolar dead space*. On the other end of the continuum, the alveolus is receiving perfusion but is not receiving any ventilation and is unable to participate in gas exchange. This situation is referred to as *intrapulmonary shunting*. In this case, the blood is returned to the left side of the heart unoxygenated.[21] Between these two extremes exist an infinite number of ventilation/perfusion mismatches. Situations in which ventilation exceeds perfusion ($\dot{V}/\dot{Q} > 0.8$) are considered to be *dead space producing*, whereas situations in which perfusion exceeds ventilation ($\dot{V}/\dot{Q} < 0.8$) are considered to be *shunt producing*. Although minor mismatching of ventilation may

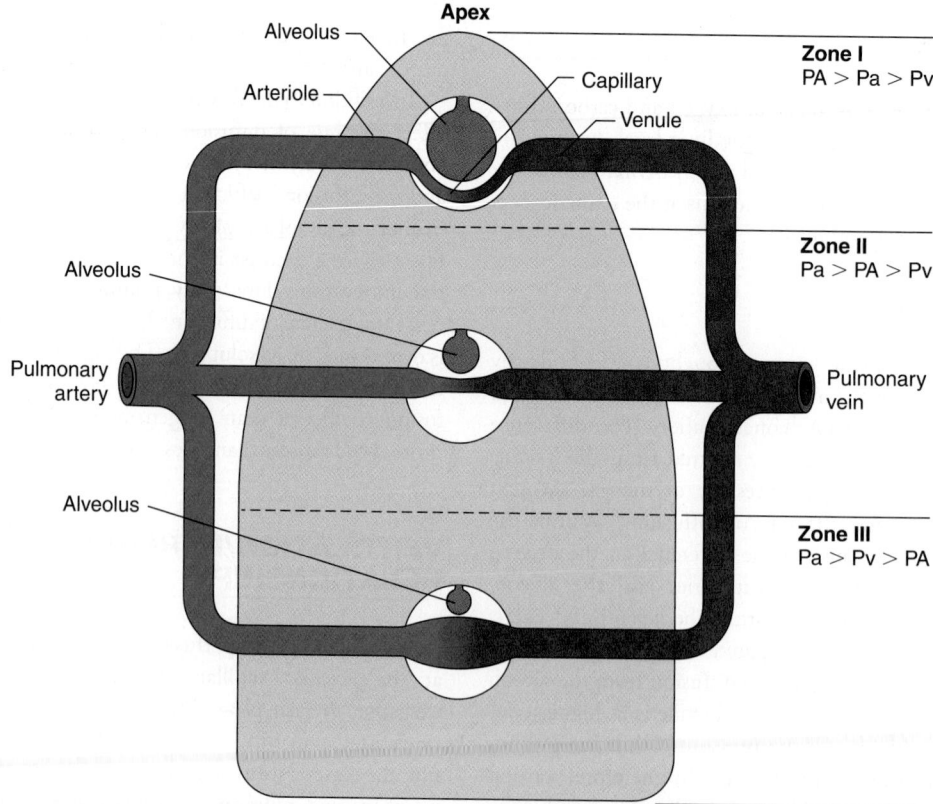

Figure 21-19 The effects of gravity and alveolar pressure on pulmonary blood flow. Notice the three lung zones. *(From McCance KL, Huether SE, editors: Pathophysiology: the biologic basis for disease in adults and children, ed 4, St Louis, 2002, Mosby.)*

not significantly affect gas exchange, significant alterations in the relationship result in hypoxemia.[15,21]

Hypoxic Vasoconstriction. The distribution of perfusion is affected by the amount of oxygen in the alveoli. Although most blood vessels in the body dilate in response to hypoxia, the pulmonary vessels constrict when the PaO_2 is less than 60 mm Hg. This event, known as *hypoxic vasoconstriction*, usually occurs when a portion of the pulmonary capillaries perfuses unventilated or underventilated alveoli. It is thought to be a compensatory response used to limit the return of unoxygenated blood to the left side of the heart. If the response is prolonged and generalized throughout the lungs, pulmonary hypertension (Box 21-2) will result.[3]

GAS TRANSPORT

Gas transport refers to the movement of oxygen and carbon dioxide to and from the tissue cells. The transportation vehicle is the bloodstream, which is moved by the pumping action of the heart (cardiac output). At the tissue level, oxygen and carbon dioxide move into and out of the cell by diffusion. Oxygen diffuses into the cell because of the pressure gradient that exists between oxygen in the capillary and oxygen in the cell (Fig. 21-21A). Carbon dioxide diffuses into the capillary because of the pressure gradient that exists between carbon dioxide in the cell and carbon dioxide in the capillary (see Fig. 21-21B).[3]

OXYGEN CONTENT

Oxygen is transported to the tissues by the blood in two ways. It is dissolved in plasma (PaO_2) or bound to hemoglobin molecules

(oxygen saturation [SaO_2]). Most of the oxygen is transported by hemoglobin, with the portion of oxygen dissolved in plasma equal to approximately 3% of the total oxygen within the blood.[23] The pressure exerted by the oxygen dissolved in

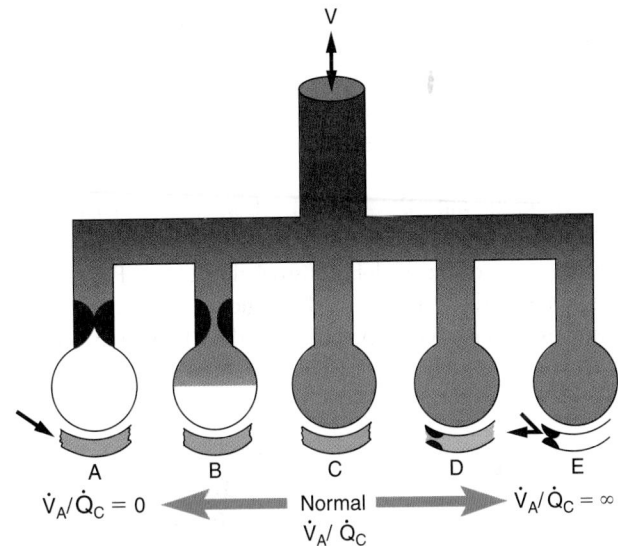

Figure 21-20 Continuum of ventilation/perfusion ($\dot{V}/\dot{Q}$) relationships. *A*, Intrapulmonary shunting. *B*, $\dot{V}/\dot{Q}$ mismatching is a shunt-producing situation. *C*, Normal $\dot{V}/\dot{Q}$ ratio. *D*, $\dot{V}/\dot{Q}$ mismatching is a dead space–producing situation. *E*, Alveolar dead space. *(From Misasi RS, Keyes JL: Matching and mismatching ventilation and perfusion in the lung,* Crit Care Nurse *16[3]:23, 1996.)*

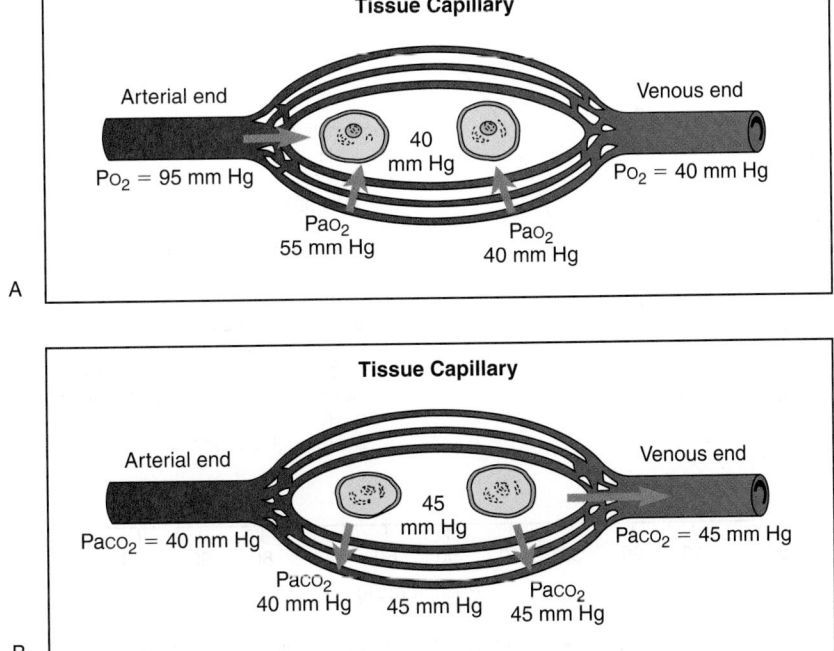

Figure 21-21 Internal respiration. *A*, Diffusion of oxygen from a tissue capillary into a tissue cell. *B*, Diffusion of carbon dioxide from a tissue cell into a tissue capillary.

plasma is important because this oxygen diffuses across the capillary membrane into the cells first and serves as the vehicle for the unloading of the oxygen from the hemoglobin molecule. As dissolved oxygen leaves the plasma and diffuses into the cells, the molecules of oxygen move off the hemoglobin molecule, dissolve into the plasma, and diffuse into the cells.[20] For this process to begin, a pressure gradient must exist between the oxygen level in the capillary and the oxygen level in the cell.

Oxygen Content Formula. The amount of oxygen in the arterial blood can be calculated using the arterial oxygen content (CaO_2) formula. The amount of oxygen in the venous blood can be calculated using the venous oxygen content (CvO_2) formula (see Appendix B).[23]

Oxyhemoglobin Dissociation Curve. The relationship between dissolved oxygen and hemoglobin-bound oxygen is plotted as the oxyhemoglobin dissociation curve (Fig. 21-22). The sigmoid shape of the oxyhemoglobin dissociation curve illustrates several essential points about the relationship between the two ways oxygen is carried. The steep lower portion of the curve, at PaO_2 levels of 10 to 60 mm Hg, shows that the peripheral tissues can withdraw large amounts of oxygen from the hemoglobin molecule with only a small change in PaO_2, preserving the gradient for the continued unloading of hemoglobin.[20,23] The area at PaO_2 levels of 60 to 100 mm Hg is called the *flat upper portion* of the curve. This portion shows that the saturation of hemoglobin remains high even as the PaO_2 declines. For example, in a healthy person, a PaO_2 of 60 mm Hg yields an oxygen saturation level of 89%, whereas a PaO_2 of 100 mm Hg yields an oxygen saturation level of 98%. The great drop in PaO_2 (from 100 to 60 mm Hg) causes only a small drop in oxygen saturation (from 98% to 89%).[21,23]

Shifts in the Oxyhemoglobin Dissociation Curve. Under normal circumstances, hemoglobin has a steady and predictable affinity for oxygen. The combination of oxygen and hemoglobin based on this affinity is responsible for the position of the oxyhemoglobin dissociation curve in which a given PaO_2

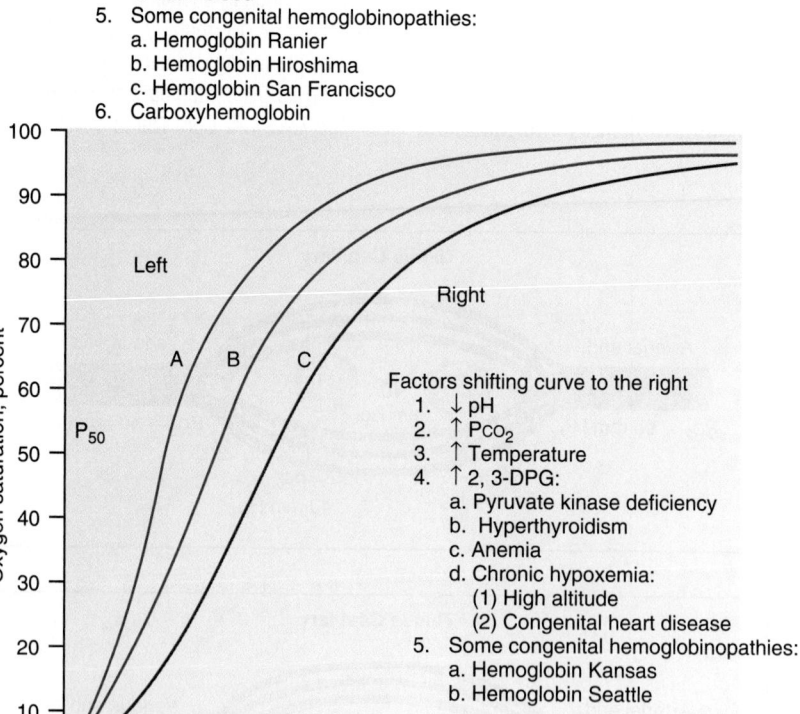

Figure 21-22 Oxyhemoglobin dissociation curve. *A,* The curve is shifted to the left because of hemoglobin's increased affinity for oxygen. *B,* The standard oxyhemoglobin dissociation curve. *C,* The curve is shifted to the right because of hemoglobin's decreased affinity for oxygen. *(Modified from Kinney MR et al, editors: AACN's clinical reference for critical care nursing, ed 4, St Louis, 1998, Mosby).*

yields a predictable oxygen saturation.[20,23] Occasionally, events occur that alter the affinity hemoglobin has for oxygen. These events include changes in pH, $PaCO_2$, temperature, and 2,3-diphosphoglycerate (2,3-DPG) levels (Box 21-4). When this affinity is altered, the position of the oxyhemoglobin dissociation curve shifts (see Fig. 21-22). Shifts in the position of the curve mean there is a change in the way oxygen is taken up by the hemoglobin molecule at the alveolar level and a change in the way oxygen is delivered at the tissue level.[21,23]

Shift to the Right. When the curve is shifted to the right (see Fig. 21-22, curve C), there is a lower oxygen saturation level for any given PaO_2; in other words, hemoglobin has less affinity for oxygen. Although the saturation level is lower than expected, a right shift enhances oxygen delivery at the tissue level because hemoglobin unloads more readily. Factors that cause this change in oxygen-hemoglobin affinity and shift the curve to the right include fever, increased $PaCO_2$, acidosis, and increased 2,3-DPG levels.[21,23]

Shift to the Left. When the curve is shifted to the left (see Fig. 21-22, curve A), the reverse occurs. There is a higher arterial saturation for any given PaO_2 because hemoglobin has an increased affinity for oxygen. Although the saturation level is higher, oxygen delivery to the tissues is impaired because hemoglobin does not unload as easily. Factors that contribute to this effect include hypothermia, alkalemia, decreased $PaCO_2$, and decreased 2,3-DPG levels.[21,23]

Abnormalities of Hemoglobin. Hemoglobin carries approximately 97% of the total amount of oxygen held within the bloodstream. This great carrying capacity depends on hemoglobin that is normal in amount and molecular structure. Most hemoglobin abnormalities affect the oxygen-carrying capability of this molecule. The most common abnormality involving hemoglobin is a decrease in amount. This can be an acute or a chronic situation (anemia). Abnormal hemoglobin structure also can pose problems, such as hemoglobin S, which is responsible for sickle cell anemia. Hemoglobin S has less affinity for oxygen than does normal hemoglobin. Normal hemoglobin can become abnormal hemoglobin under certain conditions. Methemoglobin and carboxyhemoglobin are two examples. Methemoglobin occurs when the iron atoms within the hemoglobin molecule are oxidized from the ferrous state to the ferric state. Methemoglobin does not carry oxygen. Carboxyhemoglobin occurs when carbon monoxide combines with hemoglobin. Carbon monoxide uses the same binding site as oxygen and has a much greater affinity for hemoglobin.[21]

CARBON DIOXIDE CONTENT

Carbon dioxide, one of the end products of aerobic cellular metabolism, is produced continuously within the cells. On its way from the cells to the lungs, carbon dioxide is transported within the plasma and the erythrocytes. Carbon dioxide is transported, physically dissolved as the $PaCO_2$ (5%), bound to blood proteins (including hemoglobin) in the form of carbaminohemoglobin compounds (5% to 10%), and combined with water to form carbonic acid (80% to 90%), some of which dissociates into hydrogen ions and bicarbonate. In the lungs, these methods of carbon dioxide carriage are reversed as the carbon dioxide leaves the plasma and erythrocytes for exhalation.[21]

Summary

Anatomy

- The pulmonary system consists of the thorax, conducting airways, respiratory airways, and pulmonary blood and lymph supply.
- The thorax consists of the thoracic cage, lungs, pleura, and muscles of ventilation, and its major function is to form the ventilatory pump and perform the work of breathing.
- The conducting airways consist of the upper airways, the trachea, and the bronchial tree, and their major functions are to warm and humidify the inhaled air, to prevent the entrance of foreign matter into the gas exchange areas, and to serve as a passageway for air entering and leaving the gas exchange regions of the lungs.
- The respiratory airways consist of the respiratory bronchioles and the alveoli, and their major function is gas exchange.
- The pulmonary circulation is the vascular system that forms the gas exchange network surrounding the alveoli, and the bronchial circulation is the vascular system that perfuses the tracheobronchial tree.
- The lymphatic system is responsible for removing foreign particles and cell debris from the lungs, for producing antibody- and cell-mediated immune responses, and for removing fluid from the lungs and for keeping the alveoli clear.

BOX 21-4   WHAT IS 2,3-DPG?

2,3-Diphosphoglycerate (2,3-DPG), an organic phosphate found primarily in red blood cells, has the ability to alter the affinity of hemoglobin for oxygen. When the level of 2,3-DPG increases within the red blood cells, hemoglobin's affinity for oxygen is decreased (a shift in the oxyhemoglobin curve to the right), making more oxygen available to the tissues. Increased synthesis of 2,3,-DPG is an important component of the adaptive responses in healthy persons to an acute need for more tissue oxygen. Tissue hypoxia stimulates production of 2,3-DPG, and increased amounts have been found in patients with anemia, right-to-left shunts, and congestive heart failure and in persons residing at high altitudes.

A decrease in the amount of 2,3-DPG is detrimental to tissue oxygenation because it causes hemoglobin's affinity for oxygen to increase (a shift in the oxyhemoglobin curve to the left). Decreased 2,3-DPG levels occur with hypophosphatemia, septic shock, and the use of banked blood. Blood preserved with acid citrate dextrose loses most of its red cell 2,3-DPG within several days. Blood preserved with citrate phosphate dextrose maintains its 2,3-DPG levels for several weeks. Transfusion of blood with a low level of 2,3-DPG cannot be beneficial for tissue oxygenation until the 2,3-DPG level is restored, which may take 18 to 24 hours.

Physiology

- The primary functions of the pulmonary system are ventilation and respiration.
- Ventilation is the movement of air in (inhalation) and out (exhalation) of the lungs.
- The work of breathing is the amount of work that must be performed to overcome the elastic and resistive properties of the lungs.

- Respiration is the process of gas exchange.
- External respiration takes place at the lung level through the alveolar-capillary membrane.
- Internal respiration is the diffusion of gases in and out of the cells at the tissue level.

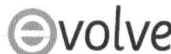 Be sure to check out the bonus material, including free self-assessment exercises, on the Evolve web site at http://evolve.elsevier.com/Urden/.

References

1. Hicks GH: The respiratory system. In Wilkins RL et al, editors: *Egan's fundamentals of respiratory care*, ed 9, St Louis, 2008, Mosby.
2. Albertine KH et al: Anatomy of the lungs. In Mason RJ et al, editors: *Murray & Nadel's textbook of respiratory medicine*, ed 4, Philadelphia, 2005, Elsevier.
3. Brashers VL: Structure and function of the pulmonary system. In McCance KL, Huether SE, editors: *Pathophysiology: the biologic basis for disease in adults and children*, ed 5, St Louis, 2006, Mosby.
4. Huggins JT, Doelken P: Pleural manometry, *Clin Chest Med* 27:229, 2006.
5. Flaminiano LE, Celli BD: Respiratory muscle testing, *Clin Chest Med* 22:661, 2001.
6. Adrich TK, Tso R: The lungs and neuromuscular diseases. In Mason RJ et al, editors: *Murray & Nadel's textbook of respiratory medicine*, ed 4, Philadelphia, 2005, Elsevier.
7. Flaminiano LE, Celli BD: Respiratory muscle testing, *Clin Chest Med* 22:661, 2001.
8. Welsh DA, Mason CM: Host defense in respiratory infections, *Med Clin North Am* 85:1329, 2001.
9. Chang AB: The physiology of cough, *Paediatr Respir Rev* 7:2, 2006.
10. Enhorning G: Surfactant in airway disease, *Chest* 133:975, 2008.
11. Polanco PM, Pinsky MR: Practical issues of hemodynamic monitoring at the bedside, *Surg Clin N Am* 86:1431, 2006.
12. Zamanian RT et al: Management strategies for patients with pulmonary hypertension in the intensive care unit, *Crit Care Med* 35:2037, 2007.
13. Wagner PD, West JB: Ventilation, blood flow, and gas exchange. In Mason RJ et al, editors: *Murray & Nadel's textbook of respiratory medicine*, ed 4, Philadelphia, 2005, Elsevier.
14. Charana NB et al: Functional anatomy of bronchial veins, *Pulm Pharmacol Ther* 20:100, 2007.
15. Misasi RS, Keyes JL: Matching and mismatching ventilation and perfusion in the lung, *Crit Care Nurse* 16(3):23, 1996.
16. Ruppel GL: Ventilation. In Wilkins RL et al, editors: *Egan's fundamentals of respiratory care*, ed 9, St Louis, 2008, Mosby.
17. Zakynthinos SG et al: Respiratory system mechanics and energetics. In Mason RJ et al, editors: *Murray & Nadel's textbook of respiratory medicine*, ed 4, Philadelphia, 2005, Elsevier.
18. Corne S, Bshouty Z: Basic principles of control of breathing, *Respir Care Clin* 11:147, 2005.
19. Eckert DJ et al: Central sleep apnea pathophysiology and treatment, *Chest* 131:595, 2007.
20. Huang YCT: Monitoring oxygen delivery in the critically ill, *Chest* 128:554S, 2005.
21. Wilkins RL: Gas exchange and transport. In Wilkins RL et al, editors: *Egan's fundamentals of respiratory care*, ed 9, St Louis, 2008, Mosby.
22. Hebert PC et al: Physiologic aspects of anemia, *Crit Care Clin* 20:187, 2004.
23. Berry BE, Pinard AE: Assessing tissue oxygenation, *Crit Care Nurse* 22(3):22, 2002.

Pulmonary Clinical Assessment

$\mathscr{A}$ssessment of the patient with pulmonary dysfunction is a systematic process that incorporates an inquiry into the chronology of the present illness, better known as a *history,* and an investigation of the current physical manifestations, better known as a *physical examination.* The purpose of the assessment is twofold: first, to recognize changes in the patient's pulmonary status that necessitate nursing or medical intervention, and second, to determine the ways in which the patient's pulmonary dysfunction is interfering with his or her self-care activities. After completion, the assessment serves as the foundation for developing the management plan for the patient. The assessment process can be brief or can involve a detailed history and examination, depending on the nature and immediacy of the patient's situation. Whatever the setting, the nurse should develop and practice a sequential pattern of assessment to avoid omitting portions of the examination.

HISTORY

Taking a thorough and accurate history is an essential part of the assessment process. The patient's history provides the foundation and direction for the rest of the assessment. The overall goal of the patient interview is to expose key clinical manifestations that will facilitate the identification of the underlying cause of the illness. This information then assists in the development of an appropriate management plan.[1]

The initial presentation of the patient determines the rapidity and direction of the interview. For a patient in acute distress (Box 22-1), the history should be curtailed to just a few questions about the patient's chief complaint and precipitating events. For a patient in no obvious distress, the history should focus on five areas: (1) review of the patient's present illness, (2) overview of the patient's general respiratory status, (3) examination of the patient's general health status, (4) survey of the patient's family and social background, and (5) description of the patient's current symptoms.[1] Specific items regarding each of these areas are outlined in the Data Collection feature on Pulmonary History.

Symptoms that are common in the pulmonary patient include dyspnea, cough, wheezing, edema, palpitations, fatigue, chest pain, hemoptysis, and sputum abnormalities. Information should be elicited regarding the location, onset and duration,

characteristics, setting, aggravating and alleviating factors, associated symptoms, and efforts to treat the symptoms. If the cough is productive, the patient should be asked questions about the color, amount, odor, and consistency of the sputum.[2-5]

PHYSICAL EXAMINATION

Four techniques are used in physical assessment: inspection, palpation, percussion, and auscultation. *Inspection* is the process of looking intently at the patient. *Palpation* is the process of touching the patient to judge the size, shape, texture, and temperature of the body surface or underlying structures. *Percussion* is the process of creating sound waves on the surface of the body to determine abnormal density of any underlying areas. *Auscultation* is the process of concentrated listening with a stethoscope to determine characteristics of body functions.[6,7]

INSPECTION

Inspection of the patient should focus on three areas: (1) observation of the tongue and sublingual area, (2) assessment of chest wall configuration, and (3) evaluation of respiratory effort. If possible, patients should be positioned upright, with their arms resting at their sides.[3] Inspection usually begins during the interview process.[2]

Tongue and Sublingual Area. The tongue and sublingual area should be observed for a blue, gray, or dark purple tint or discoloration indicating the presence of central cyanosis. *Central cyanosis* is a sign of hypoxemia, or inadequate oxygenation of the blood, and it is considered to be a life-threatening condition. It occurs when the amount of reduced hemoglobin (unsaturated hemoglobin) exceeds 5 g/dL. The fingers and toes may also appear discolored, an indication of the presence of peripheral cyanosis.[8]

Chest Wall Configuration. Assessment of chest wall configuration incorporates observations about the size and shape of the patient's chest. Normally, the ratio of anteroposterior diameter to lateral diameter ranges from 1:2 to 5:7 (Fig. 22-1A).[2,4,5] An increase in the anteroposterior diameter is suggestive of chronic obstructive pulmonary disease (COPD).[2,4,5] The shape of the chest should be inspected for any structural deviations.

BOX 22-1 MANIFESTATIONS OF RESPIRATORY DECOMPENSATION

INADEQUATE AIRWAY
- Stridor
- Noisy respirations
- Supraclavicular and intercostal retractions
- Flaring of nares
- Labored breathing with use of accessory muscles

INADEQUATE VENTILATION
- Absence of air exchange at nose and mouth (breathlessness)
- Minimal or absent chest wall motion
- Manifestations of obstructed airway
- Central cyanosis

- Decreased or absent breath sounds (bilateral, unilateral)
- Restlessness, anxiety, confusion
- Paradoxical motion involving significant portion of chest wall
- Decreased Pao_2, increased $Paco_2$, decreased pH

INADEQUATE GAS EXCHANGE
- Tachypnea
- Decreased Pao_2
- Increased dead space
- Central cyanosis
- Chest infiltrates on x-ray evaluation

Data Collection

Pulmonary History

Chief Complaint

Cough
- Onset and duration
  Sudden or gradual
  Episodic or continuous
- Characteristics
  Dry or wet
  Hacking, hoarse, barking, or congested
  Productive or nonproductive
- Sputum
  Present or absent
  Frequency of production
  Appearance—color (e.g., clear, mucoid, purulent, blood-tinged, mostly bloody), foul odor, frothy
  Amount
- Pattern
  Paroxysmal
  Related to time of day, weather, activities, talking, or deep breathing
  Change over time
- Severity
  Causes fatigue
  Disrupts sleep or conversation
  Produces chest pain
- Associated symptoms
  Shortness of breath
  Chest pain or tightness with breathing
  Fever
  Upper respiratory tract signs (sore throat, congestion, increased mucus production)
  Noisy respirations or hoarseness
  Gagging or choking
  Anxiety, stress, or panic reactions
- Efforts made to treat
  Prescription or nonprescription drugs
  Vaporizers
  Effective or ineffective

Shortness of Breath or Dyspnea on Exertion
- Onset and duration
  Sudden or gradual
  Gagging or choking episode a few days before onset
- Pattern
  Related to position—improves when sitting up or with head elevated; number of pillows used to alleviate problems
  Related to activity—exercise or eating; extent of activity that produces dyspnea
  Related to other factors—time of day, season, or exposure to something in the environment
  Harder to inhale or harder to exhale
- Severity
  Extent activity is limited
  Breathing itself causes fatigue
  Anxiety about getting enough air
- Associated symptoms
  Pain or discomfort—exact location in respiratory tree
  Cough, diaphoresis, swelling of ankles, or cyanosis
- Efforts made to treat
  Prescription or nonprescription drugs
  Oxygen
  Effective or ineffective

Chest Pain
- Onset and duration
  Gradual or sudden
  Associated with trauma, coughing, or lower respiratory tract infection
- Associated symptoms
  Shallow breathing
  Uneven chest expansion
  Fever
  Cough
  Radiation of pain to neck or arms
  Anxiety about getting enough air
- Efforts made to treat
  Heat, splinting, or pain medication
  Effective or ineffective

Data Collection—cont'd

Patient's Perception of the Problem
- Degree of concern about the symptoms
- Opinion about its cause

Patient History: Causes or Aggravating Factors Related to Respiratory Disorders
- Tobacco use—current and past
  Type of tobacco—cigarettes, cigars, pipes, or smokeless
  Duration and amount—age started, inhale when smoking, amount used in the past and present
  Pack years—number of packs per day multiplied by number of years patient has smoked
  Efforts to quit—previous attempts and current interest
- Work environment
  Nature of work
  Environmental hazards: chemicals, vapors, dust, pulmonary irritants, or allergens
  Use of protective devices
- Home environment
  Location
  Possible allergens—pets, house plants, plants and trees outside the home, or other environmental hazards
  Type of heating
  Use of air conditioning or humidifier
  Ventilation
  Stairs to climb

Medical History
- Infectious respiratory diseases
  Strep throat
  Mumps
  Tonsillitis
- Thoracic trauma or surgery
- Previous diagnosis of pulmonary disorders—dates of hospitalization

- Chronic pulmonary disease—date, treatment, and compliance with therapy
  Tuberculosis
  Bronchitis
  Emphysema
  Bronchiectasis
  Asthma
  Cystic fibrosis
  Sinus infection
- Other chronic disorders—cardiovascular, cancer, musculoskeletal, neurologic
  Nasal surgery or injury
  Obstruction of one or both nares
  Mouth breathing often necessary (especially at night)
  History of nasal discharge
- Nosebleed
  Affects one or both nostrils
  Aggravated by crusting
- Previous tests
  Allergy testing
  Pulmonary function tests
  Tuberculin and fungal skin tests
  Chest radiographs

Family History
- Tuberculosis
- Cystic fibrosis
- Emphysema
- Allergies
- Asthma
- Atopic dermatitis
- Smoking by household members
- Malignancy

Some of the more frequently seen abnormalities are pectus excavatum, pectus carinatum, barrel chest, and spinal deformities. In *pectus excavatum* (funnel chest), the sternum and lower ribs are displaced posteriorly, creating a funnel or pit-shaped depression in the chest. This causes a decrease in the anteroposterior diameter of the chest and may interfere with respiratory function. In *pectus carinatum* (pigeon breast), the sternum projects forward, causing an increase in the anteroposterior diameter of the chest. The *barrel chest* also results in an increase in anteroposterior diameter of the chest and is characterized by displacement of the sternum forward and the ribs outward (see Fig. 22-1B). Spinal deformities such as *kyphosis, lordosis,* and *scoliosis* also may be present and can interfere with respiratory function.[9]

Respiratory Effort. Evaluation of respiratory effort incorporates observations on the rate, rhythm, symmetry, and quality of ventilatory movements.[2] Normal breathing at rest is effortless and regular and occurs at a rate of 12 to 20 breaths per minute.[3] There are a number of abnormal respiratory patterns (Fig. 22-2). Some of the more commonly seen patterns in patients with pulmonary dysfunction are tachypnea, hyperventilation, and air

trapping. *Tachypnea* is manifested by an increase in the rate and decrease in the depth of ventilation. *Hyperventilation* is manifested by an increase in the rate and depth of ventilation. Patients with COPD often experience obstructive breathing, or *air trapping*. As the patient breathes, air becomes trapped in the lungs and ventilations become progressively more shallow until the patient actively and forcefully exhales.[10]

Additional Assessment Areas. Other areas of focus for the careful assessment are patient position, active effort to breathe, use of accessory muscles, presence of intercostal retractions, unequal movement of the chest wall, flaring of nares, and pausing midsentence to take a breath.[2,4,5] The presence of other iatrogenic features, such as chest tubes, central venous lines, artificial airways, and nasogastric tubes should be identified because they may affect assessment findings.

PALPATION

Palpation of the patient should focus on three aspects: (1) confirmation of the position of the trachea, (2) assessment of thoracic expansion, and (3) evaluation of fremitus. The thorax

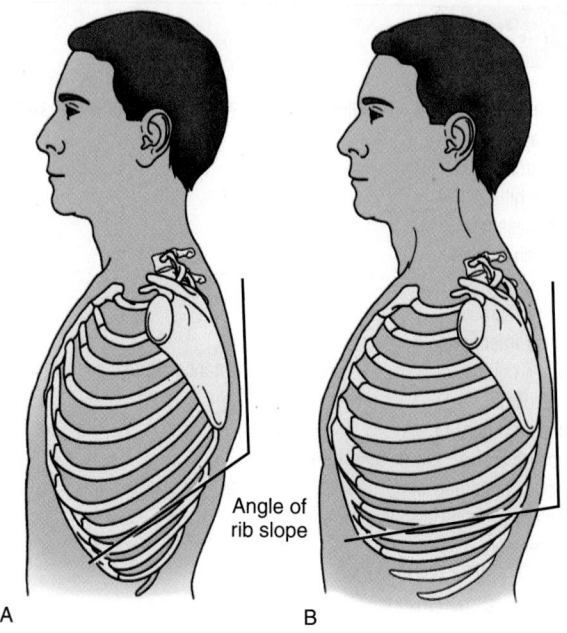

Figure 22-1 Chest wall configuration. *A,* Normal configuration. *B,* Increased anteroposterior diameter. Notice the contrast in the angle of the slope of the ribs. *(From Barkauskas V et al:* Health and physical assessment, *ed 3, St Louis, 2002, Mosby.)*

should be assessed for any areas of tenderness, lumps, or bony deformities. The anterior, posterior, and lateral areas of the chest should be evaluated in a systematic fashion.[2]

Position of the Trachea. Confirmation of the position of the trachea is performed to verify that the trachea is midline. It is assessed by placing the fingers in the suprasternal notch and moving upward (Fig. 22-3).[10] Deviation of the trachea to either side may indicate a pneumothorax, unilateral pneumonia, diffuse pulmonary fibrosis, a large pleural effusion, or severe atelectasis. With atelectasis, the trachea shifts to the same side as the problem, and with pneumothorax, the trachea shifts to the opposite side of the problem.[9]

Thoracic Expansion. Assessment of thoracic expansion involves measuring the degree and symmetry of respiratory movement. It is assessed by placing the hands on the anterolateral chest with the thumbs extended along the costal margin, pointing to the xiphoid process, or on the posterolateral chest with the thumbs on either side of the spine at the level of the 10th rib (Fig. 22-4). The patient is instructed to take a few normal breaths and then a few deep breaths. Chest movement is assessed for equality, which signifies symmetry of thoracic expansion.[3,9,10] Asymmetry is an abnormal finding that can occur with pneumothorax, pneumonia, or other disorders that interfere with lung inflation. The degree of chest movement is felt to ascertain the extent of lung expansion. The thumbs should separate 3 to 5 cm during deep inspiration.[5,10] Lung expansion of a hyperinflated chest is less than that of a normal one.[5,10]

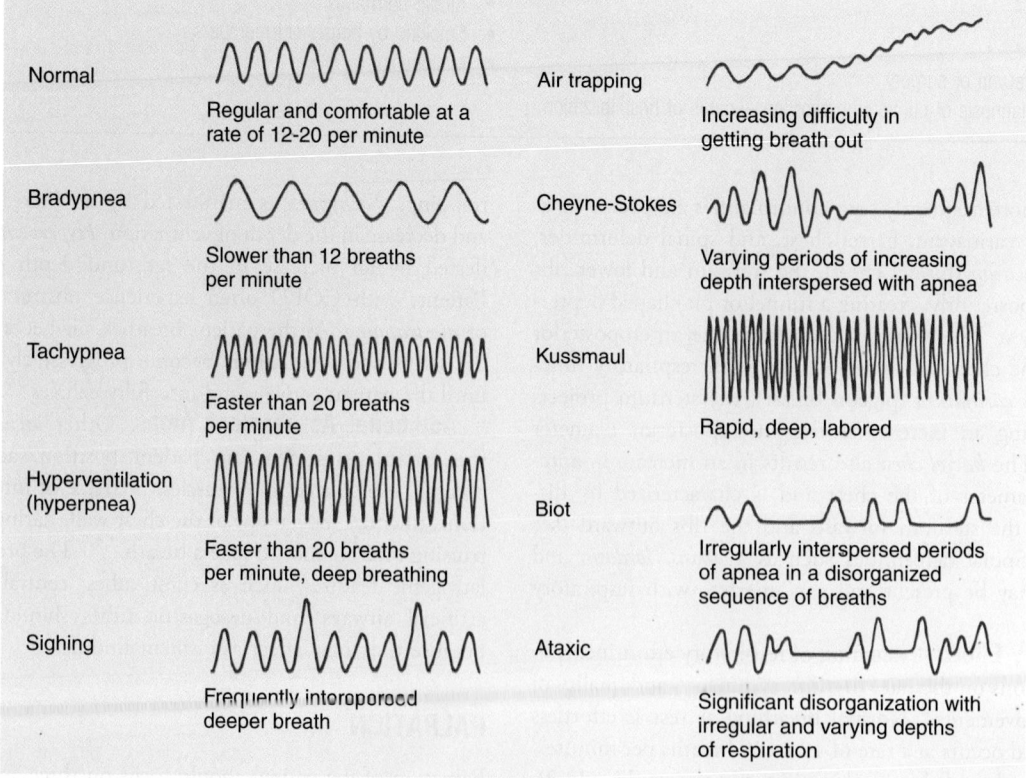

Figure 22-2 Patterns of respiration. *(From Seidel HM et al:* Mosby's guide to physical examination, *ed 6, St Louis, 2006, Mosby.)*

Tactile Fremitus. Assessment of tactile fremitus is performed to identify, describe, and localize any areas of increased or decreased fremitus. Fremitus refers to the palpable vibrations felt through the chest wall when the patient speaks. It is assessed by placing the palmar surface of the hands against opposite sides of the chest wall and having the patient repeat the word "ninety-nine" (Fig. 22-5). The hands are moved systematically around the thorax until the anterior, posterior, and both lateral areas have been assessed.[9,10] If only one hand is used, it is moved from one side of the chest to the corresponding area on the other side of the chest until all areas have been assessed.[10]

Fremitus varies from patient to patient and depends on the pitch and intensity of the voice. Fremitus is described as normal, decreased, or increased. With normal fremitus, vibrations can be felt over the trachea but are barely palpable over the periphery.[2] With decreased fremitus, there is interference with the transmission of vibrations. Examples of disorders that decrease fremitus include pleural effusion, pneumothorax, bronchial obstruction, pleural thickening, and emphysema. With increased fremitus, there is an increase in the transmission of vibrations. Examples of disorders that increase fremitus include pneumonia, lung cancer, and pulmonary fibrosis.[5]

PERCUSSION

Percussion of the patient should focus on two concerns: evaluation of the underlying lung structure and assessment of diaphragmatic excursion. Although the technique is not used often, percussion is a useful method for confirming suspected abnormalities.

Underlying Lung Structure. Evaluation of the underlying lung structure is performed to estimate the amounts of air, liquid, or solid material present. It is performed by placing the middle finger of the nondominant hand on the chest wall. The distal portion, between the last joint and the nail bed, is then struck with the middle finger of the dominant hand. The hands are moved systematically and side to side around the thorax to compare similar areas until the anterior, posterior, and both lateral areas have been assessed (Fig. 22-6). Five tones can be elicited: resonance, hyperresonance, tympany, dullness, and flatness. These tones are distinguished by differences in intensity, pitch, duration, and quality. Table 22-1 describes the different percussion tones and their associated conditions.[3,9]

Diaphragmatic Excursion. Assessment of diaphragmatic excursion is accomplished by measuring the difference in the level of the diaphragm on inspiration and expiration. It is performed by instructing the patient to inhale and hold the breath. The posterior chest is percussed downward, over the intercostal spaces, until the dull sound produced by the diaphragm is heard. The spot is marked. The patient is then instructed to take a few breaths in and out, exhale completely, and then hold his or her breath. The posterior chest is percussed again, and the new area of dullness over the diaphragm is located and marked. The difference between the two spots is identified and measured (Fig. 22-7). Normal

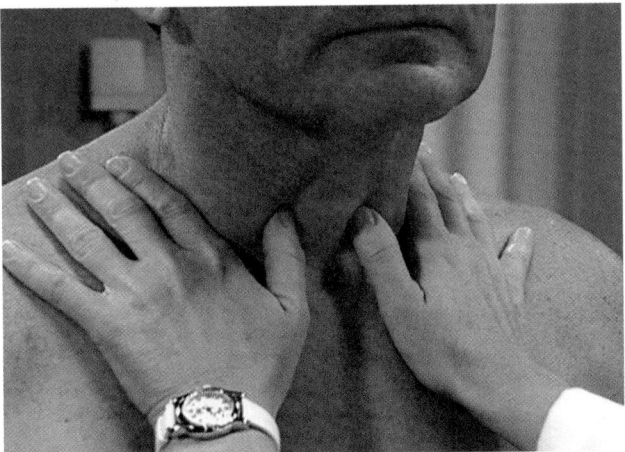

Figure 22-3 Assessment of the position of the trachea. *(From Seidel HM et al: Mosby's guide to physical examination, ed 6, St Louis, 2006, Mosby.)*

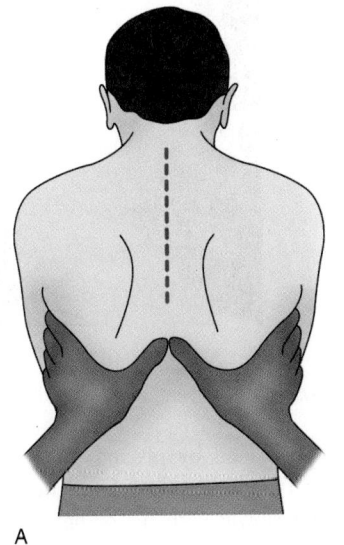
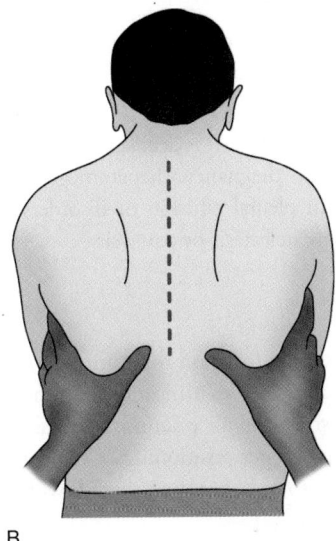

A

B

Figure 22-4 Assessment of thoracic expansion. *A,* Exhalation. *B,* Inhalation. *(From Wilkins RL et al, editors:* Egan's fundamentals of respiratory care, *ed 9, St Louis, 2008, Mosby.)*

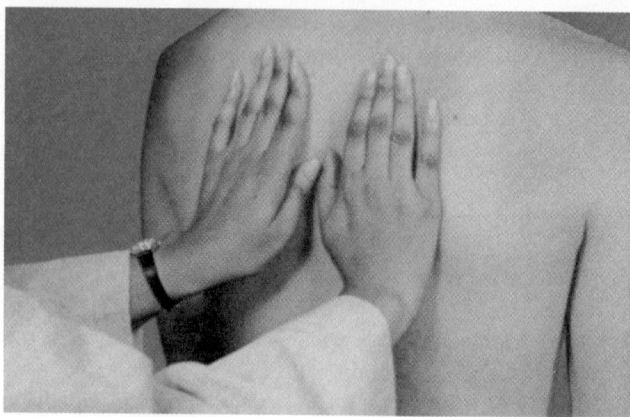

Figure 22-5 Assessment of tactile fremitus, showing simultaneous application of the fingertips of both hands to compare sides. *(From Barkauskas V et al: Health and physical assessment, ed 3, St Louis, 2002, Mosby.)*

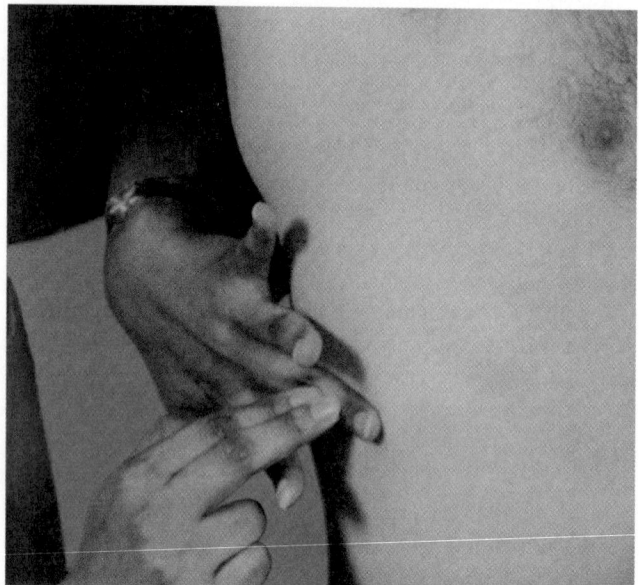

Figure 22-6 Assessment of diaphragmatic excursion. *(From Barkauskas V et al: Health and physical assessment, ed 3, St Louis, 2002, Mosby.)*

diaphragmatic excursion is 3 to 5 cm.[10] It is decreased in disorders or conditions such as ascites, pregnancy, hepatomegaly, and emphysema. It is increased in pleural effusion or disorders that elevate the diaphragm, such as atelectasis or paralysis.[9]

AUSCULTATION

Auscultation of the patient should focus on three areas: (1) evaluation of normal breath sounds, (2) identification of abnormal breath sounds, and (3) assessment of voice sounds. Auscultation requires a quiet environment, proper positioning of the patient, and a bare chest.[11] Breath sounds are best heard with the patient in the upright position.[5]

Normal Breath Sounds. Evaluation of normal breath sounds is performed to assess air movement through the pulmonary system and to identify the presence of abnormal sounds.

TABLE 22-1   Percussion Tones and Their Associated Conditions

Tone	Description	Condition
Resonance	Intensity: loud Pitch: low Duration: long Quality: hollow	Normal lung Bronchitis
Hyperresonance	Intensity: very loud Pitch: very low Duration: long Quality: booming	Asthma Emphysema Pneumothorax
Tympany	Intensity: loud Pitch: musical Duration: medium Quality: drumlike	Large pneumothorax Emphysematous blebs
Dullness	Intensity: medium Pitch: medium-high Duration: medium Quality: thudlike	Atelectasis Pleural effusion Pulmonary edema Pneumonia Lung mass
Flatness	Intensity: soft Pitch: high Duration: short Quality: extremely dull	Massive atelectasis Pneumonectomy

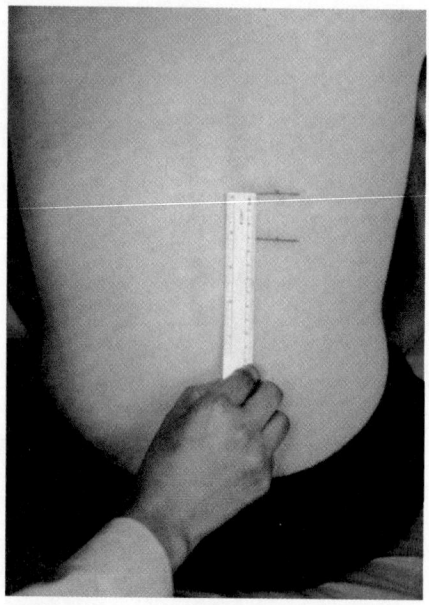

Figure 22-7 Percussion of the thorax. *(From Barkauskas V et al: Health and physical assessment, ed 3, St Louis, 2002, Mosby.)*

It is performed by placing the diaphragm of the stethoscope against the chest wall and instructing the patient to breathe in and out slowly with his or her mouth open.[2] The inspiratory and expiratory phases should be assessed. Auscultation should be done in a systematic sequence: side-to-side, top-to-bottom, posteriorly, laterally, and anteriorly (Fig. 22-8).[5]

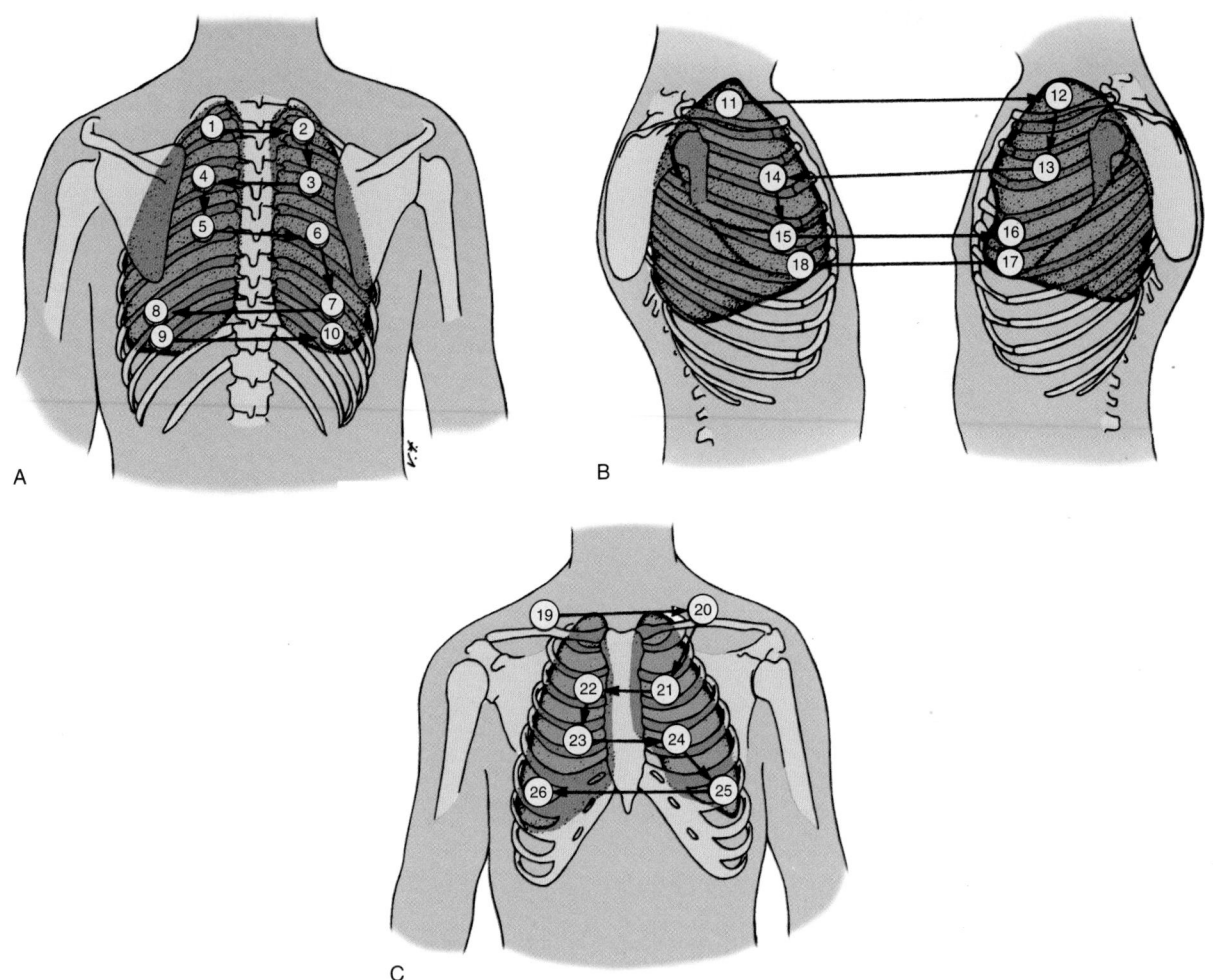

Figure 22-8 Auscultation sequence. *A*, Posterior. *B*, Lateral. *C*, Anterior. *(From Perry AG, Potter PA: Clinical nursing skills and techniques, ed 6, St Louis, 2005, Mosby.)*

TABLE 22-2 Characteristics of Normal Breath Sounds

Sound	Characteristics
Vesicular	Heard over most of lung field; low pitch; soft and short exhalation, and long inhalation
Bronchovesicular	Heard over main bronchus area and over upper right posterior lung field; medium pitch; exhalation equals inhalation
Bronchial	Heard only over trachea; high pitch; loud and long exhalation

Modified from Thompson JM et al: *Mosby's clinical nursing,* ed 5, St. Louis, 2002, Mosby.

Normal breath sounds are different, depending on their location. There are three categories: vesicular, bronchovesicular, and bronchial. Table 22-2 describes the characteristics of normal breath sounds and their associated conditions.[2,5,11]

Abnormal Breath Sounds. Identification of abnormal breath sounds occurs after the normal breath sounds have been clearly delineated. There are three categories of abnormal breath sounds: absent or diminished breath sounds, displaced bronchial breath sounds, and adventitious breath sounds. Table 22-3 describes the various abnormal breath sounds and their associated conditions.[2,5,11]

An *absent* or *diminished breath sound* indicates that there is little or no airflow to a particular portion of the lung (a small segment or an entire lung).[11] *Displaced bronchial breath sounds* are normal bronchial sounds heard in the peripheral lung fields instead of over the trachea. This condition is usually indicative of fluid or exudate in the alveoli.[11] *Adventitious breath sounds* are extra or added sounds heard in addition to the other sounds previously discussed. They are classified as crackles, rhonchi, wheezes, and friction rubs.

Crackles, also called *rales,* are short, discrete popping or crackling sounds produced by fluid in the small airways or alveoli or by the snapping open of collapsed airways during inspiration. They can be heard on inspiration and expiration

TABLE 22-3 Abnormal Breath Sounds and Their Associated Conditions

Abnormal Sound	Description	Condition
Absent breath sounds	No airflow to particular portion of lung	Pneumothorax Pneumonectomy Emphysematous blebs Pleural effusion Lung mass Massive atelectasis Complete airway obstruction
Diminished breath sounds	Little airflow to particular portion of lung	Emphysema Pleural effusion Pleurisy Atelectasis Pulmonary fibrosis
Displaced bronchial sounds	Bronchial sounds heard in peripheral lung fields	Atelectasis with secretions Lung mass with exudates Pneumonia Pleural effusion Pulmonary edema
Crackles (rales)	Short, discrete popping or crackling sounds	Pulmonary edema Pneumonia Pulmonary fibrosis Atelectasis Bronchiectasis
Rhonchi	Coarse, rumbling, low-pitched sounds	Pneumonia Asthma Bronchitis Bronchospasm
Wheezes	High-pitched, squeaking, whistling sounds	Asthma Bronchospasm
Pleural friction rub	Creaking, leathery, loud, dry, coarse sounds	Pleural effusion Pleurisy

and may clear with coughing.[2,5,11] Crackles can be further classified as fine, medium, or coarse, depending on pitch.[3,5]

Rhonchi are coarse, rumbling, low-pitched sounds produced by airflow over secretions in the larger airways or narrowing of the large airways. They are heard mainly on expiration and sometimes can be cleared with coughing. Rhonchi can be further classified as bubbling, gurgling, or sonorous, depending on the characteristics of the sound.[11]

Wheezes are high-pitched, squeaking, whistling sounds produced by airflow through narrowed small airways. They are heard mainly on expiration but may be heard throughout the ventilatory cycle. Depending on their severity, wheezes can be further classified as mild, moderate, or severe.[11]

A *pleural friction rub* is a creaking, leathery, loud, dry, coarse sound produced by irritated pleural surfaces rubbing together. It is usually heard best in the lower anterolateral chest area during inspiration and expiration. Pleural friction rubs are caused by inflammation of the pleura.[2,5]

Voice Sounds. Assessment of voice sounds is particularly useful in detecting lung consolidation or lung compression. Three abnormal types of voice sounds are bronchophony, whispering pectoriloquy, and egophony.

Bronchophony describes a condition in which the spoken voice is heard on auscultation with higher intensity and clarity than usual. Normally, the spoken word is muffled when heard through the stethoscope. It is assessed by placing the diaphragm of the stethoscope against the posterior side of the patient's chest and instructing the patient to say "ninety-nine." Bronchophony is present when the sound heard is clear, distinct, and loud.

Whispering pectoriloquy describes a condition of unusually clear transmission of the whispered voice on auscultation. Normally, the whispered word is unintelligible when heard through the stethoscope. It is assessed by placing the stethoscope against the posterior side of the patient's chest and instructing the patient to whisper "one, two, three." Whispering pectoriloquy is present when the sound heard is clear and distinct.

Egophony describes a condition in which the voice sounds increase in intensity and develop a nasal bleating quality on auscultation. It is assessed by placing the stethoscope against the posterior side of the patient's chest and instructing the patient to say "e-e-e." Egophony is present when the "e" sound changes to an "a" sound.[2,4,11]

ASSESSMENT FINDINGS OF COMMON DISORDERS

Table 22-4 presents a variety of common pulmonary disorders and their associated assessment findings.

TABLE 22-4 Assessment Findings Frequently Associated with Common Lung Conditions

Condition*	Breath Sounds	Description
NORMAL LUNG 	INSPIRATION > EXPIRATION Pitch: low Intensity: soft Adventitious sounds: none 	Tracheobronchial tree and alveoli are clear; pleurae are thin and close together; chest wall is mobile.
ASTHMA Bronchospasm	INSPIRATION = EXPIRATION Pitch: moderate Intensity: soft Adventitious sounds: expiratory sibilant wheezes 	Asthma is characterized by intermittent episodes of airway obstruction caused by bronchospasm, excessive bronchial secretion, or edema of bronchial mucosa; resultant airway resistance, especially during expiration, produces symptoms of wheezing, dyspnea, and chest tightness.
ATELECTASIS Collapsed portion of lung	INSPIRATION > EXPIRATION *Over empty area:* Pitch: low or absent Intensity: soft or absent Adventitious sounds: fine, high-pitched crackles over terminal portion of inspiration if bronchus patent *Over consolidated lung:* bronchial breath sounds, crackles, and wheezes 	Atelectasis is collapse of alveolar lung tissue, and findings reflect presence of a small, airless lung; this condition is caused by complete obstruction of a draining bronchus by a tumor, thick secretions, or an aspirated foreign body, or by compression of lung.

*Note: Although some disease conditions are bilateral, one diseased lung and one normal lung are illustrated for each condition to provide contrast. When an abnormality is illustrated, the pathologic condition is illustrated on the left side and the normal lung is on the right side of the illustration.
From Barkauskas V et al: *Health and physical assessment*, ed 3, St. Louis, 2002, Mosby.

Inspection	Palpation	Percussion	Auscultation
Good, symmetric rib and diaphragmatic movement Anteroposterior diameter < transverse diameter Respirations 12-20 breaths/min and regular	Trachea: midline Expansion: adequate, symmetric Tactile fremitus: moderate and symmetric No lesions or tenderness	Resonant Diaphragmatic excursion: 3-5 cm	Breath sounds: vesicular Vocal resonance: muffled Adventitious sounds: none, except for a few transient crackles at bases
Cyanosis Air trapping with audible wheezing Use of accessory muscles of respiration Increased respiratory rate	Tactile fremitus: decreased	Hyperresonant	Breath sounds: distant Vocal resonance: decreased Adventitious sounds: wheezes
Less chest motion on affected side Affected side retracted, with ribs appearing close together Cough Rapid, shallow breathing	Trachea: shifted to affected side Expansion: decreased on affected side Tactile fremitus: decreased or absent	Dull to flat over collapsed lung Hyperresonant over remainder of affected hemithorax	Breath sounds: decreased or absent Vocal resonance: varies in intensity, usually reduced or absent in affected area Adventitious sounds: fine, high-pitched crackles may be heard over terminal portion of inspiration

Continued

TABLE 22-4 Assessment Findings Frequently Associated with Common Lung Conditions—*cont'd*

Condition	Breath Sounds	Description
BRONCHIECTASIS 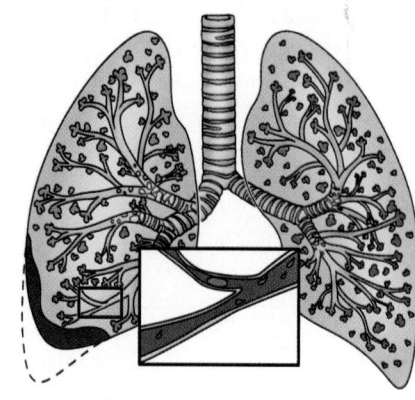	INSPIRATION > EXPIRATION Pitch: low Intensity: soft Adventitious sounds: crackles (sometimes disappear after 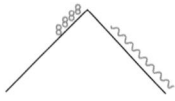	Bronchiectasis is abnormal dilation of bronchi or bronchioles, or both (coughing).
BRONCHITIS, ACUTE 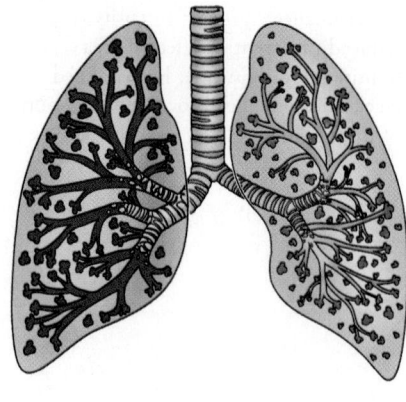	INSPIRATION ≥ EXPIRATION Pitch: low Intensity: soft Adventitious sounds: localized crackles, expiratory sibilant wheezes 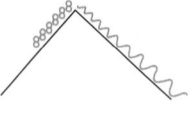	Acute bronchitis is inflammation of bronchial tree characterized by partial bronchial obstruction and secretions or constrictions; it results in abnormally deflated portions of lung.
EMPHYSEMA	INSPIRATION = EXPIRATION Pitch: low to very low Intensity: soft to very soft Adventitious sounds: occasional rhonchi and/or sibilant wheezes; fine inspiratory crackles	Emphysema is a permanent hyperinflation of lung beyond terminal bronchioles, with destruction of alveolar walls; airway resistance is increased, especially on expiration.

Inspection	Palpation	Percussion	Auscultation
If mild, respirations are normal If severe, tachypnea Less expansion of affected side Cough with purulent sputum	Trachea: midline or deviated toward affected side Expansion: decreased on affected side Tactile fremitus: increased	Resonant or dull	Breath sounds: usually vesicular Vocal resonance: usually muffled Adventitious sounds: crackles
If severe, tachypnea and cyanosis Rasping cough with mucoid sputum	Tactile fremitus: normal to increased	Resonant	Breath sounds: vesicular Vocal resonance: moderate Adventitious sounds: localized crackles, sibilant wheezes
Dyspnea with exertion Barrel chest Tachypnea Use of accessory muscles of respiration	Expansion: limited Tactile fremitus: decreased	Resonant to hyperresonant Diaphragmatic excursion: decreased	Breath sounds: decreased intensity; often prolonged expiration Vocal resonance: muffled or decreased Adventitious sounds: occasional wheezes; often fine crackles in late inspiration

Continued

TABLE 22-4　Assessment Findings Frequently Associated with Common Lung Conditions—*cont'd*

Condition	Breath Sounds	Description
PLEURAL EFFUSION AND THICKENING 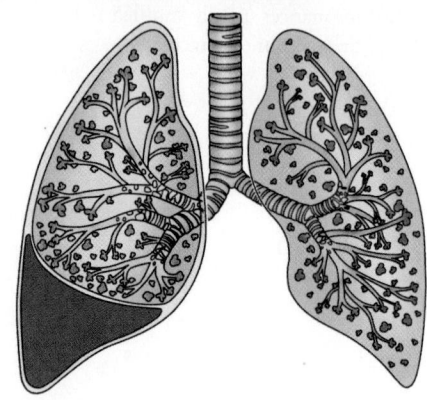	INSPIRATION > EXPIRATION Pitch: low to absent Intensity: soft to absent Adventitious sounds: occasional pleural friction rub 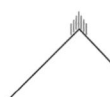	Pleural effusion is a collection of fluid in pleural space; if pleural effusion is prolonged, fibrous tissue may also accumulate in pleural space; clinical picture depends on amount of fluid or fibrosis present and rapidity of development; fluid tends to gravitate to most dependent areas of thorax, and adjacent lung is compressed.
PNEUMONIA WITH CONSOLIDATION 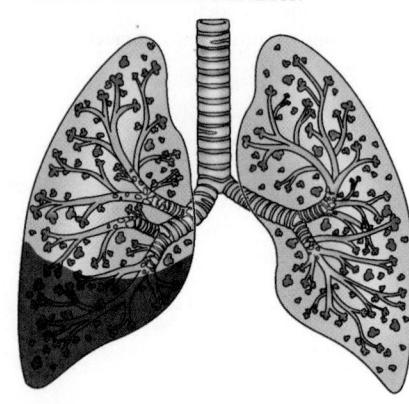	INSPIRATION = EXPIRATION Pitch: high Intensity: loud Adventitious sounds: inspiratory crackles in terminal third of inspiration 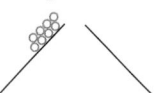	Pneumonia with consolidation occurs when alveolar air is replaced by fluid or tissue; physical findings depend on amount of parenchymal tissue involved.
PNEUMOTHORAX 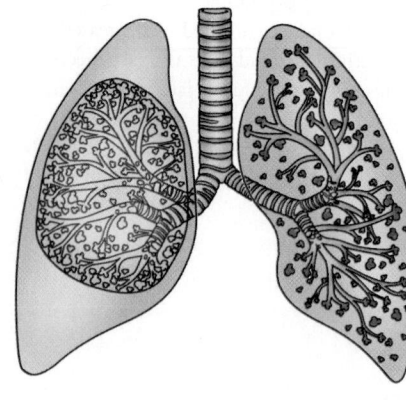	INSPIRATION > EXPIRATION Pitch: low to absent Intensity: soft to absent Adventitious sounds: none 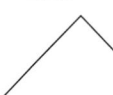	Pneumothorax implies air in pleural space: 1. Closed type: air in pleural space does not communicate with air in lung 2. Open type: air in pleural space freely communicates with air in lung; air in pleural space is atmospheric 3. Tension type: air in pleural space communicates with air in lungs only on inspiration; air pressure in pleural space is greater than atmospheric pressure Physical signs depend on degree of lung collapse and presence or absence of pleural effusion.

Inspection	Palpation	Percussion	Auscultation
Tachypnea Decreased in definition of intercostals spaces on affected side Dyspnea	Trachea: deviation toward normal side Expansion: decreased on affected side Tactile fremitus: decreased or absent	Dull to flat No diaphragmatic excursion on affected side	Breath sounds: decreased or absent Vocal resonance: muffled or absent; if fluid compresses lung, sounds may be bronchial over compression, and bronchophony, egophony, and whisper pectoriloquy may be present Adventitious sounds: pleural friction rub sometimes present
Tachypnea Guarding and less motion on affected side	Expansion: limited on affected side Tactile fremitus: usually increased, but may be weak if a bronchus leading to affected area is plugged	Dull to flat	Breath sounds: increased in intensity; bronchovesicular or bronchial breath sounds over affected area Vocal resonance: increased bronchophony, egophony, whisper pectoriloquy present Adventitious sounds: inspiratory crackles terminal third of inspiration
Restricted lung expansion on affected side If large, tachypnea Bulging in intercostal spaces on affected side Cyanosis	Trachea: deviated toward normal side Expansion: decreased on affected side Tactile fremitus: absent	Hyperresonant Decreased diaphragmatic excursion	Breath sounds: usually decreased or absent; if open pneumothorax, have an amorphous quality Vocal resonance: decreased or absent Adventitious sounds: none

Continued

TABLE 22-4 Assessment Findings Frequently Associated with Common Lung Conditions—*cont'd*

Condition	Breath Sounds	Description
PULMONARY FIBROSIS, DIFFUSE	INSPIRATION = EXPIRATION Pitch: low to absent Intensity: soft to absent Adventitious sounds: crackles	Pulmonary fibrosis is presence of excessive amount of connective tissue in lungs; consequently, lungs are smaller than normal and less compliant, lower lobes are usually affected most.

Inspection	Palpation	Percussion	Auscultation
Dyspnea on exertion Tachypnea Thoracic expansion diminished Cyanosis	Trachea: deviated to most affected side	Resonant to dull	Breath sounds: reduced or absent, bronchovesicular or bronchial Vocal resonance: increased, whisper pectoriloquy may be present Adventitious sounds: crackles on inspiration

Summary

History

- A review of the patient's current illness and symptoms, including presence or absence of shortness of breath, chest pain, and cough, is an essential part of the patient's medical history.
- As the patient's condition permits, additional information regarding his or her general respiratory status, general health status, and family and social background, including tobacco use, work environment, and home environment, should be obtained.

Clinical Assessment

- Inspection should focus on the tongue and sublingual area, chest wall configuration, and respiratory effort.

- Palpation should focus on position of the trachea, thoracic expansion, and fremitus (normal, decreased, or increased).
- Percussion (when performed) should focus on underlying lung structure and diaphragmatic excursion.
- Auscultation should focus on the presence or absence of normal breath sounds (vesicular, bronchovesicular, and bronchial), abnormal breath sounds (diminished or absent breath sounds, displaced bronchial breath sounds, and adventitious breath sounds), and voice sounds (bronchophony, whispering pectoriloquy, and egophony).
- Adventitious breath sounds are classified as crackles, rhonchi, wheezes, and friction rubs.
- Auscultation is done in a systematic fashion, side-to-side, top-to-bottom, posteriorly, laterally, and anteriorly.

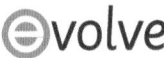 Be sure to check out the bonus material, including free self-assessment exercises, on the Evolve web site at http://evolve.elsevier.com/Urden/.

References

1. Baid H: The process of conducting a physical assessment: a nursing perspective, *Br J Nurs* 15:710, 2006.
2. Simpson H: Respiratory assessment, *Br J Nurs* 15:484, 2006.
3. Brenner M, Welliver J: Pulmonary and acid-base assessment, *Nurs Clin North Am* 25:761, 1990.
4. Finesilver C: Pulmonary assessment: what you need to know, *Prog Cardiovasc Nurs* 18:83, 2003.
5. Wilkins RL: Bedside assessment of the patient. In Wilkins RL et al, editors: *Egan's fundamentals of respiratory care*, ed 9, St Louis, 2008, Mosby.
6. Stiesmeyer JK: A four-step approach to pulmonary assessment, *Am J Nurs* 93(8):22, 1993.
7. Fitzgerald MA: The physical exam, *RN* 54(11):34, 1991.
8. DeWolfe CC: Apparent life-threatening event: a review, *Pediatr Clin North Am* 52:1127, 2005.
9. Barkauskas V et al: *Health and physical assessment*, ed 3, St Louis, 2002, Mosby.
10. Seidel HM et al: *Mosby's guide to physical examination*, ed 6, St Louis, 2006, Mosby.
11. Wilkins RL et al: *Fundamentals of lung and heart sounds*, ed 3, St Louis, 2004, Mosby.

Pulmonary Diagnostic Procedures

To complete the assessment of the critically ill pulmonary patient, a review of the patient's laboratory studies and diagnostic tests is performed. Although many procedures exist for diagnosing pulmonary disease, their application in the critically ill patient is limited. Only studies and tests that are used in the critical care setting are presented here. Bedside monitoring devices are also discussed.

LABORATORY STUDIES

ARTERIAL BLOOD GASES

Interpretation of arterial blood gas (ABG) levels can be difficult, especially if the nurse is under pressure to do it quickly and accurately. One method that can help ensure accuracy when analyzing ABG levels is to follow the same steps of interpretation each time. A specific method to be used each time that blood gas values must be interpreted is presented here (Box 23-1).

Step 1. Look at the PaO_2 level, and answer this question: Does the PaO_2 show hypoxemia? The PaO_2 is a measure of the partial pressure (P) of oxygen dissolved in arterial (a) blood plasma. Sometimes, PaO_2 is shortened to PO_2. It is reported in millimeters of mercury (mm Hg). PaO_2 reflects 3% of total oxygen in the blood.[1]

The normal range of PaO_2 values for persons breathing room air at sea level is 80 to 100 mm Hg. However, the normal range is age dependent for infants and for persons 60 years old or older. The normal level for infants breathing room air is between 50 and 70 mm Hg.[2] The normal level for persons 60 years old or older decreases with age as changes occur in the ventilation/perfusion $(\dot{V}/\dot{Q})$ matching in the aging lung.[3] The correct PaO_2 for older persons can be ascertained as follows: 80 mm Hg (the lowest normal value) minus 1 mm Hg for every year of age above 60 years. Using this formula, a 65-year-old individual can have a PaO_2 as low as 75 mm Hg (80 mm Hg − 5 mm Hg = 75 mm Hg) and still be within the normal range. An acceptable range for an 80-year-old person (20 years older than 60 years) is 60 mm Hg (80 mm Hg − 20 mm Hg = 60 mm Hg).

At any age, a PaO_2 lower than 40 mm Hg represents a life-threatening situation that necessitates immediate action.[4] A PaO_2 value less than the predicted lowest value indicates hypoxemia, which means that a lower-than-normal amount of oxygen is dissolved in plasma.[1]

The PaO_2 level should be analyzed before those of other blood gas components. A PaO_2 of less than 40 mm Hg severely compromises tissue oxygenation and calls for the immediate administration of supplemental oxygen or mechanical ventilation, or both. The test results for the PaO_2 level can be quickly analyzed. If the PaO_2 level is more than the lowest value for the patient's age, it is normal.

Step 2. Look at the pH level, and answer this question: Is the pH on the acid or alkaline side of 7.40? The pH is the hydrogen ion (H^+) concentration of plasma. Calculation of pH is accomplished by using the partial pressure of carbon dioxide $(PaCO_2)$ and the plasma bicarbonate level (HCO_3^-). The formula used is the Henderson-Hasselbalch equation (see Appendix B).[1]

The normal pH of arterial blood is 7.35 to 7.45, and the mean is 7.40. If the pH level is less than 7.40, it is on the acid side of the mean. A pH level less than 7.35 is known as *acidemia*, and the overall condition is called *acidosis*. If the pH level is greater than 7.40, it is on the alkaline side of the mean. A pH level greater than 7.45 is known as *alkalemia*, and the overall condition is called *alkalosis*.[1,5]

Step 3. Look at the $PaCO_2$ level, and answer this question: Does the $PaCO_2$ show respiratory acidosis, alkalosis, or normalcy? The $PaCO_2$ is a measure of the partial pressure of carbon dioxide dissolved in arterial blood plasma, and it is reported in millimeters of mercury (mm Hg). It is the acid-base component that reflects the effectiveness of ventilation in relation to the metabolic rate.[1] In other words, the $PaCO_2$ value indicates whether the patient can ventilate well enough to rid the body of the carbon dioxide produced as a consequence of metabolism.

The normal range for $PaCO_2$ is 35 to 45 mm Hg. This range does not change as a person ages. A $PaCO_2$ value greater than 45 mm Hg defines *respiratory acidosis*, which is caused by alveolar hypoventilation. Hypoventilation can result from chronic obstructive pulmonary disease (COPD), oversedation, head trauma, anesthesia, drug overdose, neuromuscular disease, or hypoventilation with mechanical ventilation.[1]

Ventilatory failure results when the $PaCO_2$ level exceeds 50 mm Hg. Acute ventilatory failure occurs when the $PaCO_2$ level is greater than 50 mm Hg and the pH level is less than 7.30.

BOX 23-1   STEPS FOR INTERPRETATION OF BLOOD GAS LEVELS

STEP 1
Look at the Pa_{O_2} level, and answer this question: Does the Pa_{O_2} level show hypoxemia?

STEP 2
Look at the pH level, and answer this question: Is the pH level on the acid or alkaline side of 7.40?

STEP 3
Look at the Pa_{CO_2} level, and answer this question: Does the Pa_{CO_2} level show respiratory acidosis, alkalosis, or normalcy?

STEP 4
Look at the HCO_3^- level, and answer this question: Does the HCO_3^- level show metabolic acidosis, alkalosis, or normalcy?

STEP 5
Look again at the pH level, and answer this question: Does the pH show a compensated or an uncompensated condition?

BOX 23-2   UNCOMPENSATED ARTERIAL BLOOD GAS VALUES

EXAMPLE 1
Pa_{O_2}:   90 mm Hg
pH: 7.25
Pa_{CO_2}:   50 mm Hg
HCO_3^-:   22 mEq/L
Interpretation: Uncompensated respiratory acidosis

EXAMPLE 2
Pa_{O_2}:   90 mm Hg
pH: 7.25
Pa_{CO_2}:   40 mm Hg
HCO_3^-:   17 mEq/L
Interpretation: Uncompensated metabolic acidosis

BOX 23-3   COMPENSATED ARTERIAL BLOOD GAS VALUES

EXAMPLE 1
Pa_{O_2}:   90 mm Hg
pH: 7.37
Pa_{CO_2}:   60 mm Hg
HCO_3^-:   38 mEq/L
Interpretation: Compensated respiratory acidosis with metabolic alkalosis. (The acidosis is considered the main disorder and the alkalosis the compensatory response, because the pH is on the acid side of 7.40.)

EXAMPLE 2
Pa_{O_2}:   90 mm Hg
pH: 7.42
Pa_{CO_2}:   48 mm Hg
HCO_3^-:   35 mEq/L
Interpretation: Compensated metabolic alkalosis with respiratory acidosis. (The alkalosis is considered the main disorder and the acidosis the compensatory response, because the pH is on the alkaline side of 7.40.)

It is referred to as *acute* because the pH is abnormal, not allowing enough time for the body to compensate by returning the pH to the normal range. Chronic ventilatory failure is defined as a Pa_{CO_2} value greater than 50 mm Hg and a pH level greater than 7.30.[1,6]

A Pa_{CO_2} value that is less than 35 mm Hg defines *respiratory alkalosis*, which is caused by alveolar hyperventilation. Hyperventilation can result from hypoxia, anxiety, pulmonary embolism, pregnancy, and hyperventilation with mechanical ventilation or as a compensatory mechanism for metabolic acidosis.[1]

Step 4. Look at the HCO_3 level, and answer this question: Does the HCO_3^- show metabolic acidosis, alkalosis, or normalcy? Bicarbonate (HCO_3^-) is the acid-base component that reflects kidney function. The bicarbonate level is reduced or increased in the plasma by renal mechanisms. The normal range is 22 to 26 mEq/L.[1,5,7]

A bicarbonate level of less than 22 mEq/L defines *metabolic acidosis*, which can result from ketoacidosis, lactic acidosis, renal failure, or diarrhea. The cumulative effect is a gain of acids or a loss of base. A bicarbonate level that is greater than 26 mEq/L defines *metabolic alkalosis*, which can result from fluid loss from the upper gastrointestinal tract (vomiting or nasogastric suction), diuretic therapy, severe hypokalemia, alkali administration, or steroid therapy.[1,5,7]

Step 5. Look again at the pH level, and answer this question: Does the pH show a compensated or an uncompensated condition? If the pH level is abnormal (less than 7.35 or greater than 7.45), the Pa_{CO_2} value or the HCO_3^- level, or both, will also be abnormal. This is an *uncompensated* condition because the body has not had enough time to return the pH to its normal range.[1,8] Box 23-2 provides two examples of uncompensated

ABGs. If the pH level is within normal limits and the Pa_{CO_2} value and the HCO_3^- level are abnormal, the condition is *compensated* because the body has had enough time to restore the pH to within its normal range.[1,7]

Differentiating the primary disorder from the compensatory response can be difficult. The primary disorder is the abnormality that caused the pH level to shift initially. It is determined according to the pH level; the primary disorder is considered to be the one on whichever side of 7.40 the pH level occurs.[1,8] Box 23-3 provides two examples of compensated ABGs. Partial compensation may be present and is evidenced by abnormal pH, Pa_{CO_2}, and HCO_3^- levels, indications that the body is attempting to return the pH to its normal range.[1,8]

Table 23-1 summarizes the changes in the acid-base components that accompany various acid-base disorders.[1,2] In addition to the parameters previously discussed, other factors must be considered when reviewing a patient's ABGs, including oxygen saturation, oxygen content, base excess and deficit, and anion gap analysis. Table 23-2 summarizes conditions that may potentiate acid-base abnormalities.[1]

Oxygen Saturation. Oxygen saturation is a measure of the amount of oxygen bound to hemoglobin, compared with hemoglobin's maximal capability for binding oxygen. It can be assessed as a component of the ABG (Sa_{O_2}) or can be measured noninvasively using a pulse oximeter (Sp_{O_2}).[7,9] Oxygen

TABLE 23-1 Arterial Blood Gas Assessment

Disorder	pH	Paco₂	HCO₃
Respiratory acidosis			
Uncompensated	<7.35	>45 mm Hg	22-26 mEq/L
Partially compensated	<7.35	>45 mm Hg	>26 mEq/L
Compensated	7.35-7.39	>45 mm Hg	>26 mEq/L
Respiratory alkalosis			
Uncompensated	>7.45	<35 mm Hg	22-26 mEq/L
Partially compensated	>7.45	<35 mm Hg	<22 mEq/L
Compensated	7.41-7.45	<35 mm Hg	<22 mEq/L
Metabolic acidosis			
Uncompensated	<7.35	35-45 mm Hg	<22 mEq/L
Partially compensated	<7.35	<35 mm Hg	<22 mEq/L
Compensated	7.35-7.39	<35 mm Hg	<22 mEq/L
Metabolic alkalosis			
Uncompensated	>7.45	35-45 mm Hg	>26 mEq/L
Partially compensated	>7.45	>45 mm Hg	>26 mEq/L
Compensated	7.41-7.45	>45 mm Hg	>26 mEq/L
Combined (or mixed) respiratory and metabolic acidosis	<7.35	>45 mm Hg	<22 mEq/L
Combined (or mixed) respiratory and metabolic alkalosis	>7.45	<35 mm Hg	>26 mEq/L

TABLE 23-2 Causes of Acid-Base Disorders

Disorders	Potential Cause

Respiratory acidosis	Chronic obstructive pulmonary disease
	Acute airway obstruction
	Central nervous system depression
	  Sedatives
	  Anesthetics
	  Narcotics
	Trauma
	  Spinal cord
	  Brain
	  Chest wall
	Neuromuscular disease
	  Poliomyelitis
	  Myasthenia gravis
	  Guillain-Barré syndrome
	Hypoventilation with mechanical ventilation

Respiratory alkalosis	Hypoxia Anxiety Fear Pain Stimulants Pulmonary embolism Hyperventilation with mechanical ventilation

Metabolic acidosis	High anion gap:
	  Lactic acidosis
	  Ketoacidosis
	  Renal failure (uremia)
	  Rhabdomyolysis
	  Ingestion of acids (methanol, salicylates, ethylene glycol)
	Nonanion gap:
	  Diarrhea
	  Renal tubular acidosis
	  Ureterosigmoidoscopy
	  Ileostomy
	  Pancreatic fistula

Metabolic alkalosis	Steroid therapy Vomiting Gastrointestinal suction Diuretic therapy Hypokalemia Hypovolemia Hypochloremia Sodium bicarbonate intake

saturation is reported as a percentage or as a decimal; normal values are greater than 95% when the patient is on room air. Normally, the saturation level cannot reach 100% (on room air) because of physiologic shunting.[1] However, when supplemental oxygen is administered, oxygen saturation may approach 100% so closely that it is reported as 100%.

Proper evaluation of the oxygen saturation level is vital. For example, an SaO_2 of 97% means that 97% of the available hemoglobin is bound with oxygen. The word *available* is essential to evaluating the SaO_2 level, because the hemoglobin level is not always within normal limits and oxygen can bind only with what is available. A 97% saturation level associated with 10 g/dL of hemoglobin does not deliver as much oxygen to the tissues as does a 97% saturation level associated with 15 g/dL of hemoglobin. Assessing only the SaO_2 level and finding it within normal limits does not ensure that the patient's oxygenation status is normal. The hemoglobin level must also be evaluated before a decision on oxygenation status can be made.[1,7]

Oxygen Content. Oxygen content (CaO_2) is a measure of the total amount of oxygen carried in the blood, including the amount dissolved in plasma (measured by the PaO_2) and the amount bound to the hemoglobin molecule (measured by the SaO_2). CaO_2 is reported in milliliters of oxygen carried per 100 mL of blood. The normal value is 20 mL of oxygen

TABLE 23-3 Assessing Oxygenation Status

Patient	PaO_2 Level (mm Hg)	SaO_2 Level (%)	Hgb (g/dL)	CaO_2 (mL/dL)
A	100	97	15	19.8
B	100	97	10	13.3

CaO_2, arterial oxygen content; Hgb, hemoglobin; PaO_2, arterial partial pressure of oxygen; SaO_2, arterial oxygen saturation.

BOX 23-4 ANION GAP

Formula: Concentrations (in square brackets) of extracellular fluid cations (sodium) minus extracellular fluid anions (chloride plus measured bicarbonate), or

$$[Na^+] - [Cl^-] + [HCO_3^-] = 8 \text{ to } 16 \text{ mEq/L (normal range)}$$

EXAMPLE

$$[Na^+] = 145; \ [Cl^-] = 105; \ [HCO_3^-] = 15$$

$$145 - (105 + 15) = 145 - 120 = 25 \text{ mEq/L}$$

Interpretation: High anion gap metabolic acidosis

per 100 mL of blood. To calculate the oxygen content, the PaO_2, the SaO_2, and the hemoglobin level are used (see Appendix B). A change in any one of these parameters will affect the CaO_2.[1,7]

The value of assessing the CaO_2 is best illustrated by the examples in Table 23-3. The ABG parameters that are used most commonly to evaluate oxygenation status (PaO_2 and SaO_2) are both normal. Assessing only the PaO_2 and the SaO_2 would lead to the invalid conclusion that Patient B's oxygenation status is normal. However, consideration of the hemoglobin level and the CaO_2 reveals that the oxygenation of Patient B's blood is significantly abnormal.

Base Excess and Base Deficit. Base excess and base deficit reflect the nonrespiratory contribution to acid-base balance and are reported in milliequivalents per liter (mEq/L) above or below the normal range of -2 mEq/L to $+2$ mEq/L. A negative base level is reported as a *base deficit*, which correlates with *metabolic acidosis*, whereas a positive base level is reported as a *base excess*, which correlates with *metabolic alkalosis*.[1]

Anion Gap. Calculation of the anion gap can give a more complete analysis of metabolic disturbances that occur in the critically ill patient. The anion gap is computed by subtracting the major plasma anions (chloride and bicarbonate) from the major plasma cation (sodium) (Box 23-4).[1,7] The remainder is made up of minor plasma anions such as organic ions, phosphates, and negatively charged proteins. The normal anion gap is 8 to 16 mEq/L.[4] Any process that significantly increases the minor plasma anions creates a *high anion gap metabolic acidosis*. Elevation of the anion gap is seen with processes such as

diabetic or alcoholic ketoacidosis, lactic acidosis, renal failure, and uremia and with toxins such as salicylates and methanol.[1,7] A *non-anion gap metabolic acidosis* can occur through the loss of bicarbonate and the retention of the chloride ion (hyperchloremic metabolic acidosis).[4,9] Clinically a non-anion gap acidosis is associated with diarrhea, renal failure, hyperalimentation, and ureterosigmoidoscopy.[1,7] Calculation of the anion gap therefore helps to simplify and determine the cause of metabolic acidosis.

CLASSIC SHUNT EQUATION AND OXYGEN TENSION INDICES

The efficiency of oxygenation can be assessed by measuring the degree of intrapulmonary shunting that occurs in a patient at any one time, using the classic shunt equation and oxygen tension indices. *Intrapulmonary shunting* (QS/QT [the portion of cardiac output not exchanging with alveolar blood divided by the total cardiac output]) refers to venous blood that flows to the lungs without being oxygenated because of nonfunctioning alveoli.[1] Other names for this condition include shunt effect, low $\dot{V}/\dot{Q}$, wasted blood flow, and venous admixture.[5]

Direct determination of intrapulmonary shunting requires the use of the classic shunt equation (see Appendix B), which is invasive and cumbersome. A shunt greater than 10% is considered abnormal and indicative of a shunt-producing disorder. A shunt greater than 30% is a serious and potentially life-threatening condition, which requires pulmonary intervention.[1]

Often, intrapulmonary shunting is estimated by using the oxygen tension indices. One advantage to these methods is the ease of performance, although they have been found to be unreliable in critically ill patients.[1,5] An estimate of intrapulmonary shunting can be determined by computing the difference between the alveolar and arterial oxygen concentrations. Normally, alveolar (A) and arterial (a) PO_2 values are approximately equal. When they are not, it indicates that venous blood is passing malfunctioning alveoli and returning unoxygenated to the left side of the heart.[1,5] The most common oxygen tension indices used to estimate intrapulmonary shunting are the PaO_2/FIO_2 ratio, the PaO_2/PAO_2 ratio, and the A-a gradient ($P[A - a]O_2$).

PaO_2/FIO_2 Ratio. The PaO_2/FIO_2 ratio is clinically the easiest formula to calculate because it does not call for the computation of the alveolar PO_2. Normally, the PaO_2/FIO_2 ratio is greater than 286; the lower the value, the worse the lung function.[1,10,11]

PaO_2/PAO_2 Ratio. The PaO_2/PAO_2 ratio (arterial/alveolar O_2 ratio) is normally greater than 60%. The disadvantage to using this formula is that it calls for the computation of the alveolar PO_2 (see Appendix B), but the advantage is that it is unaffected by changes in the FIO_2, as long as the underlying lung condition is stable.[1]

Alveolar-Arterial Gradient. The A-a gradient ($P[A-a]O_2$) is normally less than 20 mm Hg on room air for patients younger than 61 years. This estimate of intrapulmonary shunting is the least reliable clinically, but it is used often in clinical decision making. One of the major disadvantages to using this formula

TABLE 23-4   Calculation of Intrapulmonary Shunting

FIO₂	PaO₂ Level (mm Hg)	PAO₂ Level (mm Hg)	PaO₂/FIO₂	a/A Ratio (%)	A − a Gradient (mm Hg)
0.21	40	97	190	41	57
0.50	80	300	160	27	220
1.0	150	610	150	25	460

Modified from Murray JF, Nadel JA: *Textbook of respiratory medicine*, Philadelphia, 1988, WB Saunders.

A, alveolar; a, arterial; FIO₂, fraction of inspired oxygen; PaO₂, arterial partial pressure of oxygen.

is that it is greatly influenced by the amount of oxygen the patient is receiving.[1]

Serial determinations of the estimates of intrapulmonary shunting provide the practitioner with objective data on which to base clinical decisions.[12] Table 23-4 shows the change in intrapulmonary shunting in the hypoxemic patient using the previously described oxygen tension indices to estimate severity of shunting.

DEAD SPACE EQUATION

The efficiency of ventilation can be measured using the clinical dead space (VD/VT) equation (see Appendix B). The formula measures the fraction of tidal volume not participating in gas exchange. A dead space value greater than 0.6 indicates a dead space-producing disorder and is considered abnormal. The major limitations to using this formula are that it requires the measurement of exhaled carbon dioxide to complete and that the work of breathing by patients must remain stable during the collection.[1]

SPUTUM STUDIES

Careful analysis of sputum specimens is crucial for the rapid identification and treatment of pulmonary infections. The most difficult aspect of sputum examination is proper collection of the specimen. Collection of a good sputum sample requires a conscious, cooperative, and sufficiently hydrated patient.[13] When the patient has difficulty producing sputum, heated, nebulized saline may help to loosen secretions for expectoration.[13] Chest physiotherapy combined with nebulization improves the success rate. Collection of a sputum specimen is best done in the morning, because a greater volume of secretions is present as a result of nighttime pooling. Brushing the teeth and rinsing the oropharyngeal airway is recommended to reduce contamination before collecting a sample.[1]

Many critically ill patients cannot cough effectively, and sputum collection by other means is required. These methods include tracheobronchial aspiration, transtracheal aspiration, and the use of a fiberoptic bronchoscopy with a protected brush catheter. Because each method has its own benefits and risks,

BOX 23-5   PROCEDURE FOR COLLECTION OF TRACHEAL OR ENDOTRACHEAL SPUTUM SPECIMEN

1. Clear the endotracheal or tracheostomy tube of all local secretions, avoiding deep airway penetration.
2. Attach a sputum trap to a sterile suction catheter, and advance the catheter into the trachea while trying to avoid contact with the endotracheal tube or tracheostomy tube (Fig. 23-1).
3. After the catheter is fully advanced, apply suction until secretions return to the sputum trap. When enough secretions are collected, discontinue suctioning, and remove the catheter.
4. Do not apply suction while the catheter is being withdrawn, because this can contaminate the sample with sputum from the upper airway. Do not flush the catheter with sterile water, because this dilutes the sample.
5. If the catheter becomes plugged with secretions, place it in a sterile container, and send it to the laboratory. The specimen must be transported immediately or refrigerated if a delay is necessary.

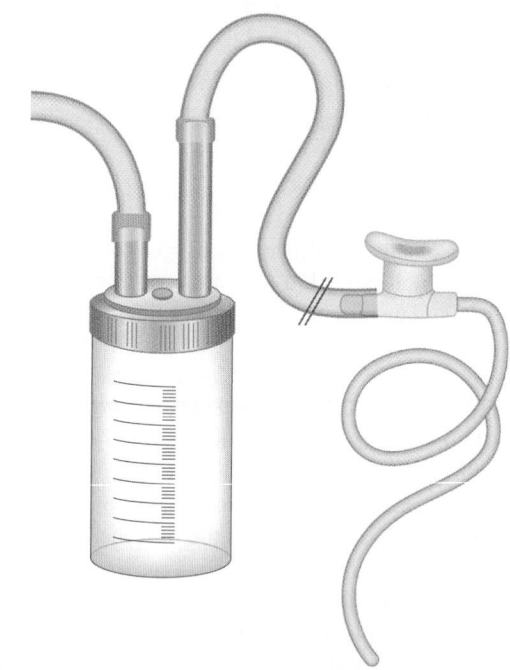

Figure 23-1 Specimen container. *(From In Wilkins RL et al, editors: Egan's fundamentals of respiratory care, ed 9, St Louis, 2008, Mosby.)*

the patient's clinical condition determines the appropriate technique.[9]

Many critically ill patients have endotracheal or tracheostomy tubes already in place. Collecting sputum specimens from these patients requires special attention to technique (Box 23-5). Deep specimens are obtained to avoid collecting specimens that contain resident upper airway flora that may have migrated down the tube. Colonization of the lower airways with upper airway flora can occur within 48 hours of intubation.[9]

After a sputum specimen is obtained, it is examined for volume, physical properties, mucopurulence, and color. Next, a microscopic examination is done to identify the source of the specimen. If a bacterial infection is suspected, a Gram stain is performed, followed by culture and sensitivity (C&S) assessments.[9]

DIAGNOSTIC PROCEDURES

BRONCHOSCOPY

Fiberoptic bronchoscopy is a relatively safe procedure done at the bedside, and it is most often used as a diagnostic and therapeutic tool. Diagnostic indications include hemoptysis, infectious pneumonia, difficult intubation, pulmonary injury after chest trauma, acute burn inhalation injury, aspiration lung injuries, and acute upper airway obstruction. Therapeutic indications include the aspiration of foreign bodies, removal of obstructing secretions, atelectasis, difficult intubation, and resection of small, benign growths from the airway.[9]

Before the bronchoscopy, a complete medical history is obtained, and a thorough examination, including a chest x-ray examination, is performed.[9] Preprocedural evaluation of the patient includes clotting studies (prothrombin time [PT], partial thromboplastin time [PTT], and platelet count) and evaluation of the ABG levels.[9] Hypoxemic patients need supplemental oxygen during the procedure. The patient must have no oral intake for 6 to 8 hours before the bronchoscopy to reduce the risk of aspiration.[9]

Although a topical anesthetic can be used alone, it is usually supplemented by an intravenous sedative or analgesic, or both. A benzodiazepine for sedative effects and a opioid analgesic are administered intravenously during the procedure.[9] Preprocedural medications for a diagnostic bronchoscopy may include atropine and intramuscular codeine. Atropine lessens the vasovagal response and reduces the secretions, whereas codeine decreases the cough reflex. When bronchoscopy is performed therapeutically to remove secretions, the patient has decreased cough and gag reflexes, which may impair secretion clearance.[9] Maintenance of the airway is essential to prevent complications.

Complications of the procedure may be related to the procedure itself, the anesthetic, or an ancillary procedure. Minor complications include laryngospasm, bronchospasm, epistaxis, fever, vomiting, altered pulmonary mechanics, and hemodynamic instability. Major complications include anaphylaxis, infection, hypotension, cardiac dysrhythmias, pneumothorax, hemorrhage, respiratory failure, hypoxemia, and cardiopulmonary arrest.[9]

THORACENTESIS

Thoracentesis is a simple, usually uncomplicated procedure done at the bedside for the removal of fluid or air from the pleural space. It is used most often as a diagnostic measure; it may also be performed therapeutically for the drainage of a pleural effusion or empyema.[9] No absolute contraindications to thoracentesis exist, although there are some risks that may contraindicate the procedure in all but emergency situations. These risk factors include unstable hemodynamics, coagulation defects, mechanical ventilation, the presence of an intraaortic balloon pump, and patients who are uncooperative. In most clinical situations, diagnostic thoracentesis can be delayed until these risk factors are eliminated.[9]

The patient is placed in a sitting position with legs over the side of the bed and with hands and arms supported on a padded overbed table. If the patient's condition precludes sitting, the side-lying position with the back flush with the edge of the bed and the affected side down can be used.[1] The patient is cautioned not to move or cough during the procedure.[9] During the thoracentesis, the site of the needle insertion is usually determined by previous chest x-ray examination, computed tomography (CT) scan, or chest percussion. A local anesthetic is used to minimize the patient's discomfort during insertion of the thoracentesis needle.[9]

Complications associated with thoracentesis include pain, pneumothorax, and reexpansion pulmonary edema. Pneumothorax can occur as a result of introduction of air into the pleural space, puncture of the lung, or rupture of the visceral pleura.[9] Reexpansion pulmonary edema can occur when a large amount of effusion fluid (approximately 1000 to 1500 mL) is removed from the pleural space. Removal of the fluid increases the negative intrapleural pressure, which can lead to edema when the lung does not reexpand to fill the space. The patient experiences severe coughing and shortness of breath. The onset of these symptoms is an indication to discontinue the thoracentesis.[9]

BEDSIDE PULMONARY FUNCTION TESTS

Pulmonary function tests (PFTs) are designed to quantify respiratory function and are an essential component of a thorough pulmonary evaluation. PFTs are used for a variety of purposes, including preoperative assessment, evaluating lung mechanics, diagnosing and tracking pulmonary diseases, and monitoring therapy. Results are individualized according to age, gender, and body size.[1]

A complete PFT consists of four components: lung volumes, mechanics of breathing, diffusion, and ABGs. PFTs may take as long as 2 hours to complete. Because of the severity of illness encountered in the critical care area, all four components are rarely completed. Most often, measurements of pulmonary function in the critically ill are limited to areas that give the practitioner information about the patient's need for or ability to wean from mechanical ventilation. This section covers the areas tested most often at the bedside of critically ill individuals.

Measurement of lung volumes and capacities (Box 23-6) provides valuable information about the origin of a disease process. Four lung volumes and four lung capacities can be measured. Measurement of volumes at the bedside is limited to tidal volume and vital capacity. A vital capacity of 10 to 15 mL/kg usually is a minimally accepted value for weaning, with a respiratory rate of less than 24 breaths/min.[1,7,14]

Assessment of the mechanics of breathing includes measurement of the flow of gas, lung and chest compliance, respiratory muscle strength, and tissue resistance. In the critical care area, dynamic and static compliance are measured at the bedside.

BOX 23-6 LUNG VOLUMES AND CAPACITIES

- *Tidal volume* (V_T): The volume of air exhaled after a normal resting inhalation: $V_T \times$ respiratory rate = minute ventilation. Normal value is 500 mL.
- *Inspiratory reserve volume* (IRV): The amount of additional air that can be taken in after a normal inhalation. Normal value is 3000 to 3100 mL.
- *Inspiratory capacity* (IC): The maximal amount of air that can be inhaled after a normal exhalation. Normal value is 3500 to 3600 mL.
- *Expiratory reserve volume* (ERV): The additional amount of air that can be exhaled after a normal resting exhalation. Normal value is 1100 to 1200 mL.
- *Vital capacity* (VC): The maximal amount of air that can be exhaled after a maximal inhalation. Normal value is 4600 to 4800 mL.
- *Residual volume* (RV): The amount of air left in the lung after maximal exhalation. Normal value is 1200 to 1300 mL.
- *Functional residual capacity* (FRC): The amount of air left in the lung after a normal exhalation, equal to the total of the ERV and RV. Normal value is 2300 to 2400 mL.
- *Total lung capacity* (TLC): The maximal volume of air in the lung after a maximal inspiration, which is the total of all lung volumes. Normal value is 5800 to 6000 mL.

TABLE 23-5 Bedside Pulmonary Function Tests

Test	Description
Respiratory rate (f)	Number of breaths per minute
Tidal volume (V_T)	Volume of air exhaled after a normal resting inhalation
Minute ventilation ($\dot{V}_E$)	Volume of air expired per minute (tidal volume respiratory rate = minute ventilation)
Maximal voluntary ventilation (MVV)	Maximal amount of air that can be moved into and out of the lungs in 1 minute
Forced vital capacity (FVC)	Maximal amount of air that can be forcefully exhaled from the lungs after maximal inhalation
Maximal inspiratory pressure (MIP)	Maximal negative pressure generated on inhalation
Maximal expiratory pressure (MEP)	Maximal positive pressure generated on exhalation
Peak expiratory flow rate (PEFR)	Maximal flow rate achieved during forced exhalation
Forced expiratory flow at midpoint of vital capacity ($FEF_{25\%-75\%}$)	Measure of the average flow rate during the middle 50% of exhalation
Forced expiratory flow at 1 second (FEV_1)	Volume of air exhaled during the first second of forced exhalation

Compliance is a measure of the distensibility of the lungs (how easily they are inflated). Dynamic compliance is measured during the breathing cycle. A value of 46 to 66 mL/cm H_2O is normal (see Appendix B). Measurement of dynamic compliance does not differentiate among resistance forces. Conditions that increase resistance therefore alter the dynamic compliance value. Dynamic compliance decreases with any decrease in lung compliance or increase in airway resistance, as occurs with bronchospasm and retained secretions. Static compliance is measured under no-flow conditions so that resistance forces are removed. Static compliance decreases with any decrease in lung compliance, as occurs with pneumothorax, atelectasis, pneumonia, pulmonary edema, and chest wall restrictions. A normal range is 57 to 85 mL/cm H_2O (see Appendix B).[1,14]

Assessment of inspiratory muscle strength can be evaluated through the measurement of maximal inspiratory pressure (MIP) and negative inspiratory pressure (NIP). Both should be more negative than -20 to -25 cm H_2O. Other names for these tests are negative inspiratory effort (NIE), peak inspiratory pressure (PIP), and peak inspiratory force (PIF). Assessing the MIP and NIP requires a cooperative patient, and the values can provide useful information about spontaneous breathing ability. Maximal expiratory pressure (MEP) can be measured to test the ability to cough in patients with neuromuscular dysfunction. Other common methods used to assess respiratory muscle strength are maximum voluntary ventilation (MVV), minute ventilation ($\dot{V}_E$), and breathing pattern.[1,9]

Dynamic PFTs are designed to evaluate the function of the respiratory muscles, thorax, and lungs. These tests are timed breathing studies that evaluate the degree of respiratory impairment and include forced vital capacity (FVC), peak expiratory flow rate (PEFR), forced expiratory volume in 1 second (FEV_1), and forced expiratory volume divided by the forced vital capacity (FEV_1/FVC). Forced expiratory flow ($FEF_{25\%-75\%}$) is the mean rate of airflow over the middle half of the FVC, and it is a good index of airway resistance. When these studies are performed at the bedside, they require the use of spirometry for volume measurement. The tests can be performed with intubated or nonintubated patients. In the intubated patient, the spirometer is attached to the end of the endotracheal tube. In the nonintubated patient, a nose clip is placed on the patient, and the patient is instructed to breathe through a spirometer tube. The patient is seated on the side of the bed if possible.[1,14] Table 23-5 provides a description of each of these parameters.

VENTILATION/PERFUSION SCANNING

Ventilation/perfusion ($\dot{V}/\dot{Q}$)scanning is indicated when a serious alteration of the normal $\dot{V}/\dot{Q}$ relationship is suspected. $\dot{V}/\dot{Q}$ studies are ordered most often to diagnose and follow a suspected pulmonary embolus. $\dot{V}/\dot{Q}$ scanning is approximately 90% accurate in determining this diagnosis. Comparing the perfusion scan with the results of a clinical examination may improve this percentage somewhat.

The V/Q scan consists of a ventilation scan and a perfusion scan. The ventilation scan is performed by having the patient inhale a radiolabeled gas and air mixture through a mask. The perfusion scan is performed by intravenously injecting the patient with a radioisotope. Scintillation cameras record the gamma radiation images produced by the isotope as it is breathed or perfused into the lung. When an obstruction of the isotope's flow into an area of the lung occurs, the diminished radioactivity is reflected in the camera image of that zone.[15,16]

Because the results are less than 100% accurate in predicting pulmonary emboli, most $\dot{V}/\dot{Q}$ scans are interpreted in one of four ways. The scan is interpreted as normal when the perfusion scan is normal, and the probability of pulmonary embolism approaches zero. A low probability interpretation is given when there are small $\dot{V}/\dot{Q}$ mismatches, focal $\dot{V}/\dot{Q}$ matches with no corresponding radiographic abnormalities, or the perfusion defects are considerably smaller than the radiographic abnormalities. This finding is associated with a 12% chance of pulmonary embolus.[15] An intermediate or indeterminate probability is assigned when there are severe diffuse airflow obstructions, perfusion defects corresponding in size and position to radiographic abnormalities, and a single, moderate $\dot{V}/\dot{Q}$ mismatch without a corresponding radiographic abnormality. A high probability interpretation is used when the perfusion defects are substantially larger than the radiographic abnormalities or when there is one or more large or two or more moderate $\dot{V}/\dot{Q}$ mismatches with no corresponding radiographic abnormalities. This finding is seen infrequently but has a highly predictive value.[9,15]

CHEST RADIOGRAPHY

Chest radiography is an important diagnostic procedure for any critically ill patient. Chest x-ray examinations aid in the diagnosis of various disorders and complications and assist in the evaluation of treatment.[9]

When interpreting a chest radiograph, a systematic method is used for viewing it (Box 23-7). Areas of the x-ray film that are assessed include bones, mediastinum, diaphragm, pleural space, and lung tissue. Fig. 23-2 provides an example of a normal chest radiograph.

Bones. The clavicles, ribs, thoracic and cervical spine, and scapulas are assessed. The clavicles should be symmetric, and the ribs should be an equal distance apart. Intervertebral disk spaces should be evident, indicating an adequately exposed inspiratory film.[17] The thoracic and cervical spine should be straight, without signs of curvature. The scapulas usually appear as areas of added density in the upper lung fields. There should be no evidence of fractures, calcification and lesions (increased density), or demineralization (decreased density).[17]

Mediastinum. The structures assessed in the mediastinal area are the aortic knob and the trachea. The trachea should be positioned in the midline, with a slight deviation to the right as it approaches the carina.[1] Shifting of the mediastinal structures can occur with atelectasis and removal of all or a portion of a lung (toward the area of involvement), pneumothorax (away from the area of involvement), pleural effusion, and tumors.[1,17]

Diaphragm. The diaphragm should be clearly visible, with sharp costophrenic angles seen where the chest wall and the tapered edges of the diaphragm meet.[17] The level of the

---

BOX 23-7 STEPS FOR INTERPRETATION OF A CHEST RADIOGRAPH

STEP 1
Look at the different densities (black, gray, and white), and answer this question: *What is air, fluid, tissue, and bone?*

STEP 2
Look at the shape or form of each density, and answer this question: *What normal anatomic structure is this?*

STEP 3
Look at the right and left sides, and answer this question: *Are the findings the same on both sides, or are there physiologic and pathophysiologic differences?*

STEP 4
Look at all the structures (bones, mediastinum, diaphragm, pleural space, and lung tissue), and answer this question: *Are any abnormalities present?*

STEP 5
Look for all tubes, wires, and lines, and answer this question: *Are the tubes, wires, and lines in the proper place?*

---

diaphragm (on deep inspiration) should appear at the 10th or 11th rib,[17] with the right side 1 to 2 cm higher than the left side.[17] A gastric air bubble may be found under the left side of the diaphragm.[17] An elevated diaphragm may be seen in pregnancy, obesity, conditions that cause air or fluid to accumulate in the peritoneal space, and intestinal obstruction.[1] An elevated hemidiaphragm is associated with several conditions, including phrenic nerve injury, previous chest surgery, subphrenic abscess, trauma, stroke, tumor, pneumonia, and radiation therapy.[1] Flattening of the diaphragm can be a sign of increased air in the lungs, as occurs with chronic COPD or a pleural effusion.[17] Obliteration or "blunting" of the costophrenic angle can occur with pleural effusion, atelectasis, or pneumothorax.[1,17]

Pleural Space. Identification of the pleural space on a chest radiograph is an abnormal finding. The pleural space is not visible unless air (pneumothorax) or fluid (pleural effusion) enters it. As fluid accumulates in the pleural space, it surrounds the lung and eventually compresses it. With a pleural effusion, blunting of the costophrenic angle may be evident first, with flattening of the diaphragm and obscuring of the heart borders occurring as the effusion grows.[18] With a pneumothorax, the pleural edges become evident as the examiner looks through and between the images of the ribs on the film. A thin line appears just parallel to the chest wall, indicating where the lung markings have pulled away from the chest wall.[17,18] The collapsed lung manifests as an area of increased density separated by an area of radiolucency (blackness).

Lung Tissue. The lung tissue is viewed for any areas of increased density or increased radiolucency that may indicate an abnormality. Increased density can be the result of accumulation of fluid in the lungs (e.g., water, pus, blood, edema fluid) or collapse of lung tissue (e.g., with atelectasis or pneumothorax). Increased radiolucency is caused by increased air in the lungs, as may occur with COPD.[18] In some patients, a fine line may be present on the right side at about the level of the sixth rib in the midlung field. This is a normal finding and represents the horizontal fissure, which separates the right upper lobe from the right middle lobe.[18]

Tubes, Wires, and Lines. The chest radiograph is assessed for proper placement of all tubes, wires, and lines. When properly positioned, an endotracheal tube is 2 to 3 cm above the carina, and a nasogastric tube runs the length of the esophagus, with the tip in the stomach.[18] The origin of a central venous catheter is observed as a thin, continuous, radiopaque line at the level of the jaw, progressing toward the superior vena cava in an internal jugular approach, whereas a subclavian approach originates in the clavicular area. A pulmonary artery catheter is viewed running through the right atrium and right ventricle into the pulmonary artery.[18] Additional items that may be present include temporary or permanent pacing wires, a permanent pacing generator, an implantable cardioverter defibrillator (ICD), a peripherally inserted central catheter (PICC), chest tubes (pleural or mediastinal), electrocardiographic (ECG) electrodes, and surgical markers and clips.[17-18]

NURSING MANAGEMENT

Nursing management of a patient undergoing a diagnostic procedure involves a variety of interventions, which include preparing the patient psychologically and physically for the procedure, monitoring the patient's responses to the procedure, and assessing the patient after the procedure. Preparing the patient includes teaching the patient about the procedure, answering any questions, and positioning the patient for the procedure. Monitoring the patient's responses to the procedure includes observing the patient for signs of pain, anxiety, or respiratory distress (see Box 23-1) and monitoring vital signs, breath sounds, and oxygen saturation. Assessing the patient after the procedure includes observing for complications of the procedure and medicating the patient for any postprocedural discomfort.

BEDSIDE MONITORING
CAPNOGRAPHY

Capnography is the measurement of exhaled carbon dioxide (CO_2) gas; it is also known as *end-tidal CO_2* monitoring. Normally, alveolar and arterial CO_2 concentrations are equal in the presence of normal $\dot{V}/\dot{Q}$ relationships. In a patient who is hemodynamically stable, the end-tidal CO_2 (P_{ETCO_2}) can be used to estimate the Pa_{CO_2}, with the P_{ETCO_2} levels 1 to 5 mm Hg less than Pa_{CO_2} levels. The practitioner must determine first that a normal $\dot{V}/\dot{Q}$ relationship exists before correlation of the P_{ETCO_2} and the Pa_{CO_2} can be assumed.[19-21] Causes of increased P_{ETCO_2} include situations in which CO_2 production is increased, such as hyperthermia, sepsis, and seizures, or in which alveolar ventilation is decreased, such as respiratory

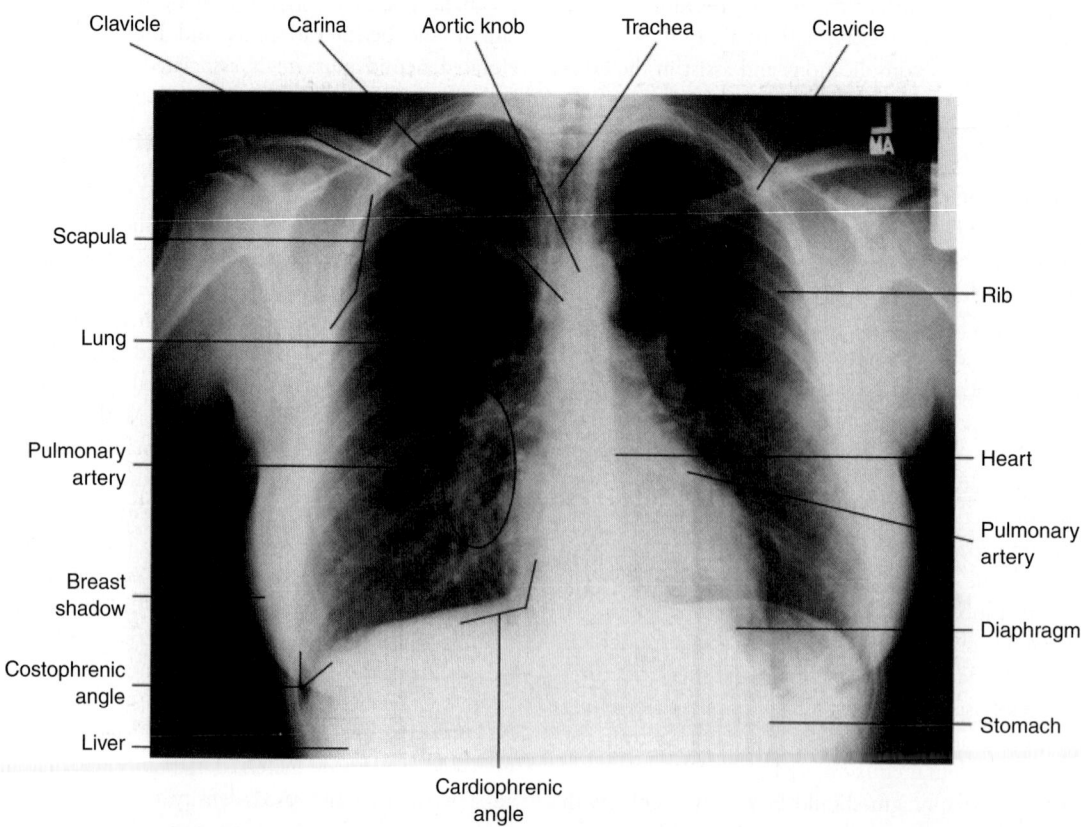

Figure 23-2 Location of structures on a normal chest radiograph. *(From Dettenmeir PA: Radiographic assessment for nurses, St Louis, 1995, Mosby.)*

depression. Causes of decreased $P_{ET}CO_2$ include situations in which CO_2 production is decreased, such as hypothermia, cardiac arrest, and pulmonary embolism, or in which alveolar ventilation is increased, such as hyperventilation.[19]

In the critical care area, continuous capnography is used for assessment and monitoring of the patient's ventilatory status in a variety of situations, including weaning from mechanical ventilation and undergoing procedural sedation. Assessment of changes in physiologic dead space can be carried out with end-tidal CO_2 monitoring, based on the degree of difference between the $Paco_2$ and the $P_{ET}CO_2$. As the severity of pulmonary impairment increases, so does the disparity between the $Paco_2$ and the $P_{ET}CO_2$, as indicated by an increased gradient. A gradient of greater than 5 mm Hg can be seen with underperfused alveolar-capillary units (dead space–producing situations) and nonperfused alveolar-capillary units (alveolar dead space). Increased dead space ventilation is a result of decreased pulmonary blood flow or cardiac output and lung disease. This leads to an abnormality in the transfer of CO_2 from the blood to the lung. The result is a $P_{ET}CO_2$ level that is lower than the $Paco_2$ because of the mixing of carbon dioxide between perfused and nonperfused units. The end result is an increased or widened $Paco_2/P_{ET}CO_2$ gradient.[20,21]

The noninvasive measurement of $P_{ET}CO_2$ enables assessment of the adequacy of cardiopulmonary resuscitation and endotracheal tube placement. Decreased pulmonary blood flow is associated with lower $P_{ET}CO_2$ values, reflected clinically by decreased cardiac output, as in the case of cardiopulmonary resuscitation.[20] During endotracheal intubation, a low $P_{ET}CO_2$ reading indicates that the tube is positioned in the stomach, because the amount of carbon dioxide in the esophagus is expected to be low.[22,23]

There are three forms of capnography: mainstream, sidestream, and microstream. All forms can be used in intubated patients, but sidestream and microstream capnography can also be used in nonintubated patients, broadening the application of end-tidal CO_2 monitoring. Mainstream capnography measures the CO_2 level directly by a sensor in the exhalation port of the ventilator tubing. During exhalation, gas passes over the sensor, and the information is transferred by an electrical cable to the display unit. The display unit produces a waveform, called a *capnogram* (Fig. 23-3), and a numerical recording ($P_{ET}CO_2$). Disadvantages to this form of capnography include the weight of the sensor on the ventilator tubing and possible

obstruction of the sensor by secretions and condensation. In sidestream capnography, the CO_2 gas is continuously aspirated through a side port in the ventilator tubing or nasal cannula and is measured and analyzed by a side unit. Disadvantages to this form of capnography include obstruction of the sampling tube with secretions and slow response time. Microstream capnography is a newer and improved version of sidestream capnography that minimizes the disadvantages (see the Patient Safety feature on Capnography).[21]

PULSE OXIMETRY

Pulse oximetry is a noninvasive method for monitoring oxygen saturation (SpO_2). It is indicated in any situation in which the patient's oxygenation status requires continuous observation. It consists of a microprocessor and a probe that attaches to the patient's forehead, finger, ear, toe, or nose. The probe consists of two light-emitting diodes and a photodetector (Fig. 23-4). The diodes transmit red and infrared light wavelengths through the pulsating arterial vascular bed to the photodetector on the other side. The percentage of oxygen saturation is determined by the difference in absorbance of the red and infrared light caused by the difference in color between oxygen-bound (bright red) and oxygen-unbound (dark red) hemoglobin. The photodetector converts the light signals into an electric signal that is sent to the microprocessor, which converts it to a digital reading. The pulse oximeter is considered very accurate; readings vary less than 4% to 5% at a saturation level greater than 70%. However, several physiologic and technical factors limit the monitoring system.[1,5,7,24]

Patient Safety Alert

Capnography

Capnography and partial pressure of end-tidal carbon dioxide ($P_{ET}CO_2$) analysis have many diverse applications in the critical care area, but the practitioner must never assume the $P_{ET}CO_2$ values reflect arterial values of the partial pressure of carbon dioxide ($Paco_2$) without waveform analysis. Any change in the waveform can indicate a change in the patient's pulmonary status and warrants further evaluation. Loss of the waveform may signal loss of effective respirations.

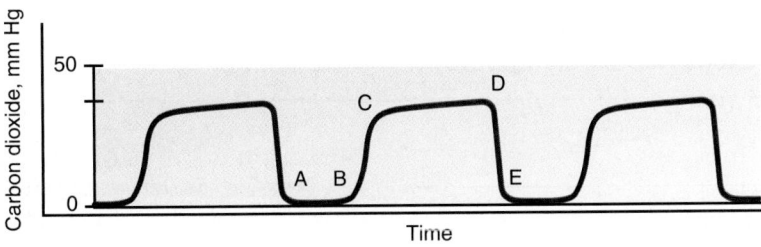

Figure 23-3 Normal findings on a capnogram. A → B indicates the baseline; B → C, the expiratory upstroke; C → D, the alveolar plateau; D, the partial pressure of end-tidal carbon dioxide; and D → E, the inspiratory downstroke. *(From Frakes M: Measuring end-tidal carbon dioxide: clinical applications and usefulness,* Crit Care Nurse *21[5]:23, 2001.)*

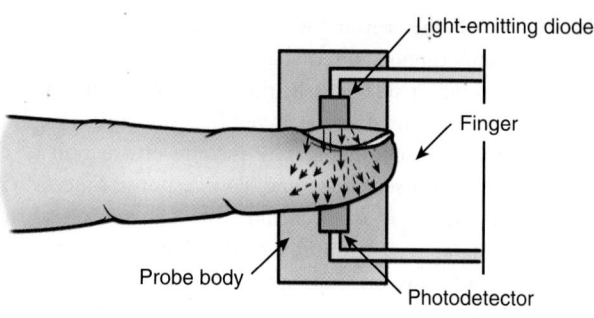

Figure 23-4 Pulse oximeter finger probe. *(From Wilkins RL et al, editors: Egan's fundamentals of respiratory care, ed 8, St Louis, 2003, Mosby.)*

Patient Safety Alert

Pulse Oximetry

In the critically ill patient, pulse oximetry is reliable only for monitoring the patient's oxygenation status. It is not a reliable method for monitoring the patient's ventilatory status. The ability of a pulse oximeter to detect hypoventilation is accurate only when the patient is breathing room air.[1] Because most critically ill patients require some form of oxygen therapy, pulse oximetry is not a reliable method of detecting hypercapnia and should *not* be used for this purpose.

[1] Witting MD et al: The sensitivity of room-air pulse oximetry in the detection of hypercapnia, *Am J Emerg Med* 23:497, 2005.

Physiologic Limitations. Physiologic limitations of pulse oximetry include elevated levels of abnormal hemoglobins, presence of vascular dyes, and poor tissue perfusion. The pulse oximeter cannot differentiate between normal and abnormal hemoglobin. Elevated levels of abnormal hemoglobin falsely elevate the SpO_2. Vascular dyes such as methylene blue, indigo carmine, indocyanine green, and fluorescein interfere with pulse oximetry and can lead to falsely low readings. Poor tissue perfusion to the area with the probe leads to loss of pulsatile flow and signal failure (see the Patient Safety feature on Pulse Oximetry).[1,7]

Technical Limitations. Technical limitations of pulse oximetry include bright lights, excessive motion, and incorrect placement of the probe. Bright lights may interfere with the photodetector and cause inaccurate results. The probe must be covered to limit optical interference. Excessive motion can mimic arterial pulsations and can lead to false readings. Incorrect placement of the probe can lead to inaccurate results, because part of the light can reach the photodetector without having passed through blood (optical shunting).[1,7] Interventions to limit these problems include using the proper probe in the appropriate spot (e.g., not using a finger probe on the ear), applying the probe according to the directions, and ensuring that the area being monitored has adequate perfusion.[24]

Summary

Laboratory Studies

- Interpretation of ABG levels involves looking at the PaO_2 (normal range, 80 to 100 mm Hg), the pH (normal range, 7.35 to 7.45), the $PaCO_2$ (normal range, 35 to 45 mm Hg), and HCO_3^- (normal range, 22 to 26 mEq/L).
- The efficiency of oxygenation can be assessed by measuring the degree of intrapulmonary shunting using the classic shunt equation and oxygen tension indices (PaO_2/FIO_2 ratio, the PaO_2/PAO_2 ratio, and the A-a gradient).
- Sputum specimens are crucial for the rapid identification and treatment of pulmonary infections.

Diagnostic Procedures

- Fiberoptic bronchoscopy and thoracentesis are often used as diagnostic and therapeutic procedures.
- PFTs are used for preoperative assessment, evaluating lung mechanics, diagnosing and tracking pulmonary diseases, and monitoring therapy.
- $\dot{V}/\dot{Q}$ scanning is indicated when a serious alteration of the normal $\dot{V}/\dot{Q}$ relationship is suspected, such as with a pulmonary embolus.
- Chest x-ray examination aids in the diagnosis of various pulmonary disorders and assists in the evaluation of treatments.

Bedside Monitoring

- Capnography is a noninvasive method used to monitor a patient's ventilatory status by measurement of exhaled carbon dioxide gas.
- Pulse oximetry is a noninvasive method used to monitor a patient oxygenation status by measurement of oxygen saturation.

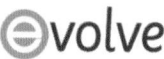 Be sure to check out the bonus material, including free self-assessment exercises, on the Evolve web site at http://evolve.elsevier.com/Urden/.

References

1. Levitzky M: *Pulmonary physiology* ed 7, New York, 2007, McGraw Hill.
2. Whitaker K: *Comprehensive perinatal and pediatric respiratory care*, Albany, NY, 2001, Delmar.
3. Ramadan F, El Solh AA: Overview of respiratory failure in older adults, *J Intensive Care Med* 21:345, 2006.
4. Scanlan CL, Wilkins RL: Gas exchange and transport. In Wilkins RL et al, editors: *Egan's fundamentals of respiratory care*, ed 9, St Louis, 2008, Mosby.
5. Ruholl L: Arterial blood gases: analysis and responses, *Medsurg Nurs* 13:343, 2006.
6. Wheeler A, Bernard G: Acute lung injury and respiratory distress syndrome, *Lancet* 369:1553, 2007.
7. Beckos V, Marini J: Monitoring the mechanically ventilated patient, *Crit Care Clin* 23:575, 2007.

8. Woodruff D: Six steps to ABG analysis, *Nursing* 2:48, 2007.

9. Bordow R et al: *Manual of clinical problems in pulmonary medicine*, ed 6, Philadelphia, 2005, Lippincott Williams & Wilkins.

10. Pruitt B: Taking an evidence-based approach to treating acute lung injury. *Nursing* 37:14, 2007.

11. Johnson KL: Diagnostic measure to evaluate oxygenation in critically ill adults: implications and limitations, *AACN Clin Issues* 15:506, 2004.

12. Bernard G: Acute respiratory distress syndrome a historical perspective, *Am J Resp Crit Care Med* 172:798, 2005.

13. Pruitt B, Jacobs M: All clear: how to keep the airways clear of secretions, *LPN* 2:46, 2006.

14. Grinnan D, Truitt J: Clinical review: respiratory mechanics in spontaneous and assisted ventilation, *Crit Care* 9:472, 2005.

15. Harris A, Bolus NE: Pulmonary embolism imaging, *Radiol Technol* 77:478, 2006.

16. Cloutier L: Diagnosis of pulmonary embolism, *Clin J Oncol* 11:343, 2007.

17. Powner D, Biebuyck J: Introduction to interpretation of chest radiographs during donor care, *Prog Transplant* 15:240, 2005.

18. Puddy E, Hill C: Interpretation of the chest radiograph, *CEACCP* 7:71, 2007.

19. Ahrens T, Sona C: Capnography application in acute and critical care, *AACN Clin Issues* 14:123, 2003.

20. Ahrens T: Monitoring carbon dioxide in critical care: the newest vital sign? *Crit Care Nurs Clin North Am* 16:445, 2004.

21. Zwernemann K: End-tidal carbon dioxide monitoring: a VITAL sign worth watching, *Crit Care Nurs Clin North Am* 18:217, 2006.

22. Thompson JE, Jaffe MB: Capnographic waveforms in the mechanically ventilated patient, *Respir Care* 50:100, 2005.

23. Castle N: Endotracheal tubes early detection of oesophageal intubation, *Emerg Nurse* 14:22, 2007.

24. Fernandez M et al: Evaluation of a new oximeter sensor, *Am J Crit Care* 16:146, 2007.

Pulmonary Disorders

$\mathcal{U}$nderstanding the pathology of the disease, the areas of assessment on which to focus, and the usual medical management allows the critical care nurse to more accurately anticipate and plan nursing interventions. This chapter focuses on pulmonary disorders commonly seen in the critical care environment.

ACUTE RESPIRATORY FAILURE

DESCRIPTION

Acute respiratory failure (ARF) is a clinical condition in which the pulmonary system fails to maintain adequate gas exchange.[1] It is the most common organ failure seen in the intensive care unit,[2,3] with a mortality rate of 22% to 75%.[2] Mortality varies directly with the number of additional organ failures.[2] Other risk factors for mortality included history of liver, renal, or hematologic dysfunction; presence of shock; and age greater than 55 years.[3]

ARF results from a deficiency in the performance of the pulmonary system (see Concept Map on Acute Respiratory Failure).[1,4] It usually is caused by another disorder that has altered the normal function of the pulmonary system in such a way as to decrease the ventilatory drive, decrease muscle strength, decrease chest wall elasticity, decrease the lung's capacity for gas exchange, increase airway resistance, or increase metabolic oxygen requirements.[5]

ARF can be classified as hypoxemic normocapnic respiratory failure (type I) or hypoxemic hypercapnic respiratory failure (type II), depending on analysis of the patient's arterial blood gases (ABGs). In type I respiratory failure, the patient presents with a low PaO_2 and a normal $PaCO_2$, whereas in type II respiratory failure, PaO_2 is low and $PaCO_2$ is high.[1,4]

ETIOLOGY

The causes of ARF may be classified as *extrapulmonary* or *intrapulmonary*, depending on the component of the respiratory system that is affected. Extrapulmonary causes include disorders that affect the brain, the spinal cord, the neuromuscular system, the thorax, the pleura, and the upper airways. Intrapulmonary causes include disorders that affect the lower airways and alveoli, the pulmonary circulation, and the alveolar-capillary membrane.[6] Table 24-1 lists the causes of ARF and their associated disorders.

PATHOPHYSIOLOGY

Hypoxemia is the result of impaired gas exchange and is the hallmark of ARF. Hypercapnia may be present, depending on the underlying cause of the problem. The main causes of hypoxemia are alveolar hypoventilation, ventilation/perfusion ($\dot{V}/\dot{Q}$) mismatching, and intrapulmonary shunting.[1,7] Type I respiratory failure usually results from $\dot{V}/\dot{Q}$ mismatching and intrapulmonary shunting, whereas type II respiratory failure usually results from alveolar hypoventilation, which may or may not be accompanied by $\dot{V}/\dot{Q}$ mismatching and intrapulmonary shunting.[1]

Alveolar Hypoventilation. Alveolar hypoventilation occurs when the amount of oxygen being brought into the alveoli is insufficient to meet the metabolic needs of the body.[6] This can be the result of increasing metabolic oxygen needs or decreasing ventilation.[5] Hypoxemia caused by alveolar hypoventilation is associated with hypercapnia and commonly results from extrapulmonary disorders.[1,7]

Ventilation/Perfusion Mismatch. $\dot{V}/\dot{Q}$ mismatching occurs when ventilation and blood flow are mismatched in various regions of the lung in excess of what is normal. Blood passes through alveoli that are underventilated for the given amount of perfusion, leaving these areas with a lower-than-normal amount of oxygen. $\dot{V}/\dot{Q}$ mismatching is the most common cause of hypoxemia and is usually the result of alveoli that are partially collapsed or partially filled with fluid.[1,7]

Intrapulmonary Shunting. The extreme form of $\dot{V}/\dot{Q}$ mismatching, intrapulmonary shunting, occurs when blood reaches the arterial system without having participated in gas exchange. The mixing of unoxygenated (shunted) blood and oxygenated blood lowers the average level of oxygen present in the blood. Intrapulmonary shunting occurs when blood passes through a portion of lung that is not ventilated. This may be the result of alveolar collapse caused by atelectasis or of alveolar flooding with pus, blood, or fluid.[1,7]

If allowed to progress, hypoxemia can result in a deficit of oxygen at the cellular level. As the tissue demands for oxygen continue and the supply diminishes, an imbalance of oxygen supply and demand occurs, and tissue hypoxia develops. Decreased oxygen to the cells contributes to impaired tissue perfusion and the development of lactic acidosis and multiple organ dysfunction syndrome.[8]

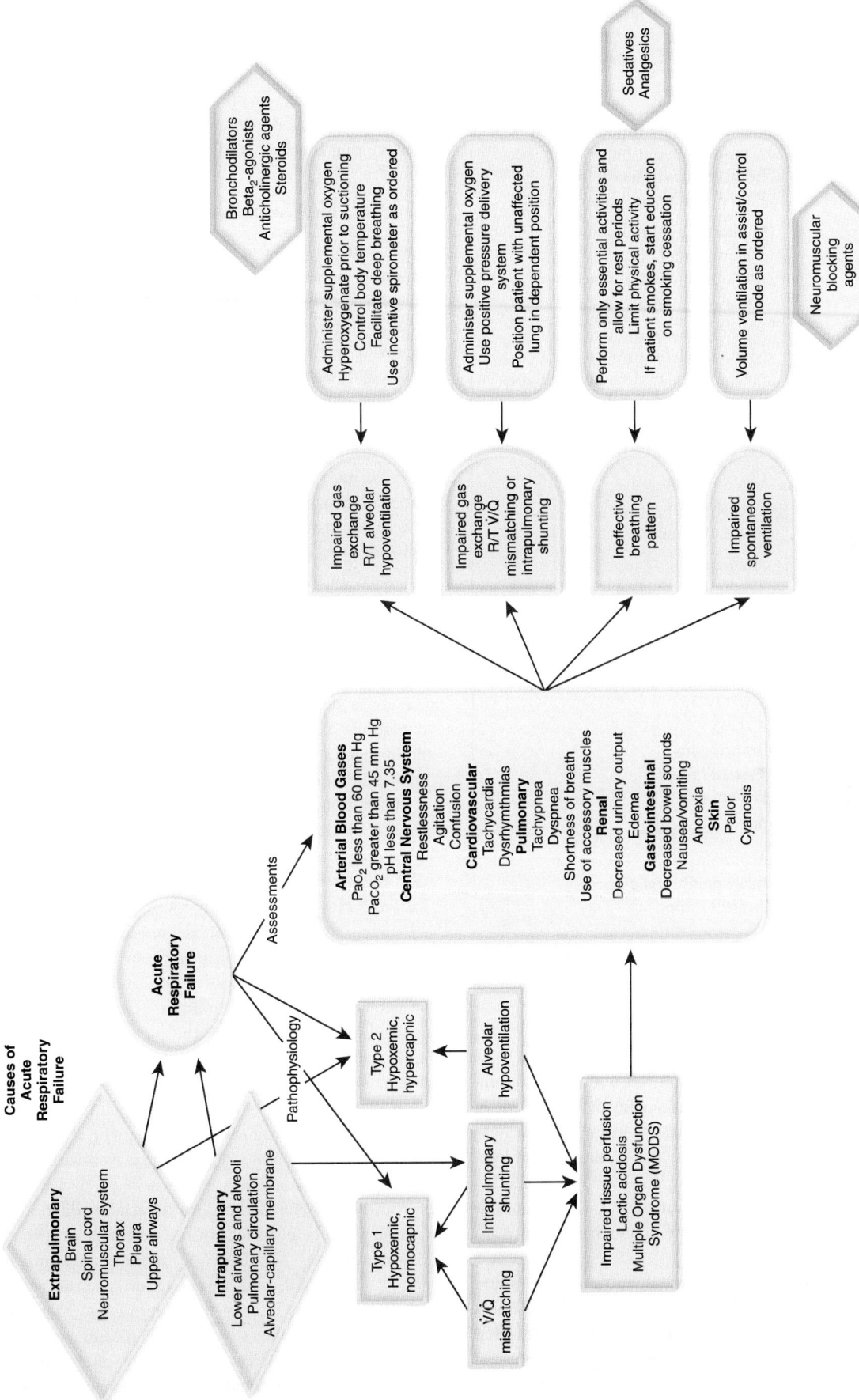

TABLE 24-1 Causes of Acute Respiratory Failure

Affected Area	Disorders*
Extrapulmonary	
Brain	Drug overdose
	Central alveolar hypoventilation syndrome
	Brain trauma or lesion
	Postoperative anesthesia depression
Spinal cord	Guillain-Barré syndrome
	Poliomyelitis
	Amyotrophic lateral sclerosis
	Spinal cord trauma or lesion
Neuromuscular system	Myasthenia gravis
	Multiple sclerosis
	Neuromuscular-blocking antibiotics
	Organophosphate poisoning
	Muscular dystrophy
Thorax	Massive obesity
	Chest trauma
Pleura	Pleural effusion
	Pneumothorax
Upper airways	Sleep apnea
	Tracheal obstruction
	Epiglottitis
Intrapulmonary	
Lower airways and alveoli	Chronic obstructive pulmonary disease (COPD)
	Asthma
	Bronchiolitis
	Cystic fibrosis
	Pneumonia
Pulmonary circulation	Pulmonary emboli
Alveolar-capillary membrane	Acute lung injury (ALI)
	Inhalation of toxic gases
	Near-drowning

*Not an inclusive list.

ASSESSMENT AND DIAGNOSIS

The patient with ARF may experience a variety of clinical manifestations, depending on the underlying cause and the extent of tissue hypoxia. The clinical manifestations commonly seen in patients with ARF are usually related to the development of hypoxemia, hypercapnia, and acidosis (Fig. 24-1 and Table 24-2).[9] Because the clinical symptoms are so varied, they are not considered reliable in predicting the degree of hypoxemia or hypercapnia[1] or the severity of ARF.[3]

Diagnosis and monitoring of the course of respiratory failure are best accomplished by ABG analysis. ABG analysis ascertains the level of $PaCO_2$, PaO_2, and blood pH. It is generally accepted that ARF is present when the PaO_2 is less than 60 mm Hg. If hypercapnia is present, the $PaCO_2$ will be greater than 45 mm Hg.

In patients with chronically elevated $PaCO_2$ levels, these criteria must be broadened to include a pH less than 7.35.[9]

A variety of additional tests are performed depending on the patient's underlying condition. These include bronchoscopy for airway surveillance or specimen retrieval, chest radiography, thoracic ultrasound, thoracic computed tomography, and selected lung function studies.[10]

MEDICAL MANAGEMENT

Medical management of ARF is aimed at treating the underlying cause, promoting adequate gas exchange, correcting acidosis, initiating nutrition support, and preventing complications. Medical interventions to promote gas exchange are aimed at improving oxygenation and ventilation.

Oxygenation. Actions to improve oxygenation include supplemental oxygen administration and the use of positive airway pressure.[8] The purpose of oxygen therapy is to correct hypoxemia. Although the absolute level of hypoxemia varies among patients, most treatment approaches aim to keep the arterial hemoglobin oxygen saturation greater than 90%.[9] The goal is to keep the tissues' needs satisfied while not producing hypercapnia or oxygen toxicity.[9] Supplemental oxygen administration is effective in treating hypoxemia related to alveolar hypoventilation and $\dot{V}/\dot{Q}$ mismatching. If intrapulmonary shunting exists, supplemental oxygen alone is ineffective.[11] In this situation, positive pressure is necessary to open collapsed alveoli and facilitate their participation in gas exchange. Positive pressure is delivered by invasive and noninvasive mechanical ventilation. To avoid intubation, positive pressure is usually administered initially noninvasively by a mask.[12,13] Chapter 25 provides additional information about noninvasive ventilation.

Ventilation. Interventions to improve ventilation include the use of noninvasive and invasive mechanical ventilation. Depending on the underlying cause and the severity of the ARF, the patient may be initially treated with noninvasive ventilation.[12] However, one study found that those patients with a pH of less than 7.25 at initial presentation had an increased likelihood of the need for invasive mechanical ventilation.[14] The selection of ventilatory mode and settings depends on the patient's underlying condition, severity of respiratory failure, and body size. Initially, the patient is started on volume ventilation in the assist control mode (discussed later). In the patient with chronic hypercapnia, the settings should be adjusted to keep the ABG values within the parameters expected to be maintained by the patient after extubation.[15] Additional information on mechanical ventilation is available in Chapter 25.

Pharmacology. Medications to facilitate dilation of the airways may also be of benefit in the treatment of ARF. Bronchodilators, such as β_2-adrenergic agonists and anticholinergic agents, aid smooth muscle relaxation and are of particular benefit to patients with airflow limitations. Methylxanthines, such as aminophylline, are no longer recommended because of their negative side effects. Steroids are often administered to decrease airway inflammation and enhance the effects of the

Subcortical Appraisal and Responsivity   **Elicited Behaviors**

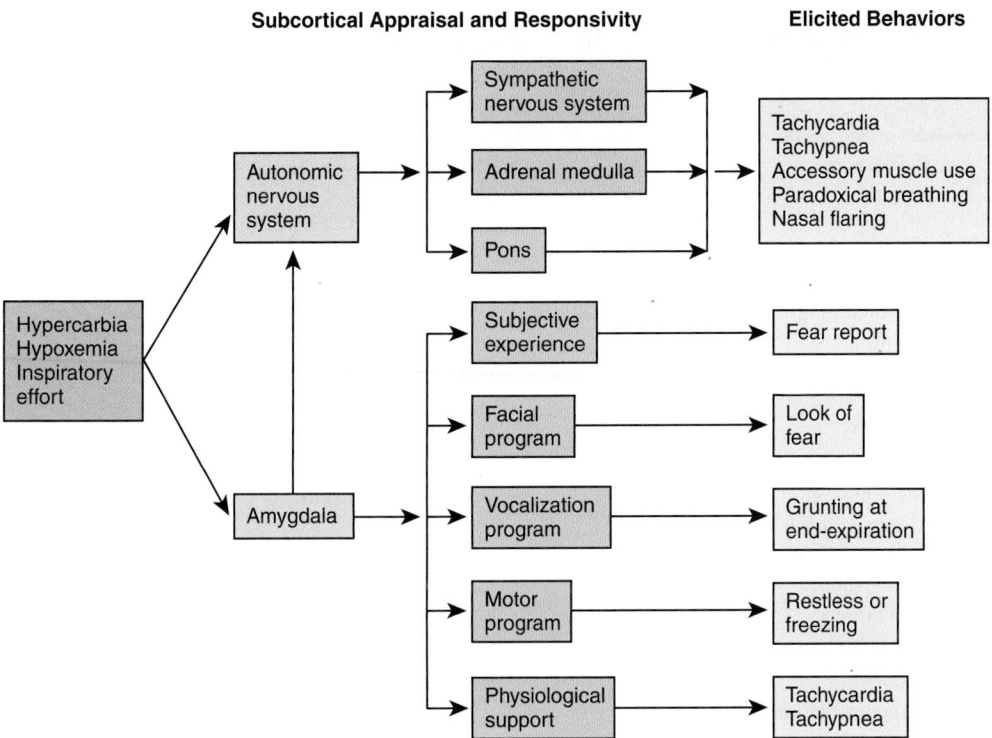

Figure 24-1 Model of respiratory distress behaviors activated from subcortical stimulation. *(From Campbell ML: Respiratory distress: a model of responses and behaviors to an asphyxial threat for patients who are unable to self-report,* Heart Lung *37:53, 2008.)*

β_2-agonists. Mucolytics and expectorants are no longer used, because they have no benefit in this patient population.[16]

Sedation is necessary in many patients to help maintain adequate ventilation. It can be used to comfort the patient and to decrease the work of breathing, particularly if the patient is fighting the ventilator. Analgesics should be administered for pain control.[17,18] In some patients, sedation does not decrease spontaneous respiratory efforts enough to allow adequate ventilation. Neuromuscular paralysis may be necessary to facilitate optimal ventilation. Paralysis may be necessary to decrease oxygen consumption in the severely compromised patient.[18]

Acidosis. Acidosis may occur for a number of reasons. Hypoxemia causes impaired tissue perfusion, which leads to the production of lactic acid and the development of metabolic acidosis. Impaired ventilation leads to the accumulation of carbon dioxide and the development of respiratory acidosis. After the patient is adequately oxygenated and ventilated, the acidosis should correct itself. The use of sodium bicarbonate to correct acidosis has been shown to be of minimal benefit and is no longer recommended as first-line treatment. Bicarbonate therapy shifts the oxygen-hemoglobin dissociation curve to the left and can worsen tissue hypoxia. Sodium bicarbonate may be used if the acidosis is severe (pH <7.1), refractory to therapy, and causing dysrhythmias or hemodynamic instability.[19]

Nutrition Support. Nutrition support is of utmost importance in the management of ARF. The goals of nutrition support are to meet the overall nutritional needs of the patient while avoiding overfeeding, to prevent nutrition delivery–related complications, and to improve patient outcomes.[20] Failure to provide the patient with adequate nutrition support results in the development of malnutrition. Malnutrition and overfeeding can interfere with the performance of the pulmonary system, further perpetuating ARF. Malnutrition decreases the patient's ventilatory drive and muscle strength, whereas overfeeding increases carbon dioxide production, which then increases the patient's ventilatory demand, resulting in respiratory muscle fatigue.[21]

The enteral route is the preferred method of nutrition administration. If the patient cannot tolerate enteral feedings or cannot receive enough nutrients enterally, parenteral nutrition is started. Because the parenteral route is associated with a higher rate of complications, the goal is to switch to enteral feedings as soon as the patient can tolerate them.[20,21] Nutrition support should be initiated before the third day of mechanical ventilation for the well-nourished patient and within 24 hours for the malnourished patient.[20,21]

Complications. The patient with ARF may experience a number of complications, including ischemic-anoxic encephalopathy,[22] cardiac dysrhythmias,[23] venous thromboembolism,[24] and gastrointestinal bleeding.[25] Ischemic-anoxic encephalopathy results from hypoxemia, hypercapnia, and acidosis.[22] Dysrhythmias are precipitated by hypoxemia, acidosis, electrolyte imbalances, and the administration of β_2-agonists.[23] Maintaining oxygenation, normalizing electrolytes, and monitoring drug levels facilitate the prevention and treatment of encephalopathy and dysrhythmias.[22,23] Venous thromboembolism is

TABLE 24-2 Clinical Manifestations of Acute Respiratory Failure

Organ System	SIGNS AND SYMPTOMS		
	Hypoxemia	Hypercapnia	Acidosis
Central nervous	Restlessness Agitation Irritability Confusion Personality changes Impaired judgment Memory loss Sleep disturbance Bizarre behavior Decreased level of consciousness	Headache Drowsiness Decreased level of consciousness Papilledema Blurred vision Confusion Seizures Sleep disturbances	Drowsiness Confusion Decreased level of consciousness
Cardiovascular	Tachycardia Bounding pulse Hypertension (systolic) Wide pulse pressure Dysrhythmias Palpitations Chest pain	Same as hypoxemia Flushing of the skin	Weak pulse Hypotension Dysrhythmias (bradycardia)
Pulmonary	Tachypnea Hyperventilation Dyspnea Shortness of breath Active accessory muscles (neck and shoulders) Active abdominal movement during respiration Ascites, edema, neck vein distention Intercostals' retractions, tracheal tugging, flaring nares	Same as hypoxemia	Same as hypoxemia
Renal	Decreased urinary output Polycythemia Hypertension Edema	Decreased urinary output Hypochloremia Edema Hypertension	Hypochloremic metabolic alkalosis
Gastrointestinal	Decreased bowel sounds Abdominal distention Anorexia Nausea Vomiting Constipation Gastrointestinal bleeding	Same as hypoxemia	Same as hypoxemia
Skin	Pallor Cyanosis Clammy Cool Plethora	Flushed Clammy	Sympathetic nervous system responses (cool, clammy, pale)

Modified from Vaughan P: Home study program: acute respiratory failure in the patient with chronic obstructive lung disease, *Crit Care Nurs* 1(6):46, 1981.

precipitated by venous stasis resulting from immobility and can be prevented through the use of graduated compression stockings or pneumatic compression devices and low-dose unfractionated heparin or low-molecular-weight heparin (LMWH).[24] Gastrointestinal bleeding can be prevented through the use of histamine H_2-antagonists, cytoprotective agents, or proton pump inhibitors.[25] The patient is at risk for the complications associated with an artificial airway, mechanical ventilation, enteral and parenteral nutrition, and peripheral arterial cannulation.

Acute Respiratory Failure

- Impaired Gas Exchange related to alveolar hypoventilation
- Impaired Gas Exchange related to ventilation/perfusion mismatching or intrapulmonary shunting
- Ineffective Breathing Pattern related to musculoskeletal fatigue or neuromuscular impairment
- Risk for Aspiration
- Imbalanced Nutrition: Less Than Body Requirements related to lack of exogenous nutrients or increased metabolic demand
- Risk for Infection
- Impaired Spontaneous Ventilation related to respiratory muscle fatigue or metabolic factors
- Acute Confusion related to sensory overload, sensory deprivation, and sleep pattern disturbance
- Anxiety related to threat to biologic, psychological, or social integrity
- Disturbed Body Image related to functional dependence on life-sustaining technology
- Compromised Family Coping related to critically ill family member
- Deficient Knowledge: Discharge Regimen related to lack of previous exposure to information (see the Patient Education special feature on Acute Respiratory Failure)

NURSING MANAGEMENT

Nursing management of the patient with ARF incorporates a variety of nursing diagnoses (see the Nursing Diagnoses feature on Acute Respiratory Failure). Nursing care is directed by the specific cause of the respiratory failure, although some common interventions are used. The nurse has a significant role in optimizing oxygenation and ventilation, providing comfort and emotional support, and maintaining surveillance for complications. Nursing interventions to optimize oxygenation and ventilation include positioning, preventing desaturation, and promoting clearance of secretions.

Positioning. Positioning of the patient with ARF depends on the type of lung injury and the underlying cause of hypoxemia. For those patients with $\dot{V}/\dot{Q}$ mismatching, positioning is used to facilitate better matching of ventilation with perfusion and thereby optimize gas exchange.[26] Because gravity normally facilitates preferential ventilation and perfusion to the dependent areas of the lungs, the best gas exchange would take place in the dependent areas of the lungs.[11] The goal of positioning is to place the least affected area of the patient's lung in the most dependent position. Patients with unilateral lung disease should be positioned with the healthy lung in a dependent position.[26,27] Patients with diffuse lung disease may benefit from being positioned with the right lung down, because it is larger and more vascular than the left lung.[27,28]

For those patients with alveolar hypoventilation, the goal of positioning is to facilitate ventilation. These patients benefit from nonrecumbent positions such as sitting or a semierect position.[29] Semirecumbency has been shown to decrease the risk of aspiration and to inhibit the development of hospital-associated pneumonia.[30] Frequent repositioning (at least every 2 hours) is beneficial in optimizing the patient's ventilatory pattern and $\dot{V}/\dot{Q}$ matching.[31]

Preventing Desaturation. A number of activities can prevent desaturation from occurring. These include performing procedures only as needed, hyperoxygenating the patient before suctioning, providing adequate rest and recovery time between procedures, and minimizing oxygen consumption. Interventions to minimize oxygen consumption include limiting the patient's physical activity, administering sedation to control anxiety, and providing measures to control fever.[29] The patient should be continuously monitored with a pulse oximeter to warn of signs of desaturation.

Promoting Secretion Clearance. Interventions to promote secretion clearance include providing adequate systemic hydration, humidifying supplemental oxygen, coughing, and suctioning. Postural drainage and chest percussion and vibration have been found to be of little benefit in the critically ill patient[32,33] and are not discussed here.

To facilitate deep breathing, the patient's thorax should be maintained in alignment, and the head of the bed should be elevated 30 to 45 degrees. This position best accommodates diaphragmatic descent and intercostal muscle action.

After the patient is extubated, deep breathing and incentive spirometry should be started as soon as possible. Deep breathing involves having the patient take a deep breath and hold it for approximately 3 seconds or longer. Incentive spirometry involves having the patient take at least 10 deep, effective breaths per hour using an incentive spirometer. These actions help prevent atelectasis and reexpand any collapsed lung tissue. The chest should be auscultated during inflation to ensure that all dependent parts of the lung are well ventilated and to help the patient understand the depth of breath necessary for optimal effect. Coughing should be avoided unless secretions are present, because it promotes collapse of the smaller airways.

Providing Patient Education. Early in the patient's hospital stay, the patient and family should be taught about ARF, its causes, and its treatment. As the patient moves toward discharge, teaching should focus on the interventions necessary to prevent reoccurrence of the precipitating disorder (see the Patient Education feature on Acute Respiratory Failure). If the patient smokes, he or she should be encouraged to stop smoking and should be referred to a smoking cessation program (see the Evidence-Based Practice feature on Smoking Cessation Guidelines). The importance of participating in a pulmonary rehabilitation program should be stressed. Additional information for the patient can be found on the American Lung Association Web site (www.lungusa.org).

Collaborative management of the patient with ARF is outlined in Box 24-1.

Patient Education: Acute Respiratory Failure

- Pathophysiology of disease
- Specific cause
- Precipitating factor modification
- Importance of taking medications
- Breathing techniques (e.g., pursed-lip breathing, diaphragmatic breathing)
- Energy conservation techniques
- Measures to prevent pulmonary infections (e.g., proper nutrition, hand washing, immunization against *Streptococcus pneumoniae* and influenza viruses)
- Signs and symptoms of pulmonary infection (e.g., sputum color change, shortness of breath, fever)
- Cough enhancement techniques (e.g., cascade cough, huff cough, end-expiratory cough, augmented cough)

BOX 24-1   COLLABORATIVE MANAGEMENT: ACUTE RESPIRATORY FAILURE

- Identify and treat underlying cause
- Administer oxygen therapy
- Intubate patient
- Initiate mechanical ventilation
- Administer medications
  - Bronchodilators
  - Steroids
  - Sedatives
  - Analgesics
- Position patient to optimize ventilation/perfusion matching
- Suction as needed
- Provide adequate rest and recovery time between procedures
- Correct acidosis
- Initiate nutritional support
- Maintain surveillance for complications
  - Encephalopathy
  - Cardiac dysrhythmias
  - Venous thromboembolism
  - Gastrointestinal bleeding
- Provide comfort and emotional support

Evidence-Based Practice: Collaborative

Smoking Cessation Guidelines

The following are the key recommendations of the updated guideline, *Treating Tobacco Use and Dependence*, based on the literature review and expert panel opinion:

1. Tobacco dependence is a chronic condition that often requires repeated intervention. However, effective treatments exist that can produce long-term or even permanent abstinence.
2. Because effective tobacco dependence treatments are available, every patient who uses tobacco should be offered at least one of these treatments:
   - Patients *willing* to try to quit tobacco use should be provided treatments identified as effective in this guideline.
   - Patients *unwilling* to try to quit tobacco use should be provided a brief intervention designed to increase their motivation to quit.
3. It is essential that clinicians and health care delivery systems (including administrators, insurers, and purchasers) institutionalize the consistent identification, documentation, and treatment of every tobacco user seen in a health care setting.
4. Brief tobacco dependence treatment is effective, and every patient who uses tobacco should be offered at least brief treatment.
5. There is a strong dose-response relation between the intensity of tobacco dependence counseling and its effectiveness. Treatments involving person-to-person contact (by individual, group, or proactive telephone counseling) are consistently effective, and their effectiveness increases with treatment intensity (e.g., minutes of contact).
6. Three types of counseling and behavioral therapies were found to be especially effective and should be used with all patients attempting tobacco cessation:
   - Provision of practical counseling (problem solving, skills training)
   - Provision of social support as part of treatment (intratreatment social support)
   - Help in securing social support outside of treatment (extratreatment social support)
7. Numerous effective pharmacotherapies for smoking cessation now exist. Except in the presence of contraindications, these should be used with all patients attempting to quit smoking.
   - Five *first-line* pharmacotherapies were identified that reliably increase long-term smoking abstinence rates:
   - Bupropion SR
   - Nicotine gum
   - Nicotine inhaler
   - Nicotine nasal spray
   - Nicotine patch
   - Two *second-line* pharmacotherapies were identified as efficacious and may be considered by clinicians if first-line pharmacotherapies are not effective:
   - Clonidine
   - Nortriptyline
   - Over-the-counter nicotine patches are effective relative to placebo, and their use should be encouraged.
8. Tobacco dependence treatments are clinically effective and cost-effective strategies compared with other medical and disease prevention interventions. Insurers and purchasers should ensure that the following occur:
   - All insurance plans include as a reimbursed benefit the counseling and pharmacotherapeutic treatments identified as effective in this guideline.
   - Clinicians are reimbursed for providing tobacco dependence treatment just as they are reimbursed for treating other chronic conditions.

From Fiore MC et al: *Treating tobacco use and dependence* (Clinical Practice Guideline), Rockville, MD, June 2000, U.S. Department of Health and Human Services, Public Health Service.

ACUTE LUNG INJURY

DESCRIPTION

Acute lung injury (ALI) is a systemic process that is considered to be the pulmonary manifestation of multiple organ dysfunction syndrome.[34] It is characterized by noncardiac pulmonary edema and disruption of the alveolar-capillary membrane as a result of injury to the pulmonary vasculature or the airways.[35]

Many different diagnostic criteria have been used to identify ALI, which has led to confusion, particularly among researchers. In an attempt to standardize the identification of this disorder, the American-European Consensus Committee on ARDS recommended the following criteria for the diagnosis of ALI[36,37]:

- Acute onset
- Ratio of partial pressure of oxygen (PaO_2) to fraction of inspired oxygen (FIO_2) less than or equal to 300 mm Hg (regardless of positive end-expiratory pressure [PEEP] level)
- Bilateral infiltrates on chest radiography
- Pulmonary artery occlusion pressure (PAOP) less than or equal to 18 mm Hg or no clinical evidence of left atrial hypertension

The most severe form of ALI is called *acute respiratory distress syndrome* (ARDS).[36] ARDS is identified by the same diagnostic criteria as ALI, except that the ratio of PaO_2 to FIO_2 is less than or equal to 200 mm Hg. Because the cause, pathophysiology, and treatment of ALI are the same as for ARDS, this discussion uses the broader term, ALI.[37]

ETIOLOGY

A wide variety of clinical conditions are associated with the development of ALI. These are categorized as *direct* or *indirect*, depending on the primary site of injury (Box 24-2).[35,38] Direct injuries are those in which the lung epithelium sustains a direct insult. Indirect injuries are those in which the insult occurs elsewhere in the body and mediators are transmitted through the bloodstream to the lungs. Sepsis, aspiration of gastric contents, diffuse pneumonia, and trauma have been found to be major risk factors for the development of ALI.[37] The mortality rate for ARDS is estimated to be 30% to 50%.[37]

BOX 24-2   RISK FACTORS FOR ACUTE LUNG INJURY

DIRECT INJURY
- Aspiration
- Near-drowning
- Toxic inhalation
- Pulmonary contusion
- Pneumonia
- Oxygen toxicity
- Transthoracic irradiation

INDIRECT INJURY
- Sepsis
- Nonthoracic trauma
- Hypertransfusion
- Cardiopulmonary bypass
- Severe pancreatitis
- Embolism—air, fat, amniotic fluid
- Disseminated intravascular coagulation (DIC)
- Shock states

PATHOPHYSIOLOGY

The progression of ALI can be described in three phases: exudative, fibroproliferative, and resolution. ALI is initiated with stimulation of the inflammatory-immune system as a result of direct or indirect injury (Fig. 24-2). Inflammatory mediators are released from the site of injury, resulting in the activation and accumulation of the neutrophils, macrophages, and platelets in the pulmonary capillaries. These cellular mediators initiate the release of humoral mediators that cause damage to the alveolar-capillary membrane.[38]

Exudative Phase. Within the first 72 hours after the initial insult, the exudative (acute) phase ensues. The mediators released cause injury to the pulmonary capillaries, resulting in increased capillary membrane permeability; this leads to leakage of fluid filled with protein, blood cells, fibrin, and activated cellular and humoral mediators into the pulmonary interstitium. Damage to the pulmonary capillaries also causes the development of microthrombi and elevation of pulmonary artery pressures. As fluid enters the pulmonary interstitium, the lymphatics become overwhelmed and are unable to drain all the accumulating fluid; this results in the development of interstitial edema. Fluid is then forced from the interstitial space into the alveoli, producing alveolar edema. Pulmonary interstitial edema also causes compression of the alveoli and small airways. Alveolar edema causes swelling of the type I alveolar epithelial cells and flooding of the alveoli. Protein and fibrin in the edema fluid precipitate the formation of hyaline membranes over the alveoli. Eventually, the type II alveolar epithelial cells are also damaged, leading to impaired surfactant production. Injury to the alveolar epithelial cells and loss of surfactant lead to further alveolar collapse.[38,39]

Hypoxemia occurs as a result of intrapulmonary shunting and $\dot{V}/\dot{Q}$ mismatching caused by compression, collapse, and flooding of the alveoli and small airways. Increased work of breathing occurs because of increased airway resistance, decreased functional residual capacity (FRC), and decreased lung compliance resulting from atelectasis and compression of the small airways. Hypoxemia and the increased work of breathing lead to patient fatigue and the development of alveolar hypoventilation. Pulmonary hypertension occurs because of damage to the pulmonary capillaries, microthrombi, and hypoxic vasoconstriction leading to the development of increased alveolar dead space and right ventricular afterload. Hypoxemia worsens as a result of alveolar hypoventilation and increased alveolar dead space. Right ventricular afterload increases and leads to right ventricular dysfunction and a decrease in cardiac output (CO).[38]

Fibroproliferative Phase. The fibroproliferative phase begins as disordered healing starts in the lungs. Cellular granulation and collagen deposition occur within the alveolar-capillary membrane. The alveoli become enlarged and irregularly shaped (fibrotic), and the pulmonary capillaries become scarred and obliterated. This leads to further stiffening of the lungs, increasing pulmonary hypertension, and continued hypoxemia.[38,39]

Resolution Phase. Recovery occurs over several weeks as structural and vascular remodeling take place to reestablish the alveolar-capillary membrane. The hyaline membranes are cleared, and intraalveolar fluid is transported out of the alveolus

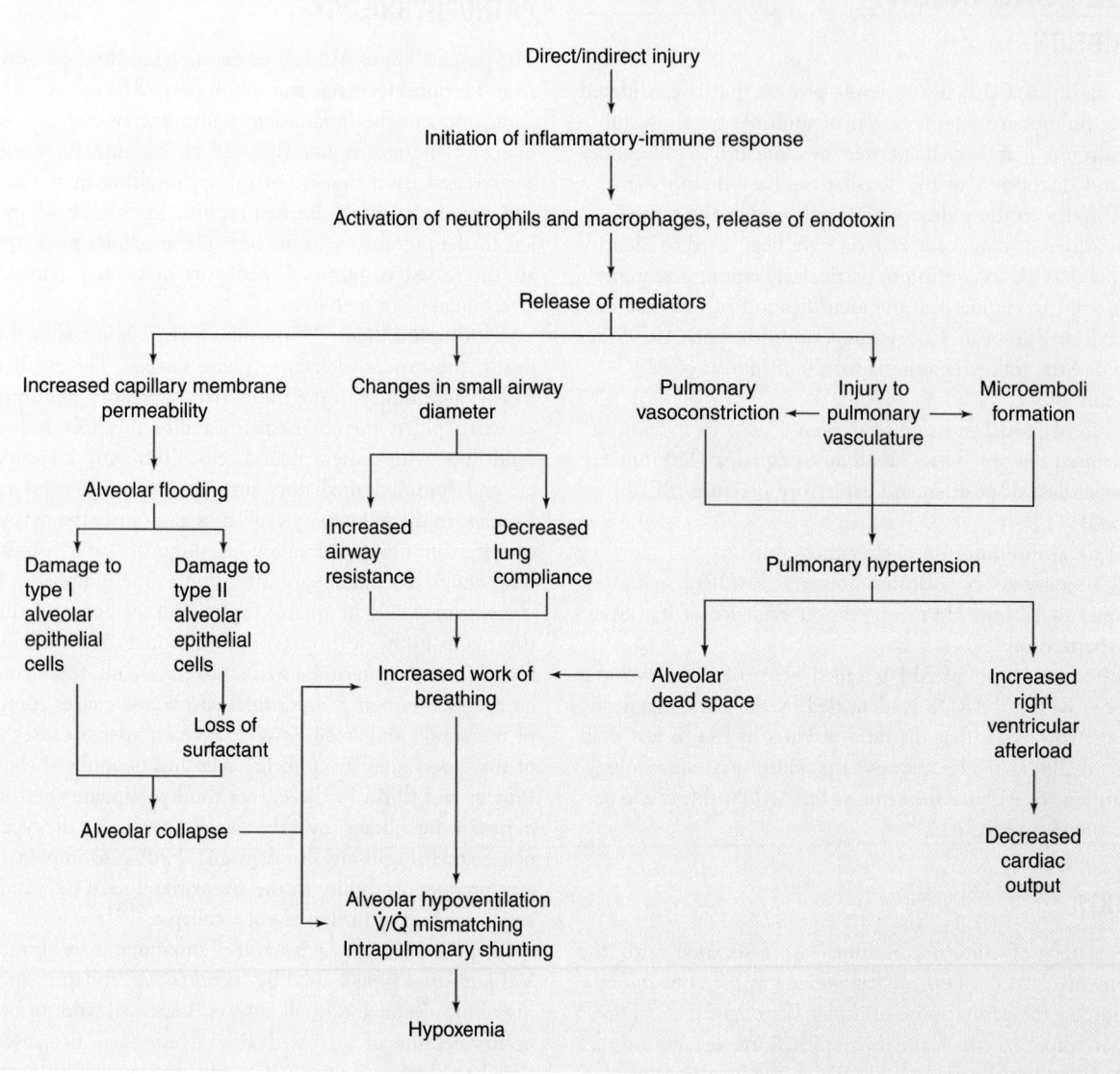

Figure 24-2 Pathophysiology of acute lung injury.

into the interstitium. The type II alveolar epithelial cells multiply, some of which differentiate to type I alveolar epithelial cells, facilitating the restoration of the alveolus. Alveolar macrophages remove cellular debris.[38,39]

ASSESSMENT AND DIAGNOSIS

Initially, the patient with ALI may have a variety of clinical manifestations, depending on the precipitating event. As the disorder progresses, the patient's signs and symptoms can be associated with the phase of ALI that he or she is experiencing (Table 24-3). During the exudative phase, the patient presents with tachypnea, restlessness, apprehension, and moderate increase in accessory muscle use. During the fibroproliferative phase, the patient's signs and symptoms progress to agitation, dyspnea, fatigue, excessive accessory muscle use, and fine crackles as respiratory failure develops.[40,41]

ABG analysis reveals a low PaO_2, despite increases in supplemental oxygen administration (refractory hypoxemia).[40] Initially, the $PaCO_2$ is low as a result of hyperventilation, but eventually the $PaCO_2$ increases as the patient fatigues. The pH is high initially but decreases as respiratory acidosis develops.[40,41]

Initially, the chest radiograph may be normal, because changes in the lungs do not become evident for up to 24 hours. As the pulmonary edema becomes apparent, diffuse, patchy interstitial and alveolar infiltrates appear. These progress to multifocal consolidation of the lungs, which appears as an area of "whiteout" on the chest radiograph.[40]

MEDICAL MANAGEMENT

Medical management of ALI involves a multifaceted approach. This strategy includes treating the underlying cause, promoting gas exchange, supporting tissue oxygenation, and preventing

TABLE 24-3 Physiology and Associated Physical Examination Findings in the Patient with Acute Lung Injury

Physiology	Physical Examination
Exudative Phase	
Parenchymal surface hemorrhage	Restless, apprehensive, tachypneic
Interstitial or alveolar edema	Respiratory alkalosis
Compression of terminal bronchioles	PaO_2 normal
Destruction of type I alveolar cells	CXR: normal
	Chest examination: moderate use of accessory muscles, lungs clear
	Pulmonary artery pressures: elevated
	Pulmonary artery occlusion pressure: normal or low
Fibroproliferative Phase	
Destruction of type II alveolar cells	Pulmonary artery pressures: elevated
Gas exchange compromised	Increased workload on right ventricle
Increased peak inspiratory pressure	Increased use of accessory muscles
Decreased compliance (static and dynamic)	Fine crackles or rales
	Increasing agitation related to hypoxia
Refractory hypoxemia	CXR: interstitial or alveolar infiltrates; elevated diaphragm
Intraalveolar atelectasis	Hyperventilation; hypercarbia
Increased shunt fraction	Decreased SvO_2
Decreased diffusion	Widening alveolar-arterial gradient
Decreased functional residual capacity	Increased work of breathing
Interstitial fibrosis	Worsening hypercarbia and hypoxemia
Increased dead space ventilation	Lactic acidosis (related to aerobic metabolism)
	Alteration in perfusion
	Increased heart rate
	Decreased blood pressure
	Change in skin temperature and color
	Decreased capillary filling
	End-organ dysfunction
	Brain: change in mentation, agitation, hallucinations
	Heart: decreased cardiac output → angina, CHF, papillary muscle dysfunction, dysrhythmias, MI
	Renal: decreased urinary or GFR
	Skin: mottled, ischemic
	Liver: elevated AST, bilirubin, alkaline phosphatase, PT/PTT; decreased albumin

Modified from Phillips JK: Management of patients with acute respiratory distress syndrome, *Crit Care Clin North Am* 11(2):233, 1999.
ALI, acute lung injury; AST, aspartate aminotransferase; CHF, congestive heart failure; CXR, chest radiograph; GFR, glomerular filtration rate; HF, heart failure; MI, myocardial infarction; PaO_2, arterial oxygen pressure; PT, prothrombin time; PTT, partial thromboplastin time; SvO_2, venous oxygen saturation.

complications. Given the severity of hypoxemia, the patient is intubated and mechanically ventilated to facilitate adequate gas exchange.[42]

Ventilation. Traditionally, the patient with ALI was ventilated with a mode of volume ventilation, such as assist control ventilation (ACV) or synchronized intermittent mandatory ventilation (SIMV), with tidal volumes adjusted to deliver 10 to 15 mL/kg. Research indicates that this approach may actually lead to further lung injury. It is now known that repeated opening and closing of the alveoli causes injury to the lung units (atelectrauma), resulting in inhibited surfactant production,

and increased inflammation (biotrauma), resulting in the release of mediators and an increase in pulmonary capillary membrane permeability. Excessive pressure in the alveoli (barotrauma) or excessive volume in the alveoli (volutrauma) leads to excessive alveolar wall stress and damage to the alveolar-capillary membrane, resulting in escape of air into the surrounding spaces.[42] Several approaches have been developed to facilitate the mechanical ventilation of the patient with ALI.

Low Tidal Volume. Low tidal volume ventilation uses smaller tidal volumes (6 mL/kg) to ventilate the patient, in an attempt to limit the effects of barotrauma and volutrauma. The goal is to provide the maximum tidal volume possible while maintaining the end-inspiratory plateau pressure at less than 30 cm H_2O. To allow for adequate carbon dioxide elimination, the respiratory rate is increased to 20 to 30 breaths/min.[42,43]

Permissive Hypercapnia.
Permissive hypercapnia uses low tidal volume ventilation in conjunction with a normal respiratory rate, in an attempt to limit the effects of atelectrauma and biotrauma. Normally, to maintain normocapnia, the patient's respiratory rate would have to be increased to compensate for the small tidal volume. In ALI, however, increasing the respiratory rate can lead to worsening alveolar damage. The patient's carbon dioxide level is allowed to rise, and the patient becomes hypercapnic. As a general rule, the patient's $PaCO_2$ should not rise faster than 10 mm Hg per hour and overall should not exceed 80 to 100 mg Hg. Because of the negative cardiopulmonary effects of severe acidosis, the arterial pH is maintained at 7.20 or greater. To maintain the pH, the patient is given intravenous sodium bicarbonate, or the respiratory rate or tidal volume, or both, are increased. Permissive hypercapnia is contraindicated in patients with increased intracranial pressure, pulmonary hypertension, seizures, or cardiac failure.[44]

Pressure Control Ventilation.
In pressure control ventilation (PCV) mode, each breath is delivered or augmented with a preset amount of inspiratory pressure (rather than tidal volume, as in volume ventilation). The actual tidal volume the patient receives varies from breath to breath. PCV is used to limit and control the amount of pressure in the lungs and decrease the incidence of volutrauma. The goal is to keep the patient's plateau pressure (end-inspiratory static pressure) lower than 30 cm H_2O. A known problem with this mode of ventilation is that, as the patient's lungs get stiffer, it becomes harder and harder to maintain an adequate tidal volume, and severe hypercapnia can occur.[42,43]

Inverse Ratio Ventilation.
Another ventilatory mode that is used in managing ALI is inverse ratio ventilation (IRV), which can be pressure controlled or volume controlled. IRV prolongs the inspiratory (I) time and shortens the expiratory (E) time, reversing the normal I:E ratio. The goal of IRV is to maintain a more constant mean airway pressure throughout the ventilatory cycle, which helps keep the alveoli open and participating in gas exchange. It also increases the FRC and decreases the work of breathing. Because the breath is delivered over a longer period of time, the peak inspiratory pressure in the lungs is decreased. A major disadvantage to IRV is the development of auto-PEEP. Because the expiratory phase of ventilation is shortened, air can become trapped in the lower airways, creating unintentional PEEP (auto-PEEP), which can cause hemodynamic compromise and worsening gas exchange. Patients on IRV usually require heavy sedation with neuromuscular blockade to prevent them from fighting the ventilator.[42,43]

High-Frequency Oscillatory Ventilation.
An alternative ventilatory mode that is used for patients who remain severely hypoxemia despite the treatments previously described is high-frequency oscillatory ventilation (HFOV). The goal of this method of ventilation is similar to that of IRV in that it uses a constant airway pressure to promote alveolar recruitment while avoiding overdistention of the alveoli. HFOV uses a piston pump to deliver very low tidal volumes at very high rates or oscillations (300 to 3000 breaths/min).[45]

Oxygen Therapy.
Oxygen is administered at the lowest level possible to support tissue oxygenation. Continued exposure to high levels of oxygen can lead to oxygen toxicity. The goal of oxygen therapy is to maintain an arterial hemoglobin oxygen saturation of 90% or greater using the lowest level of oxygen—preferably less than 0.50.[35]

Positive End-Expiratory Pressure.
Because the hypoxemia that develops with ALI is often refractory or unresponsive to oxygen therapy, it is necessary to facilitate oxygenation with PEEP. The purpose of PEEP for the patient with ALI is to improve oxygenation while reducing FIO_2 to less toxic levels. PEEP has several positive effects on the lungs, including opening collapsed alveoli, stabilizing flooded alveoli, and increasing FRC. PEEP decreases intrapulmonary shunting and increases compliance. PEEP also has several negative effects, including (1) decreased CO due to decreased venous return caused by increased intrathoracic pressure and (2) barotrauma caused by the escape of gas into the surrounding spaces as a result of alveolar rupture. The amount of PEEP a patient requires is determined by evaluating arterial hemoglobin oxygen saturation and CO. In most cases, a PEEP of 10 to 15 cm H_2O is adequate. If PEEP is too high, it can result in overdistention of the alveoli, which can impede pulmonary capillary blood flow, decrease surfactant production, and worsen intrapulmonary shunting. If PEEP is too low, it allows the alveoli to collapse during expiration, which can result in more damage to alveoli.[42]

Extracorporeal and Intracorporeal Gas Exchange.
Extracorporeal and intracorporeal gas exchanges are last-resort techniques used in the treatment of severe ALI when conventional therapy has failed. These methods allow the lungs to rest by facilitating the removal of carbon dioxide and providing oxygen external to the lungs by means of an "artificial lung," or membrane/fiber oxygenator. Extracorporeal membrane oxygenation (ECMO), extracorporeal carbon dioxide removal ($ECCO_2R$), and intravascular oxygenation (IVOX) are three techniques that employ this type of technology. ECMO is similar to cardiopulmonary bypass in that blood is removed from the body and pumped through a membrane oxygenator, where CO_2 is removed and O_2 is added, and then returned to the body. $ECCO_2R$ is a variation of ECMO in which the primary focus is removal of CO_2. IVOX facilitates oxygenation and ventilation with the use of a fiber oxygenator that is implanted in the inferior vena cava. All of these techniques pose serious bleeding problems to the patient, and none has been shown to improve patient outcome.[42,46]

Tissue Perfusion.
Adequate tissue perfusion depends on an adequate supply of oxygen being transported to the tissues. An adequate CO and a sufficient hemoglobin level are critical to oxygen transport. CO depends on heart rate, preload, afterload, and contractility. A variety of fluids and medications are used to manipulate this parameter. Newer approaches to fluid management include maintaining a very low intravascular volume (pulmonary artery occlusion pressure, 5 to 8 mm Hg) with fluid restriction and diuretics, while supporting the CO with vasoactive and inotropic medications. The goal is to decrease the amount of fluid leakage into the lungs.[47]

Nursing Diagnoses

Acute Lung Injury

- Impaired Gas Exchange related to ventilation/perfusion mismatching or intrapulmonary shunting
- Decreased Cardiac Output related to alterations in preload
- Imbalanced Nutrition: Less Than Body Requirements related to lack of exogenous nutrients or increased metabolic demand
- Risk for Aspiration
- Risk for Infection
- Anxiety related to threat to biologic, psychological, or social integrity
- Disturbed Body Image related to functional dependence on life-sustaining technology
- Compromised Family Coping related to critically ill family member

---

BOX 24-3 COLLABORATIVE MANAGEMENT: ACUTE LUNG INJURY

- Administer oxygen therapy
- Intubate patient
- Initiate mechanical ventilation
  - Permissive hypercapnia
  - Pressure control ventilation
  - Inverse ratio ventilation
- Use positive end-expiratory pressure (PEEP)
- Administer medications
  - Bronchodilators
  - Sedatives
  - Analgesics
  - Neuromuscular blocking agents
- Maximize cardiac output
  - Preload
  - Afterload
  - Contractility
- Place patient in prone position
- Suction as needed
- Provide adequate rest and recovery time between procedures
- Initiate nutritional support
- Maintain surveillance for complications
  - Encephalopathy
  - Cardiac dysrhythmias
  - Venous thromboembolism
  - Gastrointestinal bleeding
  - Atelectrauma
  - Biotrauma
  - Volutrauma
  - Barotrauma
  - Oxygen toxicity
- Provide comfort and emotional support

Investigational Therapies. A number of investigational studies of other therapies for the treatment of ALI are underway. These therapies include drugs to block or neutralize the various mediators released as part of the inflammatory-immune response and methods to limit the damage to the lungs. A variety of drugs are being tested, including corticosteroids, prostaglandin E_1, prostacyclin, lisofylline, ketoconazole, and *N*-acetylcysteine.[37] Three therapies that have been studied for the treatment of ALI are exogenous surfactant, nitric oxide, and partial liquid ventilation. None of these treatments has been shown to be effective in reducing mortality.[48-50]

NURSING MANAGEMENT

Nursing management of the patient with ALI incorporates a variety of nursing diagnoses (see the Nursing Diagnoses feature on Acute Lung Injury). Nursing interventions include optimizing oxygenation and ventilation, providing comfort and emotional support, and maintaining surveillance for complications.

Optimizing Oxygenation and Ventilation. Nursing interventions to optimize oxygenation and ventilation include positioning, preventing desaturation, and promoting secretion clearance (see "Nursing Management" in the section on ARF). An additional nursing intervention that can be used to improve oxygenation and ventilation of the patient with ALI is prone positioning.

Prone Positioning. A number of studies have shown that prone positioning the patient with ALI results in an improvement in oxygenation. Although a number of theories propose how prone positioning improves oxygenation, the discovery that with ALI there is greater damage to the dependent areas of the lungs probably provides the best explanation. It was originally thought that ALI was a diffuse, homogenous disease that affected all areas of the lungs equally. It is now known that the dependent lung areas are more heavily damaged than the nondependent lung areas. Turning the patient prone improves perfusion to less damaged parts of lungs, improves $\dot{V}/\dot{Q}$ matching, and decreases intrapulmonary shunting. Prone positioning appears to be more effective when it is initiated during the early phases of ALI.[51] More information on prone positioning is provided in Chapter 25.

Collaborative management of the patient with ALI is outlined in Box 24-3.

PNEUMONIA

DESCRIPTION

Pneumonia is an acute inflammation of the lung parenchyma that is caused by an infectious agent and can lead to alveolar consolidation. Pneumonia can be classified as community-associated (CAP) or hospital-associated (HAP). CAP is acquired outside of the hospital.[52] Severe CAP requires admission to the intensive care unit and accounts for about 10% of all patients with pneumonia. The mortality rate for this patient group is in excess of 50%.[53] HAP is acquired during a hospital stay of at least 48 hours.[54] Ventilator-associated pneumonia (VAP) is a subgrouping of HAP that refers to the development of pneumonia after the insertion of an artificial airway. VAP represents 80% of all HAP cases.[54]

ETIOLOGY

The spectrum of etiologic pathogens of pneumonia varies with the type of pneumonia, as do the risk factors for the disease.

Severe Community-Associated Pneumonia. Pathogens that can cause severe CAP include *Streptococcus pneumoniae, Legionella* spp., *Haemophilus influenzae, Staphylococcus aureus, Mycoplasma pneumoniae,* respiratory viruses, *Chlamydia pneumoniae,* and *Pseudomonas aeruginosa.*[55] A number of factors increase the risk for developing CAP, including alcoholism, chronic obstructive pulmonary disease (COPD), and comorbid conditions such as diabetes, malignancy, and coronary artery disease.[52] Impaired swallowing and altered mental status also contribute to the development of CAP, because they result in

BOX 24-4 SEVERE ACUTE RESPIRATORY SYNDROME

Severe acute respiratory syndrome (SARS) is a form of serious community-acquired pneumonia caused by the SARS-associated coronavirus (SARS-CoV). It was first reported in February 2003 and over the following months spread to more than two dozen countries before it was contained.

The virus is transmitted by respiratory droplets. The onset of symptoms usually occurs within 10 days after travel to an area with documented or suspected community transmission of SARS or close contact with a person with a respiratory illness who has traveled to a SARS area or is suspected of having SARS. The incubation period for SARS is typically 2 to 7 days, although in some cases it may be as long as 14 days. The patient may first be seen with a wide spectrum of respiratory symptoms, from mild to severe. The illness usually begins with a high fever (temperature >100.4° F [>38.0° C]), which may be accompanied with chills, headache, a general feeling of discomfort, and body aches. Respiratory symptoms may include a dry, nonproductive cough; shortness of breath; difficulty breathing; and hypoxemia.

Evidence of pneumonia (focal, unilateral area of consolidation) on chest radiograph may also be present. Laboratory findings include low white blood cell and platelet counts, raised lactate dehydrogenase concentration, and slightly raised creatinine kinase and C-reactive protein levels.

Patients with suspected SARS virus infection should be placed immediately in negative-pressure isolation. All health care personnel should wear an N-95 respirator mask and implement full barrier precautions when entering the patient's room. Antibiotics have not proved to be effective. Treatment of SARS is largely supportive, with antipyretics, supplemental oxygen, and ventilatory support administered as needed.

Data from Looney MR: Newly recognized causes of acute lung injury: transfusion of blood products, severe acute respiratory syndrome, and avian influenza, *Clin Chest Med* 27:591, 2006.

BOX 24-5 RISK FACTORS FOR HOSPITAL-ACQUIRED PNEUMONIA

HOST-RELATED FACTORS
- Advanced age
- Altered level of consciousness
- Chronic obstructive pulmonary disease
- Severity of illness
- Malnutrition
- Shock
- Trauma
- Smoking
- Dental plaque

TREATMENT-RELATED FACTORS
- Mechanical ventilation
- Unintentional extubation
- Reintubation
- Bronchoscopy
- Nasogastric tube
- Previous antibiotic therapy
- Elevated gastric pH from histamine H_2-blockers, antacid therapy, and enteral feedings
- Upper abdominal surgery
- Thoracic surgery
- Supine position

INFECTION CONTROL–RELATED FACTORS
- Poor hand-washing practices

increased exposure to various pathogens due to chronic aspiration of oropharyngeal secretions.[52] Severe acute respiratory syndrome (SARS) is discussed in Box 24-4.

Hospital-Associated Pneumonia. Pathogens that can cause HAP include *S. aureus, S. pneumoniae, P. aeruginosa, Acinetobacter baumannii, Klebsiella* spp., *Proteus* spp., *Serratia* spp., fungi, and respiratory viruses.[54] Two of the pathogens most frequently associated with VAP are *S. aureus* and *P. aeruginosa*.[30] Risk factors for HAP can be categorized as host-related, treatment-related, and infection control–related (Box 24-5).[30]

PATHOPHYSIOLOGY

Development of acute pneumonia implies a defect in host defenses, a particularly virulent organism, or an overwhelming inoculation event. Bacterial invasion of the lower respiratory tract can occur by inhalation of aerosolized infectious particles, aspiration of organisms colonizing the oropharynx, migration of organisms from adjacent sites of colonization, direct inoculation of organisms into the lower airway, spread of infection to the lungs from adjacent structures or through the blood from more distant structures, and reactivation of latent infection (usually in the setting of immunosuppression). The most common mechanism appears to be aspiration of oropharyngeal organisms.[56] Table 24-4 lists the precipitating conditions that can facilitate the development of pneumonia.

Figure 24-3 depicts the pathophysiology of HAP. Colonization of the patient's oropharynx with infectious organisms is a major contributor to the development of HAP. Normally, the oropharynx has a stable population of resident flora that may be anaerobic or aerobic. When stress occurs, such as with illness, surgery, or infection, pathogenic organisms replace normal resident flora. Previous antibiotic therapy also affects the resident flora population, making replacement by pathologic organisms more likely. The pathogens are then able to invade the sterile lower respiratory tract.[30]

Disruption of the gag and cough reflexes, altered consciousness, abnormal swallowing, and artificial airways all predispose the patient to aspiration and colonization of the lungs and subsequent infection. H_2-agonists, antacids, and enteral feedings also contribute to this problem, because they raise the pH of the stomach and promote bacterial overgrowth. The nasogastric tube then acts as a wick, facilitating movement of bacteria from the stomach to the pharynx, where the bacteria can be aspirated.[52]

TABLE 24-4 **Precipitating Conditions of Pneumonia**

Condition	Causes
Depressed epiglottal and cough reflexes	Unconsciousness, neurologic disease, endotracheal or tracheal tubes, anesthesia, aging
Decreased cilia activity	Smoke inhalation, smoking history, oxygen toxicity, hypoventilation, intubation, viral infections, aging, COPD
Increased secretion	COPD, viral infections, bronchiectasis, general anesthesia, endotracheal intubation, smoking
Atelectasis	Trauma, foreign body obstruction, tumor, splinting, shallow ventilations, general anesthesia
Decreased lymphatic flow	Heart failure, tumor
Fluid in alveoli	Heart failure, aspiration, trauma
Abnormal phagocytosis and humoral activity	Neutropenia, immunocompetent disorders, patients receiving chemotherapy
Impaired alveolar macrophages	Hypoxemia, metabolic acidosis, cigarette smoking history, hypoxia, alcohol use, viral infections, aging

COPD, chronic obstructive pulmonary disease.

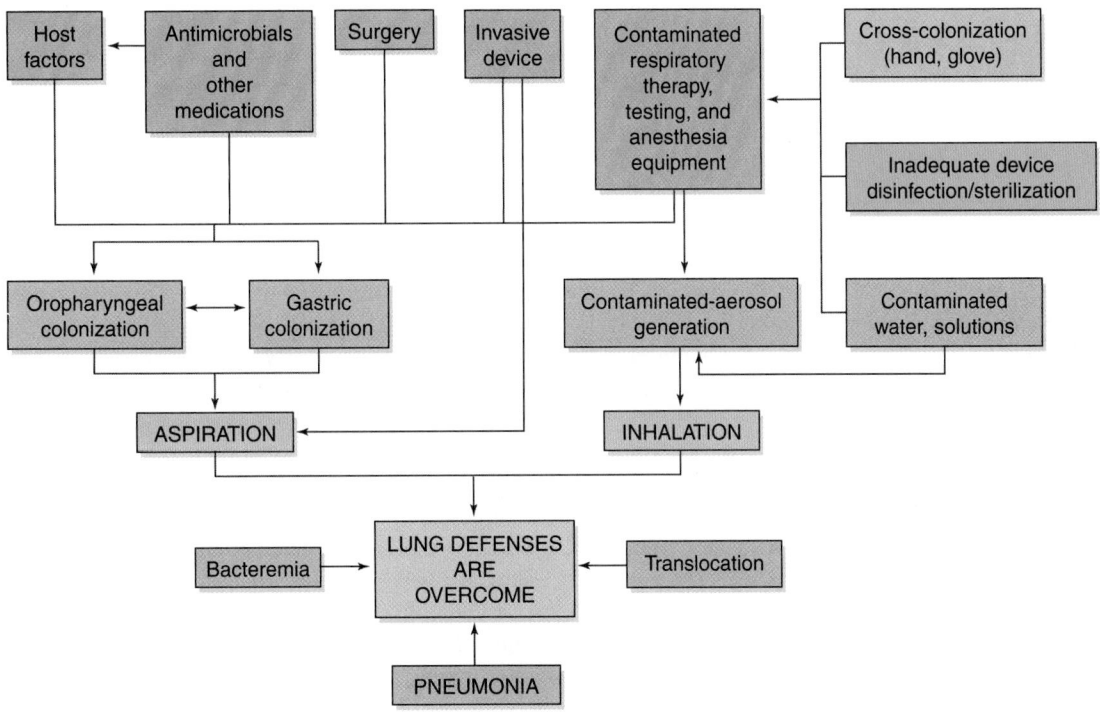

Figure 24-3 Pathophysiology of pneumonia. *(From Tablan OC et al: Guideline for prevention of nosocomial pneumonia. The Hospital Infection Control Practices Advisory Committee, Centers for Disease Control and Prevention, Am J Infect Control 22:247, 1994.)*

Infection results in pulmonary inflammation with or without significant exudates. Increased capillary permeability occurs, leading to increased interstitial and alveolar fluid. $\dot{V}/\dot{Q}$ mismatching and intrapulmonary shunting occur, resulting in hypoxemia as lung consolidation progresses. Untreated pneumonia can result in ARF and initiation of the inflammatory-immune response. The patient may develop a pleural effusion. This is a result of the vascular response to inflammation, whereby capillary permeability is increased and fluid from the pulmonary capillaries diffuses into the pleural space.[52,57] Prevention of VAP is discussed under "Invasive Mechanical Ventilation" in Chapter 25.

ASSESSMENT AND DIAGNOSIS

The clinical manifestations of pneumonia vary with the offending pathogen. The patient may first be seen with a variety of signs and symptoms including dyspnea, fever, and cough (productive or nonproductive). Coarse crackles on auscultation and dullness to percussion may also be present.[57] Manifestations in patients with severe CAP may include confusion and disorientation, tachypnea, hypoxemia, uremia, leukopenia, thrombocytopenia, hypothermia, and hypotension.[56]

Chest radiography is used to evaluate the patient with suspected pneumonia. The diagnosis is established by the presence of a new pulmonary infiltrate. The radiographic pattern of the infiltrates varies with the organism.[58] A sputum Gram stain and culture are done to facilitate identification of the infectious pathogen. In 50% of cases, however, a causative agent is not identified.[52] A diagnostic bronchoscopy may be needed, particularly if the diagnosis is unclear or current therapy is not working.[53] A complete blood count with differential, chemistry panel, blood cultures, and ABG analysis are obtained.[55]

MEDICAL MANAGEMENT

Medical management of pneumonia should include antibiotic therapy, oxygen therapy for hypoxemia, mechanical ventilation if ARF develops, fluid management for hydration, nutritional support, and treatment of associated medical problems and complications. If the patient is having difficulty mobilizing secretions, a therapeutic bronchoscopy may be necessary.[53,54]

Antibiotic Therapy. Although bacteria-specific antibiotic therapy is the goal, this may not always be possible because of difficulties in identifying the organism and the seriousness of the patient's condition. The time involved obtaining cultures should be balanced against the need to begin some treatment based on patient condition. Empiric therapy has become a generally acceptable approach. In this approach, choice of antibiotic treatment is determined based on the most likely etiologic organism and avoiding toxicity, superinfection, and unnecessary cost. If available, the results of the Gram stain should be used to guide the choice of antibiotics. Antibiotics should be chosen that offer broad coverage of the usual pathogens in the hospital or community. Failure to respond to such therapy may indicate that the chosen antibiotic regimen does not appropriately cover all of the etiologic pathogens or that a new source of infection has developed.[54,55]

The Centers for Medicare and Medicaid Services (CMS) and The Joint Commission (TJC) standards for management of CAP require that the first dose of antibiotics be administered within 6 hours after the patient's arrival at the hospital. This time frame is very controversial and has been the subject of much debate. Those in favor of the standard think that early antibiotic administration leads to improved outcomes, whereas those not in favor of the standard think that it leads to the overuse of antibiotics. More research is needed to clarify the issue.[59]

Independent Lung Ventilation. In patients with unilateral pneumonia or severely asymmetric pneumonia, independent lung ventilation (ILV), an alternative mode of mechanical ventilation, may be necessary to facilitate oxygenation. As the alveoli in the affected lung become flooded with pus, the lung becomes less compliant and more difficult to ventilate. This results in a shifting of ventilation to the good lung without a concomitant shift in perfusion, causing an increase in $\dot{V}/\dot{Q}$ mismatching.

Nursing Diagnoses

Pneumonia

- Ineffective Airway Clearance related to excessive secretions or abnormal viscosity of mucus
- Impaired Gas Exchange related to ventilation/perfusion mismatching or intrapulmonary shunting
- Imbalanced Nutrition: Less Than Body Requirements related to lack of exogenous nutrients or increased metabolic demand
- Risk for Aspiration
- Risk for Infection
- Anxiety related to threat to biologic, psychological, or social integrity
- Powerlessness related to lack of control over current situation or disease progression
- Compromised Family Coping related to critically ill family member

ILV allows each lung to be ventilated separately and the amount of flow, volume, and pressure each lung receives to be controlled. A double-lumen endotracheal tube is inserted, and each lumen is attached to a separate mechanical ventilator. The ventilator settings are then customized to the needs of each lung to facilitate optimal oxygenation and ventilation.[60]

NURSING MANAGEMENT

Nursing management of the patient with pneumonia incorporates a variety of nursing diagnoses (see the Nursing Diagnoses feature on Pneumonia). Nursing interventions include optimizing oxygenation and ventilation, preventing the spread of infection, providing comfort and emotional support, and maintaining surveillance for complications. The patient's response to the antibiotic therapy should be monitored for adverse effects.

Optimizing Oxygenation and Ventilation. Nursing interventions to optimize oxygenation and ventilation include positioning, preventing desaturation, and promoting secretion clearance (see "Nursing Management" in the section on ARF).

Preventing the Spread of Infection. Prevention should be directed at eradicating pathogens from the environment and interrupting the spread of organisms from person to person. Significant progress has been made in removing contaminants from the patient's environment through proper disinfection of respiratory equipment and increased use of disposable supplies. Other possible environmental sources of pathogens include suctioning equipment and indwelling lines. These invasive tools must be given proper aseptic care.[30]

Careful hand hygiene is the single most important measure available to prevent the spread of bacteria from person to person (see the Evidence-Based Practice feature on Hand Hygiene Guidelines). Meticulous oral care, including suctioning of the secretions pooling above the cuff of the artificial airway, is critical to decrease bacterial colonization of the oropharynx.[30]

Collaborative management of the patient with pneumonia is outlined in Box 24-6.

Evidence-Based Practice: Collaborative

Hand Hygiene Guidelines

- Wash hands with soap and water when visibly dirty or contaminated with blood and other body fluids.
  - When washing hands with soap and water, wet hands first with water, apply an amount of product recommended by the manufacturer to hands, and rub hands together vigorously for at least 15 seconds, covering all surfaces of the hands and fingers. Rinse hands with water and dry thoroughly with a disposable towel. Use towel to turn off the faucet. Avoid using hot water, because repeated exposure to hot water may increase the risk of dermatitis.
- If hands are not visibly soiled, use an alcohol-based hand rub for routinely decontaminating hands.
  - When decontaminating hands with an alcohol-based hand rub, apply product to palm of one hand and rub hands together, covering all surfaces of hands and fingers, until hands are dry (follow the manufacturer's recommendations regarding the volume of product to use).

- Decontaminate hands before and after having direct contact with patients.
- Decontaminate hands before and after donning gloves.
  - Wear gloves when contact with blood or other potentially infectious materials, mucous membranes, or nonintact skin could occur.
  - Change gloves during patient care if moving from a contaminated body site to a clean body site.
  - Remove gloves after caring for a patient. Do not wear the same pair of gloves for the care of more than one patient, and do not wash gloves between uses with different patients.
- Decontaminate hands after contact with inanimate objects (including medical equipment).
- Do not wear artificial fingernails or extenders when having direct contact with patients at high risk (e.g., those in critical care units or operating rooms).
- Keep natural nail tips less than one-quarter inch long.

From Centers for Disease Control and Prevention: Guideline for hand hygiene in health-care settings: recommendations of the Healthcare Infection Control Practices Advisory Committee and the HICPAC/SHEA/APIC/IDSA Hand Hygiene Task Force, *MMWR* 51(RR16):1, 2002.

BOX 24-6   COLLABORATIVE MANAGEMENT: PNEUMONIA

- Administer oxygen therapy
- Initiate mechanical ventilation as required
- Administer medications
  - Antibiotics
  - Bronchodilators
- Position patient to optimize ventilation/perfusion matching

- Suction as needed
- Provide adequate rest and recovery time between procedures
- Maintain surveillance for complications
  - Acute respiratory failure
- Provide comfort and emotional support

ASPIRATION PNEUMONITIS

DESCRIPTION

The presence of abnormal substances in the airways and alveoli as a result of aspiration is often referred to as *aspiration pneumonia*. This term is misleading, because the aspiration of toxic substances into the lung may or may not involve an infection. *Aspiration pneumonitis* is a more accurate title, because injury to the lung can result from the chemical, mechanical, or bacterial characteristics of the aspirate.

ETIOLOGY

A number of factors have been identified that place a patient at risk for aspiration (Table 24-5). Gastric contents and oropharyngeal bacteria (discussed earlier) are the most common things aspirated by the critically ill patient.[61,62] The effects of gastric contents on the lungs depend on the pH of the liquid. If the pH is less than 2.5, the patient will develop a severe chemical pneumonitis resulting in hypoxemia. If the pH is greater than 2.5, the immediate damage to the lungs will be lessened, but the elevated pH may have promoted bacterial overgrowth of the stomach.[61,62] After the bacteria-laden gastric contents are aspirated into the lungs, overwhelming bacterial pneumonia can develop.[62]

PATHOPHYSIOLOGY

The type of lung injury that develops after aspiration is determined by a number of factors, including the quality of the aspirate and the status of the patient's respiratory defense mechanisms.

Acid Liquid. The aspiration of acid (pH <2.5) liquid gastric contents results in the development of bronchospasm and atelectasis almost immediately. Over the next 4 hours, tracheal damage, bronchitis, bronchiolitis, alveolar-capillary breakdown, interstitial edema, and alveolar congestion and hemorrhage occur.[63] Severe hypoxemia develops as a result of intrapulmonary shunting and $\dot{V}/\dot{Q}$ mismatching. As the disorder progresses, necrotic debris and fibrin fill the alveoli, hyaline membranes form, and hypoxic vasoconstriction occurs, resulting in elevated pulmonary artery pressures.[62,63] The clinical course follows one of three patterns: (1) rapid improvement in 1 week; (2) initial improvement followed by deterioration and development of ALI or pneumonia; or (3) rapid death from progressive ARF.[63]

Acid Food Particles. The aspiration of acid (pH <2.5) nonobstructing food particles can produce the most severe pulmonary reaction because of extensive pulmonary damage.[63] Severe hypoxemia, hypercapnia, and acidosis occur.[62,63]

Nonacid Liquid. The aspiration of nonacid (pH >2.5) liquid gastric contents is similar to acid liquid aspiration initially, but minimal structural damage occurs.[63] Intrapulmonary shunting and $\dot{V}/\dot{Q}$ mismatching usually start to reverse within 4 hours, and hypoxemia clears within 24 hours.[62,63]

TABLE 24-5 **Risk Factors for Aspiration and Aspiration-Related Pneumonia**

Risk Factor	Rationale
Decreased LOC, because of CNS problems or use of sedatives	Decreases ability to protect airway from oropharyngeal secretions and regurgitated gastric contents Cough and gag reflexes diminish as LOC diminishes Slows gastric emptying Decreases tone of lower esophageal sphincter
Supine position	Increases probability of GER
Presence of a nasogastric tube	Interferes with closure of lower esophageal sphincter Biofilm on tube predisposes to aspiration of pathogenic organisms
Vomiting	Sudden and forceful entry of gastric contents into oropharynx predisposes to aspiration Predisposes to displacement of feeding tube ports into esophagus
Feeding tube ports positioned in esophagus	Infused feedings reflux into oropharynx
Tracheal intubation	Reduction in upper airway defense related to ineffective cough, desensitization of oropharynx and larynx, disuse atrophy of laryngeal muscles, and esophageal compression by inflated cuff
Mechanical ventilation	Positive abdominal pressure predisposes to aspiration of gastric contents, probably by increasing GER
Accumulation of subglottic secretions above endotracheal cuff	Secretions can leak around cuff into the lower respiratory tract, especially when cuff is deflated
Inadequate cuff inflation of tracheal devices	Persistent low cuff pressure (e.g., 20 cm H_2O) predisposes to aspiration of oropharyngeal secretions and refluxed gastric contents
Gastric feeding site when gastric emptying is significantly impaired	Accumulation of formula and gastrointestinal secretions predisposes to GER and aspiration
High GRVs	Predispose to GER and aspiration
Bolus feedings	Volume of infused formula may exceed the tolerance of patients who have poor cough and gag reflexes
Poor oral health	Colonized oropharyngeal secretions may be aspirated into respiratory tract
Advanced age	Older patients tend to have a reduced swallowing ability and are more likely to have neurologic disorders that increase aspiration risk Strong association between advanced age and probability of developing pneumonia once aspiration has occurred
Hyperglycemia	Even mild hyperglycemia can cause delayed gastric emptying by disrupting postprandial antral contractions

CNS, central nervous system; GER, gastroesophageal reflux; GRVs, gastric residual volumes; LOC, level of consciousness.
From Metheny NA: Strategies to prevent aspiration-related pneumonia in tube-fed patients, *Respir Care Clin* 12:603, 2006.

Nonacid Food Particles. The aspiration of nonacid (pH >2.5) nonobstructing food particles is similar to acid aspiration initially, with significant edema and hemorrhage occurring within 6 hours. After the initial reaction, the response changes to a foreign body–type reaction, with granuloma formation around the food particles occurring within 1 to 5 days.[63] In addition to hypoxemia, hypercapnia and acidosis occur as a result of hypoventilation.[62,63]

ASSESSMENT AND DIAGNOSIS

Clinically, the patient presents with signs of acute respiratory distress, and gastric contents may be present in the oropharynx. The patient has shortness of breath, coughing, wheezing, cyanosis, and signs of hypoxemia. Tachypnea, tachycardia, hypotension, fever, and crackles also are present. Copious amounts of sputum are produced as alveolar edema develops.[61,62]

The ABG analysis reflects severe hypoxemia. Chest radiographic changes appear 12 to 24 hours after the initial aspiration, with no one pattern being diagnostic of the event. Infiltrates appear in a variety of distribution patterns, depending on the position of the patient during aspiration and the volume of the aspirate. If bacterial infection becomes established, leukocytosis and positive sputum cultures are observed.[62]

MEDICAL MANAGEMENT

Management of aspiration lung disorder includes emergency and follow-up treatment. If the aspiration is witnessed, emergency treatment should be instituted to secure the airway and minimize pulmonary damage. The upper airway should be immediately suctioned to remove the gastric contents.[61,62] Direct visualization by bronchoscopy is indicated to remove any large particulate

Nursing Diagnoses

Aspiration Pneumonitis

- Impaired Gas Exchange related to ventilation/perfusion mismatching or intrapulmonary shunting
- Ineffective Airway Clearance related to excessive secretions or abnormal viscosity of mucus
- Risk for Aspiration
- Risk for Infection
- Anxiety related to threat to biologic, psychological, or social integrity
- Ineffective Coping related to situational crisis and personal vulnerability
- Compromised Family Coping related to critically ill family member

BOX 24-7   COLLABORATIVE MANAGEMENT: ASPIRATION PNEUMONITIS

- Administer oxygen therapy
- Secure the patient's airway
- Place patient in slight
  - Trendelenburg position
- Turn patient to right lateral decubitus position
- Suction patient's oropharyngeal area
- Initiate mechanical ventilation as required
- Maintain surveillance for complications
  - Pneumonia
  - Acute respiratory failure
  - Acute lung injury
- Provide comfort and emotional support

aspirate[61] or to confirm an unwitnessed aspiration event.[63] Bronchoalveolar lavage is not recommended, because this practice disseminates the aspirate in lungs and increases damage. Prophylactic antibiotics are not recommended.[63]

After airway clearance, attention should be given to supporting oxygenation and hemodynamics. Hypoxemia should be corrected with supplemental oxygen or mechanical ventilation with PEEP, if necessary.[61-63] Hemodynamic changes result from fluid shifts into the lungs that can occur after massive aspirations. Monitoring of the intravascular volume is essential, and judicious amounts of replacement fluids should be instituted to maintain adequate urinary output and vital signs.[63]

Initially, antibiotic therapy is not indicated. If symptoms fail to resolve within 48 hours, empiric antibiotic therapy should be initiated. Corticosteroids have not been demonstrated to be of any benefit in the treatment of aspiration pneumonitis and are not recommended.[62]

NURSING MANAGEMENT

Nursing management of the patient with aspiration lung disorder incorporates a variety of nursing diagnoses (see the Nursing Diagnoses feature on Aspiration). Nursing interventions include optimizing oxygenation and ventilation, preventing further aspiration events, providing comfort and emotional support, and maintaining surveillance for complications.

Optimizing Oxygenation and Ventilation. Nursing interventions to optimize oxygenation and ventilation include positioning, preventing desaturation, and promoting secretion clearance (see "Nursing Management" in the section on ARF).

Preventing Aspiration. One of the most important interventions for preventing aspiration is identifying the patient who is at risk for aspiration. Actions to prevent aspiration include confirming feeding tube placement, checking for signs and symptoms of feeding intolerance, elevating the head of the bed at least 30 degrees, feeding the patient through a small-bore feeding tube or gastrostomy tube, avoiding the use of a large-bore nasogastric tube, ensuring proper inflation of artificial airway cuffs, and frequent suctioning of the oropharynx of an intubated patient to prevent secretions from pooling above the cuff of the tube. For patients who are at risk for aspiration or intolerant of gastric feedings, the feeding tube should be placed in the small bowel.[64]

Collaborative management of the patient with aspiration pneumonitis is outlined in Box 24-7.

PULMONARY EMBOLISM

DESCRIPTION

A pulmonary embolism (PE) occurs when a clot (thrombotic embolus) or other matter (nonthrombotic embolus) lodges in the pulmonary arterial system, disrupting the blood flow to a region of the lungs (Fig. 24-4). Most thrombotic emboli arise from the deep leg veins, particularly the iliac, femoral, and popliteal veins.[65] Other sources include the right ventricle, the upper extremities, and the pelvic veins. Nonthrombotic emboli arise from fat, tumors, amniotic fluid, air, and foreign bodies. This section focuses on thrombotic emboli.

ETIOLOGY

A number of predisposing factors and precipitating conditions put a patient at risk for developing a PE (Box 24-8). Of the three predisposing factors that form Virchow's triad (hypercoagulability, injury to vascular endothelium, and venous stasis), endothelial injury appears to be the most significant.[65]

PATHOPHYSIOLOGY

A massive PE occurs with the blockage of a lobar or larger artery, resulting in occlusion of more than 40% of the pulmonary vascular bed. Blockage of the pulmonary arterial system has pulmonary and hemodynamic consequences.[66] The effects on the pulmonary system are increased alveolar dead space, bronchoconstriction, and compensatory shunting.[67] The hemodynamic effects include increased pulmonary vascular resistance and increased right ventricular workload.[66,67]

Increased Dead Space. An increase in alveolar dead space occurs because an area of the lung is receiving ventilation without being perfused. The ventilation to this area is known as *wasted ventilation*, because it does not participate in gas exchange. This effect leads to alveolar dead space ventilation and an increase in the work of breathing. To limit the amount of dead space ventilation, localized bronchoconstriction occurs.[67]

Bronchoconstriction. Bronchoconstriction develops as a result of alveolar hypocarbia, hypoxia, and the release of mediators. Alveolar hypocarbia occurs as a consequence of decreased carbon

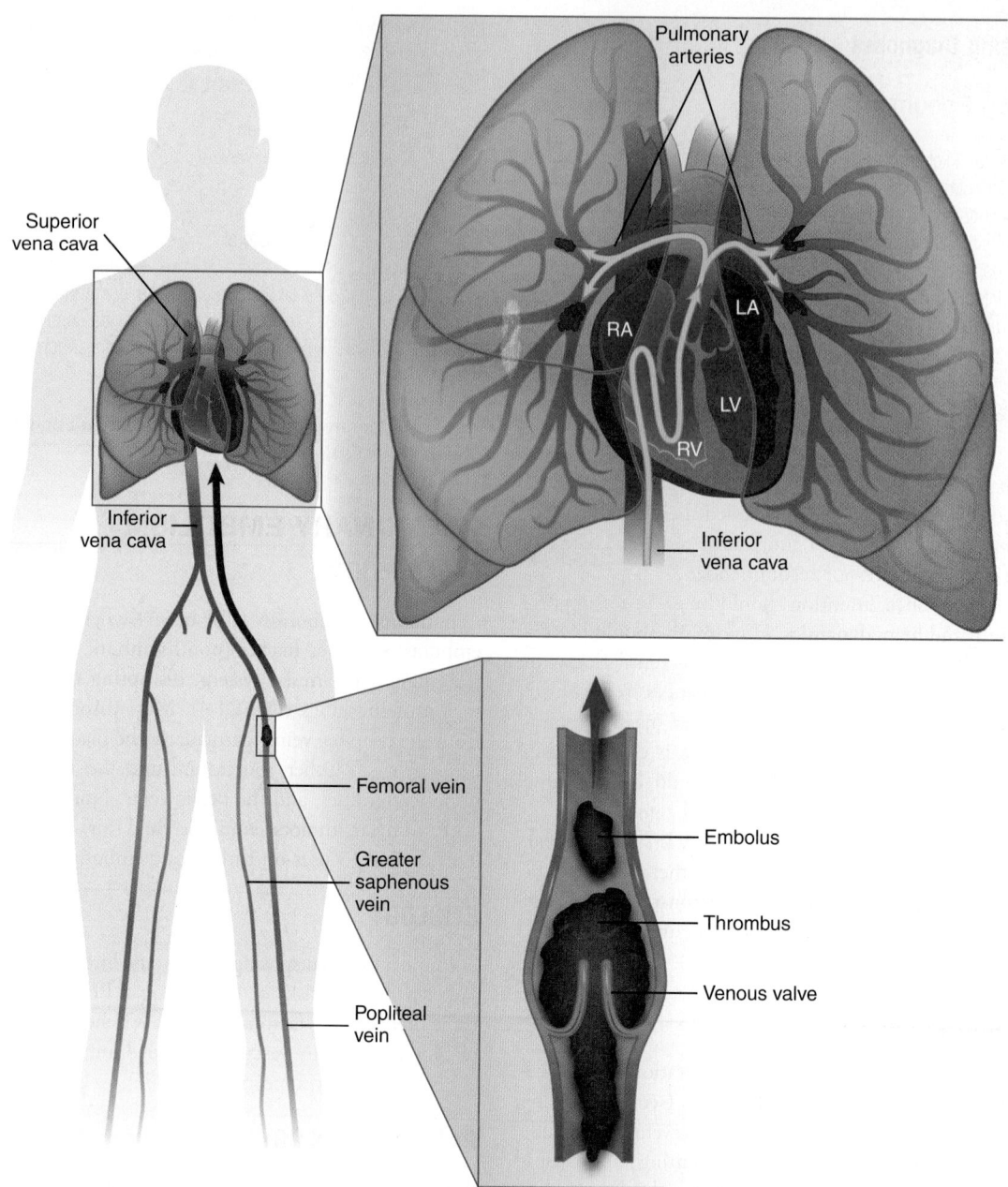

Figure 24-4 Pathophysiology of pulmonary embolism. Pulmonary embolism usually originates in the deep veins of the legs, most commonly the calf veins. These venous thrombi originate predominantly in venous valve pockets and at other sites of presumed venous stasis *(inset)*. If a clot propagates to the knee vein or above or if it originates above the knee, the risk of embolism increases. Thromboemboli travel through the right side of the heart to reach the lungs. LA, left atrium; LV, left ventricle; RA, right atrium; RV, right ventricle. *(From Tapson VF: Acute pulmonary embolism,* N Engl J Med *358:1037, 2008.)*

dioxide in the affected area and leads to constriction of the local airways, increased airway resistance, and redistribution of ventilation to perfused areas of the lungs. A variety of mediators are released at the site of the injury—from the clot or from surrounding lung tissue—and cause further constriction of the airways. Bronchoconstriction promotes the development of atelectasis.[67]

Compensatory Shunting. Compensatory shunting occurs because the unaffected areas of the lungs have to accommodate the entire CO. In this situation, perfusion exceeds ventilation, and blood is returned to the left side of the heart without having participated in gas exchange. This leads to the development of hypoxemia.[67]

Hemodynamic Consequences. The major hemodynamic consequence of a PE is the development of pulmonary hypertension, which is part of the effect of a mechanical obstruction when more than 50% of the vascular bed is occluded. The mediators released at the injury site and the development of hypoxia cause pulmonary vasoconstriction, which further exacerbates pulmonary hypertension. As the pulmonary vascular resistance increases, so does the workload of the right ventricle as reflected by a rise in pulmonary arterial pressures. Consequently, right ventricular failure occurs, which can lead to decreases in left ventricular preload, CO, and blood pressure, followed by shock.[65-67]

BOX 24-8 RISK FACTORS FOR PULMONARY THROMBOEMBOLISM

PREDISPOSING FACTORS

- Venous stasis
  - Atrial fibrillation
  - Decreased cardiac output
  - Immobility
- Injury to vascular endothelium
  - Local vessel injury
  - Infection
  - Incision
  - Atherosclerosis
- Hypercoagulability
  - Polycythemia

PRECIPITATING CONDITIONS

- Previous pulmonary embolus
- Cardiovascular disease
  - Heart failure
  - Right ventricular infarction
  - Cardiomyopathy
  - Cor pulmonale

- Surgery
  - Orthopedic
  - Vascular
  - Abdominal
- Cancer
  - Ovarian
  - Pancreatic
  - Stomach
  - Extrahepatic bile duct system
- Trauma (injury or burns)
  - Lower extremities
  - Pelvis
  - Hips
- Gynecologic status
  - Pregnancy
  - Postpartum
  - Birth control pills
  - Estrogen replacement therapy

ASSESSMENT AND DIAGNOSIS

The patient with a PE can have any number of presenting signs and symptoms, with the most common being tachycardia and tachycapnia. Additional signs and symptoms that may be present include dyspnea, apprehension, increased pulmonic component of the second heart sound (P_1), fever, rales, pleuritic chest pain, cough, evidence of a deep vein thrombosis (DVT), and hemoptysis.[65] Syncope and hemodynamic instability can occur as a result of failure of the right ventricle.[66]

Initial laboratory studies and diagnostic procedures that may be done are ABG analysis, D-dimer measurement, electrocardiography, chest radiography, and echocardiography. The ABG analysis may show a low PaO_2, indicating hypoxemia; a low $PaCO_2$, indicating hypocarbia; and a high pH, indicating a respiratory alkalosis. The hypocarbia with resulting respiratory alkalosis is caused by tachypnea.[67] An elevated D-dimer concentration occurs with a PE and with a number of other disorders. A normal D-dimer level can be used to rule PE out as the diagnosis.[66] The most frequent ECG finding in the patient with a PE is sinus tachycardia.[65] The classic ECG pattern associated with a PE—S wave in lead I and Q wave with inverted T wave in lead III—is seen in fewer than 20% of patients.[66] Other ECG findings associated with a PE include right bundle branch block, new-onset atrial fibrillation, T-wave inversion in the anterior or inferior leads,[65] and ST-segment changes.[66] Chest radiographic findings vary from normal to abnormal and are of little value in confirming the presence of a PE. Abnormal findings include cardiomegaly, pleural effusion, elevated hemidiaphragm, enlargement of the right descending pulmonary artery (Palla's sign), a wedge-shaped density above the diaphragm (Hampton's hump), and the presence of atelectasis.[67] Transthoracic or transesophageal echocardiography is useful in the identification of a PE, because it can provide visualization of emboli in the central pulmonary arteries. It can also be used to assess the hemodynamic consequences of the PE on the right side of the heart.[66]

Differentiating a PE from other illnesses can be difficult, because many of the clinical manifestations of a PE are found in a variety of other disorders as well.[65] Other tests may be necessary, including $\dot{V}/\dot{Q}$ scintigraphy, pulmonary angiography, and DVT studies.[65-67] Since the development of more sophisticated computed tomography (CT) scanners, the spiral CT has also been used to diagnose a PE.[67,68] Definitive diagnosis of a PE requires confirmation by a high-probability $\dot{V}/\dot{Q}$ scan, an abnormal pulmonary angiogram or CT, or strong clinical suspicion coupled with abnormal findings on lower extremity DVT studies.[67]

MEDICAL MANAGEMENT

Medical management of PE involves prevention and treatment strategies. Prevention strategies include the use of prophylactic anticoagulation with low-dose or adjusted-dose heparin, LMWH, or oral anticoagulants (Table 24-6). Graduated compression stockings and pneumatic compression have also been demonstrated to be effective methods of prophylaxis in low-risk patients.[69]

Treatment strategies include preventing the recurrence of a PE, facilitating clot dissolution, reversing the effects of pulmonary hypertension, promoting gas exchange, and preventing complications. Medical interventions to promote gas exchange include supplemental oxygen administration, intubation, and mechanical ventilation.[66]

Prevention of Recurrence. Interventions to prevent the recurrence of a PE include the administration of unfractionated heparin or LMWH and warfarin (Coumadin).[69] Heparin is administered to prevent further clots from forming and has no effect on the existing clot. The heparin should be adjusted to maintain the activated partial thromboplastin time (aPTT) in the range of 2 to 3 times of the upper normal value.[69] Warfarin should be started at the same time, and the heparin should be discontinued after the international normalized ratio (INR) reaches 3.0. The INR should be maintained between 2.0 and 3.0. The patient should remain on warfarin for 3 to 12 months, depending on his or her risk for thromboembolic disease.[69]

Interruption of the inferior vena cava is reserved for patients for whom anticoagulation is contraindicated or for those who still have clots despite normal therapeutic drug levels or those unable to achieve therapeutic drug levels. The procedure involves placement of a percutaneous venous filter (e.g., Greenfield filter) into the vena cava, usually below the renal arteries. The filter prevents further thrombotic emboli from migrating into the lungs.[69]

Clot Dissolution. The administration of fibrinolytic agents in the treatment of PE has had limited success. Fibrinolytic therapy is reserved for the patient with a massive PE and concomitant hemodynamic instability. Recombinant tissue-type plasminogen activator (rtPA) or streptokinase may be used. The therapeutic window for using thrombolytic therapy is 14 days.[70]

Although surgical embolectomy is often considered a last resort, it may be performed to remove the clot. It usually is performed as an open procedure with cardiopulmonary bypass.[69]

TABLE 24-6 Regimens for Venous Thromboembolism Prophylaxis

Condition	Prophylaxis
General surgery	Unfractionated heparin: 5000 units SC tid *or* Enoxaparin: 40 mg SC qd *or* Dalteparin: 2500 or 5000 units SC qd
Orthopedic surgery	Warfarin: target INR 2.0 to 3.0 *or* Enoxaparin: 30 mg SC bid *or* Enoxaparin: 40 mg SC qd *or* Dalteparin: 2500 or 5000 units SC qd *or* Fondaparinux: 2.5 mg SC qd
Neurosurgery	Unfractionated heparin: 5000 units SC bid *or* Enoxaparin: 40 mg SC qd *and* Graduated compression stockings/ intermittent pneumatic compression Consider surveillance lower extremity ultrasonography
Oncologic surgery	Enoxaparin: 40 mg SC qd
Thoracic surgery	Unfractionated heparin: 5000 units SC tid *and* Graduated compression stockings/ intermittent pneumatic compression
Medical patients	Unfractionated heparin: 5000 units SC tid *or* Enoxaparin: 40 mg SC qd *or* Dalteparin: 5000 units SC qd *or* Fondaparinux: 2.5 mg SC qd (not FDA approved) *or* Graduated compression stockings or intermittent pneumatic compression for patients with contraindications to anticoagulation Consider combination pharmacologic and mechanical prophylaxis for patients at very high risk Consider surveillance lower extremity ultrasonography for ICU patients

From Piazza G, Goldhaber SZ: Acute pulmonary embolism. Part 2: treatment and prophylaxis, *Circulation* 114:e42, 2006.
bid, twice daily; FDA, U.S. Food and Drug Administration; ICU, intensive care unit; INR, international normalized ratio; qd, daily; SC, subcutaneous; tid, three times daily.

An emerging alternative to surgical embolectomy is catheter embolectomy. The latter appears to be particularly useful if surgical embolectomy is not available or is contraindicated. It appears to be most successful when performed within 5 days after the occurrence of the PE.[71]

Reversal of Pulmonary Hypertension. To reverse the hemodynamic effects of pulmonary hypertension, additional measures may be taken. These include the administration of inotropic agents and fluid. Fluid should be administered to increase right ventricular preload, which would stretch the right ventricle and increase contractility, overcoming the elevated pulmonary arterial pressures. Inotropic agents also can be used to increase contractility and thereby facilitate an increase in CO.[66]

Nursing Diagnoses

Pulmonary Embolus

- Impaired Gas Exchange related to ventilation/perfusion mismatching or intrapulmonary shunting
- Acute Pain related to transmission and perception of cutaneous, visceral, muscular, or ischemic impulses
- Risk for Aspiration
- Anxiety related to threat to biologic, psychological, or social integrity
- Powerlessness related to lack of control over current situation or disease progression
- Compromised Family Coping related to critically ill family member
- Deficient Knowledge: Discharge Regimen related to lack of previous exposure to information (see the Patient Education special feature on Pulmonary Embolus)

NURSING MANAGEMENT

Prevention of PE should be a major nursing focus, because most critically ill patients are at risk for this disorder. Nursing actions are aimed at preventing the development of DVT, which is a major complication of immobility and a leading cause of PE. These measures include the use of graduated compression stockings or pneumatic compression devices, active/passive range-of-motion exercises involving foot extension, adequate hydration, and progressive ambulation.[24] More information about DVT is provided under "Deep Vein Thrombosis" in Chapter 19.

Nursing management of the patient with a PE incorporates a variety of nursing diagnoses (see the Nursing Diagnoses feature on Pulmonary Embolus). Nursing interventions include optimizing oxygenation and ventilation, monitoring for bleeding, providing comfort and emotional support, and maintaining surveillance for complications.

Optimizing Oxygenation and Ventilation. Nursing interventions to optimize oxygenation and ventilation include positioning, preventing desaturation, and promoting secretion clearance (see "Nursing Management" in the section on ARF).

Monitoring for Bleeding. The patient receiving anticoagulant or thrombolytic therapy should be observed for signs of bleeding. The patient's gums, skin, urine, stool, and emesis should be screened for signs of overt or covert bleeding. Monitoring of the INR or aPTT is critical to managing the anticoagulation therapy.

Patient Education. Early in the patient's hospital stay, the patient and family should be taught about PE, its causes, and its treatment (see the Patient Education feature on Pulmonary Embolus). As the patient moves toward discharge, teaching should focus on the interventions necessary to prevent reoccurrence of DVT and subsequent emboli, the signs and symptoms of DVT and of anticoagulant complications, and measures to prevent bleeding. If the patient smokes, he or she should be encouraged to stop smoking and should be referred to a smoking cessation program.

Patient Education: Pulmonary Embolus

- Pathophysiology of disease
- Specific cause
- Precipitating factor modification
- Measures to prevent deep vein thrombosis (e.g., avoid tight-fitting clothes, crossing legs, and prolonged sitting or standing; elevate legs when sitting; exercise)
- Signs and symptoms of deep vein thrombosis (e.g., redness, swelling, sharp or deep leg pain)
- Importance of taking medications
- Signs and symptoms of anticoagulant complications (e.g., excessive bruising, discoloration of the skin, changes in color of urine or stools)
- Measures to prevent bleeding (e.g., use soft-bristle toothbrush, caution when shaving)

BOX 24-9   COLLABORATIVE MANAGEMENT: PULMONARY EMBOLUS

- Administer oxygen therapy
- Intubate patient
- Initiate mechanical ventilation
- Administer medications
  - Thrombolytic therapy
  - Anticoagulants
  - Bronchodilators
  - Inotropic agents
  - Sedatives
  - Analgesics
- Administer fluids
- Position patient to optimize ventilation/perfusion matching
- Maintain surveillance for complications
  - Bleeding
  - Acute lung injury
- Provide comfort and emotional support

Collaborative management of the patient with a pulmonary embolus is outlined in Box 24-9.

STATUS ASTHMATICUS

DESCRIPTION

Asthma is a COPD that is characterized by partially reversible airflow obstruction, airway inflammation, and hyperresponsiveness to a variety of stimuli.[72] Status asthmaticus is a severe asthma attack that fails to respond to conventional therapy with bronchodilators and may result in ARF.[73]

ETIOLOGY

The precipitating cause of the attack is usually an upper respiratory tract infection, allergen exposure, or a decrease in antiinflammatory medications. Other factors that have been implicated include overreliance on bronchodilators, environmental pollutants, lack of access to health care, failure to identify worsening airflow obstruction, and noncompliance with the health care regimen.[72]

PATHOPHYSIOLOGY

An asthma attack is initiated when exposure to an irritant or trigger occurs, resulting in initiation of the inflammatory-immune response in the airways. Bronchospasm occurs, along with increased vascular permeability and increased mucus production. Mucosal edema and thick, tenacious mucus further increase airway responsiveness. The combination of bronchospasm, airway inflammation, and hyperresponsiveness results in narrowing of the airways and airflow obstruction. These changes have significant effects on the pulmonary and cardiovascular systems.[72]

Pulmonary Effects. As the diameter of the airways decreases, airway resistance increases, resulting in increased residual volume, hyperinflation of the lungs, increased work of breathing, and abnormal distribution of ventilation. $\dot{V}/\dot{Q}$ mismatching occurs and results in hypoxemia. Alveolar dead space also increases as hypoxic vasoconstriction occurs, resulting in hypercapnia.[72]

Cardiovascular Effects. Inspiratory muscle force increases in an attempt to ventilate the hyperinflated lungs. This results in a significant increase in negative intrapleural pressure, leading to an increase in venous return and pooling of blood in the right ventricle. The stretched right ventricle causes the intraventricular septum to shift, impinging on the left ventricle. The left ventricle has to work harder to pump blood from the markedly negative pressure in the thorax to elevated pressure in systemic circulation. This leads to a decrease in CO and a fall in systolic blood pressure on inspiration (pulsus paradoxus).[72]

ASSESSMENT AND DIAGNOSIS

Initially, the patient may present with a cough, wheezing, and dyspnea. As the attack continues, the patient develops tachypnea, tachycardia, diaphoresis, increased accessory muscle use, and pulsus paradoxus greater than 25 mm Hg. Decreased level of consciousness, inability to speak, significantly diminished or absent breath sounds, and inability to lie supine herald the onset of ARF.[73-75]

Initial ABG analysis indicates hypocapnia and respiratory alkalosis caused by hyperventilation. As the attack continues and the patient starts to fatigue, hypoxemia and hypercapnia develop.[73] Lactic acidosis also may occur as a result of lactate overproduction by the respiratory muscles. The end result is the development of respiratory and metabolic acidosis.[74]

Deterioration of pulmonary function test results despite aggressive bronchodilator therapy is diagnostic of status asthmaticus and indicates the potential need for intubation. A peak expiratory flow rate (PEFR) less than 40% of predicted or a 1-second forced expiratory volume (FEV_1) less than 20% of predicted indicates severe airflow obstruction, and the need for intubation with mechanical ventilation may be imminent.[75]

MEDICAL MANAGEMENT

Medical management of status asthmaticus is directed toward supporting oxygenation and ventilation. Bronchodilators, corticosteroids, oxygen therapy, and intubation and mechanical ventilation are the mainstays of therapy.[73]

Bronchodilators. Inhaled β_2-agonists and anticholinergics are the bronchodilators of choice for status asthmaticus. β_2-Agonists promote bronchodilation and can be administered by nebulizer or by metered-dose inhaler (MDI). Usually, large and frequent doses are given, and the drug is titrated to the patient's response. Anticholinergics that inhibit bronchoconstriction are not very effective by themselves, but in conjunction with β_2-agonists, they have a synergistic effect and produce a greater improvement in airflow. The routine use of xanthines is not recommended in the treatment of status asthmaticus, because they have been shown to have no therapeutic benefit.[72-75]

Several studies have focused on the bronchodilator abilities of magnesium. Although it has been demonstrated that magnesium is inferior to β_2-agonists as a bronchodilator, it may be beneficial for patients whose condition is refractory to conventional treatment. A bolus of 1 to 4 g of intravenous magnesium given over 10 to 40 minutes has been reported to produce desirable effects.[72,73,75]

A number of ongoing studies are evaluating the effects of leukotriene inhibitors such as zafirlukast, montelukast, and zileuton in the treatment of status asthmaticus. Leukotrienes are inflammatory mediators known to cause bronchoconstriction and airway inflammation. Research suggests that leukotriene inhibitors may be beneficial as bronchodilators if the status asthmaticus is refractory to β_2-agonists.[75]

Systemic Corticosteroids. Intravenous or oral corticosteroids also are used in the treatment of status asthmaticus. Their antiinflammatory effects limit mucosal edema, decrease mucus production, and potentiate β_2-agonists. It usually takes 6 to 8 hours for the effects of the corticosteroids to become evident.[73] The efficacy of inhaled corticosteroids for the treatment of status asthmaticus remains undecided at this time.[72,75] Initial studies indicate that they may be beneficial in certain patient populations.[75]

Oxygen Therapy. Initial treatment of hypoxemia is with supplemental oxygen. High-flow oxygen therapy is administered to keep the patient's SpO_2 level greater than 92%.[72]

The use of heliox is being investigated. A mixture of helium and oxygen, heliox has a lower density and higher viscosity than an oxygen and air mixture. Heliox is thought to reduce the work of breathing and to improve gas exchange because it flows more easily through constricted areas. Studies have shown that it reduces air trapping and carbon dioxide and helps relieve respiratory acidosis.[72]

Intubation and Mechanical Ventilation. Indications for mechanical ventilation include cardiac or respiratory arrest, disorientation, failure to respond to bronchodilator therapy, and exhaustion.[72,74,75] A large endotracheal tube (8 mm) should be used to decrease airway resistance and facilitate suctioning of secretions. Ventilating the patient with status asthmaticus can be very difficult. High inflation pressures should be avoided, because they can result in barotrauma. The use of PEEP should be monitored closely, because the patient is prone to developing air trapping. Patient-ventilator asynchrony also can be a major problem. Sedation and neuromuscular paralysis may be necessary to allow for adequate ventilation of the patient.[72,74]

NURSING MANAGEMENT

Nursing management of the patient with status asthmaticus incorporates a variety of nursing diagnoses (see the Nursing Diagnoses feature on Status Asthmaticus). Nursing interventions include optimizing oxygenation and ventilation, providing comfort and emotional support, and maintaining surveillance for complications.

Optimizing Oxygenation and Ventilation. Nursing interventions to optimize oxygenation and ventilation include positioning, preventing desaturation, and promoting secretion clearance (see "Nursing Management" in the section on ARF).

Patient Education. Early in the patient's hospital stay, the patient and family should be taught about asthma, its triggers, and its treatment (see the Patient Education feature on Status Asthmaticus). As the patient moves toward discharge, teaching should focus on the interventions necessary for preventing the recurrence of status asthmaticus, early warning signs of worsening airflow obstruction, correct use of an inhaler and a peak flowmeter, measures to prevent pulmonary infections, and signs and symptoms of a pulmonary infection. If the patient smokes, he or she should be encouraged to stop smoking and should be referred to a smoking cessation program. The importance of participating in a pulmonary rehabilitation program should be stressed.

Nursing Diagnoses

Status Asthmaticus

- Impaired Gas Exchange related to alveolar hypoventilation
- Impaired Gas Exchange related to ventilation/perfusion mismatching or intrapulmonary shunting
- Ineffective Breathing Pattern related to musculoskeletal fatigue or neuromuscular impairment
- Ineffective Airway Clearance related to excessive secretions or abnormal viscosity of mucus
- Risk for Infection
- Anxiety related to threat to biologic, psychological, or social integrity
- Disturbed Body Image related to actual change in body structures, function, or appearance
- Compromised Family Coping related to critically ill family member
- Deficient Knowledge: Discharge Regimen related to lack of previous exposure to information (see the Patient Education special feature on Status Asthmaticus)

Patient Education: Status Asthmaticus

- Pathophysiology of disease
- Specific cause
- Early warning signs of worsening airflow obstruction (20% drop in peak expiratory flow rate [PEFR] from predicted or personal best, increase in cough, shortness of breath, chest tightness, wheezing)
- Treatment of attacks
- Importance of taking prescribed medications and avoiding over-the-counter asthma medications
- Correct use of an inhaler (with and without spacer device)
- Correct use of a peak flow meter
- Removal or avoidance of environmental triggers (e.g., pollen; dust; mold spores; cat and dog dander; cold, dry air; strong odors; household aerosols; tobacco smoke; air pollution)
- Measures to prevent pulmonary infections (e.g., proper nutrition and hand washing, immunization against *Streptococcus pneumoniae* and influenza viruses)
- Signs and symptoms of pulmonary infection (e.g., sputum color change, shortness of breath, fever)
- Importance of participating in pulmonary rehabilitation program

Collaborative management of the patient with status asthmaticus is outlined in Box 24-10.

AIR LEAK DISORDERS

DESCRIPTION

Air leak disorders consist of those conditions that result in extraalveolar air accumulation. These disorders are commonly divided into two categories: pneumothorax[76] and barotrauma/volutrauma.[77] A pneumothorax occurs with the accumulation of air or other gas in the pleural space,[76] whereas barotrauma and volutrauma result from the accumulation of air in the interstitial space.[77] Excessive pressure in the alveoli (barotrauma) or excessive volume in the alveoli (volutrauma) can

lead to extreme alveolar wall stress and damage to the alveolar-capillary membrane, causing air to escape into the surrounding spaces.[42] The individual air leak disorders are described in Table 24-7.

ETIOLOGY

The two main causes of air leak disorders are (1) disruption of the parietal or visceral pleura, which allows air to enter the pleural space,[76] and (2) rupture of alveoli, which allows air to enter the interstitial space.[77] Disruption of the parietal pleura occurs as the result of penetrating trauma to the chest wall, which allows atmospheric air to enter the pleural space (traumatic open pneumothorax).[76] Disruption of the visceral pleura occurs as the result of entry of air into the pleural space from the lung. This may be caused by blunt chest wall trauma (traumatic closed pneumothorax), diagnostic or therapeutic procedures (traumatic iatrogenic pneumothorax), diseases of the pulmonary system (secondary spontaneous pneumothorax), or ruptured subpleural blebs (primary spontaneous pneumothorax).[76] Alveolar rupture occurs as the result of a change in the pressure gradient between the alveoli and the surrounding interstitial space. An increase in alveolar pressure or a decrease in interstitial pressure can lead to overdistention of the alveoli, rupture, and air leakage into the interstitial space. One of the most common causes of barotrauma and volutrauma is mechanical ventilation.[77]

BOX 24-10   COLLABORATIVE MANAGEMENT: STATUS ASTHMATICUS

- Administer oxygen therapy
- Intubate patient
- Initiate mechanical ventilation
- Administer medications
  - Bronchodilators
  - Corticosteroids
- Sedatives
- Maintain surveillance for complications
  - Acute respiratory failure
- Provide comfort and emotional support

TABLE 24-7 Air Leak Disorders

Type	Description
Pneumothorax	
Spontaneous	
Primary	Disruption of the visceral pleura that allows air from the lung to enter the pleural space; occurs spontaneously in patients *without* underlying lung disease
Secondary	Disruption of the visceral pleura that allows air from the lung to enter the pleural space; occurs spontaneously in patients *with* underlying lung disease
Traumatic	
Open	Laceration in the parietal pleura that allows atmospheric air to enter the pleural space; occurs as a result of penetrating chest trauma
Closed	Laceration in the visceral pleura that allows air from the lung to enter the pleural space; occurs as a result of blunt chest trauma
Iatrogenic	Laceration in the visceral pleura that allows air from the lung to enter the pleural space; occurs as a result of therapeutic or diagnostic procedures, such as central line insertion, thoracentesis, and needle aspiration
Tension	Occurs when air is allowed to enter the pleural space but not to exit it; as pressure increases inside the pleural space, the lung collapses and the mediastinum shifts to the unaffected side; may result from a spontaneous or traumatic pneumothorax
Barotrauma/Volutrauma	
Pulmonary interstitial emphysema	Air in the pulmonary interstitial space
Subcutaneous emphysema	Air in the subcutaneous tissues
Pneumomediastinum	Air in the mediastinal space
Pneumopericardium	Air in the pericardial space
Pneumoperitoneum	Air in the peritoneal space
Pneumoretroperitoneum	Air in the retroperitoneal space

PATHOPHYSIOLOGY

The pathologic consequences of pneumothorax and those of barotrauma or volutrauma are different.

Pneumothorax. Regardless of the cause, the entry of air into the pleural space compresses the affected lung. As the lung collapses, the alveoli become underventilated, causing $\dot{V}/\dot{Q}$ mismatching and intrapulmonary shunting. If the pneumothorax is large, hypoxemia ensues and ARF quickly develops. Increased pressure within the chest can lead to shifting of the mediastinum, compression of the great vessels, and decreased CO.[76]

Barotrauma and Volutrauma. After air enters the interstitial space, it travels though the pulmonary interstitium (pulmonary interstitial emphysema), out through the hilum, and into the mediastinum (pneumomediastinum), pleural space (pneumothorax),[78] subcutaneous tissues (subcutaneous emphysema),[77] pericardium (pneumopericardium),[42] peritoneum (pneumoperitoneum),[79] and retroperitoneum (pneumoretroperitoneum).[78] Except for pneumothorax, the resultant disorders are usually fairly benign. Pneumomediastinum has been associated with decreased venous return and upper airway obstruction, and pneumopericardium has been associated with cardiac tamponade.[42]

ASSESSMENT AND DIAGNOSIS

The clinical manifestations of a pneumothorax depend on the degree of lung collapse. If the pneumothorax is large, decreased respiratory excursion on the affected side may be noticed, along with bulging intercostal muscles. The trachea may deviate away from the affected side. Percussion reveals hyperresonance with decreased or absent breath sounds over the affected area. ABG analysis demonstrates hypoxemia and hypercapnia.[76] A chest radiograph confirms the pneumothorax with increased translucency evident on the affected side (Fig. 24-5).[78]

The clinical manifestations of barotrauma and volutrauma are much more subtle. Subcutaneous emphysema is manifested by crepitus, usually around the face, neck, and upper chest.[77] Stabbing substernal pain with position changes and with increased ventilation is the most commonly reported symptom of a pneumomediastinum.[80] A clicking or crunching sound synchronous with the heart sounds may be heard over the apex of the heart (Hamman's sign).[81] A friction rub may be heard with a pneumopericardium.[81] Barotrauma is also confirmed by radiography. Extraalveolar air, as evidenced by increased translucency, is present in the affected area (e.g., chest, abdomen).[78]

MEDICAL MANAGEMENT

Medical management of air leak disorders varies depending on the severity of the specific disorder. Usually, only a pneumothorax would require treatment, and that would depend on its size. A pneumothorax of less than 15% usually requires no treatment other than supplemental oxygen administration, unless complications occur or underlying lung disease or injury is present.[76]

A pneumothorax greater than 15% requires intervention to evacuate the air from the pleural space and facilitate reexpansion of the collapsed lung. Interventions include aspiration of the air with a needle and placement of a small-bore (12 to 20 Fr) or

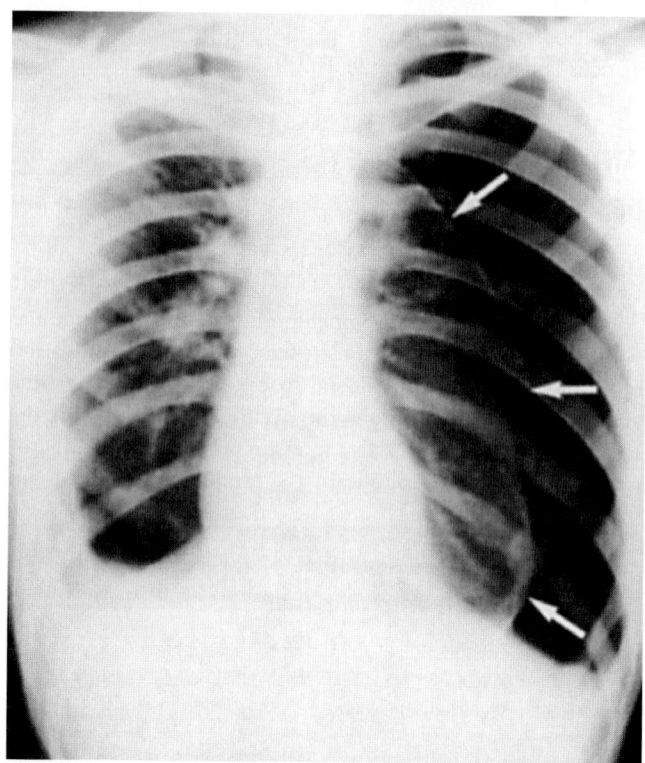

Figure 24-5 Left-sided tension pneumothorax. Notice the shift of the heart and mediastinum to the right. *(From Des Jardin T, Burton GC: Clinical management and assessment of respiratory disease, ed 3, St. Louis, 1995, Mosby.)*

large-bore (24 to 40 Fr) chest tube. Chest tubes are inserted into the pleural space to remove fluid or air, reinstate the negative intrapleural pressure, and reexpand a collapsed lung. The trend appears to be toward placement of a small-bore tube, as the smaller tubes are more comfortable for the patient and just as effective as large-bore tubes.[82] Chest tubes are usually inserted in the fourth or fifth intercostal space on the midaxillary line. After the tube is inserted, it is attached to a Heimlich valve or an underwater-seal drainage system. The Heimlich valve is a small one-way valve device that allows air to exit from the pleural space but not enter it (Fig. 24-6). It can be used alone or attached to a drainage bag. An underwater-seal drainage system is a disposable plastic unit that has three separate chambers: a water-seal chamber, a suction-control chamber, and a drainage-collection chamber (Fig 24-7). Usually the water-seal chamber is filled to the 2-cm level and the suction-control chamber is adjusted to the desired level of suction. The water-seal chamber acts as a one-way valve, allowing air to escape from the chest but not to enter it. After the chest tubes are placed, the suction-control chamber is attached to an external suction regulator, which is adjusted until the desired level of suction is established (usually 20 cm H_2O). Any fluid draining from the chest will be evident in the collection chamber. Connection points of the drainage tubing are sealed with tape, and an occlusive dressing is applied over the chest tube insertion site. After the tubes are inserted and connected to either device, a chest radiograph should be obtained to confirm reexpansion of the lung.[76]

Two conditions that require emergency intervention for immediate relief are a tension pneumothorax and a tension pneumopericardium.

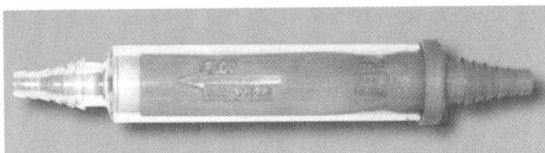

Figure 24-6 Heimlich valve. *(Courtesy BD Medical Systems, Franklin Lakes, NJ.)*

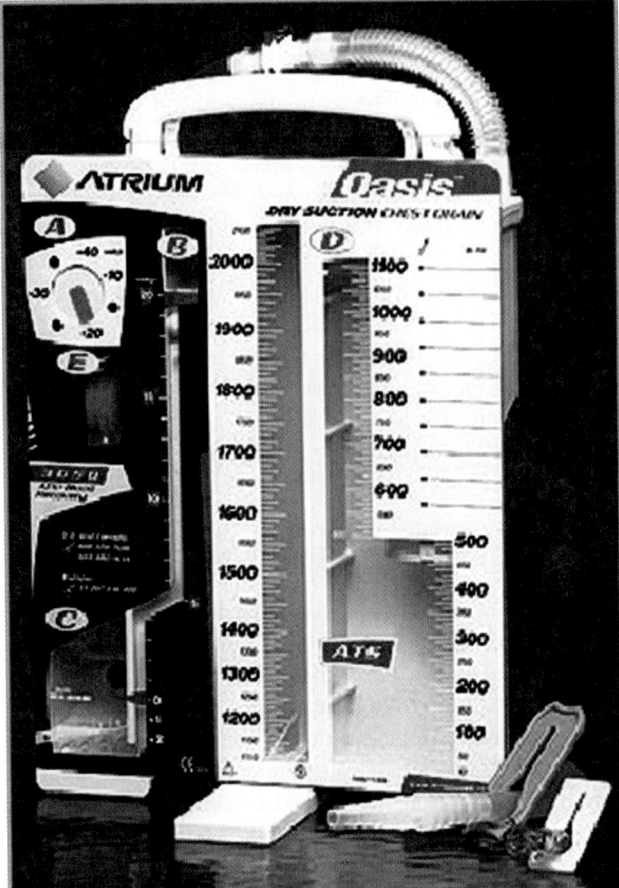

Figure 24-7 Underwater-seal drainage system. *(Courtesy Atrium Medical Corporation, Hudson, NH.)*

Tension Pneumothorax. A tension pneumothorax develops when air enters the pleural space on inhalation and cannot exit on exhalation. As pressure inside the pleural space increases, it results in collapse of the lung and shifting of the mediastinum and trachea to the unaffected side (see Fig. 24-5). The resultant effect is decreased venous return and compression of the unaffected lung. Clinical signs include diminished breath sounds, hyperresonance to percussion, tachycardia, and hypotension. Treatment comprises administration of supplemental oxygen and insertion of a large-bore needle or catheter into the second intercostal space at the midclavicular line of the affected side. This action relieves the pressure within the chest. The needle should remain in place until the patient is stabilized and a chest tube is inserted.[76]

Tension Pneumopericardium. A tension pneumopericardium develops when air enters the pericardial space and has no outlet for exiting. As pressure inside the pericardium increases, it results in compression of the heart and the development of

cardiac tamponade. A pericardiocentesis should be performed immediately to relieve the pressure within the pericardial sac.[81]

NURSING MANAGEMENT

Nursing management of the patient with an air leak disorder incorporates a variety of nursing diagnoses (see the Nursing Diagnoses feature on Air Leak Disorders). Nursing interventions should focus on optimizing oxygenation and ventilation, maintaining the chest tube system, providing comfort and emotional support, and maintaining surveillance for complications.

Optimizing Oxygenation and Ventilation. Nursing interventions to optimize oxygenation and ventilation include positioning, preventing desaturation, and promoting secretion clearance (see "Nursing Management" in the section on ARF).

Maintaining the Chest Tube System. Maintaining the chest tube system involves careful attention to the suction applied and to maintenance of unobstructed drainage tubes. Kinks and large loops of tubing should be avoided, because they impede drainage and air evacuation, which may prevent timely lung reexpansion or may result in a tension pneumothorax. Retained drainage also becomes an excellent medium for bacterial growth. The water-seal chamber must routinely be observed for unexpected bubbling caused by an air leak in the system.

If unexpected bubbling is present, the source must be identified. To determine whether the source is within the system or within the patient, systematic brief clamping of the drainage tube should be performed. The nurse should place a padded clamp on the drainage tubing as close to the occlusive dressing as possible. If the air bubbling stops, the air leak is located between the patient and the clamp. The leak can be within the patient or at the insertion site. The clamp should then be removed and the chest tube site exposed. The tube should be inspected at the site where it enters the chest to ensure that all the eyelets are within the patient. If an eyelet port is outside the chest, it can be a source of an air leak and must be occluded, which may require the attention of the physician. After the insertion site has been eliminated as a leakage source, the chest dressing should be reapplied, completely and securely covering the site. If the air bubbling does not stop when a clamp is placed on the chest tube, the leak must be located between the clamp and the drainage collector. It can be found by releasing the clamp and moving it down the tubing a few inches at a time until the bubbling stops. After the area of the leak is located, it can be taped to reestablish a seal, or the system can be replaced.

A sterile occlusive dressing and a bottle of sterile water should be available at the patient's bedside at all times. If the chest tube system is inadvertently interrupted, the tube should be placed a few centimeters into the bottle of water while the drainage system is reestablished. A sterile occlusive dressing is applied to the chest wall if the chest tube is accidentally removed. Immediate implementation of these techniques minimizes or prevents the formation of a pneumothorax and avoids greater complications.

Throughout the duration of chest tube placement, the patient should be assessed periodically for reexpansion of the lung and for complications of chest tube drainage. The nurse should assess the thorax and lungs, paying particular attention to any tracheal deviation, asymmetry of chest movement, presence of subcutaneous emphysema, characteristics of breathing, quality of lung sounds, and presence of tympany or percussion sounds, which are indicative of pneumothorax.

Collaborative management of the patient with an air leak disorder is outlined in Box 24-11.

THORACIC SURGERY

TYPES OF SURGERY

Thoracic surgery comprises a number of surgical procedures that involve opening the thoracic cavity (thoracotomy) or the organs of respiration, or both. Indications for thoracic surgery range from tumors and abscesses to repair of the esophagus and of thoracic vessels.[83] Table 24-8 describes a variety of thoracic surgical procedures and their indications. This discussion focuses only on the surgical procedures that involve the removal of lung tissue.

PREOPERATIVE CARE

Before surgery, a complete evaluation of the patient is needed to determine the appropriateness of surgery as a treatment and to determine whether lung tissue can be removed without jeopardizing respiratory function. This is especially important if a lobectomy or pneumonectomy is being considered. If resection is being undertaken for tumor treatment, preoperative care includes evaluation of the type and extent of the tumor and the physical condition of the patient.[83]

BOX 24-11 **COLLABORATIVE MANAGEMENT:**
AIR LEAK DISORDERS

- Administer oxygen therapy
- Intubate patient as needed
- Initiate mechanical ventilation as needed
- Evacuate air from the pleural space
  - Percutaneous catheter attached to Heimlich valve
  - Chest tube to water seal or suction
- Maintain surveillance for complications
  - Acute respiratory failure
- Maintain the chest drainage system
- Provide comfort and emotional support

The evaluation of the patient's physical status should focus on the adequacy of cardiopulmonary function. The preoperative evaluation should include pulmonary function tests to determine the patient's ability to manage with less lung tissue. Cardiac function also should be evaluated. Uncontrolled dysrhythmias, acute myocardial infarction, severe chronic heart failure, and unstable angina are all contraindications to surgery.[84]

SURGICAL CONSIDERATIONS

The type and location of surgery dictate the type of surgical approach that is used. The most common approach is the posterolateral thoracotomy, which allows for exposure of the lung and mediastinum. Alternative approaches include anterolateral thoracotomy and median sternotomy.[83]

Special care is taken to avoid drainage of blood or secretions into the unaffected lung during surgery, because such an occurrence could cause hypoxemia and cardiac dysfunction. A double-lumen endotracheal tube is used during the surgery to protect the unaffected lung from secretions and necrotic tumor fragments. To decrease the incidence of hypoxemia during the procedure, 5 to 10 cm H_2O of PEEP is maintained to the deflated lung. The deflated lung is intermittently ventilated during the procedure.[85]

COMPLICATIONS AND MEDICAL MANAGEMENT

A number of complications are associated with a lung resection. These include ARF, bronchopleural fistula, hemorrhage, cardiovascular disturbances, and mediastinal shift.

Acute Respiratory Failure. In the postoperative period, ARF may result from atelectasis or pneumonia. Atelectasis can occur as a result of anesthesia, the surgical procedure, immobilization, or pain. Treatment should be aimed at correcting the underlying problems and supporting gas exchange. Supplemental oxygen and mechanical ventilation with PEEP may be necessary.[85]

Bronchopleural Fistula. Development of a postoperative bronchopleural fistula is a major cause of mortality after a lung resection. A bronchopleural fistula develops when the suture line fails to secure occlusion of the bronchial stump and an opening develops into the pleural space. This can result from an imperfect stump closure, perforation of the stump (e.g., with a suction catheter), high pressure within the airways (e.g., caused by mechanical ventilation),[86] or infection.[87] During surgery, careful attention is given to isolating and closing the bronchus in an attempt to secure a lasting seal with subsequent stump healing.[83] Early extubation is encouraged to eliminate the possibility of perforation of the stump with high airway pressures.[86] Clinical manifestations of a bronchopleural fistula include shortness of breath and coughing up serosanguineous sputum. Immediate surgery is usually necessary to close the stump and prevent flooding of the remaining lung with fluid from the residual space.[87] If this occurs, the patient should be placed with the operative side down (remaining lung up), and a chest tube should be inserted to drain the residual space.[83]

TABLE 24-8 **Thoracic Operations**

Procedure	Definition	Indications
Pneumonectomy	Removal of entire lung with or without resection of the mediastinal lymph nodes	Malignant lesions Unilateral tuberculosis Extensive unilateral bronchiectasis Multiple lung abscesses Massive hemoptysis Bronchopleural fistula
Lobectomy	Resection of one or more lobes of lung	Lesions confined to a single lobe Pulmonary tuberculosis Bronchiectasis Lung abscesses or cysts Trauma
Segmental resection	Resection of bronchovascular segment of lung lobe	Small peripheral lesions Bronchiectasis Congenital cysts or blebs
Wedge resection	Removal of small wedge-shaped section of lung tissue	Small peripheral lesions (without lymph node involvement) Peripheral granulomas Pulmonary blebs
Bronchoplastic reconstruction (sleeve resection)	Resection of lung tissue and bronchus with end-to-end reanastomosis of bronchus	Small lesions involving the carina or major bronchus without evidence of metastasis May be combined with lobectomy

Continued

TABLE 24-8 Thoracic Operations—*cont'd*

Procedure	Definition	Indications
Lung volume reduction surgery	Resection of the most damaged portions of lung tissue, allowing more normal chest wall configuration	Severe emphysema
Bullectomy	Resection of a large bulla (an airspace >1 cm in diameter that formed as a result of pulmonary tissue destruction)	Severe emphysema with large bullae compressing surrounding tissue
Open lung biopsy	Resection of a small portion of the lung for biopsy	Failure of closed lung biopsy Removal of small lesions
Decortication	Removal of fibrous membrane from pleural surface of lung	Fibrothorax resulting from hemothorax or empyema
Drainage of empyema	Drainage of pus in the pleural space	Acute and chronic infections
Partial rib resection	Removal of one or more ribs to allow healing of underlying lung tissue	Chronic empyemic infections
Video-assisted thoracoscopy (VATS)	Endoscopic procedure performed through small incisions in the chest	Evaluation of pulmonary, pleural, mediastinal, or pericardial conditions Biopsy of lung, pleural, or mediastinal lesions Recurrent spontaneous pneumothorax Evacuation of emphysema, hemothorax, pleural effusion, or pericardial effusion Blebectomy or bullectomy Pleurodesis Sympathectomy Closure of bronchopleural fistula Lysis of adhesions

Hemorrhage. Hemorrhage is an early, life-threatening complication that can occur after a lung resection. It can result from bronchial or intercostal artery bleeding or disruption of a suture or clip around a pulmonary vessel.[86] Excessive chest tube drainage can signal excessive bleeding. During the immediate postoperative period, chest tube drainage should be measured every 15 minutes; the frequency is decreased as the patient stabilizes. If chest tube loss is greater than 100 mL/hr, if fresh blood is noted, or if a sudden increase in drainage occurs, hemorrhage should be suspected.

Cardiovascular Disturbances. Cardiovascular complications after thoracic surgery include dysrhythmias and pulmonary edema. Resections of a large lung area or a pneumonectomy may be followed by a rise in central venous pressure. With the loss of one lung, the right ventricle must empty its stroke volume into a vascular bed that has been reduced by 50%. This creates a higher-pressure system, which increases right ventricular workload and precipitates right ventricular failure. Depending on previous heart function, acute decompensation of both ventricles can result. Measures aimed at supporting cardiac function and avoiding intravascular volume excess are taken, including optimization of preload, afterload, and contractility with vasoactive agents.[86]

Nursing Diagnoses

Thoracic Surgery

- Ineffective Breathing Pattern related to decreased lung expansion
- Impaired Gas Exchange related to ventilation/perfusion mismatching or intrapulmonary shunting
- Impaired Gas Exchange related to alveolar hypoventilation
- Acute Pain related to transmission and perception of cutaneous, visceral, muscular, or ischemic impulses
- Anxiety related to threat to biologic, psychological, or social integrity
- Disturbed Body Image related to actual change in body structures, function, or appearance
- Compromised Family Coping related to critically ill family member

POSTOPERATIVE NURSING MANAGEMENT

Nursing care of the patient who has undergone thoracic surgery incorporates a number of nursing diagnoses (see the Nursing Diagnoses feature on Thoracic Surgery). Nursing interventions include optimizing oxygenation and ventilation, preventing atelectasis, monitoring chest tubes, assisting the patient to return to an adequate activity level, providing comfort and emotional support, and maintaining surveillance for complications.

Optimizing Oxygenation and Ventilation. Nursing interventions to optimize oxygenation and ventilation include positioning, preventing desaturation during procedures, and promoting secretion clearance.

Preventing Atelectasis. Nursing interventions to prevent atelectasis include proper patient positioning and early ambulation, deep-breathing exercises, incentive spirometry, and pain management. The goal is to promote maximal lung ventilation and prevent hypoventilation.

Patient Positioning and Early Ambulation. The nurse should consider the surgical incision site and the type of surgery when positioning the patient. After a lobectomy, the patient should be turned onto the nonoperative side to promote $\dot{V}/\dot{Q}$ matching. When the good lung is dependent and blood flow is greater to the area with better ventilation, $\dot{V}/\dot{Q}$ matching is better. $\dot{V}/\dot{Q}$ mismatching results when the affected lung is positioned down, because blood flow is increased to an area with less ventilation. The patient should be turned frequently to promote secretion removal but should have the affected lung dependent for as little time as possible. The patient who has had a pneumonectomy should be positioned supine or on the operative side during the initial period. Turning onto the operative side promotes splinting of the incision and facilitates deep-breathing exercises. Tilting the patient slightly toward the unaffected side is possible, but the surgeon should indicate when free side-to-side positioning is safe.[87]

When sitting at the bedside or ambulating, patients must be encouraged to keep the thorax in straight alignment while they breathe deeply. This position best accommodates diaphragmatic descent and intercostal muscle action. The sitting or standing position provides enhanced ventilation to areas of the lung that are dependent in the supine position, accommodating maximal inflation and promoting gas exchange. Ambulation is essential in restoring lung function and should be initiated as soon as possible.[88]

Deep Breathing and Incentive Spirometry. Deep breathing and incentive spirometry should be performed regularly by patients who have undergone a thoracotomy. Deep breathing involves taking a deep breath and holding it for approximately 3 seconds or longer. Incentive spirometry involves taking at least 10 deep, effective breaths per hour using an incentive spirometer. These activities help reexpand collapsed lung tissue, promoting early resolution of the pneumothorax in patients with partial lung resections. The chest should be auscultated during inflation to ensure that all dependent parts of the lung are well ventilated and to help the patient understand the depth of breath necessary for optimal effect. Coughing, which should be encouraged only if secretions are present, assists in mobilizing secretions for removal.[88]

Pain Management. Pain can be a major problem after thoracic surgery. Pain can increase the workload of the heart, precipitate hypoventilation, and inhibit mobilization of secretions. Clinical manifestations of pain include tachypnea, tachycardia, elevated blood pressure, facial grimacing, splinting of the incision, hypoventilation, moaning, and restlessness. Several alternatives for pain management after thoracic surgery can be used. The two most common methods are systemic opioid administration and epidural opioid administration. Systemic opioids can be administered intravenously or by means of patient-controlled analgesia (PCA). The patient should be assisted with splinting the incision with a pillow or blanket when deep breathing and coughing. Splinting stabilizes the area and reduces pain when moving, deep breathing, or coughing.[89]

Maintaining the Chest Tube System. Chest tubes are placed after most thoracic surgery procedures to remove air and fluid. The drainage initially appears bloody and becomes serosanguineous and then serous over the first 2 to 3 days postoperatively. Approximately 100 to 300 mL of drainage should occur during the first 2 hours postoperatively, decreasing to less than 50 mL/hr over the next several hours. Routine stripping of chest tubes is not recommended, because excessive negative pressure can be generated in the chest. If blood clots are present in the drainage tubing or an obstruction is present, the chest tubes may be carefully milked. The chest tube may be placed to suction or water seal.[90]

During auscultation of the lungs, air leaks should be evaluated. In the early phase, an air leak is commonly heard over the affected area, because the pleura have not yet tightly sealed. As healing occurs, this leak should disappear. An increase in an air leak or the appearance of a new air leak should prompt investigation of the chest drainage system to discover whether air is leaking into the system from outside or originating from the incision. Increased air leaks not related to the thoracic drainage system may indicate disruption of sutures.[86]

Assisting Patient to Return to an Adequate Activity Level. Within a few days after surgery, range-of-motion exercises for the shoulder on the operative side should be performed. Patients frequently splint the operative side and avoid shoulder movement because of pain. If immobility is allowed, stiffening of the shoulder joint can result. This is referred to as *frozen shoulder*, and the patient may require physical therapy and rehabilitation to regain satisfactory range of motion of the shoulder joint.[87]

Usually on the day after surgery, the patient is able to sit in a chair. Activity should be systematically increased, with attention to the patient's activity tolerance. With adequate pulmonary function before surgery and a surgical approach designed to preserve respiratory function, full return to previous activity levels is possible. This may take as long as 6 months to 1 year, depending on the tissue resected and the patient's general condition.[83]

LONG-TERM MECHANICAL VENTILATOR DEPENDENCE

DESCRIPTION

Long-term mechanical ventilator dependence (LTMVD) is a secondary disorder that occurs when a patient requires assisted ventilation longer than expected given the patient's underlying condition.[91] It is the result of complex medical problems that do not allow the weaning process to take place in a normal and timely manner. A review of the literature reveals a great deal of confusion as to the definition of LTMVD, particularly with regard to an actual time frame. In 2005, the National Association for Medical Direction of Respiratory Care (NAMDRC) consensus panel recommended that LTMVD (which they

Nursing Diagnoses

Long-Term Mechanical Ventilation Dependence

- Impaired Spontaneous Ventilation related to respiratory muscle fatigue or neuromuscular impairment
- Dysfunctional Ventilatory Weaning Response related to physical, psychosocial, or situational factors
- Risk for Aspiration
- Imbalanced Nutrition: Less Than Body Requirements related to lack of exogenous nutrients or increased metabolic demand
- Risk for Infection
- Acute Confusion related to sensory overload, sensory deprivation, and sleep pattern disturbance
- Disturbed Body Image related to functional dependence on life-sustaining technology
- Relocation Stress Syndrome related to transfer out of the intensive care unit
- Powerlessness related to lack of control over current situation or disease progression
- Compromised Family Coping related to critically ill family member

referred to as *prolonged mechanical ventilation*) be defined as the need for at least 21 consecutive days of mechanical ventilation for 6 or more hours per day.[92]

ETIOLOGY AND PATHOPHYSIOLOGY

A wide variety of physiologic and psychological factors contribute to the development of LTMVD. Physiologic factors include those conditions that result in decreased gas exchange, increased ventilatory workload, increased ventilatory demand, decreased ventilatory drive, and increased respiratory muscle fatigue (Box 24-12).[93] Psychological factors include those conditions that result in loss of breathing pattern control, lack of motivation and confidence, and delirium (Box 24-13).[94] The development of LTMVD also is affected by the severity and duration of the patient's current illness and any underlying chronic health problems.[95]

MEDICAL AND NURSING MANAGEMENT

The goal of medical and nursing management of the patient with LTMVD is successful weaning. The Third National Study Group on Weaning from Mechanical Ventilation, sponsored by the American Association of Critical-Care Nurses, proposed the Weaning Continuum Model, which divides weaning into three stages: preweaning, weaning process, and weaning outcome.[96] It is within this framework that the management of the LTMVD patient is described. The common nursing diagnoses for this patient population are listed in the Nursing Diagnoses feature on Long-Term Mechanical Ventilation.

Preweaning Stage. For the LTMVD patient, the preweaning phase consists of resolving the precipitating event that necessitated ventilatory assistance and preventing the physiologic and psychological factors that can interfere with weaning. Before any attempts at weaning are made, the patient should be assessed for weaning readiness, an approach should be determined, and a method should be selected.[92,95]

BOX 24-12 PHYSIOLOGIC FACTORS CONTRIBUTING TO LONG-TERM MECHANICAL VENTILATION DEPENDENCE

- Decreased gas exchange
  - Ventilation/perfusion mismatching
  - Intrapulmonary shunting
  - Alveolar hypoventilation
  - Anemia
  - Acute heart failure
- Increased ventilatory workload
  - Decreased lung compliance
  - Increased airway resistance
  - Small endotracheal tube
  - Decreased ventilatory sensitivity
  - Improper positioning
  - Abdominal distention
  - Dyspnea
- Increased ventilatory demand
  - Increased pulmonary dead space
  - Increased metabolic demands
- Improper ventilator mode/settings
- Metabolic acidosis
- Overfeeding
- Decreased ventilatory drive
  - Respiratory alkalosis
  - Metabolic alkalosis
  - Hypothyroidism
  - Sedatives
- Malnutrition
- Increased respiratory muscle fatigue
  - Increased ventilatory workload
  - Increased ventilatory demand
  - Malnutrition
  - Hypokalemia
  - Hypomagnesemia
  - Hypophosphatemia
  - Hypothyroidism
  - Critical illness polyneuropathy
  - Inadequate muscle rest

BOX 24-13 PSYCHOLOGICAL FACTORS CONTRIBUTING TO LONG-TERM MECHANICAL VENTILATION DEPENDENCE

- Loss of breathing pattern control
  - Anxiety
  - Fear
  - Dyspnea
  - Pain
  - Ventilator asynchrony
  - Lack of confidence in ability to breathe
- Lack of motivation and confidence
  - Inadequate trust in staff
- Depersonalization
- Hopelessness
- Powerlessness
- Depression
- Inadequate communication
- Delirium
  - Sensory overload
  - Sensory deprivation
  - Sleep deprivation
  - Pain
  - Medications

Weaning Preparedness. The patient should be physiologically and psychologically prepared to initiate the weaning process by addressing those factors that can interfere with weaning. Aggressive medical management to prevent and treat $\dot{V}/\dot{Q}$ mismatching, intrapulmonary shunting, anemia, cardiac failure, decreased lung compliance, increased airway resistance, acid-base disturbances, hypothyroidism, abdominal distention, and electrolyte imbalances should be initiated. Interventions to decrease the work of breathing should be implemented, such as replacing a small endotracheal tube with a larger tube or a tracheostomy, suctioning airway secretions, administering bronchodilators, optimizing the ventilator settings and trigger sensitivity, and positioning the patient in straight alignment with the head of the bed elevated at least 30 degrees. Enteral or parenteral nutrition should be started and the patient's nutritional state optimized. Physical therapy should be initiated for the patient with critical illness polyneuropathy, because increased mobility facilitates weaning. A means of communication should be established with the patient. Sedatives can be administered to provide anxiety control, but the avoidance of respiratory depression is critical.[97]

Weaning Readiness. Although a variety of methods for assessing weaning readiness have been developed, none has proved to be very accurate in predicting weaning success in the patient with LTMVD. One study did indicate that the presence of left ventricular dysfunction, fluid imbalance, and nutritional deficiency increased the duration of mechanical ventilation. Another study suggested that upward trending of the albumin level may be predictive of weaning success. Because so many variables can affect a patient's ability to wean, any assessment of weaning readiness should incorporate these variables. Cardiac function, gas exchange, pulmonary mechanics, nutritional status, electrolyte and fluid balance, and motivation should all be considered when making the decision to wean. This assessment should be ongoing, to reflect the dynamic nature of the process.[98]

Weaning Approach. Although weaning from short-term mechanical ventilation is a relatively simple process that can usually be accomplished with a nurse and respiratory therapist, weaning of the LTMVD patient is a much more complex process that usually requires a multidisciplinary team approach. Multidisciplinary weaning teams that use a coordinated and collaborative approach to weaning have demonstrated improved patient outcomes and decreased weaning times. The team should consist of a physician, a nurse, a respiratory therapist, a dietitian, a physical therapist, and a case manager, clinical outcomes manager, or clinical nurse specialist. Additional members, if possible, should include an occupational therapist, a speech therapist, a discharge planner, and a social worker. Working together, the team members should develop a comprehensive plan of care for the patient that is efficient, consistent, progressive, and cost-effective.[99] Several studies have demonstrated successful weaning through the use of nurse- and respiratory therapist–managed protocols.[100]

Collaborative management of the patient requiring long-term mechanical ventilation is outlined in Figure 24-8.

Weaning Method. A variety of weaning methods are available, but no one method has consistently been proven to be superior to the others. These methods include T-tube (T-piece), constant positive airway pressure (CPAP), pressure support ventilation (PSV), and SIMV. One recent multicenter study lends evidence to support the use of PSV for weaning over T-tube or SIMV weaning. Often these methods are used in combination with each other, such as SIMV with PSV, CPAP with PSV, or SIMV with CPAP.[93,95]

Weaning Process Stage. For the LTMVD patient, the weaning process phase consists of initiating the weaning method selected and minimizing the physiologic and psychological factors that can interfere with weaning.[95] It is imperative that the patient not become exhausted during this phase, because this could result in a setback in the weaning process.[97] During this phase, the patient is assessed for weaning progress and signs of weaning intolerance.[92]

Weaning Initiation. Weaning should be initiated in the morning, when the patient is rested. Before starting the weaning process, the patient is provided with an explanation of how the process works, a description of the sensations to expect, and reassurances that he or she will be closely monitored and returned to the original ventilator mode and settings if any difficulty occurs.[95] This information should be reinforced with each weaning attempt. One study showed that family presence during the weaning trial was beneficial and that the trials were longer when the family was present.[101]

T-tube and CPAP weaning are accomplished by removing the patient from the ventilator and then placing the patient on a T-tube or on CPAP mode for a specified duration of time (*weaning trial*) for a specified number of times per day. When the weaning trial is over, the patient is returned to the ACV or other mode and allowed to rest, to prevent respiratory muscle fatigue. Gradually, the duration and frequency of weaning are increased, until the patient is able to breathe spontaneously for 24 hours. If PSV is used in conjunction with CPAP, the PSV is initially set to provide the patient with an assisted tidal volume of 10 to 12 mL/kg, and this is gradually reduced until a level of 6 to 8 cm H_2O of pressure support is achieved. SIMV and PSV weaning are accomplished by gradually decreasing the number of breaths or the amount of pressure support the patient receives by a specified amount until the patient is able to breathe spontaneously for 24 hours.[95]

Weaning Progress. Weaning progress can be evaluated by various methods. With a weaning method that gradually withdraws ventilatory support, such as SIMV or PSV, progress can be evaluated by measuring the percentage of the minute ventilation requirement that is provided by the ventilator. If the percentage steadily decreases, weaning is progressing. With a weaning method that removes ventilatory support, such as T-tube or CPAP, progress can be evaluated by measuring the amount of time the patient remains free from support. If the time steadily increases, weaning is progressing.[95]

Weaning Intolerance. After the weaning process has begun, the patient should be continuously assessed for signs of intolerance. The presence of these signs indicates when to place the patient back on the ventilator or when to return the patient to the previous ventilator settings. Commonly used indicators are dyspnea, accessory muscle use, restlessness, anxiety, change in facial expression, changes in heart rate and blood pressure, rapid and shallow breathing, and discomfort.[98] Table 24-9 list the weaning intolerance indicators and actions that can be taken to control or prevent them.

Facilitative Therapies. Additional therapies may be needed to facilitate weaning if the patient is having difficulty making progress. These therapies include ventilatory muscle training and biofeedback. Inspiratory muscle training is used to enhance the strength and endurance of the respiratory muscles. Biofeedback can be used to promote relaxation and assist in the management of dyspnea and anxiety.[95]

LONG TERM DEPENDENCE ON MECHANICAL VENTILATION*

DATE Criteria —Vent >3 days —Medically stable —Unsuccessful initial weaning attempt	WEANING PHASE	EXTENDING WEANING PHASE	EXTUBATION/ DECANNULATION	POST WEANING PHASE VENTILATOR FACILITY PLACEMENT	TERMINAL WEANING
CONSULTS	Pulmonary Physician/Intensivist Wean Team assessment	Consider Psychiatric evaluation Wean Team rounds qweek	SNF Pulmonary Coordinator	Placement Coordinator	Chaplain
DIAGNOSTICS/ MONITORING	As ordered ECG monitoring Continuous SpO2 monitoring VS with weaning and q2-4h	As ordered ↑↑↑ VS with weaning and q8-12h	As ordered D/C ECG monitoring Spot check SpO2 qam VS q8-12h	As ordered D/C ECG monitoring Continuous SpO2 monitoring VS q8-12h	D/C diagnostics ECG monitoring D/C SpO2 monitoring D/C routine VS
TREATMENTS	Pressure reduction therapy or lateral rotation therapy	↑	↑	↑	↑
MEDICATIONS	Anxiety management Dyspnea management Pain management Sleep management Stress ulcer prophylaxis DVT prophylaxis Additional medications as ordered Bronchodilators as ordered	↑↑↑↑↑↑ Antidepressant therapy	↑↑↑↑↑↑↑	↑↑↑↑↑↑↑↑	Pain control Dyspnea control D/C all other medications
RESPIRATORY	Continue mechanical ventilation Maintain endotracheal tube Initiate/progress weaning trials to extubation or tracheostomy inserted Monitor for weaning intolerance Monitor for airway/cuff problems Monitor secretions/suction prn	Place tracheostomy Progress weaning trials to T-piece ↑↑↑	D/C mechanical ventilation Extubate or button trach/decannulate IS q1-2h WA; advancing to q4h WA Monitor for respiratory distress ↑↑	Place on home ventilator Tracheostomy Continue/progress weaning trials till transfer Monitor for weaning intolerance ↑↑	D/C mechanical ventilation Tracheostomy D/C weaning trials
ACTIVITY	Maintain HOB 30-45 Provide regular sleep periods Initiate PROM q4h WA Dangle/OOB in chair qd	Sleep 6-8 hours/night OOB in chair 2-3x/d Ambulate with PT/RT assist Bath patient prior to 2200 ↑	↑↑ D/C PROM Progressive ambulation ↑	↑↑ Continue PROM q4h WA ↑↑↑	↑ Complete bed rest D/C all activity
PHYSICAL THERAPY	PT evaluation Initiate/progress therapy to qd Strengthening/balance	PT reevaluation Progress therapy to 2x/d (if needed) ↑ Transfer/pre-gait training	Progress to 3h/d if going to Rehab ↑↑	Continue PT plan ↑	D/C therapy

Figure 24-8 Interdisciplinary plan of care for long-term mechanical ventilation dependence.

*This clinical pathway is a tool to assist health care providers in achieving quality patient outcomes by providing appropriate and timely patient care. It is intended to establish a community standard of care, replace a clinician's medical judgment, establish a protocol for all patients, or exclude alternative therapies.

SNF, skilled nursing facility; *ECG*, electrocardiogram; *D/C*, discontinue; *VS*, vital signs; *DVT*, deep vein thrombosis; *WA*, when awake; *HOB*, head of bed; *PT*, physical therapy; *RT*, respiratory therapy; *ST*, speech therapy; *P-M*, Passy-Muir; *OT*, occupational therapy; *M-F*, Monday through Friday; *UE*, upper extremity; *ADLs*, activities of daily living; *RD*, registered dietitian; *I&O*, intake and output; *IV*, intravenous; *PEG*, percutaneous endoscopic gastrostomy; *PICC*, peripherally inserted central catheter; *LCSW*, licensed clinical social worker; *SO*, significant other; *CM*, case manager; *WT*, weight.

Continued

LONG TERM DEPENDENCE ON MECHANICAL VENTILATION*

DATE	WEANING PHASE	EXTENDING WEANING PHASE	EXTUBATION/ DECANNULATION	POST WEANING PHASE	
				VENTILATOR FACILITY PLACEMENT	**TERMINAL WEANING**
SPEECH THERAPY		ST evaluation for P-M valve and swallowing Initiate/progress P-M valve to at least 60 min	ST reevaluation for swallowing Initiate swallowing therapy if positive for aspiration	ST reevaluation Continue ST plan	D/C therapy
OCCUPATIONAL THERAPY	OT evaluation Initiate/progress therapy to 3×/wk Initiate self-hygiene/grooming	OT reevaluation Progress therapy to qd (M-F) Hygiene, grooming, and sitting Graded UE strengthening	Dress and bathing training Stand for ADLs	Continue OT plan	D/C therapy
NUTRITION	RD evaluation Initiate/progress nutritional support to enteral feedings Monitor I&O qd Weigh patient qwk Insert small-bore feeding tube Maintain IV access	RD reevaluation Continue enteral feedings/start oral feedings if negative for aspiration Place PEG Insert PICC	Progress to total oral feedings if negative for aspiration D/C feeding tube and IV access when no longer needed	Continue RD plan Maintain PEG Maintain PICC	D/C nutritional support D/C I&O D/C weights
SOCIAL SERVICES	LCSW evaluation Identify sources of support and prior level of functioning Support for SO Conduct initial SO conferences	LCSW reevaluation Maintain communication with SO Conduct follow-up SO conference	Conduct SO conferences as needed	Continue LCSW plan Conduct transfer SO conference	
TEACHING	Orient patient/SO to environment/ procedures/equipment Explain weaning plan to patient/SO		Initiate/complete disease management education Explain discharge plan to patient/SO	Orient patient/SO to environment/procedures/equipment Explain transfer plan to patient/SO	Explain terminal weaning to patient (as appropriate)/SO
DISCHARGE PLANNING	CM evaluation Clarify payor issues Transfer to long-term ventilator unit	CM reevaluation Initiate referral process (as indicated) Initiate transfer summary form Transfer to acute care no earlier than 72h after D/C ventilator	Complete referral process Complete transfer summary form Discharge to SNF/rehab/home (with home care) no earlier than 72h after D/C tracheostomy	Arrange transportation Transfer/discharge to ventilator facility	
EXPECTED OUTCOMES To be reviewed qwk at WT rounds	• LTMV-WT evaluation completed • Skin remains intact • Anxiety controlled • Rests at regular periods • OOB in chair qd • Participates in PT qd • Participates in OT 3×/wk • Meets needs on enteral nutrition • Initial SO conference done • Transferred to 2 West • Weaned to T-piece/tracheostomy completed <21 days after intubation • Absence of complications	• Skin remains intact • Anxiety controlled • Rest 6 hours at night • OOB in chair 2×/d • Participates in PT 2×/d • Participates in OT qd (M-F) • Uses P-M valve for 60 min • Swallowing evaluated before oral feeding initiated • Meets needs on enteral nutrition • Follow-up SO conference done • Transferred to 4T • Weaned to T-piece • Absence of complications	• Extubated/decannulated without difficulty • Trach buttoned prior to decannulation • Discharged no earlier than 72h after decannulation • Patient education completed • Discharged without delay • Absence of complications	• Transferred/discharged without delay • Absence of complications	• SO conference done • Dyspnea controlled • Life support withdrawn without problems

Figure 24-8, cont'd

TABLE 24-9 Weaning Intolerance Indications and Interventions

Indicator	Cause	Intervention
Pulmonary Signs (Emotional)		
Altered breathing pattern	Inadequate understanding of weaning process	Build trust in staff; consistent care providers
Dyspnea intensity		Encouragement; concrete goals for extubation
Change in facial expression	Inability to control breathing pattern	Involve patient in process and planning daily activities
		Efficient communication established
	Environmental factors	Organize care; avoid interruptions during weaning
		Adequate sleep
		Calm, caring presence of nurse; nonsedating anxiolytics
		Measure dyspnea
		Fan; music
		Biofeedback; relaxation; breathing control
		Family involvement; normalizing daily activities
Pulmonary Signs (Physiologic)		
Accessory muscle use	Airway obstruction	Suction/air-mask bag unit ventilation; manually ventilate patient
Prolonged expiration	Secretions/atelectasis	
Asynchronous movements of chest and abdomen	Bronchospasm	Bronchodilators
	Patient position	Sitting upright in bed or chair or per patient preference
Retractions	ET tube kinked	
Facial expression changes	Increased workload or muscle	
Dyspnea	Fatigue	
Shortened inspiratory time	Caloric intake	Dietary assessment
Increased breathing frequency, decreased V_T	Electrolyte imbalances	Assess electrolytes; give replacements as necessary
	Inadequate rest	Rest between weaning trials (i.e., SIMV frequency rate >5)
	Patient/ventilator interactions	Assess ventilator settings (i.e., flow rate, trigger sensitivity)
	Increased V_E requirement	Muscle training if appropriate
	Infection	Check for infection (treat if indicated)
	Overfeeding	Appropriate caloric intake
	Respiratory alkalosis	Baseline ABGs achieved (ventilate according to pH)
	Anxiety	Coaching to regularize breathing pattern; give nonsedating anxiolytics
	Pain	Judicious use of analgesics
CNS Changes		
Restless or irritable	Hypoxemia/hypercarbia	Increase FIO_2
Decreased responsiveness		Return to mechanical ventilation
		Discern cause and treat
Cardiovascular Deterioration		
Excessive change in BP or HR	Heart failure	Diuretics as ordered
	Increase venous return	Beta-blockers
Dysrhythmias	Ischemia	Increase FIO_2
Angina		Return to mechanical ventilation
Dyspnea		Discern cause and treat

Modified from Knebel AR: When weaning from mechanical ventilation fails, *Am J Crit Care* 1(3):19, 1992.

ABGs, arterial blood gases; *BP*, blood pressure; *CNS*, central nervous system; *ET*, endotracheal; FIO_2, fraction of inspired oxygen; *HR*, heart rate; *SIMV*, synchronized intermittent mandatory ventilation; V_E, respiratory minute volume; V_T, tidal volume.

Weaning Outcome Stage. Two outcomes are possible for a patient with LTMVD: weaning completed and incomplete weaning.[95]

Weaning Completed. Weaning is deemed successful when the patient is able to breathe spontaneously for 24 hours without ventilatory support. After this occurs, the patient may be extubated or decannulated at any time, although this is not necessary for weaning to be considered successful.[91]

Incomplete Weaning. Weaning is deemed incomplete if a patient has reached a plateau in the weaning process (5 days at the same ventilatory support level without any changes) despite measures to manage the physiologic and psychological factors that impede weaning. The patient is unable to breathe spontaneously for 24 hours without full or partial ventilatory support. After this occurs, the patient should be placed in a subacute ventilator facility or discharged home on a ventilator with home care nursing follow-up.[91]

Summary

Acute Respiratory Failure

- ARF is a clinical condition in which the pulmonary system fails to maintain adequate gas exchange; it results from a deficiency in the performance of the pulmonary system.
- Hypoxemia is the hallmark of ARF and is the result of impaired gas exchange due to alveolar hypoventilation, $\dot{V}/\dot{Q}$ mismatching, or intrapulmonary shunting.
- Medical management focuses on treatment of the underlying cause, promotion of adequate gas exchange, correction of acidosis, initiation of nutrition support, and prevention of complications (i.e., ischemic-anoxic encephalopathy, cardiac dysrhythmias, venous thromboembolism, and gastrointestinal bleeding).
- Nursing actions include optimizing oxygenation and ventilation (by positioning, preventing desaturation, and promoting secretion clearance), providing comfort and emotional support, and maintaining surveillance for complications.

Acute Lung Injury

- ALI is characterized by noncardiac pulmonary edema and disruption of the alveolar-capillary membrane as a result of injury to the pulmonary vasculature or the airways.
- The hallmark of ALI is refractory hypoxemia.
- Medical management focuses on treatment of the underlying cause, promotion of gas exchange, support of tissue oxygenation, and prevention of complications.
- Nursing actions include optimizing oxygenation and ventilation, providing comfort and emotional support, and maintaining surveillance for complications.

Pneumonia

- Pneumonia is an acute inflammation of the lung parenchyma caused by an infectious agent that can lead to alveolar consolidation and can be classified as community acquired or hospital acquired.

- Medical management focuses on the initiation of antibiotic therapy, administration of oxygen and mechanical ventilation, management of fluids and nutrition support, and treatment of complications.
- Nursing actions include optimizing oxygenation and ventilation, preventing the spread of infection, providing comfort and emotional support, and maintaining surveillance for complications.

Aspiration Pneumonitis

- Aspiration pneumonitis is the presence of abnormal toxic substances in the airways and alveoli resulting in injury to the lungs.
- Medical management focuses on clearance of the toxic substance from the airways, support of oxygenation, and maintenance of hemodynamics.
- Nursing actions include optimizing oxygenation and ventilation, preventing further aspiration events, providing comfort and emotional support, and maintaining surveillance for complications.

Pulmonary Embolism

- A PE occurs when a clot (thrombotic embolus) or other matter (nonthrombotic embolus) lodges in the pulmonary arterial system, disrupting the blood flow to a region of the lungs.
- Medical management focuses on prevention of the recurrence of PE, initiation of clot dissolution, reversal of the effects of pulmonary hypertension, promotion of gas exchange, and prevention of complications.
- Nursing actions include optimizing oxygenation and ventilation, monitoring for bleeding, providing comfort and emotional support, and maintaining surveillance for complications.

Status Asthmaticus

- Status asthmaticus is a severe asthma attack that fails to respond to conventional therapy with bronchodilators; it may result in ARF.
- Medical management focuses on support of oxygenation (by bronchodilators, corticosteroids, and oxygen therapy) and ventilation.
- Nursing actions include optimizing oxygenation and ventilation, providing comfort and emotional support, and maintaining surveillance for complications.

Air Leak Disorders

- Air leak disorders consist of those conditions that result in extraalveolar air accumulation; they are classified into two categories, pneumothorax and barotrauma/volutrauma.
- Two conditions that require emergency intervention for immediate relief are a tension pneumothorax and a tension pneumopericardium.
- Nursing actions include optimizing oxygenation and ventilation, maintaining the chest tube system, providing comfort and emotional support, and maintaining surveillance for complications.

Thoracic Surgery

- Thoracic surgery refers to a number of surgical procedures that involve opening the thoracic cavity (thoracotomy) or the organs of respiration, or both; indications for thoracic surgery range from tumors and abscesses to repair of the esophagus and of thoracic vessels.
- Before surgery, a complete evaluation of the patient is needed to determine the appropriateness of surgery as a treatment and whether lung tissue can be removed without jeopardizing respiratory function.
- The most common approach is the posterolateral thoracotomy, which allows for exposure of the lung and mediastinum.
- Complications of a lung resection include ARF, bronchopleural fistula, hemorrhage, cardiovascular disturbances, and mediastinal shift.
- Nursing actions include optimizing oxygenation and ventilation, preventing atelectasis, monitoring chest tubes, assisting the patient to return to an adequate activity level, providing comfort and emotional support, and maintaining surveillance for complications.

Long-term Mechanical Ventilation Dependence

- LTMVD is a secondary disorder that occurs when a patient requires assisted ventilation for longer than expected given the patient's underlying condition.
- Weaning is can be divided into three stages: preweaning, weaning process, and weaning outcome.
- The preweaning phase consists of resolving the precipitating event that necessitated ventilatory assistance and preventing the physiologic and psychological factors that can interfere with weaning.
- The weaning process phase consists of initiating the weaning method selected and minimizing the physiologic and psychological factors that can interfere with weaning.
- Weaning is deemed successful when the patient is able to breathe spontaneously for 24 hours without ventilatory support.

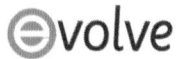 Be sure to check out the bonus material, including free self-assessment exercises, on the Evolve web site at http://evolve.elsevier.com/Urden/.

References

1. Aboussouan LS: Respiratory failure and the need for ventilatory support. In Wilkins RL, Stoller JK, Kacmarek RM, editors: *Egan's fundamentals of respiratory care*, ed 9, St Louis, 2009, Mosby.
2. Flaatten H et al: Outcome after acute respiratory failure is more dependent on dysfunction in other vital organs than on severity of the respiratory failure, *Crit Care* 7:R72, 2003.
3. Vincent JL et al: The epidemiology of acute respiratory failure in critically ill patient, *Chest* 121:1602, 2002.
4. Balk R, Bone RC: Classification of acute respiratory failure, *Med Clin North Am* 67:551, 1983.
5. Curtis JR, Hudson LD: Emergent assessment and management of acute respiratory failure in COPD, *Clin Chest Med* 15:481, 1994.
6. Raju P, Manthous CA: The pathogenesis of respiratory failure, *Respir Care Clin North Am* 6:195, 2000.
7. Wagner PD, West JD: Ventilation, blood flow and gas exchange. In Mason RJ et-al, editors: *Textbook of respiratory medicine*, ed 4, Philadelphia, 2005, Saunders.
8. Levy MM: Pathophysiology of oxygen delivery in respiratory failure, *Chest* 28(5 Suppl 2):547S, 2005.
9. Sigillito RJ, DeBlieux: Evaluation and initial management of the patient in respiratory distress, *Emerg Med Clin North Am* 21:239, 2003.
10. Dakin J, Griffiths M: The pulmonary physician in critical care 1: pulmonary investigations for acute respiratory failure, *Thorax* 57:79, 2002.
11. Misasi RS, Keyes JL: Matching and mismatching ventilation and perfusion in the lung, *Crit Care Nurse* 16(3):23, 1996.
12. Barreiro TJ, Gemmel DJ: Noninvasive ventilation, *Crit Care Clin* 23:201, 2007.
13. Peñuelas O et al: Noninvasive positive pressure ventilation in acute respiratory failure, *CMAJ*, 177:1211, 2007.
14. Soo Hoo GW et al: Hypercapnic respiratory failure in COPD patients: response to therapy, *Chest* 117:169, 2000.
15. Ward NS, Dushay KM: Clinical concise review: mechanical ventilation of patients with chronic obstructive pulmonary disease, *Crit Care Med* 36:1614, 2008.
16. Grimes GC et al: Medications for COPD: a review of effectiveness, *Am Fam Physician* 76:1141, 2007.
17. Sessler CN, Vamey K: Patient-focused sedation and analgesia in the ICU, *Chest* 133:552, 2008.
18. Luer J: Sedation and neuromuscular blockade in mechanically ventilated patients. In Burns SM, editor: *Care of mechanically ventilated patients*, ed 2, Sudbury, MD, 2007, Jones and Bartlett.
19. Kwon KT, Tsai VW: Metabolic emergencies, *Emerg Med Clin North Am* 25:1041, 2007.
20. Oltermann MH: Nutrition support in the acutely ventilated patient, *Respir Care Clin North Am* 12:533, 2006.
21. Parrish CR et al: Nutritional support for mechanically ventilated patients. In Burns SM, editor: *Care of mechanically ventilated patients*, ed 2, Sudbury, MD, 2007, Jones and Bartlett.
22. Gunther ML et al: Pathophysiology of delirium in the intensive care unit, *Crit Care Clin* 24:45, 2008.
23. Frazier SK: Cardiovascular effects of mechanical ventilation and weaning, *Nurs Clin North Am* 43:1, 2008.
24. Francis CW: Prophylaxis for thromboembolism in hospitalized medical patients, *N Engl J Med* 356:1438, 2007.
25. Martin B: Prevention of gastrointestinal complications in the critically ill patient, *AACN Adv Crit Care* 18:158, 2007.
26. Wong WP: Use of body positioning in the mechanically ventilated patient with acute respiratory failure: application of Sackett's rules of evidence, *Physiother Theory Pract* 15(1):25, 1999.
27. Force TR et al: Patient position and motion strategies, *Respir Care Clin North Am* 4:665, 1998.
28. Lasater-Erhand M: The effect of patient position on arterial saturation, *Crit Care Nurse* 15(5):31, 1995.
29. Cosenza JJ, Norton LC: Secretion clearance: state-of-the-art from a nursing perspective, *Crit Care Nurse* 6(4):23, 1986.

30. Flanders SA, Collard HR, Saint S: Nosocomial pneumonia: state of the science, *Am J Infect Control* 34:84, 2006.

31. Krishnagopalan S et al: Body positioning of intensive care patients: clinical practice versus standards, *Crit Care Med* 30:2588, 2002.

32. Stiller K: Physiotherapy in intensive care: towards an evidence-based practice, *Chest* 118:1801, 2000.

33. McCool FD, Rosen M: Nonpharmacologic airway clearance therapies: ACCP evidence-based clinical practice guidelines, *Chest* 129(1 suppl):250S, 2006.

34. Krau SD: Making sense of multiple organ dysfunction syndrome, *Crit Care Nurs Clin North Am* 19:87, 2007.

35. Crouser ED, Fahy RJ: Acute lung injury, pulmonary edema, and multiple system organ failure. In Wilkins RL, Stoller JK, Kacmarek RM, editors: *Egan's fundamentals of respiratory care*, ed 9, St Louis, 2009, Mosby.

36. Bernard GR et al: The American-European consensus conference on ARDS: definitions, mechanisms, relevant outcomes, and clinical trial coordination, *Am J Respir Crit Care Med* 149:818, 1994.

37. Jain R, DalNogare A: Pharmacological therapy for acute respiratory distress syndrome, *Mayo Clin Proc* 81:205, 2006.

38. George KJ: A systematic approach to care: adult respiratory distress syndrome, *J Trauma Nurs* 15:19, 2008.

39. Cheng IW, Matthay MA: Acute lung injury and the acute respiratory distress syndrome, *Crit Care Clin* 19:693, 2003.

40. Taylor MM: ARDS diagnosis and management, *Dimens Crit Care Nurs* 24:197, 2005.

41. Perina DG: Noncardiogenic pulmonary edema, *Emerg Med Clin North Am* 21:385, 2003.

42. Hemmila MR, Napolitano LM: Severe respiratory failure: advanced treatment options, *Crit Care Med* 34:S278, 2006.

43. Malhotra A: Low-tidal-volume ventilation in the acute respiratory distress syndrome, *N Engl J Med* 357:1113, 2007.

44. Yilmaz M, Gajic O: Optimal ventilator settings in acute lung injury and acute respiratory distress syndrome, *Eur J Anaesthesiol* 25:89, 2008.

45. Chan KP et al: High-frequency oscillatory ventilation for adult patients with ARDS, *Chest* 131:1907, 2007.

46. Peek GJ et al: CESAR: conventional ventilatory support vs extracorporeal membrane oxygenation for severe adult respiratory failure, BMC Health Serv Res 6:163, 2006.

47. Liu KD, Matthay MA: Advances in critical care for the nephrologist: acute lung injury/ARDS, *Clin J Am Soc Nephrol* 3:578, 2008.

48. Davidson WJ et al: Exogenous pulmonary surfactant for the treatment of adult patients with acute respiratory distress syndrome: results of a meta-analysis, *Crit Care* 10:R41, 2006.

49. Bream-Rouwenhorst HR et al: Recent developments in the management of acute respiratory distress syndrome in adults, *Am J Health Syst Pharm* 65:29, 2008.

50. Kacmarek RM et al: Partial liquid ventilation in adult patients with acute respiratory distress syndrome, *Am J Respir Crit Care Med* 173:882, 2006.

51. Alsaghir AH, Martin CM: Effect of prone positioning in patients with acute respiratory distress syndrome: a meta-analysis, *Crit Care Med* 36:603, 2008.

52. Pimentel L, McPherson SJ: Community-acquired pneumonia in the emergency department: a practical approach to diagnosis and management, *Emerg Med Clin North Am* 21:395, 2003.

53. Baudouin SV: The pulmonary physician in critical care. 3: critical care management of community acquired pneumonia, *Thorax* 57:267, 2002.

54. Rello J et al: Etiology of ventilator-associated pneumonia, *Clin Chest Med* 26:87, 2005.

55. Apisarnthanarak A, Mundy LM: Etiology of community-acquired pneumonia, *Clin Chest Med* 26:47, 2005.

56. Mandell LA et al: Infectious Diseases Society of America/American Thoracic Society consensus guidelines on the management of community-acquired pneumonia in adults, *Clin Infect Dis* 44(suppl 2):S27, 2007.

57. Miskovich-Riddle L, Keresztes PA: CAP management guidelines, *Nurse Pract* 31:43, 2006.

58. Tarver RD et al: Radiology of community-acquired pneumonia, *Radiol Clin North Am* 43:497, 2005.

59. Pines JM: Timing of antibiotics for acute, severe infections, *Emerg Med Clin North Am* 26:245, 2008.

60. Anantham D et al: Clinical review: independent lung ventilation in critical care, *Crit Care* 9:594, 2005.

61. Johnson JL, Hirsch CS: Aspiration pneumonia, *Postgrad Med* 113(3):99, 2003.

62. Marik PE: Aspiration pneumonitis and aspiration pneumonia, *N Engl J Med* 344:665, 2001.

63. Tietjen PA et al: Aspiration emergencies, *Clin Chest Med* 15:117, 1994.

64. Metheny NA: Strategies to prevent aspiration-related pneumonia in tube-fed patients, *Respir Care Clin* 12:603, 2006.

65. Piazza G, Goldhaber SZ: Acute pulmonary embolism. Part 1. Epidemiology and diagnosis, *Circulation* 114:e28, 2006.

66. Carlbom DJ, Davidson BL: Pulmonary embolism in the critically ill, *Chest* 132:313, 2007.

67. Dweik RA, Arroliga AC: Pulmonary vascular disease. In Wilkins RL, Stoller JK, Kacmarek, editors: *Egan's fundamentals of respiratory care*, ed 9, St Louis, 2008, Mosby.

68. Tapson AV: Acute pulmonary embolism, *N Engl J Med* 358:1037, 2008.

69. Piazza G, Goldhaber SZ: Acute pulmonary embolism. Part 2. Treatment and prophylaxis, *Circulation* 114:e42, 2006.

70. Agnelli G et al: Thrombolysis vs heparin in the treatment of pulmonary embolism: a clinical outcome–based meta-analysis, *Arch Intern Med* 162:2537, 2002.

71. Kucher N: Catheter embolectomy for acute pulmonary embolism, *Chest* 132:657, 2007.

72. Holgate ST: The mechanisms, diagnosis, and management of severe asthma in adults, *Lancet* 368:780, 2006.

73. Sims JM: An overview of asthma, *Dimens Crit Care Nurs* 25:264, 2006.

74. Cairns CB: Acute asthma exacerbations: phenotypes and management, *Clin Chest Med* 27:99, 2006.

75. Restrepo RD, Peters J: Near-fatal asthma: recognition and management, *Curr Opin Pulm Med* 14:13, 2008.

76. Strange C: Pleural diseases. In Wilkins RL, Stoller JK, Kacmarek, editors: *Egan's fundamentals of respiratory care*, ed 9, St Louis, 2008, Mosby.

77. Adams AB, Simonson DA, Dries DJ: Ventilator-induced lung injury, *Respir Care Clin North Am* 9:343, 2003.

78. Specht NL, Stoller JK: A synopsis of thoracic imaging. In Wilkins RL, Stoller JK, Kacmarek, editors: *Egan's fundamentals of respiratory care*, ed 9, St Louis, 2008, Mosby.

79. Jones R: Recognition of pneumoperitoneum using bedside ultrasound in critically ill patients presenting with acute abdominal pain, *Am J Emerg Med* 25:838, 2007.

80. Takada K et al: Management of spontaneous pneumomediastinum based on clinical experience of 25 cases, *Respir Med* 102:1329, 2008.

81. Haan JM, Scalea TM: Tension pneumopericardium: a case report and a review of the literature, *Am Surg* 72:330, 2006.

82. Horsley A et al: Efficacy and complications of small-bore, wire-guided chest drains, *Chest* 130:1857, 2006.

83. Gregory Crum BS: Thoracic surgery. In Rothrock JC, editor: *Alexander's care of the patient in surgery*, ed 13, St Louis, 2007, Mosby.

84. Wadlund DL: Prevention, recognition, and management of nursing complications in the intraoperative and postoperative surgical patient, *Nurs Clin North Am* 41:151, 2006.

85. Grichnik KP, Clark JA: Pathophysiology and management of one-lung ventilation, *Thorac Surg Clin* 15:85, 2005.

86. Kopec SE: The postpneumonectomy state, *Chest* 114:1158, 1998.

87. Brenner Z, Addona C: Caring for the pneumonectomy patient: challenges and changes, *Crit Care Nurse* 15(5):65, 1995.

88. Brooks, JA: Postoperative nosocomial pneumonia: nurse-sensitive interventions, *AACN Clin Issues* 12:305, 2001.

89. Hazelrigg SR et al: Acute and chronic pain syndromes after thoracic surgery, *Surg Clin North Am* 82:849, 2002.

90. Cerfolio RJ: Advances in thoracostomy tube management, *Surg Clin North Am* 82:833, 2002.

91. Knebel AR et al: Weaning from mechanical ventilation: concept development, *Am J Crit Care Nurs* 3:416, 1994.

92. MacIntyre NR et al: Management of patients requiring prolonged mechanical ventilation: report of a NAMDRC Consensus Conference, *Chest* 128:3937, 2005.

93. Caroleo S et al: Weaning from mechanical ventilation: an open issue, *Minerva Anesthesiol* 73:417, 2007.

94. MacIntyre NR: Psychological factors in weaning from mechanical ventilatory support, *Respir Care* 40:277, 1995.

95. Burns SM: Weaning from mechanical ventilation. In Burns SM, editor: *Care of mechanically ventilated patients*, ed 2, Sudbury, MA, 2007, Jones & Bartlett.

96. Knebel AR et al: Weaning from mechanical ventilatory support: refinement of a model, *Am J Crit Care Nurs* 7:149, 1998.

97. El-Kati MF, Bou-Khalil P: Clinical review: liberation from mechanical ventilation, *Crit Care* 12:221, 2008.

98. Cox CE, Carson SS: Prolonged mechanical ventilation. In MacIntyre NR, Branson RD, editors: *Mechanical ventilation*, ed 2, St Louis, 2009, Saunders.

99. Grap MJ et al: Collaborative practice: development, implementation, and evaluation of a weaning protocol for patients receiving mechanical ventilation, *Am J Crit Care* 12:454, 2003.

100. Tietsort J, McPeck M, Rinaldo-Gallo S: Respiratory care protocol development and impact, *Respir Care Clin North Am* 10:223, 2004.

101. Happ MB et al: Family presence and surveillance during weaning from prolonged mechanical ventilation, *Heart Lung* 36:47, 2007.

Pulmonary Therapeutic Management

OXYGEN THERAPY

Normal cellular function depends on the delivery of an adequate supply of oxygen to the cells to meet their metabolic needs. The goal of oxygen therapy is to provide a sufficient concentration of inspired oxygen to permit full use of the oxygen-carrying capacity of the arterial blood; this ensures adequate cellular oxygenation, provided the cardiac output and hemoglobin concentration are adequate.[1,2]

PRINCIPLES OF THERAPY

Oxygen is an atmospheric gas that must also be considered a drug, because—like most other drugs—it has detrimental and beneficial effects. Oxygen is one of the most commonly used and misused drugs. As a drug, it must be administered for good reason and in a proper, safe manner. Oxygen is usually ordered in liters per minute (L/min), as a concentration of oxygen expressed as a percentage, such as 40%, or as a fraction of inspired oxygen (FIO_2), such as 0.4.

The primary indication for oxygen therapy is hypoxemia.[3] The amount of oxygen administered depends on the pathophysiologic mechanisms affecting the patient's oxygenation status. In most cases, the amount required should provide an arterial partial pressure of oxygen (PaO_2) of greater than 60 mm Hg or an arterial hemoglobin saturation (SaO_2) of greater than 90% during rest and exercise.[2] The concentration of oxygen given to an individual patient is a clinical judgment based on the many factors that influence oxygen transport, such as hemoglobin concentration, cardiac output, and arterial oxygen tension.[1,2]

After oxygen therapy has begun, the patient is continuously assessed for level of oxygenation and the factors affecting it. The patient's oxygenation status is evaluated several times daily until the desired oxygen level has been reached and has stabilized. If the desired response to the amount of oxygen delivered is not achieved, the oxygen supplementation is adjusted, and the patient's condition is re-evaluated. It is important to use this dose-response method so that the lowest possible level of oxygen is administered that will still achieve a satisfactory PaO_2 or SaO_2.[2,3]

METHODS OF DELIVERY

Oxygen therapy can be delivered by many different devices (Table 25-1). Common problems with these devices include system leaks and obstructions, device displacement, and skin irritation. These devices are classified as low-flow, reservoir, or high-flow systems.[3]

Low-Flow Systems. A low-flow oxygen delivery system provides supplemental oxygen directly into the patient's airway at a flow of 8 L/min or less. Because this flow is insufficient to meet the patient's inspiratory volume requirements, it results in a variable FIO_2 as the supplemental oxygen is mixed with room air. The patient's ventilatory pattern affects the FIO_2 of a low-flow system: As the ventilatory pattern changes, differing amounts of room air gas are mixed with the constant flow of oxygen. A nasal cannula is an example of a low-flow device.[3]

Reservoir Systems. A reservoir system incorporates some type of device to collect and store oxygen between breaths. When the patient's inspiratory flow exceeds the oxygen flow of the oxygen delivery system, the patient is able to draw from the reservoir of oxygen to meet his or her inspiratory volume needs. There is less mixing of the inspired oxygen with room air than in a low-flow system. A reservoir oxygen delivery system can deliver a higher FIO_2 than a low-flow system. Examples of reservoir systems are simple face masks, partial rebreathing masks, and nonrebreathing masks.[3]

High-Flow Systems. With a high-flow system, the oxygen flows out of the device and into the patient's airways in an amount sufficient to meet all inspiratory volume requirements. This type of system is not affected by the patient's ventilatory pattern. An air-entrainment mask is an example of a high-flow system.[1,3]

COMPLICATIONS OF OXYGEN THERAPY

Oxygen, like most drugs, has adverse effects and complications resulting from its use. The adage, "If a little is good, a lot is better," does not apply to oxygen. The lung is designed to handle a concentration of 21% oxygen, with some adaptability to higher concentrations, but adverse effects and oxygen toxicity can result if a high concentration is administered for too long.[4]

TABLE 25-1 Oxygen Therapy Systems

Category	Device	Flow	FIO2 Range (%)	FIO2 Stability
Low-flow	Nasal cannula	0.25-8 L/min (adults) ≤2 L/min (infants)	22-45	Variable
	Nasal catheter	0.25-8 L/min	22-45	Variable
	Transtracheal catheter	0.25-4 L/min	22-35	Variable
Reservoir	Reservoir cannula	0.25-4 L/min	22-35	Variable
	Simple mask	5-12 L/min	35-50	Variable
	Partial rebreathing mask	6-10 L/min (prevent bag collapse on inspiration)	35-60	Variable
	Nonrebreathing mask	6-10 L/min (prevent bag collapse on inspiration)	55-70	Variable
	Nonrebreathing circuit (closed)	$3 \times V_E$ (prevent bag collapse on inspiration)	21-100	Fixed
High-flow	Air-entrainment mask (AEM)	Varies; should provide output flow >60 L/min	24-50	Fixed
	Air-entrainment nebulizer	10-15 L/min input; should provide output flow ≥60 L/min	28-100	Fixed

Modified from Wilkins RL et al, editors: *Egan's fundamentals of respiratory care*, ed 8, St Louis, 2003, Mosby.
V_E, minute volume.

Oxygen Toxicity. The most detrimental effect of breathing a high concentration of oxygen is the development of oxygen toxicity. It can occur in any patient who breathes oxygen concentrations of greater than 50% for longer than 24 hours. Patients most likely to develop oxygen toxicity are those who require intubation, mechanical ventilation, and high oxygen concentrations for extended periods.[1,3]

Hyperoxia, or the administration of higher-than-normal oxygen concentrations, produces an overabundance of oxygen free radicals. These radicals are responsible for the initial damage to the alveolar-capillary membrane. Oxygen free radicals are toxic metabolites of oxygen metabolism. Normally, enzymes neutralize the radicals, preventing any damage from occurring. During the administration of high levels of oxygen, the large number of oxygen free radicals produced exhausts the supply of neutralizing enzymes. Damage to the lung parenchyma and

vasculature occurs, resulting in the initiation of acute lung injury (ALI).[1,4]

A number of clinical manifestations are associated with oxygen toxicity. The first symptom is substernal chest pain that is exacerbated by deep breathing. A dry cough and tracheal irritation follow. Eventually, there is definite pleuritic pain on inhalation, followed by dyspnea. Upper airway changes may include a sensation of nasal stuffiness, sore throat, and eye and ear discomforts. Chest radiographs and pulmonary function tests show no abnormalities until symptoms are severe. Complete, rapid reversal of these symptoms occurs as soon as normal oxygen concentrations are restored.[4]

Carbon Dioxide Retention. In patients with severe chronic obstructive pulmonary disease (COPD), carbon dioxide (CO_2) retention may occur as a result of administration of oxygen in high concentrations. A number of theories have been proposed

TABLE 25-1 **Oxygen Therapy Systems**—*cont'd*

Advantages	Disadvantages	Best Use
Use on adults, children, infants; easy to apply; disposable, low cost; well tolerated	Unstable, easily dislodged; high flows uncomfortable; can cause dryness/bleeding; polyps, deviated septum may block flow	Stable patient needing low FIO_2; home care patient requiring long-term therapy
Use on adults, children, infants; good stability; disposable, low cost	Difficult to insert; high flows increase back pressure; needs regular changing; polyps, deviated septum may block insertion; may provoke gagging, air swallowing, aspiration	Procedures where cannula is difficult to use (bronchoscopy); long-term care for infants
Lower O_2 usage/cost; eliminates nasal/skin irritation; improved compliance; increased exercise tolerance; increased mobility; enhanced image	High cost; surgical complications; infection; mucus plugging; lost tract	Home care or ambulatory patients who need increased mobility or who do not accept nasal oxygen
Lower O_2 usage/cost; increased mobility; less discomfort because of lower flows	Unattractive, cumbersome; poor compliance; must be regularly replaced; breathing pattern affects performance	Home care or ambulatory patients who need increased mobility
Use on adults, children, infants; quick, easy to apply; disposable, inexpensive	Uncomfortable; must be removed for eating; prevents radiant heat loss; blocks vomitus in unconscious patients	Emergencies, short-term therapy requiring moderate FIO_2
Same as simple mask; moderate to high FIO_2	Same as simple mask; potential suffocation hazard	Emergencies, short-term therapy requiring moderate to high FIO_2
Same as simple mask; high FIO_2	Same as simple mask; potential suffocation hazard	Emergencies, short-term therapy requiring high FIO_2
Full range of FIO_2	Potential suffocation hazard; requires 50 psi air/O_2; blender failure common	Patients requiring precise FIO_2 at any level (21%-100%)
Easy to apply; disposable, inexpensive; stable, precise FIO_2	Limited to adult use; uncomfortable, noisy; must be removed for eating; FIO_2 >0.40 not ensured; FIO_2 varies with back-pressure	Unstable patients requiring precise low FIO_2
Provides temperature control and extra humidification	FIO_2 <28% or >0.40 not ensured; FIO_2 varies with back-pressure; high infection risk	Patients with artificial airways requiring low to moderate FIO_2

for this phenomenon. One states that the normal stimulus to breathe (i.e., increasing CO_2 levels) is muted in patients with COPD and that decreasing oxygen levels become the stimulus to breathe. If hypoxemia is corrected by the administration of oxygen, the stimulus to breathe is abolished; hypoventilation develops, resulting in a further increase in the arterial partial pressure of carbon dioxide ($PaCO_2$).[3] Another theory is that the administration of oxygen abolishes the compensatory response of hypoxic pulmonary vasoconstriction. This results in an increase in perfusion of underventilated alveoli and the development of dead space, producing ventilation/perfusion mismatching. As alveolar dead space increases, so does the retention of CO_2.[3,5] One further theory states that the rise in CO_2 is related to the ratio of deoxygenated to oxygenated hemoglobin (Haldane effect). Deoxygenated hemoglobin carries more CO_2 than oxygenated hemoglobin. Administration of oxygen increases the proportion of oxygenated hemoglobin, which

causes increased release of CO_2 at the lung level.[5] Because of the risk of CO_2 accumulation, all chronically hypercapnic patients require careful low-flow oxygen administration.[3]

Absorption Atelectasis. Another adverse effect of high concentrations of oxygen is absorption atelectasis. Breathing high concentrations of oxygen washes out the nitrogen that normally fills the alveoli and helps hold them open (residual volume). As oxygen replaces the nitrogen in the alveoli, the alveoli start to shrink and collapse. This occurs because oxygen is absorbed into the bloodstream faster than it can be replaced in the alveoli, particularly in areas of the lungs that are minimally ventilated.[1,3]

NURSING MANAGEMENT

Nursing interventions for management of the patient receiving oxygen therapy are outlined in the Nursing Interventions Classification feature on Oxygen Therapy.

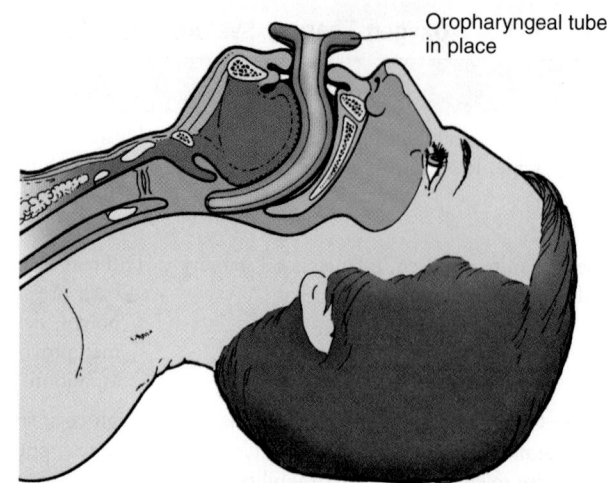

Figure 25-1 Oropharyngeal airway placement. *(From Marshak AB: Emergency life support. In Wilkins RL et al, editors:* Egan's fundamentals of respiratory care, *ed 8, St Louis, 2003, Mosby.)*

ARTIFICIAL AIRWAYS
PHARYNGEAL AIRWAYS

Pharyngeal airways are used to maintain airway patency by keeping the tongue from obstructing the upper airway. The two types of pharyngeal airways are *oropharyngeal* and *nasopharyngeal*. Complications of these airways include trauma to the oral or nasal cavity, obstruction of the airway, laryngospasm, gagging, and vomiting.[6,7]

Oropharyngeal Airway. An oropharyngeal airway is made of plastic and is available in various sizes. The proper size is selected by holding the airway against the side of the patient's face and ensuring that it extends from the corner of the mouth to the angle of the jaw. If the airway is improperly sized, it will occlude the airway.[6,7] An oral airway is placed by inserting a tongue depressor into the patient's mouth to displace the tongue downward and then passing the airway into the patient's mouth, slipping it over the patient's tongue (Fig. 25-1).[7] When properly placed, the tip of the airway lies above the epiglottis at the base of the tongue. It should be used only in an unconscious patient who has an absent or diminished gag reflex.[6,7]

Nasopharyngeal Airway. A nasopharyngeal airway is usually made of plastic or rubber and is available in various sizes. The proper size is selected by holding the airway against the side of the patient's face and ensuring that it extends from the tip of the nose to the earlobe.[6,7] A nasal airway is placed by lubricating the tube and inserting it midline along the floor of the naris into the posterior pharynx.[7] When properly placed, the tip of the airway lies above the epiglottis at the base of the tongue.[6,7]

ENDOTRACHEAL TUBES

An endotracheal tube (ETT) is the most commonly used artificial airway for providing short-term airway management. Indications for endotracheal intubation include maintenance of airway patency, protection of the airway from aspiration, application of positive-pressure ventilation, facilitation of pulmonary toilet, and use of high oxygen concentrations.[8] An ETT may be placed through the orotracheal or the nasotracheal route.[9,10] In most situations, involving emergency placement, the orotracheal route is used, because it is simpler and allows the use of a larger-diameter ETT.[10,11] Nasotracheal intubation provides greater patient comfort over time and is preferred in patients with a jaw fracture.[9,11,12] The advantages of orotracheal and nasotracheal intubation are presented in Table 25-2.

TABLE 25-2 Advantages of Orotracheal, Nasotracheal, and Tracheostomy Tubes

Orotracheal Tubes	Nasotracheal Tubes	Tracheostomy Tubes
Easier access	Easily secured and stabilized	Easily secured and stabilized
Avoids nasal and sinus complications	Reduces risk of unintentional	Reduces risk of unintentional decannulation
Allows for larger-diameter tube, which	extubation	Well tolerated by patient
facilitates	Well tolerated by patient	Enables swallowing, speech, and oral hygiene
Work of breathing	Enables swallowing and oral	Avoids upper airway complications
Suctioning	hygiene	Allows for larger-diameter tube, which
Fiberoptic bronchoscopy	Facilitates communication	facilitates
	Avoids need for bite block	Work of breathing
		Suctioning
		Fiberoptic bronchoscopy

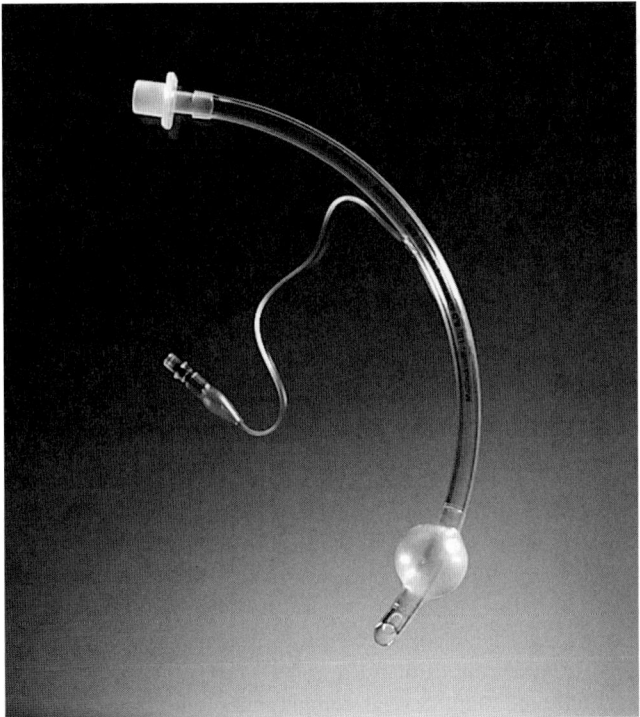

Figure 25-2 Endotracheal tube. *(Courtesy Nellcor Puritan Bennett, Pleasanton, CA.)*

ETTs are available in various sizes, based on the inner diameter of the tube, and have a radiopaque marker that runs the length of the tube. On one end of the tube is a cuff that is inflated with the use of the pilot balloon. Because of the high incidence of cuff-related problems, low-pressure, high-volume cuffs are preferred. On the other end of the tube is a 15-mm adaptor that facilitates connection of the tube to a manual resuscitation bag (MRB), T-tube, or ventilator (Fig. 25-2).[13]

Intubation. Before intubation, the necessary equipment is gathered and organized to facilitate the procedure. Readily available equipment should include a suction system with catheters and tonsil suction, an MRB with a mask connected to 100% oxygen, a laryngoscope handle with assorted blades, a variety

of sizes of ETTs, and a stylet. Before the procedure is initiated, all equipment is inspected to ensure that it is in working order. The patient should be prepared for the procedure, if possible, with an intravenous catheter in place, and should be monitored with a pulse oximeter. The patient is sedated before the procedure (as clinical condition allows), and a topical anesthetic is applied to facilitate placement of the tube. In some cases, a paralytic agent may be necessary if the patient is extremely agitated.[9,11]

The procedure is initiated by positioning the patient with the neck flexed and head slightly extended in the "sniff" position. The oral cavity and pharynx are suctioned, and any dental devices are removed. The patient is preoxygenated and ventilated using the MRB and mask with 100% oxygen. Each intubation attempt is limited to 30 seconds. After the ETT is inserted, the patient is assessed for bilateral breath sounds and chest movement. Absence of breath sounds is indicative of an esophageal intubation, whereas breath sounds heard over only one side is indicative of a main stem intubation. A disposable end-tidal CO_2 detector is used to initially verify correct airway placement, after which the cuff of the tube is inflated and the tube is secured. Finally, a chest radiograph is obtained to confirm placement.[9-11] The tip of the ETT should be approximately 3 to 4 cm above the carina when the patient's head is in the neutral position (Fig. 25-3).[10] After final adjustment of the position is complete, the level of insertion (marked in centimeters on the side of the tube) at the teeth is noted.[9,10]

A number of complications can occur during the intubation procedure, including nasal and oral trauma, pharyngeal and hypopharyngeal trauma, vomiting with aspiration, and cardiac arrest.[14,15] Hypoxemia and hypercapnia can also occur, resulting in bradycardia, tachycardia, dysrhythmias, hypertension, and hypotension.[8,12]

Complications. Several complications can occur while the ETT is in place, including nasal and oral inflammation and ulceration, sinusitis and otitis, laryngeal and tracheal injuries, and tube obstruction and displacement.

Other complications can occur days to weeks after the ETT is removed, including laryngeal and tracheal stenosis and a cricoid abscess (Table 25-3). Delayed complications usually require some form of surgical intervention.[14,15]

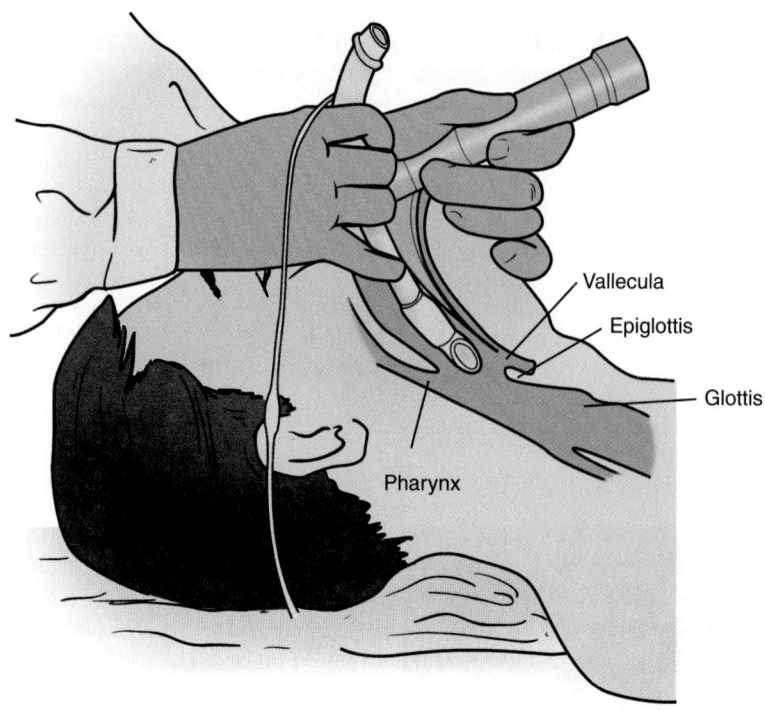

Vallecula

Epiglottis

Glottis

Pharynx

Figure 25-3 Endotracheal tube placement. *(Modified from Ellis PD, Billings DM:* Cardiopulmonary resuscitation: procedures for basic and advanced life support, *St Louis, 1980, Mosby.)*

TRACHEOSTOMY TUBES

A tracheostomy tube is the preferred method of airway maintenance in the patient who requires long-term intubation. Although no ideal time to perform the procedure has been identified, it is commonly accepted that if a patient has been intubated or is anticipated to be intubated for longer than 7 to 10 days, a tracheotomy should be performed.[16] A tracheotomy is also indicated in several other situations, such as the presence of an upper airway obstruction due to trauma, tumors, or swelling and the need to facilitate airway clearance due to spinal cord injury, neuromuscular disease, or severe debilitation.[17]

A tracheostomy tube provides the best route for long-term airway maintenance, because it avoids the oral, nasal, pharyngeal, and laryngeal complications associated with an ETT. The tube is shorter, of wider diameter, and less curved than an ETT; the resistance to air flow is less, and breathing is easier. Additional advantages of a tracheostomy tube include easier secretion removal, increased patient acceptance and comfort, capability of the patient to eat and talk if possible, and easier ventilator weaning.[11,17] Table 25-2 presents a list of the advantages of a tracheostomy tube.

Tracheostomy tubes are made of plastic or metal and may have one or two lumens. Single-lumen tubes consist of the tube; a built-in cuff, which is connected to a pilot balloon for inflation purposes; and an obturator, which is used during tube insertion. The double-lumen tubes consist of the tube with the attached cuff, the obturator, and an inner cannula that can be removed for cleaning and then reinserted or, if disposable, replaced by a new sterile inner cannula. The inner cannula can quickly be removed if it becomes obstructed, making the system safer for patients with significant

secretion problems. Single-lumen tubes provide a larger internal diameter for airflow, so airflow resistance is reduced, and the patient can ventilate through the tube with greater ease. Plastic tracheostomy tubes also have a 15-mm adaptor on the end (Fig. 25-4).[17]

Tracheotomy. A tracheostomy tube is inserted by an open procedure or a percutaneous procedure. An open procedure is usually performed in the operating room, whereas a percutaneous procedure can be done at the patient's bedside.[18]

A number of complications can occur during the tracheotomy procedure, including misplacement of the tracheal tube, hemorrhage, laryngeal nerve injury, pneumothorax, pneumomediastinum, and cardiac arrest.[15]

Complications. Several complications can occur while the tracheostomy tube is in place, including stomal infection, hemorrhage, tracheomalacia, tracheoesophageal fistula, tracheoinnominate artery fistula, and tube obstruction and displacement.

A number of complications can occur days to weeks after the tracheostomy tube is removed, including tracheal stenosis and tracheocutaneous fistula (Table 25-4). Delayed complications usually require some form of surgical intervention.[19]

NURSING MANAGEMENT

The patient with an ETT or tracheostomy tube requires some additional measures to address the effects associated with tube placement on the respiratory and other body systems (see the Nursing Interventions Classification feature on Artificial Airway Management). Nursing interventions in the management of an artificial airway include humidification, cuff management, suctioning, and communication. The tube bypasses the upper airway system, so warming

TABLE 25-3 **Complications of Endotracheal Tubes**

Complications	Causes	Prevention and Treatment
Tube obstruction	Patient biting tube Tube kinking during repositioning Cuff herniation Dried secretions, blood, or lubricant Tissue from tumor Trauma Foreign body	*Prevention:* Place bite block. Sedate patient PRN. Suction PRN. Humidify inspired gases. *Treatment:* Replace tube.
Tube displacement	Movement of patient's head Movement of tube by patient's tongue Traction on tube from ventilator tubing Self-extubation	*Prevention:* Secure tube to upper lip. Restrain patient's hands as needed. Sedate patient PRN. Ensure that only 2 inches of tube extend beyond lip. Support ventilatory tubing. *Treatment:* Replace tube.
Sinusitis and nasal injury	Obstruction of the paranasal sinus drainage Pressure necrosis of nares	*Prevention:* Avoid nasal intubations. Cushion nares from tube and tape or ties. *Treatment:* Remove all tubes from nasal passages. Administer antibiotics.
Tracheoesophageal fistula	Pressure necrosis of posterior tracheal wall, resulting from overinflated cuff and rigid nasogastric tube	*Prevention:* Inflate cuff with minimal amount of air necessary. Monitor cuff pressures every 8 hr. *Treatment:* Position cuff of tube distal to fistula. Place gastrostomy tube for enteral feedings. Place esophageal tube for secretion clearance proximal to fistula.
Mucosal lesions	Pressure at tube and mucosal interface	*Prevention:* Inflate cuff with minimal amount of air necessary. Monitor cuff pressures every 8 hr. Use appropriate size tube. *Treatment:* May resolve spontaneously. Perform surgical intervention.
Laryngeal or tracheal stenosis	Injury to area from end of tube or cuff, resulting in scar tissue formation and narrowing of airway	*Prevention:* Inflate cuff with minimal amount of air necessary. Monitor cuff pressures every 8 hr. Suction area above cuff frequently. *Treatment:* Perform tracheostomy. Place laryngeal stent. Perform surgical repair.
Cricoid abscess	Mucosal injury with bacterial invasion	*Prevention:* Inflate cuff with minimal amount of air necessary. Monitor cuff pressures every 8 hr. Suction area above cuff frequently. *Treatment:* Perform incision and drainage of area. Administer antibiotics.

PRN, as needed.

and humidifying of air must be performed by external means. Because the cuff of the tube can cause damage to the walls of the trachea, proper cuff inflation and management are imperative. The normal defense mechanisms are impaired, and secretions may accumulate; suctioning may be needed to promote secretion clearance.

Because the tube does not allow airflow over the vocal cords, development of a method of communication is also very important. Observing the patient to ensure proper placement of the tube and patency of the airway is also essential. Patient safety issues are addressed in the Patient Safety Alert feature on Artificial Airways.

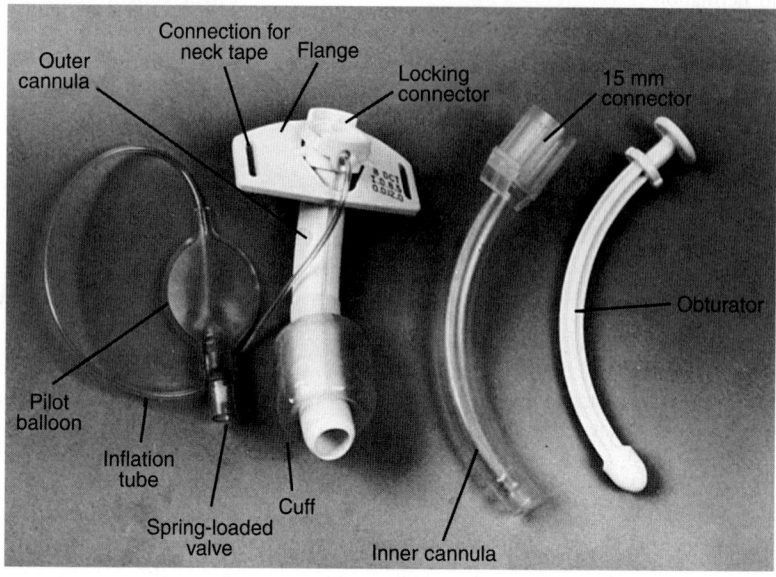

Figure 25-4 Tracheostomy tube. *(From Scanlan CL: Airway management. In Wilkins RL et al, editors:* Egan's fundamentals of respiratory care, *ed 8, St Louis, 2003, Mosby.)*

NIC

Artificial Airway Management

Definition
Maintenance of endotracheal and tracheostomy tubes and preventing complications associated with their use

Activities
Provide an oropharyngeal airway or bite block to prevent biting on the endotracheal tube, as appropriate.

Provide 100% humidification of inspired gas or air.

Provide adequate systemic hydration by oral or intravenous fluid administration.

Inflate endotracheal or tracheostoma cuff using minimal occlusive volume technique or minimal leak technique.

Maintain inflation of the endotracheal or tracheostoma cuff at 15 to 20 mm Hg during mechanical ventilation and during and after feeding.

Suction the oropharynx and secretions from the top of the tube cuff before deflating cuff.

Monitor cuff pressures every 4 to 8 hours during expiration using a three-way stopcock, calibrated syringe, and mercury manometer.

Check cuff pressure immediately after delivery of any general anesthesia.

Change endotracheal tapes or ties every 24 hours, inspect the skin and oral mucosa, and move endotracheal tube to the other side of the mouth.

Loosen commercial endotracheal tube holders at least once per day, and provide skin care.

Auscultate for presence of lung sounds bilaterally after insertion and after changing endotracheal or tracheostomy ties.

Note the centimeter reference marking on the endotracheal tube to monitor for possible displacement.

Assist with chest x-ray examination, as needed, to monitor position of tube.

Minimize leverage and traction on the artificial airway by suspending ventilator tubing from overhead support, using flexible catheter mounts and swivels, and supporting tubes during turning, suctioning, and ventilator disconnection and reconnection.

Monitor for presence of crackles and rhonchi over large airways.

Monitor for decrease in exhale volume and increase in inspiratory pressure in patients receiving mechanical ventilation.

Institute endotracheal suctioning, as appropriate.

Institute measures to prevent spontaneous decannulation: secure artificial airway with tape or ties; administer sedation and muscle paralyzing agent as appropriate; and use arm restraints, as appropriate.

Provide additional intubation equipment and Ambu bag in a readily available location.

Provide trachea care every 4 to 8 hours as appropriate; clean the inner cannula, clean and dry the area around the stoma, and change tracheostomy ties.

Inspect skin around tracheal stoma for drainage, redness, and irritation.

Maintain sterile technique when suctioning and providing tracheostomy care.

Shield the tracheostomy from water.

Provide mouth care and suction oropharynx, as appropriate.

Tape tracheostomy obturator to head of bed.

Tape a second tracheostomy tube (same type and size) and forceps to head of bed.

Institute chest physiotherapy, as appropriate.

Ensure that endotracheal or tracheostomy cuff is inflated during feedings, as appropriate.

Elevate the head of the bed or assist patient to a sitting position in a chair during feedings, as appropriate.

From Bulechek GM et al: *Nursing interventions classification (NIC),* ed 5, St Louis, 2008, Mosby.

TABLE 25-4 **Complications of Tracheostomy Tubes**

Complications	Causes	Prevention and Treatment
Hemorrhage	Vessel opening after surgery Vessel erosion caused by tube	*Prevention*: Use appropriate size tube. Treat local infection. Suction gently. Humidify inspired gases. Position tracheal window not lower than third tracheal ring. *Treatment*: Pack lightly. Perform surgical intervention.
Wound infection	Colonization of stoma with hospital flora	*Prevention*: Perform routine stoma care. *Treatment*: Remove tube, if necessary. Perform aggressive wound care and débridement. Administer antibiotics.
Subcutaneous emphysema	Positive-pressure ventilation Coughing against a tight, occlusive dressing or sutured or packed wound	*Prevention*: Avoid suturing or packing wound closed around tube. *Treatment*: Remove any sutures or packing if present.
Tube obstruction	Dried blood or secretions False passage into soft tissues Opening of cannula positioned against tracheal wall Foreign body Tissue from tumor	*Prevention*: Suction PRN. Humidify inspired gases. Use a tube with a removable inner cannula. Position tube so that opening does not press against tracheal wall. *Treatment*: Remove/replace inner cannula. Replace tube.
Tube displacement	Patient movement Coughing Traction on ventilatory tubing	*Prevention*: Use commercial tube holder. Use tubes with adjustable neck plates for patients with short necks. Support ventilatory tubing. Sedate patient PRN. Restrain patient as needed. *Treatment*: Cover stoma and manually ventilate patient by mouth. Replace tube.
Tracheal stenosis	Injury to area from end of tube or cuff, resulting in scar tissue formation and narrowing of airway	*Prevention*: Inflate cuff with minimal amount of air necessary. Monitor cuff pressures every 8 hours. *Treatment*: Perform surgical repair.
Tracheoesophageal fistula	Pressure necrosis of posterior tracheal wall, resulting from overinflated cuff and rigid nasogastric tube	*Prevention*: Inflate cuff with minimal amount of air necessary. Monitor cuff pressures every 8 hours. *Treatment*: Perform surgical repair.
Tracheoinnominate artery fistula	Direct pressure from the elbow of the cannula against the innominate artery Placement of tracheal stoma below fourth tracheal ring Downward migration of the tracheal stoma, resulting from traction on tube High-lying innominate artery	*Prevention*: Position tracheal window not lower than third tracheal ring. *Treatment*: Hyperinflate cuff to control bleeding. Remove tube and replace with endotracheal tube and apply digital pressure through stoma against the sternum. Perform surgical repair.
Tracheocutaneous fistula	Failure of stoma to close after removal of tube	*Treatment*: Perform surgical repair.

PRN, as needed.

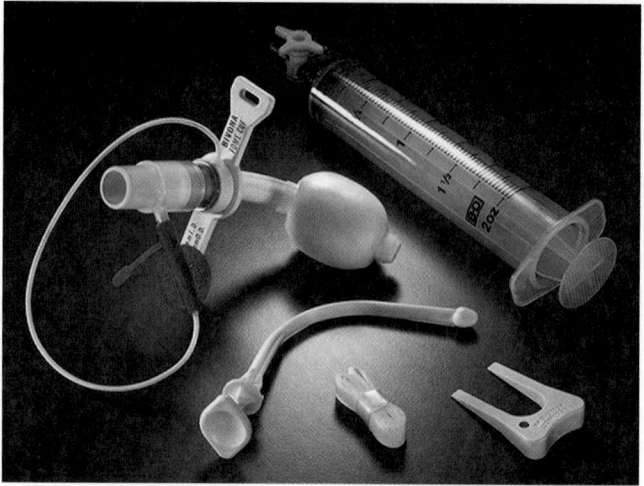

Figure 25-5 Foam cuff tracheostomy tube. *(Courtesy Smiths Medical, Inc., London, England.)*

Humidification. Humidification of air normally is performed by the mucosal layer of the upper respiratory tract. When this area is bypassed, as occurs with ETT and tracheostomy tubes, or when supplemental oxygen is used, humidification by external means is necessary. Various humidification devices add water to inhaled gas to prevent drying and irritation of the respiratory tract, to prevent undue loss of body water, and to facilitate secretion removal.[20,21] The humidification device should provide inspired gas conditioned (heated) to body temperature and saturated with water vapor.[22]

Cuff Management. Because the cuff of the ETT or tracheostomy tube is a major source of the complications associated with artificial airways, proper cuff management is essential. To prevent the complications associated with cuff design, only low-pressure, high-volume cuffed tubes are used in clinical practice.[13,23] Even with these tubes, cuff pressures can be generated that are high enough to lead to tracheal ischemia and injury. Proper cuff inflation techniques and cuff pressure monitoring are critical components of the care of the patient with an artificial airway.[10,23]

Cuff Inflation Techniques. Two cuff inflation techniques are used: the minimal leak (ML) technique and the minimal occlusion volume (MOV) technique. The ML technique consists of injecting air into the cuff until no leak is heard and then withdrawing the air until a small leak is heard on inspiration. Problems with this technique include difficulty maintaining positive end-expiratory pressure (PEEP) and aspiration around the cuff. The MOV technique consists of injecting air into the cuff until no leak is heard at peak inspiration. This technique generates higher cuff pressures than does the ML technique. The selection of one technique over the other is determined by individual patient needs. If the patient needs a seal to provide adequate ventilation or is at high risk for aspiration, the MOV technique is used. If these are not concerns, usually the ML technique is used.[10,11,23]

Cuff Pressure Monitoring. Cuff pressures are monitored at least every shift with a cuff pressure manometer. Cuff pressures should be maintained at 20 to 25 mm Hg (24 to 30 cm H_2O), because greater pressures decrease blood flow to the capillaries in the tracheal wall and lesser pressures increase the risk of aspiration. Pressures in excess of 25 mm Hg (30 cm H_2O) should be reported to the physician. Cuffs are not routinely deflated, because this increases the risk of aspiration.[10,23]

Foam Cuff Tracheostomy Tubes. One tracheostomy tube on the market has a cuff made of foam that is self-inflating

(Fig. 25-5). It is deflated during insertion, after which the pilot port is opened to atmospheric pressure (room air), and the cuff self-inflates. After inflation, the foam cuff conforms to the size and shape of the patient's trachea, thereby reducing the pressure against the tracheal wall. The pilot port can be left open to atmospheric pressure or attached to the mechanical ventilator tubing, allowing the cuff to inflate and deflate with the cycling of the ventilator. Routine maintenance of a foam cuff tracheostomy tube includes aspirating the pilot port every 8 hours to measure cuff volume, to remove any condensation from the cuff area, and to assess the integrity of the cuff. Removal is accomplished by deflating the cuff; this can be complicated if the plastic sheath covering the foam is perforated. If perforation occurs, the foam may not be deflatable because the air cannot be totally aspirated.[24]

Suctioning. Suctioning is often required to maintain a patent airway in the patient with an ETT or tracheostomy tube. Suctioning is a sterile procedure that is performed only when the patient needs it and not on a routine schedule.[10,22] Indications for suctioning include coughing, secretions in the airway, respiratory distress, presence of rhonchi on auscultation, increased peak airway pressures on the ventilator, and decreasing SaO_2 or PaO_2.[11] Complications associated with suctioning include hypoxemia, atelectasis, bronchospasms, dysrhythmias, increased intracranial pressure, and airway trauma.[11]

Complications. Hypoxemia can result because the oxygen source is disconnected from the patient or the oxygen is removed from the patient's airways when the suction is applied. Atelectasis is thought to occur when the suction catheter is larger than one half of the diameter of the ETT. Excessive negative pressure occurs when suction is applied, promoting collapse of the distal airways. Bronchospasms are the result of stimulation of the airways with the suction catheter. Cardiac dysrhythmias, particularly bradycardias, are attributed to vagal stimulation. Airway trauma occurs with impaction of the catheter in the airways and excessive negative pressure applied to the catheter.[10,11]

Suctioning Protocol. A number of protocols regarding suctioning have been developed. Several practices have been found helpful in limiting the complications of suctioning. Hypoxemia can be minimized by giving the patient three hyperoxygenation breaths (breaths at 100% FIO_2) with the ventilator before the procedure begins and again after each pass of the suction catheter.[10,25] If the patient exhibits signs of desaturation, hyperinflation (breaths at 150% tidal volume) should be added to the procedure.[10] Atelectasis can be avoided by using a suction catheter with an external diameter less than one half of the internal diameter of the ETT. Using no greater than 120 mm Hg of suction decreases the chances of hypoxemia, atelectasis, and airway trauma.[10] Limiting the duration of each suction pass to 10 to 15 seconds[10] and the number of passes to a maximum of three also help minimize hypoxemia, airway trauma, and cardiac dysrhythmias.[26] The process of applying intermittent (instead of continuous) suction has been shown to be of no benefit.[27] The instillation of normal saline to help remove secretions has not proved to be of any benefit[28] and may actually contribute to the development of hypoxemia[10,29] and lower airway colonization, resulting in hospital-acquired pneumonia (HAP).[10,30]

Closed Tracheal Suction System. One device to facilitate suctioning of a patient on a ventilator is the closed tracheal suction system (CTSS) (Fig. 25-6). This device consists of a suction catheter in a plastic sleeve that attaches directly to the ventilator tubing. It allows the patient to be suctioned while remaining on the ventilator. Advantages of the CTSS include maintenance of oxygenation and PEEP during suctioning, reduction of hypoxemia-related complications, and protection of staff members from the patient's secretions. The CTSS is convenient to use, requiring only one person to perform the procedure.

Concerns related to the CTSS include autocontamination, inadequate removal of secretions, and increased risk of unintentional

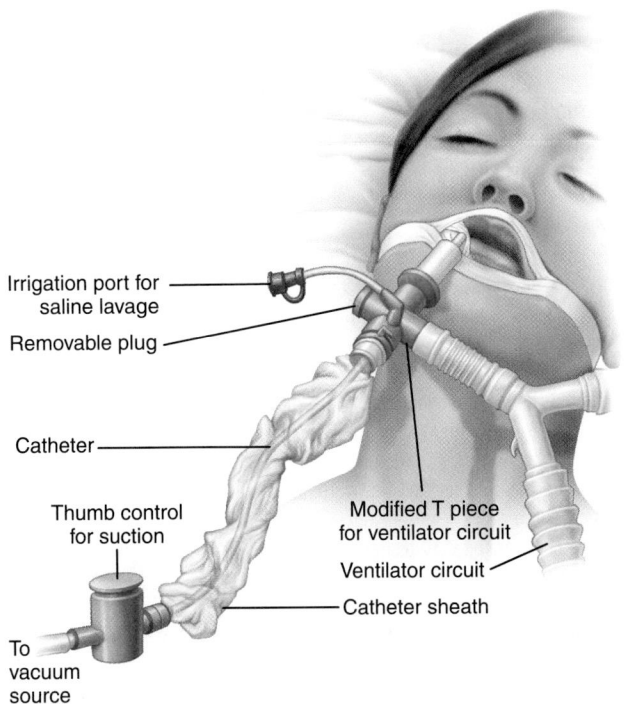

Irrigation port for saline lavage

Removable plug

Catheter

Thumb control for suction

Modified T piece for ventilator circuit

Ventilator circuit

Catheter sheath

To vacuum source

Figure 25-6 Closed tracheal suction system. *(From Sills JR: Entry-level respiratory therapist exam guide, St Louis, 2000, Mosby.)*

extubation resulting from the extra weight of the system on the ventilator tubing. Autocontamination has been shown not to be an issue if the catheter is cleaned properly after every use. Inadequate removal of secretions may or may not be a problem, and further investigation is required to settle this issue.[11] Although recommendations for changing the catheter vary, one study indicated that the catheter could be changed on an as-needed basis without increasing the incidence of HAP.[31]

Communication. One of the major stressors for the patient with an artificial airway is impaired communication. This is related to the inability to speak, insufficient explanations from staff members, inadequate understanding, fear of being unable to communicate, and difficulty with communication methods.[32] A number of interventions can facilitate communication in the patient with an ETT or tracheostomy tube. These include performing a complete assessment of the patient's ability to communicate, teaching the patient how to communicate, using a variety of methods to communicate, and facilitating the patient's ability to communicate by providing the patient with his or her eyeglasses or hearing aid.[33]

Methods to facilitate communication in this patient population include the use of verbal and nonverbal language and a variety of devices to assist the patient on short-term and long-term ventilator assistance. Nonverbal communication may include the use of sign language, gestures, lip-reading, pointing, facial expressions, or eye blinking. Simple devices available include pencil and paper; Magic Slates; magnetic boards with plastic letters; picture, alphabet, or symbol boards; and flash cards. More sophisticated devices include typewriters, computers, talking ETT and tracheostomy tubes, and external handheld vibrators. Regardless of the method selected, the patient must be taught how to use the device.[10,33]

Passy-Muir Valve. One device used to assist the mechanically ventilated patient with a tracheostomy to speak is the Passy-Muir valve. This one-way valve opens on inhalation, allowing air to enter the lungs through the tracheostomy tube, and closes on exhalation, forcing air over the vocal cords and out the mouth, permitting the patient to speak (Fig. 25-7). Before the valve can be placed on a tracheostomy tube, the cuff must be deflated to allow air to pass around the tube, and the tidal volume of the ventilator must be increased to compensate for the air leak. In addition to aiding communication, the Passy-Muir valve can assist the ventilator-dependent patient with relearning normal breathing patterns. The valve is contraindicated in patients with laryngeal or pharyngeal dysfunction, excessive secretions, or poor lung compliance.[34]

Oral Hygiene. Patients with artificial airways are extremely susceptible to developing HAP due to microaspiration of subglottic secretions. Subglottic secretions are fluids from the oropharyngeal area that pool above the inflated cuff of the ETT or tracheostomy tube. These secretions are full of microorganisms from the patient's mouth. Because the cuff of the artificial airway does not create a tight seal in the patient's airway, these secretions seep around the cuff and into the patient's lungs, promoting the development of HAP.[35] Although bacteria are normally present in a patient's mouth, in the critically ill patient there are increased amounts of bacteria and more resistant bacteria. Decreased salivary flow, poor mucosal status, and dental plaque all contribute to this problem.[36]

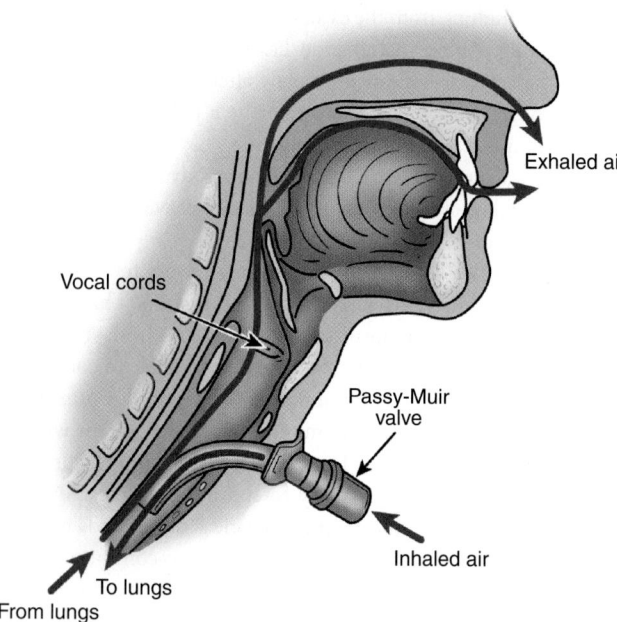

Figure 25-7 Passy-Muir valve mechanism of action. *(From Hodder RV: A 55-year-old patient with advanced COPD, tracheostomy tube, and sudden respiratory distress, Chest 121:279, 2002.)*

Proper oral hygiene has the potential to decrease the incidence of HAP.[37] However, recent studies have shown that routine oral care is not a priority intervention for many nurses.[38] Currently there is no evidence-based protocol for oral care. Research studies are lacking, particularly with regard to frequency and effectiveness of different procedures.[39] Most experts agree, however, that oral care should consist of brushing the patient's teeth with a soft toothbrush to reduce plaque, brushing the patient's tongue and gums with a foam swab to stimulate the tissue, and performing deep oropharyngeal suction to remove any secretions that have pooled above the patient's cuff.[37-39] See Box 25-1 for a sample oral care protocol. One intervention that has evidence supporting its use is rinsing the patient's mouth with chlorhexidine (15 mL of 0.12% oropharyngeal rinse applied twice daily for 30 seconds). This procedure has been shown to reduce oral colonization of bacteria and to decrease the incidence of ventilator-associated pneumonia, particularly in cardiac surgery patients.[40]

Extubation and Decannulation. After the airway is no longer needed, it is removed. Extubation is the process of removing an ETT. It is a simple procedure that can be accomplished at the bedside (see the Nursing Interventions Classification feature on Endotracheal Extubation).[10,11] Before the cuff of an ETT or tracheostomy tube is deflated in preparation for removal, it is very important to ensure that secretions are cleared from above the tube cuff. Complications of extubation include sore throat, stridor, hoarseness, odynophagia, vocal cord immobility, pulmonary aspiration, and cough.[15] Decannulation is the process of removing a tracheostomy tube. It is also a simple process that can be performed at the bedside. After removal of the tracheostomy tube, the stoma is usually covered with a dry dressing, with the expectation that it will close within several days.[10,11] Difficulty removing the tracheostomy tube because of a tight stoma is usually the only complication associated with decannulation.[15]

BOX 25-1   SAMPLE ORAL CARE PROTOCOL

STANDARD OF CARE
1. The oral cavity is assessed initially and daily by the RN.
2. Unconscious patients and those with artificial airways (endotracheal or tracheostomy tubes) are provided oral care every 4 hours and as needed.
3. Patients with cuffed artificial airways have oropharyngeal and subglottic secretions suctioned every 12 hours and before repositioning of the tube or deflation of the cuff.

PROCEDURE
1. Set up suction equipment.
2. Position patient's head to the side or place in semi-Fowler's position.
3. Provide suction, as needed, to patients with an artificial airway to remove any oropharyngeal and subglottic secretions (those secretions that migrate down the tube and settle on top of the cuff).
4. Brush teeth using suction toothbrush and small amounts of water and alcohol-free antiseptic oral rinse.
   - Brush for approximately 1 to 2 minutes.
   - Exert gentle pressure while moving in short horizontal or circular strokes.
5. Gently brush the surface of the tongue.
6. Use suction swab to clean the teeth and tongue if brushing causes discomfort or bleeding.
   - Place swab perpendicular to gum line, applying gentle mechanical action for 1 to 2 minutes.
   - Turn swab in clockwise rotation to remove mucus and debris.
7. Apply mouth moisturizer inside mouth.
8. Apply lip balm if needed.

NIC

Endotracheal Extubation

Definition
Purposeful removal of the endotracheal tube from the nasopharyngeal or oropharyngeal airway

Activities
Position the patient for best use of ventilatory muscles, usually with the head of the bed elevated 75 degrees.
Instruct the patient about the procedure.
Hyperoxygenate the patient and suction the endotracheal airway.
Suction the oral airway.
Deflate the endotracheal cuff and remove the endotracheal tube.
Encourage the patient to cough and expectorate sputum.
Administer oxygen as ordered.
Encourage coughing and deep breathing.
Suction the airway, as needed.
Monitor for respiratory distress.
Observe for signs of airway occlusion.
Monitor vital signs.
Encourage voice rest for 4 to 8 hours, as appropriate.
Monitor ability to swallow and talk.

From Bulechek GM et al: *Nursing interventions classification (NIC)*, ed 5, St Louis, 2008, Mosby.

INVASIVE MECHANICAL VENTILATION

INDICATIONS

Mechanical ventilation is the process of a using an apparatus to facilitate the transport of oxygen and carbon dioxide between the atmosphere and the alveoli for the purpose of enhancing pulmonary gas exchange. It is indicated for physiologic and clinical reasons. Physiologic objectives include supporting cardiopulmonary gas exchange (alveolar ventilation and arterial oxygenation), increasing lung volume (end-expiratory lung inflation and functional residual capacity), and reducing the work of breathing. Clinical objectives include reversing hypoxemia and acute respiratory acidosis, relieving respiratory distress, preventing or reversing atelectasis and respiratory muscle fatigue, permitting sedation and neuromuscular blockade, decreasing oxygen consumption, reducing intracranial pressure, and stabilizing the chest wall.[41]

USE OF MECHANICAL VENTILATORS

Types of Ventilators. The two main types of ventilators currently available are positive-pressure ventilators and negative-pressure ventilators. Negative-pressure ventilators are applied externally to the patient and decrease the atmospheric pressure surrounding the thorax to initiate inspiration. They generally are not used in the critical care environment. Positive-pressure ventilators use a mechanical drive mechanism to force air into the patient's lungs through an ETT or tracheostomy tube.[42]

Ventilator Mechanics. The ventilator must complete four phases of ventilation to properly ventilate the patient: (1) change from exhalation to inspiration; (2) inspiration; (3) change from inspiration to exhalation; and (4) exhalation. The ventilator uses four different variables to begin, sustain, and terminate each of these phases. These variables are described in terms of *volume, pressure, flow,* and *time.*[7,43,44]

Trigger. The phase variable that initiates the change from exhalation to inspiration is called the *trigger.* Breaths may be pressure-triggered or flow-triggered, based on the sensitivity setting of the ventilator and the patient's inspiratory effort; or they may be time-triggered, based on the rate setting of the ventilator. A breath that is initiated by the patient is known as a *patient-triggered* or *patient-assisted* breath, whereas a breath that is initiated by the ventilator is known as a *machine-triggered* or *machine-controlled* breath.

A *time-triggered breath* is a machine-controlled breath that is initiated by the ventilator after a preset length of time has elapsed. It is controlled by the rate setting on the ventilator (e.g., a rate of 10 breaths/min yields 1 breath every 6 seconds). *Flow-triggered* and *pressure-triggered* breaths are patient-assisted breaths that are initiated by decreased flow or pressure, respectively, within the breathing circuit. Flow-triggering (also known as *flow-by*) is controlled by adjusting the flow-sensitivity setting of the ventilator, whereas pressure-triggering is controlled by adjusting the pressure-sensitivity setting. Many ventilators offer the various types of triggers in combination. For example, a breath may be time-triggered and flow-triggered, depending

on the patient's ability to interact with the ventilator and initiate a breath.[7,42,43]

Limit. The variable that maintains inspiration is called the *limit* or *target.* Inspiration can be pressure-limited, flow-limited, or volume-limited. A *pressure-limited breath* is one in which a preset pressure is attained and maintained during inspiration. A *flow-limited breath* is one in which a preset flow is reached before the end of inspiration. A *volume-limited breath* is one in which a preset volume is delivered during the inspiration. However, the limit variable does not end inspiration; it only sustains it.[7,42,43]

Cycle. The variable that ends inspiration is called the *cycle.* The classification of positive-pressure ventilators is based on this variable: volume-cycled, pressure-cycled, flow-cycled, and time-cycled. *Volume-cycled ventilators* are designed to deliver a breath until a preset volume is delivered. *Pressure-cycled ventilators* deliver a breath until a preset pressure is reached within the patient's airways. *Flow-cycled ventilators* deliver a breath until a preset inspiratory flow rate is achieved. *Time-cycled ventilators* deliver a breath over a preset time interval.[7,42,43]

Baseline. The variable that is controlled during exhalation is called the *baseline.* Pressure is almost always used to adjust this variable. The patient exhales to a certain baseline pressure that is set on the ventilator. It may be set at zero (i.e., atmospheric pressure) or above atmospheric pressure (i.e., PEEP).[7,42,43]

Modes of Ventilation. The term *ventilator mode* refers to how the machine ventilates the patient. Selection of a particular mode of ventilation determines how much the patient will participate in his or her own ventilatory pattern. The choice depends on the patient's situation and the goals of treatment. The mode is determined by the combination of phase variables selected. Many modes are available (Table 25-5),[7,42-44] and some may be used in conjunction with others. Because brands of ventilators vary in their ability to perform certain functions, not all modes are available on all ventilators.[43]

Ventilator Settings. Settings on the ventilator allow the ventilator parameters to be individualized to the patient and also allow selection of the desired ventilation mode (Table 25-6). Each ventilator has a patient-monitoring system that allows all aspects of the patient's ventilatory pattern to be assessed, monitored, and displayed.[42-45]

COMPLICATIONS

Mechanical ventilation is often lifesaving, but, like other interventions, it is not without complications. Some complications are preventable, whereas others can be minimized but not eradicated. Physiologic complications associated with mechanical ventilation include ventilator-induced lung injury, cardiovascular compromise, gastrointestinal disturbances, patient-ventilator dyssynchrony, and HAP.

Ventilator-Induced Lung Injury. Mechanical ventilation can cause two different types of injury to the lungs: air leaks and biotrauma.[44,46] Air leaks related to mechanical ventilation are the result of excessive pressure in the alveoli (barotrauma), excessive volume in the alveoli (volutrauma), or shearing due to repeated opening and closing of the alveoli (atelectrauma).[44,47]

TABLE 25-5 Modes of Mechanical Ventilation

Mode of Ventilation	Clinical Application	Nursing Implications
Continuous mandatory (volume or pressure) ventilation (CMV) also known as assist-control (AC) ventilation: delivers gas at preset tidal volume or pressure (depending on selected cycling variable) in response to patient's inspiratory efforts and initiates breath if patient fails to do so within preset time	Volume-controlled (VC) CMV is used as the primary mode of ventilation in spontaneously breathing patients with weak respiratory muscles. Pressure-controlled (PC) CMV is used in patients with decreased lung compliance or increased airway resistance, particularly when the patient is at risk for volutrauma.	Hyperventilation can occur in patients with increased respiratory rates. Sedation may be necessary to limit the number of spontaneous breaths. Patient on VC-CMV should be monitored for volutrauma. Patient on PC-CMV should be monitored for hypercapnia.
Pressure-regulated volume control ventilation (PRVCV): a variation of CMV that combines volume and pressure features; delivers a preset tidal volume using the lowest possible airway pressure; airway pressure will not exceed preset maximum pressure limit	PRVCV is used in patients with rapidly changing pulmonary mechanics (airway resistance and lung compliance), limiting potential complications.	—
Pressure-controlled inverse ratio ventilation (PC-IRV): PC-CMV mode in which the inspiratory-to-expiratory (I:E) time ratio is greater than 1:1	PC-IRV is used in patients with hypoxemia refractory to positive end-expiratory pressure (PEEP); the longer inspiratory time increases functional residual capacity and improves oxygenation by opening collapsed alveoli, and the shorter expiratory time induces auto-PEEP that prevents alveoli from recollapsing.	Requires sedation or pharmacologic paralysis, or both, because of discomfort. Increased intrathoracic pressure can result in excessive air trapping and decreased cardiac output.
Intermittent mandatory (volume or pressure) ventilation (IMV), also known as synchronous intermittent mandatory ventilation (SIMV): delivers gas at preset tidal volume or pressure (depending on selected cycling variable) and rate while allowing patient to breathe spontaneously; ventilator breaths are synchronized to patient's respiratory effort	VC-IMV is used as a primary mode of ventilation in many clinical situations and as a weaning mode. PC-IMV is used in patients with decreased lung compliance or increased airway resistance when the need to preserve the patient's spontaneous effects is important.	May increase the work of breathing and promote respiratory muscle fatigue. Patient should be monitored for hypercapnia, particularly with PC-IMV.
Adaptive support ventilation (ASV): ventilator automatically adjusts settings to maintain 100 mL/min/kg of minute ventilation; pressure support	ASV is a computerized mode of ventilation that increases or decreases ventilatory support based on patient needs; can be used with any patient requiring volume-controlled ventilation.	Not intended as a weaning mode. Adapts to changes in patient position.
Constant positive airway pressure (CPAP): positive pressure applied during spontaneous breaths; patient controls rate, inspiratory flow, and tidal volume	CPAP is a spontaneous breathing mode used in patients to increase functional residual capacity and improve oxygenation by opening collapsed alveoli at end expiration; it is also used for weaning.	Side effects include decreased cardiac output, volutrauma, and increased intracranial pressure. No ventilator breaths are delivered in PEEP or CPAP mode unless used with CMV or IMV.
Airway pressure release ventilation (APRV): two different levels of CPAP (inspiratory and expiratory) are applied for set periods of time, allowing spontaneous breathing to occur at both levels	APRV is a spontaneous breathing mode used to maintain alveolar recruitment without imposing additional peak inspiratory pressures that could lead to barotrauma.	Patient needs to be monitored for hypercapnia.
Pressure support ventilation (PSV): preset positive pressure used to augment patient's inspiratory efforts; patient controls rate, inspiratory flow, and tidal volume	PSV is a spontaneous breathing mode used as the primary mode of ventilation in patients with stable respiratory drive to overcome any imposed mechanical resistance (e.g., artificial airway). PSV can also be used with IMV to support spontaneous breaths.	Patient should be monitored for hypercapnia. Advantages include reduced patient work of breathing and improved patient-ventilator synchrony.

TABLE 25-5 **Modes of Mechanical Ventilation—cont'd**

Mode of Ventilation	Clinical Application	Nursing Implications
Volume-assured pressure support ventilation (VAPSV), also known as pressure augmentation (PA): a variation of PSV with a set tidal volume to ensure that patient receives minimum tidal volume with each pressure support breath	VAPSV is a spontaneous breathing mode used to treat acute respiratory illness and to facilitate weaning	Advantages include increased patient comfort, decreased work of breathing, decreased respiratory muscle fatigue, and promotion of respiratory muscle conditioning.
Independent lung ventilation (ILV): each lung is ventilated separately	ILV is used in patients with unilateral lung disease, bronchopleural fistulas, or bilateral asymmetric lung disease.	Requires a double-lumen endotracheal tube, two ventilators, sedation, and/or pharmacologic paralysis.
High-frequency ventilation (HFV): delivers a small volume of gas at a rapid rate High-frequency positive-pressure ventilation (HFPPV): delivers 60-100 breaths/min High-frequency jet ventilation (HFJV): delivers 100-600 cycles/min High-frequency oscillation (HFO): delivers 900-3000 cycles/min	HFV is used in situations in which conventional mechanical ventilation compromises hemodynamic stability, in patients with bronchopleural fistulas, during short-term procedures, and with diseases that create a risk of volutrauma.	Patients require sedation and/or pharmacologic paralysis. Inadequate humidification can compromise airway patency. Assessment of breath sounds is difficult.

TABLE 25-6 **Ventilator Settings**

Parameter	Description	Typical Settings
Respiratory rate (f)	Number of breaths the ventilator delivers per minute	6-20 breaths/min
Tidal volume (V_T)	Volume of gas delivered to patient during each ventilator breath	10-12 mL/kg 6-8 mL/kg in acute lung injury (ALI)
Oxygen concentration (FIO_2)	Fraction of inspired oxygen delivered to patient	May be set between 21% and 100%; adjusted to maintain PaO_2 level greater than 60 mm Hg or SpO_2 level greater than 90%
Positive end-expiratory pressure (PEEP)	Positive pressure applied at the end of expiration of ventilator breaths	3-5 cm H_2O
Pressure support (PS)	Positive pressure used to augment patient's inspiratory efforts	5-10 cm H_2O
Inspiratory flow rate and time	Speed with which the tidal volume is delivered	40-80 L/min Time: 0.8-1.2 sec
I:E ratio	Ratio of duration of inspiration to duration of expiration	1:2 to 1:1.5 unless inverse ratio ventilation is desired
Sensitivity	Determines the amount of effort the patient must generate to initiate a ventilator breath; it may be set for pressure-triggering or flow-triggering	Pressure trigger: 0.5-1.5 cm H_2O below baseline pressure Flow trigger: 1-3 L/min below baseline flow
High pressure limit	Regulates the maximal pressure the ventilator can generate to deliver the tidal volume; when the pressure limit is reached, the ventilator terminates the breath and spills the undelivered volume into the atmosphere	10-20 cm H_2O above peak inspiratory pressure

Barotrauma, volutrauma, and atelectrauma can lead to excessive alveolar wall stress and damage to the alveolar-capillary membrane, resulting in air leakage into the surrounding spaces. The air then travels out through the hilum and into the mediastinum (pneumomediastinum), pleural space (pneumothorax), subcutaneous tissues (subcutaneous emphysema), pericardium (pneumopericardium), peritoneum (pneumoperitoneum), and retroperitoneum (pneumoretroperitoneum). The resultant disorders vary from the fairly benign to the potentially lethal—the most lethal of which is a pneumothorax or pneumopericardium resulting in cardiac tamponade.[44,48]

Barotrauma, volutrauma, and atelectrauma can also cause the release of cellular mediators and initiation of the inflammatory-immune response. This type of ventilator-induced injury is known as biotrauma.[44,49] Biotrauma can result in the development of ALI.[50] To limit ventilator-induced lung injury, the plateau pressure (pressure needed to inflate the alveoli) should be kept at less than 32 cm H_2O, PEEP should be used to avoid end-expiratory collapse and reopening, and the tidal volume should be set at 6 to 10 mL/kg.[46,49]

Cardiovascular Compromise. Positive-pressure ventilation increases intrathoracic pressure, which decreases venous return to the right side of the heart. Impaired venous return decreases preload, which results in a decrease in cardiac output. As a secondary consequence, hepatic and renal dysfunction may occur. Positive-pressure ventilation impairs cerebral venous return. In patients with impaired autoregulation, positive-pressure ventilation can result in increased intracranial pressure.[44,51]

Gastrointestinal Disturbances. Gastrointestinal disturbances can occur as a result of positive-pressure ventilation. Gastric distention occurs when air leaks around the ETT or tracheostomy tube cuff and overcomes the resistance of the lower esophageal sphincter.[7] Vomiting can occur as a result of pharyngeal stimulation from the artificial airway.[15] These problems can be prevented by inserting a nasogastric tube and ensuring appropriate cuff inflation. Hypomotility and constipation may occur as a result of immobility and the administration of paralytic agents, analgesics, and sedatives.[7]

Patient-Ventilator Dyssynchrony. Because the ventilatory pattern is normally initiated by the establishment of negative pressure within the chest, the application of positive pressure can lead to patient difficulties in breathing while on the ventilator. To achieve optimal ventilatory assistance, the patient should breathe in synchrony with the machine. The selected mode of ventilation, the settings, and the type of ventilatory circuitry used can increase the work of breathing and lead to breathing out of synchrony with the ventilator. Patient-ventilatory dyssynchrony can result in decreased effectiveness of mechanical ventilation, the development of auto-PEEP, and psychological distress. Patients who are not breathing in synchrony with the ventilator appear to be fighting or "bucking" the ventilator. To minimize this problem, the ventilator is adjusted to accommodate the patient's spontaneous breathing pattern and to work with the patient. If this is not possible, the patient may need to be sedated or pharmacologically paralyzed.[43,52]

Ventilator-Associated Pneumonia. Ventilator-associated pneumonia (VAP) is a subgroup of HAP that refers to the development of pneumonia while undergoing mechanical ventilation. There is great potential for the development of pneumonia after placement of an artificial airway, because the tube bypasses or impairs many of the lung's normal defense mechanisms. After an artificial airway has been placed, contamination of the lower airways follows within 24 hours. This results from a number of factors that directly and indirectly promote airway colonization. The use of respiratory therapy devices (e.g., ventilators, nebulizers, intermittent positive-pressure breathing machines) also can increase the risk of pneumonia. The severity of the patient's illness and the presence of ALI or malnutrition significantly increase the likelihood that an infection will ensue. Therapeutic measures such as nasogastric tubes and gastric alkalinization with enteral feedings or medications facilitate the development of pneumonia. Nasogastric tubes promote aspiration by acting as a wick for stomach contents, whereas enteral feedings, antacids,

histamine inhibitors, and proton-pump inhibitors increase the pH level of the stomach, promoting the growth of bacteria that can then be aspirated.[53] Additional information on managing the patient with pneumonia is provided in Chapter 24.

Prevention of VAP is critical (see the Evidence-Based Practice feature on Ventilator-Associated Pneumonia). Several strategies may assist with prevention, including semirecumbent positioning, continuous aspiration of subglottic secretions (CASS), meticulous oral hygiene with antiseptics such as chlorhexidine (discussed earlier), and proper hand hygiene (see the Evidence-Based Practice feature on Hand Hygiene Guidelines in Chapter 24).[53-55]

Semirecumbency. Positioning of the patient who requires mechanical ventilation is very important. Semirecumbent positioning (elevation of the head of the bed 30 to 45 degrees) reduces the incidence of gastroesophageal reflux and subsequent aspiration and decreases the incidence of VAP. The head of the patient's bed should be elevated to 30 to 45 degrees at all times unless contraindicated (e.g., hemodynamic instability, presence of intraaortic balloon pump, physician's order to the contrary).[53] However, this intervention does increase the risk of skin sheer on the coccyx, and extra surveillance is mandatory for prevention of pressure ulcers.

Continuous Aspiration of Subglottic Secretions. Artificial airways are a significant risk factor for the development of VAP, because they allow for aspiration of bacteria-laden oropharyngeal and gastrointestinal secretions into the lungs. This occurs as a result of pooling of secretions from the mouth and stomach above the cuff of the artificial airway and leaking of the secretions around the cuff into the patient's airways.[35] Removal of the secretions from above the cuff by continuous aspiration has been shown to decrease the incidence of VAP.[56] CASS requires the use of a specialized ETT. A CASS tube has an additional lumen, with an opening above the cuff, which is connected to continuous (−20 mm Hg) or intermittent (−100 to −150 mm Hg) suction (Fig. 25-8).[35,56] The tubes are recommended for patients who are expected to be intubated for longer than 48 hours. One problem with the CASS tube is that the aspiration lumen can become clogged with thick secretions, food particles, and clots.[35]

Other Measures to Reduce the Incidence of Ventilator-Associated Pneumonia. Recent studies have shown that use of an ETT with a polyurethane cuff may decrease the incidence of VAP. A traditional ETT has a polyvinyl low-pressure high-volume cuff. When the cuff is inflated, folds form in the cuff, allowing fluids and air to leak around the cuff and into the lungs. This is why subglottic secretion removal is so important. Polyurethane cuffs are much thinner than the traditional polyvinyl cuffs and do not form folds when they are inflated. There is no leakage of fluids into the lungs.[57]

Another recent study found that the use of silver-coated ETTs significantly reduced the incidence and delayed the onset of VAP, compared with a regular ETT. The tube decreased the incidence of VAP by preventing bacterial colonization and biofilm formation.[58] Biofilm is formed when bacteria cling to the inner lumen of the ETT and then secrete an exopolysaccharide substance. This substance forms a gelatinous matrix that allows bacteria to thrive on a nonbiologic surface (Fig. 25-9).[59]

Evidence-Based Practice: Collaborative

American Association of Critical-Care Nurses Practice Alert: Ventilator-Associated Pneumonia

Practice Alert Statements

1. All patients receiving mechanical ventilation, as well as those at high risk for aspiration (e.g., decreased level of consciousness; enteral tube in place), should have the head of the bed (HOB) elevated at an angle of 30 to 45 degrees unless medically contraindicated[1-7] (level VI).

2. Use an endotracheal tube (ETT) with a dorsal lumen above the endotracheal cuff to allow drainage by continuous suctioning of tracheal secretions that accumulate in the subglottic area[1,2,8-13] (level VI).

3. Do not routinely change, on the basis of duration of use, the patient's ventilator circuit[1,14-17] (level VI).

Supporting Evidence

- Critically ill patients who are intubated for more than 24 hours are at 6 to 21 times the risk of developing ventilator-associated pneumonia (VAP),[1,2,18-20] and those intubated for less than 24 hours are at three times the risk of VAP.[20] Other risk factors for VAP include decreased level of consciousness, supine positioning with HOB flat, use of H_2 antagonists and antacids, gastric distention, presence of gastric or small-intestine tubes, enteral feedings, and a trauma or chronic obstructive pulmonary disease (COPD) diagnosis.[1,18-22] VAP is reported to occur at rates of 10 to 35 cases per 1000 ventilator days, depending on the clinical situation.[1,19]

- Morbidity and mortality associated with the development of VAP is high, with mortality rates ranging from 20% to 41%.[20,23-25] Development of VAP increases ventilator days, critical care days, and hospital length of stay by 4, 4, and 9 days, respectively,[18,23,26] and results in more than $11,000 additional costs per VAP case.[18,25,27]

- Micro-aspiration or macro-aspiration of oropharyngeal and/or gastric fluids is presumed to be an essential step in the development of VAP.[1,2,12,28] Pulmonary aspiration is increased by supine positioning and pooling of secretions above the ETT cuff.[1,3,19]

- Compared with supine positioning, studies have shown that simple positioning with HOB elevation to 30 degrees or higher significantly reduces gastric reflux and VAP,[3-7] but national surveys and reports in the literature describe poor compliance rates with HOB elevation in critical care units.[20,29-34]

- Studies show that special ETTs that remove secretions pooled above the cuff with continuous suction decrease VAP by 45% to 50%.[8-11]

- Studies on the frequency of ventilator circuit changes have found no increase in VAP with prolonged use.[14-17]

- National regulatory and expert consensus groups include the American Association of Critical-Care Nurses (AACN) VAP Practice Alert interventions as critical to decreasing VAP rates.[1,2,35-37]

AACN Grading Level of Evidence

Level I. Manufacturer's recommendation only

Level II. Theory based—no research data to support recommendations; recommendations from expert consensus group may exist

Level III. Laboratory or bench data only—no clinical data to support recommendations

Level IV. Limited clinical studies to support recommendations

Level V. Clinical studies in more that one or two different populations or situations to support recommendations

Level VI. Clinical studies in a variety of patient populations and situations to support recommendations

Actions for Nursing Practice

- Always keep mechanically ventilated patients' HOB elevated to 30 degrees or higher, unless medically contraindicated; use an ETT with continuous suction above the cuff in patients expected to be intubated longer than 48 hours; do not routinely change ventilator circuits.

- Ensure that your critical care unit has a written practice document such as a policy, procedure, or standards of care that includes these practice alerts.[38]

- Determine your unit's rate of compliance with the HOB elevation directive and use an ETT with continuous suction above the cuff

- If compliance with HOB elevation is less than 90%, develop a plan to improve compliance.[29,38-45]

   Consider forming a multidisciplinary task force (nurses, physicians, respiratory therapists, clinical pharmacists) to address VAP practice changes.

   Educate staff about the significance of hospital-acquired pneumonias in critically ill patients and how the interventions listed in the Practice Alert can reduce VAP.

   Incorporate content into orientation programs and initial and annual competency verifications.

   Develop a variety of communication strategies to alert and remind staff of the importance of these VAP interventions and to disseminate results of audits.

   Develop documentation standards for HOB elevation that include a rationale for when HOB elevation is not done.

   Incorporate HOB elevation to at least 30 degrees for mechanically ventilated patients or patients at high risk for aspiration in any unit's standing orders. Include HOB elevation monitoring in your critical care scorecard, quality improvement (QI) plan, or performance improvement (PI) activities to ensure that compliance levels are maintained.

Expected Outcomes

- Decrease in VAP rates for the unit
- Increase in number of patients with HOB elevation to at least 30 degrees.
- Cost savings due to decreased rates of VAP and less frequent ventilator circuit changes

Resources

- Education materials
   Power Point slide program for VAP education sessions (www.aacn.org)
   Online continuing education program on prevention strategies for VAP (www.nellcor.com/educ/onlineed.aspx)
- Audit tools
   Measurement of compliance with HOB elevation in mechanically ventilated patients (www.aacn.org)
- Other resources
   Methods for estimating HOB elevation (www.aacn.org)
   For additional information or assistance, contact a clinical practice specialist with the AACN Practice Resource Network (PRN) by e-mail (practice@aacn.org) or by telephone (800-394-5995, ext 217).

Continued

Evidence-Based Practice: Collaborative—cont'd

References

1. Tablan OC et al, for the CDC; Healthcare Infection Control Practices Advisory Committee: Guidelines for preventing health-care–associated pneumonia, 2003: recommendations of CDC and the Healthcare Infection Control Practices Advisory Committee, MMWR Recomm Rep 53(RR-3):1-36, 2004.
2. American Thoracic Society; Infectious Diseases Society of America: Guidelines for the management of adults with hospital-acquired, ventilator-associated, and health-care-associated pneumonia, Am J Respir Crit Care Med 171:388-416, 2005.
3. Torres A et al: Pulmonary aspiration of gastric contents in patients receiving mechanical ventilation: the effect of body position, Ann Intern Med 116:540-542, 1992.
4. Ibanez J et al: Gastroesophageal reflux in intubated patients receiving enteral nutrition: effect of supine and semirecumbent positions, JPEN J Parenter Enteral Nutr 16:419-422, 1992.
5. Orozco-Levi M et al: Semi-recumbent position protects from pulmonary aspiration but not completely from gastroesophageal reflux in mechanically ventilated patients, Am J Respir Crit Care Me 152:1387-1390, 1995.
6. Drakulovic M et al: Supine body position as a risk factor for nosocomial pneumonia in mechanically ventilated patients: a randomized trial, Lancet 354:1851-1854, 1999.
7. Davis K Jr et al: The acute effects of body position strategies and respiratory therapy in paralyzed patients with acute lung injury, Critical Care 5:81-87, 2001.
8. Valles J et al: Continuous aspiration of subglottic secretions in preventing ventilator-associated pneumonia, Intensive Care Med 122:179-186, 1995.
9. Mahul P et al: Prevention of nosocomial pneumonia in intubated patients: respective role of mechanical subglottic secretion drainage and stress ulcer prophylaxis, Intensive Care Med 18:20-25, 1992.
10. Kollef M et al: A randomized clinical trial of continuous aspiration of subglottic secretions in cardiac surgery patients, Chest 116:1339-1346, 1999.
11. Dezfulian C et al: Subglottic secretion drainage for preventing ventilator-associated pneumonia: a meta-analysis, Am J Med 118:11-18, 2005.
12. Cook D et al: Influence of airway management on ventilator-associated pneumonia: evidence from randomized trials, JAMA 279:761-787, 1998.
13. Smulders K et al: A randomized clinical trial of intermittent subglottic secretion drainage in patients receiving mechanical ventilation. Chest 121:858-862, 2002.
14. Dreyfuss D et al: Prospective study of nosocomial pneumonia and of patient circuit colonization during mechanical ventilation with circuit changes every 48 hours versus no change. Am J Respir Crit Care Med 143:738-743, 1991.
15. Kotilainen H, Keroack M: Cost analysis and clinical impact of weekly ventilator circuit changes in patients in intensive care unit. Am J Infect Control 25:117-120, 1997.
16. Kollef M et al: Mechanical ventilation with or without 7-day circuit changes: a randomized controlled trial. Ann Intern Med 123:168-174, 1995.
17. Long M et al: Prospective, randomized study of ventilator-associated pneumonia in patients with one versus three ventilator circuit changes per week. Infect Control Hosp Epidemiol 17:14-19, 1996.
18. Rello J et al: Epidemiology and outcomes of ventilator-associated pneumonia in a large US database. Chest 122:2115-2121, 2002.
19. Craven D: Epidemiology of ventilator-associated pneumonia. Chest 117:186S-187S, 2000.
20. Kollef M: Ventilator-associated pneumonia: a multivariate analysis. JAMA 270:1965-1970, 1993.
21. Flanders SA, Collard HR, Saint S: Nosocomial pneumonia: state of the science. Am J Infect Control 34:84-93, 2006.
22. Elatrous S et al: Incidence and risk factors of ventilator-associated pneumonia: a one-year prospective study. Clin Intensive Care 20:193-198, 1996.
23. Bercault N, Boulain T: Mortality rate attributable to ventilator-associated nosocomial pneumonia in an adult intensive care unit: a prospective case-control study. Crit Care Med 29:2303-2309, 2001.
24. Heyland D et al: The attributable morbidity and mortality of ventilator-associated pneumonia in the critically ill patient. Am J Respir Crit Care Med 159:1249-1256, 1999.
25. Safdar N et al: Clinical and economic consequences of ventilator-associated pneumonia: a systematic review. Crit Care Med 33:2184-2193, 2005.
26. Chastre J, Fagon J: Ventilator-associated pneumonia. Am J Respir Crit Care Med 165:867-903, 2002.
27. Warren K et al: Outcomes and attributable cost of ventilator-associated pneumonia among intensive care unit patients in a suburban medical center. Crit Care Med 31:1312-1317, 2003.
28. Bonten M et al: Risk factors for ventilator-associated pneumonia: from epidemiology to patient management. Healthcare Epidemiol 38:1141-1149, 2004.
29. Zack J et al: Effect of an educational program aimed at reducing the occurrence of ventilator associated pneumonia. Crit Care Med 30:2407-2412, 2002.
30. Berenholtz S, Pronovost P: Barriers to translating evidence into practice. Curr Opin Crit Care 9:321-325, 2003.
31. Grap M et al: Use of backrest elevation in critical care: pilot study. Am J Crit Care 8:475-480, 1999.
32. van Nieuwenhoven CA et al: Feasibility and effects of the semirecumbent position to prevent ventilator-associated pneumonia: a randomized study. Crit Care Med 34:396-402, 2006.
33. Grap M et al: Predictors of backrest elevation in critical care. Intensive Crit Care Nurs 19:68-74, 2003.
34. Grap MJ, Munro CL: Preventing ventilator-associated pneumonia: evidence-based care. Crit Care Nurs Clin North Am 16:349-358, 2004.
35. Joint Commission on Accreditation of Healthcare Organizations (JCAHO): Specification manual for national hospital quality measures: ICU. Available at www.jointcommission.org/PerformanceMeasurement/MeasureReserveLibrary/Spec+Manual+-+ICU.htm (accessed March 2009).
36. Burns S, editor: AACN protocols for practice: care of mechanically ventilated patients, ed 2. Sudbury, MA, 2007, Jones & Bartlett.
37. Shojania K et al: Closing the quality gap: a critical analysis of quality improvement strategies. Volume 6: prevention of healthcare-associated infections, pp 71-105. AHRQ publication no. 04(07)-0051-6. U.S. Department of Health & Human Services, Agency for Healthcare Research and Quality, 2007. Available at www.ahcpr.gov/clinic/ptsafety/chap17a.htm (accessed March 2009).

From the American Association of Critical-Care Nurses. Available at www.aacn.org/WD/Practice/Docs/Ventilator_Associated_Pneumonia_1-2008.pdf (accessed March 2009).

WEANING

Weaning is the gradual withdrawal of the mechanical ventilator and the reestablishment of spontaneous breathing. Weaning should begin only after the original process for which ventilator support was required has been corrected and patient stability has been achieved. Other factors to consider when weaning are length of time on ventilator, sleep deprivation, and nutritional status. Major factors that affect the patient's ability to wean include the ability of the lungs to participate in ventilation and respiration, cardiovascular performance, and psychological readiness.[60] This discussion focuses on weaning of the patient from short-term (≤3 days) mechanical ventilation. Management of weaning in the patient on long-term mechanical ventilation is discussed in Chapter 24.

Readiness to Wean. Patients should be screened every day for their readiness to wean. The screen should include an evaluation of the patient's level of consciousness, physiologic and

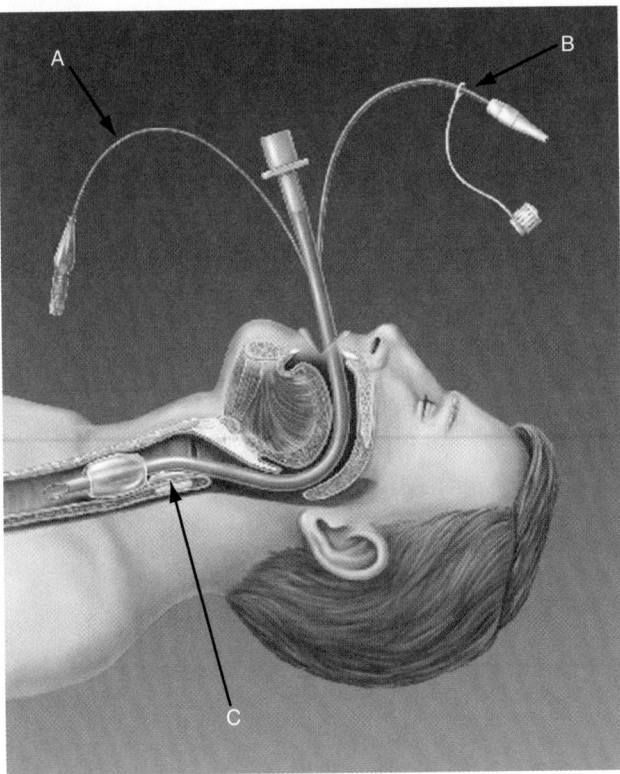

Figure 25-8 Continuous aspiration of subglottic secretions (CASS) tube. *A,* Lumen for inflation of the cuff. *B,* Lumen for aspiration of subglottic secretions. *C,* Pooling of subglottic secretions above the cuff and opening for the aspiration port. *(Courtesy Nellcor Puritan Bennett Incorporated, Pleasanton, CA.)*

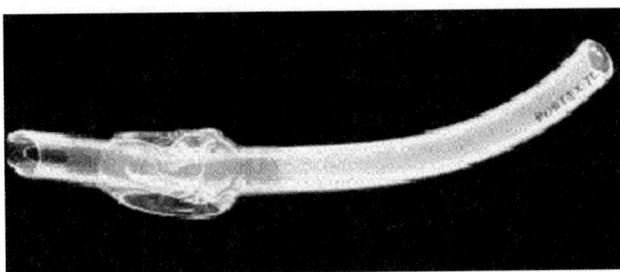

Figure 25-9 Endotracheal tube removed from a patient with respiratory failure, demonstrating thick biofilm in the tube lumen. *(From Mason CM, Nelson S:* Pulmonary host defenses and factors predisposing to lung infection, Clin Chest Med *26:11, 2005.)*

hemodynamic stability, adequacy of oxygenation and ventilation, spontaneous breathing capability, and respiratory rate and pattern. The rapid, shallow breathing index (RSBI) can predict weaning success. To calculate a RSBI, the patient's respiratory rate and minute ventilation are measured for 1 minute during spontaneous breathing. The measured respiratory rate is then divided by the tidal volume (expressed in liters). An RSBI of less than 105 is considered predictive of weaning success. If the patient is receiving sedation, the medication should be discontinued at least 1 hour before the RSBI is measured. If the patient meets criteria for weaning readiness and has a RSBI

of less than 105, a spontaneous breathing trial can be performed.[61] One study showed that implementation of a weaning program that incorporated daily spontaneous-breathing trials had a positive impact on extubation rates and no effect on reintubation rates.[62]

After readiness to wean has been established, the patient is prepared for the weaning trial. The patient is positioned upright to facilitate breathing and suctioned to ensure airway patency. The process is explained to the patient, and the patient is offered reassurance and diversional activities. Nursing activities to facilitate weaning are listed in the Nursing Interventions Classification feature on Mechanical Ventilatory Weaning. The patient is assessed immediately before the start of the trial and frequently during the weaning period for signs of weaning intolerance (Box 25-2).[60,61,63,64]

Weaning Methods. A number of methods can be used to wean a patient from the ventilator. The method selected depends on the patient, his or her pulmonary status, and length of time on the ventilator. The three main methods for weaning are (1) T-tube (T-piece) trials, (2) synchronized intermittent mandatory ventilation (SIMV), and (3) pressure support ventilation (PSV).[60,63,65]

T-Piece Trials. T-piece weaning trials consist of alternating periods of ventilatory support (usually assist control ventilation [ACV] or continuous mandatory ventilation [CMV]) with periods of spontaneous breathing. The trial is initiated by removing the patient from the ventilator and having the patient breathe spontaneously on a T-piece oxygen delivery system. After a set amount of time, the patient is placed back on the ventilator. The goal is to progressively increase the duration of time spent off the ventilator. During the weaning process, the patient is observed closely for respiratory muscle fatigue.[60-63,65] Constant positive airway pressure (CPAP) may be added to prevent atelectasis and improve oxygenation.[63,65]

Synchronized Intermittent Mandatory Ventilation Trials. The goal of SIMV weaning is the gradual transition from ventilatory support to spontaneous breathing. It is initiated by placing the ventilator in the SIMV mode and slowly decreasing the rate, usually one to three breaths at a time, until a rate of zero or near-zero is reached. An arterial blood gas (ABG) sample is usually obtained 30 minutes after the trial. This method of weaning can increase the work of breathing, and the patient must be closely monitored for signs of respiratory muscle fatigue.[60,63,65]

Pressure Support Ventilation Trials. PSV weaning consists of placing the patient on the pressure support mode and setting the pressure support at a level that facilitates the patient's achieving a spontaneous tidal volume of 10 to 12 mL/kg. PSV augments the patient's spontaneous breaths with a positive-pressure boost during inspiration. During the weaning process, the level of pressure support is gradually decreased in increments of 3 to 6 cm H_2O, while the tidal volume is maintained at 10 to 15 mL/kg, until a level of 5 cm H_2O is achieved. If the patient is able to maintain adequate spontaneous respirations at this level, extubation is considered. PSV also can be used with SIMV weaning to help overcome the resistance in the ventilator system.[60,63,65]

NIC

Mechanical Ventilatory Weaning

Definition
Assisting the patient to breathe without the aid of a mechanical ventilator

Activities
Monitor degree of shunt, vital capacity, V_D/V_T, mandatory minute ventilation, inspiratory force, and FEV_1 for readiness to wean from mechanical ventilation based on agency protocol.

Monitor to ensure that patient is free of significant infection before weaning.

Monitor for optimal fluid and electrolyte status.

Collaborate with other health team members to optimize patient's nutritional status, ensuring that 50% of the diet's nonprotein caloric source is fat rather than carbohydrate.

Position patient for best use of ventilatory muscles and to optimize diaphragmatic descent.

Suction the airway, as needed.

Administer chest physiotherapy, as appropriate.

Consult with other health care personnel in selecting a method for weaning.

Alternate periods of weaning trials with sufficient periods of rest and sleep.

Avoid delaying return of patient with fatigued respiratory muscles to mechanical ventilation.

Set a schedule to coordinate other patient care activities with weaning trials.

Promote the best use of the patient's energy by initiating weaning trials after the patient is well rested.

Monitor for signs of respiratory muscle fatigue (e.g., abrupt rise in $Paco_2$, rapid, shallow ventilation, paradoxical abdominal wall motion), hypoxemia, and tissue hypoxia while weaning is in process.

Administer medications that promote airway patency and gas exchange.

Set discrete, attainable goals with the patient for weaning.

Use relaxation techniques, as appropriate.

Coach the patient during difficult weaning trials.

Assist the patient to distinguish spontaneous breaths from mechanically delivered breaths.

Minimize excessive work of breathing that is nontherapeutic by eliminating extra dead space, adding pressure support, administering bronchodilators, and maintaining airway patency, as appropriate

Avoid pharmacologic sedation during weaning trials, as appropriate.

Provide some means of patient control during weaning.

Stay with the patient and provide support during initial weaning attempt.

Tell patient about ventilator setting changes that increase the work of breathing, as appropriate.

Provide the patient with positive reinforcement and frequent progress reports.

Consider using alternative methods of weaning as determined by patient's response to the current method.

Instruct the patient and family about what to expect during various stages of weaning.

Prepare discharge arrangements through multidisciplinary involvement with patient and family.

From Bulechek GM et al: *Nursing interventions classification (NIC)*, ed 5, St Louis, 2008, Mosby.
FEV_1, forced expiratory volume in 1 second; $Paco_2$, partial pressure of arterial oxygen; V_D/V_T, dead space volume–tidal volume ratio.

BOX 25-2   WEANING INTOLERANCE INDICATORS

- Decrease in level of consciousness
- Systolic blood pressure increased or decreased by 20 mm Hg
- Diastolic blood pressure greater than 100 mm Hg
- Heart rate increased by 20 beats/min
- Premature ventricular contractions greater than 6/min, couplets, or runs of ventricular tachycardia
- Changes in ST segment (usually elevation)
- Respiratory rate greater than 30 breaths/min or less than 10 breaths/min

- Respiratory rate increased by 10 breaths/min
- Spontaneous tidal volume less than 250 mL
- $Paco_2$ increased by 5 to 8 mm Hg and/or pH less than 7.30
- Spo_2 less than 90%
- Use of accessory muscles of ventilation
- Complaints of dyspnea, fatigue, or pain
- Paradoxical chest wall motion or chest abdominal asynchrony
- Diaphoresis
- Severe agitation or anxiety unrelieved by reassurance

NURSING MANAGEMENT

Nursing management of the patient on a ventilator is outlined in the Nursing Interventions Classification feature on Mechanical Ventilation. Routine assessment of these patients includes monitoring for patient-related and ventilator-related complications. It includes a total patient assessment, with particular emphasis on the pulmonary system, placement of the ETT, and observation for subcutaneous emphysema and dyssynchrony with the ventilator. Assessment of the ventilator includes a review of all the ventilator settings and alarms. A clear understanding of the alarms and their related problems is important (Table 25-7). The peak inspiratory pressure, exhaled tidal volume, and ABGs are also monitored. Issues regarding patient safety and patient transport are addressed, respectively, in the Patient Safety Alert feature on Invasive Mechanical Ventilation and the Evidence-Based Practice feature titled Summary of Guidelines for Intrahospital Transport of Critically Ill Patients.

Bedside evaluation of vital capacity, minute ventilation, ABG values, and other pulmonary function tests may be warranted, according to the patient's condition. The use of pulse oximetry can facilitate continuous, noninvasive assessment of oxygenation. Static and dynamic compliance should also be monitored to assess for changes in lung compliance (see Appendix B).[66]

NIC

Mechanical Ventilation

Definition
Use of an artificial device to assist a patient to breathe

Activities
Monitor for respiratory muscle fatigue.

Monitor for impending respiratory failure.

Consult with other health care personnel in selection of a ventilator mode.

Initiate setup and application of the ventilator.

Instruct the patient and family about the rationale and expected sensations associated with use of mechanical ventilators.

Routinely monitor ventilator settings.

Monitor for decrease in exhale volume and increase in inspiratory pressure.

Ensure that ventilator alarms are on.

Administer muscle-paralyzing agents, sedatives, and narcotic analgesics, as appropriate.

Monitor the effectiveness of mechanical ventilation on patient's physiologic and psychological status.

Initiate calming techniques, as appropriate.

Provide patient with a means for communication (e.g., paper and pencil or alphabet board).

Check all ventilator connections regularly.

Empty condensed water from traps, as appropriate.

Use aseptic technique, as appropriate.

Monitor ventilator pressure reading and breath sounds.

Stop NG feedings during suctioning and 30 to 60 minutes before chest physiotherapy.

Silence ventilator alarms during suctioning to decrease frequency of false alarms.

Monitor patient's progress on current ventilator settings and make appropriate changes as ordered.

Monitor for adverse effects of mechanical ventilation: infection, barotraumas, and reduced cardiac output.

Position to facilitate ventilation/perfusion matching ("good lung down"), as appropriate.

Collaborate with physician to use CPAP or PEEP to minimize alveolar hypoventilation, as appropriate.

Perform chest physical therapy, as appropriate.

Perform suctioning, based on presence of adventitious sounds and/or increased ventilatory pressures.

Promote adequate fluid and nutritional intake.

Provide routine oral care.

Monitor effects of ventilator changes on oxygenation: ABG, Sao_2, Svo_2, end-tidal CO_2, Qs/Qt, and A-ado_2 levels and patient's subjective response.

Monitor degree of shunt, vital capacity, Vd/Vt, MMV inspiratory force, and FEV_1 for readiness to wean from mechanical ventilation based on agency protocol.

From Bulechek GM et al: *Nursing interventions classification (NIC)*, ed 5, St Louis, 2008, Mosby.

A-ado_2, alveolar-arterial difference in partial pressure of oxygen; ABG, arterial blood gases; CO_2, carbon dioxide; CPAP, continuous positive airway pressure; FEV_1, forced expiratory volume in 1 second; MMV, mandatory minute ventilation; PEEP, positive end-expiratory pressure; Qs/Qt measurement of pulmonary shunt that describes the percentage of blood reaching the left side of the heart without picking up oxygen; Sao_2, arterial oxygen saturation; Svo_2, venous oxygen saturation; Vd/Vt, dead space volume–tidal volume ratio.

Evidence-Based Practice: Collaborative

Summary of Guidelines for Intrahospital Transport of Critically Ill Patients

1. Pretransport Coordination and Communication
   - Confirm receiving unit readiness to receive patient
   - Nurse to nurse handoff (if patient care responsibility is being transferred to a nurse in the receiving area)
   - Notify respiratory therapist and/or other members of the health care team of timing of transport and request equipment support as needed
   - Mechanical ventilator in receiving unit (for mechanically ventilated patients)
2. Accompanying Personnel
   - A minimum of two people should accompany a critically ill patient (one of which should be a critical care nurse).
   - Unstable patients should be accompanied by a physician.
3. Accompanying Equipment
   - Blood pressure monitor or cuff
   - Pulse oximeter

- Cardiac monitor with defibrillator
- Basic resuscitation drugs (emergency cart should be readily available in receiving unit)
- Additional sedatives and narcotic analgesics
- Additional intravenous fluids and medications
- Oxygen delivery device attached to oxygen source with at least a 30-minute reserve or manual resuscitation bag and/or transport ventilator (for mechanically ventilated patients)
- Transport ventilator must have alarms and back up battery

4. Monitoring During Transport
   - Continuous electrocardiographic monitoring
   - Continuous pulse oximetry
   - Periodic measurement of blood pressure, pulse rate, and respiratory rate

From Warren J et al: Guidelines for the inter- and intrahospital transport of critically ill patients, *Crit Care Med* 32:256, 2004.

TABLE 25-7 Troubleshooting Ventilator Alarms

Problem	Causes	Interventions
Low exhaled V_T	Altered settings; any condition that triggers high or low pressure alarm; patient stops spontaneous respirations; leak in system preventing V_T from being delivered; cuff insufficiently inflated; leak through chest tube; airway secretions; decreased lung compliance; spirometer disconnected or malfunctioning	Check settings; evaluate patient, check respiratory rate; check all connections for leaks; suction patient's airway; check cuff pressure; calibrate spirometer.
Low inspiratory pressure	Altered settings; unattached tubing or leak around ETT; ETT displaced into pharynx or esophagus; poor cuff inflation or leak; tracheal-esophageal fistula; peak flows that are too low; low V_T; decreased airway resistance resulting from decreased secretions or relief of bronchospasm; increased lung compliance resulting from decreased atelectasis; reduction in pulmonary edema; resolution of ALI; change in position	Reset alarm; reconnect tubing; modify cuff pressures; tighten humidifier; check chest tube; adjust peak flow to meet or exceed patient demand and correct for the patient's V_T; reposition or change ETT.
Low exhaled minute volume	Altered settings; leak in system; airway secretions; decreased lung compliance; malfunctioning spirometer; decreased patient-triggered respiratory rate resulting from drugs, sleep, hypocapnia, alkalosis, fatigue, change in neurologic status	Check settings; assess patient's respiratory rate, mental status, and work of breathing; evaluate system for leaks; suction airway; assess patient for changes in disease state; calibrate spirometer.
Low PEEP/CPAP pressure	Altered settings; increased patient inspiratory flows; leak; decreased expiratory flows from ventilator	Check settings and correct; observe for leaks in system; if unable to correct problem, increase PEEP settings.
High respiratory rate	Increased metabolic demand; drug administration; hypoxia; hypercapnia; acidosis; shock; pain; fear; anxiety	Evaluate ABGs; assess patient; calm and reassure patient.
High pressure limit	Improper alarm setting; airway obstruction resulting from patient fighting ventilator (holding breath as ventilator delivers V_T); patient circuit collapse; tubing kinked; ETT in right main stem bronchus or against carina; cuff herniation; increased airway resistance resulting from bronchospasm, airway secretions, plugs, and coughing; water from humidifier in ventilator tubing; decreased lung compliance resulting from tension pneumothorax, change in patient position, ALI, pulmonary edema, atelectasis, pneumonia, or abdominal distention	Reset alarms; clear obstruction from tubing; unkink and reposition patient off of tubing; empty water from tubing; check breath sounds; reassure patient and sedate if necessary; check ABGs for hypoxemia; observe for abdominal distention that would put pressure on the diaphragm; check cuff pressures; obtain chest radiograph and evaluate for ETT position, pneumothorax, and pneumonia; reposition ETT; give bronchodilator therapy.
Low-pressure oxygen inlet	Improper oxygen alarm setting; oxygen not connected to ventilator; dirty oxygen intake filter	Correct alarm setting; reconnect or connect oxygen line to a 50-psi source; clean or replace oxygen filter.
I:E ratio	Inspiratory time longer than expiratory time; use of an inspiratory phase that is too long with a fast rate; peak flow setting too low while rate too high; machine too sensitive	Change inspiratory time or adjust peak flow; check inspiratory phase, or hold; check machine sensitivity.
Temperature	Sensor malfunction; overheating resulting from too low or no gas flow; sensor picking up outside airflow (from heater, open door or window, air conditioner); improper water levels	Test or replace sensor; check gas flow; protect sensor from outside source that would interfere with readings; check water levels.

Modified from Flynn JBM, Bruce NP: *Introduction to critical care nursing skills*, St. Louis, 1993, Mosby.
ABGs, arterial blood gases; ALI, acute lung injury; CPAP, constant positive airway pressure; ETT, endotracheal tube; PEEP, positive end-expiratory pressure; V_T, tidal volume.

Patient Safety Alert

Invasive Mechanical Ventilation

Several measures are required to maintain a trouble-free ventilator system. These include maintaining a functional manual resuscitation bag connected to oxygen at the bedside, ensuring that the ventilator tubing is free of water, positioning the ventilator tubing to avoid kinking, maintaining the patency of ventilator tubing and connections, changing ventilator tubing per hospital policy, and monitoring the temperature of the inspired air. If the ventilator malfunctions, the patient is removed from the ventilator and ventilated manually with a manual resuscitation bag. Alarms should be sufficiently audible with respect to distance and competing noise within the unit.

NONINVASIVE POSITIVE-PRESSURE VENTILATION

Noninvasive positive-pressure ventilation (NPPV) is an alternative method of ventilation that uses a mask instead of an ETT to deliver the therapy. Advantages of this type of ventilation include decreased frequency of HAP, increased comfort, and the noninvasive nature of the procedure, which allows easy application and removal. It is indicated in type I and type II acute respiratory failure, cardiogenic pulmonary edema, and other situations in which intubation is not an option. Contraindications to NPPV include hemodynamic instability, dysrhythmias, apnea, uncooperativeness, intolerance of the mask, recent upper airway or esophageal surgery, and inability to maintain a patent airway, clear secretions, or properly fit the mask.[67]

NPPV can be applied with a nasal or facial mask and ventilator or with a BiPAP machine (Respironics Inc, Murrysville, PA)

(Fig. 25-10). One study found that a full-face mask is better tolerated than a nasal mask.[68] This type of ventilation uses a combination of PSV and PEEP supplied by a ventilator, or inspiratory and expiratory positive airway pressure (IPAP and EPAP, respectively) supplied by a BiPAP machine, to assist the spontaneously breathing patient with ventilation. On inspiration, the patient receives PSV or IPAP to increase tidal volume and minute ventilation, resulting in increased alveolar ventilation, a decreased $PaCO_2$ level, relief of dyspnea, and reduced accessory muscle use. On expiration, the patient receives PEEP or EPAP to increase functional residual capacity, resulting in an increased PaO_2 level. Humidified supplemental oxygen is administered to maintain a clinically acceptable PaO_2 level, and timed breaths may be added if necessary.[69]

NURSING MANAGEMENT

Routine assessment of a patient on NPPV includes monitoring the patient for patient-related and ventilator-related complications. As with invasive mechanical ventilation, the patient must be closely monitored while receiving noninvasive mechanical ventilation. Respiratory rate, accessory muscle use, and oxygenation status are continually assessed to ensure that the patient is tolerating this method of ventilation. Continuous pulse oximetry with a set alarm parameter is initiated (see the Nursing Interventions Classification feature on Respiratory Monitoring).[69,70]

The key to ensuring adequate ventilatory support is a properly fitted mask. A nasal mask or a full facemask may be used, depending on the patient. A properly fitted mask minimizes air leakage and discomfort for the patient. Transparent dressings placed over the pressure points of the face help minimize air leakage and prevent facial skin necrosis caused by the mask. The BiPAP machine is able to compensate for air leaks.[70]

NIC

Respiratory Monitoring

Definition
Collection and analysis of patient data to ensure airway patency and adequate gas exchange

Activities
Monitor rate, rhythm, depth, and effort of respirations.
Note chest movement, watching for symmetry, use of accessory muscles, and supraclavicular and intercostal muscle retractions.
Monitor for noisy respirations, such as crowing or snoring.
Monitor breathing patterns: bradypnea, tachypnea, hyperventilation, Kussmaul respirations, Cheyne-Stokes respirations, apneustic breathing, Biot respirations, and ataxic patterns.
Palpate for equal lung expansion.
Percuss anterior and posterior thorax from apices to bases bilaterally.
Note location of trachea.
Monitor for diaphragmatic muscle fatigue (paradoxical motion).
Auscultate breath sounds, noting areas of decreased/absent ventilation and presence of adventitious sounds.
Determine the need for suctioning by auscultating for crackles and rhonchi over major airways.

Auscultate lung sounds after treatments to note results.
Monitor pulmonary function test values, particularly vital capacity, maximal inspiratory force, FEV_1, and FEV_1/forced vital capacity, as available.
Monitor mechanical ventilator readings, noting increases in inspiratory pressures and decreases in tidal volume, as appropriate.
Monitor for increased restlessness, anxiety, and air hunger.
Note changes in SaO_2, SvO_2, end-tidal CO_2, and changes in arterial blood gas values, as appropriate.
Monitor patient's ability to cough effectively.
Note onset, characteristics, and duration of cough.
Monitor patient's respiratory secretions.
Monitor for dyspnea and events that improve and worsen it.
Monitor for hoarseness and voice changes every hour in patients with facial burns.
Monitor for crepitus, as appropriate.
Monitor chest x-ray reports.
Open the airway, using the head-tilt–chin-lift or jaw-thrust technique, as appropriate.
Place the patient on side, as indicated, to prevent aspiration; log roll if cervical aspiration suspected.
Institute resuscitation efforts, as needed.
Institute respiratory therapy treatments (e.g., nebulizer), as needed.

From Bulechek GM et al: *Nursing interventions classification (NIC)*, ed 5, St Louis, 2008, Mosby.
CO_2, carbon dioxide; FEV_1, forced expiratory volume in 1 second; SaO_2, arterial oxygen saturation, SvO_2, venous oxygen saturation.

The patient is positioned with the head of the bed elevated at 45 degrees to minimize the risk of aspiration and to facilitate breathing. Insufflation of the stomach is a complication of this mode of therapy and places the patient at risk for aspiration. The patient is closely monitored for gastric distention, and a nasogastric tube is placed for decompression as necessary. Often patients are very anxious and have high levels of dyspnea before the initiation of noninvasive mechanical ventilation. After adequate ventilation has been established, anxiety and dyspnea are usually sufficiently relieved. Heavy sedation should be avoided, but if it is needed,

it would constitute the need for intubation and invasive mechanical ventilation. It is important to spend 30 minutes with the patient after initiation of noninvasive ventilation, because the patient needs reassurance and must learn how to breathe on the machine.[68,70] Patient safety issues are addressed in the Patient Safety Alert on Noninvasive Mechanical Ventilation.

POSITIONING THERAPY

Positioning therapy can help match ventilation and perfusion through the redistribution of oxygen and blood flow in the lungs, which improves gas exchange. Based on the concept that there is preferential blood flow to the gravity-dependent areas of the lungs, positioning therapy is used to place the least damaged portion of the lungs into a dependent position. The least damaged portions of the lungs receive preferential blood flow, resulting in less ventilation/perfusion mismatching.[71] Currently, there are two approaches to position therapy: prone positioning and rotation therapy. Which position works best with each specific pulmonary disorder is still under investigation (see the Evidence-Based Practice feature on Recommendations for Physiotherapy in the ICU).

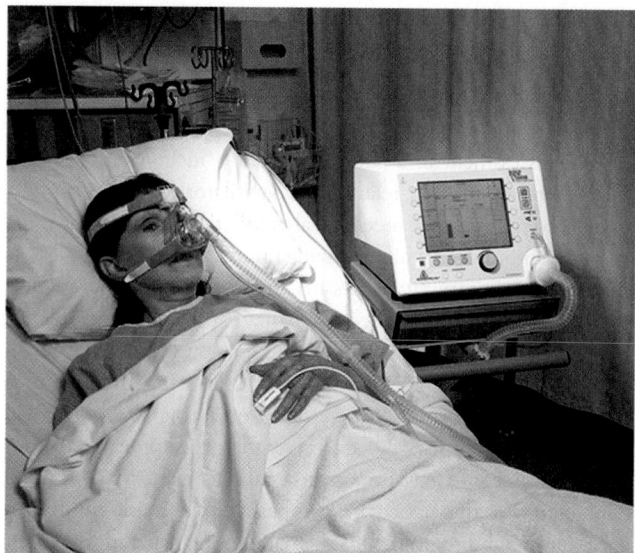

Figure 25-10 BiPAP Vision Face Mask in use. *(Courtesy Respironics Inc, Murrysville, PA.)*

Patient Safety Alert

Noninvasive Mechanical Ventilation

The patient who requires noninvasive mechanical ventilation with a full-face mask should never be restrained. The patient must be able to remove the mask if it becomes displaced or the patient vomits. A displaced mask can force the patient's bottom jaw inward and occlude the patient's airway.

Evidence-Based Practice: Collaborative

Summary of Evidence and Evidence-Based Recommendations for Physiotherapy in the Intensive Care Unit

Strong evidence for the following:
- Physiotherapy is the treatment of choice for patients with acute lobar atelectasis.
- Prone positioning improves oxygenation for some patients with severe acute respiratory failure or acute lung injury (ALI).
- Positioning in side-lying position (affected lung uppermost) improves oxygenation for some patients with unilateral lung disease.
- Hemodynamic status should be monitored during physiotherapy to detect any deleterious side effects of treatment.
- Sedation before physiotherapy will decrease or prevent adverse hemodynamic or metabolic responses.
- Preoxygenation, sedation, and reassurance are necessary before suction to avoid suction-induced hypoxemia.
- Rotation therapy (kinetic therapy) decreases the incidence of pulmonary complications.

Moderate evidence of the following:
- Multimodality physiotherapy has a short-lived beneficial effect on respiratory function.

- MH may have a short-lived beneficial effect on respiratory function, but hemodynamic status, airway pressure, or V_T should be monitored to detect any deleterious side effects of treatment.
- ICP and CPP should be monitored on appropriate patients during physiotherapy to detect any deleterious side effects of treatment.

Very limited or no evidence of the following:
- Routine physiotherapy in addition to nursing care prevents pulmonary complications commonly found in ICU patients.
- Physiotherapy is effective in the treatment of pulmonary conditions commonly found in ICU patients (with the exception of acute lobar atelectasis).
- Physiotherapy facilitates weaning, decreases length of stay in the ICU or hospital, and reduces mortality or morbidity.
- Positioning (with the exception of examples cited above), percussion, vibrations, suction, and mobilization are effective components of physiotherapy for ICU patients.
- Limb exercises prevent loss of joint range or soft-tissue length, or improve muscle strength and function, for ICU patients.

From Stiller K: Physiotherapy in intensive care: towards an evidence-based practice, *Chest* 118:1801, 2000.
ALI, acute lung injury; CPP, cerebral perfusion pressure; ICP, intracranial pressure; ICU, intensive care unit; MH, manual hyperinflation; V_T, tidal volume.

PRONE POSITIONING

Prone positioning is a therapeutic modality that is used to improve oxygenation in patients with ALI.[72] It involves turning the patient completely over onto his or her stomach in the face-down position. Although a number of theories have been proposed to explain how prone positioning improves oxygenation, the discovery that ALI causes greater damage to the dependent areas of the lungs probably provides the best explanation. It was originally thought that ALI was a diffuse, homogenous disease that affected all areas of the lungs equally. It is now known that the dependent lung areas are more heavily damaged than the nondependent lung areas. Turning the patient prone improves perfusion to less damaged areas of the lungs, improves ventilation/perfusion matching, and decreases intrapulmonary shunting. Prone positioning can be used to facilitate the mobilization of secretions and provide pressure relief. Prone positioning is contraindicated in patients with increased intracranial pressure, hemodynamic instability, spinal cord injuries, or abdominal surgery. Patients who are unable to tolerate a face-down position are also not appropriate candidates for this type of therapy.[73]

No standard has been established for the length of time a patient should remain in the prone position. A review of the research on this subject revealed a wide variation, anywhere from 30 minutes to 40 hours.[73] The therapy is considered successful if the patient has an improvement in PaO_2 of greater than 10 mm Hg within 30 minutes of being placed in the prone position.[73] The positioning schedule (length of time in prone position and frequency of turning) is usually based on the patient's tolerance of the procedure, the success of the procedure in improving the patient's PaO_2, and whether the patient is able to sustain improvements in PaO_2 when turned back to the supine position. Prone positioning is discontinued when the patient no longer demonstrates a response to the position change.[73]

The biggest limitation to prone positioning is the actual mechanics of turning the patient. A number of procedures have been discussed in the literature that advise using pillows to support the patient or using the Vollman Prone Positioner (Hill-Rom Inc, Batesville, IN). The latter is a steel frame with four cushions to support the patient's forehead, chin, chest, and pelvic area. The device is applied to the patient in the supine position and then used to turn the patient to the prone position (Fig. 25-11). Regardless of the method used, the abdomen must be allowed to hang free to facilitate diaphragmatic descent.[73]

Before the patient is turned to the prone position, his or her eyes are lubricated and taped closed, tubes and drains are secured, and the procedure is explained to the patient and family. A team is organized to implement the turning procedure, and one member is positioned at the head of the bed to maintain the patient's airway. Complications of the procedure include dislodgment or obstruction of tubes and drains, hemodynamic instability, massive facial edema, pressure ulcers, aspiration, and corneal ulcerations.[73]

ROTATION THERAPY

Automated turning beds to provide rotation therapy are often used in the critical care setting. Kinetic therapy and continuous lateral rotation therapy (CLRT) are two forms of rotation

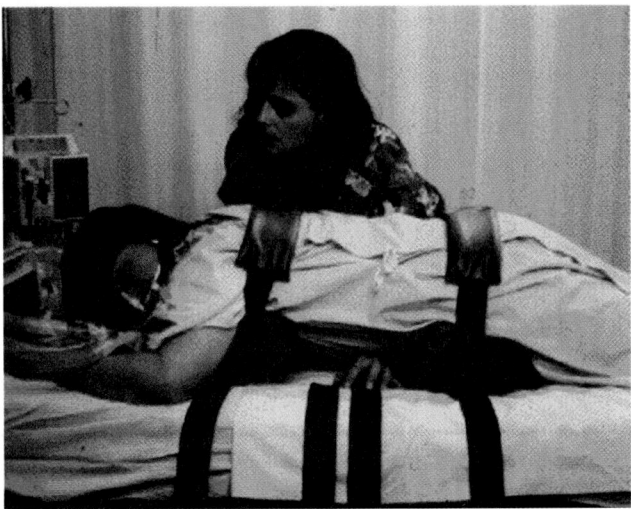

Figure 25-11 Patient in prone position. *(Courtesy Kathleen Vollman and Hill-Rom Services, Inc., Batesville, IN.)*

therapy. The patient is continuously turned from side to side with a 40-degree or greater rotation (kinetic therapy) or with a less than 40-degree rotation (CLRT).[74] Two types of beds can perform this type of therapy: an oscillation bed, one in which the mattress inflates and deflates to provide rotation, and a kinetic bed, one in which the entire platform of the bed rotates.[75]

Rotation therapy is thought to improve oxygenation through better matching of ventilation to perfusion[76] and to prevent pulmonary complications associated with bed rest and mechanical ventilation.[77] However, to achieve such benefits, rotation must be aggressive, and the patient must be turned at least 40 degrees per side, with a total arc of at least 80 degrees,[78] for at least 18 hours a day.[77] CLRT has been shown to be of minimal pulmonary benefit to the critically ill patient.[74] Kinetic therapy decreases the incidence of VAP, particularly in neurologic and postoperative patients.[78] In one study, kinetic therapy decreased the incidence of VAP and lobar atelectasis in medical, surgical, and trauma patients.[77]

Complications of the procedure include dislodgment or obstruction of tubes, drains, and lines; hemodynamic instability; and pressure ulcers. Lateral rotation does not replace manual repositioning to prevent pressure ulcers.[79] Repositioning changes the relationship of the patient's posterior surface to the mattress. This gives the skin a chance to reperfuse and to ventilate. Repositioning shifts weight-bearing points. To prevent pressure ulcers, the patient should be positioned 30 degrees from the surface of the mattress regardless of the degree of rotational turn. One study found that patients receiving rotational therapy still developed pressure ulcers of the sacrum, occiput, and heels.[80]

PHARMACOLOGY

A number of pharmacologic agents are used in the care of the critically ill patient with pulmonary dysfunction. Table 25-8 reviews these agents and the special considerations necessary for administering them.[81]

TABLE 25-8 Pharmacologic Management: Pulmonary Disorders

DRUG	DOSAGE	ACTIONS	SPECIAL CONSIDERATIONS
Neuromuscular Blocking Agents			
Vecuronium (Norcuron)	Loading dose: 0.08-0.1 mg/kg IV IV infusion: 0.8-1.2 mcg/kg/min	Used to paralyze patient to decrease oxygen demand and avoid ventilator dyssynchrony	Administer sedative and analgesic agents concurrently, because NMBAs have no sedative or analgesic properties.
Pancuronium (Pavulon)	Loading dose: 0.06-0.1 mg/kg IV IV infusion: 0.02-0.04 mg/kg/hr		Evaluate level of paralysis q4h using a peripheral nerve stimulator.
Pipecuronium (Arduan)	Loading dose: 0.8-0.1 mg/kg IV IV infusion: not recommended		Monitor patients for immobility complications.
Rocuronium (Zemuron)	Loading dose: 0.6-1 mg/kg IV IV infusion: 9-12 mcg/kg/min		Protect patients from the environment, because they are unable to respond.
Atracurium (Tracrium)	Loading dose: 0.3-0.4 mg/kg IV IV infusion: 4-12 mcg/kg/min		Prolonged muscle paralysis may occur after discontinuation of the paralytic agent.
Cisatracurium (Nimbex)	Loading dose: 0.1-0.2 mg/kg IV IV infusion: 2-8 mcg/kg/min		
Doxacurium (Nuromax)	Loading dose: 0.05-0.1 mg/kg IV IV infusion: 0.3-0.5 mcg/kg/min		
Mivacurium (Mivacron)	Loading dose: 0.15-0.25 mg/kg IV IV infusion: 3-15 mcg/kg/min		
Mucolytics			
Acetylcysteine (Mucomyst)	Nebulizer, 20% solution: 3-5 mL tid-qid Nebulizer, 10% solution: 6-10 mL tid-qid	Used to decrease viscosity and elasticity of mucus by breaking down disulfide bonds within the mucus	May be administered with a bronchodilator, because drug can cause bronchospasms and inhibit ciliary function. Treatment is considered effective when bronchorrhea develops and coughing occurs. Antidote for acetaminophen overdose.
β₂-Agonists			
Epinephrine (Adrenalin)	Nebulizer, 1% solution: 2.5-5 mg (0.25-0.5 mL) qid	Used to relax bronchial smooth muscle and dilate airways to prevent bronchospasms	May cause skeletal muscle tremors. Higher doses may cause tachycardia, palpitations, increased blood pressure, dysrhythmias, and angina.
Racemic epinephrine	Nebulizer, 2.25% solution: 5.625-11.25 mg (0.25-0.5 mL) qid		May increase serum glucose and decrease serum potassium levels.
Isoetharine 1% (Bronkosol)	Nebulizer, 1% solution: 2.5-5 mg (0.25-0.5 mL) qid		Treatment is considered effective when breath sounds improve and dyspnea is lessened.
Terbutaline (Brethaise, Brethine)	MDI, 340 mcg/puff: 1-2 puffs qid MDI, 200 mcg/puff: 2 puffs q4-6h		Only approximately 10% of the administered dose reaches the site of action within the lungs.
Metaproterenol (Alupent, Metaprel)	Nebulizer, 5% solution: 15 mg (0.3 mL) tid-qid MDI, 650 mcg/puff: 2-3 puffs tid-qid		
Albuterol (Proventil, Ventolin)	Nebulizer, 5% solution: 2.5 mg (0.5 mL) tid-qid MDI, 90 mcg/puff: 2 puffs tid-qid		
Bitolterol (Tomalate, Produral)	Nebulizer, 0.2% solution: 2.5 mg (1.25 mL) bid-qid MDI, 370 mcg/puff: 2 puffs q8h		
Levalbuterol (Xopenex)	Nebulizer: 0.63 mg q6-8h		
Anticholinergic Agents			
Ipratropium (Atrovent)	Nebulizer, 0.02% solution: 0.5 mg (2.5 mL) q6-8h	Used to block the constriction of bronchial smooth muscle and reduce mucus production	There are relatively few adverse effects, because systemic absorption is poor.

TABLE 25-8 Pharmacologic Management: Pulmonary Disorders—*cont'd*

DRUG	DOSAGE	ACTIONS	SPECIAL CONSIDERATIONS
Xanthines			
Theophylline	Loading dose: 5 mg/kg IV IV infusion: 0.5-0.7 mg/kg/hr	Used to dilate bronchial smooth muscle and reverse diaphragmatic muscle fatigue	Administer loading dose over 30 min. Monitor serum blood levels; therapeutic level is 10-20 mg/dL. Administer with caution to patients with cardiac, renal, or hepatic disease. Signs of toxicity include central nervous system excitation, seizures, confusion, irritability, hyperglycemia, headache, nausea, hypotension, and dysrhythmias.
Aminophylline	Loading dose: 6 mg/kg IV IV infusion: 0.5-0.7 mg/kg/hr		
Inhaled Corticosteroids			
Beclomethasone (Vanceril, Beclovent)	MDI, 42 mcg/puff: 2 puffs tid-qid	Used to decrease airway inflammation and enhance effectiveness of beta-agonists	Suppresses inflammatory response and interferes with ability to fight infection. Oral candidiasis is a side effect that can be minimized by having patients rinse their mouths after treatment.
Flunisolide (Aero Bid)	MDI, 250 mcg/puff: 2 puffs bid		
Triamcinolone (Azmacort)	MDI, 100 mcg/puff: 2 puffs tid-qid		

MDI, metered-dose inhaler, NMBAs, neuromuscular blocking agents.

BRONCHODILATORS AND ADJUNCTS

Medications to facilitate removal of secretions and dilate airways are of major benefit in the treatment of pulmonary disorders. Mucolytics are administered to help liquefy secretions, which facilitates their removal. Bronchodilators, such as β_2-agonists and anticholinergic agents, aid in smooth muscle relaxation and are of particular benefit to patients with airflow limitations. Steroids are often used in conjunction with β_2-agonists to enhance their effects and to decrease airway inflammation.[82-84]

NEUROMUSCULAR BLOCKING AGENTS

Sedation is necessary in many patients to assist with maintaining adequate ventilation. It can be used to comfort the patient and to decrease the work of breathing, particularly if the patient is fighting the ventilator. More information about sedation is provided in Chapter 10. In some patients, sedation does not decrease spontaneous respiratory efforts enough to allow adequate ventilation, and patient-ventilator dyssynchrony may develop. Neuromuscular paralysis may be necessary to facilitate optimal ventilation. Paralysis also may be necessary to decrease oxygen consumption in the severely compromised patient.[85-87]

Nursing management of the patient receiving a neuromuscular blocking agent should incorporate a number of additional interventions. Because paralytic agents only halt skeletal muscle movement and do not inhibit pain or awareness, they must be administered together with a sedative or anxiolytic agent. Pain medication is administered if the patient has a pain-producing illness or surgery. Providing reorientation and explanations for all procedures is critical, because the patient can still hear but cannot move or see. The patient is also at high risk for developing the complications of immobility, so interventions related to the prevention of skin breakdown, atelectasis, and deep vein thrombosis are also implemented. Patient safety is another concern, because the patient cannot react to the environment. Special precautions are taken to protect the patient at all times.[88]

Peripheral Nerve Stimulator. Long-term use of neuromuscular blocking agents can result in prolonged neuromuscular blockade and skeletal muscle weakness. To avoid this complication, the patient's level of paralysis is carefully monitored with the use of a peripheral nerve stimulator (PNS). The PNS delivers an electrical stimulus (single twitch, post-tetanic count, double-burst stimulation, or train-of-four [TOF]) to a preselected nerve (ulnar, facial, posterior tibial, or peroneal) by electrodes (needle, ball, or pregelled), and the response is monitored to gauge the level of paralysis.[88]

In most cases, the ulnar nerve is used, with pregelled electrodes being placed 2 to 3 inches proximal to the crease of the wrist (Fig. 25-12). The TOF stimulation test, which delivers four electrical stimuli in a row, is the most common test used. When the ulnar nerve is stimulated with TOF, the expected response is four twitches (adduction) of the thumb medially across the palm of the hand. The number of twitches correlates with the level of paralysis: four twitches indicates less than 75% blockade; three twitches is approximately 75% blockade; two twitches is approximately 80% blockade; one

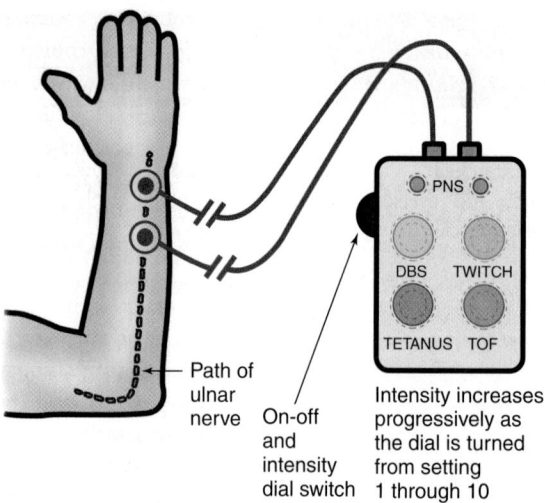

Figure 25-12 Peripheral nerve stimulator (PNS). Notice the placement of electrodes along the ulnar nerve. DBS, double-burst stimulation; TOF, train-of-four.

twitch is approximately 90% blockade; and zero twitches indicates 100% blockade. Usually, the neuromuscular blocking agent is titrated to maintain an 80% blockade (two twitches). The goal is to administer the smallest dose possible of the paralytic agent, to avoid prolonged weakness after the therapy is discontinued.[88]

Use of the PNS for estimating the degree of paralysis is not without its problems. Poor skin contact, improper electrode placement, edema in the extremity being monitored, and malfunction of the device can lead to overestimation of the degree of blockade. The patient appears to have a zero-twitch TOF response, but evidence of muscle movement is present. More problematic is underestimation of the degree of blockade. Direct stimulation of the muscle or mistaking finger responses for those of the thumb can result in a false-positive twitch response. This can result in unnecessary administration of additional doses of the paralytic agent. It is imperative that the patient's twitch response be correlated with clinical observations of patient movement.[88]

Case Study: Patient with Acute Respiratory Failure

⊖volve   Answers to the Case Study Questions can be found on the Evolve web site at http://evolve.elsevier.com/Urden/.

Brief Patient History
Mr. B is a 63-year-old, obese man. He has a long history of chronic obstructive pulmonary disease (COPD) associated with smoking two packs of cigarettes a day for 40 years. During the past week, Mr. B has experienced a flulike illness with fever, chills, malaise, anorexia, diarrhea, nausea, vomiting, and a productive cough with thick, brownish, purulent sputum.

Clinical Assessment
Mr. B is admitted to the intermediate care unit from the emergency department with acute respiratory insufficiency. He is sitting up in bed, leaning forward, with his elbows resting on the over-the-bed table. Mr. B is breathing through his mouth, taking rapid shallow breathes, using his accessory muscles to ventilate. On inhalation, his nostrils flare and his intercostal muscles retract. During exhalation, Mr. B. uses pursed-lip breathing and his intercostal muscles bulge. He appears anxious and irritable and is able to speak only one or two barely audible words between each breath. Auscultation reveals crackles posteriorly over the right and left lower lung fields.

Diagnostic Procedures
His admission chest radiograph reveals infiltrates in the right lower lobe and left lower lobe. Gram stain of Mr. B's sputum shows numerous

gram-positive diplococci. His baseline vital signs are as follows: blood pressure of 110/60 mm Hg, heart rate of 108 beats/min (sinus tachycardia), respiratory rate of 30 breaths/min, and temperature of 101.3° F. His baseline arterial blood gas (ABG) values on a 28% Venturi face mask are as follows: PaO_2 of 58 mm Hg, $PaCO_2$ of 33 mm Hg, pH of 7.52, HCO_3^- level of 28, and O_2 saturation of 88%.

Medical Diagnosis
Mr. B is diagnosed with community-associated pneumococcal pneumonia.

Questions
1. What major outcomes do you expect to achieve for this patient?
2. What problems or risks must be managed to achieve these outcomes?
3. What interventions must be initiated to monitor, prevent, manage, or eliminate the problems and risks identified?
4. What interventions should be initiated to promote optimal functioning, safety, and well-being of the patient?
5. What possible learning needs do you anticipate for this patient?
6. What cultural and age-related factors may have a bearing on the patient's plan of care?

Summary

Oxygen Therapy
- Oxygen is a drug, and its primary indication is hypoxemia.
- Oxygen can be delivered by various methods, including low-flow systems, reservoir systems, and high-flow systems.
- Complications of oxygen therapy include oxygen toxicity, carbon dioxide retention, and absorption atelectasis.

Artificial Airways
- Artificial airways (oropharyngeal and nasopharyngeal) are used to maintain airway patency by keeping the tongue from obstructing the upper airway.
- ETTs (oral and nasal) are used to maintain airway patency, to protect the airway from aspiration, to facilitate access to invasive positive-pressure ventilation, and to aid in secretion removal.

- Complications of ETTs include tube obstruction, tube displacement, sinusitis and nasal injury, tracheoesophageal fistula, mucosal lesions, laryngeal or tracheal stenosis, and cricoid abscess.
- Tracheostomy tubes provide the best method of long-term airway maintenance.
- Complications of tracheostomy tubes include hemorrhage, wound infection, subcutaneous emphysema, tube obstruction, tube displacement, tracheal stenosis, tracheoesophageal fistula, tracheoinnominate artery fistula, and tracheocutaneous fistula.
- Cuff pressure should be monitored every shift and should be maintained at 20 to 25 mm Hg (24 to 30 cm H_2O).
- Humidification is required for all ETTs and tracheostomy tubes.
- Complications associated with suctioning can be minimized if hyperoxygenation is initiated before the start of the procedure, each suction pass is limited to 10 to 15 seconds, and normal saline is not instilled.
- Oral care should consist of brushing the patient's teeth with a soft toothbrush to reduce plaque, brushing the patient's tongue and gums with a foam swab to stimulate the tissue, and performing deep oropharyngeal suction to remove any secretions that have pooled above the cuff.
- After an artificial airway is no longer needed, it should be removed.

Invasive Mechanical Ventilation

- Indications for mechanical ventilation include supporting cardiopulmonary gas exchange (alveolar ventilation and arterial oxygenation), increasing lung volume (end-expiratory lung inflation and functional residual capacity), and reducing the work of breathing.
- Complications associated with mechanical ventilation include ventilator-induced lung injury, cardiovascular compromise, gastrointestinal disturbances, patient-ventilator dyssynchrony, and VAP.
- Strategies to prevent VAP include semirecumbent positioning, CASS, meticulous oral hygiene with antiseptics such as chlorhexidine, and proper hand hygiene.
- Weaning is the gradual withdrawal of the mechanical ventilator and the reestablishment of spontaneous breathing; it should begin only after the original process for which ventilator support was required has been corrected and patient stability has been achieved.

Noninvasive Mechanical Ventilation

- Noninvasive mechanical ventilation uses a mask instead of an ETT to administer positive-pressure ventilation and is indicated in type I and type II acute respiratory failure, cardiogenic pulmonary edema, and other situations in which intubation is not an option.
- Respiratory rate, accessory muscle use, and oxygenation status are continually assessed to ensure that the patient is tolerating this method of ventilation.

Positioning Therapy

- Based on the concept that there is preferential blood flow to the gravity-dependent areas of the lungs, positioning therapy is used to place the least damaged portion of the lungs into a dependent position.
- Prone positioning involves turning the patient completely over onto his or her stomach in the face-down position; it is used to improve oxygenation in ALI.
- Kinetic therapy (continuous turning of a patient from side to side with a 40–degree or greater rotation) and CLRT (continuous turning with a less than 40–degree rotation) are two forms of rotation therapy.
- Rotation therapy is thought to improve oxygenation through better matching of ventilation to perfusion and to prevent pulmonary complications associated with bed rest and mechanical ventilation.

Pharmacology

- Mucolytics are administered to help liquefy secretions, which facilitates their removal.
- Bronchodilators, such as β_2-agonists and anticholinergic agents, aid in smooth muscle relaxation and are of particular benefit to patients with airflow limitations.
- Steroids are often used in conjunction with β_2-agonists to enhance their effects and to decrease airway inflammation.
- Sedation is necessary in many patients to assist with maintaining adequate ventilation; it can be used to comfort the patient and to decrease the work of breathing, particularly if the patient is fighting the ventilator.
- Neuromuscular paralysis may be necessary to facilitate optimal ventilation and to decrease oxygen consumption in the severely compromised patient.
- To avoid prolonged neuromuscular blockade, the patient's level of paralysis is carefully monitored by means of a PNS.

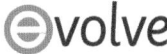 Be sure to check out the bonus material, including free self-assessment exercises, on the Evolve web site at http://evolve.elsevier.com/Urden/.

References

1. O'Connor BS, Vender JS: Oxygen therapy, *Crit Care Clin* 11:67, 1995.
2. Kruse JA: Oxygen therapy. In Kruse JA et al, editors: *Saunders manual of critical care*, Philadelphia, 2003, Saunders.
3. Heuer AJ, Scanlan CL: Medical gas therapy. In Wilkins RL et al, editors: *Egan's fundamentals of respiratory care*, ed 9, St Louis, 2009, Mosby.
4. White AC: The evaluation and management of hypoxemia in the chronic critically ill patient, *Clin Chest Med* 22:123, 2001.
5. Kim V et al: Oxygen therapy in chronic obstructive pulmonary disease, *Proc Am Thorac Soc* 5:513, 2008.

6. Barnes TA: Emergency cardiovascular life support. In Wilkins RL et al, editors: *Egan's fundamentals of respiratory care*, ed 9, St Louis, 2009, Mosby.

7. Pierce LNB: *Management of the mechanically ventilated patient*, ed 2, St Louis, 2007, Saunders.

8. McCorstin P et al: Management of the mechanically ventilated patient in the emergency department, *J Emerg Nurs* 34:121, 2008.

9. Walz JM et al: Airway management in critical illness, *Chest* 131:608, 2007.

10. St. John RE, Seckel MA: Airway management. In Burns SM, editor: *AACN protocols for practice: care of the mechanically ventilated patient*, ed 2, Sudbury, MA, 2007, Jones & Bartlett.

11. Simmons KF, Scanlan CL: Airway management. In Wilkins RL et al, editors: *Egan's fundamentals of respiratory care*, ed 9, St Louis, 2009, Mosby.

12. Chethan DB, Hughes RC: Tracheal intubation, tracheal tubes and laryngeal mask airways, *J Perioper Pract* 18:88, 2008.

13. Colice GL: Technical standards for tracheal tubes, *Clin Chest Med* 12:433, 1991.

14. Loh KS, Irish JC: Traumatic complications of intubation and other airway management procedures, *Anesthesiol Clin North Am* 20:953, 2002.

15. Feller-Kopman D: Acute complications of artificial airways, *Clin Chest Med* 24:445, 2003.

16. King C, Moores LK: Controversies in mechanical ventilation: when should a tracheotomy be placed? *Clin Chest Med* 29:253, 2008.

17. St John RE, Malen JF: Contemporary issues in adult tracheostomy management, *Crit Care Nurs Clin North Am* 16:413, 2004.

18. Rana S et al: Tracheostomy in critically ill patients, *Mayo Clin Proc* 80:1632, 2005.

19. Sue RD, Susanto I: Long-term complications of artificial airways, *Clin Chest Med* 24:457, 2003.

20. Zuchner K: Humidification: measurement and requirements, *Respir Care Clin North Am* 12:149, 2006.

21. Fink J: Humidity and bland aerosol therapy. In Wilkins RL et al, editors: *Egan's fundamentals of respiratory care*, ed 9, St Louis, 2009, Mosby.

22. Schulze A: Respiratory gas conditioning and humidification, *Clin Perinatol* 34:19, 2007.

23. Wright SE, VanDahm K: Long-term care of the tracheostomy patient, *Clin Chest Med* 24:473, 2003.

24. Bivona: *Fome-Cuf users manual*, Gary, IN, 1991, Bivona.

25. Grap MJ et al: Endotracheal suctioning: ventilator vs. manual delivery of hyperoxygenation breaths, *Am J Crit Care* 5:192, 1996.

26. Stone KS: Ventilator versus manual resuscitation bag as the method of delivering hyperoxygenation before endotracheal suctioning, *AACN Clin Issues Crit Care Nurs* 1:289, 1990.

27. Czarnik RE et al: Differential effects of continuous versus intermittent suction on tracheal tissue, *Heart Lung* 20:144, 1991.

28. Raymond SJ: Normal saline instillation before suctioning: helpful or harmful? A review of the literature, *Am J Crit Care* 4:267, 1995.

29. Kinloch D: Instillation of normal saline during endotracheal suctioning: effects on mixed venous oxygen saturation, *Am J Crit Care* 8:231, 1999.

30. Hagler DA, Traver GA: Endotracheal saline and suction catheters: sources of lower airway contamination, *Am J Crit Care* 3:444, 1994.

31. Sanja J et al: Clinical review: airway hygiene in the intensive care unit, *Crit Care* 12:209, 2008.

32. Jablonski RS: The experience of being mechanically ventilated, *Qual Health Res* 4:186, 1994.

33. Williams ML: An algorithm for selecting a communication technique with intubated patients, *Dimens Crit Care Nurs* 11:222, 1992.

34. Hodder RV: A 55-year-old patient with advanced COPD, tracheostomy tube, and sudden respiratory distress, *Chest* 120:279, 2002.

35. DePew CL, McCarthy MS: Subglottic secretion drainage: a literature review, *AACN Adv Crit Care* 18:366, 2007.

36. Yoon MN, Steele CM: The oral care imperative: the link between oral hygiene and aspiration pneumonia, *Top Geri Rehab* 23:280, 2007.

37. Munro CL, Grap MJ: Oral health and care in the intensive care unit: state of the science, *Am J Crit Care* 13:25, 2004.

38. Binkley et al: Survey of oral care practices in U.S. intensive care units, *Am J Infect Control* 32:161, 2004.

39. Garcia R: A review of the possible role of oral and dental colonization on the occurrence of health-care associated pneumonia: underappreciated risk and a call for interventions, *Am J Infect Control* 33:527, 2005.

40. Chlebicki MP, Safdar N: Topical chlorhexidine for prevention of ventilator-associated pneumonia: a meta-analysis, *Crit Care Med* 35: 595, 2007.

41. Haitsma JJ: Physiology mechanical ventilation, *Crit Care Clin* 23:117, 2007.

42. Chatburn RL, Volsko TA: Mechanical ventilators. In Wilkins RL et al, editors: *Egan's fundamentals of respiratory care*, ed 9, St Louis, 2009, Mosby.

43. Pilbeam SP, Cairo SP: *Mechanical ventilation: physiological and clinical applications*, ed 4, St Louis, 2006, Mosby.

44. MacIntyre NR, Branson RD: *Mechanical ventilation*, ed 2, St Louis, 2009, Saunders.

45. Shelledy DC: Initiating and adjusting ventilatory support. In Wilkins RL et al, editors: *Egan's fundamentals of respiratory care*, ed 9, St Louis, 2009, Mosby.

46. Adams AB et al: Ventilator-induced lung injury, *Respir Care Clin North Am* 9:343, 2003.

47. Carney D et al: Dynamic alveolar mechanics and ventilator-induced lung injury, *Crit Care Med* 33(3 suppl):S122, 2005.

48. Hemmila MR, Napolitano LM: Severe respiratory failure: advanced treatment options, *Crit Care Med* 34(9 suppl):S278, 2006.

49. Sarge T, Talmor D: Transpulmonary pressure: its role in preventing ventilator-induced lung injury, *Minerva Anesthesiol* 74:335, 2008.

50. dos Santos CC, Slutsky AS: The contribution of biophysical lung injury to the development of biotrauma, *Annu Rev Physiol* 68:585, 2006.

51. Frazier SK: Cardiovascular effects of mechanical ventilation and weaning, *Nurs Clin North Am* 43:1, 2008.

52. Ramar K, Sassoon CS: Potential advantages of patient-ventilator synchrony, *Respir Care Clin North Am* 11:307, 2005.

53. Augustyn B: Ventilator-associated pneumonia: risk factors and prevention, *Crit Care Nurse* 27(4):32, 2007.

54. Flanders SA, Collard HR, Saint S: Nosocomial pneumonia: state of the science, *Am J Infect Control* 34:84, 2006.

55. Aragon D, Sole ML: Implementing best practice strategies to prevent infection in the ICU, *Crit Care Nurs Clin North Am* 18:441, 2006.

56. Defzulian C et al: Subglottic secretion drainage for preventing ventilator-associated pneumonia: a meta-analysis, *Am J Med* 118:11, 2005.

57. Lorente L et al: Influence of an endotracheal tube with polyurethane cuff and subglottic secretion drainage on pneumonia, *Am J Respir Crit Care Med* 176: 1079, 2007.

58. Kollef MH et al: Silver-coated endotracheal tubes and incidence of ventilator-associated pneumonia: the NASCENT randomized trial, *JAMA* 300:805, 2008.

59. Ramirez P et al: Prevention measures for ventilator-associated pneumonia: a new focus on the endotracheal tube, *Curr Opin Infect Dis* 20:190, 2007.

60. Shelledy DC: Discontinuing ventilatory support. In Wilkins RL et al, editors: *Egan's fundamentals of respiratory care*, ed 9, St Louis, 2009, Mosby.

61. MacIntyre N: Discontinuing mechanical ventilatory support, *Chest* 132:1049, 2007.

62. Robertson TE et al: Improved extubation rates and earlier liberation from mechanical ventilation with implementation of a daily spontaneous-breathing trial protocol, *J Am Coll Surg* 206:489, 2008.

63. Burns SM: Weaning from mechanical ventilation. In Burns SM, editor: *AACN protocols for practice: care of the mechanically ventilated patient*, ed 2, Sudbury, MA, 2007, Jones & Bartlett.

64. Siner JM, Manthous CA: Liberation from mechanical ventilation: what monitoring matters? *Crit Care Clin* 23:613, 2007.

65. Caroleo S et al: Weaning from mechanical ventilation: an open issue, *Minerva Anesthesiol* 73:417, 2007.

66. Bekos V, Marinia JJ: Monitoring the mechanically ventilated patient, *Crit Care Clin* 23:575, 2007.

67. Garpestad E et al: Noninvasive ventilation for critical care, *Chest* 132:711, 2007.

68. Kwok H et al: Controlled trial of oronasal versus nasal mask ventilation in the treatment of acute respiratory failure, *Crit Care Med* 31:468, 2003.

69. Barreira TJ, Gemmel DJ: Noninvasive ventilation, *Crit Care Clin* 23:201, 2007.

70. Pierce LNB: Invasive and noninvasive modes and methods of mechanical ventilation. In Burns SM, editor: *AACN protocols for practice: care of the mechanically ventilated patient*, ed 2, Sudbury, MA, 2007, Jones & Bartlett.

71. Misasi RS, Keyes JL: Matching and mismatching ventilation and perfusion in the lung, *Crit Care Nurse* 16(3):23, 1996.

72. Alsaghir AH, Martin CM: Effect of prone positioning in patients with acute respiratory distress syndrome: a meta-analysis, *Crit Care Med* 36:603, 2008.

73. Vollman KM: Prone positioning in the patient who has acute respiratory distress syndrome: The art and science, *Crit Care Nurs Clin North Am* 16:319, 2004.

74. Goldhill DR et al: Rotational bed therapy to prevent and treat respiratory complications: a review and meta-analysis, *Am J Crit Care* 16:50, 2007.

75. Stiller K: Physiotherapy in intensive care: towards an evidence-based practice, *Chest* 118:1801, 2000.

76. Rance M: Kinetic therapy positively influences oxygenation in patients with ALI/ARDS, *Nurs Crit Care* 10:35, 2005.

77. Ahrens T et al: Effect of kinetic therapy on pulmonary complications, *Am J Crit Care Nurs* 13:376, 2004.

78. Collard HR: Prevention of ventilator-associated pneumonia: an evidenced-based systematic review, *Ann Intern Med* 138:494, 2003.

79. Powers J, Daniels D: Turning points: implementing kinetic therapy in the ICU, *Nurs Manage* 35(5):1, 2004.

80. Russell T, Logsdon A: Pressure ulcers and lateral rotation beds: a case study, *J Wound Ostomy Continence Nurs* 30:143, 2003.

81. MICROMEDEX

82. Grimes GC et al: Medications for COPD: a review of effectiveness, *Am Fam Physician* 76:1141, 2007.

83. Gardenhire DS: Airway pharmacology. In Wilkins RL et al, editors: *Egan's fundamentals of respiratory care*, ed 9, St Louis, 2009, Mosby.

84. Hanania NA, Sharafkhaneh A: Update on the pharmacologic therapy for chronic obstructive pulmonary disease, *Clin Chest Med* 28:589, 2007.

85. Jacobi J et al: Clinical practice guidelines for the sustained use of sedatives and analgesics in the critically ill adult, *Crit Care Med* 30:119, 2002.

86. Murray MJ: Clinical practice guidelines for sustained neuromuscular blockade in the adult critically ill patient, *Crit Care Med* 30:142, 2002.

87. Luer J: Sedation and neuromuscular blockade in mechanically ventilated patients. In Burns SM, editor: *AACN protocols for practice: care of the mechanically ventilated patient*, ed 2, Sudbury, MA, 2007, Jones & Bartlett.

88. Loyola R, Dreher HM: Management of pharmacologically induced neuromuscular blockade using peripheral nerve stimulation, *Dimens Crit Care Nurs* 22:157, 2003.

Neurologic Anatomy and Physiology

The nervous system is the "executive suite" of the human body. It directs all other systems and provides the unique ability for thought, emotion, understanding of complex information, and integration of numerous stimuli. As the recipient of all sensory information for analysis, the nervous system generates intellectual and motor responses aimed at maintaining integrity of life structures. Critical care nurses must attain a basic understanding of the anatomy and physiology of this complex system, because it serves as the basis for innervation and proper functioning of all other systems. This chapter reviews the anatomic divisions and functions of the central nervous system (CNS), including the cellular microstructure, protective encasement, networked functions, and mechanisms aimed at maintenance of structural and physiologic integrity. The cranial nerves, a component of the peripheral nervous system (PNS), are presented in tabular form.

DIVISIONS OF THE NERVOUS SYSTEM

The nervous system is the most highly organized system of the body, with all of its parts functioning as an inseparable unit. This system is usually classified by anatomic function.

ANATOMIC DIVISIONS

The CNS is made up of the brain and spinal cord. The PNS comprises the 12 pairs of cranial nerves, the 31 pairs of spinal nerves, and all other nerves serving a variety of functions throughout the body.

PHYSIOLOGIC DIVISIONS

The somatic, or voluntary, nervous system is composed of fibers that connect the CNS with structures of the skeletal muscles and the skin. The autonomic, or involuntary, nervous system is composed of fibers that connect the CNS with smooth muscle, cardiac muscle, internal organs, and glands. It includes sympathetic and parasympathetic branches.

Most activities of the nervous system originate from sensory receptors, such as visual, auditory, or tactile receptors. This sensory information is transmitted to the CNS by afferent fibers (sensory fibers). Efferent fibers (motor fibers) transmit the CNS response to the periphery to produce a motor response, such as contraction of skeletal muscles, contraction of the smooth muscles of organs, or secretion by endocrine glands. To better understand the macrostructure and functions of the nervous system, it helps to study the microstructure, or cellular level.

MICROSTRUCTURE OF THE NERVOUS SYSTEM

Two types of cells make up the nervous system: neurons and neuroglia. Neurons are the cells primarily charged with the functional work of the nervous system, including receipt of information, integration, and transmission or conduction of nerve impulses to recipient cells. Neuroglial cells serve as the support infrastructure of the nervous system, providing protection and a structural foundation for neurons and participating in neuronal repair.

NEUROGLIA

In the nervous system, there are 6 to 10 times more neuroglial cells than neurons. Neuroglial cells consist of four types: *astroglia (astrocytes), oligodendroglia, ependyma,* and *microglia* (Fig. 26-1). These cells provide the neuron with structural support, nourishment, and protection (Table 26-1).[1] They retain the ability to replicate, but they can replicate abnormally and therefore are the primary source of CNS neoplasms.[1-3]

NEURONS

Neurons are the basic functional unit within the CNS, and they are charged with the highly specialized task of data integration and signal transmission. The CNS is made up of more than 10 billion neurons.[1,3] The cellular appearance of neurons varies, but each cell contains three basic components: the cell body, dendrites, and an axon (Fig. 26-2). Neurons are structurally classified as *unipolar*, a cell body with one process that divides into a central branch (one axon) and a peripheral branch (one dendrite); as *bipolar*, a cell body with two processes (one axon

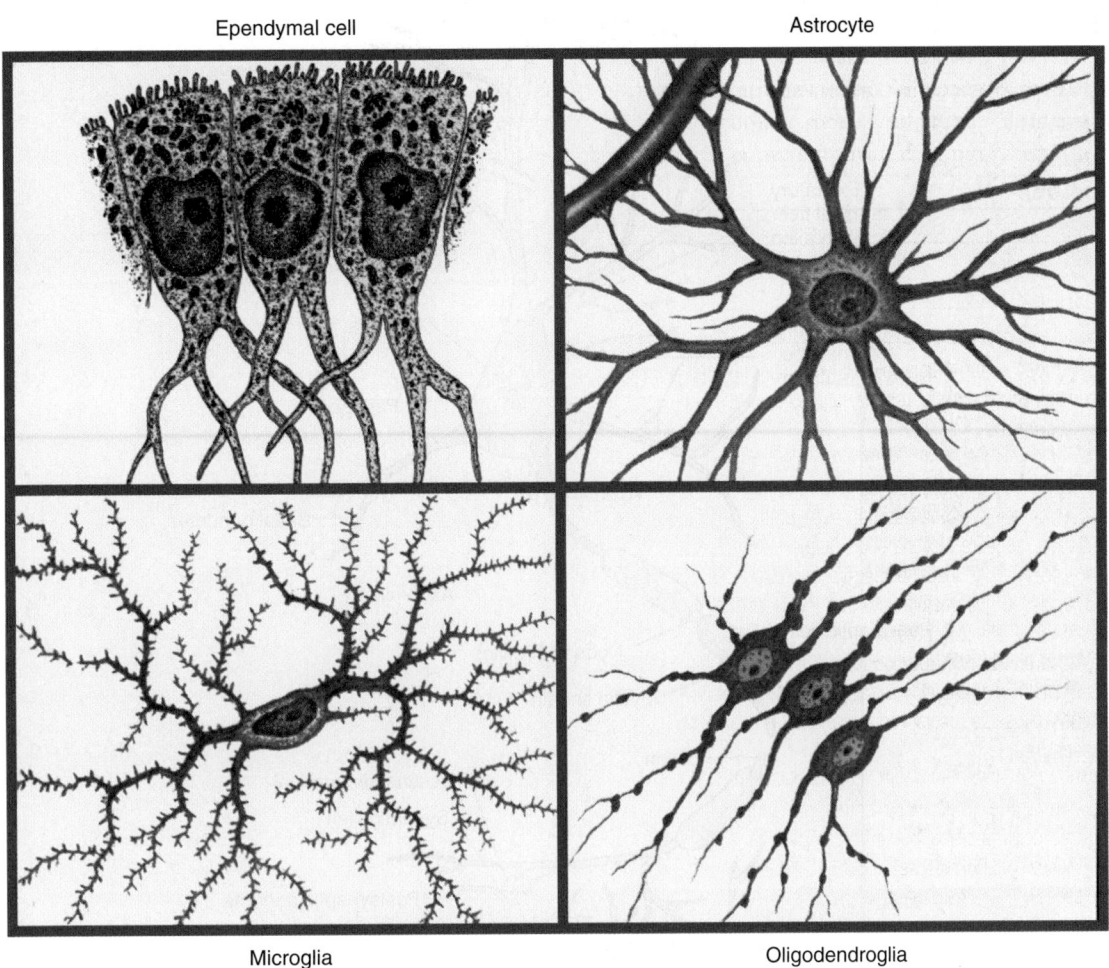

Figure 26-1 Types of neuroglial cells. *(From Thompson JM et al: Mosby's clinical nursing, ed 5. St Louis, 2002, Mosby.)*

TABLE 26-1	**Types of Neuroglial Cells**
Cell Type	**Function**
Astroglia (astrocyte)	Supplies nutrients to neuron structure and to support framework for neurons and capillaries; forms part of the blood-brain barrier
Oligodendroglia	Forms the myelin sheath in the central nervous system (CNS)
Ependyma	Lines the ventricular system; forms the choroid plexus, which produces cerebrospinal fluid (CSF)
Microglia	Occurs mainly in the white matter; phagocytizes waste products from injured neurons

and one dendrite); or *multipolar*, a cell body with one axon and several dendrites. The cell body (soma) controls the metabolic activity of the neuron and contains the organelles necessary for cellular metabolism and maintenance, such as the nucleus, mitochondria, endoplasmic reticulum, Golgi apparatus, and liposomes. Compared with other body cells, the neuron's protein-embedded membrane with its phospholipid bilayer is unique, consisting of specialized pores that work as ion-specific channels or pumps to promote passage of ions through an otherwise impermeable plasma membrane.[3]

The neuronal cell body is the life support unit of the neuron. The metabolic demands of these specialized units necessitate uninterrupted perfusion with glucose and oxygen to maintain neuronal life and optimal functioning. Until recently, it was believed that CNS neuronal repair was impossible, but research has validated that neurons are more *plastic* than was previously thought, although rates of repair (plasticity) or restoration of neuronal function are driven by factors that remain largely unknown.[4-6] Within the brain and spinal cord, neuronal cell bodies make up regions of gray matter. Outside the CNS, *ganglia* are cell bodies within the PNS that reside near and work closely with CNS neurons.[1,3]

Dendrites form the receptive component of the neuron; they are branched fibers extending only a short distance from the cell body. Each neuron may have several dendrites, which function as impulse receivers for the cell body.[1,3,7] The axon is the part of the neuron concerned with transmission of impulses away from the cell body to other neurons, muscle cells, endocrine glands, or some other effector organ. Neurons contain only one axon, whose length may be microscopic or, in some cases,

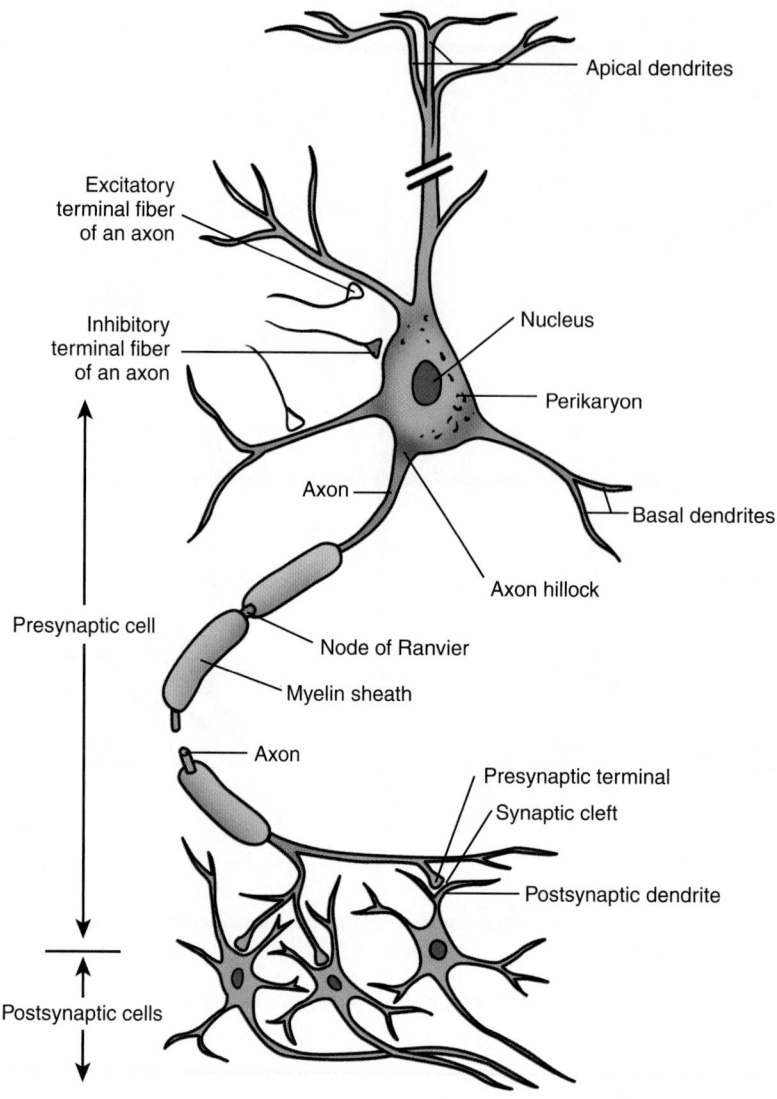

Apical dendrites

Excitatory
terminal fiber
of an axon

Inhibitory
terminal fiber
of an axon

Nucleus

Perikaryon

Axon

Basal dendrites

Axon hillock

Presynaptic cell

Node of Ranvier

Myelin sheath

Axon

Presynaptic terminal

Synaptic cleft

Postsynaptic dendrite

Postsynaptic cells

Figure 26-2 Anatomy of a neuron. *(From Layon AJ et al:* Textbook of neurointensive care, *Philadelphia, 2004, Saunders.)*

may extend up to 4 feet. Some axons are protected by a myelin sheath, a white phospholipid complex laid down by Schwann cells in the PNS and by oligodendroglia in the CNS. Myelin sheathes protect neuronal axons and provide insulation for the conduction of nerve impulses.[1,3,8] Fibers enclosed in the sheath are called *myelinated fibers;* those not enclosed are called *unmyelinated fibers.* The white matter of the CNS is composed of myelinated fiber tracts.

Myelinated fibers use a process called *saltatory conduction* to support rapid axonal transmission of nerve impulses.[1,8] Structurally, axons participating in this form of impulse transmission are laid out with a noncontinuous myelin cover, interrupted with 2-μm bare segments called the *nodes of Ranvier.* These nodes are packed with sodium channels, making them extremely sensitive to membrane depolarization. Because segments of the axon covered by myelin are impervious to sodium influx, impulse transmission is pulled down the length of the axon to the next node of Ranvier. Saltatory conduction increases transmission velocity up to 100-fold, allowing transmission at rates as high as 120 m/sec.[8]

Neuronal function is driven by depolarization-repolarization cycles, similar to that described for cardiac physiology (see Chapter 16), but what makes the nervous system so exceptional is its ability to undergo the depolarization-repolarization cycle up to 1000 times per second to ensure optimal receipt, integration, and transmission of information throughout the body.[3] The movement of ions across the neuronal membrane generates electrical action potentials (Figs. 26-3 and 26-4). Neuronal resting membrane potential (RMP) is −65 mV, approximating the equilibrium potential for potassium; on depolarization, sodium channels open, shifting the equilibrium potential in a positive direction.[1,3,8]

Mechanisms for ionic movement involve two types of neuronal channels: *voltage-gated* and *ligand-gated.* Many pharmaceutical and therapeutic agents in use or undergoing testing manipulate these ionic transport mechanisms. Voltage-gated channels become activated with changes in transmembrane electrical potential, promoting sodium and calcium influx and potassium efflux. These channels are the primary drivers of cellular action potentials.[1,2,6] Ligand-gated channels are primarily

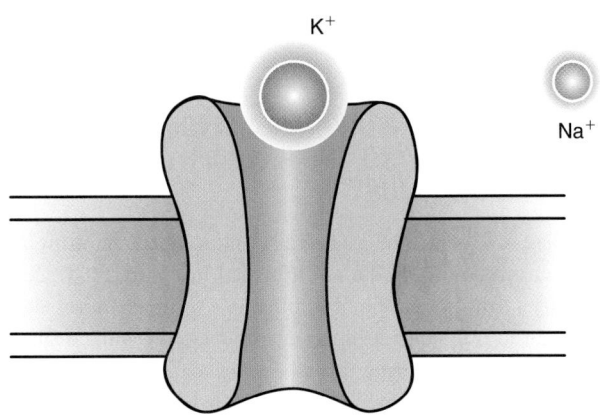

Figure 26-3 Neuronal voltage-gated channel selectivity. K^+, potassium ion; Na^+, sodium ion. *(From Layon AJ et al: Textbook of neurointensive care, Philadelphia, 2004, Saunders.)*

concerned with mitigating the response of a postsynaptic neuron to synapse and are discussed in more detail later.[2,3,9]

Action potentials begin with the influx of sodium, producing a focal zone of membrane depolarization at some level between −55 mV to −35 mV. After this critical threshold is reached, a large number of sodium channels open, resulting in fast and massive localized depolarization of the plasma membrane. Rapid sodium influx (upstroke phase) increases the membrane potential to between 70 mV and 90 mV. As the membrane potential changes locally, it stimulates adjoining regions in the neuron to begin depolarization in a self-propagating fashion until depolarization is complete. Within a millisecond of opening, sodium channels close and become inactive.[1,2,6]

Depolarization causes potassium channels to open, allowing this ion to flow out into the extracellular space, thereby promoting the onset of repolarization. Potassium efflux triggers the cell membrane to return to a potassium equilibrium potential of approximately −75 mV, allowing potassium to reenter the cell but maintaining greater polarity than RMP to hold the cell refractory to another depolarization stimulus. Cellular pumps that depend on a steady supply of adenosine triphosphate (ATP) are also activated to remove sodium and restore the −65 mV RMP, allowing the cycle to begin anew.[1,6]

After an action potential reaches the axon terminal, it initiates a cascade of events that promote interneuronal communication, or *synapse*. Two types of synapse exist: electrical and chemical. In an electrical synapse, gap junctions made up of narrow (3.5-nm) bridges allow cytoplasm and intracellular metabolites to pass in an essentially continuous fashion between neurons, facilitating impulse conduction from one neuron to the next.[1,9] In a chemical synapse, which is involved in most synaptic events, no physical bridge exists between neurons. Instead, a large synaptic cleft of 20 to 40 nm prevents direct action potential transmission from one neuron to another

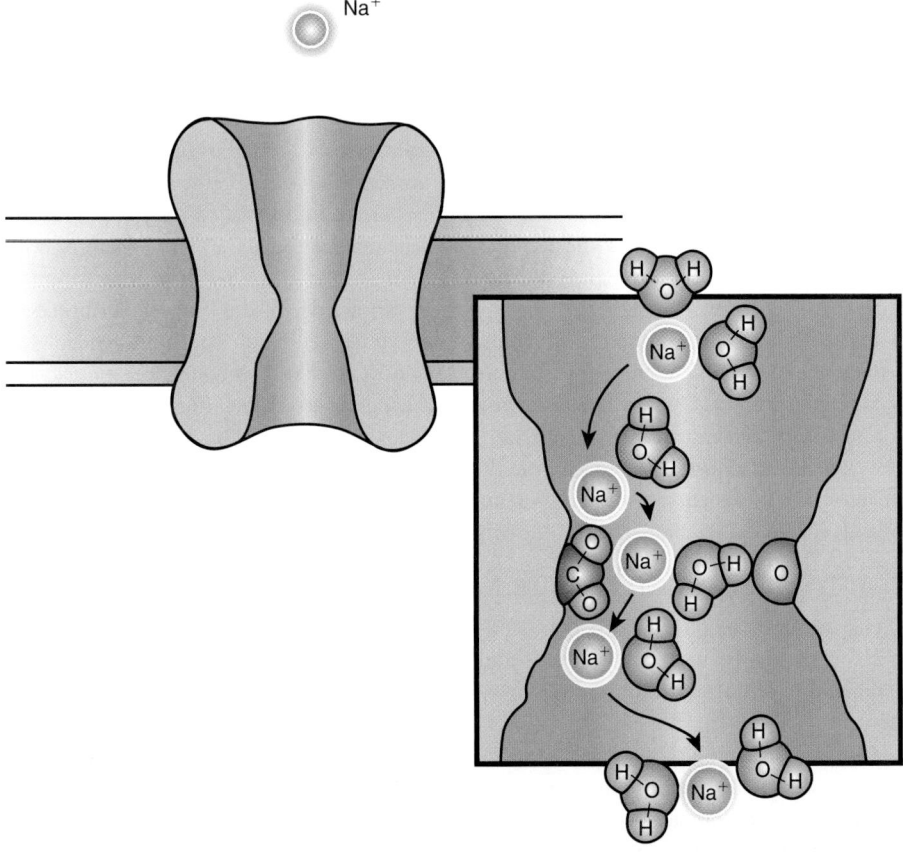

Figure 26-4 Selectivity filter of voltage-gated channels. CO_2, carbon dioxide molecule; H_2O, water molecule; Na^+, sodium ion. *(From Layon AJ et al: Textbook of neurointensive care, Philadelphia, 2004, Saunders.)*

(see Fig. 26-2).[9] When the wave of depolarization reaches the presynaptic terminal, it signals the release of neurotransmitters into the synaptic cleft.

There are two classifications of neurotransmitters: small-molecule transmitters and neuroactive peptides.[9] Examples of small-molecule transmitters include acetylcholine, dopamine, norepinephrine, epinephrine, serotonin, histamine, gamma-aminobutyric acid (GABA), glycine, and glutamate. Neuroactive peptides include substances such as pituitary peptides, hypothalamic-releasing hormones, and neurohypophyseal hormones. This chapter is primarily concerned with the small-molecule transmitters, which are stored in vesicles within the axon terminal and released into the synapse through a process called *exocytosis*. Exocytosis is stimulated by arrival of the action potential in the axon terminal and results in release of neurotransmitters into the synaptic cleft, where these molecules rapidly diffuse to interact with postsynaptic receptors.[8,9]

Ligand-gated channels are activated by binding of ligand agonists to receptors on the postsynaptic neuron.[1,9] Ions passing through ligand-gated channels promote an excitatory or inhibitory response within postsynaptic neurons. Examples of excitatory ligand-gated channel receptors include the inotropic glutamate receptors (*N*-methyl-D-aspartate [NMDA], α-amino-3-hydroxyl-5-methyl-4-isoxazolepropionic acid [AMPA], and kainite), which are primarily concerned with gating sodium, potassium, and calcium ions. Examples of inhibitory ligand-gated channel receptors include GABA receptors, glycine receptors, and nicotinic acetylcholine receptors. Most GABA receptors are found in the brain, where GABA serves as the primary inhibitory neurotransmitter, whereas glycine serves as the spinal cord's primary postsynaptic inhibitory neurotransmitter. GABA and glycine channels gate chloride ions, which inhibit by promoting repolarization to the chloride equilibrium potential (-60 mV) and by short-circuiting incoming excitatory potentials by gating anions and clamping the membrane shut to excitatory cations (shunting).[9] In other words, when inhibitor neurotransmitters are released, the neuron's internal charge becomes more negative, and the resistance to depolarization is increased.

Metabotropic receptors contribute to impulse transmission, promoting sustained effects of postsynaptic excitation or inhibition. Examples of metabotropic receptors include catecholamine receptors, neuropeptide receptors, and muscarinic receptors.[9]

Termination of the synapse reaction is most commonly accomplished through reuptake, in which transporter proteins embedded in neuron and glial cell membranes direct neurotransmitter molecules within the cleft to move back to the intracellular compartment for vesicle repackaging. Neurotransmitters may also go through enzyme degradation, with their component parts taken up for further neurotransmitter synthesis and storage.[1,9] Ultimately, remaining neurotransmitter diffuses away from the synaptic cleft.

The response in the postsynaptic neuron to synapse is an excitatory or inhibitory potential. Membrane potentials are not strong enough by themselves to generate a complete action potential within the postsynaptic neuron, but they are instead summarized or integrated by the neuronal cell body in the process of information transmission.[9] When the postsynaptic neuron is bombarded with excitatory potentials, they may combine *(summation)* to become capable of stimulating an action potential.

APPLICATION OF NEURONAL ANATOMY AND PHYSIOLOGY TO THE PATHOPHYSIOLOGY OF NEURONAL INJURY

Examples of disease- or chemically induced mechanisms that alter neuronal transmission are provided in Figure 26-5. Cellular injury begins a cascade of a multitude of biochemical events that result in immediate cellular death, delayed cellular death, or cellular recovery. During initial insult, cells are deprived of oxygen and glucose, leading to decreased levels of ATP and phosphocreatine. Anaerobic glycolysis begins, resulting in extracellular and intracellular acidosis. Calcium ions (Ca^{2+}) flow into the cell. With decreased ATP, the cell's ATP-dependent Na^+/K^+ pump fails and can no longer pump the excess Ca^{2+} out of the cell. This leads to mitochondrial and cell membrane dysfunction, causing release of excitatory amino acids, including glutamate, into the extracellular space. The release of glutamate activates *N*-methyl-D-aspartate (NMDA) receptors, facilitating more neuronal injury by promoting additional calcium influx into the cell.[10-12]

Calcium-activated proteases (such as calpains) and nucleases further the destruction. Nucleases cause breaks in deoxyribonucleic acid (DNA) strands, and elevated intracellular calcium concentrations stimulate the arachidonic acid cascade (activation of 5-lipoxygenase, prostaglandin synthase, and neuronal nitric oxide synthase), resulting in the generation of free radicals, which cause further internal cellular destruction.[6,12,13] Damage to the mitochondria liberates cytochrome C, activating proteases such as caspases that are associated with later stages of cell death.[13] Secondary injury occurs hours to weeks after the primary injury is sustained, affecting areas that neighbor the initial site of injury, called the *penumbra*. Apoptosis of penumbral cells may be triggered by the death of cells at the site of the primary insult or as a result of reperfusion injury.[12,14]

Knowledge of the intracellular processes associated with programmed cell death continues to evolve, and many other substances are likely to contribute to *apoptosis*. Biochemical events during apoptosis, including inflammatory processes, caspase cascades, genetic variation, and reperfusion injury, are being examined to further our understanding of how they contribute to cell death after trauma or ischemic injury. Neuroprotective agents are being developed to target each of these molecular processes. Hypothermia is being used to target the numerous temperature-dependent processes of ischemia and reperfusion injury. Favorable neurologic outcomes have been reported for newborn infants with perinatal asphyxia and adults after cardiac arrest.[12-14]

CENTRAL NERVOUS SYSTEM

The CNS consists of the brain and spinal cord. Serving as the control unit for all body systems, the remarkably delicate CNS requires significant protection to preserve normal function. This

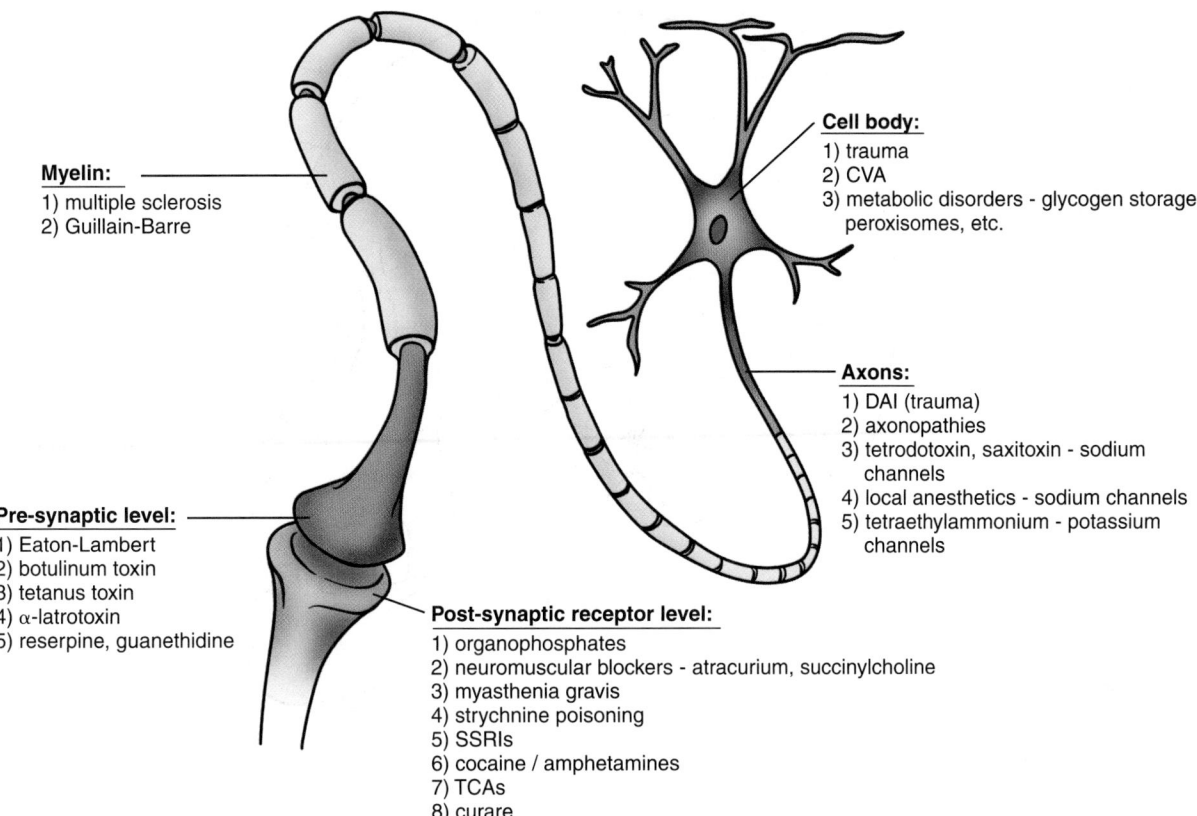

Myelin:
1) multiple sclerosis
2) Guillain-Barre

Cell body:
1) trauma
2) CVA
3) metabolic disorders - glycogen storage, peroxisomes, etc.

Axons:
1) DAI (trauma)
2) axonopathies
3) tetrodotoxin, saxitoxin - sodium channels
4) local anesthetics - sodium channels
5) tetraethylammonium - potassium channels

Pre-synaptic level:
1) Eaton-Lambert
2) botulinum toxin
3) tetanus toxin
4) α-latrotoxin
5) reserpine, guanethidine

Post-synaptic receptor level:
1) organophosphates
2) neuromuscular blockers - atracurium, succinylcholine
3) myasthenia gravis
4) strychnine poisoning
5) SSRIs
6) cocaine / amphetamines
7) TCAs
8) curare

Figure 26-5 Neuronal pathophysiology. CVA, cerebrovascular accident; DAI, diffuse axonal injury; TCAs, tricyclic antidepressants, SSRIs, selective serotonin reuptake inhibitors. *(From Layon AJ et al:* Textbook of neurointensive care, *Philadelphia, 2004, Saunders.)*

section addresses the anatomy and physiology of the brain and spinal cord, supporting the critical care nurse's understanding of pathophysiologic changes that contribute to clinical examination findings.

CRANIAL PROTECTIVE MECHANISMS

Bony Structures. The outermost protective measures underneath the integument are the bony structures that encase the CNS. The skull, or cranium, surrounds the brain and is composed of eight flat, irregular bones fused at sutures during early childhood (Fig. 26-6).[1] The skull protects the brain from direct force and superficial trauma, although excessive force may fracture the skull, destroying this protective mechanism and driving bony fragments into fragile brain tissue.

Viewing the skull from the inside, the superior surfaces form a smooth inner wall, whereas the basilar skull contains ridges and folds with sharp edges (Fig. 26-7).[1] Traumatic impact to the head often results in fracture of the basilar skull as a result of gravitational forces that displace energy in a downward fashion toward the skull base.

The cranium is a solid, nonexpanding bony vault with only one large opening at the base called the *foramen magnum,* through which the brainstem projects and connects to the spinal cord. Several other very small openings in the base of the skull allow entrance and exit of blood vessels and nerve fibers.

Meninges. Directly beneath the skull lie the meninges, which form another source of protection for the CNS. The

meninges consist of three layers: the *dura mater,* the *arachnoid mater,* and the *pia mater* (Fig. 26-8).

Dura Mater. The outermost layer of meninges directly beneath the skull is the dura mater. *Dura* is the Latin term for tough, and true to its name, this layer is made up of fibrous tissue that is double-folded to support the CNS, nerves, and vascular structures.[1,3] Within the dura mater's double layers lie venous sinuses that collect blood from intracranial and meningeal veins for drainage into the internal jugular veins.

Four extensions of the dura mater directly support and separate specific areas of the brain: the falx cerebri, the tentorium cerebelli, the falx cerebelli, and the diaphragma sellae. The falx cerebri divides the right and left hemispheres of the brain vertically through the longitudinal fissures extending from the frontal lobe to the occipital lobe. The tentorium cerebelli forms a tent between the occipital lobes and the cerebellum and separates the cerebral hemispheres from the brainstem and cerebellum. Structures within the brain that are located above the tentorium are often referred to as *supratentorial,* while those located below the tentorium are referred to as *infratentorial* and make up the region of the brain referred to as the *posterior fossa.* The falx cerebelli forms the division between the two lateral lobes of the cerebellum, and the diaphragma sellae forms a roof over the sella turcica, which houses the pituitary gland.[1,3]

The main blood supply for the dura mater is the middle meningeal artery. This artery lies on the surface of the dura in the epidural space and within grooves formed on the inside of the parietal bone.[1] Traumatic disruption of the parietal bone

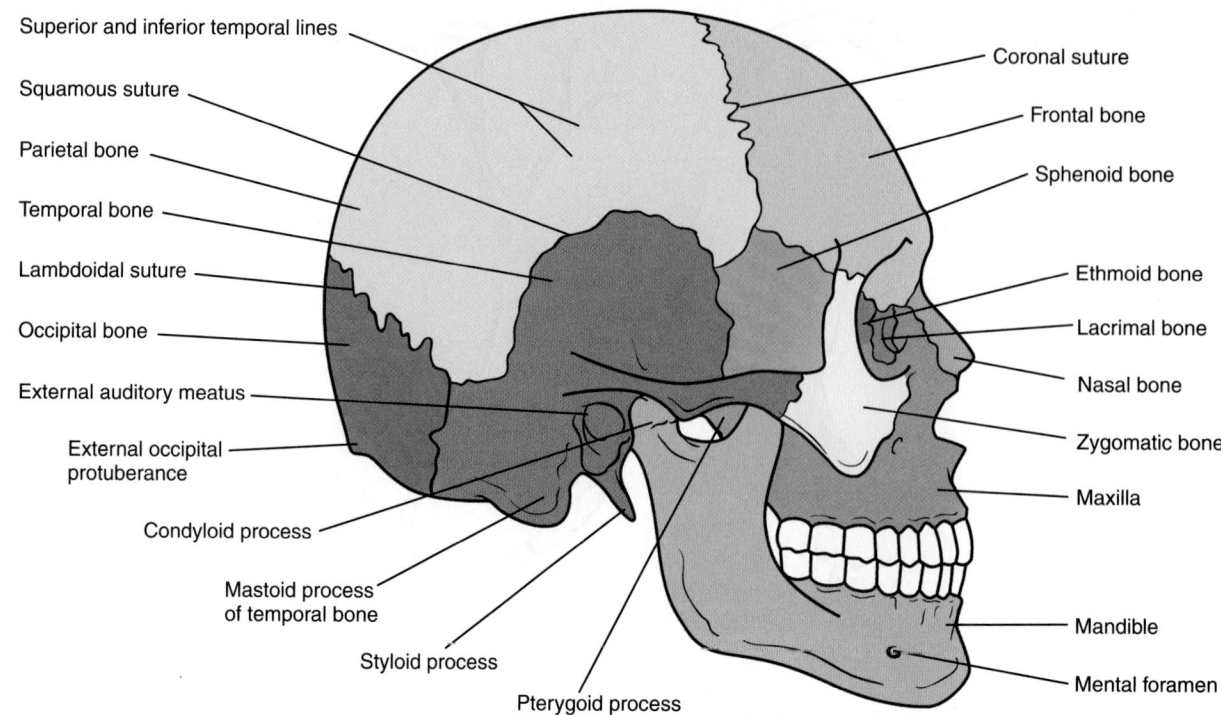

Superior and inferior temporal lines
Squamous suture
Parietal bone
Temporal bone
Lambdoidal suture
Occipital bone
External auditory meatus
External occipital protuberance
Condyloid process
Mastoid process of temporal bone
Styloid process
Pterygoid process

Coronal suture
Frontal bone
Sphenoid bone
Ethmoid bone
Lacrimal bone
Nasal bone
Zygomatic bone
Maxilla
Mandible
Mental foramen

Figure 26-6 Skull. *(From Thibodeau GF, Patton KT:* Anatomy & physiology, *ed 7, Philadelphia, 2010, Mosby.)*

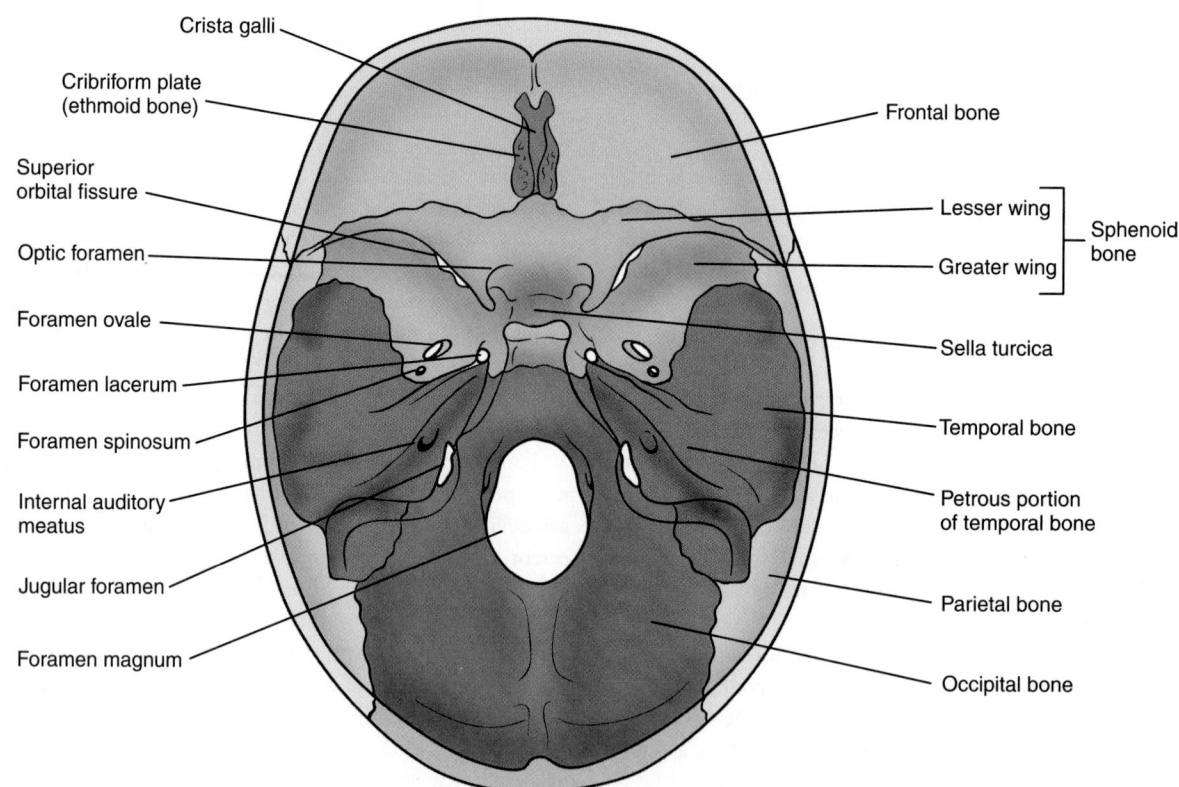

Crista galli
Cribriform plate (ethmoid bone)
Superior orbital fissure
Optic foramen
Foramen ovale
Foramen lacerum
Foramen spinosum
Internal auditory meatus
Jugular foramen
Foramen magnum

Frontal bone
Lesser wing
Greater wing
Sphenoid bone
Sella turcica
Temporal bone
Petrous portion of temporal bone
Parietal bone
Occipital bone

Figure 26-7 Basilar skull. *(From Thibodeau GF, Patton KT:* Anatomy & physiology, *ed 7, Philadelphia, 2010, Mosby.)*

may result in tearing of the middle meningeal artery and development of an epidural hematoma.

A potential space exists between the dura mater and the arachnoid mater. This area contains a large number of unsupported small veins that may become disrupted and torn when traumatic head injury occurs, leading to development of a subdural hematoma.[3]

Arachnoid Mater. The arachnoid membrane is a delicate, fragile membrane that loosely surrounds the brain. Fine threads of elastic tissue called *trabeculae* connect the arachnoid to the

Corpus callosum

Dura mater

Superior sagittal sinus

Pineal body

Tentorium cerebelli

Anterior commissure

Optic chiasm

Pituitary gland

Pons

Medulla oblongata

Cerebellum

Arachnoid villi

Superior sagittal sinus

Skin

Bone

Dura mater

Subdural space

Arachnoid

Subarachnoid space

Pia mater

G.J.Wassilchenko

Figure 26-8 Meningeal layers of the brain.

pia mater, creating a spongy, weblike structure called the *subarachnoid space*. Cerebrospinal fluid (CSF) circulates freely in the subarachnoid space, which also contains the origins of the brain's large arteries where they enter the skull and differentiate into anterior and posterior circulatory branches.[1,3,15,16] Rupture of an artery within the subarachnoid space allows for blood to mix with CSF, producing a *subarachnoid hemorrhage*.

At the base of the brain, widened areas of subarachnoid space form cisterns, or spaces, that are filled with CSF. The largest of these cisterns, the cisterna magna, lies between the medulla and the cerebellum, and it communicates with the fourth ventricle.[1]

Tufts of arachnoid membrane, called *arachnoid villi,* or granulations, project into the superior sagittal and transverse venous sinuses. Absorption of CSF by arachnoid villi allows its removal by the venous drainage system. The delicate structure of the arachnoid villi places them at risk for obstruction by blood in subarachnoid hemorrhage, resulting in *communicating hydrocephalus*.[2,3,15]

Pia Mater. The pia mater adheres directly to brain tissue. Rich in small blood vessels that supply a large volume of arterial blood to the CNS, this membrane closely follows all folds and convolutions of the brain's surface. Tufts or folds of the pia mater in the lateral, third, and fourth ventricles form a portion of the choroid plexus that is responsible for the production of CSF.[1,3]

Ventricular System. The *ventricular system* consists of four CSF-filled canals lined with ependymal cells, a type of neuroglial cell (Fig. 26-9). This system is made up of two large *lateral ventricles* that each lie within a hemisphere of the cerebral cortex. Extending from the frontal lobes to the occipital lobe, the lateral ventricles consist of a body, an atrium, and frontal, temporal, and occipital horns.[1,17] When cannulation of the ventricular system is required for intracranial pressure monitoring, CSF drainage, or placement of a CSF shunt, the frontal horn of the lateral ventricle on the nondominant side of the brain is most often selected.

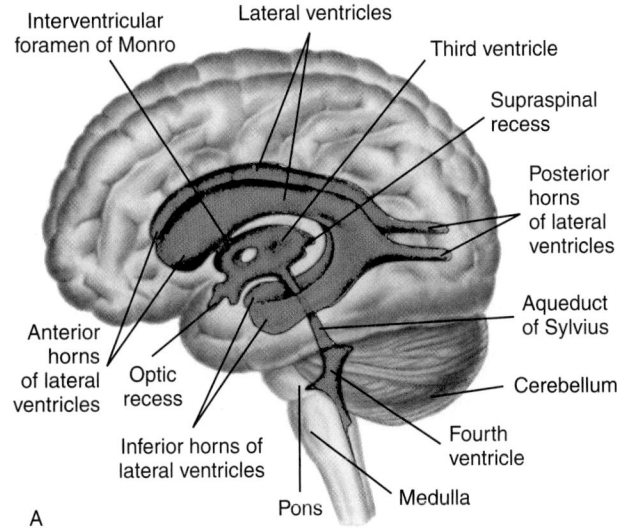

Interventricular foramen of Monro

Lateral ventricles

Third ventricle

Supraspinal recess

Posterior horns of lateral ventricles

Aqueduct of Sylvius

Cerebellum

Fourth ventricle

Medulla

Pons

Anterior horns of lateral ventricles

Optic recess

Inferior horns of lateral ventricles

A

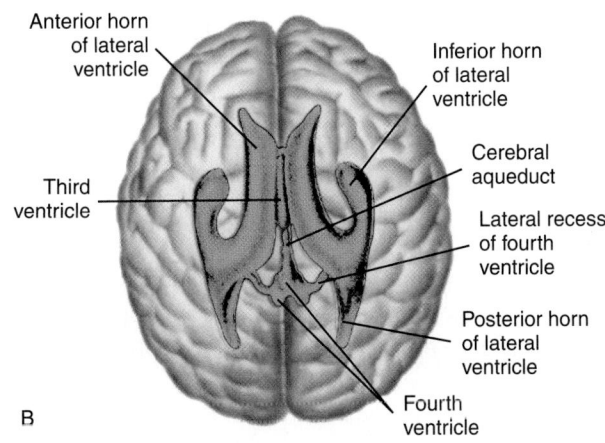

Anterior horn of lateral ventricle

Inferior horn of lateral ventricle

Cerebral aqueduct

Lateral recess of fourth ventricle

Posterior horn of lateral ventricle

Third ventricle

Fourth ventricle

B

Figure 26-9 Ventricular system. *A,* Lateral view. *B,* Superior view. *(From Thompson JM et al: Mosby's clinical nursing, ed 5, St Louis, 2002, Mosby.)*

TABLE 26-2 Normal Values for Cerebrospinal Fluid

Property	Values
pH	7.35-7.45
Specific gravity	1.007
Appearance	Clear and colorless
Cells	0 white blood cells (WBCs)/mm^3 0 red blood cells (RBCs)/mm^3 0-10 lymphocytes/mm^3
Glucose	50-75 mg/dL (two thirds of blood sugar value)
Protein	5-25 mg/dL
Volume	135-150 mL
Pressure	70-200 mm H$_2$O (lumbar puncture) 3-15 mm Hg (ventricular)

The foramen of Monro connects the two lateral ventricles with a central cavity, the *third ventricle*. Located directly above the midbrain, the walls of the third ventricle are formed by the thalami. The *cerebral aqueduct* (aqueduct of Sylvius) is the canal between the third and *fourth ventricle,* which lies between the brainstem and the cerebellum. At the base of the fourth ventricle, two openings—the *foramen of Luschka* and the *foramen of Magendie*—open into the subarachnoid space.[1,3] Blockage of CSF flow occurring within the ventricular system obstructs the normal circulation of CSF, causing dilation of the ventricles, a condition called *noncommunicating hydrocephalus.*[2,3]

Cerebrospinal Fluid. CSF fills the ventricular system and surrounds the brain and spinal cord in the subarachnoid space. Protection of the CNS is further provided by CSF, which acts as a shock absorber when energy is displaced in traumatic injury.

CSF is normally clear, colorless, and odorless. It is secreted by the choroid plexuses of the ventricular system, although small amounts are also synthesized by capillaries of the pia mater. Believed to be a filtrate of blood, CSF contains some unique properties that make its synthesis a mystery (Table 26-2).[1,3]

The production of CSF occurs at a rate of approximately 20 mL/hr, or 500 mL/day. With a circulating volume of 135 to 150 mL, CSF must be regularly resorbed to prevent development of hydrocephalus. Resorption through intact arachnoid villi is favored by increased hydrostatic pressure mechanics that maintain CSF volume within normal limits.[1] The flow of CSF begins in the lateral ventricles, moves through the foramina of Monro into the third ventricle, moves through the cerebral aqueduct into the fourth ventricle, and moves out the foramen of Magendie and the foramina of Luschka into the subarachnoid space of the brain and spinal cord (Fig. 26-10).

Blood-Brain Barrier. The blood-brain barrier is a physiologic mechanism that helps maintain the delicate metabolic balance in the CNS. The blood-brain barrier regulates the transport of nutrients, ions, water, and waste products through selective permeability.[3]

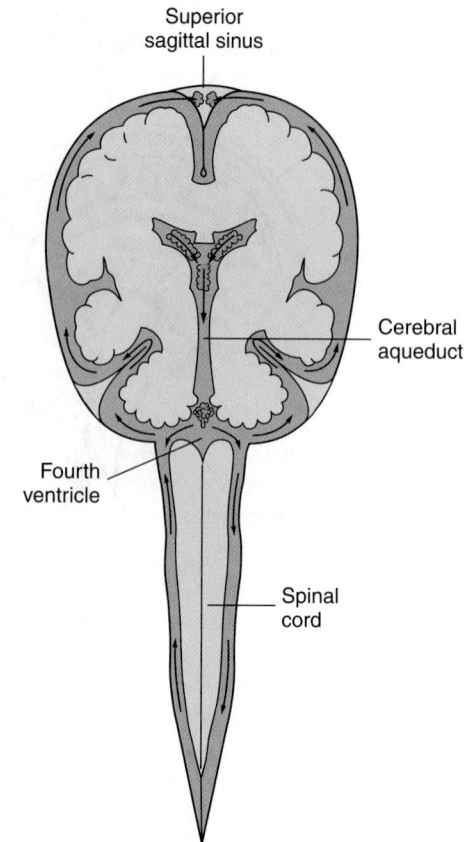

Figure 26-10 Path of circulation of cerebrospinal fluid from its formation in the ventricles to its absorption into the superior sagittal sinus. *(Adapted from Waxman SG, deGroot J: Correlative neuroanatomy, ed 23, Norwalk, CT, 1996, Appleton & Lange.)*

Stabilization of the physical and chemical environment surrounding the neurons of the CNS is the task of the blood-brain barrier. Many substances, such as metabolites or toxic compounds, cannot cross the blood-brain barrier. Other substances, such as antibiotics, cross slowly, resulting in lower concentrations of them in the brain than in other areas of the body.

The blood-brain barrier operates on the concept of *tight junctions* between adjacent cells, and it consists of three separate barriers.[1,3] The vascular endothelial barrier is formed by tight junctions between the endothelial cells of cerebral blood vessels. The blood-CSF barrier consists of tight junctions between the epithelial cells of the choroid plexus. The arachnoid barrier is created by tight junctions between the cells that form the outermost layer of the arachnoid mater. The selective permeability of the blood-brain barrier keeps out toxic or harmful compounds and protects neuronal function.

Passage of substances across the blood-brain barrier is a function of particle size, lipid solubility, and protein-binding potential.[1,3] Most drugs or compounds that are lipid soluble and stable at body pH rapidly cross the blood-brain barrier. The blood-brain barrier is also very permeable to water, oxygen, carbon dioxide, and glucose.

The blood-brain barrier exists only in certain areas of the CNS. The areas in which it does not exist—the pineal region, the basal hypothalamus, and the floor of the fourth ventricle—require contact with plasma to sense changes in concentration of glucose and carbon dioxide and the changes in serum osmolality.[1] Initiation of feedback mechanisms by the hypothalamus in response to these changes regulates the internal environment of the remainder of the body.

Of clinical significance, disruption or alteration of blood-brain barrier permeability occurs with injury to brain tissue from trauma, toxic insults, and ischemic injury. Brain irradiation also may alter the permeability of the blood-brain barrier, although intravenously administered chemotherapeutic agents have been shown to have little effect on blood-brain barrier permeability.

CEREBRUM

The cerebrum is the largest portion of the brain, comprising 80% of its weight. It is composed of two cerebral hemispheres (right and left), separated by the longitudinal fissure and connected at the base by the *corpus callosum.*

The outermost aspect of the cerebrum is called the *cerebral cortex* and is made up of *gray matter,* consisting of neuronal cell bodies. Directly below the cerebral cortex lies *white matter,* consisting of myelinated axons, which communicate impulses from the cerebral cortex to other areas of the brain. White matter tracts consist of three types of fibers: *commissural* (transverse), *projection,* and *association.*[1,3] Commissural fibers are tracts that communicate between the two cerebral hemispheres, and the corpus callosum is the largest commissural tract. Projection fibers communicate between the cerebral cortex and lower regions of the brain and spinal cord. Association fibers communicate between various regions of the same hemisphere.

The cerebral hemispheres are divided into the *frontal, parietal, temporal,* and *occipital* lobes (Fig. 26-11). The *rhinencephalon* is often labeled as a fifth lobe of the cerebral cortex. Lying deep inside the cerebrum and anatomically associated with the temporal lobe, the rhinencephalon is sometimes referred to as the *limbic lobe.*[1,18]

The primary functions of the cerebral cortex include sensory, motor, and intellectual (cognitive) functions, making this area of the brain vital to normal human functioning and providing capabilities that make humans unique as a species.[1] Brodmann's classification of cerebral cortical cytoarchitecture identifies more than 100 unique areas and provides a useful way to localize specific cortical functions within the brain (Fig. 26-12). This section covers the areas within Brodmann's classification that are commonly assessed in relation to the development of specific neurologic pathology.

Frontal Lobe. The frontal lobe lies underneath the frontal bone of the skull and is separated posteriorly from the parietal lobe by the central sulcus (fissure of Rolando) and inferiorly from the temporal lobe by the lateral fissure (Sylvian fissure). The major functions of the frontal lobe are voluntary motor function, cognitive function (orientation, memory, insight, judgment, arithmetic, and abstraction), and expressive language (verbal and written).[1,3]

The prefrontal areas (Brodmann's areas 9 to 12), located just behind the frontal bone's distribution over the forehead, are concerned with cognition.[1-3,11] These areas work in concert with other areas of the brain to intellectually appraise and respond to environmental information or stimuli. They augment intellect with socially trained emotional responses learned over the course of childhood and young adulthood, and they participate in triggering autonomic nervous system responses such as tachycardia in relation to situational needs. The location of the prefrontal cortex makes it vulnerable to traumatic injury, often resulting in profound changes in cognitive capacity and social responses to environmental stimuli after brain injury.[10]

The motor strip of the frontal cortex is represented by Brodmann's area 4 and consists of cell bodies for neurons associated with *voluntary (pyramidal) motor* functions. Because most voluntary motor tracts cross over to the opposite side as they descend through the brainstem, the right motor strip represents voluntary motor function for the left side of the body and vice versa.[1-3] The motor *homunculus* (Fig. 26-13B) is a graphic representation of the distribution of voluntary motor function throughout area 4. Appearing as an upside-down man, the foot of the homunculus is illustrated on the superior medial aspects of the frontal lobes, with the knees, hips, trunk, and shoulders extending along the lateral surfaces and with the hands, thumb, head, face, and tongue represented in a lateral inferior distribution extending to the Sylvian fissure. The homunculus demonstrates larger body part size to denote areas with greater representation because of the amount of dexterity associated with the part's function. The large surface area of the trunk occupies a relatively small part of the motor strip, whereas smaller body areas, such as the thumb or tongue that involve a great deal of dexterity and fine motor movement, occupy a larger area of the motor strip. Damage to the motor strip results in compromise of motor function on the opposite side of the body.

Broca's area (area 44) is located at the inferior frontal gyrus close to the motor strip's facial distribution (see Fig. 26-12). Most commonly, Broca's area is located on the left side of the frontal lobe, although it occasionally is located in the right frontal hemisphere. Broca's area is responsible for expressive language, and it is used in the formation of verbal and written communication.[1] Damage occurring to this area results in disability ranging from word-finding difficulties to an expressive or nonfluent aphasia, in which verbal and written communication are significantly compromised, although verbal language reception and comprehension may remain intact.[3,11,15]

Parietal Lobe. The parietal lobe lies directly behind the frontal lobe on the opposite side of the central sulcus. The posterior border of the parietal lobe is the parieto-occipital fissure, which separates it from the occipital lobe. The parietal lobes are primarily concerned with sensory functions, including integration of sensory information; awareness of body parts; interpretation of touch, pressure, and pain; and recognition of object size, shape, and texture.[1]

The parietal lobe contains a sensory strip (areas 1, 2, and 3) that lies opposite the motor strip of the frontal lobe (see Fig. 26-12). Similar to the homunculus of the motor strip, a

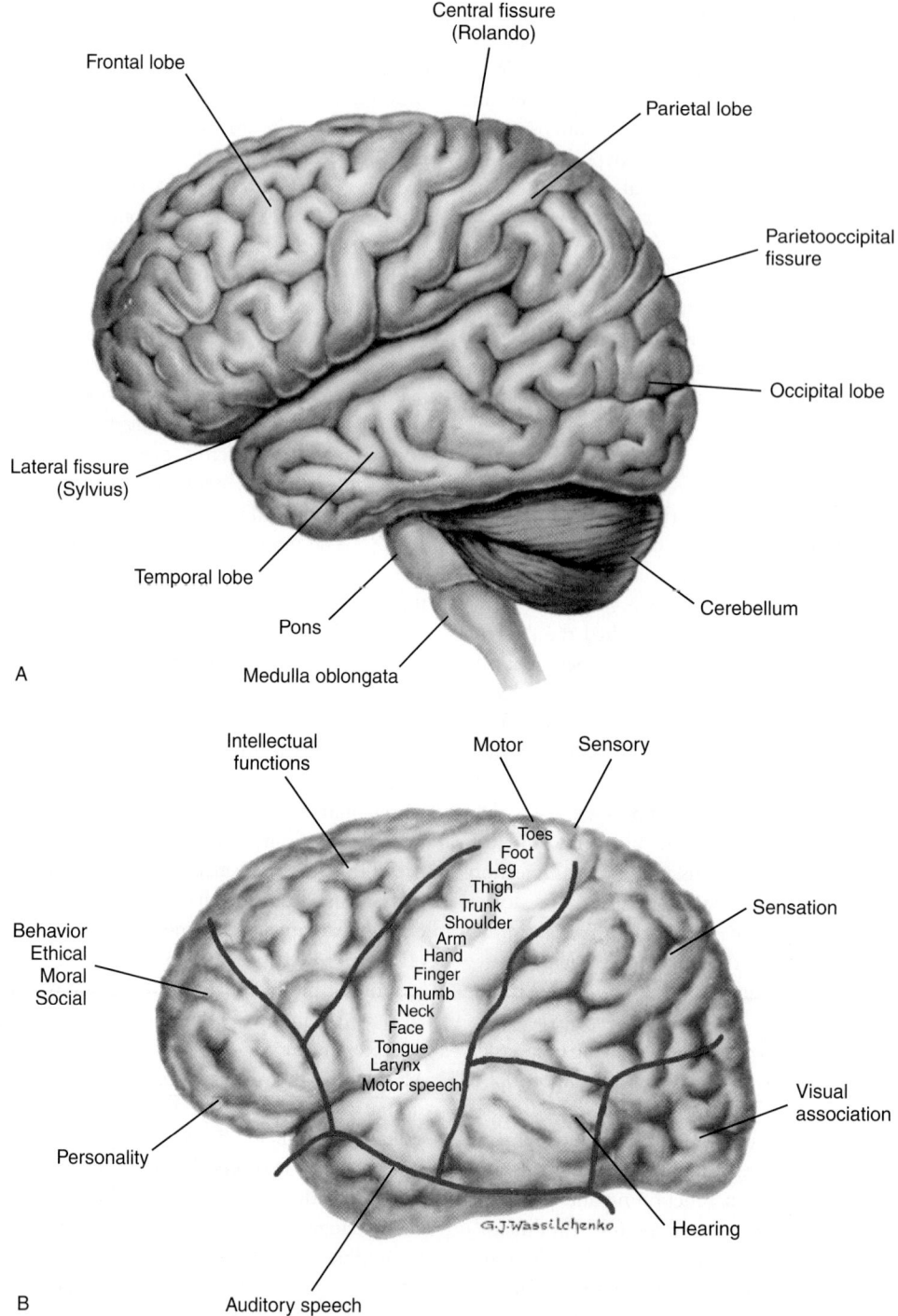

Figure 26-11 *A,* Lateral view of the cerebral hemispheres (showing lobes and principal fissures), cerebellum, pons, and medulla oblongata. *B,* Principal functional subdivisions of the cerebral hemisphere.

sensory homunculus recreates a caricature of an upside-down man (see Fig. 26-13A) representing areas that account for receipt and initial analyses of sensory information from different areas of the body. Areas of the body with greater sensory needs occupy larger areas on the sensory strip, which is concerned with deep or internal sensations and with cutaneous sensations such as touch, pressure, position, and vibration. Injury to these areas may result in tactile sensory loss on the opposite side of the body.

Associative areas of the parietal lobe (areas 5 and 7) further assessment of sensory stimuli, promoting an ability to determine size, shape, texture, locality of stimuli, temperature, vibration, and precise purpose of familiar objects based solely on tactile discrimination. Interpretive aspects of the parietal lobe's response to stimuli include awareness of body parts, perceptual orientation in space, and recognition of environmental spatial relationships.[1] Injury to these areas may result in perceptual neglect or inattention.[11,15]

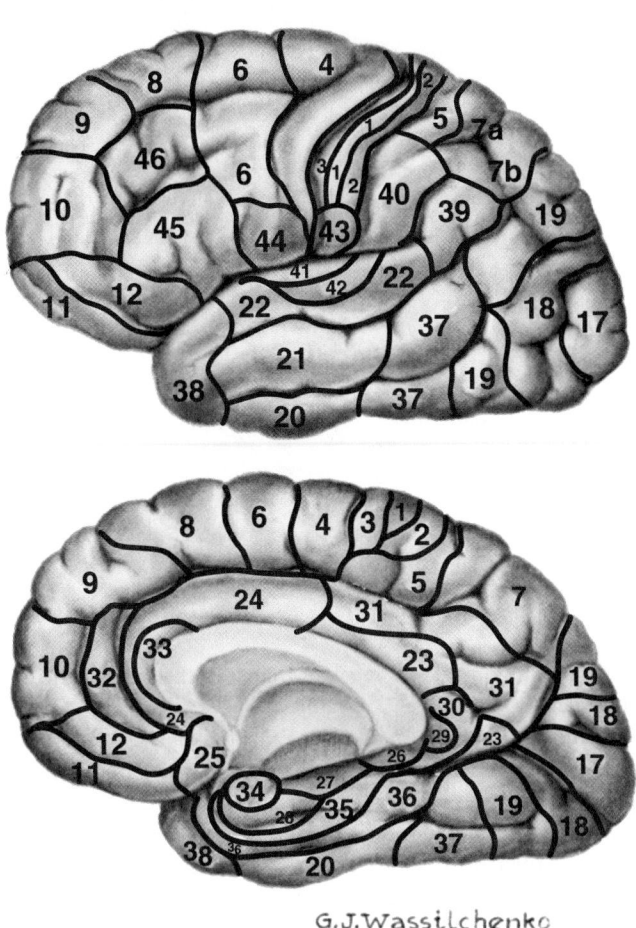

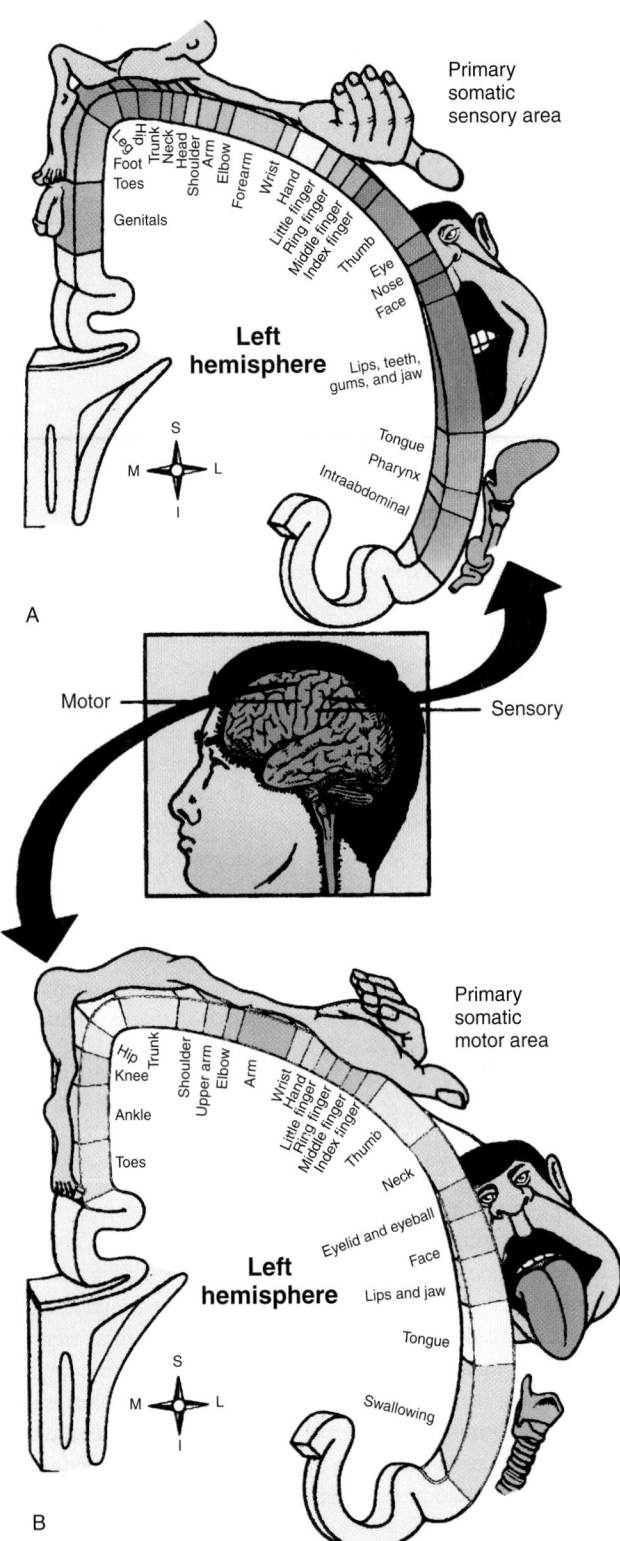

G.J.Wassilchenko

Figure 26-12 Cytoarchitectural map of the lateral and medial surface of the human cortex according to Brodmann's primary somatic sensory *(A)* and motor *(B)* areas of the cortex. *(From Thibodeau GA, Patton KT: Anatomy & physiology, ed 7, St Louis, 2010, Mosby.)*

Wernicke's area (Brodmann's area 22) is partially located within the parietal lobe and partially in the temporal lobe, most commonly on the left side of the cerebral cortex (see Fig. 26-12). This area is concerned with reception of written and verbal language and includes many intricate connections to other parts of the brain associated with auditory and visual functions, cognitive appraisal, and expressive language.[1] Injury to this area of the brain may result in disability ranging from minor receptive language dysfunction to *receptive* or *fluent aphasia*, in which expressive language function remains but is illogical in content or a "word salad." When brain injury includes the areas important to language reception and expression, *global aphasia* may result, significantly limiting receipt and expression of language.[11,15]

Temporal Lobe. The temporal lobe lies beneath the temporal bone in the lateral portion of the cranium. The anterior, lower border of the temporal lobe is encased in the sphenoid wing. With a strong blow to the head, the temporal lobe is easily contused and lacerated as it moves against this hard, irregular surface. Separated from the frontal and parietal lobes by the lateral fissure, this lobe has the primary functions of hearing, speech, behavior, and memory.[1,3]

Figure 26-13 Primary somatic sensory *(A)* and motor *(B)* areas of the cortex. *(From Thibodeau GA, Patton KT: Anatomy & physiology, ed 7, St Louis, 2010, Mosby.)*

The primary auditory areas (areas 41 and 42) receive sound impulses and assist in determining the source of sound and the meaning of sound. Injury to these areas may result in auditory perceptual loss (see Fig. 26-12). Auditory centers in the temporal lobe are closely linked with Wernicke's area.

In the superior portion of the temporal lobe, where the frontal, parietal, and temporal lobes meet, is an essential interpretive area in which auditory, visual, and somatic association areas are integrated into complex thought and memory.[1,3] Seizures in this region of the temporal lobe cause auditory, visual, and sensory hallucinations.[2]

Occipital Lobe. The occipital lobe forms the most posterior aspects of the cerebral cortex and is concerned with interpretation of visual stimuli. The primary visual cortex (area 17) receives impulses from projections of the optic nerve (cranial nerve II). These impulses are then referred to the visual associative areas (areas 18 and 19) for interpretation and integration (see Fig. 26-12). Injury to the occipital lobes may result in cortical blindness, in which the eye structures remain intact but the ability to receive and interpret visual stimuli is lost.[11,15]

Limbic Lobe. The rhinencephalon, or limbic lobe, lies medially along the inner aspects of the temporal lobe. The core of the limbic system consists of the hippocampus and the amygdaloid nucleus.[1,18] Compared with animals living in the wild, the limbic lobe is poorly developed in humans as a result of the sophisticated cognitive capabilities of the frontal lobe, which mediate many of the protective strategies used by humans in everyday life. The limbic lobe's primary functions are related to self-preservation and include functions such as recall of pleasurable and unpleasant or potentially dangerous events, modification of mood and emotional responses in relation to perceived events, interpretation of smell, and augmentation of visceral processes (e.g., heart rate, respiration) associated with emotion. When the injured prefrontal cortex results in cognitive disability, this controversial area of the brain may take on increased control to support self-preservation needs[18]; unfortunately, this may result in significantly aberrant behavior that is frequently judged as socially unacceptable.

INTERNAL CAPSULE

Fiber tracts from many portions of each half of the cerebrum converge in the area of the brain known as the internal capsule as they progress toward the brainstem and spinal cord. The internal capsule contains afferent and efferent fibers (Fig. 26-14). Afferent (sensory) impulses destined for the cortex travel through the internal capsule in the following succession: brainstem to thalamus to internal capsule to cerebral cortex. Efferent (motor) fibers leaving the cortex also pass through the internal capsule.[1] Injury to a portion of the internal capsule may result in pure sensory or motor loss, or both, on the opposite side of the body with preservation of cortical function.[11]

BASAL GANGLIA

The basal ganglia participate in regulating extrapyramidal (involuntary) motor function.[1-3] Located deep within the white matter of the cerebral hemispheres, the basal ganglia consist of four nuclei: the corpus striatum (caudate nucleus, putamen, and nucleus accumbens); the globus pallidus; the substantia nigra; and the subthalamic nucleus[1] (see Fig. 26-14). The basal ganglia are considered a telencephalic, or cerebral, structure, and

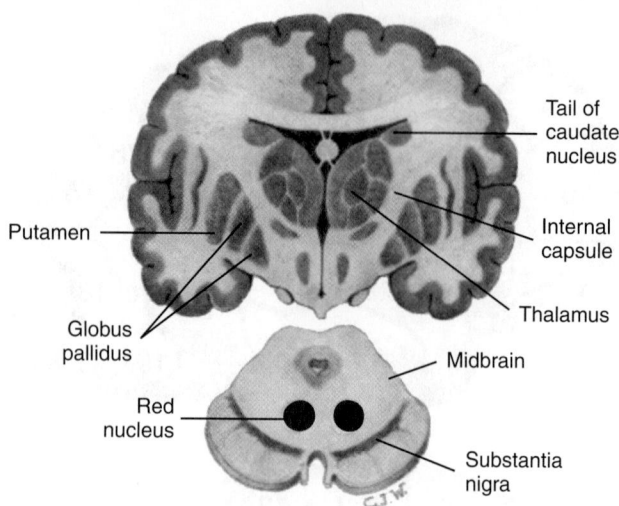

Figure 26-14 Coronal section of brain.

they are embryologically separate from the thalamus, which is considered a diencephalic structure.[1,2]

Although the basal ganglia play a major role in regulating voluntary motor function, they do not provide direct input to motor tracts through the spinal cord. Instead, input from the cerebral cortex stimulates basal ganglia output, which is sent to the brainstem and the thalamus for relay back to the frontal cortex.[1] Ultimately, the basal ganglia integrate associated movements and postural adjustments with voluntary motor movement, suppressing skeletal muscle tone as needed to provide fluid, smooth motor function. Dysfunction of the basal ganglia may result in tremor or other involuntary movements; rigid, nonfluid muscle tone; and slowness of movement without paralysis.[2]

DIENCEPHALON

The diencephalon lies below the cerebral cortex and consists of two structures: the thalamus and the hypothalamus (Fig. 26-15). Although structurally wedded to the hypothalamus, the pituitary gland is considered an endocrine organ and is not a part of the CNS.[1-3] A complete discussion of pituitary gland anatomy and physiology is found in Chapter 35.

Thalamus. The thalamus consists of two connected ovoid masses of gray matter and forms the lateral walls of the third ventricle (see Figs. 26-14 and 26-15). The two thalami serve as a relay station and gatekeeper for motor and sensory stimuli, preventing or enhancing transmission of impulses based on the behavioral needs of the person. More than 50 nuclei support thalamic function and are divided into specific, relay nuclei and nonspecific, diffusely projecting nuclei.[1] Relay nuclei have a specific relationship or trajectory within the cerebral cortex, whereas diffusely projecting nuclei are thought to mediate cortical arousal. Thalamic injury may result in sensory or motor dysfunction, or both, when normal impulse pathways are interrupted.[2,11]

Hypothalamus. The hypothalamus is located below the thalamus and is connected to the pituitary gland by the

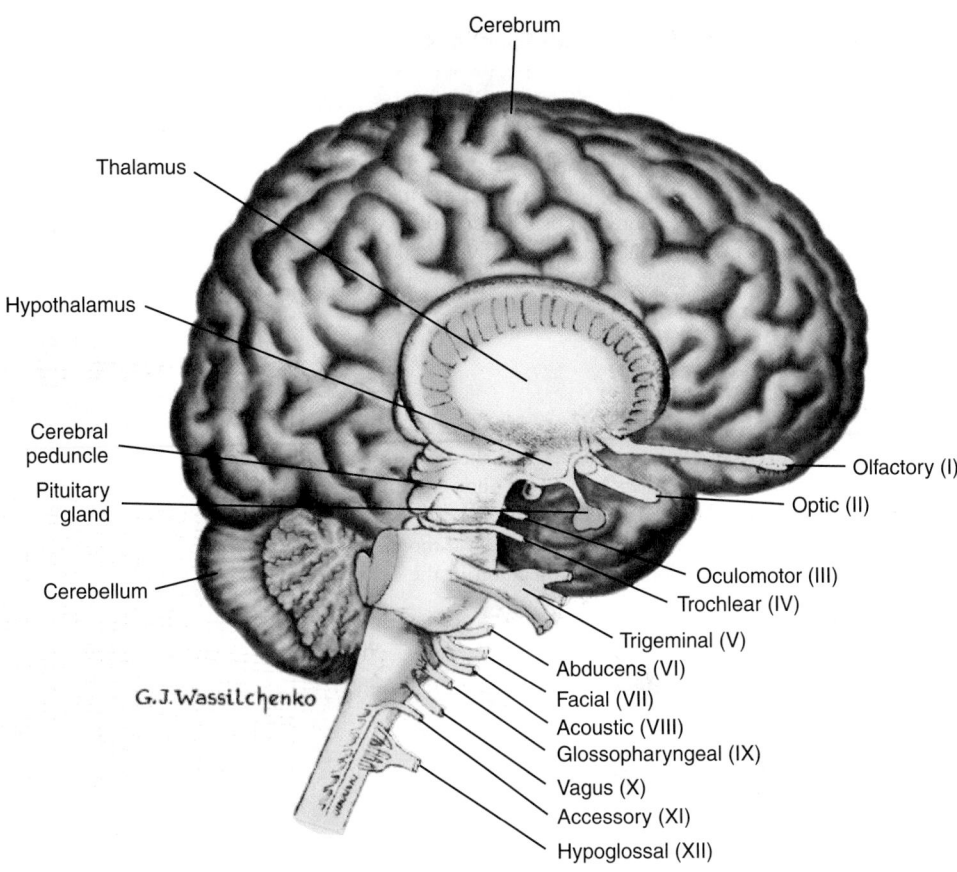

Cerebrum

Thalamus

Hypothalamus

Cerebral peduncle

Pituitary gland

Cerebellum

G.J.Wassilchenko

Olfactory (I)

Optic (II)

Oculomotor (III)

Trochlear (IV)

Trigeminal (V)

Abducens (VI)

Facial (VII)

Acoustic (VIII)

Glossopharyngeal (IX)

Vagus (X)

Accessory (XI)

Hypoglossal (XII)

Figure 26-15 Lateral view of the brain, showing the brainstem, diencephalon, and cranial nerves.

hypothalamic or pituitary stalk (see Fig. 26-15). Neural control of emotion involves many regions of the brain, including the amygdala and limbic associations with the prefrontal cortex, but to ensure homeostasis, these systems all work through the hypothalamus to coordinate the body's behavioral responses to emotion. The hypothalamus maintains internal homeostasis through its ability to stimulate autonomic nervous system response and endocrine system function in relation to body needs, giving the hypothalamus a role in temperature regulation, regulation of food and water intake, control of pituitary hormone release, and augmentation of overall autonomic nervous system output to a sympathetic or parasympathetic state.[1]

CEREBELLUM

The cerebellum (see Fig. 26-15), or hindbrain, is separated from the cerebrum by the dural fold called the *tentorium cerebelli.* Accounting for one fifth of the brain's size, the cerebellum consists of two lateral hemispheres connected by the *vermis.* The cerebellum is composed of an outer layer of gray matter, or cortex, with a core of white matter tracts lying beneath.[1,3]

Cerebellar impulses are communicated to descending motor pathways to integrate spatial orientation and equilibrium with posture and muscle tone, ensuring synchronized adjustments in movement that maintain overall balance and motor coordination.[1,2] Cerebellar monitoring and adjustment of motor activity occurs simultaneously with movement, enabling significant control of fine motor function. The cerebellum is bombarded with information related to the goals of movement and disparities between actual and intended movements. There are 40 times more axons projecting into the cerebellum than the number of axons leaving the cerebellum to ensure adequate receipt of motor information.[2] Injury to the cerebellum produces *ataxia,* defined as preservation of motor strength with lack of control (coordination) over fine motor function.[2,11]

BRAINSTEM

The brainstem consists of three major divisions: the midbrain, the pons, and the medulla oblongata. It is packed with sensory and motor pathways traveling between the spinal cord and the brain, and it contains a number of centers that regulate vital mechanisms throughout the body (see Fig. 26-15).

Midbrain. The midbrain forms the junction between the pons and the diencephalon. The cell bodies of cranial nerves III and IV originate in the midbrain (Table 26-3). The midbrain is divided by a sagittal plane into the two cerebral peduncles (see Fig. 26-15), and anatomically, it constitutes the location of the aqueduct of Sylvius. The major function of the midbrain is to relay stimuli to and from the brain through ascending sensory tracts and descending motor pathways.[1,2]

TABLE 26-3 Cranial Nerves, Origins, Course, and Functions

Cranial Nerve	Origin and Course	Function
I Olfactory Sensory	Found in the mucosa of the nasal cavity; only cranial nerves with cell body are located in peripheral structure (nasal mucosa). It passes through the cribriform plate of the ethmoid bone and goes on to olfactory bulbs at the floor of the frontal lobe. Final interpretation is in the temporal lobe.	Smell. However, the system is more than receptor and interpreter for odors; perception of smell also sensitizes other body systems and responses, such as salivation, peristalsis, and even sexual stimulus. Loss of sense of smell is called *anosmia*.
II Optic Sensory	Ganglion cells of the retina converge to the optic disc and form the optic nerve. Nerve fibers pass to the optic chiasm, which is above the pituitary gland. Some fibers decussate; others do not. The two tracts go to the lateral geniculate body near the thalamus and then on to the end station for interpretation in the occipital lobe.	Vision

A-Total blindness of right eye
B-Bitemporal hemianopsia
C-Left nasal hemianopsia
D-Left homonymous hemianopsia
E-Left homonymous hemianopsia inferior quadrant
F-Left homonymous hemianopsia superior quadrant

TABLE 26-3 Cranial Nerves, Origins, Course, and Functions—*cont'd*

Cranial Nerve	Origin and Course	Function
III Oculomotor		
Motor	Originates in the midbrain and emerges from the brainstem at the upper pons	Extraocular movement of eyes
Motor	Motor fibers go to superior, medial, and inferior recti and to the inferior oblique for eye movement and levator muscle of the eyelid.	Raises eyelid
Parasympathetic	Parasympathetic fibers go to ciliary muscles and iris of eye.	Constricts pupil; changes shape of lens

Superior rectus tested by gaze up and out

Inferior oblique tested by gaze up and in

Medial rectus tested by gaze directed in toward nose (medial)

Inferior rectus tested by gaze down and out

G.J.Wassilchenko

A   B   C

Continued

TABLE 26-3 Cranial Nerves, Origins, Course, and Functions—*cont'd*

Cranial Nerve	Origin and Course	Function
IV Trochlear Motor	Midbrain origin near oculomotor nerve, emerges at upper pons near cerebral peduncle; motor fibers go to superior oblique muscle of the eyeball	Extraocular movement of eyes

Superior oblique tested by gaze down and in

A　　　　　　　　B　　　　　　　　C

G.J. Wassilchenko

Cranial Nerve	Origin and Course	Function
V Trigeminal Sensory	Originates in the fourth ventricle and emerges at lateral parts of the pons; has three branches to face: ophthalmic, maxillary, and mandibular	*Ophthalmic branch:* sensation to cornea, ciliary body, iris, lacrimal gland, conjunctiva, nasal mucosal membranes, eyelids, eyebrows, forehead, and nose *Maxillary branch:* sensation to skin of cheek, lower lid, side of nose and upper jaw, teeth, mucosa of mouth, sphenopalatine-pterygoid region, and maxillary sinus *Mandibular branch:* sensation to skin of lower lip, chin, ear, mucous membrane, teeth of lower jaw, and tongue
Motor	Goes to temporalis, masseter, pterygoid gland, anterior part of digastric muscles (all for mastication), and the tensor tympani and tensor veli palatine muscles (clench jaw)	Supplies muscles for chewing (mastication) and opening jaw

Ophthalmic branch

Trigeminal nerve

Maxillary branch

Mandibular branches

G.J. Wassilchenko

TABLE 26-3 Cranial Nerves, Origins, Course, and Functions—*cont'd*

Cranial Nerve	Origin and Course	Function
VI Abducens Motor	Posterior part of pons goes to lateral rectus muscle for eye movement.	Extraocular eye movement; rotates eyeball outward

Lateral rectus tested by gaze directed outward away from nose (lateral)

G.J. Wassilchenko

A   B   C

Cranial Nerve	Origin and Course	Function
VII Facial Sensory	Lower portion of pons goes to anterior two thirds of tongue and soft palate.	Taste in anterior two thirds of tongue; sensation to soft palate
Motor	Pons to muscles of forehead, eyelids, checks, lips, ears, nose, and neck	Movement of facial muscles to produce facial expressions, close eyes
Parasympathetic	Pons to salivary gland and lacrimal glands	Secretory for salivation and tears
VIII Acoustic Sensory	Nerve has two divisions.	
	Cochlear division originates in spinal ganglia of the cochlea, with peripheral fibers to the organ of Corti in the internal ear. It goes to the pons, and impulses are transmitted to the temporal lobe.	Hearing
	Vestibular division originates in the otolith organs of the semicircular canals in the inner ear and in the vestibular ganglion. It terminates in the pons, with some fibers continuing to cerebellum. It is the only cranial nerve that originates wholly within a bone, the petrous portion of the temporal bone.	Equilibrium
IX Glossopharyngeal Sensory	Posterior one third of tongue for taste sensation and sensations from soft palate, tonsils, and opening to mouth in back of oral pharynx (fauces). Fibers go to the medulla and then to the temporal lobe for taste and sensory cortex for other sensations.	Taste in posterior one third of tongue; sensation in back of throat; stimulation elicits gag reflex
Motor	Medulla to constrictor muscles of pharynx and stylopharyngeal muscles.	Voluntary muscles for swallowing and phonation
Parasympathetic	Medulla to parotid salivary gland through the otic ganglia	Secretory, salivary glands; carotid reflex

Continued

TABLE 26-3 Cranial Nerves, Origins, Course, and Functions—*cont'd*

Cranial Nerve	Origin and Course	Function
X Vagus		
Sensory	Sensory fibers in back of the ear and posterior wall of the external ear go to the medulla oblongata and on to the sensory cortex.	Sensation behind ear and part of external ear meatus
Motor	Fibers go from the medulla oblongata through the jugular foramen with glossopharyngeal nerve and on to the pharynx, larynx, esophagus, bronchi, lungs, heart, stomach, small intestine, liver, pancreas, and kidneys.	Voluntary muscles for phonation and swallowing; involuntary activity of visceral muscles of heart, lungs, and digestive tract
Parasympathetic	Medulla oblongata to the larynx, trachea, lungs, aorta, esophagus, stomach, small intestines, and gallbladder	Carotid reflex; autonomic activity of respiratory tract and digestive tract, including peristalsis and secretion from organs
XI Spinal Accessory		
Motor	The nerve has two roots: cranial and spinal. Cranial portion arises at several rootlets at the side of medulla, runs below the vagus, and is joined by the spinal portion from motor cells in cervical cord. Some fibers go along with vagus nerve to supply motor impulse to the pharynx, larynx, uvula, and palate. Major portion goes to the sternomastoid and trapezius muscles, branches to cervical spinal nerves C2-C4.	Some fibers for swallowing and phonation. Turn head and shrug shoulders.
XII Hypoglossal		
Motor	Arises in the medulla oblongata and goes to the muscles of the tongue	Movement of tongue necessary for swallowing and phonation

Pons. Located above the medulla, the pons relays information to and from the brain through sensory and motor pathways. The posterior aspects of the pons make up the upper surface of the fourth ventricle (see Fig. 26-15). Two respiratory control centers are located in the pons: the apneustic and pneumotaxic centers. The apneustic center controls the length of inspiration and expiration, whereas the pneumotaxic center controls respiratory rate.[1-3]

The cell bodies of cranial nerves V (trigeminal), VI (abducens), VII (facial), and VIII (acoustic) are located in the pons (see Table 26-3).[1] The medial longitudinal fasciculus (MLF) is an important fiber tract in the pons that connects cranial nerves III, IV, and VI with the vestibular portion of the acoustic nerve and pontine paramedian reticular formation, allowing coordinated and appropriate movements of the eyes in response to noise, motion, position, and arousal. The structural integrity of the brainstem may be assessed through clinical stimulation of the MLF in caloric testing.[2]

Medulla Oblongata. The medulla oblongata forms the last section of the brainstem, situated between the pons and the spinal cord (see Fig. 26-15). In the pyramids of the medulla, decussation (crossing) of voluntary motor fibers occurs, lending the name *pyramidal* to voluntary motor function. Below the point of decussation, stimuli from the right side of the brain control movement for the left side of the body and vice versa.[1]

Centers for control of involuntary functions such as swallowing, vomiting, hiccupping, coughing, heart rate, arterial vasoconstriction, and respiration are located within the medulla oblongata. The medullary respiratory center works in conjunction with the apneustic and pneumotaxic centers in the pons to control respiratory function and is responsible for the rhythm of respiration. The cell bodies of cranial nerves IX (glossopharyngeal), X (vagus), XI (spinal accessory), and XII (hypoglossal) are located in the medulla oblongata (see Fig. 26-15 and Table 26-3).[1,2]

Reticular Formation. The reticular formation (RF) of the brainstem is located at the core of the brainstem and is active in modulating sensation, movement, consciousness, reflexive behaviors, and the activities of the cranial nerves arising from the brainstem (III through XII). The RF extends from the upper pons to the diencephalon.[1] The ascending RF is referred to as the reticular activating system (RAS), and it is responsible for increasing wakefulness, vigilance, and responsiveness of cortical and thalamic neurons to sensory stimuli. In the thalamus, the RAS activates relay and diffuse projection nuclei to increase distribution of sensory stimuli throughout the cerebral cortex.[1,2] The RAS also works through activation of the hypothalamus, which results in diffuse cortical stimulation and autonomic stimulation.[1] Damage to the thalamic or hypothalamic RAS pathways results in impaired consciousness.[19]

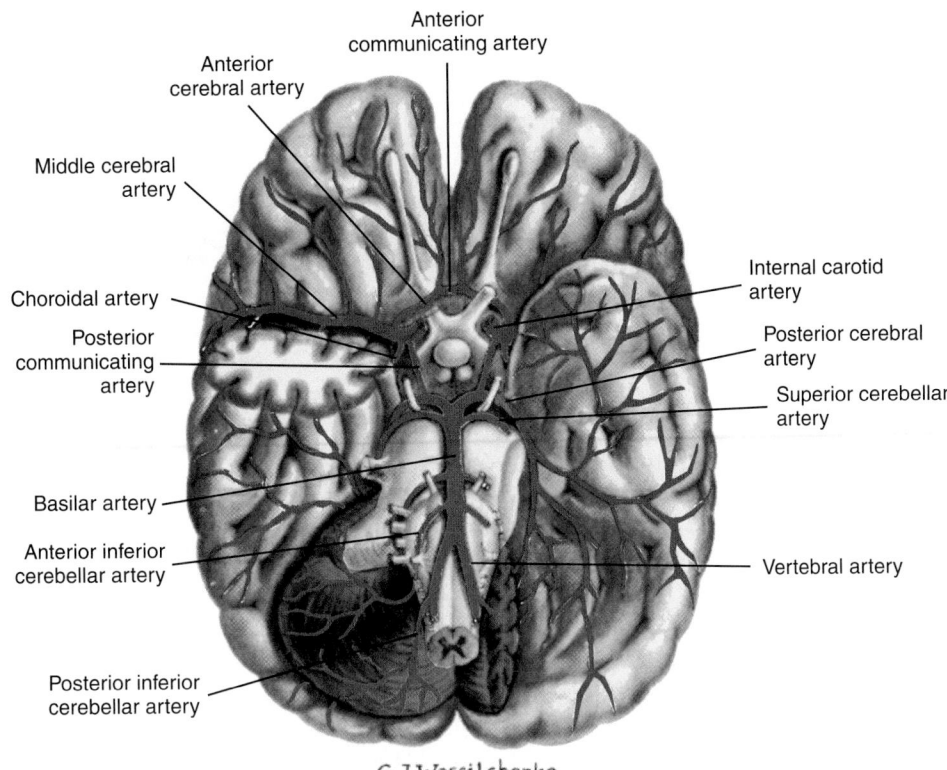

Anterior
communicating artery

Anterior
cerebral artery

Middle cerebral
artery

Choroidal artery

Posterior
communicating
artery

Internal carotid
artery

Posterior cerebral
artery

Superior cerebellar
artery

Basilar artery

Anterior inferior
cerebellar artery

Vertebral artery

Posterior inferior
cerebellar artery

G.J.Wassilchenko

Figure 26-16 Blood supply of the brain.

ARTERIAL CIRCULATION

The brain constitutes 2% of the body's weight but uses 20% of the body's total resting cardiac output.[1,15] It requires approximately 750 mL of blood flow per minute and can extract as much as 45% of arterial oxygen to meet normal metabolic needs.[1,15,16] It has no reserve of oxygen or glucose, making reductions of these substances critical to the disruption of normal cellular function. Two pairs of arteries, the internal carotids and the vertebral arteries, provide blood to the brain and are anatomically separated into the anterior and posterior circulations that connect at the base of the brain to form the circle of Willis (Fig. 26-16).[1,16] Knowledge of the brain's arterial supply as it correlates to neurologic function is an essential aspect of neuroscience critical care nursing, especially in the care of stroke patients. Arterial distribution for the cerebral cortex is illustrated in Figure 26-17.

Anterior Circulation. The anterior circulation of the brain is supplied by the right and left internal carotid arteries and their branches. Originating as the common carotids, the left common carotid takes off from the arch of the aorta, whereas the right common carotid originates from the innominate artery. At the level of the cricothyroid junction, the common carotid splits to form the external and internal carotid arteries. The external carotid feeds the face, the scalp, and the skull and includes the branch called the *middle meningeal artery,* which lies between the skull and the dura.[1]

The internal carotid artery continues upward through the carotid siphon and enters the base of the skull through an opening in the petrous bone. At the base of the brain, the internal carotid gives off the right and left middle cerebral arteries (MCAs); the right and left anterior cerebral arteries (ACAs), which are connected by the anterior communicating artery (ACoA); and the two posterior communicating arteries (PCoAs).[16] The anterior circulation provides 80% of the blood flow to the cerebral hemispheres, covering the needs of the frontal lobes and most of the parietal and temporal lobes and supplying the subcortical structures residing above the brainstem.[1,11,16]

The internal carotid artery gives rise to the ophthalmic artery at the siphon before bifurcating into the anterior cerebral and middle cerebral arteries. The ophthalmic artery supplies blood to the optic nerve and eye and may reverse its course to supplement the anterior circulation's arterial blood volume in the case of internal carotid artery occlusion.[16]

Posterior Circulation. The posterior circulation begins with the two vertebral arteries, which originate from the subclavian arteries and travel posteriorly through small openings in the lateral spinous processes of the cervical spine. They enter the skull through the foramen magnum, and at the level of the pons, the two vertebral arteries fuse to form the basilar artery.[1] The terminal portion of the vertebral arteries gives rise to two important arterial branches before basilar artery fusion the posterior inferior cerebellar arteries (PICAs).[11,16] Two major infratentorial branches of the basilar artery include the anterior inferior cerebellar arteries (AICAs) and the superior cerebellar arteries (SCAs), which together with the PICA supply the cerebellum.[11] The distal basilar artery gives rise to the two posterior cerebral arteries (PCAs), which emerge in the supratentorial region to supply the posterior aspects of the cerebral cortex.[1,11,16]

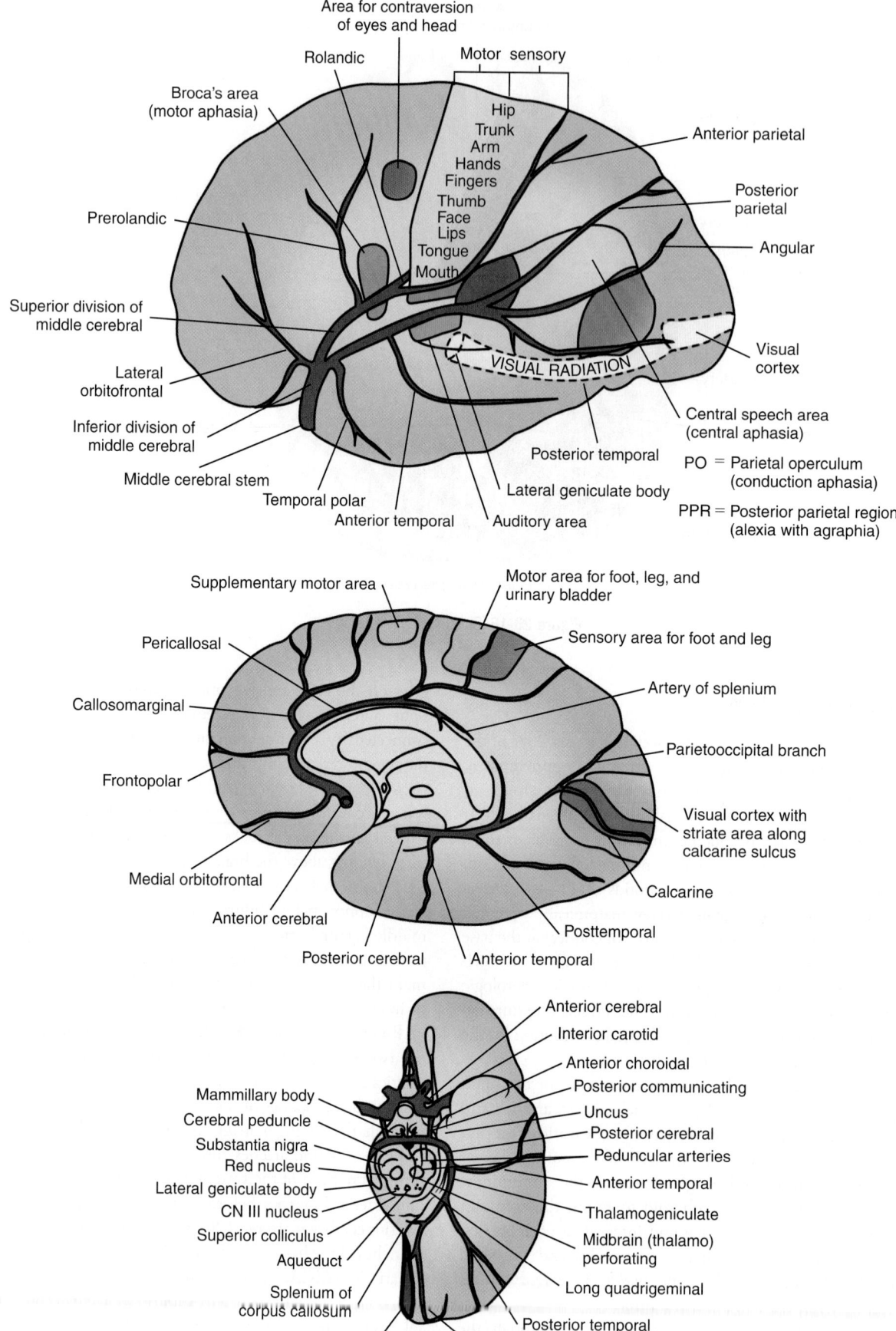

Figure 26-17 Arterial distribution. *(Modified from Adams RD, Victor M: Principles of neurology, ed 6, New York, 1997, McGraw-Hill.)*

Circle of Willis. The circle of Willis is a vascular supply system unique to the brain's circulation (see Fig. 26-16). Located above the optic chiasm in the subarachnoid space, the circle is fed by branches of the internal carotid and basilar arteries. The anterior circulation is connected between the two ACAs by the ACoA and to the posterior circulation by the two PCoAs.[1] Approximately 50% of the population has a complete or "ideal" circle of Willis. In others, atretic (small and nonfunctional or hypoplastic) segments often are found in the first branch of the ACAs, called A1; in the first branch of the PCAs, called P1; and in the PCoAs.[16] When complete, the circle of Willis is capable of supporting some degree of collateral blood flow in the case of arterial occlusion, although a sufficient arterial supply in the face of arterial obstruction is not guaranteed.

Venous Circulation. Venous drainage occurs through venous sinuses, many of which are housed in the double-folded membrane of the dura mater. Capillaries drain into venules, which then flow into cerebral veins, ultimately emptying into sinuses located throughout the cranium. Blood from these sinuses empties into the internal jugular vein, which empties into the superior vena cava (Fig. 26-18). Cerebral veins have thinner walls relative to veins in the general circulation and lack a muscular layer or valves.[1,2,15]

SPINAL CORD

The spinal cord, one division of the CNS, extends from the medulla below the foramen magnum.[1,3] Similar to the brain, the spinal cord is composed of gray and white matter, although the cord's gray matter is located internally, and the white matter is located on its surface. The distal end of the spinal cord tapers to the *conus medullaris,* which is situated at the level of the first or second lumbar vertebra. Exiting from the spinal cord are 31 pairs of spinal nerves, which exit through intervertebral foramina. Because the spinal cord ends at vertebrae L1 and the final nerve roots do not exit until the coccyx, long lengths of nerves, called the *cauda equina,* extend below the conus medullaris toward their associated intervertebral foramina to exit the spinal canal (Fig. 26-19). Protective mechanisms similar to those listed for the brain provide protection to the spinal cord.[1]

Protective Mechanisms

Bony Structures. The bony structure that encases the spinal cord is the vertebral column. Comprising 33 vertebrae and 24 intervertebral disks, this column is held together by ligaments and tendons. It provides support and protection for the spinal cord and the structure and flexibility required for body movement. The vertebrae are divided into sections in relation to their appearance. There are 7 cervical vertebrae, 12 thoracic vertebrae, 5 lumbar vertebrae, 5 sacral vertebrae (fused together as one), and 4 coccygeal vertebrae (fused together as one).[1]

Although differences in vertebral appearance exist, the basic structure includes a vertebral body connected by two pedicles to the transverse processes (Fig. 26-20). Two laminae connect the transverse processes to the posterior segment of the vertebra, the spinous process, forming a ring. The center of the spinal foramen is the canal housing the spinal cord.

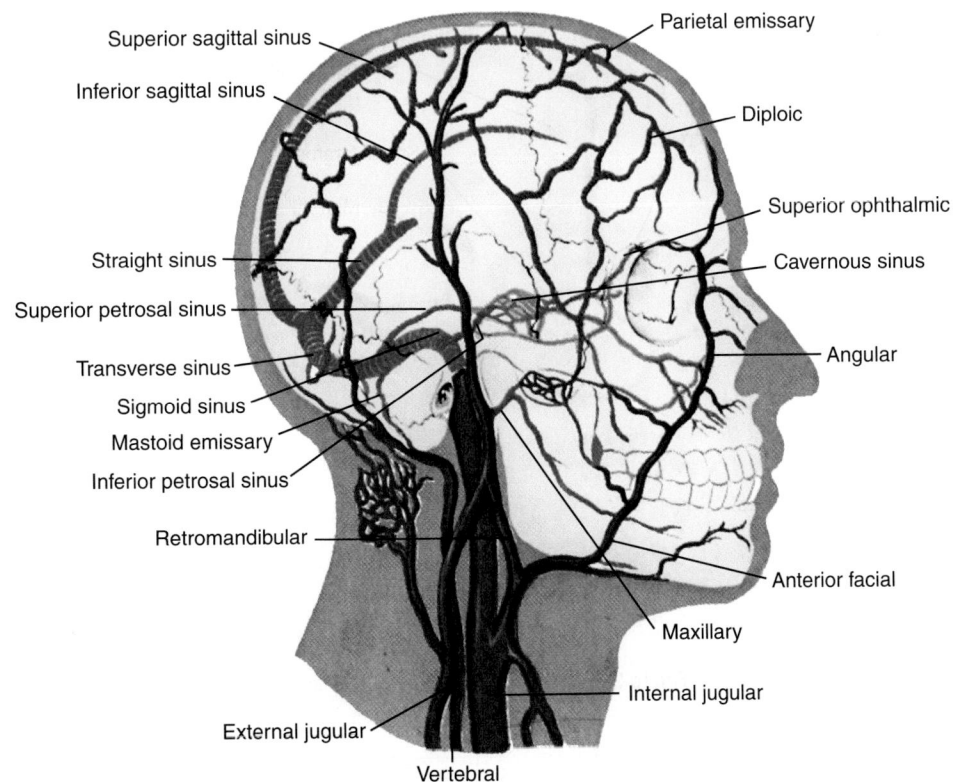

Figure 26-18 Venous circulation.

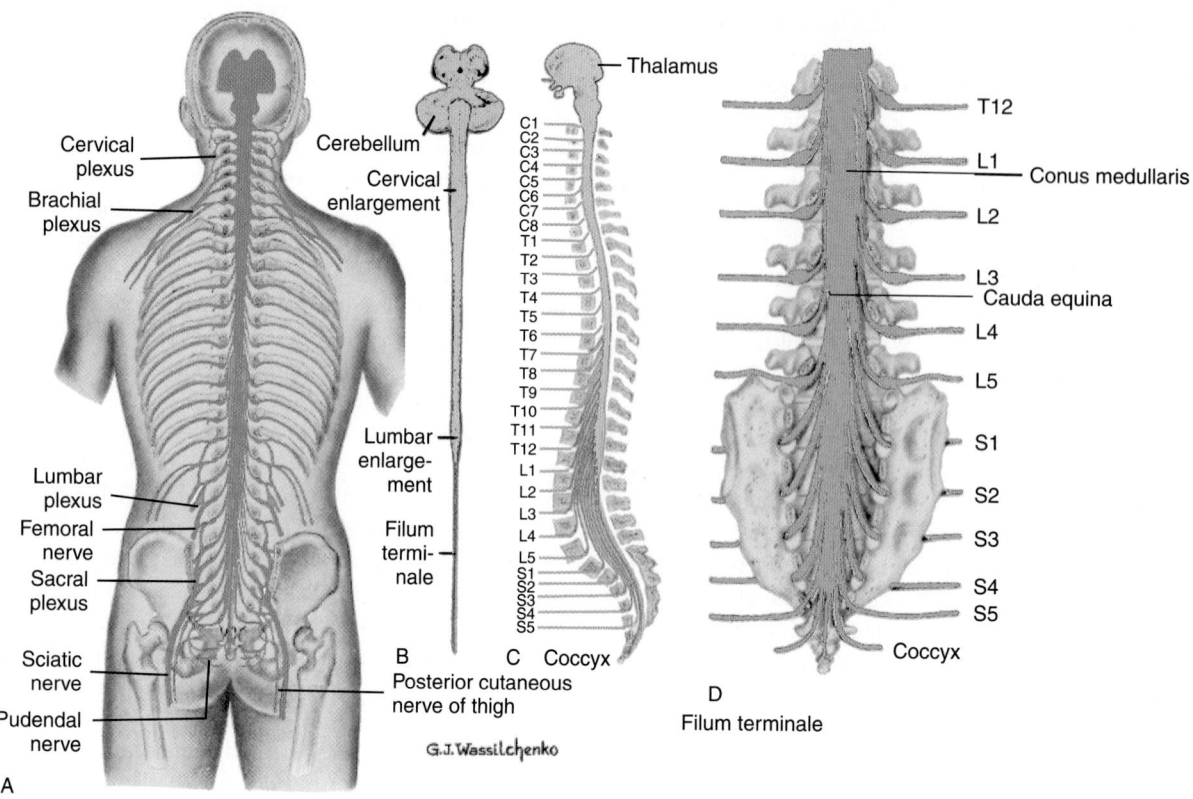

Figure 26-19 Spinal cord within the vertebral canal and exiting spinal nerves. *A*, Posterior view in situ. *B*, Anterior view. *C*, Lateral view. *D*, Cauda equina.

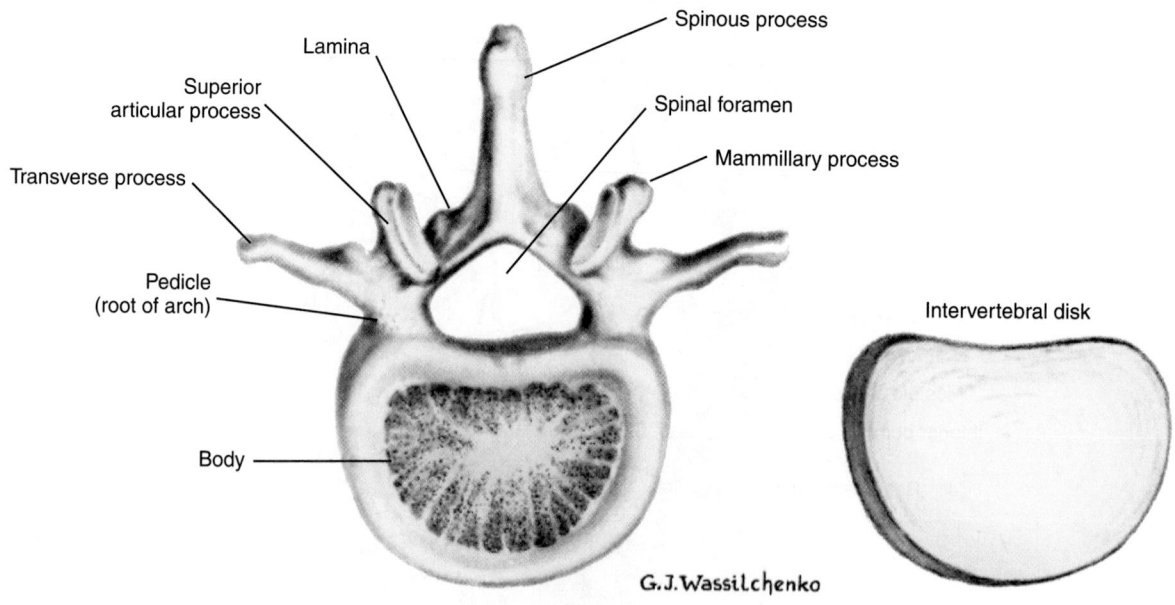

Figure 26-20 Vertebra and intervertebral disk.

Intervertebral Disk. Vertebral bodies are separated by an intervertebral disk. These fibrocartilaginous structures lie between each vertebral body, extending from the cervical vertebra to the beginning of the sacrum. Intervertebral disks are composed of two layers. The inner core, called the nucleus pulposus, is a soft, gelatinous material that assists in shock absorbency. Surrounding the nucleus pulposus is the annulus fibrosus, a thick, tough outer layer.[1] The diagnosis of herniated disk refers to dislocation of the normal anatomic position of an intervertebral disk that compromises or puts pressure on a spinal nerve.

Meninges. The meninges of the spinal cord are similar to those in the cranium (Fig. 26-21). The dura is a continuation of the intracranial dura mater, and it encases the cord, the nerve roots, and the spinal nerves until they exit from the vertebral column. The dura extends to the level of the second sacral vertebra, even though the spinal cord itself ends at the L1 or L2 level.[1]

The arachnoid mater provides the same weblike, delicate structure as in the cranium, with CSF flow within the subarachnoid space.[1] Because the spinal cord terminates at L2 and the meninges continue to S2, a volume of CSF is contained in the lumbar cistern, and it constitutes the site targeted for a lumbar puncture.[2,20] The pia mater of the spinal cord is a thicker, firmer, less vascular membrane than that in the cranium.[1]

Spinal Nerves. There are 31 pairs of spinal nerves: 8 cervical, 12 thoracic, 5 lumbar, 5 sacral, and 1 coccygeal (see Fig. 26-19).[1] In the cervical region, the first seven pairs of nerves exit the cord above the corresponding vertebrae. The C8 nerve pair exits the spinal cord below the C7 vertebra. From this point on, all thoracic, lumbar, and sacral nerves exit below the corresponding vertebrae. In other words, spinal cord segments associated with each spinal nerve and the corresponding vertebra do not directly line up.

The spinal nerve has two roots: the dorsal root and the ventral root. The dorsal root is an afferent pathway that carries sensory impulses from the body into the spinal cord. The ventral root is an efferent pathway that carries motor information from the spinal cord to the body. The dorsal and ventral roots join together as they exit the spinal foramen and become a spinal nerve (see Fig. 26-21).[1] Distribution of the sensory components of each spinal nerve are illustrated as dermatomes. Dermatome diagrams facilitate identification of sensory innervation throughout the body (Fig. 26-22).

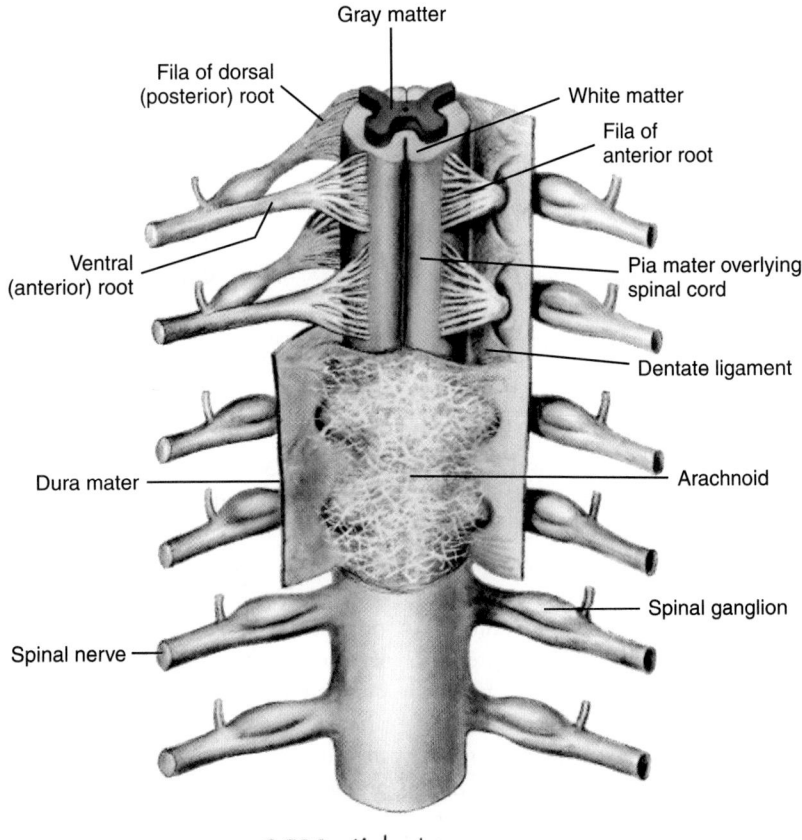

G.J.Wassilchenko

Figure 26-21 Meningeal layers of the spinal cord.

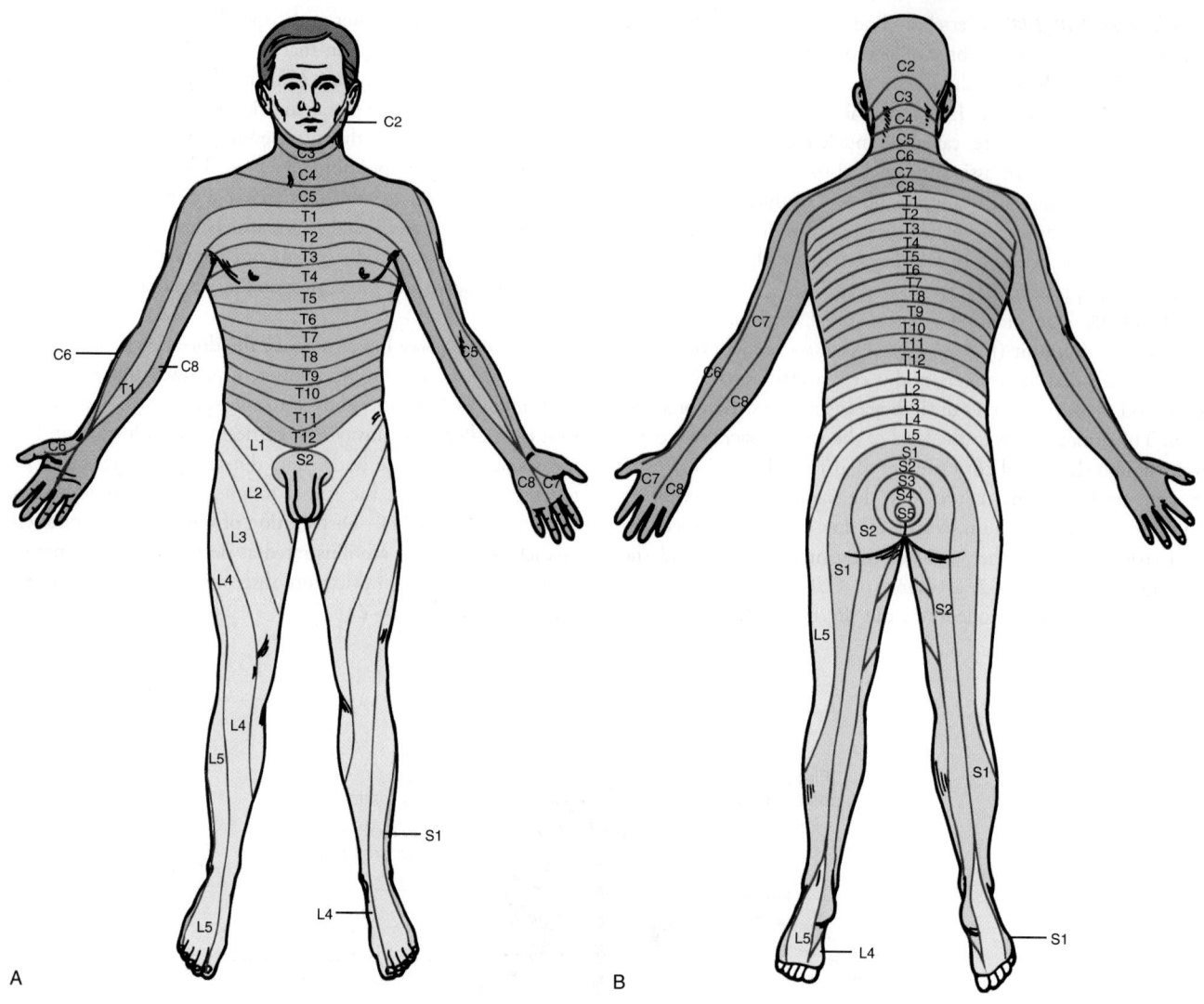

Figure 26-22 Dermatomes. *A*, Anterior view. *B*, Posterior view.

Cross Section of the Spinal Cord. The spinal cord is composed of gray matter and white matter. The central gray matter, which appears in the shape of an H, consists of cell bodies, small projection fibers, and glial support cells. The gray matter of the spinal cord has been divided into areas based on cell body type and location. The three main divisions are the anterior horn, the lateral horn, and the posterior horn. The anterior horn contains motor neurons and is the final junction for motor information before it exits the CNS. The lateral horn contains preganglionic fibers of the autonomic nervous system: sympathetic fibers T1 to L2 and parasympathetic fibers S2 to S4. The posterior horn contains sensory neurons and becomes the entry point for afferent impulses to the CNS.[1,3]

The white matter, which surrounds the gray matter, contains the myelinated ascending and descending tracts, which carry information to and from the brain (Fig. 26-23). Spinal tracts are named so that the prefix denotes the origin of the tract and the suffix is the destination, promoting easy identification of sensory or motor

tracts. Sensory tracts begin with the prefix *spino,* and motor tracts end with the suffix *spinal* (Box 26-1). The complexity of spinal cord tracts is beyond the scope of this chapter, which is limited to the tracts that are most clinically significant and easily tested.

Vascular Supply. Arterial blood supply to the spinal cord is provided by branches of the vertebral arteries and small radicular arteries that enter through intervertebral foramina. They combine to form the anterior spinal and two posterior spinal arteries. These three arteries, along with some additional radicular arterial flow from cervical, intercostal, lumbar, and sacral arteries, feed the entire length of the spinal cord (Fig. 26-24).

Arterial supply to the spinal cord is segmented at best, making portions of the spinal cord that receive blood supply from two separate sources vulnerable to low flow states. The most vulnerable of these areas are C2 to C3, T1 to T4, and L1 to L2. Evidence of this tenuous blood supply is occasionally evident after surgical procedures that involve cross-clamping of the aorta, resulting in spinal cord infarction.

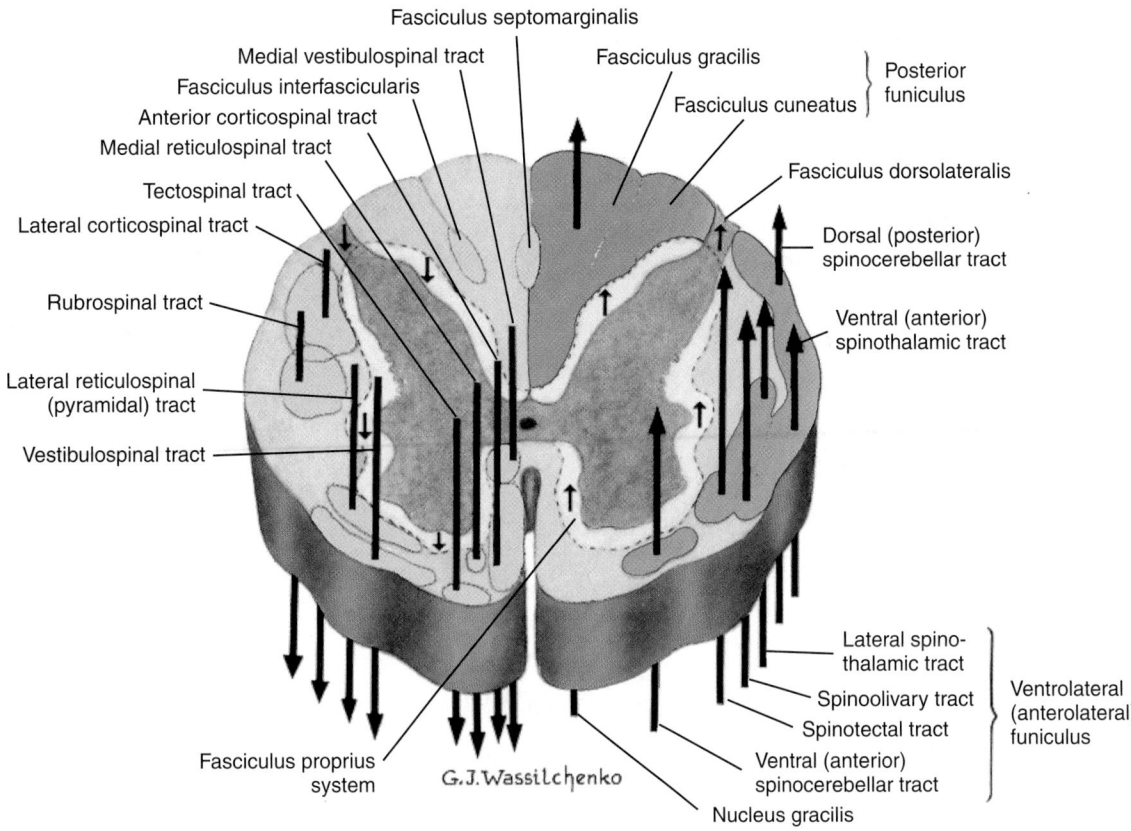

Figure 26-23 Spinal cord tracts of the white matter.

- The autonomic nervous system (sympathetic and parasympathetic) is composed of fibers that connect the CNS with smooth muscle, cardiac muscle, internal organs, and glands.
- The brain is contained within the cranial vault, the spinal cord is contained within the vertebral column, and both are surrounded by the meninges (dura mater, arachnoid mater, and pia mater).
- CSF fills the ventricular system and surrounds the brain and spinal cord in the subarachnoid space.
- Two pairs of arteries (internal carotids and vertebral arteries) provide blood to the brain and are anatomically separated into the anterior (right and left ACAs and the ACoA) and posterior (right and left PCoAs) circulations that connect at the base of the brain to form the circle of Willis.
- The PNS comprises the cranial nerves, the spinal nerves, and all other nerves serving a variety of functions throughout the body.

Summary

Anatomy

- Nervous tissue is composed of neurons and neuroglial cells.
- The CNS is made up of the brain and spinal cord.
- The somatic nervous system is composed of fibers that connect the CNS with structures of the skeletal muscles and the skin.

Physiology

- Neurons perform the functional work of the nervous system, including receipt of information, integration, and transmission of nerve impulses to recipient cells.
- Neuroglial cells (astrocytes, oligodendroglia, ependyma, and microglia) serve as the support infrastructure of the nervous system, providing protection, structural support, and neuronal repair.

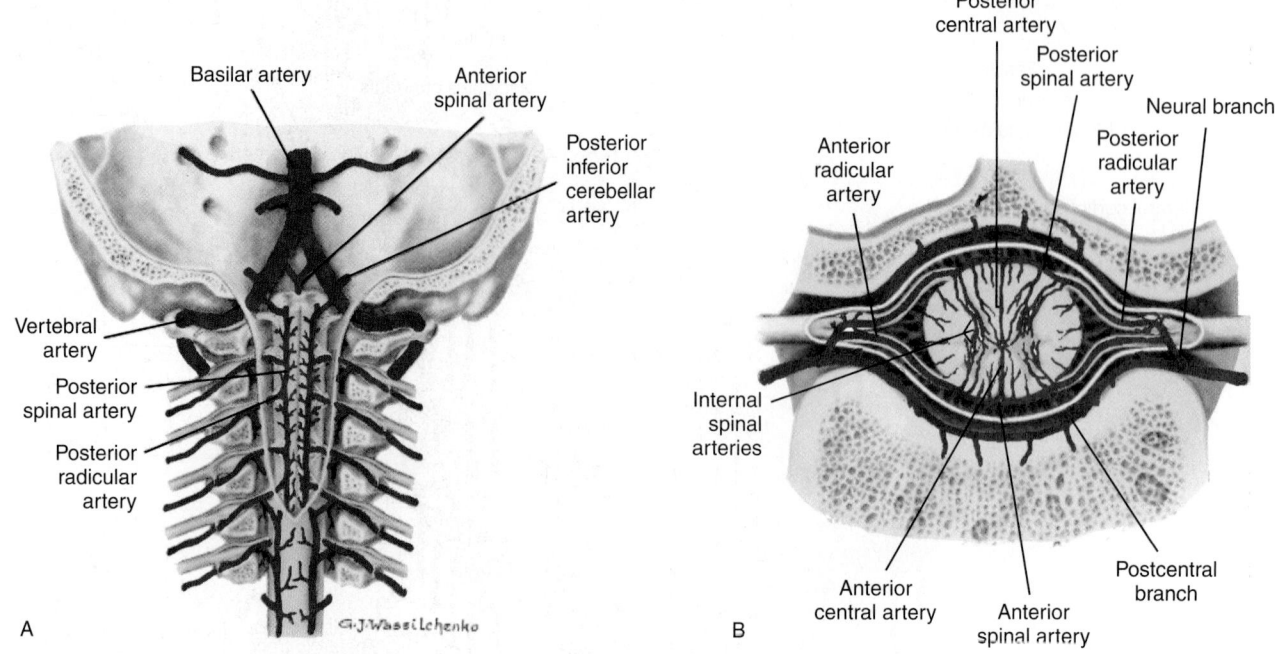

Figure 26-24 Arteries of spinal cord. *A*, cervical cord arteries. *B*, vascular distribution in the spinal cord.

- Most activities of the nervous system originate from sensory receptors, such as visual, auditory, or tactile receptors, and are transmitted to the CNS by afferent fibers (sensory fibers).
- Efferent fibers (motor fibers) transmit the CNS response to the periphery to produce a motor response, such as contraction of skeletal muscles, contraction of the smooth muscles of organs, or secretion by endocrine glands.
- The flow of CSF begins in the lateral ventricles, moves through the foramina of Monro into the third ventricle, moves through the cerebral aqueduct into the fourth ventricle, and moves out the foramen of Magendie and the oramina of Luschka into the subarachnoid space of the brain and spinal cord.
- The primary functions of the cerebral cortex include sensory, motor, and cognitive functions.
- The primary functions of the cerebellum include balance and motor coordination.

- The primary function of the brainstem (midbrain, pons, and medulla) is the regulation of vital functions such as breathing.
- Voluntary motor movement is controlled by the motor strip in the frontal cortex, and as the tracts descend through the brainstem, they cross over to the opposite side. The right motor strip controls the left side of the body and vice versa.
- Broca's area is located in the left frontal lobe and is responsible for expression of written and verbal language. Damage to the area can result in expressive aphasia.
- Wernicke's area is located in the left parietal lobe and is responsible for reception of written and verbal language. Damage to the area can result in receptive aphasia.
- The circle of Willis is provides collateral blood flow to the brain.

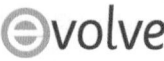 Be sure to check out the bonus material, including free self-assessment exercises, on the Evolve web site at http://evolve.elsevier.com/Urden/.

References

1. Standring S: *Gray's anatomy: the anatomical basis for clinical practice*, ed 39, London, 2004, Churchill Livingstone.
2. Kandel ER et al: *Principles of neural science*, ed 5, New York, 2008, McGraw Hill.
3. Waxman SG: *Correlative neuroanatomy*, ed 25, New York, 2003, Lange.
4. Fouad K, Tse A: Adaptive changes in the injured spinal cord and their role in promoting functional recovery, *Neurol Res* 30:17, 2008.
5. Chopp M et al: Plasticity and remodeling of the brain, *J Neurol Sci* 265 (1-2):97, 2008.
6. Povlishock JT: Pathophysiology of neural injury: therapeutic opportunities and challenges, *Clin Neurosurg* 46:113, 2000.

7. Stuart G et al: *Dendrites*, ed 2, New York, 2008, Oxford University Press.

8. Waxman SG et al: *The axon: structure, function, and pathophysiology*, Oxford, England, 1995, Oxford University Press.

9. Cowan WM et al: *Synapses*, Baltimore, 2003, Johns Hopkins University Press.

10. Harukuni I, Bhardwaj A: Mechanisms of brain injury after global cerebral ischemia, *Neurol Clin* 24:1, 2006.

11. Mohr JP et al, editors: *Stroke: pathophysiology, diagnosis, and management*, ed 4, New York, 2004, Churchill Livingstone.

12. Polderman KH: Induced hypothermia for neuroprotection: understanding the underlying mechanisms. In Vincent JL, editor: *Yearbook of intensive care and emergency medicine 2006*, Berlin, 2006, Springer-Verlag.

13. Springer JE: Apoptotic cell death following traumatic injury to the central nervous system, *J Biochem Mol Biol* 35:94, 2002.

14. MacDonald JF et al: Paradox of Ca^{2+} signaling, cell death and stroke, *Trends Neurosci* 29:75, 2006.

15. Sugerman RA: Structure and function of the neurologic system. In McCance KL, Huether SE, editors: *Pathophysiology: the biologic basis for disease in adults and children*, ed 5, St Louis, 2006, Mosby.

16. Alexandrov AV: *Cerebrovascular ultrasound in stroke prevention and treatment*, Armonk, NY, 2004, Blackwell-Futura.

17. Frackowiak RSD et al: Functional neuroimaging. In Bradley WG et al, editors: *Neurology in clinical practice*, ed 5, Boston, 2007, Butterworth-Heinemann.

18. Gloor P: *The temporal lobe and limbic system*, New York, 1997, Oxford University Press.

19. Bleck TP: Levels of consciousness and attention. In Goetz CG, editor: *Textbook of clinical neurology*, ed 3, Philadelphia, 2007, Saunders.

20. Chernecky CC, Berger BJ, editors: *Laboratory tests and diagnostic procedures*, ed 5, St Louis, 2008, Saunders.

Neurologic Clinical Assessment and Diagnostic Procedures

*A*ssessment of the critically ill patient with neurologic dysfunction includes a review of the patient's health history, a thorough physical examination, and an analysis of the patient's laboratory data. Numerous invasive and noninvasive diagnostic procedures may be performed to assist in the identification of the patient's disorder. This chapter focuses on clinical assessments, laboratory studies, and diagnostic procedures for the critically ill patient with a neurologic dysfunction.

CLINICAL ASSESSMENT

A thorough clinical assessment of the patient with neurologic dysfunction is imperative for the early identification and treatment of neurologic disorders. The completed assessment is used for developing the management plan for the patient. The assessment process can be brief or can involve a detailed history and examination, depending on the nature and immediacy of the patient's situation.

HISTORY

Neurologic assessment encompasses a wide variety of applications and a multitude of techniques. This chapter focuses on the type of assessment performed in a critical care environment. Common to all neurologic assessments is the need to obtain a comprehensive history of events preceding hospitalization. An adequate neurologic history includes information about clinical manifestations, associated complaints, precipitating factors, progression, and familial occurrences (see the Data Collection feature on Neurologic History). If the patient is incapable of providing this information, family members or significant others should be contacted as soon as possible. An ideal historian is able to provide detailed information with emphasis on the chronology of events. Valuable information is gained through medical history that assists the patient's clinical assessment.[1]

When someone other than the patient is the source of the history, it should be an individual who was in contact with the patient on a daily basis. Frequently, valuable information is gained that directs the caregiver to focus on certain aspects of the patient's clinical assessment.[1]

PHYSICAL EXAMINATION

Five major components make up the neurologic evaluation of the critically ill patient: (1) level of consciousness, (2) motor function, (3) pupillary function, (4) respiratory function, and (5) vital signs. A complete neurologic examination requires assessment of all five components.[1]

Level of Consciousness. Assessment of the level of consciousness is the most important aspect of the neurologic examination. In most situations, a patient's level of consciousness deteriorates before any other neurologic changes are noticed. These deteriorations often are subtle and must be monitored carefully. Assessment of level of consciousness focuses on two areas: evaluation of arousal or alertness and appraisal of content of consciousness or awareness.[1] Although universally accepted definitions for various levels of consciousness do not exist, the categories outlined in Box 27-1 are often used to describe the patient's level of consciousness.[1-4]

Evaluation of Arousal. Assessment of the arousal component of consciousness is an evaluation of the reticular activating system and its connection with the thalamus and the cerebral cortex. Arousal is the lowest level of consciousness, and observation centers on the patient's ability to respond to verbal or noxious stimuli in an appropriate manner. To stimulate the patient, the nurse should begin with verbal stimuli in a normal tone. If the patient does not respond, the nurse should increase the stimuli by shouting at the patient. If the patient still does not respond, the nurse should further increase the stimuli by shaking the patient. Noxious stimuli should follow if previous attempts to arouse the patient are unsuccessful. To assess arousal, central stimulation should be used (Box 27-2).

Appraisal of Awareness. Content of consciousness is a higher-level function, and appraisal of awareness is concerned with assessment of the patient's orientation to person, place, and time. Assessment of content of consciousness requires the patient to give appropriate answers to a variety of questions. Changes in the patient's answers that indicate increasing degrees of confusion and disorientation may be the first sign of neurologic deterioration.[1,3-4]

Glasgow Coma Scale. The most widely recognized level of consciousness assessment tool is the Glasgow Coma Scale (GCS).[5] This scored scale is based on evaluation of three categories: eye opening, verbal response, and best motor response

Data Collection

Neurologic History

Common Neurologic Symptoms
- Fainting
- Dizziness
- Blackouts
- Seizures
- Headache
- Memory loss
- Weakness
- Paralysis
- Tremors or other involuntary movements
- Pain
- Numbness
- Tingling
- Speech disturbances
- Vision disturbances

Events Preceding Onset of Symptoms
- Travel
- Animal contact
- Falls
- Infection
- Dental problems or procedures
- Sinus or middle ear infections
- Prodromal symptoms
- Food or drugs ingested

Progression of Symptoms
- Initial onset
- Evolution
- Frequency
- Severity
- Duration
- Associated activities/aggravating factors

Family History
- Stroke (arteriovenous malformation, aneurysm)
- Diabetes mellitus
- Hypertension
- Seizures
- Tumors
- Headaches
- Emotional problems or depression

Medical History
Child
- Birth injuries, congenital defects, encephalitis, meningitis, bedwetting, fainting, seizures, trauma

Adult
- Diabetes; hypertension; cardiovascular, pulmonary, kidney, liver, or endocrine disease; tuberculosis; tropical infection; sinusitis; visual problems; tumors; psychiatric disorders

Surgical History
- Neurologic, ear-nose-throat, dental, eye

Traumatic History
- Motor vehicle accidents, falls, blows to the head, neck or back, being knocked out

Allergies
- Drug, food, environment

Patient Profile
- Personal habits
  - Use of alcohol, recreational drugs, over-the-counter medications, smoking, dietary habits, sleeping patterns, elimination patterns, exercise habits
- Recent life changes
- Living conditions
- Working conditions
- Exposure to toxins, chemicals, fumes; occupational duties
- General temperament

Current Medication Use
- Sedatives, tranquilizers
- Anticonvulsants
- Psychotropics
- Anticoagulants
- Antibiotics
- Calcium channel blockers
- Beta-blockers
- Nitrates
- Oral contraceptives

(Table 27-1). The best possible score on the GCS is 15, and the lowest score is 3. A score of 7 or less on the GCS usually indicates coma. Originally, the scoring system was developed to assist in general communication concerning the severity of neurologic injury. Recent testing of the GCS revealed a moderate to high agreement rating among physicians and nurses.[6,7] Several points should be kept in mind when the GCS is used for serial assessment. It provides data about level of consciousness only, and it never should be considered a complete neurologic examination. It is not a sensitive tool for evaluation of an altered sensorium, nor does it account for possible aphasia. The GCS is also a poor indicator of lateralization of neurologic deterioration.[7] Lateralization involves decreasing motor response on one side or unilateral changes in pupillary reaction.

Motor Function. Assessment of motor function focuses on muscle size and tone and on an estimation of muscle strength. Each side should be assessed individually and then compared with the other.[1,8]

Evaluation of Muscle Size and Tone. Initially, the muscles should be inspected for size and shape. The presence of atrophy

BOX 27-1   CATEGORIES OF CONSCIOUSNESS

Alert	Patient responds immediately to minimal external stimuli.
Confused	Patient is disoriented to time or place but usually oriented to person, with impaired judgment and decision making and decreased attention span.
Delirious	Patient is disoriented to time, place, and person with loss of contact with reality and often has auditory or visual hallucinations.
Lethargic	Patient displays a state of drowsiness or inaction in which the patient needs an increased stimulus to be awakened.
Obtunded	Patient displays dull indifference to external stimuli, and response is minimally maintained. Questions are answered with a minimal response.
Stuporous	Patient can be aroused only by vigorous and continuous external stimuli. Motor response is often withdrawal or localizing to stimulus.
Comatose	Vigorous stimulation fails to produce any voluntary neural response.

From Barker E: *Neuroscience nursing: a spectrum of care*, ed 3, St Louis, 2008, Mosby.

BOX 27-2   STIMULATION TECHNIQUES IN PATIENT AROUSAL

CENTRAL STIMULATION
- *Trapezius pinch:* Squeeze trapezius muscle between thumb and first two fingers.
- *Sternal rub:* Apply firm pressure to sternum with knuckles, using a rubbing motion.

PERIPHERAL STIMULATION
- *Nail bed pressure:* Apply firm pressure, using object such as a pen, to nail bed.
- *Pinching of inner aspect of arm or leg:* Firmly pinch small portion of patient's tissue on sensitive inner aspect of arm or leg.

TABLE 27-1 Glasgow Coma Scale

Category	Score	Response
Eye opening	4	Spontaneous: eyes open spontaneously without stimulation
	3	To speech: eyes open with verbal stimulation but not necessarily to command
	2	To pain: eyes open with noxious stimuli
	1	None: no eye opening regardless of stimulation
Verbal response	5	Oriented: accurate information about person, place, time, reason for hospitalization, and personal data
	4	Confused: answers not appropriate to question, but use of language is correct
	3	Inappropriate words: disorganized, random speech, no sustained conversation
	2	Incomprehensible sounds: moans, groans, and incomprehensible mumbles
	1	None: no verbalization despite stimulation
Best motor response	6	Obeys commands: performs simple tasks on command; able to repeat performance
	5	Localizes to pain: organized attempt to localize and remove painful stimuli
	4	Withdraws from pain: withdraws extremity from source of painful stimuli
	3	Abnormal flexion: decorticate posturing spontaneously or in response to noxious stimuli
	2	Extension: decerebrate posturing spontaneously or in response to noxious stimuli
	1	None: no response to noxious stimuli; flaccid

is noted. Muscle tone is assessed by evaluating the opposition to passive movement. The patient is instructed to relax the extremity while the nurse performs passive range-of-motion movements and evaluates the degree of resistance. Muscle tone is appraised for signs of flaccidity (no resistance), hypotonia (little resistance), hypertonia (increased resistance), spasticity, or rigidity.[8]

Estimation of Muscle Strength. Having the patient perform a number of movements against resistance assesses muscle strength. The strength of the movement is then graded on a 6-point scale (Box 27-3). Ask the patient to extend both arms with the palms turned upward and to hold that position with the eyes closed. If the patient has a weaker side, that arm will drift downward and pronate. The lower extremities are tested by asking the patient to push and pull the feet against resistance or to elevate the legs.[9,10]

Abnormal Motor Responses. If the patient is incapable of comprehending and following a simple command, noxious stimuli are necessary to determine motor responses. The stimulus is applied to each extremity separately to allow evaluation of individual extremity function. Peripheral stimulation is used to assess motor function (see Box 27-2).[1,2] Motor responses elicited by noxious stimuli are interpreted differently from those elicited by voluntary demonstration. These responses may be classified as shown in Box 27-4.[8]

Abnormal flexion also is known as *decorticate posturing* (Fig. 27-1A). In response to painful stimuli, the upper extremities

BOX 27-3   MUSCLE STRENGTH GRADING SCALE

- 0 No movement or muscle contraction
- 1 Trace contraction
- 2 Active movement with gravity eliminated
- 3 Active movement against gravity
- 4 Active movement with some resistance
- 5 Active movement with full resistance

BOX 27-4   CLASSIFICATION OF ABNORMAL MOTOR FUNCTION

Spontaneous	Occurs without regard to external stimuli and may not occur by request
Localization	Occurs when the extremity opposite the extremity receiving pain crosses midline of the body in an attempt to remove the noxious stimulus from the affected limb
Withdrawal	Occurs when the extremity receiving the painful stimulus flexes normally in an attempt to avoid the noxious stimulus
Decortication	Abnormal flexion response that may occur spontaneously or in response to noxious stimuli (see Fig. 27-1A and C)
Decerebration	Abnormal extension response that may occur spontaneously or in response to noxious stimuli (see Fig. 27-1B and C)
Flaccid	No response to painful stimuli

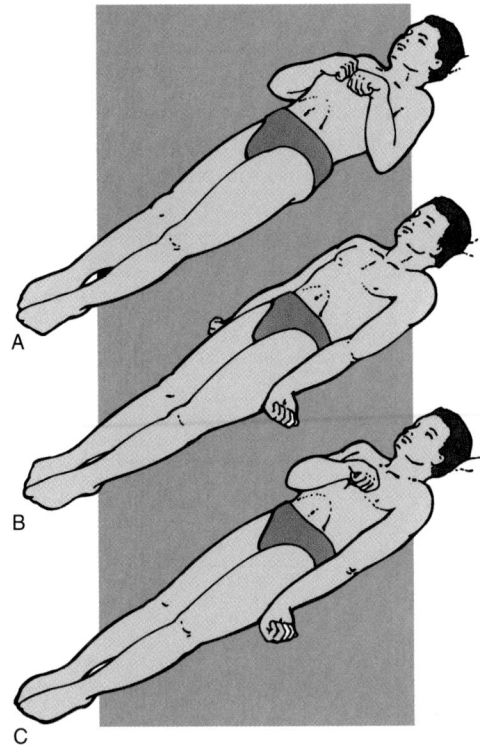

Figure 27-1 Abnormal motor responses. *A,* Decorticate posturing. *B,* Decerebrate posturing. *C,* Decorticate posturing on right side and decerebrate posturing on left side of body.

exhibit flexion of the arm, wrist, and fingers with adduction of the limb. The lower extremity exhibits extension, internal rotation, and plantar flexion. Abnormal flexion occurs with lesions above the midbrain, located in the region of the thalamus or cerebral hemispheres. Abnormal extension also is known as *decerebrate rigidity* or *posturing* (Fig. 27-1B); when the patient is stimulated, teeth clench, and the arms are stiffly extended, adducted, and hyperpronated. The legs are stiffly extended with plantar flexion of the feet. Abnormal extension occurs with lesions in the area of the brainstem. Because abnormal flexion and extension appear similar in the lower extremities, the upper extremities are used to determine the presence of these abnormal movements. It is possible for the patient to exhibit abnormal flexion on one side of the body and extension on the other (Fig. 27-1C).[1-3] Outcome studies indicate that abnormal flexion or decorticate posturing has a less serious prognosis than does extension, or decerebrate posturing. Onset of posturing or a change from abnormal flexion to abnormal extension requires immediate physician notification.[3]

Evaluation of Reflexes. Deep tendon reflexes (DTRs) are usually evaluated by a physician when a complete neurologic evaluation is performed. DTRs are tested by tapping the appropriate tendon using a reflex or percussion hammer. The muscle needs to be relaxed and the joint at midposition for reflex testing to be accurate. The four reflexes tested are the Achilles (ankle jerk), the quadriceps (knee jerk), the biceps, and

the triceps. DTRs are graded on a scale from 0 (absent) to 4 (hyperactive). A DTR grade of 2 is normal (Fig. 27-2). Hyperreflexia is associated with upper motor neuron interruption, and areflexia is associated with lesions of the lower motor neurons.[2]

Superficial reflexes are normal if present and abnormal if absent. Superficial reflexes are tested by stimulating cutaneous receptors of the skin, cornea, or mucous membrane. Stroking, scratching, or touching can be used as the stimulus (Table 27-2). The corneal reflex is present if the eyelids quickly close when the cornea is lightly stroked with a wisp of cotton. An alternative approach is to drop a small amount of water or saline onto the cornea.[1] The pathway for the corneal reflex is formed by the trigeminal cranial nerve V (CN V), facial nerve (CN VII), and the pons. The pharyngeal reflex is present if retching or gagging occurs with stimulation of the back of the pharynx.[1-3] The gag reflex is often stimulated during routine oral and pulmonary hygiene in the critical care environment. The presence of these reflexes should be documented during completion of these activities.

The presence of pathologic reflexes is an abnormal neurologic finding. The grasp reflex is present when tactile stimulation of the palm of the hand produces a grasp response that is not a conscious voluntary act. The grasp reflex is a primitive reflex that normally disappears with maturational development. Presence of the grasp reflex in the adult indicates cortical damage. Babinski's reflex is a pathologic sign in any individual older than 2 years. The presence of this reflex is tested by slow, deliberate stroking of the lateral half of the sole of the foot. Sustained extensor response of the big toe is indicative of a positive Babinski's reflex. This response is sometimes accompanied by the fanning out of the other four toes. Flexor response of all the toes in response to the same stimuli is a normal finding and indicates absence of Babinski's reflex (Fig. 27-3). Babinski's reflex is a significant neurologic finding because it indicates an upper motor neuron lesion in the brain, brainstem, or spinal cord. The disease may be degenerative, neoplastic,

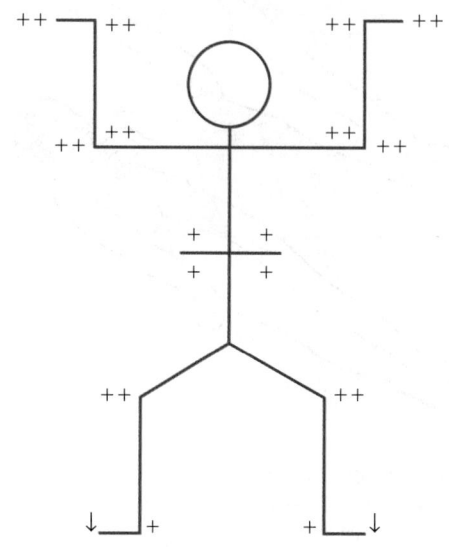

Scoring Deep Tendon Reflexes

Grade	Deep Tendon Reflex Response
0	No response
1+	Sluggish or diminished
2+	Active or expected response
3+	More brisk than expected, slightly hyperactive
4+	Brisk, hyperactive, with intermittent or transient clonus

Figure 27-2 The patient's reflex scores are recorded by entering the correct scores at the correct location on the stick figure. *(From Barker E: Neuroscience nursing: a spectrum of care, ed 3, St Louis, 2008, Mosby.)*

inflammatory, vascular, or posttraumatic. Babinski's reflex may also become positive during transtentorial herniation.[1]

Pupillary Function. Assessment of pupillary function focuses on three areas: (1) estimation of pupil size and shape, (2) evaluation of pupillary reaction to light, and (3) assessment of eye movements. Pupillary function is an extension of the autonomic nervous system. Parasympathetic control of the pupil occurs through innervation of the oculomotor nerve (CN III), which exits from the brainstem in the midbrain area. When the parasympathetic fibers are stimulated, the pupil constricts. Sympathetic control originates in the hypothalamus and travels down the entire length of the brainstem. When the sympathetic fibers are stimulated, the pupil dilates. Pupillary changes provide a valuable assessment tool because of pathway locations. The oculomotor nerve lies at the junction of the midbrain and the tentorial notch. Any increase of pressure that exerts force down through the tentorial notch compresses the oculomotor nerve. Oculomotor nerve compression results in a dilated, nonreactive pupil. Sympathetic pathway disruption occurs with involvement in the brainstem. Loss of sympathetic control leads to pinpoint, nonreactive pupils. Control of eye movements occurs with interaction of three cranial nerves: oculomotor (CN III), trochlear (CN IV), and abducens (CN VI). The pathways for these cranial nerves provide integrated function through the internuclear pathway of the medial longitudinal fasciculus (MLF) located in the brainstem. The MLF provides coordination of eye movements with the vestibular nerve (CN VIII) and the reticular formation.[3]

Estimation of Pupil Size and Shape. Pupil diameter should be documented in millimeters with the use of a pupil gauge to reduce the subjectivity of description. Most people have pupils of equal size, between 2 and 5 mm. A discrepancy up to 1 mm between the two pupils is normal; it is called anisocoria and occurs in 16% to 17% of the human population.[11] Change or inequality in pupil size, especially in patients who previously have not shown this discrepancy, is a significant neurologic sign. It may indicate impending danger of herniation and should be reported immediately. With the location of the oculomotor nerve (CN III) at the

TABLE 27-2 Superficial Reflexes

Reflex	Nerves Involved	Normal Reaction
Corneal	CN V and VII	Prompt closure of both eyelids when cornea touched with wisp of cotton
Pharyngeal	CN IX and X	Gagging response to pharyngeal stimulation
Abdominal	Epigastric (T6-T9); midabdominal (T9-T11); hypogastric (T11-L1)	Contraction of abdominal muscle when stroked, so that there is a brief, brisk movement of umbilicus toward stimulus
Cremasteric	L1, L2	Elevation of testicle when inner aspect of thigh stroked
Anal		Contraction of anal ring as perineum is stroked or scratched
Bulbocutaneous	S4, S5	
Anocutaneous	S5	
Plantar	L5, S1	Flexion of toes from stimulation of sole of foot

From Barker E: *Neuroscience nursing: a spectrum of care,* ed 3, St Louis, 2008, Mosby.
CN, cranial nerve.

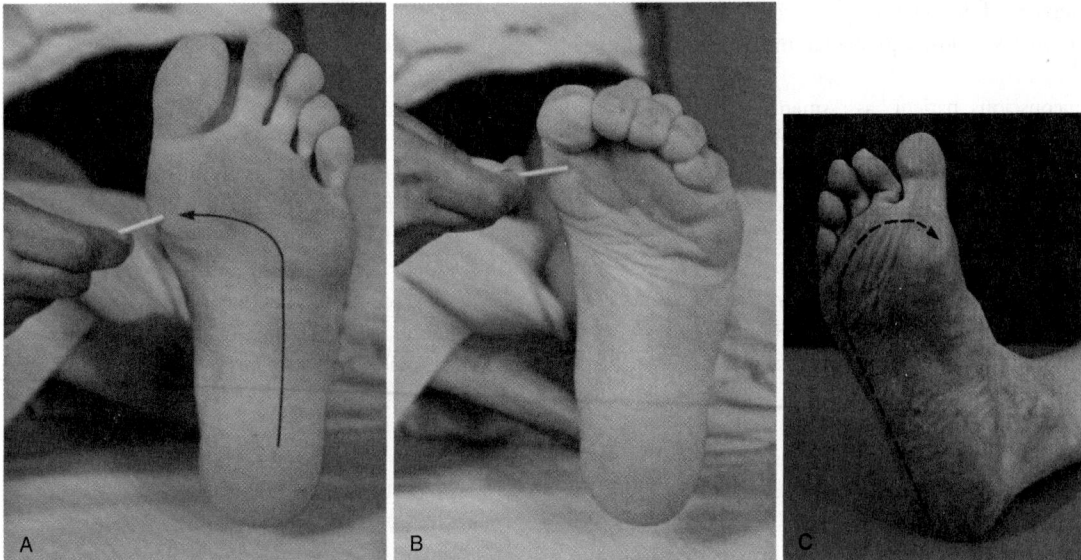

Figure 27-3 Elicitation of the plantar reflex. *A*, A hard object is applied to the lateral surface of the sole, starting at the heel, going over the ball of the foot, and ending beneath the great toe. *B*, Normal response to plantar stimulation: flexion of all toes. *C*, Babinski's sign: dorsiflexion of the great toe and fanning of the other toes. *(A and B from Barkauskas VH et al:* Health & physical assessment, *ed 3, St Louis, 2002, Mosby; C from Seidel HM, et al:* Mosby's guide to physical examination, *ed 6, St Louis, 2006, Mosby.)*

notch of the tentorium, pupil size and reactivity play a key role in the physical assessment of intracranial pressure (ICP) changes and herniation syndromes. In addition to CN III compression, changes in pupil size occur for other reasons. Large pupils can result from the instillation of cycloplegic agents, such as atropine or scopolamine, or can indicate extreme stress. Extremely small pupils can indicate opioid overdose, lower brainstem compression, or bilateral damage to the pons.[11,12]

Pupil shape is included in the assessment of pupils. Although the pupil is normally round, an irregularly shaped or oval pupil may be observed in patients who have undergone eye surgery. Initial stages of CN III compression from elevated ICP can cause the pupil to have an oval shape.[1,11]

Evaluation of Pupillary Reaction to Light. The pupillary light reflex depends on optic nerve (CN II) and oculomotor nerve (CN III) function (Fig. 27-4).[3,11] The technique for evaluation of the pupillary light response involves use of a narrow-beamed bright light shined into the pupil from the outer canthus of the eye. If the light is shined directly onto the pupil, glare or reflection of the light may prevent the assessor's proper visualization. Pupillary reaction to light is identified as brisk, sluggish, or nonreactive or fixed.[1] Each pupil should be evaluated for direct light response and for consensual response. The consensual pupillary response is constriction in response to a light shined into the opposite eye. This reflex occurs as a result of the crossing of nerve fibers at the optic chiasm.[1] Evaluation of consensual response is necessary to rule out optic nerve dysfunction as a cause for lack of a direct light reflex. Because the optic nerve is the afferent pathway for the light reflex, shining a light into a blind eye produces neither a direct light response in that eye nor a consensual response in the opposite eye. A consensual response in the blind eye produced by shining a light into the opposite eye demonstrates an intact

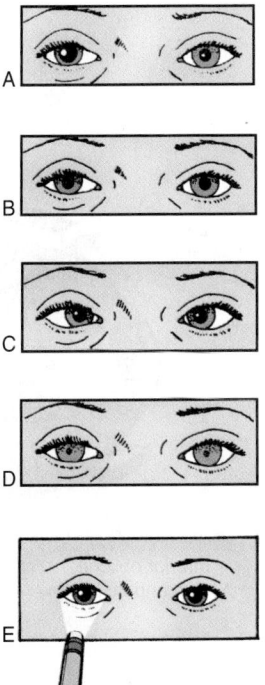

Figure 27-4 Abnormal pupillary responses. *A*, Oculomotor nerve compression. *B*, Bilateral diencephalon damage. *C*, Midbrain damage. *D*, Pontine damage. *E*, Dilated, nonreactive pupils.

oculomotor nerve. Oculomotor compression associated with transtentorial herniation affects the direct light response and the consensual response in the affected pupil.[1,2,11,12]

Assessment of Eye Movement. In the conscious patient, the function of the three cranial nerves of the eye and their MLF innervation can be assessed by asking the patient to follow the full range of eye motion. If the eyes move ... six fields, extraocular movements are intact ... unconscious patient, assessment of ocular function ... innervation of the MLF is performed by eliciting the doll's eyes reflex. If the patient is unconscious as a result of trauma, the nurse must ascertain the absence of cervical injury before performing this examination. To assess the oculocephalic reflex, the nurse holds the patient's eyelids open and briskly turns the head to one side while observing the eye movements and then briskly turns the head to the other side and observes. If the eyes deviate to the opposite direction in which the head is turned, the doll's eyes reflex is present, and the oculocephalic reflex arc is intact (Fig. 27-6A). If the oculocephalic reflex arc is not intact, the reflex is absent. This lack of response, in which the eyes remain midline and move with the head, indicates significant brainstem injury (see Fig. 27-6C). The reflex may also be absent in severe metabolic coma. An abnormal oculocephalic reflex is present when the eyes rove or move in opposite directions from each other (see Fig. 27-6B). Abnormal oculocephalic reflex indicates some degree of brainstem injury.[1-3]

The oculovestibular reflex is performed by a physician, often as one of the final clinical assessments of brainstem function. After confirmation that the tympanic membrane is intact,

the head is raised to a 30-degree angle, and 20 to 100 mL of ice water is injected into the external auditory canal. The normal eye movement response is a conjugate, slow, tonic nystagmus deviating toward the irrigated ear and lasting 30 to 120 seconds. This response indicates brainstem integrity. Rapid nystagmus returns the eyes back to the midline only in a conscious patient with cortical functioning (Fig. 27-7).[1] An abnormal response is disconjugate eye movement, which indicates a brainstem lesion, or no response, which indicates little or no brainstem function. The oculovestibular reflex may be temporarily absent in reversible metabolic encephalopathy.[3] This test is an extremely noxious stimulation and may produce a decorticate or decerebrate posturing response in a comatose patient. In the conscious patient, this procedure may produce nausea, vomiting, or dizziness.[1,12]

Respiratory Function. Assessment of respiratory function focuses on two areas: observation of respiratory pattern and evaluation of airway status. The activity of respiration is a highly integrated function that receives input from the cerebrum, brainstem, and metabolic mechanisms. In clinical assessment, correlations exist among altered levels of consciousness, the level of brain or brainstem injury, and the patient's respiratory pattern. Under the influence of the cerebral cortex and the diencephalon, three brainstem centers control respirations.

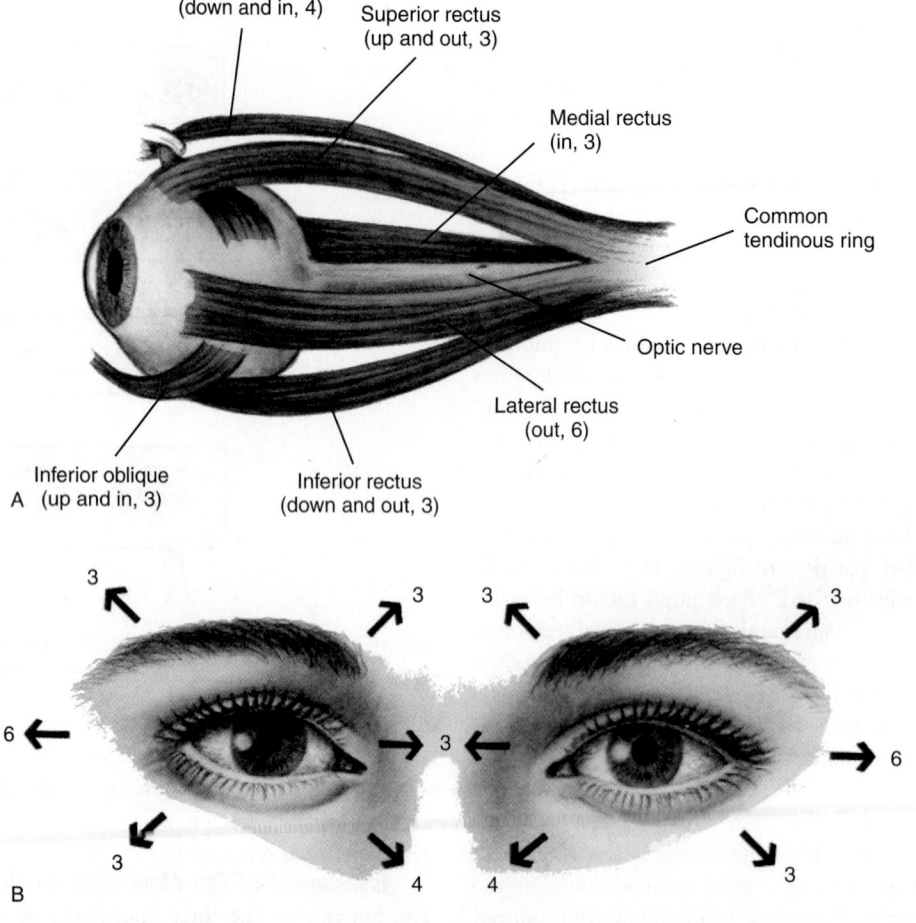

Figure 27-5 Extraocular eye movements. *A,* Extraocular muscles. *B,* The six cardinal directions of gaze with each associated cranial nerve supply.

The lowest center, the medullary respiratory center, sends impulses through the vagus nerve to innervate muscles of inspiration and expiration. The apneustic and pneumotaxic centers of the pons are responsible for the length of inspiration and expiration and the underlying respiratory rate.[1-3]

Observation of Respiratory Pattern. Changes in respiratory patterns assist in identifying the level of brainstem dysfunction or injury (Fig. 27-8 and Table 27-3). Evaluation of the respiratory pattern must include assessment of the effectiveness of gas exchange in maintaining adequate oxygen and carbon dioxide

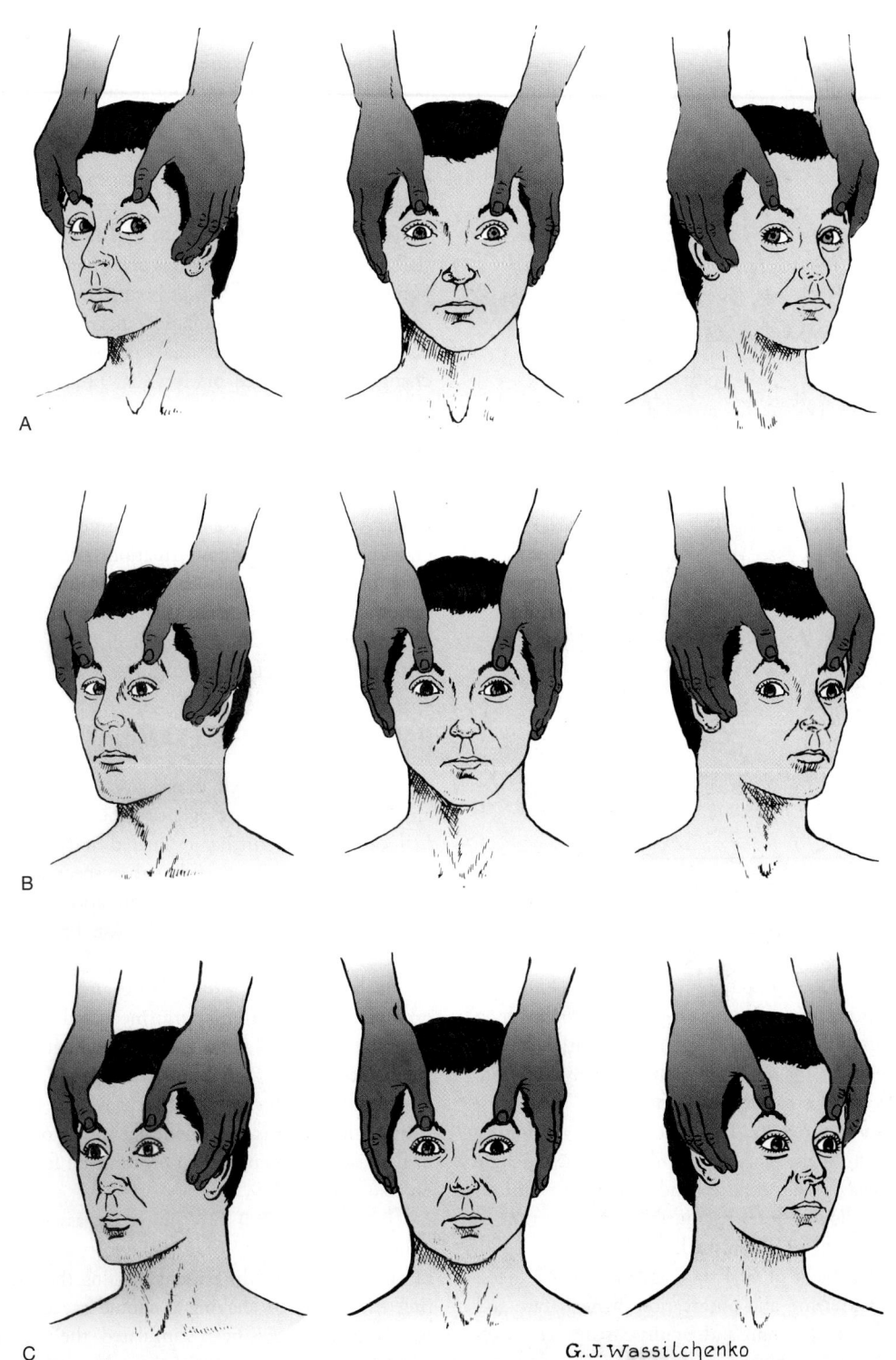

G. J. Wassilchenko

Figure 27-6 Oculocephalic reflex (doll's eyes). *A,* Normal. *B,* Abnormal. *C,* Absent.

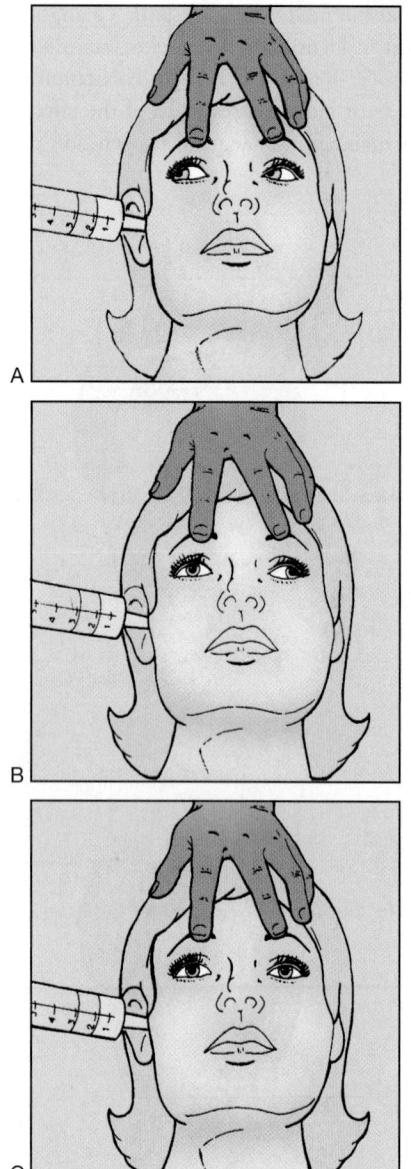

Figure 27-7 Oculovestibular reflex (cold caloric test). *A,* Normal. *B,* Abnormal. *C,* Absent.

levels. Hypoventilation is not uncommon in the patient with an altered level of consciousness. Alterations in oxygenation or carbon dioxide levels can result in further neurologic dysfunction. ICP increases with hypoxemia or hypercapnia.[1-3]

Evaluation of Airway Status. Evaluation of the respiratory function in a patient with a neurologic deficit must include assessment of airway maintenance and secretion control. Cough, gag, and swallow reflexes responsible for protection of the airway may be absent or diminished.[13]

Vital Signs. Assessment of vital signs focuses on two areas: evaluation of blood pressure and observation of heart rate and rhythm. As a result of the brain and brainstem influences on cardiac, respiratory, and body temperature functions, changes in vital signs can indicate deterioration in neurologic status.

Evaluation of Blood Pressure. A common manifestation of intracranial injury is systemic hypertension. Cerebral autoregulation, responsible for the control of cerebral blood flow (CBF), frequently is lost with any type of intracranial injury. After cerebral injury, the body often is in a hyperdynamic state (increased heart rate, blood pressure, and cardiac output) as part of a compensatory response. With the loss of autoregulation as blood pressure increases, CBF and cerebral blood volume increase, and ICP therefore increases. Control of systemic hypertension is necessary to stop this cycle, but caution must be exercised. The mean arterial pressure must be maintained at a level sufficient to produce adequate CBF in the presence of elevated ICP. Attention must also be paid to the pulse pressure because widening of this value may occur in the late stages of intracranial hypertension.[13]

Observation of Heart Rate and Rhythm. The medulla and the vagus nerve provide parasympathetic control to the heart. When stimulated, this lower brainstem system produces bradycardia. Sympathetic stimulation increases the rate and contractility.[14] Various intracranial pathologies and abrupt ICP changes can produce bradycardia, premature ventricular contractions (PVCs), QT changes, and myocardial damage.[14,15]

Cushing's Triad. Cushing's triad is a set of three clinical manifestations (bradycardia, systolic hypertension, and widening pulse pressure) related to pressure on the medullary area of the brainstem. These signs often occur in response to intracranial hypertension or a herniation syndrome. The appearance of Cushing's triad is a late finding that may be absent in patients with neurologic deterioration. Attention should be paid to alteration in each component of the triad and intervention initiated accordingly.[3]

RAPID NEUROLOGIC EXAMINATION

An adequate neurologic examination should focus on covering all major areas of neurologic control. Any abnormalities identified can then be further evaluated and investigated. Findings should always be evaluated with respect to those of previous examinations. A neurologic examination should be organized, thorough, and simple so that it can be performed accurately and easily at each assessment point.[1]

The Conscious Patient. An example of a rapid neurologic examination that can be performed in the critical care unit on a conscious patient with known or potential neurologic deficit is outlined in Box 27-5. This examination, which usually takes less than 4 minutes, is meant to provide a starting point. If any neurologic deficit is identified that is new or different from that of the last assessment, attention must be focused in more detail on that abnormality.[1]

The Unconscious Patient. In the assessment of the unconscious patient (Box 27-6), initial efforts are directed at achieving maximal arousal of the patient. Calling the patient's name, patting the chest, or shaking a shoulder accomplishes this task. After the patient has been stimulated, the examiner can proceed with the neurologic examination. As in the assessment of the conscious patient, if any abnormalities or changes from previous

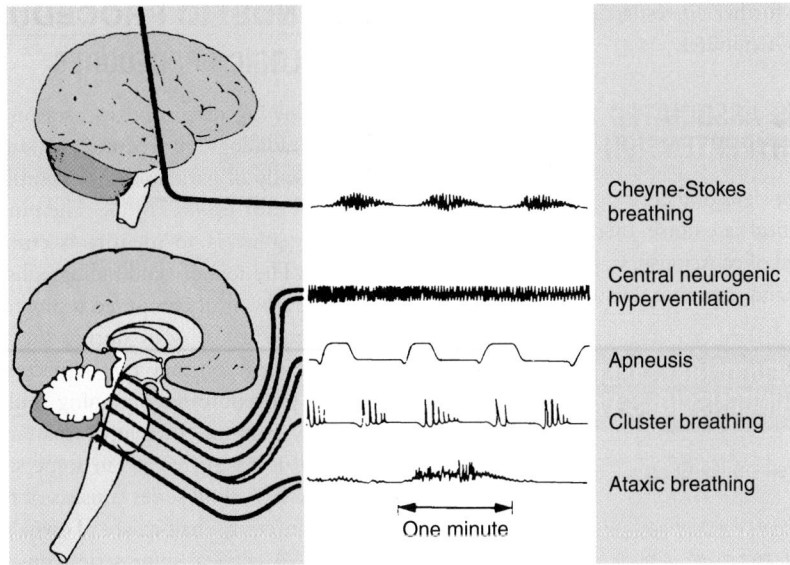

Cheyne-Stokes breathing

Central neurogenic hyperventilation

Apneusis

Cluster breathing

Ataxic breathing

One minute

Figure 27-8 Abnormal respiratory patterns with corresponding levels of central nervous system activity.

TABLE 27-3 Respiratory Patterns

Pattern of Respiration	Description of Pattern	Significance
Cheyne-Stokes	Rhythmic crescendo and decrescendo of rate and depth of respiration; includes brief periods of apnea	Usually seen with bilateral deep cerebral lesions or some cerebellar lesions
Central neurogenic hyperventilation	Very deep, very rapid respirations with no apneic periods	Usually seen with lesions of the midbrain and upper pons
Apneustic	Prolonged inspiratory and/or expiratory pause of 2-3 sec	Usually seen in lesions of the middle to lower pons
Cluster breathing	Clusters of irregular, gasping respirations separated by long periods of apnea	Usually seen in lesions of the lower pons or upper medulla
Ataxic respirations	Irregular, random pattern of deep and shallow respirations with irregular apneic periods	Usually seen in lesions of the medulla

BOX 27-5   RAPID NEUROLOGIC ASSESSMENT OF THE CONSCIOUS PATIENT

1. *Level of consciousness:* Address the patient, and ask a variety of orientation questions; avoid the obvious, overused questions about name, date, and place, and focus on questions about recent and past events from the patient's experiences, such as spouse's name, home address, what was eaten at the previous meal. As examiner, you should be aware of the correct answers to all questions asked.
2. *Facial movements:* During assessment of level of consciousness, observe the patient's facial movements for symmetry, and listen to speech patterns for evidence of slurred speech.
3. *Pupillary function and eye movements:* Perform pupil check, and assess extraocular eye movements.
4. *Motor assessment:* Assess upper and lower extremity movement and strength.
5. *Sensory:* With a finger, stroke the patient bilaterally on the face, upper aspect of the arm, hand, leg, and foot; ask the patient to identify what is touched and whether there is any difference in sensation between the two sides.
6. *Vital signs:* Observe alterations in blood pressure, heart rate or rhythm, respiratory pattern, or temperature.
7. *Change in status:* Ask the patient if he or she feels any differences between this and the previous examination.

assessment are noticed, further investigation must occur. This assessment takes 3 to 4 minutes.[1]

NEUROLOGIC CHANGES ASSOCIATED WITH INTRACRANIAL HYPERTENSION

Assessment of the patient for signs of increasing ICP is an important responsibility of the critical care nurse. Increasing ICP can be identified by changes in level of consciousness, pupillary reaction, motor response, vital signs, and respiratory patterns (Fig. 27-9).

BOX 27-6 RAPID NEUROLOGIC ASSESSMENT OF THE UNCONSCIOUS PATIENT

1. *Level of consciousness:* Perform the Glasgow Coma Scale assessment.
2. *Pupillary assessment:* Perform pupillary assessment with special attention to size, reactivity, and shape of pupil compared with the opposite eye.
3. *Motor examination:* Assess each extremity individually by means of a predetermined coding score of motor movement.
4. *Respiratory pattern:* If the patient is not receiving mechanical ventilation, observe respiratory patterns for evidence of deteriorating level of function.
5. *Vital signs:* Include a comparison of preassessment vital signs with postassessment vital signs, paying special attention to arterial blood pressure and intracranial pressure (ICP) if these parameters are being monitored.

DIAGNOSTIC PROCEDURES

RADIOLOGIC PROCEDURES

The following discussion focuses on the more commonly performed radiologic procedures that are used for the diagnosis of the critically ill patient with a neurologic dysfunction.

Skull and Spine Films. The purpose of radiographs of the skull or spine is to identify fractures, anomalies, or possible tumors. The role of skull radiographs in trauma has diminished with the advent of computed tomography (CT). If the patient is to undergo a CT scan during the initial assessment process, a skull radiograph may not be necessary.[1]

The procedure for obtaining skull and spine radiographs is relatively painless. In many situations, a single lateral view of the skull is adequate, but in some situations, a full skull series is required. A skull series consists of four different views: lateral, posteroanterior, half-axial (Towne's), and submentovertical (base).[16] A cervical spine series consists of four views: atlas and axial, anteroposterior, lateral, and oblique. Thoracic and lumbar spine series consists of two views: anteroposterior and lateral.[16]

Proper patient positioning is essential, especially for spine radiographs. Spinal precautions (e.g., cervical collar, strict maintenance of head alignment) must be maintained until lateral films confirm the integrity of the cervical structures. Nursing care involves positioning the patient to obtain adequate films. In any situation in which traumatic injury, especially head injury, is the cause of the patient's admission to the critical care unit, the cervical spine must be treated as unstable until proven otherwise.[2]

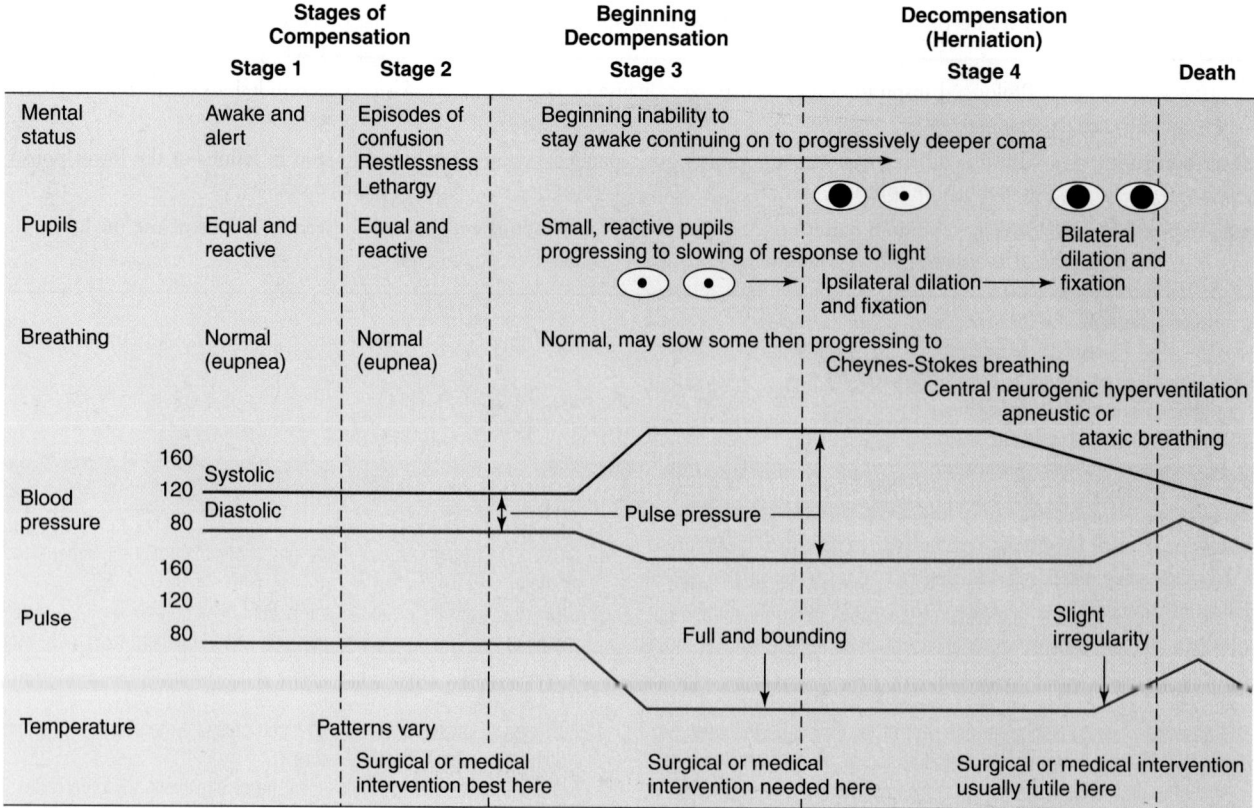

Figure 27-9 Clinical correlates of compensated and decompensated phases of intracranial hypertension. *(From Beare PG, Myers JL: Principles and practice of adult health nursing, ed 3, St Louis, 1998, Mosby.)*

Computed Tomography. CT scanning provides the clinician with a mathematically reconstructed view of multiple sections of the head and body. This is accomplished by passage of intersecting x-ray beams through the examined area and measurement of the density of substances through which the x-ray beams pass. The denser the substance through which an x-ray beam passes, the whiter it appears on the finished film. The less dense a substance is, the blacker it appears. With normal findings for a CT scan of the head, bone appears white, blood appears off-white, brain tissue appears shaded gray, cerebrospinal fluid (CSF) appears off-black, and air appears black (Fig. 27-10).[16]

CT scanning offers rapid, convenient, noninvasive visualization of structures and is the diagnostic study of choice for an acute head injury. Serial evaluations may be obtained to verify midline shift and increasing ICP.[18] CT scanning also is used in the diagnostic workup of space-occupying lesions, hemorrhage, and vascular abnormalities; cerebral edema; hydrocephalus; and severe headache. CT scan is the preferred method for diagnosing subarachnoid hemorrhage and for differentiating intracranial hemorrhage and infarction.[17,18]

CT scans can be conducted with and without the use of a contrast medium. Without contrast, the scan is noninvasive, requires no premedication of the patient, and is good for analysis and location of normal brain structures. A non–contrast-enhanced CT scan of the head is appropriate for trauma patients when the goal is to view the intracranial area for evidence of intracranial hemorrhage, cerebral edema, or shift of structures. Non–contrast-enhanced CT also is appropriate in the diagnosis of hydrocephalus.[19] The use of an intravenously injected contrast medium enhances the vascular areas and enables detection of vascular lesions or further definition of lesions identified on a non–contrast-enhanced scan. The letter *C* is evident on the film when contrast has been used.[17]

Nursing management of the patient undergoing CT can be divided into two areas of focus: observation of the patient's tolerance of the procedure and observation of the patient's reaction to the dye used in contrast-enhanced scanning. Because of the associated activity and positioning, transporting and scanning of a critically ill patient with known or suspected intracranial hypertension can cause deterioration in the patient's condition. The nurse must always remain with the patient during CT scanning and closely observe the neurologic status, vital signs, and if monitored, ICP.

If the patient is scheduled to receive contrast for CT scanning, questions about possible sensitivity to iodine-based dye must be asked beforehand if possible. During infusion of the dye and for 10 to 30 minutes afterward, the patient is observed closely for an anaphylactic reaction. Less than 1% of all patients undergoing contrast-enhanced CT have severe anaphylactic reactions, shock, or cardiac arrest. Another potential complication of the dye is acute tubular necrosis (ATN). Two measures reported to reduce the incidence and severity of ATN after contrast-enhanced CT are antihistamine administration and adequate hydration before and after the study.[17]

Magnetic Resonance Imaging. Magnetic resonance imaging (MRI) has replaced CT as the diagnostic study of choice for many conditions. MRI produces images with greater detail than CT scanning and provides views of several planes (sagittal, coronal, axial, and oblique) not possible with CT scanning.[17] No ionizing radiation is used. For MRI, the patient is placed in a large magnetic field that stimulates the nuclei of the atoms of the body. Introduction of radiofrequency waves causes resonance of the nuclei, which is emitted as the nuclei relax. A computer then constructs an image of the tissue (Fig. 27-11). Intravenous administration of a non–iodine-based contrast medium enhances the images by influencing the magnetic environment and signal intensity.[18,19]

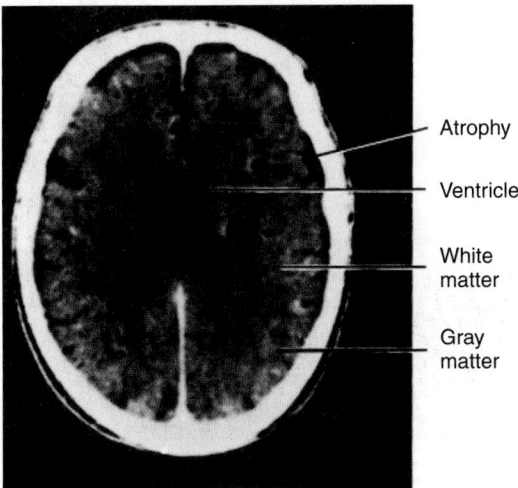

Figure 27-10 CT scan of the brain. *(From Ballinger PW: Merrill's atlas of radiographic positions and radiologic procedures, ed 7, St Louis, 1991, Mosby.)*

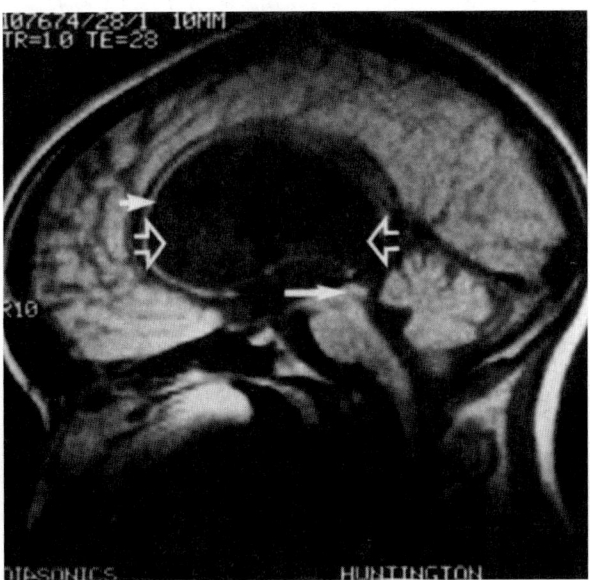

Figure 27-11 MRI of the brain. The sagittal section shows marked enlargement of the lateral ventricle *(open arrows)* and stretching of the corpus callosum *(arrowhead)* as a result of aqueductal stenosis *(arrow)*. *(From Stark DD, Bradley WG: Magnetic resonance imaging, ed 2, St Louis, 1992, Mosby.)*

With MRI, small tumors, whose tissue densities are different from those of the surrounding cells, can be identified before they would be visible by any other radiographic test. MRI also can identify small hemorrhages deep in the brain that are invisible on CT. MRI can detect areas of cerebral infarct within a few hours of the incident and can identify small areas of plaque in patients with multiple sclerosis. MRI with contrast is the preferred study for detection of infectious and inflammatory processes of the central nervous system, malignancy, and metastatic lesions; cervical spine imaging; and postoperative evaluation of tumor recurrence.[17] MRI also is the diagnostic study of choice in the evaluation of spinal cord injury.[20] Nursing management for the patient undergoing MRI is focused on the patient's tolerance of the procedure. Concerns related to transport of the neurologic patient for MRI are identical to those discussed for CT.

Teaching and preparation of the patient are essential for successful MRI. The procedure is lengthy and requires the patient to lie motionless in a tight, enclosed space. Many patients experience anxiety, panic, and an acute sense of claustrophobia. Mild sedation or a blindfold, or both, may be necessary. The neurologically impaired patient may not be able to comprehend the instructions, and sedation, possibly combined with neuromuscular blockade, is required. Removal of all metal from the patient's body and clothing is essential because the basis of MRI is a strong magnetic field. In the past, it was thought that any metal material, such as dental filling, prostheses, or internal clips or staples, would prevent scanning. Further study and changes in the type of metals used for many procedures have made the test safer. Any questions about specific devices or metals must be directed to the neuroradiologist before testing. The test is considered relatively safe and noninvasive, but all risks of this procedure have not been identified.[1]

Cerebral Angiography

Conventional Angiography. Conventional angiography involves the injection of radiopaque contrast medium into the intracranial or extracranial vasculature (Fig. 27-12).[21] With the use of serial radiologic filming, an angiogram traces the flow of blood from the arterial circulation through the capillary bed to the venous circulation. Cerebral angiography allows visualization of the lumen of vessels to provide information about patency, size (narrowing or dilation), irregularities, or occlusion. Angiography is used in the diagnosis of cerebral aneurysm, vasospasm, arteriovenous malformation (AVM), carotid artery disease, and some vascular tumors. Angiography also is used to evaluate cerebral vasculature in the stroke patient. Information obtained from the angiogram guides the surgeon in choosing the operative approach or provides information on which to make medical management decisions other than surgery.[1]

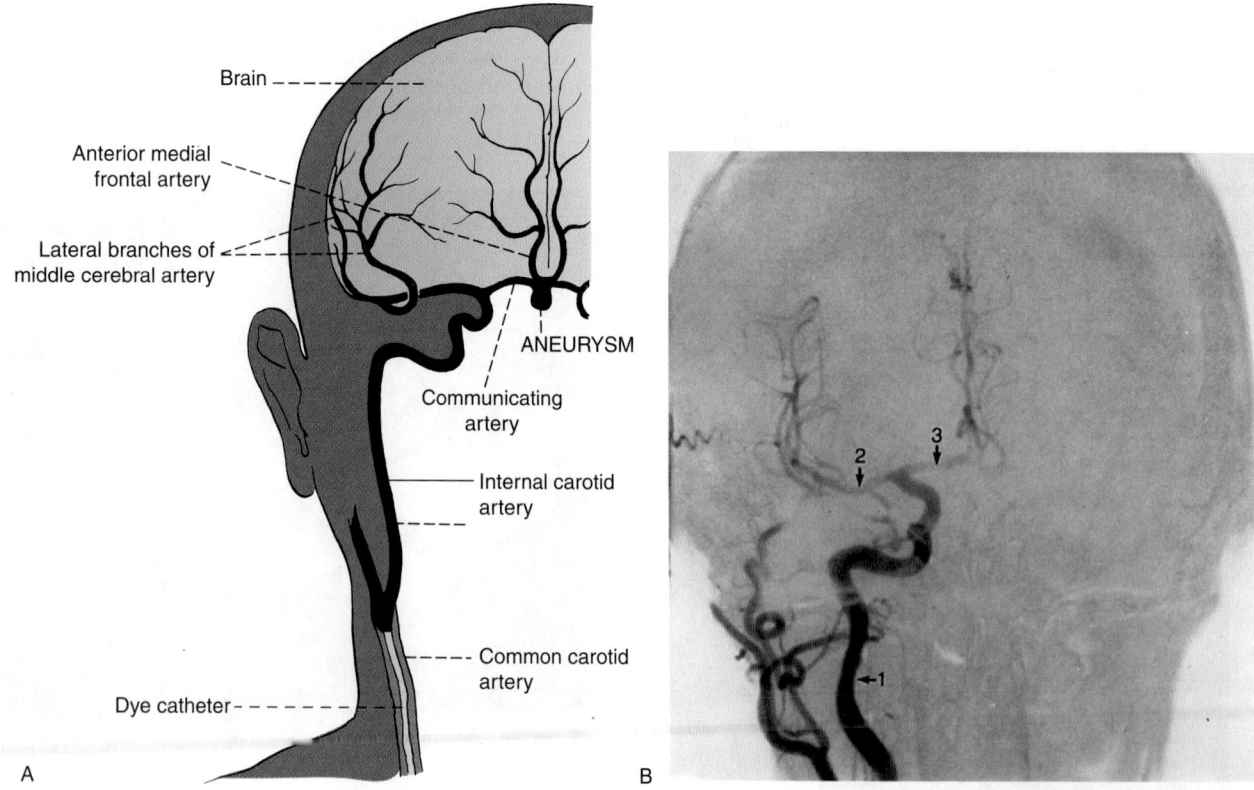

Figure 27-12 Cerebral angiography. *A,* Insertion of contrast through a catheter in the common carotid. *B,* View of the vessels. 1, internal carotid artery; 2, middle cerebral artery; 3, middle meningeal artery. *(From Black JM, Hawks JH: Medical-surgical nursing: clinical management for positive outcomes, ed 8, Philadelphia, 2009, WB Saunders.)*

The procedure involves placement of a catheter in the femoral artery and threading it up the aorta and into the origin of the cerebral circulation. Other injection sites include direct carotid or vertebral artery puncture or placement of a catheter in the brachial, the axillary, or the subclavian artery. Several views of vessels can be studied by means of angiography. A four-vessel angiogram involves injections into the right and left internal carotid arteries and the right and left vertebral arteries. If the area of suspected disease already has been identified, a single-vessel study may be all that is required. This is particularly true when angiography is used as a follow-up in the evaluation of intracranial vascular surgery. If carotid artery disease is a working diagnosis, the angiographic study may include views of the arch of the aorta and of the external and internal carotid arteries.[21]

After the catheter is appropriately placed, the contrast medium is injected. A rapid succession of radiographs is taken as the contrast medium progresses through the cerebral circulation. Separate injections of the contrast medium are administered for each vessel being studied.[2]

Nursing management associated with this invasive procedure is comprehensive. Renal insufficiency, bleeding, and cardiac instability are contraindications to cerebral angiography and must be assessed before the procedure.[2] As with contrast-enhanced CT, the nurse must assess the patient for possible sensitivity to iodine-based contrast before angiography. Instruction and education of the patient are essential to patient preparation. The patient's complete understanding of the role this procedure plays in diagnosis, as well as the process itself, relieves anxiety about the unknown and ensures cooperation in what is commonly an uncomfortable procedure.[1]

Before the procedure, the patient receives no oral intake (NPO status) for at least 4 hours. Sedation is administered immediately before the procedure. Discomforts during the procedure include the need to lie still on a cold, hard table and the possibility of pain during preparation and insertion of the groin catheter. The patient often experiences a hot, burning sensation when the contrast medium is injected, especially if it is injected into the external carotid system. Preparation of patients for this burning sensation assures them that it is not an abnormal occurrence.[1]

The patient must be made aware of the postprocedure assessment. After the procedure, adequate hydration is necessary to assist the kidneys in clearing the heavy dye load. Inadequate hydration may lead to ATN and renal shutdown. If the patient cannot tolerate oral fluids, an intravenous line is placed before the procedure is begun. Postprocedure assessment involves measurement of vital signs, neurologic evaluation, observation of the puncture site, and assessment of neurovascular integrity distal to the puncture site every 15 minutes for the first hour. Any abnormalities must be reported immediately. The patient should be kept on bed rest for 8 to 12 hours.[1] Complications associated with cerebral angiography include (1) cerebral embolus caused by the catheter dislodging a segment of atherosclerotic plaque in the vessel, (2) hemorrhage or hematoma formation at the insertion site, (3) vasospasm of a vessel caused by the irritation of catheter placement, (4) thrombosis of the extremity distal to the injection site, and (5) allergic or adverse reaction to the contrast medium, including renal impairment.[2]

Digital Subtraction Angiography. Digital subtraction angiography is a newer method of visualizing the arteriovenous circulation of the intracranial space. It can be used to identify tumors, AVMs, and vascular abnormalities. Radiographic dye is injected into either the venous or the arterial circulation, but significantly less dye is necessary for this procedure than for arterial angiography. Films taken before and after dye injection are superimposed on each other, and all matching images are subtracted. Only the dye-enhanced cerebral vessels are left for study and evaluation. Digital subtraction angiography eliminates the shadows and distortions of bone or other material that sometimes block the viewing of the cerebral vessels.[22] The major disadvantage of digital subtraction angiography involves the patient's ability to remain motionless during the entire procedure. Even swallowing interferes significantly with the imaging process. Complications and nursing management are similar to those described for cerebral angiography. The risk of embolism is decreased with the intravenous route.[1]

Magnetic Resonance Angiography. Magnetic resonance angiography (MRA) is a technique that offers noninvasive visualization of the cerebrovascular system.[18,23] It uses MRI technology to evaluate CBF and provide details about cerebral vessels. MRA of the carotid arteries has become an established complement to preoperative ultrasound evaluation.[17] It helps determine the area of salvageable tissue (or penumbra) after acute stroke and head injury.[18] MRA is also being used to identify intracranial aneurysms, AVMs, and vasospasm.[19] A contrast-enhanced MRA (CEMRA) may be performed to improve image resolution and reduce artifact. The most commonly used agent is gadolinium, a nonnephrotoxic contrast medium that is injected intravenously.[22]

Computed Tomography Angiography. Computed tomography angiography (CTA) is a technique that uses high-speed helical CT technology with the administration of contrast to visualize the cerebrovascular system. It is used to assess the carotid arteries for stenosis and to evaluate cerebral aneurysms. CTA is becoming a well-accepted substitute for conventional cerebral angiography.[23] The downside to this procedure is that it requires large doses of contrast and radiation.[22]

Myelography. Myelography is radiographic examination of the spinal cord and vertebral column after injection of a contrast material into the subarachnoid space through the lumbar region of the spine between L2 and L3 or L3 and L4 or by cisternal puncture.[4] Myelography allows visualization of the spinal canal, the subarachnoid space around the spinal cord, and the spinal nerve roots (Fig. 27-13). MRI has replaced myelography in most cases, but myelography may be necessary in postoperative patients with multiple clips or metallic hardware. Myelography is superior to MRI in identifying nerve root avulsions and dural tears.[24] Possible risks involved with the use of myelography include injection of the dye outside the subarachnoid space, arachnoiditis as a result of irritation of the arachnoid membranes from a foreign material, and allergic reaction. Other adverse reactions include confusion, hallucinations, headache, grand mal seizure, chest pain, and dysrhythmias.[24] Postprocedure care includes keeping the patient's

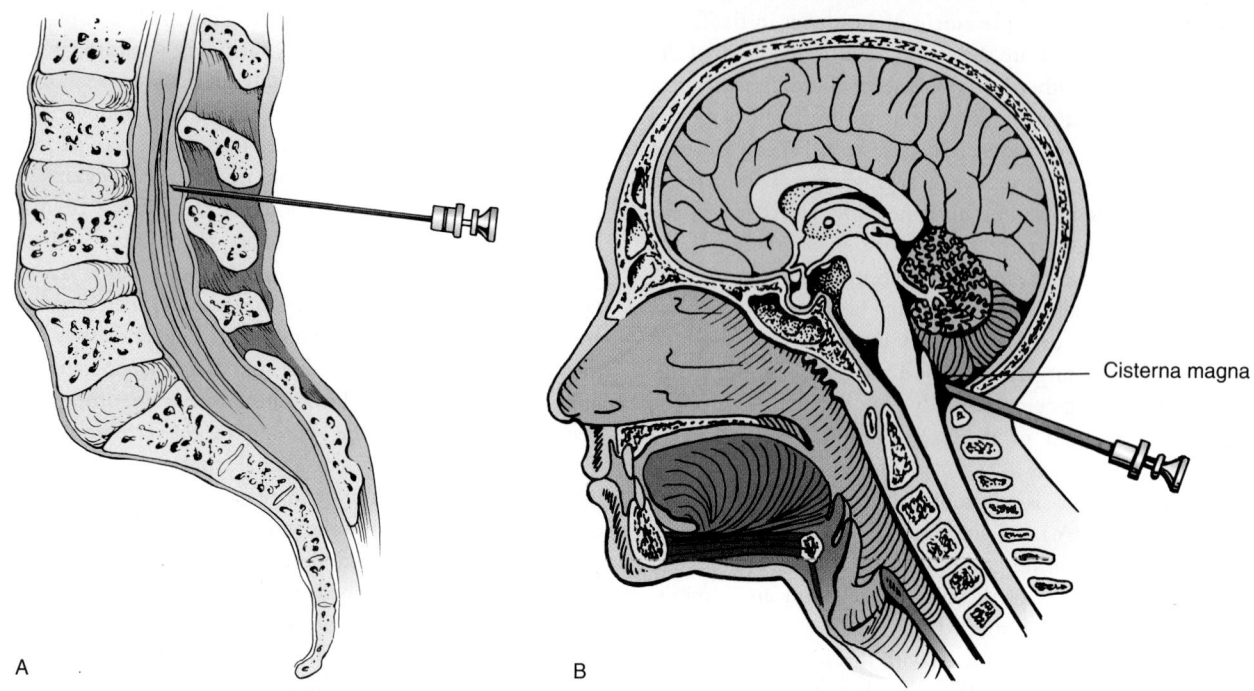

A

B

Cisterna magna

Figure 27-13 *A,* Lumbar puncture. *B,* Cisternal puncture. *(Modified from Phipps WJ et al:* Medical-surgical nursing: health and illness perspectives, *ed 7, St Louis, 2003, Mosby.)*

head elevated 45 degrees for 8 hours, monitoring neurologic status, and encouraging oral fluids.[1]

CEREBRAL BLOOD FLOW STUDIES

The following discussion focuses on the more commonly performed cerebral blood studies that are used in diagnosis of the critically ill patient with neurologic dysfunction.

Perfusion Computed Tomography. Perfusion CT is a relatively new technique that allows rapid evaluation of cerebral perfusion. A perfusion CT scan is made by passing x-rays through the brain, just like a regular CT scan, but in addition to revealing the structure of brain tissue, it measures CBF, cerebral blood volume, and mean transit time. This is done by scanning the patient several times every few seconds before, during, and after the intravenous delivery of an iodine-containing contrast agent that absorbs the x-rays. Perfusion CT has been found to be useful for diagnosis of cerebral ischemia and infarction associated with stroke and for evaluation of cerebral ischemia associated with vasospasm after subarachnoid hemorrhage.[25,26]

Xenon Computed Tomography. Xenon CT is used to study regional CBF. The scan is a computerized x-ray study of the brain that is performed while the patient breathes a carefully regulated flow of xenon, which is a colorless, odorless gas. It has higher resolution in blood flow measurements than other techniques such as positron emission tomography (PET). Xenon CT has been used in the evaluation of a wide variety of disorders and has been most useful in the evaluation of cerebrovascular disease and brain metabolism. Xenon CT studies are occasionally used to determine brain death.[26]

Carotid Duplex Sonography. Ultrasound technology, although not an absolute measure of CBF, uses a noninvasive technique to provide information about the flow velocity of blood through carotid vessels. Carotid duplex studies are used as a routine screening procedure for intraluminal narrowing of the common and internal carotid arteries as a result of atherosclerotic plaques. A Doppler probe is placed externally over the vessel, where high-frequency sound waves (ultrasound) are generated and blood flow velocities calculated. As the diameter of the vessel changes, the velocity of the flow of blood through the vessel changes; the higher the flow velocity, the narrower the vessel. Carotid duplex studies are noninvasive, relatively inexpensive, and painless. When changes in flow velocities are identified that may indicate significant occlusion of the vessel, CTA or MRA can be used to verify the degree of severity of the narrowed vessel. If necessary, cerebral angiography is performed to confirm ambiguous or equivocal findings.[1,15]

Transcranial Doppler Studies. Transcranial Doppler (TCD) studies monitor CBF velocity through cranial windows (thinned areas) of the skull. Three areas commonly used are the temporal bone (transtemporal), the eye (transorbital), and the foramen magnum (transoccipital). Depending on the angle of the Doppler probe, flow velocities can be measured in the anterior, middle, or posterior cerebral arteries and the vertebral and basilar arteries. Numerous clinical applications for TCD have been identified.[27]

TCD studies often are used in critical care for patients after an intracranial aneurysm rupture when there is concern about vasospasm development. The noninvasive technique and portability of the equipment allow frequent bedside monitoring of flow velocity and therefore of vascular diameter. Use of serial transcranial Doppler studies for the detection of cerebral vasospasm greatly reduces the need for cerebral angiograms to verify and follow postsubarachnoid hemorrhage vasospasm.[28]

Additional uses of TCD include identification of intracranial lesions in the stroke patient, evaluation of flow-velocity changes during carotid endarterectomy, and detection of CBF changes associated with increased ICP. TCD has been used to detect cerebral circulatory arrest in brain death determination, but it must be accompanied by clinical evaluation and additional diagnostic tests, because intracranial circulation may be preserved in brain-dead patients.[28]

Limitations of the TCD study must be understood. Its accuracy is operator-dependent. Correct location and angle of the probe are essential. A few patients have temporal bones too thick for ultrasound penetration. A normal TCD study does not completely rule out the presence of vasospasm, because vasospasm may not be evident in the particular vessel examined. TCD results are always evaluated in conjunction with clinical assessment findings.[28]

During the TCD study, the patient experiences only mild pressure at the transducer site. No pain is involved. The patient must remain still during the study, which lasts 15 to 90 minutes.[1]

Transcranial Color-Coded Duplex Sonography. Transcranial color-coded duplex sonography (TCCS) is a noninvasive ultrasound study that enables the visualization of the intracranial structures and basal cerebral arteries and the measurement of blood flow velocities through the arteries. The color component of the study provides more reliable data than the traditional TCD. TCCS is becoming a reliable tool for detecting narrowing or occlusion of cerebral arteries, screening for vasospasm, and monitoring changes in intracranial dynamics. AVMs can also be detected with TCCS.[29]

Emission Tomography. PET and single photon emission computed tomography (SPECT) are nuclear medicine scans used to calculate global and regional CBF. SPECT and PET scanners measure cerebral metabolic use of oxygen and glucose, enabling them to distinguish between brain tumor recurrence and brain or tumor necrosis. The PET scan uses positron-emitting radionuclotides, whereas the SPECT scan uses gamma emitters. PET scanning can quantify blood flow and can be used to evaluate the fraction of oxygen extracted from arterial blood by the cerebral tissue.

Clinical use of PET is extremely limited because of the significant cost, lack of portability, and unavailability of the technology at many hospitals. SPECT is less expensive and more available in clinical practice. SPECT offers a qualitative, rather than an absolute, measure of CBF. Results are described as normal, hypoperfused, or hyperperfused.[3,30] Nursing management of the patient undergoing PET or SPECT involves transportation of the patient to the scanning area and observation during the procedure.

Regional Cerebral Blood Flow Study. Regional CBF studies used to be the gold standard for clinical bedside evaluation of CBF. Xenon 133 is administered by inhalation or injection into a peripheral vein. Scintillation detectors, or probes, placed on the outside of the skull monitor the uptake and clearance, or washout,

of the xenon from the cerebral circulation. Information from the probes is then passed to a computer that calculates global or regional CBF. One difficulty with this method is that all body tissues take up xenon and then clear it, including the skin and muscles of the scalp under detectors. Although mathematical calculations are factored in, CBF results are an estimated value at best.[1]

ELECTROPHYSIOLOGY STUDIES

The following discussion focuses on the more commonly performed electrophysiology studies that are used in the diagnosis of the critically ill patient with a neurologic dysfunction.

Electroencephalography. Electroencephalography (EEG) records electrical impulses, commonly called *brain waves,* generated by the brain. This test has been in existence for many years and is well known to the general public. The nurse caring for a patient with a neurologic dysfunction must be aware of the appropriate indications for use and the limitations of this diagnostic procedure. The purpose of EEG is to detect and localize abnormal electrical activity. This abnormal activity can be defined as *slowing,* which occurs in areas of injury or infarct, or as the *spikes* and *waves* seen in irritated tissue. Indications for the use of EEG include suspected seizure activity, cerebral infarct, metabolic encephalopathies, altered consciousness, infectious disease, some head injuries, and confirmation of brain death.[19,31]

Noninvasive electrodes are placed on the head, and the electrical impulses detected are transferred to a central recording device that records the information in wave form. Six types of waves or rhythms may be present (Table 27-4). Intermittent slowing with triphasic wave morphology is associated with metabolic encephalopathy. Continuous, generalized slowing in the delta or theta range is associated with anoxic damage. The combination of alpha waves that do not change with stimulation and a coma state is called *alpha coma,* and it is associated with a poor prognosis.[19]

TABLE 27-4 Types of Electrical Brain Waves

Wave	Duration	Description
Delta	1-4 cycles/sec	Normal; seen in stages 3 and 4 of sleep
Alpha	8-13 cycles/sec	Normal; relaxed state with eyes closed; often seen in occipital leads
Theta	4-7 cycles/sec	Less common in adults than in children; characteristic of coma in brain injury
Beta	12-40 cycles/sec	Fast waves indicating mental or physical activity
Sleep spindles	12-14 cycles/sec	Seen in stage 2 sleep, not rapid eye movement (REM)
Spike and slow waves	Variable	Seen in irritable brain tissue (e.g., seizure)

Other EEG abnormalities associated with poor prognosis are *burst suppression* (occasional generalized bursts of activity with intervening inactivity or severe voltage depression) and *periodic patterns* (generalized spikes at fixed intervals of one to two per second).[19] Absence of electrical activity on EEG, *electrocerebral silence,* can occur transiently in the period immediately after cardiopulmonary resuscitation, severe hypothermia, and central nervous system depressant overdose.[19] Enduring electrocerebral silence provides evidence for the clinical determination of brain death.

The limitations of EEG are noteworthy. Only electrical activity involving large areas of cortex is recorded on EEG.[19] Accuracy of EEG depends on the location of electrophysiologic activity. Abnormal EEG findings are not cause specific.[19] Similar EEG changes occur with a variety of conditions. The EEG result can be normal even when significant pathology is present.[2,19]

In preparing the patient for an EEG, the nurse must stress the noninvasive aspects of this procedure. The awake patient may be asked to perform certain simple tasks during the procedure, such as blinking, closing the eye, or swallowing. Occasionally, testing must be performed during sleep or after a period of sleep deprivation.[1]

Evoked Potentials. Evoked potentials are cerebral electrical impulses generated in response to a sensory stimulus.[19] Impulses are recorded as they travel through the brainstem and into the cerebral cortex. Measuring evoked potentials is a sophisticated way of observing the status of sensory pathways as they enter the central nervous system, travel through the brainstem, and reach the cerebral cortex. Evoked potential studies are used in the determination of prognosis in coma and the existence and extent of brainstem or spinal cord injury in the traumatically injured patient. Evaluation of evoked potentials is valuable during therapeutically induced comas, such as barbiturate coma, inasmuch as these sensory pathways are unaffected by the depressive activity of such drugs.[19] Evoked potentials are monitored intraoperatively during spinal surgery and cerebral tumor dissection.[32]

The four types of evoked potential tests are (1) visual evoked responses (VERs), (2) brainstem auditory evoked responses (BAERs), (3) somatosensory evoked responses (SSERs), and (4) motor evoked potentials (MEPs). VERs involve monitoring the visual pathways through the brainstem and cortex in response to the patient's viewing a shifting geometric pattern on a screen or a flashing light stimulus emitted from a mask placed over the eye. BAERs involve monitoring the auditory pathway through the brainstem and cortex in response to a rhythmic clicking sound sent through earphones placed over the patient's ears. BAERs are useful in assessing brainstem integrity in the critical care unit when cranial nerve testing cannot be performed or is inconclusive. SSERs involve monitoring of sensory pathways from the extremities ascending the spinal cord through the brainstem and into the cortex. This is performed by administering a small electrical shock to a nerve root in the periphery, such as the ulnar or radial nerve.[19] SSERs can be used to evaluate cortical functioning after cardiac arrest or head trauma.[33] SSERs also are used routinely during spinal surgery.[32] MEPs assess the functional integrity of descending motor pathways. The motor cortex is stimulated by direct high-voltage electrical stimulation through the scalp or use of a magnetic field to induce an electrical current within the brain.[34]

Electrical stimulation is a painful procedure and must be reserved for anesthetized patients. Magnetic stimulation is painless.

NURSING MANAGEMENT

The nursing management of a patient undergoing a diagnostic procedure involves a variety of interventions. Nursing activities are directed toward preparing the patient psychologically and physically for the procedure, monitoring the patient's responses to the procedure, and assessing the patient after the procedure. Preparation includes teaching the patient about the procedure, answering questions, and transporting and positioning the patient for the procedure. During the procedure, the nurse observes the patient for signs of pain, anxiety, or hemorrhage and monitors vital signs. After the procedure, the nurse observes for complications of the procedure and medicates the patient for any postprocedure discomfort. Any evidence of increasing ICP should be immediately reported to the physician, and emergency measures to maintain circulation must be initiated.

LABORATORY STUDIES: LUMBAR PUNCTURE

The major laboratory study performed in the patient with neurologic dysfunction is analysis of CSF obtained by a lumbar puncture or a ventriculostomy.[1-3] The main purpose of a lumbar puncture is to obtain CSF for analysis. CSF opening pressure may also be obtained. CSF samples are evaluated for the presence of subarachnoid blood or infection, or they are sent for laboratory analysis (Table 27-5).

A lumbar puncture involves the introduction of a 20- to 22-gauge hollow needle into the subarachnoid space at L3 to L4 or L4 to L5, below the end of the spinal cord, which usually is at L1 or L2 (Fig. 27-13A). The patient can be placed in the lateral decubitus position with the knees and head tightly tucked or in the sitting position leaning over a bedside table or some other support. Before initiating the procedure, the patient's coagulation profile should be checked for abnormalities.[3]

Two life-threatening risks associated with lumbar puncture include possible brainstem herniation, if the ICP is elevated, and respiratory arrest associated with neurologic deterioration. During the procedure, the nurse must monitor the patient's neurologic and respiratory status. If the patient is not fully alert and cooperative, the nurse may need to assist the patient in maintaining the position necessary for the lumbar puncture.[1] The long-standing routine of keeping the patient flat in bed for several hours after a lumbar puncture to prevent a headache has been refuted by scientific study.[35]

Cisternal puncture, which is the introduction of a needle into the cisterna magna between C1 and C2 (see Fig. 27-13B), is another method for obtaining access to the subarachnoid space. Risks of cisternal puncture are slightly higher than those associated with a lumbar puncture, but cisternal puncture is necessary if the lumbar space cannot be entered because of scar tissue or some other physical barrier or if the CSF pathway is totally blocked somewhere along the spinal column.[3]

TABLE 27-5 Analysis of Cerebrospinal Fluid

Characteristic	Normal Findings	Abnormal Findings	Possible Causes and Comments
Pressure	<200 mm H_2O	<60 mm H_2O	Faulty needle placement Dehydration Spinal block along subarachnoid space Block of foramen magnum Hydrocephalus
		>200 mm H_2O	Muscle tension Abdominal compression Brain tumor Subdural hematoma Brain abscess Brain cyst Cerebral edema (any cause)
Color	Clear, colorless	Cloudy or turbid	Cloudy as a result of microorganisms (e.g., WBCs) Turbid as a result of increased cell count
		Yellow (xanthochromic)	Breakdown of RBCs with RBC pigments, high protein count
		Smoky	RBCs
Blood	None	Red blood cells: blood tinged	Traumatic tap: bloody in first sample
		Grossly bloody	Traumatic tap: bloody in all samples
Volume	150 mL	Increase	Hydrocephalus
Specific gravity	1.007	Increase	Infection, presence of cells or protein
WBCs	0-5 cells/mm^3	<500 cells/mm^3	Bacterial or viral infections of meninges, neurosyphilis, subarachnoid hemorrhage, infarction, abscess, tuberculous meningitis, metastatic lesions
		>500 cells/mm^3	Purulent infection
Glucose	50-75 mg/dL or 60%-70% of blood glucose	<40 mg/dL	Bacterial meningitis, tuberculosis, parasitic, fungal carcinomatous, subarachnoid hemorrhage
		>80 mg/dL	May not be of neurologic significance
Chloride	700-750 mg/dL	Decreased (<625 mg/dL)	Meningeal infection, tuberculosis meningitis, hypochloremia
		Increased (>800 mg/dL)	May not be of neurologic significance; correlated with blood levels of chloride and not routine; done only on request
Culture and sensitivity	No organisms present	*Neisseria* or *Streptococcus*	Identify organisms to begin therapy; Gram stain for some cultures may take several weeks.
Serology for syphilis	Negative	Positive	Syphilis
Protein*	15-50 mg/dL	Increased (>60 mg/dL)	Bacterial meningitis, brain tumors (benign and malignant), complete spinal block, ALS, Guillain-Barré syndrome, subarachnoid hemorrhage, infarction, CNS trauma, CNS degenerative diseases, herniated disk, DM with polyneuropathy
		Decreased (<10 mg/dL)	May not be of neurologic significance
Osmolality	295 Osm/L	Increased	Protein, WBCs, microorganisms, RBCs
Lactate	10-20 mg/dL	Increased	Bacterial, seizure activity, fungal meningitis, CNS trauma, coma related to toxic or metabolic causes

From Barker E: *Neuroscience nursing; a spectrum of care,* ed 3, St Louis, 2008, Mosby.

*Blood in the CSF will raise the protein level.

ALS, amyotrophic lateral sclerosis; CNS, central nervous system; CSF, cerebrospinal fluid; DM, diabetes mellitus; RBC, red blood cell; WBC, white blood cell.

BEDSIDE MONITORING

INTRACRANIAL PRESSURE MONITORING

In the patient with suspected intracranial hypertension, a monitoring device may be placed within the cranium to quantify ICP. Under normal physiologic conditions, mean ICP is maintained below 15 mm Hg. It is used to monitor serial ICPs and assist with the management of intracranial hypertension. An increase in ICP can decrease blood flow to the brain, causing brain damage. It can also provide sterile access for draining excess CSF.

Monitoring Sites. The four sites for monitoring ICP are the intraventricular space, the subarachnoid space, the epidural space, and the parenchyma (Fig. 27-14). Each site has advantages and disadvantages for monitoring ICP (Table 27-6). The type of monitor chosen depends on the suspected pathologic condition and physician's preferences.[36,37] Nursing considerations for each type of device are discussed in Table 27-6.

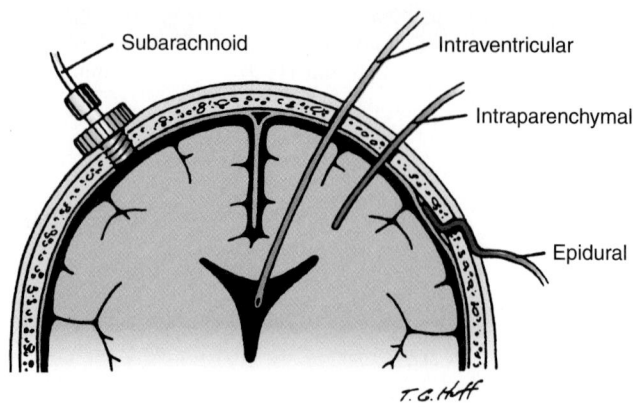

Figure 27-14 Intracranial pressure monitoring sites. *(From Lee KR, Hoff JT: Youman's neurological surgery, ed 4, Philadelphia, 1996, Saunders.)*

TABLE 27-6 Advantages, Disadvantages, and Nursing Considerations of ICP Monitoring Techniques

Monitoring Device	Advantages	Disadvantages	Nursing Considerations
Intraventricular catheter (ventriculostomy)	Allows accurate ICP measurement Provides access to CSF for drainage or sampling Provides access for instillation of contrast media Allows reliable evaluation of intracranial compliances (volume-pressure relationships)	Provides an additional site for infection Is most invasive ICP monitoring technique Requires frequent transducer balancing or recalibration Catheter may be occluded by blood clot or tissue debris Insertion difficult if ventricles are small, compressed, or displaced Is associated with risk for CSF leakage around insertion site Is associated with increased risk for infection	Provide appropriate sedatives or analgesics during catheter insertion. Do baseline and serial neurologic assessments. Measure patient's temperature at least every 4 hours. Notice character, amount, and turbidity of CSF drainage. Document ICP and CPP measurements, response to stimulation, and nursing care activities per hospital or unit protocol. Monitor quality of ICP waveform. Monitor system and tubing for air bubbles, and flush or purge system as appropriate. Drain CSF as indicated for treatment of ICP elevation. Notify physician if CSF drainage is not within prescribed parameters. Monitor insertion site for bleeding, drainage, swelling, and CSF leakage. Zero or calibrate device per hospital or unit protocol. Level transducer at the foramen of Monro; external landmarks include the tragus of the patient's ear and the external auditory canal, among others; all ICP measurements should be made with the transducer at a consistent level relative to external landmarks. Administer sedatives or analgesics as appropriate to decrease risk of catheter being dislodged by patient's movements. Educate patient's family as indicated. Notify physician if ICP or CPP is not within specified parameters.
Subarachnoid bolt or Screw	Is associated with lower infection rates than is ventriculostomy Is quickly and easily placed	Has potential for dampened waveform (cerebral edema, blood or tissue debris)	Administer appropriate sedatives or analgesics during insertion. Do baseline and serial neurologic assessments. Measure patient's temperature at least every 4 hours.

TABLE 27-6 Advantages, Disadvantages, and Nursing Considerations of ICP Monitoring Techniques—*cont'd*

Monitoring Device	Advantages	Disadvantages	Nursing Considerations
	Can be used with small or collapsed ventricles Requires no penetration of brain tissue	Is less accurate at high ICP elevations Requires frequent balancing or recalibration (e.g., with position changes) Provides no access for CSF sampling	Monitor insertion site for bleeding, drainage, swelling, and CSF leakage. Monitor quality of ICP waveform. Document ICP and CPP measurements and response to stimulation per hospital or unit protocol. Administer sedatives or analgesics as appropriate to decrease risk of catheter being dislodged by patient's movements. Zero or calibrate device per hospital or unit protocol. Level transducer at the foramen of Monro; external landmarks include the tragus of the patient's ear and the external auditory canal, among others; all ICP measurements should be made with the transducer at a consistent level relative to external landmarks. Educate patient's family as indicated. Notify physician if ICP or CPP is not within specified parameters.
Subdural or epidural catheter or sensor	Is least invasive Is associated with decreased risk of infection Is easily and quickly placed	Increase in baseline drift over time means possible loss of reliability or accuracy Provides no access for CSF drainage or sampling	Administer appropriate sedatives or analgesics during insertion. Do baseline and serial neurologic assessments. Measure patient's temperature at least every 4 hours. Monitor insertion site for bleeding, drainage, and swelling. Monitor quality of ICP waveform and drift over time. Document ICP and CPP measurements and response to stimulation per hospital or unit protocol. Administer sedatives or analgesics as appropriate to decrease risk of catheter being dislodged or damaged by patient's movements. Educate patient's family as indicated. Notify physician if ICP or CPP is not within specified parameters.
Fiberoptic transducer-tipped catheter	Can be placed in subdural or subarachnoid space, in a ventricle, or directly within brain tissue Is easily transported Requires zeroing only once (during insertion) Has baseline drift of up to 1 mm Hg per day Is associated with decreased risk for infection when brain tissue is not penetrated Provides good-quality ICP waveforms (less artifact than with other devices) Requires no adjustment in level of transducer with patient's change of position	Provides no access for CSF sampling or drainage Cannot be recalibrated after placement Requires periodic replacement of probe Is easily damaged	Administer appropriate sedatives or analgesics during insertion. Do baseline and serial neurologic assessments. Measure patient's temperature at lest every 4 hours. Monitor insertion site for bleeding, drainage, swelling, and CSF leakage. Monitor quality of ICP waveform and drift over time. Document ICP and CPP measurements and response to stimulation per hospital or unit protocol. Administer sedatives or analgesics as appropriate to decrease risk of catheter being dislodged or damaged by patient's movements. Educate patient's family as indicated. Notify physician if ICP or CPP is not within specified parameters.

From Arbour R: Intracranial hypertension: monitoring and nursing assessment, *Crit Care Nurse* 24(5):19, 2004.
CPP, cerebral perfusion pressure; CSF, cerebrospinal fluid; ICP, intracranial pressure.

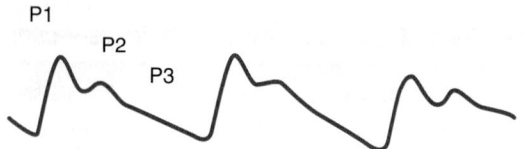

Figure 27-15 Normal intracranial pressure waveform. *(From Bader MK, Littlejohns LR: AANN core curriculum for neuroscience nursing, ed 4, St Louis, 2004, Elsevier.)*

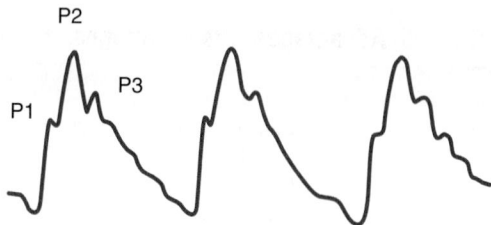

Figure 27-16 Abnormal intracranial pressure waveform. *(From Bader MK, Littlejohns LR: AANN core curriculum for neuroscience nursing, ed 4, St Louis, 2004, Elsevier.)*

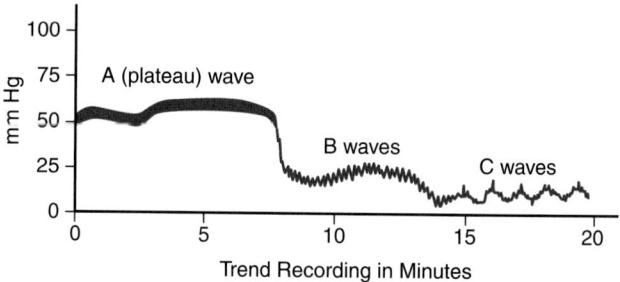

Figure 27-17 Intracranial pressure waves. Composite diagram of A (plateau) waves, B (sawtooth) waves, and C (small rhythmic) waves. *(From Barker E: Neuroscience nursing: a spectrum of care, ed 3, St Louis, 2008, Mosby.)*

Intraventricular Space. ICP monitoring is accomplished by placing a small catheter into the ventricular system; this procedure is known as a *ventriculostomy*. The catheter is inserted through a burr hole with the patient under local anesthesia, and it usually is placed in the anterior horn of the lateral ventricle. If possible, the side chosen for placement of the ventriculostomy is the nondominant hemisphere.[36,37]

Subarachnoid Space. ICP monitoring is accomplished by placing a small hollow bolt or screw into the subarachnoid space. It is inserted though a burr hole, usually located in the front of the skull behind the hairline, with the patient under local anesthesia. Inserting this device is easier than inserting the ventriculostomy catheter.[36,37]

Epidural Space. ICP monitoring is accomplished by placing a small fiberoptic sensor into the epidural space. It is inserted through a burr hole while the patient is under local anesthesia. The physician strips the dura away from the inner table of the skull before inserting the epidural monitor.[36,37]

Intraparenchymal Site. ICP monitoring is accomplished by placing a small fiberoptic catheter into the parenchymal tissue. After placing a subarachnoid bolt (as previously described), a hole is punched in the dura, and the catheter is inserted approximately 1 cm into the brain's white matter.[36,37]

Intracranial Pressure Waves. The ICP pulse waveform is observed on a continuous, real-time pressure display, and it corresponds to each heartbeat. The waveform arises primarily from pulsations of the major intracranial arteries but also receives retrograde venous pulsations.[36,37]

Normal Intracranial Pressure Waveform. The normal ICP wave has three or more defined peaks (Fig. 27-15). The first peak (P1) is called the *percussion wave*. Originating from the pulsations of the choroid plexus, it has a sharp peak and is fairly consistent in its amplitude. The second peak (P2) is called the *tidal wave*. The tidal wave varies more in shape and amplitude, ending on the dicrotic notch. The P2 portion of the pulse waveform has been most directly linked to the state of decreased compliance. When the P2 component is equal to or higher than P1, decreased compliance occurs (Fig. 27-16). Immediately after the dicrotic notch is the third wave (P3), which is called the *dicrotic wave*. After the dicrotic wave, the pressure usually tapers down to the diastolic position, unless retrograde venous pulsations add a few more peaks.[36-39]

A, B, and C pressure waves are not true waveforms (Fig. 27-17). Rather, they are the graphically displayed trend data of ICP over time. These waves reflect spontaneous alterations in ICP associated with respiration, systemic blood pressure, and deteriorating neurologic status.

A Waves. Also called *plateau waves* because of their distinctive shape, A waves are the most clinically significant of the three types. They usually occur in an already elevated baseline ICP (>20 mm Hg) and are characterized by sharp increases in ICP of 30 to 69 mm Hg, which plateau for 2 to 20 minutes and then return to baseline. The cause of A waves is unknown, but they may result from vasodilation and increased CBF, decreased venous outflow (and therefore increased cerebral blood volume), fluctuations in $PaCO_2$ (and therefore changes in cerebral blood volume), or decreased CSF absorption. B waves often precede A waves. Plateau waves are considered significant because of the reduced cerebral perfusion pressure associated with ICP, in the range of 50 to 100 mm Hg. Transient signs of intracranial hypertension, such as a decreased level of consciousness, bradycardia, pupillary changes, or respiratory changes, may accompany these waves. Some research suggests that prolonged increases in ICP associated with plateau waves may result in transient and permanent cell damage from ischemia.[2,36]

B Waves. B waves are sharp, rhythmic oscillations with a sawtooth appearance that occur every 30 seconds to 2 minutes and that can raise the ICP from 5 to 70 mm Hg. They are a normal physiologic phenomenon that can occur in any patient, but they are amplified in states of low intracranial compliance. B waves appear to reflect fluctuations in cerebral blood volume.

Decompensation of normal intracranial volume compensatory capacity is indicated by B waves with a high amplitude (>15 mm Hg pressure change from peak to trough of the wave).[2,37]

C Waves. C waves are small, rhythmic waves that occur every 4 to 8 minutes at normal levels of ICP. They are related to normal fluctuations in respiration and systemic arterial pressure. C waves are considered clinically insignificant.[2,37]

Cerebral Perfusion Pressure. Measuring CBF in the clinical setting is difficult, but at the bedside, an estimated pressure of cerebral perfusion can be derived. Cerebral perfusion pressure (CPP) is the blood pressure gradient across the brain, and it is calculated as the difference between the incoming mean arterial pressure (MAP) and the opposing ICP on the arteries:

$$CPP = MAP - ICP$$

The CPP in the average adult is approximately 80 to 100 mm Hg, with a range of 60 to 150 mm Hg. The CPP must be maintained near 80 mm Hg to provide adequate blood supply to the brain. If the CPP drops below this point, ischemia may develop. A sustained CPP of 30 mm Hg or less usually results in neuronal hypoxia and cell death. When the mean systemic arterial pressure equals the ICP, CBF may cease.[1-3]

CEREBRAL OXYGENATION MONITORING

Cerebral Metabolism. The measurements of CBF and CPP do not address the brain's metabolic need for oxygen. Active neurons require greater amounts of oxygen than those that are inactive. The determination that CBF matches the brain's metabolic needs is expressed as *cerebral metabolic rate* ($CMRo_2$), the normal value of which is 3.4 mL per 100 g of brain tissue per minute. Neuronal demand for oxygen is governed by the metabolic rate. For technical reasons, this value is not easily attained, although it can be calculated. It is the product of the measured CBF and calculated arteriojugular oxygen difference ($ajDo_2$)[40]:

$$CMRO_2 = CBF \times ajDO_2$$

CBF can be measured using a variety of complex techniques (e.g., PET, SPECT). Most recently, continuous bedside monitoring of regional cerebrocortical blood flow has become available.[8] Arteriojugular oxygen difference is the amount of oxygen extracted by the brain, and it is reflected in the difference between the arterial oxygen content and the jugular venous oxygen content. The normal value is 5.0 to 7.5 vol%.[40]

Jugular Venous Oxygen Saturation. One method of measuring CBF allows continuous measurement of oxygenation within the jugular venous system through the use of the jugular bulb monitor. Jugular venous oxygen saturation ($Sjvo_2$) can be used to reflect cerebral oxygen supply-and-demand balance. Any disorder that increases $CMRo_2$ or decreases oxygen delivery may decrease $Sjvo_2$, and conversely, any disorder that that decreases $CMRo_2$ or increases oxygen delivery may increase $Sjvo_2$.[40,41]

To measure $Sjvo_2$ a fiberoptic catheter is placed retrograde through the internal jugular vein into the jugular bulb and attached to a bedside monitor. The normal value is 60% to 80%. Patients with values less than 50% and 55% are hypoxemic or oligemic (low CBF compared with metabolic rate). Oligemia occurs as a result of decreased blood flow due to hypotension, vasospasm, or intracranial hypertension or as a result of increased brain metabolic requirements due to fever or seizures.[40,41] $Sjvo_2$ values below 45% are indicative of severe cerebral hypoxia.[40] Patients with values above 75% to 80% are considered hyperemic (high CBF compared with metabolic need). $Sjvo_2$ also increases if the brain is so severely injured the neurons are unable to extract oxygen.[40,41]

$Sjvo_2$ monitoring has several limitations. $Sjvo_2$ is a global measure of cerebral oxygenation, and a normal $Sjvo_2$ value does not rule out localized areas of cerebral ischemia.[40,41] Readings are affected by the movement of the patient's head.[41] Up to 50% of low $Sjvo_2$ readings are false, which may be caused by technical issues with the catheter, particularly catheter migration.[42] For accurate reading, the tip of the catheter must be within 1 cm of the jugular bulb.[41]

Brain Tissue Oxygen Pressure. Over the past few years, a new device has become available to measure the partial pressure of oxygen within brain tissue ($Pbto_2$). The device consists of a monitoring probe on the end of a catheter, which is inserted into the brain parenchyma and attached to a bedside monitor. The probe may be inserted into the damaged portion of the brain to measure regional oxygenation or inserted into the undamaged portion of the brain to measure global oxygenation. One risk associated with insertion of the catheter is bleeding with hematoma formation.[43] Although there is no consensus on normal values because they vary from device to device, it has been concluded that the probability of death increases with prolonged periods of $Pbto_2$ less than 15 mm Hg and any episode of $Pbto_2$ less than 6 mm Hg.[43]

In the head-injured patient, the goal of treatment is to maintain the $Pbto_2$ greater than 20 mm Hg. Factors that decrease $Pbto_2$ include tissue hypoxia, hypocapnia, hypovolemia, decreased blood pressure, low hemoglobin levels, intracranial hypertension, and hyperthermia.[44] Treatment is directed at the underlying cause.

Summary

Clinical Assessment

- A neurologic history includes information about clinical manifestations, associated complaints, precipitating factors, progression of symptoms, familial occurrences, and events preceding the onset of symptoms.
- The five major components of a neurologic examination are evaluation of (1) level of consciousness, (2) motor function, (3) pupillary function, (4) respiratory function, and (5) vital signs.
- Assessment of the level of consciousness focuses on evaluation of arousal and appraisal of awareness.
- Assessment of motor function focuses on the evaluation of muscle size and tone and estimation of muscle strength.

- Assessment of papillary function focuses on estimation of pupil size and shape, evaluation of papillary reaction to light, and appraisal of eye movements.
- Assessment of respiratory functions focuses on observation of respiratory pattern and evaluation of airway status.
- Assessment of vital signs focuses on evaluation of blood pressure and observation of heart rate.
- Increasing ICP can be identified by changes in the level of consciousness, pupillary reaction, motor response, vital signs, and respiratory patterns.

Diagnostic Procedures

- Radiologic procedures are often performed to identify abnormalities of the brain, spinal cord, and the surrounding bone and tissue. These tests include skull and spine radiography, CT, MRI, cerebral angiography, and myelography.
- CBF studies are often performed to evaluate the adequacy of flow of cerebral blood and to identify any abnormalities of the vascular system. These tests include perfusion CT, xenon CT, carotid Duplex sonography, transcranial Doppler studies, PET, and SPECT.

- Electrophysiology studies are often performed to evaluate the electrical impulses of the brain. These tests include electroencephalography, VERs, BAERs, SSERs, and MEPs.

Laboratory Studies

- Cerebrospinal fluid analysis is performed (by lumbar puncture or ventriculostomy) to look for the presence of blood or infection in the subarachnoid space.

Bedside Monitoring

- ICP monitoring is used in the patient with suspected intracranial hypertension. The four sites for monitoring ICP are the intraventricular space, the subarachnoid space, the epidural space, and the parenchyma.
- Jugular venous oxygen saturation is monitored (by jugular blub venous catheter) to assess the adequacy of cerebral metabolism.
- Brain tissue oxygen saturation is monitored, and the method can be used to directly measure the partial pressure of oxygen within brain tissue.

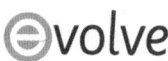 Be sure to check out the bonus material, including free self-assessment exercises, on the Evolve web site at http://evolve.elsevier.com/Urden/.

References

1. Barker E: *Neuroscience nursing: a spectrum of care*, ed 3, St Louis, 2008, Mosby.
2. Bader MK, Littlejohns LR: *AANN core curriculum for neuroscience nursing*, ed 4, St Louis, 2004, Elsevier.
3. Goetz CG: *Textbook of clinical neurology*, ed 3, St Louis, 2007, Saunders.
4. Haymore J: A neuron in a haystack: advanced neurologic assessment, *AACN Clin Issues* 15:568, 2002.
5. Teasdale G, Jennett W: Assessment of coma and impaired consciousness—a practical scale, *Lancet* 2:81, 1974.
6. Holdgate A et al: Variability in agreement between physicians and nurses when measuring the Glasgow Coma Scale in the emergency department limits its clinical usefulness, *Emerg Med Australas* 18:379, 2006.
7. Fischer J, Mathieson C: The history of the Glasgow Coma Scale: implications for practice, *Crit Care Nurs Q* 23(4):52, 2001.
8. Barnwell P: Assessing motor and sensory function—a focused survey, *Aust Emerg Nurs J* 2(3):16, 1999.
9. O'Hanlon-Nichols T: Neurologic assessment, *Am J Nurs* 99(6):44, 1999.
10. Seidel HM et al: *Mosby's guide to physical examination*, ed 6, St Louis, 2006, Mosby.
11. Adoni A, McNett M: The pupillary response in traumatic brain injury: a guide for trauma nurses, *J Trauma Nurs* 14:191, 2007.
12. Bishop BS: Pathologic papillary signs: self-learning module. Part II, *Crit Care Nurs* 11(7):58, 1991.
13. Chesnut RM: Management of brain and spine injuries, *Crit Care Clin* 20:25, 2005.
14. Keller C, Williams A: Cardiac dysrhythmias associated with central nervous system dysfunction, *J Neurosci Nurs* 25: 349, 1993.
15. MA Samuels: The brain-heart connection, *Circulation* 116:77, 2007.
16. Grainger RG et al: *Grainger & Allison's diagnostic radiology: a textbook of medical imaging*, ed 4, London, 2001, Churchill Livingstone.
17. Shpritz DW: Neurodiagnostic studies, *Nurs Clin North Am* 34:593, 1999.
18. Lindsay KW, Bone I: *Neurology and neurosurgery illustrated*, ed 4, New York, 2004, Churchill Livingstone.
19. Bradley WG et al: *Neurology in clinical practice*, ed 7, St Louis, 2007, Elsevier.
20. Selden NR et al: Emergency magnetic resonance imaging of cervical spinal cord injuries: clinical correlation and prognosis, *Neurosurgery* 44:785, 1999.
21. Fink JN, Caplan LR: Cerebrovascular cases, *Med Clin North Am* 87:755, 2003.
22. Rowe VL, Tucker SW: Advances in vascular imaging, *Surg Clin North Am* 84:1189, 2004.
23. Phillips CD, Bubash LA: CT angiography and MR angiography in the evaluation of extracranial carotid vascular disease, *Radiol Clin North Am* 40:783, 2002.
24. Humphreys SC et al: Neuroimaging in low back pain, *Am Fam Physician* 65:2299, 2002.
25. Hoeffner EG et al: Cerebral perfusion CT: technique and clinical applications, *Radiology* 231:632, 2004.
26. Perez-Arjona EA et al: New techniques in cerebral imaging, *Neurol Res* 24 (suppl 1):S17, 2002.
27. Miller RD: *Miller's anesthesia*, ed 6, St Louis, 2005, Elsevier.
28. Sloan MA et al: Assessment: transcranial Doppler ultrasonography: report of the Therapeutics and Technology Assessment Subcommittee of the American Academy of Neurology, *Neurology* 62:1468, 2004.
29. Krejza J: Clinical applications of transcranial color-coded duplex sonography, *J Neuroimaging* 14:215, 2004.
30. Alavi A et al: PET: a revolution in medical imaging, *Radiol Clin North Am* 42:983, 2004.
31. Cascino GD: Use of routine and video electroencephalography *Neurol Clin* 19:271, 2001.
32. Soriano SG et al: Neuroanesthesia. Innovative techniques and monitoring, *Anesthesiol Clin North Am* 20:137, 2002.
33. Robinson LR et al: Predictive value of somatosensory evoked potentials for awakening from coma, *Crit Care Med* 31:960, 2003.

34. Papworth D: Intraoperative monitoring during vascular surgery, *Anesthesiol Clin North Am* 22:223, 2004.

35. Thoennissen J et al: Does bed rest after cervical or lumbar puncture prevent headache? A systematic review and meta-analysis, *CMAJ* 165:1311, 2001.

36. American Association of Neuroscience Nurses: *Guide to the care of the patient with intracranial pressure monitoring: AANN reference series for clinical practice*, Chicago, 2005, The Association.

37. Arbour R: Intracranial hypertension: monitoring and nursing assessment, *Crit Care Nurse* 24(5):19, 2004.

38. Rangel-Castillo L, Robertson CS: Management of intracranial hypertension, *Crit Care Clin* 22:713, 2006.

39. Bhatia A, Gupta AK: Neuromonitoring in the intensive care unit. I. Intracranial pressure and cerebral blood flow monitoring, *Intensive Care Med* 33:1263, 2007.

40. Smith M: Perioperative uses of transcranial perfusion monitoring *Clin* 25(3):557, 2007.

41. Stevens WJ: Multimodal monitoring: head injury managen $SjvO_2$ and LICOX, *J Neurosci Nurs* 36:332, 2004.

42. Coplin WM et al: Accuracy of continuous jugular bulb oximetry in the intensive care unit, *Neurosurgery* 42:533, 1998.

43. Bader MK: Recognizing and treating ischemic insults to the brain: the role of brain tissue oxygen monitoring, *Crit Care Nurs Clin North Am* 18:243, 2006.

44. Wartenberg KE et al: Multimodality monitoring in neurocritical care, *Crit Care Clin* 23:507, 2007.

Neurologic Disorders and Therapeutic Management

$\mathcal{T}$o accurately anticipate and plan nursing interventions, the critical care nurse must have an understanding of the disease pathology, determine the areas of focused assessment, and be well acquainted with the medical management of the neurologic patient. Fortunately, despite a wide array of neurologic disorders, only a few routinely require the critical care environment.

COMA

DESCRIPTION

Normal consciousness requires awareness and arousal. Awareness is the combination of cognition (mental and intellectual) and affect (mood) that can be construed based on the patient's interaction with the environment. Alterations of consciousness may be the result of deficits in awareness, arousal, or both.[1] Box 28-1 lists the descending states of consciousness.

Coma is the deepest state of unconsciousness; arousal and awareness are lacking.[1,2] The patient cannot be aroused and does not demonstrate any purposeful response to the surrounding environment. Coma is a symptom rather than a disease, and it occurs as a result of some underlying process.[1] The incidence of coma is difficult to ascertain because a wide variety of conditions can induce coma.[2] This state of unconsciousness is unfortunately very common in critical care, and it is the focus of the following discussion.

ETIOLOGY

The causes of coma can be divided into two general categories: structural or surgical and metabolic or medical. Structural causes of coma include ischemic stroke, intracerebral hemorrhage (ICH), trauma, and brain tumors.[3] Metabolic causes of coma include drug overdose, infectious diseases, endocrine disorders, and poisonings.[3] Coma demands immediate attention, resulting in a high percentage of admissions to all hospital services.[4] Table 28-1 provides a list of the possible causes of coma.

PATHOPHYSIOLOGY

Consciousness involves arousal, or wakefulness, and awareness. Neither of these functions is present in the patient in coma. Ascending fibers of the reticular activating system (ARAS) in the pons, hypothalamus, and thalamus maintain arousal as an autonomic function. Neurons in the cerebral cortex are responsible for awareness. Diffuse dysfunction of both cerebral hemispheres and diffuse or focal dysfunction of the reticular activating system can produce coma.[4-6] Structural causes usually produce compression or dysfunction in the area of the ARAS, whereas most medical causes lead to general dysfunction of both cerebral hemispheres.[7] Trauma, hemorrhage, and tumor can damage ARAS, leading to coma. Destruction of large regions of bilateral cerebral hemispheres can be the result of seizures or viral agents. Toxic drugs, toxins, or metabolic abnormalities can suppress cerebral function.[3,4]

ASSESSMENT AND DIAGNOSIS

The clinical diagnosis of the coma state is readily established by assessment of the level of consciousness. However, determining the full nature and cause of coma requires a thorough history and physical examination. A medical history is essential, because events immediately preceding the change in level of consciousness can often provide valuable clues to the origin of the coma. When limited information is available and the coma is profound, the response of the patient to emergent treatment may provide clues to the underlying diagnosis; for example, the patient who becomes responsive with the administration of naloxone can be presumed to have ingested some type of opiate.[4]

Detailed serial neurologic examinations are essential for all patients in coma. Assessment of pupillary size and reaction to light (normal, sluggish, or fixed), extraocular eye movements (normal, asymmetric, or absent), motor response to pain (normal, decorticate, decerebrate, or flaccid), and breathing pattern yields important clues for determining whether the cause of the coma is structural or metabolic.[3,5]

The areas of the brainstem that control consciousness and pupillary responses are anatomically adjacent. The sympathetic and parasympathetic nervous systems control pupillary dilation and constriction, respectively. The anatomic directions of these pathways are known, and changes in pupillary responses can help identify where a lesion may be located (Fig. 28-1). For example, if damage occurs in the midbrain region, pupils will be slightly enlarged and unresponsive to light. Lesions that compress the third nerve result in a fixed and dilated pupil on the same side as the neurologic insult. Pupillary responses are

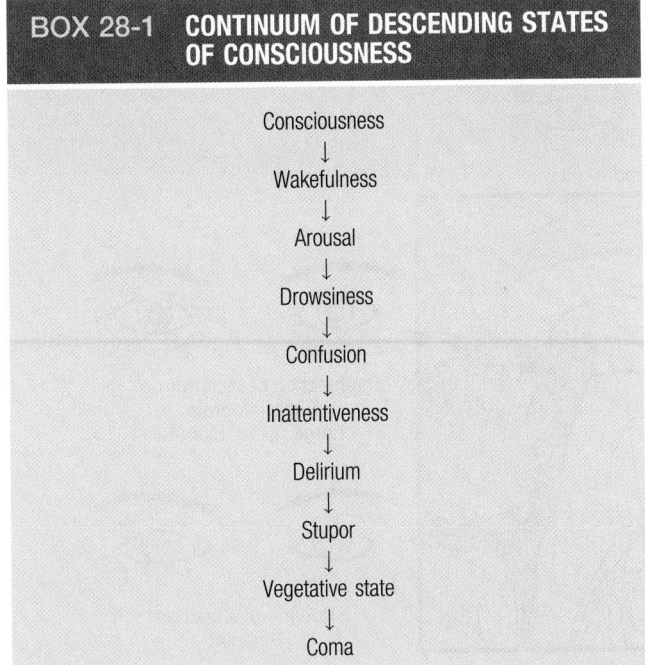

BOX 28-1   CONTINUUM OF DESCENDING STATES OF CONSCIOUSNESS

Consciousness
↓
Wakefulness
↓
Arousal
↓
Drowsiness
↓
Confusion
↓
Inattentiveness
↓
Delirium
↓
Stupor
↓
Vegetative state
↓
Coma

TABLE 28-1   Causes of Coma

Structural or Surgical Coma	Metabolic or Medical Coma
Trauma	Infection
Epidural hematoma	Meningitis
Subdural hematoma	Encephalitis
Diffuse axonal injury	Metabolic encephalopathy
Brain contusion	Metabolic conditions
Intracerebral hemorrhage	Hypoglycemia
Subarachnoid hemorrhage	Hyperglycemia
Posterior fossa hemorrhage	Hyperosmolar states
Supratentorial hemorrhage	Uremia
Hydrocephalus	Hepatic encephalopathy
Ischemic stroke	Hypertensive encephalopathy
Tumor	Hypoxic encephalopathy
Other causes	Hyponatremia
	Hypercalcemia
	Myxedema
	Intoxication
	Opioid overdose
	Alcohol
	Poisonings
	Psychogenic causes

usually preserved when the cause of the coma is metabolic in origin. Pupillary light responses are often the key to differentiating between structural and metabolic causes of coma.[3-5,8]

Areas of the brainstem adjacent to those responsible for consciousness also control the oculomotor eye movement. The ability to maintain conjugate gaze requires preservation of the internuclear connections of cranial nerves III, VI, and VIII by means of the medial longitudinal fasciculus (MLF).[8] As with pupillary responses, structural lesions that impinge on these pathways cause oculomotor dysfunction such as a disconjugate gaze. Deficits in extraocular eye movements usually accompany a structural cause.[3,5,8]

Focal or asymmetric motor deficits usually indicate structural lesions.[3,5] Abnormal motor movements may also help pinpoint the location of a lesion. Decorticate posturing (abnormal flexion) can be seen with damage to the diencephalon. Decerebrate posturing (abnormal extension) can be seen with damage to the midbrain and pons. Flaccid posturing is an ominous sign and can be seen with damage to the medulla.[8]

Abnormal breathing patterns may also assist in differentiating structural from metabolic causes of coma. Cheyne-Stokes respirations are seen in patients with cerebral hemispheric dysfunction or metabolic suppression. Central neurogenic hyperventilation, or Kussmaul breathing, occurs with metabolic acidosis or damage to the midbrain and upper pons. Apneustic breathing may occur with damage to the pons, hypoglycemia, and anoxia. Ataxic breathing occurs with damage to the medulla. Agonal breathing occurs with failure of the respiratory centers in the medulla.[4,8]

In addition to physical assessment, laboratory studies and diagnostic procedures are done. Structural causes of coma are usually readily apparent with computed tomography (CT) or magnetic resonance imaging (MRI). Laboratory studies are also used to identify metabolic or endocrine abnormalities.[6] Occasionally, the cause of coma is never clearly determined.

MEDICAL MANAGEMENT

The goal of medical management of the patient in a coma is identification and treatment of the underlying cause of the condition. Initial medical management includes emergency measures to support vital functions and prevent further neurologic deterioration. Protection of the airway and ventilatory assistance are often needed. Administration of thiamine (at least 100 mg), glucose, and a opioid antagonist is suggested when the cause of coma is not immediately known.[4,5] Thiamine is administered before glucose, because the coma produced by thiamine deficiency, Wernicke's encephalopathy, can be precipitated by a glucose load.[5]

The patient who remains in coma after emergent treatment requires supportive measures to maintain physiologic body functions and prevent complications. Intubation for continued airway protection and nutritional support are essential. Fluid and electrolyte management is often complex because of alterations in the neurohormonal system. Anticonvulsant therapy may be necessary to prevent further ischemic damage to the brain.[3-5]

The health care team and the patient's family make decisions jointly regarding the level of medical management to be provided. Family members require informational support in terms of probable cause of the coma and prognosis for recovery of consciousness and function. Prognosis depends on the cause of the coma and the length of time unconsciousness persists. Sixty percent of patients in nontraumatic coma persisting for 6 or more hours die; 12% remain in a vegetative state.[9] The recovery rate for patients who are in coma for more than 1 week is only 3%.[9] Metabolic coma usually has a better prognosis than coma caused by a structural lesion, and traumatic coma usually has a better outcome than nontraumatic coma.[3]

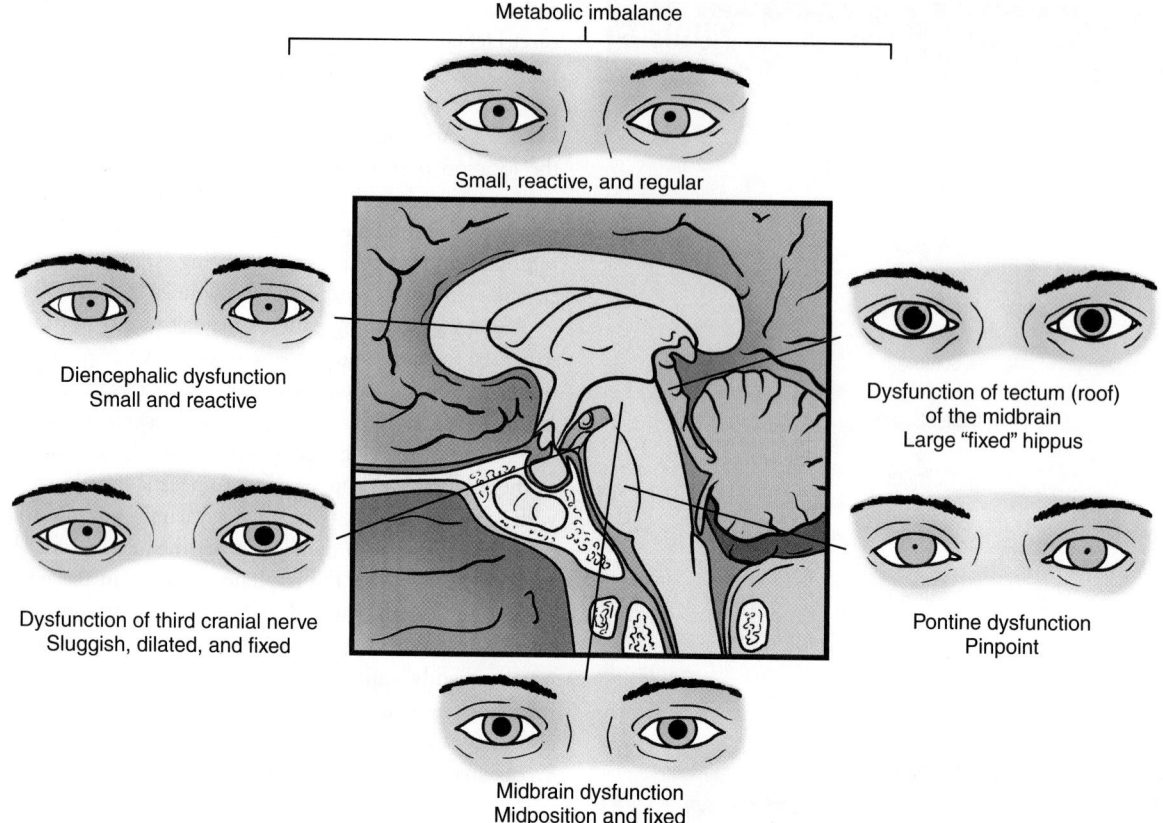

Metabolic imbalance

Small, reactive, and regular

Diencephalic dysfunction
Small and reactive

Dysfunction of tectum (roof)
of the midbrain
Large "fixed" hippus

Dysfunction of third cranial nerve
Sluggish, dilated, and fixed

Pontine dysfunction
Pinpoint

Midbrain dysfunction
Midposition and fixed

Figure 28-1 Pupils at different levels of consciousness. *(From McCance KL, Huether SE:* Pathophysiology: the biologic basis for disease in adults and children, *ed 5, St Louis, 2006, Mosby.)*

Much research has been directed toward identifying prognostic indicators for the patient in a coma after a cardiopulmonary arrest. In a meta-analysis, the best predictors of poor outcome after cardiac arrest were lack of corneal or papillary response at 24 hours and lack of motor movement at 72 hours. However, regardless of the cause or duration of coma, outcome for an individual cannot be predicted with 100% accuracy.[5,10] Research has focused on induced hypothermia in patients after cardiac arrest. The use of hypothermia has improved neurologic outcomes and survival rates. When a patient remains comatose after return of spontaneous circulation, the body is cooled to 32° C to 34° C for up to 24 hours.[11,12]

NURSING MANAGEMENT

Nursing management of the patient in a coma incorporates a variety of nursing diagnoses (see the Nursing Diagnoses feature on Coma) and is directed by the specific cause of the coma, although some common interventions are used. The patient in a coma totally depends on the health care team. Nursing interventions are directed toward assessing changes in neurologic status and clues to the origin of the coma, supporting all body functions, maintaining surveillance for complications, providing comfort and emotional support, and initiating rehabilitation measures.[5] Measures to support body functions include promoting pulmonary hygiene, maintaining skin integrity, initiating range-of-motion exercises, and ensuring adequate nutritional support.[5]

Nursing Diagnoses

Coma

- Ineffective Airway Clearance related to excessive secretions or abnormal viscosity of mucus
- Ineffective Breathing Pattern related to decreased lung expansion
- Imbalanced Nutrition: Less Than Body Requirements related to lack of exogenous nutrients or increased metabolic demand
- Risk for Aspiration
- Risk for Infection
- Compromised Family Coping related to critically ill family member

Eye Care. The blink reflex is often diminished or absent in the comatose patient. The eyelids may be flaccid and may depend on body positioning to remain in a closed position, and edema may prevent complete closure. Loss of these protective mechanisms results in drying and ulceration of the cornea, which can lead to permanent scarring and blindness.[5]

Two interventions that are commonly used to protect the eyes are instilling saline or methylcellulose lubricating drops and taping the eyelids in the shut position. Evidence suggests that an alternative technique may be more effective in preventing corneal epithelial breakdown. In addition to instilling saline drops every 2 hours, a polyethylene film is taped over the eyes, extending beyond the orbits and eyebrows. The film creates a moisture chamber around the cornea and assists in keeping the eyes moist

- Identify and treat the underlying cause.
- Protect the airway.
- Provide ventilatory assistance, as required.
- Support circulation, as required.
- Initiate nutritional support
- Provide eye care.
- Protect skin integrity.
- Initiate range-of-motion exercises.
- Maintain surveillance for complications.
  - Infections
  - Metabolic alterations
  - Cardiac dysrhythmias
  - Temperature alterations
- Provide comfort and emotional support.
- Plan for the rehabilitation program.

and in the closed position. This technique also prevents damage to the eyes that results from tape or gauze being placed directly on the delicate skin of the eyelids.[13] Collaborative management of the patient in a coma is outlined in Box 28-2.

STROKE

Stroke is a descriptive term for the sudden onset of acute neurologic deficit persisting for more than 24 hours and caused by the interruption of blood flow to the brain. Stroke is the third leading cause of death in the United States, preceded by heart disease and cancer, and the leading cause of adult disability.[14] Approximately 795,000 people have a stroke each year; 610,000 of these are first attacks, and 185,000 are recurrent attacks.[14]

Strokes are classified as ischemic or hemorrhagic (see the Concept Map on Stroke, p. 734). Hemorrhagic strokes can be further categorized as subarachnoid hemorrhages (SAHs) and ICHs. Approximately 87% of all strokes are ischemic, 10% are ICHs, and 3% are SAHs. Although less common, hemorrhagic strokes (ICHs and SAHs) have a higher mortality rate than ischemic strokes. Approximately 8% to 12% of ischemic strokes and 37% to 38% of hemorrhagic strokes result in death within 30 days.[14] The annual cost for care and loss of productivity was estimated to be $68.9 billion in 2009.[14]

The national concern for the incidence and effects of stroke is illustrated by the inclusion of emergent stroke care in the American Heart Association guidelines for basic and advanced life support. Major public education programs, stroke appraisal screening programs, development of stroke centers, and algorithms for stroke management are based on the success these same approaches have had with coronary artery disease.

ISCHEMIC STROKE

Description. Ischemic stroke results from reduction or blockage of blood flow to the brain. The occlusion can be thrombotic or embolic. Thrombosis can form in large or small

vessels. Embolic sources include the heart and atherosclerotic plaques in larger vessels.[15]

Strokes are preventable. Most thrombotic strokes are the result of the accumulation of atherosclerotic plaque in the vessel lumen, especially at bifurcations or curves of the vessel. The pathogenesis of cerebrovascular disease is identical to that of coronary vasculature. The greatest risk factor for ischemic stroke is hypertension.[6,15] Other risk factors are dyslipidemia, diabetes, smoking, and carotid atherosclerotic disease.[14,16] Common sites of atherosclerotic plaque are the bifurcation of the common carotid artery, the origins of the middle and anterior cerebral arteries, and the origins of the vertebral arteries.[6] Ischemic strokes resulting from vertebral artery dissection have been reported after chiropractic manipulation of the cervical spine.[17]

Etiology. An embolic stroke occurs when an embolus from the heart or lower circulation travels distally and lodges in a small vessel, obstructing the blood supply. At least 30% of ischemic strokes are attributed to a cardioembolic phenomenon.[6,15] The most common cause of cardiac emboli is atrial fibrillation. It is responsible for about 50% of all cardiac emboli. Other sources of cardiac emboli are from mitral stenosis, mechanical valves, atrial myxoma, endocarditis, and recent myocardial infarction. Researchers hypothesize that a patent foramen ovale or atrial septal aneurysms may be the cause of cryptogenic stroke.[18]

Pathophysiology. Ischemic stroke is a cerebral hemodynamic insult. When cerebral blood flow is reduced to a level insufficient to maintain neuronal viability, ischemic injury occurs. In focal stroke, an area of hypoperfused tissue, the ischemic penumbra, surrounds a core of ischemic cells.[6,15] The ischemic penumbra can be salvaged with return of blood flow. However, sustained anoxic insult initiates a chain of biochemical events leading to apoptosis, or cellular death.[15]

The phenomenon of a focal ischemic stroke is identical to that associated with myocardial infarction, which is why the term *brain attack* is used in public education strategies. Often, a history of transient ischemic attacks (TIAs), brief episodes of neurologic symptoms that last less than 24 hours, offers a warning that stroke is likely to occur. Sudden onset indicates embolism as the final insult to flow.[6,14] The size of the stroke depends on the size and location of the occluded vessel and the availability of collateral blood flow. Global ischemia results when severe hypotension or cardiopulmonary arrest provokes a transient drop in blood flow to all areas of the brain.[19,20]

Cerebral edema sufficient to produce clinical deterioration develops in 10% to 20% of patients with ischemic stroke and can result in intracranial hypertension. The edema results from a loss of normal metabolic function of the cells and peaks at 3 to 5 days. This process is commonly the cause of death during the first week after a stroke.[19] Secondary hemorrhage at the site of the stroke lesion, known as *hemorrhagic conversion*,[19] and seizures[21] are the two other major acute neurologic complications of ischemic stroke.

Assessment and Diagnosis. The characteristic sign of an ischemic stroke is the sudden onset of focal neurologic signs persisting for more than 24 hours. These signs usually occur in combination. Box 28-3 lists common patterns of neurologic symptoms associated with an ischemic stroke. Hemiparesis, aphasia, and

BOX 28-3 NEUROLOGIC ABNORMALITIES IN ACUTE ISCHEMIC STROKES

LEFT (DOMINANT) HEMISPHERE
Aphasia, right hemiparesis, right-sided sensory loss, right visual field defect, poor right conjugate gaze, dysarthria, difficulty in reading, writing, or calculating

RIGHT (NONDOMINANT) HEMISPHERE
Neglect of the left visual space, left visual field defect, left hemiparesis, left-sided sensory loss, poor left conjugate gaze, extinction of left-sided stimuli, dysarthria, spatial disorientation

BRAINSTEM, CEREBELLUM, AND POSTERIOR HEMISPHERE
Motor or sensory loss in all four limbs, crossed signs, limb or gait ataxia, dysarthria, disconjugate gaze, nystagmus, amnesia, bilateral visual field defects

SMALL SUBCORTICAL HEMISPHERE OR BRAINSTEM (PURE MOTOR STROKE)
Weakness of face and limbs on one side of the body without abnormalities of higher brain function, sensation, or vision

SMALL SUBCORTICAL HEMISPHERE OR BRAINSTEM (PURE SENSORY STROKE)
Decreased sensation of face and limbs on one side of the body without abnormalities of higher brain function, motor function, or vision

From Adams HP et al: Guidelines for the management of patients with acute ischemic stroke. A statement for healthcare professionals from a special writing group of the Stroke Council, American Heart Association, *Circulation* 90(3):1588-1601, 1994.

hemianopia are common. Changes in the level of consciousness usually occur only with brainstem or cerebellar involvement, seizure, hypoxia, hemorrhage, or elevated intracranial pressure (ICP). These changes may be exhibited as stupor, coma, confusion, and agitation.[5] The reported frequency of seizures in patients with ischemic stroke ranges from 3% to 8%. If seizures occur, they are usually seen within 24 hours of an insult.[21]

The National Institutes of Health Stroke Scale (NIHSS) is often used as the basis of the focused neurologic examination (Table 28-2). The score ranges from 0 to 42 points; the higher the score, the more neurologically impaired the patient. A change of 4 points on the scale indicates significant neurologic change. The components of the NIHSS include level of consciousness (LOC); LOC questions; LOC commands; gaze; visual fields; face, arm, and leg strength; sensation; limb ataxia; and language function.[5,22]

Confirmation of the diagnosis of ischemic stroke is the first step in the emergent evaluation of these patients. Differentiation from intracranial hemorrhage is vital. Noncontrast CT scanning is the method of choice for this purpose, and it is considered the most important initial diagnostic study. In addition to excluding intracranial hemorrhage, CT can assist in identifying early neurologic complications and the cause of the insult.[15,19] MRI can demonstrate infarction of cerebral tissue earlier than CT but is less useful in the emergent differential diagnosis. Because of the strong correlation between acute ischemic stroke and heart disease, 12-lead electrocardiography, chest radiography, and continuous cardiac monitoring are suggested to detect a cardiac cause or coexisting condition. Echocardiography is valuable in identifying a cardioembolic phenomenon when a sufficient index of suspicion warrants its use.[5] Laboratory evaluation of hematologic function, electrolyte and glucose levels, and renal and hepatic function is also recommended. Arterial blood gas analysis is performed if hypoxia is suspected, and an electroencephalogram is obtained if seizures are suspected. Lumbar puncture is performed only if SAH is suspected and the CT scan is normal.[19]

TABLE 28-2 National Institutes of Health Stroke Scale

Administer stroke scale items in the order listed. Record performance in each category after each subscale examination. Do not go back and change scores. Follow directions provided for each examination technique. Scores should reflect what the patient does, not what the clinician thinks the patient can do. The clinician should record answers while administering the examination and work quickly. Except where indicated, the patient should not be coached (i.e., repeated requests to patient to make a special effort). If any item is left untested, a detailed explanation must be clearly written on the form. All untested items will be reviewed by the medical monitor and discussed with the examiner by telephone.

Instructions	Scale Definition	Score
1A. Level of Consciousness (LOC) The investigator must choose a response, even if a full evaluation is prevented by obstacles such as an endotracheal tube, language barrier, orotracheal trauma, or bandages. A 3 is scored only if the patient makes no movement (other than reflexive posturing) in response to noxious stimulation.	0 = Alert; keenly responsive 1 = Not alert, but arousable by minor stimulation to obey, answer, or respond 2 = Not alert, requires repeated stimulation to attend, or is obtunded and requires strong or painful stimulation to make movements (not stereotyped) 3 = Responds only with reflex motor or autonomic effects or totally unresponsive, flaccid, areflexic	

TABLE 28-2 National Institutes of Health Stroke Scale—*cont'd*

Instructions	Scale Definition	Score

1B. LOC Questions

The patient is asked the month and his or her age. The answer must be correct; there is no partial credit for being close. Aphasic and stuporous patients who do not comprehend the questions receive a score of 2. Patients unable to speak because of endotracheal intubation, orotracheal trauma, severe dysarthria from any cause, language barrier, or any other problem not resulting from aphasia are given a score of 1. Only the initial answer should be graded, and the examiner must not "help" the patient with verbal or nonverbal cues.

0 = Answers both questions correctly
1 = Answers one question correctly
2 = Answers neither question correctly

1C. LOC Commands

The patient is asked to open and close the eyes and then to grip and release the nonparetic hand. Substitute another one-step command if the hands cannot be used. Credit is given if an unequivocal attempt is made but not completed due to weakness. If the patient does not respond to a command, the task should be demonstrated to them (pantomime) and the result scored (i.e., follows none, one, or two commands). Patients with trauma, amputation, or other physical impediments should be given suitable one-step commands. Only the first attempt is scored.

0 = Performs both tasks correctly
1 = Performs one task correctly
2 = Performs neither task correctly

2. Best Gaze

Only horizontal eye movements are tested. Voluntary or reflexive (oculocephalic) eye movements are scored, but caloric testing is not done. If the patient has a conjugate deviation of the eyes that can be overcome by voluntary or reflexive activity, the score is 1. If the patient has an isolated peripheral nerve paresis (CN III, IV, or VI), the score is 1. Gaze is testable in all aphasic patients. Patients with ocular trauma, bandages, preexisting blindness, or other disorder of visual acuity or fields should be tested with reflexive movements and a choice made by the investigator. Establishing eye contact and then moving about the patient from side to side occasionally clarifies the presence of a partial gaze palsy.

0 = Normal
1 = Partial gaze palsy; this score is given when gaze is abnormal in one or both eyes, but forced deviation or total gaze paresis is not present
2 = Forced deviation or total gaze paresis not overcome by the oculocephalic maneuver

3. Visual

Visual fields (upper and lower quadrants) are tested by confrontation, using finger counting or visual threat as appropriate. Patient must be encouraged, but if he or she looks at the side of the moving fingers appropriately, it can be scored as normal. If there is unilateral blindness or enucleation, visual fields in the remaining eye are scored. Score 1 only if a clear-cut asymmetry, including quadrantanopia, is found. If the patient is blind from any cause, score 3. Double simultaneous stimulation is performed at this point. If there is extinction, the patient receives a score of 1, and the results are used to answer question 11.

0 = No visual loss
1 = Partial hemianopia
2 = Complete hemianopia
3 = Bilateral hemianopia (blind including cortical blindness)

Continued

TABLE 28-2 National Institutes of Health Stroke Scale—*cont'd*

Instructions	Scale Definition	Score

4. Facial Palsy

Ask for or use pantomime to encourage the patient to show teeth or raise eyebrows and close eyes. Score symmetry of grimace in response to noxious stimuli in the poorly responsive or noncomprehending patient. If facial trauma or bandages, orotracheal tube, tape, or other physical barrier obscures the face, they should be removed to the extent possible.

0 = Normal symmetric movement
1 = Minor paralysis (flattened nasolabial fold, asymmetry on smiling)
2 = Partial paralysis (total or near total paralysis of lower face)
3 = Complete paralysis of one or both sides (absence of facial movement in the upper and lower face)

5 and 6. Motor Arm and Leg

The limb is placed in the appropriate position: extend the arms (palms down) 90 degrees (if sitting) or 45 degrees (if supine) and the leg 30 degrees (always tested supine). Drift is scored if the arm falls before 10 seconds or the leg before 5 seconds. The aphasic patient is encouraged using urgency in the voice and pantomime but not noxious stimulation. Each limb is tested in turn, beginning with the nonparetic arm. Only in the case of amputation or joint fusion at the shoulder or hip may the score be 9, and the examiner must clearly write the explanation for scoring as a 9.

0 = No drift, limb holds 90 (or 45) degrees for full 10 seconds
1 = Drift, limb holds 90 (or 45) degrees but drifts down before full 10 seconds; does not hit bed or other support
2 = Some effort against gravity, limb cannot get to or maintain (if cued) 90 (or 45) degrees, drifts down to bed, but has some effort against gravity
3 = No effort against gravity, limb falls
4 = No movement
9 = Amputation, joint fusion; explain:
5a. Left arm
5b. Right arm
0 = No drift, leg holds 30 degrees position for full 5 seconds.
1 = Drift, leg falls by the end of the 5 second period but does not hit bed
2 = Some effort against gravity; leg falls to bed by 5 seconds, but has some effort against gravity
3 = No effort against gravity, leg falls to bed immediately
4 = No movement
9 = Amputation, joint fusion; explain:
6a. Left leg
6b. Right leg
0 = Absent
1 = Present in one limb
2 = Present in two limbs

7. Limb Ataxia

This test seeks evidence of a unilateral cerebellar lesion. Test with eyes open. In case of a visual defect, ensure that testing is done in the intact visual field. The finger-nose-finger and heel-shin tests are performed on both sides, and ataxia is scored only if present out of proportion to weakness. Ataxia is absent in the patient who cannot understand or is paralyzed. Only in the case of amputation or joint fusion may the item be scored 9, and the examiner must clearly write the explanation for not scoring. In case of blindness, test by touching the nose from an extended arm position.

If present, is ataxia in the
Right arm
1 = Yes
2 = No
9 = Amputation or joint fusion; explain:
Left arm
1 = Yes
2 = No
9 = Amputation or joint fusion; explain:
Right leg
1 = Yes
2 = No
9 = Amputation or joint fusion; explain:
Left leg
1 = Yes
2 = No
9 = Amputation or joint fusion; explain:

TABLE 28-2 National Institutes of Health Stroke Scale—*cont'd*

Instructions	Scale Definition	Score

8. Sensory

Sensation or grimace to pinprick when tested or withdrawal from noxious stimulus in the obtunded or aphasic patient. Only sensory loss attributed to stroke is scored as abnormal, and the examiner should test as many body areas (arms [not hands], legs, trunk, face) as needed to accurately check for hemisensory loss. A score of 2 (severe or total) should be given only when a severe or total loss of sensation can be clearly demonstrated. Stuporous and aphasic patients likely will receive a score of 1 or 0. The patient with brainstem stroke who has bilateral loss of sensation is scored 2. If the patient does not respond and is quadriplegic, score 2. Patients in coma (item 1a = 3) are arbitrarily given a 2 on this item.

0 = Normal; no sensory loss
1 = Mild to moderate sensory loss; patient feels pinprick is less sharp or is dull on the affected side, or there is a loss of superficial pain with pinprick but patient is aware of being touched.
2 = Severe to total sensory loss; patient is not aware of being touched on the face, arm, and leg.

9. Best Language

Much information about comprehension is obtained during the preceding sections of the examination. The patient is asked to describe what is happening in the attached picture, to name the items on the attached naming sheet, and to read from the attached list of sentences. Comprehension is judged from these responses here and from all of the commands in the preceding general neurologic examination. If visual loss interferes with the tests, ask the patient to identify objects placed in the hand, repeat, and produce speech. The intubated patient should be asked to write. The patient in coma (question 1a = 3) arbitrarily scores 3 on this item. The examiner must choose a score for the patient with stupor or limited cooperation, but a score of 3 should be used only if the patient is mute and follows no one-step commands.

0 = No aphasia; normal
1 = Mild to moderate aphasia; some obvious loss of fluency or facility of comprehension, without significant limitation on ideas expressed or form of expression. Reduction of speech and comprehension makes conversation about provided material difficult or impossible. For example, in conversation about provided materials, examiner can identify picture or naming card from patient's response.
2 = Severe aphasia; all communication is through fragmentary expression; great need for inference, questioning, and guessing by the listener. Range of information that can be exchanged is limited; listener carries burden of communication. Examiner cannot identify materials provided from patient response.
3 = Mute, global aphasia; no usable speech or auditory comprehension

10. Dysarthria

If the patient is thought to be normal, an adequate sample of speech must be obtained by asking him or her to read or repeat words from a list. If the patient has severe aphasia, the clarity of articulation of spontaneous speech can be rated. Only if the patient is intubated or has other physical barriers to producing speech may the item be scored 9, and the examiner must clearly write an explanation for not scoring. Do not tell the patient why he or she is being tested.

0 = Normal
1 = Mild to moderate; patient slurs at least some words and, at worst, can be understood with some difficulty.
2 = Severe; patient's speech is so slurred as to be unintelligible in the absence of or out of proportion to any dysphasia, or the patient is mute or anarthric.
9 = Intubated or other physical barrier; explain:

11. Extinction and Inattention (Formerly Neglect)

Sufficient information to identify neglect may be obtained during the prior testing. If the patient has a severe visual loss preventing visual double, simultaneous stimulation and the cutaneous stimuli are normal, the score is normal. If the patient has aphasia but does appear to attend to both sides, the score is normal. The presence of visual spatial neglect or anosognosia may be taken as evidence of abnormality. Because the abnormality is scored only if present, the item is never untestable.

0 = No abnormality
1 = Visual, tactile, auditory, spatial, or personal inattention or extinction to bilateral simultaneous stimulation in one of the sensory modalities
2 = Profound hemiinattention or hemiinattention to more than one modality; does not recognize own hand or orients to only one side of space

Additional Item, Not a Part of the NIH Stroke Scale Score

A. Distal Motor Function

The patient's hand is held up at the forearm by the examiner, and the patient is asked to extend his or her fingers as much as possible. If the patient cannot or does not extend the fingers, the examiner places the fingers in full extension and observes for any flexion movement for 5 seconds. Only the patient's first attempts are graded. Repetition of the instructions or of the testing is prohibited.

0 = Normal (no flexion after 5 seconds)
1 = At least some extension after 5 seconds but not fully extended; any movement of the fingers that is not commanded is not scored.
2 = No voluntary extension after 5 seconds; movements of the fingers at another time are not scored.
   a. Left arm
   b. Right arm

BOX 28-4 INDICATIONS AND CONTRAINDICATIONS TO THROMBOLYTIC THERAPY IN ACUTE ISCHEMIC STROKE

INDICATIONS
- Acute ischemic stroke within 3 hours from symptom onset
- Age older than 18 years (rtPA has not been studied in pediatric stroke)

CONTRAINDICATIONS
- Evidence of intracranial hemorrhage on pretreatment evaluation
- Suspicion of subarachnoid hemorrhage
- Recent stroke, intracranial or intraspinal surgery, or serious head trauma in the past 3 months
- Major surgery or serious trauma in the previous 14 days*
- Arterial puncture at a noncompressible site or lumbar puncture in the last 7 days
- Major symptoms that are rapidly improving or only minor stroke symptoms (NIHSS <4)*

- History of intracranial hemorrhage
- Uncontrolled hypertension at the time of treatment
- Seizure at the stroke onset
- Active internal bleeding
- Intracranial neoplasm, arteriovenous malformation, or aneurysm
- Known bleeding diathesis, including but not limited to
  - Current use of anticoagulants or an international normalized ratio (INR) >1.7 or a prothrombin time (PT) >15 seconds
  - Administration of heparin within 48 hours preceding the onset of stroke and an elevated activated partial thromboplastin time at presentation
  - Platelet count <100,000 mm³

From Thurman RJ, Jauch EC: Acute ischemic stroke: emergent evaluation and management, *Emerg Med Clin North Am* 20:609, 2002.
*In the NINDS trial, not present in current package insert.
NIHSS, National Institutes of Health Stroke Scale; rtPA, recombinant tissue-type plasminogen activator.

Medical Management. Major changes have taken place in the medical management of ischemic stroke since 1996. Based on results of the National Institute of Neurologic Disorders and Stroke (NINDS) rtPA Stroke Study, thrombolytic therapy with intravenous rtPA is recommended within 3 hours of onset of ischemic stroke.[18] Indications and contraindications to thrombolysis are listed in Box 28-4. Confirmation of diagnosis with CT must be accomplished before rtPA administration. The recommended dose of rtPA is 0.9 mg/kg up to a maximum dose of 90 mg. Ten percent of the total dose is administered as an initial intravenous bolus, and the remaining 90% is administered by intravenous infusion over 60 minutes.[5,18] A recent European study demonstrated that thrombolysis could be given up to 4.5 hours after the onset of symptoms with the same results.[23]

The desired result of thrombolytic therapy is to dissolve the clot and reperfuse the ischemic brain. The goal is to reverse or minimize the effects of stroke. The major risk and complication of rtPA therapy is bleeding, especially intracranial hemorrhage. Unlike thrombolytic protocols for acute myocardial infarction, subsequent therapy with anticoagulant or antiplatelet agents is *not* recommended after rtPA administration in ischemic stroke. Patients receiving thrombolytic therapy for stroke should not receive aspirin, heparin, warfarin, ticlopidine, or any other antithrombotic or antiplatelet drugs for at least 24 hours after treatment.[18,24]

The major barriers to effective application of thrombolytic therapy for ischemic stroke are prehospital and in-hospital delays.[25] To help decrease delays, the public needs to be educated about stroke symptoms and activation of emergency medical system (EMS). EMS responders need adequate education and training on managing a patient with an acute ischemic stroke, focusing on stabilization and transport of the patient quickly to the emergency department. The receiving hospital should ideally be primary stroke certified and have expert staff and the infrastructure to care for the complex stroke patient.[18]

Other emergent care of the patient with ischemic stroke must include airway protection and ventilatory assistance to maintain adequate tissue oxygenation.[15] Hypertension is often present in the early period as a compensatory response, and in most cases, blood pressure (BP) must not be lowered (Table 28-3). For the patient who has not received thrombolytic therapy, antihypertensive therapy is considered only if the diastolic blood pressure is greater than 120 mm Hg or the systolic blood pressure is greater than 220 mm Hg.[18] Criteria are different for patients who have received rtPA. Their blood pressure is kept below 180/105 mm Hg to prevent intracranial hemorrhage. Intravenous labetalol or nicardipine is used to achieve blood pressure control.[18] Body temperature and glucose levels also must be normalized.[18,20]

Medical management also includes the identification and treatment of acute complications such as cerebral edema or seizure activity. Prophylaxis for these complications is not recommended. Surgical decompression is recommended if a large cerebellar infarction compresses the brainstem.[26]

SUBARACHNOID HEMORRHAGE

Description. SAH is bleeding into the subarachnoid space, which usually is caused by rupture of a cerebral aneurysm or arteriovenous malformation (AVM). At the time of autopsy, approximately 2% of the population has been found to have one or more aneurysms. With improvements in imaging techniques, an increased number of incidental intracranial aneurysms has been found. Computed tomographic angiography (CTA) and magnetic resonance angiography (MRA) can detect up to 95% of all aneurysms. Among people younger than

TABLE 28-3 Blood Pressure Management for Stroke According to the American Stroke Association Guidelines

Blood Pressure*	Treatment
Nonthrombolytic Candidates	
DBP >140 mm Hg	Sodium nitroprusside (0.5 mcg/kg/min); aim for 10%-20% reduction in DBP
SBP >220 mm Hg, DBP 121-140 mm Hg, or MAP[†] >130 mm Hg	10-20 mg of labetalol[‡] given by IVP over 1-2 min; may repeat or double labetalol every 20 min to a maximum dose of 300 mg
SBP <220 mm Hg, DBP = 120 mm Hg, or MAP[†] <130 mm Hg	Emergency antihypertensive therapy is deferred in the absence of aortic dissection, acute myocardial infarction, severe congestive heart failure, or hypertensive encephalopathy.
Thrombolytic Candidates	
Pretreatment	
SBP >185 mm Hg or DBP >110 mm Hg	1-2 inches of nitroglycerine paste (Nitropaste) or 1-2 doses of 10-20 mg of labetalol[‡] given by IVP; if BP is not reduced and maintained to <185/110 mm Hg, the patient should not be treated with tPA
During and After Treatment	
Monitor BP	BP is monitored every 15 min for 2 hr, then every 30 min for 6 hr, and then hourly for 16 hr
DBP >140 mm Hg	Sodium nitroprusside (0.5 mcg/kg/min)
SBP >230 mm Hg or DBP 121-140 mm Hg	10 mg of labetalol[‡] given by IVP over 1-2 min; may repeat or double labetalol every 10 min to a maximum dose of 300 mg or give initial labetalol bolus and then start a labetalol drip at 2-8 mg/min If BP not controlled by labetalol, consider sodium nitroprusside
SBP 180-230 mm Hg or DBP 105-120 mm Hg	10 mg of labetalol[‡] given by IVP; may repeat or double labetalol every 10-20 min to a maximum dose of 300 mg or give initial labetalol bolus and then start a labetalol drip at 2-8 mg/min

From Bader MK, Littlejohns LR: *AANN core curriculum for neuroscience nursing*, ed 4, St Louis, 2004, Elsevier.

*All initial blood pressures should be verified before treatment by repeating reading in 5 minutes.

[†]As estimated by one third of the sum of systolic and double diastolic pressure.

[‡]Labetalol should be avoided in patients with asthma, cardiac failure, or severe abnormalities in cardiac conduction. For refractory hypertension, alternative therapy may be considered with sodium nitroprusside or enalapril.

BP, blood pressure; DBP, diastolic blood pressure; IVP, intravenous push; MAP, mean arterial pressure; SBP, systolic blood pressure; tPA, tissue-type plasminogen activator.

40 years, more men than women are likely to have an SAH, whereas among those older than 40 years, more women have SAHs. Aneurysmal SAH is associated with a mortality rate of 30%, with most patients dying on the first day after the insult. Hemorrhage due to AVM rupture has a better chance of survival and is associated with an overall mortality rate of 10% to 15%.[27,28] Known risk factors for SAH include hypertension, smoking, and alcohol or stimulant use.[28,29]

Etiology. Cerebral aneurysm rupture accounts for approximately 85% of all cases of spontaneous SAH.[5] An aneurysm is an outpouching of the wall of a blood vessel that results from weakening of the wall of the vessel (Table 28-4). Ninety percent of aneurysms are congenital—the cause of which is unknown. The other 10% can be the result of traumatic injury (that stretches and tears the muscular middle layer of the arterial vessel) or infectious material (most often from infectious vegetation on valves of the left side of the heart after bacterial endocarditis) that lodges against a vessel wall and erodes the muscular layer, or they are of undetermined cause.[5] Multiple aneurysms occur in approximately 30% of the cases and often are bilateral, occurring in the same location on both sides of the cerebral vascular system.[28]

AVM rupture is responsible for roughly 6% of all SAHs.[28] An AVM is a tangled mass of arterial and venous blood vessels that shunt blood directly from the arterial side into the venous side, bypassing the capillary system. They may be small, focal lesions or large, diffuse lesions that occupy almost an entire hemisphere. AVMs are always congenital, although the exact embryonic cause for these malformations is unknown. They also occur in the spinal cord and the renal, gastrointestinal, and integumentary systems. Small, superficial AVMs are seen as port-wine stains of the skin. In contrast to the middle-aged population with SAH from aneurysm, SAH from an AVM usually occurs in the second to fourth decades of life.[5,22]

Pathophysiology. The pathophysiology of the two most common causes of SAH is distinctly different.

Cerebral Aneurysm. As the individual with a congenital cerebral aneurysm matures, blood pressure rises, and more stress is placed on the poorly developed and thin vessel wall. Ballooning of the vessel occurs, giving the aneurysm a berry-like appearance. Most cerebral aneurysms are saccular or berry-like with a stem or neck. Aneurysms are usually small, 2 to 7 mm in diameter, and often occur at the base of the brain on the circle of

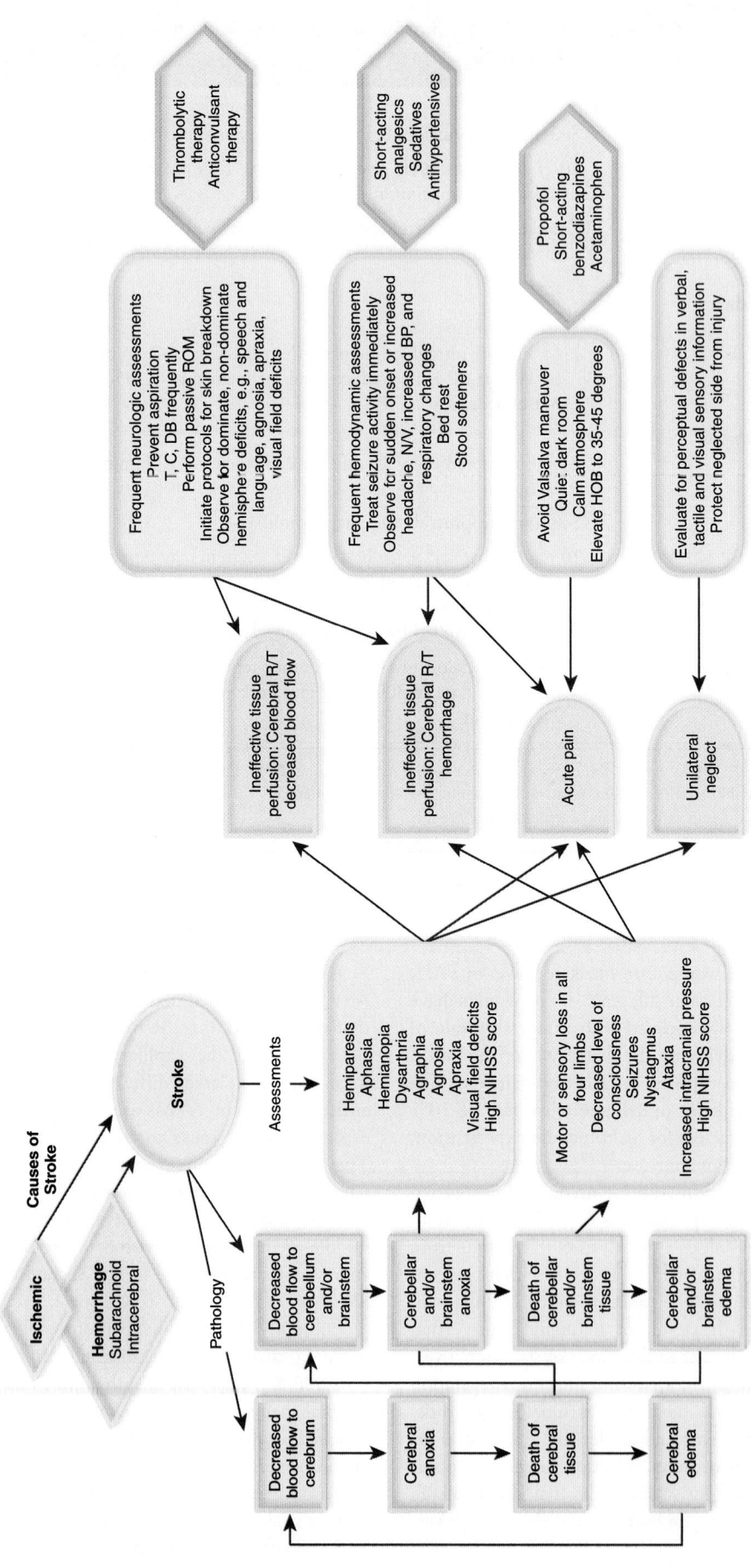

TABLE 28-4 Aneurysm Classification According to Type, Shape, Location, and Common Characteristics

Types of Aneurysms	Characteristics
Berry or saccular 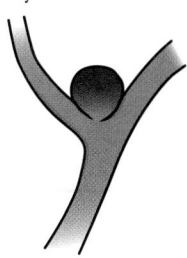	Most common type, usually congenital; appears at a bifurcation in the anterior circulation, primarily at the base of the brain or the circle of Willis and its branches; grows from the base of the arterial wall with a neck or stem; contains blood; thinned dome is usually the site of rupture
Giant or fusiform 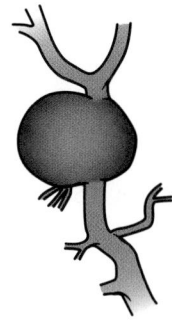	Can have an irregular shape and be larger than 2.5 cm and atherosclerotic; involves mainly the internal carotid or vertebrobasilar artery; rarely ruptures; has no stem; can act like a space-occupying lesion in the brain; difficult to manage
Mycotic 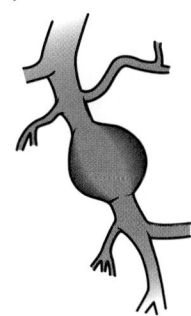	Rare form; usually occurs from septic emboli, usually results from bacterial infection, which weaken the vessel wall, causing dilation involving the distal branches of the middle cerebral arteries
Dissecting 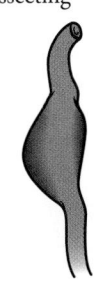	May occur during angiography; caused by trauma, syphilis, arteriosclerosis, or when blood is forced between layers of the arterial wall; intima is pulled away from the medial layer, allowing blood to enter
Traumatic	Sometimes called a *pseudoaneurysm*, which may resolve after trauma
Charcot-Bouchard	Small aneurysm that can be seen in the area of the basal ganglia or the brainstem in individuals with a history of hypertension; chronic hypertension causes fibrinoid necrosis in the penetrating and subcortical arteries, weakening the arterial walls and causing formation of small aneurismal outpouching

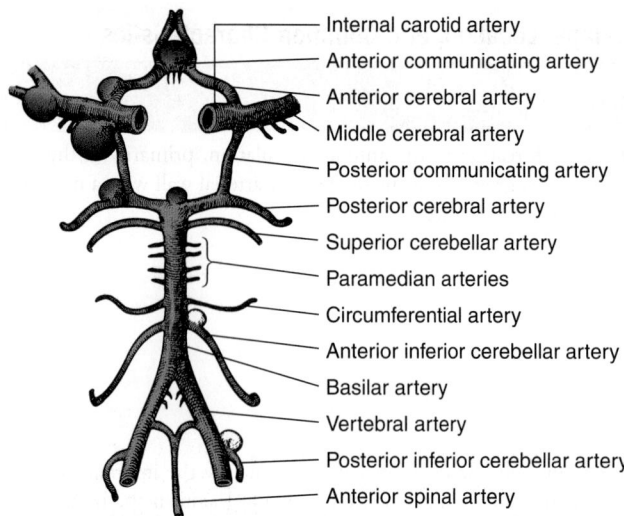

- Internal carotid artery
- Anterior communicating artery
- Anterior cerebral artery
- Middle cerebral artery
- Posterior communicating artery
- Posterior cerebral artery
- Superior cerebellar artery
- Paramedian arteries
- Circumferential artery
- Anterior inferior cerebellar artery
- Basilar artery
- Vertebral artery
- Posterior inferior cerebellar artery
- Anterior spinal artery

Figure 28-2 Common sites of berry aneurysms. The size of the aneurysm in the drawing is proportional to the frequency of occurrence at the various sites. *(From Goldman L, Ausiello D, editors: Cecil's textbook of medicine, ed 22, Philadelphia, 2004, Saunders.)*

Willis. Figure 28-2 illustrates the usual distribution between the vessels. Most cerebral aneurysms occur at the bifurcation of blood vessels.[5,22]

The aneurysm becomes clinically significant when the vessel wall becomes so thin that it ruptures, sending arterial blood at a high pressure into the subarachnoid space. For a brief moment after the aneurysm ruptures, ICP is thought to approach mean arterial pressure, and cerebral perfusion decreases. In other situations, the unruptured aneurysm expands and places pressure on surrounding structures. This is particularly true with posterior communicating artery aneurysms, because they put pressure on the oculomotor nerve (cranial nerve III), causing ipsilateral pupil dilation and ptosis.[5,22]

Arteriovenous Malformation. The pathophysiologic features of an AVM are related to the size and location of the malformation. One or more cerebral arteries, also known as *feeders*, supply an AVM. These feeder arteries tend to enlarge over time and increase the volume of blood shunted through the malformation and increase the overall mass effect. Large, dilated, tortuous draining veins develop as a result of increasing arterial blood flow being delivered at a higher than normal pressure. Normal vascular flow has a mean arterial pressure of 70 to 80 mm Hg, a mean arteriole pressure of 35 to 45 mm Hg, and a mean capillary pressure that drops from 35 to 10 mm Hg as it connects with the venous side. Lack of this capillary bridge allows blood with a mean pressure of 35 to 45 mm Hg to flow into the venous system. Unlike arteries, veins have no muscular layer, and the veins become extremely engorged and rupture easily. Some patients with AVMs also have cerebral atrophy. It is the result of chronic ischemia because of the shunting of blood through the AVM and away from normal cerebral circulation.[5,22]

Assessment and Diagnosis. The patient with an SAH characteristically has an abrupt onset of pain, described as the "worst headache of my life." A brief loss of consciousness, nausea, vomiting, focal neurologic deficits, and a stiff neck may accompany the headache.[26,28] The SAH may result in coma or death.

The patient's history may reveal one or more incidences of sudden onset of headache with vomiting in the weeks preceding a major SAH. These are small "warning leaks" of an aneurysm in which small amounts of blood ooze from the aneurysm into the subarachnoid space. The presence of blood is an irritant to the meninges, particularly the arachnoid membrane, and the irritation causes headache, stiff neck, and photophobia. These warning leaks seldom are detected because the condition is not severe enough for the patient to seek medical attention. If a neurologic deficit, such as third cranial nerve palsy, develops before aneurysm rupture, medical intervention is sought, and the aneurysm may be surgically secured before the devastation of a rupture can occur. Symptoms of unruptured AVM—headaches with dizziness or syncope or fleeting neurologic deficits—also may be found in the history.[6]

Diagnosis of SAH is based on clinical presentation, CT findings, and lumbar puncture results. Noncontrast CT is the cornerstone of definitive SAH diagnosis.[28-30] In 95% of the cases, CT can demonstrate blood in the subarachnoid space if performed within 48 hours the hemorrhage.[28] On the basis of the appearance and the location of the SAH, diagnosis of the cause—aneurysm or AVM—may be made from the CT scan. MRI is not routinely used, but it may provide greater sensitivity for detecting areas of SAH clot and potential location of bleed.[28]

If the initial CT finding is negative, a lumbar puncture is performed to obtain cerebrospinal fluid (CSF) for analysis. CSF after SAH appears bloody and has a red blood cell count greater than 1000 cells/mm^3. If the lumbar puncture is performed more than 5 days after the SAH, the CSF fluid is xanthochromic (dark amber) because the blood products have broken down.[29] Cloudy CSF usually indicates some type of infectious process, such as bacterial meningitis, not SAH.[6]

After the SAH has been documented, cerebral angiography is necessary to identify the exact cause of the hemorrhage (Fig. 28-3). If a cerebral aneurysm rupture is the cause, angiography is essential for identifying the exact location of the aneurysm in preparation for surgery.[28-30] After the aneurysm has been located, it is graded using the Hunt and Hess classification scale. This scale categorizes the patient based on the severity of the neurologic deficits associated with the hemorrhage (Box 28-5).[31] If AVM rupture is the cause, angiography is necessary to identify the feeding arteries and draining veins of the malformation.

Medical Management. SAH is a medical emergency, and time is of the essence. Preservation of neurologic function is the goal, and early diagnosis is crucial. Initial treatment must always support vital functions. Airway management and ventilatory assistance may be necessary. A ventriculostomy is performed to control ICP if the patient's level of consciousness is depressed.[28,30]

Evidence suggests that only 19% of the deaths attributable to aneurysmal SAH are related to the direct effects of the initial

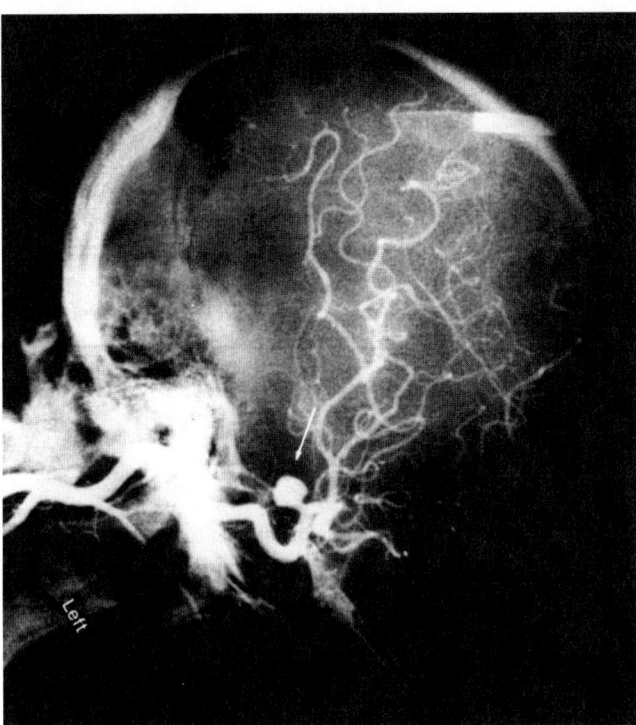

Figure 28-3 Cerebral angiography shows the location of aneurysm *(arrow)* at the posterior communicating artery. *(From Tortorici M:* Fundamentals of angiography, *St Louis, 1982, Mosby.)*

BOX 28-5 CLASSIFICATION OF SUBARACHNOID HEMORRHAGE

- *Grade I:* asymptomatic or minimal headache and slight nuchal rigidity
- *Grade II:* moderate to severe headache, nuchal rigidity, but no neurologic deficit other than cranial nerve palsy
- *Grade III:* drowsiness, confusion, or mild focal deficit
- *Grade IV:* stupor, moderate to severe hemiparesis, possible early decerebrate rigidity, and vegetative disturbances
- *Grade V:* deep coma, decerebrate rigidity, moribund appearance

---

hemorrhage.[32] Rebleeding accounts for 22% of deaths from aneurysmal SAH, cerebral vasospasm for 23%, and nonneurologic medical complications for 23%.[32] Principal nonneurologic causes of death are systemic inflammatory response syndrome (SIRS) and secondary organ dysfunction.[33] After initial intervention has provided necessary support for vital physiologic functions, medical management of acute SAH is aimed primarily toward prevention and treatment of the complications of SAH that can produce further neurologic damage and death.[5]

Rebleeding. Rebleeding is the occurrence of a second SAH in an unsecured aneurysm or, less commonly, an AVM.[6] The incidence of rebleeding during the first 24 hours after the first bleed is 4%, with a 1% to 2% chance per day for the following month. The mortality rate associated with aneurysmal rebleeding is approximately 70%.[27,28]

Historically, conservative measures to prevent rebleeding have included blood pressure control and SAH precautions (see "Nursing Management"). An elevation in blood pressure is a normal compensatory response to maintain adequate cerebral perfusion after a neurologic insult. In the belief that hypertension contributes to rebleeding, nitroprusside, metoprolol, or hydralazine has been commonly used to maintain a systolic blood pressure no greater than 150 mm Hg.[34] Individualized guidelines must be determined based on the clinical condition and preexisting values of the patient. Evidence suggests that rebleeding has more to do with variations in blood pressure than it does with absolute values and that blood pressure control does not lower the incidence of rebleeding.[30] Prophylactic anticonvulsant therapy is recommended to prevent seizures.[27,30]

Surgical Clipping of Aneurysms. Definitive treatment for the prevention of rebleeding is surgical clipping or endovascular coiling with complete obliteration of the aneurysm. Timing of the operation is a key medical management issue. Since the introduction of microsurgery and improved surgical techniques, patients commonly are taken to the operating room within the first 48 hours after rupture. This early surgical intervention to secure the aneurysm eliminates the risk of rebleeding and allows more aggressive therapy to be used in the postoperative period for the treatment of vasospasm.[28,29] Early surgery also allows the neurosurgeon to flush out the excess blood and clots from the basal cisterns (reservoir of CSF around the base of the brain and circle of Willis) to reduce the risk of vasospasm.[33] Early surgery is recommended for patients with a grade I or II SAH and some patients with a grade III SAH. In patients with a grade III SAH, the initial hemorrhage does not produce significant neurologic deficit, but the risk of rebleeding with a tragically high incidence of mortality exists until the aneurysm is secured.

Because of the patient's clinical condition and the technical difficulty of the operation, early surgical repair of the aneurysm is not always possible. Early surgery continues to be controversial for patients with grade IV or grade V SAH and those with vasospasm. However, study findings have not supported the fear of worse ischemic sequelae with early surgery in these patients.[36] Careful consideration of the patient's clinical situation is necessary in determining the optimal time for surgery.

The surgical procedure involves a craniotomy to expose and isolate the area of aneurysm. A clip is placed over the neck of the aneurysm to eliminate the area of weakness (Fig. 28-4). This is a technically difficult procedure that requires the skill of an experienced neurosurgeon. It is not uncommon, particularly in early surgery, for the clot to break away from the aneurysm as it is surgically exposed. Extensive hemorrhage into the craniotomy site results, and cessation of the hemorrhage often causes increased neurologic deficits. Deficits also may occur as a result of surgical manipulation to gain access to the site of the aneurysm.[5]

Surgical Excision of Arteriovenous Malformations. Management of AVM has traditionally involved surgical excision or conservative management of such symptoms as seizures and headache. The decision for surgical excision depends on the location and size of the AVM. Some malformations are located so deep in

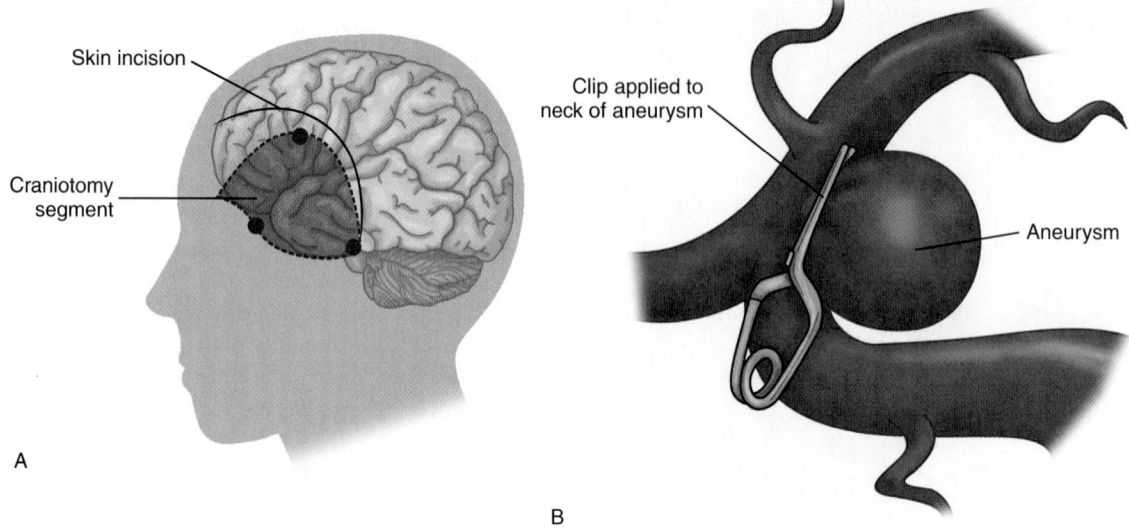

A

B

Figure 28-4 Clipping of a posterior communicating artery aneurysm. *A,* The *solid curved line* shows the typical skin incision, and the *dashed lines* show the craniotomy location. *B,* Application of the clip to the aneurysm.

the cerebral structures (thalamus or midbrain) that attempts to remove the AVM would cause severe neurologic deficits. History of a previous hemorrhage and the patient's age and overall condition are also taken into account when making the decision regarding surgical intervention.

Surgical excision of large AVMs includes the risk of reperfusion bleeding. As feeding arteries of the AVM are clamped off, the arterial blood that usually flowed into the AVM is diverted into the surrounding circulation. In many cases, the surrounding tissue has been in a state of chronic ischemia, and the arterial vessels feeding these areas are maximally dilated. As arterial blood begins to flow at a higher volume and pressure into these dilated arteries, blood may seep from the vessels. Evidence of reperfusion bleeding in the operating room is an indication that no more arterial blood can be diverted from the AVM without risk of serious ICH. In the postoperative phase, a low blood pressure is maintained to prevent further reperfusion bleeding. For large AVMs, two to four stages of surgery may be required over 6 to 12 months.[5,22]

Embolization. Embolization is used to secure a cerebral aneurysm or AVM that is surgically inaccessible because of size, location, or medical instability of the patient. Embolization involves several new interventional neuroradiology techniques. All of the techniques use a percutaneous transfemoral approach in a manner similar to an angiogram. Under fluoroscopy, the catheter is threaded up to the internal carotid artery. Specially developed microcatheters are then manipulated into the area of the vascular anomaly, and embolic materials are placed endovascularly. Three embolization techniques are used, depending on the underlying pathologic derangement.[5,22]

The first type of embolization is used to embolize an AVM. Small Silastic beads or glue is slowly introduced into the vessels feeding the AVM. Blood flow carries the material to the site, and embolization is achieved. This procedure may be used in combination with surgery. One to three sessions of embolization

of the feeding vessels are performed to reduce the size of the lesion before a craniotomy is performed for total excision. The primary risk of this procedure is lodging of the embolic substance in a vessel that feeds normal tissue, which creates an embolic stroke with the immediate onset of neurologic symptoms.[5,22]

The second type of embolization involves placement of one or more detachable coils into an aneurysm to produce an endovascular thrombus (Fig. 28-5). The advantage of this technique is that an electrical current creates a positive charge on the coil, which induces electrothrombosis. Complications include embolic stroke, coil migration, overproduction of the clot, subtotal occlusion and intraprocedural rupture of the vasculature, and death.[5]

Cerebral Vasospasm. The presence or absence of cerebral vasospasm significantly affects the outcome of aneurysmal SAH. This complication does not occur with SAH resulting from AVM rupture. Cerebral vasospasm is a narrowing of the lumen of the cerebral arteries, possibly in response to subarachnoid blood clots coating the outer surface of the blood vessels. Because aneurysms usually occur at the circle of Willis, the major vessels responsible for feeding the cerebral circulation are affected by vasospasm. Depending on the arterial vessels involved in the vasospasm reaction, decreased arterial flow occurs in large areas of the cerebral hemispheres.[6]

It is estimated that 70% of all SAH patients develop vasospasm, which is demonstrable by angiography.[36] Thirty-two percent of these patients develop symptomatic vasospasm, resulting in ischemic stroke or death for 15% to 20% of them despite the use of maximal therapy. The onset of vasospasm is usually 4 to 12 days after the initial hemorrhage.[37] Three treatments are commonly used: induced hypertensive, hypervolemic, hemodilution therapy (HHH); oral nimodipine; and transluminal cerebral angioplasty.[38]

Hypertensive, Hypervolemic, Hemodilution Therapy. HHH therapy involves increasing the patient's blood pressure and cardiac output with vasoactive medications and diluting the patient's

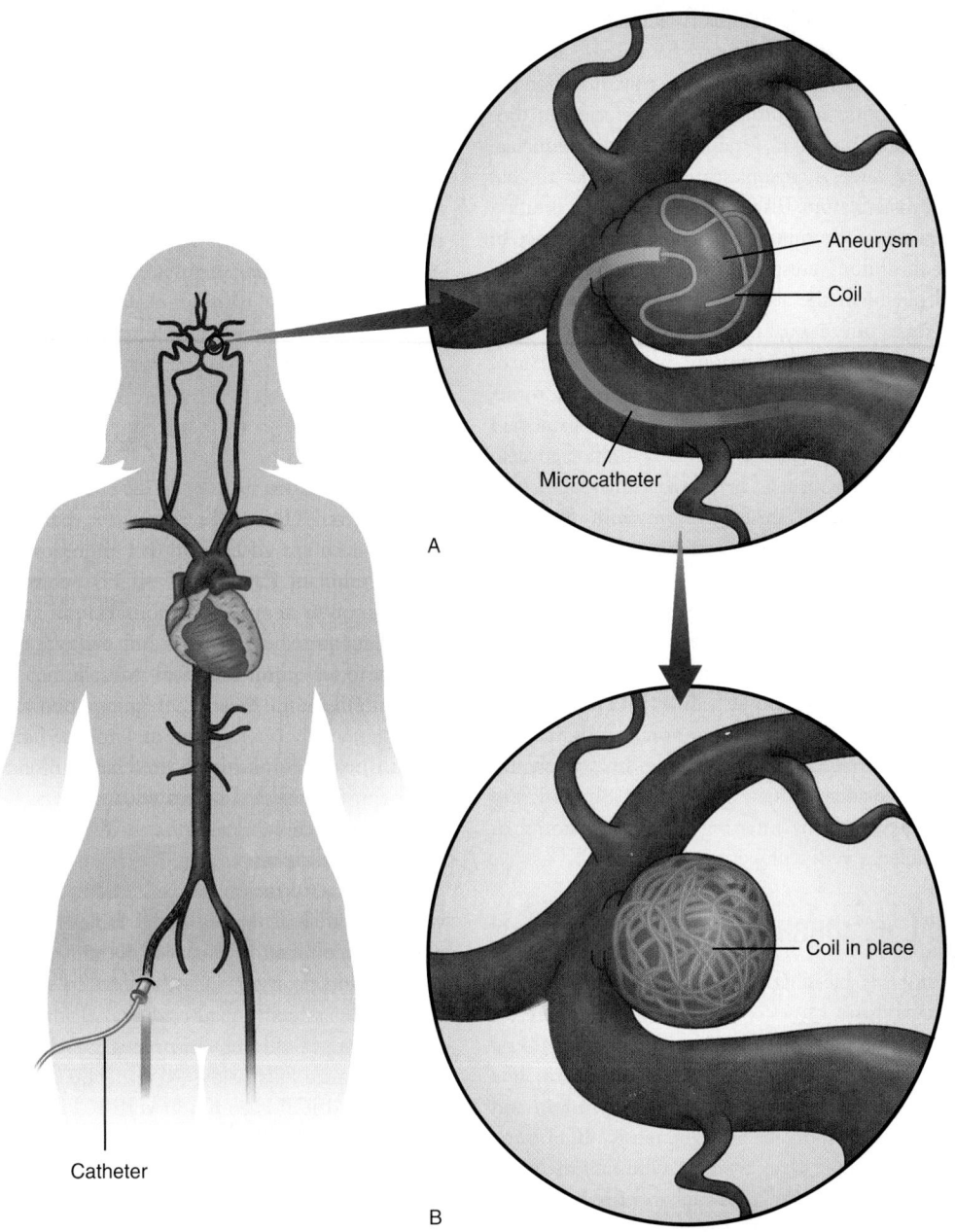

Figure 28-5 Endovascular occlusion of a posterior communicating artery aneurysm. *A,* Insertion of the microcatheter into the aneurysm through the right femoral artery, aorta, and left carotid artery. *B,* Occlusion of the aneurysm with coils.

blood with fluid and volume expanders. Systolic blood pressure is maintained between 150 and 160 mm Hg. The increase in volume and pressure forces blood through the vasospastic area at higher pressures. Hemodilution facilitates flow through the area by reducing blood viscosity. Many anecdotal reports exist of patients' neurologic deficits improving as systolic pressure increases from 130 mm Hg to between 150 and 160 mm Hg.[38] The Stroke Council of the American Heart Association (AHA) has recommended this therapy for prevention and treatment of vasospasm.[30]

The obvious deterrent to the use of induced hypertension is the risk of rebleeding in an unsecured aneurysm. Surgical clipping of the aneurysm before HHH therapy is preferred.

Cerebral edema, elevated ICP, cardiac failure, and electrolyte imbalance are also risks of HHH therapy. Careful monitoring of the patient's neurologic status, hemodynamic parameters, ICP, and serum electrolytes is necessary.[38]

Nimodipine. Nimodipine is strongly recommended to reduce the poor outcomes associated with vasospasm. The exact nature of the effect of nimodipine is not clear, but use of the drug has demonstrated consistently positive effects on outcome without any demonstrable effect on the incidence or severity of vasospasm.[28,30] A dose of 60 mg of nimodipine is given orally every 4 hours for 21 days.[38] Nimodipine may produce hypotension, especially when administered concurrently with other antihypertensive agents.

Cerebral Angioplasty. Cerebral angioplasty is used when pharmacologic management of cerebral vasospasm has failed.[39] It is performed only when CT or MRI provides evidence that infarction has not occurred. An interventional neuroradiologist performs the procedure, and the patient is under local, general, or neuroleptic analgesia. The technique of cerebral angioplasty is very similar to that used in the coronary vasculature. Risks include intimal perforation or rupture, cerebral artery thrombosis or embolism, recurrence of stenosis, and severe, diffuse vasospasm unresponsive to therapy. Hemorrhage at the femoral site also may occur. This procedure is recommended when conventional therapy is unsuccessful.[30,39]

Hyponatremia. Hyponatremia develops in 10% to 43% of patients with SAH as the result of a central salt-wasting syndrome. It usually occurs during the same period as vasospasm, several days after the initial hemorrhage.[27] The use of fluid restriction to treat hyponatremia in the SAH patient is associated with a poor outcome. The AHA Stroke Council strongly recommends that fluid restriction not be used in this instance and instead recommends sodium replenishment with isotonic fluids.[30]

Hydrocephalus. Hydrocephalus is a late complication that occurs in approximately 25% of patients after SAH.[30] Blood that has circulated in the subarachnoid space and has been absorbed by the arachnoid villi may obstruct the villi and reduce the rate of CSF absorption. Over time, increasing volumes of CSF in the intracranial space produce communicating hydrocephalus. Treatment consists of placing a drain to remove CSF. This can be accomplished temporarily by inserting a ventriculostomy or permanently by placing a ventriculoperitoneal shunt.[28,30]

INTRACEREBRAL HEMORRHAGE

Description. ICH is bleeding directly into cerebral tissue. ICH destroys cerebral tissue, causes cerebral edema, and increases ICP. The source of intracerebral bleeding is usually a small artery, but it can result also from rupture of an AVM or aneurysm. The most important cause of spontaneous ICH is hypertension, and this section concentrates on spontaneous hypertensive ICH.[40]

Spontaneous ICH is more than twice as common as SAH. The likelihood of death or disability is higher with ICH than with ischemic stroke or SAH.[40-42] The mortality rate for hemorrhagic stroke is 35% to 52% within 1 month, and half of these patients die in the first 2 days. Only 20% of ICH patients will return to a functional life at 6 months.[41] The key risk factors for ICH are age-associated cerebral amyloid angiopathy and hypertension.[28]

Etiology. ICH is most often caused by hypertensive rupture of a cerebral vessel, resulting from a long-standing history of hypertension. Other possible causes of spontaneous ICH are anticoagulation or thrombolytic therapy, coagulation disorders, drug abuse, and hemorrhage into cerebral infarct or brain tumors.[28,42] Many patients develop headache and neurologic symptoms after straining to have a bowel movement. Often on questioning, the patient with a hypertensive hemorrhage admits to having discontinued antihypertensive medication 2 to 3 weeks before the hemorrhage.

Pathophysiology. The pathophysiology of ICH is caused by continued elevated blood pressure exerting force against smaller arterial vessels that have become damaged from arteriosclerotic changes. Eventually, these arteries break, and blood bursts from the vessels into the surrounding cerebral tissue, creating a hematoma. ICP rises precipitously in response to the increase in overall intracranial volume.[5,6]

Assessment and Diagnosis. Initial assessment usually reveals a critically ill patient who often is unconscious and requires ventilatory support. History from a relative or significant other describes a sudden onset of focal deficit often accompanied by severe headache, nausea, vomiting, and rapid neurologic deterioration. Approximately 50% of patients sustain early loss of consciousness, a key feature that differentiates ICH from ischemic stroke.[40,41] More than one half of the patients with ICH present with a smooth progression of neurologic symptoms, an uncommon finding in cases of ischemic stroke or SAH.[41] One third of the patients have maximal symptoms at onset. Assessment of vital signs usually reveals a severely elevated blood pressure (200/100 to 250/150 mm Hg). Signs of increased ICP are often present by the time the patient arrives in the emergency department. Diagnosis is established easily with CT. Angiography is recommended only in patients considered surgical candidates without a clear cause of hemorrhage.[40-42]

Medical Management. ICH is a medical emergency. Initial management requires attention to airway, breathing, and circulation. Intubation is usually necessary. Blood pressure management must be based on individual factors. Reduction in blood pressure is usually necessary to decrease ongoing bleeding, but lowering blood pressure too much or too rapidly may compromise cerebral perfusion pressure (CPP), especially in the patient with elevated ICP. National guidelines recommend keeping the *mean* arterial blood pressure below 130 mm Hg in patients with a history of hypertension by moderate blood pressure reduction to a mean arterial pressure below 110 mm Hg.[41] Vasopressor therapy after fluid replenishment is recommended if systolic blood pressure falls below 90 mm Hg.[40,42]

Increased ICP is common with ICH and is a major contributor to mortality. Recommended management includes mannitol when indicated, hyperventilation, and neuromuscular blockade with sedation. Steroids are avoided. The CPP must be kept higher than 70 mm Hg.[40-42]

The goal for fluid management is euvolemia, with a recommended pulmonary artery occlusion pressure (PAOP) of 10 to 14 mm Hg. Body temperature is maintained at less than 38.5° C using acetaminophen or cooling blankets. Euglycemia, a blood glucose level less than 140 mg/dL, is maintained using insulin therapy, but hypoglycemia should be avoided. Use of short-acting benzodiazepines or propofol is recommended to treat agitation or hyperactivity. Pneumatic compression devices are used to decrease risk of pulmonary embolism. Prophylactic anticonvulsant therapy is sometimes used.[40-42]

The benefit of surgical treatment of spontaneous ICH is unclear. Recommendations for surgical removal of the clot depend on the size and location of the hematoma, the patient's ICP, and other neurologic symptoms. Medical treatment is recommended if the hemorrhage is small (<10 cm) or neurologic deficit is minimal.[40,41] Likewise, surgery offers no improvement in outcome for patients with a Glasgow Coma

Scale (GCS) score of 4 or less. Surgical evacuation of the clot is recommended for patients with cerebellar hemorrhage greater than 3 cm with neurologic deterioration or hydrocephalus with brainstem compression, as well as for young patients with moderate or large lobar hemorrhage with clinical deterioration.[40,41] Numerous techniques are being investigated to lessen the risk of brain damage associated with craniotomy for ICH.

NURSING MANAGEMENT

Nursing management of the patient with stroke incorporates a variety of nursing diagnoses (see the Nursing Diagnoses feature on Stroke). Nursing interventions are directed toward performing frequent neurologic and hemodynamic assessments and maintaining surveillance for complications.

Performing Frequent Assessments. The goal of frequent assessments is early recognition of neurologic or hemodynamic deterioration. Close monitoring of the patient's neurologic signs and vital signs is essential and requires almost continuous observation. Automatic noninvasive devices such as a blood pressure cuff and a pulse oximeter are helpful. Seizure activity must be identified and treated immediately. It is essential that all personnel working with the patient be aware of the desired hemodynamic and neurologic parameters set by the physician and that the physician be notified at the first sign of any changes.

Maintaining Surveillance for Complications. The patient with stroke should be monitored closely for signs of bleeding, vasospasm, and increased ICP. Other complications of stroke include aspiration, malnutrition, pneumonia, deep vein thrombosis (DVT), pulmonary embolism, pressure ulcers, contractures, and joint abnormalities.[5] Nursing measures to prevent these complications are well known.

Additional complications that may be seen in the patient with stroke are related to the area of the brain that has been damaged. Damage to the temporoparietal area can create a variety of disturbances that affect the patient's ability to interpret sensory information. Damage to the dominant hemisphere (usually left) produces problems with speech and language and abstract and analytic skills. Damage to the nondominant hemisphere (usually right) produces problems with spatial relationships. The resulting deficits include agnosia, apraxia, and visual field defects. Perceptual deficits are not as readily noticeable as are motor deficits, but they may be more debilitating and can lead to the inability to perform skilled or purposeful tasks. The patient also may develop impaired swallowing.[5]

Bleeding and Vasospasm. In the patient with a cerebral aneurysm, sudden onset of or an increase in headache and nausea and vomiting, increased blood pressure, and changes in respiration herald the onset of rebleeding. The first indication of vasospasm is usually the appearance of new focal or global neurologic deficits.

SAH precautions must be implemented to prevent any stress or straining that could potentially precipitate rebleeding. Precautions include blood pressure control; bed rest; a dark, quiet environment; and stool softeners. Short-acting analgesics and sedatives are used to relieve pain and anxiety. The patient must be kept calm. Limb restraints cause straining and must be avoided. The head of the bed should be elevated to 35 to 45 degrees at all times. The patient is taught to avoid any activities that correspond to performance of the Valsalva maneuver, such as pushing with the legs to move up in bed, straining for a bowel movement, or holding his or her breath during procedures or discomfort. DVT precautions are routinely implemented. Collaboration with the patient and family is used to establish a visitation plan to meet patient and family needs. Often, family members at the bedside can assist the patient to remain calm.[5,15]

Increased Intracranial Pressure. Numerous signs and symptoms of increased ICP can be observed. A change in the level of consciousness is the most sensitive indicator. Others include unequal pupil size, decreased pupillary response to light, headache, projectile vomiting, altered breathing patterns, Cushing's triad (bradycardia, systolic hypertension, and bradypnea), diminished brainstem reflexes, papilledema, and abnormal extension (decerebrate posturing) or flexion (decorticate posturing).[5,15]

Damage to the Nondominant Hemisphere. Patients with nondominant hemispheric pathologic conditions may exhibit emotional lability, with periods of euphoria, impulsiveness, and inattention. A short attention span, lack of insight, and poor judgment may lead to injuries as the patient attempts to perform activities beyond his or her capabilities. These patients also may suffer from agnosia, visual field defects, and apraxia.

Agnosia. Agnosia is a disturbance in the perception of familiar sensory (e.g., verbal, tactile, visual) information. Unilateral neglect is a form of agnosia characterized by an unawareness or denial of the affected half of the body. This denial may range from inattention to refusing to acknowledge a paralysis by neglecting the involved side of the body or by denying ownership of the side, attributing the paralyzed arm or leg to someone else.

Nursing Diagnoses

Stroke

- Ineffective Cerebral Tissue Perfusion related to decreased cerebral blood flow
- Ineffective Cerebral Tissue Perfusion related to hemorrhage
- Acute Pain related to transmission and perception of cutaneous, visceral, muscular, or ischemic impulses
- Unilateral Neglect related to perceptual disruption
- Impaired Verbal Communication related to cerebral speech center injury
- Impaired Swallowing related to neuromuscular impairment, fatigue, and limited awareness
- Risk for Aspiration
- Risk for Infection
- Anxiety related to threat of biologic, psychological, or social integrity
- Disturbed Body Image related to actual change in body structure, function, or appearance
- Compromised Family Coping related to critically ill family member
- Deficient Knowledge: Discharge Regimen related to lack of previous exposure to information (see the Patient Education feature on Stroke)

The neglect also may extend to extrapersonal space. This defect most often results from right hemispheric brain damage that causes left hemiplegia.

Other types of agnosia exist in addition to unilateral neglect. Some patients are unable to recognize objects visually (visual object agnosia), whereas others cannot recognize faces (prosopagnosia) and may have to rely on the voice or characteristic mannerisms of a familiar person to identify that person. Tactile agnosia is a perceptual disorder in which a patient is unable to recognize by touch alone an object that has been placed in his or her hand. This may occur even in the presence of an intact sense of touch. If allowed to see or hear the object, the patient usually recognizes it.

Spatial orientation is affected, resulting in interference with the patient's ability to judge position, distance, movement, form, and the relationship of his or her body parts to surrounding objects. Patients may confuse concepts such as up and down or forward and backward. They may have difficulty following a route from one place to another and may even get lost in areas that were once familiar. Stroke patients may also experience reading and writing problems related to visual perception and visuospatial deficits. One type of spatial dyslexia is related to unilateral spatial neglect. The patient may not look at the beginning of a line of written material that appears on the left. Instead, the patient fixes attention on a point to the right of the beginning of the line and reads to the end of the line. If asked to draw a design, the person completes only half of a design or drawing.

Visual Field Defects. Visual field defects may accompany agnosia, although they do not cause it. A hemispheric lesion can interrupt the visual pathways, with the resulting visual defect dependent on the location and extent of the lesion. At the optic chiasm, nerve fibers coming from the nasal half of each retina cross to the opposite side, whereas fibers coming from the temporal half of each retina do not cross. This partial crossing allows binocular vision. In the optic chiasm, fibers from the nasal half of each retina join the uncrossed fibers from the temporal half of the retina to form the optic tract. Impulses conducted to the right hemisphere by the right optic tract represent the left field of vision, and those conducted to the left hemisphere by the left optic tract represent the right field of vision. Optic radiations extend back to the occipital lobes. Visual defects restricted to a single field, right or left, are called *homonymous hemianopsia.*

The nurse may be the first person to notice that the patient has this defect. The patient with hemianopsia may neglect all sensory input from the affected side and initially may appear unresponsive if approached from the affected side. If the nurse approaches the patient from the healthy side, the patient actually may be quite alert. Another clue to hemianopsia is observing that the patient eats food only from half of the tray. Hemianopsia may recede gradually with time. Many patients can learn to scan their environment visually to compensate for the defect, although in the acute stage of stroke, the patient may be too lethargic to follow instructions in methods of visual scanning. This visual defect can lead to fear and confusion and can present a risk to the patient's safety.

Apraxia. Lesions in the parietal lobe and in other cortical structures can result in apraxia, an inability to perform a learned movement voluntarily. Even though the patient may understand the task to be performed and may have intact motor ability, he or she cannot perform the task and often fumbles and makes mistakes. The patient suffering from dressing apraxia, for example, may not be able to orient clothing in space, becoming tangled in his or her clothes when attempting to dress.

Damage to Dominant Hemisphere. Damage to the dominant hemisphere produces problems with speech and language. Impaired communication is a condition that results from a patient's difficulty in expressing and exchanging thoughts, ideas, or desires. The posterior temporoparietal area contains the receptive speech center known as *Wernicke's area.* The center for the perception of written language lies anterior to the visuoreceptive areas. Located at the base of the frontal lobe's motor strip and slightly anterior to it is *Broca's area*, also known as the *motor speech center.* These sensory and motor areas are connected by a large bundle of nerve fibers. Rather than receptive and motor language functions being entirely within discrete areas, it is thought that language is an integrated sensorimotor process, control of which is roughly located in these areas in the dominant cerebral hemisphere. It also is recognized that the elaborately complex functions of speech and language depend on other associative areas of the cerebrum and their thalamic connections. Consequently, much inconsistency exists in the degree of communication impairment among patients with lesions located in the same area of the brain.

Aphasia is a loss of language abilities caused by brain injury, usually to the dominant hemisphere. It involves more than just understanding speech or expressing oneself through verbal means. Language is a much broader term, referring to what the individual is attempting to interpret or convey through listening, speaking, reading, writing, and gesturing. Most cases of aphasia are partial rather than complete. The severity of the disorder depends on the area and the extent of the cerebral damage.

Receptive Aphasia. Receptive aphasia, also referred to as *sensory, Wernicke's,* or *fluent aphasia,* occurs when the connection between the primary auditory cortex in the temporal lobe and the angular gyrus in the parietal lobe is destroyed. The patient's comprehension of speech is impaired, but he or she can still talk if the motor area for speech (Broca's area) is intact. The patient may talk excessively, with many errors in the use of words. The patient can hear the examiner but cannot comprehend what is being said and cannot repeat the examiner's words. These patients may talk nonsense, with rambling speech that gives little information. Patients with receptive aphasia also cannot read words, although they can see them.

Expressive Aphasia. Expressive aphasia, also known as *motor, Broca's,* or *nonfluent aphasia,* is primarily a deficit in language output or speech production. Depending on the lesion's size and exact location, wide variation in the motor deficit can result. Expressive aphasia can range from a mild dysarthria (imperfect articulation as a result of weakness or lack of coordination of speech musculature) to incorrect intonation and phrasing and, in its most severe form, to complete loss of ability to communicate through verbal and written means. In this severe form of aphasia, the patient also has a loss of ability to communicate through conventional gestures, such as nodding or shaking the head for *yes* or *no.* In most cases of expressive aphasia, the muscles of articulation are intact. If speech is possible at all, the word *yes* or *no* is occasionally uttered, sometimes appropriately. In some cases, the words of well-known songs may be sung. Other patients, when excited or angered, may utter expletives. Some patients with expressive aphasia struggle or hesitate in trying to express words. They struggle to form words while using motor musculature (verbal apraxia), an articulatory disorder that is a feature of some expressive types of aphasia. All these difficulties lead to exasperation and despair for the patient. Most patients with expressive aphasia also have severely impaired writing ability. Even though penmanship may be intact, they are unable to express themselves through writing—a deficit called *agraphia*. If the right hand is paralyzed, as is often the case, the patient still cannot write or print with the left hand. In the recovery phase of severe expressive aphasia, patients become able to speak aloud to some degree, although words are uttered slowly and laboriously. Many patients, however, are able to learn to communicate ideas to some extent.

Global Aphasia. Global aphasia results when a massive lesion affects the motor and sensory speech areas. The patient cannot transform sounds into words and cannot comprehend spoken words. All language modalities are affected, and impairment may be so severe that the patient may be unable to communicate on any level. These patients usually have severe hemiplegia and homonymous hemianopsia. Their language function rarely recovers to a significant degree unless the lesion is caused by some transient disorder, such as cerebral edema or a metabolic derangement.

Impaired Swallowing. Normal swallowing occurs in four phases that are controlled by the cranial nerves. Damage to the brain, brainstem, or cranial nerves can result in a variety of swallowing deficits that can place the patient at risk for aspiration. The stroke patient is observed for signs of dysphagia, including drooling; difficulty handling oral secretions; absence of gag, cough, or swallowing reflexes; moist, gurgling voice quality; decreased mouth and tongue movements; and the presence of dysarthria. A speech therapy consult is initiated if any of these signs are present, and the patient must not be orally fed. In the absence of these warning signs, the patient may be fed, as ordered by the physician, although he or she must be continually monitored for signs of aspiration.[6]

Patient Education. Rehabilitation starts in the critical care area, with a multidisciplinary team designing and implementing an individualized plan for maximizing the patient's potential for neurologic rehabilitation. Early in the patient's hospital stay, the patient and family must be taught about stroke, its causes, and its treatment (see the Patient Education feature on Stroke). As the patient moves toward discharge, teaching focuses on the interventions necessary for preventing the recurrence of the event and on maximizing the patient's rehabilitation potential. The patient's family must be encouraged to participate in the patient's care; learn how to feed, dress, and bathe the patient; and learn some basic rehabilitation techniques. The importance of participating in a neurologic rehabilitation program or a support group, or both, must be stressed. Collaborative management of the patient with a stroke is outlined in Box 28-6.

Patient Education: Stroke

- Pathophysiology of disease
- Specific cause
- Risk factor modification
- Importance of taking medications
- Activities of daily living
- Measures to prevent injuries of impaired limbs
- Measures to compensate for residual deficits
- Basic rehabilitation techniques
- Importance of participating in neurologic rehabilitation program or support group

BOX 28-6 COLLABORATIVE MANAGEMENT: STROKE

- Differentiate the cause of the stroke.
  - Ischemic
  - Subarachnoid hemorrhage
  - Cerebral aneurysm
  - Arteriovenous malformation (AVM)
  - Intracerebral bleed
- Implement treatment according to cause of bleed.
  - Ischemic
  - Thrombolytic therapy
  - Blood pressure control
  - Subarachnoid hemorrhage
  - Surgical aneurysm clipping or AVM excision
  - Embolization
  - Intracerebral bleed
  - Blood pressure control
- Protect patient's airway.
- Provide ventilatory assistance as required.
- Perform frequent neurologic assessments.
- Maintain surveillance for complications.
  - Cerebral edema
  - Cerebral ischemia/vasospasm
  - Rebleeding
  - Impaired swallowing
  - Neurologic deficits
- Provide comfort and emotional support.
- Design and implement appropriate rehabilitation program.
- Educate patient and family.

GUILLAIN-BARRÉ SYNDROME

DESCRIPTION

Guillain-Barré syndrome (GBS), once thought to be a single entity characterized by inflammatory peripheral neuropathy, is a combination of clinical features with various forms of presentation and multiple pathologic processes. A full discussion of this complex condition is beyond the scope of this chapter. Most cases of GBS do not require admission to a critical care unit. However, the prototype of GBS, known as *acute inflammatory demyelinating polyradiculoneuropathy* (AIDP), involves a rapidly progressive, ascending peripheral nerve dysfunction leading to paralysis that may produce respiratory failure. Because of the need for ventilatory support, AIDP is one of the few peripheral neurologic diseases that necessitates care in a critical care environment.[43] In this discussion, all references to GBS pertain to the AIDP prototype.

The annual incidence of GBS is 1.8 cases per 100,000 persons.[43] It occurs more often in males and is the most commonly acquired demyelinating neuropathy.[44] Occasionally, clusters of cases are reported, such as occurred following the 1977 swine flu vaccinations.[45]

ETIOLOGY

The precise cause of GBS remains unknown, but the syndrome involves an immune-mediated response involving cell-mediated immunity and development of IgG antibodies. Most patients report a viral infection 1 to 3 weeks before the onset of clinical manifestations, usually involving the upper respiratory tract.[43]

Numerous antecedent causes, or triggering events, have been associated with GBS. They include viral infections (e.g., influenza; cytomegalovirus; hepatitis A, B, or C; Epstein-Barr virus; human immunodeficiency virus), bacterial infections (e.g., gastrointestinal *Campylobacter jejuni*, *Mycoplasma pneumoniae*), vaccines (e.g., rabies, tetanus, influenza), lymphoma, surgery, and trauma.[43,44]

PATHOPHYSIOLOGY

GBS affects the motor and sensory pathways of the peripheral nervous system, as well as the autonomic nervous system functions of the cranial nerves. The major finding in AIDP-type GBS is a segmental demyelination process of the peripheral nerves. GBS is thought to be an autoimmune response to antibodies formed in response to a recent physiologic event. T cells migrate to the peripheral nerves, resulting in edema and inflammation. Macrophages then invade the area and break down the myelin. Inflammation around this demyelinated area causes further dysfunction. Some axonal damage also occurs.[43,44]

The myelin sheath of the peripheral nerves is generated by Schwann cells and acts as an insulator for the peripheral nerve. Myelin promotes rapid conduction of nerve impulses by allowing the impulses to jump along the nerve by means of the nodes of Ranvier. Disruption of the myelin fiber slows and may eventually stop the conduction of impulses along the peripheral nerves. In GBS, the more thickly myelinated fibers of motor pathways and the cranial nerves are more severely affected than are the thinly myelinated sensory fibers of cutaneous pain, touch, and temperature.[6]

After the temporary inflammatory reaction stops, myelin-producing cells begin the process of reinsulating the demyelinated portions of the peripheral nervous system. When remyelination occurs, normal neurologic function should return. In some instances, the axon may be damaged during the inflammatory process. The degree of axonal damage is responsible for the degree of neurologic dysfunction that persists after recovery.[43]

ASSESSMENT AND DIAGNOSIS

Symptoms of GBS include motor weakness, paresthesias and other sensory changes, cranial nerve dysfunction (especially oculomotor, facial, glossopharyngeal, vagal, spinal accessory, and hypoglossal), and some autonomic dysfunction. The usual course of GBS begins with an abrupt onset of lower extremity weakness that progresses to flaccidity and ascends over a period of hours to days. Motor loss usually is symmetric, bilateral, and ascending. In the most severe cases, complete flaccidity of all peripheral nerves, including spinal and cranial nerves, occurs.[6]

The patient is admitted to the hospital when lower extremity weakness prevents mobility. Admission to the critical care unit is necessary when progression of the weakness threatens respiratory muscles. As the patient's weakness progresses, close observation is essential. Frequent assessment of the respiratory system, including ventilatory parameters such as inspiratory force and tidal volume, is necessary. The most common cause of death of patients with GBS is respiratory arrest. As the disease progresses and respiratory effort weakens, intubation and mechanical ventilation are necessary. Frequent assessment of neurologic deterioration is continued until the patient reaches the peak of the disease, and a plateau occurs.[46]

The diagnosis of GBS is based on clinical findings plus CSF analysis and nerve conduction studies. The diagnostic finding is elevated CSF protein with normal cell count.[46] The increased protein count usually occurs after the first week but does not occur in approximately 10% of all cases. Nerve conduction studies that test the velocity at which nerve impulses are conducted show significant reduction, as the demyelinating process of the disease suggests.

MEDICAL MANAGEMENT

With no curative treatment available, the medical management of GBS is limited. The disease must run its course, which is characterized by ascending paralysis that advances over 1 to 3 weeks and then remains at a plateau for 2 to 4 weeks.[46] The plateau stage is followed by descending paralysis and return to normal or near-normal function. The main focus of medical management is the support of bodily functions and the prevention of complications.

Plasmapheresis and intravenous immune globulin (IVIG) are used to treat GBS.[43,44,46] They have been shown to be equally effective.[47] Plasmapheresis involves the removal of venous blood through a catheter, separation of plasma from blood cells, and reinfusion of the cells plus autologous plasma or another replacement solution. Although the number of exchanges may vary, four to six exchanges usually are performed over a 5- to 8-day period.[43]

NURSING MANAGEMENT

The nursing management of the patient with GBS incorporates a variety of nursing diagnoses and interventions (see the Nursing Diagnoses feature on Guillain-Barré syndrome). The goal of nursing management is to support all normal body functions until the patient can do so on his or her own. Although the condition is reversible, the patient with GBS requires extensive long-term care, because recovery can be a long process. Nursing priorities are directed toward maintaining surveillance for complications, initiating rehabilitation, facilitating nutritional support, and providing comfort and emotional support.

Nursing Diagnoses

Guillain-Barré Syndrome

- Ineffective Breathing Pattern related to musculoskeletal fatigue or neuromuscular impairment
- Acute Pain related to transmission and perception of cutaneous, visceral, muscular, or ischemic impulses
- Activity Intolerance related to prolonged immobility or deconditioning
- Risk for Aspiration
- Imbalanced Nutrition: Less Than Body Requirements related to lack of exogenous nutrients or increased metabolic demand
- Risk for Infection
- Anxiety related to threat of biologic, psychological, or social integrity
- Powerlessness related to lack of control over current situation or disease progression
- Ineffective Coping related to situational crisis and personal vulnerability
- Compromised Family Coping related to critically ill family member
- Deficient Knowledge: Discharge Regimen related to lack of previous exposure to information (see the Patient Education feature on Guillain-Barré Syndrome)

Patient Education: Guillain-Barré Syndrome

- Pathophysiology of disease
- Importance of taking medications
- Measures to compensate for residual deficits
- Basic rehabilitation techniques
- Importance of participating in neurologic rehabilitation program, if necessary

BOX 28-7   COLLABORATIVE MANAGEMENT: GUILLAIN-BARRÉ SYNDROME

- Support bodily functions.
  - Protect airway.
  - Provide ventilatory assistance, as required.
- Initiate treatments to limit duration of the syndrome.
  - Plasmapheresis
  - Intravenous immunoglobulin
- Initiate nutritional support.
- Maintain surveillance for complications.
  - Infections
  - Cardiac dysrhythmias
  - Blood pressure alterations
  - Temperature alterations
- Provide comfort and emotional support.
- Design and implement appropriate rehabilitation program.
- Educate patient and family.

Maintaining Surveillance for Complications. Continuous assessment of the progressive paralysis associated with GBS is essential to timely intervention and the prevention of respiratory arrest and further neurologic insult. After the patient is intubated and placed on mechanical ventilation, close observation for pulmonary complications, such as atelectasis, pneumonia, and pneumothorax, is necessary. Autonomic dysfunction (dysautonomia) in the GBS patient can produce variations in heart rate and blood pressure that can reach extreme values.[48,49] Hypertension and tachycardia may require beta-blocker therapy. All GBS patients must be observed for this phenomenon.

Initiating Rehabilitation. In patients with GBS, immobility may last for months. The usual course of GBS involves an average of 10 days of symptom progression and 10 days of maximal level of dysfunction, followed by 2 to 48 weeks of recovery. Although GBS usually is completely reversible, the patient will require physical and occupational rehabilitation because of the problems of long-term immobility. Rehabilitation starts in the critical care area, with a multidisciplinary team designing and implementing an individualized plan for maximizing the patient's potential for rehabilitation.

Facilitating Nutritional Support. Nutritional support is implemented early in the course of the disease. Because GBS recovery is a long process, adequate nutritional support will be a problem for an extended period. Nutritional support usually is accomplished through the use of enteral feeding.

Providing Comfort and Emotional Support. Pain control is another important component in the care of the patient with GBS. Although patients may have minimal to no motor function, most sensory functions remain, causing patients considerable muscle aching and pain. Because of the length of this illness, a safe, effective, long-term solution to pain management must be identified. These patients also require extensive psychological support. Although the illness is almost 100% reversible, lack of control over the situation, constant pain or discomfort, and the long-term nature of the disorder create coping difficulties

for the patient. GBS does not affect the level of consciousness or cerebral function. Patient interaction and communication are essential elements of the nursing management plan.

Patient Education. Early in the patient's hospital stay, the patient and family must be taught about GBS and its different treatments (see the Patient Education feature on Guillain-Barré syndrome). As the patient moves toward discharge, teaching focuses on the interventions to maximize the patient's rehabilitation potential. The patient's family must be encouraged to participate in the patient's care and to learn some basic rehabilitation techniques. The importance of participating in a neurologic rehabilitation program (if necessary) must be stressed. Collaborative management of the patient with Guillain-Barré syndrome is outlined in Box 28-7.

CRANIOTOMY

TYPES OF SURGERY

A craniotomy is performed to gain access to portions of the central nervous system (CNS) inside the cranium, usually to allow removal of a space-occupying lesion such as a brain tumor (Table 28-5). Common procedures include tumor resection or removal, cerebral decompression, evacuation of hematoma or abscess, and clipping or removal of an aneurysm or AVM. Most patients who undergo craniotomy for tumor resection or removal do not require care in a critical care unit. Patients who do usually need intensive monitoring or are at greater risk for complications

TABLE 28-5 Tumor Types and Characteristics

Tumor	Clinical Features	Treatment/Prognosis
Glioblastoma multiforme	Often manifests with nonspecific complaints and increased ICP As tumor grows, focal deficits develop	Rapidly progressive course, with poor prognosis Total surgical removal usually not possible; response to radiation poor
Astrocytoma	Presentation similar to GM, but course more protracted, often over several years; cerebellar astrocytoma, especially in children, may have more benign course	Variable prognosis By diagnosis, total excision usually impossible; tumor often not radiosensitive In cerebellar astrocytoma, total excision often possible
Medulloblastoma	Glioma most often seen in children Usually arises from roof of fourth ventricle and leads to increased ICP, with brainstem and cerebellar signs; may seed subarachnoid space	Treatment consists of surgery with radiation therapy and chemotherapy
Ependymoma	Glioma arising from ependyma of ventricle, especially fourth; leads early to signs of increased ICP; arises also from central canal of spinal cord	Tumor not radiosensitive and best treated surgically, if possible
Oligodendroglioma	Slow-growing glioma, usually arises in cerebral hemisphere in adults Calcification may be visible on radiograph	Treatment is surgical and usually successful
Brainstem glioma	Manifests in childhood with cranial nerve palsies, then long-tract signs in limbs; signs of increased ICP occur late in course	Tumor is inoperable Treatment with irradiation and with shunt for increased ICP
Cerebellar hemangioblastoma	Manifests with disequilibrium, ataxia of trunk or limbs, and signs of increased ICP; sometimes familial; may be associated with retinal and spinal lesions, polycythemia, and hypernephroma	Treatment is surgical
Pineal tumor	Manifests with increased ICP, sometimes associated with impaired upward gaze (Parinaud's syndrome) and other deficits indicating midbrain lesion	Ventricular decompression by shunting, followed by surgical approach to tumor Irradiation if tumor malignant Prognosis depends on histopathologic findings and tumor extent
Craniopharyngioma	Originates from remnants of Rathke's pouch above sella turcica, depressing optic chiasm May manifest at any age but usually in childhood with endocrine dysfunction and bitemporal field deficits	Treatment is surgical, but total removal may not be possible
Acoustic neuroma	Most common initial symptom is ipsilateral hearing loss; subsequent symptoms may include tinnitus, headache, vertigo, facial weakness or numbness, and long-tract signs May be familial and bilateral when related to neurofibromatosis Most sensitive screening tests are MRI and brainstem AEP	Treatment is by excision using a translabyrinthine approach, craniectomy, or combination Prognosis usually good
Meningioma	Originates from dura mater or arachnoid; compresses rather than invades adjacent neural structures Increasingly common with advancing age Tumor size varies greatly; symptoms vary with tumor site* Tumor usually benign; readily detected by CT; may lead to calcification and bone erosion visible on plain skull radiographs	Treatment is surgical Tumor may recur if removal is incomplete; patient may receive irradiation with incomplete excision to decrease risk of recurrence
Primary central lymphoma	Associated with AIDS and other immunodeficiency states May manifest with focal deficits or disturbances of cognition and consciousness; may be indistinguishable from cerebral toxoplasmosis	Treatment is by whole-brain irradiation Chemotherapy may have adjunctive role Prognosis depends on CD4 cell count at diagnosis

From Gawlinski A, Hamwi D, editors: *Acute care nurse practitioner: clinical curriculum and certification review*, Philadelphia, 1999, Saunders.
AEP, auditory-evoked potential; AIDS, acquired immunodeficiency syndrome; CT, computed tomography; GM, glioblastoma multiforme; ICP, intracranial pressure; MRI, magnetic resonance imaging.
*For example, unilateral exophthalmos (sphenoidal ridge), anosmia, and optic nerve compression (olfactory groove).

BOX 28-8 OPERATIVE TERMS

- *Burr hole:* hole made into the cranium using a special drill
- *Craniotomy:* surgical opening of the skull
- *Craniectomy:* removal of a portion of the skull without replacing it
- *Cranioplasty:* plastic repair of the skull
- *Supratentorial:* above the tentorium, separating the cerebrum from the cerebellum
- *Infratentorial:* below the tentorium; includes the brainstem and the cerebellum; an infratentorial surgical approach may be used for temporal or occipital lesions

because of underlying cardiopulmonary dysfunction or the surgical approach used. Box 28-8 provides definitions of common neurosurgical terms.[50]

PREOPERATIVE CARE

Protection of the integrity of the CNS is a major priority of care for the patient awaiting a craniotomy. Optimal arterial oxygenation, hemodynamic stability, and cerebral perfusion are essential for maintaining adequate cerebral oxygenation. Management of seizure activity is essential for controlling metabolic needs.

Detailed assessment and documentation of the patient's preoperative neurologic status are imperative for accurate postoperative evaluation. Attention is focused on identifying and describing the nature and extent of any preoperative neurologic deficits. When pituitary surgery is planned, a thorough evaluation of endocrine function is necessary to prevent major intraoperative and postoperative complications.[51]

Trends in health care demand judicious use of routine preoperative studies. Depending on the type of surgery to be performed and the general health of the patient, preoperative screening may include a complete blood cell count (CBC); tests for blood urea nitrogen (BUN), creatinine, and fasting blood sugar (FBS); a chest radiograph, and an electrocardiogram. A blood type and crossmatch may also be ordered.[52]

Preoperative teaching is necessary to prepare the patient and family for what to expect in the postoperative period. A description of the intravascular lines and intracranial catheters used during the postoperative period allows the family to focus on the patient, rather than be overwhelmed by masses of tubing. Some or all of the patient's hair is shaved off in the operating room, and a large, bulky, turban-like craniotomy dressing is applied. Most patients experience some degree of postoperative eye or facial swelling and periorbital ecchymosis. An explanation of these temporary changes in appearance helps alleviate the shock and fear many patients and families experience in the immediate postoperative period.

All craniotomy patients require instruction to avoid activities known to provoke sudden changes in ICP. These activities include bending, lifting, straining, and the Valsalva maneuver. Patients commonly elicit the Valsalva maneuver during repositioning in bed by holding their breath and straining with a closed epiglottis. Teaching the patient to continue to breathe deeply through the mouth during all position changes is an effective deterrent.

The patient undergoing transsphenoidal surgery requires preparation for the sensations associated with nasal packing. The patient often awakens with alarm because of the inability to breathe through the nose. Preoperative instruction in mouth breathing and avoidance of coughing, sneezing, or blowing of the nose facilitates postoperative cooperation.

The psychosocial issues associated with the prospect of neurosurgery cannot be overemphasized. Few procedures are as threatening as those involving the brain or spinal cord. For some patients, the fear of permanent neurologic impairment may be as or more ominous than the fear of death. Steps to meet the needs of the patient and the family include collaboration with clergy and social services personnel, patient-controlled visitation, and provision of as much privacy as the patient's condition permits. The patient and family must be provided with the opportunity to express their fears and concerns jointly and apart from each other.[50]

SURGICAL CONSIDERATIONS

Whereas the emphasis in the surgical approach for most other types of surgery is to gain adequate exposure of the surgical site, the neurosurgeon must select a route that also produces the least amount of disruption to the intracranial contents. Neural tissue is unforgiving. A significant portion of neurologic trauma and postoperative deficits is related to the surgical pathway through the brain tissue, rather than to the procedure performed at the site of pathology. Depending on the location of the lesion and the surgical route chosen, a transcranial or a transsphenoidal approach is used to open the skull.

Transcranial Approach. In the transcranial approach, a scalp incision is made, and a series of burr holes is drilled into the skull to form an outline of the area to be opened (Fig. 28-6). A special saw is then used to cut between the holes. In most cases, the bone flap is left attached to the muscle to create a hinge effect. In some cases, the bone flap is removed completely and placed in the abdomen for later retrieval and implantation or discarded and replaced with synthetic material. Next, the dura is opened and retracted. After the intracranial procedure, the dura and the bone flap are closed, the muscles and scalp are sutured, and a turban-like dressing is applied.[50]

Transsphenoidal Approach. The transsphenoidal approach is the technique of choice for removal of a pituitary tumor without extension into the intracranial vault (Fig. 28-7).[51] This approach involves making a microsurgical entrance into the cranial vault through the nasal cavity. The sphenoid sinus is entered to reach the anterior wall of the sella turcica. The sphenoid bone and the dura are then opened to gain intracranial access. After removal of the tumor, the surgical bed is packed with a small section of adipose tissue grafted from the patient's abdomen or thigh. After closure of the intranasal structures, nasal splints and soft packing or nasal tampons impregnated with antibiotic ointment are placed in the nasal cavities. Occasionally, epistaxis balloons are used instead. A nasal drip pad or mustache-type dressing is placed at the base of the nose to catch surgical drainage.[50]

The patient may be placed in a supine, prone, or sitting position for a craniotomy procedure. A skull clamp connected to

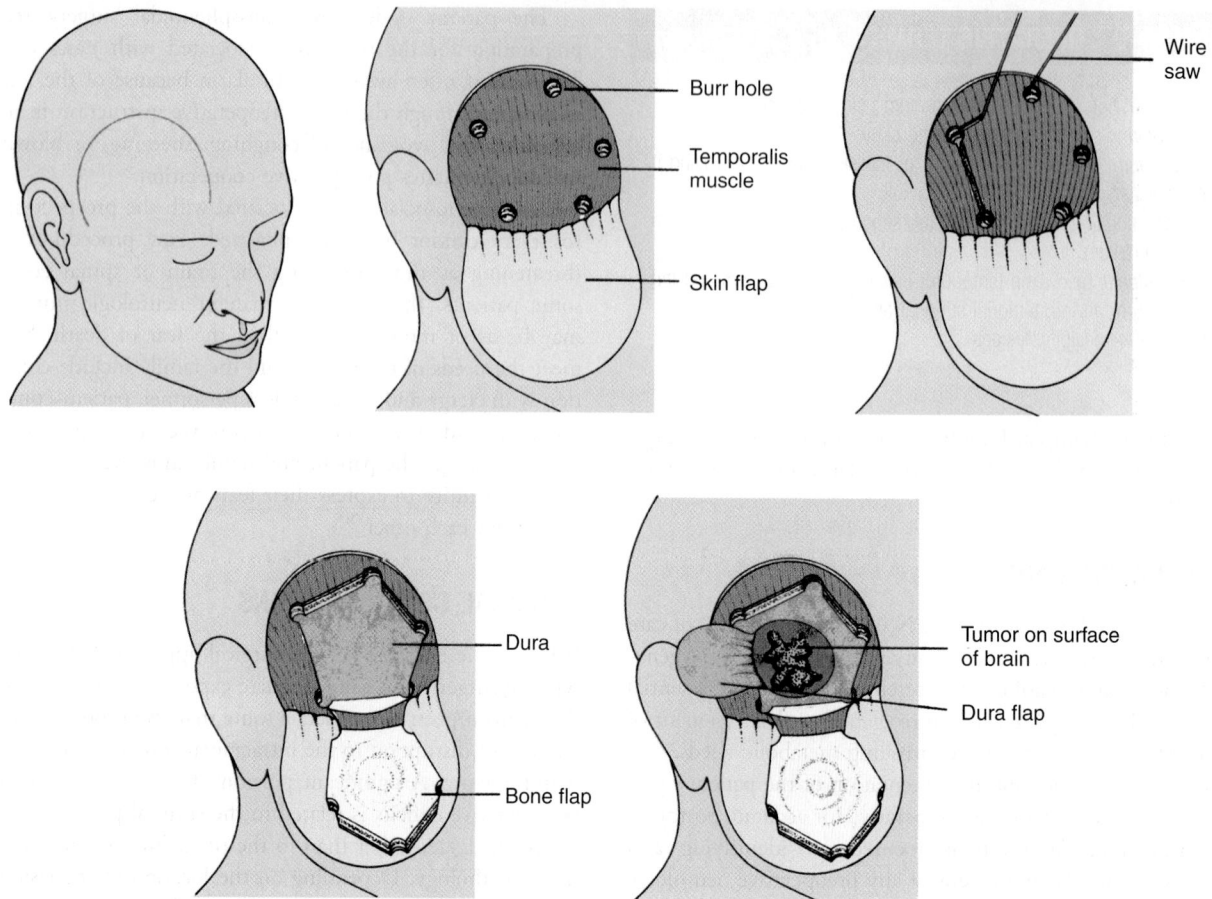

Figure 28-6 Craniotomy. *(From Beare PG, Myers JL: Principles and practice of adult health nursing, ed 2, St Louis, 1994, Mosby.)*

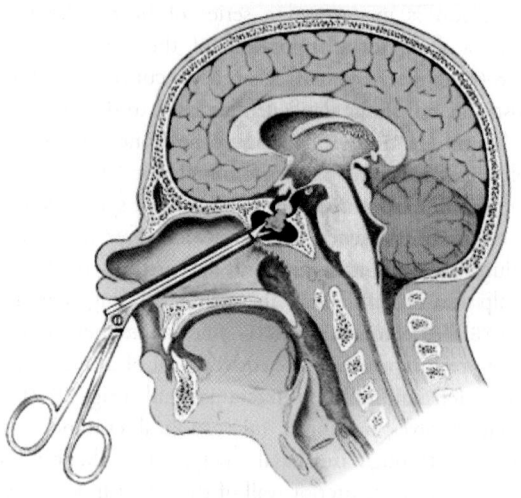

Figure 28-7 Transsphenoidal hypophysectomy.

skull pins is used to position and secure the patient's head throughout the operation. During a transsphenoidal approach or a transcranial approach into the infratentorial area, the patient's head is elevated during surgery. This position places the patient at risk for an air embolism. Air can enter the vascular system through the edges of the dura or a venous opening. Continuous monitoring of the patient's heart sounds by

Doppler signal allows immediate recognition of this complication. If it occurs, an attempt may be made to withdraw the embolus from the right atrium through a central line. Flooding the surgical field with irrigation fluid and placing a moistened sterile surgical sponge over the surgical site creates an immediate barrier to any further air entrance.[50]

POSTOPERATIVE MEDICAL MANAGEMENT

Definitive management of the postoperative neurosurgical patient varies, depending on the underlying reason for the craniotomy. During the initial postoperative period, management is usually directed toward the prevention of complications. Complications associated with a craniotomy include intracranial hypertension, surgical hemorrhage, fluid imbalance, CSF leak, and DVT.

Intracranial Hypertension. Postoperative cerebral edema is expected to peak 48 to 72 hours after surgery. If the bone flap is not replaced at the time of surgery, intracranial hypertension will produce bulging at the surgical site. Close monitoring of the surgical site is important so that integrity of the incision can be maintained. Postcraniotomy management of intracranial hypertension is usually accomplished through CSF drainage, patient positioning, and steroid administration.[5]

Surgical Hemorrhage. Surgical hemorrhage after a transcranial procedure can occur in the intracranial vault and is manifested by signs and symptoms of increasing ICP.

Hemorrhage after a transsphenoidal craniotomy may be evident from external drainage, the patient's complaint of persistent postnasal drip, or excessive swallowing. Loss of vision after pituitary surgery indicates an evolving hemorrhage. Postoperative hemorrhage requires surgical reexploration.[51]

Fluid Imbalance. Fluid imbalance in the postcraniotomy patient usually results from a disturbance in production or secretion of antidiuretic hormone (ADH). ADH is secreted by the posterior pituitary (neurohypophysis) gland. It stimulates the renal tubules and collecting ducts to retain water in response to low circulating blood volume or increased serum osmolality. Inoperative trauma or postoperative edema of the pituitary gland or hypothalamus can result in insufficient ADH secretion. The outcome is unabated renal water loss even when blood volume is low and serum osmolality is high. This condition is known as *diabetes insipidus* (DI). The polyuria associated with DI is often more than 200 mL/hour. Urine specific gravity of 1.005 or less and elevated serum osmolality provide evidence of insufficient ADH. The loss of volume may provoke hypotension and inadequate cerebral perfusion. DI is usually self-limiting, and fluid replacement is the only required therapy. In some cases, however, it may be necessary to administer vasopressin intravenously to control the loss of fluid.[5]

The syndrome of inappropriate antidiuretic hormone (SIADH) commonly occurs with neurologic insult and results from excessive ADH secretion. SIADH is manifested by inappropriate water retention with hyponatremia in the presence of normal renal function. Urine specific gravity is elevated, and urine osmolality is greater than serum osmolality. The dangers associated with SIADH include circulating volume overload and electrolyte imbalance, both of which may impair neurologic functioning. SIADH is usually self-limiting, with the mainstay of treatment being fluid restriction.[5]

Cerebrospinal Fluid Leak. Leakage of CSF results from an opening in the subarachnoid space, as evidenced by clear fluid draining from the surgical site. When this complication occurs after transsphenoidal surgery, it is evidenced by excessive, clear drainage from the nose or persistent postnasal drip. To differentiate CSF drainage from postoperative serous drainage, a specimen is tested for glucose content. A CSF leak is confirmed by glucose values of 30 mg/dL or greater. Management of the patient with a CSF leak includes bed rest and head elevation. Lumbar puncture or placement of a lumbar subarachnoid catheter may be used to reduce CSF pressure until the dura heals. The risk of meningitis associated with CSF leak often necessitates surgical repair to reseal the opening.[5,51]

Deep Vein Thrombosis. DVT occurs in 29% to 46% of all neurosurgical patients, compared with a 25% incidence among general surgical patients. Early research demonstrated a greater risk after removal of a supratentorial tumor and a twofold risk in patients whose surgery lasted for more than 4 hours.[52] Research has demonstrated numerous additional risk factors significantly associated with DVT development: preoperative leg weakness, longer preoperative critical care unit stay, longer recovery room time, longer postoperative critical care unit stay, more days on bed rest, and delay of postoperative mobility and activity.[53] Clinical manifestations of

DVT include leg or calf pain, edema, localized tenderness, and pain with dorsiflexion or plantar flexion (Homans' sign). Unfortunately, the patient with a DVT is often asymptomatic, and the diagnosis is not made until the patient experiences a pulmonary embolus.

The primary treatment for DVT is prophylaxis (see the Evidence-Based Practice feature on Deep Vein Thrombosis Prevention). In the neurosurgery patient, sequential (intermittent) pneumatic compression boots or stockings are effective in reducing the incidence of DVT. Effectiveness is enhanced when these devices are initiated in the preoperative period. Low-dose unfractionated heparin or low-molecular-weight heparin may also be used prophylactically in high-risk patients.[34]

POSTOPERATIVE NURSING MANAGEMENT

The nursing management of the neurosurgical patient incorporates a variety of nursing diagnoses (see the Nursing Diagnoses feature on Craniotomy). As in preoperative care, the primary goal of postcraniotomy nursing management is protection of the integrity of the CNS. Nursing interventions are directed toward preserving adequate CPP, promoting arterial oxygenation, providing comfort and emotional support, maintaining surveillance for complications, and initiating early rehabilitation. Frequent neurologic assessment is necessary to evaluate accomplishment of these objectives and to identify problems and quickly intervene if complications do arise. Often, a ventriculostomy is placed to facilitate ICP monitoring and CSF drainage.

Preserving Adequate Cerebral Perfusion. Nursing interventions to preserve cerebral perfusion include patient positioning, fluid management, and avoidance of postoperative vomiting and fever.

Positioning. Patient positioning is an important component of care for the craniotomy patient. The head of the bed should be elevated 30 to 45 degrees at all times to reduce the incidence of hemorrhage, facilitate venous drainage, and control ICP. Other positioning measures to control ICP include maintaining the patient's head in a neutral position at all times and avoiding neck or hip flexion. These rules of positioning must be followed throughout all nursing activities, including linen changes and transporting the patient for diagnostic evaluation. Most craniotomy patients can be turned from side to side within these restrictions, using pillows for support, except in some cases of extensive tumor removal, cranioplasty, and when the bone flap is not replaced. Specific orders from the surgeon must be obtained in these instances. The patient with an infratentorial incision may be restricted to only a very small pillow under the head to prevent strain on the incision. Avoidance of anterior or lateral neck flexion also protects the integrity of this type of incision.

Fluid Management. Fluid management is another important component of postcraniotomy care. Hourly monitoring of fluid intake and output facilitates early identification of fluid imbalance. Urine specific gravity must be measured if DI is suspected. Fluid restriction may be ordered as a routine measure to lessen the severity of cerebral edema or as treatment for the fluid and electrolyte imbalances associated with SIADH.

Evidence-Based Practice: Collaborative

American Association of Critical-Care Nurses Practice Alert: Deep Vein Thrombosis Prevention

Expected Practice

- Assess all patients on admission to the intensive care unit (ICU) for risk factors of deep vein thrombosis (DVT) and anticipate orders for DVT prophylaxis based on the risk assessment. Clinical eligibility and regimens for DVT prophylaxis include

  Moderate-risk patients, including medically ill and postoperative patients, may be placed on low-dose unfractionated heparin or low-molecular-weight heparin (LMWH).

  Higher-risk patients, including major trauma or orthopedic surgery patients, may be placed on LMWH.

  Patients at high risk for bleeding may be placed on mechanical prophylaxis, including graduated compression stockings or intermittent pneumatic compression devices.

  Mechanical prophylaxis may also be anticipated in conjunction with anticoagulant-based prophylaxis regimens.

- Review daily with the physician and during multidisciplinary rounds each patient's current DVT risk factors, including clinical status, necessity for a central venous catheter (CVC), current status of DVT prophylaxis, risk for bleeding, and response to treatment.
- Maximize patient mobility whenever possible, and take measures to reduce the amount of time the patient is immobile because of the effects of treatment (e.g., pain, sedation, neuromuscular blockade, mechanical ventilation).
- Ensure that mechanical prophylaxis devices are fitted properly and in use at all times, except when being removed for cleaning or inspection of skin.

Supporting Evidence

- Multiple medical and surgical risk factors leading to DVT formation have been identified.[1] Iatrogenic risk factors for DVT include immobilization, sedation or neuromuscular blockade, CVCs, surgery, sepsis, mechanical ventilation, vasopressor administration, heart failure, stroke, malignancy, previous DVT, and renal dialysis; most patients in critical care units have one or more major risk factors.[1-4] In five prospective studies, the rate of DVT in patients in critical care not receiving prophylaxis ranged from 13% to 31%.[5-8] Because signs and symptoms of DVT are frequently silent and can lead to fatal pulmonary embolism, the Agency for Healthcare Research and Quality (AHRQ) and American College of Chest Physicians (ACCP) recommend DVT prophylaxis for at-risk patients.[1,9-17]
- Randomized trials indicate that low-dose unfractionated heparin and LMWH are efficacious in preventing DVT in moderate-risk critical care patients.[5-8,18] For patients at higher risk, such as those who have major trauma or have had orthopedic surgery, LMWH has been shown to provide superior protection over low-dose unfractionated heparin.[1] Direct thrombin inhibitors can be used in place of low-molecular-weight heparin or unfractionated heparin for patients with documented or suspected heparin-induced thrombocytopenia.[1,19,20] Numerous studies suggest that aspirin alone is not an effective means of DVT prophylaxis for any patient group.[21-25]
- Although examined less rigorously than anticoagulant based methods, mechanical methods of prophylaxis (e.g., graduated compression stockings, intermittent compression devices, venous foot pumps) have been shown to reduce the risk of DVT.[26-36] One study involving non–lower extremity trauma patients compared the efficacy of intermittent

pneumatic compression devices and venous foot pumps. DVT rates for the venous foot pump group were three times greater than the rates for the intermittent pneumatic compression group. The researchers concluded that intermittent pneumatic compression devices provided superior prophylaxis in this patient population.[34]

- Mechanical prophylaxis usually is less efficacious compared with anticoagulation-based therapy.[31-33,35,36] Reduction in risk of death or pulmonary embolism has not been attributed to mechanical methods of prophylaxis.[1] In one study involving below-the-knee graded stockings, 98% of commercially available stockings failed to produce an ideal pressure gradient, and 54% were found to produce a dangerous reverse pressure gradient.[37] Mechanical prophylaxis methods are a desirable option because they do not pose bleeding concerns.[1] A combination of mechanical prophylaxis and chemoprophylaxis is thought to potentiate overall efficacy, but this combination has not been tested in the critical care setting.[3]
- Written policies for DVT prophylaxis in conjunction with preprinted or computerized ICU admission orders have been shown to increase compliance with prophylaxis measures.[39] One study found that implementation of a daily goals form, which included DVT prophylaxis in the ICU, resulted in a significant improvement in the percentage of residents and nurses who understood the patient's daily goals for care and decreased ICU length of stay by 1.1 days.[40]
- The presence of a CVC is an independent risk factor for upper extremity DVT in the general population.[41]
- Several studies involving a variety of patient populations with diagnostically confirmed DVT have identified immobility as a comorbidity or independent risk factor.[42-44]
- Improperly fitted graduated compression stockings producing a reversed pressure gradient were associated with a statistically significantly higher incidence of DVT compared with stockings that produced a proper gradient.[35] Studies evaluating compliance with intermittent pneumatic compression devices demonstrated rates of noncompliance ranging from 22% to 81% among at-risk patients.[37,45-46]

What You Should Do

- Ensure that your unit has a written policy for DVT prophylaxis that is updated regularly to reflect emerging evidentiary findings in addition to preprinted or computerized ICU admission orders.
- Ensure that your unit has an organized process for developing and communicating patient goals (which include DVT prophylaxis) to members of the multidisciplinary team.
- Establish a process to educate and routinely evaluate all staff in the use of mechanical prophylaxis devices.
- Review orders of patients discharged from the ICU to ensure that transfer orders include a plan for DVT prophylaxis.
- Monitor your unit's compliance with DVT prophylaxis policies and rates of DVT and pulmonary embolism. Initiate quality improvement initiatives involving a multidisciplinary team as necessary.

Need More Information or Help?

- Talk with a clinical practice specialist for additional information or assistance at www.aacn.org.

References

1. Geerts WH et al: Prevention of venous thromboembolism: the seventh ACCP conference on antithrombotic and thrombolytic therapy, *Chest* 126(suppl): 338S-400S, 2004.
2. Geerts W et al: Venous thromboembolism and its prevention in critical care, *J Crit Care* 17:95-104, 2002.
3. Cook D et al: Venous thromboembolic disease: an observational study in medical-surgical intensive care unit patients, *J Crit Care* 15,127-132, 2000.
4. Cook DJ et al: Deep venous thrombosis in medical-surgical ICU patients: prevalence, incidence and risk factors [abstract], *Crit Care* 7(suppl):S54, 2003.
5. Cade JF: High risk of the critically ill for venous thromboembolism, *Crit Care Med* 10:448-450, 1982.
6. Fraisse F et al: Nadroparin in the prevention of deep vein thrombosis in acute decompensated COPD, *Am J Respir Crit Care Med* 161:1109-1114, 2000.
7. Kapoor M et al: Subcutaneous heparin prophylaxis significantly reduces the incidence of venous thromboembolic events in the critically ill [abstract], *Crit Care Med* 27(suppl):A69, 1999.
8. Goldhaber SZ et al: Low molecular weight heparin versus minidose unfractionated heparin for prophylaxis against venous thromboembolism in medical intensive care unit patients: a randomized controlled trial [abstract], *J Am Coll Cardiol* 35(suppl):325A, 2000.
9. Lindblad B et al: Autopsy-verified pulmonary embolism in a surgical department: analysis of the period from 1951 to 1968, *Br J Surg* 78:849-852, 1991.
10. Sandler DA, Martin JF: Autopsy proven pulmonary embolism in hospital patients: are we detecting enough deep vein thrombosis? *J R Soc Med* 82:203-205, 1989.
11. Geerts WH et al: Prevention of venous thromboembolism, *Chest* 119 (suppl):132S-175S, 2001.
12. Prevention of fatal pulmonary embolism by low doses of heparin: International Multicentre Trial, *Lancet* 2:45-51, 1975.
13. Sevitt S, Gallagher NG: Prevention of venous thrombosis and pulmonary embolism in injured patients: a trial of anticoagulant prophylaxis with phenindione in middle-aged and elderly patients with fractured necks of femur, *Lancet* 2:981-989, 1959.
14. Sagar S et al: Low-dose heparin prophylaxis against fatal pulmonary embolism, *BMJ* 2:257-259, 1975.
15. Halkin H et al: Reduction of mortality in general medical inpatients by low-dose heparin prophylaxis, *Ann Intern Med* 96:561-565, 1982.
16. Collins R et al: Reduction in fatal pulmonary embolism and venous thrombosis by perioperative administration of subcutaneous heparin: overview of results of randomized trials in general, orthopedic, and urologic surgery, *N Engl J Med* 318:1162-1173, 1988.
17. Agency for Healthcare Research and Quality: Making health care safer: a critical analysis of patient safety practices. Evidence Report/Technology Assessment No. 43. Available at www.ahrq.gov/clinic/ptsafety (accessed September 2006).
18. Iorio A, Agnelli G: Low-molecular-weight and unfractionated heparin for prevention of venous thromboembolism in neurosurgery: a meta-analysis, *Arch Intern Med* 160:2327-2332, 2000.
19. Heit JA: The potential role of direct thrombin inhibitors in the prevention and treatment of venous thromboembolism, *Chest* 124(suppl):40S-48S, 2003.
20. DiNisio M et al: Direct thrombin inhibitors, *N Engl J Med* 353:1028-1040, 2005.
21. Pulmonary Embolism Prevention Trial: Prevention of pulmonary embolism and deep vein thrombosis with low dose aspirin, *Lancet* 355:1295-1302, 2000.
22. Butterfield WJ et al: Effect of aspirin on postoperative venous thrombosis, *Lancet* 2:441-445, 1972.
23. McKenna R et al: Prevention of venous thromboembolism after total knee replacement by high-dose aspirin or intermittent calf and thigh compression, *BMJ* 280:514-517, 1980.
24. Powers PJ et al: A randomized trial of less intense postoperative warfarin or aspirin therapy in the prevention of venous thromboembolism after surgery for fractured hip, *Arch Intern Med* 149:771-774, 1989.
25. Westrich GH, Sculco TP: Prophylaxis against deep venous thrombosis after total knee arthroplasty: pneumatic planter compression and aspirin compared with aspirin alone, *J Bone Joint Surg Am* 78:826-834, 1996.
26. Coe NP et al: Prevention of deep vein thrombosis in urological patients: a controlled, randomized trial of low-dose heparin and external pneumatic compression boots, *Surgery* 83:230-234, 1978.
27. Turpie AG et al: Prevention of deep vein thrombosis in potential neurosurgical patients: a randomized trial comparing graduated compression stockings alone or graduated compression stockings plus intermittent pneumatic compression with control, *Arch Intern Med* 149:679-681, 1989.
28. Vanek VW: Meta-analysis of effectiveness of intermittent pneumatic compression devices with a comparison of thigh-high to knee-high sleeves, *Am Surg* 64:1050-1058, 1998.
29. Warwick D et al: Comparison of the use of a foot pump with the use of low-molecular-weight heparin for the prevention of deep-vein thrombosis after total hip replacement, *J Bone Joint Surg Am* 80:1158-1166, 1998.
30. Agu O et al: Graduated compression stockings in the prevention of venous thromboembolism, *Br J Surg* 86:992-1004, 1999.
31. Freedman KB et al: A meta-analysis of thromboembolic prophylaxis following elective total hip arthroplasty, *J Bone Joint Surg Am* 82:929-938, 2000.
32. Westrich GH et al: Meta-analysis of thromboembolic prophylaxis after total knee arthroplasty, *J Bone Joint Surg Br* 82:795-800, 2000.
33. Amaragiri SV, Lees TA: Elastic compression stockings for prevention of deep vein thrombosis [abstract]. *Cochrane Database Syst Rev* (3):CD001484, 2000.
34. Elliot CG et al: Calf-thigh sequential pneumatic compression compared with plantar venous pneumatic compression to prevent deep-vein thrombosis after non-lower extremity trauma, *J Trauma* 47(1):25-32, 1999.
35. Hull RD et al: Effectiveness of intermittent pneumatic leg compression for preventing deep vein thrombosis after total hip replacement, *JAMA* 263:2313-2317, 1990.
36. Blanchard J et al: Prevention of deep-vein thrombosis after total knee replacement: randomised comparison between a low-molecular-weight heparin (nadroparin) and mechanical prophylaxis with a foot-pump system, *J Bone Joint Surg Br* 81:654-659, 1999.
37. Best AJ et al: Graded compression stockings in elective orthopaedic surgery: an assessment of the in vivo performance of commercially available stockings in patients having hip and knee arthroplasty, *J Bone Joint Surg Br* 82:116-118, 2000.
38. Geerts WH, Selby R: Prevention of venous thromboembolism in the ICU, *Chest* 124(suppl):357S-363S, 2003.
39. Levi D et al: Computerized order entry sets and intensive education improve the rate of prophylaxis for deep vein thrombophlebitis [abstract], *Chest* 114 (suppl):280S, 1998.
40. Pronovost P et al: Improving communication in the ICU using daily goals, *J Crit Care* 18(2):71-75, 2003.
41. Heit JA et al: Risk factors for deep vein thrombosis and pulmonary embolism: a population-based case-control study, *Arch Intern Med* 160:809-815, 2000.
42. Goldhaber SZ, Tapson VF: Prospective registry of 5,451 patients with ultrasound confirmed deep vein thrombosis, *Am J Cardiol* 15;93(2):259-262, 2004.
43. Weill-Engerer S et al: Risk factors for deep vein thrombosis in inpatients aged 65 and older: a case-control multicenter study, *J Am Geriatr Soc* 52(8): 1299-1304, 2004.
44. Landefeld CS et al: Clinical findings associated with acute proximal deep vein thrombosis: a basis for quantifying clinical judgment, *Am J Med* 88(4): 382-388, 1990.
45. Cornwell EE et al: Compliance with sequential compression device prophylaxis in at risk trauma patients: a prospective analysis, *Am Surg* 68:470-473, 2002.
46. Comerota AJ et al: Why does prophylaxis with external pneumatic compression for deep vein thrombosis fail? *Am J Surg* 164:265-268, 1992.

Modified from the American Association of Critical-Care Nurses (AACN): Available at www.AACN.org (accessed April 2009).

Nursing Diagnoses

Craniotomy

- Decreased Intracranial Adaptive Capacity related to failure of normal intracranial compensatory mechanisms
- Ineffective Cerebral Tissue Perfusion related to decreased blood flow
- Ineffective Cerebral Tissue Perfusion related to hemorrhage
- Acute Pain related to transmission and perception of cutaneous, visceral, muscular, or ischemic impulses
- Disturbed Body Image related to actual change in body structure, function, or appearance
- Deficient Knowledge: Discharge Regimen related to lack of previous exposure to information (see the Patient Education feature on Craniotomy)

Vomiting and Fever. Postoperative vomiting must be avoided to prevent sharp spikes in ICP and possibly surgical hemorrhage. Antiemetics are administered as soon as nausea is apparent. Early nutrition in the neurosurgical patient is beneficial. If the patient is unable to eat, enteral hyperalimentation delivered through a feeding tube is the preferred method of nutritional support and can be initiated as early as 24 hours after surgery.[50] Postoperative fever may also adversely affect ICP and increase the metabolic needs of the brain. Acetaminophen is administered orally, rectally, or through a feeding tube. External cooling measures, such as a hypothermia blanket, may be necessary.

Promoting Arterial Oxygenation. Routine pulmonary care is used to maintain airway clearance and prevent pulmonary complications. To prevent dangerous elevations in ICP, this care must be performed using proper technique and at time intervals that are adequately spaced from other patient care activities. If pulmonary complications do arise, consideration must be given to maintaining adequate oxygenation during repositioning. It may be necessary to restrict turning to only the side that places the good lung down.

Providing Comfort and Emotional Support. Pain management in the postcraniotomy patient primarily involves control of headache. Small doses of intravenous morphine are used in the critical care setting. As soon as oral analgesics can be tolerated, acetaminophen with codeine is used. Both analgesics cause constipation. Administration of stool softeners and initiation of a bowel program are important components of postcraniotomy care. Constipation is hazardous, because straining to have a bowel movement can create significant elevations in blood pressure and ICP.

Maintaining Surveillance for Complications. The postoperative neurosurgical patient is at risk for infection, corneal abrasions, and injury from falls or seizures.

Infection. Care of the incision and surgical dressings is specific to the institution and physician. The rule of thumb for a craniotomy dressing is to reinforce it as needed and change it only with a physician's order. Often, a drain is left in place to facilitate decompression of the surgical site. If a ventriculostomy is present, it is treated as a component of the surgical site. All drainage devices must be secured to the dressing to prevent unintentional displacement with patient movement. Sterile technique is required to prevent infection and resultant meningitis.

Corneal Abrasions. Routine eye care may be necessary to prevent corneal drying and ulceration. Periorbital edema interferes with normal blinking and eyelid closure, which are essential to adequate corneal lubrication. Saline drops are instilled every 2 hours. If the patient remains in a coma state, covering the eyes with a polyethylene film extending over the orbits and eyebrows may be beneficial.[13]

Injury. The postcraniotomy patient may experience periods of altered mentation. Protection from injury may require the use of restraint devices. The side rails of the bed must be padded to protect the patient from injury. Having a family member stay at the bedside or use of music therapy is often helpful to keep the patient calm during periods of restlessness. In rare circumstances, neuromuscular blockade and sedation may be necessary to control patient activity and metabolic needs on a short-term basis.

Initiating Early Rehabilitation. Increased activity, including ambulation, is begun as soon as tolerated by the patient in the postoperative period. Rehabilitation measures and discharge planning may begin in the critical care unit but are beyond the scope of this chapter. Transfer to a general care or rehabilitation unit is usually accomplished as soon as the patient is considered to be stable and free of complications.

Patient Education. Preoperatively, the patient and family should be taught about the precipitating event necessitating the need for the craniotomy and its expected outcome (see the Patient Education feature on Craniotomy). The severity of the disease and the need for critical care management postoperatively must be stressed. As the patient moves toward discharge, teaching focuses on medication instructions; incisional care, including the signs of infection; and the signs and symptoms of increased ICP. If the patient has neurologic deficits, teaching focuses on the interventions to maximize the patient's rehabilitation potential, and the patient's family members must be encouraged to participate in the patient's care and to learn some basic rehabilitation techniques. The importance of participating in a neurologic rehabilitation program must be stressed.

Patient Education: Craniotomy

Before Surgery
- Pathophysiology and expected outcome of underlying disease
- Need for intensive care management after surgery
- Routine preoperative surgical care

After Surgery
- Routine postoperative surgical care
- Discharge medications—purpose, dose, and side effects
- Incisional care
- Signs and symptoms of infection
- Signs and symptoms of increased intracranial pressure
- Measures to compensate for residual deficits
- Basic rehabilitation techniques
- Importance of participating in neurologic rehabilitation program

INTRACRANIAL HYPERTENSION

PATHOPHYSIOLOGY

The intracranial space comprises three components: brain substance (80%), CSF (10%), and blood (10%). Under normal physiologic conditions, the mean ICP is maintained below 15 mm Hg.[5,6,22] Essential to understanding the pathophysiology of ICP, the Monro-Kellie hypothesis proposes that an increase in volume of one intracranial component must be compensated by a decrease in one or more of the other components so that total volume remains fixed. This compensation, although limited, includes displacing CSF from the intracranial vault to the lumbar cistern, increasing CSF absorption, and compressing the low-pressure venous system.[54] Pathophysiologic alterations that can elevate ICP are outlined in Table 28-6.

Volume-Pressure Curve. When capable of compliance, the brain can tolerate significant increases in intracranial volume without much increase in ICP. The amount of intracranial compliance, however, does have a limit. After this limit has been reached, a state of decompensation with increased ICP results. As the ICP rises, the relationship between volume and pressure changes, and small increases in volume may cause major elevations in ICP (Fig. 28-8).[28,54] The exact configuration of the volume-pressure curve and the point at which the

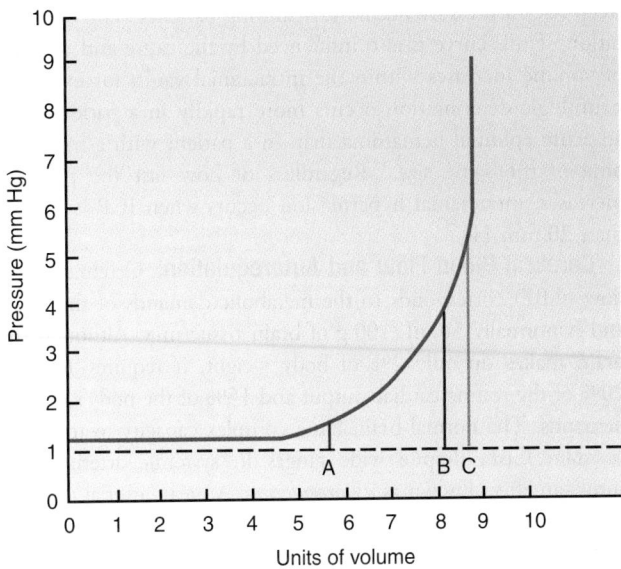

Figure 28-8 Intracranial volume-pressure curve. Pressure is normal (A) and increases in intracranial volume are tolerated without increases in intracranial pressure. Increases in volume (B) may cause increases in pressure. Small increases in volume (C) may cause larger increases in pressure.

TABLE 28-6 Mechanisms of Intracranial Pressure Elevation

Pathophysiology	Example	Treatment
Disorders of CSF Space		
Overproduction of CSF	Choroid plexus papilloma	Diuretics, surgical removal
Communicating hydrocephalus from obstructed arachnoid	Old subarachnoid hemorrhage	Surgical drainage from lumbar drain
Noncommunicative hydrocephalus	Posterior fossa tumor obstructing aqueduct	Surgical drainage by ventricular drain
Interstitial edema	Any of above	Surgical drainage of CSF
Disorders of Intracranial Blood		
Intracranial hemorrhage causing increased ICP	Epidural hematoma	Surgical drainage
Vasospasm	Subarachnoid hemorrhage	Hypervolemia and hypertensive therapy
Vasodilation	Elevated $Paco_2$	Hyperventilation
Increasing cerebral blood volume and ICP	Hypoxia	Adequate oxygenation
Disorders of Brain Substance		
Expanding mass lesion with local vasogenic edema causing increased ICP	Brain tumor	Steroids Surgical removal
Ischemic brain injury with cytotoxic edema increasing ICP	Anoxic brain injury from cardiac or respiratory arrest	Resistant to therapy
Increased cerebral metabolic rate increasing cerebral blood flow and ICP	Seizures, hyperthermia	Anticonvulsant medications to control fever

Modified from Helfaer MA, Kirsch JR: Intracranial vault pathophysiology, *Crit Care Rep* 1:12, 1989.
CSF, cerebrospinal fluid; ICP, intracranial pressure.

steep rise in pressure occurs vary among patients. The configuration of this curve is also influenced by the cause and the rate of volume increases within the intracranial vault; for example, neurologic deterioration occurs more rapidly in a patient with an acute epidural hematoma than in a patient with a meningioma of the same size.[5] Regardless of how fast the pressure increases, intracranial hypertension occurs when ICP is greater than 20 mm Hg.[54]

Cerebral Blood Flow and Autoregulation. Cerebral blood flow (CBF) corresponds to the metabolic demands of the brain and is normally 50 mL/100 g of brain tissue/min. Although the brain makes up only 2% of body weight, it requires 15% to 20% of the resting cardiac output and 15% of the body's oxygen demands. The normal brain has a complex capacity to maintain constant CBF, despite wide ranges in systemic arterial pressure—an effect known as *autoregulation*. A mean arterial pressure of 50 to 150 mm Hg does not alter CBF when autoregulation is functioning. Outside the limits of this autoregulation, CBF becomes passively dependent on the perfusion pressure.[54]

Factors other than arterial blood pressure that affect CBF are conditions that result in acidosis, alkalosis, and changes in metabolic rate. Conditions that cause acidosis (e.g., hypoxia, hypercapnia, ischemia) result in cerebrovascular dilation. Conditions causing alkalosis (e.g., hypocapnia) result in cerebrovascular constriction. Normally, a reduction in metabolic rate (e.g., from hypothermia or barbiturates) decreases CBF, and increases in metabolic rate (e.g., from hyperthermia) increase CBF.[28,55]

Arterial blood gases exert a profound effect on CBF. Carbon dioxide, which affects the pH of the blood, is a potent vasoactive substance. Carbon dioxide retention (hypercapnia) leads to cerebral vasodilation, with increased cerebral blood volume, whereas hypocapnia leads to cerebral vasoconstriction and a reduction in cerebral blood volume. Prolonged hypocapnia, however, especially at an arterial partial pressure of carbon dioxide ($PaCO_2$) level lower than 20 mm Hg, can lead to cerebral ischemia. Low arterial partial pressure of oxygen (PaO_2) levels, especially below 40 mm Hg, lead to cerebral vasodilation, which increases the intracranial blood volume and can contribute to increased ICP. High PaO_2 levels have not been shown to affect CBF in either direction.[6,55]

ASSESSMENT AND DIAGNOSIS

The numerous signs and symptoms of increased ICP include decreased level of consciousness, Cushing's triad (bradycardia, systolic hypertension, and widening pulse pressure), diminished brainstem reflexes, papilledema, decerebrate posturing (abnormal extension), decorticate posturing (abnormal flexion), unequal pupil size, projectile vomiting, decreased pupillary reaction to light, altered breathing patterns, and headache.[28] Patients may exhibit one or all of these symptoms, depending on the underlying cause of the elevation in ICP. One of the earliest and most important signs of increased ICP is a decrease in the level of consciousness. This change must be reported immediately to the physician.[55]

In the patient with suspected intracranial hypertension, a monitoring device may be placed within the cranium to quantify ICP. Under normal physiologic conditions, the mean ICP is maintained below 15 mm Hg. The device is used to monitor serial ICPs and assist with the management of intracranial hypertension. An increase in ICP can decrease blood flow to the brain, causing brain damage. The monitoring device can also provide a sterile access for draining excess CSF. The four sites for monitoring ICP are the intraventricular space, the subarachnoid space, the epidural space, and the parenchyma. Each site has advantages and disadvantages for monitoring ICP. The type of monitor chosen depends on the suspected pathologic condition and the physician's preferences.[55-57] Chapter 27 provides a more detailed discussion of ICP monitoring.

MEDICAL AND NURSING MANAGEMENT

After intracranial hypertension is documented, therapy must be prompt to prevent secondary insults (see the Concept Map on Intracranial Hypertension). Although the exact pressure level denoting intracranial hypertension remains uncertain, most current evidence suggests that ICP generally must be treated when it exceeds 20 mm Hg.[28,55] All therapies are directed toward reducing the volume of one or more of the components (e.g., blood, brain, CSF) that lie within the intracranial vault. A major goal of therapy is to determine the cause of the elevated pressure and, if possible, to remove the cause.[28,55] In the absence of a surgically treatable mass lesion, intracranial hypertension is treated medically. Nurses play an important role in rapid assessment and implementation of appropriate therapies for reducing ICP (see the Nursing Interventions Classification features on Cerebral Perfusion Promotion and Cerebral Edema Management).

Positioning and Other Nursing Activities. Positioning of the patient is a significant factor in the prevention and treatment of intracranial hypertension. Head elevation has long been advocated as a conventional nursing intervention to control ICP, presumably by increasing venous return. However, this may decrease CPP. Close monitoring of ICP and CPP should be done with positioning, customizing positioning to maximize CPP, and minimize ICP.[58]

Positions that impede venous return from the brain cause elevations in ICP. Obstruction of jugular veins or an increase in intrathoracic or intraabdominal pressure is communicated as increased pressure throughout the open venous system, thereby impeding drainage from the brain and increasing ICP. Positions that decrease venous return from the head (e.g., Trendelenburg, prone, extreme flexion of the hips, angulation of the neck) must be avoided if possible. If changes to positions such as Trendelenburg are necessary to provide adequate pulmonary care, critical care nurses must closely monitor ICP and vital signs.[5]

Some routine nursing activities do affect ICP and can be harmful. Use of positive end-expiratory pressures (PEEP) greater than 20 cm H_2O, coughing, suctioning, tight tracheostomy tube ties, and the Valsalva maneuver have been associated with increases in ICP. Cumulative increases in ICP have been reported when care activities are performed one after another. Conversely, family contact and gentle touch have been associated with decreases in ICP.[5,57,59]

Cerebral Perfusion Promotion

Definition
Promotion of adequate perfusion and limitation of complications for a patient experiencing or at risk for inadequate cerebral perfusion

Activities
Consult with physician to determine hemodynamic parameters, and maintain hemodynamic parameters within this range.

Induce hypertension with volume expansion or inotropic or vasoconstrictive agents, as ordered, to maintain hemodynamic parameters and maintain or optimize cerebral perfusion pressure (CPP).

Administer and titrate vasoactive drugs, as ordered, to maintain hemodynamic parameters.

Administer agents to expand intravascular volume, as appropriate (e.g., colloid, blood products, and crystalloid).

Administer volume expanders to maintain hemodynamic parameters, as ordered.

Monitor prothrombin time (PT) and partial thromboplastin time (PTT), if using hetastarch as a volume expander.

Administer rheologic agents (e.g., low-dose mannitol or low-molecular-weight dextrans [LMDs]), as ordered.

Keep hematocrit level around 33% for hypervolemic hemodilution therapy.

Maintain serum glucose level within normal range.

Consult with physician to determine optimal head of bed (HOB) placement (e.g., 0, 15, or 30 degrees) and monitor patient's responses to head positioning.

Avoid neck flexion or extreme hip or knee flexion.

Keep P_{CO_2} level at 25 mm Hg or greater.

Administer calcium channel blockers, as ordered.

Administer vasopressin, as ordered.

Administer and monitor effects of osmotic and loop-active diuretics and corticosteroids.

Administer pain medication, as appropriate.

Administer anticoagulant medication, as ordered.

Administer antiplatelet medications, as ordered.

Administer thrombolytic mediations, as ordered.

Monitor patient's prothrombin time (PT) and partial thromboplastin time (PTT) to keep one to two times normal, as appropriate.

Monitor for anticoagulant therapy side effects

Monitor for signs of bleeding (e.g., test stool and nasogastric tube drainage for blood).

Monitor neurologic status.

Calculate and monitor cerebral perfusion pressure (CPP).

Monitor patient's ICP and neurologic responses to care activities.

Monitor mean arterial pressure (MAP).

Monitor central venous pressure (CVP).

Monitor pulmonary artery occlusion pressure (PAOP) and pulmonary artery pressure (PAP).

Monitor respiratory status (e.g., rate, rhythm, and depth of respirations; P_{O_2}, P_{CO_2}, pH, and bicarbonate levels).

Auscultate lung sounds for crackles or other adventitious sounds.

Monitor for signs of fluid overload (e.g., rhonchi, jugular venous distention [JVD], edema, increase in pulmonary secretions).

Monitor determinants of tissue oxygen delivery (e.g., $Paco_2$, Sao_2, hemoglobin levels, cardiac output), if available.

Monitor laboratory values for changes in oxygenation or acid-base balance, as appropriate.

Monitor intake and output.

From Bulechek GM et al: *Nursing interventions classification (NIC)*, ed 5, 2008, St Louis, Mosby.

Cerebral Edema Management

Definition
Limitation of secondary cerebral injury resulting from swelling of brain tissue

Activities
Monitor for confusion, changes in mentation, complaints of dizziness, and syncope.

Monitor neurologic status closely, and compare with baseline.

Monitor vital signs.

Monitor CSF drainage characteristics: color, clarity, consistency.

Record CSF drainage.

Monitor CVP, PAWP, and PAP, as appropriate.

Monitor ICP and CPP.

Analyze ICP waveform.

Monitor respiratory status: rate, rhythm, and depth of respirations and Pao_2, Pco_2, pH, and bicarbonate levels.

Allow ICP to return to baseline between nursing activities.

Monitor patient's ICP and neurologic responses to care activities.

Decrease stimuli in patient's environment.

Plan nursing care to provide rest periods.

Give sedation, as needed.

Note patient's change in response to stimuli.

Screen conversation within patient's hearing.

Administer anticonvulsants, as appropriate.

Avoid neck flexion or extreme hip or knee flexion.

Avoid Valsalva maneuver.

Administer stool softeners.

Position with head of bed up 30 degrees or greater.

Avoid use of PEEP.

Administer paralyzing agent, as appropriate.

Encourage family or significant other to talk to patient.

Restrict fluids.

Avoid use of hypotonic IV fluids.

Adjust ventilator settings to keep $Paco_2$ at prescribed level.

Limit suction passes to less than 15 seconds.

Monitor laboratory values: serum and urine osmolality, sodium, and potassium.

Monitor volume pressure indices.

Perform passive range-of-motion exercises.

Monitor intake and output.

Maintain normothermia.

Administer loop-active or osmotic diuretics.

Implement seizure precautions.

Titrate barbiturate to achieve suppression or burst-suppression of EEG, as ordered.

Establish means of communication: ask yes or no questions, and provide magic slate, paper and pencil, picture board, flashcards, and VOCAID device.

CPP, cerebral perfusion pressure; CSF, cerebrospinal fluid; CVP, central venous pressure; EEG, electroencephalogram; ICP, intracranial pressure; IV, intravenous; PAP, pulmonary artery pressure; PAWP, pulmonary artery wedge pressure; PEEP, positive end-expiratory pressure.

From Bulechek GM et al: *Nursing interventions classification (NIC)*, ed 5, 2008, St Louis, Mosby.

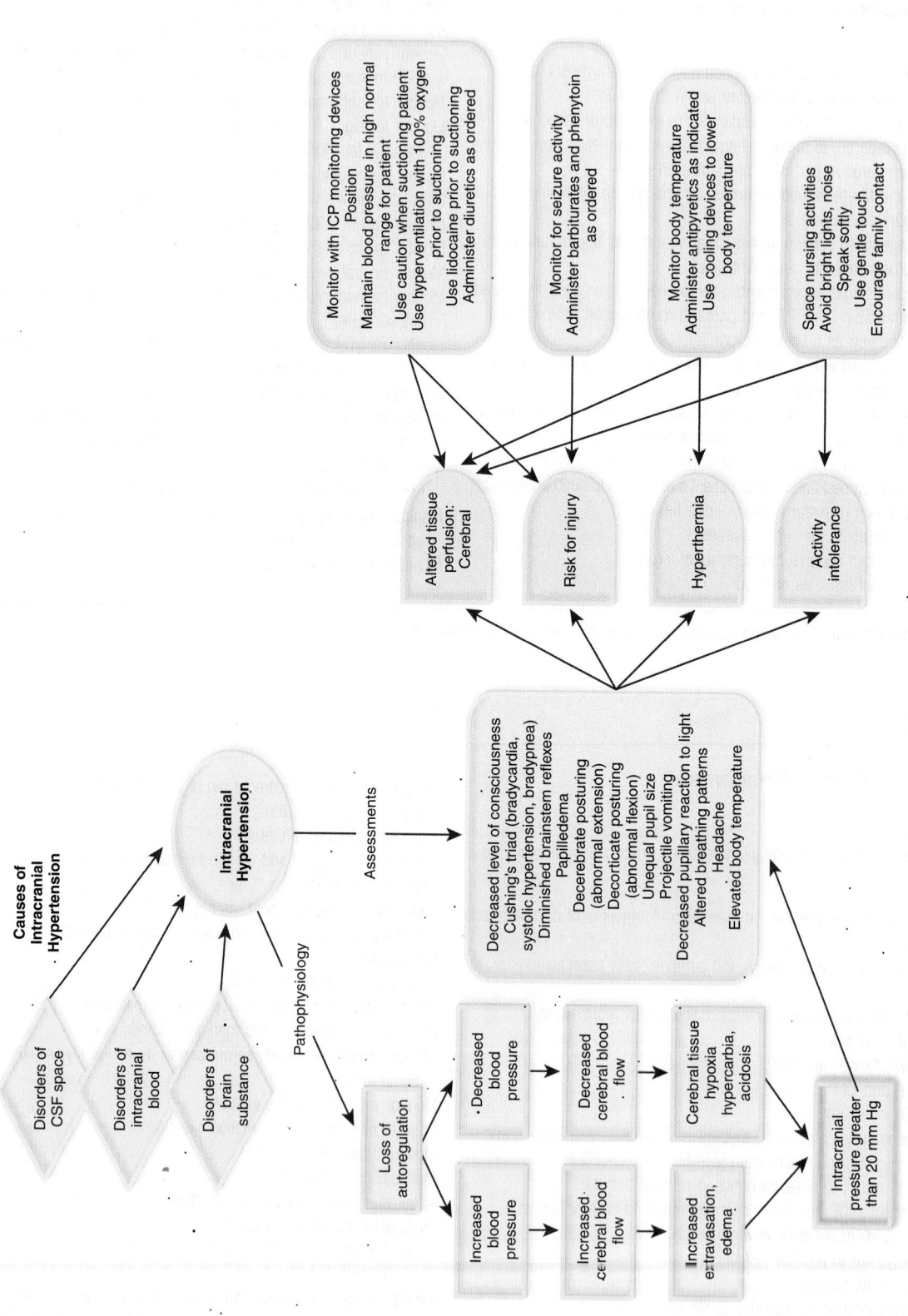

Causes of Intracranial Hypertension

Disorders of CSF space

Disorders of intracranial blood

Disorders of brain substance

Intracranial Hypertension

Assessments

Pathophysiology

Decreased level of consciousness
Cushing's triad (bradycardia, systolic hypertension, bradypnea)
Diminished brainstem reflexes
Papilledema
Decerebrate posturing (abnormal extension)
Decorticate posturing (abnormal flexion)
Unequal pupil size
Projectile vomiting
Decreased pupillary reaction to light
Altered breathing patterns
Headache
Elevated body temperature

Loss of autoregulation

Decreased blood pressure → Decreased cerebral blood flow → Cerebral tissue hypoxia hypercarbia, acidosis

Increased blood pressure → Increased cerebral blood flow → Increased extravasation, edema

Intracranial pressure greater than 20 mm Hg

Altered tissue perfusion: Cerebral

Risk for injury

Hyperthermia

Activity intolerance

Monitor with ICP monitoring devices
Position
Maintain blood pressure in high normal range for patient
Use caution when suctioning patient
Use hyperventilation with 100% oxygen prior to suctioning
Use lidocaine prior to suctioning
Administer diuretics as ordered

Monitor for seizure activity
Administer barbiturates and phenytoin as ordered

Monitor body temperature
Administer antipyretics as indicated
Use cooling devices to lower body temperature

Space nursing activities
Avoid bright lights, noise
Speak softly
Use gentle touch
Encourage family contact

Hyperventilation. Controlled hyperventilation has been an important adjunct of therapy for the patient with increased ICP. The rationale employed in hyperventilation is that if the $PaCO_2$ can be reduced from its normal level of 35 to 40 mm Hg to a range of 25 to 30 mm Hg in the patient with intracranial hypertension, vasoconstriction of cerebral arteries, reduction of CBF, and increased venous return will result. This practice is being reexamined. Additional research has indicated that severe or prolonged hyperventilation can reduce cerebral perfusion and lead to cerebral ischemia and infarction. The current trend is to maintain $PaCO_2$ levels on the lower side of normal (35 ± 2 mm Hg) by carefully monitoring arterial blood gas measurements and by adjusting ventilator settings.[54,60,61]

Although hypoxemia must be avoided, excessively high levels of oxygen offer no benefits, and increasing inspired oxygen concentrations above 60% may lead to toxic changes in lung tissue. The use of pulse oximetry has led to greater awareness of the circumstances, such as pain and anxiety, that can cause oxygen desaturation and therefore elevate ICP.[5,22]

Temperature Control. Directly proportional to body temperature, cerebral metabolic rate increases 7% per 1° C of increase in body temperature.[61] This fact is significant because as the cerebral metabolic rate increases, blood flow to the brain must increase to meet the tissue demands. To avoid the increase in blood volume associated with an increased cerebral metabolic rate, nurses must prevent hyperthermia in the patient with a brain injury. Antipyretics and cooling devices must be used when appropriate while the source of the fever is being determined.[41,61,62]

Conversely, hypothermia reduces the cerebral metabolic rate. Research done in patients with severe head injury who were unresponsive to barbiturate therapy for control of intractable intracranial hypertension demonstrated a significant decrease in ICP when subjected to mild hypothermia between 32° C and 35° C.[61]

Blood Pressure Control. Maintenance of arterial blood pressure in the high-normal range is essential in the brain-injured patient. Inadequate perfusion pressure decreases the supply of nutrients and oxygen requirements for cerebral metabolic needs. However, a blood pressure that is too high increases cerebral blood volume and may increase ICP.[55,61] Figure 28-9 shows the relationship between blood pressure and ICP.

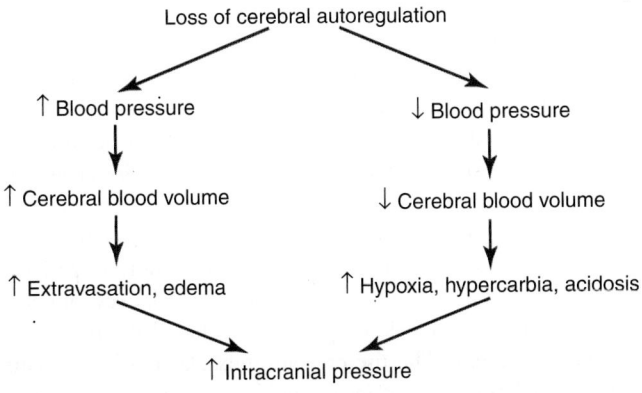

Figure 28-9 Loss of pressure autoregulation.

Control of systemic hypertension may require nothing more than the administration of a sedative agent. Small, frequent doses may be sufficient to blunt noxious stimuli and prevent them from triggering increases in blood pressure. When sedation proves inadequate in controlling systemic arterial hypertension, antihypertensive agents are used. Care must be taken in choosing these agents because many of the peripheral vasodilators (e.g., nitroprusside, nitroglycerin) also are cerebral vasodilators. All antihypertensives are believed to cause some degree of cerebral vasodilation. To reduce this vasodilating effect, concurrent treatment with beta-blockers (e.g., metoprolol, labetalol) may be beneficial.[5]

Systemic hypotension should be treated aggressively with fluids to maintain a systolic blood pressure greater than 90 mm Hg.[5] Crystalloids, colloids, and blood products can be used, depending on the patient's condition.[59] Studies have demonstrated a positive effect on ICP and CPP with hypertonic saline.[63] If fluids fail to adequately elevate the patient's blood pressure, the use of inotropic agents may be necessary.[61]

Seizure Control. The incidence of posttraumatic seizures in the head-injured population has been estimated at 5%. Because of the risk of a secondary ischemic insult associated with seizures, many physicians prescribe anticonvulsant medications prophylactically. Seizures cause metabolic requirements to increase, which results in elevation of CBF, cerebral blood volume, and ICP, even in paralyzed patients. If blood flow cannot match demand, ischemia develops, cerebral energy stores are depleted, and irreversible neuronal destruction occurs. The usual anticonvulsant regimen for seizure control includes phenytoin or phenobarbital, or both, in therapeutic doses.[62] Fast-acting, short-duration agents such as lorazepam may be indicated for breakthrough seizures until therapeutic drug levels can be achieved.

Cerebrospinal Fluid Drainage. CSF drainage for intracranial hypertension may be used with other treatment modalities. CSF drainage is accomplished by the insertion of a pliable catheter into the anterior horn of the lateral ventricle (ventriculostomy), preferably on the nondominant side. This drainage can help support the patient through periods of cerebral edema by controlling spikes in ICP. One of the major advantages of the ventriculostomy is its dual role as a monitoring device and a treatment modality. Care should be taken to avoid infection. However, cleansing ointment such as bacitracin or povidone is not recommended. Ventriculitis occurs in 10% to 17% (Figs. 28-10 and 28-11).[28,57]

Diuretics

Osmotic Agents. Clinicians have known for decades that osmotic agents effectively reduce ICP. The mechanism by which these diuretics reduce ICP continues to be a subject of investigational interest. One theory is that these agents act by remaining relatively impermeable to the blood-brain barrier, thereby drawing water from normal brain tissue to plasma. The direction of flow is from the hypoconcentrated tissue to the hyperconcentrated cerebral vasculature. If the situation becomes reversed and the tissue becomes hyperconcentrated in relation to the cerebral vasculature, a rebound phenomenon may occur. These agents have little direct effect on edematous

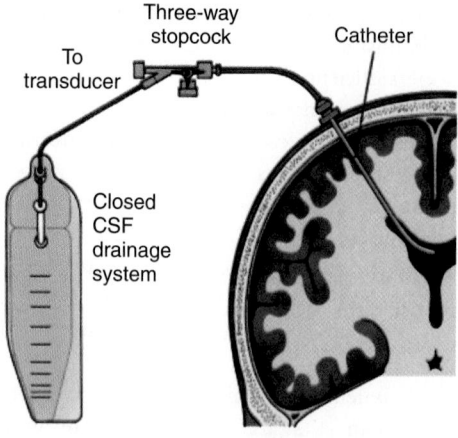

INTRAVENTRICULAR CATHETER

Figure 28-10 Intermittent drainage system. Intermittent drainage involves draining cerebrospinal fluid (CSF) through a ventriculostomy when intracranial pressure (ICP) exceeds the upper pressure parameter set by the physician. Intermittent drainage is achieved by opening the three-way stopcock to allow CSF to flow into the drainage bag for brief periods (30 to 120 seconds) until the pressure is below the upper pressure parameter. *(From Barker E:* Neuroscience nursing, *ed 3, St Louis, 2008, Mosby.)*

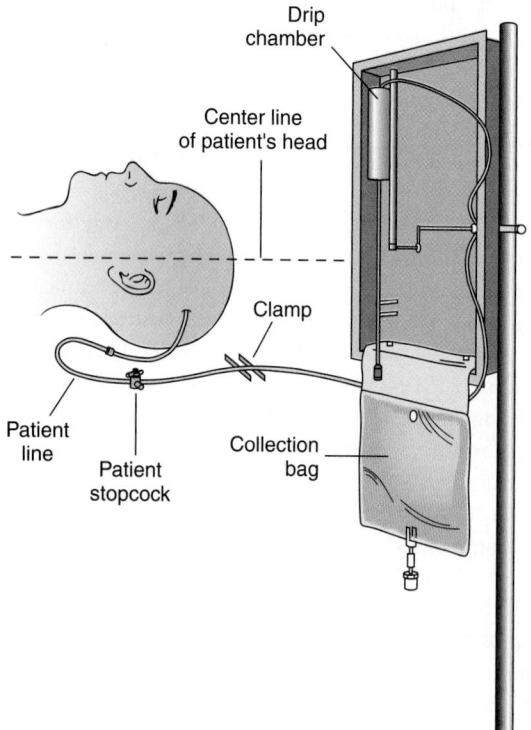

Figure 28-11 Continuous drainage system. Continuous drainage involves placing the drip chamber of the drainage system at a specified level above the foramen of Monro (usually 15 cm). The system is left open to allow continuous drainage of cerebrospinal fluid (CSF) into the chamber (which drains into a collection bag) against a pressure gradient that prevents excessive drainage and ventricular collapse. *(Courtesy Codman/ Johnson & Johnson Professional, Inc., Raynham, MA.)*

cerebral tissue situated in an area of defective blood-brain barrier; instead, they require an intact blood-brain barrier for osmosis to occur.[54,64]

The most widely used osmotic diuretic is mannitol, a large-molecule agent that is retained almost entirely in the extracellular compartment and has little or none of the rebound effect observed with other osmotic diuretics. Mannitol may improve perfusion to ischemic areas of the brain, producing cerebral vasoconstriction and resulting in a reduction of ICP.[54,64]

Perhaps the most common difficulty associated with the use of osmotic agents is the provocation of electrolyte disturbances. Careful attention must be paid to body weight and fluid and electrolyte stability. Serum osmolality must be kept between 300 and 320 mOsm/L. Hypernatremia and hypokalemia often are associated with repeated administration of osmotic agents. Central venous pressure readings must be monitored to prevent hypovolemia. Smaller doses of mannitol simplify fluid and electrolyte management, and their use is encouraged whenever possible.[62,64]

Nonosmotic Agents. Loop diuretics have been used to decrease ICP. Furosemide, one such nonosmotic diuretic, may act differently from osmotic agents by pulling sodium and water from edematous areas and perhaps by decreasing CSF production. One advantage of furosemide administration over the use of osmotic diuretics is that its effect is not generally associated with increases in serum osmolality. Electrolyte imbalances may not be as severe with the use of nonosmotic diuretics.[57,62]

Volume Maintenance. Administration of osmotic and loop diuretics can contribute to dehydration, precipitating a decrease in CPP. In the most favorable scenario, the patient is maintained in an euvolemic state to optimize cerebral perfusion. Volume replacement strategies include fluid boluses, fluid replacements, and albumin administration. Intravenous fluids administered are typically isotonic and low in glucose to prevent gradient shifts across the blood-brain barrier in the traumatically brain-injured patient.[59]

Control of Metabolic Demand. Any treatment modality that increases the incidence of noxious stimulation to the patient carries with it the potential for increasing ICP. Noxious stimuli include pain, the presence of an endotracheal tube, coughing, suctioning, repositioning, bathing, and many other routine nursing interventions. Agents used to reduce metabolic demands include the use of benzodiazepines such as midazolam and lorazepam, intravenous sedative-hypnotics such as propofol, opioid narcotics such as fentanyl and morphine, and neuromuscular blocking agents such as vecuronium and atracurium. These agents may be administered separately or in combination by continuous drip or as an intravenous bolus on an as-needed basis.

The preferred treatment regimen begins with the administration of benzodiazepines for sedation and narcotics for analgesia. If these agents fail to blunt the patient's response to noxious stimuli, propofol or a neuromuscular blocking agent is added. The use of these medications is recommended only in patients who have an ICP monitor in place, because sedatives, opioids, and neuromuscular blocking agents affect the reliability of neurologic assessment. The use of neuromuscular blocking agents without sedation is not recommended because these agents can cause skeletal muscle paralysis and because they have no analgesic effect and do not adequately protect the patient from pain and the physiologic responses that can occur from pain-producing procedures.[59,62] If these agents fail to control the patient's ICP, barbiturate therapy is considered.

Barbiturate Therapy. Barbiturate therapy is a treatment protocol developed for the management of uncontrolled intracranial hypertension that has not responded to the conventional treatments previously described.[54] The two most commonly used drugs in high-dose barbiturate therapy are pentobarbital and thiopental. The goal with either drug is a reduction of ICP to 15 to 20 mm Hg while a mean arterial pressure of 70 to 80 mm Hg is maintained. Patients are maintained on high-dose barbiturate therapy until ICP has been controlled within the normal range for 24 hours. Barbiturates must never be stopped abruptly; they are tapered slowly over approximately 4 days. Despite the theoretical reasons for barbiturate use, clinical trials of its use have not shown improved outcome.[5,28]

Complications of high-dose barbiturate therapy can be disastrous unless a specific and organized approach is used. The most common complications are hypotension, hypothermia, and myocardial depression. If any complications occur and are allowed to persist unchecked, they may cause secondary insults to an already damaged brain. Hypotension, the most common complication, results from peripheral vasodilation and can be compounded in an already dehydrated patient who has received large doses of an osmotic diuretic in an attempt to control ICP. Careful monitoring of fluid status by central venous pressure or a pulmonary artery catheter can help prevent this complication. Myocardial depression results from cardiac muscle suppression and can be avoided by frequent monitoring of fluid status, cardiac output, and serum drug levels. If an adequate cardiac output cannot be maintained in the presence of normothermia, barbiturates must be reduced, regardless of serum levels.[5,55] Collaborative management of the patient's intracranial hypertension is outlined in Box 28-9.

HERNIATION SYNDROMES

The goal of neurologic evaluation, ICP monitoring, and treatment of increased ICP is to prevent herniation. Herniation of intracerebral contents results in the shifting of tissue from one compartment of the brain to another and places pressure on cerebral vessels and vital function centers of the brain. If

unchecked, herniation rapidly causes death as a result of the cessation of CBF and respirations.

Supratentorial Herniation. The four types of supratentorial herniation syndrome are uncal; central, or transtentorial; cingulate; and transcalvarial (Fig. 28-12).

Uncal Herniation. Uncal herniation is the most common herniation syndrome. In uncal herniation, a unilateral, expanding mass lesion, usually of the temporal lobe, increases ICP, causing lateral displacement of the tip of the temporal lobe (uncus). Lateral displacement pushes the uncus over the edge of the tentorium, puts pressure on the oculomotor nerve (cranial nerve III) and the posterior cerebral artery ipsilateral to the lesion, and flattens the midbrain against the opposite side. Clinical manifestations of uncal herniation include ipsilateral pupil dilation, decreased level of consciousness, respiratory pattern changes leading to respiratory arrest, and contralateral hemiplegia leading to decorticate or decerebrate posturing. If no intervention occurs, uncal herniation results in fixed and dilated pupils, flaccidity, and respiratory arrest.[5,28,65]

Central Herniation. In central, or transtentorial, herniation, an expanding mass lesion of the midline, frontal, parietal, or occipital lobe results in downward displacement of the hemispheres, basal ganglia, and diencephalon through the tentorial notch. Central herniation often is preceded by uncal and cingulate herniation. Clinical manifestations of central herniation include loss of consciousness; small, reactive pupils progressing to fixed, dilated pupils; respiratory changes leading to respiratory arrest; and decorticate posturing progressing to flaccidity. In the late stages, uncal and central herniation syndromes affect the brainstem similarly.[5,28,65]

Cingulate Herniation. Cingulate herniation occurs when an expanding lesion of one hemisphere shifts laterally and forces the cingulate gyrus under the falx cerebri. Cingulate herniation occurs often. When a lateral shift is observed on the CT scan, cingulate herniation has occurred. Little is known about the effects of cingulate herniation, and there are no accompanying clinical manifestations that assist in its diagnosis. Cingulate herniation is not in itself a life-threatening condition, but if the expanding mass lesion that caused cingulate herniation is not controlled, uncal or central herniation will follow.[5,28,65]

BOX 28-9   COLLABORATIVE MANAGEMENT: INTRACRANIAL HYPERTENSION

- Position patient to achieve maximal intracranial pressure (ICP) reduction.
- Reduce environmental stimulation.
- Maintain normothermia.
- Control ventilation to ensure a normal $PaCO_2$ level (35 ± 2 mm Hg).
- Administer diuretic agents, anticonvulsants, sedation, analgesia, paralytic agents, and vasoactive medications to ensure cerebral perfusion pressure (CPP) >70 mm Hg.
- Drain cerebrospinal fluid for ICP >20 mm Hg.

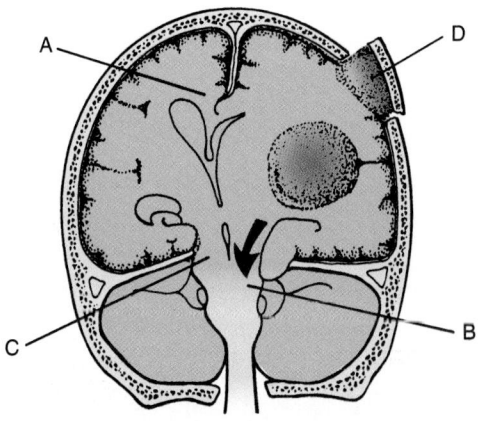

Figure 28-12 Supratentorial herniation: cingulate (A), uncal (B), central (C), and transcalvarial (D).

Transcalvarial Herniation. Transcalvarial herniation is the extrusion of cerebral tissue through the cranium. In the presence of severe cerebral edema, transcalvarial herniation occurs through an opening from a skull fracture or craniotomy site.[5]

Infratentorial Herniation.

The two infratentorial herniation syndromes are upward transtentorial herniation and downward cerebellar herniation.

Upward Transtentorial Herniation. Upward transtentorial herniation occurs when an expanding mass lesion of the cerebellum causes protrusion of the vermis (central area) of the cerebellum and the midbrain upward through the tentorial notch. Compression of the third cranial nerve and diencephalon occurs. Blockage of the central aqueduct and distortion of the third ventricle obstruct CSF flow. Deterioration progresses rapidly.[5,28,65]

Downward Cerebellar Herniation. Downward cerebellar herniation occurs when an expanding lesion of the cerebellum exerts pressure downward, sending the cerebellar tonsils through the foramen magnum. Compression and displacement of the medulla oblongata occur, rapidly resulting in respiratory and cardiac arrest.[5,28,65]

PHARMACOLOGIC AGENTS

Many pharmacologic agents are used in the care of patients with neurologic disorders. Table 28-7 reviews the various agents used and any special considerations necessary for administering them.[66,67]

TABLE 28-7 Pharmacologic Management: Neurologic Disorders

DRUG	DOSAGE	ACTIONS	SPECIAL CONSIDERATIONS
Anticonvulsants			
Phenytoin (Dilantin)	Loading dose: 10-20 mg/kg IV Maintenance dose: 100 mg q6-8h IV	Prevents the influx of sodium at the cell membrane	Monitor serum levels closely; therapeutic level is 5-20 mcg/mL Infuse phenytoin no faster than 50 mg/min; administer with normal saline only because it precipitates with other solutions
Fosphenytoin (Cerebyx)	Loading dose: 15-20 mg/kg IV Maintenance dose: 4-6 mg/kg/24 hr IV	Prevents the influx of sodium at the cell membrane	Monitor serum levels closely; therapeutic level is 5-20 mcg/mL Dosage, concentration, and infusion rate of fosphenytoin is expressed as phenytoin sodium equivalents (FE)
Barbiturates			
Phenobarbital	Loading dose: 6-8 mg/kg IV Maintenance dose: 1-3 mg/kg/24 hr IV	Produces CNS depression and reduces the spread of an epileptic focus	May depress cardiac and respiratory function Administer phenobarbital at a rate of 60 mg/min; monitor serum level closely; therapeutic level is 20-40 mcg/mL
Pentobarbital	Loading dose: 3-10 mg/kg over 30 min Maintenance dose: 0.5-3 mg/kg/hr IV	Induces barbiturate coma	Monitor serum level of pentobarbital closely; therapeutic level for coma is 20-40 mcg/mL
Osmotic Diuretics			
Mannitol	1-2 g/kg IV	Treats cerebral edema by pulling fluid from the extravascular space into the intravascular space; requires intact blood-brain barrier	Side effects include hypovolemia and increased serum osmolality Monitor serum osmolality and notify the physician if >310 mOsm/L Warm and shake before administering to ensure crystals are dissolved
Loop Diuretics			
Furosemide	0.1-2 mg/kg IV	Decreases sodium transport within the brain and thereby reduces cerebral edema; may inhibit CSF production	Side effects include hypovolemia and hypokalemia

TABLE 28-7 Pharmacologic Management: Neurologic Disorders—*cont'd*

DRUG	DOSAGE	ACTIONS	SPECIAL CONSIDERATIONS
Calcium Channel Blockers			
Nimodipine (Nimotop)	60 mg q4h NG or PO for 21 days	Decreases cerebral vasospasm	Side effects include hypotension, palpitations, headache, and dizziness Monitor blood pressure frequently when implementing therapy
Local Anesthetics			
Lidocaine	50-100 mg IV or 2 mL of 4% solution	Blunts the effects of tracheal stimulation on intracranial pressure	Must be administered not longer than 5 minutes before suctioning
Thrombolytics			
Tissue-type plasminogen activator (tPA)	0.9 mg/kg total, with 10% of the dose administered as IV bolus over 1 min and 90% of the dose administered as continuous IV infusion over 1 hr	Converts plasminogen to plasmin to dissolve clot	Treatment must start within 3 hr of the onset of the symptoms Do not exceed 90 mg Do not use anticoagulants during the first 24 hr Monitor patient for bleeding

CNS, central nervous system; CSF, Cerebrospinal fluid; IV, intravenous; NG, nasogastric; PO, by mouth.

Summary

Coma

- The two main causes of coma are structural (e.g., ischemic stroke, ICH, trauma, brain tumors) and metabolic (e.g., drug overdose, infectious diseases, endocrine disorders, poisonings).
- Coma is the deepest state of unconsciousness; arousal and awareness are lacking as a result of diffuse dysfunction of both cerebral hemispheres or diffuse or focal dysfunction of the reticular activating system.
- Medical management focuses on identification and treatment of the underlying cause of the condition and support of vital functions.
- Nursing actions include supporting all body functions, maintaining surveillance for complications, providing comfort and emotional support, and initiating rehabilitation measures.

Stroke

- The sudden onset of an acute neurologic deficit persisting for more than 24 hours is known as a *stroke*, and it is caused by the interruption of blood flow to the brain.
- Strokes are classified as ischemic or hemorrhagic. Hemorrhagic strokes can be further categorized as SAHs (cerebral aneurysms and AVMs) and ICHs.
- Nursing actions include monitoring for changes in neurologic status, maintaining surveillance for complications, providing comfort and emotional support, initiating rehabilitation measures, and educating the patient and family.

Ischemic Stroke

- The two main causes of ischemic stroke are thrombosis and embolism, and it results in a neuronal tissue injury due to decreased or absent blood flow.
- The characteristic sign of an ischemic stroke is the sudden onset of focal neurologic signs persisting for more than 24 hours. The signs depend on the affected portion of the brain.
- Medical management focuses on preservation of brain tissue through thrombolytic therapy, management of blood pressure, and treatment of complications.

Subarachnoid Hemorrhagic

- SAH is bleeding into the subarachnoid space, and it is usually caused by rupture of a cerebral aneurysm or AVM.
- Medical management focuses on preservation of neurologic function, support of vital functions, and treatment of complications (rebleeding, vasospasm, hyponatremia, and hydrocephalus).

Intracerebral Hemorrhage

- ICH is bleeding directly into cerebral tissue, and it is usually caused by rupture of a small artery in the brain resulting from hypertension.
- Medical management focuses on preservation of neurologic function, control of blood pressure, support of vital functions, and management of intracranial hypertension.

Guillain-Barré

- Guillain-Barré is a syndrome that involves a rapidly progressive, ascending peripheral nerve dysfunction leading to paralysis that may produce respiratory failure.

- Medical management focuses on support of vital functions and the administration of treatments to limit the duration of the syndrome.
- Nursing actions include maintaining surveillance for complications, initiating rehabilitative measures, providing comfort and emotional support, and educating the patient and family regarding the disorder.

Craniotomy

- A craniotomy is performed to gain access to portions of the CNS inside the cranium for the purposes of tumor resection or removal, cerebral decompression, evacuation of hematoma or abscess, or repair of an aneurysm or AVM.
- Postoperative medical management focuses on preventing complications, including intracranial hypertension, hemorrhage, fluid imbalances, CSF leaks, and DVT.
- Nursing actions include positioning the patient's head in accordance with the physician's orders, monitoring the patient's intake and output, administering medications to control vomiting and fever, promoting postoperative pulmonary care, providing comfort and emotional support, maintaining surveillance for complications, initiating rehabilitative measures, and education of the patient and family.

Intracranial Hypertension

- One of the earliest signs of increased ICP is a decrease in level of consciousness.
- ICP can be measured using an ICP monitor, and it should be treated when it exceeds 20 mm Hg.
- Medical and nursing management is directed toward reducing the volume of one or more of the components (e.g., blood, brain, CSF) that lie within the intracranial vault.
- Herniation of intracerebral contents results in the shifting of tissue from one compartment of the brain to another and places pressure on cerebral vessels and vital function centers of the brain. If unchecked, it rapidly causes death.

Case Study: Patient with a Neurologic Problem

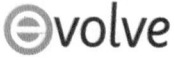 Answers to the Case Study Questions can be found on the Evolve web site at http://evolve.elsevier.com/Urden/.

Brief Patient History
Mr. P is a 24-year-old man. While he was water skiing, he was hit by a boat. He was rescued from the water by friends. He was immobilized and transported to the hospital by paramedics called to the scene.

Clinical Assessment
Mr. P is admitted to the emergency department with abrasions and bruising to his head and shoulders. He is having difficulty breathing and is unable to move his extremities. He complains of neck pain, and he has a cervical collar in place. He has urinary and fecal incontinence. There is no response to motor, sensory, or deep tendon reflexes from the neck to the feet. He is awake and able to talk.

Diagnostic Procedures
The admission MRI showed an incomplete spinal cord transection. Baseline vital signs include the following: blood pressure of 85/60 mm Hg, heart rate of 48 beats/min (sinus bradycardia), respiratory rate of 8 breaths/min, temperature of 99.3° F, and O$_2$ saturation of 88%. The Glasgow Coma Scale score was 10.

Medical Diagnosis
Mr. P is diagnosed with an incomplete spinal cord transection and neurogenic shock.

Questions
1. What major outcomes do you expect to achieve for this patient?
2. What problems or risks must be managed to achieve these outcomes?
3. What interventions must be initiated to monitor, prevent, manage, or eliminate the problems and risks identified?
4. What interventions should be initiated to promote optimal functioning, safety, and well-being of the patient?
5. What possible learning needs do you anticipate for this patient?
6. What cultural and age-related factors may have a bearing on the patient's plan of care?

Be sure to check out the bonus material, including free self-assessment exercises, on the Evolve web site at http://evolve.elsevier.com/Urden/.

References

1. Hoesch RE et al: Coma after global ischemic brain injury: pathophysiology and emerging therapies, *Crit Care Clin* 24:25, 2008.
2. Laureys S et al: Brain function in coma, vegetative state, and related disorders, *Lancet Neurol* 3:537, 2004.
3. Stevens RD, Bhardwaj A: Approach to the comatose patient, *Crit Care Med* 34:31, 2006.
4. Fauce K et al: *Harrison's principles of internal medicine*, ed 17, Philadelphia, 2008, McGraw-Hill.
5. Barker E: *Neuroscience nursing: a spectrum of care*, ed 3, St Louis, 2008, Mosby.
6. Goetz CG: *Textbook of clinical neurology*, ed 3, St Louis, 2007, WB Saunders.
7. Berger JR: Clinical approach to stupor and coma. In Bradley WG et al, editors: *Neurology in clinical practice*, ed 3, Boston, 2000, Butterworth-Heinemann.
8. Boss BJ, Wilkerson RR: Concepts of neurologic dysfunction. In McCance KL, Huether SE, editors: *Pathophysiology: the biologic basis for disease in adults and children*, ed 5, St Louis, 2006, Mosby.

9. Stubgen JP, Plum F: Evaluation of coma. In Grenvik A et-al, editors: *Textbook of critical care*, ed 4, Philadelphia, 2000, WB Saunders.

10. Booth CM, et al: Is this patient dead, vegetative, or severely neurologically impaired? Assessing outcome for comatose survivors of cardiac arrest, *JAMA* 291:870, 2004.

11. Cushman L et al: Bringing research to the bedside: the role of induced hypothermia in cardiac arrest, *Crit Care Nurs Q* 30:143, 2007.

12. Holden M, Makic MB: Clinically induced hypothermia: why chill your patient? *AACN Adv Crit Care* 17:125, 2006.

13. Cortese D et al: Moisture chamber versus lubrication for the prevention of corneal epithelial breakdown, *Am J Crit Care* 4:425, 1995.

14. Writing Group Members: Heart disease and stroke statistics—2009 update: a report from the American Heart Association Statistics Committee and Stroke Statistics Subcommittee, *Circulation* 119:e21, 2009.

15. American Association of Neuroscience Nurses: *Guide to the care of the patient with ischemic stroke: AANN reference series for clinical practice*, Chicago, 2005, The Association.

16. Romano JG, Sacco RL: Progress in secondary stroke prevention, *Ann Neurol* 63:418, 2008.

17. Chen WL et al: Vertebral artery dissection and cerebellar infarction following chiropractic manipulation. *Emerg Med J* 23(1):e1, 2006.

18. Albers GW et al: Antithrombotic and thrombolytic therapy for ischemic stroke: American College of Chest Physicians Evidence-Based Clinical Practice Guidelines (8th Edition), *Chest* 133(6 suppl):630S, 2008.

19. Finley Caulfield A, Wijman CA: Critical care of acute ischemic stroke, *Crit Care Clin* 22:581, 2006.

20. Somes J, Bergman DL: ABCDs of acute stroke intervention, *J Emerg Nurs* 33:228, 2007.

21. Szaflarski JP et al: Incidence of seizures in the acute phase of stroke: a population-based study, *Epilepsia* 49:974, 2008.

22. Bader MK, Littlejohns LR: *AANN core curriculum for neuroscience nursing*, ed 4, St Louis, 2004, Elsevier.

23. Hacke W et al: Thrombolysis with alteplase 3 to 4.5 hours after acute ischemic stroke, *N Engl J Med* 359:1317, 2008.

24. Adams HP: Emergent use of anticoagulation for treatment of patients with ischemic stroke, *Stroke* 33:856, 2002.

25. Advisory Working Group on Stroke Center Identification Options of the American Stroke Association: Recommendations for improving the quality of care through stroke centers and systems: an examination of stroke center identification options: multidisciplinary consensus recommendations from the Advisory Working Group on Stroke Center Identification Options of the American Stroke Association, *Stroke* 33:e1, 2002.

26. Swadron SP et al: The acute cerebrovascular event: surgical and other interventional therapies, *Emerg Med Clin North Am* 21:847, 2003.

27. Fahy BG, Sivaraman V: Current concepts in neurocritical care, *Anesthesiol Clin North Am* 20:441, 2002.

28. Lindsay KW, Bone I: *Neurology and neurosurgery illustrated*, ed 4, 2004, Churchill Livingstone.

29. Manno EM: Subarachnoid hemorrhage, *Neurol Clin* 22:347, 2004.

30. Benderson JB et al: Guidelines for the management of aneurysmal subarachnoid hemorrhage: a statement for healthcare professionals from a special writing group of the Stroke Council, American Heart Association, *Circulation* 40:994, 2009.

31. Hunt WE, Hess RM: Surgical risks as related to time of intervention in the repair of intracranial aneurysms, *J Neurosurg* 28:14, 1968.

32. Solenski NJ et al: Medical complications of aneurysmal subarachnoid hemorrhage: a report of the multicenter, cooperative aneurysm study, *Crit Care Med* 23:1007, 1995.

33. Classen J et al: Effect of acute physiologic derangements on outcome after subarachnoid hemorrhage, *Crit Care Med* 32:832, 2004.

34. Lefevre F, Woolger JM: Surgery in the patient with neurologic disease, *Med Clin North Am* 87:257, 2003.

35. Oyama K, Criddle L: Vasospasm after aneurysmal subarachnoid hemorrhage, *Crit Care Nurse* 24(5):58, 2004.

36. Bendo AA: Intracranial vascular surgery, *Anesthesiol Clin North Am* 20:377, 2002.

37. Treggiari-Venzi MM et al: Review of medical prevention of vasospasm after aneurysmal subarachnoid hemorrhage: a problem of neurointensive care, *Neurosurgery* 48:249, 2001.

38. Sen J et al: Triple-H therapy in the management of aneurysmal subarachnoid haemorrhage, *Lancet Neurol* 2:614, 2003.

39. Fahy BG, Sivaraman V: Current concepts in neurocritical care, *Anesthesiol Clin North Am* 20:441, 2002.

40. Hsieh PC et al: Current updates in perioperative management of intracerebral hemorrhage, *Neurol Clin* 24:745, 2006.

41. Broderick JP et al: Guidelines for the management of spontaneous intracerebral hemorrhage in adults 2007 update, *Stroke* 38:2001, 2007.

42. Mayer SA; Rincon F: Treatment of intracerebral haemorrhage, *Lancet Neurol* 4:662, 2005.

43. Chitnis T, Khoury SJ: Immunologic neuromuscular disorders, *J Allergy Clin Immunol* 111:S659, 2003.

44. Newswanger DL, Warren CR: Guillain-Barré syndrome, *Am Fam Physician* 69:2405, 2004.

45. Keenlyside R, Brezman D: Fatal Guillain-Barré syndrome after the national influenza immunization program, *Neurology* 30:929, 1980.

46. Marinelli WA, Leatherman JW: Neuromuscular disorders in the intensive care unit, *Crit Care Clin* 18:915, 2002.

47. Hughes RA et al: Intravenous immunoglobulin for Guillain-Barré syndrome, *Cochrane Database Syst Rev* (1):CD002063, 2004.

48. Kihara M et al: A dysautonomia case of Guillain-Barré syndrome with recovery: monitored by composite autonomic scoring scale, *J Auton Nerv Syst* 73:186, 1998.

49. Pfeiffer G et al: Indicators of dysautonomia in severe Guillain-Barré syndrome, *J Neurol* 246:1015, 1999.

50. Rothrock JC: *Alexander's care of the patient in surgery*, ed 13, St Louis, 2007, Mosby.

51. Vance ML: Perioperative management of patients undergoing pituitary surgery, *Endocrinol Metab Clin North Am* 32:355, 2003.

52. Valladeres JB, Hankinson J: Incidence of lower extremity deep vein thrombosis in neurosurgical patients, *Neurosurgery* 6:138, 1980.

53. Chibbaro S, Tacconi L: Safety of deep venous thrombosis prophylaxis with low-molecular-weight heparin in brain surgery. Prospective study on 746 patients, *Surg Neurol* 70:117, 2008.

54. Eigsti J, Henke K: Anatomy and physiology of neurological compensatory mechanisms, *Dimens Crit Care Nurs* 25:197, 2006.

55. Rangel-Castillo L, Robertson CS: Management of intracranial hypertension, *Crit Care Clin* 22:713, 2006.

56. Bhatia A, Gupta AK: Neuromonitoring in the intensive care unit. 1. Intracranial pressure and cerebral blood flow monitoring, *Intensive Care Med* 33:1263, 2007.

57. American Association of Neuroscience Nurses: Guide *to the care of the patient with intracranial pressure monitoring: AANN reference series for clinical practice*, Chicago, 2005, The Association.

58. Arbour R: Intracranial hypertension: monitoring and nursing assessment, *Crit Care Nurse* 24(5):19, 2004.

59. Bader MK, Palmer S: Keeping the brain in the zone: applying the severe head injury guidelines to practice, *Crit Care Nurs Clin North Am* 12:413, 2000.

60. Rauen CA et al: Seven evidence-based practice habits: putting some sacred cows out to pasture, *Crit Care Nurse* 28(2):98, 2008.

61. Wong FWH: Prevention of secondary brain injury, *Crit Care Nurse* 20(5):18, 2000.

62. Arbour R: Aggressive management of intracranial dynamics, *Crit Care Nurse* 18(3):30, 1998.

63. Qureshi AI, Suarez JI: Use of hypertonic saline solutions in treatment of cerebral edema and intracranial hypertension, *Crit Care Med* 28:3301, 2000.

64. Paczynski RP: Osmotherapy: basic concepts and controversies, *Crit Care Clin* 13:105, 1997.

65. Morrison CAM: Brain herniation syndromes, *Crit Care Nurs* 7(5):34, 1987.

66. Gahart BL, Nazareno AR: *2008 Intravenous medications*, ed 24, St Louis, 2008, Mosby.

67. Stewart-Amidei C: Pharmacology advances in the neuroscience intensive care unit, *Crit Care Nurs Clin North Am* 14:31, 2002.

Renal Anatomy and Physiology

The kidneys are complex organs responsible for numerous functions and substances necessary to maintain homeostasis. The primary roles of the kidneys are to remove metabolic wastes, maintain fluid and electrolyte balance, and help achieve acid-base balance. Because hormones are produced by the kidneys, they also have an important role in blood pressure control, red blood cell production, and bone metabolism. The kidneys are important in maintaining the intracellular and extracellular environment required by all cells to function effectively. When a patient experiences kidney dysfunction, some or all of the functions of the kidneys may be decreased or absent, leading to altered homeostasis.

This chapter provides an overview of the anatomy and physiologic processes of the kidneys. An understanding of normal kidney function is essential to understanding the pathophysiology, symptoms, and therapeutic management of kidney disease and failure.

MACROSCOPIC ANATOMY

The kidneys are paired organs located retroperitoneally, one on each side of the vertebral column between T12 and L3. The right kidney is slightly lower than the left because of the position of the liver. The kidneys are approximately 12 cm long, 6 cm wide, and 2.5 cm thick in the adult and weigh about 120 g.[1] The kidneys are protected anteriorly and posteriorly by the rib cage and by a tough fibrous capsule that encloses each kidney. Additional protection is provided by a cushion of perirenal fat and the support of the kidney fascia.[1]

Internally, the kidneys are made up of two distinct areas: the cortex and the medulla. The cortex is the outer layer and contains the glomeruli, proximal tubules, cortical portions of the loops of Henle, distal tubules, and cortical collecting ducts.[2] The medulla is the inner kidney layer, made up of the pyramids, which contain the medullary portions of the loops of Henle, the vasa recta, and the medullary portions of the collecting ducts. Numerous pyramids taper and join to form a minor calyx; several minor calyces join to form a major calyx. The major calyces then join and enter the funnel-shaped kidney pelvis, a 5- to 10-mL conduit that directs urine into the ureter (Fig. 29-1).[1,2]

The renal system also includes the urinary drainage system—the ureters, bladder, and urethra (Fig. 29-2). The ureters are fibromuscular tubes that exit the central part of the kidney pelvis and enter the urinary bladder at an oblique angle. As urine is formed by the kidneys, the urine flows through the ureters by peristalsis. The peristaltic action of the ureters and the angle at which the ureters enter the bladder help prevent reflux of urine from the bladder back up into the kidneys. The bladder is a muscular sac within the pelvis and has a capacity of 280 to 500 mL.[1] Urine leaves the bladder through the urethral orifice and is excreted from the body through the urethra. The male urethra is about 20 cm long; the female urethra is 3 to 5 cm long.[1,2]

VASCULAR ANATOMY

The kidneys are highly vascular and receive 20% to 25% of the cardiac output—about 1200 mL/min. Blood enters the kidneys through the renal arteries, which branch bilaterally from the abdominal aorta. The renal artery divides into arterial branches that become progressively smaller vessels, eventually ending with the afferent arterioles.[1,2] A single afferent arteriole supplies blood to each glomerulus, a tuft of capillaries that is the first structure of the nephron, the functional unit of the kidneys.

Blood exits the glomerulus by the efferent arteriole, which divides into the vasa recta and the peritubular capillaries. The vasa recta extend into the medulla to supply the long medullary loops of Henle; the peritubular capillaries provide blood to the cortical portions of the nephron tubules. The intricate capillary network maintains the intracapillary pressure that allows water and solutes to move between the tubules and the capillaries for urine formation and the concentration and dilution of urine.[1] The capillaries then rejoin the gradually enlarging venous vessels until the blood leaves each kidney through the renal vein and returns to the general circulation by the inferior vena cava.

MICROSCOPIC STRUCTURE AND FUNCTION

Each kidney is made up of about one million nephrons, the functional units of the kidneys. Because of the vast number of nephrons, the kidneys can continue to function even when

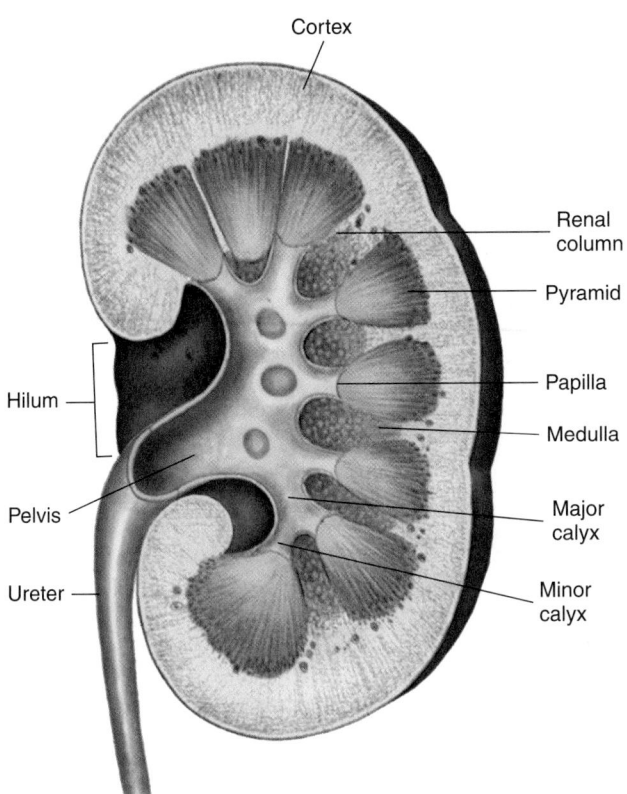

Figure 29-1 Cross section of the kidney. *(From Thompson JM et al: Mosby's clinical nursing, ed 5, St Louis, 2002, Mosby.)*

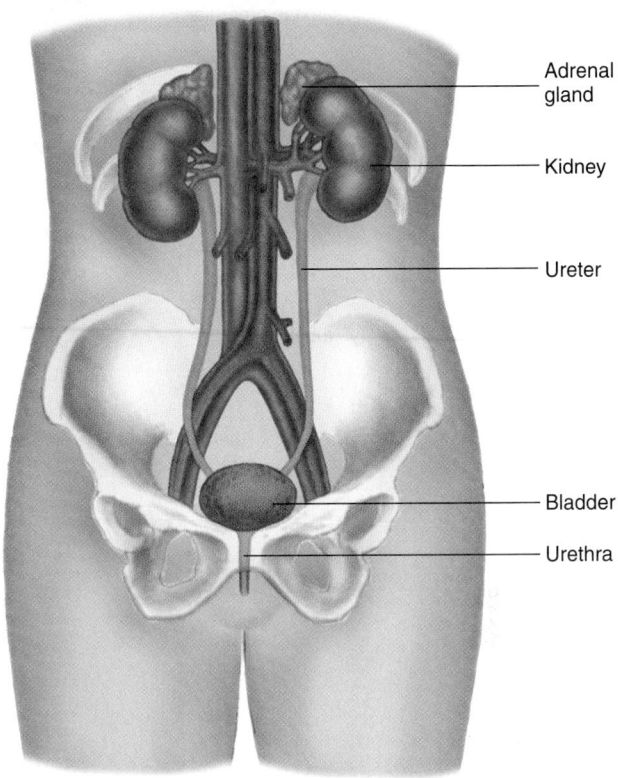

Figure 29-2 Structures of the urinary system. *(From Thompson JM et al: Mosby's clinical nursing, ed 5, St Louis, 2002, Mosby.)*

several thousand nephrons are damaged or destroyed by disease or injury. Each nephron has the ability to perform all of the individual functions of the kidneys. The nephron is made up of several distinct structures: the glomerulus, Bowman's capsule, the proximal convoluted tubule, the loop of Henle, the distal convoluted tubule, and the collecting duct (Fig. 29-3).

Two types of nephrons make up each kidney: the cortical nephrons and the juxtamedullary nephrons.[1-3] Approximately 85% of the nephrons are cortical nephrons, which are superficial or midcortical nephrons.[1] The superficial cortical nephrons have glomeruli located in the outer cortex and have short loops of Henle. The midcortical nephrons are located lower in the cortex and have loops of Henle that may be short or long. Both types of cortical nephrons perform excretory and regulatory functions. The remaining 15% of the nephrons are juxtamedullary nephrons with glomeruli located deep in the cortex and extending into the medullary layer of the kidney. The juxtamedullary nephrons have long loops of Henle that have an important role in the concentration and dilution of urine.[1-3] The vasa recta structures of the juxtamedullary nephrons maintain the concentration gradient that concentrates the urine.

GLOMERULUS

The first structure of each nephron is the glomerulus, a high-pressure capillary bed that serves as the filtering point for the blood. Positive filtration pressure in the glomerulus is achieved as a result of the high arterial pressure as the blood enters the

afferent arteriole and the resistance created by the smaller efferent arteriole as the blood exits the glomerulus. As a result of the positive-pressure gradient, fluid and solutes are filtered through the glomerular capillary walls. The glomerulus has 3 layers: the endothelium, the basement membrane, and the epithelium.[1] The inner endothelial layer lines the glomerulus and contains numerous pores that allow filtration of fluid and small solutes from the blood. The middle basement membrane layer also controls filtration according to the size, electrical charge, protein-binding capability, and shape of the molecules.[1] Large molecules such as albumin and red blood cells are prevented from entering the filtrate. The presence of large molecules in the urine is a signal that the glomerular membrane is damaged or affected by disease. The outer epithelium layer contains pores that allow the filtered blood, or filtrate, into Bowman's space.

BOWMAN'S CAPSULE

The filtrate, often called the *ultrafiltrate*, enters Bowman's space, which is surrounded by Bowman's capsule, a tough, membranous layer of epithelial cells that completely surrounds the glomerular capillary bed.[2] Bowman's space is located between the capillary walls of the glomerulus and the inner layer of Bowman's capsule and contains the initial filtrate from the blood. Fluid, solutes, and other substances filtered by the glomerulus collect in the space. Bowman's space is a continuous structure that joins the first portion of the nephron's tubular system—the proximal convoluted tubule.[1]

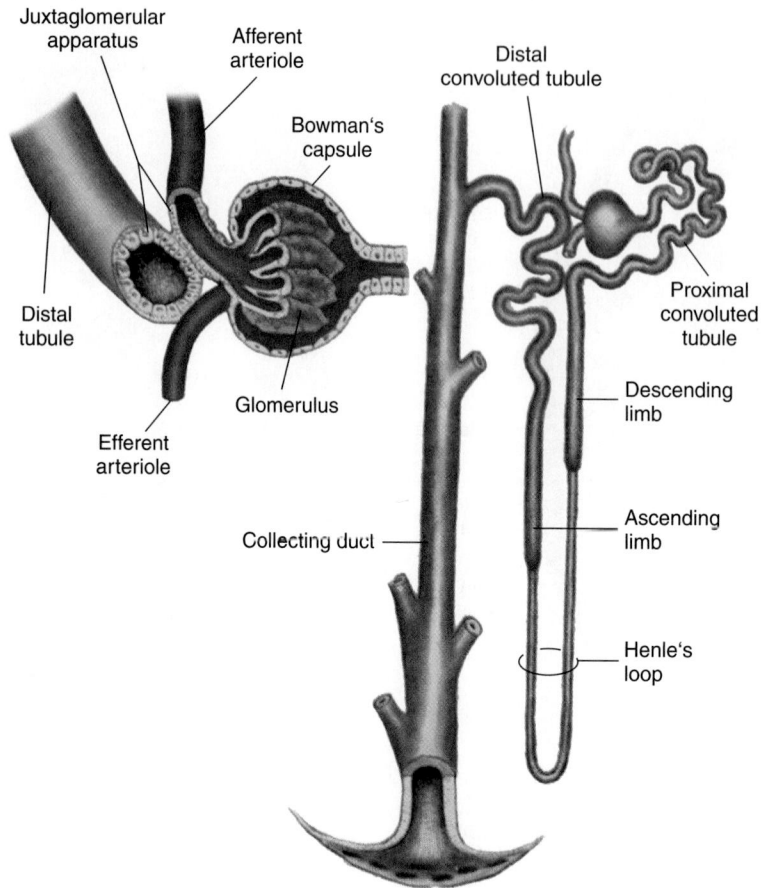

Figure 29-3 Components of the nephron. *(From Thompson JM et al: Mosby's clinical nursing, ed 5, St Louis, 2002, Mosby.)*

PROXIMAL CONVOLUTED TUBULE

The proximal convoluted tubule is located in the cortex of the kidney and has a large surface area available for solute and fluid transportation.[1,2] The proximal tubule resorbs (takes back) most of the filtered water and sodium and many of the solutes the body does not routinely excrete in the urine. Solutes that are usually resorbed include all of the glucose and amino acids, some of the water-soluble vitamins, most phosphate and bicarbonate, and much of the potassium, chloride, and calcium that is filtered by the glomerulus. Creatinine is minimally resorbed and is excreted in the urine. In addition to a major role in resorbing water and solutes from the filtrate, the proximal convoluted tubule secretes organic anions and cations into the tubular lumen. Because of the large amount of solutes in the filtrate created by the glomerulus, the fluid that enters the proximal tubule is hyperosmotic. When the filtrate leaves the proximal tubule and enters the loop of Henle, it is isosmotic (equivalent to plasma) as a result of the resorption of solutes and water.[1]

LOOP OF HENLE

After selective resorption in the proximal convoluted tubule, the isosmotic filtrate enters the loop of Henle. The loop of Henle consists of a thin descending limb, a thin ascending limb, and a thick ascending limb.[1,2] There are two types of nephrons: the cortical nephrons with short loops of Henle and the juxtamedullary nephrons with long loops of Henle. The nephrons with short loops of Henle do not have a thin ascending limb.[1] As a result, the cortical nephrons perform excretory and regulatory functions but play only a minor role in the concentration or dilution of urine. The juxtamedullary nephrons have glomeruli that are next to (juxtaposed to) the medulla near where the cortex and medulla sections of the kidney join and contain a thin ascending limb.[1] These nephrons with the thin ascending limbs are critical for concentrating and diluting the urine by means of the countercurrent mechanism. The thin descending limb is very permeable to water but fairly impermeable to urea, sodium, and other solutes. As a result, water (but not solute) is resorbed into the general circulation, and a more concentrated filtrate is produced. The filtrate then moves up the thin ascending limb, which is impermeable to water but allows movement of sodium, chloride, and urea back into the filtrate. The thick ascending limb is also impermeable to water but allows resorption of sodium, chloride, potassium, calcium, and bicarbonate. Because of the low water and high solute resorption in the loop of Henle, the filtrate leaves the ascending limb hypo-osmotic (more dilute than plasma).[1]

DISTAL CONVOLUTED TUBULE

The hypo-osmotic filtrate enters the distal convoluted tubule located in the cortex of the kidney. The first portion of the distal tubule contains the cells of the macula densa, which are specialized cells that are a component of the juxtaglomerular apparatus important in blood pressure control. The first section of the distal tubule is impermeable to water and transports solutes such as sodium, bicarbonate, calcium, and potassium.[1,2] The later section of the distal tubule further regulates sodium, bicarbonate, potassium, and calcium according to hormonal influences and the acid-base and electrolyte balance needs of the body. The permeability of the late distal tubule is influenced by antidiuretic hormone (ADH). In the presence of ADH, the late distal tubule is impermeable to water but resorbs some solutes, and the filtrate remains hypo-osmotic. In the absence of ADH, the late distal tubule is more permeable to water, and the filtrate may become isosmotic.

COLLECTING DUCT

Several distal tubules join to form a collecting duct that begins in the cortex and extends through the medulla to empty into the papilla.[1] The final composition of the urine occurs in the collecting duct, primarily because of the transport of potassium, sodium, and water. Water permeability is determined by the absence or presence of ADH.[2] In the absence of or with small amounts of ADH, the urine becomes dilute, whereas larger amounts of ADH result in concentrated urine. The filtrate usually is more concentrated when it leaves the collecting duct than it was when it entered. Acidification of the urine is accomplished by the transport of bicarbonate and hydrogen in the collecting duct. Several collecting ducts then combine to form the pyramids. After the urine leaves the collecting ducts, no change in the composition of the filtrate occurs. Box 29-1 summarizes tubular resorption and secretion in the various structures of the nephron.[1,2]

NERVOUS SYSTEM INNERVATION

The autonomic nervous system provides the primary innervation to the kidneys and the urinary drainage system. The kidneys receive messages from the lowest splanchnic and inferior splanchnic nerves, which form the renal plexus. The inferior mesenteric plexus, the hypogastric plexus, and the pudic nerve from the sacral region serve the urinary bladder, the ureters, and the urethra.[4]

Nervous system control in the urinary tract is reflected in the process of micturition, or the release of urine. Bladder fullness stimulates stretch receptors in the bladder wall and a portion of the urethra. Signals are carried through nerves in the sacral area and return as parasympathetic messages to contract the detrusor muscle of the bladder. With a full bladder, contractions usually are powerful enough to relax the external sphincter. Sympathetic stimulation returns the external sphincter to contraction after the urine is released. The cerebral cortex and brainstem portions of the central nervous system also exert control over the urinary bladder. The central nervous system regulates the micturition reflex, frequency, and external sphincter tone and allows conscious control over release of urine from the bladder.[4]

BOX 29-1 TUBULAR RESORPTION AND SECRETION

GLOMERULUS
- Filters fluid and solutes from blood

PROXIMAL CONVOLUTED TUBULE
- Resorbs Na^+, K^+, Cl^-, HCO_3^-, urea, glucose, and amino acids
- Filtrate leaves isosmotic

LOOP OF HENLE
- Resorbs Na^+, K^+, CL^-
- Blocks resorption of H_2O from ascending limb
- Countercurrent mechanism dilutes or concentrates urine
- Filtrate leaves hypo-osmotic

DISTAL TUBULE
- Na^+, K^+, Ca^{2+}, PO_4^{3-} selectively resorbed
- H_2O resorbed in the presence of antidiuretic hormone (ADH)
- Na^+ resorbed in the presence of aldosterone
- Filtrate leaves hypo-osmotic

COLLECTING DUCT
- Resorption similar to that in distal tubule
- H_2O resorbed in the presence of ADH
- HCO_3^- and H^+ resorbed or secreted to acidify urine
- Filtrate leaves hyperosmotic or hypo-osmotic, depending on body needs

---

URINE FORMATION

The nephrons are responsible for removing metabolic substances and waste products from the blood and retaining essential electrolytes and water as needed by the body. The entire blood volume of an individual is filtered by the kidneys 60 to 70 times each day, resulting in about 180 L of filtrate.[1] The glomerular filtration rate (GFR), or the amount of filtrate formed in the nephrons, is therefore about 125 mL/min. The kidneys must reduce the 180 L of filtrate to an average of 1 to 2 L of urine per day. Although 180 L of filtrate is formed, 99% of it is resorbed, and only 1% is excreted as urine. The three processes necessary for changing the 180 L of filtrate into 1 to 2 L of urine are glomerular filtration, tubular resorption, and tubular secretion.[1-3]

GLOMERULAR FILTRATION

The first process in urine formation, glomerular filtration, depends on glomerular blood flow, the pressure in Bowman's space, and plasma oncotic pressure.[1-3] Glomerular blood flow is the most important of these three factors and is maintained through an autoregulatory mechanism (ARM) within the kidneys.[1] The ARM maintains consistent kidney blood flow and perfusion at a constant level as long as the mean arterial pressure remains between 80 and 100 mm Hg. The ARM is maintained by the afferent and efferent arterioles of the glomeruli, which have the ability to increase or decrease the glomerular blood flow rate through selective dilation and constriction.[1] When the mean arterial blood pressure is decreased, the afferent arteriole dilates, and the efferent arteriole constricts to maintain a higher pressure in the glomerular capillary bed and maintain the GFR at 125 mL/min. The ability of the kidneys to autoregulate blood flow begins to fail when the mean arterial blood pressure is less than 80 mm Hg or greater than 180 mm Hg.[1]

The second factor that influences the GFR is the pressure in Bowman's space. An increase in pressure in this space decreases filtration because the increased pressure resists the movement of solutes and water from the capillaries into the space. For example, if the tubules of the nephrons are blocked by cellular debris, backward pressure is exerted on Bowman's space, the GFR drops below 125 mL/min, and urine output decreases.

The third factor that influences GFR is plasma oncotic pressure. When the oncotic pressure in the blood is decreased (as in disease states that result in low plasma protein levels), pressure in the glomerular capillary bed is decreased. Although the mean arterial pressure in the glomerulus favors filtration, decreased amounts of fluid and solutes leave the capillaries and enter Bowman's space because the oncotic pressure gradient in the plasma that encourages movement of fluid and solutes out of the plasma is less favorable. Filtration still occurs, but it is decreased from the normal 125 mL/min, resulting in a decrease in the amount of filtrate and therefore urine.

The status of the glomerular filtration system is assessed by measuring the GFR. Creatinine is used as a measure of the GFR because it is a waste product produced at a fairly constant rate by the muscles, is freely filtered by the glomerulus, and is minimally resorbed or secreted by the tubules.[5] Most of the creatinine produced by the body is excreted by the kidneys, making the creatinine clearance a good screening and follow-up test for estimating the GFR. Creatinine clearance usually mirrors the GFR, so that a normal creatinine clearance rate is approximately 125 mL/min. A creatinine clearance rate less than 100 mL/min reflects a GFR of less than 100 mL/min and is a signal of decreased kidney function. A creatinine clearance rate (and GFR) less than 20 mL/min results in symptoms of kidney failure.[5]

As kidneys age, the GFR declines by approximately 8 mL/min per decade after age 40 years.[6] However, despite the gradual decrease in the GFR and the associated reduction in clearance of creatinine, serum creatinine levels may not rise. This occurs because the reduced muscle mass associated with aging produces less creatinine to be excreted by the kidneys, essentially masking the overall effects of aging on the kidneys. As a result, relatively low levels of creatinine in elders may be associated with reductions in the GFR and creatinine clearance. The gradual decline in kidney function that occurs with aging usually is not a threat to homeostasis because the remaining GFR is adequate.[6] However, when elders become ill, the decline in kidney function can be accelerated, making elders especially susceptible to acute and chronic kidney dysfunction.

TUBULAR RESORPTION

The second process in the formation of urine is tubular resorption—the movement of a substance from the tubular lumen (filtrate) into the peritubular capillaries (blood).[1]

Tubular resorption allows the 180 L of solutes and water filtered by the glomerulus to be taken back into the circulation, decreasing the 180 L of filtrate to 1 to 2 L of urine per day. Most tubular resorption takes place in the proximal convoluted tubule and occurs by passive and active transport processes.[1-3]

Passive Transport. Passive transport of substances in the tubule depends on changes in concentration gradients and does not require energy. Diffusion and osmosis are the primary passive transport processes in the nephrons.[1] Diffusion is the spontaneous movement of molecules or solutes from an area of higher concentration to an area of lower concentration across a semipermeable membrane (not all substances cross, particularly large molecules). For example, when water is reabsorbed by the tubules, the concentration of urea in the tubules is increased. Urea then diffuses across the semipermeable membrane of the tubule and reenters the plasma to achieve balance in the concentration gradient.

Osmosis is the movement of water from an area of lower solute concentration to an area of higher solute concentration. Osmosis occurs any time the concentration of solutes on one side of a semipermeable membrane is greater than the concentration of solutes on the other side of the membrane. For example, when the concentration of sodium is greater in the peritubular capillaries than in the tubules, water passively moves from the tubules into the capillaries to balance the concentration gradient.

Active Transport. Active transport of substances into or out of the tubules requires substances to move against an electrochemical gradient, and it takes energy in the form of adenosine triphosphate (ATP).[1,2] In active transport, the substance combines with a carrier and then diffuses across the semipermeable tubular membrane. Substances that are actively resorbed include glucose, amino acids, calcium, potassium, and sodium. The rate at which substances can be actively resorbed depends on the availability of the carriers, saturation of the carriers, and availability of energy. The transport maximum refers to the maximum rate at which substances can be resorbed and varies according to each substance.[2]

The threshold concentration of a substance is important in active transport. The threshold of a substance is the plasma level of a substance at which none of the substance appears in the urine.[2] When the threshold of a substance in the plasma is exceeded, progressively larger amounts of the substance appear in the urine because the large amounts cannot be resorbed. For example, the threshold concentration for glucose is about 180 mg/dL. At or below a plasma glucose concentration of 180 mg/dL, all glucose is actively resorbed from the tubules back into the circulation, and none is excreted in the urine. When the plasma glucose concentration is above 180 mg/dL, the threshold concentration is exceeded, and some of the glucose cannot be resorbed from the tubules and is excreted in the urine.[2]

TUBULAR SECRETION

The third process in urine formation is tubular secretion, the transport of substances from the peritubular capillaries into the lumen of the tubules.[1] Tubular secretion allows the body to remove excess substances; it occurs by diffusion and by active transport, and it depends on the needs of the body. For example, potassium, hydrogen, and drugs or drug metabolites are secreted into the tubules to decrease their concentration in the body. Tubular secretion plays a lesser role than tubular resorption in changing the filtrate into urine.

FUNCTIONS OF THE KIDNEYS

The formation of urine through the processes previously described is a major function of the kidneys. The kidneys are also responsible for other functions essential to maintaining homeostasis, including the elimination of metabolic wastes, blood pressure regulation, the regulation of erythrocyte production, the activation of vitamin D, prostaglandin synthesis, acid-base balance, and fluid-electrolyte balance.[1,2]

ELIMINATION OF METABOLIC WASTES

Metabolic processes in the body produce waste products that are selectively filtered out of the circulation by the kidneys. Urea, uric acid, and creatinine are by-products of protein metabolism that the kidneys filter out of the circulation and excrete in the urine. Metabolic acids, bilirubin and drug metabolites are also eliminated as waste products.[2]

Urea. Urea and creatinine are the primary waste products that are measured in determining kidney function. Urea is measured as blood urea nitrogen (BUN) and is the end product of protein metabolism and results from the breakdown of ammonia in the liver. The level of urea in the blood is influenced by protein breakdown, the amount of protein in the diet, fluid volume, and excretion from the kidneys.[5] The body forms approximately 25 to 28 g of urea per day.[2] More urea is formed if protein intake is high or if the individual is in a catabolic state and is breaking down body protein stores. Urea is primarily excreted in the urine and therefore accumulates if the glomerulus is unable to filter it from the blood.

Creatinine. Creatinine is an end product of protein metabolism produced by the muscles. Creatinine is normally completely filtered and minimally reabsorbed by the kidneys. As a result, creatinine is excreted in the urine. Like urea, creatinine accumulates if the glomerulus is unable to filter it from the blood. The level of creatinine in the blood provides an indicator of kidney function.

BLOOD PRESSURE REGULATION

The kidneys regulate arterial blood pressure by maintaining the circulating blood volume by means of fluid balance and by altering peripheral vascular resistance through the renin-angiotensin-aldosterone system (RAAS). Regulation by the RAAS occurs in the juxtaglomerular apparatus (JGA), a group of specialized cells located around the afferent arteriole where the distal convoluted tubule and afferent arteriole make contact (see Fig. 29-3). This group of specialized cells, called the *macula densa*, provides a feedback message system from the distal tubule to control blood flow through the afferent arteriole.[1,2]

An increase in tubular filtrate in the macula densa causes the afferent arteriole to constrict and therefore decrease the GFR and the amount of filtrate produced. Conversely, a decrease in the amount of tubular filtrate results in afferent arteriole dilation, an increased GFR, and an increased amount of filtrate.

The JGA synthesizes, stores, and releases renin.[2] Renin is released in response to reduced pressure in the glomerulus, sympathetic stimulation of the kidneys, and a decrease in the amount of sodium in the distal convoluted tubule.[1,7] Renin enters the lumen of the afferent arteriole and is released into the general circulation. Renin is then converted to angiotensin I, which is further converted to angiotensin II as the blood circulates through the lungs. Angiotensin II is an active compound that causes afferent and efferent arteriole vasoconstriction, resulting in an increased vascular resistance, and it therefore maintains hydrostatic pressure within the kidneys.[1] A powerful vasoconstrictor, angiotensin II also causes increased systemic vascular resistance and therefore increased arterial blood pressure.

Angiotensin II also stimulates the release of aldosterone by the adrenal cortex. Aldosterone acts on the distal tubule to facilitate sodium and water resorption, resulting in an expanded circulating blood volume and increased blood pressure. When the arterial blood pressure increases, the JGA stops releasing renin, and the RAAS is no longer in effect. Figure 29-4 summarizes the major aspects of the renin-angiotensin-aldosterone mechanism.

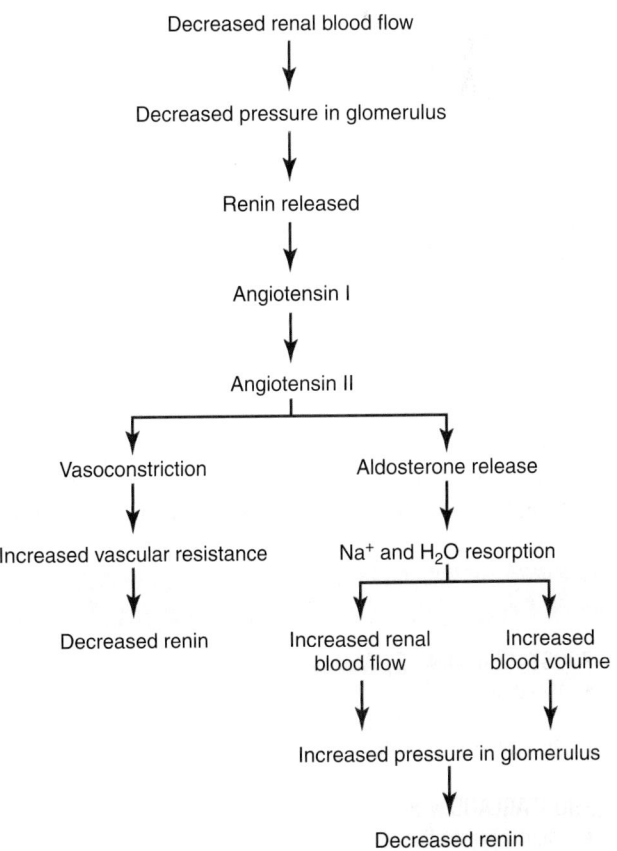

Figure 29-4 Renin-angiotensin-aldosterone system.

ERYTHROCYTE PRODUCTION

The kidneys secrete erythropoietin, the hormone that controls erythrocyte (red blood cell) production in the bone marrow. Erythropoietin is released in response to a decrease in the amount of oxygen delivered to the kidneys, such as in anemia or prolonged hypoxia.[8] The hormone remains active for about 24 hours after release and stimulates the bone marrow to increase the production of erythrocytes. The absence of erythropoietin, which occurs in individuals with kidney failure, results in a profound anemia that is treated by administering synthetic erythropoietin or by blood transfusion therapy.[8,9]

VITAMIN D ACTIVATION

The kidneys convert vitamin D from food sources into an active form for use by the body. Active vitamin D stimulates the absorption of calcium by the intestine and resorption of calcium by the tubules so that calcium is available for bone and tooth metabolism and blood clotting functions.[8] When the kidneys fail, the body is unable to convert dietary vitamin D to its active form, calcium is poorly absorbed, and bone disease results.

PROSTAGLANDIN SYNTHESIS

Prostaglandins are vasoactive substances that dilate or constrict the arteries. The kidney produces two vasodilatory prostaglandins (PGs): E and I; they are typically abbreviated PGE_1 and PGI_2. The prostaglandins produced by the kidneys have only local renal blood flow effects and have minimal or no systemic effects.[1,8] The primary prostaglandins produced by the kidneys are the vasodilators PGE_1 and PGI_2, which act on the afferent arteriole to maintain blood flow and glomerular perfusion and filtration. The vasodilating effects of the prostaglandins also counteract the effects of angiotensin II and the sympathetic nervous system on the kidneys and maintain blood flow to the kidney despite systemic vasoconstriction.[1] Another prostaglandin that may affect kidney function is PGF_2, which contributes to vasoconstriction in times of volume depletion. Box 29-2 lists the effects of prostaglandins.

ACID-BASE BALANCE

The kidneys are actively involved in acid-base regulation by resorbing or excreting acids and bases in the kidney tubules.[1,2,10] For example, bicarbonate, the principal blood buffer, is resorbed

---

BOX 29-2   EFFECTS OF PROSTAGLANDINS

PROSTAGLANDINS E_1 AND I_2
- Vasodilation
- Increased sodium and water excretion
- Stimulation of renin release

PROSTAGLANDIN F_2
- Bronchoconstriction
- Vasoconstriction (PGF_2 in volume depletion)

---

from the tubules, and hydrogen, a potent organic acid, is secreted into the tubules. However, the tubules do not function as rapidly in altering acid-base concentrations as do the lungs; the kidneys therefore regulate the day-to-day balance rather than coping with emergencies requiring quick response.

FLUID BALANCE

Regulation of the total amount of water in the body is vital for homeostasis, and it is one of the most important functions of the kidneys. In the absence of effective kidney function, fluid volume overload occurs and threatens homeostasis. Similarly, if the kidneys are unable to preserve adequate amounts of fluid, a severe volume deficit occurs that also disrupts homeostasis.

FLUID COMPARTMENTS

The fluid of the body is present in distinct internal spaces or compartments. The compartments are separated from each other by semipermeable membranes with openings (pores) that allow molecules of specific size and molecular weight to pass through while preventing larger, heavier molecules from doing so. As a result of the semipermeable membrane, fluid movement between the compartments is dynamic and constant.

The body has two main fluid compartments: intracellular and extracellular.[4,10,11] The *intracellular compartment* is the fluid inside each of the body's cells, and it accounts for 40% of a person's total body weight and therefore most of the water in the body. The remaining fluid is outside the body's cells and makes up the *extracellular compartment*. The extracellular compartment is composed of two distinct subcompartments: intravascular and interstitial. The intravascular compartment, the fluid within the blood vessels, accounts for 5% of the body's weight. The interstitial compartment corresponds to the fluid in the tissue spaces outside of the body cells and the blood vessels and accounts for 15% of the body weight. Approximate amounts of fluid contained in each compartment are shown in Figure 29-5A.

The percentage of total body weight that is made up of water varies slightly from person to person according to gender, age, and body fat content. A man has a body water content of approximately 60%, whereas a woman has closer to 50%. Infants have an estimated body fluid content of 77%, whereas body fluids may represent only 46% to 52% of body weight in older persons.[11] With an increase in body fat, the body fluid percentage decreases because fat contains a smaller and less significant amount of water than muscle.

COMPOSITION

Any information about body fluids must include a description of the substances contained within the fluids. When fluids move within the body, the substances contained in the fluids also move.

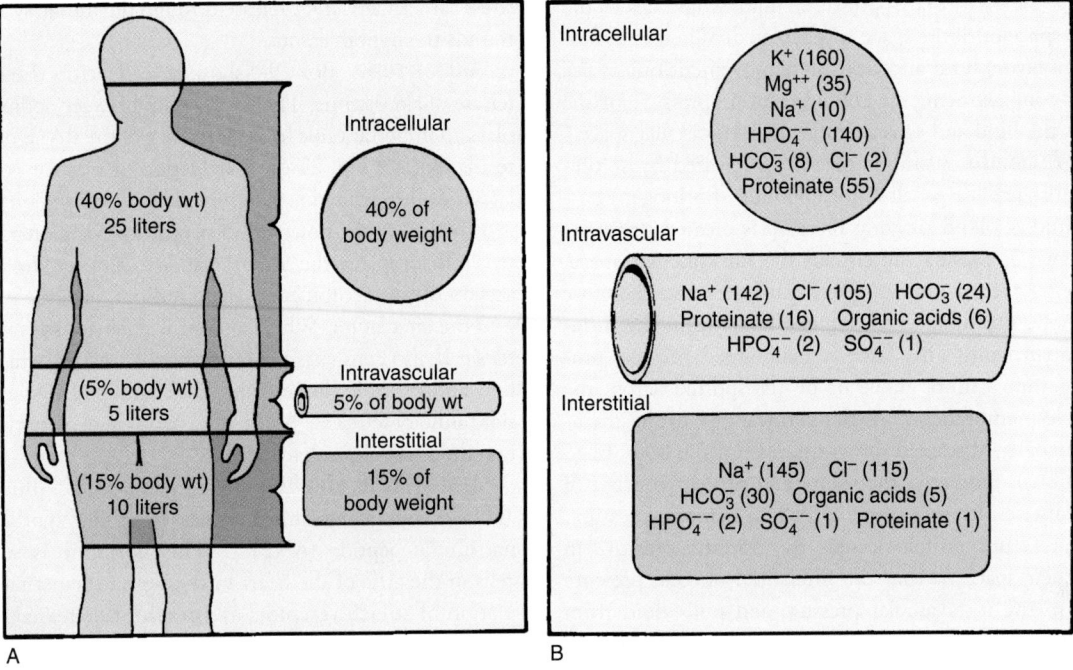

Figure 29-5 *A*, Fluid compartments. *B*, Electrolytes by fluid compartment.

Electrolytes are elements or compounds that when dissolved in water, dissociate into ions, electrically charged atomic particles. Ions in solution in the fluid allow the fluid to conduct an electrical current. A balance exists between cations (positively charged ions), anions (negatively charged ions), and other substances in the fluid compartments. Maintaining this balance is important to the normal function of all body systems. Electrolytes exist in differing amounts in each of the fluid compartments.[10,11] The primary electrolytes and other substances of importance in fluid and electrolyte balance are shown by fluid compartment in Figure 29-5B.

FLUID PHYSIOLOGY

An overall understanding is needed of the structures containing or balancing fluids and electrolytes and the physiologic forces that govern their movement and balance. Knowledge of factors that inhibit or enhance the transfer of fluids and electrolytes is required.

Tonicity. The terms *isotonic, hypotonic,* and *hypertonic* all refer to tonicity, or the osmolality of body fluids.[2] Osmolality is a measure of the number of particles (solute) in a solution, and the value is stated in milliosmoles. The normal osmolality of body fluids is 275 to 295 mOsm/kg of body weight.[11] Different hospital laboratories may use slightly different numbers, but all fall within a range of 270 to 300 mOsm/kg.

Figure 29-6 shows the effects of the tonicity of fluid in the body. An isotonic solution has roughly the same concentration of particles as the blood plasma; cells within an isotonic solution maintain consistency and do not lose or gain fluid to their surroundings. A hypertonic solution contains a greater concentration of particles than that inside the cell and causes fluid to be drawn out of the cells. Used inappropriately, too much fluid

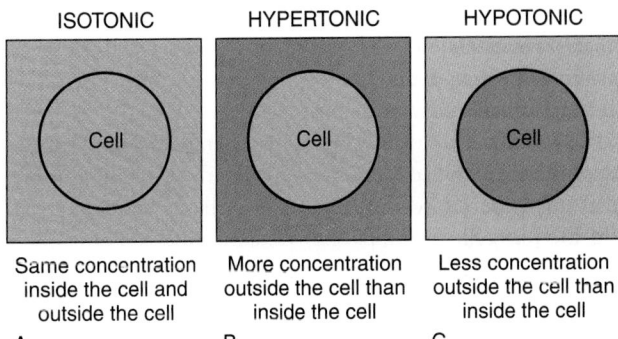

Figure 29-6 *A*, Isotonic solution. The extracellular solute concentration is the same as the intracellular concentration, with no movement of water into or out of the cell. *B*, Hypertonic solution. The extracellular solute concentration is greater than the intracellular concentration. Water moves from the cell into the extracellular compartment. *C*, Hypotonic solution. The extracellular solute concentration is less than the intracellular concentration. Water moves from the extracellular compartment into the cell.

may be withdrawn, causing a withering of the cell (crenation). A hypotonic solution contains a lesser concentration of particles than that inside the cell and causes fluid to be drawn into the cells. If used incorrectly, a hypotonic solution can cause too much fluid to enter the cell, causing the cells to swell and burst (hemolysis).

Hydrostatic Pressure. The force of left ventricular contraction of the heart propels the blood through the circulatory system, causing the blood to exert pressure against the vessel walls. This hydrostatic pressure creates the tendency for fluids and dissolved substances to move into the interstitial spaces by filtration (movement of fluid and substances from an area of high pressure to one of low pressure). Without opposing forces counteracting the hydrostatic pressure, fluid would leave the intravascular space until the space was depleted. Whereas hydrostatic pressure favors fluid and electrolyte movement out of the intravascular compartment, the colloid osmotic pressure of the plasma holds the fluid and substances in the intravascular space.[4]

Osmotic Pressure. Osmotic pressure is created by solutes and other substances (e.g., albumin, globulin, fibrinogen) suspended in fluid. Colloid osmotic pressure is created primarily by the presence of plasma proteins in the intravascular space. Plasma proteins exert a pull on water molecules and therefore produce osmotic pressure, which retains fluid within the intravascular compartment. This force is maintained because proteins are large and cannot move or be transported across the semipermeable membrane unless the permeability of the membrane is changed by disease or other assaults on the body (e.g., burns, infections). Similarly, the solute and protein content of the interstitium results in interstitial colloid osmotic pressure. A decrease in serum protein lessens the osmotic pressure in the intravascular space so that the interstitial oncotic pressure is greater than the intravascular pressure and pulls fluid from the vascular space into the interstitial space, causing edema.

Diffusion, Osmosis, and Active Transport. Fluid balance within the compartments is achieved through the processes of diffusion, osmosis, and active transport. Just as in the kidney tubule cells, these three processes are constantly at work in other parts of the body to facilitate the movement of water and solutes to maintain homeostasis between the intracellular and extracellular compartments.

Movement of Water. The forces generated by left ventricular contraction, the colloid osmotic pressure in the intravascular space, and the solute content of the extracellular fluid (ECF) and the intracellular fluid (ICF) results in the constant movement and balance of fluid throughout the fluid compartments. An increase in plasma volume results in increased capillary hydrostatic pressure, forcing fluid into the interstitial space and creating edema. A decrease in plasma volume causes the movement of fluid from the interstitium into the vascular space because the interstitial hydrostatic pressure is greater than the capillary hydrostatic pressure.

FACTORS CONTROLLING FLUID BALANCE

Antidiuretic Hormone. ADH is secreted by the posterior pituitary gland and functions as the primary controller of ECF volume.[1,3] Messages for release of ADH are sent by the osmoreceptors located in the hypothalamus and liver.[1,4] As serum osmolality rises above 285 mOsm/kg (normal range, 275 to 295 mOsm/kg), ADH is released and carried through the circulation to the nephrons. ADH acts on the late distal convoluted tubule and the collecting ducts to resorb water.[1] In the presence of ADH, water is resorbed, and the ECF volume remains high; in the absence of ADH, water resorption does not occur, and the ECF volume is diminished.[1,2] ADH can sustain the effect on the kidney tubules to a urinary osmolality of 1200 to 1400 mOsm/kg (normal range, 500 to 800 mOsm/kg).[11] Box 29-3 identifies several additional mechanisms that stimulate the release of ADH. In addition to the usual stimuli, the presence of severe emotional or physical

stress can initiate ADH release through the limbic system that surrounds the hypothalamus.

Aldosterone. Box 29-4 shows several factors that stimulate the release of aldosterone. The relationship between sodium and water plays an important role in the influence of the RAAS on body water regulation (see Fig. 29-4). A reduction in vascular volume stimulates the release of renin. Renin is converted to angiotensin I, which is converted to the powerful vasoconstrictor angiotensin II. Angiotensin II stimulates the adrenal glands to secrete aldosterone, which acts on the distal tubules to resorb sodium from the tubular lumen into the circulation. When sodium is retained, so is water. Angiotensin II also constricts the renal vasculature, reducing renal blood flow and available glomerular filtrate, sending a signal to the posterior pituitary to release ADH. The two systems intertwine to maintain fluid and electrolyte balance.[1,4]

Atrial Natriuretic Peptide. An additional influence on fluid and electrolyte regulation comes from the synthesis of atrial natriuretic peptide (ANP).[1,3] This hormone is secreted from cells in the atria of the heart in response to hypernatremia, stimulation of stretch receptors as a result of increased volume, and increased pressure in the heart (Box 29-5).[1] ANP affects sodium and water balance by blocking aldosterone and ADH

BOX 29-3　FACTORS STIMULATING RELEASE OF ANTIDIURETIC HORMONE

- Hyperosmolality of extracellular fluid (ECF)
- Hypovolemia
- Increased body temperature
- Medications
  - Opioids
  - Antineoplastics
  - Oral hypoglycemics
  - Beta-adrenergics
- Severe emotional or physical stress

BOX 29-4　FACTORS STIMULATING RELEASE OF ALDOSTERONE

- Hypovolemia
- Hyponatremia
- Hyperkalemia
- Stress—emotional, physical

BOX 29-5　FACTORS STIMULATING RELEASE OF ATRIAL NATRIURETIC PEPTIDE

- Hypernatremia
- Hypervolemia
- Vasoconstriction
- Decreased cardiac output
- Increased cardiac preload and afterload
- Increased systemic vascular resistance

production, initiating vasodilation, and stimulating increased sodium and water excretion by the collecting ducts of the kidneys. The physiologic effects of ANP include a reduction in fluid overload through diuresis, decreased cardiac workload, and reduction in cardiac preload and afterload.

ELECTROLYTE BALANCE

POTASSIUM

Potassium is the primary intracellular electrolyte and is responsible for numerous physiologic functions (Box 29-6). As with many solutes, diffusion and active transport across the cell membrane maintain potassium balance. Potassium leaves the cell by diffusion, moving toward the area of lesser concentration outside the cell, but it must be actively transported back into the cell to maintain cellular stability. One of the most important potassium functions in the body—that of aiding nervous impulse conduction and muscle contraction—is accomplished with the movement of potassium across the cell membrane.[1,10]

The gastrointestinal tract and skin excrete small amounts of potassium, but the major controllers of potassium stores are the kidneys. Potassium is resorbed by the proximal tubules and secreted into the distal tubules as needed to maintain balance. Resorption and secretion of potassium are influenced by many factors (Box 29-7). Of the estimated 60 to 100 mEq/day ingested by an individual, 90% of the potassium is resorbed before arriving at the distal convoluted tubule, where the remainder is usually excreted.[1,10]

Potassium and sodium are in a constant state of competition within the body despite the need for electrolytes and their different functions. Because both electrolytes are cations, one intracellular and one extracellular, potassium and sodium must remain in balance to preserve electrical neutrality at the cell membrane. When the sodium level is elevated, the potassium level decreases and vice versa. In the presence of aldosterone, potassium is excreted by the tubules, and sodium is retained. Potassium wasting therefore may occur despite the body's need for potassium. If potassium stores are low within the cell, the other intracellular electrolytes (magnesium and phosphorus) are often similarly depleted.[12]

SODIUM

Sodium is the most abundant extracellular electrolyte in the body and is primarily responsible for shifts in body water and the amount of water retained or excreted by the kidneys. In addition to water regulation, sodium plays a role in the transmission of nerve impulses through the sodium pump, or active transport mechanism, at the cellular level. Like potassium, sodium is key to a number of physiologic functions (Box 29-8).[10,11]

The body contains a complex system of safeguards and feedback mechanisms to protect the level of sodium in the ECF. Sodium balance is regulated by the kidneys, the adrenal glands (aldosterone secretion), and the posterior pituitary gland (ADH secretion). Most sodium resorption occurs in the proximal tubule under the influence of aldosterone. Because of the extremely sensitive mechanism for retaining sodium, ingestion of large amounts of sodium is unnecessary.

CALCIUM

Calcium is the electrolyte of greatest quantity in the body, with stores estimated at 1200 g.[4] Of the total body calcium, 99% is contained in the bones.[1,10] The remaining 1% is contained primarily in the ECF in the vascular space. The calcium contained within bone is in an inactive form that maintains bone strength and is a ready storehouse for mobilization of calcium to the serum in cases of depletion. In addition to bone metabolism,

---

BOX 29-6 FUNCTIONS OF POTASSIUM

NORMAL SERUM VALUE
- 3.5-4.5 mEq/L

FUNCTIONS
- Transmission of nerve impulses
- Intracellular osmolality
- Enzymatic reactions
- Acid-base balance
- Myocardial, skeletal, and smooth muscle contractility

BOX 29-7 FACTORS AFFECTING RESORPTION AND SECRETION OF POTASSIUM

- Sodium balance: sodium deficit results in potassium loss
- Acid-base balance: acidosis moves hydrogen into the cell and potassium out, with potassium being excreted in the urine
- Diuretics: increased loss of potassium in distal tubule
- Gastrointestinal losses: vomiting, gastric suction may remove potassium
- Insulin: promotes movement of potassium into the cell
- Epinephrine: enhances potassium resorption from distal tubule

---

BOX 29-8 FUNCTIONS OF SODIUM

NORMAL SERUM VALUE
- 135-145 mEq/L

FUNCTIONS
- Body fluid movement and retention
- Extracellular osmolality
- Active transport mechanism (with potassium)
- Neuromuscular activity
- Enzyme activities
- Acid-base balance

calcium is responsible for numerous other important functions, including myocardial contractility, coagulation, and neuromuscular activity (Box 29-9).[1,10]

The mobilization of calcium from bone stores is accomplished through the influence of parathyroid hormone (PTH). The calcium in the intravascular space (plasma calcium) exists in three general forms: ionized, protein bound, or complexed.[1] Ionized calcium is the active form and functions in cell membrane stability and blood clotting. Protein-bound calcium, which ionizes more quickly than the calcium in the bone, is readily put to use during an immediate crisis. Complexed calcium is combined with other anions such as chloride, citrate, or phosphate and is available for filtration by the glomerulus for potential removal in the urine. Ionized calcium not needed for physiologic functions is returned to the bone under the influence of the hormone *calcitonin*.

In the ionized (active) form, calcium plays an important role in maintaining the internal integrity of the cell. The amount of ionized calcium in the serum depends on changes in serum pH and on the availability of plasma protein, primarily albumin. Because changes in pH and albumin levels occur with relative frequency, the measurement of total serum calcium alone can be deceptive. To accurately determine the ionized calcium, it is necessary to measure it with a laboratory test because the results of calculated values are unreliable. Estimation of ionized calcium levels—calculated from the serum albumin and total serum calcium—were inaccurate in 38% of cases in one study of critically ill patients.[16] Often, the total serum calcium and the ionized calcium values are measured. Increasingly, the ionized calcium value is the one used to accurately guide calcium management in critically ill patients.[13]

Calcium levels depend on individual dietary intake and on a variety of physiologic mechanisms related to absorption.[1,12] The uptake of calcium is influenced by the levels of phosphorus, magnesium, vitamin D and its breakdown products, PTH, and calcitonin.

PHOSPHORUS

As with calcium and magnesium, the serum values of phosphorus represent a minute portion of the actual body stores.[11] Approximately 75% of the phosphorus is found in the bones, and part of the remaining amount is intracellular, making it difficult to measure. The primary function of phosphorus is the formation of ATP, which provides intracellular energy for active transport mechanisms across the cell membrane. Additional functions of phosphorus include cell membrane structure, acid-base balance, oxygen delivery to the tissues, cellular immunity, and bone strength (Box 29-10).[1]

Absorption of phosphorus takes place in the gastrointestinal tract, and serum phosphorus levels change frequently and dramatically, particularly in response to the ingestion of phosphate-rich foods such as milk, red meats, poultry, and fish. Most excretion occurs in the kidneys. More than 90% of the phosphorus in the plasma is filtered by the glomerulus, and about 80% is resorbed by the proximal convoluted tubules. Resorption by the kidneys is increased when body stores are low, and it is combined with sodium and excess hydrogen ions to maintain acid-base balance.[1,2,10]

Phosphorus abnormalities are evident early in the course of kidney failure. The Third National Health and Nutrition Examination Survey (NHANES III, 1988-1994, which included 14,722 adults) revealed that people with mild or moderate kidney dysfunction—defined as a urinary creatinine clearance rate (CrCl) between 50 and 60 mL/min—already have elevations of serum phosphorus and potassium levels.[12] In contrast, serum ionized calcium remains relatively unchanged until the creatinine clearance rate is extremely low (CrCl <20 mL/min) and kidney failure is advanced.[12] In kidney failure, hyperphosphatemia may contribute to lower serum calcium levels because phosphate and calcium are deposited in bone and soft tissues.[1,10]

MAGNESIUM

Magnesium is the second most important and abundant intracellular electrolyte; about 60% of it is located in the bone.[1,11] The ECF contains only about 1% of the body's magnesium, and the remaining amount resides in the ICF. The levels of other intracellular electrolytes, such as calcium and potassium, are affected by the level of magnesium. For example, calcium and magnesium compete for absorption in the gastrointestinal tract. If the dietary intake of calcium is higher than that of magnesium, calcium is preferentially resorbed and vice versa. The most important functions of magnesium are ensuring the transport of sodium and potassium across the cell membrane and as a cofactor in many intracellular enzyme reactions.[1] Depletion of magnesium liberates potassium to the ECF, which causes an increase in the excretion of potassium by the kidney and

---

BOX 29-9   FUNCTIONS OF CALCIUM

NORMAL SERUM VALUE
- 8.5-10.5 mg/dL

FUNCTIONS
- Hardness of bone and teeth
- Skeletal muscle contraction
- Blood coagulation
- Cellular permeability
- Heart muscle contraction

BOX 29-10   FUNCTIONS OF PHOSPHORUS

NORMAL SERUM VALUE
- 2.5-4.5 mg/dL

FUNCTIONS
- Intracellular energy production (ATP)
- Bone hardness
- Structure of cellular membrane
- Oxygen delivery to tissues
- Enzyme regulation (ATPase)

hypokalemia. Magnesium also plays a role in transmitting central nervous system messages, maintaining neuromuscular activity, protein synthesis, and intracellular energy production (Box 29-11).[11]

CHLORIDE

Chloride is rarely found in the body unless in combination with one of the major cations, especially sodium. Changes in serum chloride levels usually indicate changes in the other electrolytes or in acid-base balance. Because of its frequent combination with sodium, chloride plays a major role in maintaining serum osmolality, water balance, and acid-base balance because of competition with bicarbonate for combination with sodium. Additional functions of chloride are listed in Box 29-12.

Chloride is usually ingested with sodium in the form of salt and is resorbed or excreted in the proximal tubules of the kidney. Chloride is actively transported out of the tubules into he interstitium with sodium to help maintain the high tubular interstitial osmolality and the mechanism for concentrating the urine.[2]

BOX 29-11   FUNCTIONS OF MAGNESIUM

NORMAL SERUM VALUE
- 1.3-2.1 mEq/L

FUNCTIONS
- Neuromuscular transmission
- Contraction of heart muscle
- Activation of enzymes for cellular metabolism
- Active transport at cellular level
- Transmission of hereditary information

BOX 29-12   FUNCTIONS OF CHLORIDE

NORMAL SERUM VALUE
- 97-110 mEq/L

FUNCTIONS
- Body fluid osmolality (with sodium)
- Body water balance (with sodium)
- Acid-base balance
- Acidity of body fluids, especially gastric secretions
- Red blood cell oxygenation and carbon dioxide transport

BICARBONATE

Bicarbonate (HCO_3^-) is an anion in the ECF, and it performs the essential function of maintaining the acid-base balance. Although bicarbonate is not solely responsible for the acid-base balance, it is the major ECF buffer. Bicarbonate levels in the body are in balance with carbonic acid (H_2CO_3) levels. The ratio between the two must remain proportional at 1 mEq of carbonic acid to 20 mEq of bicarbonate; otherwise, acid-base disturbances will result. When the carbonic acid level is elevated, acidosis results. When the bicarbonate level is high, alkalosis results.

The amount of bicarbonate available in the ECF is regulated by the kidneys.[2] Resorption of bicarbonate occurs primarily from the proximal tubule into the peritubular capillaries. Bicarbonate is also produced in the distal tubule and resorbed into the blood in response to acid-base balance and body requirements. The kidneys resorb or excrete bicarbonate in response to the number of hydrogen ions present as part of the body's buffer system. More bicarbonate is resorbed when a large number of hydrogen ions are present, and more is excreted when few hydrogen ions are present.

EFFECTS OF AGING

Kidney function declines gradually with age, but this usually does not affect homeostasis in the healthy older adult. Electrolyte and acid-base parameters do not specifically change with advancing age.[6] However, in critical illness, the ability of aging kidneys to respond quickly to changes in electrolyte alterations, especially sodium and potassium imbalances, is reduced.

The kidneys carry out many functions that assist in the maintenance of homeostasis. Although fluid balance is one of the most important functions, an understanding of the numerous other roles the kidneys play provides clues to total body function.

Summary

- The kidneys play a major role in maintaining homeostasis.
- Important functions of the kidneys include waste product removal, fluid electrolyte balance, and acid-base balance.
- Hormone functions of the kidneys support red blood cell production, blood pressure regulation, and bone metabolism.
- Kidney function declines gradually with age, making elders more susceptible to kidney dysfunction during illness.

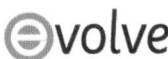 Be sure to check out the bonus material, including free self-assessment exercises, on the Evolve web site at http://evolve.elsevier.com/Urden/.

References

1. Chmielewski C et al: Renal physiology. In Molzahn A, Butera E, editors: *Contemporary nephrology nursing: Principles and practice*, ed 2, Pitman, NJ, 2006, American Nephrology Nurses Association.

2. Schira M, section editor: Kidney anatomy and physiology. In Counts C, editor: *Core curriculum for nephrology nursing*, ed 5, Pitman, NJ, 2008, American Nephrology Nurses Association.

3. Briggs J et al: Overview of kidney function and structure. In Greenberg A, editor: Primer on kidney diseases, ed 4, Philadelphia, 2005, Saunders.

4. Guyton A, Hall J: *Textbook of medical physiology*, ed 10, Philadelphia, 2000, Saunders.

5. Schira M, section editor: Assessment of kidney structure and function. In Counts C, editor: *Core curriculum for nephrology nursing*, ed 5, Pitman, NJ, 2008, American Nephrology Nurses Association.

6. Yuan F, Anderson S: The kidney in aging. In Greenberg A, editor: *Primer on kidney diseases*, ed 4, Philadelphia, 2005, Saunders.

7. Wilcox C: Pathogenesis of hypertension. In Greenberg A, editor: *Primer on kidney diseases*, ed 4, Philadelphia, 2005, Saunders.

8. Counts C, section editor: Chronic kidney disease. In Counts C, editor: *Core curriculum for nephrology nursing*, ed 5, Pitman, NJ, 2008, American Nephrology Nurses Association.

9. Himmelfarb J: Hematologic manifestations of chronic kidney disease. In Greenberg A, editor: *Primer on kidney diseases*, ed 4, Philadelphia, 2005, Saunders.

10. Parker K: Alterations in fluid, electrolyte, and acid-base balance. In Molzahn A, Butera E, editors: *Contemporary nephrology nursing: Principles and practice*, ed 2, Pitman, NJ, 2006, American Nephrology Nurses Association.

11. Metheny N: Fluid and electrolyte balance: nursing considerations, ed 4, Philadelphia, 2000, Lippincott.

12. Hsu CY, Chertow GM: Elevations of serum phosphorous and potassium in mild-to-moderate chronic renal insufficiency, *Nephrol Dial Transplant* 17 (8):1419-1425, 2002.

13. Brynes MC et al: A comparison of corrected serum calcium levels to ionized calcium levels among critically ill surgical patients, *Am J Surg* 189(3): 310-314, 2005.

Renal Clinical Assessment and Diagnostic Procedures

$\mathcal{U}$nderstanding the anatomic structures and physiologic workings of the kidneys provides the basis for understanding the clinical manifestations that signal kidney or renal system dysfunction. The body produces many clinical signs and symptoms that indicate kidney disorders. However, these signs and symptoms are often subtle, and although some symptoms point directly to the kidneys, many are exhibited by other body systems. A detailed history and careful physical examination help focus on the kidneys as the source of symptoms and often uncover the cause of the problem.

HISTORY

The history begins with a description of the chief complaint, stated in the patient's own words. A description of the chief complaint includes the onset, location, duration, and factors or strategies that lessen or aggravate the problem.[1] The individual should be encouraged to describe the effects of any treatment for the problem, prescription and nonprescription medications taken to alleviate symptoms, efforts taken to determine the cause of the problem, and procedures performed to improve the problem. A careful history that explores symptoms fully is an essential component of the clinical assessment.

Predisposing factors for acute kidney dysfunction are obtained during the history, including the use of over-the-counter medicines, recent infections requiring antibiotic therapy, antihypertensive medicines, and any diagnostic procedures performed using radiopaque contrast.[2] Nonsteroidal antiinflammatory drugs (e.g., ibuprofen), antibiotics (especially aminoglycosides), antihypertensives (especially medicines that block angiotensin), and iodine-based dyes may cause an acute or chronic decline in kidney function. A history of recent onset of nausea and vomiting or appetite loss caused by taste changes (uremia often causes a metallic taste) may provide clues to the rapid onset of kidney problems.[2] Symptoms that indicate rapid fluid volume gains are explored. For example, weight gains of more than 2 pounds per day, sleeping on additional pillows, and sitting in a chair to sleep are signals of volume overload and potential cardiac stress related to kidney dysfunction.

In addition to determining the immediate reason for admission to the critical care unit, compiling a complete medical and social history is important. Similar symptoms, problems, or treatment for similar complaints in the past may help establish the cause of the current problem or provide clues for treatment. For example, a history of obstructive urologic problems, frequent kidney infections, or previous acute kidney injury or failure may signal risk factors for current kidney problems. The patient, family member, or significant other should be encouraged to provide as much detail as possible during the history.

The family history may provide important information that points to the kidneys as the source of the patient's symptoms. For example, the patient may reveal that one or two close family members have always had swelling of the extremities or high blood pressure. These symptoms should lead to questions about a history of kidney problems in the family. The Data Collection feature summarizes the information gained from a kidney history.

PHYSICAL EXAMINATION

In the critical care area, nursing assessment does not routinely include a full physical examination of the kidneys and urologic system. However, many of the assessment parameters for the kidneys provide information related to the volume status of the individual and are helpful in a large number of patients regardless of kidney function or status. Although not often performed in the depth described in the following sections, the critical care nurse must be aware of how to perform a thorough kidney assessment in stable patients and as needed in patients with kidney dysfunction.

INSPECTION

Bleeding. Visual inspection related to the kidneys focuses on the patient's flank and abdomen. Kidney trauma is suspected if a purplish discoloration is present on the flank (Grey-Turner sign) or near the posterior 11th or 12th ribs.[1] Bruising, abdominal distention, and abdominal guarding may also signal kidney trauma or a hematoma around a kidney. Individuals who have experienced a traumatic injury should be carefully assessed for signs of kidney trauma.

Volume. Inspection is especially helpful in looking for signs of volume depletion or overload that may signal or lead to kidney problems. Fluid volume assessment begins with an inspection of

---

Data Collection

Renal History

Common Kidney-Related Symptoms
- Dyspnea
- Peripheral dependent edema
- Nocturia
- Nausea
- Metallic taste in mouth
- Loss of appetite
- Headache
- Rapid weight gain
- Itching
- Dry, scaly skin
- Weakness, fatigue
- Cognitive function changes
- Mental status changes

Patient Profile
- Personal habits
- Use of over-the-counter drugs, herbs, vitamins, and dietary supplements
- Illicit drug use
- Change in employment caused by illness
- Financial problems resulting from illness (e.g., cost, time off work)
- Sexual function (e.g., decreased libido, amenorrhea)

Risk Factors
- Family history
- Hypertension
- Diabetes mellitus
- Prior acute kidney failure

Family History
- Hypertension
- Diabetes mellitus

- Polycystic kidney disease
- Kidney disease
- Chronically swollen extremities

Past Kidney Studies
- Urinalysis with proteinuria
- Creatinine clearance
- Kidney-ureter-bladder (KUB) radiograph
- Intravenous pyelogram
- Kidney ultrasound
- Renal arteriography
- Kidney biopsy

Medical History
Childhood
- Nephrotic syndrome, streptococcal infection, hypoplastic kidneys, obstructive uropathy

Adult
- Frequent urinary tract infections
- Calculi
- Vasculitis
- Use of iodine-based radiographic contrast media
- Use of nonsteroidal antiinflammatory drugs

Current Medication Use
- Nonsteroidal antiinflammatory drugs
- Antibiotics
- Antihypertensives
- Diuretics

---

the patient's jugular neck veins. The supine position facilitates normal jugular venous distention. An absence of distention (flat neck veins) indicates hypovolemia. Assessment continues with the head of the bed elevated 45 to 90 degrees.[1] Fluid overload exists when the neck veins remain distended more than 2 cm above the sternal notch when the bed is at 45 degrees.[3]

Hand vein inspection may be helpful in assessing volume status, and it is performed by observing for venous distention when the hand is held in the dependent position. Venous filling that takes longer than 5 seconds suggests hypovolemia. When the hand is elevated, the distention should disappear within 5 seconds. If distention does not disappear within 5 seconds after the hand is elevated, fluid overload is suspected.

Assessment of skin turgor provides additional data for identifying fluid-related problems. To assess turgor, the skin over the forearm is picked up and released. Normal elasticity and fluid status allow an almost immediate return to shape after the skin is released. In fluid volume deficit, however, the skin remains raised and does not return to its normal position for several seconds. Because of the loss of skin elasticity in older persons, skin turgor assessment is not an accurate fluid assessment for this age group.

Inspection of the oral cavity provides clues to fluid volume status. When a fluid volume deficit exists, the mucous membranes of the mouth become dry. However, mouth breathing and some medicines (e.g., antihistamines) can also dry the mucous membranes temporarily. A more accurate way to assess the oral cavity is to inspect the mouth using a tongue blade. Dryness of the oral cavity is more indicative of fluid volume deficit than are complaints of a dry mouth.[3]

Edema. Edema is the presence of excess fluid in the interstitial space, and it can be a sign of volume overload. In the presence of volume excess, edema may develop in dependent areas of the body, such as the feet and legs of an ambulatory person or the sacrum of an individual confined to bed. However, edema does not always indicate fluid volume overload. A loss of albumin from the vascular space can cause peripheral edema despite hypovolemia or normal fluid states. A critically ill

TABLE 30-1 Pitting Edema Scale

Rating	Approximate Equivalent
+1	2-mm depth
+2	4-mm depth (lasting up to 15 sec)
+3	6-mm depth (lasting up to 60 sec)
+4	8-mm depth (lasting longer than 60 sec)

patient may have a low serum albumin level (hypoalbuminemia) because of inadequate nutrition after surgery, a burn, or a head injury and may exhibit edema as a result of the loss of plasma oncotic pressure and not as a result of volume overload. Edema also may signal circulatory difficulties. An individual who is fluid balanced but who has poor venous return may experience pedal edema after prolonged sitting in a chair with the feet dependent. Similarly, an individual with heart failure may experience edema because the left ventricle is unable to pump blood effectively through the vessels. A key feature that distinguishes edema due to excess volume or hypoalbuminemia from circulatory compromise is that the edema does not reverse with elevation of the extremity.

Edema can be assessed by applying fingertip pressure on the swollen area over a bony prominence, such as the ankles, pretibial areas (shins), and sacrum. If the indentation made by the fingertip does not disappear within 15 seconds, pitting edema exists. Pitting edema indicates increased interstitial volume, and it usually is not evident until significant weight gain has occurred.[4] Edema also may appear in the hands and feet, around the eyes, and in the cheeks. Dependent areas, such as the feet and sacrum, are the areas most likely to demonstrate edema in patients confined to a wheelchair or bed. One way of measuring the extent of edema is by using a subjective scale of 1 to 4, with 1 indicating only minimal pitting and 4 indicating severe pitting (Table 30-1).[1] Other scales for assessing and measuring edema can be used (see Table 17-3).

AUSCULTATION

Auscultation of the kidneys yields virtually no useful information. However, the renal arteries are auscultated for a bruit, a blowing or swishing sound that resembles a cardiac murmur (Fig. 30-1). The examiner listens for bruits above and to the left and right of the umbilicus.[1] A renal artery bruit usually indicates stenosis, which may lead to acute or chronic kidney dysfunction due to compromised blood flow to one or both kidneys. A bruit over the upper portion of the abdominal aorta may indicate an aneurysm or a stenotic area that can decrease blood flow to the kidneys.

Auscultation is especially helpful in providing information about extracellular fluid (ECF) volume status. Listening for specific sounds in the heart and lungs provides information about the presence or absence of increased fluid in the interstitium or vascular space.

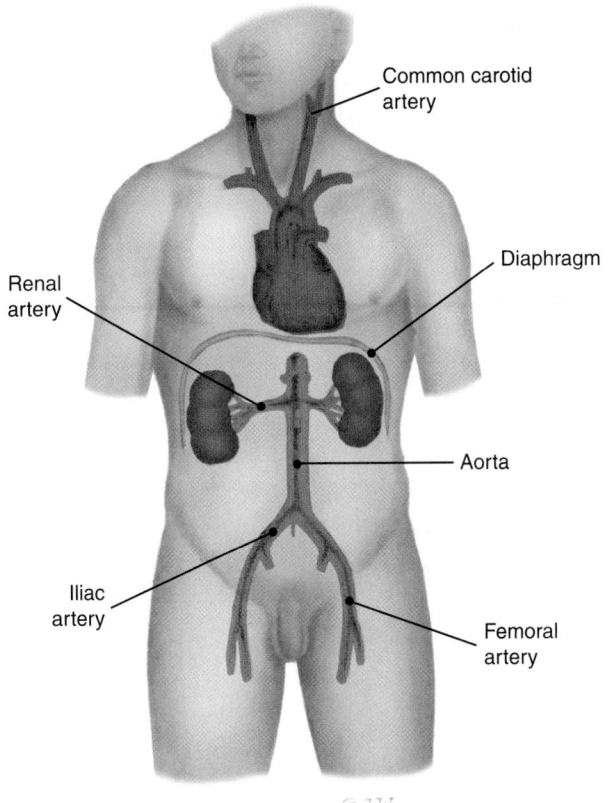

Figure 30-1 Sites for auscultation of bruits.

Heart. Auscultation of the heart requires assessing the rate and rhythm and listening for extra sounds. Fluid overload is often accompanied by a third or fourth heart sound, which is best heard with the bell of the stethoscope.[1] Increased heart rate alone provides little information about fluid volume, but combined with a low blood pressure, it may indicate hypovolemia.

The heart is auscultated for the presence of a pericardial friction rub. A rub can best be heard at the third intercostal space to the left of the sternal border while the individual leans slightly forward.[1] A pericardial friction rub indicates pericarditis, and it may result from uremia in a patient with kidney failure.

Blood Pressure. Blood pressure and heart rate changes are very useful in assessing fluid volume deficit. In stable critically ill patients or in patients on a telemetry unit, orthostatic vital sign measurements provide clues to blood loss, dehydration, unexplained syncope, and the effects of some antihypertensive medications.[4,5] A drop in systolic blood pressure of 20 mm Hg or more, a drop in diastolic blood pressure of 10 mm Hg or more, or a rise in pulse rate of more than 15 beats/min from lying to sitting or from sitting to standing indicates orthostatic hypotension. Box 30-1 describes how to assess for orthostatic hypotension. The drop in blood pressure occurs because a sufficient preload is not immediately available when the patient changes position. The heart rate increases in an attempt to maintain cardiac output and circulation. Orthostatic hypotension produces subjective feelings of weakness, dizziness, or faintness. Although orthostatic hypotension is often a sign of hypovolemia, peripheral vascular disease also may be responsible. Damage to the

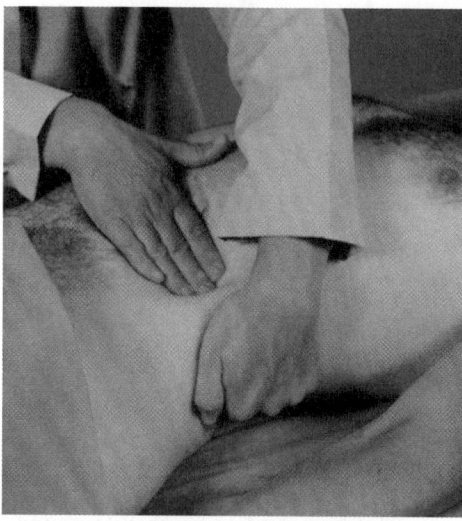

Figure 30-2 Palpation of the kidney. *(From Barkauskas V et al: Health & physical assessment, ed 3, St Louis, 2002, Mosby.)*

venous circulation of the lower extremities decreases blood return to the heart, leading to a blood pressure drop in a normovolemic individual.

Lungs. Lung assessment is essential in gauging fluid status. Crackles indicate fluid overload. Dyspnea with mild exertion, dyspnea at night that prevents sleeping in a supine position (orthopnea), or dyspnea that awakens the individual from sleep (paroxysmal nocturnal dyspnea) may indicate pooling of fluid in the lungs. Shallow, gasping breaths with periods of apnea reflect severe acid-base imbalances.

PALPATION

Although rarely performed in critically ill patients, palpation of the kidneys in stable patients provides information about the kidneys' size and shape. Palpation of the kidneys is achieved through the bimanual capturing approach. Capturing is accomplished by placing one hand posteriorly under the flank of the supine patient with the examiner's fingers pointing to the midline and placing the opposite hand just below the rib cage anteriorly.[1,2] The patient is asked to inhale deeply while pressure is exerted to bring the hands together (Fig. 30-2). As the patient

exhales, the examiner may feel the kidney between the hands. After each kidney is palpated in this manner, the two should be compared for size and shape. Each kidney should be firm and smooth, and the two organs should be of equal size. The examiner is usually unable to palpate a normal left kidney. The right kidney is more easily palpated because of its lower position, caused by downward displacement by the liver. Problems should be suspected if a mass (cancer) or an irregular surface (polycystic kidneys) is palpated, a size difference is detected, the kidney extends significantly lower than the rib cage on either side, or there is evidence of recent blunt trauma.[1,6]

PERCUSSION

Percussion is performed to detect pain in the area of a kidney or to determine excess accumulation of air, fluid, or solids around the kidneys. Percussion of the kidneys also provides information about kidney location, size, and possible problems. Like palpation, percussion of the kidneys is not a routine part of a nursing assessment in critical care. However, the information gained through percussion can provide important patient care data.

Kidneys. Percussion of a kidney is performed with the patient in a side-lying or sitting position, with the examiner's hand placed over the costovertebral angle (lower border of the rib cage on the flank).[1] Striking the back of the hand with the opposite fist produces a dull thud, which is normal. Pain may indicate infection (e.g., urinary tract infection that has extended into the kidneys) or injury resulting from trauma. Traumatic injury to the kidneys should be assessed in the presence of a penetrating abdominal wound, with blunt abdominal trauma, or with a fractured pelvis or ribs.[6,7]

Abdomen. Observation and percussion of the abdomen may help in assessing fluid status. Percussing the abdomen with the patient in the supine position generally yields a dull sound (solid bowel contents or fluid) or a hollow sound (gaseous bowel).[1]

Ascites, or excess fluid accumulation and distention of the abdominal cavity, is an important observation in determining fluid overload. Differentiating ascites from distortion caused by solid bowel contents is accomplished by producing a fluid wave. A fluid wave is elicited by exerting pressure to the abdominal midline while one hand is placed on the right or left flank.[1,4] Tapping the opposite flank produces a wave in the accumulated fluid that can be felt under the hands (Fig. 30-3). Other signs of ascites include a protuberant, rounded abdomen and abdominal striae.[1]

Individuals with kidney failure may have ascites caused by volume overload, which forces fluid into the abdomen due to increased capillary hydrostatic pressures. However, ascites may or may not represent fluid volume excess. Severe ascites in persons with compromised liver function may result from decreased plasma proteins. The ascites occurs because the increased vascular pressure associated with liver dysfunction forces fluid and plasma proteins from the vascular space into the interstitial space and abdominal cavity. Although the individual may exhibit marked edema, the intravascular space is volume depleted, and the patient is hypovolemic.

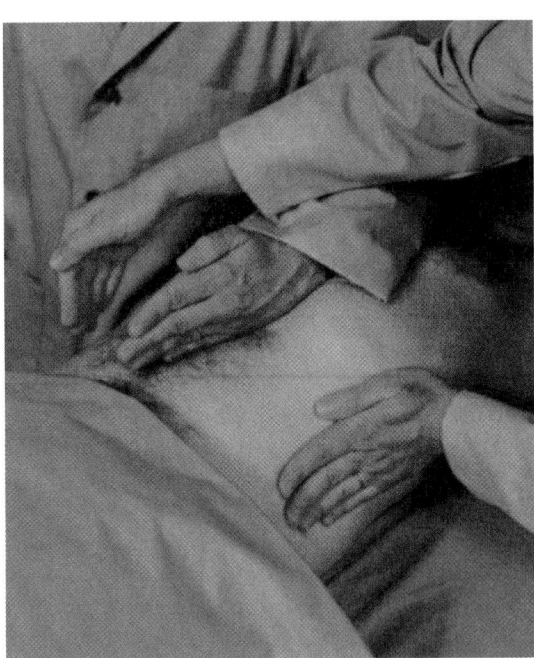

Figure 30-3 Test for the presence of a fluid wave. *(From Barkauskas V et al: Health & physical assessment, ed 3, St Louis, 2002, Mosby.)*

ADDITIONAL ASSESSMENTS

WEIGHT MONITORING

One of the most important assessments of kidney and fluid status is the patient's weight. In the critical care unit, weight is monitored for each patient every day and is an important vital signs measurement. Significant fluctuations in body weight over a 1- to 2-day period indicate fluid gains and losses. Rapid weight gains or losses of more than 2 pounds per day usually indicate fluid rather than nutritional factors. One liter of fluid equals 1 kg, or approximately 2.2 pounds.

Whenever possible, the patient is weighed during admission to the critical care unit. It is important to document whether the current weight differs significantly from the weight 1 to 2 weeks before admission to the hospital. The patient is weighed daily for comparison with the previous day's weight. The weight is obtained at the same time each day, with the patient wearing the same amount of clothing and using the same scales. The individual's weight is of critical importance to the dialysis nurse caring for a patient with acute or chronic kidney failure. The differences in weight from day to day are used to calculate the amount of fluid to remove during a dialysis treatment.[8]

INTAKE AND OUTPUT MONITORING

Like patient weight, intake and output are monitored for all patients in the critical care unit. Intake and output can be compared with the patient's weight to more accurately evaluate fluid gains or losses. Urinary output plus insensible fluid losses (perspiration, stool, and water vapor from the lungs) can vary by 750 to 2400 mL/day. When intake exceeds output

(e.g., excessive intravenous fluid, decreased urine output), a positive fluid balance exists. In impaired kidney function, the positive fluid balance results in fluid volume overload. Conversely, if output exceeds intake (e.g., fever, increased respiration, profuse sweating, vomiting, diarrhea, gastric suction, diuretic therapy), a negative fluid balance exists, and volume deficit results. During a 24-hour period, fever can increase skin and respiratory losses by as much as 75 mL per 1° F increase in temperature.

Individuals with *acute kidney injury* (AKI) often exhibit a decrease in urine output, or oliguria (<0.5 mL/kg/hr in adults; <1 mL/kg/hr in infants and young children). However, there may be a fairly normal or only slightly decreased urine output that reflects water removal without solute removal in the early phases of AKI. Although urine output is a sensitive indicator, kidney function cannot be accurately determined by urine output alone.

Abnormal output of body fluids creates fluid imbalances and causes electrolyte and acid-base disturbances. For example, gastrointestinal suction or loss by diarrhea can result in fluid deficit, sodium and potassium deficits, and metabolic acidosis from excessive loss of bicarbonate.

In maintaining daily records of intake and output, all gains or losses must be recorded. A standard list of the fluid volume held in various containers (e.g., milk cartons, juice containers) expedites this process. Discussions about the importance of accurate intake and output with the patient and family or friends are necessary and can improve the accuracy of intake and output volumes assessment.

HEMODYNAMIC MONITORING

Body fluid status is accurately reflected in measurements of cardiovascular hemodynamics. Measurements such as central venous pressure (CVP), pulmonary artery occlusion pressure (PAOP), cardiac index (CI), and mean arterial pressure (MAP) provide a clear picture of the increases or decreases in vascular volume returning to and being ejected from the heart.[9] Volume depletion and volume overload are easily detected by use of central venous or arterial catheters, from which pressure measurements can be obtained (Table 30-2).

TABLE 30-2 Hemodynamic Assessment of Fluid Status

Measurement	Volume Depletion	Volume Overload
Central venous pressure (CVP)	<2 mm Hg	>5 mm Hg
Pulmonary artery occlusion pressure (PAOP)	<5 mm Hg	>12 mm Hg
Cardiac index (CI)	<2.2 L/min/m²	>4 L/min/m²
Mean arterial pressure (MAP)	Decreased	Increased

A central venous catheter often is inserted to evaluate fluid volume status and to measure the CVP. The CVP represents the filling pressure of the right atrium and is a measurement of right ventricular preload. The CVP changes with fluctuations in volume status. A normal CVP is 2 to 5 mm Hg. In volume depletion, the CVP is less than 2 mm Hg, whereas volume overload is reflected by readings of more than 5 mm Hg (see "Bedside Hemodynamic Monitoring" in Chapter 18 for more information on CVP interpretation).

If the patient has coexisting cardiopulmonary disease or if more information about hemodynamic function is required, a pulmonary artery catheter may be inserted. This catheter provides information about left ventricular filling pressures and cardiac output. The PAOP represents the left atrial pressure required to fill the left ventricle. When the left ventricle is full at the end of diastole, it represents the volume of blood available for ejection. It is also known as left ventricular preload and is measured by the PAOP. The normal PAOP is 5 to 12 mm Hg. In fluid volume excess, the PAOP increases. In fluid volume deficit, the PAOP is low.[9]

The CI demonstrates the cardiac output, or amount of blood ejected by the left ventricle over 1 minute, standardized for body size. The normal CI is 2.2 to 4 L/min/m^2. Compensatory mechanisms in early hypovolemic shock maintain the CI at or near normal. With prolonged fluid loss, the CI decreases. Fluid volume overload increases heart rate, which increases cardiac output, but only to a point. Left ventricular failure may result from massive volume overload, such as with acute heart failure resulting from kidney failure, in which case the CI decreases. The most common cause of AKI in which hemodynamic monitoring is indicated is severe sepsis.[9]

MAP is regulated by cardiac output and systemic vascular resistance (SVR), and it represents an averaged blood pressure within the arterial system. Changes in cardiac output or SVR inevitably result in corresponding MAP changes. For example, an increase in SVR during the early stages of hypovolemic shock leads to elevation of the MAP. Ongoing fluid losses eventually lead to a decreased cardiac output, which leads to a reduction in MAP. The net effect of a decreased MAP to the kidneys is a reduction in effective blood flow, which may lead to AKI.

OTHER OBSERVATIONS

Kidney system dysfunction often leads to fluid and electrolyte imbalances and the retention of metabolic waste products. Some of the disturbances in fluid, electrolyte, and waste product levels are accompanied by clinical manifestations less observable or measurable than those previously mentioned but that indicate a change from normal function. Box 30-2 summarizes important aspects to consider during kidney and fluid and electrolyte assessment.

Sudden or slowly developing changes in cognitive function and mental status must be investigated. For example, acidosis often results in disorientation. Lethargy, decreased attention or memory, coma, and confusion may result from sodium, calcium, or magnesium excess or deficit or retained waste products. Apprehension or anxiety may result from sodium deficit, a shift of fluid from the plasma to the interstitium, or respiratory changes caused by fluid volume overload. In elders, new-onset confusion or a fall incurred by a previously mobile, alert individual may signal volume deficit in the absence of apparent acute illness.[10]

Apathy and withdrawal may accompany hypovolemic states. Patients with kidney failure and the accompanying systemic increases in electrolytes, fluids, and nitrogenous waste products may exhibit apathy, restlessness, confusion, and withdrawal.[2] The speed of onset depends on how rapidly or slowly the kidney failure progresses and alters homeostasis. In some patients, it may be difficult to separate the emotional component of critical illness from the physiologic mechanism; therefore both mechanisms are considered by the critical care nurse.

BOX 30-2   FLUID AND ELECTROLYTE ASSESSMENT

FLUID STATUS
- Skin turgor
- Mucous membranes
- Intake and output
- Presence of edema or ascites
- Neck and hand vein engorgement
- Lung sounds (crackles)
- Dyspnea
- Central venous pressure (CVP) <2 mm Hg or >5 mm Hg
- Pulmonary artery occlusive pressure (PAOP) <5 mm Hg or >12 mm Hg
- Tachycardia
- Hypertension, hypotension
- Cardiac index (CI) < 2.2 L/min/m^2
- S$_3$, S$_4$ heart sounds
- Headache
- Blurred vision
- Vertigo on rising
- Papilledema
- Mental changes
- Serum osmolality

ELECTROLYTE AND WASTE PRODUCT STATUS
- Complete blood cell count (CBC)
- Serum electrolyte levels
- Nitrogen waste products (BUN)
- Electrocardiogram tracings (potassium, calcium, magnesium levels)
- Behavioral and mental changes (sodium, BUN levels)
- Chvostek and Trousseau signs (calcium levels)
- Changes in peripheral sensation (numbness, tremor—sodium, potassium, calcium levels)
- Muscle strength (potassium, BUN)
- Gastrointestinal changes (nausea and vomiting—BUN)
- Itching (calcium, phosphorus, BUN)
- Therapies that can alter electrolyte status (gastrointestinal suction, diuretics, antihypertensives, calcium channel blockers)

LABORATORY ASSESSMENT

There is no single or ideal laboratory test or marker that detects a decrease in kidney function.[11] Laboratory tests (serum and urine) used to detect and diagnose kidney dysfunction have limitations, but when reviewed daily for changes or trends, they provide valuable information concerning the status of the kidneys. Small changes in kidney function have been associated with short- and long-term outcomes for hospitalized patients.[12] In addition to the history and physical examination, laboratory data are extremely helpful in the diagnosis, management, and ongoing evaluation of kidney system dysfunction.

SERUM COMPONENTS

Blood Urea Nitrogen. Blood urea nitrogen (BUN) is a by-product of protein and amino acid metabolism.[13] The normal value for BUN is 5 to 25 mg/dL, which is increased when kidney function deteriorates.[14] With kidney dysfunction, the BUN is elevated because of a decrease in the glomerular filtration rate (GFR) and resulting decrease in urea excretion. Elevations in the BUN can be correlated with the clinical manifestations of uremia; as the BUN rises, symptoms of uremia become more pronounced.[2] However, a drop in the GFR with an increase in the BUN also may be caused by hypovolemia and dehydration,[15] nephrotoxic drugs, or a sudden hypotensive episode. In these cases, the rise in BUN is caused by a decreased GFR in the presence of normal kidney function.[15] BUN is also increased by changes in protein metabolism that occur with excessive protein intake and catabolism.[13] A catabolic state may occur with starvation (or chronic poor nutrition in a critically ill patient), severe infection, surgery, or trauma. The BUN level also may be elevated as the result of hematoma resorption, gastrointestinal bleeding, excessive licorice ingestion, or steroid or tetracycline therapy. A decrease in the BUN level may indicate volume overload, liver damage, severe malnutrition (as a result of depleted protein stores), use of phenothiazines, or pregnancy.[14]

Creatinine. Creatinine is a by-product of muscle and normal cell metabolism, and it appears in serum in amounts generally proportional to the body muscle mass. Although slightly higher in males than females, the normal serum creatinine level is about 0.5 to 1.5 mg/dL.[14] Creatinine is freely filtered by the glomerulus, easily excreted by the renal tubules, and minimally resorbed or secreted in the tubules.[2] Creatinine levels are fairly constant and are affected by fewer factors than BUN. As a result, the serum creatinine level is a more sensitive and specific indicator of kidney function than BUN. Creatinine excess occurs most often in persons with kidney failure resulting from impaired excretion. However, the body's production and release of creatinine may vary greatly, especially during muscle wasting in acute illness, leading to a falsely low serum level of creatinine. Elevated levels of creatinine may occur in muscle growth disorders such as acromegaly with skeletal muscle injury (e.g., in a trauma patient) or with some medications that decrease creatinine removal (e.g., trimethoprim, cimetidine) in the absence of kidney dysfunction.[11] Malnutrition can result in transient increases in creatinine levels as the rapid muscle catabolism associated with malnutrition causes "dumping" of increased amounts of creatinine into the circulation.

Another useful diagnostic parameter in kidney disease is the ratio of serum urea nitrogen to creatinine. The usual ratio of BUN to creatinine is 10 to 1, and a change in the ratio may indicate kidney dysfunction and is often useful in identifying the cause of the acute kidney dysfunction.[14,17] For example, if BUN and creatinine levels are elevated and maintained at an approximate ratio of 10 to1, the disorder is intrarenal, or affecting the tubules of the kidneys. If the ratio of BUN to creatinine levels is greater than 10 to 1, the cause is most likely prerenal (e.g., hypovolemia).[13,15] In prerenal kidney failure, the creatinine is excreted by functioning tubules, but the urea nitrogen is retained because of the poor GFR and hemoconcentration, leading to the increased ratio.[13] In the diagnosis of prerenal failure, the ratio is a more useful indicator of kidney function than the separate tests of BUN and creatinine.

Creatinine Clearance. The most useful kidney function parameter is the creatinine clearance, a measure of how well the kidneys remove creatinine. Because of the relatively constant rate at which creatinine is produced and the nearly complete removal of creatinine by normal kidneys, the ability of the kidneys to remove (clear) creatinine from the blood is an indication of how well the glomeruli and tubules are working. Measuring the creatinine clearance—the amount of creatinine in the excreted urine and the amount of creatinine in the blood over 24 hours—provides a reliable and accurate estimate of glomerular filtration and therefore of kidney function.[2] The normal value for creatinine clearance is 110 to 120 mL/min; values less than 50 mL/min indicate significant kidney dysfunction. The creatinine clearance is best measured using a 12- or 24-hour urine collection and blood sample. Newer methods use a random, smaller-volume urine specimen and blood sample. Creatinine clearance can also be estimated from the serum creatinine level (Box 30-3), which is commonly used in clinical practice.[16,17] As kidney function decreases, creatinine clearance decreases and is useful in monitoring the severity, progression, and recovery of kidney function. The estimated or calculated creatinine clearance is widely used to determine changes in drug dosing with kidney dysfunction because many drugs are excreted by the kidneys.[17]

Cystatin C. Although not widely used in practice, cystatin C is another serum marker for kidney function. Cystatin C is a substance synthesized and released by most cells in the body at a constant rate.[11] Like creatinine, cystatin C is filtered easily by the glomerulus and not secreted or resorbed by the tubules. The advantage of cystatin C is that it is metabolized by the tubules. In normal kidney function, cystatin C levels are very low because the glomerulus filters it and the tubules metabolize it. In kidney dysfunction, the glomerular filtration of cystatin C is reduced and therefore not provided to the tubules for metabolism. Cystatin C is affected by fewer factors (e.g., age, gender, muscle mass) than creatinine, and a change in its level can be detected earlier during AKI than creatinine.[11] Cystatin C may become more widely used as a kidney function marker as additional clinical validation studies are completed.

BOX 30-3   CREATININE CLEARANCE CALCULATIONS

MEASURED: 24-HOUR URINE*

(Urine creatinine × Volume of urine)/Serum creatinine

ESTIMATED: ADULTS—COCKCROFT-GAULT FORMULA

[(140 − Age) × Body weight (kg)]/[72 × Plasma creatinine (mg/dL)]
For women, multiply the result by 0.85.

ESTIMATED: ADULTS—MODIFIED MODIFICATION OF DIET IN RENAL DISEASE (MDRD) FORMULA

186 × (Plasma creatinine) − 1.154 × (Age in years) − 0.203
For women, multiply the result by 0.742.
For African Americans, multiply the result by 1.210.[†]

ESTIMATED: CHILDREN

≤10 kg:	0.45 × Height (cm)/Serum creatinine (mg/dL)
>10, <70 kg:	0.55 × Height (cm)/Serum creatinine (mg/dL)
≥70 kg:	[1.55 × Age (yr)] + 0.5 × Height (cm)/Serum creatinine (mg/dL)

---

*Calculations available from the National Kidney Foundation (www.kidney.org/professionals).
Both risk factor assessments apply for African American women. The number would be multiplied by both 0.742 (woman) and 1.210 (African American).

Osmolality. The serum osmolality reflects the concentration or dilution of vascular fluid and measures the dissolved particles in the serum. The normal serum osmolality is 275 to 295 mOsm/L.[3] An elevated osmolality level indicates hemoconcentration or dehydration, and a decreased osmolality level indicates hemodilution or volume overload. When the serum osmolality level increases, antidiuretic hormone (ADH) is released from the posterior pituitary gland and stimulates increased water resorption in the kidney tubules. This expands the vascular space, returns the serum osmolality level back to normal, and results in more concentrated urine and an elevated urine osmolality level. The opposite occurs with a decreased serum osmolality level, which inhibits the production of ADH. The decreased ADH results in increased excretion of water in the tubules, producing dilute urine with a low osmolality, and returns the serum osmolality level back to normal. Sodium accounts for 85% to 95% of the serum osmolality value; doubling the serum sodium level gives an estimate of the serum osmolality level in healthy individuals.[14] Other particles in the serum can increase the osmolality and need to be considered in individuals with common comorbid conditions. A more precise estimation of serum osmolality can be calculated from the following formula:

$$2 \times Na(mmol/L) + BUN/3(mg/dL) + Glucose/18(mg/dL)$$

The calculated serum osmolality level is a useful tool while awaiting full laboratory results. Measured serum osmolality is a useful parameter in determining fluid balance and fluid replacement therapy for critically ill patients. Serum osmolality is also a useful parameter in determining disorders of ADH secretion that may occur in critically ill individuals. A decreased serum osmolality level may indicate syndrome of inappropriate ADH secretion (SIADH), or too much ADH, whereas an elevation of the serum osmolality level may indicate diabetes insipidus (DI), or too little ADH.

Anion Gap. The *anion gap* is a calculation of the difference between the measurable extracellular plasma cations (sodium and potassium) and the measurable anions (chloride and bicarbonate).[3] The value represents the remaining unmeasurable ions present in the extracellular fluid (phosphates, sulfates, ketones, lactate). In plasma, sodium is the predominant cation and chloride is the predominant anion. The extracellular potassium concentration in plasma is so small that it is generally ignored, leaving the following equation for calculation of the anion gap:

$$[Na^+] - ([Cl^-] + [HCO_3^-])$$

The normal anion gap is above 11 mEq/L and should not exceed 14 mEq/L. An increased anion gap level reflects overproduction or decreased excretion of acid products and indicates metabolic acidosis; a decreased anion gap indicates metabolic alkalosis.

Acute and chronic kidney failure can increase the anion gap because of retention of acids and altered bicarbonate resorption. The anion gap is also increased in diabetic ketoacidosis caused by ketone production. The measurement of the anion gap is a rapid method for identifying acid-base imbalance but cannot be used to pinpoint the source of the acid-base disturbance specifically.

Hemoglobin and Hematocrit. The hemoglobin and hematocrit levels can indicate increases or decreases in intravascular fluid volume.[13] Hemoglobin and hematocrit values vary between genders; the hemoglobin level in males is normally 13.5 to 17.5 g/dL, and in females, it is 12 to 16 g/dL. The hematocrit level is 40% to 54% in males and 37% to 47% in females. Hematocrit levels are higher in newborns (up to 65%) and decrease to adult ranges between the ages of 4 and 10 years.[14] Hemoglobin transports oxygen and carbon dioxide and is important in maintaining cellular metabolism and acid-base balance.[3]

The hematocrit value is the proportion or concentration of red blood cells (RBCs) in a volume of whole blood and is expressed as a percentage.[14] The hematocrit level is approximately three times the hemoglobin level if the individual is in a normal fluid balance. An increase in the hematocrit value often indicates a fluid volume deficit, which results in hemoconcentration. Although rare, true disorders of RBC production, such as polycythemia, can result in an increased hematocrit level.

Conversely, a decreased hematocrit value can indicate fluid volume excess because of the dilutional effect of the extra fluid load. Decreases also can result from anemias, blood loss, liver damage, or hemolytic reactions.[14] In individuals with acute kidney failure, anemia may occur early in the disease, and a decreased hematocrit level may indicate the anemia of kidney failure or may reflect fluid volume overload. If the hematocrit value is decreasing but the hemoglobin concentration remains constant, the cause is fluid volume overload. Decreased hematocrit values and hemoglobin concentrations indicate a true loss of RBCs. The history and bedside assessment, including hemodynamic monitoring data, aid in determining whether fluid imbalances or disease states, or both, are responsible for changes in hematocrit levels in the critically ill patient.

Albumin. Slightly more than 50% of the total plasma protein is serum albumin. It is manufactured in the liver, and a normal blood level is 3.5 to 5 g/dL.[14] Albumin is primarily responsible for the maintenance of colloid osmotic pressure, which functions to hold fluid in the vascular space. The blood vessel walls, because of their impermeability to plasma proteins, prevent albumin from leaving the vascular space. However, in some disease states such as severe burns (cell membrane destruction) or nephrotic syndrome (increased glomerular capillary permeability to protein and protein loss in the urine), albumin is lost from the vascular space.

Decreased albumin levels in the vascular space result in a fluid shift from the plasma to the interstitium, creating peripheral edema. A decreased albumin level can result from protein-calorie malnutrition, which occurs in many critically ill patients in whom available stores of albumin are depleted. A decrease in the plasma oncotic pressure results, and fluid shifts from the vascular space to the interstitial space. Liver disease or severe injury to the liver also causes a decrease in albumin levels as the diseased liver fails to synthesize sufficient albumin. Severe portal hypertension can force albumin and other plasma proteins into the abdominal cavity, resulting in ascites.

Increased albumin levels are rare. The body uses a fixed amount of protein for energy and body cell replacement and converts excess protein into stored fat. If all plasma protein levels are elevated, fluid volume deficit (hemoconcentration) is suspected.

URINANALYSIS

Analysis of the urine provides excellent information about the patient's kidney function and condition relative to fluids and electrolytes. Specific tests and abnormal indications are presented in Table 30-3.[14,18-20] In many cases, urinalysis in the critically ill patient aids in locating the site of kidney damage or disease and therefore guides therapeutic management of the patient's care. Although often considered routine, collecting and preserving the urine specimen is important to ensure that results are accurate and not the result of contamination or changes in urine sediment. For most accurate results, the specimen should be collected using a clean or sterile technique (midstream versus catheter collection) and examined within 30 minutes of collection.[20]

Appearance. Physical examination of the urine focuses on a general inspection of the urine's color, clarity, and odor.[19] Normal urine is pale yellow, but it may vary due to food intake (carrots, beets, rhubarb), drugs (phenytoin, nitrofurantoin, phenazopyridine), or metabolic by-products (bilirubin, methemoglobin).[14] Clarity of the urine may be affected by bacteria, white blood cells (WBCs), pus, or urates. Normal urine has minimal odor; a strong odor may be caused by concentrated urine (as in dehydrated states), infection, medicines (especially vitamins), or foods (broccoli, asparagus).

Urine pH. Urine pH indicates the acidity or alkalinity of the urine. The normal urinary pH is acidic but has a range from 4.5 to 8.0.[19,20] The kidneys regulate acid-base balance; more hydrogen ions are excreted than bicarbonate ions, causing the acidity of the urine. Changes in kidney function produce changes in urinary pH.

An increase in urinary acidity (decreased pH) indicates retention of sodium and acids by the body, which occurs in intrarenal AKI. A decrease in urinary acidity (increased pH or more alkaline) means the body is retaining bicarbonate. In the presence of normal kidney function, urinary pH levels are greatly affected by diet and medications. Certain food groups, such as citrus fruits and vegetables, lead to alkaline urine, whereas a diet high in protein can produce acid urine. In the critical care unit, patients receiving total parenteral nutrition or a high-protein tube-feeding formula may have acidic urine because of high protein intake.

Urine Specific Gravity. Specific gravity measures the density or weight of urine compared with that of distilled water. The normal urinary specific gravity is 1.005 to 1.030, and the normal specific gravity of distilled water is 1.000.[14] Because urine is composed of many solutes and substances suspended in water, the specific gravity should always be higher than that of water.

The specific gravity reflects hydration status and indicates the ability of the kidneys to dilute or concentrate the urine.[19] Decreases in specific gravity reflect the inability of the kidneys to excrete the usual solute load into the urine (less dense with fewer solutes). Increases in specific gravity (a more concentrated urine) occur with fluid volume deficit as the result of fever, vomiting, or diarrhea. An increased specific gravity can also occur with diabetes or glomerular membrane disease, both of which allow glucose and protein to pass into the urine, thereby increasing urine density. A fixed specific gravity (does not vary with fluid intake) suggests early kidney dysfunction because the kidneys are unable to excrete or resorb water and solutes.

Urine Osmolality. The urine osmolality more accurately pinpoints fluid balance than does the urine specific gravity or the serum osmolality value. The serum osmolality reflects serum sodium concentration and therefore is subject to more influences than the urine osmolality. The simultaneous measurement of the serum and urine osmolality levels provides an accurate assessment of fluid status. The normal urine osmolality level is 500 to 1200 mOsm/kg and depends on resorption or excretion of water in the kidney tubules.[14,19] The urine osmolality level increases (and urine output decreases) during fluid volume deficit because of the retention of fluid by the body. The urine osmolality level decreases (and urine output increases) during volume excess because fluid is excreted by the kidneys. However, in intrarenal AKI, the urine osmolality value and urine output are both decreased because solutes and fluids are being retained.[2]

Glucose. Glucose normally is completely resorbed by the kidney tubules, and the urine should be free of glucose. The appearance of glucose in the urine (glycosuria) may be transient, brought on by ingestion of a heavy carbohydrate load (as in patients on

TABLE 30-3 Urinalysis Results

Test	Normal	Possible Causes for Increased Values	Possible Causes for Decreased Values
pH	4.5-8.0	Alkalosis	Acidosis Intrarenal AKI
Specific gravity	1.003-1.030*	Volume deficit Glycosuria Proteinuria Prerenal AKI (>1.020)	Volume overload Intrarenal AKI
Osmolality	300-1200 mOsm/kg	Volume deficit Prerenal AKI (urine > serum osmolality)	Volume excess Intrarenal AKI (urine < serum osmolality)
Protein	30-150 mg/24 hr†	Trauma Infection Intrarenal AKI Transient with exercise Glomerulonephritis	
Sodium	40-220 mEq/24 hr	High-sodium diet Intrarenal AKI	Prerenal AKI
Creatinine	1-2 g/24 hr		Intrarenal AKI Chronic kidney failure
Urea	6-17 g/24 hr		Intrarenal AKI Chronic kidney failure
Myoglobin	Absent	Crush injury Rhabdomyolysis	
RBCs	0-5‡	Trauma Intrarenal AKI Infection Strenuous exercise Renal artery thrombus	
WBCs	0-5‡	Infection	
Bacteria	None to few	Infection	
Casts	None to few	RBC: glomerular disease WBC: pyelonephritis Glomerular disease Nephrotic syndrome Epithelial: glomerular disease	

*Adult value; newborn value is slightly lower at 1.001-1.020.
†Higher values usually apply for persons after exercise; lower values apply for persons at rest.
‡Cells per low-power field.
AKI, acute kidney injury; RBCs, red blood cells; WBCs, white blood cells.

total parenteral nutrition) or stress (trauma, surgery), or it may occur because of changes in the kidneys during pregnancy.

Consistent glycosuria occurs during hyperglycemic episodes of diabetes when the kidney tubule threshold for glucose is exceeded and the excess glucose spills into the urine. Glucose is usually detected in the urine when serum glucose level exceeds 180 mg/dL.[18,19] In the presence of acute or chronic kidney failure, glycosuria is not a reliable indicator of the level of hyperglycemia because of the erratic excretion of glucose by the damaged nephrons.

Protein. Protein, like glucose, normally is absent from urine because protein molecules are too large to be filtered across the intact glomerular capillary membrane. Consistent appearance of protein in urine in amounts greater than 150 mg/day suggests compromise of the glomerular membrane and possible intrinsic kidney damage that requires further evaluation.[21,22] The amount of protein in the urine often directly correlates with the severity of the damage and may exceed 4 g/day.

Transient appearance of protein in the urine can occur as the result of efferent arteriole constriction caused by extreme exercise but should decrease within 24 hours. Transient proteinuria can occur after ingestion of a high-protein meal or can accompany the kidney changes associated with pregnancy. Protein also may be found in the urine of individuals without apparent evidence of kidney dysfunction and has been detected in patients admitted to critical care units, elders, and patients in shock. In a prospective study of more than 6000 men, the risk of stroke and coronary heart disease was greater for individuals with persistent proteinuria (and normal kidney function) at the beginning of the 27-year study than those without proteinuria, suggesting proteinuria may predict future cardiovascular disease.[23]

Measuring the amount of protein in the urine through a 24-hour urine collection is the most accurate method to quantify urinary protein. Because of the challenges in collecting urine for 24 hours, a randomly collected urine specimen is more commonly used, and a ratio of protein to creatinine or albumin to creatinine is used to estimate a 24-hour value.[22] In both cases, the amount of protein (or albumin) and the amount of creatinine in the specimen are measured. As the ratio increases, the amount of protein being excreted is greater. A normal protein-to-creatinine ratio is less than 0.2 (albumin-to-creatinine ratio is less than 20); a protein-to-creatinine ratio of 3.5 indicates approximately 3.5 g of protein excretion per day and severe protein loss by the kidneys. Albumin shows a similar pattern and is often detected before the larger protein molecule is apparent.[22]

Electrolytes. With the exception of sodium, levels of electrolytes in the urine are not measured as often as levels in serum, but they can yield information about kidney function. To measure urinary electrolyte levels, a 24-hour urine sample may be needed, although potassium and sodium are frequently measured in a randomly collected specimen. Urine electrolyte levels vary widely, and the electrolytes depend on the kidneys for adequate excretion. Consequently, changes in urinary electrolyte levels strongly suggest kidney failure and usually indicate intrarenal AKI.

The most commonly measured electrolyte in the urine is sodium. Urinary sodium is a reflection of the action of aldosterone and subsequent retention or excretion of sodium by the kidney tubules to maintain fluid balance. In the presence of hypovolemia, the tubules retain sodium (and therefore water), and the amount of sodium in the urine and the fractional excretion of sodium are very low.[9] The opposite is true with volume overload and with kidney diseases that cause sodium wasting. The amount of sodium in the urine can help in determining the pathology of AKI. In cases of AKI due to ineffective circulation reaching the kidneys, the urine sodium level is very low. If the AKI results from damage to the tubules, the urine sodium level is elevated or normal.

Sediment. The presence of sediment such as epithelial cells and casts in urine aids in identifying problems related to the kidneys. A fresh urine specimen (<30 minutes since collection) is important. Urine becomes more alkaline after it has been collected, resulting in a change in the urine sediment (e.g., casts dissolve, cells lyse).[20] The presence or absence of urine sediment can be helpful in identifying the cause of AKI.[18,20] In prerenal AKI, the kidneys are not damaged, and urinary sediment is absent, which is a normal finding. However, in intrarenal AKI, the kidney glomeruli or tubules are damaged, and urinary sediment is abnormal, containing casts and epithelial cells.

Casts are cylindrical structures composed mainly of mucoprotein (Tamm-Horsfall protein), which is secreted by epithelial cells lining the loops of Henle, the distal tubules, and the collecting ducts. Casts may form in the presence of epithelial cells,

RBCs, or WBCs in the tubular lumen. These cells or clumps of cellular breakdown products can adhere to and be surrounded by the fibrillar mucoprotein matrix, and the resulting casts are washed out of the renal tubular system in the urinary flow. Casts differ in composition and size and correlate with the severity and type of renal damage. For example, WBC casts indicate pyelonephritis, or they may occur during acute glomerulonephritis. RBC casts indicate glomerulonephritis. Hyaline casts, which consist of Tamm-Horsfall protein, are associated with renal parenchymal disease and glomerular capillary membrane inflammation. Consistent appearance of epithelial cells shed by the lining of the nephron may indicate nephritis. Although small numbers of epithelial cells normally appear in the urine and an occasional cast may be found, their consistent appearance is abnormal.[18-20]

Hematuria. Obvious and microscopic hematuria may signal kidney damage. Although a few RBCs in the urine are normal, discernibly bloody urine usually indicates bleeding within the urinary tract or renal trauma.[7] Microscopic hematuria may occur normally after strenuous exercise or the insertion of a retention catheter but should disappear within 48 hours.

The presence of myoglobin can make the urine appear red. Microscopic examination of the urine fails to reveal RBCs, with myoglobin being present instead.[24] Myoglobin in the urine may result from skeletal muscle damage (e.g., traumatic crush injury) or rhabdomyolysis. Rhabdomyolysis may develop in patients admitted to a critical care unit for many reasons, including cocaine abuse, status epilepticus, and heat prostration or collapse during intense physical exercise (e.g., running a marathon race on a hot day). Myoglobin is released by the muscle cells and blocks the tubules, resulting in intrarenal AKI.[24]

IMAGING STUDIES

Although laboratory assessment is used most often in diagnosing kidney problems in the critically ill patient, imaging studies can confirm or clarify causes of particular disorders. Imaging assessment includes the use of ultrasound and radiologic techniques. Ultrasound is a noninvasive imaging technique that is available in most hospitals. Kidney ultrasound is especially useful in determining the size, shape, and contour of the kidneys, the presence of masses or cysts, and the presence of renal artery stenosis.[27] Radiologic assessment ranges from basic to more complex (Table 30-4) and provides information about abnormal masses, abnormal fluid collections, obstructions, vascular supply alterations, and other disorders of the kidneys and urinary tract.[2,25-27]

Some radiologic studies require the use of contrast or injection of a radiopaque dye. Because many of the dyes used in radiology are potentially nephrotoxic, they must be used carefully in patients with AKI or chronic kidney disease. For example, an individual with AKI undergoing a test using contrast may experience further worsening of kidney function caused by the dye. To prevent nephrotoxicity, adequate hydration before and after the test and careful monitoring of kidney function are indicated any time contrast is used.

TABLE 30-4 Kidney Imaging Tests

Test	Comments
Kidney-ureter-bladder (KUB) radiograph	Flat-plate x-ray film of the abdomen; determines position, size, and structure of the kidneys, urinary tract, and pelvis; useful for evaluating the presence of calculi and masses; usually followed by additional tests
Intravenous pyelogram (IVP)	Intravenous injection of contrast with radiography; allows visualization of internal kidney tissues
Angiography	Injection of contrast into arterial blood perfusing the kidneys; allows visualization of renal blood flow; may also visualize stenosis, cysts, clots, trauma, and infarctions
Computed tomography (CT)	Radioisotope is administered by intravenous route and absorbed by the kidneys; scintillation photography is then performed in several planes; spiral or helical CT allows rapid imaging; density of the image helps evaluate kidney vessels, perfusion, tumors, cysts, stones/calculi, hemorrhage, necrosis, and trauma
Ultrasound	High-frequency sound waves are transmitted to the kidneys and urinary tract, and the image is viewed on an oscilloscope; noninvasive; identifies fluid accumulation or obstruction, cysts, stones/calculi, and masses; useful for evaluating kidney before biopsy
Magnetic resonance imaging (MRI)	A scanner produces three-dimensional images in response to the application of high-energy radiofrequency waves to the tissues; produces clear images; density of the image may indicate trauma, cysts, masses, malformation of the vessels or tubules stones/calculi, and necrosis

KIDNEY BIOPSY

Kidney biopsy is the definitive tool for diagnosing disease processes of the kidney. Two methods are used: closed biopsy and open biopsy. Percutaneous needle biopsy (closed method) involves inserting a needle through the flank to obtain a specimen of cortical and medullary kidney tissue. An open biopsy is a surgical procedure and is rarely done in critically ill patients. In either case, biopsy is often the last choice for diagnostic assessment in the critically ill patient because of the postprocedural risks of bleeding, hematoma formation, and infection.

Summary

- Careful evaluation of volume status is important in assessing kidney function.
- Urine output may be decreased or normal, depending on the cause of the kidney dysfunction.
- Serum parameters used to detect and evaluate kidney function can be affected by nonrenal factors.
- Creatinine clearance is the best estimation of glomerular filtration and therefore of kidney function.
- Urinalysis is a valuable tool in determining the presence and cause of kidney dysfunction.

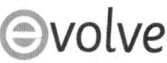 Be sure to check out the bonus material, including free self-assessment exercises, on the Evolve web site at http://evolve.elsevier.com/Urden/.

References

1. Seidel HM et al: *Mosby's guide to physical examination,* ed 5, St Louis, 2003, Mosby.
2. Schira M, section editor: Assessment of kidney structure and function. In Counts C, editor: *Core curriculum for nephrology nursing,* ed 5, Pitman, NJ, 2008, American Nephrology Nurses Association.
3. Parker K: Alterations in fluid, electrolyte, and acid-base balance. In Molnahn A, Butera E, editors: *Contemporary nephrology nursing: principles and practice,* ed 2, Pitman, NJ, 2006, American Nephrology Nurses Association.
4. Ejaz AA et al: Characteristics of 100 consecutive patients presenting with orthostatic hypotension, *Mayo Clin Proc* 79(7):890-894, 2004.
5. Irvin D: The importance of accurately assessing orthostatic hypotension, *Geriatr Nurs* 25(2):99, 2004.
6. Bozeman C et al: Selective operative management of major blunt renal trauma, *J Trauma* 57(2):305-309, 2004.
7. Knudson MM et al: Outcome after major renovascular injuries: a Western trauma association multicenter report, *J Trauma* 49(6): 1116-1122, 2000.
8. Purcell W et al: Accurate dry weight assessment: reducing the incidence of hypertension and cardiac disease in patients on hemodialysis, *Nephrol Nurs J* 31(6):631-636, 2004.
9. Subramanian S, Ziedalski TM: Oliguria, volume overload, Na⁺ balance, and diuretics, *Crit Care Clin* 21(20):291-303, 2005.
10. Faes M et al: Dehydration in geriatrics. *Geriatrics Aging* 10(9):590-596, 2007.
11. Bagshaw S, Gibney N: Conventional markers of kidney function. *Crit Care Med* 36(4 suppl):S152-158, 2008.
12. Kellum J: Acute kidney injury. *Crit Care Med* 36(4 suppl):S141-145, 2008.

13. Robinson BE, Weber H: Dehydration despite drinking: beyond the BUN/creatinine ratio, *J Am Med Dir Assoc* 5(2 suppl):S67-S71, 2004.

14. Kee J: *Laboratory & diagnostic tests with nursing implications*, ed 7, Upper Saddle River, NJ, 2006, Pearson Prentice-Hall.

15. Thomas DR et al: Physician misdiagnosis of dehydration in older adults, *J Am Med Dir Assoc* 5(2 suppl):S30-S34, 2004.

16. Miller D et al: Challenges for nephrology nurses in the management of children with chronic kidney disease, *Nephrol Nurs J* 31(3):287, 2004.

17. Simonson M: Measurement of glomerular filtration rate. In Hricik et al, editors: *Nephrology secrets*, ed 2, Philadelphia, 2003, Hanley & Belfus.

18. Ganz M: Urinalysis. In Hricik et al, editors: *Nephrology secrets*, ed 2, Philadelphia, 2003, Hanley & Belfus.

19. Hanson K: Laboratory studies in the evaluation of urologic disease. Part I, *Urol Nurs* 23(6):400, 2004.

20. Sreenarasimhavah V: Art and science of urinalysis. In Agha et al, editors: *The Washington manual. Nephrology subspecialty consult*, Philadelphia, 2004, Lippincott Williams & Wilkins.

21. Simonson M: Measurement of urinary protein. In Hricik et al, editors: *Nephrology secrets*, ed 2, Philadelphia, 2003, Hanley & Belfus.

22. Ramanujam S: Approach to proteinuria. In Agha et al, editors: *The Washington manual. Nephrology subspecialty consult*, Philadelphia, 2004, Lippincott Williams & Wilkins.

23. Madison J et al: Proteinuria and risk for stroke and coronary heart disease during 27 years of follow-up: The Honolulu heart program, *Arch Intern Med* 166(8):884-889, 2006.

24. Russell T: Acute renal failure related to rhabdomyolysis: pathophysiology, diagnosis, and collaborative management, *Nephrol Nurs J* 32(4):409, 2005.

25. Hanson K: Diagnostic tests and tools in the evaluation of urologic disease. Part II, *Urol Nurs* 23(6):405, 2004.

26. Elashi E et al: Renal imaging techniques. In Hricik et al, editors: *Nephrology secrets*, ed 2, Philadelphia, 2003, Hanley & Belfus.

27. Poole B: Imaging in renal disease. In Agha et al, editors: *The Washington manual. Nephrology subspecialty consult*, Philadelphia, 2004, Lippincott Williams & Wilkins.

Renal Disorders and Therapeutic Management

ACUTE KIDNEY INJURY

Acute kidney injury (AKI) is a relatively new term used to describe the spectrum of acute-onset kidney disorders that can range from mild impairment of kidney function through acute renal failure (ARF) that requires renal replacement therapy (dialysis).[1] Severe AKI is characterized by a sudden decline in glomerular filtration rate (GFR), with subsequent retention of products in the blood that are normally excreted by the kidneys; this disrupts electrolyte balance, acid-base homeostasis, and fluid volume equilibrium.[1,2] A transition to greater use of the word *kidney* rather than *renal* reflects a trend in the nephrology literature that emphasizes the vulnerability of the kidney during critical illness.

CRITICAL ILLNESS AND ACUTE KIDNEY INJURY

The estimated incidence of AKI is between 2000 and 3000 cases per 1 million people per year.[3] Researchers estimate that AKI accounts for 1% of acute hospital admissions and complicates more than 7% of inpatient episodes, especially for older individuals and those with preexistent chronic kidney disease.[2]

Critical care patients with AKI have a longer length of hospital stay and more complications.[3] After AKI has occurred in the critically ill patient, the risk of death rises dramatically.[3,4] The mortality rate ranges from 38% to 80%.[5] One of the reasons for the high mortality rate is that critical care patients often have coexisting nonrenal health problems that increase their susceptibility to the development of AKI. High-risk conditions include heart failure, shock, respiratory failure, and sepsis, and this situation has altered the spectrum of AKI.[4,5] An observational study that examined the incidence and course of severe AKI that resulted in ARF in six academic medical centers in the United States found that AKI was accompanied by multiorgan failure in most patients, even those who did not require dialysis.[4] In this study of 618 patients with ARF, 64% of patients required dialysis, the in-hospital mortality rate was 37%, and the rate of nonrecovery of kidney function or death was 50%.[4] The clinicians' conclusion is that death of the critically ill patient with AKI-related ARF is related to the severity of coexisting nonrenal diseases.[4] Mortality rates exceeded 50% when four or more body systems had failed.[4]

Cohort studies suggest that the incidence of AKI is increasing, whereas the mortality rate is declining.[6] Patients with AKI often have associated multiple organ dysfunction syndrome (MODS) and have more complex illnesses and comorbidities compared with patients 40 years ago, and more critical care patients are receiving dialysis therapies in the critical care unit.

Typically, a patient is not admitted to the critical care unit with a diagnosis of AKI alone; there is always coexisting hemodynamic, cardiac, pulmonary, or neurologic compromise. Many individuals come into the hospital with underlying changes in kidney function, such as an elevated serum creatinine level, although the patient is not symptomatic and is often unaware of their compromised kidney.[7] The lack of kidney reserve places them at increased risk for AKI if complications occur in any of the other major organ systems. As a result, the picture of AKI in the modern critical care unit has changed to encompass patients with kidney injury who also have multisystem dysfunction that complicates their clinical course.[3]

DEFINITIONS OF ACUTE KIDNEY INJURY AND ACUTE RENAL FAILURE

One of the challenges of estimating the incidence of AKI or ARF in the critical care unit has been the wide variation in definitions that have been used. Measurement of kidney function is necessarily indirect, and the diagnosis of AKI is predominantly derived from changes in urine output and serum creatine level, with the assumption that changes in these values reflect changes in the GFR.[8] Urine output is sometimes a problematic measure to use because diuretics artificially increase the urine output but do not alter the course of kidney failure. The clinical insult may have direct effects on the kidney, such as the inflammation associated with sepsis, which accounts for 50% of the AKI seen in critical care units.[9]

RIFLE Criteria. The risk of critically ill patients developing AKI has been classified by a multinational group of nephrologists.[10] The classification uses the acronym RIFLE (*r*isk, *i*njury, *f*ailure, *l*oss, and *e*nd-stage kidney disease [ESKD]).[11] The RIFLE system classifies AKI in three categories of increasing severity (R, I, F) and two outcome criteria (L, E) based on GFR status reflected by the change in urine output or loss of kidney function[11] (Table 31-1). If AKI is superimposed on a kidney that is already compromised, the term *chronic* is added to the RIFLE criteria to denote the cause as acute-on-chronic kidney failure.[11]

TABLE 31-1 RIFLE Criteria for Acute Kidney Dysfunction

RIFLE	Serum Creatinine Criteria*	Urine Output Criteria
*R*isk	Serum Cr increased 1.5 times above normal *or* Serum Cr increase ≥0.3 mg/dL	UO <0.5 mL/kg/hr for 6 hr
*I*njury	Serum Cr increased 2 times above normal	UO <0.5 mL/kg/hr for 12 hr
*F*ailure	Serum Cr increased 3 times above normal *or* Serum Cr ≥4 mg/dL *or* Serum Cr acute rise ≥0.5 mg/dL	UO <0.3 mL/kg/hr for 24 hr *or* anuria for 12 hr (oliguria)
*L*oss	Persistent AKI = complete loss of kidney function for more than 4 wk	
*E*SKD	End-stage kidney disease	

Data from Kellum JA et al: Definition and classification of acute kidney injury, *Nephron Clin Pract* 109(4):c182-c187, 2008.
*All serum creatinine references are based on changes from baseline.
AKI, acute kidney injury; Cr, creatinine; UO, urine output.

BOX 31-1 ACUTE KIDNEY INJURY NETWORK (AIKN) CRITERIA FOR THE DIAGNOSIS OF ACUTE KIDNEY INJURY.

- *Definition:* Acute kidney injury (AKI) is an abrupt (within 48 hours) reduction in kidney function defined as:
  - An absolute increase in the serum creatinine level of more than or equal to 0.3 mg/dL (≥26.4 μmol/L)
  - A percentage increase in serum creatinine of more than or equal to 50% (1.5-fold from baseline)
  - A reduction in urine output (documented oliguria of less than 0.5 mL/kg/hr for more than 6 hours)

EXPLANATORY NOTES

- *Serum creatinine:* These criteria include an absolute and a percentage change in creatinine to accommodate variations related to age, gender, and body mass index and to reduce the need for a baseline creatinine level, but they do require at least two serum creatinine values within 48 hours.

- *Urine output:* The urine output criterion was included based on the predictive importance of this measure but with the awareness that urine outputs may not be measured routinely in non–intensive care unit settings. It is assumed that the diagnosis based on the urine output criterion alone will require exclusion of urinary tract obstructions that reduce urine output or of other easily reversible causes of reduced urine output.
- *Clinical context:* These criteria should be used in the context of the clinical presentation and after adequate fluid resuscitation when applicable. Many acute kidney diseases exist, and some may result in AKI. Because diagnostic criteria are not documented, some cases of AKI may not be diagnosed.
- *Physiologic state:* AKI may be superimposed on or lead to chronic kidney disease.

Data from Mehta RL et al, for the Acute Kidney Injury Network: Report of an initiative to improve outcomes in acute kidney injury, *Critical Care* 11(2):R31, 2007.

Acute Kidney Injury Network Criteria. The Acute Kidney Injury Network (AKIN) criteria are listed in Box 31-1. These criteria are similar to those proposed by the RIFLE group, and both groups intend to make the point that in the acutely ill patient, small changes in the serum creatinine level and urine output may signal important declines in the GFR and kidney function. A conceptual model that combines the features of the RIFLE criteria and AKIN criteria is shown in Fig. 31-1.[11]

TYPES OF ACUTE KIDNEY INJURY

Previously, ARF was predominantly classified by the location of the insult relative to the kidney: *prerenal* (before), *intrarenal* (within), and *postrenal* (after) (Box 31-2). This remains a useful way to imagine the relationship between anatomy and functional insults to the kidney, although it is not evident that insults classified in this manner have any impact on outcomes of patients with AKI.[11]

Prerenal Acute Kidney Injury. Any condition that decreases blood flow, blood pressure, or kidney perfusion before

arterial blood reaches the renal artery that supplies the kidney may be anatomically described as *prerenal AKI.* When arterial hypoperfusion due to low cardiac output, hemorrhage, vasodilation, thrombosis, or other cause reduces the blood flow to the kidney, glomerular filtration decreases, and consequently, urine output decreases (see Box 31-2). This is a major reason the critical care nurse monitors the urine output on an hourly basis. Initially, in prerenal states, the integrity of the kidney's nephron structure and function may be preserved. If normal perfusion and cardiac output are restored quickly, the kidney will not suffer permanent injury. However, if the prerenal insult is not corrected, the GFR will decline, the blood urea nitrogen (BUN) concentration will rise (prerenal azotemia),[9] and the patient will develop oliguria and be at risk for significant kidney damage. *Oliguria* (urine output <400 mL/day) is a classic finding in AKI.[5] Prerenal AKI is seen frequently in the critically ill. In a study of hospitalized older patients with kidney failure, prerenal AKI occurred in 58% of the patients.[5] This compares with rates of 34% for intrarenal AKI and 8% for postrenal AKI in the same study.[5]

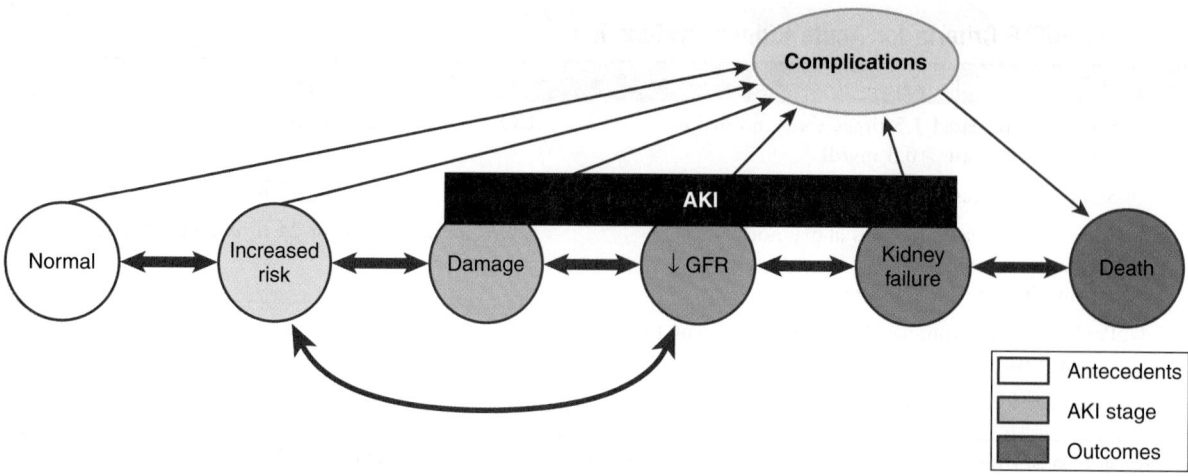

Figure 31-1 Model of the components of acute kidney injury. *(Modified from AKI conceptual model developed by AKIN [the Acute Kidney Injury Network] at the Vancouver Summit 2006 [www.akinet.org.]).*

BOX 31-2   ACUTE KIDNEY INJURY

PRERENAL ACUTE KIDNEY INJURY
- Prolonged hypotension (sepsis, vasodilation)
- Prolonged low cardiac output (heart failure, cardiogenic shock)
- Prolonged volume depletion (dehydration, hemorrhage)
- Renovascular thrombosis (thromboemboli)

INTRARENAL ACUTE KIDNEY INJURY
- Kidney ischemia (advanced stage of prerenal acute kidney injury)
- Endogenous toxins (rhabdomyolysis, tumor lysis syndrome)
- Exogenous toxins (radiocontrast dye, nephrotoxic drugs)
- Infection (acute glomerulonephritis, interstitial nephritis)

POSTRENAL ACUTE KIDNEY INJURY
- Obstruction (urethra, prostate, or bladder)
- Rare as a cause of acute kidney injury in critical care

Intrarenal Acute Kidney Injury. Any condition that produces an ischemic or toxic insult directly at the site of the nephron places the patient at risk for development of *intrarenal AKI* (see Box 31-2). Ischemic damage may be caused by prolonged hypotension or low cardiac output. Toxic injury reaction may occur in response to substances that damage the kidney tubular endothelium, such as some antimicrobial drugs and the contrast dye used in radiologic diagnostic studies. The insult may involve the glomeruli and the tubular epithelium. When the internal filtering structures are pathologically affected, the condition is called *acute tubular necrosis* (ATN).

Postrenal Acute Kidney Injury. Any obstruction that hinders the flow of urine from beyond the kidney through the remainder of the urinary tract may lead to *postrenal AKI.* This is not a common cause of kidney failure in the critically ill. When monitoring of the urine output reveals a sudden decrease in the patient's urine output from the urinary catheter, a blockage may be responsible. Sudden development of *anuria* (urine output < 100 mL/24 hr) should prompt verification that the urinary catheter is not occluded.

AZOTEMIA

The term *azotemia* is used to describe an acute rise in the BUN level.[9] *Uremia* is another term used to describe an elevated BUN value.

ACUTE TUBULAR NECROSIS

ATN results from nephrotoxic or ischemic injury that damages the kidney tubular epithelium and, in severe cases, extends to the collagen of the basement membrane. Injury that is limited to the epithelial layer recovers sooner than injury that also involves the basement membrane. ATN is a histologic diagnosis that must be verified with a kidney biopsy, a diagnostic test that is rarely performed or warranted.[12] The term *ATN* is used when describing severe AKI and ARF that requires hemodialysis support.

EPIDEMIOLOGY AND ETIOLOGY

Damage to the cells in the glomerular and tubular structures prevents normal concentration of urine, filtration of wastes, and regulation of acid-base, electrolyte, and water balance. The kidney tubular cells are constantly at risk for damage because of their normally high blood flows, high oxygen requirements, and the constant resorption and secretion of metabolites. A number of disorders can result in ATN, and several contributing factors often work together to produce tubular damage. Common causes of ATN are traditionally divided into two categories: ischemic injury and nephrotoxic injury (Box 31-3). Overall, ATN accounts for 76% of cases of AKI in the critically ill.[6]

Ischemic Acute Tubular Necrosis. Ischemic damage from inadequate perfusion impairs tubular endothelial function, causing patchy areas of tubular cell damage and cast formation. Ischemic necrosis occurs as a result of vasodilation associated with sepsis and when hypotension or an episode of low cardiac output is prolonged; it may be worsened by kidney hypoperfusion or dehydration. In other words, prerenal low perfusion can develop

BOX 31-3   ISCHEMIC VERSUS NEPHROTOXIC ACUTE TUBULAR NECROSIS

ISCHEMIC INJURY
- Advanced stage of prerenal acute kidney injury
  - Massive hemorrhage
  - Severe volume loss
  - Severe dehydration
  - Severe, prolonged hypotension
  - Shock: cardiogenic, hypovolemic, septic
  - Sepsis
  - Anaphylaxis

NEPHROTOXIC INJURY
Endogenous Toxins*
- Rhabdomyolysis
- Tumor lysis syndrome

Exogenous Toxins*
- Radiopaque contrast dye

Nephrotoxic Antimicrobials
- Aminoglycosides: gentamicin, tobramycin
- Cephalosporins: cefazolin
- Antifungals: amphotericin B
- Antivirals: acyclovir

Nephrotoxic Immunosuppressants
- Cyclosporin
- Tacrolimus (FK506)

Nephrotoxic Chemotherapeutics
- 5-Azacitidine
- Cisplatin
- Methotrexate

Nephrotoxic Street Drugs
- Heroin
- Amphetamines
- Phencyclidine (PCP)

Nephrotoxic Analgesics
- Nonsteroidal antiinflammatory drugs (NSAIDs)

---

*Represents only a partial list of potential nephrotoxic medications.

---

procedure. Although patients with normal kidney function are not considered to be at risk, those with elevated serum creatinine levels, diabetes, or microvascular disease are highly vulnerable (see Box 31-3).[13]

PATHOPHYSIOLOGY

Several mechanisms are responsible for tubular dysfunction in ischemic ATN. When cellular debris accumulates in the nephron tubular lumen, obstruction occurs if there is not adequate flow of filtrate through the nephron. The obstruction is made up of casts and sloughing tissue and is exacerbated by interstitial edema. Filtration ceases when tubular hydrostatic pressure increases to match the GFR. This decreases the formation of urine because of the lack of filtrate to process. The result is more tubular cell swelling, obstruction, decreased capillary blood flow, and further ischemia and cell injury. The clinical course of ATN is thought to progresses through four phases.

PHASES OF ACUTE TUBULAR NECROSIS

Onset Phase. The onset (initiating) phase of ATN is the period from the initial insult until cell injury occurs. Ischemic injury is evolving during this time. The GFR is decreased because of impaired blood flow to the kidney and decreased glomerular ultrafiltration pressure. This disrupts the integrity of the tubular epithelium, which leaks the glomerular filtrate back into the kidney. This phase lasts hours to days, depending on the cause, with toxic factors causing the phase to last longer. If treatment is initiated during this time, irreversible damage can be alleviated. A longer course of recovery reflects the presence of more extensive tubular injury.

Oliguric or Anuric Phase. The oliguric or anuric phase, the second phase of ATN, lasts 5 to 8 days in the nonoliguric patient and 10 to 16 days in the oliguric patient.[14] The accumulation of necrotic cellular debris in the tubular space blocks the flow of urine and causes damage to the tubular wall and basement membranes. Backleak occurs because damage in the tubular wall causes the glomerular filtrate to flow passively into the kidney tissue rather than be passed out as urine through the ureters and bladder. Oliguria is encountered more often in ischemic damage and is a sign that the damage is extensive and severe. During the oliguric or anuric phase, the GFR is greatly reduced, which leads to increased levels of BUN (azotemia), elevated serum creatinine levels, electrolyte abnormalities (hyperkalemia, hyperphosphatemia, hypocalcemia), and metabolic acidosis.

Diuretic Phase. The third phase, the diuretic phase of ATN, lasts 7 to 14 days and is characterized by an increase in the GFR and sometimes by polyuria with a urine output as high as 2 to 4 L/day. For the patient receiving hemodialysis during this phase, the polyuria is not evident because excess volume is removed by dialysis. During the diuretic phase, the tubular obstruction has passed, but edema and scarring remain. In this situation, the GFR returns before the ability of the tubules to function normally. The kidneys can clear fluid volume but not solutes, and with a large diuresis, this can lead to volume depletion.

into intrinsic ischemic ATN (see Box 31-3). In the multicenter study of critical care patients with AKI by Mehta and colleagues, 50% of the patients had ischemic ATN, which was largely precipitated by hypotension (20%), and sepsis (19%).[4]

Toxic Acute Tubular Necrosis. Nephrotoxic damage results from injury by drugs and chemical agents. A common cause of toxic ATN is the radiopaque (contrast) dye administered during an interventional or diagnostic radiologic studies. Complications from the contrast cause AKI in 9% to 14% of patients.[4] In affected patients, the serum creatinine levels typically begin to rise 48 to 72 hours after the study, peak at 3 to 5 days, and return to baseline within another 3 to 5 days.[13] Kidney dysfunction can persist up to 3 weeks after the

TABLE 31-2 Initial Urine Laboratory Analysis Findings in Acute Kidney Injury*

Assessment	Prenatal[†]	Intrarenal[‡]	Postrenal[§]
Urine volume	Normal	Oliguria or nonoliguria	Oliguria to anuria
Urine specific gravity	>1.020	1.010	1.000-1.010
Urine osmolality (mOsm/kg)	>350	<300	300-400
Urine sodium (mEq/L)	<20	>30	20-40
FENa (%)	<1%	>2-3%	1%-3%
BUN/Cr ratio	20:1	Ischemic: 20:1 Toxic: 10:1	10:1
Urine microscopy (sediment)	Normal	ATN: dark granular casts, hyaline casts, kidney epithelial cells	Normal

*Results of urine laboratory tests are valid only in the absence of diuretics.
[†]Urine in prerenal failure is concentrated, with low sodium.
[‡]Urine in intrarenal failure shows kidney damage because the nephron cannot concentrate urine or conserve sodium, and evidence of kidney damage (casts) is seen.
[§]Urine test results in postrenal failure vary because the findings initially depend on the hydration status of the patient rather than the status of the kidney.
Anuria, urine volume less than 100 mL/24 hr; ATN, acute tubular necrosis; Cr, creatinine; BUN, blood urea nitrogen; FENa, fractional excretion of sodium; oliguria, urine volume of 100-400 mL/24 hr; polyuria, urine volume excessive over 24 hours.

Recovery Phase. The last phase of ATN is the recovery phase. Animal-based research suggests that the kidney tubular cells that have survived prior injury contribute to the healing process through proliferation and migration to denuded (damaged) areas.[15] Kidney stem cells and related growth factors are also involved in cellular recovery.[15]

Patients who were oliguric or nonoliguric may have increased urine output when they enter the recovery stage. During this stage, kidney function slowly returns to normal or near normal, with a GFR that is 70% to 80% of normal within 1 to 2 years.[16] However, if significant kidney parenchymal damage has occurred, BUN and creatinine levels may never return to normal. For patients who survive ATN, approximately 62% eventually recover normal kidney function, 33% have residual kidney damage, and at least 5% require long-term hemodialysis.[16]

ASSESSMENT AND DIAGNOSIS

LABORATORY ASSESSMENT

After acute kidney disease is suspected, the presence or degree or AKI is assessed using urinalysis and blood analysis. Table 31-2 lists the initial urinanalysis findings for patients with AKI. Most serum levels of electrolytes become increasingly elevated as AKI develops (Table 31-3). Clinical findings associated with AKI are listed in Table 31-4. Normal and abnormal urinalysis findings and reasons for their significance are summarized in Chapter 30.

Acidosis. Acidosis (pH <7.35) is one of the trademarks of severe acute kidney insult.[17] Metabolic acidosis occurs as a result of the accumulation of unexcreted waste products. The acid waste products consist of strong negative ions (anions), elevated serum phosphorus levels (hyperphosphatemia), and other normally unmeasured ions (e.g., sulfate, urate, lactate) that decrease the serum pH.[17] A low serum albumin concentration, which often occurs in AKI, has a slight alkalinizing effect, but it

TABLE 31-3 Normal Serum Electrolyte Values

Electrolyte	Normal Value
Sodium	135-145 mEq/L
Potassium	3.5-4.5 mEq/L
Chloride	98-108 mEq/L
Calcium	8.5-10.5 mg/dL or 4.5-5.8 mEq/L
Phosphorus	2.7-4.5 mg/dL
Magnesium	1.5-2.5 mEq/L
Bicarbonate	24-28 mEq/L

is not enough to offset the metabolic acidosis.[17] Even respiratory compensation and mechanical ventilatory support are rarely sufficient to reverse the metabolic acidosis. Acidosis in AKI is complex, as evidenced by the fact that many AKI patients maintain a normal anion gap.[17] The reasons for this remain unknown.[17] Information on acidosis and arterial blood gas interpretation is found in Chapter 23. Anion gap measurement is discussed in Chapter 30.

Blood Urea Nitrogen. The BUN level is not a reliable indicator of kidney damage.[9,18] The BUN concentration is changed by protein intake, blood in the gastrointestinal tract, and cell catabolism, and it is diluted by fluid administration. A BUN-to-creatinine ratio may be calculated to determine the cause of the AKI (see Table 31-2). The BUN-to-creatinine ratio is most useful in diagnosing prerenal AKI (often described as prerenal azotemia), in which the BUN level is greatly elevated relative to the serum creatinine value.

Serum Creatinine. Creatinine is a by-product of muscle metabolism that is formed from nonenzymatic dehydration of creatine in the liver[18]; 98% of creatine is in the muscles,[18] and it is almost totally excreted by the kidney tubules. If the kidneys are not working, the serum creatinine level will

TABLE 31-4 Serum Electrolytes in Acute Kidney Failure

Electrolyte Disturbance	Serum Value	Clinical Findings
Potassium		
Hypokalemia	<3.5 mEq/L	Muscular weakness Cardiac irregularities on ECG Abdominal distention and flatulence Paresthesia Decreased reflexes Anorexia Dizziness, confusion Increased sensitivity to digitalis
Hyperkalemia	>4.5 mEq/L	Irritability and restlessness Anxiety Nausea and vomiting Abdominal cramps Weakness Numbness and tingling (fingertips and circumoral) Cardiac irregularities on ECG
Sodium		
Hyponatremia	<135 mEq/L	Disorientation Muscle twitching Nausea, vomiting, abdominal cramps Headaches, dizziness Seizures, postural hypotension Cold, clammy skin Decreased skin turgor Tachycardia Oliguria
Hypernatremia	>145 mEq/L	Extreme thirst Dry, sticky mucous membranes Altered mentation Seizures (later stages)
Calcium		
Hypocalcemia	<8.5 mg/dL or <4.5 mEq/L	Irritability Muscular tetany, muscle cramps Decreased cardiac output (decreased contractions) Bleeding (decreased ability to coagulate) Changes on ECG Positive Chvostek or Trousseau signs
Hypercalcemia	>10.5 mg/dL or >5.8 mEq/L	Deep bone pain Excessive thirst Anorexia Lethargy, weakened muscles
Magnesium		
Hypomagnesemia	<1.4 mEq/L	Choroid or athetoid muscle activity Facial tics, spasticity Cardiac dysrhythmias
Hypermagnesemia	>2.5 mEq/L	CNS depression Respiratory depression Lethargy Coma Bradycardia Changes on ECG

Continued

TABLE 31-4   Serum Electrolytes in Acute Kidney Failure—cont'd

Electrolyte Disturbance	Serum Value	Clinical Findings
Phosphate		
Hypophosphatemia	<3.0 mg/dL	Hemolytic anemias
		Depressed white blood cell function
		Bleeding (decreased platelet aggregation)
		Nausea, vomiting
		Anorexia
Hyperphosphatemia	>4.5 mg/dL	Tachycardia
		Nausea, diarrhea, abdominal cramps
		Muscle weakness, flaccid paralysis
		Increased reflexes
Chloride		
Hypochloremia	<98 mEq/L	Hyperirritability
		Tetany or muscular excitability
		Slow respirations
Hyperchloremia	>108 mEq/L	Weakness, lethargy
		Deep, rapid breathing
		Possible unconsciousness (later stages)
Albumin		
Hypoalbuminemia	<3.8 g/dL	Muscle wasting
		Peripheral edema (fluid shift)
		Decreased resistance to infection
		Poorly healing wounds

CNS, central nervous system; ECG, electrocardiogram.

increase. When the serum creatinine doubles (e.g., from 0.75 to 1.5 mg/dL), the increase reflects a decrease of approximately 50% in the GFR.[18] Serum creatinine level is assessed daily to follow the trend of kidney function and to determine whether the kidney function stable, getting better, or getting worse.[18]

Creatinine Clearance. If the patient is making sufficient urine, the urinary creatinine clearance can be measured. A normal urinary creatinine clearance rate is 120 mL/min, but this value decreases with kidney failure. Critical care patients with severe AKI are oliguric, and the urinary creatinine clearance rate is infrequently measured.

Fractional Excretion of Sodium. The fractional excretion of sodium (FENa) in the urine is measured early in the AKI course to differentiate between a prerenal condition and ATN (intrarenal). An FENa value below 1% (in the absence of diuretics) suggests prerenal compromise, because *resorption* of almost all the filtered sodium is an appropriate response to decreased perfusion to the kidneys. If diuretics are administered, the test is meaningless. An FENa value above 2% implies the kidney cannot concentrate the sodium and that the damage is intrarenal (ATN).

Urinary sodium is measured in milliequivalents per liter (mEq/L). The interpretation of results is similar to the FENa. A urinary sodium concentration less than 10 mEq/L (low) suggests a prerenal condition. A urinary sodium level greater than 40 mEq/L (in the presence of an elevated serum creatinine and the absence of a high salt load) suggests intrarenal damage has occurred (see Table 31-2). As with other urinalysis tests, the use of diuretics invalidates any results. Because the diuretics alter resorption of water and produce dilute urine, the test result will not reflect actual kidney function.

AT-RISK DISEASE STATES AND ACUTE KIDNEY INJURY

Many patients come into the critical care unit with disease states that predispose them to the development of AKI. Many others already have kidney damage but are unaware of this condition.[7]

UNDERLYING CHRONIC KIDNEY DISEASE

The incidence of chronic kidney disease (CKD) in United States is estimated to be 11% (19.2 million adults).[19] Clinical practice guidelines for the management of ESKD organize kidney dysfunction in five stages.[20] Because of the large numbers of adults with kidney dysfunction (diagnosed or not), kidney function must be assessed on all critically ill patients at risk for fluid and electrolyte imbalance. The GFR associated with each stage and the numeric population estimates for each stage of kidney dysfunction are shown in Table 31-5.

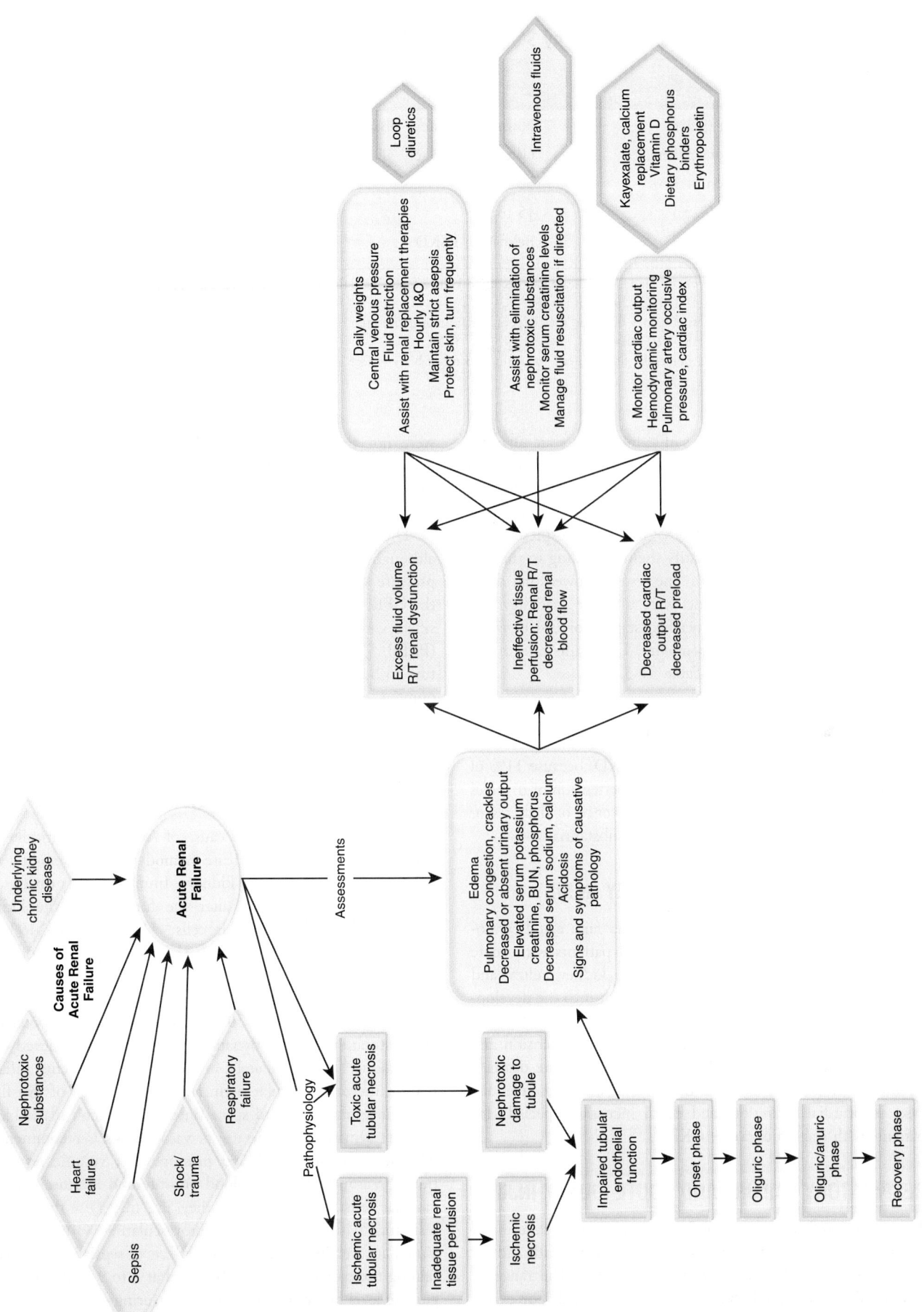

TABLE 31-5 **Decreased Kidney Function by Stage in Adult U.S. Population**

Stage*	Population Affected*	GFR and Diagnosis*	Percentage Who Know They Have Kidney Dysfunction (%)†
1	9 million (3.3%)	Normal; persistent albuminuria	40.5
2	5.3 million (3.0%)	60 to 89; persistent albuminuria	29.3
3	7.6 million (4.3%)	30 to 59	22.0
4	400,000 (0.2%)	15 to 29	44.5
5	300,000 (0.2%)	Below 15: ESKD	100

*Data from Coresh J et al: Prevalence of chronic kidney disease and decreased kidney function in the adult US population: Third National Health and Nutrition Examination Survey, *Am J Kidney Dis* 41(1):1-12, 2003.

†Data from Nickolas TL et al: Awareness of kidney disease in the US population: findings from the National Health and Nutrition Examination Survey (NHANES) 1999 to 2000, *Am J Kidney Dis* 44(2):185-197, 2004.

ESKD, end-stage kidney disease; GFR, glomerular filtration rate (mL/min/1.73 m² of body surface area).

Most people in the early stages of kidney disease are unaware of their condition.[7] A national health survey queried individuals about whether they had ever been told by their physician that they had "weak or failing kidneys." The answer to this question was correlated with the individual's GFR and the presence of albuminuria by urine test to stratify them according to the five stages of CKD (see Table 31-5). The results showed that more than one half of the respondents were unaware that they had kidney dysfunction until they reached stage 5 or ESKD when they would become dialysis dependent.[7] The results categorized by stage of CKD are listed in Table 31-5.

OLDER AGE AND ACUTE KIDNEY INJURY

Older age appears to be a risk factor for CKD, because 11% of individuals older than 65 years *without* hypertension or diabetes have stage 3 or worse CKD.[19] In the presence of diabetes or hypertension, the risk for CKD increases substantially.

HEART FAILURE AND ACUTE KIDNEY INJURY

There is a strong association between kidney failure and cardiovascular disease. In studies of critically ill patients with acute kidney failure, 54%[4] to 63%[5] have acute kidney failure and heart failure. Hypertension, a major contributor to the development of heart failure, is also a major risk factor for the development of CKD.[21] Unfortunately, people with hypertension and diabetes are at increased risk for CKD and premature death.[21] As the patient's GFR declines, the risks of cardiovascular disease, myocardial infarction, and death increase, especially for patients with stage 3 or worse CKD.[22,23]

RESPIRATORY FAILURE AND ACUTE KIDNEY INJURY

There is a significant association between respiratory failure and kidney failure. In studies of critically ill patients with kidney failure, 54% to 88% have respiratory failure.[4,5] The range in values reflects how the kidney failure was classified. For example, in one study, 57% had respiratory and kidney failure but

were not treated with dialysis,[4] and in another study, 88% had respiratory and kidney failure and were given dialysis treatment with continuous renal replacement therapy (discussed later).[5]

The process of mechanical ventilation affects the kidney, although it is not known whether it is deleterious.[24] Positive-pressure ventilation reduces blood flow to the kidney, lowers the GFR, and decreases urine output.[24] These effects are intensified with the addition of positive end-expiratory pressure (PEEP).[24] AKI increases inflammation, causes the lung vasculature to become more permeable, and contributes to the development of acute respiratory failure.[25] Prolonged mechanical ventilation in critical illness is associated with an increased incidence of AKI and dialysis.[26]

SEPSIS AND ACUTE KIDNEY INJURY

Sepsis is the most common cause of AKI in the critically ill.[9] Sepsis and septic shock create hemodynamic instability and reduce perfusion to the kidney. Immunologic, toxic, and inflammatory factors may alter the function of the kidney microvasculature and tubular cells.[27] Sepsis caused 19% of AKI in one study[4] and 55% of AKI in a population of older hospitalized patients.[5] Clinical guidelines for hemodynamic support in sepsis emphasize the need for adequate fluid resuscitation, because in 40% to 50% of cases, reversal of hypotension and restoration of hemodynamic stability can be achieved with fluids alone.[28] Unfortunately, in severely septic patients, inflammation increases vascular permeability, and much of this fluid may move into the third space (interstitial space). If the blood pressure remains low, the use of vasopressors is recommended to raise refractory low blood pressure after volume resuscitation.[28] Vasopressors raise blood pressure and increase systemic vascular resistance (SVR), but they also may raise the vascular resistance within the kidney microvasculature. Other practices aimed at reversing the deleterious effects of sepsis include maintaining the patient's hemoglobin level at 7 to 9 g/dL and blood glucose level below 150 mg/dL and ensuring optimal hydration as evidenced by a central venous pressure above 8 mm Hg.[28]

TRAUMA AND ACUTE KIDNEY INJURY

Trauma Admissions. Trauma patients have different demographics from those of other critical care populations. They are always emergency admissions, are younger, are more often male, and have fewer coexisting illnesses.[29] A 5-year retrospective study of 9449 trauma admissions to critical care units in Australia and New Zealand used the RIFLE criteria to determine incidence of AKI in the first 24 hours after admission; 18% of trauma patients developed AKI.[29] However, if patients were older or had preexisting comorbid illnesses, their risk of AKI rose to 35%.[29] Although these AKI numbers are high, they likely underestimate the true incidence because the study did not include patients who developed AKI later than 24 hours after admission to the critical care unit.[29]

Rhabdomyolysis. Trauma patients with major crush injuries have an elevated risk of kidney failure because of the release of creatine and myoglobin from damaged muscle cells, a condition called *rhabdomyolysis*.[30] Myoglobin in large quantities is toxic to the kidney. Overall survival from rhabdomyolysis is 77%.[30]

The level of creatine kinase (CK), a marker of systemic muscle damage, increases in patients with rhabdomyolysis. One trauma service reported that of 2083 critical care trauma admissions, 85% had elevated CK levels, and 10% developed acute kidney failure resulting from rhabdomyolysis.[31] A CK level of 5000 units/L was the lowest abnormal value in patients who developed AKI associated with rhabdomyolysis.[31]

Volume resuscitation is the primary treatment for preservation of adequate kidney function and prevention of AKI. In many hospitals, the intravenous fluids are alkalinized by the addition of sodium bicarbonate, and the urine output is increased by intravenous administration of the diuretic mannitol.[30] A bicarbonate and mannitol regimen is instituted to prevent acidosis and hyperkalemia, because both are frequent complications of rhabdomyolysis. Close attention is paid to urine output, CK levels, increases in serum creatinine levels, and any signs of compartment syndrome in all patients admitted with this diagnosis.

CONTRAST-INDUCED NEPHROTOXIC INJURY AND ACUTE KIDNEY INJURY

More than 1 million radiologic studies or procedures that involve use of intravenous radiopaque contrast are performed every year.[13] Approximately 1% of those patients will require dialysis as a result of contrast-induced nephrotoxicity,[32] with prolongation of the hospital stay to an average of 17 days.[13] Patients at risk are those with chronic kidney dysfunction, baseline serum creatinine levels more than 1.5 mg/dL, and known diabetes, heart failure, or volume depletion.[33,34] A clinical definition of contrast-induced nephrotoxicity is an increase in serum creatinine concentration of 0.5 mg/dL or more or a 25% increase from the patient's baseline within 48 to 72 hours of contrast medium exposure.[13,33] The effects of reversible, contrast-induced AKI may not be limited to the immediate hospitalization; it has been linked to increased mortality in the 5-year period after the reversible AKI compared with similar patients who did not have kidney injury.[34]

Radiopaque Contrast. High-molecular-weight contrast medium is a potential cause of nephrotoxicity.[13,35] A recommended strategy to prevent contrast-induced nephrotoxicity involves use of a lower quantity of contrast per study and use of nonionic, low-osmolar or iso-osmolar (iohexol) contrast media that are less nephrotoxic.[35,36]

Promote Hydration and Avoid Dehydration. The best method of prevention is aggressive hydration with intravenous normal saline during and after the procedure.[37,38] After some diagnostic intravascular catheterization procedures, the alert patient is asked to drink several liters of water over a 12-hour period to protect the kidney. Avoiding dehydration is vital. In research studies, the addition of sodium bicarbonate or *N*-acetylcysteine did not confer additional protection to the vulnerable kidney beyond hydration with normal saline only.[37-39]

Medications. Several medications have been tried to mitigate the risk of AKI in at-risk patients who undergo diagnostic studies involving radiopaque contrast. They include oral *N*-acetylcysteine, intravenous sodium bicarbonate, and an intravenous infusion of fenoldopam.[37-40] In randomized, controlled trials, *N*-acetylcysteine has not lived up to its early promise.[37-40] For sodium bicarbonate, the picture is mixed, with some studies reporting a benefit[39,41] and other studies reporting no effect.[37,38] Because *N*-acetylcysteine and sodium bicarbonate are inexpensive and have almost no side effects, many physicians prescribe them on an empirical basis, even though the research evidence is not yet conclusive.

In summary, the mainstay measures to protect the kidney from contrast-induced AKI are to use the smallest dose of low- or iso-osmolar contrast media possible, provide vigorous fluid volume expansion, stop all nephrotoxic drugs, and avoid repeat contrast media injections within 48 hours.[42]

HEMODYNAMIC MONITORING AND FLUID BALANCE

Hemodynamic monitoring is important for the analysis of fluid volume status in the critically ill patient with AKI.

Hemodynamic Monitoring. Hemodynamic monitoring includes surveillance of the central venous pressure, pulmonary artery occlusion pressure, cardiac output, and cardiac index.[43]

Daily Weight. A less high-tech method but also important is a daily weight and focused physical assessment. The daily weight, combined with accurate intake and output monitoring, is a powerful indicator of fluid gains or losses over 24 hours. A 1-kg weight gain over 24 hours represents 1000 mL (1 liter) of additional fluid retention.

Physical Assessment. Physical signs and symptoms are used to assess fluid balance. Signs that suggest extracellular fluid (ECF) depletion include thirst, decreased skin turgor, and lethargy. Signs that imply intravascular fluid volume overload include pulmonary congestion, increasing heart failure, and rising blood pressure. The patient with untreated AKI is edematous. Several factors contribute to this state:

1. Fluid retention caused by inadequate urine output.
2. Low serum albumin levels create a lower oncotic pressure in the vasculature, and more fluid seeps out into the interstitial spaces to cause peripheral edema.

3. Inflammation associated with AKI or a coexisting nonrenal disease increases vascular permeability, facilitating fluid movement from the vessels into interstitial spaces.

In critical illness, even though there is peripheral edema, and the patient may have gained 8 L of fluid over his or her "dry-weight" baseline, the patient may remain "intravascularly dry" and hemodynamically unstable, because the retained fluid is not inside a vascular compartment and cannot contribute to maintenance of hemodynamic stability. The patient with AKI is assessed frequently for pitting edema over bony prominences and in dependent body areas.

ELECTROLYTE BALANCE

Potassium. Electrolyte levels require frequent observation, especially in the critical phases of AKI (see Table 31-4). Potassium may quickly reach levels of 6.0 mEq/L or higher. Specific electrocardiographic changes are associated with hyperkalemia: peaked T waves, a widening of the QRS interval, and ultimately, ventricular tachycardia or fibrillation. If hyperkalemia is identified, all potassium supplements are stopped.[44] If the patient is producing urine, intravenous diuretics can be administered. Acute hyperkalemia can be treated temporarily by intravenous administration of insulin and glucose. An infusion of 50 mL of 50% dextrose accompanied by 10 units of regular insulin forces potassium out of the serum and into the cells.

Sodium polystyrene sulfonate (Kayexalate), a cation-exchange resin, is mixed in water and sorbitol and given orally, rectally, or through a nasogastric tube. The resin binds potassium in the bowel, which eliminates it in the feces. Kayexalate and dialysis are the only permanent methods of potassium removal.[44]

Sodium. Dilutional hyponatremia, associated with kidney failure, is an expected finding (see Table 31-4). It can be corrected over a few days with fluid restriction. Sodium levels may be raised more rapidly during dialysis by changing the amount of sodium in the dialysate bath.

Calcium and Phosphorus. Serum calcium levels are reduced (hypocalcemia) in kidney failure (see Table 31-4). This reduction results from multiple factors, including hyperphosphatemia. Chronically elevated serum phosphorus levels (>5.5 to 6.5 mEq/L) are associated with higher mortality rates for patients in kidney failure.[20,45,46] Calcium and phosphorus are regulated in part by parathyroid hormone (PTH). Normally, PTH helps calcium be resorbed back into the bloodstream at the proximal tubule and distal nephron, and it promotes excretion of phosphorus by the kidney to maintain homeostasis. In kidney failure, this mechanism is nonfunctional; the serum phosphorus level rises, and the serum calcium level falls.

Calcium Replacement. Most calcium in the bloodstream is bound to protein. Calcium levels can be measured in two ways: total calcium (tCa) or ionized calcium (iCa).[46] Unfortunately, protein-calcium binding confounds the measurement of accurate calcium levels. In the past, calculations were used to estimate the amounts of protein-bound versus unbound calcium, but these calculations have been shown to produce inaccurate results.[47] The metabolically active, non–protein-bound portion is known as the *ionized calcium* and is the preferred method of measurement.[47] Without adequate levels of serum calcium, a compensatory mechanism "steals" calcium from the bones, making the patient with kidney failure more vulnerable to fractures.[48] Maintaining adequate calcium stores in the body is important and is achieved by administration of calcium supplements, vitamin D preparations, and synthetic calcitriol.[49]

Dietary-Phosphorus Binding Drugs. A second method used in tandem with calcium supplements to achieve normal calcium levels is to lower the level of phosphorus in the bloodstream.[46] Phosphorus occurs in many foods, and eliminating all phosphorus-containing foods from the diet would make it unpalatable.[50] Foods that contain particularly high levels of phosphorus include dairy products, processed meats, some carbonated drinks, and nuts.[50] After eating these foods, free phosphorus passes from the gastrointestinal tract into the bloodstream and raises the serum level. Medications that bind dietary phosphorus in the gastrointestinal tract are administered orally or by nasogastric tube. The binding agent must be taken at the same time as a meal.[50] After the dietary phosphorus is bound to the binding substance in the bowel, it is eliminated from the intestine with stool. This lowers the serum phosphorus level.

The types of dietary-phosphorus binders used have changed over the years. The original binders were aluminum salts (aluminum hydroxide) that bound dietary phosphorus effectively in the gastrointestinal tract but conferred aluminum toxicity because some of the aluminum metal was also absorbed.[50] For this reason, aluminum binders have largely been abandoned.[50]

The second generation of dietary-phosphorus binding agents that are most widely prescribed use calcium salts (calcium carbonate; calcium acetate [PhosLo]) to bind dietary phosphorus in the gastrointestinal tract. Calcium-based drugs are safer, but elevated serum calcium levels and calcium deposits in other areas of the body (extraosseous calcification) are a problem.[50] This category of drugs remains in widespread use.

A third generation of dietary-phosphorus binding medications is available. They are non–aluminum-, non–calcium-based medications. They include sevelamer hydrochloride (RenaGel) and lanthanum carbonate (Fosrenol).[50]

MEDICAL MANAGEMENT

Treatment Goals. Treatment goals for patients with AKI focus on prevention, compensation for the deterioration of kidney function, and regeneration of the remaining kidney functional capacity. Over the past 4 decades, the mortality rate for AKI has remained at more than 50%.[4,5] Key areas that are evaluated include prevention strategies, fluid balance, anemia, medications, and electrolyte imbalance.

Prevention. The only truly effective remedy for AKI is prevention. Effective prevention requires assessment of the patient's risk for AKI. Knowledge of the most frequent causes of AKI in the critically ill is essential if prevention strategies are to be enacted. The critical care team collaborates closely with the clinical pharmacist to avoid drugs with nephrotoxic side effects in patients with AKI or CKD.[19,20] Nonsteroidal antiinflammatory drugs (NSAIDs) for pain relief are avoided in patients with elevated creatinine levels.[2] The use of intravascular contrast dye is preferably delayed until the patient is fully rehydrated.[42]

Fluid Resuscitation. Prerenal failure is caused by decreased perfusion and flow to the kidney. It is often associated with trauma, hemorrhage, hypotension, and major fluid losses. If contrast dye is used, aggressive fluid resuscitation with normal saline (NaCl) is recommended. Fluid replacement is the only treatment shown to prevent kidney tubular injury.[51] The objectives of volume replacement are to replace fluid and electrolyte losses and to prevent ongoing loss. Maintenance intravenous fluid therapy is initiated when oral (PO) fluid intake is inadvisable. Maintenance fluids are calculated with consideration for individual body surface area. Adults require approximately 1500 mL/m^2/24 hr; fever, burns, and trauma significantly increase fluid requirements. Other important criteria when calculating fluid volume replacement include baseline metabolism, environmental temperature, and humidity. The rate of replacement depends on cardiopulmonary reserve, adequacy of kidney function, urine output, fluid balance, ongoing loss, and type of fluid replaced.

Crystalloids and Colloids. Crystalloids and colloids refer to two different types of intravenous fluids used for volume management in critically ill patients. These intravenous solutions are used on all types of patients, not just those with acute kidney failure. Adequacy of intravenous fluid replacement depends on strict, ongoing evaluation and frequent adjustment. Frequent monitoring of serum electrolyte levels is required, and strictly regulated intake and output are correlated with daily weight records. In septic shock, hemodynamic readings are frequently undertaken. After a fluid challenge, a merely minimal increase in central venous pressure implies that additional fluid replacement is required. Continued decreases in central venous pressure, pulmonary artery occlusion pressure, and the cardiac index indicate ongoing volume losses.

Which intravenous fluid to select to most successfully resuscitate hemodynamically unstable patients has been a controversial topic in critical care. The major debate centers on the differences between crystalloid and colloid solutions.

Crystalloids. Crystalloid solutions, which are balanced salt solutions, are in widespread use for maintenance infusion and replacement therapy. Crystalloid fluids include normal saline solution (0.9 NaCl), half-strength saline solution (0.45 NaCl), and lactated Ringer's (LR) solution (Table 31-6). LR solution usually is avoided in patients with kidney failure because it contains potassium. A noncrystalloid solution that may be infused is dextrose (5% or 10%) in water (D_5W, $D_{10}W$).

Colloids. Colloids are solutions containing oncotically active particles that are used to expand intravascular volume to achieve and maintain hemodynamic stability. Albumin (5% and 25%) and hetastarch are colloid solutions (see Table 31-6). Colloids expand intravascular volume, and the effect can last as long as 24 hours. The goal is to optimize the pulmonary artery occlusion pressure ("wedge" pressure), raise mean arterial pressure (MAP), and increase cardiac output and the cardiac index to a therapeutic level. However, the role of colloids in critical care volume resuscitation is discouraged because of increased cost without evidence of increased benefit.

The controversy over whether colloids or crystalloid intravenous fluids are most effective for volume resuscitation appears to have been put to rest by a series of randomized clinical trials and meta-analytic reviews. The SAFE study (*s*aline versus *a*lbumin *f*luid *e*valuation) was a randomized, prospective, double-blind trial that examined whether the selection of resuscitation fluid in the critical care unit affected survival at 28 days.[52] This was a huge study, with almost 7000 critical care patients randomized to two similar groups. One group received 4% albumin, and the other group received 0.9 normal saline (NaCl) for fluid resuscitation.[52] The patients in both groups were similar in terms of organ dysfunction, mechanical ventilator support (64% of patients), and renal replacement therapy (1% of patients). The SAFE results showed that there was that there was no difference in the mortality rate, time in the critical care unit, ventilator days, or renal replacement therapy days.[52] The researchers concluded that albumin and saline should be considered clinically equivalent treatments for intravascular volume expansion in critically ill patients.[52] The exception was for patients with traumatic brain injury (TBI), in which case albumin was associated with a higher mortality rate.[53]

The findings of the SAFE study investigators have been validated by a systematic review of randomized trials of crystalloids versus colloids that reported no difference in mortality rates for the critically ill and injured based on resuscitation fluid.[54] Consequently, colloids are not favored because of their higher cost, and crystalloids are the recommended fluid to use for resuscitation in critical care.

Fluid Restriction. Fluid restriction constitutes a large part of the medical treatment for acute kidney failure. Fluid restriction is used to prevent circulatory overload and the development of interstitial edema when the kidneys cannot remove excess volume. The fluid requirements are calculated on the basis of daily urine volumes and insensible losses. Obtaining daily weight measurements and keeping accurate intake and output records is essential. Patients with kidney failure are usually restricted to 1 L of fluid per 24 hours if the urine output is 500 mL or less. Insensible losses range from 500 to 750 mL/day.

Fluid Removal. Acute kidney failure promotes increased amounts of water, solutes, and potential toxins in the circulation, and prompt measures are needed to decrease their levels. Diuretics are used to stimulate the urine output. However, renal replacement therapy (hemodialysis or hemofiltration) is the treatment of choice, particularly if volume overload exacerbates acute lung injury and heart failure.

PHARMACOLOGIC MANAGEMENT

The first step is to eliminate all nephrotoxic medications. Second, if drugs are eliminated through the kidneys, it is important to decrease the frequency of administration (e.g., from every 6 hours to every 12 or 24 hours) or to decrease the dose and to monitor the serum concentration by measuring serum drug levels.[55]

Diuretics. Diuretics are used to stimulate urinary output in the fluid overloaded patient with functioning kidneys. Care must be taken in their use to avoid the creation of secondary

TABLE 31-6 Frequently Used Intravenous Solutions

Solution	Electrolytes	Indications
Crystalloids*		
Dextrose in water (D$_5$W), isotonic	None	Maintain volume Replace mild loss Provide minimal calories
Normal saline solution (0.9% NaCl)	Sodium: 154 mEq/L Chloride: 154 mEq/L Osmolality: 308 mEq/L	Maintain volume Replace mild loss Correct mild hyponatremia
Half-strength saline solution (0.45% NaCl)	Sodium: 77 mEq/L Chloride: 77 mEq/L	Free water replacement Correct mild hyponatremia Free water and electrolyte replacement (fluid- and electrolyte-restricted conditions)
Lactated Ringer's solution	Sodium: 130 mEq/L Potassium: 4 mEq/L Calcium: 2.7 mEq/L Chloride: 107 mEq/L Lactate: 27 mEq/L pH: 6.5	Fluid and electrolyte replacement (contraindicated for patients with kidney or liver disease or in lactic acidosis)
Colloids		
5% Albumin (Albumisol)	Albumin: 50 g/L Sodium: 130-160 mEq/L Potassium: 1 mEq/L Osmolality: 300 mOsm/L Osmotic pressure: 20 mm Hg pH: 6.4 to 7.4	Volume expansion Moderate protein replacement Achievement of hemodynamic stability in shock states
25% Albumin (salt-poor)	Albumin: 240 g/L Globulins: 10 g/L Sodium: 130-160 mEq/L Osmolality: 1500 mOsm/L pH: 6.4 to 7.4	Concentrated form of albumin sometimes used with diuretics to move fluid from tissues into the vascular space for diuresis
Hetastarch	Sodium: 154 mEq/L Chloride: 154 mEq/L Osmolality: 310 mOsm/L Colloid osmotic pressure: 30-35 mm Hg	Synthetic polymer (6% solution) used for volume expansion Hemodynamic volume replacement after cardiac surgery, burns, sepsis
Low-molecular-weight dextran (LMWD)	Glucose polysaccharide molecules with average molecular weight of 40,000; no electrolytes	Volume expansion and support (contraindicated for patients with bleeding disorders)
High-molecular-weight dextran (HMWD)	Glucose polysaccharide molecules with average molecular weight of 70,000; no electrolytes	Used prophylactically in some cases to prevent platelet aggregation; available in saline and glucose solutions

*For crystalloid solutions that contain electrolytes, specific concentrations of electrolytes and pH vary according to the manufacturer.

electrolyte abnormalities (Table 31-7). Diuretics reduce volume overload and are helpful for symptoms such as pulmonary edema, but they have not been shown to prevent AKI.[56] Diuretics are used in many patient populations other than those with incipient kidney failure.

Loop Diuretics. The loop diuretic *furosemide* (Lasix) is the most frequently used diuretic in critical care patients. It may be prescribed as a bolus dose or as a continuous infusion. Electrolytic abnormalities are frequently encountered, and close monitoring of serum potassium, magnesium, and sodium is essential.

Thiazide Diuretics. Diuretics may be prescribed in combination. A thiazide diuretic such as chlorothiazide (Diuril) or metolazone (Zaroxolyn) may be administered and followed by a loop diuretic to take advantage of the fact that these drugs work on different parts of the nephron.

Osmotic Diuretics. Osmotic diuretics (e.g., mannitol) are prescribed to decrease fluid overload and improve urine output. It is important to use an in-line 5-micron filter when administering this drug. Mannitol is frequently prescribed for patients with brain injury and increased intracranial pressure (ICP). More information on the use of mannitol in this population can be found in Chapter 27.

Heart Failure. For patients with heart failure, two of the natriuretic peptides (atrial natriuretic peptide [ANP] and brain natriuretic peptide [BNP] which acts on the ventricles) may

TABLE 31-7 Pharmacologic Management: Kidney-Related Medications

DRUG	DOSAGE	ACTIONS	SPECIAL CONSIDERATIONS
Diuretics			
Loop Diuretics			
Furosemide Bumetanide	20-80 mg/day (Lasix) 0.5-2 mg/day (Bumex)	Acts on loop of Henle to inhibit sodium and chloride	Ototoxicity if administered too rapidly or with other ototoxic drugs Monitor intake and output, hydration; watch for hypotension
Thiazide Diuretics			
Chlorothiazide (Diuril)	500 mg-1 g/day	Inhibit sodium, chloride resorption in distal tubule	Enhanced with low-sodium diet Synergistic effect with loop diuretics
Potassium-Sparing Diuretics			
Aldactone	100 mg/day for 5 days	Exert effects on collecting tubule; reduce potassium, hydrogen and increase sodium	Weak diuretic effect, so given with other diuretics Potassium supplements not required; monitor for hyperkalemia Used as an aldosterone blocker to treat heart failure
Osmotic Diuretics			
Mannitol	0.25-1.0 g/kg IV infusion as a 15%-20% solution over 30-90 min	Increases urine output because higher plasma osmolality, increases flow of water from tissues causing increased GFR Increases serum sodium, potassium levels.	Often used in head injury to decrease cerebral edema Can be used to promote urinary secretion of toxic substances At low temperatures mannitol may crystallize, use in-line 5-micron IV filter with >15% (>15 g/100 mL) solutions

BP, blood pressure; ECG, electrocardiogram; GFR Glomerular filtration rate; GI, gastrointestinal; IV, intravenous; PO, by mouth.

be prescribed. These drugs work by stimulating natriuretic receptors in the atrium (ANP) and ventricular myocardium (BNP). The potassium-sparing diuretic Aldactone (spironolactone) is also used in heart failure management, not as a diuretic but primarily as an aldosterone antagonist to lower aldosterone levels. Most heart failure patients and hypertensive patients require loop diuretics as part of their medication regimen to control fluid volume overload. More information on the use of diuretics in heart failure management is provided in Chapters 18 and 19.

Controversies. The use of diuretics in the critically ill continues to be controversial, and the topic is being actively investigated. Mehta and colleagues published an observational study showing that for critically ill patients with established AKI and oliguria, loop diuretics increased the mortality rate and delayed kidney recovery.[57] A subsequent study found that furosemide helped maintain urine output but had no more impact on survival and recovery of kidney function than a placebo.[58] A third research trial found that furosemide neither helped nor worsened AKI in the critically ill.[59] The debate and research studies will continue, but for now, it appears that loop diuretics increase the urine output, which makes clinicians feel better, but these drugs have no impact on the outcome of established oliguric AKI.[56]

Dopamine. Low-dose dopamine (2 to 3 mcg/kg/min), previously known as renal-dose dopamine, is frequently infused to stimulate blood flow to the kidney. Dopamine is effective in increasing urine output in the short term, but tolerance of the dopamine renal receptor to the drug is theorized to develop in the critically ill patients who are most at risk for AKI.[60] A meta-analysis of related research studies determined that renal-dose dopamine did not prevent onset of AKI and did not decrease the need for dialysis or reduce mortality.[61] At this point, the support for routine use of low-dose dopamine for the prevention of AKI remains anecdotal only.[62]

Acetylcysteine. *N*-Acetylcysteine (Mucomyst, Mucosil) is an *N*-acetyl derivative of the amino acid L-cysteine. It has been used for many years as a mucolytic agent to assist with expectoration of thick pulmonary secretions. It is also frequently prescribed for patients with mildly elevated serum creatinine levels before a radiologic study using contrast dye.[63] In research trials, the addition of *N*-acetylcysteine to normal saline hydration has not showed a reduction in the incidence of contrast-induced AKI.[37,39,63] In clinical trials enrolling cardiac surgery patients, prophylactic use of *N*-acetylcysteine did not decease the rate of AKI.[63,64] Most studies suggest that *N*-acetylcysteine does not prevent AKI during radiologic procedures or after cardiac surgery.

Fenoldopam. Fenoldopam mesylate (Corlopam) is a dopamine 1 (D_1) receptor agonist similar in structure to dopamine and dobutamine. It is used to lower blood pressure. Claims that this drug would prevent contrast-induced nephrotoxicity in high-risk patients have not been supported by clinical trial results.[40]

Dietary-Phosphorus Binders. Many patients with kidney failure are prescribed a dietary-phosphorus binding medication (see earlier section on "Dietary-Phosphorus Binding Drugs").[50] Many dietary-phosphorus binding drugs are available, and some important issues concern all of them. The dietary-phosphorus binder must be taken at the time of the meal. If it is taken 2 hours later, it will increase only the level of the binding substance (e.g., calcium) in the bloodstream and will not lower the serum phosphorus level. Related issues such as the quantity of phosphorus in the diet should be discussed with a clinical nutritionist (dietitian).

NUTRITION

Diet or nutritional supplementation for the patient with AKI in the critical care unit is designed to account for the diminished excretory capacity of the kidney. The recommended energy intake is between 20 and 30 kilocalories/kg per day, with 1.2 to 1.5 g/kg of protein per day to control azotemia (increased BUN level).[65] Oral nutrition is preferred, and if the patient cannot eat, enteral nutrition is recommended over parenteral (intravenous) nutrition. Fluids are limited, and tight glucose control is recommended.[65] The electrolytes potassium, sodium, and phosphorus are strictly limited.

NURSING MANAGEMENT

Nursing management of the patient with AKI patients involves a variety of nursing diagnoses (see the Nursing Diagnoses feature on Acute Kidney Dysfunction). "Prevention is the best cure" is an old saying that captures the role of the critical care nurse, who evaluates all patients for level of kidney function, risk of infection, fluid imbalance, electrolyte disturbances, anemia, readiness to learn, and need for education.

Nursing Diagnoses

Acute Kidney Dysfunction

- Excess Fluid Volume related to kidney dysfunction
- Ineffective Kidney Tissue Perfusion related to decreased renal blood flow
- Anxiety related to threat to biologic, psychological, or social integrity
- Decreased Cardiac Output related to decrease in preload
- Risk for Infection risk factors: protein-calorie malnourishment, invasive monitoring devices
- Disturbed Body Image related to functional dependence on life-sustaining technology
- Ineffective Coping related to situational crisis and personal vulnerability
- Disturbed Sleep Pattern related to fragmented sleep
- Deficient Knowledge: Fluid Restriction, Reportable Symptoms, and Medications related to lack of previous exposure to information

---

Risk Factors for Acute Kidney Injury. Some individuals are at increased risk for AKI as a complication during hospitalization, and the alert critical care nurse recognizes potential risk factors and acts as a patient advocate.[19,20] Patients at risk include older persons because their GFR may be decreased,[5] dehydrated patients with kidney hypoperfusion, patients with increased creatinine levels before their hospitalization, and patients undergoing a radiologic procedure involving contrast dye.

Infectious Complications. The critical care patient with infectious complications is at risk for AKI. Signs of infection such as an increased white blood cell (WBC) count, redness at a wound or intravenous line site, or increased temperature are always a cause for concern. A urinary catheter is inserted to facilitate accurate urine measurement and patient comfort. However, any indwelling catheter is a potential source for infection. When the patient no longer makes large quantities of urine and is hemodynamically stable, the catheter must be removed promptly. If the patient cannot void urine spontaneously, a scheduled "straight catheterization" is performed to minimize the risk of infection from an indwelling catheter and drainage system. This method allows the patient's bladder to be emptied, but the catheter does not remain in place.

Fluid Balance. Intravascular fluid balance is often assessed on an hourly basis for the critically ill patient who has hemodynamic lines inserted. Hemodynamic values (heart rate, blood pressure, central venous pressure, pulmonary artery occlusion pressure, cardiac output, and cardiac index) and daily weight measurements are correlated with the intake and output. Urine output is measured hourly by means of a urinary catheter and drainage bag throughout all phases of AKI, particularly in response to diuretics. Any fluid removed with dialysis is included the daily fluid balance. Recognition of the clinical signs and symptoms of fluid overload is important. Excess fluid moves from the vascular system into the peripheral tissues (dependent edema), abdomen (ascites), and lungs (crackles, pulmonary edema, and pulmonary effusions); around the heart (pericardial effusions); and into the brain (increased intracranial swelling).

Electrolyte Imbalance. Hyperkalemia, hypocalcemia, hyponatremia, hyperphosphatemia, and acid-base imbalances occur during AKI (see Table 31-4). Clinical manifestations of these electrolyte imbalances must be prevented and their associated side effects controlled. The more likely imbalances are hyperkalemia and hypocalcemia, which can result in life-threatening cardiac dysrhythmias. Dilutional hyponatremia may develop as fluid overload worsens in the patient with oliguria. Monitoring the serum sodium level is important to prevent this complication. Hyperphosphatemia results in severe pruritus. Nursing care is directed at soothing the itching by performing frequent skin care with emollients, discouraging scratching, and administering phosphate-binding medications.[50] The acid-base imbalances that occur with AKI are monitored by arterial blood gas (ABG) analyses. The goal of treatment is to maintain the pH within the normal range.

Preventing Anemia. Anemia is an expected side effect of kidney failure that occurs because the kidney no longer produces the hormone *erythropoietin.*[66] As a result, the bone marrow is not stimulated to produce red blood cells (RBCs). Decreased RBC production by the bone marrow also occurs as a consequence of critical illness.[67] Care is taken to prevent blood loss in the patient with AKI, and blood withdrawal is minimized as much as possible. Irritation of the gastrointestinal tract from metabolic waste accumulation is expected, and stress ulcer prophylaxis must be prescribed. Gastrointestinal bleeding remains a possibility. Stool, nasogastric tube drainage, and emesis are routinely tested for occult blood. Anemia may be treated pharmacologically by the administration of recombinant human erythropoietin (rhEPO), epoetin alfa (Procrit, Epogen), to stimulate erythrocyte production by the bone marrow and if required by RBC transfusion. Treatment of anemia early in the course of AKI (before dialysis) appears to slow the progression of the kidney failure and delays the initiation or renal replacement therapies.[68] Even in anemic, critically ill patients without kidney failure, administration of rhEPO weekly significantly decreases the number of blood transfusions.[69] However, this therapy is not recommended for anemia related to sepsis in the critically ill.[28]

PATIENT EDUCATION

Accurate and uncomplicated information must be provided to the patient and family about AKI, including its prognosis, treatment, and possible complications.[7] Education of the patient can be challenging because elevations of BUN and creatinine levels can negatively affect the level of consciousness. Sleep-rest disorders and emotional upset often occur as complications of AKI and can disrupt short-term memory. Encouraging the patient and family to voice concerns, frustrations, or fears and allowing the patient to control some aspects of the acute care environment and treatment also are essential (see the Patient Education feature on Acute Kidney Injury).

Patient Education: Acute Kidney Dysfunction

- Explain the pathophysiology.
  - Severe acute kidney injury (AKI) is a sudden decline in kidney function that causes an acute buildup of toxins in the blood.
- Explain the cause.
  - Prerenal (before the kidney)
  - Intrarenal (within the kidney)
  - Postrenal (after the kidney)
- Identify predisposing factors; explain the level of kidney function after the acute phase is over.
- Explain diet and fluid restrictions.
- Demonstrate how to check blood pressure, pulse, respirations, and weight.
- Discuss good hygiene and how to avoid infections.
- Emphasize need for exercise and rest.
- Describe medications and adverse effects.
- Explain need for ongoing follow-up with health care professional.
- Explain purpose of dialysis and importance of regular treatments.

RENAL REPLACEMENT THERAPY: DIALYSIS

Two types of renal replacement therapy are available for the treatment of AKI. They are intermittent hemodialysis (IHD) therapy and continuous renal replacement therapy (CRRT).

HEMODIALYSIS

Hemodialysis roughly translates as "separating from the blood." Indications and contraindications for hemodialysis are listed in Box 31-4. As a treatment, hemodialysis separates and removes from the blood the excess electrolytes, fluids, and toxins by mean of a hemodialyzer (Fig. 31-2). Although hemodialysis is efficient in removing solutes, it does not remove all metabolites. Levels of electrolytes, toxins, and fluids increase between treatments, necessitating hemodialysis on a regular basis. Hemodialysis therapy is always intermittent; each dialysis treatment takes 3 to 4 hours. In the acute phases of kidney failure, dialysis is performed daily.[70] The dialysis frequency gradually decreases to three times per week as the patient moves into a more chronic phase of kidney failure.

Hemodialyzer. Hemodialysis works by circulating blood outside the body through synthetic tubing to a dialyzer, which consists of hollow-fiber tubes. The dialyzer is sometimes described as an artificial kidney (Fig. 31-3). While the blood flows through the membranes, which are semipermeable, a fluid (dialysate bath) bathes the membranes and, through osmosis and diffusion, performs exchanges of fluid, electrolytes, and toxins from the blood to the bath, where toxins and dialysate then pass out of the artificial kidney. The blood and the dialysate bath are shunted in opposite directions (countercurrent flow) through the dialyzer to match the osmotic and chemical gradients at the most efficient level for effective dialysis.

BOX 31-4   INDICATIONS AND CONTRAINDICATIONS FOR HEMODIALYSIS

INDICATIONS
- Blood urea nitrogen (BUN) level exceeds 90 mg/dL
- Serum creatinine level of 9 mg/dL
- Hyperkalemia
- Drug toxicity
- Intravascular and extravascular fluid overload
- Metabolic acidosis
- Symptoms of uremia
  - Pericarditis
  - Gastrointestinal bleeding
- Changes in mentation
- Contraindications to other forms of dialysis

CONTRAINDICATIONS
- Hemodynamic instability
- Inability to anticoagulate
- Lack of access to circulation

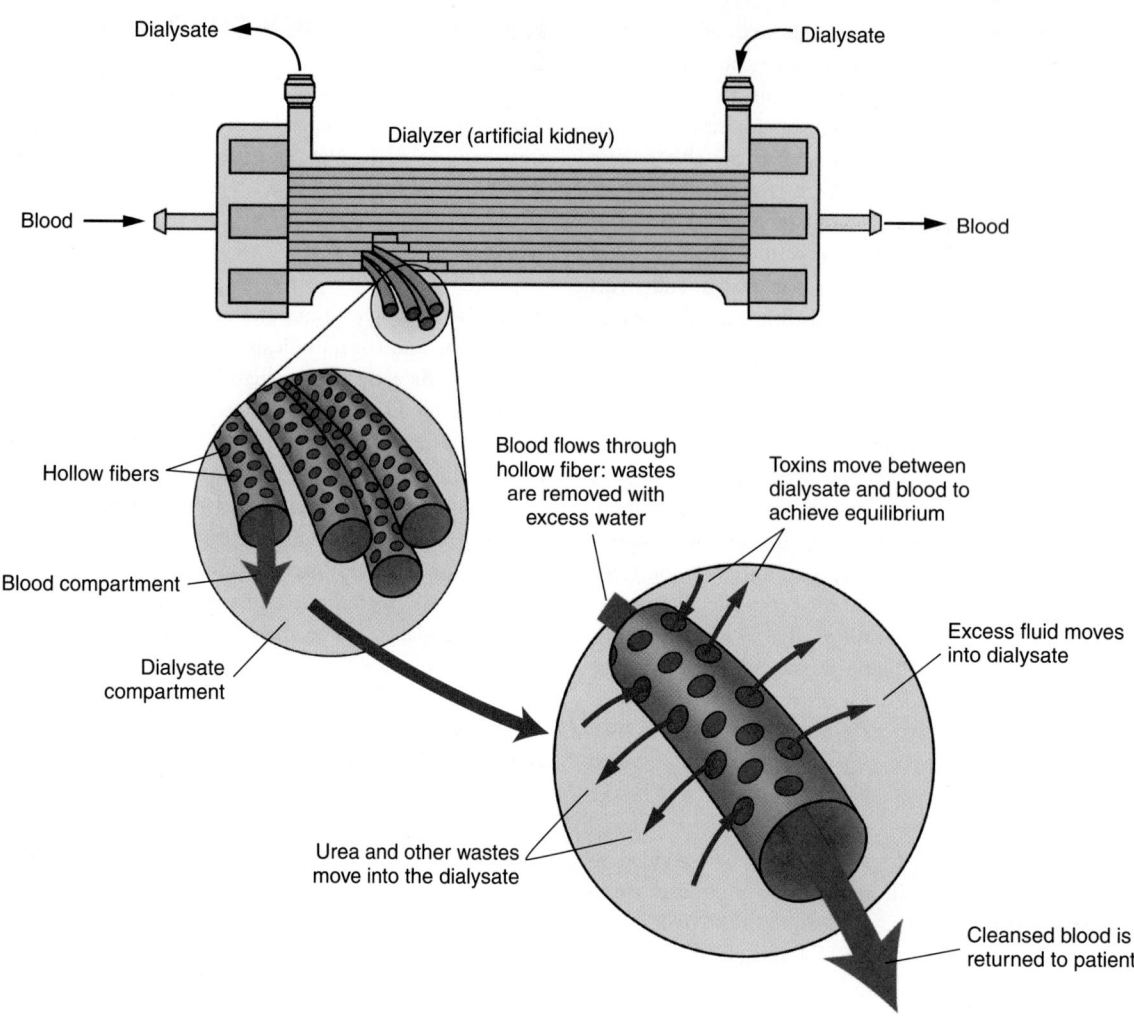

Figure 31-2 Hemodialyzer.

Ultrafiltration. To remove fluid, a positive hydrostatic pressure is applied to the blood, and a negative hydrostatic pressure is applied to the dialysate bath. The two forces together, called *transmembrane pressure*, pull and squeeze the excess fluid from the blood. The difference between the two values (expressed in millimeters of mercury [mm Hg]) represents the transmembrane pressure and results in fluid extraction, known as *ultrafiltration*, from the vascular space.

Anticoagulation. Heparin or sodium citrate is added to the system just before the blood enters the dialyzer to anticoagulate the blood within the dialysis tubing. Without an anticoagulant, the blood clots because its passage through the foreign tubular substances of the dialysis machine activates the clotting mechanism. Heparin can be administered by bolus injection or intermittent infusion. It has a short half-life, and its effects subside within 2 to 4 hours. If necessary, the effects of heparin are easily reversed with the antidote protamine sulfate. When there is concern about the development of heparin-induced thrombocytopenia (HIT),[71] alternative anticoagulants can be used. Citrate (trisodium citrate) can be infused as an anticoagulant by intermittent bolus or continuous infusion.[72]

Vascular Access. Hemodialysis requires access to the bloodstream. Various types of temporary and permanent devices are in clinical use. It is important for patient safety to be able to recognize these different vascular access devices and to properly care for them. The following section discusses temporary vascular access catheters used in the acute care hospital environment and permanent methods used for long-term hemodialysis.

Temporary Acute Access. *Subclavian* and *femoral* veins are catheterized when short-term access is required or when vascular access is nonfunctional in a patient requiring immediate hemodialysis. Subclavian and femoral catheters are routinely inserted at the bedside. Most temporary catheters are venous lines only. Blood flows out toward the dialyzer and flows back to the patient through the same vein. A dual-lumen venous catheter is most commonly used. It has a central partition running the length of the catheter. The outflow catheter section pulls the blood flow through openings that are proximal to the inflow openings on the opposite side (Fig. 31-4). This design helps prevent dialyzing the same blood just returned to the area (recirculation), which would severely reduce the procedure's efficiency. A silicone rubber, dual-lumen catheter with a polyester cuff designed to decrease catheter-related infections is also available.

Permanent Vascular Access. The common denominator in permanent vascular access devices is a connection to the arterial circulation and a return conduit to the venous circulation.

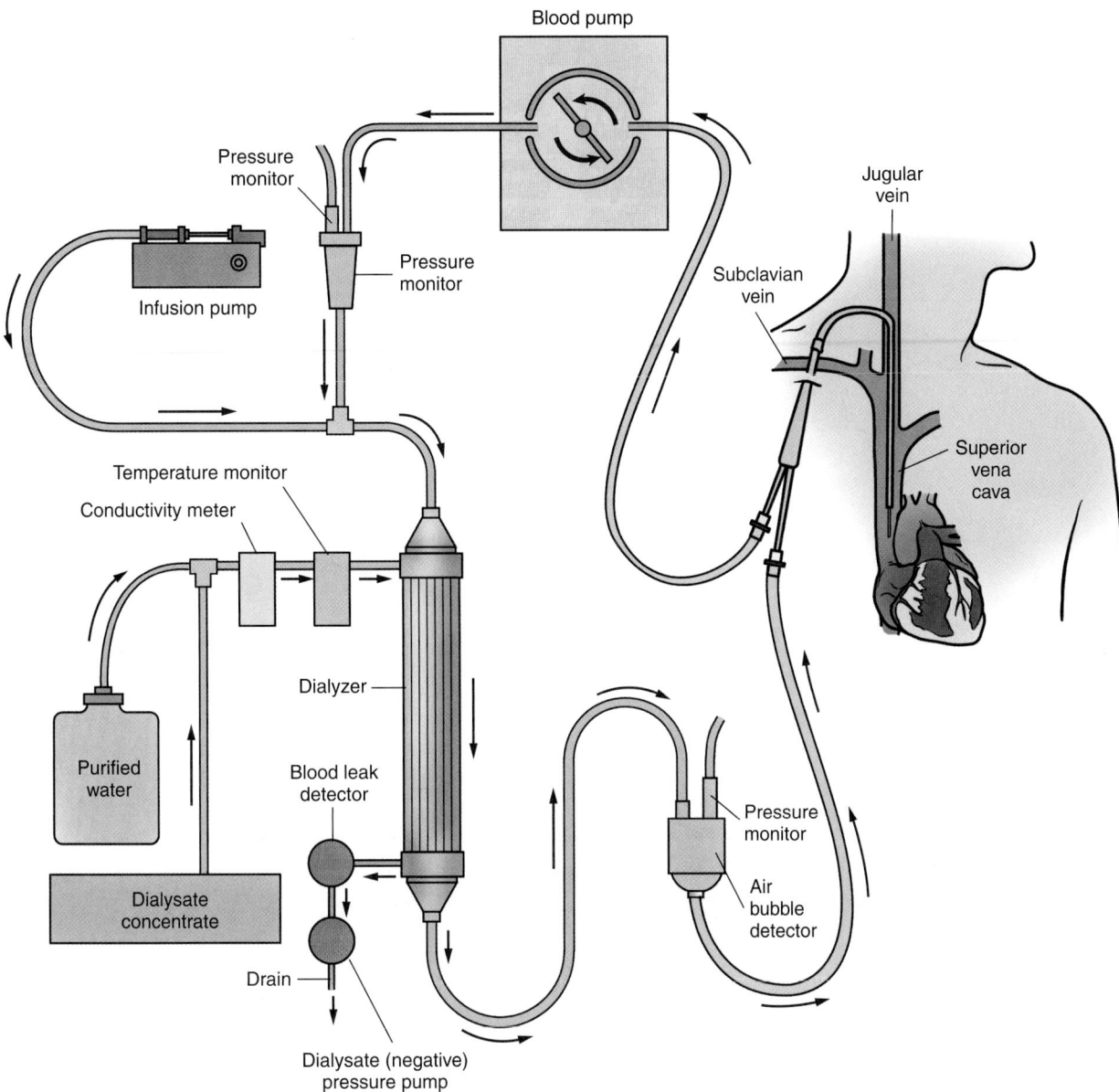

Figure 31-3 Components of a hemodialysis system.

Double Lumen Catheter

A

Distal Port
Venous

From pump
and hemofilter

To pump
and hemofilter

Proximal Port
"Arterial"

Vein

Recirculation ~10%

Direction of venous blood flow

B

Distal Port
Venous

To pump
and hemofilter

From pump
and hemofilter

Proximal Port
"Arterial"

Vein

Recirculation ~50%

Direction of venous blood flow

Figure 31-4 Temporary dialysis venous access catheter.

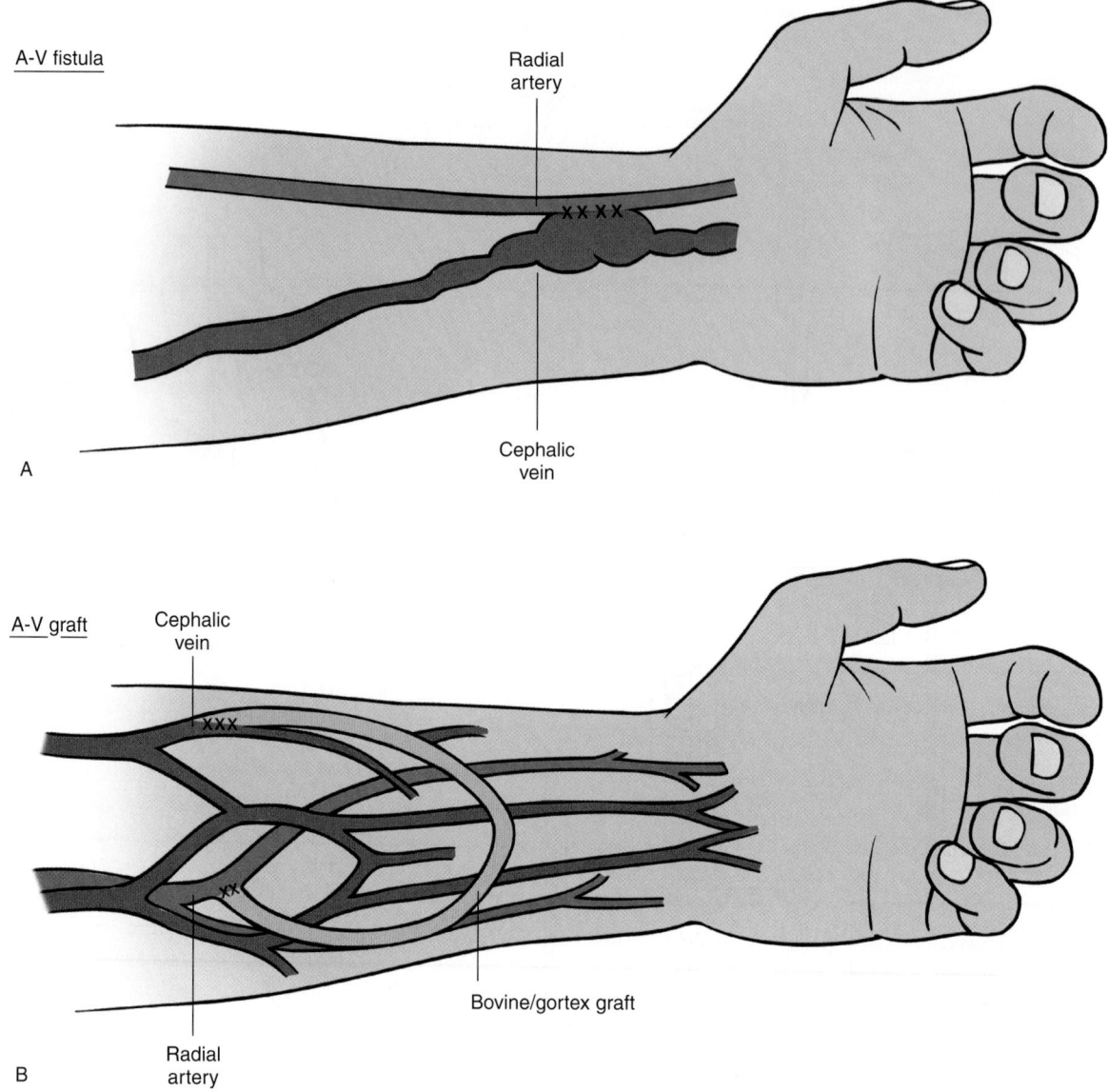

Figure 31-5 Methods of vascular access for hemodialysis. *A,* Arteriovenous fistula between the vein and artery. *B,* Internal synthetic graft corrects the artery and vein.

Arteriovenous Fistula. The arteriovenous fistula is created by surgically exposing a peripheral artery and vein, creating a side-by-side opening in the artery and the vein that joins the two vessels together. The high arterial flow creates a swelling of the vein, or a pseudoaneurysm, at which point (when healed) a large-bore needle can be inserted to obtain arterial outflow to the dialyzer. Inflow is accomplished through a second large-bore needle inserted into a peripheral vein distal to the fistula (Fig. 31-5A). If the patient's vessels are adequate, fistulas are the preferred mode of access because of the durability of blood vessels, relatively few complications, and less need for revision compared with other access methods.[20] An initial disadvantage of a fistula concerns the time required for development of sufficient arterial flow to enlarge the new access. The minimum reported length of time before a fistula can be cannulated for dialysis is 14 days,[73] but the time lag for many patients is longer, as much as weeks or months.[74]

In caring for a patient with a fistula, there are some important nursing priorities to ensure the ongoing viability of the vascular access and safety of the limb (Table 31-8). The critical care nurse frequently assesses the quality of blood flow through the fistula. A patent fistula has a thrill when palpated gently with the fingers and has a bruit if auscultated with a stethoscope. The extremity should be pink and warm to the touch. No blood pressure measurements, intravenous infusions, or laboratory phlebotomy procedures are performed on the arm with the fistula.[75]

The arteriovenous fistula is the preferred long-term access for hemodialysis.[20] However, in the United States, only 27% of hemodialysis patients have an arteriovenous fistula; 47% have a synthetic graft; and 23% have a tunneled hemodialysis catheter.[76] An arteriovenous fistula provides the most favorable long-term patency for hemodialysis access and is recommended if patients require long-term hemodialysis.[20]

TABLE 31-8 Complications and Nursing Management of Arteriovenous Fistula/Graft

Type	Complications	Nursing Management
Fistula	Thrombosis Infection Pseudoaneurysm Vascular steal syndrome Venous hypertension Carpal tunnel syndrome Inadequate blood flow	Teach patients to avoid wearing constrictive clothing on limbs containing access. Teach patients to avoid sleeping on or bending accessed limb for prolonged periods. Use aseptic technique when cannulating access. Avoid repetitious cannulation of one segment of access. Offer comfort measures, such as warm compresses and ordered analgesics, to lessen pain of vascular steal. Teach patients to develop blood flow in the fistulas through exercises (squeezing a rubber ball) while applying mild impedance to flow just distal to the access (at least once per day for 10-15 min). Avoid too-early cannulation of new access.
Graft	Bleeding Thrombosis False aneurysm formation Infection Arterial or venous stenosis Vascular steal syndrome	Teach patients to avoid wearing constrictive clothing on accessed limbs. Avoid repeated cannulation of one segment of access. Use aseptic technique when cannulating access. Monitor for changes in arterial or venous pressure while patients are on dialysis. Provide comfort measures to reduce pain of vascular steal (e.g., warm compresses, analgesics as ordered).

Arteriovenous Grafts. Arteriovenous grafts are vascular access devices for treating chronic kidney failure. The graft is a tube made of synthetic material, which is surgically implanted inside the limb. The area is surgically opened, and an artery and a vein are located. A tunnel is created in the tissue where the graft is placed. Anastomoses are made with the graft ends connected to the artery and vein. The blood is allowed to flow through the graft, and the surgical area is closed. The graft creates a raised area that looks like a large peripheral vein just under the skin and peripheral tissue layers (see Fig. 31-5B). Two large-bore needles are used for outflow from and inflow to the graft. For grafts and fistulas, after needle removal at the end of the hemodialysis treatment, firm pressure must be applied to stop any bleeding (see Table 31-8).

Tunneled Catheters. While waiting for the fistula or graft to mature to be ready for access, some patients with CKD may have a tunneled, cuffed catheter placed.[77] The cuff and tunneling are physical barriers to reduce central venous line infections. Modern catheters are made of silicone or polyurethane, tunneled under the skin, and inserted through the jugular or subclavian vein into the superior vena cava.[75,77]

MEDICAL MANAGEMENT

Medical management involves the decision to place a vascular access device and then to choose the most appropriate type and location for each patient. Patients in the critical care setting who require vascular access for hemodialysis typically use a temporary hemodialysis catheter. The exact quantity of fluid and solute removal to be achieved by hemodialysis is determined individually for each patient by clinical examination and review of all relevant laboratory results.

NURSING MANAGEMENT

A noncritical care nurse who is specially trained in dialysis manages the IHD. The dialysis nurse typically comes to the patient's bedside with the hemodialysis machine. During the acute phase of treatment, hemodialysis occurs daily. The frequency is reduced to 3 days per week as the patient becomes hemodynamically stable. The essential nursing elements to manage a patient on hemodialysis are listed in the Nursing Interventions Classification feature on Hemodialysis Therapy. The essential role of the critical care nurse during dialysis is to monitor the patient's hemodynamic status and ensure the patient remains hemodynamically stable. The AKI patient on hemodialysis depends on a viable venous access catheter. When not in use, the catheter is "heparin-locked" to preserve patency. The critical care nurse provides education about the disease process and treatment plan to patient and family.

CONTINUOUS RENAL REPLACEMENT THERAPY

CRRT is a newer mode of dialysis that has many similarities to traditional hemodialysis. CRRT is a continuous therapy that is monitored by the critical care nurse, and it may continue over many days. The venous blood is circulated through a highly porous hemofilter. As with traditional hemodialysis, access and return of blood are achieved through a large venous catheter (venovenous). The CRRT system allows the continuous removal of fluid from the plasma. The patient's blood flow is 100 to 200 mL/min, and the dialysate flow is 17 to 40 mL/min.[78] The fluid removal rate varies depending on the particular CRRT method used and removal of solutes (urea, creatinine, and electrolytes), as listed in Table 31-9. The removed fluid is described as *ultrafiltrate*. In an ideal situation, the hydrostatic pressure exerted by a MAP greater than 70 mm Hg would propel a continuous flow of blood through the hemofilter to remove fluid and solute. However, because many critically ill patients are hypotensive and cannot provide adequate flow through the hemofilter, an electric roller pump "milks" the tubing to augment flow. If large amounts of fluid are to be removed, intravenous replacement solutions are infused. Indications and contraindications for CRRT are described in Box 31-5.

Hemodialysis Therapy

Definition
Management of extracorporeal passage of the patient's blood through a dialyzer

Activities
Draw blood sample and review blood chemistries (e.g., BUN, serum creatinine, serum sodium, potassium, phosphate [PO_4] levels) before treatment.

Record baseline vital signs: weight, temperature, pulse, respirations, and blood pressure.

Explain hemodialysis procedure and its purpose.

Check equipment and solutions according to protocol.

Use sterile technique to initiate hemodialysis and for needle insertions and catheter connections.

Use gloves, eye shield, and clothing to prevent direct contact with blood.

Initiate hemodialysis according to protocol.

Anchor connections and tubing securely.

Check system monitors (e.g., flow rate, pressure, temperature, pH level, conductivity, clots, air detector, negative pressure for ultrafiltration, blood sensor) to ensure patient safety.

Monitor blood pressure, pulse, respirations, temperature, and patient response during dialysis.

Administer heparin, according to protocol.

Monitor clotting times and adjust heparin administration appropriately.

Adjust filtration pressures to remove an appropriate amount of fluid.

Institute appropriate protocol if patient becomes hypotensive.

Discontinue hemodialysis according to protocol.

Compare postdialysis vital signs and blood chemistries with predialysis values.

Avoid taking blood pressure or doing intravenous punctures in arm with fistula.

Provide catheter or fistula care according to protocol.

Work collaboratively with patient to adjust diet regulations, fluid limitations, and medications to regulate fluid and electrolyte shifts between treatments.

Teach patient to self-monitor signs and symptoms that indicate need for medical treatment (e.g., fever, bleeding, clotted fistula, thrombophlebitis, irregular pulse).

Work collaboratively with patient to relieve discomfort from side effects of the disease and treatment (e.g., cramping, fatigue, headaches, itching, anemia, bone demineralization, body image changes, role disruption).

Work collaboratively with patient to adjust length of dialysis, diet regulations, and pain and diversion needs to achieve optimal benefit of the treatment.

From Bulechek GM et al: *Nursing interventions classification (NIC)*, ed 5, 2008, St Louis, Mosby.

TABLE 31-9 Comparison of Continuous Renal Replacement Therapy Methods

Type	Ultrafiltration Rate	Fluid Replacement	Method of Solute Removal	Indication
SCUF	100-300 mL/hr	None	None	Fluid removal
CVVH	500-800 mL/hr	Predilution or postdilution, calculating hourly net loss	Convection	Fluid removal, moderate solute removal
CVVHD	500-800 mL/hr	Predilution or postdilution, subtracting dialysate, then calculating hourly net loss	Diffusion	Fluid removal, maximum solute removal
CVVHDF		Predilution or postdilution, subtracting dialysate, then calculating hourly net loss	Convection and diffusion	Maximal fluid removal, maximal solute removal

CVVH, continuous venovenous hemofiltration; CVVHD, continuous venovenous hemodialysis; CVVHDF, continuous venovenous hemodiafiltration; SCUF, slow continuous ultrafiltration.

Controversy exists about when CRRT should be started, the optimal dialysis dose, which patients can derive the greatest benefit, and when CRRT should be discontinued.[79-82] The debate over the optimal "dose" of dialysis is likely to continue because the multicenter Veterans Administration and National Institutes of Health trial showed no difference in mortality between critically ill patients receiving intensive or nonintensive dialysis regimens.[83]

Because controlled removal and replacement of fluid is possible over many hours or days with CRRT, hemodynamic stability is maintained. This makes CRRT highly advantageous for use in the hemodynamically unstable patient with multisystem problems. Several modes of CRRT are used in critical care units[81,82]:

1. Slow continuous ultrafiltration (SCUF)
2. Continuous venovenous hemofiltration (CVVH)
3. Continuous venovenous hemodialysis (CVVHD)
4. Continuous venovenous hemodiafiltration (CVVHDF)

The decision about which type of therapy to initiate is based on clinical assessment, metabolic status, severity of uremia, whether a particular treatment modality is available at that institution, and other factors.

Continuous Renal Replacement Therapy Terminology. In CRRT, solutes are removed from the blood by *diffusion* or *convection*. Both processes remove fluid, and the two methods remove molecules of different sizes.

Diffusion. Diffusion describes the movement of solutes along a *concentration gradient* from a high concentration to a low concentration across a semipermeable membrane. This is the main mechanism used in hemodialysis. Solutes such as

BOX 31-5 INDICATIONS AND CONTRAINDICATIONS FOR CONTINUOUS RENAL REPLACEMENT THERAPY

INDICATIONS
- Need for large fluid volume removal in hemodynamically unstable patient
- Hypervolemic or edematous patients unresponsive to diuretic therapy
- Patients with multiple organ dysfunction syndrome
- Ease of fluid management in patients requiring large daily fluid volume
  - Replacement for oliguria
  - Administration of total parenteral nutrition
- Contraindication to hemodialysis and peritoneal dialysis
- Inability to be anticoagulated

CONTRAINDICATIONS
- Hematocrit >45%
- Terminal illness

creatinine and urea cross the dialysis membrane from the blood to the dialysis fluid compartment.

Convection. Convection occurs when a pressure gradient is set up so that the water is pushed or pumped across the dialysis filter and carries the solutes from the bloodstream with it. This method of solute removal is known as *solvent drag*, and it is commonly employed in CRRT.

Absorption. The filter attracts solute, and molecules attach (adsorb) to the dialysis filter. The size of solute molecules is measured in *daltons*. The different sizes of molecules that can be removed by convection or diffusion methods are shown in Table 31-9. Tiny molecules such as urea and creatinine are removed by diffusion and convection (all methods). As the molecular size increases above 500 daltons, convection is the more efficient method (Table 31-10).

Ultrafiltrate Volume. The fluid that is removed each hour is not called *urine*; it is known as *ultrafiltrate*.

Replacement Fluid. Typically, some of the ultrafiltrate is replaced through the CRRT circuit by a sterile replacement fluid. The replacement fluid can be added before the filter (prefilter dilution) or after the filter (postfilter dilution). The purpose is to increase the volume of fluid passing through the hemofilter and improve convection of solute.

Anticoagulation. Because the blood outside the body is in contact with artificial tubing and filters, the coagulation cascade and complement cascades are activated. To prevent the

hemofilter from becoming obstructed by clotting, or clotting off, low-dose anticoagulation must be used.[84] The dose should be low enough to have no effect on patient anticoagulation parameters. Systemic anticoagulation is not the goal. Typical anticoagulant choices include unfractionated heparin (UFH) and sodium citrate.[72,84] Citrate is an effective prefilter anticoagulant, which has the side effect that it *chelates* (binds to and removes) calcium from the blood. Consequently, ionized calcium levels are verified, and calcium is replaced per protocol when sodium citrate is the anticoagulant.

Methods of Continuous Renal Replacement. Because of the design of the CRRT machine, it is not possible to look at the outside and follow the flow of blood and, if used, dialysate. Each of the CRRT methods is described, and diagrams are employed to clarify the mode of CRRT that is used.

Slow Continuous Ultrafiltration. SCUF slowly removes fluid (100 to 300 mL/hr) through a process of ultrafiltration (Fig. 31-6A). This consists of a movement of fluid across a semipermeable membrane. SCUF has minimal impact on solute removal. Because small amounts of fluid are removed by this process, it was initially hoped it would be a suitable choice for edematous patients with acute heart failure and diminished perfusion to the kidneys who were unresponsive to diuretics. However, SCUF is an infrequent clinical choice because it requires both arterial and venous access for effective functioning. The SCUF system is more likely to thrombose (clot off) than other CRRT methods that use higher flows.

Continuous Venovenous Hemofiltration. CVVH is indicated when the patient's clinical condition warrants removal of significant volumes of fluid and solutes. Fluid is removed by ultrafiltration in volumes of 5 to 20 mL/min or up to 7 to 30 L/24 hr. Removal of solutes such as urea, creatinine, and other small non–protein-bound toxins is accomplished by convection. The replacement fluid rate of flow through the CRRT circuit can be altered to achieve desired fluid and solute removal without causing hemodynamic instability. Replacement fluid can be added by the addition of a prehemofilter replacement fluid (see Fig. 31-6B) or posthemofilter replacement fluid.

As with other CRRT systems, the blood outside the body is anticoagulated, and the ultrafiltrate is drained off by gravity or by the addition of negative-pressure suction into a large drainage bag. Because large volumes of fluid may be removed in CVVH, some of the removed ultrafiltrate volume must be replaced hourly with a continuous infusion (replacement fluid) to avoid intravascular dehydration. Replacement fluids may consist of standard solutions of bicarbonate, potassium-free LR solution, acetate, or

TABLE 31-10 Size of Molecules Cleared by Continuous Renal Replacement Therapy

Type of Molecule	Size of Molecule	Solutes	Solute Removal Method
Small	<500 daltons	Urea, creatinine	Convection, diffusion
Middle	500-5000 daltons	Vancomycin	Convection better than diffusion
Low-molecular-weight (small) proteins	5000-50,000 daltons	Cytokines, complement	Convection or absorption onto hemofilter
Large proteins	>50,000 daltons	Albumin	Minimal removal

dextrose. Electrolytes such as potassium, sodium, calcium chloride, magnesium sulfate, and sodium bicarbonate may be added. The formula used to calculate the volume removed from the patient follows with an example:

$$\text{Ultrafiltrate in bag} + \text{Other output} -$$
$$(\text{CVVH replacement fluid} + \text{IV/oral/NG intake}) = \text{Output}$$
$$1000 \text{ mL} - 800 \text{ mL} = 200 \text{ mL/hr output}$$

Continuous Venovenous Hemodialysis. CVVHD is technically like traditional hemodialysis, and it removes solute by diffusion because of a slow (15 to 30 mL/min) countercurrent drainage flow on the membrane side of the hemofilter (see Fig. 31-6C). Blood and fluid move by countercurrent flow through the hemofilter. *Countercurrent* means the blood flows in one direction and the dialysate flows in the opposite direction. As with other types of CRRT and hemodialysis, although

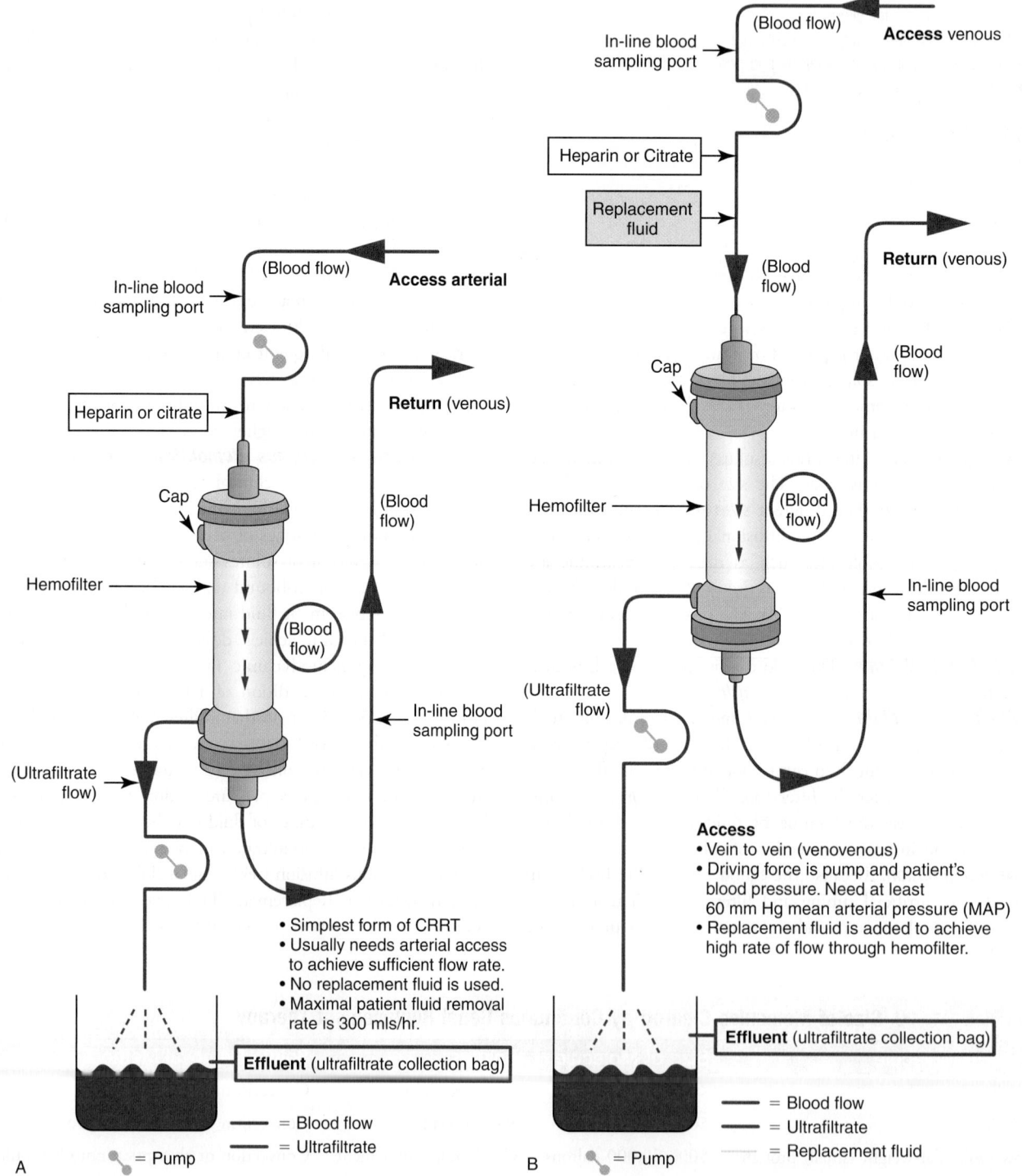

Figure 31-6 Continuous renal replacement therapy (CRRT) systems. *A,* Slow, continuous ultrafiltration (SCUF). *B,* Continuous venovenous hemofiltration (CVVH).

arterial access is always possible, venovenous vascular access is the most common choice.

CVVHD is indicated for patients who require large-volume removal for severe uremia or critical acid-base imbalances or for those who are resistant to diuretics. A MAP of at least 70 mm Hg is desirable for effective volume removal and dialysis, and it is most effective when used over days, not hours. The use of replacement fluid is optional and depends on the patient's clinical condition and plan of care. The critical care nurse is responsible for calculating the hourly intake and output, identifying fluid trends, and replacing excessive losses. This therapy is ideal for hemodynamically unstable patients in the critical care setting because they do not experience the abrupt fluid and solute changes that can accompany standard hemodialysis treatments.

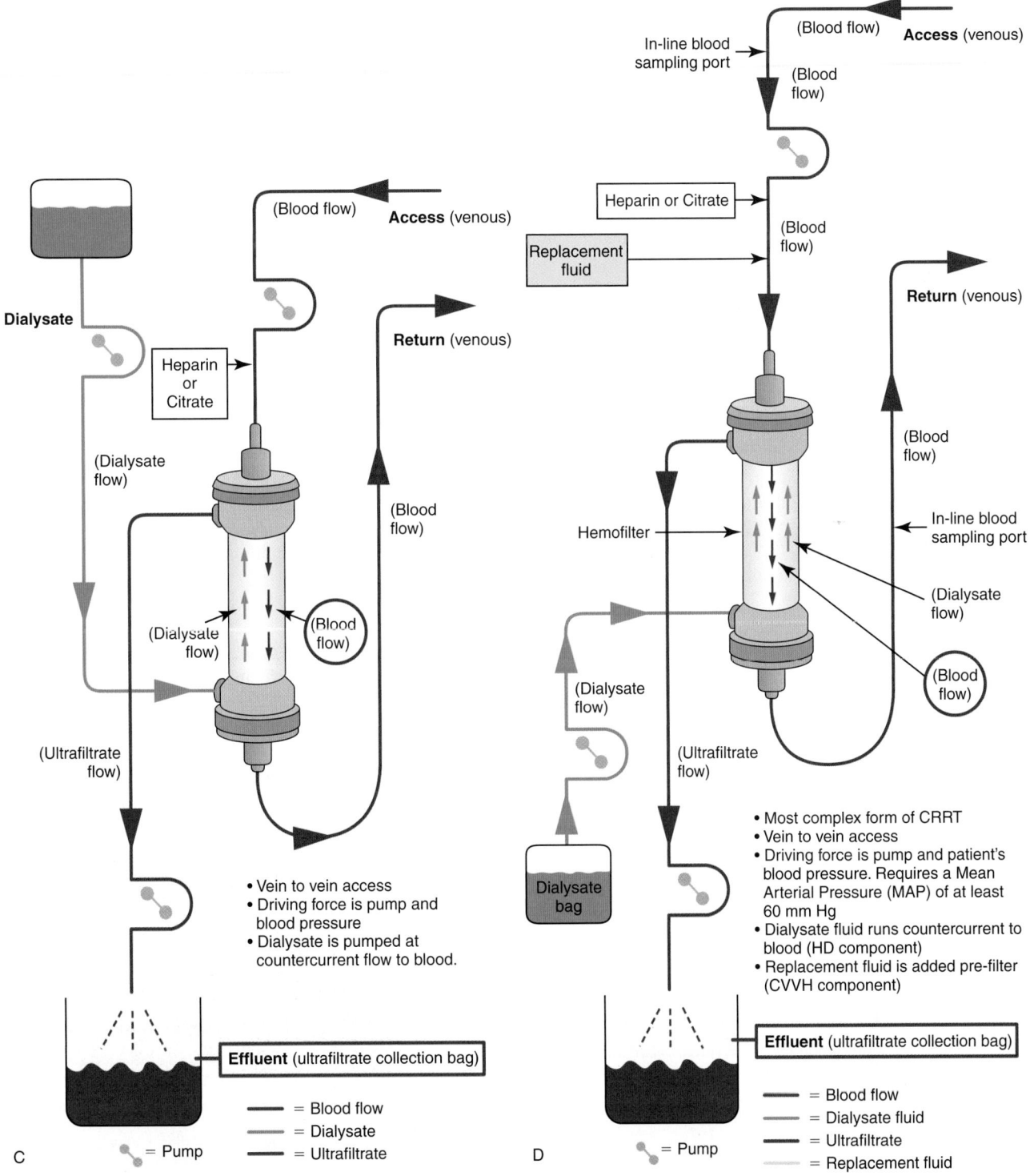

Figure 31-6, cont'd *C*, Continuous venovenous hemofiltration dialysis (CVVHD). *D*, Continuous venovenous hemodiafiltration (CVVHDF).

Continuous Venovenous Hemodiafiltration. Another CRRT option is CVVHDF, which combines two of the previously described methods (CVVH and CVVHD) to achieve maximal fluid and solute removal. A strong transmembrane pressure is applied to the hemofilter to push water across the filter, and a negative pressure is applied at the other side to pull fluid across the membrane and produce large volumes of ultrafiltrate and to create a "solvent drag" (CVVH method). The blood and the dialysate are circulated in a countercurrent flow pattern to remove fluid and solutes by diffusion (hemodialysis method). CVVHDF can remove large volumes of fluid and solute because it employs diffusion gradients and convection.

Complications. Potential problems associated with CRRT and appropriate nursing interventions are listed in Table 31-11.

TABLE 31-11 Complications Associated with Continuous Renal Replacement Therapy

Problem	Cause	Clinical Manifestations	Nursing Management
Decreased ultrafiltration rate	Hypotension Dehydration Kinked lines Bending of catheters Clotting of filter	Ultrafiltration rate decreased Minimal flow through blood lines	Observe filter and arteriovenous system Control blood flow Control coagulation time Position patient on back Lower height of collection container
Filter clotting	Obstruction Insufficient heparinization	Ultrafiltration rate decreased, despite height of collection container being lower	Control anticoagulation (heparin/citrate) Maintain continuous system anticoagulation Call physician Remove system Prime catheters with anticoagulated solution Prime new system; connect it Start predilution with 1000 mL saline 0.9% solution per hour Do not use three-way stopcocks
Hypotension	Increased ultrafiltration rate Blood leak Disconnection of one of lines	Bleeding Call physician	Control amount of ultrafiltration Control access sites Clamp lines
Fluid and electrolyte changes	To much or too little removal of fluid Inappropriate replacement of electrolytes Inappropriate dialysate	Changes in mentation ↑ or ↓ CVP ↑ or ↓ PAOP ECG change ↑ or ↓ BP and heart rate Abnormal electrolyte levels	Observe for • Changes in CVP or PAOP • Changes in vital signs • ECG changes resulting from electrolyte abnormalities Monitor output values every hour Control ultrafiltration
Bleeding	System disconnection ↑ Heparin dose	Oozing from catheter insertion site or connection	Monitor ACT no less than once every hour (heparin) Adjust heparin dose within specifications to maintain ACT Monitor serum calcium if using citrate as an anticoagulant Observe dressing on vascular access for blood loss Observe for blood in filtrate (filter leak)
Access dislodgement or infection	Catheter or connections not secured Break in sterile Technique Excessive patient movement	Bleeding from catheter site or connections Inappropriate flow or infusion Fever Drainage at catheter site	Observe access site at least once every 2 hours Ensure that clamps are available within easy reach at all times Observe strict sterile technique when dressing vascular access

ACT, activated coagulation time; BP, blood pressure; CRRT, continuous renal replacement therapy; CVP, central venous pressure; ECG, electrocardiogram; PAOP, pulmonary artery occlusion pressure or wedge pressure; ↑, increased; ↓, decreased.

Complications are often related to the rate of flow through the system. If the patient becomes hypotensive or the access lines remain kinked, the ultrafiltration rate will decrease. This can lead to increased clot formation within the hemofilter. As the surface of the hemofilter becomes more clotted, it will not provide effective fluid or solute clearance, and CRRT will be stopped; a new CRRT circuit must then be set up. The critical care nurse monitors the pressures displayed on the CRRT machine screen to monitor the positive pressure of fluid going into the hemofilter (inflow) and the pressures coming out of the hemofilter to ensure that resistance to the negative-pressure pull of the fluid across the hemofilter membrane has not developed. Other patient-related complications include fluid and electrolyte alterations, bleeding because of anticoagulation, or problems with the access site, such as dislodgement or infection.

Medical Management. The choice of the method of blood purification to use to treat AKI is a medical decision. There is no clear clinical or research consensus about whether IHD or CRRT is the most beneficial. Age, gender, and preexisting chronic conditions are of little help in determining the need for hemofiltration or hemodialysis. Often, the acute clinical diagnosis, physician's preference, availability of the CRRT machine, and knowledgeable physicians and nurses at the hospital are the deciding factors. Infectious complications are associated with a grave prognosis. Dialysis is prescribed for almost anyone who develops severe AKI, unless the patient is clearly dying.

IHD or CCRT is usually begun before the BUN level exceeds 90 mg/dL or the creatinine level exceeds 9 mg/dL. In many hospitals, the threshold to begin treatment is considerably lower. Whether daily treatment is more effective than treatment every other day is controversial. The patient's serum creatinine concentration, BUN level, and fluid volume status are the deciding factors. CCRT is often prescribed when the BUN level is approximately 60 mg/dL. CRRT is more effective in the early stages of AKI. If the patient has severe electrolyte imbalance or fluid overload, even earlier intervention may be required.

Nursing Management. Critical care nurses play a vital role in monitoring the patient receiving CRRT. In many critical care units, the CRRT system is set up by the dialysis staff but is run on a 24-hour basis by critical care nurses with additional training. Complications may be related to the CRRT circuit, the CRRT pump, or to the patient, as shown in Box 31-6. The critical care nurse monitors fluid intake and output, prevents and detects potential complications (e.g., bleeding, hypotension), identifies trends in electrolyte laboratory values, supervises safe operation of the CRRT equipment, and provides patient and family education about the patient's condition and the use of CRRT.

PERITONEAL DIALYSIS

Peritoneal dialysis (PD) is a modality used in patients with CKD.[85] Only 8.4% of patients with ESKD are treated with PD.[85,86] When a PD-dependent patient is admitted to the critical care unit with a nonrenal acute illness, PD may be continued, but the patient is more often converted to hemodialysis or CRRT because of the critical illness. PD involves the introduction of sterile dialyzing fluid through an implanted catheter into the abdominal cavity. The dialysate bathes the peritoneal membrane, which covers the abdominal organs and overlies the capillary beds that support the organs.[85] By the processes of osmosis, diffusion, and active transport, excess fluid and solutes travel from the peritoneal capillary fluid through the capillary walls, through the peritoneal membrane, and into the dialyzing fluid. After a selected period, the fluid is drained out of the abdomen by gravity (Fig. 31-7). The process is then repeated at regular, prescribed intervals.[87]

The peritoneal membrane's structure and capillary blood flow to the peritoneum account for the relatively slow nature of PD. The small capillary pores, the capillary membrane, the interstitium, the mesothelium of the peritoneum, and the fluid film layers in the capillary and the peritoneal cavity provide formidable barriers to fluid and solute passage. If needed, a peritoneal equilibration test can be performed to determine the level of solute clearance for a specific patient.[85]

The volume of dialysate instilled into the abdomen affects the clearance. Normally the PD-dependent patients are well versed in the amount, type, and frequency of dialysate to be infused into the abdomen, with subsequent drainage by gravity into a waste bag. The primary nursing consideration is to avoid contamination of the access point and monitor the patient's vital signs during this process. The dialysate should be instilled at body temperature to be comfortable, provide some vasodilation, and provide increased solute transport in the peritoneum. The length of time the solution remains in the peritoneal cavity, called the *dwell time*, and the solution composition affect the outcome. The dwell time affects the amount of fluid removed from the peritoneal capillaries, although a longer dwell time does not remove proportionately more fluid because of osmotic equilibration across the membranes. The various glucose concentrations of the dialysate provide different rates of fluid removal.[85,88]

BOX 31-6   COMPLICATIONS OF CONTINUOUS RENAL REPLACEMENT THERAPY

THE CIRCUIT
- Air embolism
- Clotted hemofilter
- Poor ultrafiltration
- Blood leaks
- Broken filter
- Recirculation or disconnection
- Access failure
- Catheter dislodgment

THE PUMP
- Circuit pressure alarm
  - Decreased inflow pressure
  - Decreased outflow pressure
- Increased outflow resistance
- Air bubble detector alarm
- Power failure
- Mechanical dysfunction

THE PATIENT
- Code or emergency situation
- Dehydration
- Hypotension
- Electrolyte imbalances
- Acid-base imbalances
- Blood loss or hemorrhage
- Hypothermia
- Infection

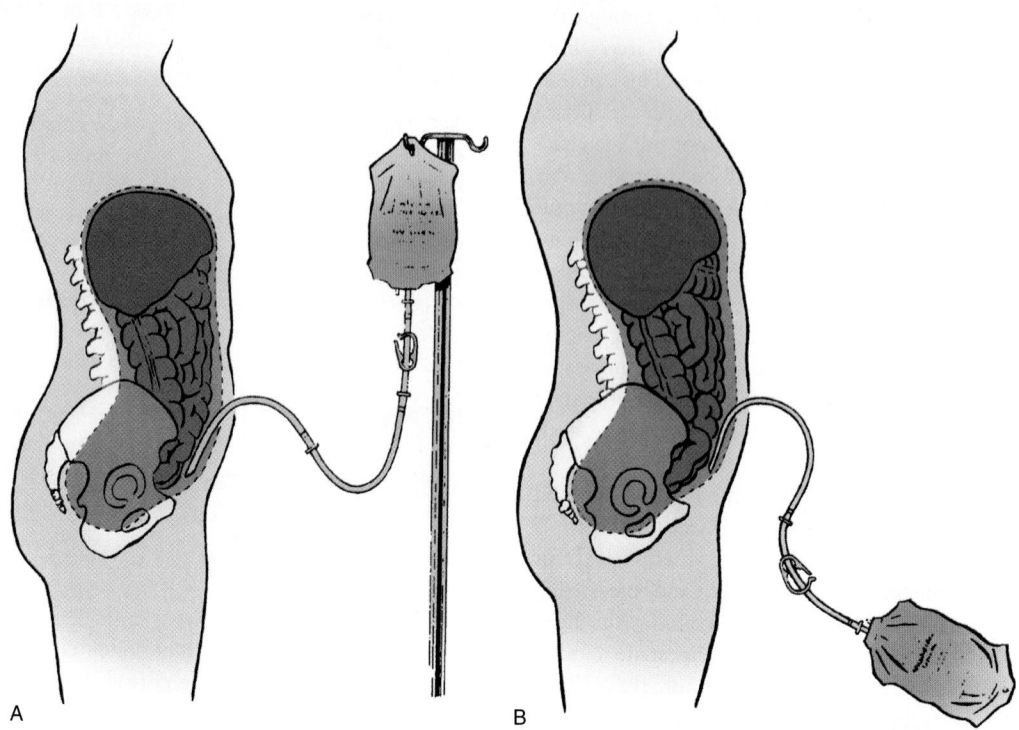

Figure 31-7 Peritoneal dialysis. *A,* Inflow. *B,* Outflow (drains by gravity). *(From Thompson JM et al:* Mosby's clinical nursing, *ed 5, St Louis, 2002, Mosby.)*

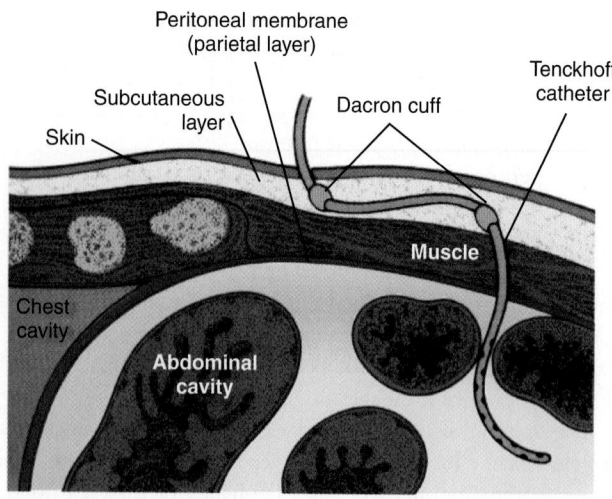

Figure 31-8 Tenckhoff catheter used in peritoneal dialysis. *(From Lewis SL et al:* Medical-surgical nursing assessment and management of clinical problems, *ed 7, St Louis, 2007, Mosby.)*

Catheter Placement. Most catheters have four segments: an external segment outside the abdomen, a tunnel segment that passes through subcutaneous tissue and muscle, a cuff for stabilization at the peritoneal membrane, and an internal segment with numerous holes for fast delivery and drainage of dialysate (Fig. 31-8). The infusion and removal of the dialysate fluid are sterile procedures.

Infection. The most significant risk to the patient with the use of PD is development of peritonitis from catheter contamination

and infection. Infection accounts for about two thirds of all PD catheter losses.[85] PD catheter infection results in peritonitis in 25% to 50% of cases.[85] Serious infection is also a reason for admitting a patient who uses PD to the hospital.[85] The critical care nurse must be acutely aware of the signs and symptoms of systemic infection, such as a sudden rise in the WBC count, increased temperature, and malaise. Clinicians must remain vigilant for signs of localized catheter or abdominal infection manifested by catheter-site redness, site swelling, cloudy dialysis effluent after the dwell time, and abdominal tenderness or pain, which occurs in 75% of patients with infection.[85]

Medical Management. PD is used for long-term end-stage kidney failure. It is never used as a first-line acute care intervention. If a patient uses PD at home, the dialysis method will continue to be used during the acute care hospitalization, provided the condition precipitating the admission is unrelated to the kidneys or abdomen.

Nursing Management. Nursing management of the patient receiving PD is complex. A comprehensive list of nursing interventions while caring for the patients with PD is provided in the Nursing Interventions Classification feature on Peritoneal Dialysis Therapy. Nurses are vigilant about prevention and detection of complications related to PD (Table 31-12). The critical care nurse observes for signs and symptoms of infection, monitors fluid volume status, infuses the dialysate fluid, observes drainage of the ultrafiltrate fluid, prevents complications associated with the PD catheter, and provides patient and family education. Patients who use PD are partners in the maintenance of their health because of the huge commitment they make in managing of their PD care.[86-90]

NIC

Peritoneal Dialysis Therapy

Definition

Administration and monitoring of dialysis solution into and out of the peritoneal cavity.

Activities

Explain the selected peritoneal dialysis procedure and purpose.

Warm the dialysis fluid before instillation.

Assess patency of catheter, noting difficulty in inflow or outflow.

Maintain record of inflow and outflow volumes and individual and cumulative fluid balances.

Have patient empty bladder before peritoneal catheter insertion.

Avoid excess mechanical stress on peritoneal dialysis catheters (e.g., coughing, dressing change, infusing large volumes).

Monitor blood pressure, pulse, respirations, temperature, and patient response during dialysis.

Ensure aseptic handling of peritoneal catheter and connections.

Draw blood samples and review blood chemistries (e.g., levels of blood urea nitrogen [BUN]; serum creatinine ; serum sodium, potassium, and phosphate [PO$_4$] levels).

Obtain cell count cultures of peritoneal effluent, if indicated.

Record baseline vital signs: weight, temperature, pulse, respirations, and blood pressure.

Measure and record abdominal girth.

Measure and record daily weight.

Anchor connections and tubing securely.

Check equipment and solutions according to protocol.

Administer dialysis exchanges (inflow, dwell, and outflow) according to protocol.

Monitor for signs of infection (e.g., peritonitis, exit-site inflammation or drainage).

Monitor for signs of respiratory distress.

Monitor for bowel perforation or fluid leaks.

Work collaboratively with patient to adjust length of dialysis, diet regulations, and pain and diversion needs to achieve optimal benefit of the treatment.

Teach patient to monitor self for signs and symptoms that indicate need for medical treatment (e.g., fever, bleeding, respiratory distress, irregular pulse, cloudy outflow, abdominal pain).

Teach procedure to patient requiring home dialysis.

From Bulechek GM et al: *Nursing interventions classification (NIC)*, ed 5, 2008, St Louis, Mosby.

TABLE 31-12 Complications Associated with Peritoneal Dialysis

Complication	Nursing Management
Peritonitis	Assess for signs and symptoms: cloudy effluent, abdominal pain, rebound tenderness, nausea and vomiting, fever. Obtain effluent sample for culture. Administer antibiotics as ordered. Teach the patient and family about signs and symptoms and prevention.
Exit site infection	Monitor the site daily for signs and symptoms of infection: induration, erythema, purulence, hyperthermia. Increase daily cleaning of site. Apply topical antibiotics as ordered (controversial). Teach the patient and family to avoid agents such as creams and lotions around exit site.
Catheter-tunnel infection	Assess for signs and symptoms of infection: pain along tunnel, induration for several centimeters away from catheter, erythema leading away from exit site, drainage at exit site or as tunnel is "milked" toward exit site. Teach the patient and family about the signs and symptoms of infection. Teach the patient and family to avoid pulls or tugs on catheter or trauma to exit site. Emphasize the need to maintain the cleansing regimen at exit site.
Fluid obstruction	Change the position of the patient (standing, lying, side-lying, knee-chest). Relieve the patient's constipation. Irrigate the catheter. Ensure that sufficient fluid is in the abdomen (sometimes requires a residual reservoir of approximately 50 mL).
Rectal pain	Ensure a sufficient reservoir of fluid. Use a slow infusion rate.
Shoulder pain	Ensure that all air is primed from infusion tubing. Attempt draining the effluent with the patient in a knee-chest position. Administer mild analgesics as ordered.
Hernia	Monitor for an increase in size of or pain in the area of the hernia. Decrease volume of exchanges as ordered. Dialyze with patients in the supine position. Use an abdominal binder or support for patients (as long as not binding on catheter exit site). Avoid initiation of peritoneal dialysis until exit site healing has taken place (approximately 1 to 2 weeks) if possible.

Continued

TABLE 31-12 Complications Associated with Peritoneal Dialysis—*cont'd*

Complication	Nursing Management
Fluid overload	Increase the use of hypertonic solutions. Decrease oral (PO) fluid intake. Shorten dwell times. Weigh patients frequently. Monitor lung sounds and peripheral edema.
Dehydration	Assess patients for decreased skin turgor, muscle cramps, hypotension, tachycardia, and dizziness. Discontinue hypertonic solutions. Increase oral fluid intake. Lengthen dwell times.
Blood-tinged effluent	Monitor for a change in effluent color (clear yellow to pink or rust). Administer heparin, as ordered, to prevent fibrin formation. Obtain a patient history about catheter trauma and patient activity before appearance of complication.

Case Study: Patient with a Renal Problem

Answers to the Case Study Questions can be found on the Evolve web site at http://evolve.elsevier.com/Urden/.

Brief Patient History
Ms. L is a 32-year-old woman found down in the street near the hospital. She is awake but confused. She unable to give any medical history and has no idea how long she has been in the street.

Clinical Assessment
Ms. L is admitted to the intensive care unit with muscle pain and minimal dark urine output. She continues to be confused, but her neurologic examination results are otherwise normal. She repeatedly tells the nurses that she is tired, has pain everywhere, and just wants to sleep. She is able to move all her extremities and has no signs of injury on skin examination.

Diagnostic Procedures
Laboratory tests show the following results: creatinine phosphokinase (CPK) level of 40,400 U/L, serum myoglobin level of 2.5 mg/L, urinary myoglobin level of 300 mg/L, and serum potassium level of 4.8 mEq/dL. Baseline vital signs were as follows: blood pressure of 85/60 mm Hg, heart rate

of 128 beats/min (sinus tachycardia), respiratory rate of 18 breaths/min, temperature of 101.3° F, and O_2 saturation of 98%.

The toxicology screen showed that the patient tested positive for cocaine. The Glasgow Coma Scale score was 14.

Medical Diagnosis
Ms. L is diagnosed with rhabdomyolysis.

Questions
1. What major outcomes do you expect to achieve for this patient?
2. What problems or risks must be managed to achieve these outcomes?
3. What interventions must be initiated to monitor, prevent, manage, or eliminate the problems and risks identified?
4. What interventions should be initiated to promote optimal functioning, safety, and well-being of the patient?
5. What possible learning needs do you anticipate for this patient?
6. What cultural and age-related factors may have a bearing on the patient's plan of care?

Summary

- Risk factors for development of AKI include being older or diabetic, or both.
- Many critically ill patients have AKI as a complication of their illness. The initial reason for admission to the critical care unit might have been sepsis, hypovolemic shock,

trauma, or major surgery. If AKI and ARF develop, mortality and morbidity rates increase.
- Vigorous hydration with normal saline remains the most effective intervention to prevent contrast-induced AKI.
- Acute-care renal replacement therapies include IHD and CRRT. Both are valuable in acute kidney failure, and one method is not superior to the other in terms of mortality outcomes or recovery of kidney function.

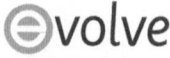 Be sure to check out the bonus material, including free self-assessment exercises, on the Evolve web site at http://evolve.elsevier.com/Urden/.

References

1. Kellum JA: Acute kidney injury, *Crit Care Med* 36(4 suppl):S141-S145, 2008.
2. Brincat S, Hilton R: Prevention of acute kidney injury, *Br J Hosp Med (Lond)* 69(8):450-454, 2008.
3. Kellum JA, Hoste EA: Acute kidney injury: epidemiology and assessment, *Scand J Clin Lab Invest Suppl* 241:6-11, 2008.
4. Mehta RL et al: Spectrum of acute renal failure in the intensive care unit: the PICARD experience, *Kidney Int* 66(4):1613-1621, 2004.
5. Sesso R et al: Prognosis of ARF in hospitalized elderly patients, *Am J Kidney Dis* 44(3):410-419, 2004.
6. Ponte B et al: Long-term functional evolution after an acute kidney injury: a 10-year study, *Nephrol Dial Transplant* 23(12):3859-3866, 2008.
7. Nickolas TL et al: Awareness of kidney disease in the US population: findings from the National Health and Nutrition Examination Survey (NHANES) 1999 to 2000, *Am J Kidney Dis* 44(2):185-197, 2004.
8. Bellomo R: Defining, quantifying, and classifying acute renal failure, *Crit Care Clin* 21(2):223-237, 2005.
9. Bellomo R et al: Pre-renal azotemia: a flawed paradigm in critically ill septic patients? *Contrib Nephrol* 156:1-9, 2007.
10. Bellomo R et al: Acute renal failure—definition, outcome measures, animal models, fluid therapy and information technology needs: the Second International Consensus Conference of the Acute Dialysis Quality Initiative (ADQI) Group, *Crit Care* 8(4):R204-212, 2004.
11. Kellum JA et al: Definition and classification of acute kidney injury, *Nephron Clin Pract* 109(4):c182-c187, 2008.
12. Abdulkader RC et al: Histological features of acute tubular necrosis in native kidneys and long-term renal function, *Ren Fail* 30(7):667-673, 2008.
13. Asif A, Epstein M: Prevention of radiocontrast-induced nephropathy, *Am J Kidney Dis* 44(1):12-24, 2004.
14. Sheridan AM, Bonventre JV: Cell biology and molecular mechanisms of injury in ischemic acute renal failure, *Curr Opin Nephrol Hypertens* 9(4):427-434, 2000.
15. Liu KD, Brakeman PR: Renal repair and recovery, *Crit Care Med* 36(4 suppl):S187-S192, 2008.
16. Liano F et al: The spectrum of acute renal failure in the intensive care unit compared with that seen in other settings. The Madrid Acute Renal Failure Study Group, *Kidney Int Suppl* 66:S16-24, 1998.
17. Rocktaeschel J et al: Acid-base status of critically ill patients with acute renal failure: analysis based on Stewart-Figge methodology, *Crit Care* 7(4):R60-R66, 2003.
18. Bellomo R et al: Defining acute renal failure: physiological principles, *Intensive Care Med* 30(1):33-37, 2004.
19. Coresh J et al: Prevalence of chronic kidney disease and decreased kidney function in the adult US population: Third National Health and Nutrition Examination Survey, *Am J Kidney Dis* 41(1):1-12, 2003.
20. K/DOQI clinical practice guidelines for chronic kidney disease: evaluation, classification, and stratification, *Am J Kidney Dis* 39(2 suppl 1):S1-S266, 2002.
21. K/DOQI clinical practice guidelines on hypertension and antihypertensive agents in chronic kidney disease, *Am J Kidney Dis* 43(5 suppl 1):S1-S290, 2004.
22. Go AS et al: Chronic kidney disease and the risks of death, cardiovascular events, and hospitalization,, *N Engl J Med* 351(13):1296-1305, 2004.
23. Anavekar NS et al: Relation between renal dysfunction and cardiovascular outcomes after myocardial infarction, *N Engl J Med* 351(13):1285-1295, 2004.
24. Pannu N, Mehta RL: Mechanical ventilation and renal function: an area for concern? *Am J Kidney Dis* 39(3):616-624, 2002.
25. Scheel PJ et al: Uremic lung: new insights into a forgotten condition, *Kidney Int* 74(7):849-851, 2008.
26. Vieira JM Jr et al: Effect of acute kidney injury on weaning from mechanical ventilation in critically ill patients, *Crit Care Med* 35(1):184-191, 2007.
27. Wan L et al: Pathophysiology of septic acute kidney injury: what do we really know? *Crit Care Med* 36(4 suppl):S198-S203, 2008.
28. Dellinger RP et al: Surviving Sepsis Campaign: international guidelines for management of severe sepsis and septic shock: 2008, *Crit Care Med* 36(1):296-327, 2008.
29. Bagshaw SM et al: A multi-center evaluation of early acute kidney injury in critically ill trauma patients, *Ren Fail* 30(6):581-589, 2008.
30. Criddle LM: Rhabdomyolysis: pathophysiology, recognition, and management, *Crit Care Nurse* 23(6):14-28, 2003.
31. Brown CV et al: Preventing renal failure in patients with rhabdomyolysis: do bicarbonate and mannitol make a difference? *J Trauma* 56(6):1191-1196, 2004.
32. Weisbord SD et al: The incidence of clinically significant contrast-induced nephropathy following non-emergent coronary angiography, *Catheter Cardiovasc Interv* 71(7):879-885, 2008.
33. Kandzari DE et al: Contrast nephropathy: an evidence-based approach to prevention, *Am J Cardiovasc Drugs* 3(6):395-405, 2003.
34. Goldenberg I et al: Reversible acute kidney injury following contrast exposure and the risk of long-term mortality, *Am J Nephrol* 29(2):136-144, 2008.
35. Aspelin P et al: Nephrotoxic effects in high-risk patients undergoing angiography, *N Engl J Med* 348(6):491-499, 2003.
36. Kuhn MJ et al: The PREDICT study: a randomized double-blind comparison of contrast-induced nephropathy after low- or iso-osmolar contrast agent exposure, *AJR Am J Roentgenol* 191(1):151-157, 2008.
37. Maioli M et al: Sodium bicarbonate versus saline for the prevention of contrast-induced nephropathy in patients with renal dysfunction undergoing coronary angiography or intervention, *J Am Coll Cardiol* 52(8):599-604, 2008.
38. Brar SS et al: Sodium bicarbonate vs sodium chloride for the prevention of contrast medium-induced nephropathy in patients undergoing coronary angiography: a randomized trial, *JAMA* 300(9):1038-1046, 2008.
39. Ozcan EE et al: Sodium bicarbonate, *N*-acetylcysteine, and saline for prevention of radiocontrast-induced nephropathy. A comparison of 3 regimens for protecting contrast-induced nephropathy in patients undergoing coronary procedures. A single-center prospective controlled trial, *Am Heart J* 154(3):539-544, 2007.
40. Stone GW et al: Fenoldopam mesylate for the prevention of contrast-induced nephropathy: a randomized controlled trial, *JAMA* 290(17):2284-2291, 2003.
41. Kanbay M et al: Sodium bicarbonate for the prevention of contrast-induced nephropathy: a meta-analysis of 17 randomized controlled trials. *Int Urol Nephrol* Pub on-line ahead of print 25 April 2009.
42. Thomsen HS et al: Contrast-induced nephropathy: the wheel has turned 360 degrees, *Acta Radiol* 49(6):646-657, 2008.
43. McGee WT: The pulmonary artery catheter in critical care, *Semin Dial* 19(6):480-491, 2006.
44. Ahee P, Crowe AV: The management of hyperkalaemia in the emergency department, *J Accid Emerg Med* 17(3):188-191, 2000.
45. Levey AS et al: National Kidney Foundation practice guidelines for chronic kidney disease: evaluation, classification, and stratification, *Ann Intern Med* 139(2):137-147, 2003.
46. K/DOQI clinical practice guidelines for bone metabolism and disease in chronic kidney disease, *Am J Kidney Dis* 42(4 suppl 3):S1-S201, 2003.
47. Gauci C et al: Pitfalls of measuring total blood calcium in patients with CKD, *J Am Soc Nephrol* 19(8):1592-1598, 2008.
48. Leavey SF, Weitzel WF: Endocrine abnormalities in chronic renal failure, *Endocrinol Metab Clin North Am* 31(1):107-119, 2002.
49. McCann L: Calcium in chronic kidney disease: recommended intake and serum targets, *Adv Chronic Kidney Dis* 14(1):75-78, 2007.
50. Emmett M: A comparison of clinically useful phosphorus binders for patients with chronic kidney failure, *Kidney Int Suppl* (90):S25-32, 2004.
51. Mehta RL et al: Techniques for assessing and achieving fluid balance in acute renal failure, *Curr Opin Crit Care* 8(6):535-543, 2002.
52. The SAFE Study Investigators: A comparison of albumin and saline for fluid resuscitation in the intensive care unit, *N Engl J Med* 350(22):2247-2256, 2004.
53. The SAFE Study Investigators: Saline or albumin for fluid resuscitation in patients with traumatic brain injury, *N Engl J Med* 357(9):874-884, 2007.

54. Perel P, Roberts I: Colloids versus crystalloids for fluid resuscitation in critically ill patients, *Cochrane Database Syst Rev* (4):CD000567, 2007.

55. M Schetz et al: Drug-induced acute kidney injury, *Curr Opin Crit Care* 11(6):555-565.

56. Karajala V et al: Diuretics in acute kidney injury, *Minerva Anestesiol* Jul 18, 2008 [Epub ahead of print].

57. Mehta RL et al: Diuretics, mortality, and nonrecovery of renal function in acute renal failure, *JAMA* 288(20):2547-2553, 2002.

58. Cantarovich F et al: High-dose furosemide for established ARF: a prospective, randomized, double-blind, placebo-controlled, multicenter trial, *Am J Kidney Dis* 44(3):402-409, 2004.

59. Uchino S et al: Diuretics and mortality in acute renal failure, *Crit Care Med* 32(8):1669-1677, 2004.

60. Ichai C et al: Prolonged low-dose dopamine infusion induces a transient improvement in renal function in hemodynamically stable, critically ill patients: a single-blind, prospective, controlled study, *Crit Care Med* 28(5):1329-1335, 2000.

61. Kellum JA, Decker JM: Use of dopamine in acute renal failure: a meta-analysis, *Crit Care Med* 29(8):1526-1531, 2001.

62. Bellomo R et al: Low-dose dopamine in patients with early renal dysfunction: a placebo-controlled randomised trial. Australian and New Zealand Intensive Care Society (ANZICS) Clinical Trials Group, *Lancet* 356(9248):2139-2143, 2000.

63. Sisillo E et al: N-acetylcysteine for prevention of acute renal failure in patients with chronic renal insufficiency undergoing cardiac surgery: a prospective, randomized, clinical trial, *Crit Care Med* 36(1):81-86, 2008.

64. Haase M et al: Phase II, randomized, controlled trial of high-dose N-acetylcysteine in high-risk cardiac surgery patients, *Crit Care Med* 35(5):1324-1331, 2007.

65. Casaer MP et al: Bench-to-bedside review: metabolism and nutrition, *Crit Care* 12(4):222, 2008.

66. KDOQI Clinical Practice Guidelines and Clinical Practice Recommendations for Anemia in Chronic Kidney Disease, *Am J Kidney Dis* 47(5 suppl 3):S11-S145, 2006.

67. Corwin HL, Eckardt KU: Erythropoietin in the critically ill: what is the evidence? *Nephrol Dial Transplant* 20(12):2605-2608, 2005.

68. Gouva C et al: Treating anemia early in renal failure patients slows the decline of renal function: a randomized controlled trial, *Kidney Int* 66(2):753-760, 2004.

69. Corwin HL et al: Efficacy of recombinant human erythropoietin in critically ill patients: a randomized controlled trial, *JAMA* 288(22):2827-2835, 2002.

70. Baldwin I et al: A pilot randomised controlled comparison of continuous veno-venous haemofiltration and extended daily dialysis with filtration: effect on small solutes and acid-base balance, *Intensive Care Med* 33(5):830-835, 2007.

71. Warkentin TE et al: Treatment and prevention of heparin-induced thrombocytopenia: American College of Chest Physicians Evidence-Based Clinical Practice Guidelines (8th Edition), *Chest* 133(6 suppl):340S-380S, 2008.

72. Fealy N et al: A pilot randomized controlled crossover study comparing regional heparinization to regional citrate anticoagulation for continuous venovenous hemofiltration, *Int J Artif Organs* 30(4):301-307, 2007.

73. Rayner HC et al: Creation, cannulation and survival of arteriovenous fistulae: data from the Dialysis Outcomes and Practice Patterns Study, *Kidney Int* 63(1):323-330, 2003.

74. Beathard GA et al: Aggressive treatment of early fistula failure, *Kidney Int* 64(4):1487-1494, 2003.

75. McCann M et al: Vascular access management 1: an overview, *J Ren Care* 34(2):77-84, 2008.

76. Asif A et al: Arteriovenous fistula creation: should US nephrologists get involved? *Am J Kidney Dis* 42(6):1293-1300, 2003.

77. Bagul A et al: Tunnelled catheters for the haemodialysis patient, *Eur J Vasc Endovasc Surg* 33(1):105-112, 2007.

78. O'Reilly P, Tolwani A: Renal replacement therapy III: IHD, CRRT, SLED, *Crit Care Clin* 21(2):367-378, 2005.

79. Gibney N et al: Timing of initiation and discontinuation of renal replacement therapy in AKI: unanswered key questions, *Clin J Am Soc Nephrol* 3(3):876-880, 2008.

80. Bagshaw SM, Gibney RT: Ideal determinants for the initiation of renal replacement therapy: timing, metabolic threshold or fluid balance? *Acta Clin Belg Suppl* 2007(2):357-361, 2007.

81. Chrysochoou G et al: Renal replacement therapy in the critical care unit, *Crit Care Nurs Q* 31(4):282-290, 2008.

82. Dirkes S, Hodge K: Continuous renal replacement therapy in the adult intensive care unit: history and current trends, *Crit Care Nurse* 27(2):61-66, 68-72, 74-80, 2007.

83. Palevsky PM et al: Intensity of renal support in critically ill patients with acute kidney injury, *N Engl J Med* 359(1):7-20, 2008.

84. Joannidis M, Oudemans-van Straaten HM: Clinical review: patency of the circuit in continuous renal replacement therapy, *Crit Care* 11(4):218, 2007.

85. Teitelbaum I, Burkart J: Peritoneal dialysis, *Am J Kidney Dis* 42(5):1082-1096, 2003.

86. Curtin RB et al: The peritoneal dialysis experience: insights from long-term patients, *Nephrol Nurs J* 31(6):615-624, 2004.

87. Kelley KT: How peritoneal dialysis works, *Nephrol Nurs J* 31(5):481-482, 488-489, 2004.

88. Crawford-Bonadio TL, Diaz-Buxo JA: Comparison of peritoneal dialysis solutions, *Nephrol Nurs J* 31(5):499-507, 520, 2004.

89. Maaz DE: Troubleshooting non-infectious peritoneal dialysis issues, *Nephrol Nurs J* 31(5):521-532, 545, 2004.

90. Perce J: Documenting peritoneal dialysis, *Nursing* 2007 37(10):28, 2007.

Gastrointestinal Anatomy and Physiology

The major function of the gastrointestinal tract is digestion. It converts ingested nutrients into simpler forms that can be transported from the tract's lumen to the portal circulation and then used in metabolic processes. The gastrointestinal system also plays a vital role in detoxification and elimination of bacteria, viruses, chemical toxins, and drugs. Disturbances of the gastrointestinal system itself or of the complex hormonal and neural controls that regulate it can severely upset homeostasis and compromise the overall nutritional status of the patient. Any circumvention of the normal feeding mechanism can alter digestive processes or contribute to malabsorption.[1]

The critical care nurse must have a comprehensive knowledge of the anatomy and normal function of the gastrointestinal tract to facilitate assessment, diagnosis, and intervention in patients with gastrointestinal dysfunction. The gastrointestinal tract consists of the mouth, the esophagus, the stomach, the small intestine, and the large intestine (Fig. 32-1).

MOUTH

The mouth and accessory organs, which include the lips, cheeks, gums, tongue, palate, and salivary glands, perform the initial phases of digestion, which are ingestion, mastication, and salivation.[1]

INGESTION AND MASTICATION

The mouth is the beginning of the alimentary canal (see Fig. 32-1) and is the means for ingestion and entry of nutrients. The teeth cut, grind, and mix food, transforming it into a form suitable for swallowing and increasing the surface area of food available to mix with salivary secretions. Healthy dentition is vital for this process. Mucous glands located behind the tip of the tongue and serous glands located at the back of the tongue aid in the lubrication of food and in its distribution over the taste buds.[2]

SALIVATION

Salivation has an important role in the first stage of digestion because saliva lubricates the mouth, facilitates the movement of the lips and the tongue during swallowing, and washes away bacteria. Saliva consists of approximately 99.5% water[3] that contains a large amount of ions such as potassium, chloride, bicarbonate,[1] thiocyanate, and hydrogen,[3] as well as immunoglobulin A, which is vital for destroying oral bacteria,[1] and mucus. Approximately 1000 to 1500 mL of saliva is produced each day by three pairs of major salivary glands: the submandibular glands, the sublingual glands, and the parotid glands. Parotid gland secretions are enzymatic, containing amylase (ptyalin), which begins the chemical breakdown of large polysaccharides into dextrins and sugars. The mouth and pharynx also are lined with minor salivary glands that provide additional lubrication.[3]

The salivary glands are regulated by the autonomic nervous system, with parasympathetic effects predominating. Increased parasympathetic stimulation results in profuse secretions of watery saliva, whereas decreased parasympathetic stimulation results in inhibition of salivation.[1,3]

ESOPHAGUS

The esophagus is a hollow muscular tube that lacks cartilage. In adults, it is 23 to 25 cm (9 to 10 inches) long and 2 to 3 cm (1 inch) wide. It is the narrowest part of the digestive tube and lies posterior to the trachea and heart, with attachments at the hypopharynx and at the cardiac portion of the stomach below the diaphragm. It begins at the level of the C6 to T1 vertebrae and extends vertically through the mediastinum and diaphragm to the level of T11.[4]

The esophagus has two sphincters, the upper esophageal (also known as *hypopharyngeal*) and the lower esophageal (also known as *cardioesophageal* or *gastroesophageal*).[4] The upper esophageal sphincter inhibits air from entering the esophagus during respiration. The lower esophageal sphincter controls the passage of food into the stomach and prevents reflux of gastric contents.[1]

SWALLOWING

The functions of the esophagus are to accept a bolus of food from the oropharynx, to transport the bolus through the esophageal body by gravity and peristalsis, and to release the bolus into the stomach through the lower esophageal sphincter. This

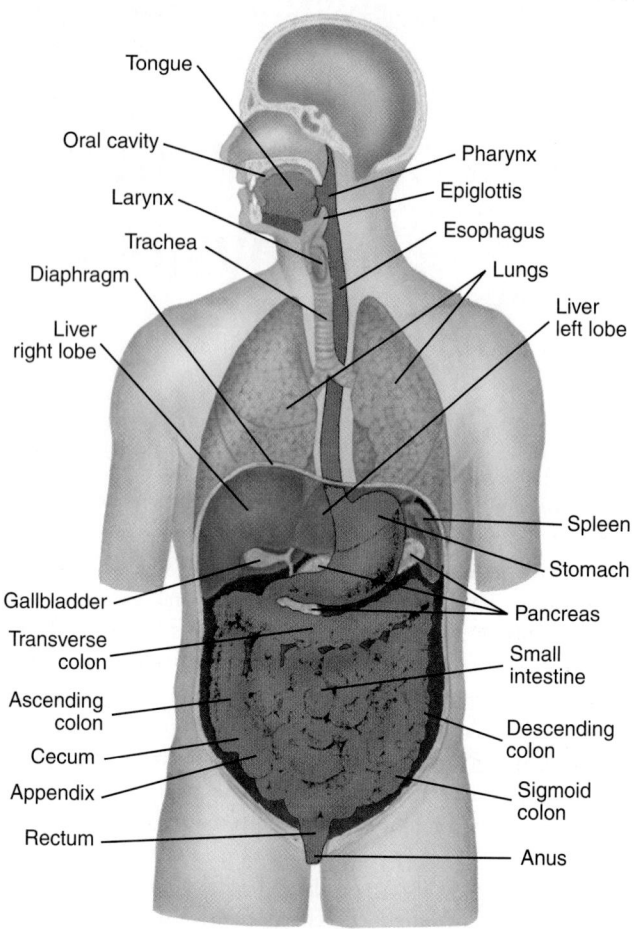

Figure 32-1 Anatomy of the gastrointestinal system. *(From Thompson JM et al: Mosby's clinical nursing, ed 5, St Louis, 2002, Mosby.)*

process is known as *swallowing.*[5] Peristalsis consists of waves of circular muscle contractions and relaxations. Peristalsis that is initiated by swallowing is known as *primary peristalsis,* whereas peristalsis that is initiated by esophageal distention is known as *secondary peristalsis.* Peristaltic waves begin in the pharynx and move distally at a rate of 2 to 6 cm per second.[1]

STOMACH

The stomach is an elongated pouch that is approximately 25 to 30 cm (10 to 12 inches) long and 10 to 15 cm (4 to 6 inches) wide at the maximal transverse diameter (Fig. 32-2). It lies obliquely beneath the cardiac sphincter at the esophagogastric junction and above the pyloric sphincter, next to the small intestine. The anatomic divisions of the stomach are the cardia (proximal end), the fundus (portion above and to the left of the cardiac sphincter), the body (middle portion), the antrum (elongated, constricted portion), and the pylorus (distal end connecting the antrum to the duodenum) (Fig. 32-3). The greater curvature, which begins at the cardiac orifice and arches backward and upward around the fundus, is in contact with the transverse colon and the pancreas at the posterior edge. The lesser curvature extends from the cardia to the pylorus. Two sphincters control the rate of food passage: the lower esophageal sphincter at the esophagogastric junction and the pyloric sphincter at the gastroduodenal junction.[6]

The stomach wall has four layers (Fig. 32-4). The outermost layer, the serous layer (serosa), consists of squamous epithelial tissue and continues as a double fold from the lower edge of the stomach to cover the intestine. The second layer, the muscular layer (muscularis), extends from the fundus to the antrum and consists of three smooth muscle layers, which are the longitudinal layer, the circular layer, and the oblique layer. The third layer, the submucous layer (submucosa), consists of connective tissue that contains blood vessels, lymphatics, and nerve plexuses.

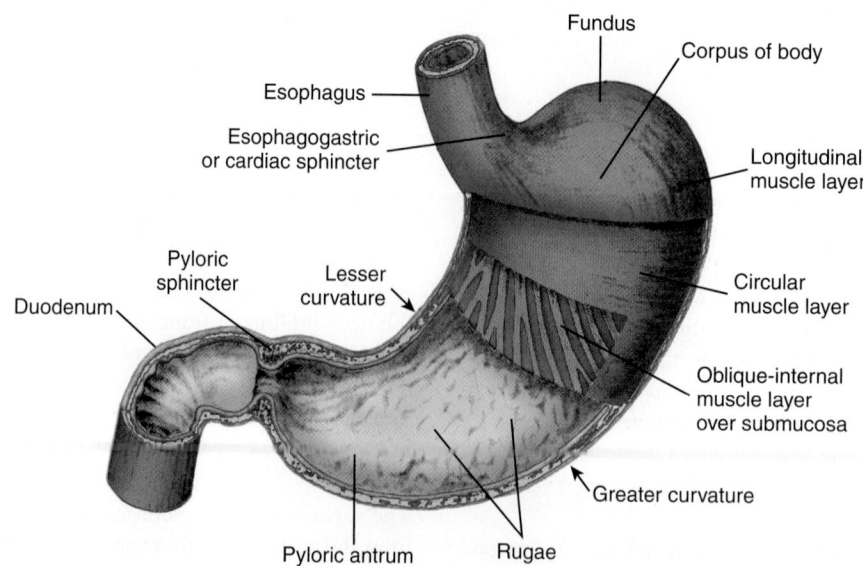

Figure 32-2 Gross anatomy of the stomach. *(From Thompson JM et al: Mosby's clinical nursing, ed 5, St Louis, 2002, Mosby.)*

The innermost layer, the mucous layer (mucosa), consists of a muscular layer that is arranged in longitudinal folds, or rugae, that can expand as the stomach fills.[6] This layer also contains glands that secrete up to 3000 mL of gastric juice per day.[7]

The celiac artery provides the blood supply required for the motor and secretory activity of the stomach. The splenic vein provides venous drainage for the right side of the stomach, and the gastric vein provides it for the left.[1] Numerous lymphatic channels arise in the submucosa and terminate in the thoracic duct. The stomach is innervated by the autonomic nervous system. Sympathetic fibers arise from the celiac plexus, and parasympathetic fibers arise from the gastric branch of the vagus nerve.[6]

The epithelial cells of the gastric mucosa are packed very close together and serve as a protective barrier, preventing diffusion of hydrogen ions into the mucosa. The surface epithelial cells produce alkaline mucus and secrete a bicarbonate-laden fluid. The mucus further protects the gastric mucosa by delaying back-diffusion of hydrogen ions and trapping them for neutralization by the secreted bicarbonate.[8] The gastric mucosal cells can compensate for cell destruction. Epithelial cells are in a constant state of growth, migration, and desquamation, and they are shed at a rate of one-half million cells per minute. The gastric mucosa also has the ability to increase blood flow, providing an additional buffer for acid neutralization and aiding in the removal of toxic metabolites and chloride ions from injured mucosa. The gastric mucosal cells synthesize a family of unsaturated fatty acids known as *prostaglandins*. Prostaglandins facilitate mucosal bicarbonate secretion and inhibit acid secretion by preventing the activation of parietal cells by histamine (a local biochemical mediator). Certain lipid-soluble substances, such as alcohol, aspirin and other nonsteroidal anti-inflammatory drugs, regurgitated bile, and uremic toxins, can break through the mucosal barrier and penetrate the cells, causing their destruction, edema, and eventual bleeding.[8]

GASTRIC SECRETION

The stomach has three types of glands—cardiac, oxyntic, and pyloric—that contain cells of various types that secrete 1500 to 3000 mL of gastric juice into the lumen per day, depending on the diet and other stimuli.[7] Gastric juice is composed of hydrochloric acid (HCl), pepsin, (necessary for the breakdown of protein), mucus, intrinsic factor (necessary for vitamin B_{12} absorption), sodium, and potassium. Pepsinogen, secreted by the chief cells of the stomach lining, is converted to its active form, pepsin, in the acidic environment of the stomach.[1] The cardiac glands secrete mucus and pepsinogen. The oxyntic glands contain parietal cells, which secrete HCl and intrinsic factor, and chief cells, which secrete pepsinogen. Pyloric glands contain mucous cells, which secrete mucus and pepsinogen, and G cells, which secrete gastrin (Table 32-1).[6] Gastric glands are stimulated by the parasympathetic stimulation and gastrin and inhibited by gastric-inhibitory peptide and enterogastrone. Histamine and entero-oxyntin also stimulate the parietal cells to produce acid, and secretin stimulates the chief cells to produce pepsinogen.[1]

The pH of gastric juice is 1.0, but when mixed with food, it rises to 2.0 to 3.0. Gastric juice dissolves soluble foods and has

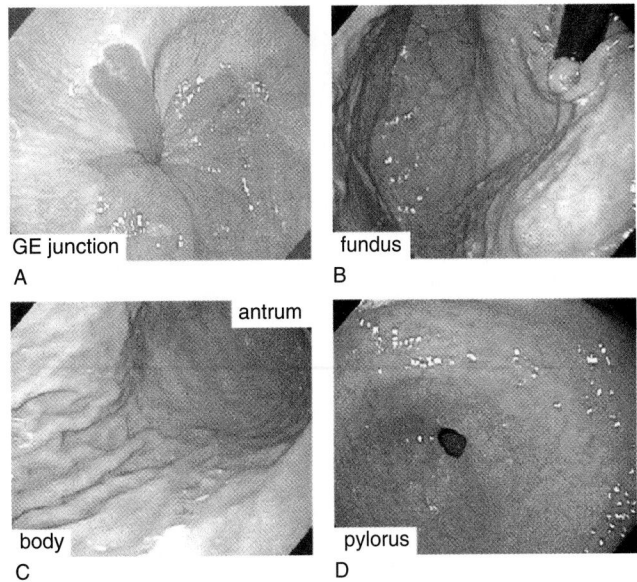

GE junction
A

fundus
B

antrum
body
C

pylorus
D

Figure 32-3 Endoscopic view of the stomach. *(From Soybel DI: Anatomy and physiology of the stomach,* Surg Clin North Am *85:875, 2005.)*

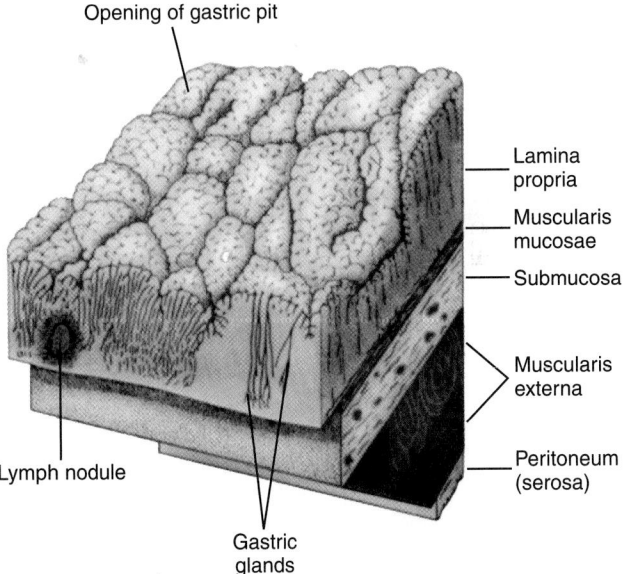

Opening of gastric pit

Lamina propria

Muscularis mucosae

Submucosa

Muscularis externa

Peritoneum (serosa)

Lymph nodule

Gastric glands

Figure 32-4 Structure of the gastric mucosa. *(From Berne RM, et al:* Physiology, *ed 5, St Louis, 2005, Mosby.)*

bacteriostatic action against swallowed microorganisms. The composition of gastric secretions depends on a variety of factors, including flow rate, volume, and the time of day. Pain, fear, or rage can inhibit gastric secretion, whereas aggression or hostility can stimulate it.[1]

GASTRIC MOTILITY

The functions of the stomach include food storage, digestion, and emptying. The stomach receives food through the lower esophageal sphincter, stores it for a period of time, and mixes

TABLE 32-1 Digestive Hormones

Source	Hormone	Stimulus for Secretion	Action
Mucosa of the stomach	Gastrin	Presence of partially digested proteins in the stomach	Stimulates gastric glands to secrete hydrochloric acid and pepsinogen
Mucosa of the small intestines	Motilin Secretion Cholecystokinin Enterogastrone Entero-oxyntin Gastric-inhibitory peptide	Presence of acid and fat in the duodenum Presence of chyme (acid, partially digested proteins, and fats) in the duodenum Same as for secretin Presence of fat in the duodenum Presence of chyme in small intestine Stretching of the duodenum and fatty acids	Increases gastrointestinal motility Stimulates pancreas to secrete alkaline pancreatic juice and liver to secrete bile; decreases gastrointestinal motility Stimulates gallbladder to eject bile and pancreas to secrete alkaline fluid; decreases gastric motility Inhibits gastric secretion and motility Stimulates gastric glands to secrete hydrochloric acid Decreases gastric motility and secretion of pepsin and hydrochloric acid (HCl)

From McCance KL et al, editors: *Pathophysiology: the biologic basis for disease in adults and children*, ed 5, St Louis, 2006, Mosby.

it with gastric secretions. The food is then ground into a semifluid consistency called *chyme*, which is delivered through the pylorus to the duodenum. Gastric motility is regulated by the autonomic nervous system, digestive hormones, and neural reflexes. Gastrin, motilin (see Table 32-1), and parasympathetic stimulation increase gastric motility, whereas secretin, cholecystokinin, enterogastrone, gastric-inhibitory peptide (see Table 32-1), and sympathetic stimulation decrease it. The ileogastric reflex inhibits gastric motility when the ileum is distended.[8]

SMALL INTESTINE

The small intestine, a coiled, folded tube that is approximately 7 m (22 to 23 feet) long, extends from the pyloric sphincter to the cecum and fills most of the abdominal cavity. It has three anatomic divisions: duodenum, jejunum, and ileum. The duodenum, shaped like the letter C, begins at the pyloric sphincter of the stomach and ends at the ligament of Treitz. It is 30 cm (12 inches) long and 4 cm (1 to 1.5 inches) wide.[9] The jejunum, which is 250 cm (8 to 9 feet) long and 4 cm (1 to 1.5 inches) wide, lies in the left iliac and umbilical regions. The ileum, which is 375 cm (12 feet) long and 2.5 cm (1 inch) wide, lies in the hypogastric, right iliac, and pelvic regions. Although the demarcating line between the jejunum and the ileum is somewhat arbitrary, the ileum is narrower than the jejunum. The ileocecal valve, located at the terminal end of the ileum at the junction of the cecum and colon, controls the flow of small bowel contents into the large intestine and prevents reflux (Fig. 32-5).[1]

The small intestine has four layers (Fig. 32-6). The outermost layer, the serous layer (serosa), is a continuation of the serous coat surrounding the stomach. The second layer, the muscular layer (muscularis), consists of two smooth muscle layers called the *longitudinal* and *circular layers*. The third layer, the submucous layer (submucosa), consists of connective tissue that contains blood vessels, lymphatics, glands, and nerve plexuses. The innermost layer, the mucous layer (mucosa), consists of simple columnar epithelium.[5] The mucosa and submucosa are arranged in circular folds (plicae circulares),[5] which are largest and most numerous in the jejunum and upper ileum.[1] These folds are covered by a second series of projectile-like folds called *villi* that are in constant motion—constricting, lengthening, and shortening (villous movement). The 4 to 5 million villi (see Fig. 32-5) give the intestine a velvety appearance; they are more numerous and larger in the jejunum than in the ileum. Villi contain a network of capillaries and blind lymphatic vessels called *lacteals*. The outer layer of the villus is composed of microvilli. The circular folds of the small intestine, along with the villi and microvilli, increase the digestive-absorptive surface of the small intestine 600 times.[9,10]

The gastroduodenal artery provides the blood supply for the duodenum, and branches of the superior mesenteric artery provide for the jejunum and the ileum. The superior mesenteric vein provides for venous drainage of the small intestine.[11] Numerous lymphatic channels arise in the submucosa and terminate in the thoracic duct. The small intestine is extrinsically innervated by the autonomic nervous system. Sympathetic fibers arise from the celiac plexus, whereas parasympathetic fibers arise from the gastric branch of the vagus nerve. Intrinsic innervation, which initiates motor functions, is provided by Auerbach's plexus and Meissner's plexus, which are located in the intestinal wall.[1]

INTESTINAL SECRETION

The small intestine has two major types of glands: Brunner's glands and intestinal glands. Brunner's glands lie in the mucosa of the duodenum and secrete mucus, an alkaline fluid (pH of 9) that neutralizes chyme and protects the mucosa.[10] Intestinal glands are found in pits of the submucosa and are called the *crypts of Lieberkühn*. These crypts secrete 2 to 3 L per day of yellow fluid containing enzymes that assist in nutrient digestion.[7]

INTESTINAL MOTILITY

Intestinal motility consists of two separate motions: peristalsis and haustral segmentation. Peristalsis is sequential contraction and relaxation of short segments of the small intestine that facilitate digestion and absorption. Haustral segmentation is rhythmic contractions that facilitate the mixing and forward

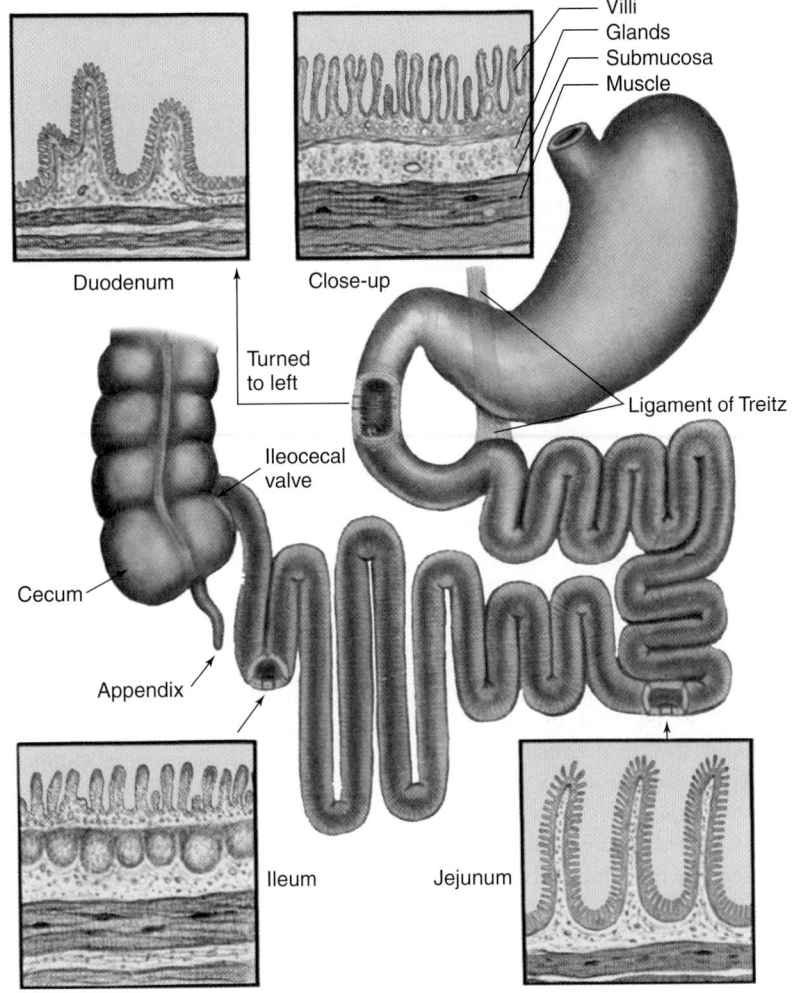

Figure 32-5 Clinical anatomy of the small intestine. *(From Thompson JM et al: Mosby's clinical nursing, ed 5, St Louis, 2002, Mosby.)*

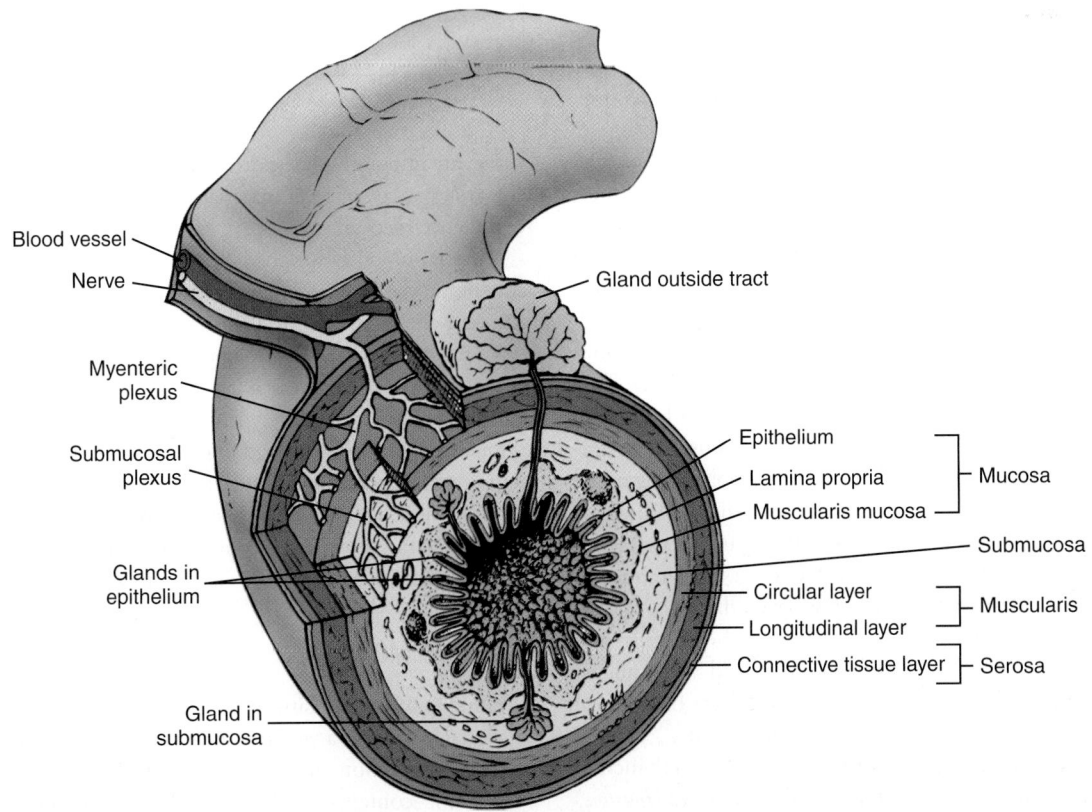

Figure 32-6 Cross section of the small intestine. *(From Moffett DF et al: Human physiology: foundations and frontiers, ed 2, St Louis, 1993, Mosby.)*

movement of chyme. It is controlled by Auerbach's plexus. Intestinal motility is also affected by neural reflexes located along the length of the small intestine. Motility is inhibited by the intestinointestinal reflex, which is activated by distention of the small intestine, and is stimulated by the gastroileal reflux, which is initiated by an increase in gastric motility.[12]

DIGESTION AND ABSORPTION

The functions of the small intestine include digestion and absorption. Digestion, which involves breaking down large molecules into small ones, is essential for nutrient absorption from the small intestine. Maintenance of pH and osmolality is crucial for digestion in the small intestine. The entry of chyme into the duodenum stimulates the production of secretin, which stimulates the pancreas to secrete a highly alkaline fluid into the duodenum. In the small intestine, the chyme mixes with pancreatic enzymes, intestinal enzymes, and bile from the liver and gallbladder, and it is then reduced to absorbable elements of proteins, fats, and carbohydrates. The nutrients are absorbed through the villi and transported to the liver by the portal system for further processing (Table 32-2). The small intestine absorbs up to 8 L of fluid per day, passing only a small part of this fluid into the large intestine. In addition to the nutrients, electrolytes, water, components of saliva, gastric juice, and bile, intestinal and pancreatic secretions are also absorbed.[1]

LARGE INTESTINE

The large intestine, which extends from the ileocecal valve to the anus, is approximately 90 to 150 cm (4 to 5 feet) long and 4 to 6 cm (2 inches) in diameter. It is divided into the ascending colon, the hepatic flexure, the transverse colon, the splenic flexure, the descending colon, the sigmoid colon, the rectum, and the anal canal (Fig. 32-7).[10]

The colon has four layers. The outermost layer, the serous layer (serosa), is formed from the visceral peritoneum and covers most of the large intestine, with the exclusion of the sigmoid colon. The second layer, the muscular layer (muscularis), consists of two smooth muscle layers: the longitudinal and the circular muscles. These muscles work together to propel fecal matter through the colon and to "knead" the stool into a compact bolus. The longitudinal muscle consists of three muscular bands that stretch from the cecum to the distal sigmoid colon. These muscular bands create sacculations of haustra, important clinical features that normally are apparent on a barium enema radiograph. Haustra aid segmentation so that absorption of fluid from the fecal bolus is achieved. The third layer, the submucous layer (submucosa), consists of connective tissue that contains blood vessels, lymphatics, glands, and nerve plexuses. The innermost layer, the mucous layer (mucosa), is lined with simple columnar epithelial cells and contains deep crypts of Lieberkühn that are lined with mucus-producing goblet cells. The mucus eases the passage of the fecal material and protects the mucosal surface from trauma.[10]

The rectum begins at the midsacrum, is 12 to 15 cm (5 inches) long, and is quite angulated. These angles, also known as *Houston's*

TABLE 32-2 Nutrient Digestion and Absorption

Digestive Enzymes	Site of Action or Absorption
Carbohydrates	
Amylase	Produced in mouth (salivary glands)
	Absorbed in stomach (limited)
	Produced in small intestine (pancreas)
	Absorbed in small intestine
Disaccharidases (sucrase, maltase isomaltase, lactase)	Produced in small intestine (brush border)
	Absorbed in small intestine
Pepsin	Produced in stomach (chief cells)
	Absorbed in small intestine
Proteins	
Trypsin, chymotrypsin	Produced in small intestine (pancreas)
	Absorbed in small intestine
Carboxypeptidase	Produced in small intestine (brush border)
Peptidases	
	Absorbed in small intestine
Bile (not enzyme)	Produced in liver and delivered to duodenum
	Absorbed in small intestine
Lipids	
Lipase	Produced in small intestine (pancreas, brush border)
	Absorbed in small intestine
Esterase	Produced in small intestine (pancreas)
	Absorbed in small intestine

From Doughty DB, Jackson DB: *Gastrointestinal disorders,* St Louis, 1993, Mosby.

valves, are important in the defecation process because they tend to slow the passage of fecal material in the rectal vault, assisting the continence mechanism.

Arterial blood is supplied to the colon from branches of the superior and inferior mesenteric arteries. Venous drainage occurs through the branches of the superior and inferior mesenteric veins into the portal system. The colon is intrinsically innervated by Auerbach's plexus, which controls secretion and motility, and is extrinsically innervated by the autonomic nervous system. The sympathetic and parasympathetic branches of the autonomic system innervate the colon, regulating motility. Sympathetic stimulation inhibits colonic activity and constricts the anal sphincters, whereas parasympathetic stimulation increases colonic activity and secretion and relaxes the anal sphincters.[9]

COLONIC MOTILITY

Colonic motility consists of haustral shuttling and peristalsis. Haustral shuttling, a variation of haustral segmentation, consists of the contraction and relaxation of the circular muscle. It moves the contents of the colon back and forth to facilitate

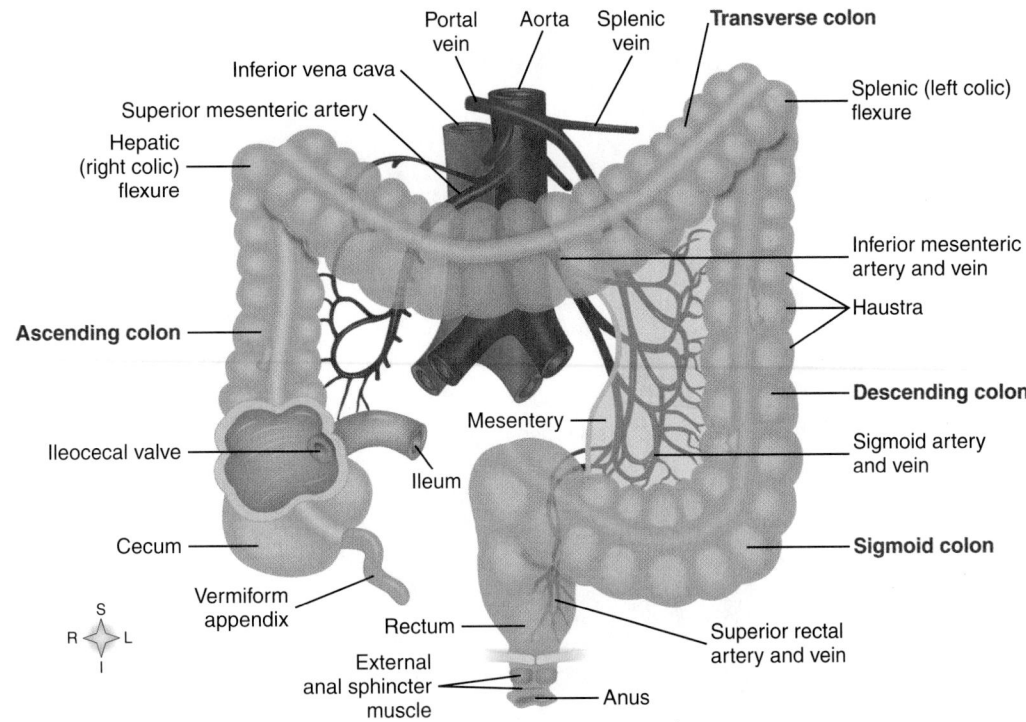

Figure 32-7 Large intestine. *(Modified from Thibodeau GA, Patton KT:* Anatomy & physiology, *ed 5, St Louis, 2003, Mosby.)*

the grinding of food masses and fluid absorption. Peristalsis is produced primarily by the longitudinal muscles and propels the fecal bolus forward. Mass peristalsis is a strong, slow contraction in which the distal left colon contracts en masse to move the fecal bolus into the rectum.[13]

RESORPTION

The major functions of the colon are resorption of water, sodium, chloride, glucose, and urea; dehydration of undigested residue; putrefaction of contents by bacteria; movement of the fecal bolus through the colon; and elimination of the fecal mass. The colon receives approximately 1000 to 2000 mL of chyme per day, and all but 50 to 250 mL of it is absorbed in the ascending and transverse colon.[5]

The colon contains billions of anaerobic bacteria that putrefy remaining proteins and indigestible residue; synthesize folic acid, vitamin K, nicotinic acid, riboflavin, and some B vitamins; and convert urea salts to ammonium salts and ammonia for absorption into the portal circulation.[1] Common colonic bacteria include *Bacteroides, Lactobacillus,* and *Clostridium.*[14]

ACCESSORY ORGANS

The accessory organs of digestion are the liver, the biliary system, and the pancreas (Fig. 32-8).

LIVER

The liver is the largest internal organ in the body. Weighing 1200 to 1600 g (3 to 4 pounds), it is friable and dark red and has a soft-solid consistency. Located in the right upper

abdominal quadrant, it fits snugly against the right interior diaphragm. The liver is surrounded by connective tissue known as *Glisson's capsule,* which is covered by serosa and contains blood vessels and lymphatics. The peritoneum covering the liver forms the falciform ligament, which attaches the liver to the anterior portion of the abdomen between the diaphragm and umbilicus and divides the liver into two main lobes, right and left (see Fig. 32-8). The right lobe, which is six times larger than the left, has three sections: the right lobe proper, the caudate lobe, and the quadrate lobe. The left lobe is divided into two sections. Each lobe is divided into numerous lobules.[10,15]

The liver receives one third of the total cardiac output from two major sources: the hepatic artery, which provides oxygenated blood; and the portal vein, which is supplied with nutrient-rich blood from the gut, pancreas, spleen, and stomach (Fig. 32-9). The portal vein, which accounts for 75% of the total liver blood flow, branches into sinusoids to transport blood to each lobule. Unlike capillaries, sinusoids lack a definite cell wall but contain a lining of phagocytic (Kupffer) cells and some nonphagocytic cells of modified epithelium. Sinusoids empty blood into an intralobular vein in the center of the lobule. Intralobular veins empty into larger veins and then into the hepatic vein, which empties on the posterior surface of the liver and eventually into the vena cava. The hepatic artery also divides and subdivides between the lobules, supplying sinusoids with oxygenated blood before emptying into the hepatic vein. Lymphatic spaces are between liver cells. Lymph drains into lymphatic vessels that surround the hepatic vein and bile ducts.[15]

Nutrient Metabolism. The liver plays a key role in metabolizing and storing carbohydrates, fats, proteins, and vitamins. Glycogen, the stored form of glucose, can be synthesized from glucose or from protein, fat, or lactic acid. Glycogen is broken

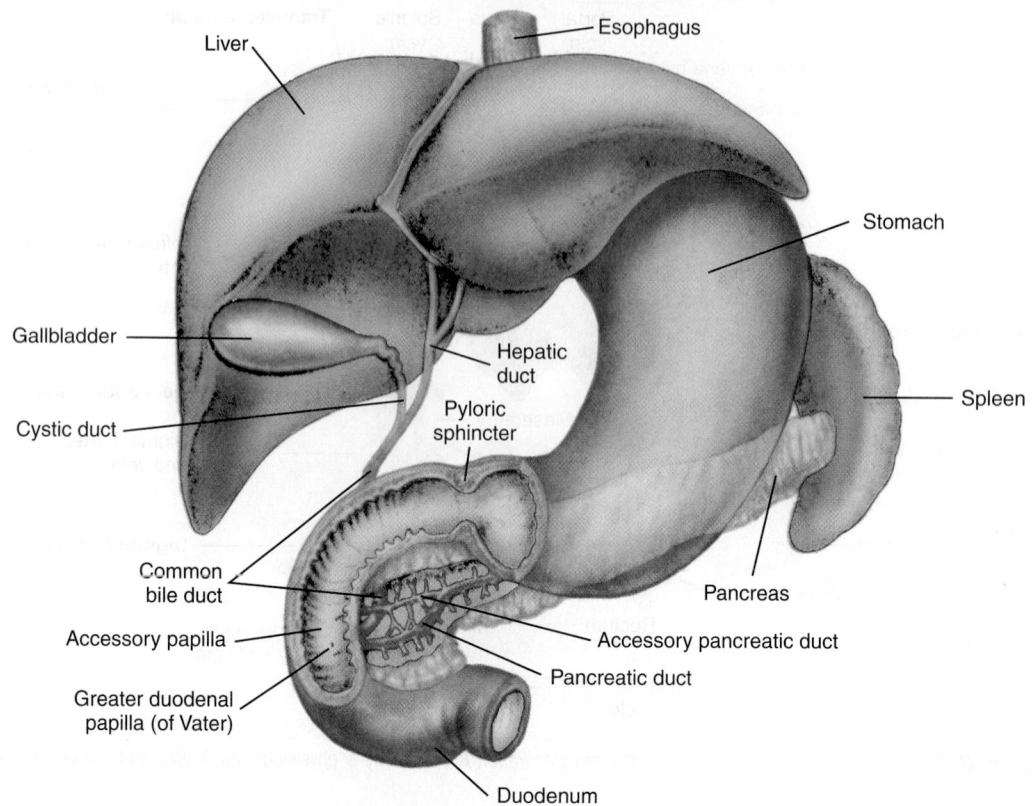

Figure 32-8 Liver, gallbladder, and pancreas. *(From Thompson JM et al:* Mosby's clinical nursing, *ed 5, St Louis, 2002, Mosby.)*

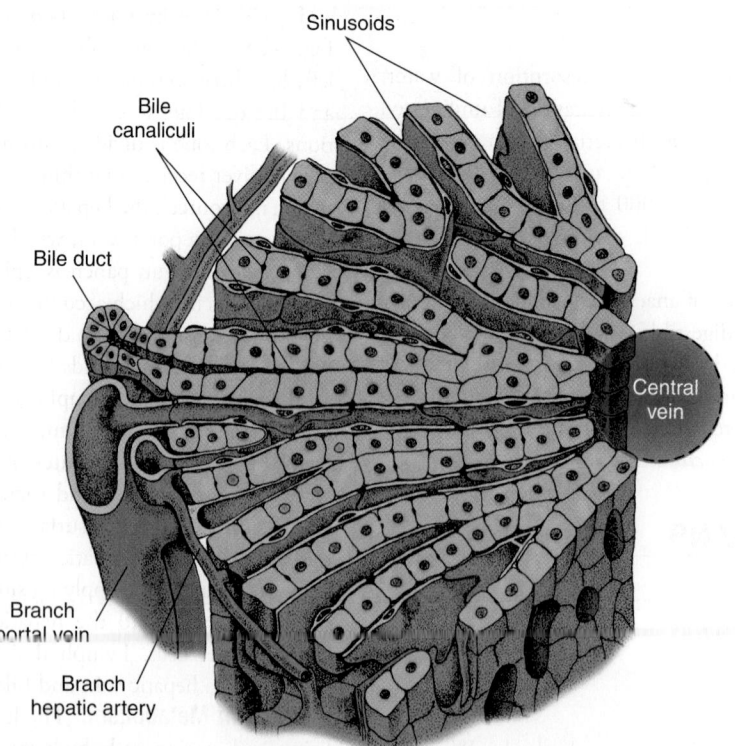

Figure 32-9 Cross section of a liver lobule. *(From Berne RM, Levy MN:* Principles of physiology, *ed 3, St Louis, 1993, Mosby.)*

down to glucose by the liver to maintain normal blood glucose levels. The liver also has a vital role in amino acid metabolism and can synthesize amino acids from metabolites of carbohydrates and fats or can deaminate amino acids to produce keto-acids and ammonia, from which urea is formed. In fat metabolism, the liver hydrolyzes triglycerides to glycerol and fatty acids in the process of ketogenesis and synthesizes phospholipids, cholesterol, and lipoproteins.[10,15]

Hematologic Function. The liver synthesizes plasma proteins, such as globulins and albumin, which are important in maintaining the normal osmotic balance of blood. It also synthesizes a number of clotting factors, including fibrinogen and prothrombin. The Kupffer cells destroy worn red blood cells, and hepatocytes conjugate bilirubin (by-product of red cell destruction) for excretion.[10,15]

Detoxification and Storage. Steroid hormones are conjugated and polypeptide hormones are inactivated by the liver. The liver stores fat-soluble vitamins, vitamin B_{12}, and the minerals iron and copper. Detoxification of drugs and toxins occurs in the Kupffer cells.[10,15]

Bile. The production of bile makes the liver a vital organ in digestion and absorption. The major components of bile are bile pigments, bile salts, cholesterol, neutral fats, phospholipids, inorganic salts, fatty acids, mucin, conjugated bilirubin, lecithin, and water. Traces of albumin, gamma globulin, urea, nitrogen, and glucose are also present in bile. The principal electrolytes of bile are sodium, chloride, and bicarbonate.[15]

Bile emulsifies fat globules and absorbs fat-soluble vitamins. Bile salts also serve as an excretion route for bilirubin, cholesterol, and various hormones. Approximately 80% of bile salts are actively resorbed in the distal ileum and are recycled to the liver through the enterohepatic circulation; only 20% are lost in the feces.[1]

Bilirubin. The primary bile pigment, bilirubin, is formed from the heme portion of hemoglobin during the degradation of red blood cells by the Kupffer cells. When released into the bloodstream, bilirubin binds to albumin as fat-soluble, unconjugated bilirubin. Taken up by liver hepatocytes, unconjugated bilirubin is conjugated with glucuronic acid to form water-soluble, conjugated bilirubin, which is then excreted through hepatic ducts into the large intestine. If the amount of bilirubin sent to the liver is in excess, the ability of the liver to conjugate the bilirubin may be taxed; free, unconjugated or indirect bilirubin appears in the blood. High levels of unconjugated bilirubin in the blood suggest hepatocellular dysfunction, whereas high levels of conjugated bilirubin suggest biliary tract obstruction.[1]

BILIARY SYSTEM

The biliary system (Fig. 32-10) consists of the gallbladder and its related ductal system, including the hepatic, cystic, and common bile ducts. The hepatic duct, from the liver, joins the cystic duct, from the gallbladder, to form the common bile duct, which empties into the duodenum. The common bile duct is surrounded by Oddi's sphincter, which pierces the wall of the duodenum and

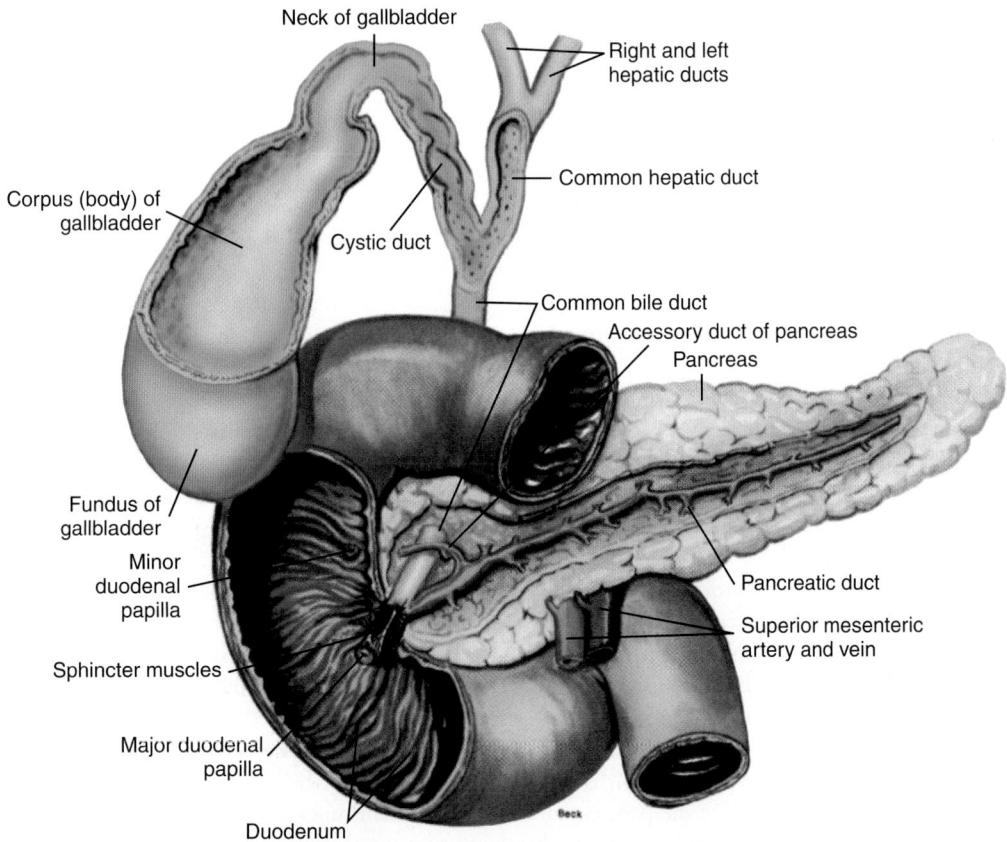

Figure 32-10 Gallbladder and pancreas. *(From McCance KL, Huether SE, editors:* Pathophysiology: the biologic basis for disease in adults and children, *ed 5, St Louis, 2006, Mosby.)*

controls the flow of bile into the duodenum. The gallbladder is a pear-shaped organ that is 7 to 10 cm (3 to 4 inches) long and 2.5 to 3.5 cm (approximately 1 inch) wide, lying on the underside of the liver (see Fig. 32-8). It is attached to the liver by connective tissue, peritoneum, and blood vessels.[10,16]

Bile. The main functions of the gallbladder are to collect, concentrate, acidify, and store bile. Bile is continuously formed in the liver and excreted into the hepatic duct for transport to the gallbladder through the cystic duct. The gallbladder can store up to 90 mL of bile and concentrate it approximately 15 to 29 times by removing approximately 90% of the water. Cholesterol and pigment are likewise concentrated. Bile, which is golden or orange-yellow in the liver, becomes dark brown when concentrated in the gallbladder. By altering its shape and volume, the gallbladder regulates pressure within the biliary system. Relaxation of the sphincter of Oddi is coordinated with gallbladder contraction through the regulatory action of cholecystokinin. Factors such as sight, smell, and taste can stimulate gallbladder contraction, whereas fear or excitement can decrease contraction. After a meal, the amount of bile entering the duodenum increases as a result of enhanced liver secretion and gallbladder contraction. Intestinal secretion of cholecystokinin and secretin, high levels of bile salts in the blood, and vagal stimulation increase biliary secretion.[15]

PANCREAS

The pancreas is a soft, lobulated, fish-shaped gland (see Fig. 32-10) lying beneath the duodenum and the spleen (see Fig. 32-8). The pinkish yellow organ is 15 to 20 cm (6 to 8 inches) long and 5 cm (1 to 1.5 inches) wide. Its anatomic divisions include the head, which lies in the C-shaped curve of the duodenum to which it is attached; the body, the main part of the gland, which extends horizontally across the abdomen and is largely hidden behind the stomach; and the tail, a thin, narrow portion in contact with the spleen. The main pancreatic duct, called the *duct of Wirsung,* traverses the entire length of the organ. Wirsung's duct empties exocrine secretions into the ampulla of Vater, which is the same lumen draining the common bile duct, at the entrance to the duodenum.[10]

The internal structural unit of the pancreas is the lobule, consisting of numerous small ducts with secretory cells called *tubuloacinar* cells. Each acinus has a small duct that empties into lobular ducts. Lobules are joined by connective tissue into lobes, which unite to form the gland. The ducts from each lobule empty into the duct of Wirsung.[10]

Arterial blood supply to the pancreas is provided by branches of the superior mesenteric artery and celiac arteries. Venous drainage of the head of the pancreas occurs through the portal vein, and drainage of the body and tail occurs through the splenic vein. The pancreas is innervated by the autonomic nervous system. Sympathetic stimulation decreases pancreatic secretion, and parasympathetic stimulation increases it.[10]

Exocrine Functions. Exocrine functions of the pancreas are limited to digestion. Acinar cells secrete pancreatic juice, which consists of water, sodium bicarbonate, and electrolytes at a highly alkaline pH. Enzymes produced in the pancreas include trypsin, chymotrypsin, carboxypeptidase, amylase, and lipase. The pancreas also produces a trypsin inhibitor that prevents activation of trypsinogen (inactive form of trypsin), which inhibits autodigestion. Autodigestion is the underlying cause of acute pancreatitis.

Pancreatic exocrine function is regulated by digestive hormones. Signals provided primarily by the intestinal hormones *secretin* and *cholecystokinin* stimulate the pancreas to secrete pancreatic juice. The two hormones potentiate each other's effects on the pancreas.[17]

Endocrine Functions. Endocrine tissue in the pancreas consists of spherical islets called *islets of Langerhans,* which are embedded within the lobules of acinar tissue throughout the pancreas, especially in the distal body and tail. Endocrine products include insulin, which is produced in beta cells; glucagon, which is produced in alpha cells; and gastrin. All of these hormones are secreted directly into the bloodstream.[17]

Summary

Anatomy

- The gastrointestinal tract consists of the mouth (lips, cheeks, gums, tongue, palate, and salivary glands), the esophagus, the stomach, the small intestine, and the large intestine.
- The accessory organs of digestion are the liver, the biliary system, and the pancreas.

Physiology

- The major function of the gastrointestinal tract is digestion.
- Digestion is the conversion of ingested nutrients into simpler forms that can be transported from the tract's lumen to the portal circulation and then used in metabolic processes.
- The mouth and accessory organs perform the initial phases of digestion, which are ingestion, mastication, and salivation.
- The functions of the stomach include food storage, digestion, and emptying.
- Gastric motility is regulated by the autonomic nervous system, digestive hormones, and neural reflexes.
- The functions of the small intestine include digestion and absorption.
- Intestinal motility consists of peristalsis and haustral segmentation.
- The major functions of the colon include resorption of water, sodium, chloride, glucose, and urea; dehydration of undigested residue; putrefaction of contents by bacteria; movement of the fecal bolus through the colon; and elimination of the fecal mass.
- Colonic motility consists of haustral shuttling and peristalsis.
- The functions of the liver include metabolism and storage of carbohydrates, fats, proteins, and vitamins; synthesis of plasma proteins; detoxification of drugs and toxins; and the production of bile.
- The main functions of the gallbladder are to collect, concentrate, acidify, and store bile.
- The main functions of the pancreas are digestion and glucose regulation.

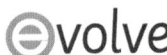 Be sure to check out the bonus material, including free self-assessment exercises, on the Evolve web site at http://evolve.elsevier.com/Urden/.

References

1. Huether SE: Structure and function of the digestive system. In McCance KL, Huether SE, editors: *Pathophysiology: the biologic basis for disease in adults and children*, ed 5, St Louis, 2006, Mosby.

2. Canaan TJ: Variations of structure and appearance of the oral mucosa, *Dent Clin North Am* 49:1, 2005.

3. Silvers AR, Som PM: Salivary glands, *Radiol Clin North Am* 36:941, 1998.

4. Achildi O, Grewal H: Congenital anomalies of the esophagus, *Otolaryngol Clin North Am* 40:219, 2007.

5. Ashley J et al: Speech, language, and swallowing disorders in the older adult, *Clin Geriatr Med* 22:291, 2006.

6. Soybel DI: Anatomy and physiology of the stomach, *Surg Clin North Am* 85:875, 2005.

7. Guyton AC, Hall JE: *Textbook of medical physiology*, ed 11, Philadelphia, 2006, Saunders.

8. Eswaran S, Roy MA: Medical management of acid-peptic disorders of the stomach, *Surg Clin North Am* 85:895, 2005.

9. Androulakis J et al: Embryologic and anatomic basis of duodenal surgery, *Surg Clin North Am* 80:171, 2000.

10. Society of Gastroenterology Nurses and Associates Core Curriculum Committee: *Gastroenterology nursing: a core curriculum*, ed 3, St Louis, 2003, Mosby.

11. Lin PH, Chaikof EL: Embryology, anatomy, and surgical exposure of the great abdominal vessels, *Surg Clin North Am* 80:417, 2000.

12. Quigley EMM: Gastric and small intestinal motility in health and disease, *Gastroenterol Clin North Am* 25:113, 1996.

13. Mazzone A, Farrugia G: Evolving concepts in the cellular control of gastrointestinal motility: neurogastroenterology and enteric sciences, *Gastroenterol Clin North Am* 36:499, 2007.

14. Kalliomaki MA, Walker WA: Physiologic and pathologic interactions of bacteria with gastrointestinal epithelium, *Gastroenterol Clin North Am* 34:383, 2005.

15. Wanless IR: Anatomy, histology, embryology, and developmental anomalies of the liver. In Feldman M et al, editors: *Sleisenger & Fordtran's gastrointestinal and liver disease: pathophysiology, diagnosis, and management*, ed 8, Philadelphia, 2006, Saunders.

16. Adkins RB et al: Embryology, anatomy, and surgical applications of the extrahepatic biliary system, *Surg Clin North Am* 80:363, 2000.

17. Kang SY, Go VLW: Pancreatic exocrine-endocrine interrelationships: clinical implication, *Gastroenterol Clin North Am* 28:551, 1999.

Gastrointestinal Clinical Assessment and Diagnostic Procedures

*A*ssessment of the critically ill patient with gastrointestinal dysfunction includes a review of the patient's history, a thorough physical examination, and analysis of the patient's laboratory data. Numerous invasive and noninvasive diagnostic procedures may also be performed to help identify the disorder.

CLINICAL ASSESSMENT

A thorough clinical assessment of the patient with gastrointestinal dysfunction is imperative for the early identification and treatment of gastrointestinal disorders. The completed assessment serves as the foundation for developing the management plan for the patient. The assessment process can be brief or can involve a detailed history and examination, depending on the nature and immediacy of the patient's situation.[1]

HISTORY

Taking a thorough and accurate history is extremely important to the assessment process. The patient's history provides the foundation and direction for the rest of the assessment. The overall goal of the patient interview is to expose key clinical manifestations that will facilitate the identification of the underlying cause of the illness. This information can then assist in the development of an appropriate management plan.[2]

The initial presentation of the patient determines the rapidity and direction of the interview. For a patient in acute distress, the history should be curtailed to a few questions about the patient's chief complaint and the precipitating events. For a patient in no obvious distress, the history should focus on current symptoms, the patient's medical history, and the family's history. Specific items regarding each of these areas are outlined in the Data Collection feature on Gastrointestinal History.[3,4]

PHYSICAL EXAMINATION

The physical examination helps to establish baseline data about the physical dimensions of the patient's situation.[3] The abdomen is divided into four quadrants (left upper, right upper, left lower, and right lower), with the umbilicus as the middle point, to help specify the location of examination findings (Fig. 33-1 and Box 33-1). The assessment should proceed when the patient is as comfortable as possible and in the supine position; however, the position may need readjustment if it elicits pain. To prevent stimulation of gastrointestinal activity, the order for the assessment should be changed to inspection, auscultation, percussion, and palpation.[4]

INSPECTION

Inspection should be performed in a warm, well-lighted environment with the patient in a comfortable position and with the abdomen exposed. Although assessment of the gastrointestinal system classically begins with inspection of the abdomen, the patient's oral cavity also must be inspected to determine any unusual findings. Abnormal findings of the mouth include joint tenderness, inflammation of the gums, missing teeth, dental caries, ill-fitting dentures, and mouth odor.[5]

Observe the skin for pigmentation, lesions, striae, scars, petechiae, signs of dehydration, and venous pattern. Pigmentation may vary considerably and still be within normal limits because of race and ethnic background, although the abdomen usually is a lighter color than other exposed areas of the skin. Abnormal findings include jaundice, skin lesions, and a tense and glistening appearance of the skin. Old striae (stretch marks) usually are silver, whereas pinkish purple striae may indicate Cushing's syndrome.[4] A bluish discoloration of the umbilicus (Cullen's sign) and of the flank (Grey Turner's sign) indicates retroperitoneal bleeding.[1]

Observe the abdomen for contour, noting whether it is flat, slightly concave, or slightly round; observe for symmetry and for movement. Marked distention is an abnormal finding. In particular, ascites may cause generalized distention and bulging flanks. Asymmetric distention may indicate organ enlargement or a mass. Peristaltic waves should not be visible except in very thin patients. In the case of intestinal obstruction, hyperactive peristaltic waves may be observed. Pulsation in the epigastric area is often a normal finding, but increased pulsation may indicate an aortic aneurysm. Symmetric movement of the abdomen with respirations is usually seen in men.[4,5]

Data Collection

Gastrointestinal History

Demographic Data
- Name, address, phone number, birth date, sex, race, marital status, occupation, education, religious preference

Chief Complaint or Reason for Visit
- In patient's own words

Current Problem or Health Status
- Description includes onset, duration, severity, associated factors, associated symptoms, exacerbating or relieving factors, patient's concerns

Medical History
- Chronic illnesses
- Previous weight gain or loss
- Tooth extractions or orthodontic work
- Gastrointestinal (GI) disorders (e.g., peptic ulcer, inflammatory bowel disease, polyps, cholelithiasis, diverticular disease, pancreatitis, intestinal obstruction)
- Hepatitis or cirrhosis
- Abdominal surgery
- Abdominal trauma
- Cancer affecting GI system
- Spinal cord injury
- Women: episiotomy or fourth-degree laceration during delivery

Family History
- Investigate for history of following disorders, and document (+ or −) responses
- Hirschsprung's disease
- Obesity
- Metabolic disorders
- Inflammatory disorders
- Malabsorption syndromes
- Familial Mediterranean fever
- Rectal polyps
- Polyposis syndromes
- Cancer of the GI tract

Personal and Social History
- Dietary habits
  - Usual number of meals or snacks per day
  - Usual fluid intake per day
- Exercise patterns
- Oral care patterns
  Frequency of toothbrushing or denture care
  Frequency of flossing
- Alcohol intake (e.g., frequency, usual amounts)
- Review of GI system

General Data
- Usual height and weight
- Nutrient intake
  - Types of food usually eaten at each meal or snack
  - Food likes and dislikes
  - Religious or medical food restrictions
  - Food intolerances
  - Patient's perceptions and concerns about adequacy of diet and appropriateness of weight
  - Effects of lifestyle on food intake, weight gain or loss
  - Vitamins or nutritional supplements (e.g., type, amount, frequency)
- Oral hygiene
  Last visit to dentist
  Presence of braces, dentures, bridges, or crowns
- Bowel elimination
  Usual frequency of bowel movements
  Usual consistency and color of stool
  Ability to control elimination of gas and stool
  Any changes in bowel elimination patterns
  Use of enemas or laxatives (e.g., reason for use, frequency, type, response)
- Medications (e.g., laxatives, stool softeners, antiemetics, antidiarrheals, antacids, frequent or high doses of aspirin, acetaminophen, corticosteroids)

Specific Data
- Oral lesions
- Appetite
- Digestion or indigestion (heartburn)
- Dysphagia
- Nausea
- Vomiting
- Hematemesis
- Change in stool color or contents (e.g., clay-colored, tarry, fresh blood, mucus, undigested food)
- Constipation
- Diarrhea
- Flatulence
- Hemorrhoids
- Abdominal pain
- Hepatitis
- Jaundice
- Ulcers
- Gallstones
- Polyps
- Tumors
- Anal discomfort
- Fecal incontinence
- Exposure to infectious agents (e.g., foreign travel, water source)

AUSCULTATION

Auscultation of the abdomen provides clinical data regarding the status of the bowel's motility. Initially, listen with the diaphragm of the stethoscope below and to the right of the umbilicus. The examination proceeds methodically through all four quadrants, lifting and then replacing the diaphragm of the stethoscope lightly against the abdomen (see Fig. 33-1). Normal bowel sounds include high-pitched, gurgling sounds that occur approximately every 5 to 15 seconds or at a rate of 5 to 34 times per minute. Colonic sounds are low-pitched and have a rumbling

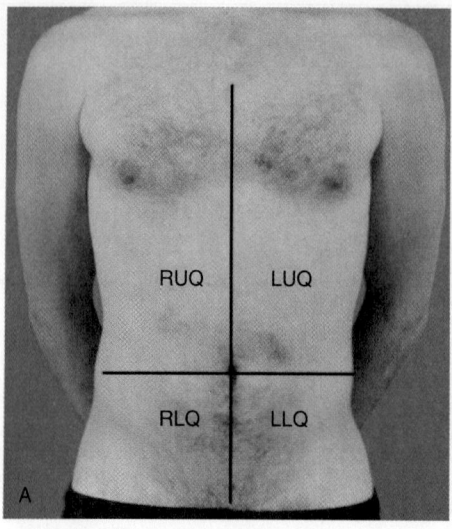
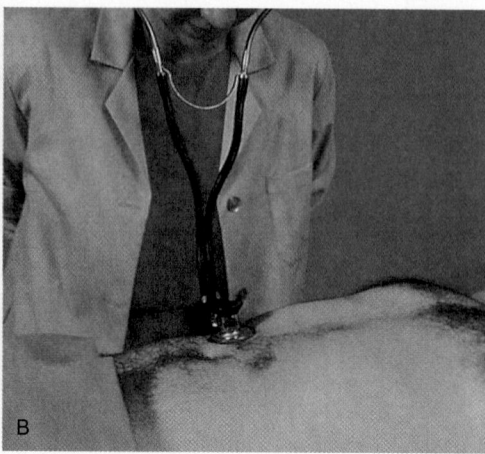

Figure 33-1 *A,* Anatomic mapping of the four quadrants of the abdomen. *B,* Auscultation for bowel sounds. *(From Barkauskas V et al:* Health & physical assessment, *ed 3, St Louis, 2002, Mosby.)*

BOX 33-1   ANATOMIC CORRELATES OF THE FOUR QUADRANTS OF THE ABDOMEN

RIGHT UPPER QUADRANT
- Liver and gallbladder
- Pylorus
- Duodenum
- Head of pancreas
- Right adrenal gland
- Portion of right kidney
- Hepatic flexure of colon
- Portion of ascending and transverse colon

LEFT UPPER QUADRANT
- Left lobe of liver
- Spleen
- Stomach
- Body of pancreas
- Left adrenal gland
- Portion of left kidney
- Splenic flexure of colon
- Portions of transverse and descending colon

RIGHT LOWER QUADRANT
- Lower pole of right kidney
- Cecum and appendix
- Portion of ascending colon
- Bladder (if distended)
- Ovary and salpinx
- Uterus (if enlarged)
- Right spermatic cord
- Right ureter

LEFT LOWER QUADRANT
- Lower pole of left kidney
- Sigmoid colon
- Portion of descending colon
- Bladder (if distended)
- Ovary and salpinx
- Uterus (if distended)
- Left spermatic cord
- Left ureter

From Barkauskas V et al: *Health & physical assessment,* ed 3, St Louis, 2002, Mosby.

---

quality. A venous hum may be audible sometimes.[6] Table 33-1 provides a list of abnormal abdominal sounds.

Abnormal findings include the absence of bowel sounds throughout a 5-minute period, extremely soft and widely separated sounds, and increased sounds with a high-pitched, loud rushing sound (peristaltic rush). Absent bowel sounds may result from inflammation, ileus, electrolyte disturbances, and ischemia. Bowels sounds may be increased with diarrhea and early intestinal obstruction.[6]

The abdomen should be auscultated for the presence of bruits, using the bell of the stethoscope (Fig. 33-2). Bruits are created by turbulent flow over a partially obstructed artery and are always considered an abnormal finding. The aorta, the right and left renal arteries, and the iliac arteries should be auscultated.[5,6]

PERCUSSION

Percussion is used to elicit information about deep organs, such as the liver, spleen, and pancreas (Fig. 33-3). Because the abdomen is a sensitive area, muscle tension may interfere with this part of the assessment. Percussion often helps relax tense

TABLE 33-1 Abnormal Abdominal Sounds

Sound	Cause
Hyperactive bowel sounds (borborygmi), loud and prolonged	Hunger, gastroenteritis, or early intestinal obstruction
High-pitched, tinkling sounds	Intestinal air and fluid under pressure; characteristic of early intestinal obstruction
Decreased (hypoactive) bowel sounds	Possible peritonitis or ileus
Infrequent and abnormally faint sounds	
Absence of bowel sounds (confirmed only after auscultation of all four quadrants and continuous auscultation for 5 min)	Temporary loss of intestinal motility, as occurs with complete ileus
Friction rubs	Pathologic conditions such as tumors or infection that cause inflammation of organ's peritoneal covering
High-pitched sounds heard over liver and spleen (RUQ and LUQ), synchronous with respiration	
Bruits	Abnormality of blood flow (requires additional evaluation to determine specific disorder)
Audible swishing sounds that may be heard over aortic, iliac, renal, and femoral arteries	
Venous hum	Increased collateral circulation between portal and systemic venous systems
Low-pitched, continuous sound	

From Doughty DB, Jackson DB: *Gastrointestinal disorders,* St Louis, 1993, Mosby.
LUQ, left upper quadrant; RUQ, right upper quadrant.

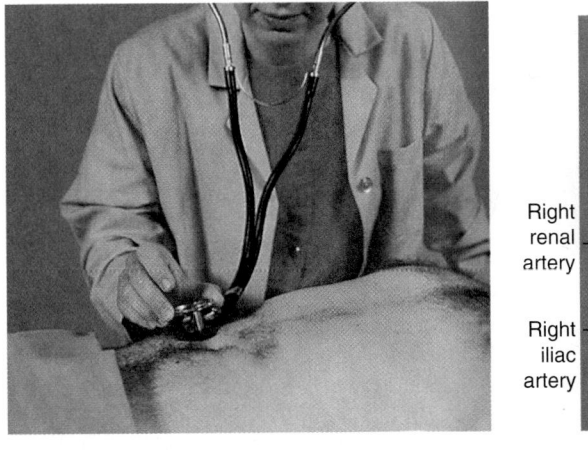 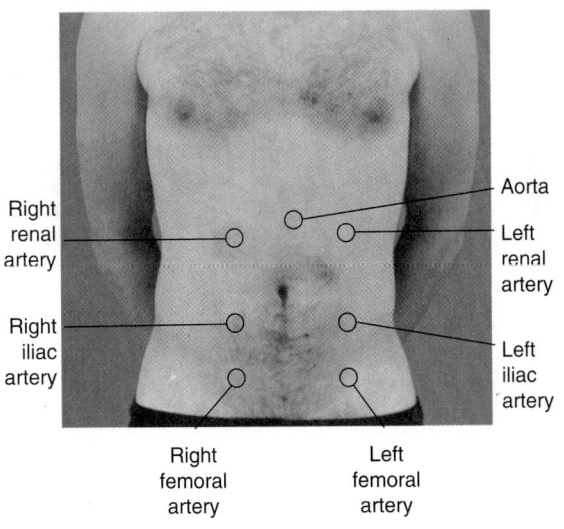

Figure 33-2 Auscultation for bruits. The left illustration shows the correct placement of the stethoscope. *(From Barkauskas V et al: Health & physical assessment, ed 3, St Louis, 2002, Mosby.)*

muscles, and it is performed before palpation. Percussion in the absence of disease helps to delineate the position and size of the liver and spleen, and it assists in the detection of fluid, gaseous distention, and masses in the abdomen.[5]

Percussion should proceed systematically and lightly in all four quadrants. Normal findings include tympany over the stomach when empty, tympany or hyperresonance over the intestine, and dullness over the liver and spleen. Abnormal areas of dullness may indicate an underlying mass. Solid masses, enlarged organs, and a distended bladder also produce areas of dullness. Dullness over both flanks may indicate ascites and necessitates further assessment.[6]

PALPATION

Palpation is the assessment technique most useful in detecting abdominal pathologic conditions. Light and deep palpation of each organ and quadrant should be completed. Light palpation, which has a palpation depth of approximately 1 cm, assesses to the depth of the skin and fascia (Fig. 33-4A). Deep palpation assesses the rectus abdominis muscle and is performed bimanually to a depth of 4 to 5 cm (see Fig. 33-4B). Deep palpation is most helpful in detecting abdominal masses. Areas in which the patient complains of tenderness should be palpated last.[6]

Normal findings include no areas of tenderness or pain, no masses, and no hardened areas. Persistent involuntary guarding may indicate peritoneal inflammation, particularly if it continues even after relaxation techniques are used. Rebound tenderness, in which pain increases with quick release of a palpated area, indicates an inflamed peritoneum.[4]

ASSESSMENT FINDINGS FOR COMMON DISORDERS

Table 33-2 presents a variety of common gastrointestinal disorders and their associated assessment findings.

LABORATORY STUDIES

The value of various laboratory studies used to diagnose and treat diseases of the gastrointestinal system has been emphasized often. However, no single study provides an overall picture of the various organs' functional state, and no single value is

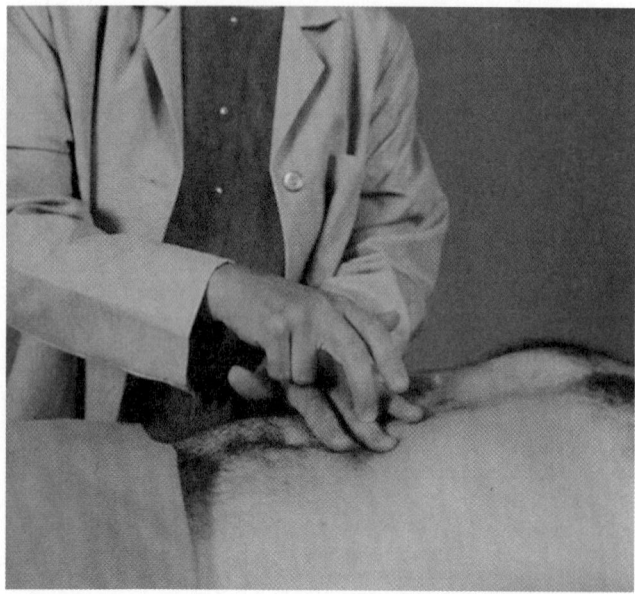

Figure 33-3 Percussion of the abdomen. *(From Barkauskas V et al:* Health & physical assessment, *ed 3, St Louis, 2002, Mosby.)*

predictive by itself. Laboratory studies used in the assessment of gastrointestinal function, liver function, and pancreatic function are found in Tables 33-3, 33-4, and 33-5, respectively.

DIAGNOSTIC PROCEDURES

To complete the assessment of the critically ill patient with gastrointestinal dysfunction, the patient's diagnostic tests are reviewed. Although many procedures exist for diagnosing gastrointestinal disease, their application in the critically ill patient is limited. Only procedures that are currently used in the critical care setting are presented here.

The nursing management of a patient undergoing a diagnostic procedure involves a variety of interventions. Nursing actions include preparing the patient psychologically and physically for the procedure, monitoring the patient's responses to the procedure, and assessing the patient after the procedure. Preparing the patient includes teaching the patient about the procedure, answering any questions, and transporting and positioning the patient for the procedure. Monitoring the patient's responses to the procedure includes observing the patient for signs of pain, anxiety, or hemorrhage and monitoring vital signs. Assessing the patient after the procedure includes observing for complications of the procedure and medicating the patient for any postprocedural discomfort. Any evidence of gastrointestinal bleeding should be immediately reported to the physician, and emergency measures to maintain circulation must be initiated.

ENDOSCOPY

Available in several forms, fiberoptic endoscopy is a diagnostic procedure for the direct visualization and evaluation of the gastrointestinal tract. Endoscopy can provide information regarding lesions, mucosal changes, obstructions, and motility dysfunction, and a biopsy specimen can be obtained during the procedure. The main difference between the various diagnostic forms is the length of the anatomic area that can be examined. Esophagogastroduodenoscopy (EGD) permits viewing of the upper gastrointestinal tract from the esophagus to

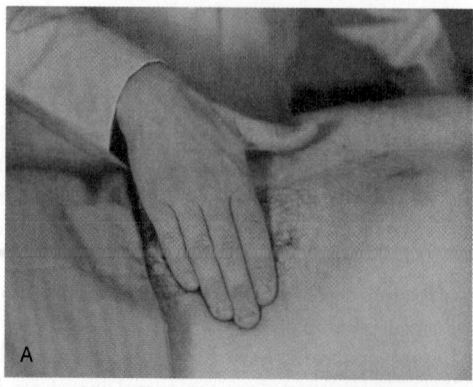
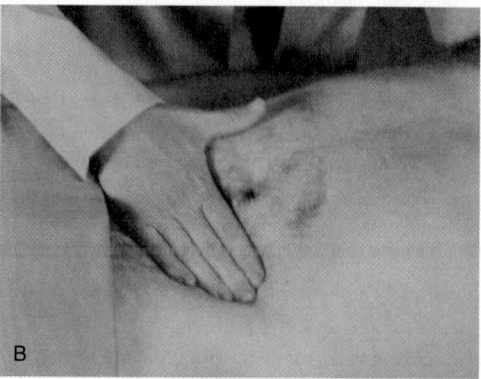

Figure 33-4 Palpation of the abdomen. *A,* Light. *B,* Deep. *(From Barkauskas V et al:* Health & physical assessment, *ed 3, St Louis, 2002, Mosby.)*

TABLE 33-2 Assessment Findings of Common Gastrointestinal Disorders

Condition	History	Symptoms	Signs
Right Lower Quadrant (RLQ) of the Abdomen			
Appendicitis	Children (except infants) and young adults	Anorexia Nausea Early vague epigastric, periumbilical, or generalized pain after 12-24 hours; RLQ at McBurney's point	Signs may be absent early Vomiting Localized RLQ guarding and tenderness after 12-24 hours Rovsing's sign: pain in RLQ with application of pressure, iliopsoas sign Obturator sign White blood cell count of 10,000/mm^3 or shift to left Low-grade fever Cutaneous hyperesthesia in RLQ Signs highly variable
Perforated duodenal ulcer	Prior history	Abrupt onset pain in epigastric area or RLQ	Tenderness in epigastric area or RLQ Signs of peritoneal irritation Heme-positive stool Increased white blood cell count
Cecal volvulus	Seen most often in older adults	Abrupt severe abdominal pain	Distention Localized tenderness Tympany
Strangulated hernia	Any age Women: femoral Men: inguinal	Severe localized pain If bowel obstructed, generalized pain	If bowel obstructed, distention
Right Upper Quadrant (RUQ) of the Abdomen			
Liver hepatitis	Any age, often young blood product user Drug addict	Fatigue Malaise Anorexia Pain in RUQ Low-grade fever May have severe fulminating disease with liver failure	Hepatic tenderness Hepatomegaly Bilirubin elevated Jaundice Lymphocytosis in one third of cases Liver enzymes elevated Hepatitis A or B or antibodies to the viruses may be found
Acute hepatic congestion	Usually older adults with acute heart failure Pericardial disease Pulmonary embolism	Symptoms of acute heart failure	Hepatomegaly Acute heart failure
Biliary stones, colic	"Fair, fat, forty" (90%) but can be 30 to 80 years old	Anorexia Nausea Pain severe in RUQ or epigastric area Episodes lasting 15 minutes to hours	Tenderness in RUQ Jaundice
Acute cholecystitis	"Fair, fat, forty" (90%) but may be 30 to 80 years old	Severe RUQ or epigastric pain Episodes prolonged up to 6 hours	Vomiting Tenderness in RUQ Peritoneal irritation signs Increased white blood cell count
Perforated peptic ulcer	Any age	Abrupt RUQ pain	Tenderness in epigastrium and/or right quadrant Peritoneal irritation signs Free air in abdomen
Left Upper Quadrant (LUQ) of the Abdomen			
Splenic trauma	Blunt trauma to LUQ of abdomen	Pain: LUQ pain of the abdomen often referred to the left shoulder (Kehr's sign)	Hypotension Syncope Increased dyspnea X-ray studies show enlarged spleen

Continued

TABLE 33-2   Assessment Findings of Common Gastrointestinal Disorders—*cont'd*

Condition	History	Symptoms	Signs
Pancreatitis	Alcohol abuse Pancreatic duct Obstruction Infection Cholecystitis	Pain in LUQ or epigastric region radiating to the back or chest	Fever Rigidity Rebound tenderness Nausea Vomiting Jaundice Cullen's sign Turner's sign Abdominal distention Diminished bowel sounds
Pyloric obstruction	Duodenal ulcer	Weight loss Gastric upset Vomiting	Increasing dullness in LUQ Visible peristaltic waves in epigastric region
Left Lower Quadrant (LLQ) of the Abdomen			
Ulcerative colitis	Family history Jewish ancestry	Chronic, watery diarrhea with bloody mucus Anorexia Weight loss Fatigue	Fever Cachexia Anemia Leukocytosis
Colonic diverticulitis	Older than 39 years Low-residue diet	Pain that recurs in LUQ	Fever Vomiting Chills Diarrhea Tenderness over descending colon

Modified from Barkauskas V et al: *Health & physical assessment,* ed 3, St Louis, 2002, Mosby.

TABLE 33-3   Selected Laboratory Studies of Gastrointestinal Function

Test	Normal Findings	Clinical Significance of Abnormal Findings
Stool studies	Resident microorganisms: clostridia, enterococci, *Pseudomonas,* a few yeasts Fat: 2-6 g/24 hr Pus: none Occult blood: none (ortho-toluidine or guaiac test) Ova and parasites: none	Detection of *Salmonella typhi* (typhoid fever), *Shigella* (dysentery), *Vibrio cholerae* (cholera), *Yersinia* (enterocolitis), *Escherichia coli* (gastroenteritis), *Staphylococcus aureus* (food poisoning), *Clostridium botulinum* (food poisoning), *Clostridium perfringens* (food poisoning), *Aeromonas* (gastroenteritis) Steatorrhea (increased values) can result from intestinal malabsorption or pancreatic insufficiency. Large amounts of pus are associated with chronic ulcerative colitis, abscesses, and anorectal fistula. Positive test results associated with bleeding Detection of *Entamoeba histolytica* (amebiasis), *Giardia lamblia* (giardiasis), and worms
D-Xylose absorption	5-hr urinary excretion: 4.5 g/L Peak blood level: >30 mg/dL	Differentiation of pancreatic steatorrhea (normal D-xylose absorption) from intestinal steatorrhea (impaired D-xylose absorption)
Gastric acid stimulation	11-20 mEq/hr after stimulation	Detection of duodenal ulcers, Zollinger-Ellison syndrome (increased values), gastric atrophy, gastric carcinoma (decreased values)
Manometry*	Values vary at different levels of the intestine	Inadequate swallowing, motility, sphincter function
Culture and sensitivity of duodenal contents	No pathogens	Detection of *Salmonella typhi* (typhoid fever)

From McCance KL, Huether SE, editors: *Pathophysiology: the biologic basis for disease in adults and children,* ed 5, St Louis, 2006, Mosby.
*Use of water-filled catheters connected to pressure transducers passed into the esophagus, stomach, colon, or rectum to evaluate contractility.

TABLE 33-4 Common Laboratory Studies of Liver Function

Test	Normal Value	Interpretation
Serum Enzymes		
Alkaline phosphatase	13-39 units/mL	Increases with biliary obstruction and cholestatic hepatitis
Aspartate amino transferase (AST; formerly serum glutamate oxaloacetate transaminase [SGOT])	5-40 units/mL	Increases with hepatocellular injury
Alanine amino transferase (ALT; formerly serum glutamate pyruvate transaminase [SGPT])	5-35 units/mL	Increases with hepatocellular injury
Lactate dehydrogenase (LDH)	200-500 units/mL	Isoenzyme LD_5 is elevated with hypoxic and primary liver injury
5'-Nucleotidase	2-11 units/mL	Increases with increase in alkaline phosphatase and cholestatic disorders
Bilirubin Metabolism		
Serum bilirubin		
Indirect (unconjugated)	<0.8 mg/dL	Increases with hemolysis (lysis of red blood cells)
Direct (conjugated)	0.2-0.4 mg/dL	Increases with hepatocellular injury or obstruction
Total	<1.0 mg/dL	Increases with biliary obstruction
Urine bilirubin	0	Decreases with biliary obstruction
Urine urobilinogen	0-4 mg/24 hr	Increases with hemolysis or shunting or portal blood flow
Serum Proteins		
Albumin	3.3-5.5 g/dL	Reduced with hepatocellular injury
Globulin	2.5-3.5 g/dL	Increases with hepatitis
Total	6-7 g/dL	
Albumin-to-globulin (A/G) ratio	1.5-2.5:1	Ratio reverses with chronic hepatitis or other chronic liver disease
Transferrin	250-300 μg/dL	Liver damage with decreased values, iron deficiency with increased values
Alpha-fetoprotein	6-20 ng/mL	Elevated values in primary hepatocellular carcinoma
Blood Clotting Functions		
Prothrombin time	11.5-14 sec or 90%	Increases with chronic liver disease (cirrhosis) or vitamin K deficiency
	100% of control	
Partial thromboplastin time	25-40 sec	Increases with severe liver disease or heparin therapy
Bromsulphalein (BSP) excretion	<6% retention in 45 min	Increased retention with hepatocellular injury

From McCance KL, Huether SE, editors: *Pathophysiology: the biologic basis for disease in adults and children*, ed 5, St Louis, 2006, Mosby.

TABLE 33-5 Common Laboratory Studies of Pancreatic Function

Test	Normal Value	Clinical Significance
Serum amylase	60-180 Somogyi units/mL	Elevated levels with pancreatic inflammation
Serum lipase	1.5 Somogyi units/mL	Elevated levels with pancreatic inflammation (may be elevated with other conditions; differentiates with amylase, isoenzyme study)
Urine amylase	35-260 Somogyi units/hr	Elevated levels with pancreatic inflammation
Secretin test	Volume 1.8 mL/kg/hr Bicarbonate concentration: >80 mEq/L Bicarbonate output: >10 mEq/L/30 sec	Decreased volume with pancreatic disease because secretin stimulates pancreatic secretion
Stool fat	2-5 g/25 hr	Measures fatty acids: decreased pancreatic lipase increases stool fat

From McCance KL, Huether SE, editors: *Pathophysiology: the biologic basis for disease in adults and children*, ed 5, St Louis, 2006, Mosby.

the upper duodenum, and it is used to evaluate sources of upper gastrointestinal bleeding (see Fig. 33-3). Colonoscopy permits viewing of the lower gastrointestinal tract from the rectum to the distal ileum, and it is used to evaluate sources of lower gastrointestinal bleeding. Enteroscopy permits viewing of the small bowel beyond the ligament of Treitz, and it is used to evaluate sources of gastrointestinal bleeding that have not been identified previously with EGD or colonoscopy. Endoscopic retrograde cholangiopancreatography (ERCP) enables viewing of the biliary and pancreatic ducts, and it is used in the evaluation of pancreatitis. During this procedure, contrast is injected into the ducts through the endoscope, and radiographs are obtained.[7] Endoscopy also provides therapeutic benefits for a variety of conditions, including the treatment of gastrointestinal bleeding.[8]

Nursing Management. The patient should take nothing by mouth (NPO) for 6 to 12 hours before endoscopy of the upper gastrointestinal tract. The patient should receive a bowel preparation before endoscopy of the lower gastrointestinal tract.[7] In some cases, the procedure is performed at the patient's bedside, particularly if the patient is actively bleeding and too unstable to be moved to the gastrointestinal suite. Fiberoptic endoscopy may present risks for the patient. Although rare, potential complications include perforation of the gastrointestinal tract, hemorrhage, aspiration, vasovagal stimulation, and oversedation.[7] Signs of perforation include abdominal pain and distention, gastrointestinal bleeding, and fever.[9]

ANGIOGRAPHY

Angiography is used as a diagnostic and a therapeutic procedure. Diagnostically, it is used to evaluate the status of the gastrointestinal circulation (Fig. 33-5).[7] Therapeutically, it is used to achieve transcatheter control of gastrointestinal bleeding.[8] Angiography is used in the diagnosis of upper gastrointestinal (UGI) bleeding only when endoscopy fails, and it is used to treat patients (approximately 15%) whose gastrointestinal bleeding is not stopped with medical measures or endoscopic treatment.[8] Angiography also is used to evaluate cirrhosis, portal hypertension, intestinal ischemia, and other vascular abnormalities.[7]

The radiologist cannulates the femoral artery with a needle and passes a guidewire through it into the aorta. The needle is removed, and an angiographic catheter is inserted over the guidewire. The catheter is advanced into the vessel supplying the portion of the gastrointestinal tract that is being studied. After the catheter is in place, contrast medium is injected, and serial radiographs are obtained. If the procedure is undertaken to control bleeding, vasopressin (Pitressin Synthetic) or embolic material (Gelfoam) is injected after the site of the bleeding is located.[8]

Nursing Management. Complications include overt and covert bleeding at the femoral puncture site, neurovascular compromise of the affected leg, and sensitivity to the contrast medium. Before the procedure, the patient should be asked about any sensitivities to contrast. Postprocedural assessment involves monitoring vital signs, observing the injection site for

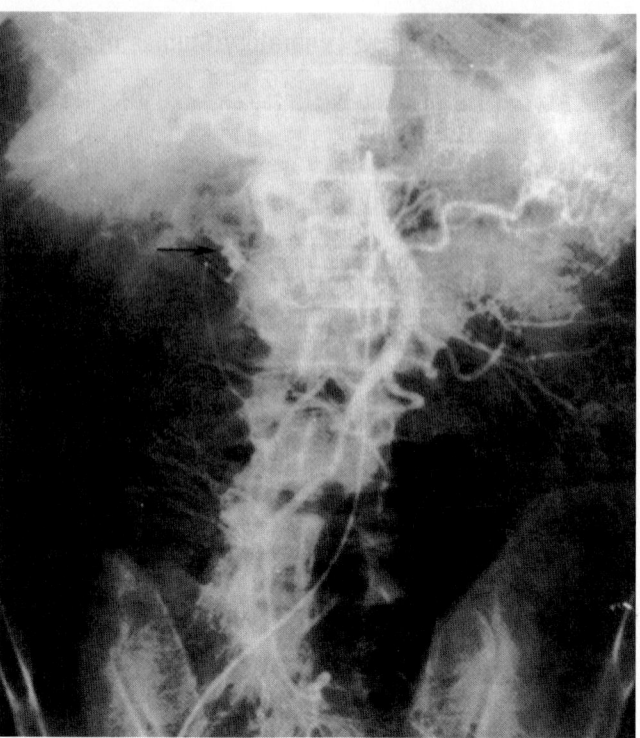

Figure 33-5 Arteriogram of superior mesenteric artery shows diverticular bleeding. Notice the area of contrast extravasation. *(From Doughty DB, Jackson DB: Gastrointestinal disorders, St Louis, 1993, Mosby.)*

bleeding, and assessing neurovascular integrity distal to the injection site every 15 minutes for the first 1 to 2 hours. Depending on how the puncture site is stabilized after the procedure, the patient may have to remain flat in bed for a specified length of time. Any evidence of bleeding or neurovascular impairment must be immediately reported to the physician.[10]

PLAIN ABDOMINAL SERIES

Although numerous radiologic studies are available to investigate gastrointestinal dysfunction further, many of these studies are not performed on the critically ill patient. The radiologic study that is performed most often is the plain abdominal series (Fig. 33-6). An abdominal film is useful in the diagnosis of a bowel obstruction and perforation.[11,12]

Air in the bowel serves as a contrast medium to aid in the visualization of the bowel. Gas patterns (the presence of gas inside or outside the bowel lumen and the distribution of gas in dilated and nondilated bowel) are best revealed by plain x-ray films. Common radiologic signs of free air in the abdomen include the presence of air on both sides of the bowel wall and the presence of air in the right upper quadrant anterior to the liver.[11,12] Table 33-6 lists common radiologic findings. The abdominal radiographs are used to verify nasogastric or feeding tube placement.

Nursing Management. An abdominal radiographic series can be obtained at the patient's bedside using a portable x-ray machine. The series includes two views of the abdomen:

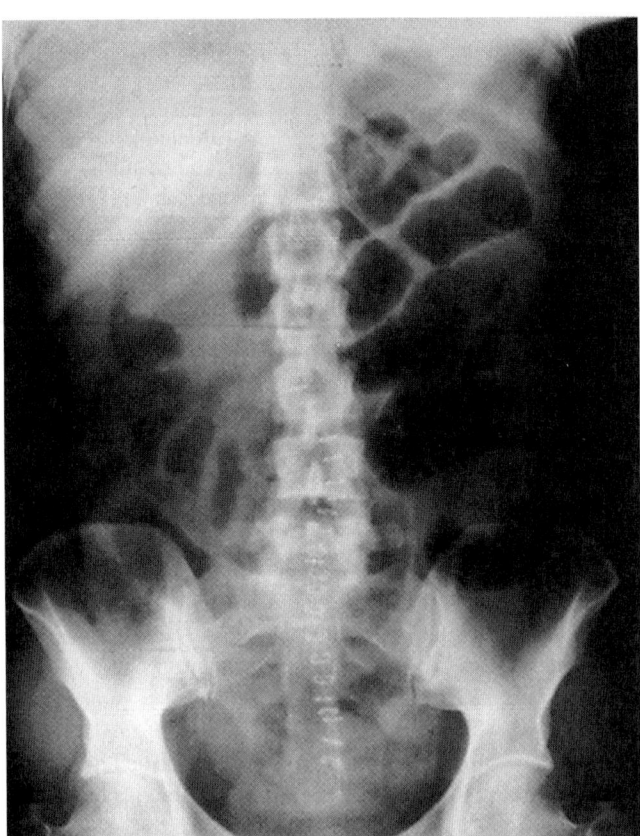

Figure 33-6 Abdominal flat plate radiograph. Notice the dilated loops of small bowel, which are consistent with the diagnosis of postoperative ileus. *(From Doughty DB, Jackson DB:* Gastrointestinal disorders, *St Louis, 1993, Mosby.)*

Ultrasound is easily performed, noninvasive, and well tolerated by critically ill patients. The procedure requires only that the patient lie still for 20 to 30 minutes. No special interventions are required before or after the procedure.[10]

COMPUTED TOMOGRAPHY OF THE ABDOMEN

Computed tomography (CT) is a radiographic examination that provides cross-sectional images of internal anatomy. It may be used to evaluate abdominal vasculature and identify focal points found on nuclear scans as solid, cystic, inflammatory, or vascular. CT detects mass lesions more than 2 cm in diameter and allows visualization and evaluation of many different aspects of gastrointestinal disease. It is particularly useful in identifying pancreatic pseudocysts, abdominal abscesses, biliary obstructions, and a variety of gastrointestinal neoplastic lesions.[14]

The procedure involves taking the patient to the CT scanner, placing the patient on the table, and inserting the area to be studied into the opening of the scanner. Multiple x-ray scans are obtained at a variety of angles, and a computer synthesizes images of the structures being studied. Intravenous or gastrointestinal contrast may be used to facilitate the imaging of the blood vessels or the gastrointestinal tract, respectively.[14]

Nursing Management. Before the procedure, the patient should be asked about any sensitivities to contrast. The procedure usually takes 30 minutes without contrast and 60 minutes with contrast, during which time the patient must lie very still. No special interventions are required before or after the procedure.[10]

one in the supine and one in the upright position. For patients unable to sit upright, a lateral decubitus film may be obtained with the patient's left side down. No special interventions are required before or after the procedure.[10]

ABDOMINAL ULTRASOUND

Abdominal ultrasound is useful in evaluating the status of the gallbladder and biliary system, the liver, the spleen, and the pancreas. It plays a key role in the diagnosis of many acute abdominal conditions, such as acute cholecystitis and biliary obstructions, because it is sensitive in detecting obstructive lesions and ascites. Ultrasound is used to identify gallstones and hepatic abscesses, candidiasis, and hematomas. Intestinal gas, ascites, and extreme obesity can interfere with transmission of the sound waves and limit the usefulness of the procedure.[13]

The procedure uses sound waves to produce echoes that are converted into electrical energy and transferred to a screen for viewing. A transducer, which emits and receives sound waves, is moved slowly over the area of the abdomen being studied. Tissues with various densities produce different echoes, which translate into the different structures on the viewing screen.[13]

Nursing Management. An ultrasound scan can be obtained at the patient's bedside using a portable scanning unit.

HEPATOBILIARY SCINTIGRAPHY

A hepatobiliary scan is a nuclear scan that is used to assess the status of the liver and the biliary system. It is valuable in detecting abnormalities such as acute and chronic cholecystitis, biliary obstruction, and bile leaks, and it yields additional information regarding organ size.[15]

The scan involves injecting an intravenous technetium 99m (^{99m}Tc)–labeled iminodiacetic agent (radiotracer), such as disofenin (DISIDA) or mebrofenin (TMBIDA). Serial images are then obtained using a gamma (scintillation) camera.[13] The liver cells take up 80% to 90% of the radiotracer, which is then secreted into the bile and transported throughout the biliary system, allowing visualization of the biliary tract, the gallbladder, and the duodenum.[7] Pooling of the iminodiacetic agent around the liver indicates poor uptake and hepatocellular dysfunction.[15]

Nursing Management. The hepatobiliary scan is relatively noninvasive and safe, although the patient must be transported to the nuclear medicine department. The patient may need to maintain NPO status for 2 to 4 hours before the procedure. Sedation is usually not required, but the patient must be able to lie flat and still for 60 minutes during the scanning procedure. No special interventions are required after the procedure.[10]

TABLE 33-6   Plain Film Findings

Finding	Appearance	Associations
Pneumoperitoneum	Air seen under diaphragm on upright chest or overlying right lobe of liver on left lateral decubitus films	Most commonly associated with bowel perforation, although other causes exist
Peritoneal fluid	Medial displacement of colon separated from flank stripes by fluid density on flat plate	Ascites or hemorrhage
Adynamic ileus	Dilatation of entire intestinal tract including stomach	Many causes, including trauma, infection (intraabdominal and extraabdominal), metabolic disease, and medications (e.g., narcotics)
Sentinel loop	Single distended loop of small bowel containing an air-fluid level	Represents localized ileus associated with localized inflammatory process such as cholecystitis, appendicitis, or pancreatitis
Small bowel obstruction	Dilated loops of small bowel (distinguished by valvulae conniventes, thin, transverse linear densities that extend completely across diameter of bowel) with air-fluid levels	Can be associated with other serious pathology such as incarcerated hernia, appendicitis, or mesenteric ischemia
Large bowel obstruction	Dilated loops, usually more peripheral in the abdomen (distinguished by haustra—short, thick indentations that do not completely cross bowel and are less frequently spaced than valvulae conniventes)	Can be associated with diverticulitis and malignancy
Cecal volvulus	Usually found in middle or upper abdomen to the left; often kidney shaped	
Sigmoid volvulus	Dilated loop of colon arising from left side of pelvis and projecting obliquely upward toward right side of abdomen	
Early ischemic bowel findings	May resemble mechanical obstruction with dilated loops and air-fluid levels	
Later ischemic bowel findings	May resemble a dynamic ileus; thumbprinting (edema of bowel wall with convex indentations of lumen) and pneumatosis intestinalis (linear or mottled gas pattern in bowel wall)	
Gallbladder emergency findings	Ring of air outlining the gallbladder Air in biliary tree combined with signs of small bowel obstruction, possibly with visible calculus in pelvis	Emphysematous cholecystitis Gallstone ileus
Abdominal aortic aneurysm (AAA)	Usually appears left of midline on supine film and anterior to spine in lateral projection; calcification in wall of aneurysm is variable	Ruptured or leaking AAA may reveal loss of psoas shadows or large soft tissue mass

From Hendrickson M, Naparst TR: Abdominal surgical emergencies in the elderly, *Emerg Med Clin North Am* 21:937, 2003.

GASTROINTESTINAL BLEEDING SCAN

A scan of gastrointestinal bleeding is used to evaluate the presence of an active bleed, to identify the site of the bleed, and to assess the need for an arteriogram.[15] The gastrointestinal bleeding scan is sensitive to low rates of bleeding (0.1 to 0.35 mL/min),[15] but it is reliable only when the patient is actively bleeding.[7]

The scan is usually performed with intravenous ^{99m}Tc-labeled sulfur colloid or ^{99m}Tc-labeled red blood cells (radiotracers). To tag the red blood cells, a blood sample is taken from the patient. The red blood cells are separated, tagged with ^{99m}Tc, and then returned to the patient. Serial images are obtained using a gamma (scintillation) camera. Extravasation and accumulation or pooling of radiotracers in the bowel lumen indicates active bleeding is occurring and facilitates identification of the site.[7,15]

Nursing Management. The gastrointestinal bleeding scan is relatively noninvasive and safe, although the patient must be transported to the nuclear medicine department. Sedation usually is not required, but the patient must be able to lie flat and still for 60 minutes or longer during the scanning procedure. No special interventions are required after the procedure.[10]

MAGNETIC RESONANCE IMAGING

Magnetic resonance imaging (MRI) is used to identify tumors, abscesses, hemorrhages, and vascular abnormalities. Small tumors, whose tissue densities are different from those of the surrounding cells, can be identified before they would be visible on any other radiographic test.[7] Magnetic resonance angiography is a form of MRI that is used to assess blood vessels and blood flow.[16] Magnetic resonance cholangiopancreatography (MRCP) is a form of MRI used to evaluate the biliary and pancreatic ducts.[17]

During MRI, the patient is placed in a large magnetic field that stimulates the protons of the body. Introduction of radiofrequency waves causes resonance of these protons, which then emit an image that a computer is able to reconstruct for viewing. Intravenous administration of a non–iodine-based contrast medium enhances the image by influencing the magnetic environment and signal intensity.[18]

Nursing Management. The MRI procedure is lengthy and requires that the patient be transported to the scanner. The patient must lie motionless in a tight, enclosed space (if a closed MRI scanner is used), and sedation may be necessary. Removal of all metal from the patient's body is essential because the basis of MRI is a magnetic field. Patients with implanted metal objects are not candidates for the procedure. No special interventions are required after the procedure.[10]

PERCUTANEOUS LIVER BIOPSY

Liver biopsy is a diagnostic procedure that is used to evaluate liver disease. Morphologic, biochemical, bacteriologic, and immunologic studies are performed on the tissue sample to diagnose liver disorders such as cirrhosis, hepatitis, infections, or cancer. The biopsy can also yield information about the progression of the patient's disease and response to therapy.[7,19]

Percutaneous liver biopsy can be performed at the bedside or in the imaging department using an imaging-guided needle. Before the test, the patient should maintain NPO status for 6 hours and have blood drawn for coagulation studies. The procedure is performed by anesthetizing the pericapsular tissue, inserting a coring or suction needle between the eighth and ninth intercostal space into the liver while the patient holds his or her breath on exhalation, withdrawing the needle with the sample, and applying pressure to stop the bleeding.[7]

Nursing Management. During the liver biopsy, the patient may experience a deep pressure sensation or dull pain that radiates to the right shoulder. Afterward the procedure, the patient is positioned on the right side for 2 hours and kept on complete bed rest for the next 6 to 8 hours.[7,19] Hemorrhage is the major complication associated with a liver biopsy, although it occurs in less than 1% of patients. Other complications include damage to neighboring organs (e.g., kidney, lung, colon, gallbladder), bile peritonitis, hemothorax, and infection at the needle site. Puncturing the gallbladder can cause leakage of the bile into the abdominal cavity, resulting in peritonitis.[19]

Summary

History

- A review of the patient's current illness and symptoms, including the presence or absence of bleeding, abdominal pain, and dysphagia, is an important part of obtaining the patient's history.

- As the patient's condition permits, additional information regarding the patient's personal and social status, general health status, and family history, including nutritional intake, oral hygiene, and bowel elimination, should be obtained.

Clinical Assessment

- To prevent stimulation of gastrointestinal activity, the order for the assessment should be changed to inspection, auscultation, percussion, and palpation.
- Inspection should focus on the oral cavity, skin, and abdomen.
- Auscultation provides clinical data regarding the status of the bowel's motility.
- Normal bowel sounds are high-pitched, gurgling sounds that occur approximately every 5 to 15 seconds, and colonic sounds are low-pitched and have a rumbling quality.
- Percussion is used to elicit information about deep organs, such as the liver, spleen, and pancreas.
- Light and deep palpation methods are used to detect pathologic conditions of the abdomen.

Laboratory Studies

- No single laboratory study provides an overall picture of the various organs' functional state.

Diagnostic Procedures

- Fiberoptic endoscopy is a diagnostic procedure for the direct visualization and evaluation of the gastrointestinal tract.
- Angiography is used diagnostically to evaluate the status of the gastrointestinal circulation and therapeutically to achieve control of gastrointestinal bleeding.
- An abdominal radiograph is useful in the diagnosis of a bowel obstruction and perforation.
- Abdominal ultrasound is useful in evaluating the status of the gallbladder and biliary system, the liver, the spleen, and the pancreas.
- CT provides cross-sectional images of the internal anatomy, and it is used to evaluate abdominal vasculature and identify focal points found on nuclear scans as solid, cystic, inflammatory, or vascular.
- A hepatobiliary scan is a nuclear scan that is used to assess the status of the liver and the biliary system.
- A gastrointestinal bleeding scan is used to evaluate the presence of an active gastrointestinal bleed, to identify the site of the bleed, and to assess the need for an arteriogram.
- MRI is used to identify tumors, abscesses, hemorrhages, and vascular abnormalities.
- Liver biopsy is a diagnostic procedure that is used to evaluate liver disease.

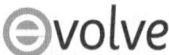 Be sure to check out the bonus material, including free self-assessment exercises, on the Evolve web site at http://evolve.elsevier.com/Urden/.

References

1. O'Toole MT: Advanced assessment of the abdomen and gastrointestinal problems, *Nurs Clin North Am* 24:771, 1990.
2. Baid H: The process of conducting a physical assessment: a nursing perspective, *Br J Nurs* 15:710, 2006.
3. Seidel HM et al: *Mosby's guide to physical examination*, ed 6, St Louis, 2006, Mosby.
4. Barkauskas V et al: *Health and physical assessment*, ed 3, St Louis, 2002, Mosby.
5. Thompson JM et al: *Mosby's clinical nursing*, ed 5, St Louis, 2002, Mosby.
6. O'Hanlon-Nicholas T: Basic assessment series: gastrointestinal system, *Am J Nurs* 98(4):48, 1998.
7. Society of Gastroenterology Nurses and Associates Core Curriculum Committee: *Gastroenterology nursing: a core curriculum*, ed 3, St Louis, 2003, Mosby.
8. Lefkovitz Z et al: Radiologic diagnosis and treatment of gastrointestinal hemorrhage and ischemia, *Med Clin North Am* 86:1357, 2002.
9. Ginzburg L: Complications of endoscopy, *Gastrointest Endosc Clin N Am* 17:405, 2007.
10. Pangana KD, Pangana TJ: *Mosby's diagnostic and laboratory test reference*, ed 8, St Louis, 2006, Mosby.
11. Flaser MH, Goldberg E: Acute abdominal pain, *Med Clin North Am* 90:481, 2006.
12. Yeh EL, McNamara RM: Abdominal pain, *Clin Geriatr Med* 23:255, 2007.
13. Puylaert JB: Ultrasonography of the acute abdomen: gastrointestinal conditions, *Radiol Clin North Am* 41:1227, 2003.
14. Kundra V, Silverman PM: Impact of multislice CT on imaging of acute abdominal disease, *Radiol Clin North Am* 41:1083, 2003.
15. Zuckier LS, Freeman LM: Selective role of nuclear medicine in evaluating the acute abdomen, *Radiol Clin North Am* 41:1275, 2003.
16. Anderson CM: GI magnetic resonance angiography, *Gastrointest Endosc* 55: S42, 2002.
17. Fulcher AS, Turner MA: MR cholangiopancreatography, *Radiol Clin North Am* 40:1363, 2002.
18. Pedrosa I, Rofsky NM: MR imaging in abdominal emergencies, *Radiol Clin North Am* 41:1243, 2003.
19. Crockett SD et al: Do we still need a liver biopsy? Are the serum fibrosis tests ready for prime time? *Clin Liver Dis* 10:513, 2006.

$\mathcal{U}$nderstanding the pathology of a disease, the areas of assessment on which to focus, and the usual medical management allows the critical care nurse to accurately anticipate and plan nursing interventions. This chapter focuses on gastrointestinal disorders commonly seen in the critical care environment.

ACUTE GASTROINTESTINAL HEMORRHAGE

DESCRIPTION

Gastrointestinal hemorrhage is a potentially life-threatening emergency that remains a common complication of critical illness[1] and results in 250,000 to 300,000 hospital admissions yearly.[2] Despite advances in medical knowledge and nursing care, the mortality rate for patients with acute gastrointestinal bleeding remains at 10%.[1,3]

ETIOLOGY

Gastrointestinal hemorrhage occurs from bleeding in the upper or lower gastrointestinal tract. The ligament of Treitz is the anatomic division used to differentiate between the two areas. Bleeding proximal to the ligament is considered to be upper gastrointestinal in origin, and bleeding distal to the ligament is considered to be lower gastrointestinal in origin.[1,4] The various causes of acute gastrointestinal hemorrhage are listed in Box 34-1.[3-5] Only the three main causes of gastrointestinal hemorrhage commonly seen in the intensive care unit (ICU) are discussed further.

Peptic Ulcer Disease. Peptic ulcer disease (gastric and duodenal ulcers), which results from the breakdown of the gastromuscosal lining, is the leading cause of upper gastrointestinal hemorrhage, accounting for approximately 21% of cases.[3,4,6] Normally, protection of the gastric mucosa from the digestive effects of gastric secretions is accomplished in several ways. First, the gastroduodenal mucosa is coated by a glycoprotein mucus barrier that protects the surface of the epithelium from hydrogen ions and other noxious substances present in the gut lumen.[7,8] Adequate gastric mucosal blood flow is necessary to maintain this mucosal barrier function. Second, gastroduodenal epithelial cells are protected structurally against damage from

acid and pepsin because they are connected by tight junctions that help prevent acid penetration. Third, prostaglandins and nitric oxide protect the mucosal barrier by stimulating mucus and bicarbonate secretion and inhibiting the secretion of acid.[8]

Peptic ulceration occurs when these protective mechanisms cease to function, allowing gastroduodenal mucosal breakdown. After the mucosal lining is penetrated, gastric secretions autodigest the layers of the stomach or duodenum, leading to injury of the mucosal and submucosal layers. This results in damaged blood vessels and subsequent hemorrhage. The two main causes of disruption of gastroduodenal mucosal resistance are nonsteroidal anti-inflammatory drugs and the bacterial action of *Helicobacter pylori.*[4,9]

Stress-Related Mucosal Disease. Stress-related mucosal disease (SRMD) is an acute erosive gastritis that covers both types of mucosal lesions that are often found in the critically ill patient: stress-related injury and discrete stress ulcers.[10,11] These abnormalities develop within hours of admission.[10] They range from superficial mucosal erosions to deep focal lesions and usually affect the upper gastrointestinal tract.[10] SRMD occurs by means of the same pathophysiologic mechanisms as peptic ulcer disease, but the main cause of disruption of gastric mucosal resistance is increased acid production and decreased mucosal blood flow, resulting in ischemia and degeneration of the mucosal lining.[10,11] Patients at risk include those in situations of high physiologic stress, such as occur with mechanical ventilation, extensive burns, severe trauma, major surgery, shock, sepsis, coagulopathy, or acute neurologic disease.[10,11] Gastroduodenal lesions are estimated to occur in 75% to 100% of ICU patients within 24 hours of admission.[10] SRMD is a leading cause of upper gastrointestinal hemorrhage, accounting for approximately 15% of cases.[3,11]

Esophagogastric Varices. Esophagogastric varices are engorged and distended blood vessels of the esophagus and proximal stomach that develop as a result of portal hypertension caused by hepatic cirrhosis, a chronic disease of the liver that results in damage to the liver sinusoids (Fig. 34-1). Without adequate sinusoid function, resistance to portal blood flow is increased, and pressures within the liver are elevated. This leads to increased portal venous pressure (portal hypertension), causing collateral circulation to divert portal blood from areas of high pressure within the liver to adjacent areas of low pressure

UPPER GASTROINTESTINAL TRACT
- Peptic ulcer disease
- Stress-related erosive syndrome
- Esophagogastric varices
- Mallory-Weiss tear
- Esophagitis
- Neoplasm
- Aortoenteric fistula
- Angiodysplasia

LOWER GASTROINTESTINAL TRACT
- Diverticulosis
- Angiodysplasia
- Neoplasm
- Inflammatory bowel disease
- Trauma
- Infectious colitis
- Radiation colitis
- Ischemia
- Aortoenteric fistula
- Hemorrhoids

TABLE 34-1 Clinical Classification of Hemorrhage

Class	Blood Loss (%)	Clinical Signs and Symptoms
1	≤15	Pulse rate: normal or <100 beats/min (supine) Capillary refill <3 sec Urine output: adequate (30-35 mL/hr) Orthostatic hypotension Apprehensive
2	15-30	Pulse rate: increased (>100 beats/min) Capillary refill: sluggish Pulse pressure: decreased Blood pressure: normal (supine) Tachypnea Urine output: low (25-30 mL/hr)
3	30-40	Pulse rate: 120+ beats/min (supine) Hypotension Skin: cool, pale Confused Hyperventilating Urine output: low (5-15 mL/hr)
4	≥40	Profoundly hypotensive Pulse rate: 140+ beats/min Confused, lethargic Urine output minimal

From Klein DG: Physiologic response to traumatic shock. *AACN Clin Issues Crit Care Nurs* 1:505-521, 1990.

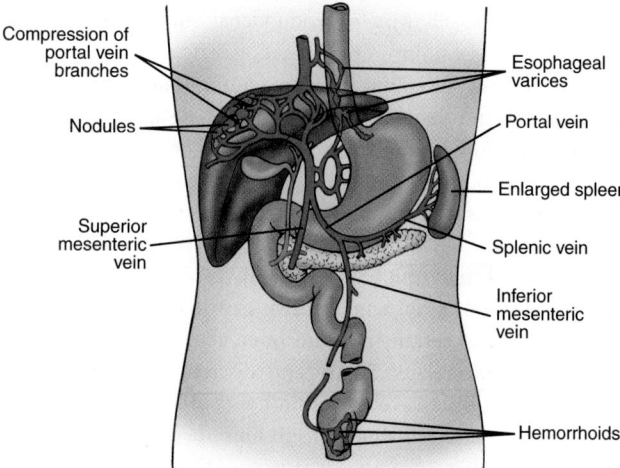

Figure 34-1 Esophageal varices caused by cirrhosis. (*Modified from Powell LW, Piper DW:* Fundamentals of gastroenterology, *Sydney, 1991, McGraw-Hill. Reproduced with permission of the McGraw-Hill Companies.*)

outside the liver, such as into the veins of the esophagus, the spleen, the intestines, and the stomach. The tiny, thin-walled vessels of the esophagus and proximal stomach that receive this diverted blood lack sturdy mucosal protection. The vessels become engorged and dilated, forming esophagogastric varices that are vulnerable to damage from gastric secretions and that may result in subsequent rupture and massive hemorrhage.[12] The risk of variceal bleeding increases with disease severity and variceal size, but overall, bleeding occurs in up to 30% of patients with medium or large varices, and only 50% of patients stop bleeding spontaneously.[12,13]

PATHOPHYSIOLOGY

Gastrointestinal hemorrhage is a life-threatening disorder that is characterized by acute, massive bleeding. Regardless of the cause, acute gastrointestinal hemorrhage results in hypovolemic

shock, initiation of the shock response, and development of multiple organ dysfunction syndrome if left untreated (see Concept Map).[8] However, the most common cause of death in cases of gastrointestinal hemorrhage is exacerbation of the underlying disease, not intractable hypovolemic shock.

ASSESSMENT AND DIAGNOSIS

The initial clinical presentation of the patient with acute gastrointestinal hemorrhage is that of a patient in hypovolemic shock, and the clinical presentation depends on the amount of blood lost (Table 34-1).[8] Hematemesis (bright red or brown, coffee grounds emesis), hematochezia (bright red stools), and melena (black, tarry, or dark red stools) are the hallmarks of gastrointestinal hemorrhage.[1,4,5]

Hematemesis. The patient who is vomiting blood is usually bleeding from a source above the duodenojejunal junction; reverse peristalsis is seldom sufficient to cause hematemesis if the bleeding point is below this area. The hematemesis may be bright red or look like coffee grounds, depending on the amount of gastric contents at the time of bleeding and the length of time the blood has been in contact with gastric secretions. Gastric acid converts bright red hemoglobin to brown hematin, accounting for the coffee grounds appearance of the emesis. Bright red emesis results from profuse bleeding with little contact with gastric secretions.[1]

Hematochezia and Melena. The presence of blood in the gastrointestinal tract results in increased peristalsis and diarrhea. Hematochezia (bright red stool) occurs from massive lower gastrointestinal hemorrhage and, if rapid enough, upper gastrointestinal hemorrhage. Melena (black, tarry, or dark red stool) occurs from digestion of blood from an upper gastrointestinal hemorrhage and may take several days to clear after the bleeding has stopped.[4]

Laboratory Studies. Laboratory tests can help to determine the extent of bleeding, although the patient's hemoglobin level and hematocrit are poor indicators of the severity of blood loss if the bleeding is acute. As whole blood is lost, plasma and red blood cells are lost in the same proportion; if the patient's hematocrit is 45% before a bleeding episode, it will be 45% several hours later.[8] It may take as long as 72 hours for the redistribution of plasma from the extravascular space to the intravascular space to occur and cause the patient's hemoglobin level and hematocrit value to decrease.[14]

Diagnostic Procedures. To isolate and treat the source of bleeding, an urgent fiberoptic endoscopy is usually undertaken. If performed within 12 hours of the bleeding event, endoscopy therapy has a 90% effectiveness rate in achieving hemostasis and reducing mortality.[1,15] Before endoscopy, the patient must be hemodynamically stabilized.[15] Tagged red blood cell scanning or angiography, or both, may be done to assist with localizing and treating a bleeding lesion in the gastrointestinal tract when it is impossible to clearly view the gastrointestinal tract because of continued active bleeding.[1,5]

MEDICAL MANAGEMENT

To reduce mortality related to gastrointestinal hemorrhage, patients at risk should be identified early, and interventions should be implemented to reduce gastric acidity and support the gastric mucosal defense mechanisms. Management of the patient at risk for gastrointestinal hemorrhage should include prophylactic administration of pharmacologic agents for gastric acid neutralization. These agents include antacids, histamine-2 (H_2) antagonists, cytoprotective agents, and proton-pump inhibitors (PPIs).[7,10,11]

Priorities in the medical management of the patient with gastrointestinal hemorrhage include airway protection, fluid resuscitation to achieve hemodynamic stability, correction of comorbid conditions (e.g., coagulopathy), therapeutic procedures to control or stop bleeding, and diagnostic procedures to determine the exact cause of the bleeding.[1,2,7]

Stabilization. The initial treatment priority is the restoration of adequate circulating blood volume to treat or prevent shock. This is accomplished with the administration of intravenous infusions of crystalloids, blood, and blood products.[13,15,16] Hemodynamic monitoring can help to guide fluid replacement therapy,[8] particularly in patients at risk for cardiac failure. Supplemental oxygen therapy is initiated to increase oxygen delivery and improve tissue perfusion.[2,5] Intubation may be necessary in the patient at risk for aspiration or to facilitate gastric lavage.[16] A large nasogastric tube may be inserted to confirm the diagnosis of active

bleeding and to prepare the esophagus, stomach, and proximal duodenum for endoscopic evaluation.[1,2] A urinary drainage catheter should be inserted to monitor urine output.[8]

Controlling the Bleeding. Interventions to control bleeding are the second priority for the patient with gastrointestinal hemorrhage.

Peptic Ulcer Disease. In the patient with gastrointestinal hemorrhage related to peptic ulcer disease, bleeding hemostasis may be accomplished by endoscopic injection therapy in conjunction with thermal or hemostatic clips.[2,17] Endoscopic thermal therapy uses heat to cauterize the bleeding vessel, and endoscopic injection therapy uses a variety of agents such as hypertonic saline, epinephrine, ethanol, and sclerosants to induce localized vasoconstriction of the bleeding vessel.[1,2,17] Intraarterial infusion of vasopressin into the gastric artery or intraarterial injection of an embolizing agent (e.g., Gelfoam pledgets, polyvinyl alcohol particles, coils) can be performed during arteriography to control bleeding after the site has been identified.[2]

Stress-Related Mucosal Disease. In the patient with gastrointestinal hemorrhage caused by SRMD, bleeding hemostasis may be accomplished by intraarterial infusion of vasopressin and intraarterial embolization. Endoscopic therapies provide minimal benefit because of the diffuse nature of the disease.[15]

Esophagogastric Varices. In acute variceal hemorrhage, control of bleeding may be initially accomplished through the use of pharmacologic agents and endoscopic therapies. Intravenous vasopressin, somatostatin, and octreotide can reduce portal venous pressure and slow variceal hemorrhaging by constricting the splanchnic arteriolar bed.[18] Two commonly used endoscopic therapies are injection therapy and variceal band ligation. Endoscopic injection therapy (also referred to as sclerotherapy) controls bleeding by the injection of a sclerosing agent in or around the varices. This creates an inflammatory reaction that induces vasoconstriction and results in the formation of a venous thrombosis. During endoscopic variceal band ligation, bands are placed around the varices to create an obstruction to stop the bleeding.[18]

If these initial therapies fail, esophagogastric balloon tamponade or transjugular intrahepatic portosystemic shunting (TIPS) may be necessary. Balloon tamponade tubes (Sengstaken-Blakemore, Linton, and Minnesota tubes) stop hemorrhaging by applying direct pressure against bleeding vessels while decompressing the stomach.[12,18-20] In a TIPS procedure, a channel between the systemic and portal venous systems is created to redirect portal blood, thereby reducing portal hypertension and decompressing the varices to control bleeding (Fig. 34-2).[1,17,18]

Surgical Intervention. The patient who remains hemodynamically unstable despite volume replacement may need urgent surgery.

Peptic Ulcer Disease. The operative procedure of choice to control bleeding from peptic ulcer disease is a vagotomy and pyloroplasty. During this procedure, the vagus nerve to the stomach is severed, eliminating the autonomic stimulus to the gastric cells and reducing hydrochloric acid production. Because

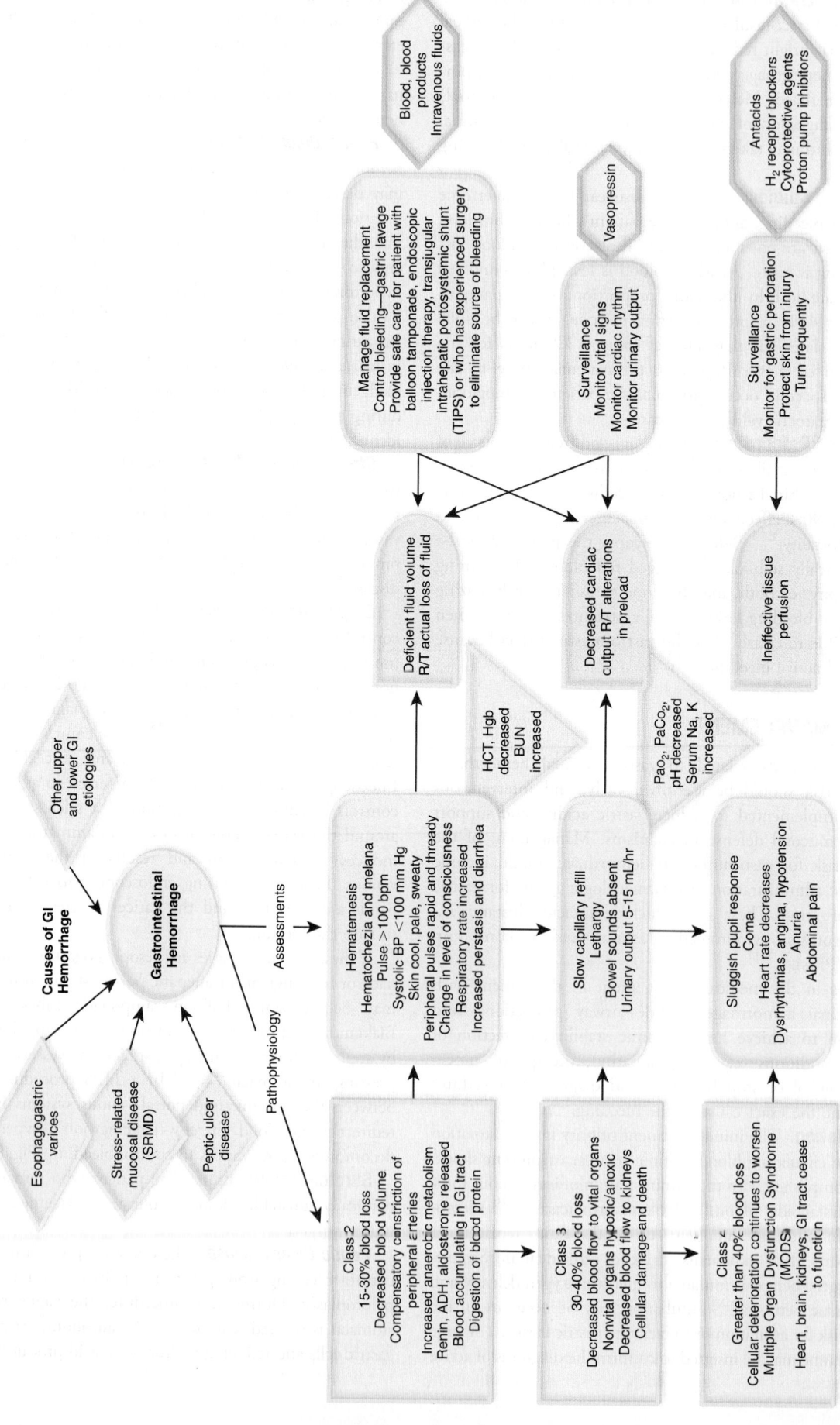

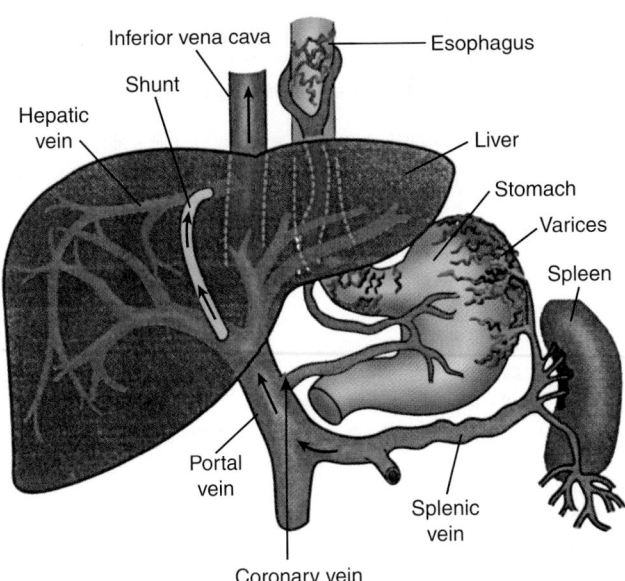

Figure 34-2 Anatomic location of the transjugular intrahepatic portosystemic shunt (TIPS). *(From Vargas HE et al: Management of portal hypertension-related bleeding,* Surg Clin North Am *79:1-22, 1999.)*

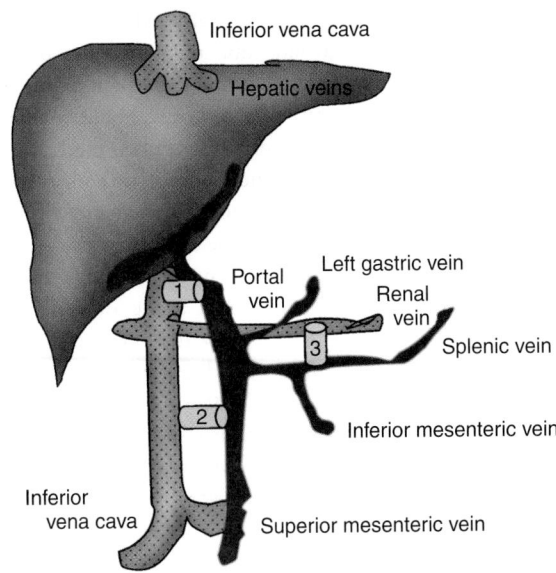

Figure 34-3 The anatomy of the portal venous system and the sites in which surgical anastomoses are made to shunt blood from the portal *(dark)* to the systemic *(light)* venous circulation. Several sites are used for surgical portal decompression: (1) portacaval shunt; (2) mesocaval shunt; (3) splenorenal shunt. *(From Luketic VA, Sanyal AJ: Esophageal varices. II. TIPS (transjugular intrahepatic portosystemic shunt) and surgical therapy,* Gastroenterol Clin North Am *29:387-421, vi, 2000.)*

the vagus nerve also stimulates motility, a pyloroplasty is performed to provide for gastric emptying.[9,16,20]

Stress-Related Mucosal Disease. Several operative procedures can be used to control bleeding from SRMD. A total gastrectomy is performed when bleeding is generalized. The ulcers are oversewn when bleeding is localized.[20] Total gastrectomy involves the complete removal of the stomach with anastomosis of the esophagus to the jejunum. During an oversew of the ulcers, the bleeding vessel is ligated, and the ulcer crater is closed.[16,20]

Esophagogastric Varices. Operative procedures to control bleeding gastroesophageal varices include portacaval shunt, mesocaval shunt, and splenorenal shunt (Fig. 34-3).[18] These shunt procedures are also referred to as decompression procedures, because they result in the diversion of portal blood flow away from the liver and decompression of the portal system. The portacaval shunt procedure has two variations. An end-to-side portacaval shunt procedure involves the ligation of the hepatic end of the portal vein with subsequent anastomosis to the vena cava. During a side-to-side portacaval shunt procedure, the side of the portal vein is anastomosed to the side of the vena cava. A mesocaval shunt procedure involves the insertion of a graft between the superior mesenteric artery and the vena cava. During a distal splenorenal shunt procedure, the splenic vein is detached from the portal vein and anastomosed to the left renal vein.[18,20]

NURSING MANAGEMENT

All critically ill patients should be considered at risk for stress ulcers and therefore gastrointestinal hemorrhage. Routine assessment of gastric fluid pH monitoring is controversial.[10] Maintaining the pH between 3.5 and 4.5 is a goal of prophylactic therapy. Gastric pH measurements made with litmus paper

---

Nursing Diagnoses

Acute Gastrointestinal Hemorrhage

- Deficient Fluid Volume related to absolute loss
- Decreased Cardiac Output related to alterations in preload
- Risk for Aspiration
- Imbalanced Nutrition: Less Than Body Requirements related to lack of exogenous nutrients and increased metabolic demand
- Risk for Infection
- Powerlessness related to health care environment or illness-related regimen
- Compromised Family Coping related to critically ill family member
- Deficient Knowledge related to lack of previous exposure to information (see the Patient Education feature on Acute Gastrointestinal Hemorrhage)

---

or direct nasogastric tube probes may be used to assess gastric fluid pH and the effectiveness or need for prophylactic agents.[11] Patients at risk also should be assessed for the presence of bright red or coffee grounds emesis, bloody nasogastric aspirate, and bright red, black, or dark red stools.[10] Any signs of bleeding should be promptly reported to the physician.

Nursing management of a patient experiencing acute gastrointestinal hemorrhage incorporates a variety of nursing diagnoses (see the Nursing Diagnoses feature on Acute Gastrointestinal Hemorrhage). Nursing interventions include administering volume replacement, controlling the bleeding, providing comfort and emotional support, maintaining surveillance for complications, and educating the patient and family.

Administering Volume Replacement. Measures to facilitate volume replacement include obtaining intravenous access and administering prescribed fluids and blood products. Two large-diameter peripheral intravenous catheters should be inserted to facilitate the rapid administration of prescribed fluids.[16,20]

Controlling the Bleeding. One measure to control active bleeding is gastric lavage. It is used to decrease gastric mucosal blood flow and evacuate blood from the stomach. Gastric lavage is performed by inserting a large-bore nasogastric tube into the stomach and irrigating it with normal saline or water until the returned solution is clear. It is important to keep accurate records of the amount of fluid instilled and aspirated to ascertain the true amount of bleeding.[1] Historically, iced saline was favored as a lavage irrigant. Research has shown, however, that low-temperature fluids shift the oxyhemoglobin dissociation curve to the left, decrease oxygen delivery to vital organs, and prolong bleeding time and prothrombin time. Iced saline also may further aggravate bleeding; therefore, room-temperature water or saline is the preferred irrigant for use in gastric lavage.[21]

Maintaining Surveillance for Complications. The patient should be continuously observed for signs of gastric perforation. Although a rare complication, gastric perforation constitutes a surgical emergency. Signs and symptoms include sudden, severe, generalized abdominal pain with significant rebound tenderness and rigidity. Perforation should be suspected when fever, leukocytosis, and tachycardia persist despite adequate volume replacement.[9]

Patient Education. Early in the hospital stay, the patient and family should be taught about acute gastrointestinal hemorrhage and its causes and treatments. As the patient moves toward discharge, teaching should focus on the interventions necessary for preventing the recurrence of the precipitating disorder. If an alcohol abuser, the patient should be encouraged to stop drinking and be referred to an alcohol cessation program (see the Patient Education feature on Acute Gastrointestinal Hemorrhage).

Collaborative management of the patient with acute gastrointestinal hemorrhage is outlined in Box 34-2.

Patient Education: Acute Gastrointestinal Hemorrhage

- Gastrointestinal hemorrhage
- Specific cause
- Precipitating factor modification
- Interventions to reduce further bleeding episodes
- Importance of taking medications
- Lifestyle changes
- Stress management
- Diet modifications
- Alcohol cessation
- Smoking cessation

BOX 34-2   COLLABORATIVE MANAGEMENT: ACUTE GASTROINTESTINAL HEMORRHAGE

- Initiate fluid resuscitation to achieve hemodynamic stability.
  - Crystalloids
  - Colloids
  - Blood and blood products
- Determine the cause of the bleeding.
  - Gastric lavage
- Control bleeding.
  - Endoscopic interventions
  - Vasopressin, somatostatin, octreotide
  - Esophagogastric balloon tube
  - Transjugular intrahepatic portosystemic shunting
  - Surgery
- Provide comfort and emotional support.
- Maintain surveillance for complications.
  - Hypovolemic shock
  - Gastric perforation

ACUTE PANCREATITIS

DESCRIPTION

Acute pancreatitis is an inflammation of the pancreas that produces exocrine and endocrine dysfunction that may also involve surrounding tissues and/or remote organ systems. The clinical course can range from a mild, self-limiting disease to a systemic process characterized by organ failure, sepsis, and death. In approximately 80% of patients, it takes the milder form of *edematous interstitial pancreatitis,* whereas the other 20% develop severe *acute necrotizing pancreatitis.*[22] Reported mortality rates for acute pancreatitis range from 2% to 15% overall and from 20% to 50% for patients with severe disease.[22,23] Several prognostic scoring systems have been developed to predict the severity of acute pancreatitis. One of the most commonly used is Ranson's criteria (Box 34-3). If the patient has 0 to 2 factors present, the predicted mortality rate is 2%; with 3 to 4 factors, the rate is 15%; with 5 to 6 factors, the rate is 40%; and with 7 to 8 factors, predicted mortality rate is 100%.[22,24]

ETIOLOGY

The two most common causes of acute pancreatitis are gallstones and alcoholism. Together, they account for approximately 80% of cases. Less common causes are quite diverse and include surgical trauma, hypercalcemia, various toxins, ischemia, infections, and the use of certain drugs (Box 34-4). In 10% to 20% of patients with acute pancreatitis, no etiologic factor can be determined.[23]

PATHOPHYSIOLOGY

In acute pancreatitis, the normally inactive digestive enzymes become prematurely activated within the pancreas itself, leading to autodigestion of pancreatic tissue. The enzymes become activated

BOX 34-3 RANSON'S CRITERIA FOR ESTIMATING THE SEVERITY OF ACUTE PANCREATITIS

AT ADMISSION

- Age >55 years
- Hypotension
- Abnormal pulmonary findings
- Abdominal mass
- Hemorrhagic or discolored peritoneal fluid
- Increased serum LDH levels (>350 units/L)
- AST >250 units/L
- Leukocytosis (>16,000/mm^3)
- Hyperglycemia (>200 mg/dL; no diabetic history)
- Neurologic deficit (confusion, localizing signs)

DURING INITIAL 48 HOURS OF HOSPITALIZATION

- Fall in hematocrit >10% with hydration or hematocrit <30%
- Necessity for massive fluid and colloid replacement
- Hypocalcemia (<8 mg/dL)
- Arterial Po$_2$ <60 mm Hg with or without acute respiratory distress syndrome
- Hypoalbuminemia (<3.2 mg/dL)
- Base deficit >4 mEq/L
- Azotemia

From Latifi R et al: Nutritional management of acute and chronic pancreatitis. *Surg Clin North Am* 71:583, 1991.
AST, aspartate aminotransferase; LDH, lactate dehydrogenase: Po$_2$, partial pressure of oxygen.

BOX 34-4 CAUSES OF ACUTE PANCREATITIS

- Toxins (ethyl alcohol, methyl alcohol, scorpion, venom, parathion)
- Biliary disease (stones, sludge, common bile duct obstruction)
- Drugs (sulfonamides, thiazide diuretics, furosemide, estrogens, tetracycline, pentamidine, procainamide, salicylates, steroids, cyclosporine, amphetamines, nonsteroidal antiinflammatory agents, valproic acid, azathioprine, allopurinol)
- Hypercalcemia (hyperparathyroidism)

- Hyperlipidemia
- Tumors
- Infections (bacterial, viral, parasitic)
- Trauma (abdominal, surgical, endoscopic)
- Ischemia
- Graft-versus-host disease
- Vasculitis
- Pregnancy
- Hypothermia
- Sphincter of Oddi dysfunction
- Systemic lupus erythematosus
- Ampullary stenosis
- Idiopathic cause

BOX 34-5 PRESENTING CLINICAL MANIFESTATIONS OF ACUTE PANCREATITIS.

- Pain
- Vomiting
- Nausea
- Fever
- Abdominal distention
- Abdominal guarding
- Abdominal tympany
- Hypoactive or absent bowel sounds

- Severe disease
  - Peritoneal signs
  - Ascites
  - Jaundice
  - Palpable abdominal mass
  - Grey-Turner's sign
  - Cullen's sign
  - Signs of hypovolemic shock

From Krumberger JM: Acute pancreatitis. *Crit Care Nurs Clin North Am* 5:185-202, 1993.

direct cell damage. It dissolves the elastic fibers of blood vessels and ducts, leading to hemorrhage. Phospholipase A, in the presence of bile, destroys the phospholipids of cell membranes, causing severe pancreatic and adipose tissue necrosis. Lipase flows into the damaged tissue and is absorbed into the systemic circulation, resulting in fat necrosis of the pancreas and surrounding tissues.[8,22]

The extent of injury to the pancreatic cells determines the type of acute pancreatitis that develops. If injury to the pancreatic cells is mild and without necrosis, edematous pancreatitis develops. The acinar cells appear structurally intact, and blood flow is maintained through small capillaries and venules. This form of acute pancreatitis is self-limiting. If injury to the pancreatic cells is severe, acute necrotizing pancreatitis develops.[22,23] Cellular destruction in pancreatic injury results in the release of toxic enzymes and inflammatory mediators into the systemic circulation and causes injury to vessels and other organs distant from the pancreas; this may result in systemic inflammatory response syndrome (SIRS), multiorgan failure, and death.[22,23] Local tissue injury results in infection, abscess and pseudocyst formation, disruption of the pancreatic duct, and severe hemorrhage with shock.[22]

ASSESSMENT AND DIAGNOSIS

The clinical manifestations of acute pancreatitis range from mild to severe and often mimic those of other disorders (Box 34-5). Acute onset of abdominal pain is a hallmark symptom.[23] Epigastric to periumbilical pain may vary from mild and tolerable to severe and incapacitating. Many patients report a twisting or knifelike sensation that radiates to the low dorsal region of the back. The patient may obtain some comfort by leaning forward or assuming a semifetal position. Nausea and vomiting are common.[23] Other clinical findings include fever, diaphoresis, weakness, tachypnea, hypotension, and tachycardia. Depending on the extent of fluid loss and hemorrhage, the patient may exhibit signs of hypovolemic shock.[22,23,25]

Physical Examination. The results of physical assessment usually reveal hypoactive bowel sounds and abdominal tenderness, guarding, distention, and tympany. Findings that may

through various mechanisms, including obstruction of or damage to the pancreatic duct system, alterations in the secretory processes of the acinar cells, infection, ischemia, and other unknown factors.[8,22]

Trypsin is the enzyme that becomes activated first. It initiates the autodigestion process by triggering the secretion of proteolytic enzymes such as kallikrein, chymotrypsin, elastase, phospholipase A, and lipase. Release of kallikrein and chymotrypsin results in increased capillary membrane permeability, leading to leakage of fluid into the interstitium and the development of edema and relative hypovolemia. Elastase is the most harmful enzyme in terms of indicate pancreatic hemorrhage include Grey Turner's sign (gray-blue discoloration of the flanks) and Cullen's sign (discoloration of the umbilical region); however, they are rare and usually seen several days into the illness.[22] A palpable abdominal mass indicates the presence of a pseudocyst or abscess.[26]

Laboratory Studies. Assessment of laboratory data usually demonstrates elevated levels of serum amylase and lipase. Serum lipase is more pancreas specific than amylase and a more accurate marker for acute pancreatitis. Amylase is present in other body tissues, and other disorders (e.g., intraabdominal emergencies, renal insufficiency, salivary gland trauma, liver disease) may contribute to an elevated level. Unlike other serum enzymes, however, amylase is excreted in urine, and this clearance increases with acute pancreatitis. Measurement of urinary versus serum amylase should be considered in light of the patient's creatinine clearance. The serum amylase level may be elevated for only 3 to 5 days; if the patient delays seeking treatment, a normal level (false-negative result) may be detected. Leukocytosis, hypocalcemia, hyperglycemia, hyperbilirubinemia, and hypoalbuminemia may also be present (Table 34-2).[8,22,23]

Diagnostic Procedures. An abdominal ultrasound scan is obtained as part of the diagnostic evaluation to determine the presence of biliary stones. A contrast-enhanced computed tomography (CT) scan is considered the gold standard for diagnosing pancreatitis and for ascertaining the overall degree of pancreatic inflammation and necrosis.[22,23]

MEDICAL MANAGEMENT

Initial management of the patient with severe acute pancreatitis includes ensuring adequate fluid and electrolyte replacement, providing nutritional support, and correcting metabolic alterations.[23] Careful monitoring for systemic and local complications is critical.[22,24,25]

Fluid Management. Because pancreatitis if often associated with massive fluid shifts, intravenous crystalloids and colloids are administered immediately to prevent hypovolemic shock and maintain hemodynamic stability. In severe forms of acute pancreatitis, a pulmonary artery catheter may be used to guide ongoing fluid management.[25,27] Electrolytes are monitored closely, and abnormalities such as hypocalcemia, hypokalemia, and hypomagnesemia are corrected.[22,25] If hyperglycemia develops, exogenous insulin may be required.[25]

Nutritional Support. Over the past 3 decades, nutritional support has shifted. Previously, conventional nutritional management was to place the patient on a no oral intake (NPO) regimen and institute intravenous hydration. The rationale was to rest the inflamed pancreas and prevent enzyme release. Oral feeding was initiated only when the attack had subsided and enzymes had normalized. Total parenteral nutrition (TPN) was started for patients anticipated to have oral feedings held for more than 5 days. Randomized clinical trials have demonstrated that enteral feeding (gastric or jejunal) is safe and cost-effective and that it is associated with fewer septic and metabolic complications than other methods.[27,28] Enteral feeding enhances immune modulation and maintenance of the intestinal barrier, and it avoid complications associated with

TABLE 34-2	Laboratory Tests and Diagnostic Procedures for Acute Pancreatitis
Study	**Finding in Pancreatitis**
Laboratory Studies	
Serum amylase	Elevated
Serum isoamylase	Elevated
Urine amylase	Elevated
Serum lipase (if available)	Elevated
Serum triglycerides	Elevated
Glucose	Elevated
Calcium	Decreased
Magnesium	Decreased
Potassium	Decreased
Albumin	Decreased or increased
White blood cell count	Elevated
Bilirubin	May be elevated
Liver enzymes	May be elevated
Prothrombin time	Prolonged
Arterial blood gases	Hypoxemia, metabolic acidosis
Diagnostic Procedures	
Abdominal ultrasonography	
Computed tomography scan	
Magnetic resonance imaging	
Endoscopic retrograde cholangiopancreatography	
Abdominal radiographs (flat plate and upright or decubitus)	
Chest radiographs (posteroanterior and lateral)	

Modified from Krumberger JM: Acute pancreatitis. *Crit Care Nurs Clin North Am* 5:185-202, 1993.

parental nutrition.[27-29] Early initiation of enteral feeding is preferred over TPN.[27-29] However, TPN still has a role for the critically ill patient with acute pancreatitis who does not tolerate enteral feeding or when nutritional goals are not reached within 2 days.[23,27] In the past, nasogastric suction was also recommended, but this intervention has not been shown to be of benefit and should be instituted only if the patient has persistent vomiting, obstruction, or gastric distention.[22]

Systemic Complications. Acute pancreatitis can affect every organ system, and recognition and treatment of systemic complications are crucial to management of the patient (Box 34-6). The most serious complications are hypovolemic shock, acute lung injury (ALI), acute renal failure (ARF), and gastrointestinal hemorrhage. Hypovolemic shock is the result of relative hypovolemia resulting from third spacing of intravascular volume and vasodilation caused by the release of inflammatory immune mediators.

BOX 34-6 COMPLICATIONS OF ACUTE PANCREATITIS

RESPIRATORY
- Early hypoxemia
- Pleural effusion
- Atelectasis
- Pulmonary infiltration
- Acute lung injury
- Mediastinal abscess

CARDIOVASCULAR
- Hypotension
- Pericardial effusion
- ST-T changes

RENAL
- Acute tubular necrosis
- Oliguria
- Renal artery or vein thrombosis

HEMATOLOGIC
- Disseminated intravascular coagulation
- Thrombocytosis
- Hyperfibrinogenemia

ENDOCRINE
- Hypocalcemia
- Hypertriglyceridemia
- Hyperglycemia

NEUROLOGIC
- Fat emboli
- Psychosis
- Encephalopathy

OPHTHALMIC
- Purtscher's retinopathy (sudden blindness)

DERMATOLOGIC
- Subcutaneous fat necrosis

GASTROINTESTINAL OR HEPATIC
- Hepatic dysfunction
- Obstructive jaundice
- Erosive gastritis
- Paralytic ileus
- Duodenal obstruction
- Pancreatic
  - Pseudocyst
  - Phlegmon
  - Abscess
  - Ascites
- Bowel infarction
- Massive intraperitoneal bleed
- Perforation
  - Stomach
  - Duodenum
  - Small bowel
  - Colon

Nursing Diagnoses

Acute Pancreatitis

- Acute Pain related to transmission and perception of cutaneous, visceral, muscular, ischemia impulses
- Deficient Fluid Volume related to relative fluid loss
- Decreased Cardiac Output related to alterations in preload
- Ineffective Breathing Pattern related to decreased lung expansion
- Imbalanced Nutrition: Less Than Body Requirements related to lack of exogenous nutrients or increased metabolic demand
- Anxiety related to threat to biologic, psychologic, and/or social integrity
- Compromised Family Coping related to critically ill family member
- Deficient Knowledge related to lack of previous exposure to information (see the Patient Education feature on Acute Pancreatitis)

These mediators also contribute to the development of ALI and ARF. Other possible pulmonary complications include pleural effusions, atelectasis, and pneumonia.

Local Complications. Local complications include the development of infected pancreatic necrosis and pancreatic pseudocyst.[23,27] The necrotic areas of the pancreas can lead to development of a widespread pancreatic infection (infected pancreatic necrosis), which significantly increases the risk of death.[27]

Prophylactic antibiotics reduce sepsis and mortality and are initiated in patients suspected of having necrotizing pancreatitis.[27] After the patient develops infected necrosis, however, surgical débridement is necessary.[23,27] The procedure of choice is a minimal invasive necrosectomy, which entails careful débridement of the necrotic tissue in and around the pancreas. A pancreatic pseudocyst is a collection of pancreatic fluid enclosed by a nonepithelialized wall.[26] Cyst formation may result from liquefaction of a pancreatic fluid collection or from direct obstruction in the main pancreatic duct.[24] A pancreatic pseudocyst may (1) resolve spontaneously; (2) rupture, resulting in peritonitis; (3) erode a major blood vessel, resulting in hemorrhage; (4) become infected, resulting in abscess; or (5) invade surrounding structures, resulting in

obstruction.[24] Treatment involves drainage of the pseudocyst surgically,[30] endoscopically, or percutaneously.[23,27]

NURSING MANAGEMENT

Nursing management of the patient with pancreatitis incorporates a variety of nursing diagnoses (see the Nursing Diagnoses feature on Acute Pancreatitis). Nursing interventions include providing pain relief and emotional support, maintaining surveillance for complications, and educating the patient and family.

Providing Comfort and Emotional Support. Pain management is a major priority in acute pancreatitis. Administration of analgesics to achieve pain relief is essential. For years, meperidine (Demerol) was considered to be the preferred agent in the patient with acute pancreatitis because morphine produced spasms at the sphincter of Oddi. However, studies have demonstrated that all opioids have a spasmogenic effect on the sphincter of Oddi. There is no evidence to indicate that morphine is contraindicated for use in acute pancreatitis, and it may provide more effective analgesia with fewer side effects than meperidine.[22,27] Relaxation techniques and positioning the patient in the knee-chest position can also assist in pain control.

Maintaining Surveillance for Complications. The patient must be routinely monitored for signs of local or systemic complications (see Box 34-6). Intensive monitoring of each of the organ systems is imperative, because organ failure is a major indicator of the severity of the disease.[31] The patient must be closely monitored for signs and symptoms of pancreatic infection, which include increased abdominal pain and tenderness, fever, and increased white blood cell count (Box 34-7).[22]

Patient Education. Early in the patient's hospital stay, the patient and family should be taught about acute pancreatitis and its causes and treatment. As the patient moves toward discharge, teaching should focus on the interventions necessary for preventing the recurrence of the precipitating disorder. If there is sustained, permanent damage to the pancreas, the patient will require teaching specific to diet modification and supplemental pancreatic enzymes. Diabetes education may also be necessary. If an alcohol abuser, the patient should be encouraged to stop drinking and be referred to an alcohol cessation program (see the Patient Education feature on Acute Pancreatitis).[25]

Patient Education: Acute Pancreatitis

- Pancreatitis
- Specific cause
- Precipitating factor modification
- Interventions to reduce further episodes
- Importance of taking medications
- Lifestyle changes
- Diet modification
- Stress management
- Alcohol cessation
- Diabetes management, if needed

BOX 34-7   SIGNS AND SYMPTOMS OF PANCREATIC INFECTION

SYMPTOMS
- Persistent abdominal pain
- Abdominal tenderness

SIGNS
- Prolonged fever
- Abdominal distention
- Palpable abdominal mass
- Vomiting

DIAGNOSTICS
- Laboratory findings
  - Increased white blood cell count

- Persistent elevation of serum amylase
- Hyperbilirubinemia
- Elevated alkaline phosphatase level
- Positive culture and Gram's stain
- Radiography or computed tomography findings
- Pancreatic inflammation or enlargement
- Necrosis
- Cystic or mass lesions
- Fluid accumulations
- Pseudocyst abscess

Modified from Krumberger JM: Acute pancreatitis. *Crit Care Nurs Clin North Am* 5:185-202, 1993.

BOX 34-8   COLLABORATIVE MANAGEMENT: ACUTE PANCREATITIS

- Ensure adequate circulating volume.
- Provide nutritional support.
- Correct metabolic alterations.
- Minimize pancreatic stimulation.
- Provide comfort and emotional support.
- Maintain surveillance for complications.
- Multiple organ dysfunction syndrome.

Collaborative management of the patient with pancreatitis is outlined in Box 34-8.

FULMINANT HEPATIC FAILURE

DESCRIPTION

Fulminant hepatic failure (FHF) is a life-threatening condition characterized by severe and sudden liver cell dysfunction, coagulopathy, and hepatic encephalopathy.[32,33] Although uncommon, FHF is associated with a mortality rate as high as 75% to 80%, and it usually occurs in patients without preexisting liver disease.[33,34] Because liver transplantation is one of the few definitive treatments, the patient with FHF should be transferred to a critical care unit and strongly considered for referral to a major medical center where transplantation services are available.[32-34]

ETIOLOGY

The causes of FHF include infections, drugs, toxins, hypoperfusion, metabolic disorders, and surgery (Box 34-9); however, viral hepatitis and drug-induced liver damage are the predominant causes in North America. Patients are usually healthy before the onset of symptoms because FHF tends to occur in patients with no known liver history. A thorough medication and health history is imperative to determine a possible cause. The patient should be questioned about exposure to environmental toxins, hepatitis, intravenous drug use, and sexual history. Viral hepatitis, drug toxicity, poisoning, and vascular and metabolic disorders such as Reye's syndrome and Wilson's disease should be considered.[32]

PATHOPHYSIOLOGY

FHF is a syndrome characterized by the development of acute liver failure over 1 to 3 weeks, followed by the development of hepatic encephalopathy within 8 weeks, in a patient with a previously healthy liver. The interval between the failure of the liver and the onset of hepatic encephalopathy usually is less than 2 weeks. The underlying cause is massive necrosis of the hepatocytes.[32,33]

Acute liver failure results in a number of derangements, including impaired bilirubin conjugation, decreased production of clotting factors, depressed glucose synthesis, and decreased lactate clearance. This results in jaundice, coagulopathies, hypoglycemia, and metabolic acidosis. Other effects of acute liver failure include increased risk of infection and altered carbohydrate, protein, and glucose metabolism. Hypoalbuminemia, fluid and electrolyte imbalances, and acute portal hypertension contribute to the development of ascites.[33,34] Hepatic encephalopathy is thought to result from failure of the liver to detoxify various substances in the bloodstream, and it may be worsened by metabolic and electrolyte imbalances.[33]

The patient may experience a variety of other complications, including cerebral edema, cardiac dysrhythmias, acute respiratory failure, sepsis, and acute renal failure. Cerebral edema and increased intracranial pressure (ICP) develop as a result of breakdown of the blood-brain barrier and astrocyte swelling. Circulatory failure that mimics sepsis is common in FHF and may exacerbate low cerebral perfusion pressure (CPP).[34] Hypoxemia, acidosis, electrolyte imbalances, and cerebral edema can precipitate the development of cardiac dysrhythmias. Acute respiratory failure, progressing to ALI, can result from pulmonary edema, aspiration pneumonia, and atelectasis. ARF may be caused by acute tubular necrosis, hypotension, or hemorrhage.[33,34]

BOX 34-9   CAUSES OF FULMINANT HEPATIC FAILURE

INFECTIONS
- Hepatitis A, B, C, D, E, non-A, non-B, non-C
- Herpes simplex virus (types 1 and 2)
- Epstein-Barr virus
- Varicella zoster
- Dengue fever virus
- Rift Valley fever virus

DRUGS OR TOXINS
- Industrial substances (chlorinated hydrocarbons, phosphorus)
- *Amanita phalloides* (mushrooms)
- Aflatoxin (a toxic metabolite of fungus)
- Medications (isoniazid, rifampin, halothane, methyldopa, tetracycline, valproic acid, monoamine oxidase inhibitors, phenytoin, nicotinic acid, tricyclic antidepressants, isoflurane, ketoconazole, trimethoprim-sulfamethoxazole, sulfasalazine, pyrimethamine, octreotide)
- Acetaminophen toxicity
- Cocaine

HYPOPERFUSION
- Venous obstructions
- Budd-Chiari syndrome
- Veno-occlusive disease
- Ischemia

METABOLIC DISORDERS
- Wilson's disease
- Tyrosinemia
- Heat stroke
- Galactosemia

SURGERY
- Jejunoileal bypass
- Partial hepatectomy
- Liver transplant failure

OTHER CAUSES
- Reye's syndrome
- Acute fatty liver of pregnancy
- Massive malignant infiltration
- Autoimmune hepatitis

BOX 34-10   STAGING OF HEPATIC ENCEPHALOPATHY

I   Euphoria or depression, mild confusion, slurred speech, disordered sleep rhythm; slight asterixis and normal electroencephalogram (EEG)

II   Lethargy, moderate confusion; marked asterixis and abnormal EEG

III Marked confusion, incoherent speech, sleeping but arousable; asterixis present and abnormal EEG

IV   Coma; initially responsive to noxious stimuli, later unresponsive; asterixis absent and abnormal EEG

ASSESSMENT AND DIAGNOSIS

Early recognition of FHF is essential. The diagnosis should include potentially reversible conditions (e.g., autoimmune hepatitis) and should differentiate FHF from decompensating chronic liver disease. Prognostic indicators such as coma grade, serum bilirubin, prothrombin time, coagulation factors, and pH should be assessed and potential causes investigated.[33,34]

Signs and symptoms of FHF include headache, hyperventilation, jaundice, mental status changes, palmar erythema, spider nevi, bruises, and edema. The patient should be evaluated for the presence of asterixis or "liver flap," best described as the inability to voluntarily sustain a fixed position of the extremities. Asterixis is best demonstrated by having the patient extend the arms and dorsiflex the wrists, resulting in downward flapping of the hands. Hepatic encephalopathy is assessed using a grading system that stages the encephalopathy according to the patient's clinical manifestations (Box 34-10).[33,34] Diagnostic findings include elevated levels of serum bilirubin, aspartate aminotransferase (AST), alkaline phosphatase, and serum ammonia and decreased levels of serum albumin. Arterial blood gases (ABGs) reveal respiratory alkalosis or metabolic acidosis, or both. Hypoglycemia, hypokalemia, and hyponatremia also may be present.[33,34]

Factors I (fibrinogen), II (prothrombin), V, VII, IX, and X are produced exclusively by the liver. Prothrombin time may be the most useful of tests of these in the evaluation of acute FHF because levels may be 40 to 80 seconds above control values. Test results show decreased levels of plasmin and plasminogen and increased levels of fibrin and fibrin-split products. Platelet counts may be less than 100,000/mm³.[33]

MEDICAL MANAGEMENT

Medical interventions are directed toward management of the multiple system impact of FHF.

Ammonia Levels. Neomycin or lactulose is administered to remove or decrease production of nitrogenous wastes in the large intestine. Neomycin, given orally or rectally, reduces bacterial flora of the colon. This aids in decreasing ammonia formation by decreasing bacterial action on protein in the feces. Side effects include renal toxicity and hearing impairment. Lactulose, a synthetic ketoanalogue of lactose split into lactic acid and acetic acid in the intestine, is given orally through a nasogastric tube or as a retention enema. The result is the creation of an acidic environment that decreases bacterial growth. Lactulose also traps ammonia and has a laxative effect that promotes expulsion.[34]

Complications. Bleeding is best controlled through prevention. Because these patients are at risk for acute gastrointestinal hemorrhage, stress ulcer prophylaxis is essential.[35] If an invasive procedure (e.g., central line placement, ICP monitor) will be performed or the patient develops active bleeding, vitamin K, fresh-frozen plasma (to maintain a reasonable prothrombin time), and platelet transfusions are necessary.[37] Metabolic disturbances such as hypoglycemia, metabolic acidosis, hypokalemia, and hyponatremia should be monitored and treated appropriately. Prophylactic antibiotic administration may be initiated because the patient is at high risk for an infection.[33,34]

The development of cerebral edema necessitates ICP monitoring. Mannitol is the only treatment shown to be of benefit in managing increased ICP in the patient with FHF, but it must be used with caution in patients with renal failure.[35] Other interventions to control intracranial hypertension include elevating the head of the bed (HOB) to 30 degrees, treating fever and hypertension, minimizing noxious stimulation, and correcting hypercapnia and hypoxemia.[35] Various experimental therapies to prevent or treat cerebral edema, such as induction of hypothermia, prophylactic phenytoin, and induction of hypernatremia, have been studied but have not improved survival.[35] If renal failure develops, continuous renal replacement therapy (CRRT) should be initiated.[35] Intubation and mechanical ventilation may be necessary as the inability to protect airway and hypoxemia develops.[34] Hemodynamic instability is a common complication necessitating fluid administration and vasoactive medications to prevent prolonged episodes of hypotension. A pulmonary artery catheter may be used to guide clinical management.[34]

If FHF continues and the patient shows no immediate signs of improvement or reversal, the patient should be considered for a liver transplant. Prompt referral to a transplantation center should be a high priority for patients experiencing FHF.[33-35]

NURSING MANAGEMENT

Nursing management of the patient with FHF incorporates a variety of nursing diagnoses (see the Nursing Diagnoses feature on Fulminant Hepatic Failure). Nursing interventions include protecting the patient from injury, providing comfort and emotional support, maintaining surveillance for complications, and educating the patient and family.

Protecting the Patient from Injury. Use of benzodiazepines and other sedatives is discouraged in the FHF patient because pertinent neurologic changes may be masked and hepatic encephalopathy may be exacerbated.[34] These patients are often very difficult to manage because they may be extremely agitated and combative. Physical restraint may be necessary to prevent patient injury.

Maintaining Surveillance for Complications. As the neurologic condition worsens, respiratory depression and arrest can occur quickly. Continuous pulse oximetry monitoring and ABG analysis are helpful in assessing adequacy of respiratory efforts. A thorough neurologic assessment should be performed at least every hour.

Patient Education. Early in the patient's hospital stay, the patient and family should be taught about FHF and its causes and treatment. As the patient moves toward discharge, teaching should focus on the interventions necessary for preventing the recurrence of the precipitating cause. If the patient is considered a candidate for liver transplantation, the patient and family will need specific information regarding the procedure and care. Liver transplant evaluation may include screening for medical contraindications, human immunodeficiency virus (HIV) serology, anticipated compliance, and assessment of the social support system. Psychiatric and other specialty team consultations are necessary for a thorough evaluation of the patient's suitability for a liver transplant (see the Patient Education feature on Fulminant Hepatic Failure). Collaborative management of the patient with FHF is outlined in Box 34-11.

Patient Education: Fulminant Hepatic Failure

- Specific cause
- Precipitating factor modification
- Interventions to reduce further episodes
- Importance of taking medications
- Lifestyle changes
- Diet modification
- Alcohol cessation

Nursing Diagnoses

Fulminant Hepatic Failure

- Ineffective Breathing Pattern related to decreased lung expansion
- Impaired Gas Exchange related to ventilation/perfusion mismatching or intrapulmonary shunting
- Decreased Cardiac Output related to alterations in preload
- Decreased Cardiac Output related to alterations in heart rate
- Decreased Intracranial Adaptive Capacity related to failure of normal compensatory mechanisms
- Ineffective Renal Tissue Perfusion related to decreased renal blood flow
- Risk for Infection
- Imbalanced Nutrition: Less Than Body Requirements related to lack of exogenous nutrients or increased metabolic demand
- Disturbed Body Image related to actual change in body structure, function, or appearance
- Compromised Family Coping related to critically ill family member
- Deficient Knowledge related to lack of previous exposure to information (see the Patient Education feature on Fulminant Hepatic Failure)

BOX 34-11 COLLABORATIVE MANAGEMENT: FULMINANT HEPATIC FAILURE

- Decrease ammonia levels.
- Control bleeding.
- Correct metabolic alterations.
- Prevent infection
- Prepare patient for liver transplantation, if necessary.
- Protect patient from injury.
- Provide comfort and emotional support.
- Maintain surveillance for complications:
  - Cerebral edema
  - Renal failure

GASTROINTESTINAL SURGERY

TYPES OF SURGERY

Gastrointestinal surgery refers to a wide variety of surgical procedures that involve the esophagus, the stomach, the intestine, the liver, the pancreas, or the biliary tract. Indications for gastrointestinal surgery are numerous and include bleeding or perforation from peptic ulcer disease, obstruction, trauma, inflammatory bowel disease, and malignancy. Patients may be admitted to the critical care unit for monitoring after gastrointestinal surgery as a result of their underlying medical condition; however, this portion of the chapter focuses only on several surgical procedures that commonly require postoperative critical care.

Esophagectomy. Esophagectomy is usually performed for cancer of the distal esophagus and gastroesophageal junction. The technically difficult procedure involves the removal of part or the entire esophagus, part of the stomach, and lymph nodes in the surrounding area. The stomach is then pulled up into the chest and connected to the remaining part of the esophagus. If the entire esophagus and stomach must be removed, part of the bowel may be used to form the esophageal replacement (Figs. 34-4 and 34-5).[36,37]

Pancreaticoduodenectomy. The standard operation for pancreatic cancer is a pancreaticoduodenectomy, also called a *Whipple procedure*. In the Whipple procedure, the pancreatic head, the duodenum, part of the jejunum, the common bile duct, the gallbladder, and part of the stomach are removed. The continuity of the gastrointestinal tract is restored by anastomosing the remaining portion of the pancreas, the bile duct, and the stomach to the jejunum (Fig. 34-6).[37,38]

Bariatric Surgery. Bariatric surgery refers to surgical procedures of the gastrointestinal tract that are performed to induce weight loss. Bariatric procedures are divided into three broad types: restrictive, malabsorptive, and combined restrictive and malabsorptive.[39] Restrictive procedures such as vertical banded gastroplasty (VBG) (Fig. 34-7A) and gastric banding (Fig. 34-7B) reduce the capacity of the stomach and limit the amount of food that can be consumed. Malabsorptive procedures such as the biliopancreatic diversion (BPD) (Fig. 34-7C) alter the gastrointestinal tract to limit the digestion and absorption of food. The Roux-en-Y gastric bypass (RYGBP) (Fig. 34-7D) combines both strategies by creating a small gastric pouch and anastomosing the jejunum to the pouch. Food then bypasses the lower stomach and duodenum, resulting in decreased absorption of digestive materials.[39,40]

PREOPERATIVE CARE

A thorough preoperative evaluation should be conducted to evaluate the patient's physical status and identify risk factors that may affect the postoperative course. Because obesity is associated with a higher incidence of comorbidities such as cardiovascular disease, hypertension, diabetes, gastroesophageal reflux, obstructive sleep apnea, and heart failure, an extensive workup may be required for the bariatric patient.[40] Before esophagectomy or pancreaticoduodenectomy, the patient may undergo multiple diagnostic tests, such as CT, positron emission tomography (PET), and endoscopic ultrasound (EUS), to determine the invasiveness of the tumor.[36]

SURGICAL CONSIDERATIONS

Two approaches may be used for esophageal resection: transhiatal or transthoracic (Figs. 34-4 and 34-5). In both approaches, the stomach is mobilized through an abdominal incision and then transposed into the chest. The anastomosis

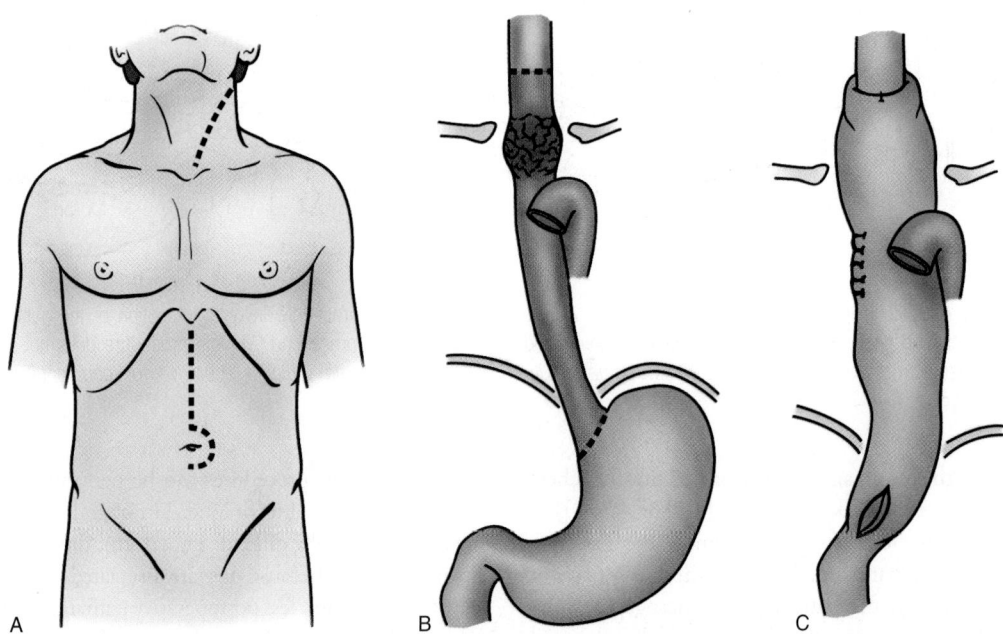

A   B   C

Figure 34-4 Overview of transhiatal esophagectomy *(A)* with gastric mobilization *(B)* and gastric pull-up *(C)* for cervical-esophagogastric anastomosis. *(A to C, Modified from Ellis F: Esophagogastrectomy for carcinoma: technical considerations based on anatomic location of lesion, Surg Clin North Am 60:265-279, 1980.)*

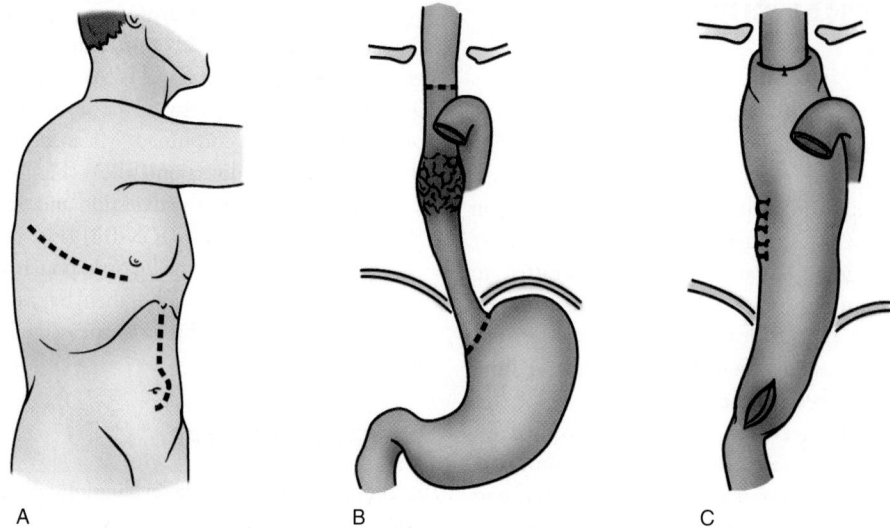

Figure 34-5 Overview of right thoracotomy *(A)* with esophageal resection, gastric mobilization *(B)*, and intrathoracic anastomosis *(C)* for a midesophageal tumor. *(A to C, Modified from Ellis FH: Esophagogastrectomy for carcinoma: technical considerations based on anatomic location of lesion, Surg Clin North Am 60:265-279, 1980.)*

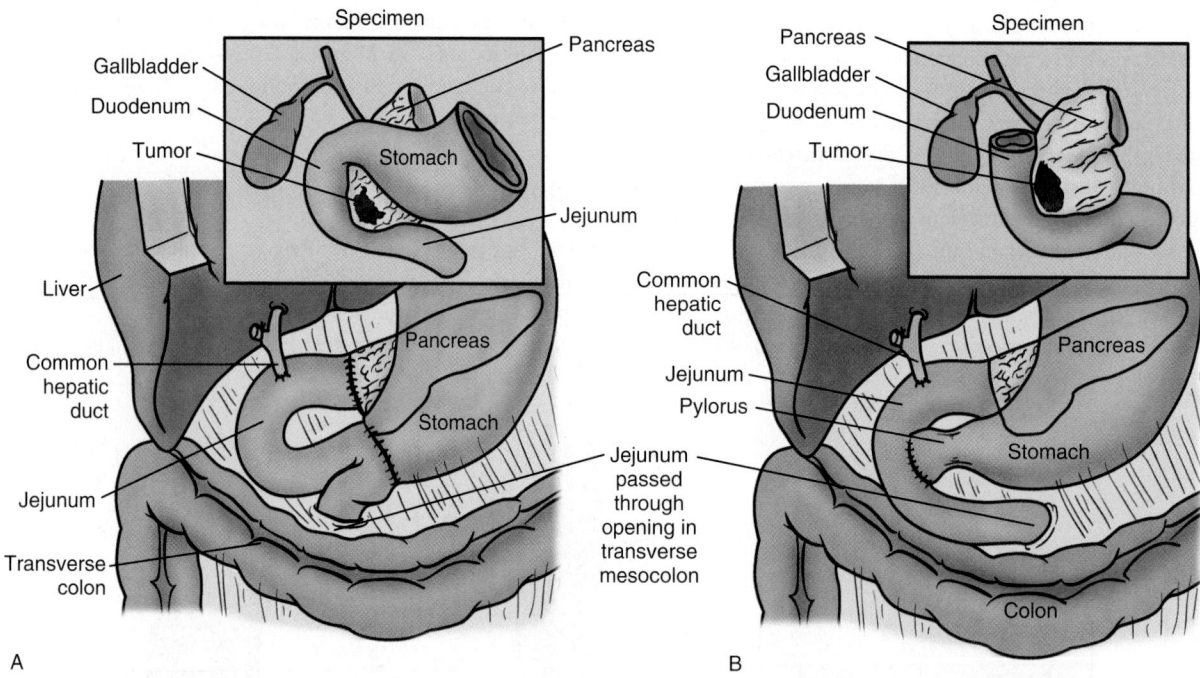

Figure 34-6 Standard and pylorus-preserving Whipple procedures. *A,* The standard Whipple procedure involves resection of the gastric antrum, head of pancreas, distal bile duct, and entire duodenum with reconstruction as shown. *B,* The pylorus-preserving Whipple procedure does not include resection of the distal stomach, pylorus, or proximal duodenum *(From Cameron JL: Current status of the Whipple operative for periampullary carcinoma, Surg Rounds:77-87, 1988.)*

of the stomach to the esophagus is performed in the chest (transthoracic) or in the neck (transhiatal). The approach selected depends on the location of the tumor, the patient's overall health and pulmonary function, and the experience of the surgeon. After surgery, the patient has an nasogastric tube in place that should not be manipulated because of the potential to damage the anastomosis. Those who undergo transthoracic esophagectomy have one or more chest tubes.[36,37]

Most bariatric procedures can be performed using an open or laparoscopic surgical technique. Although laparoscopic approaches are more technically difficult to perform, they have largely replaced open procedures because they are associated with decreased pulmonary complications, less postoperative pain, reduced length of hospital stay, fewer wound complications (e.g., infections, incisional hernia), and an earlier return to full activity.[39,41] Open procedures are performed on patients who have had prior upper abdominal

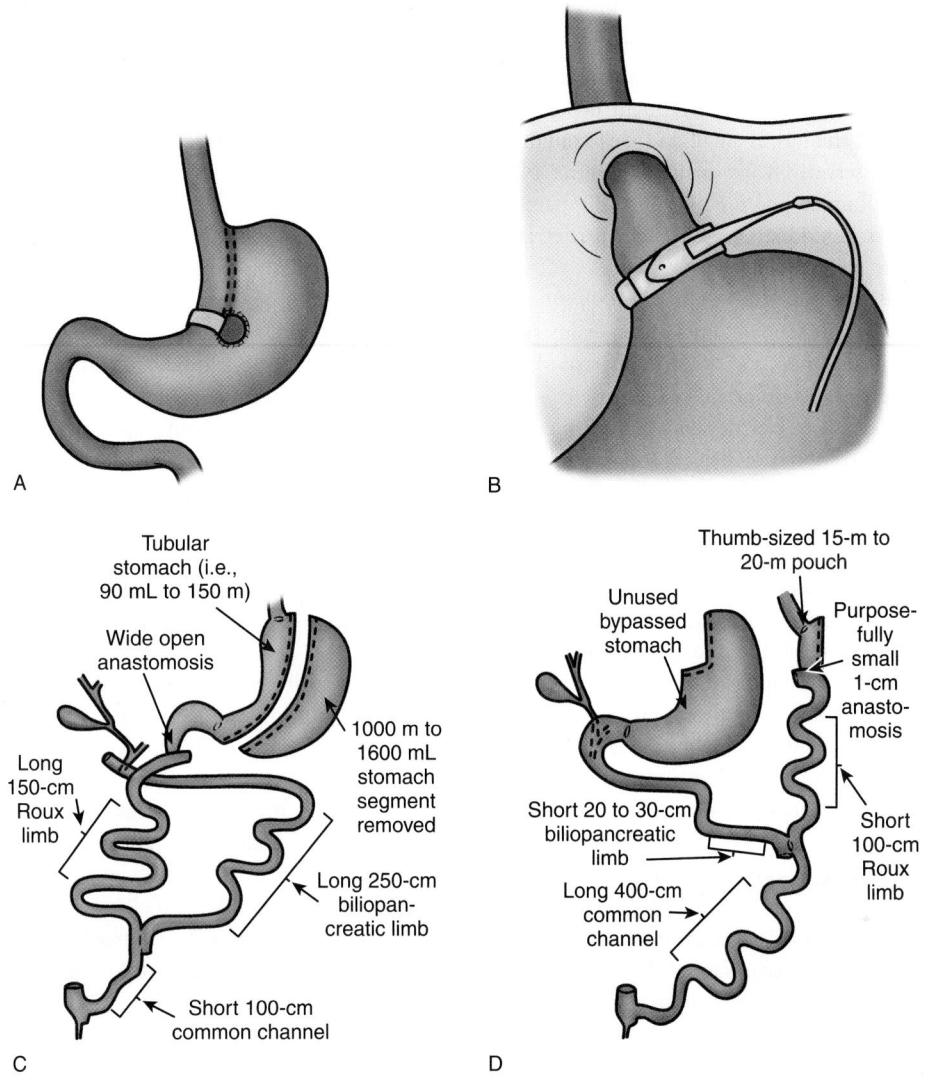

Figure 34-7 Bariatric surgical procedures. *A,* Vertical banded gastroplasty creates a tubular stomach that is restrictive. *B,* Gastric banding systems are adjustable and reversible, and they can be placed laparoscopically. *C,* Biliopancreatic diversion with duodenal switch and vertical gastroplasty/sleeve gastrectomy. *D,* Roux-en-Y proximal gastric bypass. *(From Association of Perioperative Registered Nurses:* Standards, recommended practices, and guidelines, *2005, Denver, Association of Operating Room Nurses, 2005.)*

surgery, are morbidly obese, or who may not be able to tolerate the increased abdominal pressure associated with laparoscopic procedures.[37]

COMPLICATIONS AND MEDICAL MANAGEMENT

Several complications are associated with gastrointestinal surgery, including respiratory failure, atelectasis, pneumonia, anastomotic leak, deep vein thrombosis, pulmonary embolus, and bleeding. The morbidly obese patient is at even greater risk for many postoperative complications.[39,40]

Pulmonary Complications. The risk for pulmonary complications is substantial after gastrointestinal surgery, and adverse respiratory events such as atelectasis and pneumonia are twice as likely to occur in the obese patient.[39] Aggressive pulmonary exercise should be initiated in the immediate postoperative period. Early ambulation and adequate pain control assist in reducing

the risk of atelectasis development. Suctioning, chest physiotherapy, or bronchodilators may be needed to optimize pulmonary function. Patients should be closely monitored for the development of oxygenation problems. Treatment should be aimed at supporting adequate ventilation and gas exchange. Mechanical ventilation may be required in the event of respiratory failure.

Anastomotic Leak. An anastomotic leak is a severe complication of gastrointestinal surgery. It occurs when there is a breakdown of the suture line in a surgical anastomosis and results in leakage of gastric or intestinal contents into the abdomen or mediastinum (transthoracic esophagectomy).[36,39,40] The clinical signs and symptoms of a leak can be subtle and often go unrecognized. They include tachycardia, tachypnea, fever, abdominal pain, anxiety, and restlessness.[39,40] In the patient with an esophagectomy, a leak of the esophageal anastomosis may manifest as subcutaneous emphysema in the chest and neck.[36] If undetected, a leak can result in sepsis, multiorgan failure, and death. Patients with progressive tachycardia and tachypnea should have a radiologic study (upper gastrointestinal study with Gastrografin or CT scan with contrast) to rule out an anastomotic leak.[40,42,43] The type of treatment depends on the severity of the leak. If the leak is small and well contained, it may be managed conservatively by maintaining the NPO status, administering antibiotics, and draining the fluid percutaneously. If the patient is deteriorating rapidly, an urgent laparotomy is indicated to repair the defect.[42]

Deep Vein Thrombosis and Pulmonary Embolism. Pulmonary embolism (PE) is a very serious complication of any surgical procedure. Deep vein thrombosis (DVT) prophylaxis should be initiated before surgery and continue until the patient is fully ambulatory to reduce the risk of clot development. Typically, a combination of sequential compression devices and subcutaneous unfractionated heparin or low-molecular-weight heparin is used. Patients determined to be at high risk for PE may benefit from prophylactic inferior vena cava filter placement.[36,39,42]

Bleeding. Upper gastrointestinal bleeding is an uncommon but life-threatening complication of gastrointestinal surgery. Early bleeding usually occurs at the site of the anastomosis and can usually be treated through endoscopic intervention. Surgical revision may be needed for persistent, uncontrolled bleeding. Late bleeding is usually a result of ulcer development. Medical therapy is aimed at the prevention of this complication through administration of H_2-antagonists or PPIs.[36]

POSTOPERATIVE NURSING MANAGEMENT

Nursing care of the patient who has had gastrointestinal surgery incorporates a number of nursing diagnoses (see the Nursing Diagnoses feature on Gastrointestinal Surgery). Nursing management involves interventions aimed at optimizing oxygenation and ventilation, preventing atelectasis, providing comfort and emotional support, and maintaining surveillance for complications.

Pulmonary Management. Nursing interventions in the postoperative period are focused on promoting ventilation and adequate oxygenation and preventing complications such as atelectasis and pneumonia. After the patient is extubated, deep-breathing exercises and incentive spirometry should be initiated and then performed regularly. Early ambulation is

---

Nursing Diagnoses

Gastrointestinal Surgery

- Ineffective Breathing Pattern related to decreased lung expansion
- Impaired Gas Exchange related to alveolar hypoventilation
- Decreased Cardiac Output related to alterations in preload
- Acute Pain related to transmission and perception of cutaneous, visceral, muscular, or ischemic impulses
- Anxiety related to threat to biologic, psychologic, or social integrity
- Disturbed Body Image related to actual change in body structure, function, or appearance
- Deficient Knowledge related to lack of previous exposure to information

---

encouraged to promote maximal lung inflation and thereby reduce the risk of pulmonary complications and to reduce the potential for pulmonary embolus.

Pain Management. It is imperative to appropriately manage the patient's pain after gastrointestinal surgery. Adequate analgesia is necessary to promote mobility of the patient and decrease pulmonary complications. Initial pain management may be accomplished by intravenous opioid (morphine, hydromorphone) administration by means of a patient-controlled analgesia (PCA) pump, or through continuous epidural infusion of an opioid and local anesthetic (bupivacaine).[37,39,40] Oral pain medications can be started after an anastomosis leak is ruled out. Nonpharmacologic interventions such as positioning, application of heat or cold, and distraction may also be used. If the patient's pain is not being sufficiently relieved, the pain management service should be consulted.[36,40]

THERAPEUTIC MANAGEMENT
GASTROINTESTINAL INTUBATION

Because gastrointestinal intubation is used so often in critical care units, it is important for nurses to know the clinical indications and responsibilities inherent in tube use. The four categories of gastrointestinal tubes are based on function: nasogastric suction tubes, long intestinal tubes, feeding tubes, and esophagogastric balloon tamponade tubes (see the Patient Safety Alert on Tubing Misconnections).

Nasogastric Suction Tubes. Nasogastric tubes remove fluid regurgitated into the stomach, prevent accumulation of swallowed air, may partially decompress the bowel, and reduce the patient's risk for aspiration. Nasogastric tubes also can be used for collecting specimens, assessing the presence of blood, and administering tube feedings. The most common nasogastric tubes are the single-lumen Levin tube and the double-lumen Salem sump. The Salem sump has one lumen that is used for suction and drainage and another that allows air to enter the patient's stomach and prevents the tube from adhering to the gastric wall and damaging the mucosa. The tube is passed through the nose into the nasopharynx and then down through the pharynx into the esophagus and stomach. The length of time the nasogastric tube remains in place depends on its use. The tube is then placed to gravity, low intermittent suction, or low continuous suction, and in rare instances, it is clamped.[44,45]

Nursing management focuses on preventing complications common to this therapy, such as ulceration and necrosis of the nares, esophageal reflux, esophagitis, esophageal erosion and stricture, gastric erosion, and dry mouth and parotitis from mouth breathing. Interference with ventilation and coughing, aspiration, and loss of fluid and electrolytes can be critical problems. Interventions include irrigating the tube every 4 hours with normal saline, ensuring the blue air vent of the Salem sump is patent and maintained above the level of the patient's stomach, and providing frequent mouth and nares care.[44] The Nursing Interventions Classification feature on Tube Care: Gastrointestinal outlines the nursing activities for managing a patient with a gastrointestinal tube.

Patient Safety Alert

Tubing Misconnections—A Persistent and Potentially Deadly Occurrence

Tubing and catheter misconnection errors are an important and underreported problem in health care organizations. These errors often are caught and corrected before any injury to the patient occurs. Given the reality of and potential for life-threatening consequences, increased awareness and analysis of these errors—including averted errors—can lead to dramatic improvement in patient safety.

Nine cases involving tubing misconnections have been reported to The Joint Commission's sentinel event database. These errors resulted in eight deaths and one instance of permanent loss of function, and they affected seven adults and two infants. Reports in the media and to organizations such as the ECRI Institute, the U.S. Food and Drug Administration (FDA), the Institute for Safe Medication Practices (ISMP), and the United States Pharmacopeia (USP) indicate that misconnection errors occur with significant frequency and, in a number of instances, lead to deadly consequences.

Types of Misconnections

The types of tubes and catheters involved in the cases reported to The Joint Commission included central intravenous (IV) catheters, peripheral IV catheters, nasogastric (NG) feeding tubes, percutaneous enteric feeding tubes, peritoneal dialysis catheters, tracheostomy cuff inflation tubes, and automatic blood pressure cuff insufflation tubes. The specific misconnections involved an enteric tube feeding into an IV catheter (4 cases); injection of barium sulfate (gastrointestinal contrast medium) into a central venous catheter (1 case); an enteric tube feeding into a peritoneal dialysis catheter (1 case); a blood pressure insufflator tube connected to an IV catheter (2 cases); and injection of IV fluid into a tracheostomy cuff inflation tube (1 case).

A review by the USP of more than 300 cases reported to its databases found misconnection errors involving the following:

- IV infusions connected to epidural lines and epidural solutions (intended for epidural administration) connected to peripheral or central IV catheters
- Bladder irrigation solutions using primary IV tubing connected as secondary infusions to peripheral or central IV catheters
- Infusions intended for IV administration connected to an indwelling bladder (Foley) catheter
- Infusions intended for IV administration connected to NG tubes
- IV solutions administered with blood administration sets and blood products transfused with primary IV tubing
- Primary IV solutions administered through various other functionally dissimilar catheters, such as external dialysis catheters, a ventriculostomy drain, an amnio-infusion catheter, and the distal port of a pulmonary artery catheter

Many of the misconnection cases involved Luer connectors, which are small devices used in the connection of many medical components and accessories. There are two types of Luer connectors: slips and locks. A Luer slip connector consists of a tapered "male" fitting that slips into a wider "female" fitting to create a secure connection. The Luer lock connector has a threaded collar on the male fitting and a flange on the female fitting that screw together to create a more secure connection.

Examples of misconnections involving Luer connectors include the following:

- Capnography sampling tube to an IV cannula
- Enteral feeding set to a central venous catheter
- Enteral feeding set to a hemodialysis line
- Noninvasive blood pressure (NIBP) insufflation tube to a needleless IV port
- Oxygen tubing to a needleless IV port
- Sequential compression device (SCD) hose to a needleless "piggyback" port of an IV administration set

Root Causes Identified

The basic lesson from these cases is that if it *can* happen, it *will* happen. Luer connectors are implicated in or contribute to many of these errors because they enable functionally dissimilar tubes or catheters to be connected. Other causes include the routine use of tubes or catheters for unintended purposes, such as using IV extension tubing for epidurals, irrigation, drains, and central lines; using them to extend enteric feeding tubes; and positioning functionally dissimilar tubes used in patient care close to one another. In the cases reported to the Sentinel Event Database, contributing factors included movement of the patient from one setting or service to another and staff fatigue associated with working consecutive shifts.

Risk Reduction Strategies

There are no published standards that specifically restrict the use of Luer connectors to certain medical devices. Consequently, a broad range of medical devices, which have different functions and access the body through different routes, are often outfitted with Luer fittings that can be easily misconnected. Organizations in Europe and the United States are developing standards to restrict the types of devices that use Luer fittings in an attempt to mitigate misconnection hazards. According to Jim Keller, vice president, Health Technology Evaluation and Safety for the ECRI Institute, and Stephanie Joseph, project engineer for the ECRI Institute, the solution to reducing or eliminating misconnection errors lies in engineering controls respecting how products and devices are designed ("incompatibility by design") and in re-engineering work practices.

"A well-designed device should prevent misconnections and should prompt the user to take the correct action," explained Joseph, author of a guidance article published in the March 2006 issue of the ECRI Institute's *Health Devices* journal. As a first step in prevention, Joseph urges hospitals to avoid buying non-IV equipment (e.g., nebulizers, NIBP devices, enteral feeding sets) that can mate with the Luer connectors on patient IV lines. Joseph also emphasizes that the single most important work practice solution for clinicians is to trace all lines back to their origin before connecting or disconnecting any devices or infusions.

Other solutions include specific education and training regarding this problem for all clinicians and having practitioners take simple precautions such as turning on the light in a darkened room before connecting or reconnecting tubes or devices. The risk of waking a sleeping patient is minimal by comparison. Errors have occurred when patients or family members attempted to disconnect and reconnect equipment themselves. Staff should emphasize to all patients the importance of contacting a clinical staff member for assistance when there is an identified need to disconnect or reconnect devices.

Continued

Patient Safety Alert—*cont'd*

Some approaches to reducing the risk of misconnections have significant potential for unintended consequences:

- Labeling all tubes and catheters may not always be practical and may therefore lead to inconsistent implementation. However, labeling certain high-risk catheters (e.g., epidural, intrathecal, arterial) should always be done.
- Color-coding tubes and catheters can lead users to rely on the color coding rather than having a clear understanding of which tubes and catheters are connected correctly to which body inlets. Training or educating all staff (including temporary agency and travel staff) about the institution's color-coding system requires ongoing attention. Color-coding schemes often vary across institutions in the same community, creating increased risk when agency and travel staff are used.

Joint Commission Recommendations

The Joint Commission offers the following recommendations and strategies to health care organizations to reduce tubing misconnection errors:

1. Do not purchase non-IV equipment that is equipped with connectors that can physically mate with a female Luer IV line connector.
2. Conduct acceptance testing (for performance, safety, and usability) and, as appropriate, risk assessment (e.g., failure mode and effect analysis) on new tubing and catheter purchases to identify the potential for misconnections, and take appropriate preventive measures.
3. Always trace a tube or catheter from the patient to the point of origin before connecting any new device or infusion.
4. Recheck connections, and trace all patient tubes and catheters to their sources on the patient's arrival to a new setting or service as part of the hand-off process. Standardize this "line reconciliation" process.
5. Route tubes and catheters having different purposes in different, standardized directions (e.g., IV lines routed toward the head;

enteric lines toward the feet). This is especially important in the care of neonates.
6. Inform nonclinical staff, patients, and their families that they must get help from clinical staff whenever there is a real or perceived need to connect or disconnect devices or infusions.
7. For certain high-risk catheters (e.g., epidural, intrathecal, arterial), label the catheter, and do not use catheters that have injection ports.
8. Never use a standard Luer syringe for oral medications or enteric feedings.
9. Emphasize the risk of tubing misconnections in orientation and training curricula.
10. Identify and manage conditions and practices that may contribute to health care worker fatigue, and take appropriate action.

The Joint Commission also urges product manufacturers to implement "designed incompatibility," as appropriate, to prevent dangerous misconnections of tubes and catheters.

Resources

The ECRI Institute: Fatal air embolism caused by the misconnection of a medical device hoses to needleless Luer ports on IV administration sets [hazard report], *Health Devices*, 33(6):223-235, 2004.

The ECRI Institute: Misconnected flowmeter leads to two deaths [special report], *Health Devices Alerts*, January 25, 2003.

The ECRI Institute: Preventing misconnections of lines and cables, *Health Devices*, 35 (3):81-95, 2006.

Safe systems, safe patients: common connectors pose a threat to safe practice. *Texas Board Nurs Bull* 37(2):6-7, 2006.

U.S. Food and Drug Administration: FDA patient safety news, Show #31, September 2004; Show #20, October 2003; Show #46, December 2005. Available at www.accessdata.fda.gov/psn/index.cfm (accessed May 2009).

Modified from The Joint Commission: Sentinel Event Alert, no. 36, April 3, 2006. Available at www.jointcommission.org/SentinelEvents/SentinelEventAlert/sea_36.htm (accessed May 2009).

NIC

Tube Care: Gastrointestinal

Definition

Management of a patient with a gastrointestinal tube

Activities

Monitor for correct placement of the tube per agency protocol.
Verify placement with x-ray per agency protocol.
Connect tube to suction, if indicated.
Secure tube to appropriate body part with consideration for patient comfort and skin integrity.
Irrigate tube per agency protocol.
Monitor for sensations of fullness, nausea, and vomiting.
Monitor bowel sounds.

Monitor for diarrhea.
Monitor fluid and electrolyte status.
Monitor amount, color, and consistency of nasogastric output.
Replace the amount of gastrointestinal output with the appropriate intravenous (IV) solution as ordered.
Provide nose and mouth care 3 to 4 times daily or as needed.
Provide hard candy or chewing gum to moisten mouth as appropriate
Initiate and monitor delivery of enteral tube feedings, per agency protocol, as appropriate.
Teach patient and family how to care for tube, when indicated.
Provide skin care around tube insertion site.
Remove tube when indicated.

From, Bulechek GM et al: *Nursing interventions classification (NIC)*, ed 5, St Louis, 2008, Mosby.

Long Intestinal Tubes. Miller-Abbott, Cantor, and Andersen tubes are examples of long, weighted-tip intestinal tubes that are placed preoperatively or intraoperatively. The long length allows removal of contents from the intestine to treat an obstruction that cannot be managed by an nasogastric tube. These tubes can decompress the small bowel and can splint the small bowel intraoperatively or postoperatively. Because progression of the tubes depends on bowel peristalsis, their use is contraindicated in patients with paralytic ileus and severe mechanical bowel obstructions. Older devices such as the Cantor and Miller-Abbott tubes are rarely used today because the balloon and the distal end is filled with mercury; the newer Andersen tube has a preweighted tungsten tip and is a safer option.[44,48]

Interventions used in the care of the patient with a long intestinal tube are similar to those with a nasogastric tube. The patient should be observed for (1) gaseous distention of the balloon section, which makes removal difficult; (2) rupture of the balloon or spillage of mercury into the intestine; (3) overinflation of the balloon, which can lead to intestinal rupture; and (4) reverse intussusception if the tube is removed rapidly. Intestinal tubes should be removed slowly; usually 6 inches of the tube is withdrawn every hour.[44,48]

Feeding Tubes. Small-diameter (8- to 12-Fr) flexible feeding tubes, such as Dobhoff tubes, are commonly placed at the bedside for patients who cannot take nourishment orally. The feeding tube may be inserted orally or nasally so that the tip ends up in the stomach or duodenum. To facilitate passage into the gastrointestinal tract, these tubes have a weighted tungsten tip, and a guidewire is needed to prevent them from curling up in the back of the patient's throat. An x-ray film must be obtained to verify correct placement of the tube before initiating feeding.[44-47] The tube should also be marked with indelible ink where it exits the mouth or nares so that the nurse can later verify that the tube has not been dislodged.[47]

Nursing management of the patient with a feeding tube includes prevention of complications and monitoring the tolerance of feeding. Tracheobronchial aspiration of gastric contents is a serious potential complication.[46] Before administering medications or feedings, it is important to ensure that the tube is in the patient's stomach or duodenum. Assessing the exit point marked on the tube helps to determine whether the tube has maintained the same position. Looking for coiling in the mouth or throat can help detect upward displacement that may have occurred as a result of vomiting. The traditional practice of confirming placement by auscultating air inserted through the tube over the epigastrium is not reliable and is not recommended.[45-47] If there is any doubt about the tube's position, a repeat radiograph should be obtained. During feedings, the head of bed should be elevated at least 30 degrees to minimize the risk of aspiration, and gastric residuals should be checked at least every 4 to 6 hours.[46] Large gastric residuals, cramping, and abdominal distention may indicate intolerance of feeding, and the physician should be notified.[46] Other interventions include nares and oral care and flushing the tube with normal saline or water to maintain patency.[44,45]

Esophagogastric Balloon Tamponade Tubes. Tamponading tubes may be used to stop bleeding in patients when endoscopic therapy fails or while waiting for surgical intervention.

Although effective in 80% to 90% of patients, they are only a temporizing measure until definitive treatment can occur, and more than 50% of patients will rebleed when the balloon is deflated.[12,18-20] Three different types of balloon tamponade tubes are available. The Sengstaken-Blakemore tube has three lumens: one for the gastric balloon, one for the esophageal balloon, and one for the gastric suction (Fig. 34-8 A). The Linton-Nachlas tube also has three lumens: one for the gastric balloon, one for gastric suction, and one for esophageal suction (see Fig. 34-8B). The Minnesota tube has four lumens: one for the gastric balloon, one for the esophageal balloon, one for gastric suction, and one for esophageal suction (see Fig. 34-8C).

Balloon tamponade tubes are inserted by the physician.[20] After the tube is passed into the stomach and placement is confirmed by gastric aspirate, the gastric balloon is slowly inflated to a total contents of 500 mL of air (or as specified by the tube manufacturer). After radiographic confirmation of placement, the tube is secured and placed under tension so that the gastric balloon places pressure on the gastroesophageal junction. Usually, 1 to 3 pounds of tension are applied using a helmet with a constant-traction spring device.[20,44] If bleeding continues, the esophageal balloon is inflated to a pressure of 25 to 40 mm Hg.[19] Low, intermittent suction is applied to the gastric and esophageal ports. To prevent tissue necrosis, balloons are deflated every 4 hours for 15 minutes and discontinued after 24 to 48 hours.[19,20] When discontinuing tamponade therapy, the esophageal balloon pressure should be gradually decreased, and the patient is observed for evidence of bleeding. If bleeding occurs, the physician should be consulted.[19]

Nursing management of the patient with a balloon tamponade tube includes monitoring for rebleeding and observing for complications of the tube. The most common complication is pulmonary aspiration, which can be limited by emptying the stomach and placing an endotracheal tube before passing the balloon tamponade tube.[44] Additional complications include esophageal erosion and rupture, balloon migration, and nasal necrosis (see the Patient Safety Alert on Esophagogastric Balloon Tamponade Tubes).

ENDOSCOPIC INJECTION THERAPY

Endoscopic injection therapy is used to control bleeding of varices and ulcers. It may be performed emergently, electively, or prophylactically. An endoscope is introduced through the patient's mouth, and endoscopy of the esophagus and stomach

---

Patient Safety Alert

Esophagogastric Balloon Tamponade Tubes

Balloon migration can be a potentially life-threatening complication of this type of therapy. If the gastric balloon is allowed to slowly deflate or rupture, the esophageal balloon migrates upward, where it can occlude the patient's airway. If the patient develops respiratory distress, the gastric and esophageal balloon ports must be cut immediately.

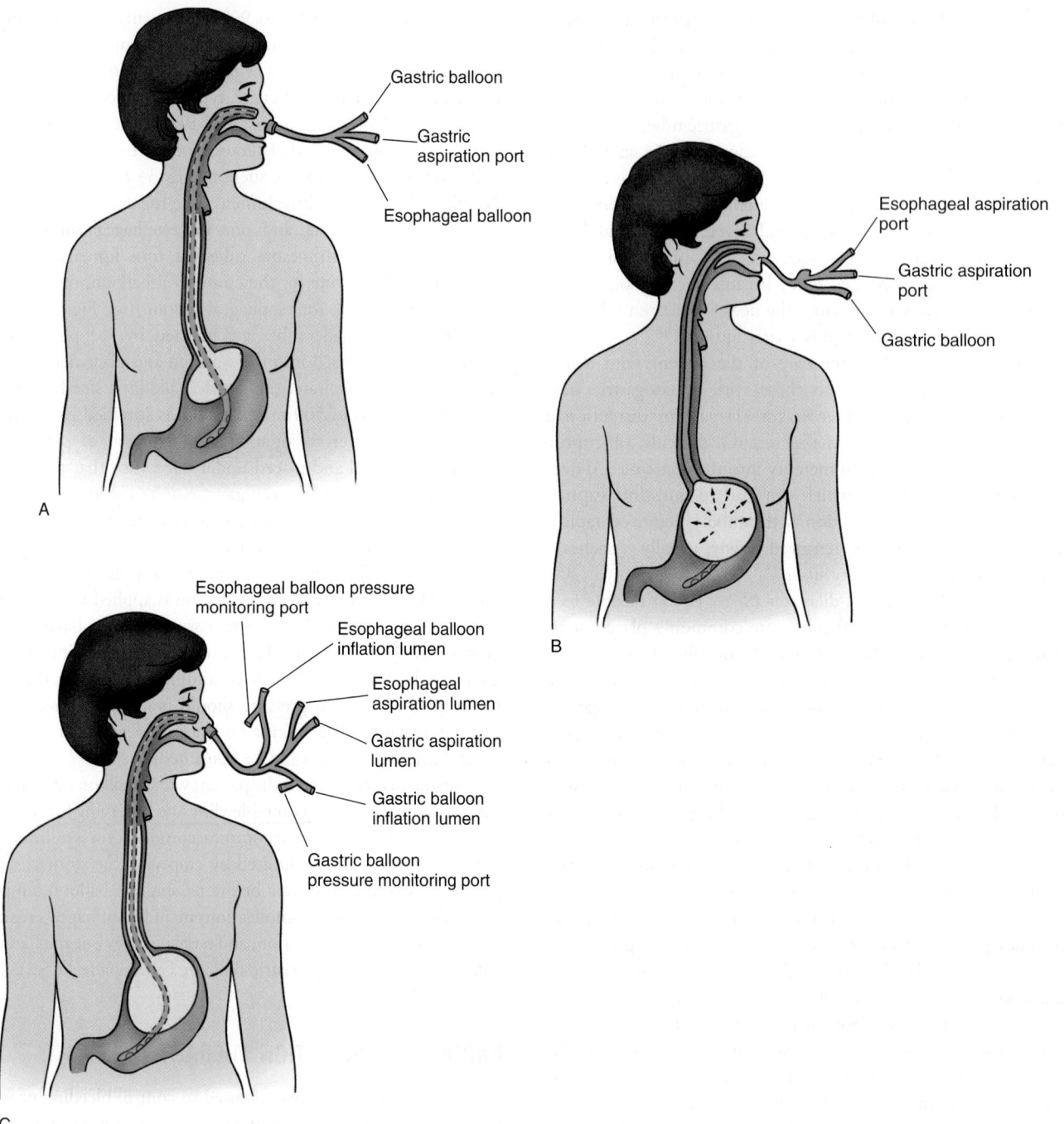

Figure 34-8 Esophageal tamponade tubes. *A,* Sengstaken-Blakemore tube. *B,* Linton-Nachlas tube. *C,* Minnesota tube.

is performed to identify the bleeding varices or ulcers. An injector with a retractable 23- to 25-gauge needle is introduced through the biopsy channel of the endoscope. The needle then is inserted in or around the varices or into the area around the ulcer, and a liquid agent is injected. The most commonly used agent is epinephrine, which results in localized vasoconstriction and enhanced platelet aggregation. Sclerosing agents such as ethanolamine, alcohol, and polidocanol also may be used. These agents cause an inflammatory reaction in the vessel that results in thrombosis and eventually produces a fibrous band. Repeated

sclerotherapy results in the development of supportive scar tissue around the varices. Other agents used include fibrinogen and thrombin, which when injected together react to form an active fibrin clot, and cyanoacrylate glue, which is used as a sealant to stop the bleeding.[2,9,12,18]

Endoscopic injection therapy controls acute variceal bleeding in as many as 70% to 90% of patients.[49] Complications can vary from mild to severe and include esophageal perforation, extravasation of the injection agent, and strictures of the esophagus.[12,18] This procedure is contraindicated in patients with severe coagulopathies.[15,18]

ENDOSCOPIC VARICEAL LIGATION

Endoscopic variceal ligation involves applying bands or metal clips around the circumference of the bleeding varices to induce venous obstruction and control bleeding. Between 1 and 2 days after the procedure, necrosis and scar formation promote band and tissue sloughing. Fibrinous deposits within the healing ulcer potentiate vessel obliteration. Band ligation is accomplished through endoscopy, with 5 to 8 bands placed per session.[12,18] The procedure may be repeated on an inpatient or outpatient basis over 2 to 3 weeks until all the varices are obliterated.[12,18]

Endoscopic variceal ligation controls bleeding in approximately 86% of the time.[50] This procedure is reported to require fewer endoscopic treatment sessions and has a lower rebleeding rate and fewer complications than endoscopic sclerotherapy.[12] The most common complication of endoscopic variceal ligation is the development of superficial mucosal ulcers. Systemic complications are rare.[50]

TRANSJUGULAR INTRAHEPATIC PORTOSYSTEMIC SHUNT

TIPS is an angiographic interventional procedure for decreasing portal hypertension. TIPS is advocated for (1) patients with portal hypertension who are also experiencing active bleeding or have poor liver reserve, (2) transplant recipients, and (3) patients with other operative risks.[12,18,20] The TIPS procedure is usually performed by a gastroenterologist, vascular surgeon, or interventional radiologist.

Portal hypertension is confirmed by direct measurement of the pressure in the portal vein (gradient greater than 10 mm Hg). Cannulation is achieved through the internal jugular vein, and an angiographic catheter is advanced into the middle or right hepatic vein. The midhepatic vein is then catheterized, and a new route is created connecting the portal and hepatic veins using a needle and guidewire with a dilating balloon. An expandable stainless steel stent is then placed in the liver parenchyma to maintain that connection (Fig. 34-9). The increased resistance in the liver is bypassed.[20]

TIPS may be performed on patients with bleeding varices, with refractory bleeding varices, or as a bridge to liver transplantation if the candidate becomes hemodynamically unstable. Postprocedural care should include observation for overt (cannulation site) or covert (intrahepatic site) bleeding, hepatic or portal vein laceration (resulting in rapid loss of blood volume), and inadvertent puncture of surrounding organs. Other complications include bile duct trauma, stent migration, and stent thrombosis.[12] Portal hypertension recurs almost universally after TIPS, whereas shunt dysfunction occurs in 50% to 60% of patients within 6 months.[12,18,20] The use of polytetrafluoroethylene-coated stents may improve shunt patency.[51]

GASTRIC TONOMETRY

Gastric tonometry is an indirect means of assessing regional perfusion of the gut by measuring the carbon dioxide (CO_2) of the gastric mucosa. Because the gut is extremely sensitive to decreased oxygen delivery and decreased blood flow results in increased hydrogen ion production, lactate formation, and CO_2 accumulation, measurement of the partial pressure of CO_2 in the stomach may enable early identification of hypoperfusion. This information provides the clinician with an enhanced clinical picture and assists with recognition and treatment of shock. This relatively noninvasive measurement is obtained with a modified nasogastric tube that has been combined with a gas-permeable silicone balloon system.[52-54]

Two types of tonometry methods are available: saline tonometry and air tonometry. In saline tonometry, the nasogastric tonometer is primed to clear all air and then is inserted as a normal nasogastric tube (Fig. 34-10). After insertion, the balloon lies close to the gastric mucosa. The balloon is then infused with anaerobic saline. The balloon is semipermeable to CO_2, which is produced by cells during the normal metabolic process. The level of CO_2 in the saline in the balloon equilibrates with the level of CO_2 in the gastric mucosal cells after 30 to 60 minutes. A sample of the saline is then withdrawn anaerobically and sent along with an ABG sample to the blood gas laboratory. The CO_2 concentration from the saline and the HCO_3^- concentration from the ABG sample are correlated using the Henderson-Hasselbalch equation to determine the intramucosal pH (pHi).

Air tonometry is a newer technique in which air from the balloon is automatically withdrawn and analyzed by an infrared sensor. The pHi and gut mucosal CO_2 ($PgCO_2$) are then displayed at 10-minute intervals.[52-54]

A normal pH value is 7.35 to 7.45, and a normal $PgCO_2$ concentration is 35 mm Hg to 45 mm Hg, the same as an ABG level. In the presence of decreased gastric or splanchnic perfusion, as occurs in shock, the $PgCO_2$ value increases, and the pHi value decreases as a result of anaerobic metabolism. The PCO_2 gap is the difference between the mucosal and the arterial CO_2 concentrations and has been proposed as a better indicator of gastrointestinal mucosal perfusion. A normal gap is less than 10 mm Hg. A widening gap indicates compromised blood flow to the splanchnic bed.[52-53]

Nursing considerations for the use of gastric tonometry monitoring include accurate user sampling procedures if using saline tonometry. Mistakes in sample drawing or timing may produce a measurement that misdirects therapy. Enteral feedings and an acidic gastric environment can also affect readings.[52,53]

PHARMACOLOGIC AGENTS

Many pharmacologic agents are used in the care of patients with gastrointestinal disorders. Table 34-3 reviews the various agents and any special considerations necessary for administering them.

Antiulcer Agents. A number of different antiulcer agents are commonly used in the critical care setting, including H_2-antagonists, gastric PPIs, and gastric mucosal agents. H_2-antagonists are used to decrease the volume and concentration of gastric secretions and control gastric pH, decreasing the incidence of stress-related upper gastrointestinal bleeding. These agents work by blocking histamine stimulation of the

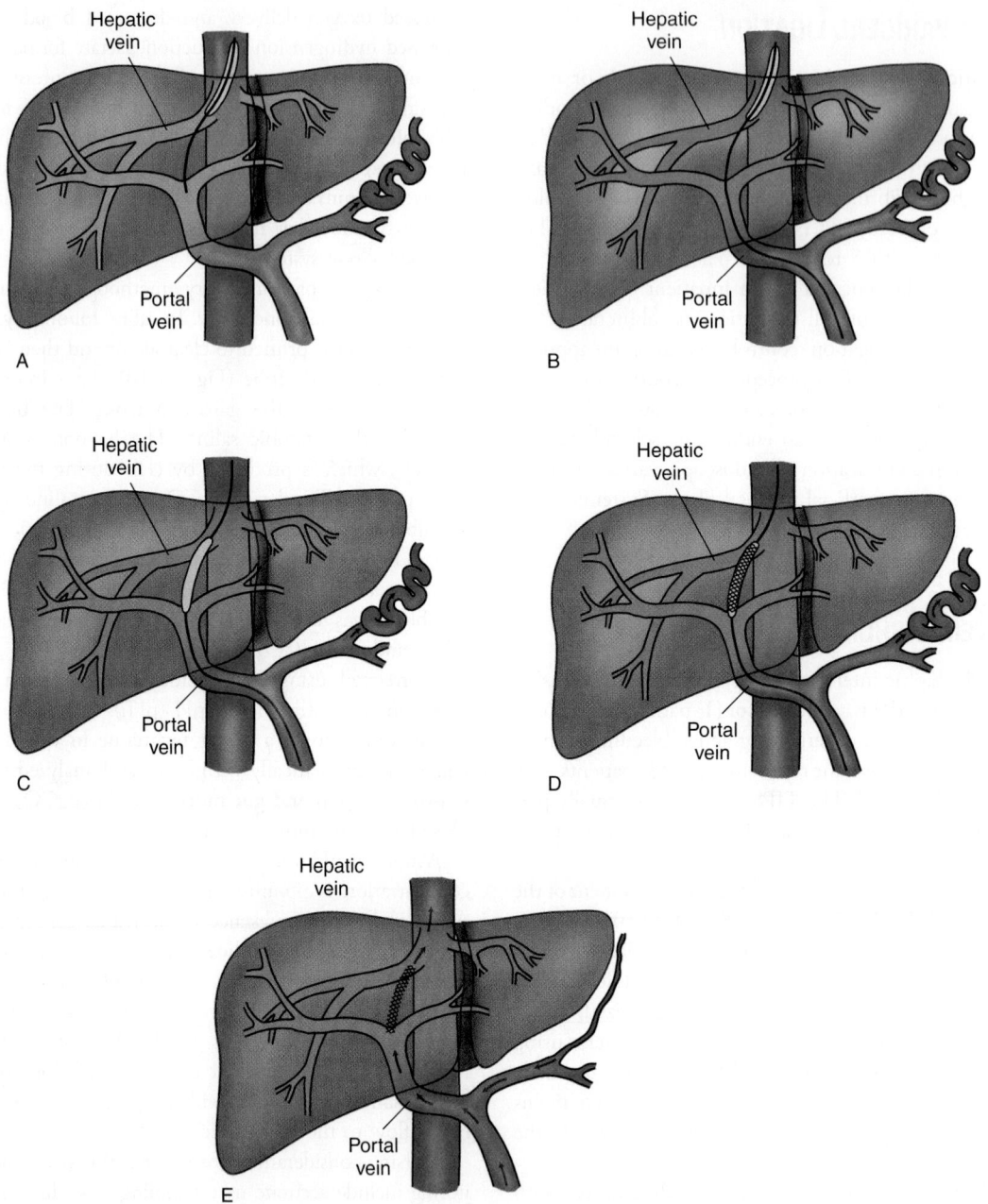

Figure 34-9 Transjugular intrahepatic portosystemic shunt (TIPS). *A,* Needle directed though liver parenchyma to portal vein. *B,* Needle and guidewire passed down to midportal vein. *C,* Balloon dilation. *D,* Deployment of stent. *E,* Intrahepatic shunt from portal to hepatic vein. *(From Zemel G et al: Percutaneous transjugular portosystemic shunt.* JAMA *266:390-393, 1991. ©1991 American Medical Association.)*

H$_2$-receptors on the gastric parietal cells, reducing acid production.[55] Although these drugs may be administered orally, intramuscularly, or intravenously, they usually are given intravenously in the critical care setting.

Proton-pump inhibitors decrease gastric acid secretion by binding to the proton pump, blocking the release of acid from the gastric parietal cells. PPIs are potent acid inhibitors and have greater suppressive ability than the H$_2$-agonists.[10,15] Pantoprazole and lansoprazole are the only PPIs available for intravenous administration.[10] The oral PPIs are formulated as enteric-coated tablets or as delayed-release capsules containing enteric-coated granules. Absorption occurs in an alkaline environment and begins only after

the granules leave the stomach and enter the duodenum.[55] For patients with an nasogastric or gastrostomy tube, administration can be time consuming and labor intensive.[10,56] The capsule can be opened and the granules mixed with 8.4% sodium bicarbonate to form a suspension or mixed with acidic juice.[56]

Unlike H$_2$-antagonists or PPIs, sucralfate does not affect gastric acid concentration but rather exerts its action locally. Sucralfate reacts with hydrochloric acid to form a sticky, paste-like substance that adheres to the surface of the ulcer and shields it from pepsin, acid, and bile. Sucralfate predominantly binds to damaged gastrointestinal mucosa, with minimal adherence to normal tissue. It is administered orally or through a

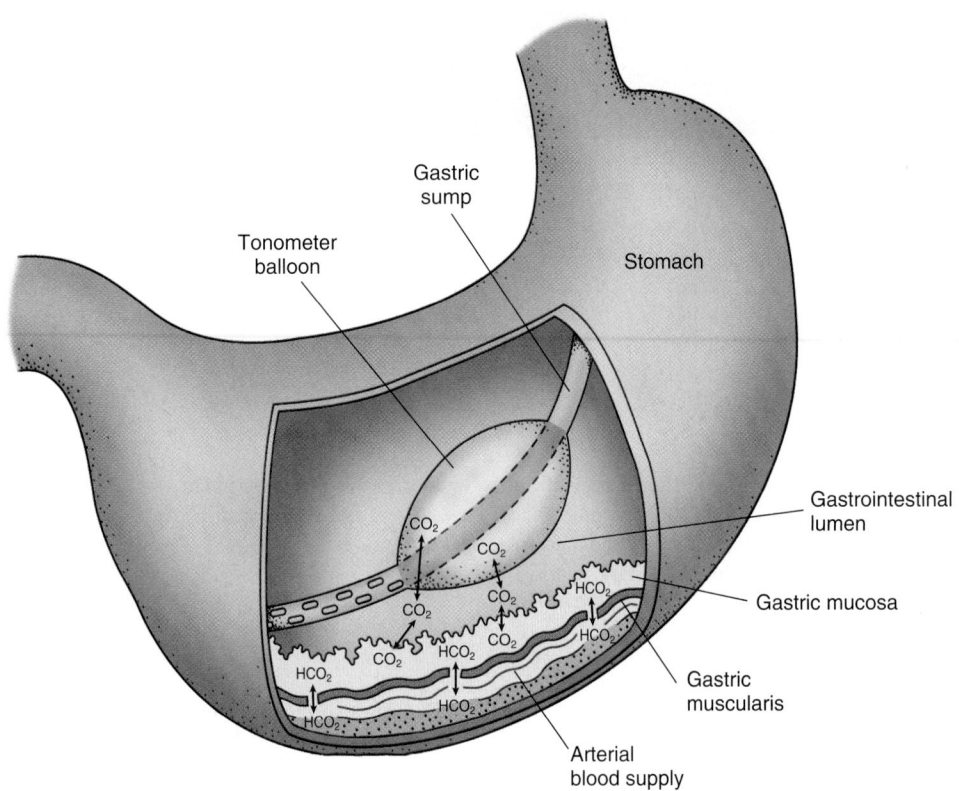

Figure 34-10 Principles of Pa_{CO_2} and HCO_3^- diffusion in gastric tonometry. *(From Clark CH, Gutierrez G: Gastric intramucosal pH: a noninvasive method for the indirect measurement of tissue oxygenation. Am J Crit Care 1:53, 1992.)*

TABLE 34-3 Pharmacologic Management: Gastrointestinal Disorders

MEDICATION	DOSAGE	ACTIONS	SPECIAL CONSIDERATIONS
Antacids	30-90 mL q1-2h PO or NG; possibly titrated to NG pH	Used to buffer stomach acid and raise gastric pH	Can cause diarrhea or constipation and electrolyte disturbances Irrigate NG tube with water after administration because antacids can clog tube.
Histamine₂ (H₂) Antagonists			
Cimetidine (Tagamet) Ranitidine (Zantac) Famotidine (Pepcid) Nizatidine (Axid)	300 mg q6h IV or PO 150 mg q12h PO or 50 mg q8h IV 40 mg daily PO or 20 mg q12h IV 150 mg q12h PO or 300 mg q 24h	Used to reduce volume and concentration of gastric secretions	Side effects include CNS toxicity (confusion or delirium) and thrombocytopenia. Separate administration of antacids and histamine blocking agents by 1 hour.
Gastric Mucosal Agents			
Sucralfate (Carafate)	1 g q6h NG or PO, given 1 hour before meals and at bedtime	Forms an ulcer-adherent complex with proteinaceous exudates Covers the ulcer and protects against acid, pepsin, and bile salts	Requires an acid medium for activation; do not administer within 30 minutes of an antacid May cause severe constipation May cause decreased absorption of certain drugs

Continued

TABLE 34-3 Pharmacologic Management: Gastrointestinal Disorders—*cont'd*

MEDICATION	DOSAGE	ACTIONS	SPECIAL CONSIDERATIONS
Gastric Proton-Pump Inhibitors			
Omeprazole (Prilosec)	20-40 mg q12h PO	Inactivates acid, or hydrogen, acid pump, blocking secretion of hydrochloric acid by gastric parietal cells	Capsules should be swallowed intact
Lansoprazole (Prevacid)	15-30 mg q24h PO		May increase levels of phenytoin, diazepam, warfarin
	30 mg over 30 min q24h IV		May administer concomitantly with antacids
Rabeprazole (Aciphex)	20-40 mg q24h PO		
Esomeprazole (Nexium)	40 mg q12-24h PO		
	20-40 mg q24h IV		
Pantoprazole (Protonix)	20-40 mg q24h PO		
	80 mg q8-12h IV		
Vasopressin			
(Pitressin Synthetic)	Loading dose of 20 units over 20 min IV, followed by 0.2-0.4 unit/min IV infusion. Doses can be increased to 0.9 unit/min if necessary.	Decreases splanchnic blood flow, reducing portal pressure	Side effects include coronary, mesenteric, and peripheral vasoconstriction. May be administered concurrently with nitroglycerin to minimize side effects
Octreotide			
(Sandostatin)	Bolus dose of 25-50 mcg followed by IV infusion of 25-50 mcg/hr for 48 hours.	Decreases splanchnic blood flow, reducing portal pressure	May cause hyperglycemia or hypoglycemia when initiating the drip and changing dosages

CNS, central nervous system IV, intravenous; NG, nasogastric; PO, by mouth.

gastric tube. Sucralfate should not be crushed but may be dissolved in 10 mL of water to form a slurry. It is also available as a suspension.[10,55]

Vasopressin. Vasopressin is used to control gastric ulcer and variceal bleeding. It is administered intraarterially, through a catheter inserted into the right or left gastric artery (through the femoral artery, aorta, and celiac trunk) or intravenously. It causes splanchnic and systemic vasoconstriction, subsequently reducing portal blood flow and pressure.[52]

A major side effect of the drug is systemic vasoconstriction, which can result in cardiac ischemia, chest pain, hypertension, acute heart failure, dysrhythmias, phlebitis, bowel ischemia, and cerebrovascular accident. These side effects can be offset with concurrent administration of nitroglycerin.[18] Other complications include bradycardia and fluid retention. Nursing responsibilities associated with the use of this therapy include maintenance of a patent infusion line and continuous monitoring for vasoconstrictive complications of therapy.[12,18]

Somatostatin and Octreotide. Somatostatin is a peptide that is administered parenterally in the acutely bleeding, cirrhotic patient. It reduces splanchnic vasodilation and portal pressure through the inhibition of secretion of various vasodilator hormones, and it is as effective as vasopressin in treating variceal bleeding with minimal side effects. Octreotide is a commonly used, long-acting synthetic analogue of somatostatin.[12,15,18]

Summary

Acute Gastrointestinal Hemorrhage

- Acute gastrointestinal hemorrhage can be caused by peptic ulcer disease or stress-related erosive syndrome, and it can result in hypovolemic shock.
- Medical management focuses on restoration of hemodynamic stability and control of bleeding.
- Nursing actions include administering volume replacement, controlling the bleeding, and maintaining surveillance for complications.

Acute Pancreatitis

- Acute pancreatitis can be caused by gallstones and alcoholism, and it can result in autodigestion of the pancreas.
- Medical management focuses on fluid management, nutritional support, and control of systemic and local complications.
- Nursing actions include providing comfort and emotional support and maintaining surveillance for complications.

Fulminant Hepatic Failure

- FHF is a syndrome characterized by the development of acute liver failure over 1 to 3 weeks, followed by the

development of hepatic encephalopathy within 8 weeks, in a patient with a previously healthy liver.
- Medical management focuses on treatment of elevated ammonia levels and control of complications such as bleeding, metabolic disturbances, and cerebral edema.
- Nursing actions include protecting the patient from injury and maintaining surveillance for complications.

Gastrointestinal Surgery
- Complications of surgery include atelectasis, pneumonia, anastomosis leak, deep vein thrombosis, and bleeding.
- Postoperative nursing actions include managing pain and preventing complications.

Therapeutic Management
- Nasogastric suction tubes and long intestinal tubes are often used in the management of gastrointestinal disorders.
- Esophagogastric balloon tamponade tubes are used to control bleeding varices when endoscopic therapy fails.
- Endoscopic procedures to control bleeding include endoscopic injection therapy and endoscopic variceal ligation.
- TIPS is a procedure for decreasing portal hypertension.
- Gastric tonometry is a method for assessing regional perfusion in the presence of shock.
- Common pharmacologic agents used in the management of gastrointestinal disorders include antacids, H_2-antagonists, gastric mucosal agents, proton pump inhibitors, vasopressin, and octreotide.

Case Study: Patient with Gastrointestinal Issues

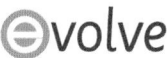 Answers to the Case Study Questions can be found on the Evolve web site at http://evolve.elsevier.com/Urden/.

Brief Patient History
Mrs. S is a 70-year-old woman with a long history of chronic back pain. She has been taking nonsteroidal antiinflammatory drugs (NSAIDs) for several years. She was recently started on warfarin for atrial fibrillation.

Clinical Assessment
Mrs. S is admitted to the intensive care unit because she is vomiting bright red blood. She is pale and diaphoretic and complains of epigastric pain.

Diagnostic Procedures
Mrs. S's vital signs include the following: blood pressure of 70/40 mm Hg, heart rate of 130 beats/min (sinus tachycardia), respiratory rate of 30 breaths/min, and temperature of 101.3° F. Her urine output is 15 mL/hr, hemoglobin level is 9 g/dL, and international normalized ratio (INR) is 5.3.

Medical Diagnosis
Mrs. S is diagnosed with upper gastrointestinal bleeding.

Questions
1. What major outcomes do you expect to achieve for this patient?
2. What problems or risks must be managed to achieve these outcomes?
3. What interventions must be initiated to monitor, prevent, manage, or eliminate the problems and risks identified?
4. What interventions should be initiated to promote optimal functioning, safety, and well-being of the patient?
5. What possible learning needs do you anticipate for this patient?
6. What cultural and age-related factors may have a bearing on the patient's plan of care?

---

evolve Be sure to check out the bonus material, including free self-assessment exercises, on the Evolve web site at http://evolve.elsevier.com/Urden/.

References

1. Tariq SH, Mekjian G: Gastrointestinal bleeding in older adults, *Clin Geriatr Med* 23:769, 2007.
2. Martins NB, Wassef W: Upper gastrointestinal bleeding, *Curr Opin Gastroenterol* 22:612, 2006.
3. Ferguson CB, Mitchell RM: Non-variceal upper gastrointestinal bleeding, *Ulster Med J* 75:32, 2006.
4. Cappell MS, Friedel D: Acute nonvariceal upper gastrointestinal bleeding: endoscopic diagnosis and therapy, *Med Clin North Am* 92:511, 2008.
5. Manning-Dimmitt LL et al: Diagnosis of gastrointestinal bleeding in adults, *Am Fam Physician* 71:1339, 2005.
6. Boonponmanee S et al: The frequency of peptic ulcer as a cause of upper-GI bleeding is exaggerated, *Gastrointest Endosc* 59:778, 2004.
7. Eswaran S, Roy MA: Medical management of acid-peptic disorders of the stomach, *Surg Clin North Am* 85:895, 2005.
8. McCance KL, Huether SE: *Pathophysiology: the biologic basis for disease in adults and children*, ed 5, St Louis, 2006, Mosby.
9. Ramakrishnan K, Salinas RC: Peptic ulcer disease, *Am Fam Physician* 76:1005, 2007.
10. Spirt MJ, Stanley S: Update on stress prophylaxis in critically ill patients, *Crit Care Nurse* 26:18, 2006.
11. Sesler JM: Stress-related mucosal disease in the intensive care unit: an update on prophylaxis, *AACN Adv Crit Care*, 18:119, 2007.
12. Dib N et al: Current management of the complications of portal hypertension: variceal bleeding and ascites, *CMAJ* 174:1433, 2006.
13. Toubia N, Sanyal AJ: Portal hypertension and variceal hemorrhage, *Med Clin North Am* 92:551, 2008.

14. Dutton RP: Current concepts in hemorrhagic shock, *Anesthesiol Clin* 25:23, 2007.

15. Rivkin K, Lyakhovetskiy A: Treatment of nonvariceal upper gastrointestinal bleeding, *Am J Health Syst Pharm* 62:1159, 2005.

16. Krumberger J: How to manage an acute upper GI bleed, *RN* 68:34, 2005.

17. Cerulli MA: *Upper gastrointestinal bleeding,* 2006. Available at http://emedicine.medscape.com/article/187857-overview (accessed April 2009).

18. Sanyal AJ: *Treatment of active variceal hemorrhage,* 2007. Available at www.uptodate.com/patients/content/topic.do?topicKey=~0lqS9r/KI33rsl (accessed May 2009).

19. Christensen, T: The treatment of oesophageal varices using a Sengstaken-Blakemore tube: considerations for nursing practice, *Nurs Crit Care* 9:58, 2004.

20. de Caestecker J, Straus J: *Upper gastrointestinal bleeding: surgical treatment,* 2006. Available at http://emedicine.medscape.com/article/196561-overview (accessed April 2009).

21. Gilbert DA, Saunders DR: Iced saline lavage does not slow bleeding from experimental canine gastric ulcers, *Dig Dis Sci* 26:1065, 1981.

22. Holcomb SS: Stopping the destruction of acute pancreatitis, *Nursing* 37:42, 2007.

23. Carroll JK et al: Acute pancreatitis: diagnosis, prognosis, and treatment, *Am Fam Physician* 75:1520, 2007.

24. Bank S et al: Evaluation of factors that have reduced mortality from acute pancreatitis over the past 20 years, *J Clin Gastroenterol* 35:50, 2002.

25. Hughes E: Understanding the care of patients with acute pancreatitis, *Nurs Stand* 18:45, 2003.

26. Cothren C, Burch JM: Acute pancreatitis. In Harken AH, Moore EE, editors: *Abernathy's surgical secrets: questions and answers reveal the secrets to successful surgery,* ed 5, Philadelphia, 2004, Hanley & Belfus.

27. Vege SS, Chari ST: *Treatment of acute pancreatitis,* 2007. Available at www.utdol.com/utd/content/topic.do?topicKey=pancdis/11212&view=print (accessed April 2009).

28. McClave SA et al: Nutrition support in acute pancreatitis: a systematic review of the literature, *J Parenter Enteral Nutr* 30:143, 2006.

29. Lugli AK et al: The importance of nutrition status assessment: the case of severe acute pancreatitis, *Nutr Rev* 65:329, 2007.

30. Gourgiotis S et al: Surgical management of chronic pancreatitis, *Hepatobiliary Pancreat Dis Int* 6:121, 2007.

31. Vege SS, Chari ST: *Predicting the severity of acute pancreatic,* 2007. Available at www.utdol.com/utd/content/topic.do?topicKey=pancdis/2975&view=print (accessed April 2009).

32. Goldberg E, Chopra S: *Fulminant hepatic failure: definition; etiology; and prognostic indicators,* 2007. Available at www.utdol.com/utd/content/topic.do?topicKey=hep_dis/14112&view=print (accessed April 2009).

33. Khan SA et al: Acute liver failure: a review, *Clin Liver Dis* 10:239, 2006.

34. Polson J, Lee WM: *AASLD guideline: the management of acute liver failure,* 2007. Available at www.aasld.org/practiceguidelines/Documents/Practice%20Guidelines/Acuteliverfailurepg.pdf (accessed May 2009).

35. O'Grady J: Modern management of acute liver failure, *Clin Liver Dis* 11:291, 2007.

36. Mackenzie DJ, Popplewell PK, Billingsley KG: Care of patients after esophagectomy, *Crit Care Nurse* 24:16, 2004.

37. Smith CE: Gastrointestinal surgery. In Rothrock JC, editor: *Alexander's care of the patient in surgery,* ed 13, St Louis, 2007, Mosby.

38. Wente MN: Pancreaticojejunostomy versus pancreaticogastrostomy: systematic review and meta-analysis, *Am J Surg* 193:171, 2007.

39. Barth MM, Jenson CE: Postoperative nursing care of gastric bypass patients, *Am J Crit Care* 15:378, 2006.

40. Harrington L: Postoperative care of patients undergoing bariatric surgery, *Med Surg Nursing,* 15:357, 2006.

41. Leslie D et al: Surgery primer for the internist: keys to the surgical consultation, *Med Clin North Am* 91:353, 2007.

42. Mun EC, Tavakkolizadeh A: Complications of bariatric surgery. Available at www.uptodate.com/patients/content/topic.do?topicKey=~PDuu_Bd7aaKphm (accessed May 2009).

43. Ukleja A, Stone RL: Medical and gastroenterologic management of the post-bariatric patient, *J Clin Gastroenterol* 38: 312, 2004.

44. Noble KA: Name that tube, *Nursing* 33:56, 2003.

45. May S: Testing nasogastric tube positioning in the critically ill: exploring the evidence, *Br J Nurs* 16:414, 2007.

46. Metheny NA: Preventing respiratory complications of tube feeding, *Am J Crit Care* 15:360, 2006.

47. American Association of Critical-Care Nurses: Verification of feeding tube placement, *AACN News* 22(5):4, 2005.

48. Quickel R, Hodin RA: Treatment of small bowel obstruction, 2008. Available at www.uptodate.com/patients/content/topic.do?topicKey=~o14460Z pAhyypE (accessed May 2009).

49. Qureshi W et al: ASGE guideline: the role of endoscopy in the management of variceal hemorrhage, *Gastrointest Endosc* 62:651, 2005.

50. Raju GS et al: Endoscopic mechanical hemostasis of GI arterial bleeding, *Gastrointest Endosc* 66:774, 2007.

51. Bureau C et al: Improved clinical outcome using polytetrafluoroethylene-coated stents for TIPS: results of a randomized study. *Gastroenterology* 126:469, 2004.

53. Marshall AP, West SH: Gastric tonometry and monitoring gastrointestinal perfusion: using research to support nursing practice, *Nurs Crit Care* 9:123, 2004.

54. Marshall AP, West SH: Gastric tonometry and enteral nutrition: a possible conflict in critical care nursing practice, *Am J Crit Care* 12:349, 2003.

55. Carlesso E et al: Gastric tonometry, *Minerva Anestesiol* 72:529, 2006.

56. Soll AH: *Pharmacology of antiulcer medications,* 2007. Available at www.utdol.com/utd.com/content/topic.do?topicKey=acidpep/8883&view=print (accessed April 2009).

57. Ziegler A: The role of proton pump inhibitors in acute stress prophylaxis in mechanically ventilated patients, *Dimens Crit Care Nurs* 24:109, 2005.

Chapter
35

Endocrine Anatomy
and Physiology

$\mathcal{M}$aintaining dynamic equilibrium among the various cells, tissues, organs, and systems of the human body is a highly complex and specialized process. Two systems regulate these critical relationships: the nervous system and the endocrine system. The nervous system communicates by nerve impulses that control skeletal muscle, smooth muscle tissue, and cardiac muscle tissue. The endocrine system controls and communicates by distributing potent hormones throughout the body. Figure 35-1 lists the endocrine glands and their hormones, target tissues, and actions. When stimulated, the endocrine glands secrete hormones into surrounding body fluids. In the circulation, these hormones travel to specific target tissues, where they exert a pronounced effect. Receptors found on or within these specialized target tissue cells are equipped with molecules that recognize the hormone and bind it to the cell, producing a specific response.

PANCREAS

ANATOMY

The pancreas is a long, triangular organ. It is clinically described as consisting of a *head, neck, body,* and *tail.* The head of the organ lies in the C-shaped curvature of the duodenum, and the tail extends behind and below the stomach toward the spleen. The pancreas is approximately 15 cm (6 inches) long and 4 cm (1.5 inches) wide.

Pancreas Blood Supply. The pancreas receives arterial blood supply from many sources. The head of the pancreas receives it blood supply from both *pancreaticoduodenal arteries*: the superior pancreaticoduodenal artery, which is a branch of the common hepatic (which comes from the celiac trunk), and the inferior pancreaticoduodenal artery, which branches from the superior mesenteric artery. These two blood supplies *anastomose*. The neck, body, and tail of the pancreas receive their blood supply from multiple branches of the splenic artery (another branch of the celiac trunk). Venous drainage occurs through the veins that correspond to the arteries and that ultimately empty into the portal vein. The pancreas has two major functions: digestive and hormonal.

Exocrine Cells. Specialized exocrine cells within the pancreas secrete digestive enzymes into a duct that is 3 mm wide that transverses the length of the pancreas. The pancreatic duct

joins with the cystic duct, carrying bile from the liver and gallbladder, before it empties into the duodenum at the major duodenal papilla. This common ductal exit for the two organs raises the danger of a gallstone lodging at the duodenal papilla and blocking the outflow of pancreatic enzymes. Pancreas exocrine anatomy is illustrated in Figure 32-8 in Chapter 32, and pancreatic digestive juices are discussed as part of the physiology of the gastrointestinal system. Most pancreatic tissue is devoted to production of exocrine digestive juices.

Endocrine Cells. The pancreas contains specialized endocrine cells that secrete hormones directly into the bloodstream. The endocrine tissue is less than 5% of the total volume of the pancreas. The function of the endocrine hormones is the focus of the following discussion.

PHYSIOLOGY

Clusters of cells that appear to form tiny islands among the exocrine cells accomplish the endocrine functions of the pancreas. These clusters are known as the *islets of Langerhans* and are composed of four distinct cell types: *alpha, beta, delta,* and *PP*. The locations of the cells that produce these hormones is shown in Figure 35-2. Alpha cells secrete glucagon, beta cells secrete insulin, delta cells secrete somatostatin, and PP cells secrete pancreatic polypeptide hormone. Glucagon, insulin, somatostatin, and polypeptide hormones are released into the surrounding capillaries to empty into the portal vein, where they are distributed to target cells in the liver. They then go into general circulation to reach other target cells.

Insulin. Insulin is a potent anabolic hormone whose production is stimulated by the presence of glucose. Insulin is produced by the beta cells of the pancreas. It is the only hormone produced in the body that directly lowers glucose levels in the bloodstream. Insulin is responsible for the storage of carbohydrate, protein, and fat nutrients. Insulin also augments the transport of potassium into the cells, decreases the mobilization of fats, and stimulates protein synthesis (Table 35-1). Box 35-1 defines the terms commonly used when discussing glucose and insulin balance. The major stimulant for insulin secretion is an elevation of serum glucose. The greater the rise in blood glucose, the more insulin the normal pancreas produces. Other hormones inhibit the release of insulin (Box 35-2).

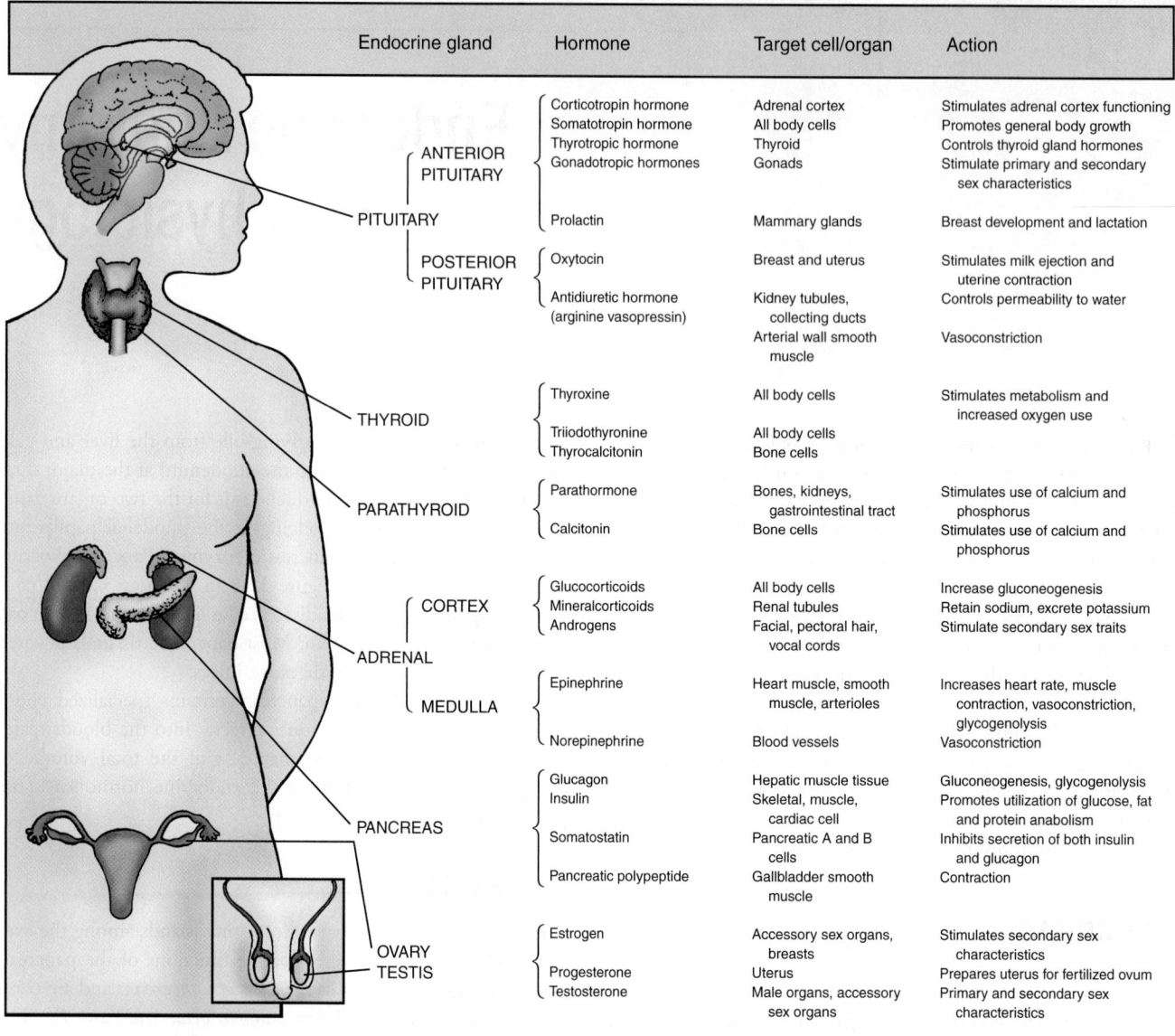

Endocrine gland	Hormone	Target cell/organ	Action
PITUITARY — ANTERIOR PITUITARY	Corticotropin hormone	Adrenal cortex	Stimulates adrenal cortex functioning
	Somatotropin hormone	All body cells	Promotes general body growth
	Thyrotropic hormone	Thyroid	Controls thyroid gland hormones
	Gonadotropic hormones	Gonads	Stimulate primary and secondary sex characteristics
	Prolactin	Mammary glands	Breast development and lactation
POSTERIOR PITUITARY	Oxytocin	Breast and uterus	Stimulates milk ejection and uterine contraction
	Antidiuretic hormone (arginine vasopressin)	Kidney tubules, collecting ducts	Controls permeability to water
		Arterial wall smooth muscle	Vasoconstriction
THYROID	Thyroxine	All body cells	Stimulates metabolism and increased oxygen use
	Triiodothyronine	All body cells	
	Thyrocalcitonin	Bone cells	
PARATHYROID	Parathormone	Bones, kidneys, gastrointestinal tract	Stimulates use of calcium and phosphorus
	Calcitonin	Bone cells	Stimulates use of calcium and phosphorus
ADRENAL — CORTEX	Glucocorticoids	All body cells	Increase gluconeogenesis
	Mineralcorticoids	Renal tubules	Retain sodium, excrete potassium
	Androgens	Facial, pectoral hair, vocal cords	Stimulate secondary sex traits
MEDULLA	Epinephrine	Heart muscle, smooth muscle, arterioles	Increases heart rate, muscle contraction, vasoconstriction, glycogenolysis
	Norepinephrine	Blood vessels	Vasoconstriction
PANCREAS	Glucagon	Hepatic muscle tissue	Gluconeogenesis, glycogenolysis
	Insulin	Skeletal, muscle, cardiac cell	Promotes utilization of glucose, fat and protein anabolism
	Somatostatin	Pancreatic A and B cells	Inhibits secretion of both insulin and glucagon
	Pancreatic polypeptide	Gallbladder smooth muscle	Contraction
OVARY	Estrogen	Accessory sex organs, breasts	Stimulates secondary sex characteristics
	Progesterone	Uterus	Prepares uterus for fertilized ovum
TESTIS	Testosterone	Male organs, accessory sex organs	Primary and secondary sex characteristics

Figure 35-1 Location of endocrine glands with the hormones they produce, target cells or organs, and hormonal actions.

Glucose Transporters. Human cells take up glucose by means of a facultative glucose transport family of proteins known as GLUTs, which are specialized in their tissue distribution and function (Table 35-2).[1,2] At the cellular level, glucose crosses the cell plasma membrane through *aqueous pores* formed by *facilitative transporters* of the GLUT family. GLUT4 plays a pivotal role in the way glucose moves from the bloodstream into the cell and is described in more detail.

GLUT4. After a meal, the levels of sugars and amino acids in the bloodstream rise. This increase signals pancreatic beta cells to release insulin into the bloodstream. As the insulin circulates in the vascular system, it activates an insulin receptor on the plasma membrane of cells, primarily peripheral muscle and adipose cells. This receptor initiates signaling cascades inside the cell to activate the glucose transporter 4 (GLUT4), which resides within the cells in clathrin-coated pits until needed. GLUT4 translocates (travels) from intracellular storage sites to the plasma membrane in response to the signal from the insulin

receptor *tyrosine kinase.*[3] At the cell surface, GLUT4 facilitates the passive transport of glucose down a concentration gradient into striated muscle and fat cells.

In the baseline state (between meals with normal blood glucose) only 4% to 10% of GLUT4 is located at the cell surface. Within 10 to 15 minutes of insulin stimulation of muscle cells, GLUT4 levels at the cell surface double as they rapidly translocate from the interior to the cell surface.[4] Between meals, the liver normally provides sufficient glucose output to maintain constant circulating glucose levels within the normal range.[3]

GLUT1 and GLUT3. The central nervous system (CNS) is freely permeable to glucose transported by GLUT1 and GLUT3, and it does not rely on insulin for the transport of glucose across the neural cell membrane.[5] The brain and other CNS cells require a constant source of glucose as they retain minimal glucose and glycogen stores.

Blood Glucose. Blood glucose is reported in millimoles per liter (mmol/L), which is the System International (SI) unit of

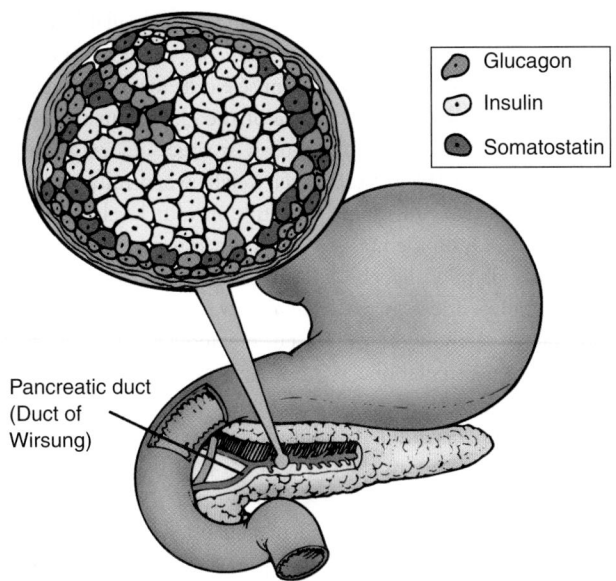

Glucagon
Insulin
Somatostatin

Pancreatic duct
(Duct of
Wirsung)

Figure 35-2 Macroscopic and microscopic structures of the pancreas and the islets of Langerhans.

BOX 35-1 TERMS USED FOR INSULIN AND GLUCOSE IMBALANCE

- **Anabolism**—constructive phase of metabolism in which the body converts simple substances into more complex compounds in the presence of energy
- **Catabolism**—destructive phase of metabolism in which the body breaks down complex substances to form simpler substances in the presence of energy
- **Gluconeogenesis**—formation of glucose from noncarbohydrate nutrients (e.g., fats, protein), which occurs in the liver
- **Glycogen**—storage form of glucose in liver and muscles
- **Glycogenesis**—formation of glycogen from glucose and ATP after a meal when both are plentiful
- **Glycogenolysis**—conversion of glycogen stored in the liver and muscles into usable glucose
- **Ketonemia**—production of ketone bodies more rapidly than the body can process them through the liver, with accumulation of acetone, β-hydroxybutyric acid, and acetoacetic acid in the bloodstream
- **Ketonuria**—excess of ketone bodies filtered from the bloodstream and excreted in the urine
- **Osmolality**—measurement of the number of particles in a solution or the concentration of a solution

measure used throughout the world. In the United States, blood glucose is measured in milligrams per deciliter (mg/dL). The normal blood glucose range is 70 to 100 mg/dL (3.9 to 5.6 mmol/L). To convert mmol/L of glucose to mg/dL, multiply the mmol/L value by 18. To convert mg/dL of glucose to mmol/L, divide the mg/dL value by 18.

In patients who have symptoms of diabetes, pancreatic beta cell destruction has already occurred. In type 1 diabetes, all of the beta cells are nonfunctional. In type 2 diabetes, about 50% of the beta cells are destroyed by the time the patient exhibits

signs and symptoms of diabetes.[6] The destruction of the beta cells disrupts homeostatic ability to regulate blood glucose.

Carbohydrate Anabolism. Glucose is admitted to the skeletal, cardiac, and adipose cells for use as energy in the presence of effective insulin facilitated by the glucose transporter GLUT4, as previously described. The movement of glucose from the circulation into the intracellular compartment reduces the concentration of glucose in the bloodstream and helps preserve the

TABLE 35-1 Pancreatic Endocrine Cells, Hormones, Stimulant Release Factor, Target Tissue, and Response or Action

Cell	Hormone	Stimulant Release Factor	Target Tissue	Response or Action
Alpha	Glucagons	↓ Glucose Exercise ↑ Amino acids SNS stimulation	Hepatocyte Myocyte	↑ Glucose in bloodstream ↑ Gluconeogenesis ↑ Glycogenolysis ↑ Fat mobilization ↑ Protein mobilization
Beta	Insulin	Glucose	Skeletal cells Muscle cells Cardiac cells	↓ Blood glucose ↓ Fat mobilization ↑ Fat storage ↓ Protein mobilization ↑ Protein synthesis ↑ Glucogenesis
Delta	Somatostatin	Hyperglycemia	A cells B cells	↓ Blood glucose ↓ Glycogen secretion ↓ Insulin secretion
PP	Pancreatic polypeptide	Acute hypoglycemia	Gallbladder Smooth muscle	↑ Gallbladder contraction ↓ Pancreatic enzyme

SNS, sympathetic nervous system; ↑, increases; ↓, decreases.

BOX 35-2 AGENTS THAT RELEASE OR INHIBIT INSULIN

Insulin Release (Major Stimulant: Elevated Blood Glucose Level)	Insulin Inhibition (Major Inhibitor: Low Blood Glucose Level)
HORMONES	
• Glucagons	• Somatostatin
• Corticotropic hormone	• Norepinephrine
• Thyrotropin	• Epinephrine
• Somatotropin	
• Glucocorticoids	
• Secretin	
• Gastrin	
DRUGS	
• β-Adrenergic stimulators	• β-Adrenergic blocking agents
• Sulfonylurea	• Diazoxide
• Theophylline	• Phenytoin
• Acetylcholine	• Thiazide or sulfonamide diuretics

TABLE 35-2 Glucose Transporters

GLUT	Anatomic Locations	Function
GLUT1	Erythrocytes, endothelial cells of brain	Basal glucose uptake Transport across blood-brain barrier
GLUT2	Pancreatic beta bells, liver, kidney, small intestine	High-capacity, low-affinity glucose transporter Can transport fructose
GLUT3	Brain cells, nerve cells	Transports glucose into neural tissue
GLUT4	Striated muscle and adipose tissue	Insulin-regulated transport in muscle and fat
GLUT5	Intestine, kidney, testis	Transports fructose
GLUT6	Spleen, leukocytes, brain	
GLUT7	Small intestine, colon, testis	Transports fructose
GLUT8	Testis, blastocyst, brain, muscle, adipocytes	Fuel supply of mature spermatozoa Insulin-responsive transport in blastocyst
GLUT9	Liver, kidney	
GLUT10	Liver, pancreas	
GLUT11	Heart, muscle	Muscle-specific fructose transporter
GLUT12	Heart, prostate, mammary gland	

GLUT, glucose transporter.

blood's osmolality. Simultaneously, glucose is available to the cell as its main energy source. Excess glucose in the form of glycogen is stored in the hepatic and muscle cells for use as fuel at a later time. In skeletal muscle, 90% of the glucose in the cell is converted to *glycogen* for longer-term storage.[7] Liver glycogen contributes up to 10% of total liver weight when fully replete.[7]

Fat Anabolism. Adequate, effective insulin levels affect fat metabolism. Dyslipidemias are strongly associated with type 2 diabetes.[8] Type 2 diabetes is characterized by overproduction of large, triglyceride-rich, *very-low-density lipoproteins* (VLDLs).[9] Disorders of carbohydrate and fat metabolism are also associated with the metabolic syndrome, a precursor to diabetes and cardiovascular disease.[10]

Protein Conservation. Insulin plus the GLUTs facilitate the transfer of glucose across the cell wall. By having glucose (carbohydrate) available as the body's fuel source, protein is spared from use as energy. Protein is then available for critical protein synthesis and for amino acid transport into the cells. Protein metabolism also benefits from an adequate insulin supply. Only in acute hyperglycemia of diabetic ketoacidosis (DKA) or in starvation states does the body use protein for energy sources.

Glucagon. Glucagon, synthesized by alpha cells in the pancreas, has the opposite effect of insulin. Glucagon is released during hypoglycemia to induce hepatic glucose output.[11] Because glucagon counterregulates insulin levels and raises blood glucose levels, it may be described as a potent *gluconeogenic hormone*. By means of gluconeogenesis, glucagon can form glucose from noncarbohydrate sources such as fat and protein when required. Glucagon release from the pancreas is stimulated by low blood glucose levels, starvation, exercise, or stimulation of the sympathetic nervous system (SNS), as listed in Box 35-3. Glucagon release protects the body from the consequences of hypoglycemia.

BOX 35-3 EFFECTS OF THE INSULIN-TO-GLUCAGON RATIO ON CARBOHYDRATE, FAT, AND PROTEIN METABOLISM

Balanced Insulin and Glucagon	Decreased Insulin and Increased Glucagon
• ↑ Use of glucose by cells	• ↓ Use of glucose by cells
• ↑ Movement of potassium intracellularly	• ↓ Movement of potassium intracellularly
• ↑ Carbohydrate metabolism	• ↑ Blood glucose
• ↓ Gluconeogenesis	• ↑ Gluconeogenesis
• ↑ Glycogen storage	• ↓ Glycogen storage
• ↓ Glycogenolysis	• ↑ Glycogenolysis
• ↓ Lipolysis	• ↑ Lipolysis
• ↓ Fat mobilization	• ↑ Fat mobilization
• ↑ Fat storage	• ↓ Fat stores
• ↓ Protein mobilization	• ↑ Hepatic metabolism fats
• ↑ Protein synthesis	• ↑ Ketogenesis
	• ↑ Mobilization of protein
	• ↑ Proteolysis
	• ↑ Lipoprotein

To meet short-term energy requirements glucagon stimulates the release of *glycogen* stores from liver and muscle cells. Through a process called *glycogenolysis,* the glycogen stored in the liver is converted into a glucose form that can be used by the cells.

For long-term energy needs, glucagon stimulates glucose release through the more complex process of *gluconeogenesis.* In gluconeogenesis, fat and protein nutrients are rapidly broken down into end products that are then changed into glucose.

A normal blood glucose level is maintained in the healthy body by the insulin-to-glucagon ratio. When the blood glucose level is high, insulin is released, and glucagon is inhibited. When blood glucose levels are low, glucagon rather than insulin is released to raise the blood glucose level. The brain has a very limited supply of glucose, and glucagon release is essential to protect the brain from the effects of hypoglycemia.[11]

Somatostatin. Somatostatin is a hormone that is produced in the pancreatic delta cells. Somatostatin decreases glucagon secretion,[11] and in high quantities, it decreases insulin release (see Table 35-1). Hyperglycemia stimulates the activity of the delta cells. It is theorized that the release of insulin enables somatostatin to control beta cell activity. Somatostatin may be involved in the regulation of the postprandial influx of glucose into cells.

Pancreatic Polypeptide. The role of pancreatic polypeptide, synthesized by the PP cells within the islets of Langerhans, is not completely understood. Pancreatic polypeptide release can be stimulated by acute hypoglycemia or by an intake that is high in protein and low in carbohydrate. The effect of hypersecretion or hyposecretion of this hormone has not been identified. The hormone represses pancreatic enzyme secretion and relaxes the smooth muscle tissue of the gallbladder.

PITUITARY GLAND AND HYPOTHALAMUS

ANATOMY

The hypothalamus is linked to the pituitary gland in two distinct ways. A vascular network connects the anterior portion of the pituitary with the hypothalamus, and a separate pathway of nerve fibers connects the posterior pituitary with the hypothalamus. Understanding the proximity of the hypothalamus and the pituitary gland is necessary to appreciate the correlation that exists between these organs.

The hypothalamus lies in the base of the brain, superior to the pituitary gland. It is composed of specialized nervous tissue responsible for the integrated functioning of the nervous system and endocrine system, which is called *neuroendocrine control.* The hypothalamus weighs approximately 4 g and forms the walls and lower portion of the third ventricle of the brain. The area composing the floor of the ventricle thickens in the center and elongates. It is from this funnel-shaped portion, called the *infundibular stalk* or *stem,* that the pituitary gland is suspended, as illustrated in Figure 35-3. The infundibular stalk contains a rich vascular supply and a network of communicating neurons that travel from the hypothalamus to the pituitary.

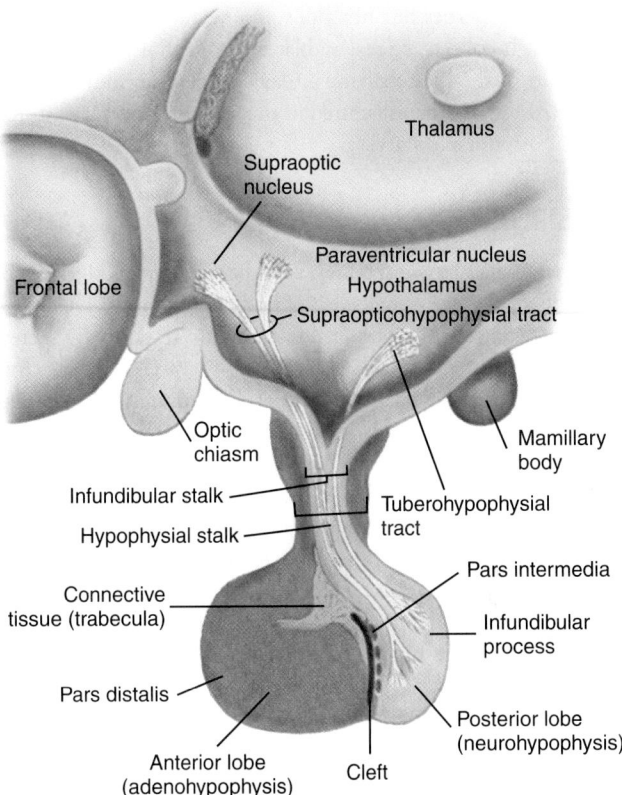

Figure 35-3 Anatomy of the hypothalamus and the pituitary gland and their locations in the skull. *(From Thompson JM et al: Mosby's clinical nursing, ed 5, St Louis, 2002, Mosby.)*

The vascular network and neural pathways transport chemical and neural signals and maintain constant communication between the nervous system and the endocrine system.

The pituitary gland is also called the *hypophysis.* It is attached below the hypothalamus and is found recessed in the base of the cranial cavity in a hollow depression of the sphenoid bone known as the *sella turcica.* Secured in such a protected environment, the pituitary is one of the most inaccessible endocrine glands in humans. However, because of this location, the pituitary gland is susceptible to injury from surgical and accidental trauma to the face and head. The pituitary is composed of the anterior lobe and the posterior lobe (see Fig. 35-3). Each component within the pituitary has its own origin, morphology, and function.

Anterior Pituitary. The anterior lobe of the pituitary, also called the *adenohypophysis,* is the largest portion of the gland. It communicates with the hypothalamus by means of a vascular network. The glandular tissue of the anterior pituitary produces several hormones, including adrenocorticotropic hormone (ACTH), thyroid-stimulating hormone (TSH), follicle-stimulating hormone (FSH), luteinizing hormone (LH), growth hormone, and prolactin. Information about all the hormones, their target tissues, and their actions is found in Figure 35-1.

Posterior Pituitary. The posterior lobe of the pituitary gland is also known as the *neurohypophysis.* It retains its continuity with the hypothalamus by means of neural fibers running through the infundibular stalk. The neurohypophysis has no glandular properties but functions as an extension of the hypothalamus. It collects, stores, and later releases hormones that are produced in the hypothalamus. Oxytocin and antidiuretic hormone (ADH) are manufactured in the hypothalamus and stored in the posterior pituitary.

PHYSIOLOGY

The hypothalamus gland is known as the master gland because of the influence it has over all areas of body functioning. The hypothalamus controls pituitary gland action and response by secreting substances called *release-inhibiting factors.* These factors control the release or inhibition of hormones. Thyrotropin-releasing hormone (TRH) is an example of a release-inhibiting factor. Virtually every function necessary to maintaining the human body in a state of dynamic equilibrium is regulated in this manner. One of the most important hormones to understand in caring for the critically ill patient is ADH.

Antidiuretic Hormone. ADH, known also as *arginine vasopressin,* is an important hormone responsible for regulating fluid balance within the body. ADH acts through specialized vasopressin receptors (V receptors) in specific target tissue[12]:

V_1 receptors in arterial walls
V_2 receptors in renal tissue
V_3 receptors in pituitary tissue

ADH has two functions. By means of the V_1 receptors, it constricts smooth muscles within the arterial wall, and through V_2 receptors, it regulates fluid balance by altering the permeability of the kidney tubule to water. ADH also contributes to control of the sodium level in the extracellular fluid by control of plasma osmolality. The sodium ion concentration in the plasma largely determines plasma osmolality. Osmoreceptors, believed to be sodium receptors, are located in the hypothalamus and are sensitive to changes in the circulating plasma osmolality.

Disorders of water metabolism are divided into *hyperosmolar* and *hypo-osmolar* states. Hyperosmolar disorders have a deficit of body water relative to body solute. Hypo-osmolar disorders have an excess of body water relative to total body solute.[13]

Sodium and water metabolism are regulated by different but complementary systems within the body. Sodium metabolism is predominately regulated by the renin-angiotensin-aldosterone system (RAAS), and water metabolism is primarily controlled by arginine vasopressin.[14]

A low sodium level is associated with a low serum osmolality (hypo-osmolar state). When sodium levels rise, plasma osmolality increases (hyperosmolar state). ADH is then released to stimulate water resorption at the nephron to maintain sodium balance. This process decreases water loss from the body and subsequently concentrates and reduces urine volume. Fluid conserved in this manner is returned to the circulating plasma, where it dilutes the concentration (osmolality) of plasma, as shown in Figure 35-4.

The release of ADH increases with hypovolemia. Primarily, the plasma osmotic pressure and the volume of circulating blood regulate the release of ADH. Stretch receptors located in the left atrium are sensitive to volume changes in the plasma that may be caused by vomiting, diarrhea, or blood loss. Hemorrhage that is sufficient to lower the blood pressure or emesis that is sufficient to reduce fluid volume stimulates the release of ADH. Other factors capable of influencing ADH secretion are pain, stress, malignant disease, surgical intervention, alcohol, and some drugs. Box 35-4 provides additional factors that affect ADH levels.

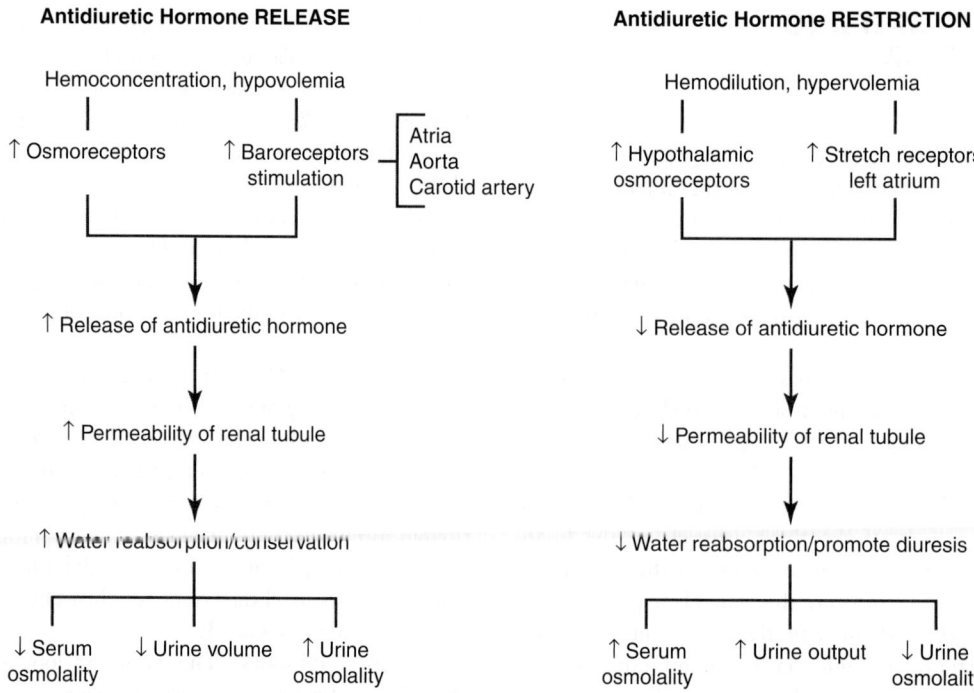

Figure 35-4 Physiology of the release and restriction of antidiuretic hormone.

THYROID GLAND

ANATOMY

The thyroid gland weighs 15 to 20 g in the adult human.[15] There is variation in the size of the adult gland according to the availability of dietary iodine in different geographic regions. The gland partially encases the trachea, is wrapped around the second to fourth tracheal rings anteriorly and laterally, and is located at the level of the sixth and seventh cervical vertebrae posteriorly. The thyroid gland lies inferior the thyroid cartilage and the articulating surface of the *cricoid cartilage*. This bow tie–shaped gland has two lateral lobes that are partially covered by the sternohyoid and sternothyroid muscles. The thyroid isthmus, the band of narrow thyroid tissue that connects the lateral lobes, lies directly inferior to the cricoid cartilage, as shown in Figure 35-5. The basic functional units

of the thyroid gland are spherical cells called *follicles*. Follicles are filled with a protein called *thyroglobulin*.

The parathyroid glands (usually four) are intimately associated with the posterior surface of the thyroid gland. The parathyroid glands derive their name from their anatomical proximity to the thyroid although they have completely different function. The parathyroid glands maintain calcium homeostasis.

Thyroid Blood Supply. The richly vascularized thyroid tissue receives about 5 mL of blood per gram of thyroid tissue per minute from the superior thyroid artery (a branch of the external carotid artery) and inferior thyroid artery (a branch of the *thyrocervical trunk* from the subclavian).

PHYSIOLOGY

Functioning of the thyroid gland depends on many factors that respond to a delicate hormonal interplay; the hypothalamus, anterior pituitary, dietary intake of iodine, and circulating protein bodies in the blood all affect thyroid gland function.

Pituitary Gland and Thyroid-Stimulating Hormone. The anterior lobe of the pituitary gland secretes TSH, also known as *thyrotropin*. TSH then stimulates the thyroid gland to produce thyroid hormones.

Iodine and Iodide. Through a complex process, dietary iodine is absorbed and concentrated in the thyroid follicles. About 100 mcg of iodide is needed on a daily basis to generate sufficient quantities of thyroid hormone.[15] In the United States, dietary ingestion of iodide ranges from 200 to 500 mcg per day.[15] The iodine is oxidized to iodide by the enzyme thyroid peroxidase.[15] Through active transport, the amino acid tyrosine binds the iodide to thyroglobulin, eventually yielding triiodothyronine (T_3) and thyroxine (T_4). More than 99% of T_3 and T_4 circulates in the bloodstream bound to transport proteins: thyroxin-binding globulin, prealbumin, and albumin. The minute amount of free thyroid hormone that is not protein bound is responsible for activating thyroid responses throughout the body. The free thyroid hormone is measured as T_3 and T_4. The unbound, physiologically active, free fraction of T_4 is only 0.02% of the total T_4 in the bloodstream. Free T_3 represents only 0.03% of the total serum level.[16]

Thyroglobulin. Thyroglobulin (Tg) is a key precursor in the biosynthesis of thyroid hormone. Thyroglobulin is stored in the thyroid follicles until needed. TSH release stimulates thyroglobulin secretion into the bloodstream.[17]

Triiodothyronine and Thyroxine. TSH prompts the thyroid cells to produce thyroid hormones (T_4 and T_3) in the presence of iodine from food that is ingested. T_4 is secreted only in the thyroid gland.[15] Most T_4 is subsequently converted into the more biologically active T_3.[18] Eighty percent of T_3 is the result of the conversion of T_4 to T_3 in peripheral tissues, and in the liver and kidneys.[15] A normal person with a healthy thyroid gland produces 90 to 100 mcg of T_4 per day and 30 to 35 mcg of T_3 per day.[15] T_3 acts more rapidly on target tissues in the body than does T_4, and it is more actively potent. Both thyroid hormones affect the rate at which oxygen is used in the body and therefore affect all metabolic processes in the body.

BOX 35-4	FACTORS AFFECTING ANTIDIURETIC HORMONE

Antidiuretic Hormone Stimulation	Antidiuretic Hormone Restriction
• Increased serum osmolality	• Decreased serum osmolality
• Emesis	• Hypervolemia
• Hypovolemia	• Water intoxication
• Hemorrhage	• Cold
• Pain	• Congenital defect
	• CO_2 inhalation

HYPOTHALAMIC-PITUITARY SYSTEM DAMAGE

• Accidental trauma	• Accidental trauma
• Surgical trauma	• Surgical trauma
• Pathologic trauma	• Pathologic trauma
• Stress	
• Physical	
• Emotional	
• Acute infections	
• Malignancies	
• Nonmalignant pulmonary disorders	
• Stimulated pulmonary baroreceptors	
• Nocturnal sleep	

DRUGS

• Nicotine	• Phenytoin
• Barbiturates	• Chlorpromazine
• Oxytocin	• Reserpine
• Glucocorticoids	• Norepinephrine
• Anesthetics	• Ethanol
• Acetaminophen	• Opioids
• Amitriptyline	• Lithium
• Carbamazepine	• Demeclocycline
• Cyclophosphamide	• Tolazamide
• Chlorpropamide	
• K^+-depleting diuretics	
• Vincristine	
• Isoproterenol	

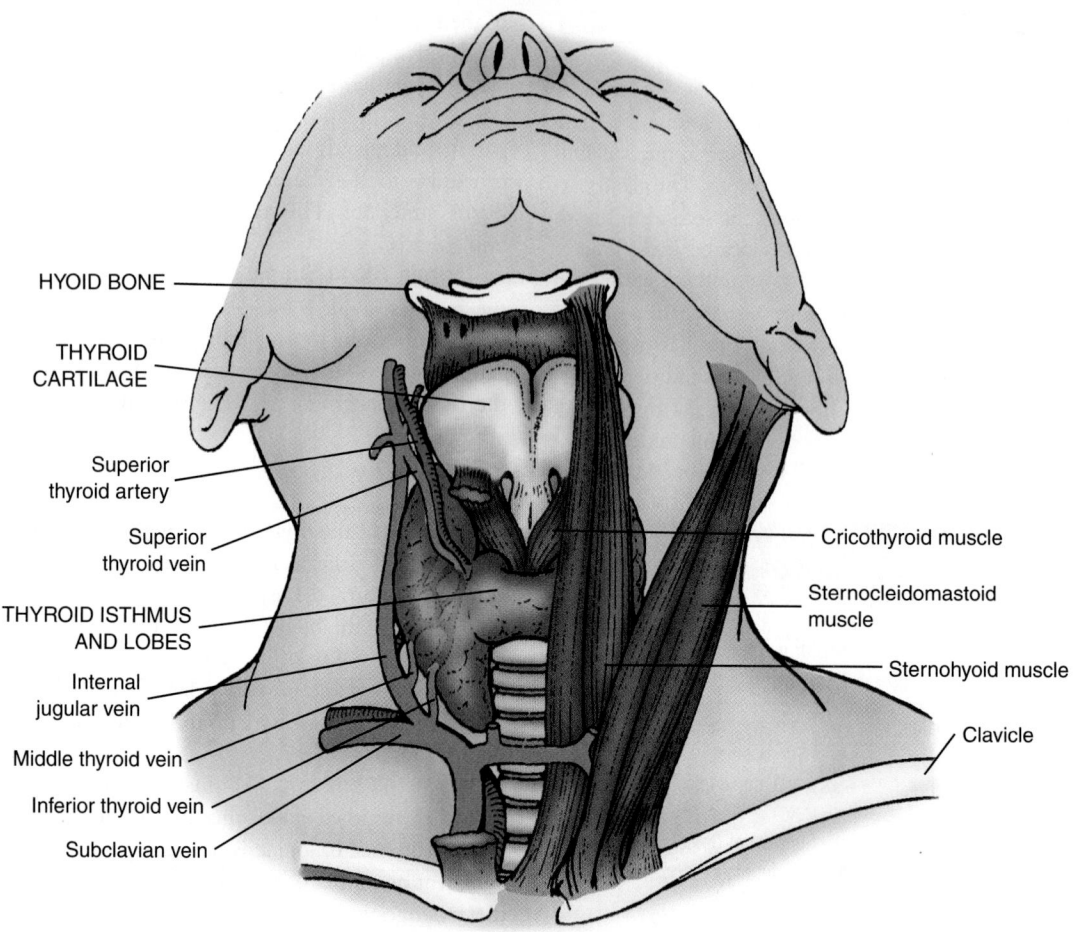

Figure 35-5 Gross anatomy of the human thyroid.

Calcitonin. The thyroid gland produces a third hormone, *thyrocalcitonin*, also called *calcitonin*. This hormone is produced by the parafollicular cells, or C cells, found scattered among the thyroid follicular cells. Calcitonin acts in concert with parathyroid hormone to maintain normal calcium blood levels. Calcitonin lowers calcium levels in the blood through urinary excretion and by promoting calcium absorption in the bone. In contrast, parathyroid hormone limits urinary loss and stimulates bones to release calcium. Throughout the remainder of this discussion, thyroid hormone refers collectively to T_3 and T_4, not calcitonin.

Hypothalamic-Pituitary-Thyroid Axis Feedback Loop. The hypothalamic-pituitary-thyroid axis regulates the mechanism for the synthesis and secretion of thyroid hormone. The production and secretion of thyroid hormone is regulated by a feedback mechanism that limits the amount of hormone circulating to the cellular need at that time, as illustrated in Figure 35-6.

In response to decreased circulating levels of T_3 and T_4, the hypothalamus releases TRH.[15] TRH then activates TSH in the anterior pituitary, and TSH stimulates the thyroid gland to manufacture and release the thyroid hormones T_3 and T_4 in the presence of iodine.[15] When serum blood levels of T_3 and T_4 become high, the pituitary inhibits the production of additional TSH. When levels of T_3 and T_4 become too low, the pituitary is stimulated to secrete additional TSH.

T_4 prompts the activation of β-adrenergic receptors in widespread areas of the body. These receptors trigger an SNS response and release norepinephrine at sympathetic nerve endings.[19] The effect is stimulation of the cardiac tissue, nervous tissue, and smooth muscle tissue, as well as an increase in metabolism and thermogenesis (increased body heat). Box 35-5 lists the major functions of thyroid hormone in more detail.

ADRENAL GLAND

ANATOMY

The adrenal glands, also called suprarenal glands, are small, yellowish, bilateral, pyramidal or semilunar-shaped organs located at the superior pole of the kidney. As a neighbor to the kidney, they are retroperitoneal and embedded in the renal fat pad. The normal adrenal gland is 3 to 4 cm in its longest axis and weighs approximately 5 g in the adult (Fig. 35-7). Functionally and histologically, two glands exist within the suprarenal gland: the outer cortex and the inner medulla. Both regions secrete hormones that are integral to the body's response to stress.

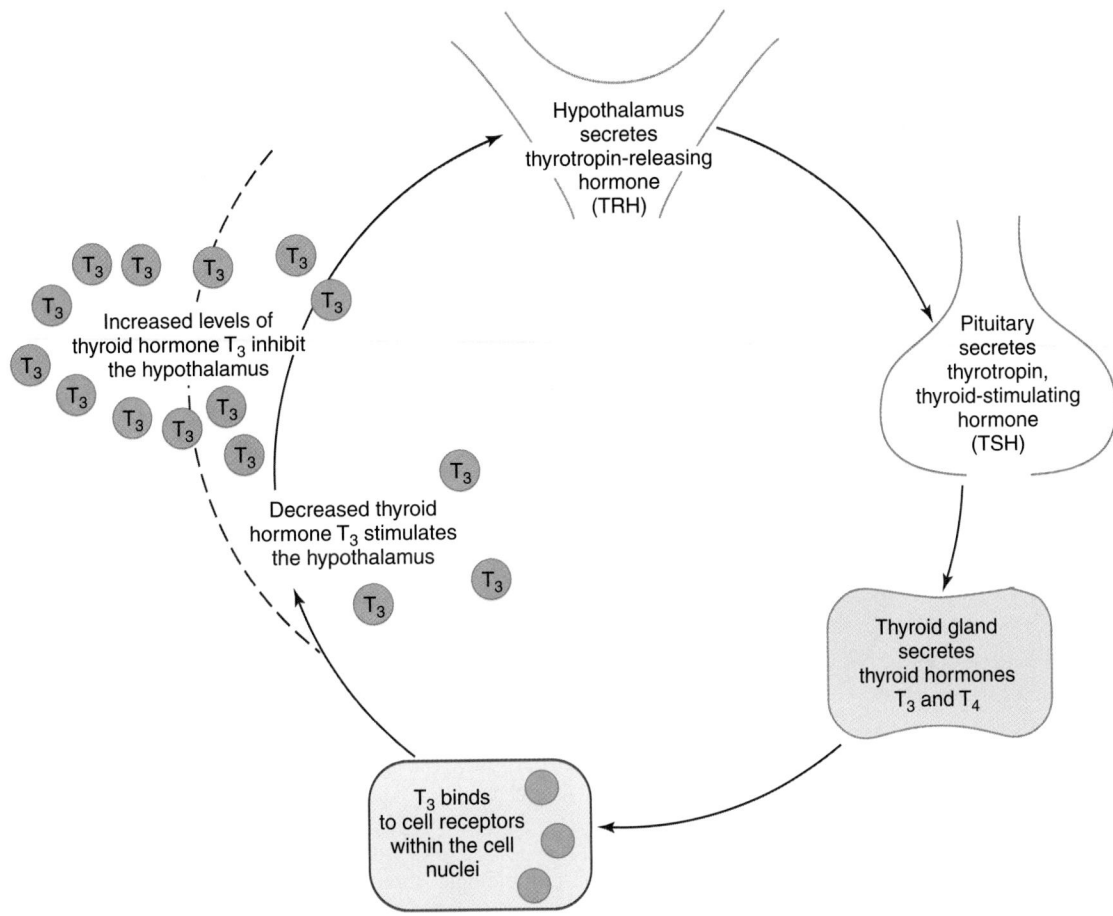

Figure 35-6 Hypothalamus-pituitary-thyroid axis feedback loop.

BOX 35-5   MAJOR FUNCTIONS OF THYROID HORMONES

- Interact with growth hormone
  - Maturation of skeletal system
  - Development of central nervous system
- Stimulate carbohydrate metabolism
  - Increase the rate of glucose absorption from the gastrointestinal tract
  - Increase the rate of glucose use by the cells
- Accelerate the rate of fat metabolism
  - Increase cholesterol degradation in the liver
  - Decrease serum cholesterol levels
- Increase protein anabolism and catabolism
  - Mobilize protein and release amino acids into circulation
  - Increase energy from protein nutrients through gluconeogenesis
- Increase the body's demand for vitamins

- Increase oxygen consumption and use
- Increase basal metabolic rate
- Have marked chronotropic and inotropic effects on heart
- Increase cardiac output
- Stimulate contractility and excitability of myocardium
- Increase blood volume
- Expand respiratory rate and depth necessary for normal hypoxic and hypercapnic drive
- Promote sympathetic overactivity
- Boost erythropoiesis
- Increase metabolism and clearance of various hormones and pharmacologic agents
- Stimulate bone resorption

Adrenal Cortex. The adrenal cortex is the thicker outer region, and it makes up 85% of the gland. The cortex is composed of three different layers of cells, each with a specific endocrine function: the zona glomerulosa, zona fasciculata, and the zona reticularis. The cortex secretes cortisol, it regulates fluid homeostasis by means of aldosterone, and it secretes androgens.

Adrenal Medulla. The inner region is called the adrenal medulla. The inner medulla is a part of the SNS, and it resembles a cluster of neurons more than an endocrine gland. The adrenal medulla contains clusters of specialized *chromaffin cells* that are modified preganglionic sympathetic neurons.[20] Different sets of chromaffin cells contain chromaffin granules that are specific for each of catecholamines epinephrine or norepinephrine.[20] The granules for each catecholamine appear in different sets of cells within the adrenal medulla. A chromaffin cell usually contains granules only for one catecholamine or the other.[20]

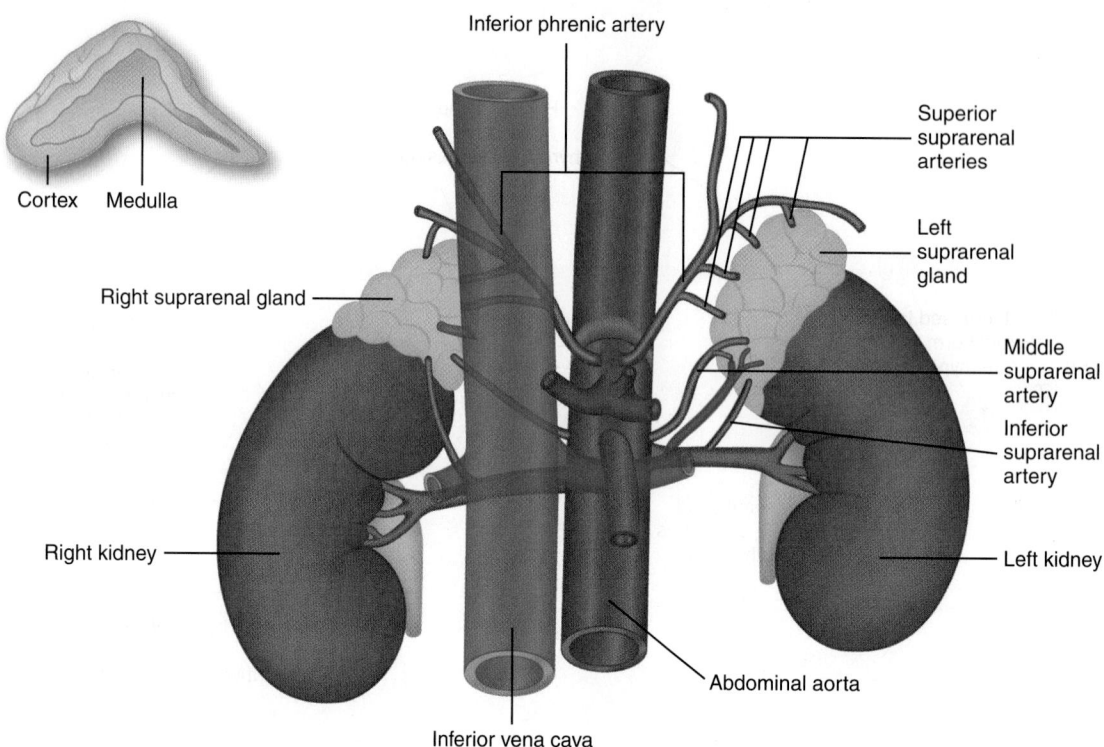

Figure 35-7 Adrenal gland.

The adrenal medulla is stimulated by the SNS by preganglionic bundles of sympathetic nerve fibers that originate in the spinal cord.[20] The role of the chromaffin cells is to secrete the catecholamines epinephrine and norepinephrine. In the bloodstream, these hormones produce a widespread excitatory effect described as a "surge of adrenaline" or as the fight-or-flight response.

Adrenal Blood Supply. The rich arterial blood supply comes to the adrenal gland from three sources (see Fig. 35-7):

1. The superior suprarenal artery is a branch of the inferior phrenic artery.
2. The middle suprarenal artery branches directly off of the aorta.
3. The inferior suprarenal artery branches off the renal artery.

Venous drainage is usually achieved through a single vein from each adrenal gland. The vein from the right adrenal gland drains into the inferior vena cava, and the vein from the left adrenal gland empties into the left renal vein.[21]

PHYSIOLOGY

The adrenal cortex and the adrenal medulla secrete important and very different hormones. Each part of the gland is functionally independent.

Hormones of the Adrenal Cortex. The adrenal cortex (outer layer) secretes three different classes of hormone, all of which are lipid-based steroid hormones. The *glucocorticoid* hormone *cortisol* is secreted from the cells of the *zona fasciculata* and *zona reticularis*. Cortisol is released in response to

physiologic stress caused by infection, trauma, and the fasting state. In hypoglycemia, the release of cortisol triggers other cells in the body to produce energy from fats and amino acids (proteins) to ensure that the brain receives a steady supply of glucose. Pharmacologic doses (high doses) of glucocorticoids are used to depress the inflammatory response and inhibit the immune system. Pharmacologic corticosteroids are administered to prevent rejection of newly transplanted solid organs (see Chapter 42). Corticosteroids are also used to treat inflammatory disorders, and they are administered when the adrenal gland is cortisol deficient.

The principal *mineralocorticoid* hormone *aldosterone* is secreted from the cells of the zona glomerulosa. Secretion of aldosterone is the final step in the RAAS. Aldosterone is secreted in response to intravascular hypovolemia, and its target of action is the distal tubules of the kidneys to retain more sodium and water in the bloodstream. In the healthy person, aldosterone contributes to the equilibrium of water and potassium in the body. Figure 19-16 in Chapter 19 illustrates the neurohormonal role of the RAAS in heart failure. In patients with heart failure, medications to block the effect of aldosterone on the kidneys often are prescribed. The most frequently used drug is Aldactone (spironolactone) (see "Neurohormonal Compensatory Mechanisms in Heart Failure" in Chapter 19). Some androgen hormones (e.g., dehydroepiandrosterone [DHEA]) are also secreted from the zona reticularis in the cortex. The function of DHEA is not fully understood.

Hormones of the Adrenal Medulla. The adrenal medulla (inner region) secretes two important catecholamines: *epinephrine,* also known as adrenaline, and *norepinephrine,* also known as noradrenaline. The adrenal medulla acts as a functional extension of the SNS. Stimulation of the SNS stimulates the chromaffin cells in the adrenal medulla to secrete predominantly epinephrine and some norepinephrine into the bloodstream. This results in an epinephrine surge described as the fight-or-flight response.[22] In the critical care unit, intravenous infusions of epinephrine and norepinephrine are used in shock states to raise the blood pressure. The pharmacologic effects of these catecholamines are described in Chapter 20 (see "Antidysrhythmic Drugs" and "Inotropic Drugs"), and the physiologic effects are listed in Table 20-10.

Hypothalamic-Pituitary-Adrenal Axis. The adrenal glands are physiologically linked to the hypothalamus and the pituitary gland. When the brain perceives a stressful or threatening situation, the hypothalamus releases *corticotropin-releasing hormone* (CRH), which acts on the anterior pituitary to release *adrenocorticotrophic hormone* (ACTH), which circulates in the bloodstream to reach the adrenal cortex and stimulate glucocorticoid hormone release. Under nonstress conditions, cortisol is secreted in a diurnal pattern, and levels are highest in the early morning and lowest in the late evening.[23] Illness or trauma disrupts this normal physiology with resultant loss of the diurnal pattern.[23]

Summary

- Insulin is released by the beta cells of the pancreas. An elevated blood glucose level is the stimulus for insulin secretion from the pancreas. The higher the blood glucose, the more insulin the normal pancreas produces.
- Glucagon is synthesized from the alpha cells in the pancreas. Its effect is the opposite of the effect of insulin. Glucagon release is stimulated by hypoglycemia, and it stimulates glucose output from the liver.
- The anterior pituitary gland secretes ACTH and TSH; the posterior pituitary gland secretes ADH, also known also as *arginine vasopressin.*
- Sodium and water metabolism are regulated by two complementary systems within the body. Sodium metabolism is regulated by the RAAS, and water metabolism is primarily controlled by arginine vasopressin.
- The thyroid hormones are T_4 and T_3. Most T_4 is converted to the more potent and biologically active T_3.
- The adrenal gland contains two functionally different endocrine regions. The adrenal cortex secretes cortisol and aldosterone. The adrenal medulla secretes epinephrine and norepinephrine.

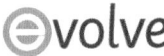 Be sure to check out the bonus material, including free self-assessment exercises, on the Evolve web site at http://evolve.elsevier.com/Urden/.

References

1. Scheepers A et al: The glucose transporter families SGLT and GLUT: molecular basis of normal and aberrant function, *JPEN J Parenter Enteral Nutr* 28(5):364-371, 2004.
2. Zhao FQ, Keating AF: Functional properties and genomics of glucose transporters, *Curr Genomics* 8(2):113-128, 2007.
3. Watson RT, Pessin JE: Bridging the GAP between insulin signaling and GLUT4 translocation, *Trends Biochem Sci* 31(4):215-222, 2006.
4. Zaid H et al: Insulin action on glucose transporters through molecular switches, tracks and tethers, *Biochem J* 413(2):201-215, 2008.
5. Simpson IA et al: Supply and demand in cerebral energy metabolism: the role of nutrient transporters, *J Cereb Blood Flow Metab* 27(11):1766-1791, 2007.
6. Rolla A: The pathophysiological basis for intensive insulin replacement, *Int J Obes Relat Metab Disord* 28(suppl 2):S3-S7, 2004.
7. Greenberg CC et al: Glycogen branches out: new perspectives on the role of glycogen metabolism in the integration of metabolic pathways, *Am J Physiol Endocrinol Metab* 291(1):E1-E8, 2006.
8. Poitout V, Robertson RP: Glucolipotoxicity: fuel excess and beta-cell dysfunction, *Endocr Rev* 29(3):351-366, 2008.
9. Adiels M et al: Overproduction of very low-density lipoproteins is the hallmark of the dyslipidemia in the metabolic syndrome, *Arterioscler Thromb Vasc Biol* 28(7):1225-1236, 2008.
10. Brunzell JD et al: Lipoprotein management in patients with cardiometabolic risk: consensus statement from the American Diabetes Association and the American College of Cardiology Foundation, *Diabetes Care* 31 (4):811-822, 2008.
11. Gromada J et al: Alpha-cells of the endocrine pancreas: 35 years of research but the enigma remains, *Endocr Rev* 28(1):84-116, 2007.
12. Maybauer MO et al: Physiology of the vasopressin receptors, *Best Pract Res Clin Anaesthesiol* 22(2):253-263, 2008.
13. Loh JA, Verbalis JG: Disorders of water and salt metabolism associated with pituitary disease, *Endocrinol Metab Clin North Am* 37(1):213-234, 2008.
14. Adler SM, Verbalis JG: Disorders of body water homeostasis in critical illness, *Endocrinol Metab Clin North Am* 35(4):873-894, 2006.
15. Demers LM: Thyroid disease: pathophysiology and diagnosis, *Clin Lab Med* 24(1):19-28, 2004.
16. Langton JE, Brent GA: Nonthyroidal illness syndrome: evaluation of thyroid function in sick patients, *Endocrinol Metab Clin North Am* 31 (1):159-172, 2002.
17. Torrens JI, Burch HB: Serum thyroglobulin measurement. Utility in clinical practice, *Endocrinol Metab Clin North Am* 30(2):429-467, 2001.
18. Fliers E et al: Hypothalamic thyroid hormone feedback in health and disease, *Prog Brain Res* 153:189-207, 2006.
19. Silva JE, Bianco SD: Thyroid-adrenergic interactions: physiological and clinical implications, *Thyroid* 18(2):157-165, 2008.
20. Díaz-Flores L et al: Histogenesis and morphofunctional characteristics of chromaffin cells, *Acta Physiol* 192(2):145-163, 2008.
21. Parnaby CN et al: Experience in identifying the venous drainage of the adrenal gland during laparoscopic adrenalectomy, *Clin Anat* 21(7):660-665, 2008.
22. de Diego AM et al. A physiological view of the central and peripheral mechanisms that regulate the release of catecholamines at the adrenal medulla, Acta Physiol 192(2):287-301, 2008.
23. Mesotten D et al: The altered adrenal axis and treatment with glucocorticoids during critical illness, *Nat Clin Pract Endocrinol Metab* 4(9):496-505, 2008.

Endocrine Clinical Assessment and Diagnostic Procedures

Chapter 36

ssessment of the patient with endocrine dysfunction is a systematic process that incorporates the history and the physical examination. Most of the endocrine glands are deeply encased in the human body. Although the placement of the glands provides security for the glandular functions, their resulting inaccessibility limits clinical examination. Nevertheless, the endocrine glands can be assessed indirectly. The critical care nurse who understands the metabolic actions of the hormones produced by endocrine glands assesses the physiology of the gland by monitoring that gland's target tissue as listed in Figure 35-1 in Chapter 35. This chapter describes clinical and diagnostic evaluation of the pancreas, the posterior pituitary, and the thyroid gland.

HISTORY

The initial presentation of the patient determines the rapidity and direction of the interview. For a patient in acute distress, the history is curtailed to only a few questions about the patient's chief complaint and precipitating events. For the patient without obvious distress, the endocrine history focuses on four areas: current health status, description of the current illness, medical history and general endocrine status, and family history. Data collection in the endocrine history for diabetes complications is outlined in the Data Collection feature on Diabetic Complications.

PANCREAS

PHYSICAL ASSESSMENT

Insulin, which is produced by the pancreas, is responsible for glucose metabolism. The clinical assessment provides information about pancreatic functioning. Clinical manifestations of abnormal glucose metabolism often include hyperglycemia, which is the initial assessment priority for the patient with pancreatic dysfunction.[1,2] Patients with hyperglycemia may ultimately be diagnosed with type 1 or type 2 diabetes[1,2] or be hyperglycemic in association with a severe critical illness.[1,3] All of these conditions have specific identifying features. More information on the specific pathophysiology and management of each condition is available in Chapter 37.

Hyperglycemia. Because severe hyperglycemia affects a variety of body systems, all systems are assessed. The patient may complain of blurred vision, headache, weakness, fatigue, drowsiness, anorexia, nausea, and abdominal pain. On *inspection,* the patient has flushed skin, polyuria, polydipsia, vomiting, and evidence of dehydration. Progressive deterioration in the level of consciousness, from alert to lethargic or comatose, is observed as the hyperglycemia exacerbates. If ketoacidosis occurs, the patient's breathing becomes deep and rapid (Kussmaul respirations), and the breath may have a fruity odor. *Auscultation* of the abdomen may reveal hypoactive bowel sounds. *Palpation* elicits abdominal tenderness. *Percussion* may reveal diminished deep tendon reflexes. Because hyperglycemia results in osmotic diuresis, the patient's fluid volume status is assessed. Signs of dehydration include tachycardia, orthostatic hypotension, and poor skin turgor. The key laboratory tests that assist in assessment are discussed in the following section.

LABORATORY STUDIES

Pertinent laboratory tests for pancreatic function measure short-term and long-term blood glucose levels, which can identify and diagnose diabetes.

Blood Glucose. The fasting plasma glucose (FPG) level is assessed by a simple blood test after the person has not eaten for 8 hours. A normal FPG level is between 70 and 100 mg/dL.[1] A fasting glucose level between 100 and 125 mg/dL identifies a person who is *prediabetic.* Even prediabetic individuals are at increased risk for complications of diabetes such as coronary heart disease and stroke. A FPG level of 126 mg/dL (7 mmol/L) or higher is diagnostic of diabetes (Table 36-1). In nonurgent settings, the test is repeated on another day to ensure the result is accurate. After a meal, the concentration of glucose increases in the bloodstream. Recommended postprandial glucose levels should not exceed 180 mg/dL (10 mmol/L).[4]

All hospitalized patients must have their blood glucose levels monitored frequently while in the hospital.[1] Clinical practice guidelines from the American Association of Clinical Endocrinologists (AACE) and the American Diabetes Association (ADA) recommend a target blood glucose level of 140-180 mg/dL in the critically ill.[5] This range was selected to increase patient safety while on continuous insulin infusions by decreasing the risk of hypoglycemia.

Data Collection

Diabetic Complications

Current Health Status
- The body may not be able to adjust to increased insulin needs resulting from sudden physiologic changes such as infection, injury, or surgery. The nurse assesses whether the patient has a severe infection, surgical wound, or traumatic injury.
- Recent or current signs and symptoms
  Unexplained changes in weight, thirst, hunger
  Headache, blurred vision
  Long-standing, unhealed infection
  Vaginitis, pruritus
  Leg pain, numbness
- Unexplained change in urinary patterns (e.g., daytime and nighttime, frequency, volume)
  Energy or stamina changes
  Endurance level
  Weakness
  Unexplained, excessive fatigue
- Behavior or mental changes (also ask family member or significant other for input)
  Memory loss
  Orientation

Assessment of Current Illness: Onset, Characteristics, and Course
- Chronic illness—Physiologic or psychologic stress can increase endogenous glucose.

- Recent treatments that could be a source of exogenous glucose
  Hyperalimentation
  Peritoneal dialysis
  Hemodialysis
- Medications, including prescription and over-the-counter preparations—Pharmacologic agents can alter pancreatic function by increasing or decreasing the release of endocrine hormones. Drugs also may interfere with hormonal action at the receptor site on the target cell.

Patient's Medical History: Questions
- Have you had prior pancreatic surgery?
- Have you ever been told that any of the following applied to you?
  Too much sugar in the urine?
  Too much sugar in the blood?
  Will probably develop too much sugar later in life?
- If you answered yes to any of these questions, what treatment, if any, was prescribed?
- Are you currently following such a treatment?

Family History: Questions
- Has a family member ever been diagnosed with diabetes or "sugar in the blood"?
- If so, how did he or she treat the condition?

TABLE 36-1 Blood Glucose Levels

Patient Status	Level (mg/dL)	Level (mmol/L)
Hypoglycemia	<70	< 3.9
Normal FPG level	70-100	>3.9-5.6
Impaired FPG level pre-diabetes*	100-125	5.6-6.9
Fasting FPG level diagnostic of diabetes	≥126	≥7.0
Non-FPG level diagnostic of diabetes	≥200	≥11.1

Data from American Diabetes Association: Standards of medical care in diabetes—2009, *Diabetes Care* 32(suppl 1):S13-S61, 2009.

FPG, fasting plasma glucose.

*Intermediate group whose FPG levels do not meet the criteria for diabetes but are too high to be considered normal.

When a continuous insulin infusion is administered, point-of-care blood glucose testing is performed hourly or according to hospital protocol by the critical care nurse to achieve and maintain the blood glucose within the target range.[1,5]

Hypoglycemia is defined as a blood glucose level below 70 mg/dl (3.9 mmol/L).[1,5,6] A complication of intensive glucose control is that hypoglycemic episodes may occur more frequently both in the hospital and with self-management of glucose levels in diabetes.[5-7]

Before discharge to home, diabetic patients should be taught to monitor their blood glucose levels.[1,4,7] Maintaining blood glucose within the normal range is associated with fewer types of diabetes-related complications and a lower rate of complications of diabetes.[4] Laboratory tests and point-of-care or self-monitoring of blood glucose represent the standard of care for management of diabetes. Unfortunately, home monitoring of blood glucose is not the norm, despite research evidence that maintaining blood glucose levels as close to normal as possible prolongs life and reduces complications. Only 40% of patients with type 1 diabetes and 26% of patients with type 2 diabetes monitor their blood glucose levels at least once daily.[4]

Urine Glucose. Testing the urine for glucose is not recommended for diabetic patients because there is too much variation in the renal threshold for glucose when diabetes-related kidney damage has occurred.[4] Urine glucose measurements are affected by variation in fluid intake, reflect an average glucose level, and not a specific point in time, and are altered by some drugs. Urine glucose testing does not offer any help in the identification of hypoglycemia.[4] For all of these reasons, urine testing is not recommended.

Glycated Hemoglobin. Blood testing of glucose is useful for daily management of diabetes. However, a different blood test is used to achieve an objective measure of blood glucose over an extended period. The glycated hemoglobin test (also known as glycosylated hemoglobin [HbA$_{1C}$ or A$_{1C}$]) provides information about the average amount of glucose that has been present in the patient's bloodstream over the previous 3 to 4 months.[4] During the 120-day life span of red blood cells (erythrocytes), the hemoglobin within each cell binds to the available blood glucose through a process known as *glycosylation.* Typically, 4% to 6% of hemoglobin contains the glucose group A$_{1C}$. A normal HbA$_{1C}$ value is 4% to 6%, with an acceptable target level for diabetic patients below 7%.[1] The HbA$_{1C}$ value correlates with specific blood glucose levels as shown in Table 36-2.[1] Not all clinical laboratories use the same analytic techniques to measure the glycated hemoglobin A$_{1C}$, and methods to standardize the reporting of results worldwide are being developed.[4,8] The American Diabetes Association recommends use of the HbA$_{1C}$ value both during initial assessment of diabetes mellitus, and for follow-up to monitor treatment effectiveness.[1]

Blood Ketones. Ketones (acetoacetate, β-hydroxybutyrate, and acetone) are by-products of fat metabolism. In most cases, when the body uses carbohydrate as its main source of energy, the liver completes fat metabolism, and minimal or no ketones are found in the blood. Ketone levels in the blood rise in acute illness, fasting, and with sustained elevation of blood glucose in type 1 diabetes when there is insufficient insulin. Home monitors to test capillary blood for elevated ketones (generally β-hydroxybutyrate) are recommended for type 1 diabetics in times or illness or stress.[4]

Elevated levels of ketones (ketonemia) are also detected by a fruity, sweet-smelling odor on the exhaled breath. This distinctive breath odor derives from the elimination of acetone as part of the compensatory response to maintain a normal pH. Ketones are also eliminated in the urine.

Urine Ketones. Urine ketone monitoring is important, particularly in patients with type 1 diabetes.[4] The presence of ketones in urine is retrospective and indicates that blood ketones were elevated. In diabetic ketoacidosis (DKA), fat breakdown (lipolysis) occurs so rapidly that fat metabolism is incomplete, and ketone bodies (acetone, β-hydroxybutyric acid, and acetoacetic acid) accumulate in the blood (ketonemia) and are excreted in the urine (ketonuria). It is recommended that all diabetic patients self-test or have their blood or urine tested for the presence of ketones during any acute illness or stress with a blood glucose level greater than 250 mg/dL, with symptoms of nausea, vomiting, or abdominal pain; and for women during pregnancy.

Normally, in healthy nonfasting individuals, only minute quantities of ketones are present in the urine, and these low levels are below the threshold of detection with routine testing methods.[4] In fasting and starvation states, ketones may be present in the urine.[4]

PITUITARY GLAND

The pituitary gland, recessed in the base of the cranium, is not accessible to physical assessment. The critical care nurse must therefore be aware of the systemic effects of a normally functioning pituitary to be able to identify dysfunction. One essential hormone formed in the hypothalamus but secreted through the posterior pituitary gland is *antidiuretic hormone* (ADH), also known as *vasopressin.*

PHYSICAL ASSESSMENT

ADH controls the amount of fluid lost and retained within the body. Acute dysfunction of the posterior pituitary or the hypothalamus can result in insufficient or excessive ADH production. The clinical signs of posterior pituitary dysfunction often manifest as fluid volume deficit (insufficient ADH production) or fluid volume excess (excessive ADH production).

Hydration Status. The nurse determines the effectiveness of ADH production by conducting a hydration assessment. A hydration assessment includes observations of skin integrity, skin turgor, and buccal membrane moisture. Moist, shiny buccal membranes indicate satisfactory fluid balance. Skin turgor that is resilient and returns to its original position in less than 3 seconds after being pinched or lifted indicates adequate skin elasticity. Skin over the forehead, clavicle, and sternum is the most reliable for testing tissue turgor because it is less affected by aging and more easily assessed for changes related to fluid balance. A well-hydrated patient has skin in the groin and axilla that is slightly moist to touch. In older patients, these typical assessment findings may be absent. Older persons, especially women, experience as much as a 50% decrease in total-body water content by age 75 years.[9]

Other indicators that the patient's hydration status is adequate for metabolic demands include a balanced intake and output and absence of thirst. Absence of thirst, however, is not a reliable indicator of dehydration in those with decreased thirst mechanisms, such as the older or critically ill patients. Absence of abrupt changes in mental status may also indicate normal hydration. Other indicators of normal hydration include absence of edema, stable weight, and urine specific gravity that falls within the normal range (1.005 to 1.030).

TABLE 36-2   Correlation between Hemoglobin A$_{1C}$ Concentration and Plasma Glucose Level

HbA$_{1C}$ (%)	Mean Plasma Glucose Level (mg/dL)	Mean Plasma Glucose Level (mmol/L)
6	126	7.0
7	154	8.6
8	183	10.2
9	212	11.8
10	240	13.4
11	269	14.9
12	298	16.5

Data from American Diabetes Association: Standards of medical care in diabetes—2009, *Diabetes Care* 32(suppl 1):S13-S61, 2009.

Vital Signs. Changes in heart rate, blood pressure, and central venous pressure (when available) are useful to determine fluid volume status. Blood pressure and pulse are monitored frequently. Decreased blood pressure with increased pulse is characteristic of hypovolemia, whereas elevated blood pressure and a rapid, bounding pulse may indicate hypervolemia. Orthostatic hypotension, which occurs when intravascular fluid volume decreases, is identified by a drop in systolic blood pressure of 20 mm Hg or a drop in diastolic blood pressure of 10 mm Hg when the patient changes position from lying to standing.

Weight Changes and Intake and Output. Daily weight changes coincide with fluid retention and fluid loss. Sudden changes in weight can result from a change in fluid balance; 1 L of fluid lost or retained is equal to approximately 2.2 pounds, or 1 kg, of weight gained or lost. To use weight as a true determinant of the fluid balance, all extraneous variables are eliminated, and the same scale is used at the same time each day. Precise measurement and notation of intake and output are used as criteria for fluid replacement therapy.

LABORATORY ASSESSMENT

No single diagnostic test identifies dysfunction of the posterior pituitary gland. Diagnosis usually is made through an array of laboratory tests combined with the clinical profile of the patient.

Serum Antidiuretic Hormone. The result of a blood test for normal levels of serum ADH is 1 to 5 pg/mL.[9] To prepare the patient for the test, all drugs that may alter the release of ADH are withheld for a minimum of 8 hours. Common medications that affect ADH levels include morphine sulfate, lithium carbonate, chlorothiazide, carbamazepine, oxytocin, and selective serotonin reuptake inhibitors (SSRIs).[10] Nicotine, alcohol, positive-pressure and negative-pressure ventilation, and emotional stress also influence ADH levels and must be considered in the interpretation of values.

The test, which is read by comparing serum ADH levels with the blood and urine osmolality, is helpful in differentiating the *syndrome of inappropriate antidiuretic hormone* (SIADH) from central *diabetes insipidus* (DI). Increased ADH levels in the bloodstream compared with a low serum osmolality and elevated urine osmolality confirms the diagnosis of SIADH. Reduced levels of serum ADH in a patient with high serum osmolality, hypernatremia, and reduced urine concentration signal central DI. Chapter 37 provides more information about SIADH and DI.

Urine and Serum Osmolality. Values for serum osmolality in the bloodstream range from 275 to 295 mOsm/kg H_2O. *Osmolality* measurements determine the concentration of dissolved particles in a solution. In a healthy person, a change in the concentration of solutes triggers a chain of events to maintain adequate serum dilution. Urine osmolality in the person with normal kidneys depends on fluid intake. With high fluid intake, particle dilution is low but will increase if fluids are restricted, and the expected range for urine osmolality therefore is wide, ranging from 50 to 1400 mOsm/kg.

Increased serum osmolality stimulates the release of ADH, which reduces the amount of water lost through the kidney.

Body fluid thereby is retained to dilute the particle concentration in the bloodstream. Decreased serum osmolality inhibits the release of ADH, the kidney tubules increase their permeability, and fluid is eliminated from the body in an attempt to regain normal concentration of particles in the bloodstream. The most accurate measures of the body's fluid balance are obtained when urine and blood samples are collected simultaneously.

Antidiuretic Hormone Test. The ADH test is used to differentiate *neurogenic* DI (central) from *nephrogenic* (kidney) DI. The patient is challenged with 0.05 to 1.0 mL of intranasally administered ADH in the form of desmopressin (1-deamino-8-D-arginine vasopressin [DDAVP]).[11] An intravenous line is inserted before ADH administration, and urine volume and osmolality are measured every 30 minutes for 2 hours before and after the ADH challenge. The patient with normal posterior pituitary function responds to the exogenous ADH by resorbing water at the kidney tubule and raising the urine osmolality slightly. In cases of severe central DI, in which the pituitary is affected, the urine osmolality shows a significant increase (becomes more concentrated), which indicates that the cell receptor sites on the kidney tubules are responsive to vasopressin. Test results in which urine osmolality remains unchanged indicate nephrogenic DI, suggesting kidney dysfunction because the kidneys are no longer responsive to ADH. This test is rarely performed in the critical care unit because of the unstable hemodynamic and volume status of most patients.[11]

DIAGNOSTIC PROCEDURES

In addition to laboratory tests, radiographic examination, computed tomography (CT), and magnetic resonance imaging (MRI) are used to diagnose structural lesions such as cranial bone fractures, tumors, or blood clots in the region of the pituitary. Although these procedures do not diagnose DI or SIADH, they are useful in uncovering the likely underlying cause.[11,12]

Radiographic Examination. A basic x-ray examination of the inferior skull views the sella turcica and surrounding bone formation. Bone fractures or tissue swelling at the base of the brain, which are apparent on a radiograph, suggest interference with the vascular supply and nerve impulses to the hypothalamic-pituitary system. Dysfunction can occur if the hypothalamus, infundibular stalk, or pituitary is impaired.

Computed Tomography. CT of the base of the skull identifies pituitary tumors, blood clots, cysts, nodules, or other soft tissue masses. This rapid procedure causes no discomfort except that it requires the patient to lie perfectly still. CT studies can be performed with radiopaque contrast (sodium iodine solution) or without contrast. The contrast dye is given intravenously to highlight the hypothalamus, infundibular stalk, and pituitary gland. This dye may cause allergic reactions in iodine-sensitive persons, and the patient must be carefully questioned about iodine allergy before the test. The size and shape of the sella turcica and the position of the hypothalamus, infundibular stalk, and pituitary are identified.

Magnetic Resonance Imaging. MRI enables the radiologist to visualize internal organs and cellular characteristics of specific tissues. MRI uses a magnetic field rather than radiation to produce high-resolution, cross-sectional images. The soft brain tissue and surrounding cerebrospinal fluid (CSF) make the brain especially suited to MRI. Although not a definitive diagnostic test for posterior pituitary hormonal imbalance, MRI may identify anatomic disruption of the gland and the surrounding area to uncover a primary cause of DI or SIADH.

THYROID GLAND
CLINICAL ASSESSMENT

History. The history of a patient in the critical care area should be as detailed as possible. Information regarding the clinical manifestations of hypothyroidism or hyperthyroidism must be obtained from the patient, family, or others with knowledge about the patient. Sample questions considered pertinent to detection of thyroid disease are provided in the Data Collection feature on Thyrotoxicosis (Hyperthyroidism) and Myxedema (Hypothyroidism).

Physical Examination. The thyroid is palpated for tenderness, nodules, and enlargement and is auscultated for bruits. The normal-size thyroid gland usually is neither visible nor palpable in the anterior neck.[13] Palpation may be done from an anterior or posterior approach. Auscultation of the thyroid is accomplished by use of the bell portion of the stethoscope to identify a bruit or blowing noise from the circulation through the thyroid gland. The presence of a bruit indicates enlargement of the thyroid, as evidenced by increased blood flow through the glandular tissue.

LABORATORY STUDIES

There is controversy about routine measurement of thyroid function in adults without clinical symptoms. The American Thyroid Association recommends thyroid function measurement in all adults beginning at age 35 years and every 5 years thereafter; more frequent screening is recommended for high-risk or symptomatic individuals.[14] The U.S. Preventive Services Task Force (USPSTF) found the research evidence insufficient to either recommend or recommend against routine screening for thyroid disease in asymptomatic adults.[15] There are no specific recommendations related to thyroid function screening for critically ill patients.

Data Collection

Thyrotoxicosis (Hyperthyroidism) and Myxedema (Hypothyroidism)

The patient is the best source for the following information. If the patient is unable to respond, the following questions can be directed to family, friends, a significant other, or those involved in admission of the patient to the intensive care unit.

- Have you ever been diagnosed with overactive thyroid, increased metabolism, or hyperthyroidism? What about underactive thyroid, slowed metabolism, or hypothyroidism?
- Have you ever been treated for hyperthyroidism or hypothyroidism?
- Have you ever had an operation for thyroid disease?
- Have you ever received radioactive iodine for thyroid disease?
- Were you taking any medicine for thyroid disease? If so, what is the name of the medicine, and what is the prescribed dose and frequency?
- When did you first notice the constant restlessness or extreme fatigue?
- Has your weight been the same or changed over the past year?
- Has your appetite changed over the past 6 months?
- Have you lost weight even though your appetite has increased (may indicate hyperthyroidism)?
- Have you gained weight or stayed at the same weight even though you have not felt like eating over the past 6 months (may indicate hypothyroidism)?
- Do you always feel warm (may indicate hyperthyroidism)?
- Do you open windows in house, even in winter months?
- Do you wear lightweight clothing, even when others are wearing layers of heavier clothing?

- Do you always feel cold (may indicate hypothyroidism)?
- Do you wear multiple layers of clothing despite warm weather or the use of a heater or furnace?
- Do you use several blankets and keep windows closed, even in warm weather?
- Do you complain about never being able to "warm up"?
- Over the past 6 months to 1 year, have you developed any of the following?

Indicators for Hypothyroidism	Indicators for Hyperthyroidism
Loss of coarse, dry scalp hair and outer edge of eyebrow	Hair thinning
Sleepiness, lethargy, depression	Swelling (face, eyes, legs)
Weight gain despite decreased appetite	Insomnia, nervousness, anxiety
Severe constipation	Weight loss despite increased appetite
Muscle and joint pain (hands, wrists, feet)	Diarrhea
Dry, itchy skin	Muscle weakness or wasting; tremors
Increased sensitivity to cold	Warm, moist skin
Bradycardia	Heat intolerance, sweating
Menstruation changes; impaired fertility	Tachycardia, atrial fibrillation
	Menstruation changes; impaired fertility

Thyroid hormone blood tests measure the levels of circulating thyroid hormone and assess the integrity of the hormonal negative feedback response within the hypothalamic-pituitary axis. Laboratory diagnosis of hyperthyroidism and hypothyroidism usually is based on the value of thyroid-stimulating hormone (TSH) and measurement of free thyroxine (T_4).[16,17] Laboratory tests developed to analyze TSH have become much more sensitive over the past decade, allowing more accurate measurement of low levels of thyroid hormone.[17] Thyroid hormone reference ranges in adults are listed in Table 36-3.[16] Because serum values vary slightly between laboratory methods, it is imperative to know the normal reference values used by the hospital laboratory.[5,18]

The upper limit of normal for some of these values is under scrutiny. A U.S. national survey found the average level of TSH in the population in all ages to be only 1.49 mIU/L, considerably lower than most cited laboratory norms.[5] The serum level of TSH increases as people grow older, which may signal declining thyroid function as more stimulation of the thyroid gland is required.[5] The average TSH level varies by age[16]:

1.60 mIU/L after age 50 years
1.79 mIU/L after age 60 years
1.98 mIU/L after age 70 years
2.08 mIU/L for those older than 80 years

Because this age-adjusted increase is predictable, it is not recommended that laboratories use age-adjusted reference values when assessing thyroid function.[5] Most asymptomatic people with a normal thyroid gland have a TSH level below 2.5 mIU/L.[5,16]

Thyroid Tests in the Critically Ill. Thyroid hormone testing in patients with nonthyroidal critical illness is often inconclusive because of the hormonal disruption caused by the illness.[5,17,18]

Drugs and Thyroid Testing. Additional measurement difficulties involve concomitant use of certain drugs that interfere with thyroid function.[16] Glucocorticoids in large doses can lower the serum level of triiodothyronine (T_3) and inhibit TSH secretion.[5] Dopamine directly inhibits TSH stimulation and consequently lowers serum levels.[17] Dobutamine infusions decrease the serum TSH concentration by 10% to 15%.[16] The antidysrhythmic drug amiodarone is an iodine-rich compound that is structurally similar to T_3 and T_4, and at usual doses,[5] it can cause iodine overload of up to 50 to 100 times the optimal daily intake.[19] Several drugs increase the serum level of T_4 by displacing protein-bound T_4.[20] Drugs that displace T_4, including unfractionated and low-molecular-weight heparins, cause an increase in serum T_4 levels.[20] Salicylates (aspirin) and furosemide (Lasix) raise T_4 serum levels by the same mechanism.[20] A more complete list of drugs that alter thyroid hormone serum levels is provided in Box 36-1. Whether it is necessary to adjust management of the critically ill patient in response to these laboratory findings is not clear.

Relationship of Thyroid-Stimulating Hormone and Thyroxine. There is an inverse, linear relationship between TSH and T_4.[5] When the hypothalamic-pituitary axis is normal, TSH production is inhibited by the presence of normal thyroid hormone.[5] It is more common to come across misleading serum T_4 results than to encounter misleading TSH results.[5] High TSH and low T_4 values are characteristic of hypothyroidism.[5] Low TSH and high serum T_4 values indicate hyperthyroidism.[5] Measurement of T_4 is recommended when the TSH level is below 10 mU/L or undetectable.[21] According to clinical practice guidelines on thyroid laboratory measurement, the sensitivity and specificity of TSH assays have improved so much that the indirect measurement of thyroid function (TSH measurement) offers better diagnostic sensitivity than does direct T_4 measurement.[5,18]

Thyrotoxicosis, the precursor of thyrotoxic crisis, is diagnosed in part by elevated serum levels of T_4 and T_3. Laboratory levels of TSH and thyrotropin-releasing hormone (TRH) are measured to confirm thyrotoxicosis and to identify the cause as intrinsically thyroid, a thyroid malignancy, or perhaps related to pituitary dysfunction.

DIAGNOSTIC PROCEDURES

Thyroid scanning involves the use of oral radioactive iodine. The preferred isotope to use in a scan to determine the cause of the hyperthyroidism is ^{123}I.[5] It is a low-energy isotope, with a short half-life to minimize the patient's exposure to radioactive material. The thyroid-scanning procedure is useful in detecting the presence of ectopic thyroid tissue and thyroid carcinomas.

TABLE 36-3 Thyroid Tests

Name of Test	Abbreviation	Reference Value*	Reference Value*
Total serum thyroxine	TT$_4$	58-160 nmol/L	4.5-12.6 mcg/dL
Free thyroxine	T$_4$	9-23 pmol/L	0.7-1.8 ng/dL
Total serum triiodothyronine	TT$_3$	1.2-2.7 nmol/L	80-180 ng/dL
Free triiodothyronine	T$_3$	3.5-7.7 pmol/L	0.2-0.5 ng/dL
Thyroid-stimulating hormone (thyrotropin)	TSH	0.4-4.0 mIU /L	
Thyroglobulin†	Tg	3.0-40 mcg/L	

*Some tests are reported with more than one reference value because different laboratories report results using several reference scales.

†Thyroglobulin (Tg) reference values should be determined locally because serum Tg concentrations are influenced by iodide intake.

Reference values from Demers LM et al: Laboratory medicine practice guidelines. Laboratory support for the diagnosis and monitoring of thyroid disease, *Thyroid* 13 (1):3-126, 2003.

BOX 36-1 DRUGS THAT INFLUENCE DIAGNOSTIC THYROID LEVELS

TRIIODOTHYRONINE (T_3)

Increase
- Methadone
- Estrogens
- Progestins
- Amiodarone

Decrease
- Anabolic steroid
- Androgens
- Salicylates
- Phenytoin
- Lithium
- Reserpine
- Propranolol
- Sulfonamides
- Propylthiouracil
- Methylthiouracil

THYROXINE (T_4)

Increase
- Oral contraceptives
- Heparin
- Aspirin
- Furosemide
- Clofibrate
- Phenylbutazone
- Some nonsteroidal antiinflam-matory drugs (NSAIDs)
- Propranolol
- Corticosteroids
- Amiodarone

Decrease
- Phenytoin
- Steroids
- Diphenylhydantoin
- Chlorpromazine
- Lithium
- Sulfonylurea
- Sulfonamides
- Reserpine
- Chlordiazepoxide

THYROID-STIMULATING HORMONE (TSH)

Increase TSH
- Metoclopramide
- Iodides
- Lithium
- Potassium iodide
- Morphine sulfate

Decrease TSH and TSH Response to TRH
- Glucocorticoids
- Dopamine
- Heparin
- Aspirin
- Carbamazepine

THYROXINE-BINDING GLOBULIN (TBG)

Increase
- Opiates
- Oral contraceptives
- Estrogens
- Clofibrate
- 5-Fluorouracil (5-FU)
- Perphenazine

Decrease
- Androgen therapy
- L-Asparaginase

TRH, thyrotropin-releasing hormone.

Thyroid scans also identify the presence and amount of viable thyroid glandular tissue after therapeutic irradiation.

ADRENAL GLAND

PRIMARY ADRENAL DISORDERS

Admission to the critical care unit with a primary adrenal disorder is rare. The term *primary* indicates that the principal problem lies within the adrenal gland. Secondary adrenal dysfunction is caused by dysfunction in another gland or by a clinical condition such as sepsis.

The adrenal gland is actually two glands in one, as described in Chapter 35, and this can make the history and presentation complex. The adrenal cortex (outer layer) secretes two classes of hormones, and if deficient or released in excess, they can cause clinical symptoms. Two hormones relevant to care of the critically ill are the glucocorticoid hormone cortisol and the mineralocorticoid hormone aldosterone. Cortisol is secreted in response to physiologic stress as a result of infection, trauma, and hypoglycemia. Aldosterone is secreted in response to intravascular hypovolemia. It is the final step in renin-angiotensin-aldosterone system (RAAS) pathway.

The adrenal medulla (inner layer) also secretes two hormones, which cause clinical symptoms if they are deficient or released in excess. They are *epinephrine* (also known as adrenalin), and *norepinephrine* (noradrenalin), and both are secreted from the adrenal gland in response to stress.[22]

CLINICAL ASSESSMENT

History. A detailed history can help to identify conditions or medications that may affect adrenal gland function. Primary endocrine disorders are rare, but a history of uncontrolled hypertension despite three or more oral medications may indicate whether endocrine-related hypertension should be investigated. The medication history can help determine whether the patient takes glucocorticoid tablets, and the patient or family should be asked about using steroid creams for dermatologic conditions and about using steroid-based inhalers for chronic obstructive lung disease (COPD).

Physical Examination. The physical examination is related to the effects of adrenal dysfunction, and the signs depend on the hormone involved and whether the problem is related to excess or deficiency. This means that the signs and symptoms are very diverse. A methodic approach to assessing all signs and symptoms is important, because adrenal disease is often missed or misdiagnosed.

The Adrenal Cortex

Primary Cushing's Syndrome. Cushing's syndrome is caused by the excess release of the glucocorticoid hormone *cortisol*. Excess cortisol produces the classic signs and symptoms listed in Box 36-2. Primary Cushing's disease is rare,[23-25] but if a patient is not taking exogenous steroids, it becomes a diagnosis of exclusion when the relevant constellation of signs and symptoms are present.

Secondary Cushing's Syndrome. Symptoms identical to those of primary Cushing's syndrome (see Box 36-2) occur in patients with the secondary form who chronically take pharmacologic doses of glucocorticoids, such as transplant recipients who take steroids to prevent solid organ rejection; patients with COPD, or those with chronic inflammatory conditions. When patients are admitted to the critical care unit, it is important to ascertain whether they are steroid dependent to avoid the deleterious effects of abrupt steroid withdrawal.

Primary Aldosteronism. In patients with primary aldosteronism, the adrenal cortex secretes excess mineralocorticoid

BOX 36-2   CAUSES OF CUSHING'S SYNDROME

PRIMARY CUSHING'S SYNDROME

Cushing's syndrome is divided into adrenocorticotropin-dependent and adrenocorticotropin-independent types. Adrenocorticotropin is also known as adrenocorticotropic hormone (ACTH) or corticotropin.

1. ACTH-dependent Cushing's syndrome

    Most (80%) cases result from a pituitary adenoma that causes the pituitary gland to produce excess ACTH. Excess secretion of ACTH stimulates the adrenal cortex to release supraphysiologic amounts of *cortisol* into the bloodstream, circumventing the normal inhibitory feedback loop.

    The other 20% of cases are caused by ectopic ACTH secretion from small-cell cancers of the lung, metastases, and endocrine tumors.

2. ACTH-independent Cushing's syndrome

    It is usually caused by a unilateral adrenal tumor: adrenal adenoma (60%) or adrenal carcinoma (40%).

3. Secondary or iatrogenic Cushing's syndrome

The patient takes pharmacologic doses of glucocorticoids, which may be prescribed to prevent rejection after solid organ transplantation or for the treatment of chronic inflammatory conditions.

CLINICAL SIGNS AND SYMPTOMS OF CUSHING'S SYNDROME

Emotional lability (can range from depression to psychosis)
Hyperglycemia and poorly controlled type 2 diabetes
Obesity or weight gain in abdomen
Rounded face
Acne
Thin skin, bruises easily, poor wound healing
Hypertension
Hirsutism (excess hair growth)
Dorsocervical fat pad ("buffalo hump")
Decreased libido
Fatigue, weakness

(aldosterone). There are several subtypes of this rare condition, but all can cause the patient to present emergently with severe hypertension and critically low serum level of potassium (hypokalemia), which can be lethal if not identified and effectively treated.

Addison's Disease. Addison's disease is a rare disorder of the adrenal cortex that involves hyposecretion of glucocorticoids (cortisol), sometimes occurring with hyposecretion of mineralocorticoids (aldosterone). Physiologically, it can be envisioned as the opposite of the disorders described previously, and the signs and symptoms are the inverse of the conditions with excess hormone secretion. An *addisonian crisis* is a life-threatening condition in which the adrenal gland is almost nonfunctional, usually due to destruction of adrenal tissue. The patient presents acutely with critical hypotension, an elevated serum potassium level (hyperkalemia), a low serum sodium level (hyponatremia), and hypoglycemia.

Critical Illness-Related Corticosteroid Insufficiency. The adrenal gland is designed to respond to acute physiologic stress. However, in prolonged critical illness and in septic shock, there is evidence that the adrenal gland may become exhausted and no longer secrete adequate amounts of stress hormones.[26] Secondary adrenal failure is also reported after traumatic brain injury (TBI).[27] The Society of Critical Care Medicine (SCCM) recommends that this condition be called *critical illness–related corticosteroid insufficiency* (CIRCI).[28] Differentiating the signs and symptoms of adrenal insufficiency caused by shock from other causes by clinical examination alone is almost impossible in the critically ill, and CIRCI was probably an overlooked diagnosis in the past. The routine use of the corticotropin stimulation test in the presence of refractory vasopressor-dependent hypotension helps to make this diagnosis.[28]

The Adrenal Medulla

Pheochromocytoma. Pheochromocytomas are rare tumors that arise from the catecholamine-producing *chromaffin cells* of the adrenal medulla.[29] Most produce norepinephrine, but some

BOX 36-3   PHEOCHROMOCYTOMA: SIGNS AND SYMPTOMS

Signs*	Symptoms*
• Hypertension	• Headaches
• Tachycardia	• Dizziness or faintness
• Tachypnea	• Palpitations, chest pain
• Pallor or flushing	• Anxiety and nervousness
• Hyperglycemia or poorly controlled type 2 diabetes	• Excessive sweating
	• Weakness, fatigue
• Decreased gastrointestinal motility	• Weight loss
	• Constipation

*Not all patients have all signs and symptoms.

produce both norepinephrine and epinephrine.[29] Less than 10% are malignant. These tumors produce a far greater quantity of catechols than normal adrenal medullary tissue. The concentrations of catecholamines are so high within the tumor that it has have been likened to a volcano that can erupt at any time.[29] When huge amounts of norepinephrine or epinephrine are released into the bloodstream, it creates a *catecholamine storm* that can be life-threatening. The body responds as if to a severe fight-or-flight threat by hypertension, tachycardia, increased respiratory rate, and hyperglycemia. The patient may describe symptoms of headache, dizziness, palpitations, chest pain, anxiety, nervousness, and fatigue (Box 36-3).[29,30] Because the body perceives the catecholamine onslaught to be a signal for the person to be ready to escape a threatening situation, it slows down the gastrointestinal tract, and constipation is another symptom. Most pheochromocytomas are detected on autopsy rather than during life, and the patients at greatest risk are those who are admitted to a critical care unit for another reason or are admitted in shock with an undiagnosed adrenal tumor.[30]

Endocrine Hypertension. *Pheochromocytoma* and *primary aldosteronism* can manifest as severe, uncontrollable hypertension. This is a rare finding, but in a youthful patient, in a patient who has uncontrolled hypertension while on multiple antihypertensive medications, or in a patient with coexisting symptoms of sympathetic nervous system stimulation (pheochromocytoma) or severe hyperkalemia (excess aldosterone), the diagnosis of endocrine hypertension may be considered.[31]

LABORATORY STUDIES

Adrenal Insufficiency and Critical Illness. For critically ill patients with refractory hypotension, especially if septic and hypotensive while on vasopressors after adequate fluid resuscitation, a diagnosis of CIRCI should be considered. To determine whether the adrenal gland can to respond to stress, the diagnosis is facilitated by the *cosyntropin stimulation test* (CST). Cosyntropin is the name for synthetic adrenocorticotropic hormone (ACTH). An initial measurement of total serum cortisol is obtained to establish a baseline value. If the baseline value is below 10 mcg/dL (in the presence of the clinical signs described previously), the patient is considered to have adrenal insufficiency. If after intravenous administration of a stimulation dose of 250 mcg of cosyntropin, the rise from baseline is less than 9 mcg/dL, the patient is considered to have adrenal insufficiency related to critical illness.[28] This test is invalid if the patient has recently received steroids.[28]

Summary

- Assessment of the patient with endocrine dysfunction is a systematic process that incorporates the medical and family history, physical examination, and laboratory test results.
- A normal fasting blood glucose level is between 70 and 100 mg/dL. A fasting glucose level between 110 and 126 mg/dL identifies prediabetes. A glucose level greater than 126 mg/dL is diagnostic of diabetes. Hyperglycemia is a frequent finding in the critically ill patient.
- Hypothyroidism is identified by high TSH and low T_4 values.
- Hyperthyroidism is identified by low TSH and high T_4 values.
- The adrenal gland is designed to respond to acute physiologic stress. In prolonged critical illness and in septic shock, the adrenal gland may become exhausted and no longer secrete adequate amounts of stress hormones. The cosyntropin stimulation test is used to evaluate adrenal gland function.

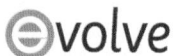 Be sure to check out the bonus material, including free self-assessment exercises, on the Evolve web site at http://evolve.elsevier.com/Urden/.

References

1. American Diabetes Association: Standards of medical care in diabetes—2009, *Diabetes Care* 32(suppl 1):S13-S61, 2009.
2. American Diabetes Association: Diagnosis and classification of diabetes mellitus, *Diabetes Care* 32(suppl 1):S62-S67, 2009.
3. ACE/ADA Task Force on Inpatient Diabetes: American College of Endocrinology and American Diabetes Association Consensus statement on inpatient diabetes and glycemic control, *Diabetes Care* 29(8):1955-1962, 2006.
4. Goldstein DE et al: Tests of glycemia in diabetes, *Diabetes Care* 27(7):1761-1773, 2004.
5. Moghissi ES et al: American Association of Clinical Endocrinologists and American Diabetes Association consensus statement on inpatient glycemic control, *Endocr Pract* 15(4):1-17, 2009.
6. Cryer PE et al: Evaluation and management of adult hypoglycemic disorders: An endocrine society clinical practice guideline, *J Clin Endocrinol Metab* 94(3):709-728, 2009.
7. Funnell MM et al: National standards for diabetes self-management education, *Diabetes Care* 32 Suppl 1:S87-94, 2009.
8. Weykamp C et al: The IFCC Reference Measurement System for HbA1c: a 6-year progress report, *Clin Chem* 54(2):240-248, 2008. Endo
9. Janicic N, Verbalis JG: Evaluation and management of hypo-osmolality in hospitalized patients, *Endocrinol Metab Clin North Am* 32(2):459-481, 2003.
10. Rottmann CN: SSRIs and the syndrome of inappropriate antidiuretic hormone secretion, *Am J Nurs* 107(1):51-58, 2007.
11. Holcomb S: Diabetes insipidus, *Dimens Crit Care Nurs* 21(3):94-97, 2002.
12. Hadjizacharia P et al: Acute diabetes insipidus in severe head injury: a prospective study, *J Am Coll Surg* 207(4):477-484, 2008.
13. Ellis H: The clinical examination of the thyroid gland, *Br J Hosp Med (Lond)* 68(9):M154-M155, 2007.
14. U.S. Preventive Services Task Force Screening for Thyroid Disease (USPSTF): Screening for thyroid disease: recommendation statement, *Ann Intern Med* 140(2):125-127, 2004.
15. Gharib H et al: Consensus statement: subclinical thyroid dysfunction: a joint statement on management from the American Association of Clinical Endocrinologists, the American Thyroid Association, and The Endocrine Society, *Thyroid* 15(1):24-28, 2005.
16. Ross DS: Serum thyroid-stimulating hormone measurement for assessment of thyroid function and disease, *Endocrinol Metab Clin North Am* 30(2):245-264, 2001.
17. Demers LM et al: Laboratory medicine practice guidelines. Laboratory support for the diagnosis and monitoring of thyroid disease, *Thyroid* 13(1):3-126, 2003.
18. Langton JE, Brent GA: Nonthyroidal illness syndrome: evaluation of thyroid function in sick patients, *Endocrinol Metab Clin North Am* 31(1):159-172, 2002.
19. Piga M et al: Amiodarone-induced thyrotoxicosis. A review, *Minerva Endocrinol* 33(3):213-228, 2008.
20. Stockigt JR: Free thyroid hormone measurement. A critical appraisal, *Endocrinol Metab Clin North Am* 30(2):265-289, 2001.

21. Stockigt J: Assessment of thyroid function: towards an integrated laboratory-clinical approach, *Clin Biochem Rev* 24(4):109-122, 2003.

22. de Diego AM et al: A physiological view of the central and peripheral mechanisms that regulate the release of catecholamines at the adrenal medulla, *Acta Physiol* (Oxf) 192(2):287-301, 2008.

23. Newell-Price J, Bertagna X, Grossman AB, et al: Cushing's syndrome, *Lancet* 367(9522):1605-1617, 2006.

24. Biller BM et al: Treatment of adrenocorticotropin-dependent Cushing's syndrome: a consensus statement, *J Clin Endocrinol Metab* 93(7):2454-2462, 2008.

25. Nieman LK et al: The diagnosis of Cushing's syndrome: an Endocrine Society Clinical Practice Guideline, *J Clin Endocrinol Metab* 93(5):1526-1540, 2008.

26. Marik PE: Mechanisms and clinical consequences of critical illness associated adrenal insufficiency, *Curr Opin Crit Care* 13(4):363-369, 2007.

27. Rossi GP et al: Primary aldosteronism: an update on screening, diagnosis and treatment, *J Hypertens* 26(4):613-621, 2008.

28. Marik PE et al: Recommendations for the diagnosis and management of corticosteroid insufficiency in critically ill adult patients: consensus statements from an international task force by the American College of Critical Care Medicine, *Crit Care Med* 36(6):1937-1949, 2008.

29. Pacak K: Preoperative management of the pheochromocytoma patient, *J Clin Endocrinol Metab* 92(11):4069-4079, 2007.

30. Eisenhofer G et al: Adverse drug reactions in patients with phaeochromocytoma: incidence, prevention and management, *Drug Saf* 30(11):1031-1062, 2007.

31. Young WF Jr: Adrenal causes of hypertension: pheochromocytoma and primary aldosteronism, *Rev Endocr Metab Disord* 8(4):309-320, 2007.

Endocrine Disorders and Therapeutic Management

The endocrine system is almost invisible when it functions well, but it causes widespread upset when an organ is suppressed, hyperstimulated, or under physiologic stress. This results in a wide spectrum of possible disorders; some are rare, and others are frequently encountered in the critical care unit. This chapter focuses on the neuroendocrine stress associated with critical illness and on disorders of three major endocrine glands: the pancreas, the thyroid gland, and the posterior pituitary gland.

NEUROENDOCRINOLOGY OF STRESS AND CRITICAL ILLNESS

Major neurologic and endocrine changes occur when an individual is confronted with physiologic stress caused by any critical illness,[1,2] sepsis,[3-5] trauma, major surgery, or underlying cardiovascular disease.[5,6] The normal "fight or flight" response that is initiated in times of physiologic or psychological stress is exacerbated in critical illness through activation of the neuroendocrine system, specifically the hypothalamic-pituitary-adrenal axis (HPA),[3,7] thyroid,[8] and pancreas.[1,2] The influence of the HPA on the course of critical illness is just beginning to be understood. Hormonal neuroendocrine output is very active at the beginning of a critical insult but greatly diminishes if the critical illness is prolonged.[9,10] All endocrine organs are affected by acute critical illness, as shown in Table 37-1. How much influence hormonal fluctuations have on morbidity and mortality remains the focus of ongoing research.

ACUTE NEUROENDOCRINE RESPONSE TO CRITICAL ILLNESS

The fight or flight acute response to physiologic threat is a rapid discharge of the catecholamines *norepinephrine* and *epinephrine* into the bloodstream.[6] Norepinephrine is released from the nerve endings of the sympathetic nervous system (SNS).[6]

Hypothalamic-Pituitary-Adrenal Axis in Acute Stress.
Epinephrine (Adrenalin) is released from the medulla of the adrenal glands. Epinephrine increases cerebral blood flow and cerebral oxygen consumption and may be the trigger for recruitment of the hypothalamic-pituitary axis.[6]

The pituitary gland has two parts (anterior and posterior) that function under control of the hypothalamus, as described

in Chapter 35. As a response to stress, the *posterior pituitary gland* releases antidiuretic hormone (ADH), also known as *vasopressin* (pitressin). This hormone is an antidiuretic with a powerful vasoconstrictive effect on blood vessels.[6] The combination of epinephrine and vasopressin raises blood pressure quickly; it also decreases gastric motility.[6] Epinephrine increases heart rate, causes ventricular dysrhythmias in susceptible patients, and provides some analgesia or lack of pain awareness during acute physical stress.[6]

The *anterior pituitary gland* is under the control of the hypothalamus (see Chapter 35). In acute physiologic stress, "pulses" of growth hormone (GH) are released from the anterior pituitary gland to boost serum GH levels.[10] In critical illness, the anterior pituitary actively secretes hormone, but the quantity may be insufficient for extreme physiologic needs. A different problem is that peripheral tissues may be resistant and unable to use the anabolic GH.[11] The anterior pituitary gland also produces *corticotropin* (also called ACTH), which stimulates release of *cortisol* from the adrenal cortex.[12]

Cortisol release is an important protective response to stress, and serum levels increase sixfold with normal adrenal function.[12] High cortisol levels alter carbohydrate, fat, and protein metabolism so that energy is immediately and selectively available to vital organs such as the brain.[10] However, if critical illness is prolonged, the HPA may not be able to respond adequately to the prolonged physiologic stress.[7]

Liver and Pancreas in Acute Stress.
The liver releases the hormone *glucagon* to stimulate the liver to pour additional glucose into the bloodstream. This greatly raises blood glucose levels.[3] Paradoxically, the pancreas does not produce more insulin, and serum insulin levels remain normal, even with the increased metabolic demand associated with critical illness or sepsis. Peripheral tissues become *insulin resistant*.[3] In other words, the tissues are unable to use the available insulin to transport glucose inside the cells for normal metabolism. This raises blood glucose levels, causing persistent hyperglycemia. There is a second metabolic system that enables insulin to enter the cell (see Chapter 35). Although the insulin-independent *glucose transporters* (GLUT 1, GLUT 2, and GLUT 3) are active during physiologic stress, they cannot keep up with the massive increase in glucose production by the liver.[13] Continuous infusion of insulin to return and maintain blood glucose levels within a safe, near-normal range reduces morbidity and

TABLE 37-1 Endocrine Responses to Stress

Gland or Organ	Hormone	Response or Physical Examination
Adrenal cortex	Cortisol	↑ Insulin resistance → ↑ glycogenolysis → ↑ glucose circulation
		↑ Hepatic gluconeogenesis → ↑ glucose available
		↑ Lipolysis
		↑ Protein catabolism
		↑ Sodium → ↑ water retention to maintain plasma osmolality by movement of extravascular fluid into the intravascular space
		↓ Connective tissue fibroblasts → poor wound healing
	Glucocorticoid	↓ Histamine release → suppression of immune system
		↓ Lymphocytes, monocytes, eosinophils, basophils
		↑ Polymorphonuclear leukocytes → ↑ infection risk
		↑ Glucose
		↓ Gastric acid secretion
	Mineralocorticoids	↑ Aldosterone → ↓ sodium excretion → ↓ water excretion → ↑ intravascular volume
		↑ Potassium excretion → hypokalemia
		↑ Hydrogen ion excretion → metabolic acidosis
Adrenal medulla	Epinephrine	↑ Endorphins → ↓ pain
	Norepinephrine, epinephrine	↑ Metabolic rate to accommodate stress response
		↑ Live glycogenolysis → ↑ glucose
		↑ Insulin (cells are insulin resistant)
		↑ Cardiac contractility
		↑ Cardiac output
		↑ Dilation of coronary arteries
		↑ Blood pressure
		↑ Heart rate
		↑ Bronchodilation → ↑ respirations
		↑ Perfusion to heart, brain, lungs, liver, and muscle
		↓ Perfusion to periphery of body
		↓ Peristalsis
	Norepinephrine	↑ Peripheral vasoconstriction
		↑ Blood pressure
		↑ Sodium retention
		↑ Potassium excretion
Pituitary	All hormones	↑ Endogenous opioids → ↓ pain
Anterior pituitary	Corticotropin	↑ Aldosterone → ↓ sodium excretion → ↓ water excretion → ↑ intravascular volume
		↑ Cortisol → ↑ blood volume
	Growth hormones	↑ Protein anabolism of amino acids to protein
		↑ Lipolysis → ↑ gluconeogenesis
Posterior pituitary	Antidiuretic hormone	↑ Vasoconstriction
		↑ Water retention → restoration of circulating blood volume
		↓ Urine output
		↑ Hypo-osmolality
Pancreas	Insulin	↑ Insulin resistance → hyperglycemia
	Glucagon	↑ Glycolysis (directly opposes action of insulin)
		↑ Glucose for fuel
		↑ Glycogenolysis
		↑ Gluconeogenesis
		↑ Lipolysis
Thyroid	Thyroxine	↓ Routine metabolic demands during stress
Gonads	Sex hormones	Energy and oxygen supply diverted to brain, heart, muscles, and liver

↑, Increased; →, causes; ↓, decreased.

mortality.[1,2] Management of hyperglycemia for the nondiabetic critically ill patient is discussed in detail in a later section.

Thyroid Gland in Acute Stress. Within 2 hours after trauma or surgery, serum levels of triiodothyronine (T_3) decrease.[10] The greater the decrease of T_3 in the first 24 hours, the more severe the critical illness.[8] Thyroid-stimulating hormone (TSH) and thyroxine (T_4) briefly increase and then return to normal levels. In the acute phase of critical illness, a low serum T_3 is associated with a poor prognosis.[10]

Systemic illnesses that do not directly involve the thyroid gland but alter thyroid gland metabolism are referred to as *nonthyroidal illness syndromes* or *sick euthyroid syndromes*.[14] The significance of altered thyroid function in critical illness is unknown,[14] and there is ongoing debate as to whether this condition requires treatment.[15]

PROLONGED NEUROENDOCRINE RESPONSE TO CRITICAL ILLNESS

If critical illness is prolonged, the neuroendocrine response changes dramatically. The initially high hormonal levels are greatly reduced, and output is decreased from all the major endocrine glands.

Hypothalamic-Pituitary-Adrenal Axis in Prolonged Stress. If critical illness is prolonged for more 7 to 10 days, the production of hormones from the pituitary gland is significantly lessened.

The posterior pituitary gland produces ADH. The impact of prolonged critical illness on vasopressin production has not been reported.

GH from the anterior pituitary is greatly decreased and lacks the pulses or bolus doses delivered during the initial acute phase.[10] GH levels are low compared with the high levels observed during the initial stress response (described earlier). Unexpectedly, when critically ill patients were given high-dose GH as part of a large multicenter study, the morbidity increased and the mortality rate doubled.[10] Because of this finding, exogenous administration of GH is not recommended.

Adrenal dysfunction is common in critical illness that lasts longer than 7 to 10 days. The serum corticotropin level decreases, whereas the cortisol level remains high.[10] The reason for this paradoxical effect is unknown. Some researchers believe that an alternative metabolic pathway, as yet unidentified, may be stimulating the adrenal cortex to produce cortisol outside the normal channels. With prolonged illness, all pathways fail, as indicated by a 20-fold increase in adrenal failure observed in critically ill patients older than 50 years who spend more than 14 days in a critical care unit.[10] If the critical illness is prolonged and the patient remains hypotensive, vasopressor-dependent, and mechanically ventilated, adequacy of adrenal function must be evaluated. Even if a corticotropin test was performed earlier in the hospitalization, it is important to repeat the test, because the an initially normal adrenal gland may have failed due to the stress of the critical illness.[12] Older patients are particularly susceptible to adrenal failure.[16]

Liver-Pancreas in Prolonged Stress. Hyperglycemia is often persistent. Gluconeogenesis (the metabolism of glucose from

fat or protein) and proteolysis (protein breakdown) continue throughout the catabolic phase of critical illness.[11] Critically ill patients can lose up to 10% of their lean body mass per week.[11] The addition of adequate supplemental nutrition is recommended, in addition to an intravenous insulin infusion, to reduce hyperglycemia and provide additional substrate other than the patient's own body tissues.[1,2] Insulin is an anabolic hormone and can improve protein synthesis and reduce protein breakdown.[11] While the critical illness is ongoing, nutrition and insulin seem to limit rather than stop the loss of lean body mass.

Thyroid Gland in Prolonged Stress. The thyroid gland appears to follow a pattern similar to that of the pituitary gland when critical illness is prolonged. The serum levels of T_3, T_4, and TSH are greatly reduced, and the normal pulses of TSH are flattened.[10]

Gonads in Prolonged Stress. If critical illness is prolonged, hypogonadism develops. This is measured as a low serum testosterone concentration in men. Testosterone is an endogenous anabolic steroid (i.e., it builds muscle), and its level is decreased in catabolic states such as starvation, acute myocardial infarction, burns, and prolonged critical illness.[10] Again, the significance of this finding is unknown.

If critical illness is prolonged beyond 7 to 10 days, there is profound suppression of pituitary, thyroid, adrenal, and gonadal gland function. This occurs is in addition to the initial clinical problem and any other organ dysfunction that may be present. Research is ongoing to understand the neuroendocrine pathways in acute and prolonged critical illness, with a view to blocking counterproductive metabolic pathways. The critical care nurse who understands the pathophysiology of the stress response in critical illness is in a better position to recognize the neuroendocrine symptoms and collaborate with the multidisciplinary team to return the patient to physiologic normalcy.

ADRENAL DYSFUNCTION IN CRITICAL ILLNESS

Diminished adrenal gland function may result from one or more causes during critical illness:

- *Primary hypoadrenalism* describes an intrinsic failure of the adrenal gland to produce normal endogenous glucocorticosteroid hormones (e.g., cortisol) and mineralocorticosteroids (e.g., aldosterone). Primary adrenal failure is rare and occurs in only 0.01% to 3% of critically ill patients.[17,18]
- *Secondary adrenal dysfunction, or Cushing's syndrome,* occurs as a result of the administration of therapeutic steroids. In response to exogenous glucocorticosteroids, the adrenal glands stop production of intrinsic hormones. Patients who have taken steroids before their admission to the hospital need their dosage increased. One recommendation is to double the dose for a febrile illness.[12]
- *Critical illness–related corticosteroid insufficiency* (CIRCI) describes a situation in which the adrenal gland produces glucocorticosteroids but the quantity is insufficient for the disease process. Estimates of the frequency of CIRCI range from about 20% in medical patients to 60% in septic patients.[19]

- *Peripheral cortisol resistance* is thought to occur in severe sepsis and septic shock.[7,17] In septic patients, inflammatory cytokines induce cellular resistance to cortisol; low-dose, short-term replacement corticosteroids may be provided to patients with CIRCI.[7,17]

Assessment of Adrenal Function. Clinical assessment of adrenal dysfunction is difficult in the critically ill, and a specialized laboratory assay is necessary for an accurate diagnosis. First, a baseline serum cortisol level is obtained. Adrenal failure is likely if the cortisol level is less than 10 mcg/dL.[7]

Cosyntropin Stimulation Test. Further confirmation of adrenal dysfunction may be obtained by performance of a corticotropin stimulation test *(cosyntropin test)*. Cosyntropin is a medication made from the first 24 amino acids of corticotropin.[12] In the test, 250 mcg cosyntropin is administered by the intravenous route, and serum blood levels are measured 30 minutes later. A serum cortisol rise from baseline of less than 9 mcg/dL after 30 minutes denotes inability of the adrenal gland to respond to a stress stimulus (nonresponder).[7,12] If the cortisol rise is greater than 9 mcg/dL in response to corticotropin stimulation, the adrenal glands are functioning normally (responder).[7] Corticosteroids are given only to nonresponders. The combination of a low baseline cortisol value (<10 mcg/dL) with minimal or no rise (<9 mcg/dL) after cosyntropin stimulation is evidence of corticosteroid deficiency.[7]

Corticosteroid Replacement. Clinical practice guidelines[7] recommend short-term provision of low-dose hydrocortisone for patients who have a diagnosis of septic shock with refractory vasopressor-dependent hypotension. Hydrocortisone is the recommended replacement because it is the pharmacologic steroid that most resembles endogenous cortisol.

The guidelines recommend use of the cosyntropin stimulation test as described previously. However, the test is not recommended as a stand-alone method to identify patients who might receive low-dose steroids. This apparent contradiction is explained by the fact that several clinical trials of low-dose steroid replacement in sepsis have demonstrated a faster resolution of the shock symptoms but no difference in overall mortality compared with placebo.[7] The controversy continues. The most recently published randomized control trial of low-dose steroids versus placebo in 499 patients with septic shock did not show any mortality benefit, even among responders to the cosyntropin stimulation test. Nor was there any difference in survival between those who responded to the 250 mg cosyntropin and received steroids and those who responded and received a placebo.[20]

High-dose steroid replacement is never recommended in the management of sepsis. Corticosteroids are never discontinued abruptly and must be tapered gradually over several days.[7]

HYPERGLYCEMIA IN CRITICAL ILLNESS

Normal fasting blood glucose levels range between 70 and 100 mg/dL in a healthy person. Critically ill patients frequently have much higher blood glucose levels, and several retrospective analyses have reported that hyperglycemic patients have a higher mortality rate than patients with normal blood glucose values.[21] In 2001, a landmark prospective, randomized study showed a significant reduction in morbidity and mortality among critically ill surgical patients whose blood glucose concentration was maintained between 80 and 110 mg/dL with a continuous insulin infusion, compared with those whose blood glucose was only treated if it was greater than 180 mg/dL.[1] A study of medical critical care patients by the same group with the same protocol demonstrated a mortality benefit after 3 days of tight glucose control with an insulin infusion.[2] These initial studies were greeted with tremendous enthusiasm and many critical care units adopted stringent glucose control standards to reduce hyperglycemia-associated morbidity and mortality. However, these earlier studies have now been challenged.

The NICE-SUGAR trial was a prospective randomized trial of 6,014 critically ill patients.[22] It compared continuous insulin infusion to achieve tight glucose control (target 80-108 mg/dL) with a conventional glucose control range (target below 180 mg/dL).[22] In the tight glucose control group 6.8% had episodes of severe hypoglycemia (below 40 mg/dL); in the conventional control group only 0.5% experienced severe hypoglycemia.[22] There was a 2.6% higher risk of death in the intensive glucose control group (27.5% died) compared with the conventional control group (24.9% died).[22] Other prospective, randomized trials[23,24] and meta-analysis[25] were unable to demonstrate a reduction in mortality with tight glucose control. These research studies suggest that the risks of hypoglycemia with the use of intensive insulin protocols outweigh the benefits of tight glucose control in the critically ill.[22-25]

Clinical Practice Guidelines Related to Blood Glucose Management in Critically Ill Patients. As a result of the studies just described, clinical practice guidelines were developed by the American Association of Clinical Endocrinologists (AACE) and the American Diabetes Association (ADA) that recommend the use of continuous insulin infusions to maintain blood glucose in critical care patients between 140-180 mg/dL, with frequent monitoring of blood glucose.[5] The 140-180 mg/dL level was selected to minimize the risk of hypoglycemia.

Other glucose-control guidelines relevant to critical illness have also been published. The Society of Critical Care Medicine (SCCM) Surviving Sepsis guideline recommends maintaining the blood glucose concentration lower than 150 mg/dL in critically ill septic patients after initial stabilization.[4] The American Heart Association recommends a target range of 90 to 140 mg/dL while avoiding hypoglycemia.[26] More liberal glucose control represents the current trend of targeted values.

Hyperglycemia and the Cardiovascular System. Many patients who are admitted to the hospital with acute complications of atherosclerotic disease are diabetic; 65% of individuals with diabetes die from coronary artery disease or a stroke.[27] Risk of coronary artery disease is two to three times higher in diabetics compared with nondiabetics.[28] Hyperglycemia is present in 25% to 50% of patients with acute coronary syndrome (ACS) who are admitted to the hospital, and the higher the blood glucose level, the greater the risk of death.[26] Diabetic patients who were admitted to the hospital for an acute myocardial infarction and had an admission blood glucose level greater than 180 mg/dL had a 70% relative increase in the risk of in-hospital death compared with similar patients who had a normal glucose value on admission.[26] Retrospective analyses of blood glucose levels of cardiac surgery patients show a higher in-hospital mortality rate for patients with elevated blood glucose concentrations.[29,30] Patients who were unaware of their diabetes before hospital admission and nondiabetic patients who were hyperglycemic during their critical illness also had higher mortality rates.[31,32]

Hypoglycemia and Brain Injury. The brain does not store glucose and is dependent on a continuous supply of glucose from the peripheral bloodstream. It is essential to avoid hypoglycemia in any brain-injured patient. However, there are no published guidelines as what the correct target glucose range should be for this population. Experts favor a less restrictive target, because blood glucose concentrations lower than 135 mg/dL (6 mmol/L) have been shown to increase brain metabolic distress.[33]

INSULIN MANAGEMENT IN THE CRITICALLY ILL

A profound shift in the management of the hyperglycemic critically ill ventilated patient has recently taken place. As a result of the research that has highlighted the deleterious effects of hyperglycemia in critical illness, most hospitals have developed an institution-specific tight glucose control algorithm to lower blood glucose into the targeted range. The vigilance of the critical care nurse is pivotal to the success of any intervention to lower blood glucose using a continuous insulin infusion. As discussed earlier, many glucose control protocols are becoming less restrictive due to concerns about iatrogenic hypoglycemia.

Some clinical interventions increase the likelihood that the patient will receive exogenous insulin. Infusion of total parental nutrition (TPN) typically requires a continuous insulin infusion to normalize blood glucose. In a study of critically ill surgical patients with preexisting type 2 diabetes who did not previously require insulin, 77% of patients needed insulin to control blood sugar while receiving TPN.[34] Some enteral nutrition formulas are high in carbohydrates and increase blood sugar in the same way. In this situation, the composition of the enteral feeding is altered, or the insulin dosage is increased to achieve target blood glucose levels. It is important to provide nutrition, and insulin can be a powerful adjunct to nutritional support.

Frequent Blood Glucose Monitoring. Monitoring the blood glucose with a point-of-care glucometer is the basis of targeted glucose control. As part of the comprehensive initial assessment, the blood sugar is measured by a standard laboratory sample or by a finger-stick capillary blood sample. In many institutions, if the blood sugar is greater than 180 mg/dL (an initial value that may vary among hospitals), the patient is started on a continuous intravenous insulin infusion. In critically ill catabolic patients, the initial blood glucose level can be well above 200 mg/dL. While the glucose is elevated, blood sample measurements are usually obtained hourly, to allow titration of the insulin drip to lower blood glucose. After the patient is stable, blood glucose measurements can be spaced approximately every 2 hours, based on individual hospital protocols.[21]

Several different blood-sampling methods are available. A capillary finger-stick is perhaps the easiest initial option, although the fingers can become noticeably marked if there are numerous sticks over several days. Trauma to the fingers is also exacerbated if peripheral perfusion is diminished. If a central venous catheter (CVC) or an arterial line with a blood conservation system attached is in place, this can be a highly efficient system for sampling, because there is no blood wastage. If a blood conservation setup is not attached, use of the venous or arterial catheter for access is unacceptable because of the amount of waste blood that would be discarded.

Continuous Insulin Infusion. Many hospitals use insulin infusion protocols for management of stress-induced hyperglycemia that are implemented by the critical care nurse.[5] Effective glucose protocols gauge the insulin infusion rate based on two parameters: (1) the immediate blood glucose result and (2) the rate of change in the blood glucose level since the last hourly measurement. The following three examples illustrate this concept:

- Patient A receives 3 units of continuous intravenous regular insulin per hour and has a blood glucose measurement of 110 mg/dL, but 1 hour ago it was 190 mg/dL; the insulin rate must be decreased to avoid sudden hypoglycemia.
- Patient B receives 3 units of continuous IV regular insulin per hour and has a blood glucose measurement of 110 mg/dL, but 1 hour ago it was 112 mg/dL; in this situation, no change is made in the insulin infusion rate.
- Patient C receives 3 units of continuous intravenous regular insulin per hour and has a blood glucose measurement of 190 mg/dL, and 1 hour ago it was 197 mg/dL; the insulin rate must be increased to more rapidly move the patient's blood sugar toward the targeted glucose range (i.e., 140-180 mg/dL, although this range will vary by hospital and protocol).

The important point to emphasize is that the *rate of change* of the blood glucose is as important as the *most recent* blood glucose measurement. Each of the patients described in the examples may have the same insulin infusion rate, depending on their catabolic state, but individualization among patients with different diagnoses can be safely achieved as long as the rate of change is also considered.

A person's insulin requirement often fluctuates over the course of an illness. This occurs in response to changes in the clinical condition, such as development of an infection, caloric alterations caused by stopping or starting enteral nutrition or TPN, or administration of therapeutic steroids, or because the person is less catabolic.[34] A method to allow for corrective incremental changes (up or down) to adapt to the reality of clinical developments and maintain the glucose within the target range is essential.[34] Some protocols alter only the infusion rate, whereas others incorporate bolus insulin doses if the glucose concentration is greater than a preestablished threshold (e.g., 180 mg/dL). Typically, after the blood glucose has remained within the target range for a number of hours (4 to 12 hours, depending on the hospital protocol), the time interval between measurements for blood glucose monitoring is extended to every 2 hours.

Transition from Continuous to Intermittent Insulin Coverage. The transition from a continuous insulin infusion to intermittent insulin coverage must be handled with care to avoid large fluctuations in blood glucose levels. Before the conversion, the regular insulin infusion should be at a stable and preferably low rate, and the patient's blood glucose level should be maintained consistently within the target range.

The transition from intravenous to subcutaneous administration depends on numerous factors, especially whether the patient is able to eat a normal diet.[34]

Clinicians use various methods to calculate the quantity of insulin to prescribe during the transition from intravenous to subcutaneous insulin to maintain stable blood glucose levels. Figure 37-1 depicts hypothetical examples of how a combination of basal and bolus insulin regimens (prandial insulin) can

work in clinical practice.[21,35] The following paragraphs describe the application of one calculation method for a 67-year-old patient, Alice Smith, who is recovering from critical illness and has recently been extubated.

1. Ms. Smith is in stable condition on a regular insulin drip at 1 unit per hour. She is ready to be transitioned to subcutaneous insulin and will be taking food and liquids by mouth. Her total insulin requirement over the previous

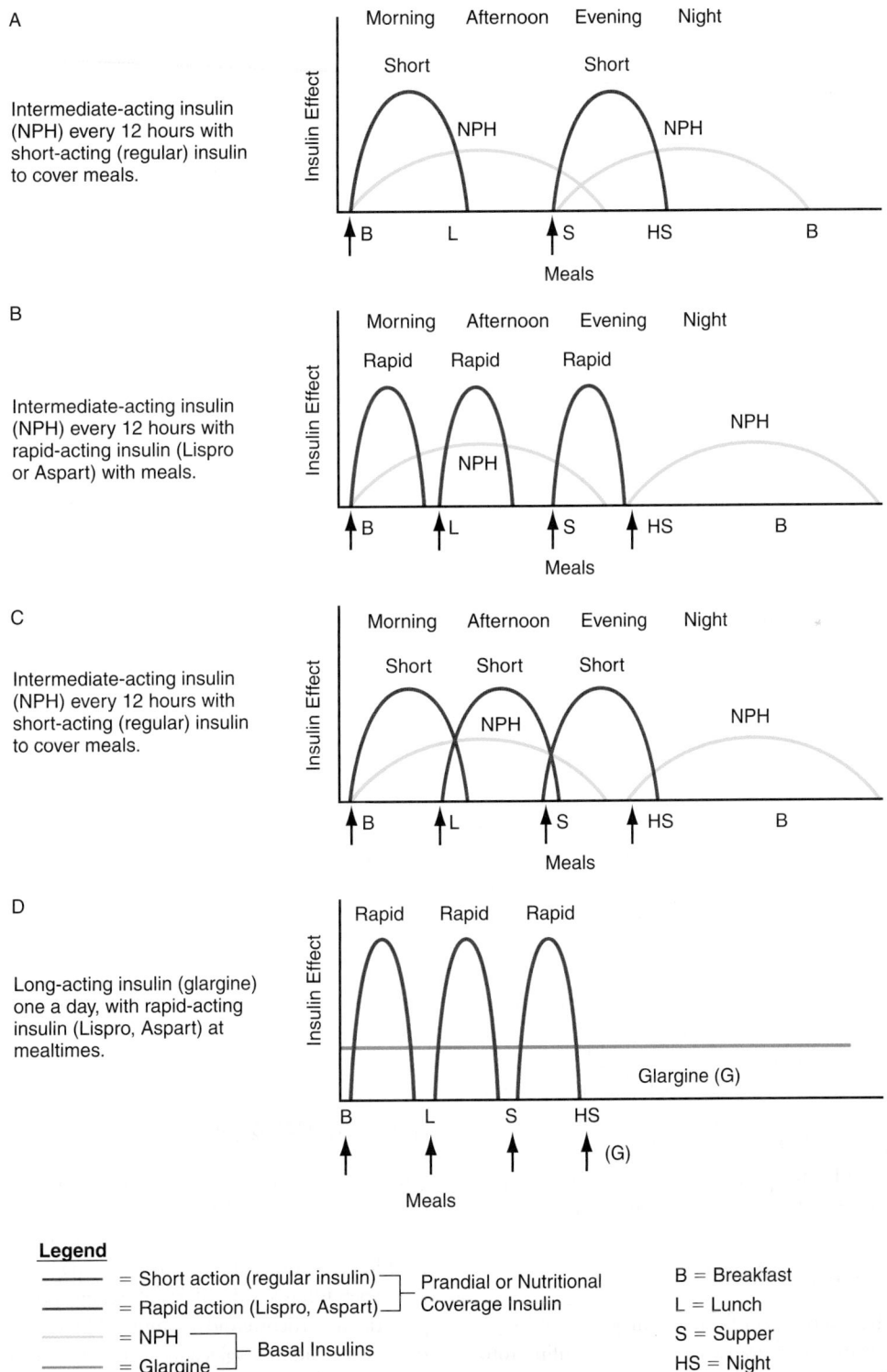

Figure 37-1 Basal and nutritional bolus insulin combinations.

24 hours was 24 units. Ms. Smith will now require basal coverage (provided by subcutaneous intermediate or long-acting insulin) and nutritional coverage for mealtimes (provided by short-acting subcutaneous insulin).

2. The 24 units of insulin infused during the previous 24 hours is Ms. Smith's required daily insulin dose. To transition to subcutaneous insulin, a proportion of this amount (i.e., 75%-80%) will be divided between basal and prandial components.[5] In this situation, 75% of the 24 units = 18 units. Half of this amount (9 units) will be administered subcutaneously as intermediate or long-acting insulin; the other half will be administered as short-acting insulin to coincide with meals (i.e., 3 units with each of three meals).

3. The options for insulin administration for Ms. Smith are as follows[34-36]:

Basal insulin: 9 units of glargine once daily, *or* 4.5 units twice daily of Neutral Protamine Hagedorn (NPH) administered subcutaneously

Prandial/nutritional insulin: 3 units regular insulin given subcutaneously before each meal (short-acting), *or* 3 units Lispro or Aspart given subcutaneously with each meal (ultra–short-acting insulin), verify current blood glucose level.

Supplemental correction dosages: A supplemental correction scale can be used to cover any hyperglycemia above the target range, and administration can be combined with scheduled blood glucose measurements; verify current blood glucose level.

After the transition to subcutaneous insulin, the dosage is adjusted to the individual patient's needs. In a stable *insulin-sensitive* patient, 1 unit of short-acting insulin will lower the blood glucose by 50 to 100 mg/dL.[21] In a critical care patient, more insulin is typically required to reduce blood glucose levels, because of the stress of the critical illness.[36]

Table 37-2 for a description of describes the various types of insulin available for use. These include ultra–short-acting, short-acting, intermediate-acting, long-acting, and combination insulin replacement options. Even after the transition to subcutaneous insulin is completed, blood glucose is monitored frequently to maintain blood glucose within the target range and detect hyperglycemia or hypoglycemia.

Intermittent Insulin Coverage. A patient may be prescribed supplemental "correctional" doses of insulin in addition to the basal/prandial insulin combination. The use of the trio of basal, prandial, and correctional insulin is designed to eliminate the use of the traditional sliding scale.[35] A frequent criticism of sliding scale therapy is that the dosages are rarely reevaluated or adjusted once established.[34] A second criticism is that the scales treat hyperglycemia only after it has occurred; they are not proactive in the manner of continuous insulin infusions.[34]

HYPOGLYCEMIA MANAGEMENT

It is important to have a protocol for the management of hypoglycemia. The major drawback to use of intensive insulin protocols, as described earlier, is the potential for hypoglycemia. Whenever hypoglycemia is detected, it is important to *stop*

any continuous infusion of insulin. An example of one protocol to reverse hypoglycemia follows:

- Blood glucose level lower than 40 mg/dL: administer 50 mL dextrose (50%) in water ($D_{50}W$) as an intravenous bolus.
- Blood glucose level between 40 and 70 mg/dL: administer 25 mL of $D_{50}W$ as an intravenous bolus.

In all cases of hypoglycemia, the blood glucose concentration is monitored every 15 to 20 minutes until the blood sugar has risen into a safe range. The ADA recommends incorporation of level of consciousness plus the blood glucose result as a guide to glucose replacement with hypoglycemia,[37] with the administration of 15 to 20 g of glucose to the conscious hypoglycemic patient.[37] A different protocol suggests the following response to a blood glucose concentration of less than 60 mg/dL[36]:

- Blood glucose level lower than 60 mg/dL and patient is awake and responsive: administer intravenous push of 25 mL of $D_{50}W$.
- Blood glucose level lower than 60 mg/dL and patient is unresponsive: administer intravenous push of 50 mL of $D_{50}W$.

NURSING MANAGEMENT

Nursing management of the patient with neuroendocrine stress resulting from critical illness incorporates a variety of nursing diagnoses (see the Nursing Diagnosis feature on Stress of Critical Illness). The goals of nursing management are to monitor the hyperglycemic side effects of vasopressor therapy; administer prescribed corticosteroids; monitor blood glucose, insulin effectiveness, avoid hypoglycemia; provide nutrition; and provide education to the patient's family and supportive others (see the Patient Education feature on Stress of Critical Illness).

TABLE 37-2 Pharmacologic Management: Insulin*

INSULIN	ROUTE†	ACTION	ONSET/PEAK/DURATION	SPECIAL CONSIDERATIONS
Ultra–Short-Acting Insulins				
Aspart (NovoLog)	SQ	Insulin replacement, rapid onset	5-15 min/30-90 min/<5 hr	Insulin analogue almost *immediately* absorbed; must be taken with food. Insulin appearance should be clear. Must be used in combination with intermediate-acting or long-acting basal insulin regimen. See Fig. 37-1.
Lispro (Humalog)	SQ	Insulin replacement, rapid onset	5-15 min/30-90 min/<5 hr	First available synthetic insulin (analogue); almost *immediately* absorbed; must be taken with food. Shorter duration of action than regular insulin; should be used with basal longer-acting insulin. See Fig. 37-1.
Glulisine (Aprida)	SQ	Insulin replacement, rapid onset	5-15 min/30-90 min/<5 hr	New insulin analog
Short-Acting Insulin				
Regular	IV or SQ	Insulin replacement therapy	IV: <15 min SQ: 30-60 min/2-3 hr/5-8 hr	Only type of insulin suitable for IV continuous infusion or bolus administration.
Intermediate-Acting Basal Insulin				
Neutral Protamine Hagedorn (NPH)	SQ	Insulin replacement, intermediate action	2-4 hr/4-10 hr/10-16 hr	
Long-Acting Basal Insulins				
Glargine (Lantus)	SQ	Long-acting basal insulin analogue; longer-acting than NPH or Ultralente	2-4 hr until steady state/No peak. Concentration relatively constant over 20-24 hr	Synthetic insulin (analogue); differs from human insulin by three amino acids, slowing release over 24 hr; no peak. Decrease dose by 20% if switching from NPH to glargine. Must not be diluted or mixed with other insulins. See Fig. 37-1.
Detemir (Levemir)	SQ	Long-acting basal analog	3-8 hr until steady state/No peak/5-23 hr	
Combination (Premixed) Insulins				
Various	SQ	Rapid plus intermediate or long-acting insulin combination	Varies according to combination used	Many combinations exist; examples (long-acting component/short-acting component) include 70/30 regular (70% NPH with 30% Regular), NovoLog mix 70/30 (70% aspart-protamine suspension with 30% aspart), and Humalog mix 75/25 (75% lispro-protamine suspension with 25% lispro).

*Dosages are individualized according to patient's age and size.
†Only regular insulin is suitable for intravenous use.
IV, intravenous; SQ, subcutaneous.
Data from AACE Diabetes Mellitus Clinical Practice Guidelines Task Force, *Endocr Pract*, 13(suppl 1) 13(5):3-68, 2007.

Monitor Hyperglycemic Side Effects of Vasopressor Therapy. Two vasopressors frequently used as continuous infusions to counteract hypotension in the critically ill also raise blood glucose. Epinephrine and, to a lesser extent, norepinephrine stimulate an increase in gluconeogenesis (creation of new glucose), an increase of skeletal muscle and hepatic glycogenolysis (increased glucose production), an increase in lipolysis (increased fat breakdown), direct suppression of insulin secretion, and an increase in peripheral insulin resistance.[13] All of these actions serve to raise the serum glucose level in the bloodstream.

Administer Prescribed Corticosteroids. Critically ill patients with below-normal cortisol levels may be prescribed intravenous hydrocortisone.[4] Therapeutic steroids raise blood glucose levels and make glycemic control more difficult. Frequent monitoring of the blood glucose concentration is necessary to guide treatment of hyperglycemia in the patient receiving intravenous corticosteroids. Short-term use of low-dose steroids confers greater benefit than harm in the septic patient with hypotension refractory to volume and vasopressor resuscitation therapies.[4] Ongoing monitoring for the presence of new infection is mandatory.

Monitor Blood Glucose, Insulin Effectiveness, Avoid Hypoglycemia. The critical care nurse is responsible for the hourly monitoring of blood glucose and titration of the insulin infusion according to the hospital's established protocol while the patient is hyperglycemic. The use of standardized protocols makes possible a systematic approach to the control of blood glucose. This results in improved glycemic control and lower rates of hypoglycemia. It is essential and recommended that nurses receive effective and ongoing education about the anabolic impact of insulin therapy in critical illness.[5] Hospital protocols to minimize development of hypoglycemia, such as using the 140-180 mg/dL target range,[5] and rapid reversal of any occurrence of severe hypoglycemia (below 40 mg/dL) by provision of intravenous dextrose ($D_{50}W$) are mandatory.

Provide Nutrition. Whenever an insulin infusion is started to lower blood glucose, nutritional support (enteral or TPN) should be considered. In the absence of nutrition, a 10% dextrose solution may temporarily be infused. The 10% dextrose offers the advantage of carbohydrate calories for metabolism, limits fluctuations in the blood sugar, and reduces the risk of hypoglycemia. After the patient's metabolic condition is stable, introduction of non-glucose nutrition (protein and fat) is recommended.[38]

Patient Education. While the patient is acutely ill, most of the educational interventions are directed to the family at the bedside. Numerous explications are required to describe the intravenous medications, the nutritional needs, the purpose of insulin, the role of steroids (if applicable), the ongoing nursing care, prevention of complications, risk of multiorgan system dysfunction (MODS) and management of the underlying disease process. Educational issues that may be discussed are listed in the Patient Education feature on Stress of Critical Illness.

COLLABORATIVE MANAGEMENT

It is well established that standardized protocols designed to manage the complications of critical illness result in lower morbidity and mortality for the patients. Optimally, all disciplines concerned with the endocrine status of the patient will have participated in the design of these guidelines in each critical care area. The guideline that applies to most patients relates to targeted glucose control. Many professional organizations have endorsed the importance of monitoring blood glucose in the critically ill patient, as described in the Evidence-Based Practice feature on Hyperglycemia Management in Critical Illness.[5,34]

DIABETES MELLITUS

Diabetes mellitus is a progressive endocrinopathy associated with carbohydrate intolerance and insulin dysregulation.

Morbidity and Mortality Associated with Diabetes Mellitus. According to the U.S. Centers for Disease Control and Prevention (CDC), diabetes is the sixth most common cause of death among U.S. adults. Heart disease and stroke are the first and third leading causes of death among U.S. adults.[39] These data must be interpreted in light of the knowledge that adults with diabetes have a risk for dying from cardiovascular diseases that is two to four times greater than in adults without diabetes.[27] Diabetes is also associated with an increased risk of cancer. Malignant neoplasms are the second leading cause of death in the United States.[39] The CDC reports that diabetes is also an independent predictor of mortality from cancer of the colon, the pancreas, the female breast and, in men, the liver and the bladder.[40] The annual cost for hospital care per capita for persons with diabetes is $6309, compared with $2971 for persons without diabetes.[34] This represents a cost ratio of 2:1.[34]

Diagnosis of Diabetes. Diabetes mellitus is diagnosed by measurement of the fasting plasma glucose (FPG) laboratory test. The blood glucose may also called a fasting blood glucose (FBG) or fasting blood sugar (FBS) level. The benchmarks for a normal FPG value have been progressively lowered as more knowledge has been gained about the benefits of maintaining the plasma glucose level as close to normal as possible.

Evidence-Based Practice: Collaborative

Hyperglycemia Management in Critical Illness

Summary of evidence and evidence-based recommendations for controlling hyperglycemic symptoms related to physiologic stress of critical illness

Strong Evidence to Support
- Initiate insulin therapy for persistent hyperglycemia beginning at a threshold of no greater than 180 mg/dL.
- Once a continuous insulin infusion is initiated, maintain the target blood glucose level between 140 and 180 mg/dL.
- Frequent blood glucose monitoring to avoid hypoglycemia (hypoglycemia is defined as a blood glucose below 70 mg/dL; severe hypoglycemia <40 mg/dl).

- For patients who are eating, maintain preprandial blood glucose below 110 mg/dL; maintain 2-hour post-postprandial blood glucose below 140 mg/dL.
- A multidisciplinary team approach to implement institutional guidelines, protocols, and standardized order-sets results in fewer hypoglycemic and hyperglycemic events.

References
ACE/ADA task force on inpatient diabetes, *Endocr Pract* 12(4):458-68, 2006.

Moghissi ES et al: American Association of Clinical Endocrinologists and American Diabetes Association consensus statement on inpatient glycemic control, *Endocr Pract* 15(4):1-17, 2009.

The current values endorsed by the American Diabetes Society are as follows[41]:

- An FPG level 70-100 mg/dL (5.6 mmol/L) signifies normal fasting glucose.
- An FPG level between 100 and 125 mg/dL (5.6 and 6.9 mmol/L) denotes impaired fasting glucose (IFG).
- An FPG level greater than 126 mg/dL (7 mmol/L) provides a diagnosis of diabetes (result is verified by testing more than once).

Two FPG values of 126 mg/dL or higher confirm the diagnosis of diabetes. For the acutely ill patient, hyperglycemia is actively treated with insulin to lower the blood sugar to a safe target range.[5] There are differences in the values of plasma versus whole blood glucose measurements. Plasma glucose values are 10% to 15% higher than whole blood glucose values, and it is essential that health care clinicians and people with diabetes know whether their monitor and strips provide whole blood or plasma results, especially when results from more than one setting (laboratory or monitor) are being compared. Although most laboratories measure plasma glucose levels, most home-monitoring units and point-of-care units measure glucose using whole blood from capillary blood obtained by a finger-stick.[42]

The benefit and importance of maintaining blood glucose at levels as close to normal as possible has been conclusively demonstrated in patients with type 1 and type 2 diabetes.[42] The Diabetes Control and Complications Trial (DCCT) of 1995 on type 1 diabetes and the United Kingdom Prospective Diabetes Study (UKPDS), published in 1998, on type 2 diabetes demonstrated that lifestyle changes and use of medications that lead to consistently normal glucose levels reduce microvascular diabetes-related complications and decrease mortality.[42]

Types of Diabetes. Two distinct types of diabetes are discussed in this chapter[41]:

- Type 1 diabetes results from beta-cell destruction, usually leading to absolute insulin deficiency.
- Type 2 diabetes results from a progressive insulin secretory defect in addition to insulin resistance.

The two diseases are different in nature, cause, treatment, and prognosis.[41] A further category of *prediabetes* has more recently been added to describe patients with impaired fasting glucose (FPG between 100 and 125 mg/dL) who are likely to develop diabetes at some time in the future and are at increased risk for coronary artery disease and stroke.[41] Other conditions, such as gestational diabetes, are not discussed in this chapter.

Glycated Hemoglobin. For individuals with diabetes, maintenance of blood glucose within a tight normal range is fundamental to avoid the development of microvascular and neuropathic secondary conditions. Although the FPG produces a snapshot of the blood glucose concentration at a single point in time, the *glycated hemoglobin* (HbA$_{1C}$), also known as a *glycosylated hemoglobin,* identifies the percentage of glucose that the red cells have absorbed from the plasma over the previous 3-month period. A normal HbA$_{1c}$ falls between 4% and 6%.[41] The target for diabetic patients is an A$_{1C}$ value lower than 7%.[41] Currently, the HbA$_{1C}$ measurement is not recommended as a diagnostic tool for new diabetics, but only for those with known diabetes as a means to track the degree of glycemic control.[41]

TYPE 1 DIABETES

Type 1 diabetes mellitus accounts for only about 5% to 10% of the diabetic population.[37] Older names for this condition included insulin-dependent diabetes (IDDM) and juvenile diabetes. Type 1 diabetes is a cellular-mediated autoimmune disease that causes progressive destruction of the beta cells of the islets of Langerhans in the pancreas. Autoantibodies that falsely identify self as a foreign invader to be destroyed can now be identified by laboratory analysis. Many responsible autoantibodies contribute to pancreatic destruction, including autoantibodies to the islet cell, to insulin, to glutamic acid decarboxylase (GAD65), and to the tyrosine phosphatases IA-2 and IA-2β.[37] One or more of these autoantibodies are present in 85% to 90% of individuals with type 1 diabetes when fasting hyperglycemia is initially detected.[37] Over time, the autoantibodies render the pancreatic beta cells incapable of secreting insulin and regulating intracellular glucose. In type 1 diabetes, the rate of beta-cell destruction is highly variable. It occurs rapidly in some individuals (mainly children) and slowly in others (mainly adults). Some patients, particularly children and adolescents, may have ketoacidosis as the first manifestation of their disease.

Genetic predisposition and unknown environmental factors are also believed to play an important role.[37] Patients with type 1 diabetes are prone to development of other autoimmune disorders such as Graves' disease (hyperthyroidism), Hashimoto's thyroiditis, Addison's disease, autoimmune hepatitis, myasthenia gravis, and pernicious anemia.[37] Lack of insulin impairs carbohydrate, protein, and fat metabolism.

Management of Type 1 Diabetes. Patients with type 1 diabetes must receive intravenous or subcutaneous insulin therapy. Treatment with exogenous insulin replacement restores normal entry of glucose into the cells. The range of insulin replacements available is expanding, and it is essential that critical care nurses be knowledgeable about this class of medications (see Table 37-2). Insulin is manufactured with the use of human-based recombinant DNA technology.[43] Without insulin, the rapid breakdown of noncarbohydrate substrate, particularly fat, leads to ketonemia, ketonuria, and diabetic ketoacidosis (DKA), a life-threatening complication associated with type 1 diabetes (see later discussion).

TYPE 2 DIABETES

An estimated 8.7% of the population in the United States have diabetes, almost all of them have type 2.[44] Most affected individuals are older and obese, and many have a condition known as *metabolic syndrome*.[45] Up to one third of people with diabetes are undiagnosed. Patients at high risk for type 2 diabetes include those who meet the following criteria[44-46]:

- A family history of type 2 diabetes in a first-degree relative
- Member of racial or ethnic groups known to be at greater risk for type 2 diabetes (Native Americans, African Americans, Hispanic Americans, Asians/South Pacific Islanders)

- Signs of *insulin resistance syndrome* or conditions associated with insulin resistance, such as hypertension, dyslipidemia, polycystic ovary syndrome, and metabolic syndrome

In type 2 diabetes, pancreatic beta cells are present and functioning; however, the amount of insulin they produce varies greatly among patients:

- In some patients, the pancreatic beta cells do not produce sufficient insulin to meet the metabolic need. In these patients, there is evidence that the beta cells may have been in decline for years before the appearance of clinical symptoms. This is called an *inadequate insulin response.*
- In other patients, the pancreas may produce sufficient insulin or even more than is needed (hyperinsulinemia), but the tissues are resistant to the effects of the insulin. This is known as *insulin resistance syndrome.*[47]
- Some patients have a combination of conditions—a lower than normal level of insulin production and a heightened insulin resistance at the cellular level.

Insulin resistance describes a complex metabolic situation in which organ and tissue cells deny entry to insulin and glucose. This creates the clinical paradox in which elevated serum insulin levels and hyperglycemia are present at the same time. Obesity increases insulin resistance.[41] Insulin resistance has a strong association with type 2 diabetes. Until researchers clarify the exact nature of insulin resistance, many labels will continue to be used to describe similar clusters of symptoms, including *insulin resistance syndrome* and *metabolic syndrome.*[45,47]

Metabolic Syndrome.
The major known stimuli for development of metabolic syndrome are obesity and disorders of insulin resistance.[45] Specific measurable factors are diagnostic of metabolic syndrome. These include abdominal adiposity, as demonstrated by a waist measurement greater than 40 inches in men or 35 inches in women; triglyceride levels higher than 150 mg/dL; high-density lipoprotein (HDL) cholesterol levels lower than 40 mg/dL in men or 35 mg/dL in women; blood pressure higher than 130/85 mg Hg; and an FPG value higher than 100 mg/dL. The ADA uses the FPG cutoff point of 100 mg/dL to identify individuals who are prediabetic.[45] Metabolic syndrome is strongly associated with the development of heart disease and is also discussed in Chapter 19.

Screening for Type 2 Diabetes.
The ADA recommends screening individuals who are at risk for type 2 diabetes at 3-year intervals, beginning at 45 years of age, especially those who are overweight (defined as a body mass index [BMI] ≥ 25 kg/m^2) or obese (BMI ≥ 30 kg/m^2).[44] With the rise of obesity in the United States, the incidence of type 2 diabetes in children and adolescents has also increased dramatically in the last decade.[41]

Lifestyle Management for Type 2 Diabetes.
Most adults with type 2 diabetes are overweight or obese based on their BMI. For most patients with type 2 diabetes, a program of weight reduction, increased physical exercise, and a change in diet pattern are recommended. Diets that contain large quantities of carbohydrate are discouraged.[48] The diet should contain less than 30% of calories from fat, reduced sugar intake, low levels of saturated and trans fats, and an increased quantity of whole grains, vegetables, and fruits. Crash diets are discouraged,

and a gradual program of weight loss, if needed, is recommended.[48] The exercise program is tailored to the individual but might start with 30 minutes of brisk walking each day if the person was previously sedentary.

Pharmacologic Management of Type 2 Diabetes.
If lifestyle changes are unsuccessful in reversing the pattern of type 2 diabetes, oral antihyperglycemic medications are prescribed (Table 37-3). These drugs are not oral forms of insulin, because insulin would be destroyed by gastric juices. There are five major classes of oral agents: sulfonylureas, glinides, biguanides, thiazolidinediones, and alpha-glucosidase inhibitors. These oral antidiabetic drugs work to lower plasma glucose levels by several different mechanisms: increasing insulin secretion, increasing sensitivity to insulin, or delaying carbohydrate absorption[49-52] (Box 37-1).

Insulin secretagogues stimulate secretion of insulin from the pancreatic beta cells and decrease hyperglycemia.[50] Two classes of drugs have this action: the *sulfonylureas* (glyburide, glipizide, glimepiride, and gliclazide), and the *glinides* (repaglinide and nateglinide).[51] Both classes of drugs reduce the HbA$_{1C}$ by about 1.5 percentage points and have a long duration of action. Side effects include hypoglycemia and weight gain.[50,51]

Insulin sensitizers work at two locations in the body. They increase insulin sensitivity in the liver, thereby increasing the ability of insulin to suppress endogenous glucose production, and they increase insulin sensitivity at the peripheral cellular level, to increase glucose uptake.[51] Two separate classes of drugs work in different ways to increase insulin sensitivity.

The *biguanides* (metformin) increase insulin sensitivity in the liver and have only a minor effect on skeletal muscle. Metformin is considered first-line therapy for patients with type 2 diabetes.[50] Metformin is associated with a rare risk of metabolic acidosis; gastrointestinal side effects are common.[50,51]

The *thiazolidinediones* (TZDs), also known as *glitazones* (pioglitazone and rosiglitazone), belong to a class of drugs called *peroxisome proliferator–activated receptor gamma modulators.*[51] These drugs increase the sensitivity of muscle, fat, and liver cells to endogenous and exogenous insulin (insulin sensitizers).[51] The TZDs cause fluid gain and pedal edema in 3% to 5% of patients and heart failure in less than 1%.[51] Of greater concern is use of TZDs in combination with insulin therapy: the incidence of heart failure rises to between 2% and 3%.[53] Caution is recommended when using these drugs with patients who have risk factors for heart failure (pioglitazone and rosiglitazone), or risk factors for myocardial infarction (rosiglitazone).[52]

A third mechanism of action is exhibited by the *alpha-glucosidase inhibitors.* They slow digestion of ingested carbohydrates, delay glucose absorption, and reduce postprandial (after meals) hyperglycemia. The drugs in this class are acarbose and miglitol.[49] A review of the physiology of carbohydrate digestion is helpful to understand how these drugs work. Carbohydrates are broken down to absorbable components in the duodenum and upper jejunum. The carbohydrates are digested to oligosaccharides in the small intestine by pancreatic lipase, after which the oligosaccharides are cleaved to monosaccharides by the alpha-glucosidase group of enzymes. The monosaccharides are then available to be absorbed from the intestine into the

TABLE 37-3 Pharmacologic Management: Oral Medications for Type 2 Diabetes

DRUG	DOSAGE*	ACTION	ONSET/PEAK/ DURATION	SPECIAL CONSIDERATIONS
Insulin Secretagogues				
First-Generation Sulfonylureas				
Tolbutamide (Orinase)	0.5-2.0 g bid-tid	Stimulates release of insulin	Rapid absorption 30-60 min/3-5 hr/ 6-12 hr	Metabolized in liver, excreted in kidneys. In renal insufficiency, start with lower dose and observe for signs of hypoglycemia. Contraindicated in pregnancy. Numerous drug interactions.
Tolazamide (Tolinase)	0.1-1.0 g single dose or bid	Stimulates release of insulin	4 hr/4 hr/10 hr	
Chlorpropamide (Diabinese)	0.1-0.5 g single dose	Stimulates release of insulin Antidiuretic	1 hr/2-4 hr/48 hr	Frequent monitoring is needed for patients with fluid retention or cardiac dysfunction.
Second-Generation Sulfonylureas				
Glipizide (Glucotrol, Glucotrol XL)	5-10 mg bid 5-20 mg bid	Stimulates release of insulin	1 hr/1-3 hr/12-24 hr	
Glyburide (Micronase, DiaBeta, Glynase PresTab)	5 mg single dose or bid	Stimulates release of insulin	1 hr/4 hr/18-24 hr	3-6 mg daily
Glimepiride (Amaryl)	1-4 mg daily	Stimulates release of insulin	Duration 24 hr	
Glinides				
Nateglinide (Starlix)	120 mg tid (15-30 min before meals)	Stimulates release of insulin	Peak <1 hr	Contraindicated in pregnant or breast-feeding women, children, and patients with hepatic disorders. Dose may need to be adjusted with increased glucose during times of stress (infection, surgery, trauma).
Repaglinide (Prandin)	0.5-4.0 mg (15-30 min before meals)	Binds to potassium on pancreatic beta cells; increases insulin secretion	Useful in patients with sulfa allergies	

Continued

TABLE 37-3 Pharmacologic Management: Oral Medications for Type 2 Diabetes—cont'd

DRUG	DOSAGE*	ACTION	ONSET/PEAK/ DURATION	SPECIAL CONSIDERATIONS
Insulin Sensitizers				
Biguanides				
Metformin (Glucophage)	Max: 500-2550 mg in 3 divided doses	Sensitizer Antihyperglycemic Suppresses hepatic glucose production	1-3 hr/24 hr/24-48 hr	Lowers serum glucose by reducing hepatic glucose output. Decreases peripheral insulin resistance. Temporarily withhold if patient is having contrast radiography. Adverse effects: lactic acidosis, GI upset. Promotes weight loss. Contraindicated in pregnancy, kidney dysfunction, acute or chronic acidosis, DKA, hepatic dysfunction, and excessive alcohol intake.
Thiazolidinediones (TZDs)				
Pioglitazone (Actos)	15-45 mg	Enhances insulin action by increasing cell receptors to exogenous and endogenous insulin	Peak 2-3 hr	Decreases insulin resistance and decreases hepatic glucose production. Take with meals to increase absorption.
Rosiglitazone (Avandia)	4-8 mg			Reduces blood pressure and triglycerides. Administration with oral contraceptives reduces efficacy of both drugs by 30%.
Carbohydrate Inhibitors				
Alpha-Glucosidase Inhibitors				
Acarbose (Precose)	100 mg tid with meals	Inhibits activity of intestinal enzymes that metabolize carbohydrate Reduces postprandial glucose mobilization	Peak 2-3 hr	Take with "first bite" of each meal. First drug to effectively reduce postprandial glucose. Delays carbohydrate digestion by blocking absorption of complete carbohydrates in small intestine. Does not promote weight loss; carbohydrate is absorbed in distal small intestine and perhaps in the colon. No apparent effect on lactose absorption, so lactose (not sucrose) substances should be used to treat hypoglycemia. Side effects (flatulence, abdominal pain, diarrhea) are minimized with slow titration. Not recommended in severe renal impairment; safety in pregnancy not established.

Miglitol (Glyset)	50-100 mg tid Initially 25 mg daily; adjust to biweekly based on GI tolerance	Peak 2-3 hr	Same as for acarbose Administration with digoxin reduces average plasma concentration of digoxin. Administration with propranolol or ranitidine greatly reduces bioavailability of these two drugs. Do not take concomitantly with digestive enzymes (e.g., amylase, pancreatin).
Combination Drug			
Glyburide and metformin (Glucovance)	1.25 mg/250 mg 2.5 mg/500 mg 5.0 mg/500 mg	Initial or second-line therapy; glyburide stimulates insulin secretion, and metformin decreases glucose production and absorption	See glyburide and metformin Common side effects include diarrhea, nausea, upset stomach. Gradually increase dose over several weeks.

*Second-generation oral hypoglycemics in this table are more potent than the first-generation hypoglycemics. Dosage is lower than for the first-generation drugs, and fewer side effects are associated with the second-generation agents.

bid, twice daily; DKA, diabetic ketoacidosis; GI, gastrointestinal; LDL, low-density lipoprotein; tid, three times daily.

BOX 37-1   ORAL ANTIHYPERGLYCEMIC DRUG ACTIONS

- Drugs that stimulate the pancreas to make more insulin (insulin secretagogues)
  - Sulfonylureas
  - Glinides
  - Drugs that sensitize the body to insulin (insulin sensitizers)
  - Biguanides
  - Thiazolidinediones
- Drugs that delay carbohydrate absorption from small intestine
  - Alpha-glucosidase inhibitors

bloodstream. The alpha-glucosidase inhibitor drugs work by decreasing the conversion of carbohydrates from oligosaccharides to monosaccharides, limiting the rise in blood glucose that occurs after eating. The most frequently prescribed drug in this class is acarbose, which is nonabsorbable.[49]

Monotherapy versus Combination Therapy for Type 2 Diabetes. The goal of long-term oral therapy is to reduce the HbA$_{1C}$ level to less than 7% while avoiding hypoglycemia. This frequently requires prescription of drugs from more than one class or use of a drug that combines two different methods of action.[51,52] Table 37-3 provides for more specific details related to these oral antihyperglycemic drugs.

Pancreatic beta cell decline occurs as type 2 diabetes progresses, and eventually, in many patients, oral agents alone fail to control hyperglycemia. Insulin may then be added to the drug regimen to maintain normal blood sugar levels.[51,52] At this stage, many patients with type 2 diabetes take a combination of oral medications and subcutaneous insulin. Some patients convert entirely to type 1 diabetes. When a patient with type 2 diabetes is admitted to the critical care unit, he or she is switched to subcutaneous or intravenous insulin, and the oral medications are temporarily stopped.

Patients who have type 2 diabetes are prone to a wide range of other complications that increase morbidity and mortality. In addition to drugs to control blood glucose, these patients often require medications to lower their blood pressure, lower their cholesterol and triglyceride levels, treat ischemic heart disease, and manage symptoms of heart failure.[41]

A serious complication of type 2 diabetes that, when present, mandates admission to a critical care unit, is hyperglycemic, hyperosmolar nonketotic syndrome, also called hyperglycemic hyperosmolar state (HHS). This severe, sustained elevation of glucose levels leads to a serum hyperosmolality, and if left untreated, it progresses toward cellular dehydration, coma, and death (discussed later).

DIABETIC KETOACIDOSIS
EPIDEMIOLOGY AND ETIOLOGY

DKA is a life-threatening complication of diabetes mellitus. Type 1 diabetics who are dependent on insulin are typically affected.[54] Some older patients with type 2 diabetes can develop DKA, but this is not as frequently encountered.[55,56]

The diagnostic criteria for DKA are as follows[54]:
- Blood glucose >250 mg/dL
- pH <7.3
- Serum bicarbonate <15 mEq/L
- Moderate or severe ketonemia or ketonuria

The annual incidence of DKA ranges from 4.6 to 8 episodes per 1000 patients with diabetes, and the annual hospital costs for patients with DKA exceed $1 billion per year.[54]

Infection is the major reason that diabetic patients progress to DKA. Symptoms of fatigue and polyuria may precede full-blown DKA, which can develop in less than 24 hours in a person with type 1 diabetes.[54] In an undiagnosed diabetic patient, it is unknown how long it may take for DKA to develop as the pancreatic beta cells gradually fail. About 20% of hospital admissions for DKA are related to diagnosis of new-onset type 1 diabetes.[55] With management by clinicians experienced in treatment of DKA, the mortality rate from this disorder in type 1 diabetics is less than 5%.[54]

Changes in the type of insulin, change in dosage, or increased metabolic demand can precipitate DKA in individuals with type 1 diabetes.[54] Life cycle changes, such as growth spurts in the adolescent, require an increase in insulin intake, as do surgery, infection, and trauma. In young persons with diabetes, psychological problems combined with eating disorders are a contributing factor in up to 20% of cases of recurrent ketoacidosis.[54]

Ketoacidosis also occurs with acute pancreatitis. In addition to elevated glucose and acidosis, the serum amylase and lipase are abnormally high, which helps to establish the diagnosis as separate from type 1 diabetes.[55] Other nondiabetes causes of ketoacidosis are starvation and alcoholism. These cases are distinguished from classical DKA by clinical history and usually by a plasma glucose concentration of less than 250 mg/dL.[54]

PATHOPHYSIOLOGY

Insulin Deficiency. Insulin is the metabolic key to the transfer of glucose from the bloodstream into the cell, where it can be used immediately for energy or stored for use at a later time. Without insulin, glucose remains in the bloodstream, and cells are deprived of their energy source. A complex pathophysiologic chain of events follows (Fig. 37-2). The release of glucagon from the liver is stimulated when insulin is ineffective in providing the cells with glucose for energy. Glucagon increases the amount of glucose in the bloodstream by breaking down stored glucose (glycogenolysis). Noncarbohydrates (fat and protein) are converted into glucose (gluconeogenesis). Blood glucose levels for the patient in DKA typically range from 300 to 800 mg/dL of blood. The reason the plasma glucose concentration is not higher is because of the short time period during which DKA develops. Elevated serum glucose levels alone do not define DKA; the major determining factor is the presence of ketoacidosis.

Hyperglycemia. Hyperglycemia increases the plasma osmolality, and the blood becomes hyperosmolar. Cellular dehydration occurs as the hyperosmolar extracellular fluid draws the more dilute intracellular and interstitial fluid into the vascular space in an attempt to return the plasma osmolality to normal.

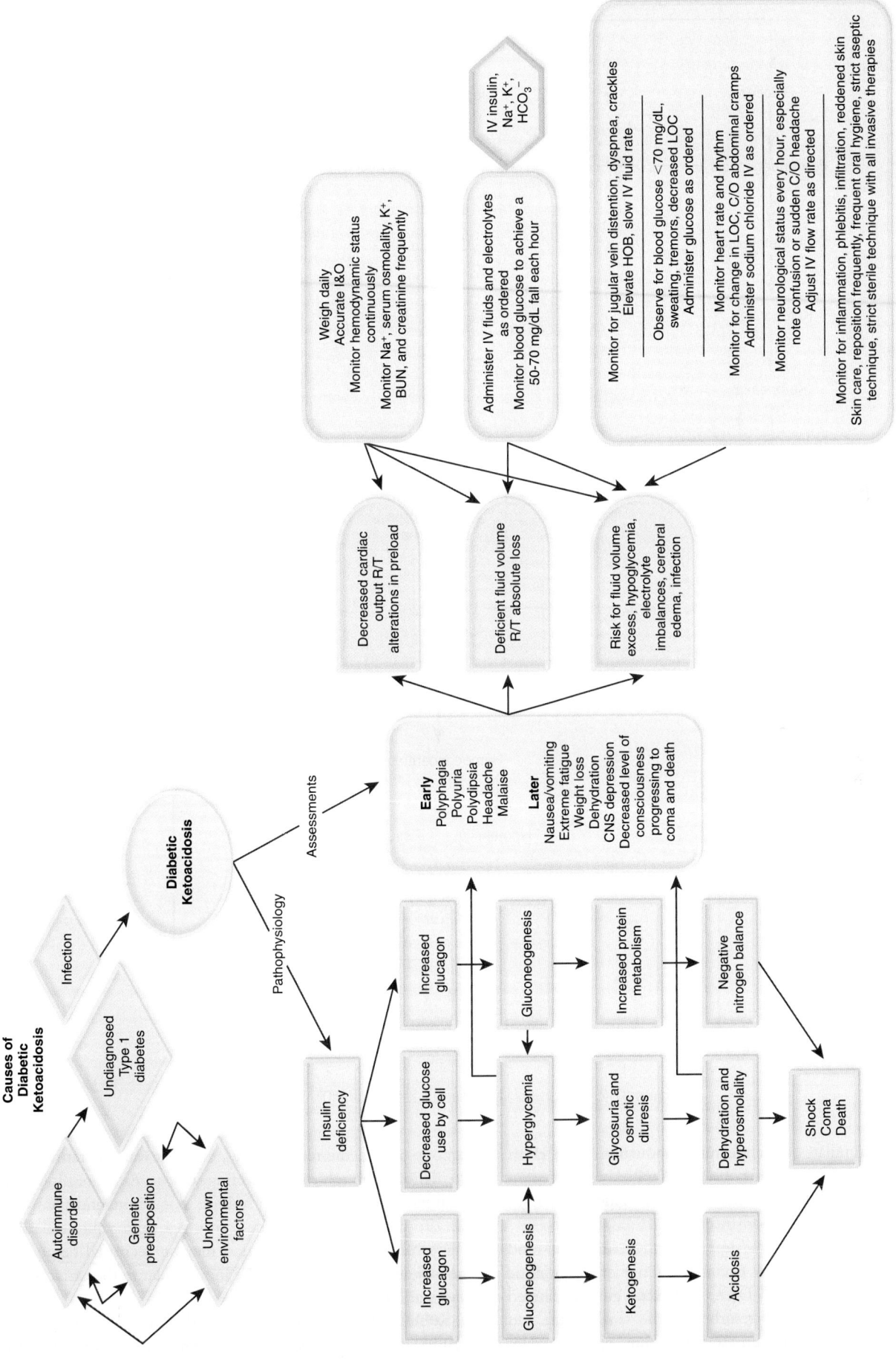

Causes of Diabetic Ketoacidosis

Autoimmune disorder

Genetic predisposition

Unknown environmental factors

Undiagnosed Type 1 diabetes

Infection

Diabetic Ketoacidosis

Pathophysiology

Assessments

Insulin deficiency

Increased glucagon

Decreased glucose use by cell

Increased glucagon

Gluconeogenesis

Gluconeogenesis

Hyperglycemia

Increased protein metabolism

Glycosuria and osmotic diuresis

Ketogenesis

Negative nitrogen balance

Dehydration and hyperosmolality

Acidosis

Shock Coma Death

Early
Polyphagia
Polyuria
Polydipsia
Headache
Malaise

Later
Nausea/vomiting
Extreme fatigue
Weight loss
Dehydration
CNS depression
Decreased level of consciousness progressing to coma and death

Decreased cardiac output R/T alterations in preload

Deficient fluid volume R/T absolute loss

Risk for fluid volume excess, hypoglycemia, electrolyte imbalances, cerebral edema, infection

IV insulin, Na⁺, K⁺, HCO₃⁻

Weigh daily
Accurate I&O
Monitor hemodynamic status continuously
Monitor Na⁺, serum osmolality, K⁺, BUN, and creatinine frequently

Administer IV fluids and electrolytes as ordered
Monitor blood glucose to achieve a 50-70 mg/dL fall each hour

Monitor for jugular vein distention, dyspnea, crackles
Elevate HOB, slow IV fluid rate

Observe for blood glucose <70 mg/dL, sweating, tremors, decreased LOC
Administer glucose as ordered

Monitor heart rate and rhythm
Monitor for change in LOC, C/O abdominal cramps
Administer sodium chloride IV as ordered

Monitor neurological status every hour, especially note confusion or sudden C/O headache
Adjust IV flow rate as directed

Monitor for inflammation, phlebitis, infiltration, reddened skin
Skin care, reposition frequently, frequent oral hygiene, strict aseptic technique, strict sterile technique with all invasive therapies

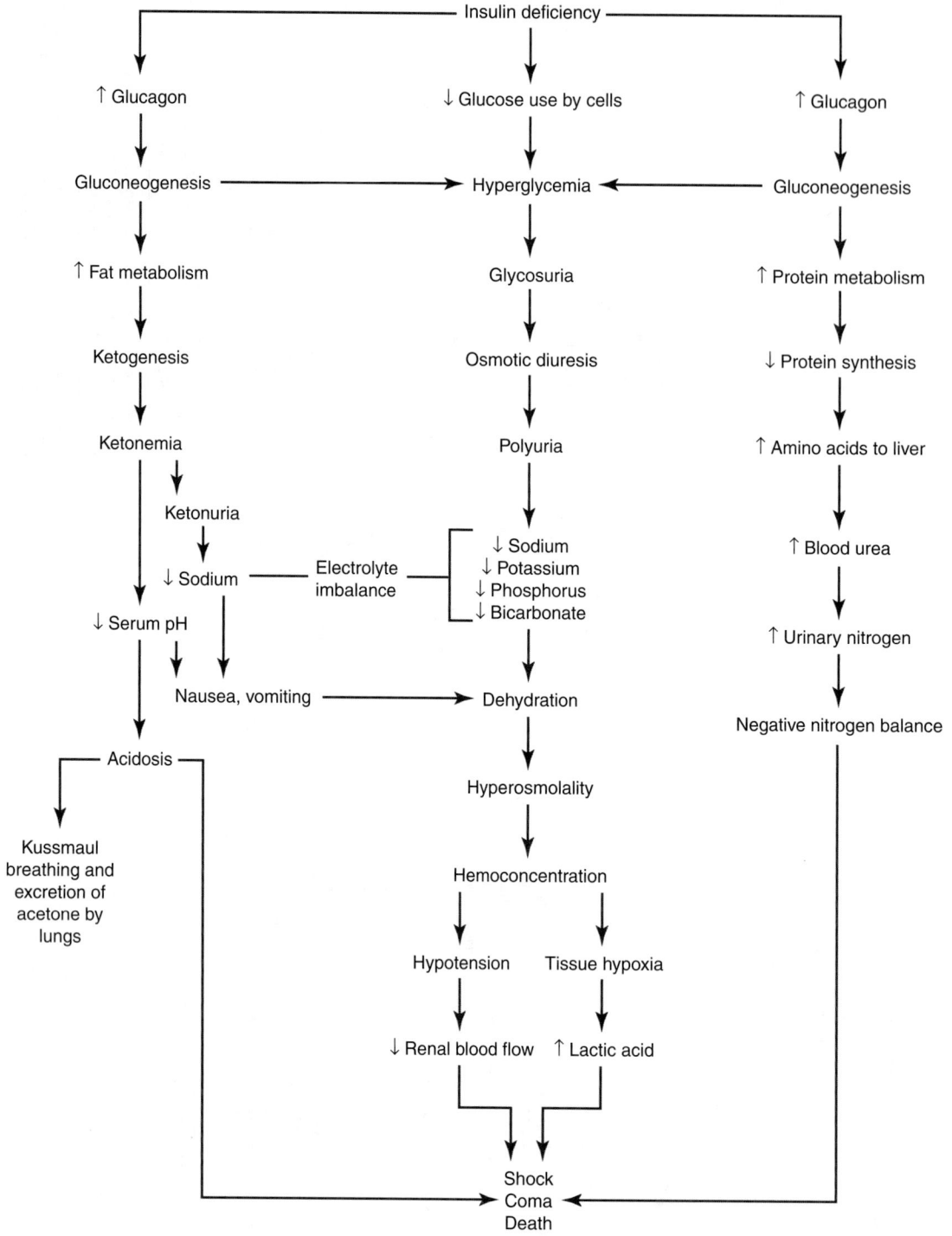

Figure 37-2 Pathophysiology of diabetic ketoacidosis (DKA).

Dehydration stimulates catecholamine production in an effort to provide emergency support. Catecholamine output stimulates further glycogenolysis, lipolysis, and gluconeogenesis, pouring glucose into the bloodstream.

Fluid Volume Deficit. *Polyuria* (excessive urination) and *glycosuria* (sugar in the urine) occur as a result of the osmotic particle load that occurs with DKA. The excess glucose, filtered at the glomeruli, cannot be resorbed at the renal tubule and spills into the urine. The unresorbed solute exerts its own osmotic pull in the renal tubules, and less water is returned to circulation through the collecting ducts. As a result, large volumes of water, along with sodium, potassium, and phosphorus, are excreted in the urine, causing a fluid volume deficit. The serum sodium concentration may be decreased because of the movement of water from the intracellular to the extracellular (vascular) space.[54]

Ketoacidosis. In the healthy individual, the presence of insulin in the bloodstream suppresses the manufacture of ketones. In insulin deficiency states, fat is rapidly converted into glucose (gluconeogenesis). Ketoacidosis occurs when free fatty acids are metabolized into ketones: acetoacetate, β-hydroxybutyrate, and acetone are the three ketone bodies that are produced.[56] During normal metabolism, the ratio of β-hydroxybutyrate to acetoacetate is 1:1, with acetone present in only small amounts. In insulin deficiency, the quantities of all three ketone bodies increase substantially, and the ratio of β-hydroxybutyrate to acetoacetate increases to as much as 10:1.[56] β-Hydroxybutyrate and acetoacetate are the ketones responsible for acidosis in DKA. Acetone does not cause acidosis and is safely excreted in the lungs, causing the characteristic fruity odor.

Ketones are measurable in the bloodstream (ketonemia). Blood tests that measure the quantity of β-hydroxybutyric acid, the predominant ketone body in the blood, are the most useful.[54] Because ketones are excreted by the kidney, they are also measurable in the urine *(ketonuria)*. Ketone blood tests are preferred over urine tests for diagnosis and monitoring of DKA in critical care. When the blood and urine become clear of ketones, the DKA is resolved.

Acid-Base Balance. The acid-base balance varies depending on the severity of the DKA. The patient with mild DKA typically has a pH between 7.25 and 7.30. In moderate to severe DKA, the pH can drop as low as 7.00.[54] Acid ketones dissociate and yield hydrogen ions (H^+), which accumulate and precipitate a fall in serum pH. The level of serum bicarbonate also decreases, consistent with a diagnosis of metabolic acidosis. Breathing becomes deep and rapid (Kussmaul respirations) to release carbonic acid in the form of carbon dioxide. Acetone is exhaled, giving the breath its characteristic fruity odor.

Gluconeogenesis. Gluconeogenesis is the process of breaking down fat or protein to make new glucose. Fat is metabolized to ketones, as described earlier. Protein used for gluconeogenesis leaves no reserve protein available for synthesis and repair of vital body tissues. Nitrogen accumulates as protein is metabolized to urea. Urea, added to the bloodstream, increases the osmotic diuresis and accentuates the dehydration.

ASSESSMENT AND DIAGNOSIS

Clinical Manifestations. DKA has a predictable clinical presentation. It is usually preceded by patient complaints of malaise, headache, polyuria (excessive urination), polydipsia (excessive thirst), and polyphagia (excessive hunger). Nausea, vomiting, extreme fatigue, dehydration, and weight loss follow. Central nervous system depression, with changes in the level of consciousness, can lead quickly to coma.[41,54]

The patient with DKA may be stuporous or unresponsive, depending on the degree of fluid-balance disturbance. The physical examination reveals evidence of dehydration, including flushed dry skin, dry buccal membranes, and skin turgor that takes longer than 3 seconds to return to its original position after the skin has been lifted. Often, "sunken eyeballs," resulting from lack of fluid in the interstitium of the eyeball, are observed. Tachycardia and hypotension may signal profound

fluid losses. Kussmaul respirations are present, and the fruity odor of acetone may be detected.

Laboratory Studies. Considering the complexity and potential seriousness of DKA, the laboratory diagnosis is straightforward. With a known diabetic patient, the presence of urine ketones and hyperglycemia on bedside finger-stick samples provides rapid diagnostic confirmation of DKA. If a blood gas sample is obtained, it can confirm the acid-base imbalance. Other clues may be gleaned from the venous blood chemistry panel. CO_2, if measured, is low in the presence of uncompensated metabolic acidosis, and the anion gap is elevated. Serum sodium may be low as a result of the movement of water from the intracellular space into the extracellular (vascular) space.[54] The serum potassium level is often normal; a low serum potassium level indicates a severe total-body potassium deficiency.[54]

MEDICAL MANAGEMENT

Diagnosis of DKA is based on the combination of presenting symptoms, patient history, medical history (type 1 diabetes), precipitating factors (if known), and results of serum glucose and urine ketone testing. After diagnosis, DKA requires aggressive clinical management to prevent progressive decompensation. The goals of treatment are to reverse dehydration, replace insulin, reverse ketoacidosis, and replenish electrolytes.

Reversing Dehydration. The patient with DKA is dehydrated and may have lost 5% to 10% of body weight in fluids. A fluid deficit of up to 6 L can exist in severe dehydration.[54] Aggressive fluid replacement is provided to rehydrate the intracellular and extracellular compartments and prevent circulatory collapse (Fig. 37-3).[54] Assessment of hydration is an important first step in the treatment of DKA.

Intravenous isotonic normal saline (0.9% NaCl) is infused to replenish the vascular deficit and to reverse hypotension. For the severely dehydrated patient, 1 L of normal saline is infused immediately.[54] Laboratory assessment of serum osmolality and the serum sodium concentration can help guide the subsequent interventions. If the serum osmolality is elevated and serum sodium is high (hypernatremia), infusions of hypotonic sodium chloride (0.45) follow the initial saline replacement. The replacement infusion typically includes 20 to 30 mEq of potassium per liter to restore the intracellular potassium debt, provided kidney function is normal.[54] In patients without normally functioning kidneys and in those with cardiopulmonary disease, careful attention must be paid to the volume of fluid replacement to avoid fluid overload.

After the serum glucose level decreases to 200 mg/dL, the infusing solution is changed to a 50/50 mix of hypotonic saline and 5% dextrose.[54] Dextrose is added to replenish depleted cellular glucose as the circulating serum glucose level falls. Dextrose infusion also prevents unexpected hypoglycemia when the insulin infusion is continued but the patient cannot take in sufficient carbohydrate from an oral diet.

Replacing Insulin. In moderate to severe DKA, an initial intravenous bolus of regular insulin at 0.1 unit for each kilogram of body weight is administered.[54] Subsequently, a continuous infusion of regular insulin at 0.1 unit/kg/hr is infused

Management of Adult Patients with DKA

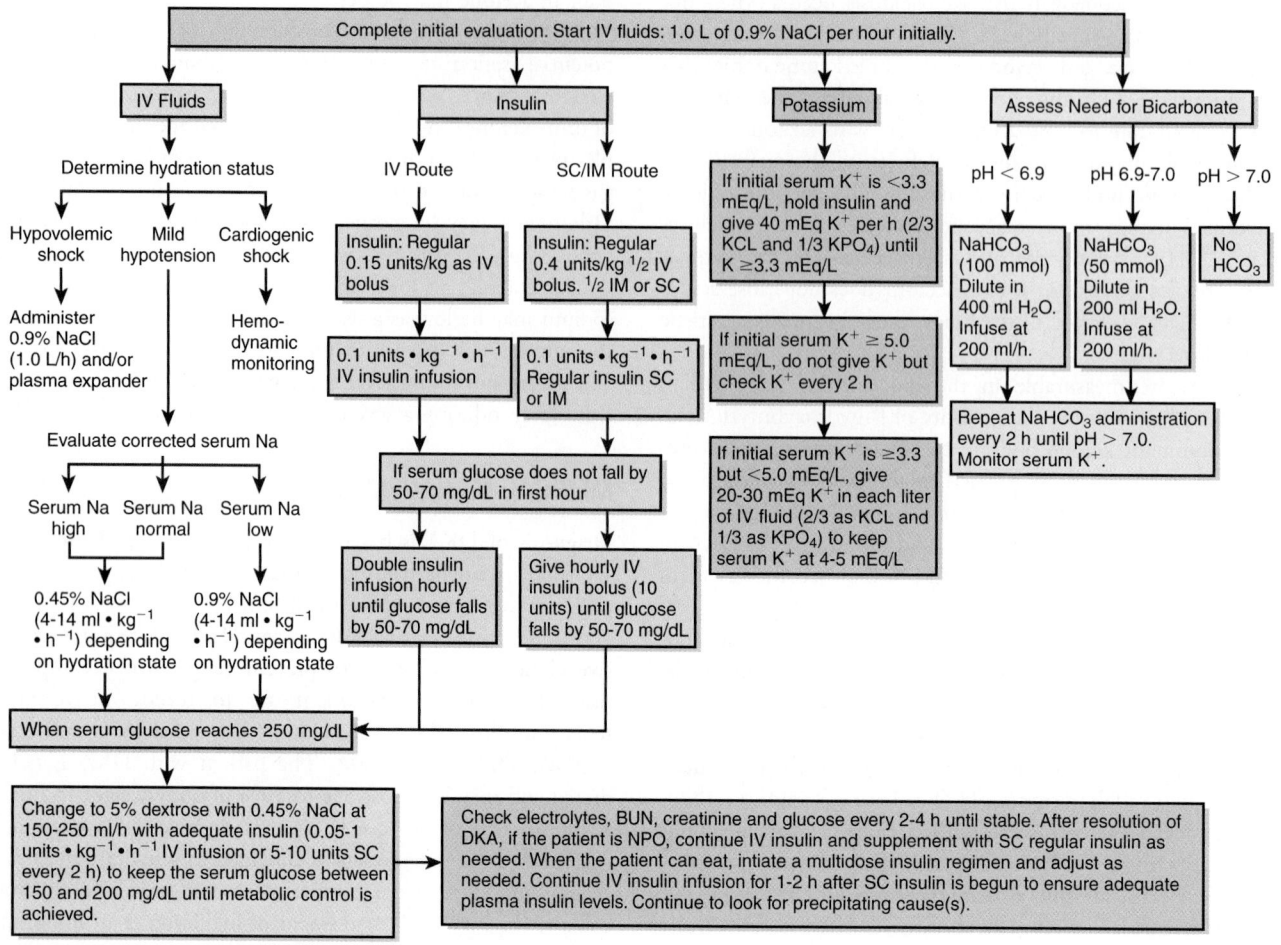

Figure 37-3 Protocol for the management of diabetic ketoacidosis (DKA) in adult patients. *(From Kitabchi AE et al: Hyperglycemic crises in adult patients with diabetes: a consensus statement from the American Diabetes Association,* Diabetes Care, *29[12]:2739, 2006.)*

simultaneously with intravenous fluids.[54] For example, in a 70-kg adult, 7 units of insulin would be infused per hour. If the plasma glucose concentration does not fall by 50 to 70 mg/dL during the first hour of treatment, the glucose measurement should be rechecked and the hydration status of the patient re-evaluated. If the plasma glucose level is decreasing as expected, the insulin infusion may be doubled every hour until a steady glucose decline of between 50 and 70 mg/dL is achieved.[54] Figure 37-3 is a diagrammatic representation of intravenous and subcutaneous insulin administration options in DKA.

Frequent assessment of the patient's blood glucose concentration is mandatory in moderate to severe DKA. Initially, blood glucose tests are performed hourly. The frequency then decreases to every 2 to 4 hours as the patient's blood glucose level stabilizes and approaches normal. After the level has decreased to 200 mg/dL, the acidosis has been corrected, and rehydration has been achieved, the insulin infusion rate may be decreased to 0.05 to 0.1 unit/kg/hr. This usually represents 3 to 6 units per hour in an adult receiving a continuous intravenous insulin infusion.[54] It is important to verify that the serum potassium concentration is not lower than 3.3 mEq/L

and to replace potassium if necessary, before administering the initial insulin bolus.[54]

Reversing Ketoacidosis. Replacement of fluid volume and insulin interrupts the ketotic cycle and reverses the metabolic acidosis. In the presence of insulin, glucose enters the cells, and the body ceases to convert fats into glucose.

Adequate hydration and insulin replacement usually correct the acidosis, and this treatment is sufficient for many patients with DKA. As shown in Figure 37-3, replacement of bicarbonate is no longer routine except for the severely acidotic patient with a serum pH value lower than 7.0.[54] An indwelling arterial line provides access for hourly sampling of arterial blood gases (ABGs) to evaluate pH, bicarbonate, and other laboratory values in the patient with severe DKA. If an arterial line is not available, the pH can be assessed by using the venous pH.[54]

Hyperglycemia usually resolves before the ketoacidemia does. In one clinical report, patients with previously diagnosed type 1 diabetes in DKA took an average of 21 hours after being started on an intravenous insulin protocol to clear ketones from the urine; the infusion was continued for 36 hours until the patients could tolerate an oral diet; and the patients received a total of 9.5 L of normal saline for rehydration.[55] Patients who

Nursing Diagnoses

Diabetic Ketoacidosis

- Decreased Cardiac Output related to alterations in preload
- Deficient Fluid Volume related to absolute loss
- Anxiety relate to threat to biologic, psychological, and social integrity
- Disturbed Body Image related to functional dependence on life-sustaining technology
- Ineffective Coping related to situational crisis and personal vulnerability
- Powerlessness related to lack of control over current situation and/or disease progression
- Deficient Knowledge: Discharge Regimen related to lack of previous exposure to information (see Patient Education feature on Diabetic Ketoacidosis)

BOX 37-2 HYDRATION ASSESSMENT

- Hourly intake
- Blood pressure changes
  - Orthostatic hypotension
  - Pulse pressure
  - Pulse rate, character, rhythm
- Neck vein filling
- Skin turgor
- Skin moisture
- Body weight
- Central venous pressure
- Pulmonary arterial occlusion pressure
- Hourly output
- Complaints of thirst

are newly diagnosed with type 1 diabetes take longer to clear urine ketones and require more insulin to achieve normal glycemic control, compared with long-term diabetics.[55]

Replenishing Electrolytes. Low serum potassium (hypokalemia) occurs as insulin promotes the return of potassium into the cell and metabolic acidosis is reversed. Replacement of potassium by administration of potassium chloride (KCl) begins as soon as the serum potassium falls below normal. Frequent verification of the serum potassium concentration is required for the DKA patient receiving fluid resuscitation and insulin therapy.

The serum phosphate level is sometimes low (hypophosphatemia) in DKA. Insulin treatment may make this more obvious as phosphate is returned to the interior of the cell. If the serum phosphate level is less than 1 mg/dL, phosphate replacement is recommended.[54] See Figure 37-3 for further information about potassium replacement options.

NURSING MANAGEMENT

Nursing management of the patient with DKA incorporates a variety of nursing diagnoses (see the Nursing Diagnoses feature on Diabetic Ketoacidosis). The goals of nursing management are to administer prescribed fluids, insulin, and electrolytes; monitor response to therapy; maintain surveillance for complications; and provide patient education.

Administering Fluids, Insulin, and Electrolytes. Rapid intravenous fluid replacement requires the use of a volumetric pump. Insulin is administered intravenously to patients who are severely dehydrated or have poor peripheral perfusion, to ensure effective absorption. Patients with DKA are kept on NPO status (nothing by mouth) until the hyperglycemia is under control. Throughout the insulin therapy, the patient's response and the laboratory data are assessed for changes relating to blood glucose levels. The critical care nurse is responsible for monitoring the rate of plasma glucose decline in response to insulin. The goal is to achieve a fall in glucose levels of approximately 50 to 70 mg/dL each hour.[54] The coordination involved in monitoring blood glucose, potassium, and often blood gases on an hourly basis is considerable.

When the blood glucose level falls to 200 mg/dL, a 5% dextrose solution (D_5W) with 0.45% NaCl solution is infused to prevent hypoglycemia.[54] At this time, it is likely that the insulin dose per hour will also be decreased. The regular insulin drip is not discontinued until the ketoacidosis subsides, as identified by absence of ketones and a normal pH by arterial or venous blood gas analysis.[54]

Insulin is given subcutaneously after glucose levels, dehydration, hypotension, and acid-base balance are normalized and the patient is in stable condition and taking an oral diet.

Monitoring Response to Therapy. Accurate intake and output (I&O) measurements must be maintained to monitor reversal of dehydration. Hourly urine output is an indicator of kidney function and provides information to prevent overhydration or underhydration. Vital signs, especially heart rate (HR), hemodynamic values, and blood pressure (BP), are continuously monitored to assess response to the fluid replacement. Evidence that fluid replacement is effective includes normal central venous pressure (CVP), decreased HR, and normal BP. Box 37-2 lists the standard features to be included in an assessment of hydration status. More invasive hemodynamic monitoring, such as a pulmonary artery catheter, is rarely needed. Further evidence of hydration improvement includes a change from a previously weak, thready pulse to a pulse that is strong and full, and a change from hypotension to a gradual elevation of systolic BP. Respirations are assessed frequently for changes in rate, depth, and presence of the fruity acetone odor.

Blood glucose is measured each hour in the initial period. Sometimes, potassium is measured just as frequently. The serum osmolality and serum sodium concentration are evaluated, and blood urea nitrogen (BUN) and creatinine levels are assessed for possible kidney impairment related to decreased renal perfusion. The purpose of these frequent assessments is to determine that the patient's clinical status is improving. After the patient has stable laboratory indicators and is awake and alert, the transition to subcutaneous insulin and an oral diet can be made. Hypoglycemia is a risk during the transition period. For example, in anticipation of discontinuing the insulin and intravenous dextrose infusion, a patient receives a subcutaneous dose of insulin and is expected to eat a meal.

However, if the patient is then unable to eat an adequate amount, hypoglycemia results from the administration of subcutaneous insulin without adequate glucose.[55]

The markers for resolution of DKA include a blood glucose level lower than 200 mg/dL, a serum bicarbonate level greater than 18 mEq/L, and a venous pH level greater than 7.3.[54]

Surveillance for Complications. The patient in DKA can experience a variety of complications, including fluid volume overload, hypoglycemia, hypokalemia or hyperkalemia, hyponatremia, cerebral edema, and infection.

Fluid Volume Overload. Fluid overload from rapid volume infusion is a serious complication that can occur in the patient with a compromised cardiopulmonary system or kidneys. Neck vein engorgement, dyspnea without exertion, and pulmonary crackles on auscultation signal circulatory overload. Reduction in the rate and volume of infusion, elevation of the head of the bed, and provision of oxygen may be required to manage the increased intravascular volume. Hourly urine measurement is mandatory to assess renal output and adequacy of fluid replacement.

Hypoglycemia. Hypoglycemia is defined as a serum glucose level lower than 70 mg/dL.[41] Most acute care hospitals have specific procedures for management of the hypoglycemic patient (see the Nursing Interventions Classification feature on Hypoglycemia Management). For example, if hypoglycemia is detected by finger-stick point-of-care testing at the bedside, a blood sample is sent to the laboratory for verification, the physician is notified immediately, and replacement glucose is given intravenously or orally, depending on the patient's clinical condition, diagnosis, and level of consciousness.

Unexpected behavior change or decreased level of consciousness, diaphoresis, and tremors are physical warning signs that the patient has become hypoglycemic. These symptoms are especially important to recognize if the frequency of glucose testing has lengthened to 2- to 4-hour intervals. A comparison between the physical symptoms expected with hypoglycemia and those of hyperglycemia is provided in Box 37-3.

Hypokalemia and Hyperkalemia. Hypokalemia can occur within the first 4 hours of rehydration and insulin treatment. Continuous cardiac monitoring is required, because low serum potassium (hypokalemia) can cause ventricular dysrhythmias.

Hyperkalemia occurs with acidosis or with overaggressive administration of potassium replacement in patients with renal insufficiency. Severe hyperkalemia is demonstrated on the cardiac monitor by a large, peaked T wave; flattened P wave; and widened QRS complex. See Figure 18-75 in Chapter 18. Ventricular fibrillation can follow.

Hyponatremia. Sodium elimination from the body results from the osmotic diuresis and is compounded by the vomiting and diarrhea that occur during DKA. Clinical manifestations of hyponatremia include abdominal cramping, apprehension, postural hypotension, and unexpected behavioral changes. Sodium chloride is infused as the initial intravenous solution. Maintenance of the saline infusion depends on clinical manifestations of sodium imbalance and serum laboratory values.

NIC

Hypoglycemia Management

Definition
Preventing and treating low blood glucose levels

Activities
Identify patient at risk for hypoglycemia.
Determine recognition of hypoglycemia signs and symptoms.
Monitor blood glucose levels, as indicated.
Monitor for signs and symptoms of hypoglycemia (e.g., shakiness, tremor, sweating, nervousness, anxiety, irritability, impatience, tachycardia, palpitation, chills, clamminess, lightheadedness, pallor, hunger, nausea, headache, tiredness, drowsiness, weakness, warmth, dizziness, faintness, blurred vision, nightmares, crying out in sleep, paresthesias, difficulty concentrating, difficulty speaking, incoordination, behavior change, confusion, coma, seizure).
Provide simple carbohydrate, as indicated.
Provide complex carbohydrate and protein, as indicated.
Administer glucagons, as indicated.
Contact emergency medical services, as necessary.
Administer intravenous glucose, as indicated.
Maintain IV access, as appropriate.
Maintain patent airway, as necessary.
Protect from injury, as necessary.

Review events prior to hypoglycemia to determine probable cause.
Provide feedback regarding appropriateness of self-management of hypoglycemia.
Instruct patient and significant others on signs and symptoms, risk factors, and treatment of hypoglycemia.
Instruct patient to have simple carbohydrates available at all times.
Instruct patient to obtain and carry or wear appropriate emergency identification.
Instruct significant others on the use and administration of glucagons, as appropriate.
Instruct on interaction of diet, insulin or oral agents, and exercise.
Provide assistance in making self-care decisions to prevent hypoglycemia (e.g., reducing insulin/oral agents and/or increasing food intake for exercise).
Encourage self-monitoring of blood glucose levels.
Encourage ongoing telephone contact with diabetes care team for consultation regarding adjustments in treatment regimen.
Collaborate with patient and diabetes care team to make changes in insulin regimen (e.g., multiple daily injections), as indicated.
Modify blood glucose goals to prevent hypoglycemia in the absence of hypoglycemia symptoms.
Inform patient of increased risk of hypoglycemia with intensive therapy and normalization of blood glucose levels.
Instruct patient regarding probable changes in hypoglycemia symptoms with intensive therapy and normalization of blood glucose levels.

From Bulechek GM et al: *Nursing interventions classification (NIC)*, ed 5, St Louis, 2008, Mosby.

Risk for Cerebral Edema. Changes in the patient's neurologic status may be insidious. Alterations in level of consciousness, pupil reaction, and motor function may be the result of fluctuating glucose levels and cerebral fluid shifts. Confusion and sudden complaints of headache are ominous signs that may signal cerebral edema. These observations require immediate action to prevent neurologic damage. Neurologic assessments are performed every hour or as needed during the acute phase of hyperglycemia and rehydration. Assessment of level of consciousness serves as the index of the patient's cerebral response to the rehydration therapy.

Risk for Infection. Skin care takes on new dimensions for the patient with DKA. Dehydration, hypovolemia, and hypophosphatemia interfere with oxygen delivery at the cell site and contribute to inadequate perfusion and tissue breakdown. Patients must be repositioned frequently to relieve capillary pressure and promote adequate perfusion to body tissues. The typical patient with type 1 diabetes is of normal weight or underweight. Bony prominences must be assessed for tissue breakdown, and the patient's body weight must be repositioned every 1 to 2 hours. Irritation of skin from adhesive tape, shearing force, and detergents should be avoided. Maintenance of skin integrity prevents unwanted portals of entry for microorganisms.

Oral care, including tooth brushing and use of lip balm, helps keep lips supple and prevents cracking. Prepared sponge sticks or moist gauze pads can be used to moisten oral membranes of the unconscious patient. Swabbing the mouth moistens the tissue and displaces the bacteria that collect when saliva, which has a bacteriostatic action, is curtailed by dehydration. The conscious patient must be provided the means to self-remove oral bacteria by tooth brushing and frequent oral rinsing.

Strict sterile technique is used to maintain all intravenous systems. All venipuncture sites are checked every 4 hours for signs of inflammation, phlebitis, or infiltration. Strict surgical asepsis is used for all invasive procedures. Sterile technique is used if urinary catheterization is necessary to obtain urine samples for testing. Urinary catheter care is provided every 8 hours.

Patient Education. It is important to be aware of the knowledge level and compliance history of patients with previously diagnosed diabetes to formulate an appropriate teaching plan. Learning objectives include a discussion of target glucose levels, definition of hyperglycemia and its causes, harmful effects, symptoms, and how to manage insulin and diet when one is unwell and unable to eat.[55] Additional objectives include a definition of DKA and its causes, symptoms, and harmful consequences. The patient and family are also expected to learn the principles of diabetes management. Universal precautions must be emphasized for all family caregivers.[34] The patient and family must also learn the warning signs to report to the attention of a health care practitioner. Education of the patient, family, or other support persons to achieve knowledge-based, independent self-management of blood glucose level and avoidance of diabetes-related complications are the ultimate goals of the teaching process (see the Patient Education feature on Diabetic Ketoacidosis).

COLLABORATIVE MANAGEMENT

In all aspects of patient care management, health care professionals work as a team with the major collaborative goal of providing the best possible outcome for each patient. Current guidelines related to Collaborative Management of patients with hyperglycemia crisis are listed in the Evidence-Based Practice feature on Diabetic Ketoacidosis.

BOX 37-3 CLINICAL MANIFESTATIONS OF HYPOGLYCEMIA AND HYPERGLYCEMIA

Hypoglycemia	Hyperglycemia
• Restlessness	• Excessive thirst
• Apprehension	• Excessive urination
• Irritability	• Hunger
• Trembling	• Weakness
• Weakness	• Listlessness
• Diaphoresis	• Mental fatigue
• Pallor	• Flushed, dry skin
• Paresthesia	• Itching
• Pallor	• Headache
• Headache	• Nausea
• Hunger	• Vomiting
• Difficulty thinking	• Abdominal cramps
• Loss of coordination	• Dehydration
• Difficulty walking	• Weak, rapid pulse
• Difficulty talking	• Postural hypotension
• Visual disturbances	• Hypotension
• Blurred vision	• Acetone breath odor
• Double vision	• Kussmaul respirations
• Tachycardia	• Rapid breathing
• Shallow respirations	• Changes in level of consciousness
• Hypertension	• Stupor
• Changes in level of consciousness	• Coma
• Seizures	
• Coma	

Patient Education: Diabetic Ketoacidosis

- Acute phase
  - Explain rationale for critical care unit admission
  - Reduce anxiety associated with critical care unit
- Predischarge
  - Assess knowledge level
  - Assess compliance history
  - Diabetes disease process
  - Target glucose levels
  - Causes of diabetic ketoacidosis (DKA)
  - Pathophysiology of DKA
  - Self-care monitoring of blood glucose level
  - Insulin regimen
  - Sick-day management
  - Universal precautions for caregivers
  - Signs and symptoms to report to health care practitioner

HYPERGLYCEMIC HYPEROSMOLAR STATE

EPIDEMIOLOGY AND ETIOLOGY

HHS is a potentially lethal complication of type 2 diabetes. The hallmarks of HHS are extremely high levels of plasma glucose with resultant elevation in hyperosmolality causing osmotic diuresis. Ketosis is absent or mild. Inability to replace fluids lost through diuresis leads to profound dehydration and changes in level of consciousness. The overall mortality rate from HHS is 11%.[54] However, because patients with HHS have type 2 diabetes as an underlying disorder, they are older and have associated illnesses, which increase their mortality risk. When the mortality rate for diabetic patients is stratified by age, there is no difference based on the underlying hyperglycemic crisis (HHS or DKA). For HHS patients younger than 75 years, the mortality rate is 10%; for those age 75 to 84 years, it is 19%; and for those older than 85 years, it is 35%.[56]

The diagnostic criteria for HHS are as follows[54]:
- Blood glucose >600 mg/dL
- Arterial pH >7.3
- Serum bicarbonate >15 mEq/L
- Serum osmolality >320 mOsm/kg H_2O (320 mmol/kg)
- Absent or mild ketonuria

Most patients with this level of metabolic disruption experience visual changes, mental status changes, and potentially hypovolemic shock.

HHS occurs when the pancreas produces a relatively insufficient amount of insulin for the high levels of glucose that flood the bloodstream. HHS primarily affects older, obese persons with underlying cardiovascular conditions. Infection is the primary reason that type 2 diabetics develop HHS; the most common infections are pneumonia and urinary tract infections. The patient may have type 2 diabetes treated with diet and oral hypoglycemic agents that is destabilized by an infection. Other precipitating causes of HHS include stroke, myocardial infarction, trauma, burns, and the stress of a major illness. Many classes of medications have been associated with the development of HHS, including corticosteroids, phenytoin, thiazide diuretics, beta-blockers, dobutamine, terbutaline, and antipsychotics.[54,55]

Differences between Hyperglycemic Hyperosmolar State and Diabetic Ketoacidosis. Clinically, HHS is distinguished from DKA by the presence of extremely elevated serum glucose, more profound dehydration, and minimal or absent ketosis (Table 37-4). Another major difference is that protein and fats are not used to create new supplies of glucose in HHS as they are in DKA; as a result, the ketotic cycle is never started or does not occur until the glucose level is extremely elevated. Patients with type 1 diabetes do not develop HHS, whereas some patients with type 2 diabetes do develop DKA.[54,55]

PATHOPHYSIOLOGY

HHS represents a deficit of insulin and an excess of glucagon (Fig. 37-4). Reduced insulin levels prevent the movement of glucose into the cells, allowing glucose to accumulate in the plasma. The decreased insulin triggers glucagon release from the liver, and hepatic glucose is poured into the circulation. As the number of glucose particles increases in the blood, serum hyperosmolality increases. In an effort to decrease the serum osmolality, fluid is drawn from the intracellular compartment (inside the cells) into the vascular bed. Profound intracellular volume depletion occurs if the patient's thirst sensation is absent or decreased. HHS may evolve over days or even weeks.[54]

Hemoconcentration persists despite removal of large amounts of glucose in the urine (glycosuria). The glomerular filtration and elimination of glucose by the kidney tubules is ineffective in reducing the serum glucose level sufficiently to maintain normal glucose levels. The hyperosmolality and reduced blood volume stimulate release of ADH to increase the tubular resorption of water. ADH, however, is powerless to overcome the osmotic pull exerted by the glucose load. Excessive fluid volume is lost at the kidney tubule, with simultaneous loss of potassium, sodium, and phosphate in the urine. This chain of events results in progressively worsening hypovolemia.

Hypovolemia reduces renal perfusion and oliguria develops. Although this process conserves water and preserves the blood volume, it prevents further glucose loss, and hyperosmolality increases. Ketosis is absent or mild in HHS. However, the patient with HHS who had an extremely elevated serum glucose level (>1000 mg/dL) can develop a metabolic acidosis from dehydration, poor tissue perfusion, and lactic acid accumulation.

The SNS reacts to the body's stress response to try to restore homeostasis. Epinephrine, a potent stimulus for gluconeogenesis, is released, and additional glucose is added to the bloodstream.

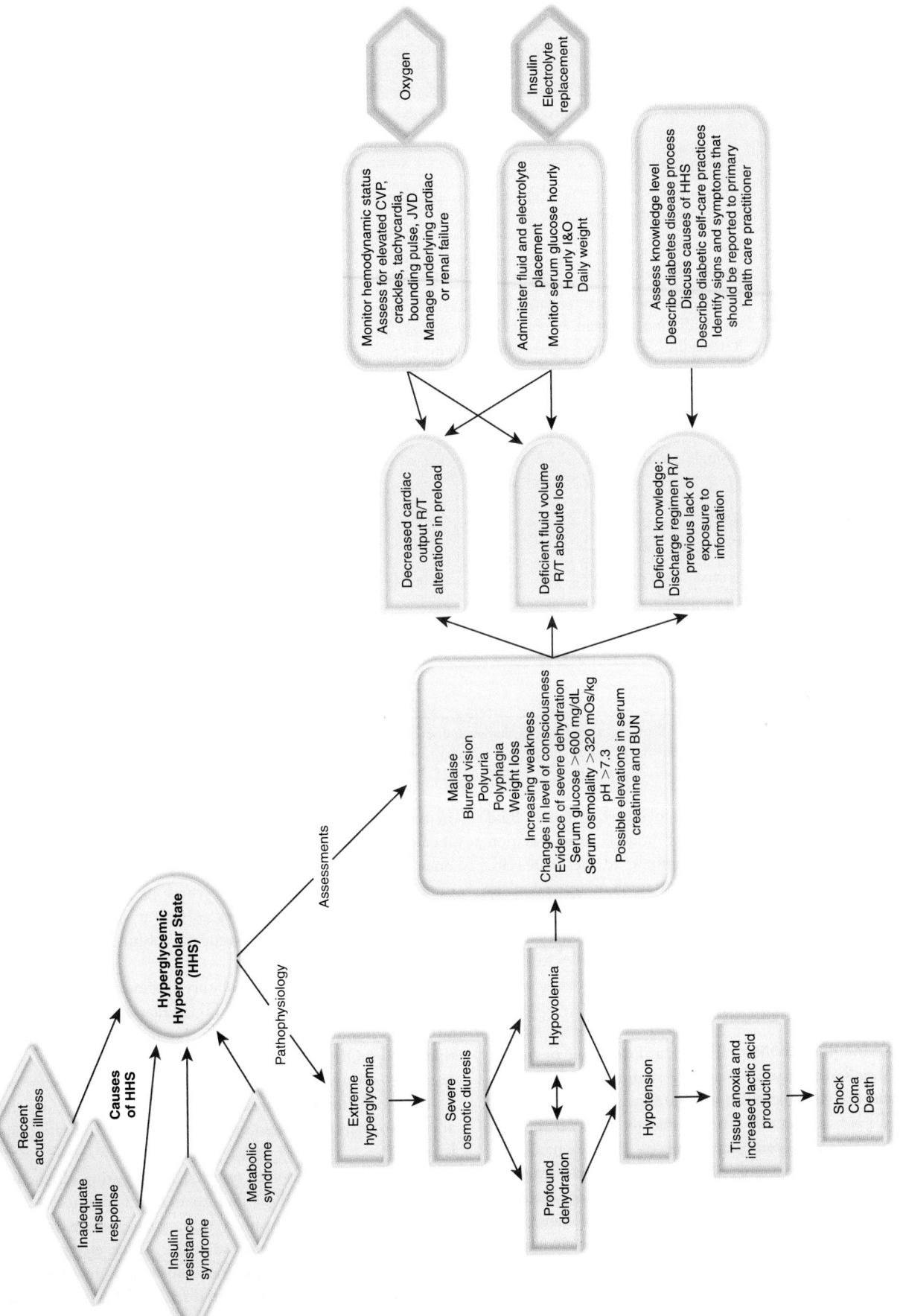

TABLE 37-4 Comparison of Diabetic Ketoacidosis and Hyperglycemic Hyperosmolar State

Characteristics and Laboratory Tests	DKA	HHS
Cause	Insufficient exogenous glucose for glucose needs	Insufficient exogenous/endogenous insulin for glucose needs
Onset	Sudden (hours)	Slow, insidious (days, weeks)
Precipitating factors	Noncompliance with type 1 diabetes therapy, illness, surgery, decreased activity	Recent acute illness in an older patient; therapeutic procedures
Mortality (%)	9-14	10-50
Population affected	Type 1 diabetics	Type 2 diabetics
Clinical manifestations	Dry mouth, polydipsia, polyuria, polyphagia, dehydration, dry skin, hypotension, weakness Ketoacidosis; air hunger, acetone breath odor, respirations deep and rapid, nausea, vomiting	Mental confusion, tachycardia, changes in level of consciousness No ketosis, no breath odor, respirations rapid and shallow, usually mild nausea/vomiting
Laboratory tests		
Glucose (mg/dL)	300-800	600-2000
Ketones	Strongly positive	Normal or mildly elevated
pH	<7.3	Normal*
Osmolality (mOsm/L)	<350	>350
Sodium	Normal or low	Normal or elevated
Potassium (K$^+$)	Normal, low, or elevated (total body K$^+$ depleted)	Low, normal, or elevated
Bicarbonate	<15 mEq/L	Normal
Phosphorus	Low, normal, or elevated (may decrease after insulin therapy)	Low, normal, or elevated (may decrease after insulin therapy)
Urine acetone	Strong	Absent or mild

*Exception: In severe HHS, lactic acidosis may develop as a result of dehydration and severe tissue hypoperfusion and ischemia.
DKA, diabetic ketoacidosis; HHS, hyperglycemic hyperosmolar state.

Unless the glycemic diuresis cycle is broken by aggressive fluid replacement and insulin administration, intracellular dehydration negatively affects fluid and oxygen transport to the brain cells. Central nervous system dysfunction may result and may lead to coma. Hemoconcentration increases the blood viscosity, which may result in clot formation, thromboemboli, and cerebral, cardiac, and pleural infarcts.

ASSESSMENT AND DIAGNOSIS

Clinical Manifestations. HHS has a slow, subtle onset and develops over several days. Initially, the symptoms may be non-specific and may be ignored or attributed to the patient's concurrent disease processes. History reveals malaise, blurred vision, polyuria, polydipsia (depending on the patient's thirst sensation), weight loss, and advancing weakness.[56] Medical attention may not be obtained for these nonspecific, nonacute symptoms until the patient is unable to take sufficient fluids to offset the fluid losses. Progressive dehydration follows and leads to mental confusion, convulsions, and eventually coma, especially in older patients.

The physical examination may reveal a profound fluid deficit. Signs of severe dehydration include longitudinal wrinkles in the tongue, decreased salivation, and decreased CVP, with increases in HR and rapid respirations (Kussmaul air hunger does not occur). In older patients, assessment of clinical signs of dehydration is challenging. Neurologic status is affected as the serum glucose climbs, especially at levels greater than 1500 mg/dL. Without intervention, obtundation and coma occur.

Laboratory Studies. Laboratory findings are used to establish the definitive diagnosis of HHS. Plasma glucose levels are strikingly elevated (>600 mg/dL). Serum osmolality is greater than 320 mOsm/kg. Acidosis is absent (arterial pH >7.3), and the serum bicarbonate concentration is greater than 15 mEq/L. Ketonuria is absent or mild.[54] The patient may have an elevated hematocrit and depleted potassium and phosphorus levels.

Point-of-care finger-stick or arterial-line testing of glucose at the bedside is the usual method for frequent monitoring of the serum blood glucose. Insulin replacement is then prescribed according to the blood glucose result. Some electrolytes also can be tested at the bedside (potassium, sodium, ionized calcium), but usually an arterial line is required for frequent blood access. If point-of-care testing is not available, traditional serial laboratory tests keep the clinician apprised of the fluctuating

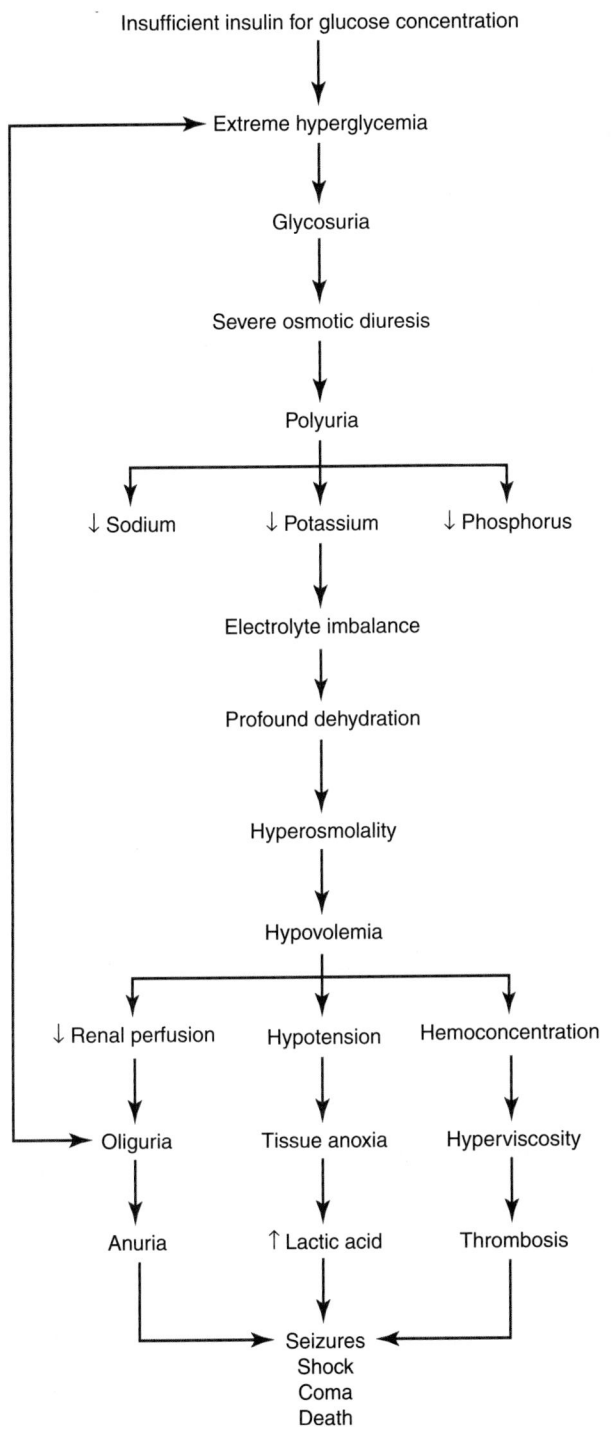

Insufficient insulin for glucose concentration

↓

Extreme hyperglycemia

↓

Glycosuria

↓

Severe osmotic diuresis

↓

Polyuria

↓ Sodium   ↓ Potassium   ↓ Phosphorus

↓

Electrolyte imbalance

↓

Profound dehydration

↓

Hyperosmolality

↓

Hypovolemia

↓ Renal perfusion   Hypotension   Hemoconcentration

Oliguria   Tissue anoxia   Hyperviscosity

Anuria   ↑ Lactic acid   Thrombosis

Seizures
Shock
Coma
Death

Figure 37-4 Pathophysiology of hyperglycemic hyperosmolar state (HHS).

serum electrolyte levels and provide the basis for electrolyte replacement. Intracellular potassium and phosphate levels usually are depleted as a result of dehydration.[54]

Elevated BUN and creatinine levels suggest kidney impairment as a result of the severe reduction in renal circulation. Metabolic acidosis usually is absent at lower glucose levels. Acidosis may result from starvation ketosis or from an increase in lactic acid production caused by poor tissue perfusion.

MEDICAL MANAGEMENT

The goals of medical management are rapid rehydration, insulin replacement, and correction of electrolyte abnormalities, specifically potassium replacement. The underlying stimulus of HHS must be discovered and treated. The same basic principles used to treat DKA are used for the patient with HHS.

Rapid Rehydration. The primary intervention for HHS is rapid rehydration to restore the intravascular volume. The fluid deficit may be as much as 150 mL/kg of body weight. The average 150-pound adult can lose more than 7 to 10 L of fluid. The total body deficit of sodium and potassium may be as high as 500 to 700 mEq.[54] Physiologic saline solution (0.9%) is infused at 1 L/hr, especially for the patient in hypovolemic shock. Between 6 and 10 L of fluid replacement in the first 10 hours may be required to achieve a BP and CVP within normal range.[54] This may necessitate an initial infusion rate of 250 to 500 mL/hour with infusion volumes adjusted according to the patient's hydration state and sodium level.[54]

The serum sodium concentration is the parameter that is monitored to determine whether to change from isotonic (0.9%) to hypotonic (0.45%) saline. For example, patients with sodium levels equal to or less than 140 mEq/L may be given 0.9% normal saline solution, whereas those with levels greater than 140 mEq/L are given 0.45% saline solution (Fig. 37-5). In reality, it is difficult to assess the serum sodium level in the presence of hemoconcentration. Another recommendation is to calculate a *corrected sodium value.* This involves adding 1.6 mEq to the sodium laboratory value for each 100 mg/dL plasma glucose above normal.[54] Sodium input should not exceed the amount required to replace the losses. Careful monitoring of the serum sodium level is recommended to avoid a sodium-water imbalance and hemolysis as the hemoconcentration is reduced.

To prevent hypoglycemia, when the serum glucose decreases to 200 to 250 mg/dL range, the hydrating solution is changed to D₅W with 0.45% NaCl at 250 to 500 mL/hr.[54]

Insulin Administration. Volume resuscitation lowers the serum glucose level and improves symptoms even without insulin administration.[56] However, insulin replacement is recommended in the treatment of HHS because of clinical reports that acidosis can develop if insulin is withheld.[56] Insulin is given to facilitate the cellular use of glucose.

Methods to lower the blood glucose level vary. One method is to administer an intravenous bolus of regular insulin (0.15 unit/kg of body weight) initially, followed by a continuous insulin drip. Regular insulin, infusing at an initial rate calculated as 0.1 unit/kg hourly (e.g., 7 units/hr for a person weighing 70 kg) should lower the plasma glucose concentration by 50 to 70 mg/dL during the first hour of treatment. If the measured glucose level does not decrease by this amount, the insulin infusion rate may be doubled until the blood glucose is declining at a rate of 50 to 70 mg/dL per hour.[54]

Insulin Resistance. Patients with HHS have underlying type 2 diabetes; many have metabolic syndrome and exhibit signs of insulin resistance.[48] In critical illness, the presence of *counter-regulatory hormones,* also known as *stress hormones*

Management of Adult Patients with HHS

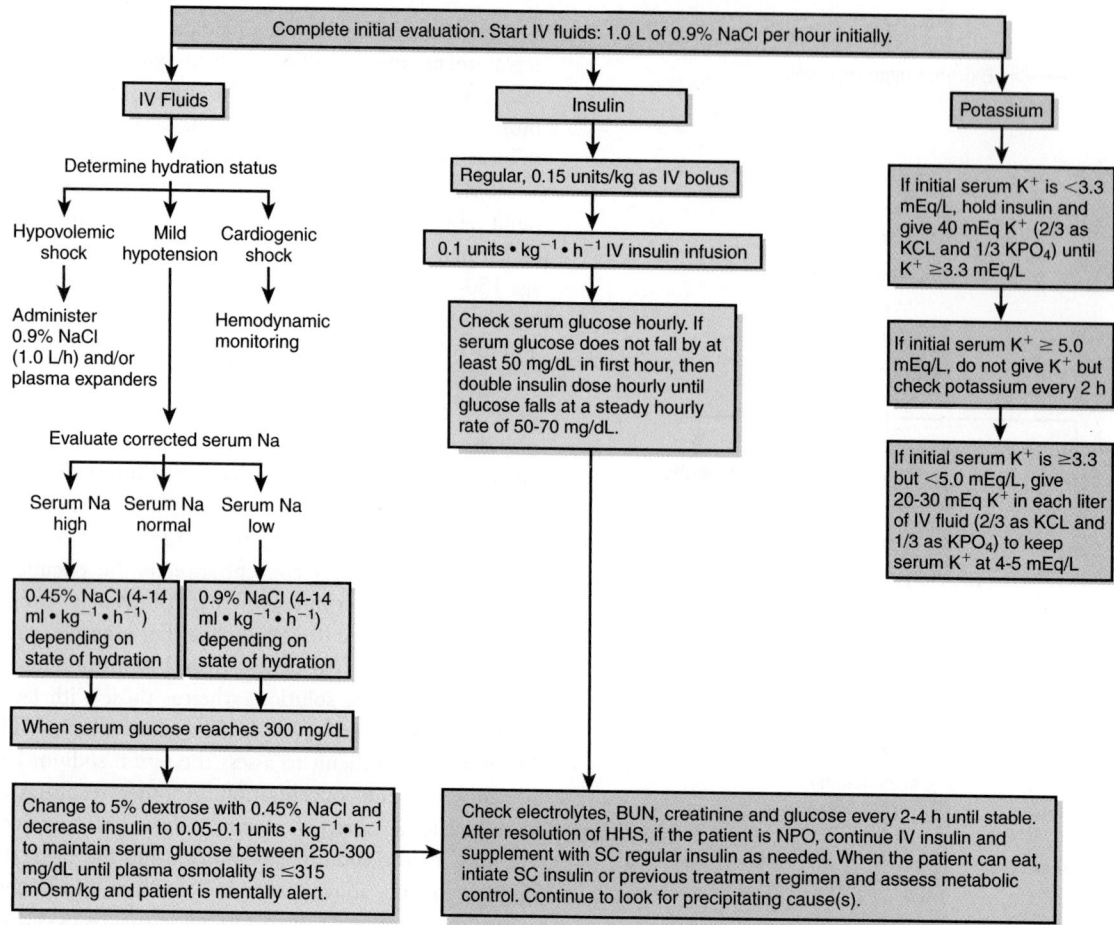

Figure 37-5 Protocol for the management of adult patients with hyperglycemic hyperosmolar state (HHS). *(From Kitabchi AE et al: Hyperglycemic crises in adult patients with diabetes: a consensus statement from the American Diabetes Association,* Diabetes Care *29[12]:2739, 2006.)*

(cortisol, glucagon, GH, epinephrine) increases glucose production and also induces insulin resistance.[56] Patients with HHS may require supraphysiologic doses of insulin initially to overcome the hyperglycemia and insulin resistance.[56] Hourly serial monitoring of the blood glucose level permits safe glycemic management and avoids the most common complication, which is hypoglycemia caused by overzealous insulin administration.[54] After the patient is over the hyperglycemic crisis and insulin has been discontinued, oral agents designed to decrease insulin resistance in type 2 diabetics are prescribed (see Table 37-3).

Electrolyte Replacement. Increasing the circulating levels of insulin with therapeutic doses of intravenous insulin promotes the rapid return of potassium and phosphorus into the cell. Serial laboratory tests keep the clinician apprised of the serum electrolyte levels and provide the basis for electrolyte replacement. Potassium typically is added to the intravenous infusion (see Fig. 37-5). If the serum potassium concentration is lower than 3.3 mEq/L, it is essential to replenish the serum potassium before giving insulin.[54] Many hospitals have potassium replacement algorithms that are used to treat hypokalemia. Serum phosphate levels are carefully monitored, and phosphate replaced if the level is lower than 1.0 mg/dL.[54]

Nursing Diagnoses

Hyperglycemic Hyperosmolar State

- Decreased Cardiac Output related to alterations in preload
- Deficient Fluid Volume related to absolute loss
- Anxiety related to threat to biologic, psychological, and social integrity
- Deficient Knowledge: Discharge Regimen related to previous lack of exposure to information (see Patient Education feature on Hyperglycemic Hyperosmolar State)

NURSING MANAGEMENT

Nursing management of the patient with HHS incorporates a variety of nursing diagnoses (see the Nursing Diagnoses feature on Hyperglycemic Hyperosmotic State). Nursing management goals are similar to those outlined for DKA. The critical care nurse administers prescribed fluids, insulin, and electrolytes; monitors the response to therapy; maintains surveillance for complications; and provides patient education.

NIC

Hyperglycemia Management

Definition
Preventing and treating above-normal blood glucose levels

Activities
Monitor blood glucose levels, as indicated.

Monitor for signs and symptoms of hyperglycemia: polyuria, polydipsia, polyphagia, weakness, lethargy, malaise, blurring of vision, or headache.

Monitor urine ketones, as indicated.

Monitor ABG, electrolyte, and beta-hydroxybutyrate levels, as available.

Monitor orthostatic blood pressure and pulse, as indicated.

Administer insulin, as prescribed.

Encourage oral fluid intake.

Monitor fluid status (including intake and output).

Maintain IV access, as appropriate.

Administer IV fluids, as needed.

Administer potassium, as prescribed.

Consult physician if signs and symptoms of hyperglycemia persist or worsen.

Assist with ambulation if orthostatic hypotension is present.

Provide oral hygiene, if necessary.

Identify possible causes of hyperglycemia.

Anticipate situations in which insulin requirements will increase (e.g., intercurrent illness).

Restrict exercise when blood glucose levels are greater than 250 mg/dL, especially if urine ketones are present.

Instruct patient and significant others on prevention, recognition, and management of hyperglycemia.

Encourage self-monitoring of blood glucose levels.

Instruct on urine ketone testing, as appropriate.

Instruct on indications for, and significance of, urine ketone testing, if appropriate.

Instruct patient to report moderate or high urine ketone levels to the health professional.

Instruct patient and significant others on diabetes management during illness, including use of insulin and/or oral agents, monitoring fluid intake; carbohydrate replacement; and when to seek health professional assistance, as appropriate.

Provide assistance in adjusting regimen to prevent and treat hyperglycemia (e.g., increasing insulin or oral agent), as indicated.

Facilitate adherence to diet and exercise regimen.

Test blood glucose levels of family members.

From Bulechek GM et al: *Nursing interventions classification (NIC)*, ed 5, St Louis, 2008, Mosby.
ABG, arterial blood gas; IV, intravenous.

Administering Fluids, Insulin, and Electrolytes. Rigorous fluid replacement and continuous intravenous insulin replacement must be controlled with an electronic volumetric pump. Accurate I&O measurements are maintained to monitor fluid balance. I&O measurements include the total of all fluids administered minus hourly losses, typically urine output and sometimes emesis. Hemodynamic monitoring may include use of an arterial line and measurements of CVP if the patient manifests signs of hypovolemic shock. Arterial line access is very helpful in monitoring serial blood glucose and electrolyte values. The use of a blood conservation system on the arterial line is essential to avoid iatrogenic exsanguination of the patient. Most critical care units have developed protocols or guidelines to ensure that patients in hyperglycemic crisis are managed safely (see Fig. 37-3). The major responsibility for delivery of insulin, hourly monitoring of blood glucose, and infusion of appropriate crystalloid solutions lies with the critical care nurse (see the Nursing Interventions Classification on Hyperglycemia Management). Many hospitals mandate a double-check procedure for medications such as insulin that have the potential to cause harm if wrongly administered.

Monitoring Response to Therapy. The BP, HR, and CVP are monitored to evaluate the degree of dehydration, the effectiveness of hydration therapy, and the patient's fluid tolerance. Because patients with HHS have underlying type 2 diabetes and, if older, are likely have preexisting illnesses such as heart failure and kidney failure, it is important to monitor for symptoms of circulatory overload. Symptoms to anticipate include elevated CVP, tachycardia, bounding pulse, dyspnea, tachypnea, lung crackles, and engorged neck veins. The astute critical care nurse is aware of the clinical manifestations of fluid overload and observes for potential complications when rehydrating the patient with HHS and cardiac, pulmonary, or renal disease.

The serum glucose level should decrease by 50 to 70 mg/dL per hour with insulin administration.[54] This decrease is monitored by hourly blood glucose determinations. Based on the result, the critical care nurse can alter the infusion of insulin according to hospital protocol (see Fig. 37-5).

Surveillance for Complications. The potential complications of HHS are similar to those described for DKA: hypoglycemia, hypokalemia or hyperkalemia, and infection. The patient with HHS is at risk for other complications specific to associated disease entities. A history of cardiovascular, pulmonary, or kidney disease, whether known or latent, places HHS patients at high risk for complications.

Patient Education. As the patient's condition improves and the patient demonstrates readiness to learn, education about type 2 diabetes and avoiding a recurrence of HHS becomes a priority (see the Patient Education feature on Hyperglycemic Hyperosmolar State). Most teaching occurs after the patient has left the critical care unit. Teaching topics include a description of type 2 diabetes and how it relates to HHS, dietary restrictions, exercise requirements, medication protocols, home testing of blood glucose, signs and symptoms of hyperglycemia and hypoglycemia, foot care, and lifestyle modifications if cardiovascular disease is present.

COLLABORATIVE MANAGEMENT

Because HHS is an acute condition superimposed on the chronic health problem of type 2 diabetes, many health professionals provide care and work collaboratively to restore homeostasis for each patient (see the Evidence-Based Practice feature on Hyperglycemic Hyperosmolar State).

DIABETES INSIPIDUS

Diabetes insipidus (DI) is recognized by the vast quantities of very dilute urine that are produced in susceptible patients. In the critically ill patient, the extreme diuresis is most likely to be caused by a lack of ADH (vasopressin). Any patient who has head trauma or has undergone neurosurgery has an increased risk of developing DI. Normally, ADH is produced in the hypothalamus and stored in the posterior pituitary gland (see Chapter 35). Physiologically, ADH is released primarily in response to even small elevations in serum osmolality and secondarily in reaction to hypovolemia or hypotension.[57] DI can occur if (1) the hypothalamus produces insufficient ADH, (2) the posterior pituitary fails to release ADH, or (3) the kidney nephron is resistant (unresponsive) to ADH.[58]

Patient Education: Hyperglycemic Hyperosmolar State

- Acute phase
  - Explain rationale for critical care unit admission
- Predischarge
  - Assess knowledge level
  - Assess compliance history
  - Diabetes disease process
  - Definition of hyperglycemic hyperosmotic state (HHS)
  - Causes of HHS
  - Self-care for diabetes
  - Signs and symptoms to report to health care practitioner

ETIOLOGY

DI is divided into three types according to cause: central, nephrogenic, and psychogenic (Box 37-4). Only central DI, also known as neurogenic DI because of its association with the brain, is encountered with any frequency in the critical care unit.

BOX 37-4   CAUSES OF DIABETES INSIPIDUS

CENTRAL DIABETES INSIPIDUS
Primary (Rare in Critical Care)
- ADH deficiency caused by hypothalamic-hypophyseal malformation
  - Congenital defect
  - Idiopathic

Secondary (Most Common in Critical Care)
- ADH deficiency caused by damage to the hypothalamic-hypophyseal system
  - Trauma
  - Infection
  - Surgery
  - Primary neoplasms
  - Metastatic malignancies

NEPHROGENIC DIABETES INSIPIDUS
- Inability of kidney tubules to respond to circulating ADH
  - Decrease or absence of ADH receptors
  - Cellular damage to nephron, especially loop of Henle
  - Kidney damage (e.g., hydronephrosis, pyelonephritis, polycystic kidney)
  - Untoward response to drug therapy (e.g., lithium carbonate, demeclocycline)

PSYCHOGENIC DIABETES INSIPIDUS
- Rare form of water intoxication
- Compulsive water drinking

ADH, antidiuretic hormone.

Evidence-Based Practice: Collaborative

Hyperglycemic Hyperosmolar State

Summary of evidence and evidence-based recommendations for controlling symptoms related to hyperglycemic hyperosmolar state (HHS)

Strong Evidence to Support
Regular insulin by continuous infusion is recommended to normalize blood glucose to 80 to 110 mg/dL (euglycemic levels).
Replace serum phosphate if the level is less than 1 mg/dL.
A multidisciplinary team approach to care reduces length of stay and improves clinical outcomes.
Close follow-up after discharge is recommended to maintain glycosylated hemoglobin (HbA$_{1c}$) at less than 7% and to prevent diabetes-related complications.

Weak Evidence to Support
Use of a sliding insulin scale alone is discouraged, because it is associated with hyperglycemia and hypoglycemia in hospitalized patients.

References
Clement S et al: Management of diabetes and hyperglycemia in hospitals, *Diabetes Care* 27(2):553-591, 2004.
Garber AJ et al: American College of Endocrinology position statement on inpatient diabetes and metabolic control, *Endocr Pract* 10(suppl 2):4-9, 2004.
Kitabchi AE et al: Hyperglycemic crises in adult patients with diabetes: a consensus statement from the American Diabetes Association, *Diabetes Care* 29(12):2731, 2006.

Central Diabetes Insipidus. In central DI, there is an inability to secrete an adequate amount of arginine vasopressin in response to an osmotic or nonosmotic stimuli, resulting in inappropriately dilute urine.[59,60] The synthesis of ADH is incomplete in the hypothalamus, or the release of ADH from the pituitary is interrupted. Central DI can be congenital or idiopathic. In critical care, the most likely acute cause of central DI is neurosurgery, traumatic head injury, tumors, increased intracranial pressure, brain death, and infections such as encephalitis or meningitis. Among patients undergoing surgery on the pituitary gland, DI occurs in approximately 12% and is permanent in 3%.[61] The degree of hormone replacement required after surgery depends the quantity of pituitary tissue removed.[61] One prospective study reported the incidence of central DI to be 15% among patients with traumatic brain injury.[62]

Nephrogenic Diabetes Insipidus. Nephrogenic DI is a rare congenital or an acquired disorder that occurs when the V_2 receptors on the kidney tubule become nonresponsive to the action of ADH. Some drugs cause nephrogenic DI by decreasing the responsiveness of the kidney tubules to ADH. Long-term use of lithium carbonate, prescribed for bipolar disorder, was a frequent culprit in the past.[63]

Psychogenic Diabetes Insipidus. Psychogenic DI is a rare form of the disease that occurs with compulsive drinking of more than 5 L of water daily. Long-standing psychogenic DI closely mimics nephrogenic DI because the kidney tubules become less responsive to ADH as a result of prolonged conditioning to hypotonic urine. This condition is uncommonly seen in the critical care unit.

PATHOPHYSIOLOGY

The purpose of ADH is to maintain normal serum osmolality and circulating blood volume. Normally, ADH binds to the V_2 receptors on the kidney collecting tubules, causing insertion of water channels, known as aquaporins, along the luminal surface.[57] Even small (1% to 2%) increases in plasma osmolality are sufficient to stimulate ADH release.[57] Although there are several types of DI, this discussion focuses on neurogenic (central) DI, the condition encountered in the critical care unit after neurosurgery or head injury[56] (Fig. 37-6).

In DI, as free water is eliminated, the urine osmolality and specific gravity decrease (dilute urine). At the same time, in the bloodstream, the serum sodium concentration and serum osmolality rise. Normally, a rise in the serum osmolality to greater than 290 mOsm per kilogram of H_2O (290 mmol/L) triggers the synthesis and release of ADH.[57] At 295 mOsm/kg H_2O, the thirst sensors are activated in the hypothalamus.[57] In central DI, however, no ADH is released, or the ADH released is insufficient. Without ADH, the kidney collecting tubules are incapable of concentrating urine and retaining water.

As extracellular dehydration ensues, hypotension and hypovolemic shock occur. If the person is alert, extreme thirst will lead to replacement of lost fluids by drinking lots of water. This excessive intake of water reduces the serum osmolality to a more normal level and prevents dehydration. In the person with decreased level of consciousness, the polyuria leads to severe hypernatremia, dehydration, decreased cerebral perfusion, seizures, loss of consciousness, and death.

ASSESSMENT AND DIAGNOSIS

Clinical Manifestations. The clinical diagnosis is made based on the dramatic increase in dilute urine output occurring in the absence of diuretics, a fluid challenge, or hyperglycemia. Central DI is anticipated in conditions in which the underlying disease process is likely to disrupt pituitary function. Central DI that occurs because of increasing intracranial pressure is life-threatening. It is imperative that the underlying condition be recognized and treated appropriately. In this situation, medications that treat DI are not sufficient.

Laboratory Studies. The core diagnostic tests used to establish the presence of DI and that evaluate the body's ability to balance fluid and electrolytes are not specific to the endocrine system. The most common tests are serum sodium concentration, serum osmolality, and urine osmolality (Table 37-5). The combination of an obvious clinical picture with high volumes of hypotonic urine, in the presence of the following laboratory criteria, is sufficient to diagnose central DI[60]:

- Serum sodium level >145 mEq/L
- Serum osmolality >295 mOsm/kg H_2O (>295 mmol/L).
- Urine osmolality <200 mOsm/kg H_2O (<200 mmol/L),
- Urine specific gravity <1.005.

Serum Sodium. The normal serum sodium concentration is 140 mEq/L (range, 135 to 145 mEq/L). In central DI, the serum sodium level can rise precipitously because of the loss of free water. Hypernatremia is always associated with serum hyperosmolality.[64]

Serum Osmolality Test. Serum osmolality has a narrow normal range, 275 to 295 mOsm/kg. Severe DI can raise serum osmolality to greater than 320 mOsm/kg.[57]

Urine Osmolality. Urine osmolality is low, less than 300 mOsm/kg H_2O (300 mmol/L) in patients with central DI. For greatest accuracy, the urine sample should be collected and tested simultaneously with the blood sample. Normal urine ADH ranges from 500 to 1400 mOsm/L of H_2O and varies with fluid intake and hydration status.

Measurement of Antidiuretic Hormone. Measurement of the baseline serum ADH level is an additional diagnostic step. This is not typically performed in critical care if the clinical circumstances (e.g., head injury with raised intracranial pressure) make further testing unnecessary. Normal ADH levels range from 1 to 5 pg/mL. Most hydrated people have a morning fasting serum level lower than 4 pg/mL.[65]

To test for the underlying cause of DI, exogenous ADH may be administered. An ADH plasma concentration of approximately 1 pg/mL increases urinary concentration and decrease urine flow. Maximum antidiuresis occurs at an ADH concentration of approximately 5 pg/mL.[59] ADH administration (1 mcg of desmopressin given subcutaneously) is used to distinguish between central DI and nephrogenic DI.[64] A urine output that is greatly decreased in response to ADH administration diagnoses central DI. A urine output that is unchanged in response to ADH administration suggests nephrogenic DI.

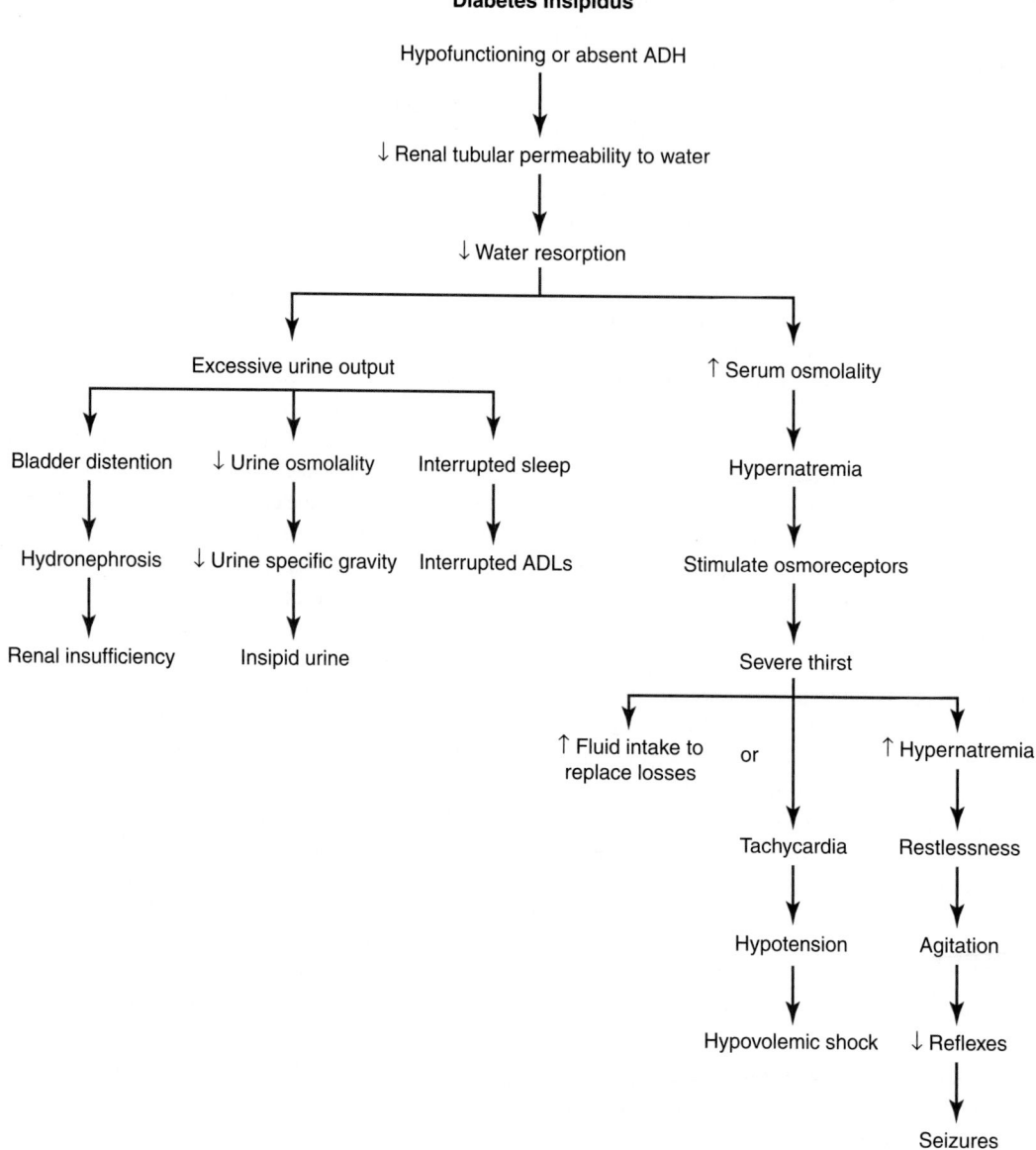

Diabetes Insipidus

Hypofunctioning or absent ADH

↓ Renal tubular permeability to water

↓ Water resorption

Excessive urine output | ↑ Serum osmolality

Bladder distention | ↓ Urine osmolality | Interrupted sleep

Hydronephrosis | ↓ Urine specific gravity | Interrupted ADLs

Renal insufficiency | Insipid urine

Hypernatremia

Stimulate osmoreceptors

Severe thirst

↑ Fluid intake to replace losses — or — ↑ Hypernatremia

Tachycardia | Restlessness

Hypotension | Agitation

Hypovolemic shock | ↓ Reflexes

Seizures

Figure 37-6 Pathophysiology of diabetes insipidus (DI). ADH, antidiuretic hormone; ADLs, activities of daily living.

MEDICAL MANAGEMENT

Immediate management of DI requires an aggressive approach. Treatment goals include restoration of circulating fluid volume, pharmacologic ADH replacement, and treatment of the underlying condition.

Volume Restoration. Fluid replacement is provided in the initial phase of the treatment to prevent circulatory collapse. Patients who are able to drink are given voluminous amounts of fluid orally to balance output. For those who are unable to take sufficient fluids orally, hypotonic intravenous solutions are infused and carefully monitored to restore the hemodynamic balance.

Medications. Central DI requires immediate pharmacologic management. Table 37-6 presents the medications most frequently prescribed to treat central DI and replace ADH.

Medications Used for Central Diabetes Insipidus. Patients with central DI who are unable to synthesize ADH require replacement with ADH *(vasopressin)* or an ADH analogue. The most commonly prescribed drug is the synthetic analogue of ADH, *desmopressin* (DDAVP). It is preferred over vasopressin (Pitressin) because it has a stronger antidiuretic action with little effect on blood pressure. DDAVP can be given intravenously, subcutaneously, or as a nasal spray. A typical DDAVP dose is 1 to 2 mcg given intravenously or subcutaneously every 12 hours.[66] Sometimes, only 0.5 mcg is given intravenously. The dosage is subsequently titrated according to the patient's antidiuretic response to the drug. To avoid a medication error, it is important to be aware that DDAVP is also used to control hemorrhage caused by platelet disorders and that the dose ranges for all of these conditions are different.

Vasopressin (Pitressin), 5 to 10 units given intramuscularly every 3 to 4 hours, produces a reduction in urine output.[66] Vasopressin acts on the V_1 receptors in vascular smooth muscle and can elevate systemic blood pressure. Water intoxication also

TABLE 37-5 Laboratory Values for Patients with Diabetes Insipidus and Syndrome of Inappropriate Antidiuretic Hormone

Value	Normal	DI	SIADH
Serum ADH	1-5 pg/mL	Decreased in central DI	Elevated
Serum osmolality (mOsm/L)	275-295*	>295*	<270
Serum sodium (mEq/L)	135-145	>145	<120
Urine osmolality (mOsm/L)	300-1400	<300	Increased
Urine specific gravity	1.005-1.030	<1.005	>1.030
Urine output	1.0-1.5 L/day	1.0-1.5 L/hr	Below normal

*Some hospitals use 280-300 mOsm/L as their normal reference value.
ADH, antidiuretic hormone; DI, diabetes insipidus; SIADH, syndrome of inappropriate antidiuretic hormone.

TABLE 37-6 Pharmacologic Management: Diabetes Insipidus

DRUG	DOSAGE*	ACTIONS	SPECIAL CONSIDERATIONS
Central Diabetes Insipidus			
DDAVP (available IV, as nasal spray, Rhinal tube, Rhinyle drops, Stimate)	Nasal: 10-40 µg at bedtime or in divided doses Parenteral: 2-4 µg twice daily	Central DI Antidiuretic Increases water resorption in nephron. Prevents and controls polydipsia, polyuria.	Few side effects Observe for nasal congestion, upper respiratory infection, allergic rhinitis. Monitor intake and output, urine osmolality, serum sodium level.
Vasopressin (Pitressin Synthetic, Pressyn)	Intramuscular, intravenous, subcutaneous, intra-arterial Topical: nasal mucosa	Central DI Antidiuretic Promotes resorption of water at kidney tubule. Decreases urine output. Increases urine osmolality. Diagnostic aid Increases gastrointestinal peristalsis.	Monitor fluid volume often, especially in older patients. Assess cardiac status. May precipitate angina, hypertension, or myocardial infarction if increased dose is given to patient with cardiac history. Parenteral extravasation can cause skin necrosis.
Lypressin (Diapid)	Intranasal: 1-2 sprays (7-14 µg) in each nostril four times daily	Central DI Synthetic ADH Increases resorption of sodium and water in nephron.	Proper instillation is important for absorption and action. Patient sits upright while holding bottle upright for administration. Repeat sprays (>2-3) are ineffective and wasteful; if dose is increased to 2-3 sprays, shorten time between dosing. Cough, chest tightness, shortness of breath
Nephrogenic Diabetes Insipidus			
Thiazide diuretics	Varies according to diuretic chosen, patient's size, and age.	Nephrogenic DI Leads to mild fluid depletion. Increases resorption of water and sodium in proximal nephron; less fluid travels to distal nephron, excreting less water.	Varies according to diuretic chosen.
Psychogenic Diabetes Insipidus			
Anti-compulsive disorder drugs, anxiolytics, psychopharmacologic agents	Dosage varies	Psychogenic DI	Varies according to medication chosen.

*Parenteral indicates intravenous or subcutaneous administration.
ADH, antidiuretic hormone; DI, diabetes insipidus; DDAVP, desmopressin acetate; IV, intravenous.

can occur if the dosage is higher than the therapeutic level. Because of the risk of hypertension, this is not typically the first drug of choice for treating central DI. Vasopressin can also be prescribed for septic shock states as an intravenous infusion and for cardiac arrest as an intravenous push. Dosages for these conditions are very different from that used to treat central DI. Extreme care must be taken to ensure that all drug dosages are accurate for each specific diagnosis.

Medications Used for Nephrogenic Diabetes Insipidus. The mainstay of therapy is to stop any medications that are inducing the ADH resistance. Nephrogenic DI is not a diagnosis frequently encountered in critical care. It is treated with hydrochlorothiazide, 12.5 to 25 mg administered once or twice daily. The dosage is then titrated according to the patient's antidiuretic response.

NURSING MANAGEMENT

Nursing management of the patient with DI incorporates a variety of nursing diagnoses (see the Nursing Diagnoses feature on Diabetes Insipidus). Nursing management is directed toward administration of prescribed fluids and medications, evaluation of response to therapy, surveillance for complications, and provision of patient education.

Administration of Fluids and Medications. Rapid intravenous fluid replacement requires the use of a volumetric pump. Initially, a hypotonic intravenous solution is used to replace fluids lost and lower the serum hyperosmolality. ADH replacement is accomplished with extreme caution in the patient with a history of cardiac disease, because ADH may cause hypertension and overhydration. At the first signs of cardiovascular impairment, the drug is discontinued and fluid intake is restricted until urine specific gravity is less than 1.015 and polyuria resumes.

Evaluation of Response to Therapy. Critical assessment and management of fluid status are the most important initial concerns for the patient with DI. Monitoring of HR, BP, CVP, and pulmonary artery pressures (if a pulmonary artery catheter is in place) provides early indications of response to fluid volume replacement. I&O measurement, condition of buccal membranes, skin turgor, daily weight measurements, presence of thirst, and temperature provide a basic assessment list that is vital for the patient who is unable to regulate fluid needs and losses. Placement of a urinary catheter is essential to accurately monitor the urinary output. Simultaneous urine and blood specimens for determination of osmolality and sodium and potassium levels are collected, and the results are relayed to the physician as necessary. The patient who is unable to satisfy sensations of thirst or to complete any task or self-care activity without the need to urinate may be confused and frightened. For patients who are able to verbalize their fears, having a caring nurse who is interested and nonjudgmental helps to reduce the emotional turmoil associated with their condition.

Surveillance for Complications. The most dangerous potential complication is hypertension and vasospasm of cardiac, cerebral, or mesenteric arterial vessels in response to vasopressin replacement. In most cases, DDAVP is selected for ADH replacement to avoid this complication. A less serious complication of DI is constipation due to fluid loss; it is treated with dietary fiber, stool softeners, or both. Conversely, diarrhea, abdominal cramping, and intestinal hyperactivity may accompany vasopressin therapy. Untoward effects can be mitigated by modification of the vasopressin dose.

Patient Education. Educating the patient and the family about the disease process and how it affects thirst, urination, and fluid balance encourages patients to participate in their care and reduces the feelings of hopelessness (see the Patient Education feature on Diabetes Insipidus). For most critical care patients, central DI is a temporary condition that resolves as the underlying medical condition (e.g., brain injury) improves. Patients who are discharged with DI are taught, along with their families, the signs and symptoms of dehydration and overhydration and procedures for accurate daily weight and urine specific gravity measurements. Printed information pertaining to drug actions, side effects, dosages, and timetable is provided, as well as an outline of factors that must be reported to the physician.

COLLABORATIVE MANAGEMENT

Central DI is a life-threatening condition. The collaborative assessment and clinical skills of all health care professionals and use of a clear plan of care are essential to achieve optimal outcomes for each patient.

Nursing Diagnoses

Diabetes Insipidus

- Deficient Fluid Volume related to compromised regulatory mechanism
- Decreased Cardiac Output related to alterations in preload
- Anxiety related to threat to biologic, psychological, and social integrity
- Deficient Knowledge: Discharge Regimen related to lack of previous exposure to information (see Patient Education feature on Diabetes Insipidus)

Patient Education: Diabetes Insipidus

- Acute phase
  - Explain rationale for critical care unit admission
- Predischarge
  - Assess knowledge base
  - Measurement of fluid intake and output
  - Urine specific gravity
  - Causes of diabetes insipidus
  - Disease process of diabetes insipidus
  - Nutritional information to prevent constipation and diarrhea
  - Medications: explain purpose, side effects, dosage, and how often to use
  - Signs and symptoms to report to health care professional

SYNDROME OF INAPPROPRIATE SECRETION OF ANTIDIURETIC HORMONE

The opposing syndrome to DI is the syndrome of inappropriate secretion of antidiuretic hormone (SIADH), also known as the *syndrome of antidiuresis* (SIAD).[67] The patient with SIADH has an excess of ADH secreted into the bloodstream, more than the amount needed to maintain normal blood volume and serum osmolality. Excessive water is resorbed at the kidney tubule, leading to dilutional hyponatremia.

ETIOLOGY

Numerous causes of SIADH are observed in patients who are critically ill (Box 37-5). Central nervous system injury, tumors, and diseases that interfere with the normal functioning of the hypothalamic-pituitary system can cause SIADH.[67] A common cause is malignant bronchogenic small cell carcinoma.[68] This type of malignant cell is capable of synthesizing and releasing ADH regardless of the body's needs.[57,69] With much less frequency, other cancers that involve the brain, head and neck, gastroenteral, gynecologic, and hematologic systems are capable of autonomous production of ADH.[57] Levels of ADH rise with the use of positive-pressure ventilators that decrease venous return to the thorax, because they stimulate pulmonary baroreceptors to release and increase levels of circulating ADH.

PATHOPHYSIOLOGY

ADH is a powerful, complex polypeptide compound. When released into the circulation by the posterior pituitary gland, ADH regulates water and electrolyte balance in the body. In SIADH, profound fluid and electrolyte disturbances result from

---

BOX 37-5 CAUSES OF SYNDROME OF INAPPROPRIATE SECRETION OF ANTIDIURETIC HORMONE

- *Malignant disease* associated with autonomous production of ADH
  - Bronchogenic small cell carcinoma
  - Pancreatic adenocarcinoma
  - Duodenal, bladder, ureter, and prostatic carcinomas
  - Lymphosarcoma, Ewing's sarcoma
  - Acute leukemia, Hodgkin's disease
  - Cerebral neoplasm, thymoma
- *Central nervous system diseases* that interfere with the hypothalamic-hypophyseal system and increase the production or release of ADH
  - Head injury
  - Brain abscess
  - Hydrocephalus
  - Pituitary adenoma
  - Subdural hematoma
  - Subarachnoid hemorrhage
  - Cerebral atrophy
  - Guillain-Barré syndrome
- *Neurogenic stimuli* capable of increasing ADH
  - Decreased glomerular filtration rate
  - Physical or emotional stress
  - Pain
  - Fear
  - Trauma
  - Surgery
  - Myocardial infarction
  - Acute infection
  - Hypotension
  - Hemorrhage
  - Hypovolemia
- *Pulmonary diseases* believed to stimulate the baroreceptors and increase ADH
  - Pulmonary tuberculosis
  - Viral and bacterial pneumonia
  - Empyema
  - Lung abscess

- Chronic obstructive lung disease
- Status asthmaticus
- Cystic fibrosis
- *Endocrine disturbances* that hormonally influence ADH
  - Myxedema
  - Hypothyroidism
  - Hypopituitarism
  - Adrenal insufficiency—Addison's disease
- *Medications* that mimic, increase the release of, or potentiate ADH
  - Hypoglycemics
    - Insulin
    - Tolbutamide
    - Chlorpropamide
  - Potassium-depleting thiazide diuretics
  - Tricyclic antidepressants
    - Imipramine
    - Amitriptyline
  - Phenothiazine
    - Fluphenazine
    - Thioridazine
  - Thioxanthenes
    - Thiothixene
    - Chlorprothixene
  - Chemotherapeutic agents
    - Vincristine
    - Cyclophosphamide
  - Opiates
  - Carbamazepine
  - Clofibrate
  - Acetaminophen
  - Nicotine
  - Oxytocin
  - Vasopressin
  - Anesthetics

ADH, antidiuretic hormone.

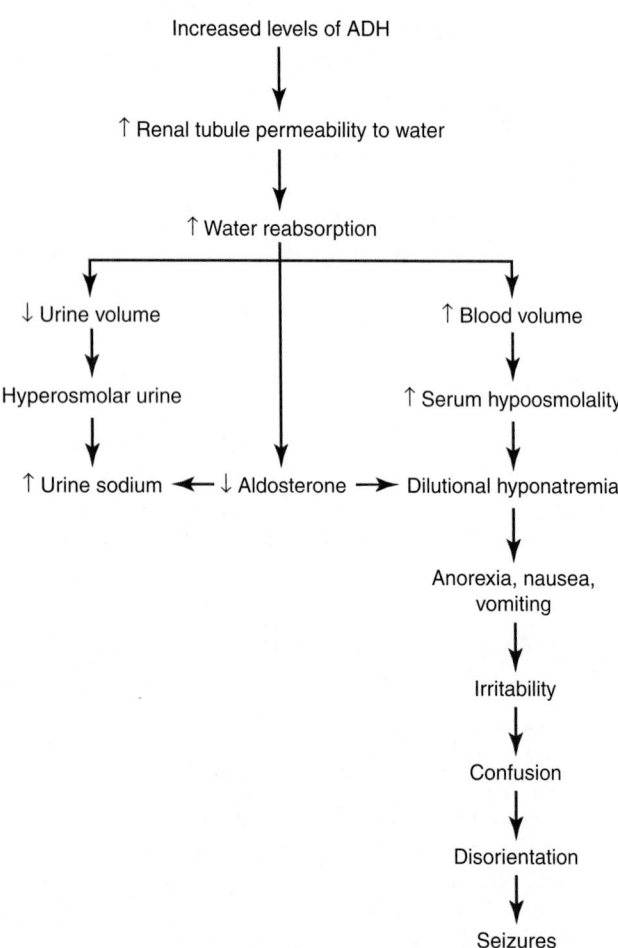

Increased levels of ADH

↓

↑ Renal tubule permeability to water

↓

↑ Water reabsorption

↓ Urine volume   ↑ Blood volume

↓   ↓

Hyperosmolar urine   ↑ Serum hypoosmolality

↓   ↓

↑ Urine sodium ← ↓ Aldosterone → Dilutional hyponatremia

↓

Anorexia, nausea, vomiting

↓

Irritability

↓

Confusion

↓

Disorientation

↓

Seizures

Figure 37-7 Pathophysiology of syndrome of inappropriate secretion of antidiuretic hormone (SIADH). ADH, antidiuretic hormone.

the unsolicited, continuous release of the hormone into the bloodstream (Fig. 37-7). Excessive ADH stimulates the kidney tubules to retain fluid regardless of need. This results in severe overhydration.

Excessive ADH dramatically alters the sodium balance in the extracellular vascular compartment. The overhydration causes a dilutional hyponatremia and reduces the sodium concentration to critically low levels. In the healthy adult, hyponatremia inhibits the release of ADH; in SIADH, however, the increased levels of circulating ADH are unrelated to the serum sodium concentration. Aldosterone production from the adrenal glands is also suppressed. Serum hypo-osmolality leads to a shift of fluid from the extracellular fluid space into the intracellular fluid compartment (inside the cells) in an attempt to equalize osmotic pressure. Because minimal sodium is present in this fluid, edema usually does not result. Without ADH and aldosterone, water is retained, urine output is diminished, and further sodium is excreted in the urine. The urine has an increased osmolality from the decreased water excretion. Urinary concentration is also elevated by excess sodium in the urine. It is believed that, despite the serum hyponatremia, the increased release of ADH promotes sodium loss through the kidneys into the urine.

ASSESSMENT AND DIAGNOSIS

Clinical Manifestations. The clinical manifestations of SIADH relate to the excess fluids in the extracellular compartment and the proportionate dilution of the circulating sodium. Edema usually is not present, although slight weight gain may occur from the expanded extracellular fluid volume. Early clinical manifestations of dilutional hyponatremia include lethargy, anorexia, nausea, and vomiting. Severe neurologic symptoms usually do not develop until the serum sodium concentration drops to less than 120 mEq/L.[70] Progressively deteriorating neurologic signs of hyponatremia then predominate, and the patient is admitted to the critical care unit. Symptoms of severe hyponatremia include inability to concentrate, mental confusion, apprehension, seizures, decreased level of consciousness, coma, and death.

Laboratory Values. Patients with SIADH present with very dilute serum and very concentrated urine output. Laboratory values confirm this clinical picture. In SIADH, the serum is hypoosmolar (<275 mOsm/kg H_2O), with low serum sodium concentration and a urine osmolality greater than would be expected with such hypotonic blood (>100 mOsm/kg has been suggested).[67] A serum sodium concentration of less than 125 mEq/L (<120 mEq/L according to some authorities) is associated with increasing severity of neurologic symptoms.[64,70] An elevated urine sodium concentration, greater than 30 to 40 mEq/L, is congruent with the concentrated urine output of SIADH.[64,67,70] Use of diuretics negates the reliability of the urine sodium and urine osmolality levels.[70] Table 37-5 compares the typical laboratory values associated with SIADH with those of DI.

MEDICAL MANAGEMENT

In the critical care unit, SIADH often occurs as a secondary disease. Ideally, recognition and treatment of the primary disease will reduce the production of ADH. If the patient is receiving any of the medications suspected of causing SIADH, discontinuing the drug may return ADH levels to normal. Some of the drugs that alter ADH levels are listed in Box 37-5. The goals of medical management are to restore fluid and sodium balance.

Fluid Restriction. The medical therapy that is the most effective (along with treatment of the primary disease) is simple reduction of fluid intake.[64] This is achieved most successfully in the patient with a moderate increase in body fluid volume and hyponatremia. Although fluid restrictions are calculated on the basis of individual needs and losses, a general criterion is to restrict fluids to 500 mL less than average daily output.[57]

Sodium Replacement. Patients with severe hyponatremia (<125 mEq/L serum sodium) experience severe neurologic symptoms, even seizures. How rapidly the sodium should be corrected and which sodium concentration to use remain controversial.[71] One recommended regimen is an intravenous rate that provides sufficient sodium to raise serum sodium levels by up to 12 mEq/day for the first 24 hours (no more than 0.5 mEq each hour), with a total rise of 18 mEq/L in the initial

48 hours.[64] Another option is to add furosemide (Lasix) to increase the diuresis of free water.

If hyponatremia is severe (<120 mEq/L), an infusion of 3% hypertonic saline solution may be used to replenish the serum sodium without adding extra volume. It is imperative to be aware that hypertonic saline solution is dangerous if administered too quickly, and calculation of the quantity of sodium that will be administered is advised. An example of one sodium replacement regimen is an infusion of 3% saline infusion at 35 mL/hr in a 70-kg patient, which will increase the serum sodium level by approximately 0.5 mEq/L per hour (12 mEq/day).[64] Suggested end points at which to stop the acute sodium repletion include the following: (1) the patient's symptoms are abolished; (2) a safe serum sodium level is achieved (usually >120 mEq/L); (3) a total correction of 20 mEq/L is achieved.[64]

Too-rapid serum sodium correction must be avoided to reduce the risk of *osmotic demyelination,* previously known as *central pontine myelinolysis.* The demyelination occurs in the pons and in other areas of the brain's white matter.[57] The lesions may be detected on imaging studies (computed tomography and magnetic resonance imaging), and severe neurologic damage or death can result.[57] Patients with a baseline serum sodium level lower than 120 mEq/L are most at risk.[57] Serum sodium levels must be evaluated at least every 4 hours during the acute phase of sodium replacement.[64]

Medications. Medications are prescribed only if water restriction is ineffective in correcting the SIADH. Certain drugs decrease the output of ADH from the pituitary gland, and others increase the action of ADH on the V_2 kidney tubule receptors so that more water is excreted.

Medications That Increase Kidney Water Excretion. Two classes of drugs are available to treat SIADH. Until recently, the only medication used to treat SIADH was demeclocycline, a derivative of tetracycline.[64] The dosage range is from 600 to 1200 mg per day, and several days of therapy are necessary to achieve maximal effects.[64] It is advisable to wait several days before changing the initial dose regimen.[64]

The vasopressin receptor antagonists are a newer class of drugs, not yet in widespread use. Conivaptan (Vaprisol), at a dosage of 20 to 40 mg/day given intravenously, is approved for management of hypervolemic hyponatremia, such as SIADH. It is available in oral and intravenous forms and is approved for use only in hospitalized patients. Conivaptan is a nonselective vasopressin receptor antagonist, which means that it blocks V_1 receptors in the vasculature and V_2 receptors in the kidney.[67] The patient must be observed carefully to avoid hypotension (caused by V_1 receptor blockade), and hypovolemia is a contraindication. Several V_2 receptor–selective drugs are currently in clinical trials.

NURSING MANAGEMENT

Nursing management of the patient with SIADH incorporates a variety of nursing diagnoses (see the Nursing Diagnoses feature on Syndrome of Inappropriate Secretion of Antidiuretic Hormone). Nursing management is directed toward restriction of fluids, surveillance for complications, and provision of patient education.

Nursing Diagnoses

Syndrome of Inappropriate Secretion of Antidiuretic Hormone

- Excess Fluid Volume related to comprised regulation mechanism
- Anxiety related to lack of control over current situation or disease progression
- Deficient Knowledge: Discharge Regimen related to lack of previous exposure to information (see Patient Education feature on Syndrome of Inappropriate Secretion of Antidiuretic Hormone)

Restriction of Fluids. Thorough, astute nursing assessments are required for care of the patient with SIADH while an attempt is made to correct the fluid and sodium imbalance; the systemic effects of hyponatremia occur rapidly and can be lethal. Frequent assessment of the patient's hydration status is accomplished with serial measurements of urine output, serum sodium levels, and serum osmolality. Accurate measurement of I&O is required to calculate fluid replacement for the patient with SIADH. All fluids are restricted. Intake that equals urine output may be given until the serum sodium level returns to normal. Frequent mouth care (moistening of the buccal membrane) may give comfort during the period of fluid restriction. The patient is weighed daily to gauge fluid retention or loss. Weight gain signifies continual fluid retention, whereas weight loss indicates loss of body fluid.

Constipation is a frequent complication of decreased fluid intake. Cathartics or low-volume hypertonic enemas may be given to stimulate peristalsis. Tap water or hypotonic enemas should never be given, because the water in the enema solution may be absorbed through the bowel and potentiate water intoxication.

Surveillance for Complications. The patient's neurologic status, especially level of consciousness, should be evaluated on an hourly basis if the serum sodium level is critically low (<125 mEq/L). Seizure precautions for the patient with SIADH are provided regardless of the degree of hyponatremia. Serum sodium levels may fluctuate rapidly, and neurologic impairment may occur with no apparent warning. The patient's altered neurologic response also may be influenced by the acuteness of the primary disease (central nervous system disease) and not solely by the low sodium levels. Seizure precautions include nursing actions to protect the patient from injury (padded side rails, bed in low position when patient is unattended) and to provide an open airway (oral airway, head turned to the side without forcible restraint of the patient, suction apparatus). Oxygen may be required to maintain a saturation level greater than 92% if there is pulmonary congestion or edema that interferes with alveolar gas exchange.

Patient Education. Rapidly occurring changes in the patient's neurologic status may worry visiting family members. Sensitivity to the family's unspoken fears can be shown by words that express empathy and by providing time for the patient and family to ask questions and express their concerns. The nurse may discuss the course of SIADH, its effect on water balance, and the reasons for fluid restrictions (see the Patient Education feature on Syndrome of Inappropriate Secretion of Antidiuretic Hormone).

Patient Education: Syndrome of Inappropriate Secretion of Antidiuretic Hormone

- Acute phase
  - Explain reasons for admission to the critical care unit
  - Explain reasons for neurologic changes
- Predischarge
  - Assess knowledge level
  - Causes of inappropriate secretion of antidiuretic hormone (SIADH)
  - Disease process of SIADH
  - Measuring intake and output
  - Measuring urine specific gravity
  - Signs and symptoms to report to health care professional

BOX 37-6   CONDITIONS ASSOCIATED WITH HYPERTHYROIDISM

- Iodine-induced hyperthyroidism (e.g., related to amiodarone therapy)
- Excessive pituitary production of thyroid-stimulating hormone (TSH) or trophoblastic disease
- Excessive ingestion of thyroid hormone
- Toxic diffuse goiter (Graves' disease)
- Toxic adenoma
- Toxic multinodular goiter (Plummer's disease)
- Painful subacute thyroiditis
- Silent thyroiditis, including lymphocytic and postpartum variations

---

COLLABORATIVE MANAGEMENT

At this time, there are no published guidelines that discuss acute collaborative care management of the patient with SIADH. This is a complex condition, and effective clinical management requires the skills of many health care professionals working as a team, with goals that are clearly communicated to all team members.

THYROID STORM

DESCRIPTION

Thyroid storm always occurs as a complication of preexisting hyperthyroidism. Hyperthyroidism, also called *thyrotoxicosis,* occurs when the thyroid gland produces thyroid hormone in excess of the body's need.[72] The most common cause of primary hyperthyroidism is *Graves' disease,* an autoimmune disease that affects 0.4% of the U.S. population, with a 5:1 ratio favoring women to men.[73,74] The antidysrhythmic drug amiodarone (Cordarone) is known to cause thyroid dysfunction in 14% to 18% of patients.[72,75] Hyperthyroid conditions also may result from ingestion of excessive thyroid replacement drugs. Conditions associated with hyperthyroidism are presented in Box 37-6.[72]

Thyroid storm, also called *thyroid crisis,* is a critical stage of hyperthyroidism. It is a rare and life-threatening condition. The pathophysiology underlying the transition from hyperthyroidism to thyroid storm is not fully understood. Activation of the SNS and enhanced sensitivity to the effects of thyroid hormone are apparent. Major stressors, such as infection, surgery, trauma, pregnancy, or critical illness, can precipitate thyroid storm in the hyperthyroid patient.[76,77]

ETIOLOGY

In hyperthyroidism, excessive thyroid hormone causes increased metabolic activity and stimulates the β-adrenergic receptors, which results in a heightened SNS response. There is hyperactivity of cardiac tissue, nervous tissue, and smooth muscle tissue and tremendous heat production.[78]

PATHOPHYSIOLOGY

Thyroid hormone increases cellular oxygen consumption in almost all metabolically active cells. Energy in the form of heat is lost rather than used by the cell. Excess metabolism generates heat, and the body temperature may rise to as high as 41 °C (105.8 °F). Cellular oxygen demands are dramatically increased. The cardiac response is to increase cardiac output and pump more blood more rapidly to deliver oxygen and expel carbon dioxide. Hypertension and tachycardia follow.[76,79] The oxygen demands in the hypermetabolic state are so great that the cardiac system cannot compensate adequately. A critically high fever is typically present.[76,79]

The increased metabolic rate requires increased oxygen and sufficient energy sources. Catabolism and a negative nitrogen balance occur. Metabolic acidosis is a potential problem. Intestinal peristalsis increases, often resulting in diarrhea, nausea, and vomiting. These symptoms all lead to dehydration and compound the problem of malnutrition and weight loss. Muscular contraction and relaxation increase more rapidly and are referred to as the *hyperreflexia of hyperthyroidism.* Muscular weakness occurs and is compounded by the excessive protein breakdown.

Hypersensitivity to the increased adrenergic-binding sites potentiates the cardiovascular and nervous system responses to the hypermetabolic state. Atrial fibrillation or flutter is reported in 8.3% of patients with hyperthyroidism.[80] Tachydysrhythmias may are to be anticipated in thyroid storm, especially in patients with underlying heart disease.[81] Pulmonary edema and acute heart failure also can occur. Increased β-adrenergic activity manifests in emotional lability, fine muscular tremors, agitation, and even delirium. Clinical manifestations of thyroid storm are listed in Box 37-7.

ASSESSMENT AND DIAGNOSIS

Thyroid storm is a potentially lethal complication of thyrotoxicosis. Early symptoms may be missed and insidious, creating a paradoxically abrupt presentation of a cluster of symptoms. Thyroid storm lacks a textbook profile to signal its presence, and it may be masked by another presenting condition.[76] The presenting symptoms and severity of the disease differ from one patient to another and change during the course of the disease, posing a profound threat to the patient's survival. The patient with

CLINICAL MANIFESTATIONS OF THYROID STORM

CARDIOVASCULAR SYSTEM
Prompted by Increased Affinity of β-Adrenergic Receptors in the Heart
- Tachycardia
- Systolic murmur
- Increased stroke volume
- Increased cardiac output
- Increased systolic blood pressure
- Decreased diastolic blood pressure
- Extra systoles
- Paroxysmal atrial tachycardia
- Premature ventricular contraction
- Palpitations
- Chest pain
- Increased cardiac contractility
- Congestive heart failure
- Pulmonary edema
- Cardiogenic shock

CENTRAL NERVOUS SYSTEM
Resulting from an Increased Catecholamine Response
- Hyperkinesis
- Nervousness
- Muscle weakness
- Confusion
- Convulsions
- Heat intolerance
- Fine tremor
- Emotional lability

- Frank psychosis
- Apathy
- Stupor
- Diaphoresis

GASTROINTESTINAL SYSTEM
- Nausea
- Vomiting
- Diarrhea
- Liver enlargement
- Abdominal pain
- Weight loss
- Increased appetite

INTEGUMENTARY SYSTEM
- Pruritus
- Hyperpigmentation of skin
- Fine, straight hair
- Alopecia

THERMOREGULATORY SYSTEM
- Hyperthermia
- Heat dissipation
- Diaphoresis

SERUM OR URINE
- Hypercalcemia
- Hyperglycemia
- Hypoalbuminemia
- Hypoprothrombinemia
- Hypocholesterolemia
- Creatinuria

undiagnosed or previously controlled thyrotoxicosis who is hospitalized for a major illness is at high risk for thyroid storm.

Laboratory findings are used to confirm the suspicion raised by the clinical signs. The TSH value is extremely low, and the free T_4 is high, compared with the norms of the hospital laboratory (see Table 36-3 in Chapter 36 for normal reference values).[76] These results, in combination with the clinical picture, provide the diagnosis.

No diagnostic test is available to differentiate thyroid storm from its predecessor, thyrotoxicosis, for which the laboratory values may be similar. Thyroid storm is identified by a combination of the patient's medical history and current clinical manifestations.[73]

MEDICAL MANAGEMENT

The goal of acute medical management of thyroid storm is to reduce the clinical effects of thyroid hormone as rapidly as possible. This includes preventing cardiac decompensation, reducing hyperthermia, and reversing dehydration caused by pyrexia or gastrointestinal losses.

Preventing Cardiovascular Collapse. The body's heightened sensitivity to the increased adrenergic and catecholamine receptors must be suppressed. Cardiac irregularities need to be controlled and progression of heart failure halted. Beta-blockers are the mainstay of therapy for cardiac protection.[82]

Reducing Hyperthermia. Reduction in body temperature is achieved by use of a cooling blanket and the antipyretic agent acetaminophen. Salicylates (aspirin) are contraindicated because they prevent protein binding of T_3 to T_4, increasing the level of free, metabolically active, thyroid hormone.[76]

Reversing Dehydration. Vigorous fluid replacement must be instituted to treat or prevent dehydration. Antibiotic therapy may be warranted in the presence of systemic infection. Other existing pathologic conditions are treated appropriately. If dehydration and metabolic acidosis are present, they are treated with large volumes of glucose and sodium solutions to replace circulating fluid and sodium losses caused by hypermetabolism.

PHARMACOLOGIC MANAGEMENT

Pharmacologic treatment is essential in treatment of thyroid storm. Drug administration is divided into three phases.[76,82] Initially prescribed are drugs that block the synthesis and release of thyroid hormone into circulation. Second, drugs that block and inhibit the peripheral conversion of T_4 to T_3 are given. Third, drugs (beta-blockers) are used to decrease the peripheral cellular sensitivity to catecholamines.

Drugs That Block Thyroid Synthesis. The synthesis of new thyroid hormone is blocked by the administration of *antithyroid drugs* in the *thiouracil* class.[82] Two drugs are frequently used: propylthiouracil (PTU) and methimazole.[83] Neither drug is available in parenteral form; they must be given by mouth or through a nasogastric tube. PTU is especially therapeutic because it also blocks the de-iodination conversion of T_4 to T_3. Methimazole has a slower action rate but is more potent than PTU. Both drugs act within 1 to 2 hours after absorption from the gastrointestinal tract. These drugs have no impact on previously released thyroid hormone.

Drugs That Block Release of Thyroid Hormone. Administration of inorganic iodine blocks the release of any preformed thyroxine that is already in the thyroid gland but not yet released.[82] It is essential that iodine therapy not be administered until adequate inhibition of new hormone synthesis has occurred. The iodide preparations are rapid-acting and have a short duration. They are given approximately 1 hour after administration of the antithyroid drugs (described in the previous section) to prevent the iodide from being used for thyroid hormone production and possible worsening of the clinical state.

Orally or nasogastrically administered *iodides* are given in large amounts to decrease thyroid hormone production.[83] The iodides maintain and increase the level of protein-bound thyroid hormone, thereby decreasing the level of free active thyroid hormone. The iodide most commonly used for thyroid storm is sodium iodide. Potassium iodide, saturated solution of potassium iodide, or strong iodide solution also may be used.

Drugs That Block the Catecholamine Effect. To decrease the catecholamine effects of excessive thyroid hormone, β-adrenergic blocking agents are used. Propranolol is the most frequently used drug.[82] Beta-blockers have no effect on thyroid hormone but reduce the exaggerated myocardial stimulation and contractile force and slow the atrioventricular (AV) conduction rate. Therapeutic doses vary from patient to patient, but higher doses are typically required to effectively control the symptoms.[82] Esmolol, a short-acting beta-blocker administered by intravenous infusion, may also be used.[82] Calcium channel blockers may be effective in controlling the heart rate in patients for whom beta-blockers are contraindicated.[83]

Some patients with thyroid storm have concomitant adrenal insufficiency, and they may be prescribed dexamethasone or hydrocortisone during the initial stages of thyroid storm management.[82] Table 37-7 lists the most commonly used medications and their nursing implications for the patient in thyroid storm.

NURSING MANAGEMENT

Nursing management of the patient with thyroid storm incorporates a variety of nursing diagnoses (see the Nursing Diagnoses feature on Thyroid Storm). Nursing interventions are directed toward safe administration and monitoring of the effects of prescribed medications, normalizing body temperature, rehydration with correction of other metabolic derangements, and provision of patient education.

Medication Administration. The timely and ordered sequence of medication administration is essential in the management of thyroid storm (see previous sections on pharmacologic management). The patient in thyroid storm is agitated, anxious, and unable to rest and benefits from an environment that is calm. The effects of the antithyroid medications, iodides, and β-adrenergic blocking drugs gradually decrease the neurologic symptoms related to the catecholamine sensitivity. Heart rate should decrease with beta-blockade.

The patient and family need to be reassured that this extreme agitation is the result of the disease process and that the medications will help control the nonstop fidgeting and tremors.

Frequent reassurance and clear, simple explanations of the patient's condition help decrease the fear brought on by the onset of thyroid storm.

Normalizing Body Temperature. In thyroid storm, the patient has hyperthermia related to a hypermetabolic state, as evidenced by a critically high body temperature; diaphoresis; hot, flushed skin; intolerance to heat; tachycardia; and tachypnea. Temperature is assessed frequently until safe levels are attained. Nursing measures to provide comfort while the patient is intolerant to heat include a room with a cool environment and a fan to circulate air, lightweight bed coverings, and comfortable, nonrestrictive bedclothes. A tepid sponge bath helps to reduce heat by evaporation, and cold-pack applications to the groin and axilla increase heat loss at major blood vessels. If antipyretic drugs are required, acetaminophen is the agent of choice, and salicylates are avoided.[82]

Rehydration and Correction of Metabolic Derangements. Hyperthermia, tachypnea, diaphoresis, vomiting, and diarrhea predispose the patient to a fluid volume deficit. Fluids and electrolytes are as vigorously replaced as the decompensated cardiovascular system can tolerate. Glucose solutions are given to replace glycogen stores, which are depleted. Insulin is administered to treat the hyperglycemia that results from mobilization of nutrients and glucocorticoids. Point-of-care (bedside) blood glucose measurements are performed frequently and used as reference points for insulin dosing. Hyponatremia from active loss (e.g., vomiting) is monitored by means of laboratory serum values. Hyponatremia can be prevented or treated with isotonic intravenous fluid replacement. Additional nursing measures focus on frequent hydration assessments (see Box 37-2). I&O assessment includes estimating diaphoretic fluid loss through the number of gown and linen changes, checking buccal membranes for moisture, and recording the patient's weight daily.

Patient Education. During the critical events surrounding the thyroid storm, the patient and family are given information according to their emotional state and cognitive level of understanding. The cause of the high fever, anxiety, and cardiac dysrhythmias is explained in understandable terms (see the Patient Education feature on Thyroid Storm). Often, the patient and family are relieved to know that the agitation and nervousness result from circulating chemicals that may be decreased by taking daily medications.

Nursing Diagnoses

Thyroid Storm

- Hyperthermia related to increased metabolic rate
- Imbalanced Nutrition: Less Than Body Requirements related to lack of exogenous nutrients or increased metabolic demand
- Decreased Cardiac Output related to alterations in heart rate
- Anxiety related to threat to biologic, psychological, and social integrity
- Disturbed Sleep Pattern related to fragmented sleep
- Deficient Knowledge: Discharge Regimen related to lack of previous exposure to information (see Patient Education feature on Thyroid Storm)

Patient Education: Thyroid Storm

- Acute phase
  - Explain reasons for critical care unit admission
  - Explain reasons for extreme hypermetabolism
- Predischarge
  - Assess knowledge level
  - Disease process of thyrotoxicosis
  - Causes of thyrotoxic crisis
  - Medications: explain purpose, side effects, dosage, and how often to use
  - Signs and symptoms to report to health care professional

TABLE 37-7 Pharmacologic Management: Thyroid Storm

DRUG	DOSAGE	ACTIONS	SPECIAL CONSIDERATIONS
Blocks Synthesis of Thyroid Hormone			
Propylthiouracil	Loading dose: 800-1200 mg Maintenance dose: 100-400 mg q4-6h PO or gavage	Blocks synthesis of thyroid hormone Blocks conversion of T_3 to T_4	Monitor thyrotoxic response (heart rate, nervousness, fever, diarrhea, diaphoresis). Observe for sudden conversion to hypothyroidism: headache, sluggish responses. Assess for skin rash. Administer with meals to reduce GI effects. May cause rash, nausea, vomiting, agranulocytosis, skin hyperpigmentation, prothrombin deficiency.
Methimazole	10-20 mg q6-8h PO or gavage	Blocks synthesis of thyroid hormone	More toxic than propylthiouracil Presence of rash may be reason to discontinue drug. Monitor signs listed for propylthiouracil. May cause rash, agranulocytosis.
Suppresses Release of Thyroid Hormone			
Sodium iodide	1 g/L q12h IV	Suppresses releases of thyroid hormone	Give iodide 1 hr after propylthiouracil or methimazole. Signs of toxic iodinism poisoning: edema, mucosal stomatitis, hemorrhage, metallic taste, skin lesions, severe GI upset
Potassium iodide, Saturated solution of potassium iodide (SSKI)	KI: 2-5 gtt q8h PO SSKI: 10 gtt q8h PO	Suppresses release of thyroid hormone	Discontinue if rash appears. Signs of toxic iodinism as above Give through a straw to prevent teeth discoloration. Mix with juice or milk to lessen GI upset.
Dexamethasone	2 mg q6h (variable) IV	Suppresses release of thyroid hormone Blocks conversion of T_4 to T_3	Monitor intake and output; monitor serum glucose levels. May cause hypertension, nausea, vomiting, anorexia, increased susceptibility to infection.
Beta-Blockers			
Propranolol	1-3 mg q1-4h IV 40-80 mg q4-6h PO	β-Adrenergic blocking agent to counter sympathetic activity	Monitor cardiac activity, CVP, PAOP, bradycardia, hypotension, pending CHF. Hold if heart rate <50 beats/min Have atropine available; may cause GI upset, weakness, fatigue
Esmolol	500 mcg/kg/min for first minute, then 50 mcg/kg/min for 4 min IV	β-Adrenergic blocker	Monitor for bradycardia, orthostatic hypotension, dysrhythmia. Measure intake and output. May cause edema, diarrhea, diaphoresis, vertigo.
Alpha-Blockers			
Reserpine	1-2.5 mg q24h PO	Depletes stores of catecholamine in sympathetic nerve endings	Monitor BP, heart rate changes in hyperthyroid conditions. May cause bradycardia, drowsiness, GI bleeding, diarrhea.
Guanethidine sulfate	50-150 mg q24h PO	Antiadrenergic Inhibits norepinephrine release in response to sympathetic nerve stimulation	Monitor orthostatic hypotension. Measure and record intake and output. Monitor diarrhea. May cause GI upset, edema, fatigue, drowsiness.

BP, blood pressure; CHF, congestive heart failure; CVP, central venous pressure; GI, gastrointestinal; gtt, drops; IV, intravenous; PAOP, pulmonary artery occlusion pressure; PO, by mouth.

Side effects of drug therapy are taught before discharge. Patients treated with beta-blockers are taught to report signs of bradycardia, unexplained fatigue, and orthostatic hypotension, among other untoward effects. Patients discharged with antithyroid drugs are alerted to the main side effect, agranulocytosis. Symptoms of agranulocytosis include sudden cough, fever, rash, and inflammation. These symptoms must be brought to the attention of the primary care provider. Patients are instructed to use acetaminophen rather than salicylates, because salicylates increase the amount of free thyroid hormone in circulation.

COLLABORATIVE MANAGEMENT

There are no published guidelines that discuss acute collaborative care management of the patient with thyroid storm. Guidelines do exist for non-acute care of the patient with hyperthyroidism.[72] The patient with thyroid storm requires interventions by many health care professionals, with clearly communicated goals to facilitate rapid recovery.

MYXEDEMA COMA

DESCRIPTION

A severe deficiency or absence of thyroid hormone produces hypothyroidism. Hypothyroidism, as defined by laboratory tests and clinical symptoms, ranges from mild to severe. Mild hypothyroidism has no symptoms.[84] Severe hypothyroidism leads to a comatose state called *myxedema coma,* which can be fatal.[85,86] Discussion of myxedema coma necessitates frequent reference to its precursor state, hypothyroidism. The term *myxedema* is used only when referring to myxedema coma, as a description of the progressive worsening or terminal stage of hypothyroidism.

ETIOLOGY

Hypothyroidism is caused by a deficiency of circulating thyroid hormone. In 95% of cases this is the result of a problem with the thyroid gland, and in 5% of cases it is related to dysfunction of the pituitary gland. Insufficient thyroid hormone affects all body cells and organs and slows the metabolic rate and response times in every system.[73] Subclinical hypothyroidism is underdiagnosed and is present in up to 20% of the adult U.S. population older than 60 years.[72]

Myxedema coma is rare, more commonly afflicts older patients, and affects many more women than men.[85,86] Early recognition of symptoms and prompt treatment decrease the mortality rate associated with myxedema, although it remains high compared with many other diseases—35%[85] and 52%[86] in two case series. Myxedema coma is rarely seen as a single disease entity in the critical care unit. Its underlying presence often is revealed by an acute primary disease, by surgery, or as a consequence of increased metabolic demands. Cardiopulmonary disease, systemic infection, and exposure to extreme cold are a few of the physiologic stressors that increase metabolic demand.[87]

PATHOPHYSIOLOGY

The effects of hypothyroidism are widespread and varied. When the basal metabolic rate of oxygen consumption is reduced, the cell is unable to maintain the processes necessary to sustain life. Without thyroid hormone, protein synthesis is severely curtailed, and amino acid production, manufacture of blood proteins, and repair of tissues are halted. Metabolism of carbohydrate and fat is incomplete, and gluconeogenesis cannot supply additional sources of glucose. Lipolysis is ineffective, and cholesterol collects in the bloodstream. All systems are affected.

Skin. The composition of the skin changes as deposits of *hyaluronic acid* (a gel-like substance capable of holding large amounts of fluid) accumulate in the interstitial spaces, giving rise to a full, puffy appearance of face, hands, and feet. The facial expression is dull and mask-like. The skin is pale, with an overall yellowish appearance resulting from increased carotene deposits. The nails and hair are thin and brittle. Absence of thyroid hormone also leads to decreased or absent sweat production. The hyaluronic acid deposits are evident in heart muscle, skeletal muscles, and muscles of the tongue, pharynx, and proximal esophagus. These striated muscular changes of the tongue, pharynx, and esophagus probably contribute to the hoarse, husky voice and dull facial expression of patients with hypothyroidism.

Cardiopulmonary System. Interstitial edema impairs cardiac myocytes, resulting in bradycardia and diminished cardiac output. The heart appears to be enlarged, but its size may be exaggerated by serous fluid accumulation in the pericardial sac. Cardiac output decreases by 30% to 50% in severe hypothyroidism. A decreased sensitivity to catecholamines is present even though serum catecholamine levels are elevated. Resting heart rate and stroke volume are reduced. The force of myocardial contraction is weakened. There is a decrease in the systolic blood pressure and an increase in the diastolic pressure, causing a narrowed pulse pressure. Electrocardiography (ECG) typically reveals low-voltage QRS complexes and nonspecific ST-segment changes.[87]

Pulmonary System. Pleural effusions and muscular changes affect gas exchange. The basal rate of oxygen consumption decreases, with a resulting insensitivity to CO_2. Hypoventilation increases the CO_2 serum content, which increases cerebral hypoxia. Hypoxic and hypercapnic ventilatory drives are severely impaired.[87] Respiratory acidosis can occur.[88] Pleural effusion, reduced vital capacity, and shallow respirations occur with any exertion. Respiratory muscle weakness, sleep apnea, and upper airway obstruction may be present.

Patients with myxedema are a high-risk category for any surgical procedure or critical care admission because of their limited ventilatory capacity.[87] Respiratory failure and requirement for mechanical ventilation may be the reason the patient is admitted to the critical care unit.

Kidneys and Fluid and Electrolyte Balance. Renal blood flow is reduced, and the glomerular filtration rate (GFR), urine specific gravity, and urine osmolality are decreased. The ADH level is increased (fluid retention), and sodium is decreased. Urea production is diminished. Elimination of drugs by the kidneys is severely slowed in hypothyroidism.[87] Coexisting adrenal insufficiency should also be considered.[88]

Nutrition and Elimination. Decreased gastric motility or even ileus is an expected complication for the patient with severe hypothyroidism.[87] Food utilization and nutrient mobilization decrease with insufficient thyroid hormone. Intestinal hypomotility and abdominal distention prevent absorption of food nutrients in the small intestine. Lipolysis decreases, and serum cholesterol increases. Abdominal distention, decreased intestinal peristalsis, and eventual paralytic ileus lead to extreme constipation. These findings make the provision of enteral nutrition a challenge. In the more alert patient, a lack of appetite and inability to eat coexist.

Thermoregulation. Heat production decreases as a result of insufficient energy to maintain the base metabolic rate within the cells. The ability to maintain body heat is further restricted by the hypoglycemia. Sweating and insensible water loss diminish. In one clinical series, cold exposure and resultant hypothermia precipitated critical care admission for myxedema coma in 25% of cases.[86]

Anemia. Anemia is present in 25% to 50% of patients with hypothyroidism. Symptoms of fatigue and depression are associated. Erythropoiesis (red cell production) is impaired and inadequate. Coagulation abnormalities may coexist.[87]

ASSESSMENT AND DIAGNOSIS

The diagnosis of myxedema coma is based on the clinical manifestations of end-stage hypothyroidism. A comparison of severe hyperthyroidism (thyroid storm) and severe hypothyroidism (myxedema) is provided in Box 37-8.

Clinical Presentation. The diagnosis of end-stage hypothyroidism is based on the clinical presentation. Increasing signs of somnolence, depression, and diminished mental acuity signal diminished cellular function. Interstitial edema collects in almost all tissues. Organs become infiltrated with the mucoid-rich mucopolysaccharides, compromising organ function. Patients manifest cardiovascular collapse, hypothermia, decreased kidney function, fluid excess, hypoventilation, and severe metabolic disorders.

Weight gain is attributed to the collection of mucopolysaccharides in the interstitium, the increase in fluid retention, and the decrease in metabolism. Paresthesias of hands and feet are caused by the hyaluronic acid accumulation in the synovial sacs, which leads to compression of nerves and carpal tunnel syndrome. Compression of nerves interferes with the simplest hand grasp and the ability to raise one's hands. Reflexes contract briskly but take extended seconds to relax.

BOX 37-8 CLINICAL MANIFESTATIONS OF HYPERTHYROIDISM COMPARED WITH HYPOTHYROIDISM

Hyperthyroidism (Thyrotoxicosis, Thyroid Storm)	Hypothyroidism (Myxedema, Myxedema Coma)
• Elevated T_4, T_3	• Decreased T_4, T_3
• Decreased TSH	• Elevated TSH
• Hypercalcemia	• Hyponatremia
• Hyperglycemia	• Hypoglycemia
• Metabolic acidosis	• Respiratory acidosis, metabolic acidosis
	• Hypercholesterolemia
	• Anemia
• Tachycardia, palpitations, atrial fibrillation	• Bradycardia
• Angina	• Peripheral vasoconstriction
• ST wave changes	• Flattened, inverted T waves
• Shortened QT	• Prolonged QT and PR intervals
• Hypertension	• Decreased stroke volume, decreased cardiac output
• AV block, acute heart failure	• Enlarged heart, pericardial effusion
• Hypovolemia	• Increased total body fluid with decreased effective arterial blood volume
• Shortness of breath, tachypnea	• Hypoventilation, possible CO_2 retention
• Hypermetabolism	• Depressed metabolism
• Polyphagia	• Decreased lipolysis, increased cholesterol
• Weight loss	• Weight gain
• Nausea, vomiting, increased peristalsis	• Constipation
• Tremor	• Seizures
• Extreme restlessness, insomnia, uneasiness, anxiety	• Slowness, depression
• Emotional instability, despondency	• Impaired short-term memory
	• Slow, deliberate speech
	• Thickened tongue
• Diaphoresis	• Coarse, dry, scaly, edematous skin
• Heat intolerance	• Hypothermia
	• Frank delirium (myxedema madness)
	• Lethargy → stupor → coma (myxedema coma)
• Increased DTRs	• Diminished DTRs
• Muscle weakness or muscle wasting	• Paresthesia of hands
• Oligomenorrhea	• Menorrhagia

AV, atrioventricular; DTRs deep tension reflexes; TSH, thyroid-stimulating hormone.

Hypothermia is a very distressing symptom. The patient is unable to keep warm. Temperatures have been reported to fall to less than 35° C (95.9° F).[88] Most cases of myxedema are diagnosed in the winter months. The myxedematous patient has hypotension, reduced total blood volume, decreased cardiac output, and bradycardia—all related to a decrease in β-adrenergic stimulation. Neuropsychiatric symptoms of depression, confusion, and decreased mental acuity may degenerate to a psychosis aptly called *myxedema madness*.

Laboratory Studies. Laboratory test results do not differentiate between hypothyroidism and myxedema coma. The blood test results simply confirm the clinical picture. Typically, patients with myxedema have primary hypothyroidism with a high TSH level and a low T_4 level. If the TSH level is normal or low, other causes of the hypothyroidism must be investigated.[88] TSH is released by the pituitary gland (see Table 36-3 in Chapter 36 for normal reference values); endocrine studies to evaluate the level of pituitary function should be undertaken.

MEDICAL MANAGEMENT

The patient's primary admitting diagnosis may mask an underlying hypothyroidism. However, clinical manifestations can trigger the alert clinician to suspect a hypofunctioning thyroid. The primary disease condition and the myxedema coma must be treated immediately to improve the patient's chances for recovery. A complete blood cell count and differential are evaluated to establish the presence of infection. Hypothyroidism produces a characteristically low white blood cell count. A normal white blood cell count and a differential with elevated and immature neutrophils indicate an ongoing acute infection. Severe systemic infection, often a precipitating factor for the myxedema coma, must be treated to decrease the stress on the thyroid-pituitary axis. Empirical antibiotic therapy may be required.

The goal for the treatment of end-stage or decompensated hypothyroidism is to restore the patient to a euthyroid (normal thyroid function) condition. This is accomplished with thyroid hormone replacement and support measures for the multisystem involvement.

PHARMACOLOGIC MANAGEMENT

Methods of treating end-stage hypothyroidism with medications vary among practitioners. A common method is to replete T_4 levels with an initial dose of levothyroxine (100 to 500 mcg given intravenously) to saturate the previously empty T_4 binding sites. The thyroid-binding globulin must be saturated before any free thyroxine can circulate. The loading dose is followed by daily administration of 75 to 100 mcg of levothyroxine.[88] If an older patient with concurrent heart disease is treated with replacement hormones, it is necessary to start the treatment slowly so as not to precipitate heart failure or angina.

A serum cortisol level is obtained to evaluate adrenal gland function. Glucocorticoids may be necessary to assist the patient to respond to the stress state of hypothyroidism, until a coexisting adrenal insufficiency is ruled out.

NURSING MANAGEMENT

Nursing care of the patient with myxedema coma focuses on management of the precipitating disease and on the severe impact of hypothyroidism on multiple organ systems. Many nursing diagnoses are associated with management of myxedema coma and are listed in the Nursing Diagnoses feature on Myxedema Coma.

Pulmonary Care. The patient with myxedema coma who is admitted to the critical care unit may require intubation and mechanical ventilatory support. Individuals who are not intubated are monitored for development of respiratory failure. Arterial blood gas measurements are evaluated to monitor for CO_2 retention and respiratory acidosis.

Cardiac Concerns. Dysrhythmias are common in the myxedematous patient with impaired myocardial contraction and can quickly be identified by continuous ECG monitoring. Expected signs of myxedema, such as flattened or inverted T waves or prolonged QT and PR intervals, resolve in a positive response to thyroxine replacement therapy. Hypotension management requires cautious fluid replacement of 5% to 10% glucose in 0.45% sodium chloride or 0.9% sodium chloride, depending on the serum sodium level.

Thermoregulation. Hypothermia gradually improves as the patient is treated with thyroid hormone. Several warm blankets comfortably wrapped around the patient with mild hypothermia may be sufficient to help raise the body temperature to normal. Active warming devices are also used. Continuous assessments are important to avoid too-rapid heating and vasodilation. Electronic devices that can measure accurately at the extreme lower range of body temperatures are used.

Thyroid Replacement Therapy. Older patients and those with a cardiac history receive intravenous thyroxine with due precautions. Thyroxine can precipitate angina and dysrhythmias. Hemodynamic monitoring includes HR, BP, ECG, CVP, and in rare situations, information from a pulmonary artery catheter. Improvements in the patient's cardiopulmonary and neurologic status, together with changes in T_4 and TSH laboratory values, are used to gauge the success of the thyroid hormone replacement therapy.

Skin Care. Patients with myxedema coma have rough, dry skin. Measures are taken to avoid skin breakdown related to decreased circulation and widespread edema. Soap is used sparingly and is followed by an emollient. Frequent repositioning minimizes pressure against capillary beds over bony prominences.

Nursing Diagnoses

Myxedema Coma

- Hypothermia related to decreased metabolic rate
- Impaired Spontaneous Ventilation related to respiratory fatigue or metabolic factors
- Activity Intolerance related to prolonged immobility or deconditioning
- Disturbed Body Image related to functional dependence on life-sustaining technology
- Deficient Knowledge: Discharge Regimen related to lack of previous exposure to information (see Patient Education feature on Myxedema Coma)

Elimination. Constipation is managed on a daily basis to avoid impaction. Use of fiber-enriched enteral nutrition may be helpful. Food choices for oral intake include sources of increased fiber, such as fresh fruits and vegetables. Fluids are encouraged as the hypovolemia is corrected and blood pressure stabilizes. Increased fiber is preferable to use of enemas. Enemas are to be avoided, because insertion of the rectal tube may stimulate the vagal nerve.

Patient Education. Patients with myxedema coma have decreased comprehension and mental acuity. All instructions, procedures, and activities are to be explained slowly and provided in written form. The patient and family members may experience myriad emotions with one constant: fear of the unknown. Before any teaching, the nurse evaluates the family's ability to accept the patient's slowed thinking and slowed response time. The family may benefit from a referral to the hospital's social service department for assistance in dealing with the patient's neuropsychiatric symptoms.

All instructions given to the patient or family are given verbally and in writing. A written copy of all schedules is given as a reference for home care before discharge. The nurse discusses the medication schedule and the frequency of the drug doses with the patient and family. Side effects of each drug are described. The patient and family need to know the side effects of drugs, including over-the-counter drugs, so that they can deal with them at home, and they need to know which signs or symptoms are to be reported to their health care provider (see the Patient Education feature on Myxedema Coma).

COLLABORATIVE MANAGEMENT

There are no published guidelines that discuss acute collaborative care management of the patient with myxedema coma. Guidelines do exist for non-urgent care of the patient with

hypothyroidism.[72] Collaborative management is required to decrease mortality in myxedema coma. Early recognition of symptoms and a willingness to request laboratory tests to confirm the diagnosis allow therapy to be instituted as early as possible by the clinical team.

Summary

- The endocrine system is complex, and assessment relies heavily on laboratory tests for confirmation of disease processes. To fully participate in the care of patients with these complex conditions, the critical care nurse must be aware of the intricacies of the endocrine system.
- Physiologic stress associated with critical illness causes increased secretion of stress hormones by the hypothalamic-pituitary-adrenal pathway. This results in secretion of cortisol, stimulation of the SNS, and release of norepinephrine and epinephrine to mobilize glucose. If critical illness is prolonged beyond 7 to 10 days, profound suppression of pituitary, thyroid, and adrenal gland function occurs.
- The diagnostic criteria for DKA include a blood glucose concentration greater than 250 mg/dL, an arterial pH value of less than 7.3, a serum bicarbonate level lower than 15 mEq/L, and moderate or severe ketonemia or ketonuria.
- The diagnostic criteria for HHS include a blood glucose concentration greater than 600 mg/dL, an arterial pH value higher than 7.3, a serum bicarbonate level greater than 15 mEq/L, a serum osmolality greater than 320 mOsm/kg H_2O (320 mmol/kg), and absent or mild ketonuria.
- Central DI occurs when ADH is not released from the posterior pituitary gland. The excretion of large quantities of hypotonic urine creates the following alterations in serum and urinary laboratory values: serum sodium greater than 145 mEq/L, serum osmolality greater than 295 mOsm/kg H_2O (295 mmol/L), urine osmolality lower than 200 mOsm/kg H_2O (200 mmol/L), and urine specific gravity lower than 1.005.
- Thyroid storm is identified by clinical signs such as high fever, tachycardia, hypertension, tremor—evidence of the rapid metabolic rate. The laboratory values are similar to those seen in hyperthyroidism: low TSH and elevated T_4.
- Myxedema is characterized by hypothermia, hypoventilation, bradycardia, depression, and decreased mental acuity, reflecting a slowed metabolic rate. The laboratory values are similar to those seen with hypothyroidism: high TSH and low T_4 levels.

Patient Education: Myxedema Coma

- Acute phase
  - Explain reasons for critical care unit admission
  - Explain reasons for extreme hypermetabolism
- Predischarge
  - Assess knowledge level
  - Disease process of thyrotoxicosis
  - Causes of thyrotoxic crisis
  - Medications: explain purpose, side effects, dosage, and how often to use
  - Signs and symptoms to report to health care professional

Case Study: Patient with an Endocrine Disorder

⊝volve Answers to the Case Study Questions can be found on the Evolve web site at http://evolve.elsevier.com/Urden/.

Brief Patient History

Ms. S is a 72-year-old woman with a history of hypertension treated with an angiotensin-converting enzyme (ACE) inhibitor and thiazide diuretics. She has a past 100-pack-year history of tobacco abuse but quit 2 years

ago. Ms. S lives independently in a senior apartment. She was brought to the hospital by friends because of a fall. Ms S states that she has a severe headache but cannot recall whether she hit her head during the fall. She is also having difficulty recalling recent events.

Continued

Case Study: Patient with an Endocrine Disorder—cont'd

Clinical Assessment

Ms. S is admitted to the intensive care unit from the emergency department because of nonspecific ECG changes suggestive of inferior wall ischemia and electrolyte abnormalities. She is awake; alert; oriented to person, time, place; and unable to recall the events leading to her hospitalization. She states that her headache is severe and feels like someone is hitting her head with a hammer. Her skin is warm and dry. Ms. S's gait is visibly unsteady.

Diagnostic Procedures

Ms. S's vital signs include the following: blood pressure of 180/92 mm Hg, heart rate of 100 beats/min (sinus rhythm), respiratory rate of 24 breaths/min, and temperature of 98.8° F.

Ms. S reports that her headache is a 10 on the Baker-Wong faces scale. Laboratory findings include the following: sodium level of 116 mmol/L, potassium level of 3.3 mmol/L, chloride level of 88 mmol/L, carbon dioxide level of 22 mEq/L, magnesium level of 1.8 mg/dL, urinary sodium level of 30 mmol/L, and urine osmolality value of 118 mOsm/L. The test result for troponin I on admission was negative. ECG testing shows a normal sinus rhythm, T wave inversion in leads II, III, and AVF, and a change from prior ECG findings, suggestive of inferior wall ischemia. Chest radiography identified a mass in the right upper lobe that strongly suggested a neoplasm.

Medical Diagnosis

Ms. S is diagnosed with syndrome of inappropriate diuretic hormone (SIADH).

Questions

1. What major outcomes do you expect to achieve for this patient?
2. What problems or risks must be managed to achieve these outcomes?
3. What interventions must be initiated to monitor, prevent, manage, or eliminate the problems and risks identified?
4. What interventions should be initiated to promote optimal functioning, safety, and well-being of the patient?
5. What possible learning needs do you anticipate for this patient?
6. What cultural and age-related factors may have a bearing on the patient's plan of care?

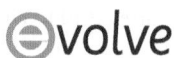 Be sure to check out the bonus material, including free self-assessment exercises, on the Evolve web site at http://evolve.elsevier.com/Urden/.

References

1. van den Berghe G et al: Intensive insulin therapy in the critically ill patients, *N Engl J Med* 345(19):1359-1367, 2001.
2. van den Berghe G et al: Intensive insulin therapy in the medical ICU, *N Engl J Med* 354(5):449-461, 2006.
3. Marik PE, Raghavan M: Stress-hyperglycemia, insulin and immunomodulation in sepsis, *Intensive Care Med* 30(5):748-756, 2004.
4. Dellinger RP et al: Surviving Sepsis Campaign: international guidelines for management of severe sepsis and septic shock, 2008, *Crit Care Med* 36(1):296-327, 2008.
5. Moghissi ES et al: American Association of Clinical Endocrinologists and American Diabetes Association consensus statement on inpatient diabetes control, *Endocr Pract* 15(4):1-17, 2009.
6. Wortsman J: Role of epinephrine in acute stress, *Endocrinol Metab Clin North Am* 31(1):79-106, 2002.
7. Marik PE et al: Recommendations for the diagnosis and management of corticosteroid insufficiency in critically ill adult patients: consensus statements from an international task force by the American College of Critical Care Medicine, *Crit Care Med* 36(6):1937-1949, 2008.
8. Peeters RP et al: Changes within the thyroid axis during critical illness, *Crit Care Clin* 22(1):41-55, 2006.
9. van den Berghe G: Neuroendocrine pathobiology of chronic critical illness, *Crit Care Clin* 18(3):509-528, 2002.
10. van den Berghe G: Endocrine evaluation of patients with critical illness, *Endocrinol Metab Clin North Am* 32(2):385-410, 2003.
11. Weekers F, Van den Berghe G: Endocrine modifications and interventions during critical illness, *Proc Nutr Soc* 63(3):443-450, 2004.
12. Cooper MS, Stewart PM: Corticosteroid insufficiency in acutely ill patients. *N Engl J Med* 348(8):727-734, 2003.
13. Collier B et al: Glucose control and the inflammatory response, *Nutr Clin Pract* 23(1):3-15, 2008.
14. Langton JE, Brent GA: Nonthyroidal illness syndrome: evaluation of thyroid function in sick patients, *Endocrinol Metab Clin North Am* 31 (1):159-172, 2002.
15. Wyne KL: The role of thyroid hormone therapy in acutely ill cardiac patients, *Crit Care* 9(4):333-334, 2005.
16. Rivers EP et al: Adrenal insufficiency in high-risk surgical ICU patients, *Chest* 119(3):889-896, 2001.
17. Keh D, Sprung CL: Use of corticosteroid therapy in patients with sepsis and septic shock: an evidence-based review, *Crit Care Med* 32(11):S527-S533, 2004.
18. Axelrod L: Perioperative management of patients treated with glucocorticoids, *Endocrinol Metab Clin North Am* 32(2):367-383, 2003.
19. Marik PE: Mechanisms and clinical consequences of critical illness associated adrenal insufficiency, *Curr Opin Crit Care* 13(4):363-369, 2007.
20. Sprung CL et al: Hydrocortisone therapy for patients with septic shock, *N Engl J Med* 358(2):111-124, 2008.
21. Clement S: Better glycemic control in the hospital: beneficial and feasible, *Cleve Clin J Med* 74(2):111-112, 114-120, 2007.
22. NICE_SUGAR Study Investigators: Intensive versus conventional glucose control in critically ill patients *N Eng J Med* 360(13): 1283-97
23. De La Rosa GD et al: Strict glycaemic control in patients hospitalised in a mixed medical and surgical intensive care unit: a randomised clinical trial, *Crit Care* 12(5):R120, 2008.
24. Gandhi GY et al: Intensive intraoperative insulin therapy versus conventional glucose management during cardiac surgery: a randomized trial, *Ann Intern Med* 146(4):233-243, 2007.
25. Wiener RS et al: Benefits and risks of tight glucose control in critically ill adults: a meta-analysis, *JAMA* 300(8):933-944, 2008.
26. Deedwania P et al: Hyperglycemia and acute coronary syndrome: a scientific statement from the American Heart Association Diabetes Committee of the Council on Nutrition, Physical Activity, and Metabolism, *Circulation* 117(12):1610-1619, 2008.
27. Prevalence of self-reported cardiovascular disease among persons aged > or =35 years with diabetes—United States, 1997–2005, *MMWR Morb Mortal Wkly Rep* 56(43):1129-1132, 2007.
28. Ryden L et al: Guidelines on diabetes, pre-diabetes, and cardiovascular diseases: executive summary. The Task Force on Diabetes and Cardiovascular Diseases of the European Society of Cardiology (ESC) and of the European Association for the Study of Diabetes (EASD), *Eur Heart J* 28(1):88-136, 2007.

29. Ascione R et al: Inadequate blood glucose control is associated with in-hospital mortality and morbidity in diabetic and nondiabetic patients undergoing cardiac surgery, *Circulation* 118(2):113-123, 2008.

30. Jones KW et al: Hyperglycemia predicts mortality after CABG: postoperative hyperglycemia predicts dramatic increases in mortality after coronary artery bypass graft surgery, *J Diabetes Complications* 22(6):365-370, 2008.

31. Whitcomb BW et al: Impact of admission hyperglycemia on hospital mortality in various intensive care unit populations, *Crit Care Med* 33 (12):2772-2777, 2005.

32. Egi M et al: Blood glucose concentration and outcome of critical illness: the impact of diabetes, *Crit Care Med* 36(8):2249-2255, 2008.

33. Oddo M et al: Glucose control after severe brain injury, *Curr Opin Clin Nutr Metab Care* 11(2):134-139, 2008.

34. Clement S et al: Management of diabetes and hyperglycemia in hospitals, *Diabetes Care* 27(2):553-591, 2004.

35. Braithwaite SS: Inpatient insulin therapy, *Curr Opin Endocrinol Diabetes Obes* 15(2):159-166, 2008.

36. Moghissi E: Hospital management of diabetes: beyond the sliding scale, *Cleve Clin J Med* 71(10):801-808, 2004.

37. American Diabetes Association: Diagnosis and classification of diabetes mellitus, *Diabetes Care* 31(suppl 1):S55-S60, 2008.

38. American Diabetes Association: Nutrition recommendations and interventions for diabetes: a position statement of the American Diabetes Association, *Diabetes Care* 31(suppl 1):S61-S78, 2008.

39. Heron MP: Deaths: leading causes for 2004, *National Vital Statistics Reports* 56(5), Hyattsville, MD: National Center for Health Statistics, 2007.

40. Coughlin SS et al: Diabetes mellitus as a predictor of cancer mortality in a large cohort of US adults, *Am J Epidemiol* 159(12):1160-1167, 2004.

41. American Diabetes Association: Standards of medical care in diabetes—2009, *Diabetes Care* 32(suppl 1):S13-S61, 2009.

42. Blake DR, Nathan DM: Point-of-care testing for diabetes, *Crit Care Nurs Q* 27(2):150-161, 2004.

43. Richter B et al: Human versus animal insulin in people with diabetes mellitus: a systematic review, *Endocrinol Metab Clin North Am* 31(3):723-749, 2002.

44. Screening for type 2 diabetes, *Diabetes Care* 27(suppl 1):S11-S14, 2004.

45. Grundy SM et al: Diagnosis and management of the metabolic syndrome: an American Heart Association/National Heart, Lung, and Blood Institute Scientific Statement, *Circulation* 112(17):2735-2752, 2005.

46. Rosenzweig JL et al: Primary prevention of cardiovascular disease and type 2 diabetes in patients at metabolic risk: an Endocrine Society clinical practice guideline, *J Clin Endocrinol Metab* 93(10):3671-3689, 2008.

47. American College of Endocrinology position statement on the insulin resistance syndrome, *Endocr Pract* 9(suppl 2):5-21, 2003.

48. Grundy SM et al: Clinical management of metabolic syndrome: report of the American Heart Association/National Heart, Lung, and Blood Institute/American Diabetes Association conference on scientific issues related to management, *Circulation* 109(4):551-556, 2004.

49. Lebovitz HE: Oral antidiabetic agents: 2004, *Med Clin North Am* 2004;88 (4):847-863.

50. Krentz AJ et al: New drugs for type 2 diabetes mellitus: what is their place in therapy? *Drugs* 68(15):2131-2162, 2008.

51. Nathan DM et al: Management of hyperglycemia in type 2 diabetes—a consensus algorithm for the initiation and adjustment of therapy. A consensus statement from the American Diabetes Association and the European Association for the Study of Diabetes, *Diabetes Care* 29(8):1963-1972, 2006.

52. Nathan DM et al: Management of hyperglycemia in type 2 diabetes—a consensus algorithm for the initiation and adjustment of therapy: update regarding thiazolidinediones. A consensus statement from the American Diabetes Association and the European Association for the Study of Diabetes, *Diabetes Care* 31(1):173-175, 2008.

53. Nesto RW et al: Thiazolidinedione use, fluid retention, and congestive heart failure: a consensus statement from the American Heart Association and American Diabetes Association, *Circulation* 108(23):2941-2948, 2003.

54. Kitabchi AE et al: Hyperglycemic crises in adult patients with diabetes: a consensus statement from the American Diabetes Association, *Diabetes Care* 29(12):2739-2748, 2006.

55. Newton CA, Raskin P: Diabetic ketoacidosis in type 1 and type 2 diabetes mellitus: clinical and biochemical differences, *Arch Intern Med* 164 (17):1925-1931, 2004.

56. Gaglia JL et al: Acute hyperglycemic crisis in the elderly, *Med Clin North Am* 88(4):1063-1084, 2004.

57. Janicic N, Verbalis JG: Evaluation and management of hypo-osmolality in hospitalized patients, *Endocrinol Metab Clin North Am* 32(2):459-481, 2003.

58. Holcomb S: Diabetes insipidus, *Dimens Crit Care Nurs* 21(3):94-97, 2002.

59. Wong LL, Verbalis JG: Systemic diseases associated with disorders of water homeostasis, *Endocrinol Metab Clin North Am* 31(1):121-140, 2002.

60. Loh JA, Verbalis JG: Disorders of water and salt metabolism associated with pituitary disease, *Endocrinol Metab Clin North Am* 37(1):213-234, 2008.

61. Vance ML: Perioperative management of patients undergoing pituitary surgery, *Endocrinol Metab Clin North Am* 32(2):355-365, 2003.

62. Hadjizacharia P et al: Acute diabetes insipidus in severe head injury: a prospective study, *J Am Coll Surg* 207(4):477-484, 2008.

63. Khanna A: Acquired nephrogenic diabetes insipidus, *Semin Nephrol* 26(3):244-248, 2006.

64. Verbalis JG: Disorders of body water homeostasis, *Best Pract Res Clin Endocrinol Metab* 17(4):471-503, 2003.

65. Holmes CL et al: Science review: vasopressin and the cardiovascular system part 2—clinical physiology, *Crit Care* 8(1):15-23, 2004.

66. DDAVP. In *Mosby's Drug Consult*. St. Louis, Mosby, 2004.

67. Ellison DH, Berl T: Clinical practice: the syndrome of inappropriate antidiuresis, *N Engl J Med* 356(20):2064-2072, 2007.

68. Gustafsson BI et al: Bronchopulmonary neuroendocrine tumors, *Cancer* 113(1):5-21, 2008.

69. Seute T et al: Neurologic disorders in 432 consecutive patients with small cell lung carcinoma, *Cancer* 100(4):801-806, 2004.

70. Freda BJ et al: Evaluation of hyponatremia: a little physiology goes a long way, *Cleve Clin J Med* 71(8):639-650, 2004.

71. Johnson AL, Criddle LM: Pass the salt: indications for and implications of using hypertonic saline, *Crit Care Nurse* 24(5):36-48, 2004.

72. American Association of Clinical Endocrinologists: Medical guidelines for clinical practice for the evaluation and treatment of hyperthyroidism and hypothyroidism, *Endocr Pract* 8(6):458-469, 2002.

73. Demers LM: Thyroid disease: pathophysiology and diagnosis, *Clin Lab Med* 24(1):19-28, 2004.

74. Brent GA: Clinical practice: Graves' disease, *N Engl J Med* 358(24): 2594-2605, 2008.

75. Porsche R, Brenner ZR: Amiodarone-induced thyroid dysfunction, *Crit Care Nurse* 26(3):34-41, 2006.

76. Wilkinson JN: Thyroid storm in a polytrauma patient, *Anaesthesia* 63 (9):1001-1005, 2008.

77. Waltman PA et al: Thyroid storm during pregnancy: a medical emergency, *Crit Care Nurse* 24(2):74-79, 2004.

78. Silva JE, Bianco SD: Thyroid-adrenergic interactions: physiological and clinical implications, *Thyroid* 18(2):157-165, 2008.

79. Bagtharia S et al: Ruptured ectopic pregnancy concealing thyroid storm, *J Obstet Gynaecol* 27(2):213-214, 2007.

80. Frost L et al: Hyperthyroidism and risk of atrial fibrillation or flutter: a population-based study, *Arch Intern Med* 164(15):1675-1678, 2004.

81. Nadkarni PJ et al: Thyrotoxicosis-induced ventricular arrhythmias, *Thyroid* 18(10):1111-1114, 2008.

82. Wald DA, Silver A: Cardiovascular manifestations of thyroid storm: a case report, *J Emerg Med* 25(1):23-28, 2003.

83. Holcomb SS: Thyroid diseases: a primer for the critical care nurse, *Dimens Crit Care Nurs* 21(4):127-133, 2002.

84. Surks MI et al: Subclinical thyroid disease: scientific review and guidelines for diagnosis and management, *JAMA* 291(2):228-238, 2004.

85. Rodriguez I et al: Factors associated with mortality of patients with myxoedema coma: prospective study in 11 cases treated in a single institution, *J Endocrinol* 180(2):347-350, 2004.

86. Dutta P et al: Predictors of outcome in myxedema coma: a study from a tertiary care centre, *Crit Care* 12(1):R1, 2008.

87. Stathatos N, Wartofsky L: Perioperative management of patients with hypothyroidism, *Endocrinol Metab Clin North Am* 32(2):503-518, 2003.

88. Wall CR: Myxedema coma: diagnosis and treatment, *Am Fam Physician* 62 (11):2485-2490, 2000.

Trauma

$\mathcal{T}$rauma is the leading cause of death for all age groups younger than 44 years. Injury costs the United States hundreds of billions of dollars annually. It is one of the most pressing health problems in the United States today, but the problem continues to go largely unrecognized.

Injury as a result of trauma is no longer considered to be an accident. The term *motor vehicle accident* (MVA) has been replaced with *motor vehicle crash* (MVC), and the term *accident* has been replaced with *unintentional injury*. Unintentional injury is no accident. Accident traditionally has implied an act of God or an unpredictable event. Domestic violence and alcohol-related issues are priority prevention areas with which health care providers must be actively involved.

Intimate partner violence (IPV) constitutes a major public health issue in the United States. IPV is the leading cause of injury to women in the United States, and it has been estimated that 1.5 million women and 834,700 men every year are raped or physically assaulted each year.[1] IPV and alcohol abuse have a high prevalence among female trauma patients admitted to trauma centers.[2] Health care providers should consider routinely inquiring about domestic violence as part of the history for all female adolescents and adult patients.[3] Key points in prevention, recognition, and treatment of domestic violence have been summarized by Sisley and colleagues[4] (1999) and are listed in Box 38-1.

An alcohol-related MVC kills someone every 30 minutes and nonfatally injures someone every 2 minutes.[5] Each year, alcohol-related crashes in the United States cost about $51 billion.[6] To further decrease alcohol-related crashes, communities need to implement and enforce effective strategies, such as sobriety checkpoints, 0.08% blood alcohol levels, minimum legal drinking age laws, and zero tolerance for young drivers.[5] Alcohol screening and intervention have been recommended as routine components of trauma care.[7] The Alcohol Use Disorders Identification Test (AUDIT) is a screening questionnaire that has been recommended (Table 38-1) because it can be used to identify frequency of alcoholic drinking and problem drinking.[8]

Over the past few decades, major advances have been made in the management of patients with traumatic injuries, and significant improvements have been made in their care in the prehospital and emergency department settings. Patients with complex, multisystem trauma are admitted to critical care units, and these patients require complex nursing care. This chapter reviews nursing management of patients with traumatic injuries, particularly in the critical care setting.

MECHANISMS OF INJURY

Trauma occurs when an external force of energy impacts the body and causes structural or physiologic alterations, or *injuries*. External forces can be radiation, electrical, thermal, chemical, or mechanical forms of energy. This chapter focuses on trauma from mechanical energy. Mechanical energy can produce blunt or penetrating traumatic injuries. Understanding the mechanism of injury helps health care providers anticipate and predict potential internal injuries.

BLUNT TRAUMA

Blunt trauma is seen most often with MVCs, contact sports, blunt force injuries (e.g., trauma caused by a baseball bat), or falls. Injuries occur because of the forces sustained during a rapid change in velocity (deceleration). To estimate the amount of force sustained in an MVC, multiply the person's weight by the miles per hour (speed) the vehicle was traveling. A 130-pound woman in a vehicle traveling at 60 miles per hour that hits a brick wall, for example, would sustain 7800 pounds of force within milliseconds. As the body stops suddenly, tissues and organs continue to move forward. This sudden change in velocity causes injuries that result in lacerations or crush injuries of internal body structures.

PENETRATING TRAUMA

Penetrating injuries occur with stabbings, firearms, or impalement—injuries that penetrate the skin and result in damage to internal structures. Damage is created along the path of penetration. Penetrating injuries can be misleading inasmuch as the condition of the outside of the wound does not determine the extent of internal injury. Bullets can create internal cavities 5 to 30 times larger than the diameter of the bullet.[9]

Several factors determine the extent of damage sustained as a result of penetrating trauma. Different weapons cause different types of injuries. The severity of a gunshot wound depends on the type of gun, type of ammunition used, and the distance and angle from which the gun was fired. Pellets from a shotgun blast expand on impact and cause multiple injuries to internal structures. Handgun bullets usually damage what is directly in the bullet's path. Inside the body, the bullet can ricochet off bone and create further damage along its pathway. With penetrating stab wounds, factors that determine the extent of injury include the type and length of object used and the angle of insertion.

BOX 38-1   PREVENTION, RECOGNITION, AND TREATMENT OF DOMESTIC VIOLENCE

- Development of a curriculum on domestic violence for health care providers and students
- Support for a policy of universal screening of all female patients for domestic violence
- Promotion of hospital-based domestic violence programs
- Advocacy for an increase in the number of beds available in battered women's shelters
- Development of intervention programs for children who witness domestic violence
- Treatment programs for batterers
- Development of a research agenda
- Support for the establishment of a national database for compiling incidence and other epidemiologic data on domestic violence

---

PHASES OF TRAUMA CARE

Care of trauma victims during wartime enhanced principles of triage and rapid transport of the injured to medical facilities. The military experience has demonstrated that more lives can be saved by decreasing the time from injury to definitive care. It also has enhanced incentives and models for improvements in civilian trauma care, such as emergency medical service (EMS) systems and trauma care centers. The goal with critically injured patients is to minimize the time from initial insult to definitive care and to optimize prehospital care so that the patient arrives at the hospital alive.

Statistics demonstrate that deaths as a result of trauma occur in a trimodal distribution (Fig. 38-1).[9] The first peak includes victims who die before medical attention can be provided. The second peak occurs within a few hours after injury. This

---

TABLE 38-1 AUDIT Alcohol Screening Questionnaire

Question	Score*
How often do you have a drink containing alcohol?	Never Monthly or less 2-4 times per month 2-3 times per week 4 or more times per week
How many standard drinks containing alcohol do you have on a typical day when drinking?	1 or 2 3 or 4 5 or 6 7 to 9 10 or more
How often do you have six or more drinks on one occasion?	
During the past year, how often have you found that you were not able to stop drinking once you had started?	
During the past year, how often have you failed to do what was normally expected of you because of drinking?	Never Less than monthly Monthly Weekly Daily or almost daily
During the past year, how often have you needed a drink in the morning to get yourself going after a heavy drinking session?	
During the past year, how often have you had a feeling of guilt or remorse after drinking?	
During the past year, have you been unable to remember what happened the night before because you had been drinking?	
Have you or someone else been injured as a result of your drinking?	No Yes, but not in the past year Yes, during the past year
Has a relative or friend, doctor or other health worker been concerned about your drinking or suggested you cut down?	

*Scores for each question range from 0 to 4, with the first response for each question (never) scoring 0, the second (less than monthly) scoring 1, the third (monthly) scoring 2, the fourth (weekly) scoring 3, and the fifth response (daily or almost daily) scoring 4. For the last two questions, which only have three responses, the scoring is 0, 2, and 4. A score of 8 or more is associated with harmful or hazardous drinking, and a score of 13 or more by women or 15 or more by men is likely to indicate alcohol dependence.

AUDIT, Alcohol Use Disorders Identification Test.

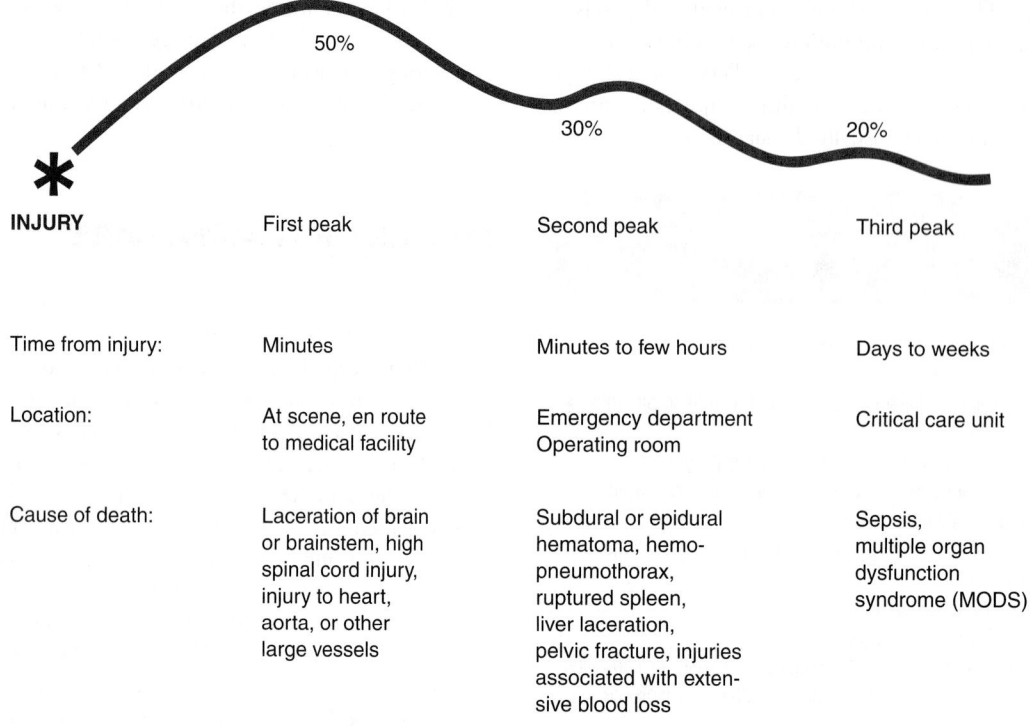

50%

30%

20%

	First peak	Second peak	Third peak
Time from injury:	Minutes	Minutes to few hours	Days to weeks
Location:	At scene, en route to medical facility	Emergency department Operating room	Critical care unit
Cause of death:	Laceration of brain or brainstem, high spinal cord injury, injury to heart, aorta, or other large vessels	Subdural or epidural hematoma, hemo- pneumothorax, ruptured spleen, liver laceration, pelvic fracture, injuries associated with exten- sive blood loss	Sepsis, multiple organ dysfunction syndrome (MODS)

Figure 38-1 Trimodal distribution of trauma deaths.

peak commonly is referred to as the *golden hour* for those critically injured. The golden hour is a 60-minute time frame that incorporates activation of the EMS system, stabilization in the prehospital setting, transportation to a medical facility, rapid resuscitation on arrival in the emergency department, and provision of definitive care. For the critically injured patient, the primary goal is to minimize the time from injury to definitive care. The third death peak occurs days to weeks after injury as a result of complications, including infection or multiple organ dysfunction syndrome (MODS). It is a nursing challenge to influence the quality of care the trauma patient receives in an attempt to "beat" the trimodal distribution of trauma deaths.

Nursing management of the patient with traumatic injuries begins the moment a call for help is received and continues until the patient's death or return to the community.[10] Care of the trauma patient is seen as a continuum that includes six phases: prehospital resuscitation, hospital resuscitation, definitive care and operative phase, critical care, intermediate care, and rehabilitation.

PREHOSPITAL RESUSCITATION

The goal of prehospital care is immediate stabilization and transportation. This is achieved through airway maintenance, control of external bleeding and shock, immobilization of the patient, and immediate transport (ground or air) to the closest appropriate medical facility.[9] Prehospital personnel should communicate information needed for triage at the hospital. Advanced planning for the injured patient is essential.

EMERGENCY DEPARTMENT RESUSCITATION

The American College of Surgeons developed guidelines (advanced trauma life support [ATLS]) for rapid assessment, resuscitation, and definitive care for trauma patients in the emergency department.[9] These guidelines delineate a systematic approach to care of the trauma patient: rapid primary survey, resuscitation of vital functions, more detailed secondary survey, and initiation of definitive care. This process constitutes the ABCDEs of trauma care and assists in identifying injuries.

Primary Survey. On arrival of the trauma patient in the emergency department, the primary survey is initiated. During this assessment, life-threatening injuries are discovered and treated. The five steps in the trauma primary survey are performed in ABCDE sequence (Table 38-2):

Airway maintenance with cervical spine protection
Breathing and ventilation
Circulation with hemorrhage control
Disability: neurologic status
Exposure or environmental control

Airway. The patient's airway is assessed for ineffective airway clearance and airway obstruction. The trauma patient is at risk for ineffective airway clearance, especially in the presence of altered consciousness, drugs and alcohol, and maxillofacial or thoracic injuries. Airway obstruction can be caused by foreign bodies, blood clots, or broken teeth. Airway patency should be assessed by inspecting the oropharynx for foreign body obstruction, listening for air movement at the nose and mouth, and auscultation of lung fields. Airway assessment must incorporate cervical spine immobilization. The patient's head should not be rotated,

TABLE 38-2 Primary Survey of the Trauma Patient

Survey Component	Nursing Diagnosis	Nursing Assessment, Care
Airway	Ineffective Airway Clearance related to obstruction or actual injury	Immobilize cervical spine Look • Is there obvious airway trauma, tachypnea, accessory muscle use, tracheal shift? Listen • Stridor, hyperresonance, dullness to percussion? Feel • For air exchange over the mouth; insert finger sweep to clear foreign bodies Secure airway • Oropharyngeal • Nasopharyngeal • Endotracheal tube • Cricothyrotomy
Breathing	Ineffective Breathing Pattern related to actual injury Impaired Gas Exchange related to actual injury or disrupted tissue perfusion	Assess for • Spontaneous breathing • Respiratory rate, depth, symmetry • Chest wall integrity For absent breathing • Intubate, mechanical ventilation If breathing but ineffective • Assess life-threatening conditions (e.g., tension pneumothorax, flail chest) • Administer supplemental oxygen • Initiate pulse oximetry
Circulation	Decreased Cardiac Output related to actual injury Alteration in Tissue Perfusion related to actual injury or shock Deficient Fluid Volume related to actual loss of circulating volume	Assess pulse quality and rate Use ECG monitoring If no pulse • Initiate ACLS If pulse but ineffective • Assess and treat life-threatening conditions (uncontrolled bleeding, shock) Initiate two large-bore IVs or central catheter; obtain serum samples for laboratory tests Provide fluid replacement
Disability	Ineffective Cerebral Tissue Perfusion Risk for Injury related to actual injury of brain or spinal cord	Determine Glasgow Coma Scale score Assess pupil size and reactivity
Exposure or environmental control	Risk for Imbalanced Body Temperature	Remove all clothing to inspect all body regions Prevent hypothermia

ACLS, advanced cardiac life support; ECG, electrocardiogram; IV, intravenous line.

hyperflexed, or hyperextended to establish and maintain an airway. The cervical spine must be immobilized in all trauma patients until a cervical spinal cord injury has been definitively ruled out. If the patient can verbally communicate, it is likely that the airway is patent. Patients who display nonpurposeful motor movements or who have a Glasgow Coma Scale (GCS) score of 8 or less usually require the placement of a definitive airway.[9]

Breathing. The patient is assessed for ineffective breathing patterns and impaired gas exchange; an open, clear airway does not ensure adequate ventilation and gas exchange. Assessment includes chest wall integrity and respiratory rate, depth, and symmetry. Auscultation is performed to assess gas flow in the lungs. Air or blood in the chest may be identified by percussion. Decreased breath sounds or alteration in chest wall integrity necessitate chest tube placement. Endotracheal intubation may be required for patients who have compromised airways caused by mechanical factors, who are unconscious, or who have ventilatory problems.[9] Supplemental oxygen is administered to all injured patients.[9]

Circulation. The next step is to assess for decreased cardiac output, impaired tissue perfusion, and deficient fluid volume. External exsanguination is identified and controlled by direct manual pressure on the wound. Rapid assessment of the circulatory status includes assessment of level of consciousness, skin color, and pulse.[9] Level of consciousness provides data on cerebral perfusion. Ashen, gray facial skin color or white, pale extremities may be ominous signs of hypovolemia.[9] Central pulses (femoral or carotid artery) are assessed bilaterally for rate, regularity, and quality. If a pulse is not present, advanced cardiac life support (ACLS) protocols are instituted. Electrocardiographic (ECG) monitoring is initiated to assess for rhythm disturbances. Life-threatening dysrhythmias are treated according to ACLS protocols.

Disability. A rapid neurologic assessment is performed. During this step, the nurse assesses the potential for injury by completing a brief neurologic assessment to establish the patient's level of consciousness and pupil size and reaction. The AVPU method can be used to quickly describe the patient's level of consciousness:

A: alert
V: responds to verbal stimuli
P: responds to painful stimuli
U: unresponsive

The patient's GCS score can be used if time allows (see Table 27-1).

Exposure. The final step in the primary survey is exposure and environmental control. All clothing is removed to facilitate a thorough examination of all body surfaces for the presence of injury. After all clothing is removed, the patient must be protected from hypothermia. This can be accomplished through external blankets, warm ambient room temperature, and warmed intravenous fluids.

Resuscitation Phase. After the primary survey the resuscitation phase begins. Hypovolemic shock is the most common type of shock that occurs in trauma patients.[9] Hemorrhage must be identified and treated rapidly. Two large-bore (14- to 16-gauge), peripheral intravenous catheters or a central venous catheter is inserted. During the initiation of intravenous lines, blood samples are drawn (Box 38-2). Intravenous therapy with Ringer's lactate solution should be administered rapidly. High-flow fluid warmers may be used to deliver warmed intravenous solutions at rates greater than 1000 mL/min. If the patient remains unresponsive to bolus intravenous therapy, O-negative blood or type-specific blood may be administered.[9] Transfusion of autologous salvaged blood (autotransfusion) may be used to replace intravascular volume and to provide oxygen-carrying capacity.

Placement of urinary and gastric catheters is part of the resuscitation phase. An indwelling urinary catheter can help evaluate urine output as an indicator of volume status and kidney perfusion. A gastric tube is inserted to reduce gastric distention and lower the risk of aspiration.[9]

The resuscitation phase begins in the emergency department and may continue well into the critical care phase. Resuscitation is aimed at ensuring adequate perfusion of tissues with oxygen and nutrients to support cellular function. The patient's response to resuscitation efforts is a priority nursing assessment because the patient's response to these efforts is key to determining subsequent therapy. Resuscitation end points (variables or parameters) must be viewed across the continuum of resuscitation from shock. During resuscitation from traumatic hemorrhagic shock, normalization of standard clinical parameters such as blood pressure, heart rate, and urine output are not adequate.[11] The optimal resuscitation end point is a major focus of research in trauma care. Current guidelines recommend that during resuscitation, attempts should be made to improve oxygen delivery to normalize base deficit, lactate, or gastric pH during the first 24 hours after injury.[12]

Secondary Survey. The secondary survey begins when the primary survey is completed, resuscitation is well established, and the patient is demonstrating normalization of vital signs. During the secondary survey, a head-to-toe approach is used to thoroughly examine each body region. The history is one of the most important aspects of the secondary survey. Often, head injury, shock, or the use of drugs or alcohol may preclude a good history, so the history must be pieced together from other sources. The prehospital providers (paramedics, emergency medical technicians) usually can provide most of the vital information pertaining to the *unintentional injury*. Specific information that must be elicited pertaining to the mechanism of injury is summarized in Box 38-3. This information can help predict internal injuries and facilitate rapid intervention.

BOX 38-2 SERUM SAMPLES TO OBTAIN WITH INTRAVENOUS PLACEMENT

- Complete blood cell (CBC) count
- Electrolyte profile (Na^+, K^+, Cl^-, CO_2, glucose, blood urea nitrogen [BUN] creatinine [Cr])
- Coagulation parameters: prothrombin time (PT); partial thromboplastin time (PTT)
- Type and screen (ABO compatibility)
- Amylase
- Toxicology screens
- Liver function studies
- Pregnancy test (for females of childbearing age)
- Lactate

BOX 38-3 HISTORY OF MECHANISM OF INJURY

PENETRATING TRAUMA
- Weapon used (handgun, shotgun, rifle, knife)
- Caliber of weapon
- Number of shots fired
- Gender of assailant
- Position of victim and assailant when injury occurred

BLUNT TRAUMA
- Height of fall
- Motor vehicle crash extrication time

- Ejection
- Steering wheel deformation
- Location in automobile (passenger, driver, front seat, back seat)
- Restraint status (lap belt, shoulder harness, or combination; unrestrained)
- Speed of automobiles, direction of impact
- Occupants (number and morbidity status)

The patient's pertinent past history can be assessed by use of the mnemonic AMPLE:

*A*llergies,

*M*edications currently used,

*P*ast medical illnesses/pregnancy,

*L*ast meal, and

*E*vents/environment related to the injury.

During the secondary survey the nurse ensures the completion of special procedures, such as an electrocardiogram (ECG); radiographic studies (chest, cervical spine, thorax, and pelvis); and ultrasonography and diagnostic peritoneal lavage (DPL). Throughout this survey the nurse continuously monitors the patient's vital signs and response to medical therapies. Emotional support to the patient and family also is imperative.

DEFINITIVE CARE AND OPERATIVE PHASE

After the secondary survey has been completed, specific injuries usually have been diagnosed. Definitive care related to specific injuries is described throughout this chapter. Trauma is often referred to as a "surgical disease" because the nature and extent of injuries usually requires operative management. After surgery, depending on the patient's status, transfer to the intensive care unit may be indicated.

CRITICAL CARE PHASE

Critically ill trauma patients are admitted into the intensive care unit (ICU) as direct transfers from the emergency department or operating room. Information the ICU nurse must obtain from the emergency department or operating room nurse, or both, is summarized using the SBAR method: **S**ituation, **B**ackground, **A**ssessment, and **R**ecommendations (Box 38-4). This information must be obtained before the patient's admission to the ICU to ensure availability of needed personnel, equipment, and supplies. This information also helps the ICU nurse to assess the impact of trauma resuscitation on the patient's ICU presentation and course. Table 38-3 summarizes the prehospital, emergency department, and operating room resuscitative measures that can affect the trauma patient's care in the ICU.

After the patient's arrival to the ICU, the nurse uses the primary and secondary surveys and resuscitative measures in accordance with ATLS guidelines to assess the trauma patient's status. Priority nursing care during the critical care phase includes ongoing physical assessments and monitoring the patient's response to medical therapies. The ICU nurse constantly is aware that the third peak of the trimodal distribution of trauma deaths occurs in the ICU setting as a result of complications, including acute respiratory distress syndrome (ARDS), sepsis, prolonged shock states, and MODS. Ongoing nursing assessments are imperative for early detection and treatment of complications.

One of the most important nursing roles is assessment of the balance between oxygen delivery and oxygen demand. Oxygen delivery must be optimized to prevent further system damage. Assessment of circulatory status includes the use of noninvasive

BOX 38-4	**NURSING REPORT FROM A REFERRING AREA USING THE SBAR METHOD**
S: Situation	Age
	Gender
	Mechanism of injury/injuries sustained
	Admission diagnosis/chief complaint; any loss of consciousness and its duration with current Glasgow Coma Scale score
	Diagnostic tests and procedures completed and results
	Laboratory results
	Medications administered (particularly opiates, sedatives)
	Current issues, including derangements in any physical assessments requiring acute interventions
B: Background	Significant medical and surgical history
	Home medications
A: Assessments	Current assessment findings, including vital signs, level of consciousness, established airway and mechanical ventilation settings
	Family members present and their assessment of coping and current knowledge of nature and extent of injuries and treatment plan
R: Recommendations	Description of the plan, including fluid volume and blood products

TABLE 38-3 Effects of Trauma Resuscitation

Aspect of Injury or Resuscitation	Effect on ICU Course
Prolonged extrication time	Gives an indication of length of time patient may have been hypotensive and/or hypothermic before medical care
Period of respiratory or cardiac arrest	Effects of loss of perfusion to brain (anoxic injury), kidneys, and other vital organs
Time on backboard	Potentiates risk of sacral or occipital breakdown
Number of units of blood; whether any were not fully cross-matched; packed cells versus whole blood used	Potentiates risk of ARDS, MODS

ARDS, acute respiratory distress syndrome; *ICU,* intensive care unit; *MODS,* multiple organ dysfunction syndrome.

and invasive techniques. The trauma patient is at high risk for impaired oxygenation as a result of a variety of factors (Table 38-4). These risk factors must be promptly identified and treated to prevent life-threatening sequelae. Prevention and treatment of hypoxemia depend on accurate assessment of the adequacy of pulmonary gas exchange, oxygen delivery, and oxygen consumption.

TABLE 38-4 Factors Predisposing the Trauma Patient to Impaired Oxygenation

Factor	Impairment
Impaired ventilation	Injury to airway structures, loss of central nervous system regulation of breathing, impaired level of consciousness
Impaired pulmonary gas diffusion	Pneumothorax, hemothorax, aspiration of gastric contents Shifts to the left of the oxyhemoglobin dissociation curve (can result from infusion of large volumes of banked blood, hypocarbia or alkalosis, or hypothermia)
Decreased oxygen supply	Reduced hemoglobin (from hemorrhage) Reduced cardiac output (cardiovascular injury, decreased preload)
Increased oxygen supply	Increased metabolic demands (associated with the stress response to injury)

Frequent and thorough nursing assessments of all body systems are important because these assessments are the cornerstone to the medical and nursing management of the critically ill trauma patient. The nurse can detect subtle changes and facilitate the implementation of timely therapeutic interventions to prevent complications often associated with trauma. The nurse must be knowledgeable about specific organ injuries and their associated sequelae.

SPECIFIC TRAUMA INJURIES

TRAUMATIC BRAIN INJURIES

More than 1.4 million traumatic brain injuries (TBIs) occur annually, with approximately 235,000 of patients hospitalized as a result of their injury, and approximately 50,000 Americans die each year of TBI.[13] At least 5.3 million Americans are living with disabilities resulting from TBI.[14]

Mechanism of Injury. TBIs occur when mechanical forces are transmitted to brain tissue. Mechanisms of injury include penetrating or blunt trauma to the head. The leading causes of TBI include falls (28%), MVCs (20%), struck by or against events (19%), and assaults (11%).[13] Penetrating trauma can result from the penetration of a foreign object such as a bullet, which causes direct damage to cerebral tissue. Blunt trauma can be the result of deceleration, acceleration, or rotational forces. Deceleration causes the brain to crash against the skull after it has hit something such as the dashboard of a car. Acceleration injuries occur when the brain has been forcefully hit, such as with a baseball bat. In many instances, TBIs can be caused by acceleration and deceleration. Acceleration injuries occur when the skull is hit by a force that causes the brain to move forward to the point of impact, and then as the brain reverses direction and hits the other side of the skull, deceleration injuries occur.

Pathophysiology. Review of the pathophysiology of a TBI can be divided into two categories: primary injury and secondary injury. The critical care nurse must understand this pathophysiology, because goals of ICU care include efforts to reduce morbidity and mortality from primary and secondary injuries.

Primary Injury. The primary injury occurs at the moment of impact as a result of mechanical forces to the head. The extent of and recovery from injury are related to whether the primary injury was localized to an area or whether it was diffuse or widespread throughout the brain. Primary injuries may include direct damage to the parenchyma or as injury to the vessels that causes hemorrhage, compressing nearby structures. Examples of primary injuries include contusion, laceration, shearing injuries, and hemorrhage. Primary injury may be mild, with little or no neurologic damage, or severe, with major tissue damage. Immediately after the injury, a cascade of neural and vascular processes is activated.

Secondary Injury. Secondary injury is the biochemical and cellular response to the initial trauma that can exacerbate the primary injury and cause loss of brain tissue not originally damaged.[15] Secondary injury can be caused by ischemia, hypercapnia, hypotension, cerebral edema, sustained hypertension, calcium toxicity, or metabolic derangements. Hypoxia or hypotension, the best known culprits for secondary injury, typically are the result of extracranial trauma.[15] A self-perpetuating cycle develops that may cause the expansion of a relatively focal primary injury as a result of uncontrolled, refractory secondary injury.[9,15]

Tissue ischemia occurs in areas of poor cerebral perfusion as a result of hypotension or hypoxia. The cells in ischemic areas become edematous. Extreme vasodilation of the cerebral vasculature occurs in an attempt to supply oxygen to the cerebral tissue. This increase in blood volume increases intracranial volume and raises intracranial pressure (ICP).

Significant hypotension causes inadequate perfusion to neural tissue. Hypotension rarely is associated with TBI. Hypotension typically is not caused by brain injury unless terminal medullary failure occurs.[15] If a trauma patient is unconscious and hypotensive, a detailed assessment of the chest, abdomen, and pelvis is performed to rule out internal injuries.

Hypercapnia is a powerful vasodilator. Most often caused by hypoventilation in an unconscious patient, hypercapnia results in cerebral vasodilation and increased cerebral blood volume and ICP.

Cerebral edema occurs as a result of the changes in the cellular environment caused by contusion, loss of autoregulation, and increased permeability of the blood-brain barrier. Cerebral edema can be focal as it localizes around the area of contusion or diffuse as a result of hypotension or hypoxia. The extent of cerebral edema can be minimized by controlling the other aspects of secondary injury, such as oxygenation, ventilation, and perfusion.

Initial hypertension in the patient with severe TBI is common. As a result of the loss of autoregulation, increased blood pressure results in increased intracranial blood volume and ICP. Every effort must be made to control hypertension to prevent the secondary injury caused by increased ICP (see "Increased Intracranial Pressure" in Chapter 28). The effects of increased ICP may be varied. As pressure increases inside the closed skull vault, cerebral perfusion decreases, which further compromises the brain. The combined effects of increasing pressure and decreasing perfusion precipitate a downward spiral of events.

Classification. Injuries of the brain are described by the functional changes or losses that occur. Some of the major functional abnormalities seen in head injury are described here.

Skull Fracture. Skull fractures are common, but they do not by themselves cause neurologic deficits. Skull fractures can be classified as open (dura is torn) or closed (dura is not torn), or they can be classified as those of the vault or those of the base. Common vault fractures occur in the parietal and temporal regions. Basilar skull fractures usually are not visible on conventional skull films and a computed tomography (CT) is typically required. Assessment findings may include cerebral spinal fluid otorrhea (from nose) or rhinorrhea (from ear), Battle's sign (ecchymosis overlying the mastoid process behind the ear), "raccoon eyes" (subconjunctival and periorbital ecchymosis), or palsy of the seventh cranial nerve.

The significance of a skull fracture is that it identifies the patient with a higher probability of having or developing an intracranial hematoma. Open skull fractures require surgical intervention to remove bony fragments and to close the dura. The major complications of basilar skull fractures are cranial nerve injury and leakage of cerebrospinal fluid (CSF). CSF leakage may result in a fistula, which increases the possibility of bacterial contamination and resultant meningitis. Because fistula formation may be delayed, patients with a basilar skull fracture are admitted to the hospital for observation and possible surgical intervention.

Concussion. A concussion is a brain injury accompanied by a brief loss of neurologic function, especially loss of consciousness.[14] When loss of consciousness occurs, it may last for seconds to an hour. The neurologic dysfunctions include confusion, disorientation, and sometimes a period of antegrade or retrograde amnesia. Other clinical manifestations that occur after concussion are headache, dizziness, nausea, irritability, inability to concentrate, impaired memory, and fatigue. The diagnosis of concussion is based on the loss of consciousness inasmuch as the brain remains structurally intact despite functional impairment.

Contusion. Contusion, or bruising of the brain, usually is related to acceleration-deceleration injuries, which result in hemorrhage into the superficial parenchyma, often the frontal and temporal lobes. Frontal or temporal contusions are most common and can be seen in a coup-contrecoup mechanism of injury (Fig. 38-2). Coup injury affects the cerebral tissue directly under the point of impact. Contrecoup injury occurs in a line directly opposite the point of impact.

The clinical manifestations of contusion are related to the location of the contusion, the degree of contusion, and the presence of associated lesions. Contusions can be small, in which localized areas of dysfunction result in a focal neurologic deficit. Larger contusions can evolve over 2 to 3 days after injury as a result of edema and further hemorrhaging. A large contusion can produce a mass effect that can cause a significant increase in ICP. Contusions are almost always associated with subdural hematoma.[9]

Contusions of the tips of the temporal lobe are a common occurrence and are of particular concern. Because the inner aspects of the temporal lobe surround the opening in the tentorium where the midbrain enters the cerebrum, edema in this area can cause rapid deterioration of the patient's condition and can

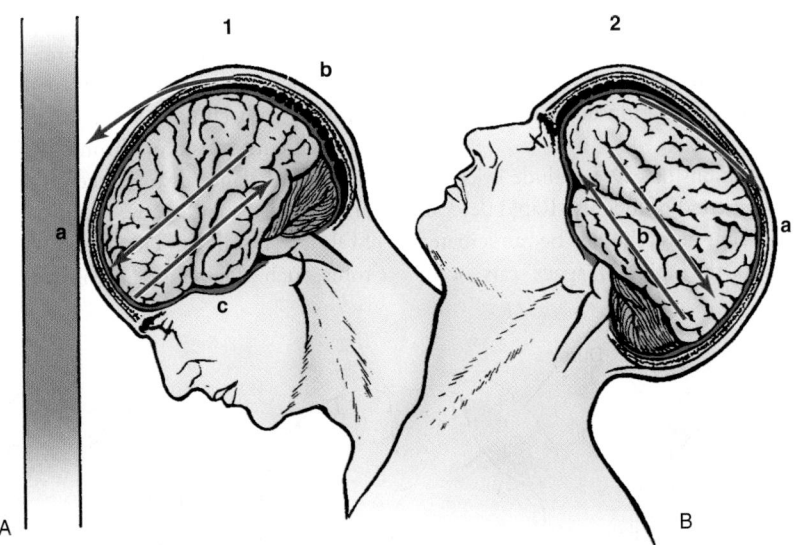

Figure 38-2 Coup and contrecoup head injury after blunt trauma. *A,* Coup injury: impact against object, showing the site of impact and direct trauma to brain (a), shearing of subdural veins (b), and trauma to the base of the brain (c). *B,* Contrecoup injury: impact within skull, showing the site of impact from brain hitting opposite side of skull (a) and shearing forces throughout brain (b). These injuries occur in one continuous motion; the head strikes the wall (coup) and then rebounds (contrecoup).

lead to herniation. Because of the location, this deterioration can occur with little or no warning at a deceptively low ICP.

Diagnosis of contusion is made by CT. If the CT scan indicates contusion, especially in the temporal area, the nurse must pay particular attention to neurologic assessments and look for subtle changes in pupillary signs or vital signs, irrespective of a stable ICP.

Medical management of cerebral contusions may consist of medical or surgical therapies. Because a contusion can progress over 3 to 5 days after injury, secondary injury may occur. If contusions are small, focal, or multiple, they are treated medically with serial neurologic assessments and possibly with ICP monitoring. Larger contusions that produce considerable mass effect require surgical intervention to prevent the increased edema and ICP as the contusion matures. Outcome of cerebral contusion varies, depending on the location and the degree of contusion.

Cerebral Hematomas. Extravasation of blood creates a space-occupying lesion within the cranial vault that can lead to increased ICP. Three types of hematomas are discussed here (Fig. 38-3). The first two, epidural and subdural hematomas, are extraparenchymal (outside of brain tissue) and produce injury by pressure effect and displacement of intracranial contents. The third type, intracerebral hematoma, directly damages neural tissue and can produce further injury as a result of pressure and displacement of intracranial contents.

Epidural Hematoma. Epidural hematoma (EDH) is a collection of blood between the inner table of the skull and the outermost layer of the dura. EDHs are most often associated with patients with skull fractures and middle meningeal artery lacerations (two thirds of patients) or skull fractures with venous bleeding.[9] A blow to the head that causes a linear skull fracture on the lateral surface of the head may tear the middle meningeal artery. As the artery bleeds, it pulls the dura away from the skull, creating a pouch that expands into the intracranial space.

The incidence of EDH is relatively low. EDH can occur as a result of low-impact injuries (e.g., falls) or high-impact injuries (e.g., MVCs). EDH occurs from trauma to the skull and meninges rather than from the acceleration-deceleration forces seen in other types of head trauma.

The classic clinical manifestations of EDH include brief loss of consciousness followed by a period of lucidity. Rapid deterioration in the level of consciousness should be anticipated because arterial bleeding into the epidural space can occur

quickly. A dilated and fixed pupil on the same side as the impact area is a hallmark of EDH.[9] The patient may complain of a severe, localized headache and may be sleepy. Diagnosis of EDH is based on clinical symptoms and evidence of a collection of epidural blood identified on the CT scan. Treatment of EDH involves surgical intervention to remove the blood and to cauterize the bleeding vessels.

Subdural Hematoma. Subdural hematoma (SDH), which is the accumulation of blood between the dura and underlying arachnoid membrane, most often is related to a rupture in the bridging veins between the cerebral cortex and the dura.[16] Acceleration-deceleration and rotational forces are the major causes of SDH, which often is associated with cerebral contusions and intracerebral hemorrhage. SDH is common, representing about 30% of severe head injuries. The three types of SDH— acute, subacute, and chronic—are based on the time frame from injury to clinical symptoms.

Acute Subdural Hematoma. Acute SDHs are hematomas that occur after a severe blow to the head. The clinical presentation of acute SDH is determined by the severity of injury to the underlying brain at the time of impact and the rate of blood accumulation in the subdural space. In other situations, the patient has a lucid period before deterioration. Careful observation for deterioration of the level of consciousness or lateralizing signs, such as inequality of pupils or motor movements, is essential. Rapid surgical intervention, including craniectomy, craniotomy, or burr hole evacuation, and aggressive medical management can reduce mortality.

Subacute Subdural Hematoma. Subacute SDHs are hematomas that develop symptomatically 2 days to 2 weeks after trauma. In subacute SDHs, the expansion of the hematoma occurs at a rate slower than that in acute SDH, and it takes longer for symptoms to become obvious. Clinical deterioration of the patient with a subacute SDH usually is slower than with an acute SDH, but treatment by surgical intervention, when appropriate, is the same.

Chronic Subdural Hematoma. Chronic SDH is diagnosed when symptoms appear days or months after injury. Most patients with chronic SDH usually are older or in late middle age. Patients at risk for chronic SDH include those with coordination or balance disturbances, older adults, and those receiving anticoagulation therapy. Clinical manifestations of chronic SDH are insidious. The patient may report a variety of symptoms, such as lethargy, absent-mindedness, headache, vomiting,

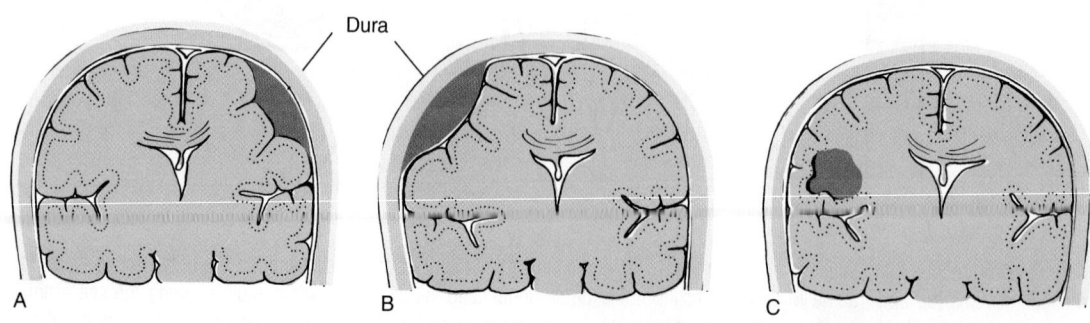

Figure 38-3 Types of hematomas. *A,* Subdural hematoma. *B,* Epidural hematoma. *C,* Intracerebral hematoma.

stiff neck, and photophobia and may show signs of transient ischemic attack, seizures, pupillary changes, or hemiparesis. Because a history of trauma often is not significant enough to be recalled, chronic SDH seldom is seen as an initial diagnosis. CT evaluation can confirm the diagnosis of chronic SDH.

If surgical intervention is required, evacuation of the chronic SDH may occur by craniotomy, burr holes, or catheter drainage. Evacuation by burr hole involves drilling a hole in the skull over the site of the chronic SDH and draining the fluid. Drains or catheters are left in place for at least 24 hours to facilitate total drainage. Outcome after chronic SDH evacuation varies. Return of neurologic status often depends on the degree of neurologic dysfunction before removal. Because this condition is most common in older or debilitated patient, recovery is a slow process. Recurrence of chronic SDH is not infrequent.

Intracerebral Hematoma. Intracerebral hematoma (ICH) results when bleeding occurs within cerebral tissue. Traumatic causes of ICH include depressed skull fractures, penetrating injuries (bullet, knife), or sudden acceleration-deceleration motion. The ICH can act as a rapidly expanding lesion; however, late ICH into the necrotic center of a contused area also is possible. Sudden clinical deterioration of a patient 6 to 10 days after trauma may be the result of ICH.

Medical management of ICH may include surgical or non-surgical management. It is thought that hemorrhages that do not cause significant ICP problems should be treated without surgery. Over time, the hemorrhage may be reabsorbed. If significant problems with ICP occur as a result of the ICH producing a mass effect, surgical removal is necessary. The outcome of a patient with an ICH depends greatly on the location of the hemorrhage. Size, mass effect, and displacement of other intracranial structures also affect the outcome.

Missile Injuries. Missile injuries are caused by objects that penetrate the skull to produce a significant focal damage but little acceleration-deceleration or rotational injury. The injury may be depressed, penetrating, or perforating (Fig. 38-4). Depressed injuries are caused by fractures of the skull, with penetration of bone into cerebral tissue. Penetrating injury is caused by a missile that enters the cranial cavity but does not exit. A low-velocity penetrating injury (knife) may involve only focal damage and no loss of consciousness. A high-velocity missile (bullet) can produce shock waves that are transmitted throughout the brain in addition to the injury caused by the bullet. Perforating injuries are missile injuries that enter and then exit the brain. Perforating injuries have much less ricochet effect but are still responsible for significant injury.

Risk of infection and cerebral abscess is a concern in cases of missile injuries. If fragments of the missile are embedded within the brain, careful consideration of the location and risk of increasing neurologic deficit is weighed against the risk of abscess or infection. The outcome after missile injury is based on the degree of penetration, the location of the injury, and the velocity of the missile.

Diffuse Axonal Injury. Diffuse axonal injury (DAI) is a term used to describe prolonged posttraumatic coma that is not caused by a mass lesion, although DAI with mass lesions have been reported.[16] DAI covers a wide range of brain dysfunction typically caused by acceleration-deceleration and rotational forces. DAI occurs as a result of damage to the axons or disruption of axonal transmission of the neural impulses.

The pathophysiology of DAI is related to the stretching and tearing of axons as a result of movement of the brain inside the cranium at the time of impact. The stretching and tearing of axons result in microscopic lesions throughout the brain, but especially deep within cerebral tissue and the base of the cerebrum. Disruption of axonal transmission of impulses results in loss of consciousness. Unless surrounding tissue areas are significantly injured, causing small hemorrhages, DAI may not be visible on CT or magnetic resonance imaging (MRI). DAI can be classified as one of three grades based on the extent of lesions: mild, moderate, or severe. The patient with mild DAI may be in a coma for 24 hours and may exhibit periods of decorticate and decerebrate posturing. Patients with moderate DAI may be in a coma for longer than 24 hours and exhibit periods of decorticate and decerebrate posturing. Severe DAI usually manifests as a prolonged, deep coma with periods of hypertension, hyperthermia, and excessive sweating. Treatment of DAI includes support of vital functions and maintenance of ICP within normal limits. The outcome after severe DAI is poor because of the extensive dysfunction of cerebral pathways.

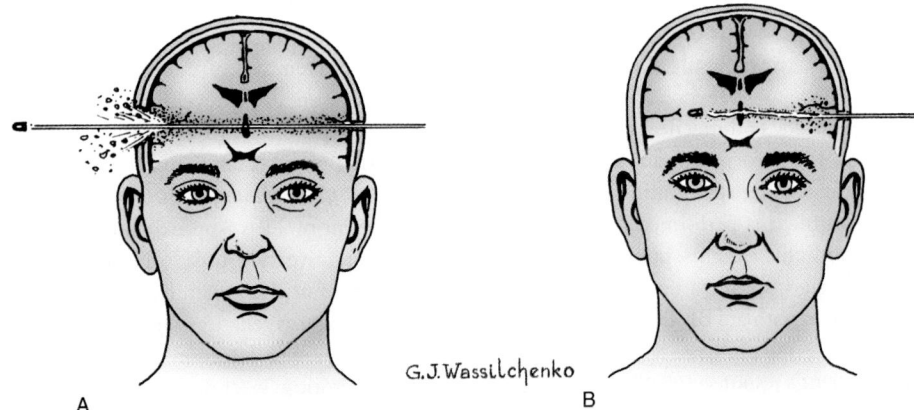

G.J.Wassilchenko

A   B

Figure 38-4 Bullet wounds of the head. A bullet wound or other penetrating missile wounds cause an open (compound) skull fracture and damage to brain tissue. Shock wave effects are transmitted throughout the brain. *A,* Perforating injury. *B,* Penetrating injury.

Neurologic Assessment of Traumatic Brain Injury. The neurologic assessment is the most important tool for evaluating the patient with a severe TBI, because it can indicate the severity of injury, provide prognostic information, and dictate the speed with which further evaluation and treatment must proceed.[14] The cornerstone of the neurologic assessment is the GCS,[15] although it is not a complete neurologic examination. Pupils and motor strength assessment must be incorporated into the early and ongoing assessments. After injuries are specifically identified, a more thorough, focused neurologic assessment, such as examination of the cranial nerves, is warranted. To assist with the initial assessment, TBIs are divided into three descriptive categories— mild, moderate, or severe—on the basis of the patient's GCS score and length of the unconscious state.

Degree of Injury

Mild Injury. Mild TBI is described as a GCS score of 13 to 15, with a loss of consciousness that lasts up to 15 minutes. Patients with mild injury often are seen in the emergency department and discharged home with a family member who is instructed to evaluate the patient routinely and to bring the patient back to the hospital if any further neurologic symptoms appear.

Moderate Injury. Moderate TBI is described as a GCS score of 9 to 12, with a loss of consciousness for up to 6 hours. Patients with this type of TBI usually are hospitalized. They are at high risk for deterioration from increasing cerebral edema and ICP, and serial clinical assessments are an important function of the nurse. Hemodynamic and ICP monitoring and ventilatory support may not be required for these patients unless other systemic injuries make them necessary. A CT scan usually is obtained on admission. Repeat CT scans are indicated if the patient's neurologic status deteriorates.

Severe Injury. Patients with a GCS score of 8 or less after resuscitation or those who deteriorate to that level within 48 hours of admission have a severe TBI. Patients with severe TBI often receive ventilatory support along with ICP and hemodynamic monitoring. A CT scan is performed to rule out any mass lesions that can be surgically removed. Patients are placed in a critical care setting for continual assessment, monitoring, and management.

Nursing Assessment of the Patient with Traumatic Brain Injury.

As in all traumatic injuries, evaluation of the airway, breathing, and circulation (ABCs) is the first step in the assessment of the patient with TBI in the ICU. Patients with moderate primary injury may deteriorate as a result of diffuse swelling or bleeding.[14] A patient with severe TBI who is breathing spontaneously may require prophylactic endotracheal or nasotracheal intubation with mechanical ventilatory support to reduce the risk of hypoxia and hypercapnia. After stabilization of the ABCs is ensured, a neurologic assessment is performed.

Level of consciousness, motor movements, pupillary response, respiratory function, and vital signs are all part of a complete neurologic assessment in the patient with a TBI. Level of consciousness can be elicited to assess wakefulness. Consciousness is assessed by obtaining the patient's response to verbal and painful stimuli. Determination of orientation to person, place, and time assesses mental alertness. Pupils are assessed for size, shape, equality, and reactivity. Asymmetry must be reported immediately.

Pupils are also assessed for constriction to a light source (parasympathetic innervation) or dilation (sympathetic innervation). Because parasympathetic fibers are present in the brainstem, pupils that are slow to react to light may indicate a brain stem injury. A "blown" pupil can be caused by compression of the third ocular nerve or transtentorial herniation. Bilateral fixed pupils can indicate midbrain involvement (see "Pupillary Function" in Chapter 27).

Neurologic assessments are ongoing throughout the patient's critical care stay as part of the initial shift assessment and as part of ongoing assessments to detect subtle deterioration. Serial assessments include monitoring hemodynamic status and ICP. The use of muscle relaxants and sedation for ICP control may mask neurologic signs in the patient with a severe head injury. In these situations, observations for changes in pupils and vital signs become extremely important. Newer shorter-acting sedatives with a very short half-life, such as propofol, can be turned off, and within minutes, a neurologic examination can be performed.

Diagnostic Procedures.

The cornerstone of diagnostic procedures for evaluation of TBI is the CT scan.[15] CT is a rapid, noninvasive procedure that can provide invaluable information about the presence of mass lesions and cerebral edema. Serial CT scans may be used over a period of several days to assess areas of contusion and ischemia and to detect delayed hematomas. A nurse must always remain with a TBI patient during a CT scan to provide continued observation and monitoring and during transport to and from the scanner. Transporting the patient, moving the patient from the bed to the CT table, and positioning the head flat during the CT scan are all stressful events and can cause severe increases in ICP. Continuous monitoring enables rapid intervention.

Electrophysiology studies can aid in ongoing assessments of neurologic function. Somatosensory evoked potentials may be used to evaluate injures deep in the brain structures to gain prognostic information.[15] MRI produces more detailed images of the brain and is useful in detecting more subtle injuries, hematomas, and cerebral edema (see Chapter 27).

Medical Management

Surgical Management. If a lesion identified on CT is causing a shift of intracranial contents or increasing ICP, surgical intervention is necessary. A craniotomy is performed to remove the EDH, SDH, or large ICH. Occasionally, if an area of contusion is large, hemorrhagic, and associated with an elevated ICP, a craniotomy for removal of the contused area may be performed to relieve pressure and prevent herniation. Patients who have had surgery for penetrating head trauma have an increased incidence of posttraumatic seizures, and they may receive anticonvulsants.

Nonsurgical Management. No longer is surgery the mainstay of treatment of TBIs Approximately 95% of management occurs in the intensive care unit.[15] Nonsurgical management includes management of ICP, maintenance of adequate cerebral perfusion pressure and oxygenation, and treatment of any complications (e.g., pneumonia, infection). The decision of when to initiate ICP monitoring is critical. ICP monitoring may be required for patients with a GCS score less than 8 and abnormal findings on a head CT scan.[17] Brain tissue oxygen monitoring may also be used.

Nursing Management. Nursing diagnoses for the patient with TBI are listed in the Nursing Diagnoses feature on Traumatic Brain Injury. Priority nursing goals include stabilization of vital signs, prevention of further injury, and reduction of increased ICP. Ongoing nursing assessments are the cornerstone to the care of patients with TBI. These assessments are the primary mechanism for determining secondary brain injury from cerebral edema and increased ICP. If secondary injury is to be prevented, the ICU nurse must respond immediately to hypotensive events and, in collaboration with physicians, maximize cerebral perfusion pressure through reduction of ICP and restoration of mean arterial pressure.[17]

All aspects of care, including hemodynamic management, pulmonary care, maintenance of body temperature, and control of the environment, can impact outcome after TBI.[17] Hemodynamic and fluid management are vital. Arterial blood pressure should be monitored because hypotension in a patient with TBI is rare and may indicate additional injuries. *Cerebral perfusion pressure* (CPP) should be maintained at a minimum of 60 mm Hg.[17] In the absence of cerebral ischemia, aggressive attempts to keep CPP above 70 mm Hg with intravenous fluids and vasopressors should be avoided secondary to the risk of ARDS.[17]

Close monitoring of hemodynamic status is of paramount importance in patients with TBI because in addition to fluid management, changes in cardiovascular function and circulating catecholamines contribute to hemodynamic instability.[15] Pulmonary artery catheterization may be required to optimize fluid status and cardiac output. Capnography (monitoring of exhaled carbon dioxide levels) is suggested to prevent inadvertent hypocapnia or hypercapnia.[15] Aggressive pulmonary care must be instituted. However, endotracheal suctioning can elevate ICU. Techniques to eliminate elevation in ICP with suctioning are outlined in Box 38-5. Cerebral oxygen consumption is increased during periods of increased body temperature, and therefore euthermia (36° to 37° C) may be achieved with early workup and intervention for infection, use of antipyretics, and cooling measures such as evaporative cooling.

In the early postinjury phase, the patient's environment must be controlled. Stimuli that produce pain, agitation, or discomfort can increase ICP. Analgesics and sedatives should be administered, and patients should be given rest periods.

After ICP stabilization, stimulation programs for patients in a coma may be employed. These programs provide stimulation to the tactile, kinesthetic, olfactory, gustatory, auditory, and visual senses. Several methods have been used to stimulate coma patients with various degrees of intensity:

- Intense Multisensory Stimulation Program: stimulatory cycles lasting approximately 15 to 20 minutes, repeated every hour for 12 to 14 hours per day, 6 days per week
- Formalized Not-Intensive Stimulation Program: cycles of stimulation of 10 to 60 minutes twice daily
- Sensory Regulation Program: single brief sessions of stimulation in a quiet environment completely free of noise[18]

Whatever program is used, a stimulation schedule should be established, and accurate documentation of the stimulus and response is essential. Coma stimulation programs should be individualized and family members encouraged to participate.

SPINAL CORD INJURIES

Approximately 12,000 new spinal cord injuries (SCIs) occur annually. Since 2005, the average age at injury has been 39.5 years.[19] This age has increased compared with data before 1980, likely as a result of the aging population.[19] Of the new cases of SCI each year, about 4000 patients will die before arrival to the hospital, and 1000 patients will die of complications of their SCI during hospitalization.[20] The diagnosis of SCI begins with a detailed history of events surrounding the incident, precise evaluation of sensory and motor function, and radiographic studies of the spine.

Mechanism of Injury. The type of primary injury sustained depends on the mechanism of injury. Mechanisms of injury can

---

Nursing Diagnoses

Traumatic Brain Injury

- Ineffective Breathing Pattern related to neuromuscular impairment, perceptual or cognitive impairment
- Risk for Aspiration risk factors: impaired laryngeal sensation or reflex; impaired pharyngeal peristalsis or tongue function; impaired laryngeal closure or elevation; increased gastric volume; decreased lower esophageal sphincter pressure
- Impaired Gas Exchange related to ventilation-perfusion mismatching
- Imbalanced Nutrition: Less Than Body Requirements related to lack of exogenous nutrients and increased metabolic demand
- Disturbed Sensory Perception related to altered sensory reception or transmission (neurologic trauma)
- Powerlessness related to lack of control over current situation
- Decreased Intracranial Adaptive Capacity related to failure of normal compensatory mechanisms
- Impaired Physical Mobility related to perceptual or cognitive impairment
- Ineffective Cerebral Tissue Perfusion related to hemorrhage, cerebral edema

---

BOX 38-5 RECOMMENDATIONS FOR SUCTIONING PATIENTS WITH TRAUMATIC BRAIN INJURY

- Pass the suction catheter for no longer than 10 seconds.
- Limit the number of suction catheter passes, preferably to no more than two passes per suctioning episode.
- Hyperoxygenate the patient before and after each passage of the suction catheter (e.g., deliver 4 ventilator breaths at 135% of the patient's tidal volume on 100% FiO_2, at a rate of 4 breaths in 20 seconds).
- Minimize airway stimulation (e.g., stabilize endotracheal tube, avoid passing the suction catheter all the way to the carina).

From McQuillan KA, Thurman P: Traumatic brain injuries. In McQuillan K et al, editors: *Trauma: from resuscitation through rehabilitation.* St. Louis, 2009, p 491, Elsevier.

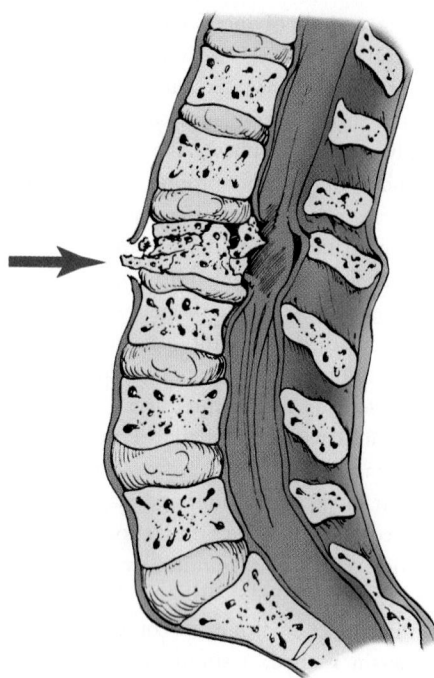

Figure 38-5 Spinal cord compression burst fracture. Compression injuries cause burst fractures of the vertebral body that often send bony fragments into the spinal canal or directly into the spinal cord.

Nursing Diagnoses

Spinal Cord Injury

- Decreased Cardiac Output related to lack of sympathetic innervation
- Risk for Autonomic Dysreflexia related to spinal cord injury above T6
- Impaired Gas Exchange related to alveolar hypoventilation
- Ineffective Breathing Pattern related to impairment of innervation of diaphragm (lesion above C5), complete or mixed loss of intercostal muscle function
- Impaired Physical Mobility related to neuromuscular impairment, immobilization by traction, paralysis
- Risk for Impaired Skin Integrity related to immobility, traction, tissue pressure, altered peripheral circulation, and sensation
- Bowel Incontinence related to disruption of innervation to bowel and rectum, perceptual impairment, altered fluid and food intake
- Constipation related to disruption of innervation to bowel and rectum, perceptual impairment, altered fluid and food intake
- Impaired Urinary Elimination related to disruption in bladder innervation, bladder atony
- Disturbed Body Image related to actual change in body structure, function, or appearance
- Ineffective Coping related to situational crisis and personal vulnerability

---

include hyperflexion, hyperextension, rotation, axial loading (vertical compression), and missile or penetrating injuries.

Hyperflexion. Hyperflexion injury most often is seen in the cervical area, especially at the level of C5 to C6, because this is the most mobile portion of the cervical spine. This type of injury most often is caused by sudden deceleration motion, as in head-on collisions. Injury occurs from compression of the cord as a result of fracture fragments or dislocation of the vertebral bodies. Instability of the spinal column occurs because of the rupture or tearing of the posterior muscles and ligaments.

Hyperextension. Hyperextension injuries involve backward and downward motion of the head. With this injury, often seen in rear-end collisions or MVCs, the spinal cord is stretched and distorted. Neurologic deficits associated with this injury are often caused by contusion and ischemia of the cord without significant bony involvement. A mild form of hyperextension is the *whiplash* injury.

Rotation. Rotation injuries often occur in conjunction with a flexion or extension injury. Severe rotation of the neck or body results in tearing of the posterior ligaments and displacement (rotation) of the spinal column.

Axial Loading. Axial loading, or vertical compression, injuries occur from vertical force along the spinal cord. This most commonly is seen in a fall from a height in which the person lands on the feet or buttocks. Compression injuries cause burst fractures of the vertebral body that often send bony fragments into the spinal canal or directly into the spinal cord (Fig. 38-5).

Penetrating Injuries. Penetrating injury to the spinal cord can be caused by a bullet, knife, or any other object that penetrates the cord. These types of injury cause permanent damage by anatomically transecting the spinal cord.

Pathophysiology. SCIs are the result of a mechanical force that disrupts neurologic tissue or its vascular supply, or both. Much like the pathophysiology of TBI, the injury process includes primary and secondary injury mechanisms. Primary injury is the neurologic damage that occurs at the moment of impact. Secondary injury refers to the complex biochemical processes affecting cellular function. Secondary injury can occur within minutes of injury and can last for days to weeks.[20]

Several events after an SCI lead to spinal cord ischemia and loss of neurologic function. A cascade of events is initiated that includes systemic and local vascular changes, electrolyte and biochemical changes, neurotransmitter accumulation, and local edema (Box 38-6). Collectively, these pathophysiologic events result in worsening of the injury, potentially extending the level of functional deficit and worsening long-term outcome.[20] Knowledge of the pathophysiology of secondary processes has led to the development of new drugs, which target the cellular changes contributing to injury.[20] Despite ongoing research efforts at repairing the primary injury, minimizing damage by reducing secondary injury has shown the most promise.

Functional Injury of the Spinal Cord. Functional injury of the spinal cord refers to the degree of disruption of normal spinal cord function. This depends on what specific sensory and motor structures within the cord are damaged. SCIs are classified as complete or incomplete (see the Nursing Diagnoses feature on Spinal Cord Injury). Since 2000, the most frequent category at discharge has been incomplete tetraplegia (34.1%) followed by complete tetraplegia.[19] SCI cannot be classified until spinal shock has resolved.

BOX 38-6 PRIMARY AND SECONDARY MECHANISMS OF ACUTE SPINAL CORD INJURY

PRIMARY INJURY MECHANISMS
- Acute compression
- Impact
- Missile
- Distraction
- Laceration
- Shear

SECONDARY INJURY MECHANISMS
- Systemic effects
- Heart rate: brief increase, then prolonged bradycardia
- Blood pressure: brief hypertension, then prolonged hypotension
- Decreased
- Peripheral resistance
- Decreased cardiac output
- Increased catecholamines, then decreased
- Hypoxia
- Hyperthermia
- Injudicious movement of the unstable spine leading to worsening compression
- Local vascular changes
- Loss of autoregulation
- Systemic hypotension (neurogenic shock)
- Hemorrhage (especially gray matter)
- Loss of microcirculation

- Reduction in blood flow
- Vasospasm
- Thrombosis
- Electrolyte changes
- Increased intracellular calcium
- Increased intracellular sodium
- Increased sodium permeability
- Increased intracellular potassium

BIOCHEMICAL CHANGES
- Neurotransmitter accumulation
- Catecholamines (e.g., norepinephrine, dopamine)
- Excitotoxic amino acids (e.g., glutamate)
- Arachidonic acid release
- Free radical production
- Eicosanoid production
- Prostaglandins
- Lipid peroxidation
- Endogenous opioids
- Cytokines
- Edema
- Loss of energy metabolism
- Decreased adenosine triphosphate production
- Apoptosis

Adapted from Sekhon LHS, Fehlings MG: Epidemiology, demographics, and pathophysiology of acute spinal cord injury. *Spine* 26(24S):S2-S12, 2001.

Complete Injury. Complete SCI results in a total loss of sensory and motor function below the level of injury. Regardless of the mechanism of injury, the result is a complete dissection of the spinal cord and its neurochemical pathways, resulting in one of two conditions: tetraplegia or paraplegia.

Tetraplegia. With tetraplegia, the injury occurs from the C1 to T1 level. Residual muscle function depends on the specific cervical segments involved. The potential functional status resulting from different neurologic levels of injury is described in Table 38-5.

Paraplegia. With paraplegia, the injury occurs in the thoracolumbar region (T2 to L1). Patients with injuries in this area may have full use of the arms and may need a wheelchair, although some may have limited ability to ambulate short distances with crutches and orthoses. Thoracic L1 and L2 injuries produce paraplegia with variable innervation to intercostal and abdominal muscles.

Incomplete Injury. Incomplete SCI results in a mixed loss of voluntary motor activity and sensation below the level of the lesion. Incomplete SCI exists if any function remains below the level of injury. Incomplete injuries can result in a variety of syndromes, which are classified according to the degree of motor and sensory loss below the level of injury. Some of the more common syndromes are described here.

Brown-Séquard Syndrome. The Brown-Séquard syndrome is associated with damage to only one side of the cord. This produces loss of voluntary motor movement on the same side

TABLE 38-5 Quadriplegia Functional Status

Neurologic Level (Vertebrae) of Complete Injury	Functional Ability
C1-C4	Requires electric wheelchair with breath, head, or shoulder controls
C5	Needs electric wheelchair with hand control and/or manual wheelchair with rim projections; may require adaptive devices to assist with ADLs
C6	Independent in manual wheelchair on level surface; may need hand controls; adaptive devices may be needed for ADLs
C7	Requires manual wheelchair on most surfaces
C8-T1	May need adaptive devices

ADLs, activities of daily living.

as the injury, with loss of pain, temperature, and sensation on the opposite side. Functionally, the side of the body with the best motor control has little or no sensation, whereas the side of the body with sensation has little or no motor control.

Central Cord Syndrome. Central cord syndrome is associated with cervical hyperextension-hyperflexion injury and hematoma formation in the center of the cervical cord. This injury produces a motor and sensory deficit more pronounced in the upper extremities than in the lower extremities. Various degrees of bowel and bladder dysfunction may be present.

Anterior Cord Syndrome. The anterior cord syndrome is associated with injury to the anterior gray horn cells (motor), the spinothalamic tracts (pain), anterior spinothalamic tract (light touch), and the corticospinal tracts (temperature). The result is a loss of motor function and loss of the sensations of pain and temperature below the level of injury. However, below the level of injury, position sense and sensations of pressure and vibrations remain intact. Anterior cord syndrome is commonly caused by flexion injuries or acute herniation of an intervertebral disk.

Posterior Cord Syndrome. Posterior cord syndrome is associated with cervical hyperextension injury with damage to the posterior column. This results in the loss of position sense, pressure, and vibration below the level of injury. Motor function and sensation of pain and temperature remain intact. These patients may not be able to ambulate because the loss of position sense impairs spontaneous movement.

Spinal Shock. Spinal shock is a condition that can occur shortly after traumatic injury to the spinal cord. Spinal shock is the complete loss of all muscle tone and normal reflex activity below the level of injury.[9] Patients with spinal shock may appear completely without function below the area of the injury, although all of the area may not necessarily be destroyed.

Neurogenic Shock. Neurogenic shock results from injury to the descending sympathetic pathways in the spinal cord. This results from loss of vasomotor tone and sympathetic innervation to the heart. A relative hypovolemia and hypovolemic shock ensues, causing hypotension and decreased systemic vascular resistance. Patients with SCI at T6 or above may have profound neurogenic shock as a result of interruption of the sympathetic nervous system and loss of vasoconstrictor response below the level of the injury. Blood vessels cannot constrict, and the heart rate is slow, which results in hypotension, venous pooling, and decreased cardiac output. Cellular oxygenation is threatened as cardiac output declines because of a decrease in stroke volume (hypovolemia) and heart rate (bradycardia). The duration of this shock state can persist for up to 1 month after injury. Blood pressure support may be required with the use of sympathomimetic drugs. Because hypotension is a problem, the nurse must be cautious when adjusting backrest position or when repositioning a patient in bed because orthostatic blood pressure changes can occur (see "Neurogenic Shock" in Chapter 39).

Autonomic Dysreflexia. Autonomic dysreflexia is a life-threatening complication that may occur with SCI. This condition is caused by a massive sympathetic response to a noxious stimuli (e.g., full bladder, line insertions, fecal impaction) that results in bradycardia, hypertension, facial flushing, and headache. Immediate intervention is needed to prevent cerebral hemorrhage, seizures, and acute pulmonary edema. Treatment is aimed at alleviating the noxious stimuli. A clinical algorithm for treatment of autonomic dysreflexia is provided in Box 38-7.[21] If symptoms persist, antihypertensive agents can

BOX 38-7   AUTONOMIC DYSREFLEXIA

- If patient is supine, immediately sit the patient up.
- Begin frequent vital sign monitoring, and perform every 5 minutes.
- Survey for instigating causes; begin with urinary system.
- Loosen clothing, constrictive devices.
- If indwelling catheter is not placed, catheterize the patient.
  - Lidocaine jelly may be instilled 5 minutes before catheter insertion.
- If indwelling catheter is present, do the following:
  - Check system for kinks and obstructions to flow.
  - Irrigate the bladder with small sterile amount of fluid, utilizing strict aseptic technique.
  - If not draining, remove the catheter and replace.
- If systolic blood pressure is greater than 150 mm Hg, consider rapid-onset, short-duration antihypertensive agent.
- If acute symptoms persist, suspect fecal impaction:
  - Instill lidocaine jelly into rectum; wait at least 5 minutes.
  - Perform digital examination to check for presence of stool; if present, gently remove. If signs of autonomic dysreflexia persist, stop examination; instill additional lidocaine jelly, and wait 20 minutes to re-examine.
- If no stool is found and the abdomen is distended, consider administration of laxative.

be administered to reduce blood pressure. Prevention of autonomic dysreflexia is imperative and can be accomplished through the use of a good bowel and bladder program.

Assessment. On admission to the ICU, attention to the ABCs is imperative in the patient with known or suspected SCI. Stabilization of the spinal cord is mandatory to prevent further injury, and spinal precautions are maintained until the spine is cleared of injury. Stabilization in the ICU may include the use of bed rest with log-rolling maneuvers and a hard cervical collar until definitive stabilization is achieved. After the ABCs have been evaluated and interventions for life-threatening complications have been initiated, a full physical assessment is made to determine the extent of injury.

Airway. Assessment of ABCs is essential to ensure optimal oxygenation and perfusion to all vital organs, including the spinal cord. Complete cardiovascular and respiratory assessments are essential to the patient's survival and prognosis. The primary assessment begins with an evaluation of airway clearance. In an unresponsive person, an oral airway is inserted while the patient's neck is maintained in a neutral position. The patient must undergo intubation before severe hypoxia can occur, which could further damage the spinal cord.

Breathing. Assessment of breathing patterns and gas exchange is made after an airway has been secured. The level of injury dictates the degree of altered breathing patterns and gas exchange (Table 38-6). Because complete injuries above the C3 level result in paralysis of the diaphragm, patients with these injuries require ventilatory assistance.

Circulation. Assessment of cardiac output and tissue perfusion is imperative to detect life-threatening injuries and promote recovery of injured spinal cord tissue. The patient with SCI is at high risk for developing alterations in cardiac output

TABLE 38-6 **Effects of Spinal Cord Injury on Ventilatory Functions**

Neurologic Level (Vertebrae) of Complete Injury	Respiratory Function	Comment
C1-C2	Paralysis of diaphragm	Ventilator dependent
C3-C5	Various degrees of diaphragm paralysis	Some diaphragm control; may need ventilatory support; weaning depends on preinjury pulmonary status
C6-T11	Various degrees of impaired intercostal muscles and abdominal muscles	Compromised respiratory function; reduced inspiratory ability; paradoxical breathing patterns; ineffective cough, sneeze

Modified from Moore EE et al: Organ injury scaling, *Surg Clin North Am* 74:293-303, 1995.

TABLE 38-7 **Muscle Strength Scale**

Active movement against maximal resistance
Active movement through range of motion against resistance
Active movement through range of motion against gravity
Active movement through range of motion with gravity eliminated
Flicker or trace of contraction
No contraction; total paralysis

and tissue perfusion because the cardiovascular system is subjected to a variety of serious and potential physiologic alterations, including dysrhythmias, cardiac arrest, orthostatic hypotension, emboli, and thrombophlebitis.

The patient with an SCI is assessed for adequate tissue perfusion by means of invasive and noninvasive hemodynamic monitoring techniques. Cardiac monitoring is required to detect bradycardia and other dysrhythmias that occur in response to reflex vagus activity mediated by the dominant parasympathetic nervous system, as well as changes in cardiac rhythm as a result of hypothermia or hypoxia.

Neurologic Assessment for Spinal Cord Injury. The initial neurologic assessment may not be an accurate indication of eventual motor and sensory loss. It focuses on the rapid and accurate identification of present, absent, or impaired functioning of the motor, sensory, and reflex systems that coordinate and regulate vital functions. A detailed motor and sensory examination includes the assessment of all 32 spinal nerves for evidence of dysfunction. Carefully mapped pathways for the sensory portion of the spinal nerves, called *dermatomes,* can assist in localizing the functional sensory level of injury. Motor function may be graded on a 6-point scale (Table 38-7). Initial assessment must be performed correctly and findings thoroughly documented in detail so that subsequent serial assessments can rapidly identify deterioration. The American Spinal Injury Association (ASIA) has developed a form that outlines the required assessments for initial and ongoing classification of SCIs (Fig. 38-6). Ongoing spinal cord assessments must be documented during the critical care phase.

Diagnostic Procedures. Diagnostic radiographic evaluations can identify the severity of damage to the spinal cord. Initial evaluation includes anteroposterior and lateral views for all areas of the spinal cord. CT scan of all seven cervical vertebrae and the top of T1 must be obtained to rule out cervicothoracic junction injury. Flexion and extension views can identify subtle ligament injuries. CT, tomography, myelography, and MRI also may be used.

Screening for Spinal Cord Injury. About 15% of trauma patients with an SCI have a cervical spine injury.[15] Screening of the spinal cord for injury becomes an integral part of the assessment for all trauma patients. The degree of trauma, alteration in mentation, intoxication, and distracting injuries dictate the type and extent of examination required to clear the cervical spine. The Eastern Association of Surgeons in Trauma (EAST) developed guidelines for the clearance of the cervical spine (Table 38-8). In these guidelines CT scan has replaced plain radiography as the principal modality for cervical spine assessment following trauma. On admission, the spine is palpated for obvious deformity, and the patient is assessed for the subjective response of pain to palpation. If the patient has distracting injuries, such as rib fractures, is intoxicated, or has received analgesics, examination of the spinal cord may be deferred.[15] MRI may be warranted to definitively diagnose an SCI when the patient is stabilized.

Medical Management. After assessment and diagnosis of the SCI, medical management begins. The primary treatment goal is to preserve remaining neurologic function with pharmacologic, surgical, and nonsurgical interventions.

Pharmacologic Management. Methylprednisolone can improve neurologic outcome after SCI, although it has been called into question because of the infection risk in these patients.[21] Current guidelines cite the use of methylprednisolone as an option for the management of acute cervical spine injury.[22] When it is used, patients receive a methylprednisolone bolus followed by a continuous infusion for at least 24 hours (preferably 48 hours) if their treatment began 3 to 8 hours after their injury.[22] Although the exact mechanism is not completely understood, it is thought that methylprednisolone directly affects the changes that occur within the spinal cord after injury, primarily by preventing posttraumatic spinal cord ischemia, improving energy metabolism, restoring extracellular calcium, and improving nerve impulse conduction.

Surgical Management. Surgical intervention provides spinal column stability in the presence of an unstable injury.

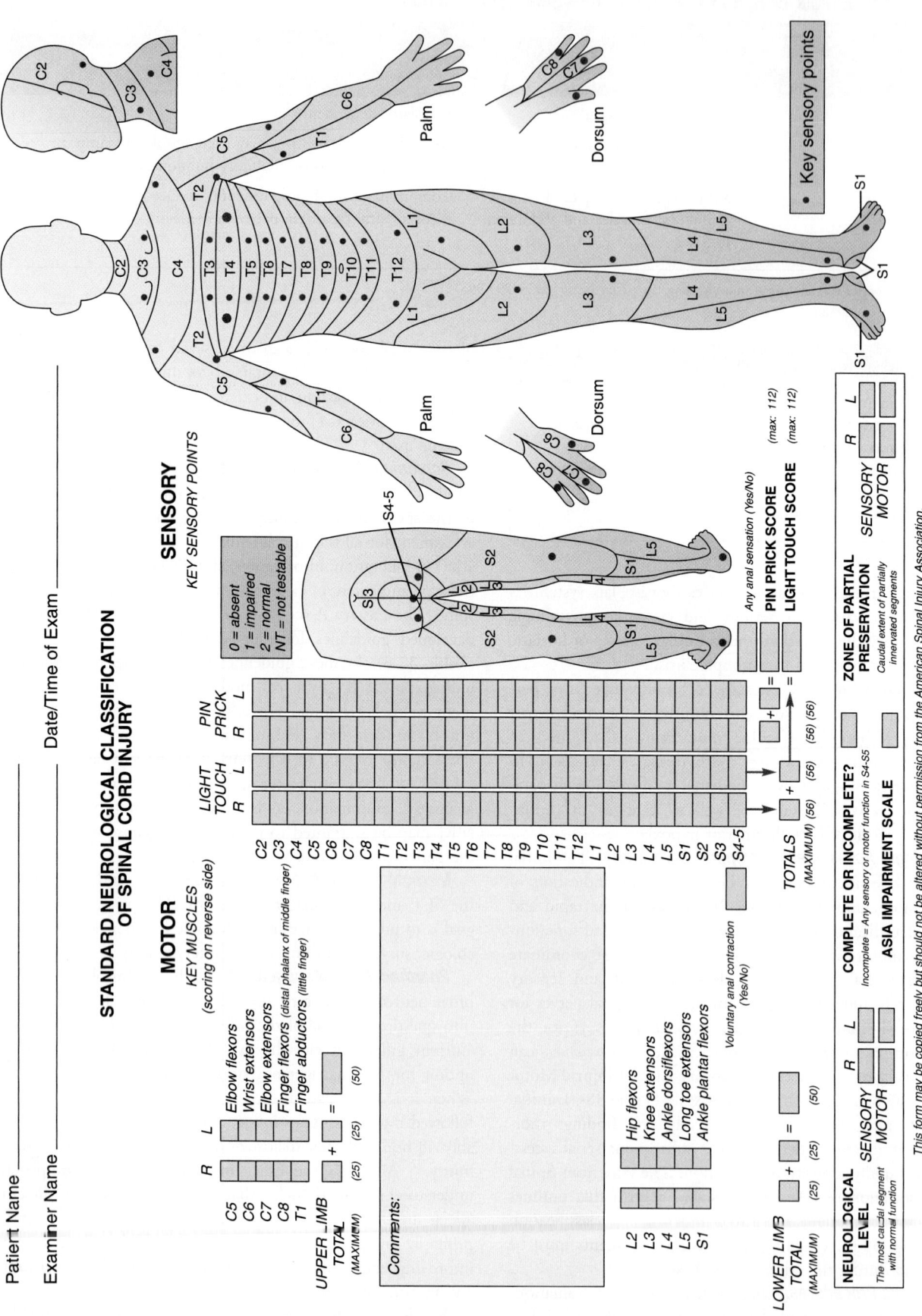

Figure 38-6 American Spinal Injury Association classification of spinal cord injuries.

MUSCLE GRADING

0 total paralysis

1 palpable or visible contraction

2 active movement, full range of motion, gravity eliminated

3 active movement, full range of motion, against gravity

4 active movement, full range of motion, against gravity and provides some resistance

5 active movement, full range of motion, against gravity and provides normal resistance

5* muscle able to exert, in examiner's judgement, sufficient resistance to be considered normal if identifiable inhibiting factors were not present

NT not testable. Patient unable to reliably exert effort or muscle unavailable for testing due to factors such as immobilization, pain on effort or contracture.

ASIA IMPAIRMENT SCALE

☐ **A = Complete:** No motor or sensory function is preserved in the sacral segments S4-S5.

☐ **B = Incomplete:** Sensory but not motor function is preserved below the neurological level and includes the sacral segments S4-S5.

☐ **C = Incomplete:** Motor function is preserved below the neurological level, and more than half of key muscles below the neurological level have a muscle grade less than 3.

☐ **D = Incomplete:** Motor function is preserved below the neurological level, and at least half of key muscles below the neurological level have a muscle grade of 3 or more.

☐ **E = Normal:** Motor and sensory function are normal.

CLINICAL SYNDROMES (OPTIONAL)

☐ Central Cord
☐ Brown-Sequard
☐ Anterior Cord
☐ Conus Medullaris
☐ Cauda Equina

STEPS IN CLASSIFICATION

The following order is recommended in determining the classification of individuals with SCI.

1. Determine sensory levels for right and left sides.

2. Determine motor levels for right and left sides.
   Note: in regions where there is no myotome to test, the motor level is presumed to be the same as the sensory level.

3. Determine the single neurological level.
   This is the lowest segment where motor and sensory function is normal on both sides, and is the most cephalad of the sensory and motor levels determined in steps 1 and 2.

4. Determine whether the injury is Complete or Incomplete. (sacral sparing).
   *If voluntary anal contraction = **No** AND all S4-5 sensory scores = **0** AND any anal sensation = **No**, then injury is COMPLETE. Otherwise injury is incomplete.*

5. Determine ASIA Impairment Scale (AIS) Grade:
   Is injury Complete? If **YES**, AIS=A Record ZPP
          (For ZPP record lowest dermatome or myotome on each side with some (non-zero score) preservation)
   NO ↓
   Is injury motor incomplete? If **NO**, AIS=B
   YES ↓
       (Yes=voluntary anal contraction OR motor function more than three levels below the motor level on a given side.)

   Are at least half of the key muscles below the (single) neurological level graded 3 or better?
   NO ↓   YES ↓
   AIS=C   AIS=D

   If sensation and motor function is normal in all segments, AIS=E
   Note: AIS E is used in follow up testing when an individual with a documented SCI has recovered normal function. If at initial testing no deficits are found, the individual is neurologically intact; the ASIA Impairment Scale does not apply.

Figure 38-6, cont'd

TABLE 38-8 EAST Guidelines for Cervical Spine Clearance

Trauma Patient Population	Recommendation
Trauma patients that are awake, alert, not intoxicated, neurologically normal, no complaints of neck pain or tenderness with full range of motion of the cervical spine.	Neck is palpated in all directions for tenderness or pain. If physical examination is negative for pain or tenderness, CT imaging of the cervical spine is not required and the cervical collar may be removed.
All other trauma patients with suspected cervical injury must be radiologically evaluated. This includes patients with neck pain or tenderness, whether alert or with altered mental status / neurological deficit, or distracting injury.	Axial CT from occiput to T1 with sagital and coronal reconstructions. If CT is positive for injury, continue cervical collar, obtain spine consultation and obtain MRI. In the neurologically intact awake patient with neck pain, if the CT is negative (no injury seen), MRI is negative, and adequate flexion/extension films are negative, discontinue cervical collar.
Trauma patients that are obtunded with gross motor function of extremities	Axial CT from occiput to T1 with sagital and coronal reconstructions. If the CT is negative (no injury seen), the risk/benefit of an additional MRI, must be determined in each hospital. Options are: A. Continue cervical collar until a clinical exam can be performed. B. Remove the cervical collar on the basis of negative CT alone. C. Obtain MRI. If MRI is negative collar can be safely removed. Flexion/Extension radiography should not be performed.

CT, computed tomography; MRI, magnetic resonance imaging; EAST, Eastern Association of Surgeons in Trauma.

Eastern Association of Surgeons in Trauma: EAST guidelines: determination of cervical spine stability in trauma patients, Chicago, Eastern Association of Surgeons in Trauma, 2000. Available at www.east.org/tpg/cspine2009.pdf (accessed May 2009).

Unstable injuries include disrupted ligaments and tendons and a vertebral column that cannot maintain normal alignment. Identification and immobilization of unstable injuries are particularly important for the patient with incomplete neurologic deficit. Without adequate stabilization, movement and dislocation of the vertebral column may cause a complete neurologic deficit. A variety of surgical procedures may be performed to achieve decompression and stabilization. The question of when surgery should be performed remains controversial.

Laminectomy. The laminectomy procedure is the removal of the lamina of the vertebral ring to allow decompression and removal of bony fragments or disk material from the spinal canal.

Spinal Fusion. Spinal fusion entails the surgical fusion of two to six vertebral elements to provide stability and to prevent motion. Fusion is accomplished through the use of bone parts or bone chips taken from the iliac crest or by use of wire or acrylic glue.

Rodding. The rodding procedure stabilizes and realigns larger segments of the spinal column by means of a variety of rodding procedures, such as the use of Harrington rods. The rods are attached by screws and glue to the posterior elements of the spinal column. These types of procedures most often are performed to stabilize the thoracolumbar area.

Nonsurgical Management. If the injury to the spinal cord is stable, nonsurgical management is the treatment of choice. Nonsurgical management for cervical and thoracolumbar injuries is discussed in the following sections.

Cervical Injury. Management of cervical injuries involves the immobilization of the fracture site and realignment of any dislocation. This is accomplished through skeletal traction that involves the use of two-point tongs, which are inserted into the skull through shallow burr holes and are connected to traction weights. Several types of cervical tongs are used. Gardner-Wells and Crutchfield tongs are the most common. These tongs can be applied at the bedside with the use of a local anesthetic.

After the procedure, the patient can be immobilized on a kinetic therapy bed or a regular bed. The kinetic therapy bed is the most popular method used for cervical immobilization because it maintains spinal column alignment while providing constant turning motion to reduce pulmonary and skin breakdown. Use of cervical skeletal traction on a regular bed makes it difficult to provide adequate care to the pulmonary system and skin because of the extensive degree of immobility.

After the spinal column has been adequately realigned by means of skeletal traction, a halo traction brace often is applied. The halo vest consists of a metal ring secured to the skull with two occipital and two temporal screws. Steel bars anchor the screws to the vest to provide cervical immobilization (Fig. 38-7). The halo traction brace immobilizes the cervical spine, which allows the patient to ambulate and participate in self-care.

Thoracolumbar Injury. Nonsurgical management of the patient with a thoracolumbar injury also involves immobilization. Skeletal traction may be used in high thoracic injury. For the most part, misalignment of the spinal canal does not occur in stable injuries of the thoracolumbar spine. Immobilization to allow fractures to heal is accomplished by bed rest (with the bed flat) and the use of a plastic or fiberglass jacket, a body cast, or a brace.

Nursing Management. Nursing diagnoses and management for the patient with SCI are summarized in the Nursing

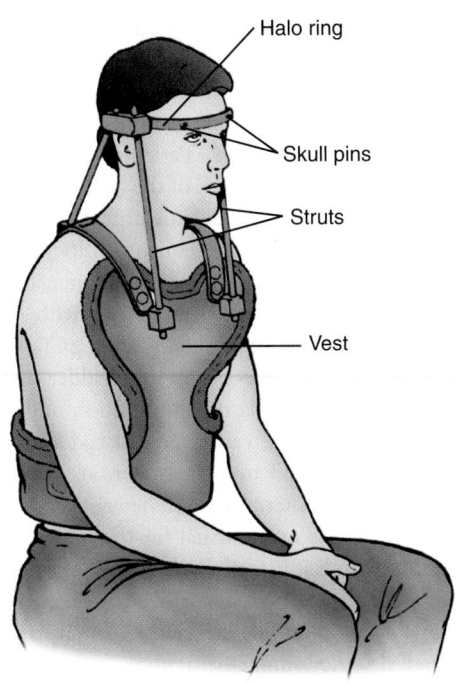

Halo ring

Skull pins

Struts

Vest

Figure 38-7 Halo vest. The halo traction brace immobilizes the cervical spine, which allows the patient to ambulate and participate in self-care.

Diagnoses feature on Spinal Cord Injury. The goal during the critical care phase is to prevent life-threatening complications while maximizing the function of all organ systems. Nursing interventions are aimed at preventing secondary damage to the spinal cord and managing the complications of the neurologic deficit. Because almost all body systems are affected by SCI, nursing management must include interventions that optimize nutrition, elimination, skin integrity, and mobility. Patients with SCIs have complex psychosocial needs that require a great deal of emotional support from the critical care nurse.

Cardiovascular Complications. The risk for cardiovascular instability is profound in patients with SCI at the C3 to C5 levels, although cardiovascular alterations can occur with most injuries above T6. Alteration in tissue perfusion because of hypotension may require the administration of intravenous fluids. Like management of TBI, the management of acute cervical SCI involves close hemodynamic monitoring. The guidelines for the management of acute cervical SCI cite as an option that hypotension (systolic blood pressure <90 mm Hg) should be avoided if possible or corrected as soon as possible after acute SCI.[22] It is also considered an option to maintain the mean arterial blood pressure at 85 to 90 mm Hg for the first 7 days after acute SCI to improve spinal cord perfusion.[22]

Astute assessment of fluid volume is required because pulmonary edema is a threat to SCI patients. Pulmonary artery catheterization may be required to assess for this complication. After the fluid volume status has been optimized, inotropic or vasopressor support, or both, may be implemented.

Another consequence of sympathetic nervous system dysfunction is loss of thermoregulation (poikilothermy), in which body temperature is regulated by the external environment. Judicious use of heat or cold for therapeutic or comfort measures is required. Profound changes in body temperature must be avoided. Hypothermia can produce bradydysrhythmias and sinus arrest. This is of concern when the patient has symptoms. Symptomatic bradydysrhythmias may be treated with inotropic drugs such as isoproterenol, or the anticholinergic drug atropine. Both medications increase the heart rate but also increase myocardial oxygen consumption. Another option is a temporary transvenous or transcutaneous pacemaker. Before antipyretics are given or a cooling blanket is used, the environment must be assessed for potential causes of hyperthermia or hypothermia.

After a prolonged period of bed rest, orthostatic hypotension may become a significant problem. It may be helpful when initially mobilizing the patient with an SCI to gradually elevate the head of the bed and dangle the legs over the side of the bed. The incidence of orthostatic hypotension may be reduced by leg elevation, antiembolic hose, or an abdominal binder.[21] As with any immobilized patient, the risk for development of deep vein thrombosis (DVT) is high. However, detection of DVT is difficult because pain and tenderness are not applicable to the patient with an SCI. Prevention of DVT is imperative and may include a combination of therapies such as low-dose heparin, low-molecular-weight heparin, sequential compression devices, and embolic hose.

Pulmonary Complications. Pulmonary complications are the most common cause of mortality in SCI patients.[19] Initial and ongoing nursing assessments of respiratory status are imperative for identifying actual or potential impairment in ventilation. These evaluations include observation of respiratory rate and rhythm, observation of symmetry of chest expansion and use of accessory muscles, inspection of quantity and character of secretions, and auscultation of breath sounds. Judicious use of serial arterial blood gas (ABG) values provides information on the adequacy of gas exchange.

Depending on the level of SCI, the patient's breathing pattern may be ineffective (see Table 38-6). Intubation and mechanical ventilation may be required. Patients with lesions at C3 to C5 may be able to be weaned from mechanical ventilation. Some patients with C3 injuries may require mechanical ventilation only at night. Weaning can be a complex process because of physical requirements of the diaphragm and the psychological effects of the fear of the inability to breathe. A variety of weaning methods are available, but a well-coordinated approach by the nurse, physician, respiratory therapist, and patient is essential (see "Invasive Mechanical Ventilation" in Chapter 25). Setbacks are common and reintubation may be required. The critical care nurse must be aware that the neuromuscular blocking agent *succinylcholine* (Suxamethonium) must never be administered to an SCI patient any time after 72 hours post-injury. Use of this depolarizing agent can produce hyperkalemic arrest.

Alternative modes of ventilation may include the *pneumobelt*. The corset-like device produces ventilation by assisting with expiration. Another assist device is the abdominal binder. It is thought to support the sagging diaphragm in patients with higher-level SCI with loss of abdominal muscle innervation.

Ineffective airway clearance is a particular problem for the SCI patient as a result of hypoventilation (paralysis of respiratory muscles), increased bronchial secretions, and atelectasis secondary to decreased cough. Frequent suctioning for airway clearance is required. Caution must be used with vigorous suctioning because stimulation of the unopposed vagus nerve (which runs alongside the trachea) can cause profound bradycardia. Bradycardia exacerbated by hypoxia is likely to develop in patients with cervical SCI. Use of hyperventilation breaths with 100% oxygen before suctioning may help. Chest percussion and drainage facilitate removal of secretions. Kinetic therapy beds, which can rotate up to 60 degrees on each side, may provide continual postural drainage and mobilization of secretions. To further aid in mobilizing secretions in the presence of an ineffective cough, a technique of cough assistance can be used (Fig. 38-8). This procedure is similar to abdominal thrusts (formerly known as the Heimlich maneuver). Exact hand placement may vary, and it is important to assess which placement works best for the patient.

Impaired gas exchange can occur in the SCI patient as a result of hypoventilation (paralysis of respiratory muscles), increased bronchial secretions that interfere with adequate gas diffusion, shunting resulting from atelectasis and associated pulmonary injuries, and pulmonary complications (pulmonary embolism). Nursing interventions are directed at improving and maintaining adequate gas exchange.

Musculoskeletal Complications. Immobilized patients are at high risk for contractures. When a muscle is denervated, as in the case of SCI, the muscle fibers shorten and produce a contracture. Irreversible contractures may result in skin breakdown, inability to perform activities of daily living, poor wheelchair posture, and inability to use adaptive devices.[21] Physical therapy and occupational therapy personnel should be consulted early in the patient's ICU course. Range-of-motion exercises are initiated as soon as the spine has been stabilized. Footdrop splints should be applied on admission to prevent contractures and prevent skin breakdown of the heels.[21] Hand splints should be applied for quadriplegics. Hand and foot splints should be removed every 2 hours. Nursing management of the patient in a halo vest includes inspection of pins and traction for

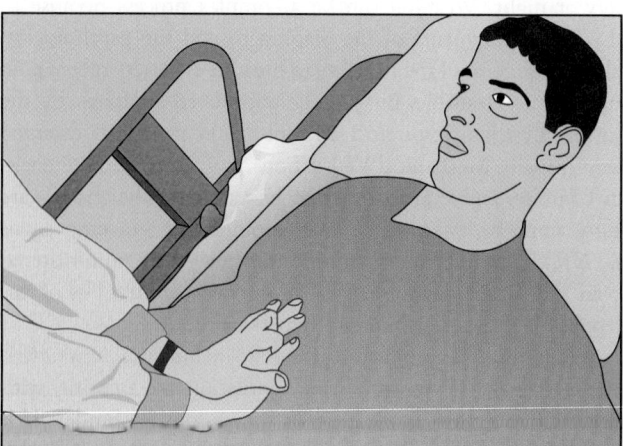

Figure 38-8 Cough assistance. A hand or both hands are placed over the upper diaphragm. After the patient inhales, pressure is directed inward and upward as the patient attempts to cough.

security, correct positioning and turning (traction bars or the halo ring must never be used to lift or reposition the patient), placement of wrenches on the front of the vest in case of cardiac arrest, and maintenance of skin integrity inside the halo vest.

Integumentary Complications. Patients with an SCI are at high risk for pressure ulcers because of the lack of motor control and sensation. Prevention is the best treatment. Diligent assessments, meticulous skin care, and frequent position changes are required. Specialty surfaces or low-air-loss beds may be necessary for the prevention of pressure ulcers in patients with an SCI.[21]

Elimination Complications. Initially after SCI, bowel and bladder tone are flaccid. The degree of bladder and urinary sphincter dysfunction depends on the location and completeness of the injury. A Foley catheter is placed on admission, but it should be removed 3 to 4 days later, at which time the patient is placed on an intermittent catheterization schedule of every 4 to 6 hours. It is not unusual for the male patient with an upper motor neuron injury to experience a reflexogenic erection when being catheterized.[21] An overdistended bladder in the patient with an injury at T6 or above may trigger autonomic dysreflexia. Abdominal distention, constipation, and fecal impaction are major problems encountered in care of the SCI patient. Innervation between the brain and defecation center in the sacral cord has been disrupted. A bowel program to prevent fecal impaction and encourage normal, regular bowel function must be instituted. The patient should not go longer than 3 to 4 days without a bowel movement. Laxatives and stool softeners may be needed, especially if the patient is receiving opiates. Aspects of a successful bowel program include consistent timing of evacuation, proper positioning, physical activity, appropriate fluid intake, a high-fiber diet, and reflex stimulation for those with upper motor neuron injuries.[21]

Maximizing Psychosocial Adaptation. Nursing management of the patient with SCI must include the provision of dedicated emotional support. In the critical care unit, the patient and family experience anxiety, grief, denial, anger, frustration, and hopelessness, because long-term neurologic deficits remain unknown.

Nursing interventions include the promotion of coping mechanisms, support systems, and adaptive skills. Simple, accurate, and consistent information can alleviate fear and anxiety. Feelings of powerlessness may be reduced by including the patient and family in care and decision making. Further psychosocial support can be given by social workers, occupational therapists, psychiatric clinical nurse specialists, and pastors.

MAXILLOFACIAL INJURIES

Trauma to the face results in complex physiologic and psychological sequelae. Vital functions that depend on facial integrity include mastication, deglutination, perception of the environment (e.g., vision, hearing, speech, olfaction), and respiration. The face also represents a direct link to self and to expression by playing a major role in personal identity, appearance, and communication. Consequently, maxillofacial trauma has the potential to produce long-term sequelae, with emotional, sensory, and disfigurement implications.

Mechanism of Injury. Maxillofacial injury results from blunt or penetrating trauma. Blunt trauma may occur from motor vehicle, industrial, or athletic injuries; violent blows to the head; or falls. The mechanism for this injury is exemplified by the unbelted driver or passenger who is thrown into the dashboard or windshield. Associated injuries may include concussion, skull fracture, rhinorrhea, SCI, and fractures of other bones. The facial skeleton serves as an energy-absorbing shield to protect the brain, spinal cord, eyes, and pharynx. Nasal bones, the zygoma, and the mandibular condyle are the most susceptible to fracture. Bullet wounds can be life-threatening injuries because of hemorrhage and airway obstruction. Maxillofacial trauma can result in soft tissue injury ranging from abrasions to destruction of most of the face and maxillofacial skeletal fractures. This discussion is limited to maxillofacial skeletal injuries.

Maxillofacial Skeletal Injuries. Fractures of the maxilla are diagnosed according to the *Le Fort classification*. Le Fort fractures are classified in three broad categories, depending on the level of the fracture (Fig. 38-9). The most common, Le Fort I, consists of horizontal fractures in which the entire maxillary arch moves separately from the upper facial skeleton. Le Fort II fractures are an extension of Le Fort I fractures, and they involve the orbit, ethmoid, and nasal bones. Le Fort III fractures are associated with craniofacial disruption. CSF frequently leaks with Le Fort II and III fractures because there is usually communication between the cranial base and the cribriform plate.[23]

Assessment and Diagnostic Procedures. Patients with maxillofacial trauma are especially prone to ineffective airway clearance, deficient fluid volume related to hemorrhage, and risk for injury. Life-threatening complications associated with maxillofacial trauma include airway obstruction and head and cervical spine injuries. Major or minor facial deformities should not distract the trauma team from the standard assessments and interventions needed to stabilize the airway, breathing, and circulation of the patient.

Patients with maxillofacial trauma are at high risk for ineffective airway clearance. The tongue, edema, hemorrhage, foreign objects, vomit, broken teeth, or bone fragments can obstruct the airway. The "look, listen, and feel" methods (see Table 38-2) should be used to assess airway obstruction. An artificial airway may be required. An oral endotracheal tube is used unless there is a laryngeal fracture. Nasotracheal or nasogastric intubation is contraindicated in the presence of unstable facial fractures because a fracture of the cribriform plate may exist, and the tube could be inadvertently placed through the fractured base of the cranium and into the brain.[9] A tracheostomy may be required for patients with hypopharynx swelling or hemorrhage.

Patients with maxillofacial trauma are at risk for deficient fluid volume related to massive hemorrhage as a result of bleeding from the ethmoid or maxillary sinuses. Profuse bleeding through the nares may occur with nasal fractures, maxillary fractures, or cranial base fractures, and nasal packing may be required to control the bleeding.[23] Intravenously administered fluids are given to correct the deficient fluid volume.

After life-saving interventions are initiated, the comprehensive examination of facial structures is begun as part of the

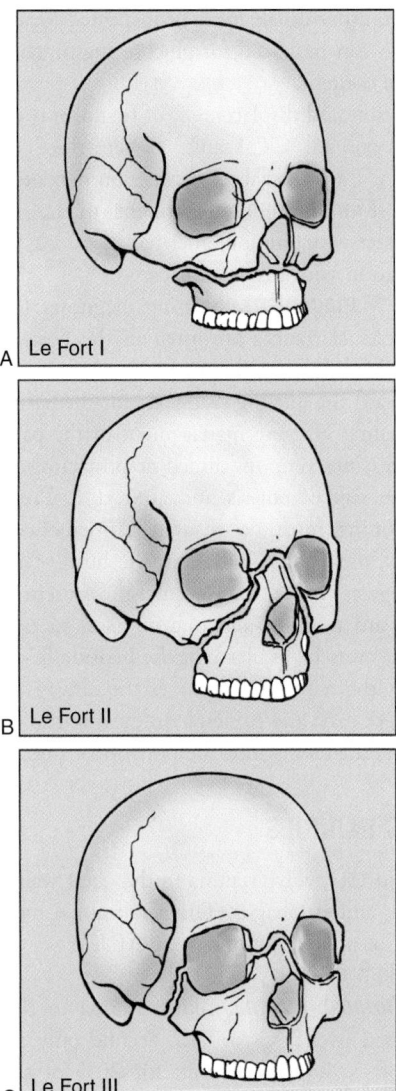

Figure 38-9 Fractures of the maxillae are diagnosed according to the Le Fort classification, which consists of three broad categories based on the level of the fracture. *A,* Le Fort I. *B,* Le Fort II. *C,* Le Fort III.

general head-to-toe sequence of assessment. Assessment of the face involves a careful inspection and palpation of the soft tissues. A small abrasion or contusion of the face may seem unobtrusive, but the impact to the underlying structures might have disrupted facial bone integrity, the parotid gland, or facial nerve.[23] The mouth is inspected for traumatic tooth dislodgement, recognizing that some teeth may intrude into the underlying alveolar bone. The ear canal is inspected for occult lacerations of the tympanic membrane. Because many of the facial structures enter from the cranium through the eye orbit, careful inspection and palpation of the orbit is required.

Maxillofacial trauma often is associated with cervical SCI. An altered level of consciousness in the presence of maxillofacial fractures strongly suggests neurotrauma. Fractures involving the cranium and dura mater may enable oral bacterial flora to enter CSF, placing the patient at risk for meningitis.

Nasal and auditory canals must be inspected for discharge. The drainage also can be tested for glucose inasmuch as CSF has a high glucose content.

The location and displacement of fractures is determined by axonal and coronal CT scans.[9] When true coronal CT is unavailable, CT with facial reconstruction may be substituted.[23]

Medical Management. Treatment of Le Fort fractures includes direct visualization and reduction of the fragments and stabilization with plates and screws.[24]

Nursing Management. Nursing diagnoses for the patient with maxillofacial trauma are listed in the Nursing Diagnoses feature on Maxillofacial Trauma. Nursing interventions are directed toward the nursing diagnoses for the patient with maxillofacial trauma. Nursing management of the patient with jaw wires requires interventions aimed at protecting the airway by reducing the risk of emesis and aspiration. Proper orogastric tube functioning must be ensured. Antiemetics may be administered. Unless contraindicated, the head of the bed is elevated 30 degrees. If vomiting occurs, the patient is placed in a side or forward position and oral or nasal suctioning is used. Wire cutters must be available at the bedside in case the vomit cannot clear the wires and occludes the airway. Although this seldom is necessary, the principle in cutting the wires is to cut the vertical attachments, not the horizontal ones.

THORACIC INJURIES

Thoracic injuries involve trauma to the chest wall, lungs, heart, great vessels, and esophagus. Thoracic trauma most commonly is the result of a violent crime or an MVC.

Mechanism of Injury

Blunt Thoracic Trauma. Blunt trauma to the chest most often is caused by MVCs or falls. Second only to head injury or SCI, thoracic injuries account for 20% of trauma deaths. The underlying mechanism of injury tends to be a combination of acceleration-deceleration injury and direct transfer mechanics, as in a crush injury. Various mechanisms of blunt trauma are associated with specific injury patterns. After head-on collisions, drivers have a higher frequency of injury than do backseat passengers because the driver comes in contact with the steering assembly. Severe thoracic injuries often are seen in patients who are unrestrained. Falls from greater than 20 feet are typically associated with thoracic injury.

Nursing Diagnoses

Maxillofacial Trauma

- Risk for Aspiration risk factors: impaired pharyngeal peristalsis or tongue function; impaired laryngeal sensation or reflex; impaired laryngeal closure or elevation
- Deficient Fluid Volume related to absolute loss
- Imbalanced Nutrition: Less Than Body Requirements related to lack of exogenous nutrients and increased metabolic demands
- Acute Pain related to transmission and perception of cutaneous, visceral, muscular, or ischemic impulses

---

Penetrating Thoracic Injuries. The penetrating object involved determines the damage sustained from penetrating thoracic trauma. Low-velocity weapons (e.g., .22-caliber gun, knife) usually damage only what is in the weapon's direct path. Of particular concern, however, are stab wounds that involve the anterior chest wall between the midclavicular lines, the angle of Louis, and the epigastric region because of the proximity of the heart and great vessels.

Specific Thoracic Traumatic Injuries

Chest Wall Injuries

Rib Fractures. Fractures of certain ribs or multiple rib fractures can be serious, even life-threatening, particularly when associated with additional injuries and occurring in older patients.[25] Fractures of the first and second ribs are associated with intrathoracic vascular injuries (e.g., brachial plexus, great vessels), and because they are protected by the scapula, clavicle, humerus, and muscles, they signify a very high degree of force applied to the thorax. Fractures to the lower ribs (7th to 12th) may be associated with abdominal injuries, such as spleen and liver injuries. Fractures to the middle ribs may be associated with lung injury, including pulmonary contusion and pneumothorax. Lack of bone calcification in pediatric trauma patients results in more compliant chest walls, and rib fractures need not have occurred for a tremendous amount of force to have been absorbed by the underlying structures in these patients.[26]

The pain associated with rib fractures can be aggravated by respiratory excursion. The patient often splints, takes shallow breaths, and refuses to cough, which can result in atelectasis and pneumonia. Localized pain that increases with respiration or that is elicited by rib compression may indicate rib fractures. Definitive diagnosis can be made with a chest radiograph. Nursing diagnoses may include Pain, Ineffective Airway Clearance, Ineffective Breathing Pattern, and Impaired Gas Exchange.

Interventions include aggressive pulmonary physiotherapy and pain control to improve chest expansion efforts and gas exchange. Pain management interventions must be tailored to the patient's response to therapy. The primary goal of pain management in patients with rib fractures is prevention of pulmonary complications and patient comfort. Nonsteroidal antiinflammatory drugs (NSAIDs), intercostal nerve blocks, thoracic epidural analgesia, and opiates may be considered to assist with pain control.[27] Epidural analgesia can help increase the functional residual capacity, dynamic lung compliance, and vital capacity; decrease the airway resistance; and increase PaO_2.[27] External splints are not recommended because they further limit chest wall expansion and may add to atelectasis.[27] The patient's preexisting pulmonary status and age may dictate the course of recovery.[25]

Flail Chest. Flail chest, which is caused by blunt trauma, disrupts the continuity of chest wall structures. A flail chest occurs when two or more ribs are fractured in two or more places and are no longer attached to the thoracic cage, producing a free-floating segment of the chest wall. The segment moves independently from the rest of the thorax and causes paradoxical chest wall movement during the respiratory cycle (Fig. 38-10). During inspiration, the intact portion of the chest wall expands while the injured part is sucked in. During expiration, the chest

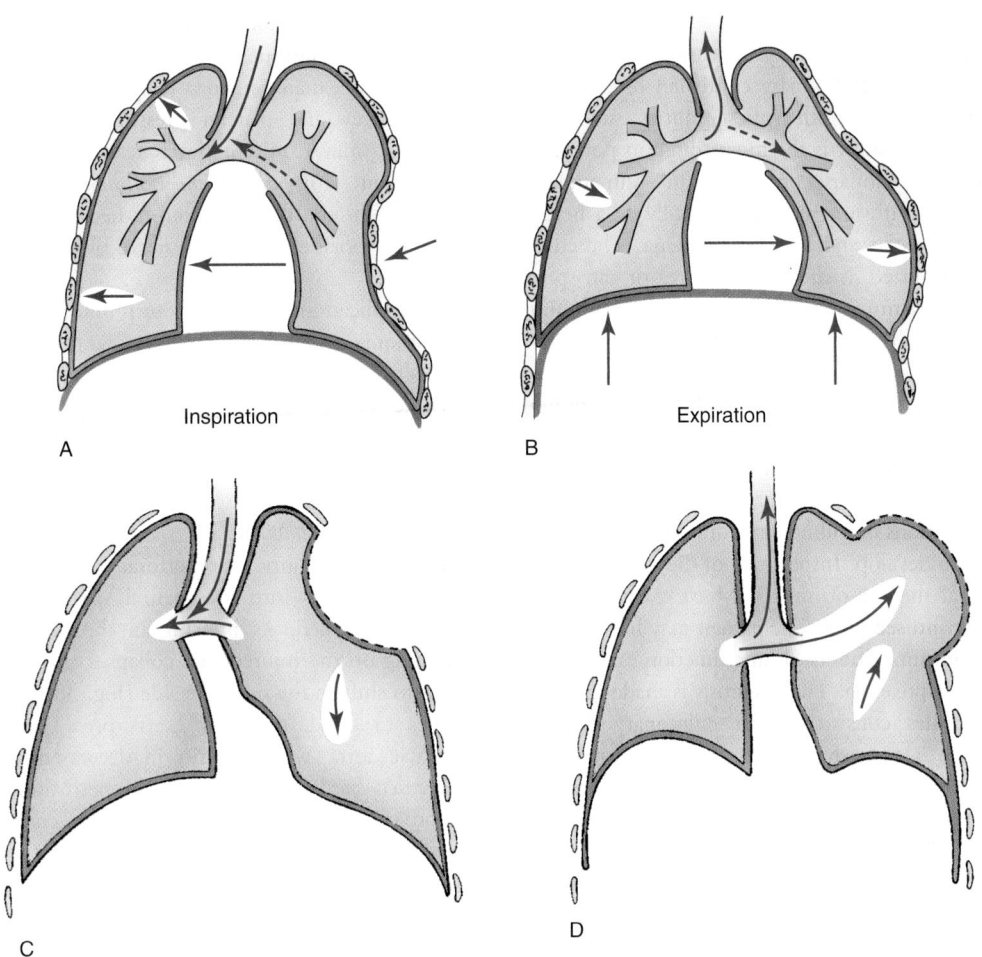

Figure 38-10 Flail chest. *A,* Normal inspiration. *B,* Normal expiration. *C,* The area of lung underlying the unstable chest wall sucks in on inspiration. *D,* The same area balloons out on expiration. Notice the movement of mediastinum toward opposite lung on inspiration.

wall moves in, and the flail segment moves out. Although the flail segment increases the work of breathing, the main cause of hypoxemia is the underlying pulmonary contusion. The physiologic effects of the impaired chest wall motion of a flail chest include decreased tidal volume and vital capacity and impaired cough, which lead to hypoventilation and atelectasis.

Inspection of the chest reveals paradoxical movement. Palpation of the chest may indicate crepitus and tenderness near fractured ribs. A chest radiograph that reveals multiple rib fractures and evidence of hypoxia demonstrated by ABG values aid in the diagnosis. Nursing diagnoses for the patient with a flail chest include Ineffective Breathing Patterns, Impaired Gas Exchange, and Pain.

Interventions focus on ensuring adequate oxygenation, judicious administration of fluids, and analgesia to improve ventilation.[27] Intubation and mechanical ventilation may be required to prevent further hypoxia.

Ruptured Diaphragm. Diagnosis of a diaphragmatic rupture is often missed in trauma patients because of the subtle and nonspecific symptoms this injury produces. The mechanism of injury appears to be a rapid rise in intraabdominal pressure as a result of compression force applied to the lower part of the chest or upper region of the abdomen. This injury can occur when a

person is thrown forward over the edge of the steering wheel in a high-speed MVC involving deceleration forces. The diaphragm, which offers little resistance to the force, can rupture or tear. Abdominal viscera then can gradually enter the thoracic cavity, moving from the positive pressure of the abdomen to the negative pressure in the thorax. Diaphragmatic rupture can be a life-threatening event. Massive herniation of abdominal contents into the thoracic cavity can compress the lungs and mediastinum, which hampers venous return and leads to decreased cardiac output. Herniated bowel can become strangulated and perforate.

Diaphragmatic herniation may produce significant compromise and changes in respiratory effort. Auscultation of bowel sounds in the chest or unilateral breath sounds may indicate a ruptured diaphragm. The patient may complain of shoulder pain, shortness of breath, or abdominal tenderness. Thoracoscopy may be helpful in evaluating the diaphragm in indeterminate cases, and multidetector CT analysis is a useful diagnostic tool for the evaluation of diaphragmatic injuries.[28] A chest radiograph may reveal the tip of a nasogastric tube above the diaphragm, a unilaterally elevated hemidiaphragm, a hollow or solid mass above the diaphragm, and a shift of the mediastinum away from the affected side. Treatment of a ruptured diaphragm includes its immediate repair.

Pulmonary Injuries

Pulmonary Contusion. A pulmonary contusion is fundamentally a bruise of the lung. Pulmonary contusion often is associated with blunt trauma and other chest injuries, such as rib fractures and flail chest, and it is the most common potentially lethal chest injury.[29] Pulmonary contusions can occur unilaterally or bilaterally. A contusion manifests initially as a hemorrhage, followed by alveolar and interstitial edema. The edema can remain rather localized in the contused area or can spread to other lung areas. Inflammation affects alveolar-capillary units. As more units are affected by inflammation, further pathophysiologic events can occur, including decreased compliance, increased pulmonary vascular resistance, and decreased pulmonary blood flow. These processes result in a ventilation-perfusion imbalance that results in progressive hypoxemia and poor ventilation over a 24- to 48-hour period.

Clinical manifestations of pulmonary contusion may take up to 24 to 48 hours to develop. Inspections of the chest wall may reveal ecchymosis at the site of impact. Moist crackles may be auscultated in the contused lung. The patient may have a cough and blood-tinged sputum. Abnormal lung function can manifest as systemic arterial hypoxemia. The diagnosis is made primarily by chest x-ray studies consistent with pulmonary infiltrate corresponding to the area of external chest impact that manifests within 12 to 24 hours of injury. Pulmonary contusions tend to worsen over a 24- to 48-hour period and then slowly resolve unless complications occur (e.g., infection, ARDS). Nursing diagnoses for the patient with pulmonary contusions may include Impaired Gas Exchange, Risk for Infection, Acute Pain, Ineffective Tissue Perfusion, and Ineffective Airway Clearance.

Aggressive respiratory care is the cornerstone for care of nonintubated patients with pulmonary contusion. Interventions include ambulation, deep-breathing exercises, turning, and incentive spirometry. Chest physiotherapy is not tolerated if there are coexisting rib fractures. Aggressive removal of airway secretions is important to avoid infection and to improve ventilation. Patients with unilateral contusions are placed with the injured side up and uninjured side down ("down with the good lung"). This positioning maximizes the match between pulmonary ventilation and perfusion. Patients with severe contusions may continue to show decompensation despite aggressive nursing management. Respiratory acidosis, increases in peak airway and plateau pressures, and increased work of breathing may require endotracheal intubation and mechanical ventilation with *positive end-expiratory pressure* (PEEP). Adequate pain control is accomplished with administration of NSAIDs, opiates, intercostal nerve blocks, or thoracic epidural analgesia.

Complications resulting from pulmonary contusions include pneumonia, ARDS, lung abscesses, emphysema, and pulmonary embolism. Factors that contribute to increased mortality rates include shock, coexisting head injury, flail chest, falls from heights greater than 20 feet, advanced age, and preexisting disease (e.g., coronary artery disease, chronic obstructive pulmonary disease).

Tension Pneumothorax. A tension pneumothorax usually is caused by an injury that perforates the chest wall or pleural space. Air flows into the pleural space with inspiration and becomes trapped. As pressure in the pleural space increases, the lung on the injured side collapses and causes the mediastinum to shift to the opposite side (Fig. 38-11). As pressure continues to build, the shift exerts pressure on the heart and thoracic aorta, which results in decreased venous return and decreased cardiac output. Tissue perfusion with oxygenated blood is further hampered because the collapsed lung cannot participate in gas exchange.

Clinical manifestations of a tension pneumothorax include dyspnea, tachycardia, hypotension, and sudden chest pain extending to the shoulders. Tracheal deviation can be observed as the trachea shifts away from the injured side. On the injured side, breath sounds may be decreased or absent. Percussion of the chest reveals a hyperresonant sound over the affected side. Diagnosis of tension pneumothorax is made by clinical assessment. Nursing diagnoses for a patient with a tension pneumothorax include Decreased Cardiac Output and Impaired Gas Exchange.

There is no time for a chest radiograph because this potentially lethal condition must be treated immediately.[9] A large-bore (14-gauge) needle or chest tube is inserted into the affected

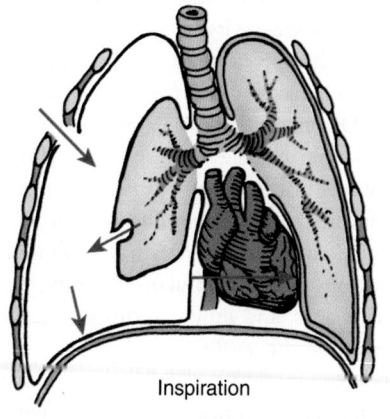
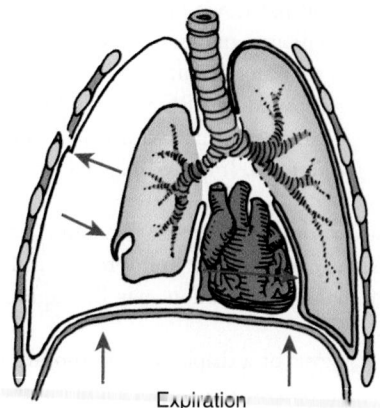

Inspiration

Expiration

Figure 38-11 A tension pneumothorax usually is caused by an injury that perforates the chest wall or pleural space. Air flows into the pleural space with inspiration and becomes trapped. As pressure in the pleural space increases, the lung on the injured side collapses and causes the mediastinum to shift to the opposite side. *(From Marx J et al: Rosen's Emergency medicine: concepts and clinical practice, ed 5, St Louis, 2002, Mosby.)*

lung. This procedure allows immediate release of air from the pleural space. A hissing sound is heard as the tension pneumothorax is converted to a simple pneumothorax.

Open Pneumothorax. An open pneumothorax ("sucking chest wound") usually is caused by penetrating trauma. Open communication between the atmosphere and intrathoracic pressure results in immediate lung deflation. Air moves in and out of the hole in the chest, producing a sucking sound heard on inspiration. An open pneumothorax produces the same symptoms as a tension pneumothorax. Subcutaneous emphysema may be palpated around the wound.

Initial management of an open pneumothorax is accomplished by promptly closing the wound at end expiration with a sterile occlusive dressing (plastic wrap or petroleum gauze) large enough to overlap the wound's edges.[9] This dressing should be taped securely on three sides. As the patient breathes in, the dressing gets sucked in to occlude the wound and prevent air from entering. A chest tube is placed as soon as possible. Surgical intervention may be required to close the wound.

Hemothorax. Blunt or penetrating thoracic trauma can cause bleeding into the pleural space, resulting in a hemothorax (Fig. 38-12). A massive hemothorax results from the accumulation of more than 1500 mL of blood in the chest cavity.[29] The source of bleeding may be the intercostal or internal mammary arteries, lungs, heart, or great vessels. Lacerations to the lung parenchyma are low-pressure bleeds and typically stop bleeding spontaneously.[29] Arterial bleeding from hilar vessels usually require immediate surgical intervention.[9] In either case, increasing intrapleural pressure results in a decrease in vital capacity. Increasing vascular blood loss into the pleural space causes decreased venous return and decreased cardiac output.

Assessment findings for patients with a hemothorax include hypovolemic shock. Breath sounds may be diminished or absent over the affected lung. With hemothorax, the neck veins are collapsed, and the trachea is at midline. Massive hemothorax can be diagnosed on the basis of clinical manifestations of hypotension associated with the absence of breath sounds or dullness to percussion on one side of the chest.[9,29] Nursing diagnoses for a patient with a hemothorax include Deficient Fluid Volume, with resulting Decreased Cardiac Output, and Impaired Gas Exchange.

This life-threatening condition must be treated immediately. Resuscitation with intravenous fluids is initiated to treat the hypovolemic shock. A chest tube is placed on the affected side to allow drainage of blood. An autotransfusion device can be attached to the chest tube collection chamber. Thoracotomy may be necessary for patients who require persistent blood transfusions or who have significant bleeding (200 mL/hr for 2 to 4 hours or more than 1500 mL on initial tube insertion) or when there are injuries to major cardiovascular structures.[29]

Cardiac and Vascular Injuries

Penetrating Cardiac Injuries. Penetrating cardiac trauma can occur from mechanical injuries as a result of bullets, knives, or impalements. The chest wall offers little protection to the heart from penetrating trauma. The most common site of injury is the right ventricle because of its anterior position. The mortality rate from penetrating trauma to the heart is high. The prehospital mortality rate for penetrating cardiac injuries is very high, and most deaths occur within minutes after injury as a result of exsanguination or tamponade.

Cardiac Tamponade. Cardiac tamponade is the progressive accumulation of blood in the pericardial sac (Fig. 38-13). With cardiac tamponade, progressive accumulation of 120 to 150 mL of blood increases the intracardiac pressure and compresses the atria and ventricles. An increase in intracardiac pressure leads to decreased venous return and decreased filling pressure, which leads to decreased cardiac output, myocardial hypoxia, cardiac failure, and cardiogenic shock.

Classic assessment findings associated with cardiac tamponade are called *Beck's triad*—presence of elevated central venous pressure with neck vein distention, muffled heart sounds, and hypotension. Pulsus paradoxus may occur. Pulseless electrical activity (PEA) in the absence of hypovolemia and tension pneumothorax suggests cardiac tamponade.[9] Ultrasonography in the emergency setting may be used in cases of penetrating cardiac injuries to identify a hemopericardium.[30] The major nursing diagnosis for this injury is Decreased Cardiac Output.

Immediate treatment is required to remove the accumulation of fluid in the pericardial sac. Pericardiocentesis involves aspiration of fluid from the pericardium by use of a large-bore needle. The inherent risk in this procedure is potential laceration of the coronary artery. Other approaches include surgical procedures

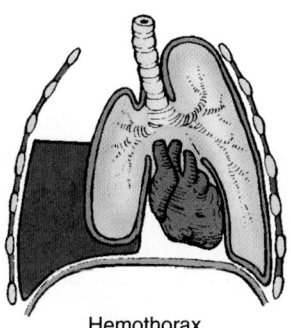

Figure 38-12 Blunt or penetrating thoracic trauma can cause bleeding into the pleural space to form a hemothorax.

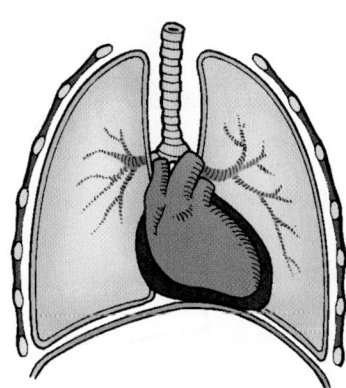

Figure 38-13 Cardiac tamponade is the progressive accumulation of blood in the pericardial sac.

such as thoracotomy or median sternotomy. The goal of these procedures is to locate and control the source of bleeding.

Blunt Cardiac Injuries. The most common causes of blunt cardiac trauma include high-speed MVCs, direct blows to the chest, and falls. Because of its mobility and its location between the sternum and thoracic vertebrae, the heart is susceptible to blunt traumatic injury. Sudden acceleration (as from contact with a steering wheel) can cause the heart to be thrown against the sternum (Fig. 38-14). Sudden deceleration can cause the heart to be thrown against the thoracic vertebrae by a direct blow to the chest, such as blows caused by a baseball, animal kick, or fall.

Blunt cardiac injury (BCI), formerly called *myocardial contusion*, covers the spectrum of myocardial contusion, concussion, and rupture. The most often injured chambers include the right atrium and ventricle because of their anterior position in the chest.[31]

Few clinical signs and symptoms are specific for BCI. Evidence of external chest trauma, such as steering wheel imprint or sternal fractures, should raise the suspicion for blunt cardiac injury. However, the presence of a sternal fracture does not predict the incidence of BCI. The patient may complain of chest pain that is similar to anginal pain, but it is not typically relieved with nitroglycerin.[31] The chest pain is usually caused by associated injuries. The EAST guidelines for screening of BCI are listed in Box 38-8. The 12-lead ECG may reveal dysrhythmias, ST changes, heart block, or unexplained sinus tachycardia.

Medical management is aimed at preventing and treating complications. This approach may include administration of antidysrhythmic medications, treatment of heart failure, or insertion of a temporary pacemaker to control conduction abnormalities. Assessment of fluid and electrolyte balance is imperative to ensure adequate cardiac output and myocardial conduction.

Aortic Injury. Blunt aortic injury is one of the most lethal blunt thoracic injuries. Disruption of the aorta in blunt chest

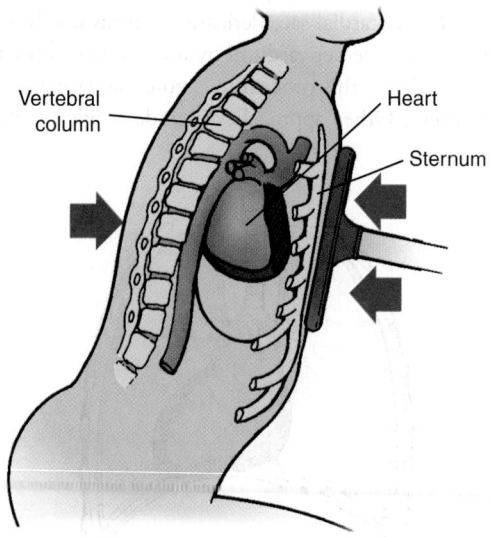
Figure 38-14 Blunt cardiac trauma. Sudden acceleration (as from contact with the steering wheel) can cause the heart to be thrown against the sternum.

Vertebral column

Heart

Sternum

BOX 38-8	EAST GUIDELINES FOR SCREENING OF BLUNT CARDIAC INJURY

- Obtain an admission ECG for all patients in whom there is suspected BCI.
- If ECG is abnormal, the patient should be admitted for continuous ECG monitoring for 24 to 48 hours.
- If the patient is hemodynamically unstable, an echocardiogram may be performed.
- Cardiac biomarkers such as cardiac troponin T values are not useful in predicting which patients will have complications related to BCI.

BCI, blunt cardiac injury; EAST, Eastern Association for the Surgery of Trauma; ECG, electrocardiogram.

---

trauma is leading cause of immediate death in trauma patients: 22% die before reaching the emergency department, 37% die during initial resuscitation or in the operating room, and 14% die postoperatively.[32] Nineteen percent of survivors develop paraplegia or paresis.[32] Injuries associated with aortic injury include a first or second rib fracture, high sternal fracture, left clavicular fracture at the level of the sternal margin, and massive hemothorax.[33] Blunt aortic injury should be suspected in all victims of trauma with a rapid deceleration or acceleration mechanism of injury.

The thoracic aorta is relatively mobile and tears at fixed anatomic points within the thorax. Sites of aortic disruption (in order of frequency) include the aortic isthmus, just distal to the subclavian artery (where the vessel is fixed to the chest by the ligamentum arteriosum); at the ascending aorta (where the aorta leaves the pericardial sac); at the descending aorta (where the aorta enters the diaphragm); and avulsion of the innominate artery from the aortic arch.

The nurse assesses blood pressure in both arms because a tear in the aortic arch may create a pressure gradient resulting in blood pressures changes between upper extremities. If aortic disruption is suspected, blood pressure is also compared between upper and lower extremities. Baroreceptors are stimulated, resulting in upper extremity hypertension with relative lower extremity hypotension. Additional clinical assessment findings include a pulse deficit anywhere, unexplained hypotension, sternal pain, precordial systolic murmur, hoarseness, dyspnea, and lower extremity sensory deficits.

An initial chest radiograph is obtained in the upright position after it is considered safe to do so. Radiograph findings suggesting aortic injury include a widened mediastinum, obscured aortic knob, deviation of the left main stem bronchus or nasogastric tube, and opacification of the aortopulmonary window.[33] Spiral or helical CT is warranted if the initial chest radiograph is inconclusive, but the definitive diagnosis is made by aortography in indeterminate cases.[33]

During the resuscitation phase for a patient with aortic disruption, blood pressure management is the primary goal to minimize injury. Patients with tears at the aortic isthmus are typically hypertensive, and minimizing stress on the vessel is achieved by maintaining the systolic blood pressure less than 90 mm Hg by using antihypertensive agents such as sodium nitroprusside.[33] The nurse anticipates definitive surgical intervention early in the resuscitation. Surgical repair may be achieved by a graft, primary anastomosis, and bypass.[33]

Postoperative care is directed toward blood pressure stabilization, with the goal of minimizing vessel stress while maintaining tissue perfusion, which typically is accomplished with the use of sodium nitroprusside. Careful assessment of postoperative paraplegia is needed because lack of blood flow to the spinal column might have occurred perioperatively. Paraplegia is closely related to the duration of clamp time intraoperatively. The critical care nurse monitors for signs of bowel ischemia (e.g., tube feeding intolerance, lactic acidosis) and renal failure (e.g., poor urinary output, rising creatinine) because mesenteric and renal blood flow might have been compromised as a result of the injury or aortic clamp time.

ABDOMINAL INJURIES

Abdominal injuries often are associated with multisystem trauma. Abdominal injuries are the third leading cause of traumatic death. Injuries to the abdomen are the result of blunt or penetrating trauma. Two major life-threatening conditions that occur after abdominal trauma are hemorrhage and hollow viscus perforation with associated peritonitis. Death occurring after 48 hours following injury is the result of sepsis and its complications. The critical care nurse must pay particular attention to complication prevention strategies throughout the trauma cycle.

Mechanism of Injury

Blunt Trauma. Blunt abdominal injuries are common. They result most often from MVCs, falls, and assaults. In MVCs, abdominal injury is more likely to occur when a vehicle is struck from the side. In the passenger position of the front seat, hepatic injury is likely when the point of impact is on the same side as the passenger. A driver is likely to sustain injury to the spleen when the impact is on the driver's side. Pedestrians hit by motor vehicles are at risk for serious abdominal injuries. Blunt trauma to the thorax can produce injuries to the liver, spleen, and diaphragm. Deceleration and direct forces can produce retroperitoneal hematomas. Blunt abdominal injuries often are hidden, requiring careful assessment and reassessment. Unrecognized abdominal trauma is a common cause of preventable deaths, and blunt abdominal injury deaths are more likely to be fatal than are penetrating abdominal injuries.

Penetrating Trauma. Penetrating abdominal trauma is caused most often by knives or bullets. The danger of penetrating abdominal trauma is that the outside appearance of the wound does not reflect the extent of internal injury. Commonly injured organs from knife wounds are the colon, liver, spleen, and diaphragm. Gunshot wounds to the abdomen usually are more serious than are stab wounds. A bullet destroys tissue along its path. Inside the abdomen, a bullet can travel in erratic paths and ricochet off bone. Death from penetrating injuries depends on the injury to major vascular structures and resultant intraabdominal hemorrhage.

Assessment. The initial assessment of the trauma patient, whether in the emergency department or the critical care unit, follows the primary and secondary survey techniques as outlined by ATLS guidelines.[9] The initial physical assessment may be unreliable given the confounding influences of alcohol, illicit drugs, analgesics, and an altered level of consciousness. Specific assessment findings associated with abdominal trauma are reviewed here.

Physical Assessment. The location of entry and exit sites associated with penetrating trauma are assessed and documented. Inspection of the patient's abdomen may reveal purplish discoloration of the flanks or umbilicus (Cullen's sign), which indicates blood in the abdominal wall. Ecchymosis in the flank area (Turner's sign) may indicate retroperitoneal bleeding or a possible fracture of the pancreas. A hematoma in the flank area suggests renal injury. A distended abdomen may indicate the accumulation of blood, fluid, or gas resulting from a perforated organ or ruptured blood vessel. Auscultation of the abdomen may reveal friction rubs over the liver or spleen and may indicate rupture. The abdomen is assessed for rebound tenderness and rigidity. These assessment findings indicate peritoneal inflammation. Referred pain to the left shoulder (Kehr's sign) may indicate a ruptured spleen or irritation of the diaphragm from bile or other material in the peritoneum. Subcutaneous emphysema palpated on the abdomen suggests free air as a result of a ruptured bowel.

Diagnostic Procedures. Insertion of a nasogastric tube and urinary catheter serves as a useful diagnostic and therapeutic aid. A nasogastric tube can decompress the stomach, and the contents can be checked for blood. Urine obtained from the urinary catheter can also be tested for the presence of blood.

Serial laboratory test results may be nonspecific for the patient with abdominal trauma. A serum amylase determination can detect pancreatic injuries. Because of hemoconcentration, hemoglobin and hematocrit results may not reflect actual values. Serial values are more valuable in diagnosing abdominal injuries.

Because of the unreliability of physical examination alone in the patient suspected of having abdominal trauma,[34] diagnostic testing may occur simultaneously during the primary and secondary surveys. Noninvasive tests include bedside ultrasound, CT, and chest and abdominal radiographs. Invasive tests such as the *diagnostic peritoneal lavage* (DPL) can exclude or confirm the presence of intraabdominal injury with a high accuracy rate.[9] After the patient's bladder has been emptied, a small incision is made in the abdomen through the skin and into the peritoneum. A small catheter is inserted (Fig. 38-15). If frank blood is encountered, intraabdominal injury is evident, and the patient is taken immediately to the operating room. If gross blood is not initially encountered, a liter of fluid (lactated Ringer's or 0.9% normal saline) is infused through the catheter into the abdomen. The intravenous bag is then placed in a dependent position, and abdominal fluid is allowed to drain into the intravenous bag. The drainage fluid is sent to the laboratory for analysis. Positive DPL results signal intraabdominal trauma and usually necessitate surgical intervention (Box 38-9). DPL is invasive, has been associated with complications, and cannot exclude retroperitoneal injuries.

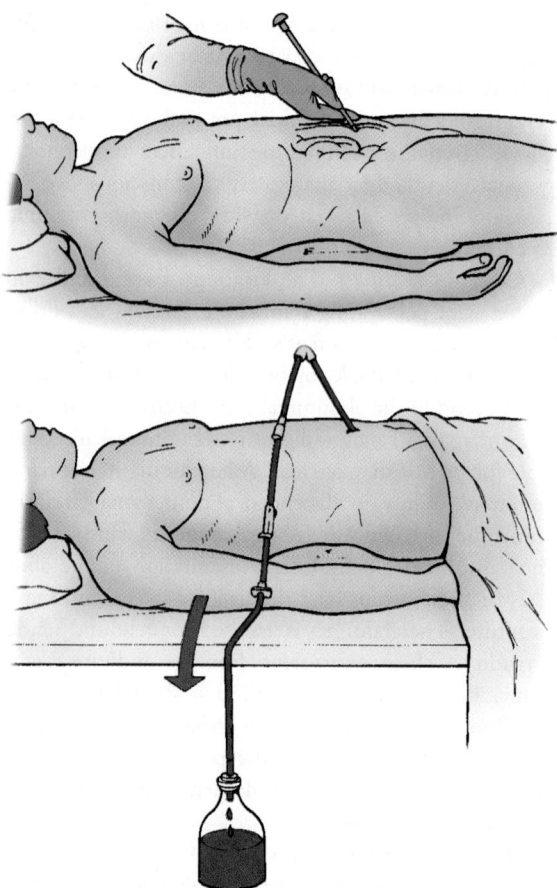

Figure 38-15 Diagnostic peritoneal lavage (DPL) can exclude or confirm the presence of intraabdominal injury with a high accuracy rate.

BOX 38-9   POSITIVE PERITONEAL LAVAGE RESULTS

- Red blood cell count: 100,000/mm^3
- White blood cell count: 500/mm^3
- Amylase: 175 units/dL
- Presence of blood, stool, bile, or bacteria

The bedside ultrasound, called the focused assessment sonography for trauma (FAST examination) is done at most trauma centers to evaluate the patient for the presence of intraabdominal blood.[34] This is a quick and noninvasive means of rapid assessment, but success depends on the skill level of the operator.[34] Bedside ultrasonography is used widely in the United States for the detection of abdominal free fluid and hemoperitoneum. Typically, the right and left upper abdominal quadrant areas are examined: the right upper quadrant (Morrison's pouch); the left upper quadrant splenorenal area; the pericardial sac; and the pelvis (Douglas' pouch).[35] The primary disadvantage of FAST is the need for free intraperitoneal fluid to produce a positive study result.[41] An initial negative FAST result may be followed by serial ultrasound examinations, abdominal CT, or DPL.[34]

BOX 38-10   DAMAGE CONTROL SEQUENCE

INITIAL OPERATION
- Control contamination
- Control hemorrhage
- Intraabdominal packing
- Temporary closure

INTENSIVE CARE UNIT (ICU) RESUSCITATION
- Correct coagulopathy
- Rewarming
- Maximize hemodynamics
- Ventilatory support
- Injury identification

PLANNED REOPERATION
- Pack removal
- Definitive repair

Although the FAST test has had good sensitivity and specificity, it is not intended to replace DPL or CT. Obese abdomens and patients with ascites may have erroneous results, and further workup for these patients is warranted.[35] Ultrasound is also limited in its ability to diagnose diaphragmatic, intestinal, or pancreas injuries.[36] Abdominal CT scanning is the mainstay of diagnostic evaluation in the hemodynamically stable trauma patient.[34,36] Abdominal CT provides information about specific organ injury, pelvic injury, and retroperitoneal hemorrhage.

Combined Abdominal Organ Injuries. Patients with multiple visceral injuries may require surgical intervention that uses somewhat nontraditional techniques ("damage control" surgery). The three phases of this treatment strategy are the *initial operation, ICU resuscitation,* and *definitive reoperation* (Box 38-10).[37] The duration of the initial operation is kept to a minimum. The decision to abbreviate the initial operation is made early during surgery. Factors that may lead the surgeon to choose an abbreviated laparotomy include hypothermia and coagulopathy in a patient who is hemodynamically unstable, an inability to control bleeding by direct pressure, and an inability to close the abdomen because of massive abdominal edema.[37] Hypothermia induced by an open visceral cavity in conjunction with massive blood transfusion can lead to coagulopathy and continued bleeding, which results in shock and metabolic acidosis. The triad of hypothermia, coagulopathy, and acidosis creates a self-propagating cycle that can eventually lead to an irreversible physiologic insult.[37] The initial operation must be completed quickly to terminate this self-propagating cycle. Reconstruction and formal closure of the wound may not be completed at this time. The patient is transferred to the ICU.

The goal of the critical care phase of this strategy is to continue aggressive resuscitation and correct hypothermia, coagulopathy, and acidosis. Rewarming techniques, described in Box 38-11, are used to correct hypothermia. Coagulation factors and platelets may be given to correct coagulopathies. Serial lactate and base deficit measurements, as well as a mixed venous oxygen saturation (S$\bar{v}$o$_2$) pulmonary artery catheter, may

BOX 38-11   INTERVENTIONS FOR REWARMING THE TRAUMA PATIENT

Intervention	External Rewarming Procedures	Internal Rewarming Procedures
Passive	Maintain a warm room temperature. Remove all wet clothing and linen. Cover the patient with blankets. Avoid bathing patient until normothermia achieved.	Administer warmed, humidified oxygen. Administer warmed intravenous fluids.
Active	Use radiant heat lamps, heating blankets or pads, and hot water bottles.	Perform gastrointestinal irrigation with warmed solutions. Perform extracorporeal rewarming for profound hypothermia. Use esophageal rewarming tubes.

Adapted from Morris J: Environmental emergencies. In Newberry L, editor: *Sheehy's emergency nursing: principles and practice*, 5 ed, St. Louis, 2003, Mosby.

TABLE 38-9   Liver Injury Scale

Grade*		Injury Description
I	Hematoma	Subcapsular, <10% surface area
	Laceration	Capsular tear, <1 cm parenchymal depth
II	Hematoma	Subcapsular, 10%-50% surface area; intraparenchymal <10 cm in diameter
	Laceration	Capsular tear, 1-3 cm parenchymal depth, <10 cm long
III	Hematoma	Subcapsular, >50% surface area or expanding; ruptured subcapsular or parenchymal hematoma; intraparenchymal hematoma >10 cm or expanding
	Laceration	>3 cm parenchymal depth
IV	Laceration	Parenchymal disruption involving 25%-75% of hepatic lobe or 1-3 Couinaud's segments within a single lobe
V	Laceration	Parenchymal disruption involving >75% of hepatic lobe or >3 Couinaud's segments within a single lobe
	Vascular	Juxtahepatic venous injuries (retrohepatic vena cava, central major hepatic veins)
VI	Vascular	Hepatic avulsion

Modified from Trunkey DD: Hepatic trauma: contemporary management. *Surg Clin North Am* 84:437-450, 2004.
*Advance one grade for multiple injuries up to grade II.

be used to guide fluid resuscitation, inotropic support, and oxygenation to prevent further development of acidosis.

Abdominal Compartment Syndrome. The patient is assessed for additional complications, including ongoing hemorrhage, intraabdominal hypertension, and abdominal compartment syndrome. Abdominal compartment syndrome is defined as end-organ dysfunction caused by intraabdominal hypertension.[38] Increased pressure can be caused by bleeding, ileus, visceral edema, or a noncompliant abdominal wall. Increased abdominal cavity pressure can impinge on diaphragmatic excursion and can affect ventilation. Clinical manifestations of abdominal compartment syndrome include decreased cardiac output, increased pulmonary vascular resistance, increased peak pulmonary pressures, decreased urine output, and hypoxia.[38] Intraabdominal pressure can be measured through a bladder catheter after the injection of 25 mL of sterile saline.[38] Measurements may be graded: grade I (12 to 15 mm Hg), grade II (16 to 20 mm Hg), grade III (21 to 25 mm Hg) and grade IV (>25 mm Hg).[38]

Surgical decompression of the abdomen may be required for abdominal pressures greater than 20 to 25 mm Hg that are associated with other assessment findings such as decreased cardiac output, hypotension, elevated peak inspiratory pressures, and decreased urine output.[39] Surgical decompression involves opening the abdomen and then temporarily closing the abdomen with a sterile perforated plastic sheet, clips, vacuum-assisted techniques, and many other options.[39] The open abdomen is then covered with towels or dressings, and closed suction drains are placed over the top and brought out through a plastic drape over the entire wound. The wound is closed permanently several weeks later, or it is allowed to heal by second intention and eventual skin grafting.

After the patient is hemodynamically stable and the triad of hypothermia, coagulopathy, and acidosis has been corrected, the patient is taken back to the operating room for the definitive surgery, if required. This usually occurs within 48 to 72 hours of the initial operation.[40] During this phase, definitive repairs and wound closure are performed. Postoperatively, the patient is transported back to the ICU for continued care.

Specific Organ Injuries. Physical assessment findings, DPL, and CT scanning aid in making a diagnosis of specific abdominal organ injury. The medical and nursing management vary according to specific organ injuries. Liver, spleen, and bowel injuries, which are seen more commonly, are discussed here.

Liver Injuries. The liver is the primary organ injured in penetrating trauma and the second most often injured organ in blunt trauma. Abdominal CT is considered to be the most reliable diagnostic tool to identify and assess the severity of the injury to the liver.[41] The severity of liver injuries is graded to provide a mechanism for determining the amount of trauma sustained by that organ, the care needed, and the possible outcomes (Table 38-9). Nonoperative management is considered the standard of care for hemodynamically stable patients with liver injury.[41] Patients are admitted to the ICU or a step-down unit and are monitored for signs of hemorrhage. Serial serum hematocrit and hemoglobin levels and vital signs are monitored over several days.

Patients with penetrating or blunt liver trauma who are hemodynamically unstable may require surgical intervention to correct the defect. Resection of the devitalized tissue is required for massive injuries. Hemorrhage is common with liver injuries, and ligation of the hepatic arteries or veins may be required to control hemorrhage. Drains may be placed intraoperatively to drain areas of blood and to prevent hematomas.

Care of the patient with severe liver injuries can be challenging for the critical care nurse. Lack of hemodynamic stability can result from hemorrhage and hypovolemic shock, leading to fluid volume deficit, decreased cardiac output, and decreased tissue perfusion. Combinations of crystalloid and colloid intravenous solutions may be used to correct hypovolemia. Fresh-frozen plasma, platelets, and cryoprecipitate may be administered to correct coagulopathies. A crucial nursing responsibility is to monitor the patient's response to medical therapies. Continued hemodynamic instability (e.g., hypotension, decreased cardiac output) despite aggressive medical intervention may indicate continued hemorrhage, in which case an exploratory laparotomy may be required to determine and correct the source of bleeding. The patient's postoperative ICU course may be complicated by coagulopathy, acidosis, and hypothermia. Jaundice may occur as a sign of hepatic dysfunction, but it may also be caused by reabsorption of hematomas or breakdown of transfused blood.

Spleen Injuries. The spleen is the organ most commonly injured by blunt abdominal trauma and is second to the liver as a source of life-threatening hemorrhage. Spleen injuries, like liver injuries, are graded for the purpose of determining the amount of trauma sustained, the care needed, and the possible outcomes (Table 38-10). Hemodynamically stable patients may be monitored in the critical care unit by means of serial hematocrit values and vital signs. Progressive deterioration may indicate the need for operative management.[41]

Patients who exhibit hemodynamic instability require operative intervention with splenectomy, partial splenectomy, or splenorrhaphy. Patients who have had a splenectomy are at risk for the development of overwhelming postsplenectomy sepsis with streptococcal pneumonia. These patients require polyvalent pneumococcal vaccine (Pneumovax) to help promote immunity against most pneumococcal bacteria. Patients with isolated spleen injuries that require surgical intervention rarely are admitted to the critical care unit. Complications after splenic trauma include wound infection, sepsis, subdiaphragmatic abscess, and fistulas of the colon, pancreas, and stomach.

Intestinal Injuries. Intestinal injuries can result from blunt or penetrating trauma. The diagnosis of small intestinal injuries is difficult. Surgical intervention is usually required in the presence of multiple CT findings (e.g., unexplained free fluid, pneumoperitoneum, bowel wall thickening, mesenteric fat streaking, mesenteric hematoma, intravenous contrast extravasation).[36] Regardless of the mechanism of injury, intestinal contents (e.g., bile, stool, enzymes, bacteria) leak into the peritoneum and cause peritonitis. Surgical resection and repair are required. The patient's postoperative course is dictated by the amount of

TABLE 38-10 Spleen Injury Scale

Grade*		Injury Description
I	Hematoma	Subcapsular, <10% surface area
	Laceration	Capsular tear, <1 cm, parenchymal depth
II	Hematoma	Subcapsular, 10%-50% surface area; intraparenchymal <5 cm in diameter
	Laceration	Capsular tear: 1-3 cm parenchymal depth, which does not involve a trabecular vessel
III	Hematoma	Subcapsular, >50% surface area or expanding; ruptured subcapsular or parenchymal hematoma; intraparenchymal hematoma >5 cm or expanding
IV	Laceration	>3 cm parenchymal depth or involving trabecular vessels
	Laceration	Laceration involving segmental or hilar vessels producing major devascularization (>25% of spleen)
V	Laceration	Completely shattered spleen
	Vascular	Hilar vascular injury that devascularizes spleen

*Advance one grade for multiple injuries up to grade II.

spillage of intestinal contents. The patient is observed for signs of sepsis and for abscess or fistula formation.

GENITOURINARY INJURIES

Trauma to the genitourinary tract seldom occurs as an isolated injury. A genitourinary injury must be suspected in any patient with penetrating trauma to the torso; pelvic fracture; blunt trauma to the lower chest or flank; contusions, hematoma, tenderness over the flank, lower abdomen, or perineum; genital swelling or discoloration; blood at the urethral meatus; hematuria after Foley catheter placement; or difficulty with micturition.[9]

Mechanism of Injury. Genitourinary injuries, like all other traumatic injuries, can result from blunt or penetrating trauma.

Assessment. Evaluation of genitourinary trauma begins after the primary survey has been conducted and immediate life-threatening conditions have been effectively managed. The conscious patient may complain of flank pain or colic pain. Rebound tenderness can be elicited if intraperitoneal extravasation of urine has occurred. Inspection may reveal blood at the urethral meatus. Bluish discoloration of the flanks may indicate retroperitoneal bleeding, whereas perineal discoloration may indicate a pelvic fracture and possible bladder or urethral injury. Hematuria is the most common assessment finding with genitourinary trauma; however, the absence of gross or microscopic hematuria does not exclude a urinary tract injury.[9]

Specific Genitourinary Injuries

Kidney Trauma. Most renal trauma is caused by blunt trauma, resulting in contusions or lacerations without urinary extravasation. Injury to the kidneys may be reflected by flank ecchymosis and fracture of inferior ribs or spinous processes. Gross or microscopic hematuria may be present; however, the extent of kidney damage is often incongruous with the degree of hematuria.[42] Gross hematuria can exist with minor injuries and usually clears within a few hours. CT is the most accurate modality available for diagnosing renal injuries because it can assess the extent of parenchymal laceration, urine extravasation, surrounding hemorrhage, and the presence of vascular injury.[42]

Contusions and minor lacerations can usually be treated with observation. The success of nonoperative management may be enhanced by using angiographic embolization. Nonoperative treatment of patients with major lacerations and vascular injuries may be achieved in those who are hemodynamically stable.[43] Operative interventions may be performed in patients with kidney injuries with a devascularized segment of the kidney. Postoperative and postinjury complications can include infection, hemorrhage, infarction, extravasation, calcification, acute tubular necrosis, and hypertension.

Bladder Trauma. A large percentage of bladder injuries result from pelvic fractures.[42] Physical findings may include lower abdominal bruising, distention, and pain. More definitive findings include difficulty in voiding or incomplete recovery of irrigation fluids from catheterized patients.[42] Bladder injuries are classified as contusions, extraperitoneal ruptures, intraperitoneal ruptures, or combined injuries. The type of injury depends on the location and strength of the blunt force and volume of urine in the bladder at the time of injury. Extraperitoneal rupture of the bladder may be managed conservatively with catheterization and antibiotics for 7 to 10 days.[43] Unresolved extravasation may require surgical intervention.

Nursing Management. Nursing diagnoses that can be applicable in caring for a patient with genitourinary trauma include Ineffective Tissue Perfusion, Pain, Risk for Infection, and Risk for Deficient Fluid Volume.

After the patient is admitted to the critical care unit, the nurse makes an assessment according to the ATLS guidelines. After the patient's condition has stabilized, nursing management of postoperative renal trauma is similar to that for genitourinary surgery. The primary nursing interventions include assessment for hemorrhage, maintenance of fluid and electrolyte balance, and maintenance of patency of drains and tubes. Measurement of urinary output includes drainage from the urinary catheter and the nephrostomy or suprapubic tubes. Drainage from these areas is recorded separately. Urine output is measured frequently until bloody drainage and clots have cleared. Gentle irrigation of drainage tubes may be required to clear clots and maintain the patency of the tubes.

PELVIC FRACTURES

The pelvis is a ring-shaped structure composed of the hip bones, sacrum, and coccyx. Because the pelvis protects the lower urinary tract and major blood vessels and nerves of the lower extremities, pelvic trauma can result in life-threatening hemorrhage and in urologic and neurologic dysfunction. The pelvis is highly vascular and can sequester a large volume of blood; the patient with pelvic fractures is at high risk for hemorrhagic shock.

Mechanism of Injury. Blunt trauma to the pelvis can be caused by MVCs, falls, or a crushing injury. One study found that motor cycle crashes have the highest prevalence of pelvic fractures.[44] Pelvic injuries may be associated with damage to underlying tissues and about 15% to 20% of patients with pelvic fractures may have concomitant abdominal or urogenital injuries.[44]

Assessment. Signs of pelvic fracture include perianal ecchymosis (scrotum or vulva) indicating extravasation of urine or blood, pain on palpation or "rocking" of the iliac crests, lower limb paresis or hypesthesia, hematuria. Lower extremity rotation or leg shortening is also cause for suspicion of a pelvic injury. Patients with a suspected pelvic injury should have a rectal examination to assess for SCI or presence of occult or obvious rectal bleeding.

The diagnosis of pelvic fracture is made by an anteroposterior pelvic radiograph with the patient in the supine position.[45] Additional x-ray films may be required for definitive treatment, but the timing depends on the patient's hemodynamic stability.

Classification of Pelvic Fractures. Pelvic fractures constitute a spectrum of complexity ranging from a single nondisplaced fracture of a pubic ramus to a life-threatening condition in which there are multiple fractures and crush injuries associated with significant hemorrhage and internal injuries.

Lateral Compression. The lateral compression (LC) vector of pelvic injury is the most common type.[46] This fracture produces a shortening of the pelvic diameter and typically does not involve ligamentous injury. Although this type of fracture is forgiving to the pelvic ring vessels, localized bleeding may occur, particularly to the posterior pelvis. There are three types of LC fractures. Type I includes the posterior compression of the sacroiliac joint without ligament disruption or an oblique pubic ramus fracture. Type II includes rupture of the posterior sacroiliac ligament or internal rotation of the hemipelvis with a crush injury of the sacrum and an oblique pubic ramus fracture. Type III includes the findings of type II LC injury with additional evidence of anteroposterior (AP) compression to the contralateral hemipelvis.

Anteroposterior Compression. When force is applied in the AP direction, the pelvic diameter widens. In this case, the injury can be completely ligamentous, which manifests as an open sacroiliac joint or open pubic symphysis.[46] This type of injury is commonly associated with vascular injury. There are three types of AP compression fractures. Type I includes disruption of the pubic symphysis with less than 2.5 cm of diastasis and with insignificant posterior pelvic involvement. Type II includes the disruption of the pubic symphysis of more than 2.5 cm with tearing of associated ligaments. Type III is a complete disruption of the pubic symphysis, posterior ligament complexes, and hemipelvic involvement.

Vertical Shear. A vertical shear pelvic injury includes a complete disruption of a hemipelvis associated with a hemipelvic displacement. This type of injury typically occurs in people who fall from a great height and land on one extremity.

Open Fractures. Open pelvic fractures involve an open wound with direct communication between the site of the fracture and a laceration involving the vagina, rectum, or perineum. The mortality rate for these injuries is high, because unlike closed pelvic fractures that bleed into the peritoneum, open pelvic fractures result in external exsanguinations.[46]

Medical Management.
The priority of the medical management of pelvic fractures is to prevent or to control life-threatening hemorrhage. External exsanguination is an immediate threat to patients with an open pelvic fracture. Current guidelines suggest that as a level 2 recommendation, patients with evidence of unstable fractures of the pelvis who are hypotensive should be considered for external pelvic stabilization.[47] This temporary pelvic stabilization may be accomplished by wrapping the pelvis with a sheet between the greater trochanter and the iliac crests. Advantages of this technique are that it is quick, does not involve specialized training, allows continued access to the patient during the resuscitation, and does not require specialized equipment.[45] Temporary external fixation is performed concurrently with resuscitation to reduce further bleeding of the vessels in the pelvis. In the event patients require a laparotomy (e.g., multiple trauma), the pelvis should be stabilized before the laparotomy incision to control blood loss.[47] If there are no obvious intraabdominal injuries, the pelvis is stabilized, and the patient may be considered for angiography and possible embolization to achieve hemostasis.[47]

Patients who are hemodynamically stable and have stable closed pelvic fractures are usually treated conservatively with bed rest. These patients may receive elective orthopedic stabilization after it is deemed safe to operate.[46] Definitive management of pelvic fracture may include placement of internal or external fixation devices.

Nursing Management.
Initial assessment of the patient with a pelvic fracture in the critical care unit proceeds according to ATLS guidelines. Nursing diagnoses include Ineffective Tissue Perfusion, Pain, Risk for Infection, and Risk for Injury.

Massive blood loss contributes to alteration in tissue perfusion. On admission to the critical care unit, the patient may have hemodynamic instability with abnormal coagulation factors. Interventions include intravenously administered crystalloid and colloid fluids. The nurse must ensure that an appropriate amount of blood remains cross-matched and available if needed. Adequate oxygenation is assessed by means of pulse oximetry and $S\bar{v}o_2$ and by monitoring serial hematocrit and hemoglobin levels.

The patient is at high risk for injury caused by neurovascular compromise, development of abdominal compartment syndrome, fat embolism syndrome, and wound infection. These syndromes are discussed further later in this chapter. Before the patient is moved, the nurse should know whether the physician has classified the closed pelvic fracture as *stable* or *unstable*. A stable pelvic injury implies that no further pathologic displacement of the pelvis can occur with turning or moving. An unstable pelvic fracture means that further pathologic displacement of the pelvis can occur with turning or moving.

Routine nursing assessments include neurovascular assessments of the lower extremities. Neurologic injury as a result of pelvic fracture may be transient and temporary. Open pelvic fractures may necessitate complex, time-consuming dressing changes. Aggressive pain management strategies should be employed during these dressing changes, because they can be quite painful.

Patients with open pelvic fractures usually have a prolonged critical care course with various degrees of complications. The patient with pelvic fractures is at risk for infection because of associated injuries and internal or external fixation devices. Nursing management of external fixation insertion sites is directed at preventing infection. Most institutions have protocols for pin care that require strict compliance.

COMPLICATIONS OF TRAUMA

In the trimodal distribution of trauma deaths, the third peak of death often occurs in the critical care unit as a result of complications days to weeks after the initial injury. Ongoing nursing assessments are imperative for early detection of complications associated with traumatic injuries. A single complication can increase hospital length of stay and the associated costs of treating the complication.

HYPERMETABOLISM

Nutritional support is an essential component in the care of critically ill trauma patients. Within 24 to 48 hours after traumatic injury, a predictable hypermetabolic response occurs. The metabolic response to injury mobilizes amino acids and accelerates protein synthesis to support wound healing and the immunologic response to invading organisms.[48] Stress hypermetabolism occurs after any major injury and is characterized by increases in metabolic rate and oxygen consumption. Energy requirements accelerate to promote immune function and tissue repair. The goal of early aggressive nutrition is to maintain host defenses by supporting this hypermetabolism and to preserve lean body mass.[48]

Most nutrition experts advocate beginning enteral nutrition as early as possible. Current guidelines recommend enteral feedings be initiated within 72 hours for patients with blunt and penetrating abdominal injuries and those with severe head injuries.[48] Enteral feeding sites can include the gastric route or any site beyond the pylorus of the stomach, including the duodenum and jejunum. Prompt feeding tube placement by the ICU nurse must be a priority, unless contraindicated. Diminished or absent bowel sounds do not mean the small bowel is not working. Small bowel function and the ability to absorb nutrients remain intact, despite the presence of gastroparesis and absent bowel sounds. Because access to the stomach can be obtained more quickly and easily than the duodenum, early gastric feeding is possible.[48] Patients at risk for pulmonary aspiration due to gastric retention or gastroesophageal reflux should receive enteral feedings into the jejunum.[48] If enteral feeding is not successful, parenteral nutrition should be initiated by day 7.[48]

INFECTION

Infection remains a major source of mortality and morbidity in critical care units. The trauma patient is at risk for infection because of contaminated wounds, invasive therapeutic and diagnostic catheters, intubation and mechanical ventilation, host susceptibility, and the critical care environment. Nursing management must include interventions to decrease and eliminate the trauma patient's risk of infection. The patient with multiple trauma is at risk for infection because of host susceptibility (including preexisting medical conditions) and the adverse effect of trauma on the immune system (see Chapter 40).

Wound contamination poses an infection risk for the trauma patient, especially with injuries resulting from deep or penetrating trauma. Exogenous bacteria (from the external environment) can enter through open wounds. Exogenous bacteria can be introduced by dirt, grass, and debris inoculated into the wound at the time of injury, or they can be introduced by personnel during wound care. Endogenous bacteria (from the internal environment) can be released as a result of gastrointestinal or genitourinary perforation, which spills bacteria into the internal environment.

Meticulous wound care is essential. The goals of wound care include minimizing infection risks, removing dead and devitalized tissue, allowing for wound drainage, and promoting wound epithelialization and contraction. Wound healing also is accomplished through interventions that promote tissue perfusion of well-oxygenated blood and that ensure adequate nutritional support for wound healing.

Standard interventions for the prevention of ventilator-associated pneumonia and catheter-related bloodstream infection apply to the trauma patient. Proper hand hygiene, invasive catheter care, patient positioning, sterile technique for all invasive procedures, and tight glucose control are paramount to optimal to patient outcome.

SEPSIS

The patient with multiple injuries is at risk for overwhelming infections and sepsis. The source of sepsis in the trauma patient can be invasive therapeutic and diagnostic catheters or wound contamination with exogenous or endogenous bacteria. The source of the septic nidus must be promptly evaluated. Gram stain and cultures of blood, urine, sputum, invasive catheters, and wounds are obtained (see Chapter 39).

PULMONARY COMPLICATIONS

Respiratory Failure. Posttraumatic respiratory failure often leads to the development of ARDS.[49] ARDS can be caused by direct injury to the lungs or indirect injury (see "Acute Respiratory Failure" in Chapter 24).[49] Primary direct injuries in the trauma patient can include aspiration, inhalation, and pulmonary contusion.[50] The indirect injuries include sepsis, massive transfusion, fat emboli, and missed injury.[50] ARDS in the trauma patient can develop 24 to 72 hours after initial injury. The patient receiving multiple blood products, particularly fresh-frozen plasma, must also be monitored for *transfusion-related acute lung injury*

(TRALI).[51] Signs of TRALI are similar to those of ARDS, although there is a temporal relationship between the new onset of respiratory distress and the transfusion of blood products.[51]

Fat Embolism Syndrome. Fat embolism syndrome can occur as a complication of orthopedic trauma. The clinical onset of fat embolism syndrome ranges from 12 to 72 hours after injury, although 90% of patients develop it within 24 hours after injury.[52] Fat embolism syndrome appears to develop as a result of fat droplets that leak from fractured bone and embolize to the lungs. The droplets are broken down into free fatty acids that are toxic to the pulmonary microvascular membranes. Pulmonary fat emboli alter pulmonary hemodynamics and pulmonary vascular permeability. The lung becomes highly edematous and hemorrhagic. The clinical presentation is almost indistinguishable from that of ARDS. Early stabilization of unstable extremity fractures may limit the seeding of fat droplets into the pulmonary system.[52]

PAIN

Pain in the ICU may come from many sources, including surgery, procedures, and trauma. Trauma may contribute to cellular death and inflammation that leads to pain. Relief of pain is a major component in the care of trauma patients.

An issue that often complicates pain management is the high incidence of substance abuse among patients who sustain traumatic injury. The Society of Critical Care Medicine proposed guidelines for the optimal use of analgesia and sedatives[53] (see Chapters 9 and 10).

KIDNEY COMPLICATIONS

Acute Kidney Injury. Assessment and ongoing monitoring of kidney function is critical to the survival of the trauma patient. The cause of posttraumatic renal failure is complex and may involve a variety of factors, as listed in Box 38-12.

BOX 38-12 ETIOLOGIC FACTORS IN POSTTRAUMATIC ACUTE KIDNEY INJURY

- Preexisting disease
  - Hypertension
  - Heart failure
  - Diabetes
  - Chronic kidney disease
  - Chronic liver disease
- Prolonged shock states
- Profound acidosis
- SIRS or reperfusion injury
- Abdominal compartment syndrome
- Muscle ischemia; myoglobinuria
- Microemboli
- Nephrotoxic drugs
- Radiocontrast dye

SIRS, systemic inflammatory response syndrome.

Prevention of kidney failure is the best treatment, and it begins with ensuring adequate renal perfusion. Serial assessments of blood urea nitrogen (BUN) and creatinine levels commonly are used to evaluate kidney function. Urine output as a measurement to determine kidney function can be misleading because posttraumatic renal insufficiency can manifest as nonoliguric renal failure. Progressive kidney failure requires prompt diagnosis and treatment (see "Acute Kidney Injury" in Chapter 31).

Myoglobinuria. Patients with a crush injury are susceptible to the development of myoglobinuria, with subsequent secondary kidney failure. Crush injuries can compromise blood flow. Loss of arterial blood flow, particularly to the extremities, results in the loss of oxygen transport to distal tissues and ischemia. This initiates a cascade of events that leads to the necrosis of skeletal muscle cells. As cells die, intracellular contents—particularly potassium and myoglobin—are released. Myoglobin, a muscular pigment, is a large molecule. Circulating myoglobin can lead to the development of kidney failure by three mechanisms: decreased renal perfusion, cast formation with tubular obstruction, and direct toxic effects of myoglobin in the renal tubules.[54]

Dark tea–colored urine suggests myoglobinuria. Testing for myoglobin in the urine can be done, but may take several days, depending on laboratory resources available for this test. The most rapid screening test is a serum creatine kinase level. Urine output and serial creatine kinase levels should be monitored.

After myoglobinuria is diagnosed, treatment is aimed at prevention of subsequent kidney failure. Aggressive administration of intravenous fluids increases renal blood flow and decreases the concentration of nephrotoxic pigments. Continuous infusion of mannitol and sodium bicarbonate ($NaHCO_3$) maybe used. Mannitol and $NaHCO_3$ are thought to alkalinize the urine and prevent myoglobin crystallization in the renal tubules. Acetazolamide (Diamox) may be given to prevent metabolic alkalosis that may be caused by the continuous $NaHCO_3$ infusion. Nursing management is directed toward achievement of fluid and electrolyte balance. The patient should be assessed for hypernatremia, hyperosmolarity, and volume overload. Assessment parameters may include maintaining urine output greater than or equal to 200 mL/hr and maintaining urine pH between 6.0 and 7.0 and serum pH at less than 7.5.[54]

VASCULAR COMPLICATIONS

Compartment Syndrome. Compartment syndrome is a condition in which increased pressure within a limited space compromises circulation, resulting in ischemia and necrosis of tissues within that space. Among those at high risk for the development of compartment syndrome are patients with lower extremity trauma, including fractures, penetrating trauma, vascular ruptures, massive tissue injuries, or venous obstruction. Clinical manifestations of compartment syndrome include obvious swelling and tightness of an extremity, paresis, and pain of the affected extremity. Diminished pulses and decreased capillary refill do not reliably identify compartment syndrome because they may be intact until after irreversible changes have occurred. Elevated intracompartmental pressures confirm the

diagnosis. The treatment can consist of simple interventions, such as removing an occlusive dressing, to more complex interventions, including a fasciotomy.

Deep Venous Thrombosis. Despite improvements in the care of the trauma patient, deep venous thrombosis (DVT) and the attendant risk of pulmonary embolism remain important causes of morbidity and mortality in the multiply injured trauma patient. Major trauma patients have a DVT risk that exceeds 50%.[55] The factors that form the basis of DVT pathophysiology are blood stasis, injury to the intimal surface of the vessel, and hypercoagulopathy. Trauma patients are at risk for DVT because of endothelial injury, coagulopathy, and immobility.

Trauma patients are at the greatest risk for developing thromboembolism early in their hospitalization. Prevention is key. Practice guidelines for the prevention and management of thromboembolism recommend that trauma patients at high risk for DVT receive sequential compression devices for prophylaxis against DVT.[56] High-risk patients include those with an SCI, lower extremity or pelvic fractures, need for a surgical procedure, increasing age, central venous catheters or venous injury, and prolonged immobility or hospital stay.[55] For patients in whom the lower leg is inaccessible, foot pumps may act as an effective alternative to lower the rate of DVT. Low-molecular-weight heparin (e.g., enoxaparin) is recommended for DVT prophylaxis in trauma patients with the following injury patterns:

- Pelvic fractures requiring operative fixation or prolonged bed rest (longer than 5 days);
- Complex lower extremity fractures requiring operative fixation or prolonged bed rest;
- SCI with complete or incomplete motor paralysis.

The selection of DVT prophylaxis for trauma patients is often challenging because of the need to achieve balance between DVT risk and bleeding risk. For high-risk trauma patients who cannot receive anticoagulation because of their risk of bleeding, the prophylactic placement of an inferior vena cava filter is considered when following patterns of injury are present:[56]

- Severe closed head injury with a GCS below 8, intracranial hemorrhage, or intraocular (eye) injury with associated hemorrhage
- Incomplete SCI with paraplegia or quadriplegia
- Complex pelvic fractures with associated long-bone fractures, retroperitoneal hematoma requiring transfusions
- Multiple long bone fractures

The purpose of inferior vena cava filter placement is to reduce the risk of fatal pulmonary embolism. Filter placement does not negate the requirement to use sequential compression devices for prophylaxis against DVT.

MISSED INJURY

Nursing assessment of the multiply injured patient in the critical care unit may reveal missed diseases or missed injuries. Missed injuries have a reported incidence of 2% to 14% and

HEMODYNAMIC INSTABILITY
- Shock states in the emergency department
- Aggressive resuscitation
- Emergent surgery taking precedence over thorough secondary surveys

ALTERATIONS IN CONSCIOUSNESS
- Presence of drugs or alcohol intoxication confuses physical assessments and masks physical findings.
- Disoriented patients are challenging to assess.
- Agitation makes diagnostic testing challenging.
- Patients with altered consciousness cannot provide a history of the injury.

are a cause of morbidity and mortality.[57] Missed disorders may include preexisting undiagnosed medical illnesses, such as endocrine disorders (diabetes, hypothyroidism); myocardial infarction; hypertension; decreased respiratory reserve; undiagnosed kidney failure; or malnutrition.

Occasionally, injuries may not be diagnosed in the pre-critical care phases. Missed injuries are commonly discovered in the first 24 to 48 hours of the hospital stay during the routine assessments of the trauma tertiary survey. Injuries are missed for a variety of reasons,[57,58] as summarized in Box 38-13. In the critical care unit, a missed injury may be suspected if the patient fails to show appropriate response to medical or surgical intervention. Change in the character of drainage from wounds or catheters may represent biliary or duodenal injuries. Hypotension and a falling hematocrit level despite aggressive fluid administration may indicate an expanding hematoma. As the patient begins to mobilize, small bone fractures and sprains may manifest. The critical care nurse must be alert to the possibility of a missed injury, especially when the patient does not appear to be responding appropriately to interventions. The physician must be notified immediately because potential complications of infection and hemorrhage may be life-threatening. Nurses play a key role in identifying missed injuries, particularly when patients regain consciousness and begin to increase their activity.

MULTIPLE ORGAN DYSFUNCTION SYNDROME

MODS is a clinical syndrome of progressive dysfunction of organ systems. Trauma patients are at high risk for systemic inflammatory response syndrome (SIRS) and MODS. Organ dysfunction can be the result of primary MODS, which is caused by direct traumatic injury, as may occur with acute lung dysfunction because of pulmonary contusion. Organ dysfunction that occurs later in the trauma patient's ICU course, secondary MODS, results from uncontrolled systemic inflammation with resultant organ dysfunction. Trauma patients may experience primary and secondary MODS. Treatment is aimed at controlling or eliminating the source of inflammation, maintenance of oxygen delivery and consumption, and nutritional and metabolic support for individual organs (see Chapter 40).

SPECIAL CONSIDERATIONS

MEETING THE NEEDS OF FAMILY MEMBERS AND SIGNIFICANT OTHERS

The impact of traumatic injury can be devastating for patients and for family members and significant others. They are faced with a crisis situation for which they have had little time to prepare. Trauma can precipitate a crisis within the family. Families may exhibit physical and sociocultural reactions and a combination of emotional reactions, including anger, fear, powerlessness, confusion, and mistrust. Recovery from traumatic injury can be long and frustrating for families. There may be many peaks and valleys of good days and bad days. During this time, the family may exhaust its social and financial support systems. Nurses should recognize this and facilitate supportive relationships for families.

A trend has evolved to move away from a paternalistic model of care to one that incorporates the family into all aspects of care, including resuscitation. Review of the literature suggests that many family members wish to remain close to their loved ones during these times, and there has been demonstrated benefit to the patient and the family in this model of care delivery.[59,60] Not surprisingly, this continues pose a dilemma—ethically, morally, and medicolegally—for health care providers.[59,60] Regardless of the specific system of care delivery, the nurse ensures the family is supported during all aspects of care.

A valuable intervention is to bring families of trauma patients together in support groups. Trauma family support groups can offer sharing of experiences, expression of emotions, mutual support, sharing of coping strategies, and education about hospital and community services.

TRAUMA IN THE OLDER PATIENT

Trauma affects people of all ages. Older patients are predisposed to traumatic injuries because of the inevitable consequences of aging. The ability to react to or avoid environmental hazards is impaired because of age-related deterioration of the senses and changes in motor strength, postural stability, balance, and coordination (see Chapter 14).

Older persons experience most of the falls that result in injuries, and these falls are likely to occur from level surfaces or steps.[61] Factors that predispose older persons to falls are summarized in Box 38-14.[61] Because many of the falls may be caused by an underlying medical condition (e.g., syncope, myocardial infarction, dysrhythmias), management of the older patient who has fallen must include an evaluation of events and conditions immediately preceding the fall.

The exposure of older adults to MVC trauma is a consequence of the increasing growth of the older population and the growing number of older drivers and occupants of motor

BOX 38-14   RISK FACTORS FOR FALLS IN OLDER ADULTS

ACUTE ILLNESS
- Cerebrovascular accidents
- Dysrhythmias
- Syncope
- Diabetes

COGNITIVE IMPAIRMENT
- Dementia

NEUROMUSCULAR DISORDERS
- Arthritis
- Lower extremity weakness
- Unstable gait

MEDICATIONS
- Antidepressants
- Benzodiazepines
- Diuretics
- Phenothiazines

BOX 38-15   FACTORS THAT PREDISPOSE OLDER ADULTS TO MOTOR VEHICLE CRASHES

- Alterations in visual and auditory acuity
- Deterioration in strength and slower reaction times
- Diminution of cerebral skills
- Diminution of motor skills
- Exacerbation of acute or chronic medical conditions
- Medications that may interfere with safe driving

vehicles. Factors that predispose older adults to MVCs are summarized in Box 38-15.[61] A pedestrian struck by a motor vehicle receives one of the most devastating injuries. Many deaths of older individuals occur in crosswalks. Physiologic deterioration of cerebral and motor skills and alterations in visual and auditory acuity cause older pedestrians to walk directly into the path of oncoming vehicles.

Trauma in older adults is associated with higher mortality rates, even when the injuries are less severe. Older adults have a higher complication rate and a higher mortality rate, starting at age 40 years, because of preexisting medical conditions, decreased physiologic reserves, and decreased ability to compensate for severe injury.[62] Older patients who do survive traumatic injury are often faced with changes in their preinjury functional status. Relatively minor trauma can be the event that changes the lifestyle of an older person from one of relative independence to one that requires prolonged rehabilitation or skilled nursing care. Discharge planning early in the patient's hospitalization is necessary.

The concept of *limited physiologic reserve* in the older trauma patient highlights the key difference between the average younger trauma patient with normal physiologic reserve and the older patient with underlying physiologic derangements. Age-related changes that occur in virtually every organ system may not produce evidence of organ dysfunction in the resting state. However, the ability of organs to augment function in response to traumatic stress may be greatly compromised. Fluid resuscitation is an integral part of trauma resuscitation. Patients on chronic diuretic therapy may require more volume and potassium supplementation as a result of chronic volume and potassium depletion. The assessment and management of hypovolemic shock is more complex in the older trauma patient. Older adults have limited ability to increase their heart rate in response to blood loss, obscuring one of the earliest signs of hypovolemia—tachycardia.[9] Loss of physiologic reserve and the presence of preexisting medical conditions are likely to produce further conflicting hemodynamic data. The older patient's lack of physiologic reserve makes it imperative that early nutritional support is initiated.

Trauma protocols are well established for the management of young patients after injury. Clinicians increasingly are recognizing that these protocols must be individualized for the older trauma patient. The best outcomes for this patient population have been achieved through early, appropriate, aggressive trauma care, including early hemodynamic monitoring in high-risk older trauma patients (those with a high-risk mechanism of injury, unknown cardiovascular status, preexisting cardiac or kidney disease).[63]

Summary

- Trauma is costly in lives lost and in dollars.
- Traumatic injuries may be caused by blunt or penetrating mechanisms.
- Assessment of the trauma patient is performed in a systematic fashion, moving from the brief primary survey to the head-to-toe secondary survey to the very detailed tertiary survey.
- Resuscitation of the trauma patient involves hemostasis to control hemorrhage, goal-directed volume support to restore cellular oxygenation, maintenance of normothermia, and prevention and correction of acidosis and coagulopathy.
- Management of severe TBIs and SCIs focuses on the prevention of secondary injury by ensuring that healthy tissue remains intact through maintaining oxygen delivery to the brain and spinal cord.
- Airway compromise is a major focus of care for the patient who has sustained maxillofacial injuries.
- Rib fractures are a cause of morbidity and mortality and require that care be balanced between pain relief and respiratory sufficiency through the use of multimodal pain management.
- Pelvic fractures may result in tremendous volume loss, and the nurse must remain alert to the possibility of hemorrhagic shock.
- Complication prevention involves early enteral nutrition, DVT prophylaxis, and prevention of infection.

Case Study: Patient with Trauma

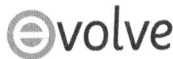 Answers to the Case Study Questions can be found on the Evolve web site at http://evolve.elsevier.com/Urden/.

Brief Patient History

Mr. G is a 21-year-old man. He was traveling in the back of a pickup truck that collided with another vehicle. He was ejected onto the side of the road and now is not awake and is barely breathing. He was intubated by emergency services, placed in a collar, and immobilized.

Clinical Assessment

Mr. G is admitted to the emergency department with minimal signs of external injury except for some small abrasions to the side of his face.

Diagnostic Procedures

Admission CT scan shows a large subdural hematoma.
Chest x-ray confirms appropriate placement of the endotracheal tube.
Baseline vital signs are blood pressure (BP) 110/60, heart rate (HR) 108 (sinus tachycardia), respiratory rate (RR) 30, temperature (T) 98.3° F, O_2 saturation 88%, Glasgow Coma Scale 7.

Medical Diagnosis

Mr. G is diagnosed with subdural hematoma secondary to trauma.

Questions

1. What major outcomes do you expect to achieve for this patient?
2. What problems or risks must be managed to achieve these outcomes?
3. What interventions must be initiated to monitor, prevent, manage, or eliminate the problems and risks identified above?
4. What interventions should be initiated to promote optimal functioning, safety, and well-being of the patient?
5. What possible learning needs would you anticipate for this patient?
6. What cultural and age-related factors might have a bearing on the patient's plan of care?

⊜ volve Be sure to check out the bonus material, including free self-assessment exercises, on the Evolve web site at http://evolve.elsevier.com/Urden/.

References

1. Centers for Disease Control and Prevention: Preventing violence against women: program activities guide. Available at www.cdc.gov/ncipc/dvp/vawguide.htm (accessed April 2009).
2. Melnick DM et al: Domestic violence and alcohol abuse in female trauma patients admitted to trauma centers, *J Trauma* 53:33, 2002.
3. Sheridan DJ, Nash KR: Acute injury patterns of intimate partner violence victims, *Trauma Violence Abuse* 8:281-289, 2007.
4. Sisley A et al: Violence in America: a public health crisis—domestic violence, *J Trauma* 46:1105, 1999.
5. Dept of Transportation (US), National Highway Traffic Safety Administration (NHTSA): *Traffic safety facts 2005: alcohol*, Washington, DC, 2006, National Highway Traffic Safety Safety Administration. Available at www-nrd.nhtsa.dot.gov/Pubs/TSF2005.PDF (accessed May 2009).
6. Blincoe L et al: *The economical impact of motor vehicle crashes: 2000.* Washington, DC, 2002, Department of Transportation, National Highway Traffic Safety Administration.
7. Committee on Trauma, American College of Surgeons: *Resources for optimal care of the injured patient*, Chicago, 2006, American College of Surgeons.
8. Saitz R: Unhealthy alcohol use, *N Engl J Med* 352:596-607, 2005.
9. American College of Surgeons: *Advanced trauma life support*, ed 8, Chicago, 2008, American College of Surgeons.
10. Beachley M: Evolution of the trauma cycle. In McQuillan KA et al, editors: *Trauma nursing: from resuscitation through rehabilitation*, ed 4, Philadelphia, 2009, Saunders.
11. Englehart MS, Schreiber MA: Measurement of acid–base resuscitation endpoints: lactate, base deficit, bicarbonate or what? *Curr Opin Crit Care* 12:569-574, 2006.
12. Tisherman SA et al: Clinical practice guideline: endpoints of resuscitation, *J Trauma* 57(4):898-912, 2004.
13. Center for Disease Control and Prevention, National Center on Injury Prevention and Control: Traumatic brain injury. Available at www.cdc.gov/ncipc/tbi/TBI.htm (accessed April 2009).
14. McQuillan KA, Thurman PA: Traumatic brain injuries. In McQuillan KA et al, editors: *Trauma nursing: from resuscitation through rehabilitation*, ed 4, Philadelphia, 2009, Saunders.
15. Chestnut RM: Management of brain and spinal cord injuries, *Crit Care Clin* 20(1):25-56, 2004.
16. Letarte P: The brain. In Feliciano DV et al, editors: *Trauma*, ed 6, New York, 2007, McGraw-Hill.
17. Brain Trauma Foundation: Guidelines for the management of severe traumatic brain injury, *J Neurotrauma* 24(suppl 1):1-106, 2007.
18. Lombardi F et al: Sensory stimulation for brain injured individuals in coma or vegetative state. *Cochrane Database Syst Rev* (2):CD001427, 2002.
19. National Spinal Cord Injury Statistical Center, Spinal Cord Injury Information Network: Facts and figures at a glance, January 2008. Available at www.spinalcord.uab.edu/show.asp?durki=116979&site=1021&return=19775 (accessed April 2009).
20. Sekhon LHS, Fehlings MG: Epidemiology, demographics, and pathophysiology of acute spinal cord injury, *Spine* 26(24S):S2-S12, 2002.
21. Russo-McCourt TA: Spinal cord injuries. In McQuillan KA et al, editors: *Trauma nursing: from resuscitation through rehabilitation*, ed 4, Philadelphia, 2009, Saunders.
22. Hadley MN et al: Guidelines for the management of acute cervical spine and spinal injuries, *Clin Neurosurg* 49:409-498, 2002.
23. Sherwood SF, McQuillan KA: Maxillofacial injuries. In McQuillan KA et al, editors: *Trauma nursing: from resuscitation through rehabilitation*, ed 4, Philadelphia, 2009, Saunders.
24. Kellman RM, Rontal ML: Face. In Feliciano DV et al, editors: *Trauma*, ed 6, New York, 2007, McGraw-Hill.
25. Brasel KJ et al: Rib fractures: relationship with pneumonia and mortality, *Crit Care Med* 34:1642-1646, 2006.
26. Holmes JF et al: A clinical decision rule for identifying children with thoracic injuries after blunt torso trauma, *Ann Emerg Med* 39(5):492-499, 2002.
27. Karmakar MK, Ho AM: Acute pain management of patients with multiple fractured ribs, *J Trauma* 54(3):615-625, 2003.
28. Stein DM et al: Accuracy of computed tomography (CT) scan in the detection of penetrating diaphragm injury, *J Trauma* 63(3):538-543, 2007.

29. Yamamoto L et al: Thoracic trauma: the deadly dozen, *Crit Care Nurs Q* 28(1):22-40, 2005.

30. Asencio JA et al: Trauma to the heart. In Feliciano DV et al, editors: *Trauma*, ed 6, New York, 2007, McGraw-Hill.

31. Schultz JM, Trunkey DD: Blunt cardiac injury. *Crit Care Clin* 20(1): 57-70, 2004.

32. Morgan PB, Buetchter KJ: Blunt thoracic aortic injuries: initial evaluation and management, *South Med J* 93(2):173-175, 2004.

33. Eastern Association of Surgeons in Trauma: Guidelines for the diagnosis and management of blunt aortic injury, 2000. Available at www.east.org (accessed April 2009).

34. Hoff WS et al: Practice management guidelines for the evaluation of blunt abdominal trauma, *J Trauma* 53(3):602-615, 2002.

35. Jones KM: Abdominal injuries. In McQuillan KA et al, editors: *Trauma nursing: from resuscitation through rehabilitation*, ed 4, Philadelphia, 2009, Saunders.

36. Todd SR: Critical concepts in abdominal injury, *Crit Care Clin* 20:119-134, 2004.

37. Germanos S et al: Damage control surgery in the abdomen: an approach for the management of severe injured patients, *Int J Surg* 6:246-252, 2008.

38. Malbrain MLNG et al: Results from the International Conference of Experts on Intra-abdominal Hypertension and Abdominal Compartment Syndrome: definitions, *Intensive Care Med* 32:1722-1732, 2006.

39. Cheatham MLA et al: Results from the International Conference of Experts on Intra-abdominal Hypertension and Abdominal Compartment Syndrome: Recommendations, *Intensive Care Med* 33:951-962, 2007.

40. Schreiber MA: Damage control surgery, *Crit Care Clin* 20:119-134, 2004.

41. Eastern Association of Surgeons in Trauma: Practice management guidelines for the nonoperative management of blunt injury to the liver and spleen, 2000. Available at www.east.org (accessed April 2009).

42. Snyder KA, Veronese V: Genitourinary injuries and renal management. In McQuillan KA et al, editors: *Trauma nursing: from resuscitation through rehabilitation*, ed 4, Philadelphia, 2009, Saunders.

43. Eastern Association of Surgeons in Trauma: Practice management guidelines for the management of genitourinary trauma, 2004. Available at www.east.org (accessed April 2009).

44. Demetriades D et al: Pelvic fractures: epidemiology and predictors of associated abdominal injuries and outcomes, *J Am Coll Surg* 195:1-10, 2002.

45. Mirza A, Ellis T: Initial management of pelvic and femoral fractures in the multiply injured patient, *Crit Care Clin* 20:159, 2004.

46. Burgess AR et al: Pelvic ring disruptions: effective classification system and treatment protocols, *J Trauma* 30:848-856, 1990.

47. EAST Practice Management Guidelines Work Group: Practice management guidelines for hemorrhage in pelvic fracture, 2001, Eastern Association for the Surgery of Trauma. Available at www.east.org (accessed April 2009).

48. Jacobs DG et al: Practice management guidelines for nutritional support of the trauma patient, *J Trauma* 57(3):660-679, 2004.

49. Chirag SV et al: The impact of development of acute lung injury on hospital mortality in critically ill trauma patients, *Crit Care Med* 36:2309-2315, 2008.

50. Micheals AJ: Management of post-traumatic respiratory failure, *Crit Care Clin* 29:83, 2004.

51. Wallis JP: Transfusion-related acute lung injury (TRALI): presentation, epidemiology and treatment, *Intensive Care Med* 33(suppl 1):S12-S16, 2007.

52. Husebye EE et al: Bone marrow fat in the circulation: clinical entities and pathophysiological mechanisms, *Injury* 37(suppl 4):S8-S18, 2006.

53. Jacobi F et al: Clinical practice guidelines for the sustained use of sedatives and analgesics in the critically ill adult, *Crit Care Med* 30:119, 2002.

54. Malinowski DJ et al: Crush injury and rhabdomyolysis. *Crit Care Clin* 20:171, 2004.

55. Geerts WH, Heit JA: Prevention of venous thromboembolism, *Chest* 119:1325, 2001.

56. Eastern Association for the Surgery of Trauma: Practice management guidelines for the management of venous thromboembolism in trauma patients, 1998. Available at www.east.org (accessed April 2009).

57. Clarke DL et al: Applying modern error theory to the problem of missed injuries in trauma, *World J Surg* 32:1176-1182, 2008.

58. Sommers MS: Missed injuries: a case of trauma hide and seek, *AACN Clin Issues* 6:187, 1995.

59. Alvarez GF, Kirby AS: The perspective of families of the critically ill patient: their needs. *Curr Opin Crit Care* 12:614-618, 2006.

60. Moreland P: Family presence during invasive procedures and resuscitation in the emergency department: a review of the literature, *J Emerg Nurs* 31(1):58-72, 2005.

61. Aschkenasy MT, Rothenhaus TC: Trauma and falls in the elderly, *Emerg Med Clin North Am* 24:413-432, 2006.

62. Victorino G et al: Trauma in the elderly, *Arch Surg* 138:1093, 2003.

63. Eastern Association for the Surgery of Trauma: Practice management guidelines for geriatric trauma, 2001. Available at www.east.org (accessed April 2009).

Shock is an acute, widespread process of impaired tissue perfusion that results in cellular, metabolic, and hemodynamic alterations. Ineffective tissue perfusion occurs when an imbalance develops between cellular oxygen supply and cellular oxygen demand. This imbalance can occur for a variety of reasons and eventually results in cellular dysfunction and death. This chapter presents an overview of the general shock response, or shock syndrome, followed by a discussion of the various shock states.

SHOCK SYNDROME

DESCRIPTION

Shock is a complex pathophysiologic process that often results in multiple organ dysfunction syndrome (MODS) and death. All types of shock eventually result in ineffective tissue perfusion and acute circulatory failure. The shock syndrome is a pathway involving a variety of pathologic processes that may be categorized as four stages: initial, compensatory, progressive, and refractory. Progression through each stage varies with the patient's prior condition, duration of initiating event, response to therapy, and correction of underlying cause.

ETIOLOGY

Shock can be classified as hypovolemic, cardiogenic, or distributive, depending on the pathophysiologic cause and hemodynamic profile. Hypovolemic shock results from a loss of circulating or intravascular volume. Cardiogenic shock results from the impaired ability of the heart to pump. Distributive shock results from maldistribution of circulating blood volume and can be further classified as septic, anaphylactic, or neurogenic. Septic shock is the result of microorganisms entering the body. Anaphylactic shock is the result of a severe antibody-antigen reaction. Neurogenic shock is the result of the loss of sympathetic tone.

PATHOPHYSIOLOGY

During the initial stage, cardiac output (CO) is decreased, and tissue perfusion is threatened. Almost immediately, the compensatory stage begins as the body's homeostatic mechanisms attempt to maintain CO, blood pressure, and tissue perfusion. The compensatory mechanisms are mediated by the sympathetic nervous system (SNS) and consist of neural, hormonal, and chemical responses. The neural response includes an increase in heart rate and contractility, arterial and venous vasoconstriction, and shunting of blood to the vital organs. Hormonal compensation includes activation of the renin response and stimulation of the anterior pituitary and adrenal medulla. Activation of the renin response results in the production of angiotensin II, which causes vasoconstriction and the release of aldosterone and antidiuretic hormone (ADH), leading to sodium and water retention. Stimulation of the anterior pituitary results in the secretion of adrenocorticotropic hormone (ACTH), which stimulates the adrenal cortex to produce glucocorticoids, causing a rise in blood glucose levels. Stimulation of the adrenal medulla causes the release of epinephrine and norepinephrine, which further enhance the compensatory mechanisms.

During the progressive stage, the compensatory mechanisms begin failing to meet tissue metabolic needs, and the shock cycle is perpetuated (see Concept Map). As tissue perfusion becomes ineffective, the cells switch from aerobic to anaerobic metabolism to produce energy. Anaerobic metabolism produces small amounts of energy but large amounts of lactic acid, producing lactic acidemia. Increased vascular permeability from endothelial and epithelial hypoxia and inflammatory mediators results in intravascular hypovolemia, tissue edema, and further decline in tissue perfusion.[1,2] A systemic release of inflammatory mediators in response to tissue hypoxia, especially in gut tissue, produces microcirculatory impairment and derangement of cellular metabolism, facilitating progression of the shock cycle.[1-3] The patient is experiencing the systemic inflammatory response syndrome (SIRS), and irreversible damage begins to occur. Some cells die as a result of apoptosis, an injury-activated, preprogrammed cellular suicide. Others die as the sodium-potassium pump in the cell membrane fails, causing the cell and its organelles to swell. Cellular energy production comes to a complete halt as the mitochondria swell and rupture. At this point, the problem becomes one of oxygen use instead of oxygen delivery. Even if the cell were to receive more oxygen, it would be unable to use it because of damage to the mitochondria. The cell's digestive organelles swell and leak destructive enzymes into the cell, accelerating cell death.

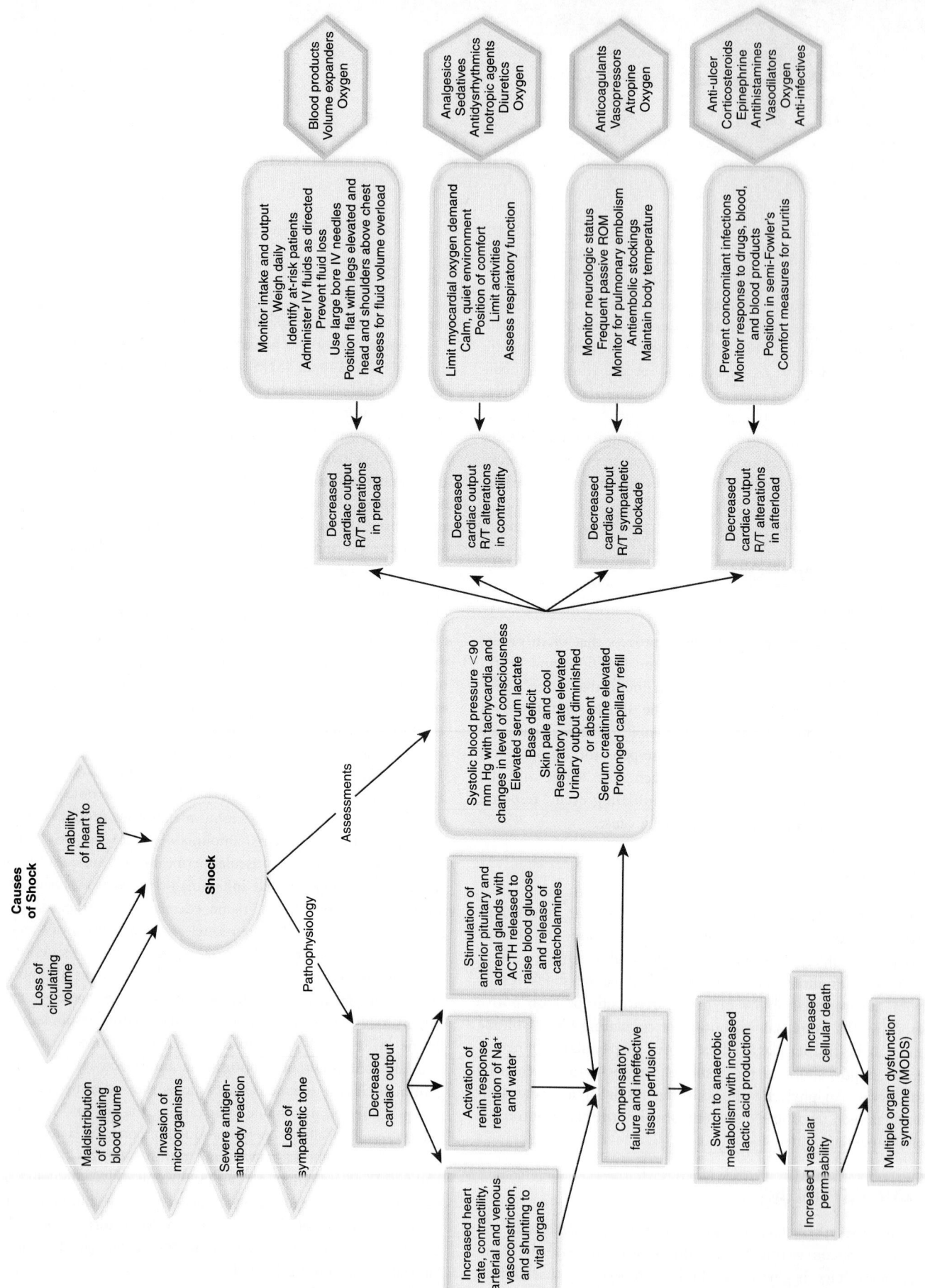

BOX 39-1   CONSEQUENCES OF SHOCK

CARDIOVASCULAR
- Ventricular failure
- Microvascular thrombosis

NEUROLOGIC
- Sympathetic nervous system dysfunction
- Cardiac and respiratory depression
- Thermoregulatory failure
- Coma

PULMONARY
- Acute respiratory failure
- Acute lung injury (ALI)

RENAL
- Acute tubular necrosis (ATN)

HEMATOLOGIC
- Disseminated intravascular coagulation (DIC)

GASTROINTESTINAL
- Gastrointestinal tract failure
- Hepatic failure
- Pancreatic failure

Every system in the body is affected by this process (Box 39-1). Cardiac dysfunction develops as a result of the release of myocardial depressant cytokines.[1,2] Ventricular failure eventually occurs, further perpetuating the entire process. Central nervous system (CNS) dysfunction develops as a result of cerebral hypoperfusion, leading to failure of the SNS, cardiac and respiratory depression, and thermoregulatory failure. Endothelial injury from hypoxia and inflammatory cytokines and impaired blood flow result in microvascular thrombosis. Hematologic dysfunction occurs as a result of consumption of clotting factors, release of inflammatory cytokines, and dilutional thrombocytopenia. Disseminated intravascular coagulation (DIC) eventually may develop. Pulmonary dysfunction occurs as a result of increased pulmonary capillary membrane permeability, pulmonary microemboli, and pulmonary vasoconstriction. Ventilatory failure and acute lung injury (ALI) develop. Renal dysfunction develops as a result of renal vasoconstriction and renal hypoperfusion, leading to acute tubular necrosis (ATN). Gastrointestinal dysfunction occurs as a result of splanchnic vasoconstriction and hypoperfusion and leads to failure of the gut organs. Disruption of the intestinal epithelium releases gram-negative bacteria into the system, which further perpetuates the entire shock syndrome.[4]

During the refractory stage, shock becomes unresponsive to therapy and is considered irreversible. As the individual organ systems die, MODS—defined as failure of two or more body systems—occurs (see Chapter 40). Death is the final outcome. Regardless of the etiologic factors, death occurs from ineffective tissue perfusion because of the failure of the circulation to meet the oxygen needs of the cell.

ASSESSMENT AND DIAGNOSIS

The patient with a mean arterial blood pressure (MAP) less than 60 mm Hg or with evidence of multisystem organ hypoperfusion is considered to be in a shock state.[1,5] Because shock is a dynamic physiologic phenomenon, hypotension may occur late in the process.[6] Clinical manifestations vary according to the underlying cause of shock, the stage of the shock, and the patient's response to shock.

Compensatory mechanisms may produce normal hemodynamic values even when tissue perfusion is compromised.[4-7] Global indicators of systemic perfusion and oxygenation include serum lactate, arterial base deficit, serum bicarbonate, and central or mixed venous oxygen saturation levels. Inadequate cellular oxygenation with anaerobic metabolism and increased metabolic lactate production increase the serum lactate level.[8] The level and duration of this hyperlactatemia are predictive of morbidity and mortality.[7-11] The base deficit derived from arterial blood gas (ABG) values also reflects global tissue acidosis and is frequently used to assess the severity of shock.[6-7,9] Studies have demonstrated serum bicarbonate to be an equivalent alternative to arterial base deficit in predicting mortality in surgical and trauma patients.[12,13] The use of mixed venous oxygen saturation ($S\bar{v}O_2$) measured by means of a pulmonary artery catheter or central venous oxygen saturation ($ScvO_2$) measured with a central venous catheter allows assessment of the balance of oxygen delivery and oxygen consumption and the ratio of oxygen extraction.[14-16] After years of recommended use to guide the care of patients with severe sepsis, this measure of global oxygen balance is being evaluated for use in other critically ill populations.[15-21] The sections on different types of shock discuss clinical assessment and diagnosis of the patient in shock.

MEDICAL MANAGEMENT

The major focus of the treatment of shock is the improvement and preservation of tissue perfusion. Adequate tissue perfusion depends on an adequate supply of oxygen being transported to the tissues and the cell's ability to use it. Oxygen transport is influenced by pulmonary gas exchange, CO, and hemoglobin level. Oxygen use is influenced by the internal metabolic environment. Management of the patient in shock focuses on supporting oxygen delivery.[1,22]

Adequate pulmonary gas exchange is critical to oxygen transport. Establishing and maintaining an adequate airway are the first steps in ensuring adequate oxygenation. After the airway is patent, emphasis is placed on improving ventilation and oxygenation. Therapies include administration of supplemental oxygen and mechanical ventilatory support.

An adequate CO and hemoglobin level are crucial to oxygen transport. CO depends on heart rate, preload, afterload, and contractility. A variety of fluids and drugs are used to manipulate these parameters. The types of fluids used include crystalloids and colloids. The categories of drugs used include vasoconstrictors, vasodilators, positive inotropes, and antidysrhythmics.

Fluid administration is indicated for decreased preload related to intravascular volume depletion, and it can be accomplished by use of a crystalloid or colloid solution, or both. Crystalloids are balanced electrolyte solutions that may be hypotonic, isotonic, or hypertonic. Examples of crystalloid solutions used in shock situations are normal saline and lactated Ringer's solution. Colloids are protein- or starch-containing solutions. Examples of colloid solutions are blood and blood components, such as albumin, and pharmaceutical plasma expanders, such as hetastarch, dextran, and mannitol.

The choice of fluid is a subject of debate and depends on the situation.[15,23-25] Fluid resuscitation with normal saline or with albumin produces similar outcomes regardless of baseline serum albumin level, and both are considered safe.[26,27] Crystalloid solutions are inexpensive and effective. Advantages of colloids include faster restoration of intravascular volume and use of smaller amounts. Colloids are believed to stay in the intravascular space, unlike crystalloids, which readily leak into the extravascular space. Disadvantages include expense, allergic reactions, and difficulties in typing and cross-matching blood. Colloids also can leak out of damaged capillaries and cause a variety of additional problems, particularly in the lungs.

Blood should be considered to augment oxygen transport if the patient's hemoglobin level is critically low, although controversy exists about what threshold value should be used.[4,15] Transfusion of stored red blood cells does not substantially increase oxygen consumption and has been associated with immunosuppression, infection, impairment of microcirculatory flow, coagulopathy, and increased mortality, and restrictive transfusion practice has demonstrated lower mortality.[4,16,28] Transfusion-related acute lung injury (TRALI) resulting from immune and nonimmune neutrophil activation has become the leading cause of transfusion-related death and may occur with transfusion of any plasma-containing blood or blood product.[28-31]

Vasoconstrictor agents are used to increase afterload by increasing the systemic vascular resistance (SVR) and improving the patient's blood pressure level. Vasodilator agents are used to decrease preload or afterload, or both, by decreasing venous return and SVR. Positive inotropic agents are used to increase contractility. Antidysrhythmic agents are used to influence heart rate. Box 39-2 provides examples of each of these agents.

Sodium bicarbonate is not recommended in the treatment of shock-related lactic acidosis.[16,32,33] No overall benefit has been found, and the risks associated with its use are significant. They include shifting of the oxyhemoglobin dissociation curve to the left, rebound increase in lactic acid production, development of hyperosmolar state, fluid overload resulting from excessive sodium, and rapid cellular electrolyte shifts.[11,32,33]

The patient should be started on nutritional support therapy as early as possible. The type of nutritional supplementation initiated varies according to the cause of shock, and it should be tailored to the individual patient's need, as indicated by the underlying condition and laboratory data. The enteral route is preferred over the parenteral, although parenal nutrition should be considered when enteral feeding is contraindicated.[3,25,34-37] Supplementation of enteral feeding with parenteral nutrition to increase caloric intake has not been shown to improve patient outcomes.[3,36]

BOX 39-2 AGENTS USED IN THE TREATMENT OF SHOCK

VASOCONSTRICTORS
- Epinephrine (Adrenalin)
- Norepinephrine (Levophed)
- Alpha-range dopamine (Intropin)
- Metaraminol (Aramine)
- Phenylephrine (Neo-Synephrine)
- Ephedrine
- Vasopressin (Pitressin)

VASODILATORS
- Nitroprusside (Nipride, Nitropress)
- Nitroglycerin (Nitrol, Tridil)
- Hydralazine (Apresoline)
- Labetalol (Normodyne, Trandate)

INOTROPES
- Beta-range dopamine (Intropin)
- Dobutamine (Dobutrex)
- Epinephrine (Adrenalin)
- Isoproterenol (Isuprel)
- Norepinephrine (Levophed)

ANTIDYSRHYTHMICS
- Lidocaine (Xylocaine)
- Adenosine (Adenocard)
- Procainamide (Pronestyl)
- Labetalol (Normodyne, Trandate)
- Verapamil (Calan, Isoptin)
- Esmolol (Brevibloc)
- Diltiazem (Cardizem)
- Amiodarone (Cordarone)

Tight glucose control is recommended for all critically ill patients.[38,39] Benefits of glucose control in the critically ill include lower incidences of infection, renal failure, sepsis, polyneuropathy, need for blood transfusion, prolonged mechanical ventilation, and death.[38-42]

NURSING MANAGEMENT

The nursing management of a patient in shock is a complex and challenging responsibility. It requires an in-depth understanding of the pathophysiology of the disease and the anticipated effects of each intervention, as well as a solid understanding of the nursing process. Later sections discuss specific interventions for the patient in shock.

The psychosocial needs of the patient and family dealing with shock are extremely important. These needs are based on situational, familial, and patient-centered variables. Nursing interventions for the psychosocial stress of critical illness include providing information on patient status, explaining procedures and routines, supporting the family, encouraging the expression of feelings, facilitating problem solving and shared decision making, individualizing visitation schedules, involving the

- Support oxygen transport.
  - Establish a patent airway.
  - Initiate mechanical ventilation.
  - Administer oxygen.
  - Administer fluids (crystalloids, colloids, blood and other blood products).
  - Administer vasoactive medications.
  - Administer positive inotropic medications.
  - Ensure sufficient hemoglobin and hematocrit.
- Support oxygen use.
  - Identify and correct cause of lactic acidosis.
  - Ensure adequate organ and extremity perfusion.
  - Initiate nutritional support therapy.
- Identify underlying cause of shock and treat accordingly.
- Maintain surveillance for complications.
- Provide comfort and emotional support.

ABSOLUTE FACTORS
- Loss of whole blood
  - Trauma or surgery
  - Gastrointestinal bleeding
- Loss of plasma
  - Thermal injuries
  - Large lesions
- Loss of other body fluids
  - Severe vomiting or diarrhea
  - Massive diuresis
  - Loss of intravascular integrity
  - Ruptured spleen
  - Long bone or pelvic fractures
  - Hemorrhagic pancreatitis
  - Hemothorax or hemoperitoneum
  - Arterial dissection or rupture

RELATIVE FACTORS
- Vasodilation
  - Sepsis
  - Anaphylaxis
  - Loss of sympathetic stimulation
- Increased capillary membrane permeability
  - Sepsis
  - Anaphylaxis
  - Thermal injuries
- Decreased colloidal osmotic pressure
  - Severe sodium depletion
  - Hypopituitarism
  - Cirrhosis
  - Intestinal obstruction

family in the patient's care, and establishing contacts with necessary resources.[43] Patients and families should be given the option of family presence during invasive procedures and resuscitation.[43-45] Collaborative management of the patient with shock is outlined in Box 39-3.

HYPOVOLEMIC SHOCK

DESCRIPTION

Hypovolemic shock occurs from inadequate fluid volume in the intravascular space. The lack of adequate circulating volume leads to decreased tissue perfusion and initiation of the general shock response. Hypovolemic shock is the most commonly occurring form of shock.

ETIOLOGY

Hypovolemic shock can result from absolute or relative hypovolemia. Absolute hypovolemia occurs when there is a loss of fluid from the intravascular space. This can result from an external loss of fluid from the body or from internal shifting of fluid from the intravascular space to the extravascular space. Fluid shifts can result from a loss of intravascular integrity, increased capillary membrane permeability, or decreased colloidal osmotic pressure. Relative hypovolemia occurs when vasodilation produces an increase in vascular capacitance relative to circulating volume (Box 39-4).

PATHOPHYSIOLOGY

Hypovolemia results in a loss of circulating fluid volume. A decrease in circulating volume leads to a decrease in venous return, which results in a decrease in end-diastolic volume or preload. Preload is a major determinant of stroke volume (SV) and CO. A decrease in preload results in a decrease in SV and CO. The decrease in CO leads to inadequate cellular oxygen supply and ineffective tissue perfusion (Fig. 39-1).

ASSESSMENT AND DIAGNOSIS

The clinical manifestations of hypovolemic shock depend on the severity of fluid loss and the patient's ability to compensate for it. Clinical classes have been developed by the American College of Surgeons to describe the levels of severity of hypovolemic shock. Class I indicates a fluid volume loss up to 15% or an actual volume loss up to 750 mL. Compensatory mechanisms maintain CO, and the patient appears free of symptoms other than slight anxiety.[4,46]

Class II hypovolemia occurs with a fluid volume loss of 15% to 30% or an actual volume loss of 750 to 1500 mL. Falling CO activates more intense compensatory responses. The heart rate increases to more than 100 beats/min in response to increased SNS stimulation unless blocked by preexisting beta-blocker therapy. The pulse pressure narrows as the diastolic blood pressure increases because of vasoconstriction. The respiratory rate increases to 20 to 30 breaths/min, and respiratory depth increases in an attempt to improve oxygenation. ABG specimens drawn during this phase reveal respiratory alkalosis and hypoxemia, as evidenced by a low partial pressure of carbon dioxide ($PaCO_2$) and a low partial pressure of oxygen (PaO_2), respectively. Urine output starts to decline to 20 to 30 mL/hr

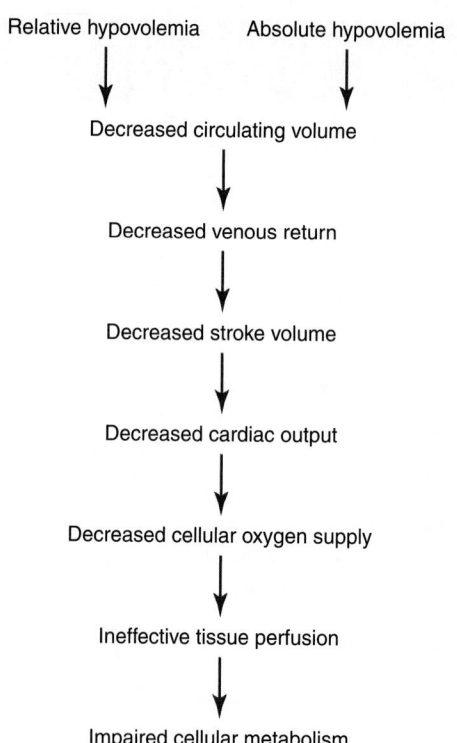

Relative hypovolemia   Absolute hypovolemia

↓   ↓

Decreased circulating volume

↓

Decreased venous return

↓

Decreased stroke volume

↓

Decreased cardiac output

↓

Decreased cellular oxygen supply

↓

Ineffective tissue perfusion

↓

Impaired cellular metabolism

Figure 39-1 The pathophysiology of hypovolemic shock.

as renal perfusion decreases. The urine sodium level decreases, whereas urinary osmolality and specific gravity increase as the kidneys start to conserve sodium and water. The patient's skin becomes pale and cool with delayed capillary refill because of peripheral vasoconstriction. Jugular veins appear flat as a result of decreased venous return.[4,46]

Hypovolemic shock that is class III occurs with a fluid volume loss of 30% to 40% or an actual volume loss of 1500 to 2000 mL. This level of severity produces the progressive stage of shock as compensatory mechanisms become overwhelmed and ineffective tissue perfusion develops. Blood pressure decreases. The heart rate increases to more than 120 beats/min, and dysrhythmias develop as myocardial ischemia ensues. Respiratory distress occurs as the pulmonary system deteriorates. ABG values during this phase reveal respiratory and metabolic acidosis and hypoxemia, as evidenced by a high $PaCO_2$, low bicarbonate (HCO_3^-), and low PaO_2, respectively. Decreased renal perfusion results in the development of oliguria. Blood urea nitrogen (BUN) and serum creatinine levels start to rise as the kidneys begin to fail. The patient's skin becomes ashen, cold, and clammy, with marked delayed capillary refill. The patient appears confused as cerebral perfusion decreases and the level of consciousness deteriorates.[4,7,46]

Class IV hypovolemic shock is usually refractory in nature. It occurs with a fluid volume loss of greater than 40% or an actual volume loss of more than 2000 mL. The compensatory mechanisms of the body completely deteriorate, and organ failure occurs.[5,7] Severe tachycardia and hypotension ensue. Peripheral pulses are absent, and because of marked peripheral vasoconstriction, capillary refill does not occur. The skin

appears cyanotic, mottled, and extremely diaphoretic. Urine output ceases. The patient becomes lethargic and unresponsive, and various clinical manifestations associated with failure of the different body systems develop.[4,7,46]

Assessment of the hemodynamic parameters of a patient in hypovolemic shock varies by stage but commonly reveals a decreased CO and cardiac index (CI). Loss of circulating volume leads to a decrease in venous return to the heart, which results in a decrease in the preload of the right and left ventricles. This is evidenced by a decline in the central venous pressure (CVP) or right atrial pressure (RAP) and pulmonary artery occlusion pressure (PAOP). Vasoconstriction of the arterial system results in an increase in the afterload of the heart, as evidenced by an increase in the SVR. This vasoconstriction may produce a falsely elevated systolic blood pressure when measured by arterial catheter. MAP is more accurate in this low-flow state.[7]

MEDICAL MANAGEMENT

The major goals of therapy for the patient in hypovolemic shock are to correct the cause of the hypovolemia, restore tissue perfusion, and prevent complications. This approach includes identifying and stopping the source of fluid loss and administering fluid to replace circulating volume. Fluid administration can be accomplished with use of a crystalloid solution, a colloid solution, blood products, or a combination of fluids. The type of solution used depends on the type of fluid lost, the degree of hypovolemia, the severity of hypoperfusion, and the cause of hypovolemia.

Aggressive fluid resuscitation in trauma and surgical patients is the subject of great debate. The benefit of limited or hypotensive (systolic blood pressure >80 mm Hg) volume resuscitation in patients with uncontrolled hemorrhage is postulated to lessen bleeding and improve survival.[22,47-49] The type and amount of solutions used for fluid resuscitation and the rate of administration influence immune function, inflammatory mediator release, coagulation, and the incidence of cardiac, pulmonary, and gastrointestinal complications.[23,24,50-52] Consensus on the optimal resuscitative strategy for hypovolemic shock is lacking.[23,24,48]

NURSING MANAGEMENT

Prevention of hypovolemic shock is one of the primary responsibilities of the nurse in the critical care area. Preventive measures include the identification of patients at risk and frequent assessment of the patient's fluid balance. Accurate monitoring of intake and output and daily weights are essential components of preventive nursing care. Early identification and treatment result in decreased mortality.

Management of the patient in hypovolemic shock requires continuous evaluation of intravascular volume, tissue perfusion, and response to therapy. The patient in hypovolemic shock may have any number of nursing diagnoses, depending on the progression of the process (see the Nursing Diagnoses feature on Hypovolemic Shock). Nursing interventions also include minimizing fluid loss, administering volume replacement, providing comfort and emotional support, and maintaining surveillance for complications.

Measures to minimize fluid loss include limiting blood sampling, observing lines for accidental disconnection, and applying direct pressure to bleeding sites. Measures to facilitate the administration of volume replacement include insertion of large-bore peripheral intravenous catheters, rapid administration of prescribed fluids, and positioning the patient with the legs elevated, trunk flat, and head and shoulders above the chest. Monitoring the patient for clinical manifestations of fluid overload or complications related to fluid and blood product administration is essential for preventing further problems.

CARDIOGENIC SHOCK

DESCRIPTION

Cardiogenic shock is the result of failure of the heart to effectively pump blood forward. It can occur with dysfunction of the right or the left ventricle, or both. The lack of adequate pumping function leads to decreased tissue perfusion and circulatory failure. It occurs in approximately 5% to 8% of the patients with an ST-segment myocardial infarction (MI), and it is the leading cause of death of patients hospitalized with MI.[53,54] The mortality rate for cardiogenic shock has decreased with the advent of early revascularization therapy and is currently about 50% to 60%.[53-56]

ETIOLOGY

Cardiogenic shock can result from primary ventricular ischemia, structural problems, and dysrhythmias.[53,54] The most common cause is acute MI resulting in the loss of 40% or more of the functional myocardium. It can occur with ST-elevation or non–ST-elevation MI.[54,57] The damage to the myocardium may occur after one massive MI (usually of the anterior wall), or it may be cumulative as a result of several smaller MIs or a small MI in a patient with preexisting ventricular dysfunction.[53,57] Structural problems of the cardiopulmonary system and dysrhythmias also may cause cardiogenic shock if they disrupt the forward motion of the blood through the heart (Box 39-5).[53,54,57]

BOX 39-5	**ETIOLOGIC FACTORS IN CARDIOGENIC SHOCK**

PRIMARY VENTRICULAR ISCHEMIA
- Acute myocardial infarction
- Cardiopulmonary arrest
- Open heart surgery

STRUCTURAL PROBLEMS
- Septal rupture
- Papillary muscle rupture
- Free wall rupture
- Ventricular aneurysm
- Cardiomyopathies
  - Congestive
  - Hypertrophic
  - Restrictive
- Intracardiac tumor
- Pulmonary embolus
- Atrial thrombus
- Valvular dysfunction
- Acute myocarditis
- Cardiac tamponade
- Myocardial contusion
- Prolonged septic shock
- Recent hemorrhage

DYSRHYTHMIAS
- Bradydysrhythmias
- Tachydysrhythmias

PATHOPHYSIOLOGY

Cardiogenic shock results from the impaired ability of the ventricle to pump blood forward, which leads to a decrease in SV and an increase in the blood left in the ventricle at the end of systole. The decrease in SV results in a decrease in CO, which leads to decreased cellular oxygen supply and ineffective tissue perfusion. Typically, myocardial performance spirals downward as compensatory vasoconstriction increases myocardial afterload and low blood pressure worsens myocardial ischemia. Evidence of SIRS has been observed in a substantial number of patients with cardiogenic shock.[55,57-59] Activation of inflammatory cytokines induce systemic vasodilation, defective cellular oxygen use, and occasionally, normalization of the CO. Whether this process contributes to the genesis or the outcome of cardiogenic shock is uncertain, but it is thought to be activated by acute MI and to facilitate development of sepsis.[55,57,58] As left ventricular contractility declines and ventricular compliance decreases, an increase in end-systolic volume results in blood backing up into the pulmonary system and the subsequent development of pulmonary edema. Pulmonary edema causes impaired gas exchange and decreased oxygenation of the arterial blood, which further impair tissue perfusion (Fig. 39-2). Death due to cardiogenic shock may result from multiple organ failure or cardiopulmonary collapse.[55,58]

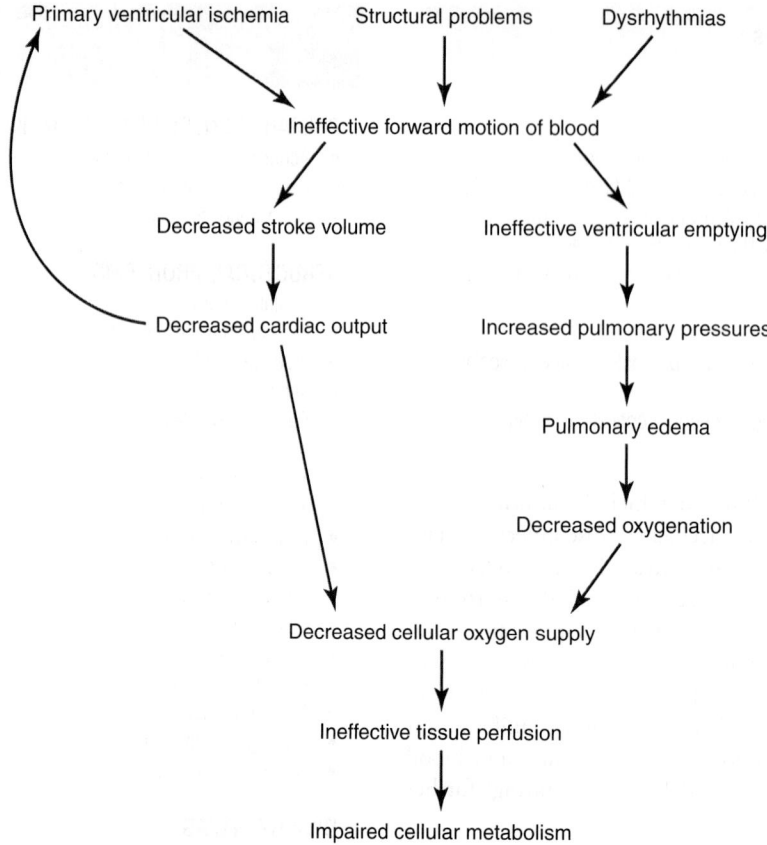

Figure 39-2 The pathophysiology of cardiogenic shock.

ASSESSMENT AND DIAGNOSIS

A variety of clinical manifestations occur in the patient in cardiogenic shock, depending on etiologic factors in pump failure, the patient's underlying medical status, and the severity of the shock state. Some clinical manifestations are caused by failure of the heart as a pump, whereas many are related to the overall shock response (Box 39-6).

Initially, clinical manifestations reflect the decline in CO. These signs and symptoms include systolic blood pressure less than 90 mm Hg or an acute drop in systolic or mean blood pressure of 30 mm Hg or more; decreased sensorium; cool, pale, moist skin; and urine output of less than 30 mL/hr.[57,60] The patient also may complain of chest pain. Tachycardia develops to compensate for the decrease in CO. A weak, thready pulse develops, and diminished S_1 and S_2 heart sounds may occur as a result of the decreased contractility. The respiratory rate increases to improve oxygenation. ABG values at this point indicate respiratory alkalosis, as evidenced by a decrease in $Paco_2$. Urinalysis findings demonstrate a decrease in urine sodium level and an increase in urine osmolality and specific gravity as the kidneys start to conserve sodium and water. The patient also may experience a variety of dysrhythmias, depending on the underlying problem.[54]

As the left ventricle fails, auscultation of the lungs may disclose crackles and rhonchi, indicating the development of

BOX 39-6   CLINICAL MANIFESTATIONS OF CARDIOGENIC SHOCK

- Systolic blood pressure <90 mm Hg
- Acute drop in blood pressure >30 mm Hg
- Heart rate >100 beats/min
- Weak, thready pulse
- Diminished heart sounds
- Change in sensorium
- Cool, pale, moist skin
- Urine output <30 mL/hr
- Chest pain
- Dysrhythmias
- Tachypnea
- Crackles
- Decreased cardiac output
- Cardiac index <2.2 L/min/m²
- Increased pulmonary artery occlusion pressure
- Increased right atrial pressure
- Increased systemic vascular resistance

pulmonary edema. Hypoxemia occurs, as evidenced by a fall in Pao_2 and Sao_2 as measured by ABG values. Heart sounds may reveal an S_3 and S_4. Jugular venous distention is evident with right-sided failure.

Assessment of the hemodynamic parameters of a patient in cardiogenic shock reveals a decreased CO with a CI less than 2.2 L/min/m^2 in the presence of an elevated PAOP of more than 15 to 18 mm Hg.[53,54,57,59] Increased filling pressures are necessary to rule out hypovolemia as the cause of circulatory failure. The increase in PAOP reflects an increase in the left ventricular end-diastolic pressure (LVEDP) and left ventricular end-diastolic volume (LVEDV) resulting from decreased SV. With right ventricular failure, the RAP also increases. Compensatory vasoconstriction results in an increase in the afterload of the heart, as evidenced by an increase in the SVR. Echocardiography confirms the diagnosis of cardiogenic shock and rules out other causes of circulatory failure.[53,54,57]

As compensatory mechanisms fail and ineffective tissue perfusion develops, other clinical manifestations appear. Myocardial ischemia progresses, as evidenced by continued increases in heart rate, dysrhythmias, and chest pain. Pulmonary function deteriorates, which leads to respiratory distress. ABG values during this phase reveal respiratory and metabolic acidosis and hypoxemia, as indicated by a high $PaCO_2$, low HCO_3^-, and low PaO_2, respectively. Renal failure occurs, as exhibited by the development of anuria and increases in BUN and serum creatinine levels. Cerebral hypoperfusion manifests as decreasing level of consciousness.

MEDICAL MANAGEMENT

Treatment of the patient in cardiogenic shock requires an aggressive approach. The major goals of therapy are to treat the underlying cause, enhance the effectiveness of the pump, and improve tissue perfusion. This approach includes identifying the etiologic factors of pump failure and administering pharmacologic agents to enhance CO. Inotropic agents are used to increase contractility and maintain adequate blood pressure and tissue perfusion. A vasopressor may be necessary to maintain blood pressure when hypotension is severe.[57,60] Diuretics are used for preload reduction. After blood pressure has been stabilized, vasodilating agents are used for preload and afterload reduction. Antidysrhythmic agents should be used to suppress or control dysrhythmias that can affect CO.[53] Intubation and mechanical ventilation may be necessary to support oxygenation.

Intraaortic balloon pump (IABP) support should be instituted if drug therapy does not quickly reverse the shock state.[54-57] The IABP is a temporary measure to decrease myocardial workload by improving myocardial supply and decreasing myocardial demand. It achieves this goal by improving coronary artery perfusion and reducing left ventricular afterload. Chapter 20 provides more information about IAPB therapy.

After the cause of pump failure has been identified, measures should be taken to correct the problem if possible. If the problem is related to an acute MI, early revascularization by coronary angioplasty or coronary artery bypass surgery provides significant survival benefit.[53-57,61] Thrombolytic agents may be used in select patients. When conventional therapies fail, a ventricular assist device (VAD) or extracorporeal life support with a membrane oxygenator may be used to support the patient in acute cardiogenic shock.[54,57,62,63] These mechanical circulatory assist devices provide an external means to sustain effective organ perfusion, allowing time for the patient's ventricle to heal or for cardiac transplantation to take place.

NURSING MANAGEMENT

Prevention of cardiogenic shock is one of the primary responsibilities of the nurse in the critical care area. Preventive measures include the identification of patients at risk, facilitation of early reperfusion therapy for acute MI, and frequent assessment and management of the patient's cardiopulmonary status.

The patient in cardiogenic shock may have any number of nursing diagnoses, depending on the progression of the process (see the Nursing Diagnoses feature on Cardiogenic Shock). Nursing interventions include limiting myocardial oxygen demand, enhancing myocardial oxygen supply, providing comfort and emotional support, and maintaining surveillance for complications. Measures to limit myocardial oxygen demand include administering analgesics, sedatives, and agents to control afterload and dysrhythmias; positioning the patient for comfort; limiting activities; providing a calm and quiet environment and offering support to reduce anxiety; and teaching the patient about the condition. Measures to enhance myocardial oxygen supply include administering supplemental oxygen, monitoring the patient's respiratory status, and administering prescribed medications.

Effective nursing management of cardiogenic shock requires precise monitoring and management of heart rate, preload, afterload, and contractility. This is accomplished through accurate measurement of hemodynamic variables and controlled administration of fluids and inotropic and vasoactive agents. Close assessment and management of respiratory function is also essential to maintain adequate oxygenation. Dysrhythmias are common and require immediate recognition and treatment.

Patients who require IABP therapy need to be observed frequently for complications. Complications include embolus formation, infection, rupture of the aorta, thrombocytopenia, improper balloon placement, bleeding, improper timing of the balloon, balloon rupture, and circulatory compromise of the cannulated extremity.

Nursing Diagnoses

Cardiogenic Shock

- Ineffective Cardiopulmonary Tissue Perfusion related to acute myocardial ischemia
- Decreased Cardiac Output related to alterations in contractility
- Decreased Cardiac Output related to alterations in heart rate
- Imbalanced Nutrition: Less Than Body Requirements related to increased metabolic demands or lack of exogenous nutrients
- Risk for Infection
- Disturbed Body Image related to functional dependence on life-sustaining technology
- Compromised Family Coping related to a critically ill family member

ANAPHYLACTIC SHOCK

DESCRIPTION

Anaphylactic shock, a type of distributive shock, is the result of an immediate hypersensitivity reaction. It is a life-threatening event that requires prompt intervention. The severe antibody-antigen response leads to decreased tissue perfusion and initiation of the general shock response.[64,65]

ETIOLOGY

Anaphylactic shock is caused by an antibody-antigen response. Almost any substance can cause a hypersensitivity reaction. These substances, known as *antigens*, can be introduced by injection or ingestion or through the skin or respiratory tract. A number of antigens have been identified that can cause a reaction in a hypersensitive person. This list includes foods, food additives, diagnostic agents, biologic agents, environmental agents, drugs, and venoms (Box 39-7).[65-67] In the hospital environment latex is an extremely problematic antigen for patients and health care providers (see the Patient Safety feature on Latex Allergy).

BOX 39-7   ETIOLOGIC FACTORS IN ANAPHYLACTIC SHOCK

FOODS
- Eggs and milk
- Fish and shellfish
- Nuts and seeds
- Legumes and cereals
- Soy
- Wheat
- Citrus fruits
- Chocolate
- Strawberries
- Tomatoes
- Avocados
- Bananas
- Kiwi fruit
- Other

FOOD ADDITIVES
- Food coloring
- Preservatives

DIAGNOSTIC AGENTS
- Iodinated contrast dye
- Sulfobromophthalein (Bromsulphalein [BSP])
- Dehydrocholic acid (Decholin)
- Iopanoic acid (Telepaque)

BIOLOGIC AGENTS
- Blood and blood components
- Insulin and other hormones
- Gamma globulin
- Seminal plasma

- Enzymes
- Vaccines and antitoxins

ENVIRONMENTAL AGENTS
- Pollens, molds, and spores
- Sunlight
- Animal hair
- Latex

DRUGS
- Antibiotics
- Aspirin
- Nonsteroidal antiinflammatory drugs
- Narcotics
- Dextran
- Vitamins
- Local anesthetic agents
- Muscle relaxants
- Neuromuscular blocking agents
- Barbiturates
- Protamine
- Other

VENOMS
- Bees, hornets, yellow jackets, and wasps
- Snakes
- Jellyfish
- Spiders
- Deer flies
- Fire ants

Anaphylactic reactions can be IgE-mediated or non–IgE-mediated responses. IgE is an antibody that is formed as part of the immune response. The first time an antigen enters the body, an antibody IgE, specific for the antigen, is formed. The antigen-specific IgE antibody is then stored by attachment to mast cells and basophils. This initial contact with the antigen is known as a *primary immune response.* The next time the antigen enters the body, the preformed IgE antibody reacts with it,

---

Patient Safety Alert

Latex Allergies

Latex is the milky sap of the rubber tree *Hevea brasilliensis*. It is treated with preservatives, accelerators, stabilizers, and antioxidants to make a more elastic, stable rubber. Reactions to products containing latex can be triggered by the latex protein or by an additive used in the manufacturing process.

Latex reactions can be classified in three categories: *irritation* (nonallergic inflammation occurring when the skin is abraded), *type IV delayed hypersensitivity* (non–IgE-mediated response to the chemical agents added during the manufacturing process), or *type I immediate sensitivity* (IgE-mediated response to latex proteins). Although the overall prevalence of latex allergy in the general population is only 1%, it is much higher (10% to 55%) in selected groups, such as patients with neural tube defects (e.g., spina bifida, myelomeningocele, lipomyelomeningocele) or congenital urologic disorders; those who have undergone multiple operations or who have a history of allergy to anesthetic drugs; and health care, rubber industry, or glove-manufacturing plant workers.

Five routes of exposure to latex proteins have resulted in systemic reactions: cutaneous (contact with moist skin); mucous membrane (mouth, vagina, urethra, or rectum); internal tissue (during surgery and other invasive procedures); intravascular; and inhalation (exposure to anesthesia equipment or endotracheal tubes or through the aerosolization of glove powder). It has been postulated that the latex allergen adheres to the cornstarch or powder and is released into the air with the manipulation of rubber gloves.

The American Academy of Allergy and Immunology has published guidelines for providing care to persons with latex allergy. All persons at risk for latex allergy should have a careful history and should complete a standardized latex allergy questionnaire. A history suggestive of reactivity to latex includes local swelling or itching after blowing up balloons, dental examinations, contact with rubber gloves, vaginal or rectal examinations, using condoms or diaphragms, and contact with other rubber products. Other historical information that may suggest increased risk of latex allergy includes hand eczema; previous, unexplained anaphylaxis; oral itching after eating bananas, chestnuts, kiwis, or avocados; and multiple surgical procedures in infancy. Patients at high risk should be offered clinical testing for latex allergy.

To minimize the risk of exposure to latex the use of powder-free latex gloves and nonlatex gloves should be adopted when caring for all patients. The patient with a latex allergy should be cared for in a latex free environment, an environment in which no latex gloves are used and there is no direct patient contact with other latex devices.

From Reines DH, Seifert PC: Patient safety: latex allergy, *Surg Clin North Am* 85:1329, 2005.

and a secondary immune response occurs. This reaction triggers the release of biochemical mediators from the mast cells and basophils and initiates the cascade of events that precipitates anaphylactic shock.[65,68,69]

Some anaphylactic reactions are non–IgE-mediated responses in that they occur in the absence of activation of IgE antibodies. These responses occur as a result of direct activation of the mast cells to release biochemical mediators. Direct activation of mast cells can be triggered by humoral mediators, such as the complement system and the coagulation-fibrinolytic system. Biochemical mediators can be released as a direct or indirect response to many drugs. This type of reaction, formerly known as *anaphylactoid reaction,* is produced in persons not previously sensitized, and it can occur with the first exposure to an antigen.[65,67,69]

PATHOPHYSIOLOGY

The antibody-antigen response (immunologic stimulation) or the direct triggering (nonimmunologic activation) of the mast cells results in the release of biochemical mediators. These mediators include histamine, eosinophil chemotactic factor of anaphylaxis (ECF-A), neutrophil chemotactic factor of anaphylaxis (NCF), platelet-activating factor (PAF), proteinases, heparin, serotonin,

leukotrienes (also known as *slow-reacting substance of anaphylaxis*), and prostaglandins. The activation of the biochemical mediators causes vasodilation, increased capillary permeability, laryngeal edema, bronchoconstriction, excessive mucus secretion, coronary vasoconstriction, inflammation, cutaneous reactions, and constriction of the smooth muscle in the intestinal wall, bladder, and uterus. Coronary vasoconstriction causes severe myocardial depression. Cutaneous reactions cause stimulation of nerve endings, followed by itching and pain.[64,65,68]

ECF-A promotes chemotaxis of eosinophils, facilitating the movement of eosinophils into the area. During allergic reactions, eosinophils phagocytose the antibody-antigen complex and other inflammatory debris and release enzymes that inhibit vasoactive mediators, such as histamine and leukotrienes. Secondary mediators such as bradykinin and plasmin are produced that enhance or inhibit the already released biochemical mediators. Peripheral vasodilation results in relative hypovolemia and decreased venous return. Increased capillary membrane permeability results in the loss of intravascular volume, worsening the hypovolemic state. Decreased venous return results in decreased end-diastolic volume and SV. The decline in SV leads to decreased CO and ineffective tissue perfusion. Death may result from airway obstruction or cardiovascular collapse, or both (Fig. 39-3).[64,65,68,69]

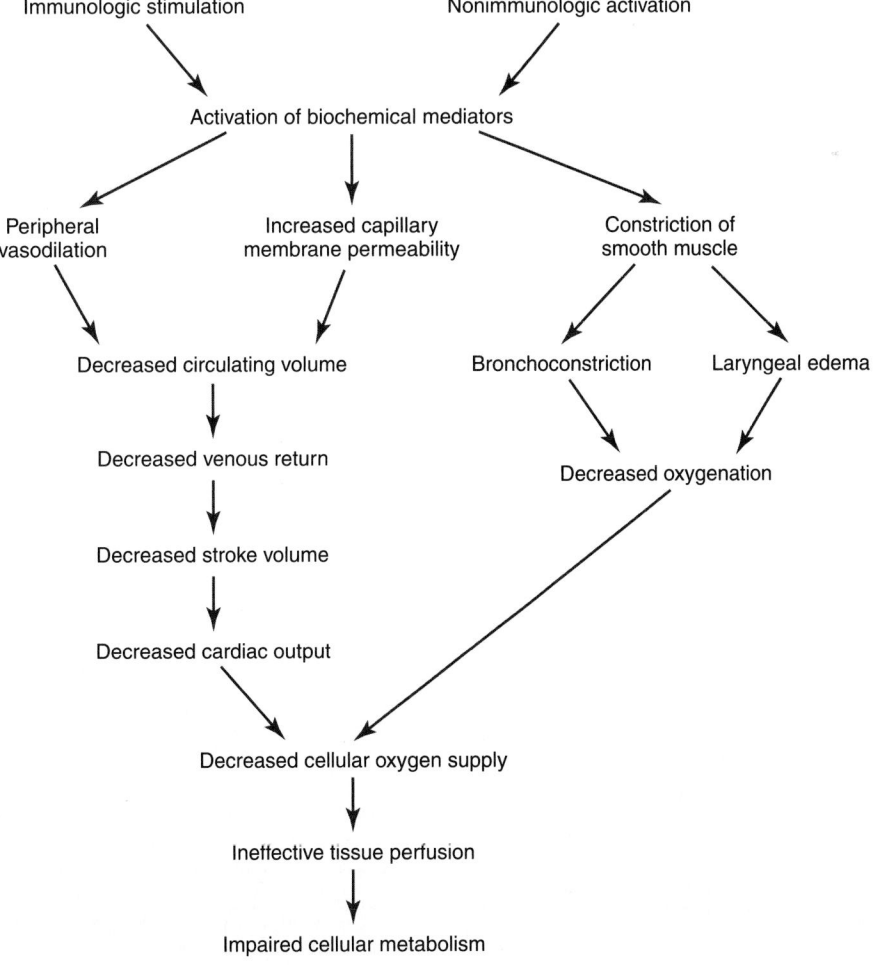

Figure 39-3 The pathophysiology of anaphylactic shock.

ASSESSMENT AND DIAGNOSIS

Anaphylactic shock is a severe systemic reaction that can affect multiple organ systems. A variety of clinical manifestations occur in the patient in anaphylactic shock, depending on the extent of multisystem involvement. The symptoms usually start to appear within minutes of exposure to the antigen, but they may not occur for up to 1 hour (Box 39-8).[64] Symptoms may also reappear after a 1- to 72-hour window of resolution. These late-phase reactions may be similar to the initial anaphylactic response, milder, or more severe.[64,70]

The cutaneous effects may appear first and include pruritus, generalized erythema, urticaria, and angioedema. Commonly seen on the face and in the oral cavity and lower pharynx, angioedema develops as a result of fluid leaking into the interstitial space. The patient may appear restless, uneasy, apprehensive, and anxious and may complain of being warm. Respiratory effects include the development of laryngeal edema, bronchoconstriction, and mucous plugs. Clinical manifestations of laryngeal edema include inspiratory stridor, hoarseness, a sensation of fullness or a lump in the throat, and dysphagia. Bronchoconstriction causes dyspnea, wheezing, and chest tightness.[64,65,68] Gastrointestinal and genitourinary manifestations, which may develop as a result of smooth muscle contraction, include vomiting, diarrhea, cramping, and abdominal pain.

As the anaphylactic reaction progresses, hypotension and reflex tachycardia develop. This occurs in response to massive vasodilation and loss of circulating volume. Jugular veins appear flat as right ventricular end-diastolic volume is decreased. The eventual outcome is circulatory failure and ineffective tissue perfusion.[64,65,68] The patient's level of consciousness may deteriorate to unresponsiveness.

Assessment of the hemodynamic parameters of a patient in anaphylactic shock reveals a decreased CO and CI. Venous vasodilation and massive volume loss lead to a decrease in preload, which results in a decline in the RAP and PAOP. Vasodilation of the arterial system results in a decrease in the afterload of the heart, as evidenced by a decrease in the SVR. Box 39-9 outlines the clinical criteria for diagnosing anaphylaxis.

MEDICAL MANAGEMENT

Treatment of anaphylactic shock requires an immediate and direct approach. The goals of therapy are to remove the offending

---

BOX 39-8 CLINICAL MANIFESTATIONS OF ANAPHYLACTIC SHOCK

CARDIOVASCULAR
- Hypotension
- Tachycardia

RESPIRATORY
- Lump in throat
- Cough
- Dyspnea
- Dysphagia
- Hoarseness
- Stridor
- Wheezing
- Rales and rhonchi

CUTANEOUS
- Pruritus
- Erythema
- Urticaria
- Angioedema

NEUROLOGIC
- Restlessness
- Uneasiness
- Apprehension
- Anxiety
- Dizziness
- Headache
- Decreased level of consciousness

GASTROINTESTINAL
- Nausea
- Vomiting
- Diarrhea
- Abdominal pain

GENITOURINARY
- Incontinence
- Vaginal bleeding

SUBJECTIVE COMPLAINTS
- Sensation of warmth
- Dyspnea
- Abdominal cramping and pain
- Itching

HEMODYNAMIC PARAMETERS
- Decreased cardiac output (CO)
- Decreased cardiac index (CI)
- Decreased right atrial pressure (RAP)
- Decreased pulmonary occlusion pressure (PAOP)
- Decreased systemic vascular resistance (SVR)

BOX 39-9 CLINICAL CRITERIA FOR DIAGNOSING ANAPHYLAXIS

Anaphylaxis is highly likely when one of the following three criteria is fulfilled:

1. Acute onset of an illness (minutes to several hours) with involvement of the skin or mucosal tissue, or both (e.g., generalized hives; pruritus or flushing; swollen lips, tongue, and uvula) *and at least one of the following:*
   a. Respiratory compromise (e.g., dyspnea, wheeze [bronchospasm], stridor, reduced peak expiratory flow, hypoxemia)
   b. Reduced blood pressure or associated symptoms of end-organ dysfunction (e.g., hypotonia [collapse], syncope, incontinence)
2. Two or more of the following that occur rapidly after exposure *to a likely allergen for that patient* (minutes to several hours):
   a. Involvement of the skin-mucosal tissue (e.g., generalized hives; pruritus or flushing; swollen lips, tongue, and uvula)
   b. Respiratory compromise (e.g., dyspnea, wheeze [bronchospasm], stridor, reduced peak expiratory flow, hypoxemia)
   c. Reduced blood pressure or associated symptoms of end-organ dysfunction (e.g., hypotonia [collapse], syncope, incontinence)
   d. Persistent gastrointestinal symptoms (e.g., crampy abdominal pain, vomiting)
3. Reduced blood pressure after exposure *to known allergen for that patient* (minutes to several hours):
   a. Infants and children: low systolic blood pressure (age specific) or greater than 30% decrease in systolic blood pressure*
   b. Adults: systolic blood pressure of less than 90 mm HG or greater than 30% decrease for the person's baseline

---

*Low systolic blood pressure is defined as less than 70 mm Hg for children 1 month to 1 year old, less than (70 mm Hg + [2 × age]) for children 1 to 10 years old, and less than 90 mm Hg for children 11 to 17 years old.
From Sampson HA et al: Second symposium on the definition and management of anaphylaxis: summary report—second National Institute of Allergy and Infectious Disease/Food Allergy and Anaphylaxis Network symposium, *J Allergy Clin Immunol* 117:391, 2006.

antigen, reverse the effects of the biochemical mediators, and promote adequate tissue perfusion. When the hypersensitivity reaction occurs as a result of administration of medications, dye, blood, or blood products, the infusion should be immediately discontinued. Often, it is not possible to remove the antigen because it is unknown or has already entered the patient's system.

Reversal of the effects of the biochemical mediators involves the preservation and support of the patient's airway, ventilation, and circulation. This is accomplished through oxygen therapy, intubation, mechanical ventilation, and administration of drugs and fluids.

Epinephrine is the first-line treatment of choice for anaphylaxis. It promotes bronchodilation and vasoconstriction and inhibits further release of biochemical mediators. In mild cases of anaphylaxis, 0.3 to 0.5 mg (0.3 to 0.5 mL) of a 1:1000 dilution of epinephrine is administered by intramuscular injection into the anterolateral thigh and repeated every 5 to 15 minutes until anaphylaxis is resolved.[64,65,69-71] Subcutaneous injection is no longer recommended.[70] For anaphylactic shock with hypotension, epinephrine is administered intravenously. The intravenous dose is 0.1 (1 mL) of a 1:10,000 dilution administered over 5 minutes. If hypotension persists, a continuous infusion of epinephrine is recommended, administered at 1 to 4 mcg/min with titration up to 10 mcg/min as needed.[65,66,68,72] Patients receiving beta-blockers may have a limited response to epinephrine. Intravenous glucagon administered as a 20 to 30 mcg/kg bolus over 5 minutes followed by continuous infusion at 5 to 15 mcg/min is recommended for inotropic and vasoactive support for these patients.[64,65,70,72]

Diphenhydramine (Benadryl), which is given as 1 to 2 mg/kg (25 to 50 mg) by a slow intravenous route every 4 to 8 hours, is a second-line agent used to block the histamine response.[64,65,68,70,72] Corticosteroids also may be given with the goal of preventing a delayed reaction and stabilizing capillary membranes.[64,65,70] Fluid replacement is accomplished by use of a crystalloid or colloid solution. Positive inotropic agents and vasoconstrictor agents may be necessary to reverse the effects of myocardial depression and vasodilation.[64,65,68,70]

NURSING MANAGEMENT

Prevention of anaphylactic shock is one of the primary responsibilities of the nurse in the critical care area. Preventive measures include the identification of patients at risk and cautious assessment of the patient's response to the administration of drugs, blood, and blood products. A complete and accurate history of the patient's allergies is an essential component of preventive nursing care. In addition to a list of the allergies, a detailed description of the type of response for each one should be obtained.

The patient in anaphylactic shock may have any number of nursing diagnoses, depending on the progression of the process (see the Nursing Diagnoses feature on Anaphylactic Shock). Nursing interventions include facilitating ventilation, administering volume replacement, promoting comfort and emotional support, and maintaining surveillance for complications.

Nursing Diagnoses

Anaphylactic Shock

- Deficient Fluid Volume related to relative loss
- Decreased Cardiac Output related to alterations in preload
- Decreased Cardiac Output related to alterations in afterload
- Ineffective Breathing Pattern related to decreased lung expansion
- Impaired Gas Exchange related to ventilation/perfusion mismatching or intrapulmonary shunting
- Imbalanced Nutrition: Less Than Body Requirements related to increased metabolic demands or lack of exogenous nutrients
- Risk for Infection
- Ineffective Coping related to situational crisis and personal vulnerability
- Compromised Family Coping related to a critically ill family member

---

Measures to facilitate ventilation include positioning the patient to assist with breathing and instructing the patient to breathe slowly and deeply. Airway protection through prompt administration of prescribed medications is essential. Measures to facilitate the administration of volume replacement include inserting large-bore peripheral intravenous catheters, rapidly administering prescribed fluids, and positioning the patient with the legs elevated, trunk flat, and head and shoulders above the chest. Measures to promote comfort include administering medications to relieve itching, applying warm soaks to skin, and if necessary, covering the patient's hands to discourage scratching. Observing the patient for clinical manifestations of a delayed reaction is critical. Patient education about how to avoid the precipitating allergen is essential for preventing future episodes of anaphylaxis.

NEUROGENIC SHOCK
DESCRIPTION

Neurogenic shock, another type of distributive shock, is the result of the loss or suppression of sympathetic tone. The lack of sympathetic tone leads to decreased tissue perfusion and initiation of the general shock response. Neurogenic shock is the most uncommon form of shock.

ETIOLOGY

Neurogenic shock can be caused by anything that disrupts the SNS. The problem can occur as the result of interrupted impulse transmission or blockage of sympathetic outflow from the vasomotor center in the brain.[73-75] The most common cause is spinal cord injury. Neurogenic shock may mistakenly be referred to as *spinal shock*. The latter condition refers to loss of neurologic activity below the level of spinal cord injury, but it does not necessarily involve ineffective tissue perfusion.[76-78]

PATHOPHYSIOLOGY

Loss of sympathetic tone results in massive peripheral vasodilation, inhibition of the baroreceptor response, and impaired thermoregulation. Arterial vasodilation leads to a decrease in

SVR and a fall in blood pressure. Venous vasodilation leads to relative hypovolemia and pooling of blood in the venous circuit. The decreased venous return results in a decrease in end-diastolic volume or preload, causing a decrease in SV and CO. The fall in blood pressure and CO leads to inadequate or ineffective tissue perfusion. Loss of sympathetic tone and inhibition of the baroreceptor response result in bradycardia.[73-75,77] The slow heart rate worsens CO, which further compromises tissue perfusion. Impaired thermoregulation occurs because of loss of vasomotor tone in the cutaneous blood vessels that dilate and constrict to maintain body temperature. The patient becomes poikilothermic, or dependent on the environment for temperature regulation (Fig. 39-4).

ASSESSMENT AND DIAGNOSIS

The patient in neurogenic shock characteristically presents with hypotension, bradycardia, and warm, dry skin.[73-75] The decreased blood pressure results from massive peripheral vasodilation. The decreased heart rate is caused by inhibition of the baroreceptor response and unopposed parasympathetic control of the heart.[41] Hypothermia develops from uncontrolled peripheral heat loss. The warm, dry skin occurs as a consequence of pooling of blood in the extremities and loss of vasomotor control in surface vessels of the skin that control heat loss.

Assessment of the hemodynamic parameters of a patient in neurogenic shock reveals a decreased CO and CI. Venous

vasodilation leads to a decrease in preload, which results in a decline in the RAP and PAOP. Vasodilation of the arterial system causes a decrease in the afterload of the heart, as evidenced by a decrease in the SVR.[75]

MEDICAL MANAGEMENT

Treatment of neurogenic shock requires a careful approach. The goals of therapy are to treat or remove the cause, prevent cardiovascular instability, and promote optimal tissue perfusion. Cardiovascular instability can result from hypovolemia, bradycardia, and hypothermia. Specific treatments are aimed at preventing or correcting these problems as they occur.

Hypovolemia is treated with careful fluid resuscitation. The minimal amount of fluid is administered to ensure adequate tissue perfusion. Volume replacement is initiated for systolic blood pressure lower than 90 mm Hg, urine output of less than 30 mL/hr, or changes in mental status that indicate decreased cerebral tissue perfusion. The patient is carefully observed for evidence of fluid overload. Vasopressors are used as necessary to maintain blood pressure and organ perfusion.[73,75,77] The bradycardia associated with neurogenic shock rarely requires specific treatment, but atropine or electrical pacing can be used when necessary.[68,73] Hypothermia is treated with warming measures and environmental temperature regulation.

NURSING MANAGEMENT

Prevention of neurogenic shock is one of the primary responsibilities of the nurse in the critical care area. This includes the identification of patients at risk and constant assessment of the neurologic status. Vigilant immobilization of spinal cord injuries and slight elevation of the head of the patient's bed after spinal anesthesia are essential components of preventive nursing care. Early identification allows for early treatment and decreased mortality.

The patient in neurogenic shock may have any number of nursing diagnoses, depending on the progression of the process (see the Nursing Diagnoses feature on Neurogenic Shock). Nursing interventions include treating hypovolemia, maintaining normothermia, monitoring for dysrhythmias, promoting comfort and emotional support, and maintaining surveillance for complications.

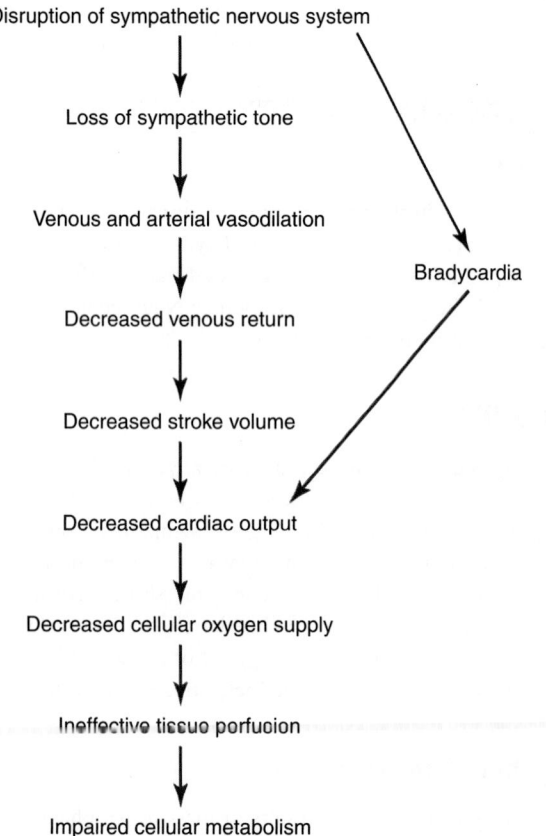

Figure 39-4 The pathophysiology of neurogenic shock.

Nursing Diagnoses
Neurogenic Shock

- Deficient Fluid Volume related to relative loss
- Decreased Cardiac Output related to sympathetic blockade
- Hypothermia related to exposure to cold environment, trauma, or damage to the hypothalamus
- Imbalanced Nutrition: Less Than Body Requirements related to increased metabolic demands or lack of exogenous nutrients
- Risk for Infection
- Anxiety related to threat to biologic, psychologic, or social integrity
- Compromised Family Coping related to a critically ill family member

Venous pooling in the lower extremities promotes the formation of deep vein thrombosis (DVT), which can result in a pulmonary embolism. All patients at risk for DVT should be started on prophylaxis therapy. DVT-prophylactic measures include monitoring of calf and thigh measurements, passive range-of-motion exercises, application of antiembolic stockings or sequential pneumatic stockings, and administration of prescribed anticoagulation therapy.

SEVERE SEPSIS AND SEPTIC SHOCK

DESCRIPTION

Sepsis occurs when microorganisms invade the body and initiate a systemic inflammatory response. This host response often results in perfusion abnormalities with organ dysfunction (severe sepsis) and eventually hypotension (septic shock). The primary mechanism of this type of shock is the maldistribution of blood flow to the tissues.[32,79] Severe sepsis is estimated to occur in more than 750,000 patients annually in the United States,[80] with an estimated mortality rate of 38% to 59%.[32,81-83] It is the leading cause of death in noncoronary critical care units.[15,84]

Specific terms are used to describe the continuum of conditions that the patient with an infection may experience. In 1991, at the American College of Chest Physicians/Society of Critical Care Medicine (ACCP/SCCM) Consensus Conference, definitions were developed to describe and differentiate these conditions (Box 39-10).[85] These definitions were clarified and reinforced in subsequent conferences in 2001 and 2007.[16,84] This discussion focuses on severe sepsis and septic shock.

ETIOLOGY

Sepsis is caused by a wide variety of microorganisms, including gram-negative and gram-positive aerobes, anaerobes, fungi, and viruses. The source of these microorganisms varies. Exogenous sources include the hospital environment and members of the health care team. Endogenous sources include the patient's skin, gastrointestinal tract, respiratory tract, and genitourinary tract. In recent years, the incidence of chest-related infections has risen dramatically, and the lungs have replaced the intraabdominal organs as the most common site of infection producing severe sepsis and septic shock.[82-83] Gram-positive bacteria are responsible for more than one half of the cases of sepsis.[80] Sepsis and septic shock are associated with a wide variety of intrinsic and extrinsic precipitating factors (Box 39-11). All of these factors interfere directly or indirectly with the body's anatomic and physiologic defense mechanisms. Several of the intrinsic factors are not modifiable or are very difficult to control. Several of the extrinsic factors may be required for diagnosis and management. All critically ill patients are therefore at risk for septic shock.

PATHOPHYSIOLOGY

The syndrome encompassing severe sepsis and septic shock is a complex systemic response that is initiated when a microorganism enters the body and stimulates the inflammatory/immune system. Shed protein fragments and the release of toxins and other substances from the microorganism activate the plasma enzyme cascades (complement, kinin/kallikrein, coagulation, and fibrinolytic factors), as well as platelets, neutrophils, monocytes, and macrophages. On activation, these systems and cells release a variety of mediators, or cytokines, that initiate a chain of complex interactions leading to a maladaptive SIRS.[86-90]

After the mediators are activated, a variety of physiologic and pathophysiologic events occur that affect clotting, the distribution of blood flow to the tissues and organs, capillary membrane permeability, and the metabolic state of the body. Subsequently, a systemic imbalance between cellular oxygen supply

---

BOX 39-10 DEFINITIONS FOR SEPSIS AND ORGAN FAILURE

- *Infection:* Microbial phenomenon characterized by an inflammatory response to the presence of microorganisms or the invasion of normally sterile host tissue by those organisms
- *Bacteremia:* Presence of viable bacteria in the blood
- *Systemic inflammatory response syndrome (SIRS):* Systemic inflammatory response to a variety of severe clinical insults, manifested by two or more of the following conditions: (1) temperature >38° C or <36° C; (2) heart rate >90 beats/min; (3) respiratory rate >20 breaths/min or $Paco_2$ <32 mm Hg; and (4) white blood cell count >12,000/mm^3, <4000/mm^3, or >10% immature (band) forms
- *Sepsis:* Systemic response to infection, manifested by two or more of the following conditions as a result of infection: (1) temperature >38° C or <36° C; (2) heart rate >90 beats/min; (3) respiratory rate >20 breaths/min or $Paco_2$ <32 mm Hg; and (4) white blood cell count >12,000/mm^3, <4000/mm^3, or >10% immature (band) forms.

- *Severe sepsis:* Sepsis associated with organ dysfunction, hypoperfusion, or hypotension. Hypoperfusion and perfusion abnormalities may include, but are not limited to, lactic acidosis, oliguria, or an acute alteration in mental status.
- *Septic shock:* Sepsis-induced shock with hypotension despite adequate fluid resuscitation, along with the presence of perfusion abnormalities that may include, but are not limited to, lactic acidosis, oliguria, or an acute alteration in mental status. Patients who are receiving inotropic or vasopressor agents may not be hypotensive at the time that perfusion abnormalities are measured.
- *Sepsis-induced hypotension:* A systolic blood pressure <90 mm Hg or a reduction of ≥40 mm Hg from baseline in the absence of other causes for hypotension
- *Multiple organ dysfunction syndrome (MODS):* Altered organ function in an acutely ill patient such that homeostasis cannot be maintained without intervention

Adapted from American College of Chest Physicians/Society of Critical Care Medicine Consensus Conference Committee: Definitions for sepsis and organ failure and guidelines for the use of innovative therapies in sepsis, *Crit Care Med* 20:864, 1992.

and demand develops that results in cellular hypoxia, damage, hibernation, and death (Fig. 39-5).[4,87,89,90]

Hallmarks of severe sepsis are endothelial damage and coagulation dysfunction.[86,87,91,92] Tissue factor is released from endothelial cells and monocytes in response to stimulation by the inflammatory cytokines.[86,87] Release of tissue factor initiates the coagulation cascade, producing widespread microvascular thrombosis and further stimulation of the systemic inflammatory pathways.[87] Diffuse endothelial damage impairs endogenous

anticlotting mechanisms.[87] Mediator-induced suppression of fibrinolysis slows clot breakdown. The result is DIC with eventual consumption of coagulation factors, bleeding, and hemorrhage.[91,93]

Significant alterations in cardiovascular hemodynamics are caused by the activation of inflammatory cytokines and endothelial damage.[32,87,92] Massive peripheral vasodilation results in the development of relative hypovolemia. Increased capillary permeability produces a loss of intravascular volume to the interstitium, which accentuates the reduction in preload and CO. These changes, coupled with the microvascular thrombosis, produce maldistribution of circulating blood volume, decreased tissue perfusion, and inadequate oxygen delivery to the cells. Microcirculatory shunting is a key feature of this distributive shock.[87,94,95] Impaired ventricular contractility results from cytokine activity.[4,32,87]

Activation of the central nervous and endocrine systems also occurs as part of the response to invading microorganisms. This activation leads to stimulation of the SNS and the release of ACTH. These events trigger the release of epinephrine, norepinephrine, glucocorticoids, aldosterone, glucagon, renin, and growth hormone resulting in the development of a hypermetabolic state and contributing to vasoconstriction of the renal, pulmonary, and splanchnic beds. Selective vasoconstriction in the splanchnic bed may contribute to hypoperfusion of the gastric mucosa. The resulting gut injury propagates the inflammatory response.[2,96]

Several metabolic alterations occur as a result of CNS, endocrine system, and cytokine activation. The hypermetabolic state increases energy expenditure and oxygen demand, and it contributes to cellular hypoxia. Lactic acid is produced as a result of increased metabolic lactate production and hypoxic anaerobic metabolism. Glucocorticoids, ACTH, epinephrine, glucagon, and growth hormone are all catabolic hormones that are

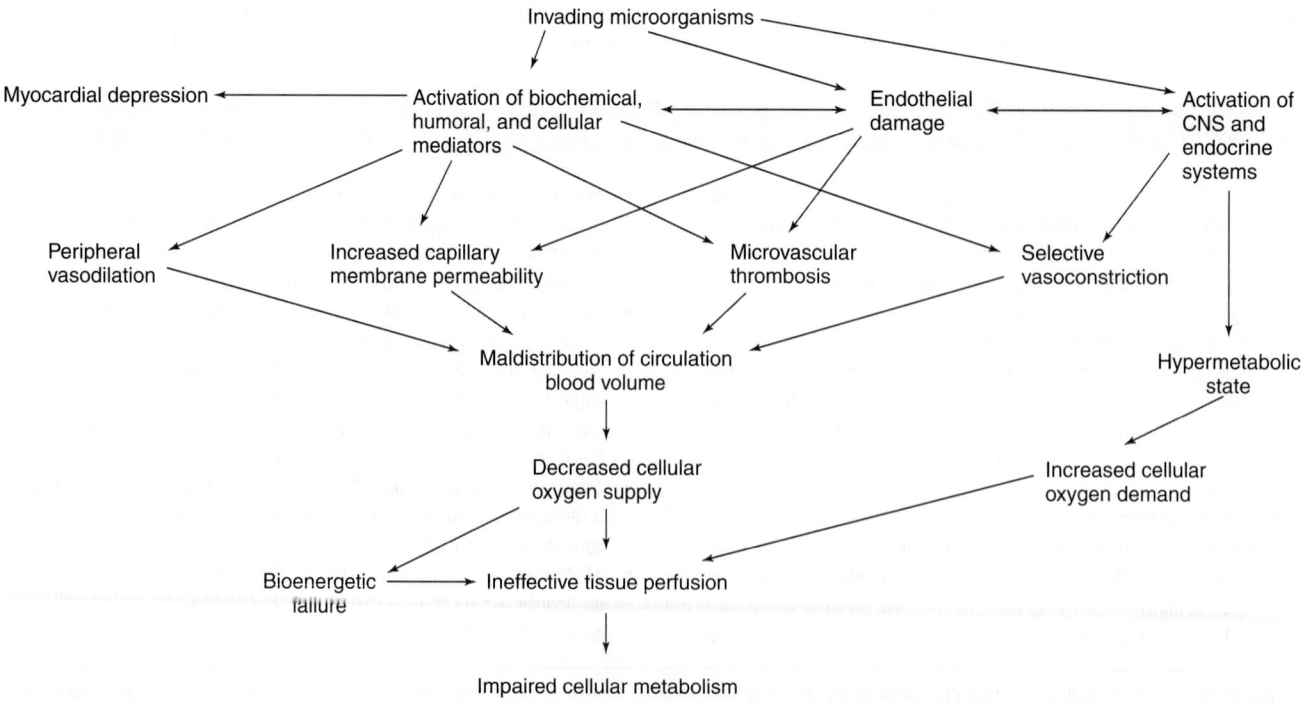

Figure 39-5 The pathophysiology of septic shock.

released as part of this response. In conjunction with the inflammatory cytokines, these hormones stimulate catabolism of protein stores in the visceral organs and skeletal muscles to fuel glucose production in the liver, hyperglycemia, and insulin resistance.[8] The cytokines also stimulate the use of fats for energy production (lipolysis).[8,90,97]

Metabolic derangements in severe sepsis and septic shock include an inability of the cells to use oxygen even if blood flow is adequate. Mitochondrial dysfunction is thought to be the underlying mechanism.[87,90,97] This bioenergetic failure plays an important role in the development of multiple organ dysfunction.[32,87,90,97] The exaggerated inflammatory response in severe sepsis results in apoptosis, a programmed cell death or cellular suicide affecting endothelial and immune cells in particular.[87,90,92]

These complex and interrelated pathophysiologic changes associated with severe sepsis and septic shock produce a pathologic imbalance between cellular oxygen demand and cellular oxygen supply and consumption. If unabated, this situation ultimately results in tissue ischemia, MODS, and death.

ASSESSMENT AND DIAGNOSIS

Effective treatment of severe sepsis and septic shock depends on timely recognition. The diagnosis of severe sepsis is based on the identification of three conditions: known or suspected infection, two or more of the clinical indications of the systemic inflammatory response, and evidence of at least one organ dysfunction. Clinical indications of systemic inflammatory response and sepsis were included in the original ACCP/SCCM consensus definitions and are listed in Box 39-10. The second consensus conference expanded this list to facilitate prompt clinical recognition (Box 39-12).[84]

Signs of individual organ dysfunction are discussed in Chapter 40. The two most common organs to demonstrate dysfunction in severe sepsis are the cardiovascular system and the lungs. The patient with persistent hypotension requiring vasopressor therapy despite adequate volume resuscitation is demonstrating cardiovascular dysfunction. Pulmonary dysfunction is manifested by a PaO_2/FIO_2 (fraction of oxygen in inspired air) ratio of less than 300, indicating ALI.[86] Signs indicating septic shock are hypotension despite adequate fluid resuscitation and the presence of perfusion abnormalities such as lactic acidosis, oliguria, or acute change in mentation.

The patient in severe sepsis or septic shock may present with a variety of clinical manifestations that may change dynamically as the condition progresses (Box 39-13). During the initial stage, massive vasodilation occurs in the venous and arterial beds. Dilation of the venous system leads to a decrease in venous return to the heart, which results in a decrease in the preload of the right and left ventricles. This is evidenced by a decline in the RAP and PAOP. Dilation of the arterial system results in a decrease in the afterload of the heart, as evidenced by a decrease in the SVR. The patient's skin becomes pink, warm, and flushed as a result of the massive vasodilation. Myocardial contractility is decreased, as evidenced by a decline in the left ventricular stroke work index (LVSWI).

The heart rate rises in response to increased SNS, metabolic, and adrenal gland stimulation. If circulating volume and preload are adequate, this results in a normal-to-high CO and CI despite impaired contractility. The pulse pressure widens as the diastolic blood pressure decreases because of the vasodilation, and the systolic blood pressure increases because of the elevated CO. A full, bounding pulse develops. The net result of these changes is a relatively normal blood pressure in severe sepsis. However, as the reduction in preload and afterload becomes overwhelming and contractility fails, hypotension ensues, resulting in septic shock.

In the lungs, ventilation/perfusion mismatching develops as a result of pulmonary vasoconstriction and the formation of pulmonary microemboli. Hypoxemia occurs, and the respiratory rate increases to compensate for the lack of oxygen. Crackles develop as increased pulmonary capillary membrane permeability leads to pulmonary edema.[79]

BOX 39-12 EXPANDED LIST OF DIAGNOSTIC CRITERIA FOR SEPSIS

GENERAL VARIABLES
- Core temperature >38.3° or <36° C
- Heart rate >90 beats/min
- Tachypnea
- Altered mental status
- Significant edema or positive fluid balance >20 mL/kg over 24 hours
- Hyperglycemia (>120 mg/dL) in absence of diabetes

INFLAMMATORY VARIABLES
- WBC count >12,000, <4000 mm^3, or >10% immature forms
- Elevated plasma C-reactive protein level
- Elevated plasma procalcitonin level

HEMODYNAMIC VARIABLES
- Systolic BP <90 mm Hg or decrease >40 mm Hg
- Mean arterial pressure <70 mm Hg
- $S\bar{v}O_2$ >70%
- CI >3.5 L/m/m^3

TISSUE PERFUSION VARIABLES
- Serum lactate level >1 mmol/L
- Decreased capillary refill or mottling

ORGAN DYSFUNCTION VARIABLES
- PaO_2/FIO_2 <300
- Urine output <0.5 mL/kg/hr
- Creatinine increase >0.5 mg/dL
- INR >1.5 or aPTT >60 sec
- Ileus
- Platelet count <100,000 mm^3
- Hyperbilirubinemia (plasma total bilirubin >4 mg/dL)

---

aPTT, activated partial thromboplastin time; BP, blood pressure; CI, cardiac index; FIO$_2$, fraction of oxygen in inspired air; INR, international normalized ratio; PaO$_2$, partial pressure of oxygen; S$\bar{v}$O$_2$, mixed venous oxygen saturation; WBC, white blood cells.

Modified from Levy MN et al: 2001 SCCM/ESICM/ACCP/ATS/SIS international sepsis definitions conference, *Crit Care Med* 31:1250, 2003.

BOX 39-13 CLINICAL MANIFESTATIONS OF SEPTIC SHOCK

- Increased heart rate
- Decreased blood pressure
- Wide pulse pressure
- Full, bounding pulse
- Pink, warm, flushed skin
- Increased respiratory rate (early) or decreased respiratory rate (late)
- Crackles
- Change in sensorium
- Decreased urine output
- Increased temperature
- Increased cardiac output and cardiac index
- Decreased systemic vascular resistance
- Decreased right atrial pressure
- Decreased pulmonary artery occlusion pressure
- Decreased left ventricular stroke work index
- Decreased Pao_2
- Decreased $Paco_2$ (early) or increased $Paco_2$ (late)
- Decreased HCO_3^-
- Increased mixed or central venous oxygen saturation ($S\bar{v}o_2$ or $Scvo_2$)

$Paco_2$, partial pressure of carbon dioxide; Pao_2, partial pressure of oxygen; $S\bar{v}o_2$, mixed venous oxygen saturation; $Scvo_2$, central venous oxygen saturation.

BOX 39-14 SEVERE SEPSIS BUNDLES

SEPSIS RESUSCITATION BUNDLE
1. Measure serum lactate.
2. Obtain blood cultures before administering antibiotics.
3. Improve time to broad-spectrum antibiotics.
4. In the event of hypotension or lactate level >4 mmol/L (36 mg/dL)
   a. Deliver an initial minimum of 20 mL/kg of crystalloid (or colloid equivalent).
   b. Apply vasopressors for ongoing hypotension.
5. In the event of persistent hypotension despite fluid resuscitation or lactate level >4 mmol/L (36 mg/dL)
   a. Achieve central venous pressure of ≥8 mm Hg.
   b. Achieve central venous oxygen saturation of ≥70%.

SEPSIS MANAGEMENT BUNDLE
1. Administer low-dose steroids.
2. Administer drotrecogin alfa (activated).
3. Maintain adequate glycemic control.
4. Prevent excessive inspiratory plateau pressures.

Adapted from Hurtado FJ, Nin N: The role of bundles in sepsis care, *Crit Care Clin* 22:521, 2006.

The level of consciousness starts to change as a result of decreased cerebral perfusion, immune mediator activation, hyperthermia, and lactic acidosis. This septic encephalopathy is demonstrated by acute onset of impaired cognitive functioning, or delirium, which may fluctuate during its course.[79] The patient may appear disoriented, confused, combative, or lethargic.

ABG values initially reveal respiratory alkalosis, hypoxemia, and metabolic acidosis. This is demonstrated by a low Pao_2, low $Paco_2$, and low HCO_3^- level, respectively. The respiratory alkalosis is caused by the patient's increased respiratory rate. As pathologic pulmonary changes progress and the patient becomes fatigued, the effectiveness of respirations decreases and the $Paco_2$ increases, resulting in respiratory acidosis. The metabolic acidosis is the result of lack of oxygen to the cells and the development of lactic acidemia. Serum lactate levels increase above 2 mmol/L because of anaerobic metabolism. The mixed venous oxygen saturation ($S\bar{v}o_2$) may increase because of microcirculatory shunting or decrease because of inadequate oxygen delivery.[87,95] The white blood cell (WBC) count is elevated as part of the immune response to the invading microorganisms. The WBC differential count reveals an increase in immature neutrophils (shift to the left). This occurs because the body has to mobilize increasing numbers of WBCs to fight the infection. An elevated procalcitonin level is a valuable indicator of significant infection.[87,98] Serum glucose levels increase as part of the hypermetabolic response and the development of insulin resistance. The patient's temperature is elevated in response to pyrogens released from the invading

microorganisms, immune mediator activation, and increased metabolic activity. Urine output declines because of decreased perfusion of the kidneys. As impaired tissue perfusion develops, a variety of other clinical manifestations appear that indicate the development of MODS.

MEDICAL MANAGEMENT

Treatment of the patient in severe sepsis or septic shock requires a multifaceted approach. The goals of treatment are to reverse the pathophysiologic responses, control the infection, and promote metabolic support. This approach includes supporting the cardiovascular system and enhancing tissue perfusion, identifying and treating the infection, limiting the systemic inflammatory response, restoring metabolic balance, and initiating nutritional therapy. Dysfunction of the individual organ systems must be prevented. Early treatment reduces mortality.[16,89,99,100] Guidelines for the management of severe sepsis and septic shock have been developed and updated under the auspices of the Surviving Sepsis Campaign (SSC), an international effort of more than 11 organizations to improve patient outcomes.[15,16] From these guidelines, a group ("bundle") of selected interventions was identified as having the most impact on patient outcomes (Box 39-14). The sepsis resuscitation bundle should be implemented within the first 6 hours, and the sepsis management bundle should be implemented within the first 24 hours. More information regarding these interventions is available at the SSC Web site (www.survivingsepsis.org).

The patient in severe sepsis or septic shock requires immediate resuscitation of the hypoperfused state. Specific interventions are aimed at increasing cellular oxygen supply and decreasing cellular oxygen demand. These treatments include administration of fluids, vasopressors, and positive inotropic agents. Early goal-directed therapy during the first 6 hours of resuscitation improves survival[60] and is recommended in the SSC guidelines.[15,16] This therapy includes aggressive fluid resuscitation to augment intravascular volume and increase preload until a CVP of 8 to 12 mm Hg (12 to 15 mm Hg in mechanically ventilated patients) is achieved. Crystalloids or colloids may be used. A fluid challenge for hypovolemia should be initiated with at least 1000 mL of crystalloids or 300 to 500 mL of colloids over 30 minutes. Vasopressors (norepinephrine or dopamine as first-choice agents) should be administered as necessary to maintain a MAP of at least 65 mm Hg. These agents reverse the massive peripheral vasodilation and increase SVR. Epinephrine is recommended as an alternative agent if response to norepinephrine or dopamine is poor.[16] Arterial line placement is recommended for any patient requiring vasopressor therapy. Intermittent or continuous monitoring of central venous or mixed venous oxygen saturation ($ScvO_2$ or $S\bar{v}O_2$) allows evaluation of the effectiveness of oxygen delivery. If the $ScvO_2$ is less than 70% or the $S\bar{v}O_2$ is less than 65% after the CVP goal is achieved, administration of packed red cells to achieve a hematocrit of at least 30%.[60] or inotropic stimulation with dobutamine (administered to a maximum of 20 mcg/kg/min) to counteract myocardial depression and maintain adequate CO is recommended to obtain this goal.[16,99] The dobutamine infusion should be reduced or discontinued if a tachycardia greater than 120 beats/min develops.[99]

Intubation and mechanical ventilatory support are usually required to optimize oxygenation and ventilation for the patient in severe sepsis or septic shock. Ventilation with lower than traditional tidal volumes (6 versus 12 mL/kg) in patients with ALI and acute respiratory distress syndrome (ARDS) decreases mortality.[101] SSC guidelines recommend the goals of 6 mL/kg of predicted body weight and plateau pressures no more than 30 cm H_2O for patients with severe sepsis or septic shock with ALI or ARDS.[16] Increased $PaCO_2$ may result from this therapy and is acceptable if tolerated as evidenced by hemodynamic stability. Ventilator settings should include positive end-expiratory pressure and be adjusted to provide the patient with a PaO_2 greater than 70 mm Hg. Patients receiving mechanical ventilation should be maintained in a semirecumbent position with the head of the bed raised to 45 degrees to decrease the incidence of ventilator-associated pneumonia.[16] Prone positioning should be considered in the septic patient with ARDS requiring high levels of oxygen.[16] Sedation protocols using intermittent bolus or continuous infusion using a standardized sedation scale and specific goals are recommended for all patients requiring mechanical ventilation. Daily interruption of sedative infusions to allow wakefulness and reevaluation of sedation needs reduces duration of mechanical ventilation and is recommended.[16] Neuromuscular blocking agents should be avoided, if possible, to prevent prolonged blockade after discontinuation.[16]

A key measure in the treatment of septic shock is finding and eradicating the cause of the infection. At least two blood cultures plus urine, sputum, and wound cultures should be obtained to find the location of the infection before antibiotic therapy is initiated.[16] Antibiotic therapy should be started within 1 hour of recognition of severe sepsis without delay for cultures.[16] Each hour of delay is associated with a substantial drop in the survival rate.[100] If the microorganism is unknown, antiinfective therapy with one or more agents known to be effective against likely pathogens should be initiated, with daily reassessment of the regimen. Combination therapy is recommended for known or suspected *Pseudomonas* infection and for neutropenic patients but should be limited to less than 3 to 5 days.[16] A specific source of infection should be established within 6 hours of presentation.[16] Surgical intervention to débride infected or necrotic tissue or to drain abscesses may be necessary to facilitate removal of the septic source.[16] Intravascular devices that may be the source of the infection should be removed after establishment of alternative vascular access.

Recombinant human activated protein C (rhAPC) administration has been demonstrated to improve survival of patients with severe sepsis at high risk for death.[102,103] In consideration of recent trial results after U.S. Food and Drug Administration (FDA) approval and an associated risk of bleeding, Xigris (drotrecogin alfa [activated]) is recommended only for adult patients with sepsis-induced multiple organ failure or a clinical determination of high risk for death.[16,87] Although its specific mechanisms for improving survival are not fully understood, drotrecogin alfa has anticoagulant, profibrinolytic, and antiinflammatory properties.[102] The proposed mechanisms of action of endogenous activated protein C are illustrated in Figure 39-6. Guidelines for patient selection and appropriate administration of this agent must be strictly followed for safe and effective use. It is administered intravenously at an infusion rate of 24 mcg/kg/hr for a total infusion duration of 96 hours. Interruption of the infusion is necessary for invasive procedures. The most common serious side effect of drotrecogin alfa is bleeding. Contraindications for use include active internal bleeding, recent hemorrhagic stroke (within 3 months) or intracranial or intraspinal surgery (within 2 months); severe head trauma, trauma with an increased risk of life-threatening bleeding, or presence of an epidural catheter; and intracranial neoplasm or mass lesion or evidence of cerebral herniation.[103] Studies of numerous other drugs thought to block or alter the effects of immune mediators have failed to demonstrate effectiveness or have been associated with unacceptable adverse effects.[91,105]

Intravenous corticosteroids reduce mortality in catecholamine-dependent septic shock patients with relative adrenal insufficiency.[106] Intravenous hydrocortisone is recommended only for the patient in septic shock who is poorly responsive to fluid resuscitation and vasopressor therapy.[16] Doses greater than 300 mg/day may be harmful and should not be used and steroid therapy should be weaned when vasopressors are no longer required.[16]

Continuous infusion of insulin and glucose to maintain a blood glucose level of less than 150 mg/dL improves outcomes[42] and is recommended by SSC guidelines after initial stabilization. Glucose levels should be monitored every 1 to 2 hours until stable and then every 4 hours. Low glucose levels measured by capillary testing may be inaccurate in this population.[16] Platelets should be administered when counts are less than 5000/mm^3 and red blood cell transfusions are recommended when the hemoglobin level is less than 7.0 g/dL to obtain a target value of 7 to 9 g/dL.[16] Stress ulcer prophylaxis

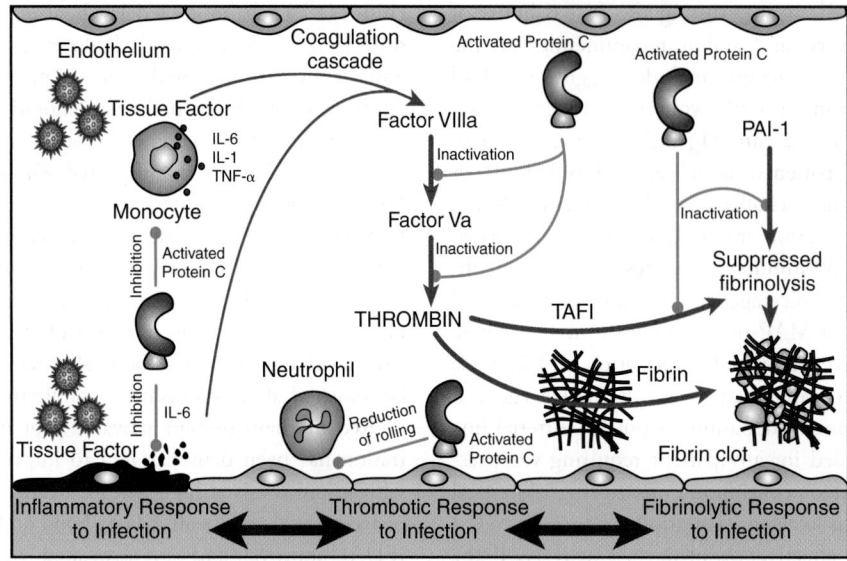

Figure 39-6 Proposed mechanisms of action of endogenous activated protein C in severe sepsis. IL, interleukin; PAI-1, plasminogen activator inhibitor 1; TAFI, thrombin activatable fibrinolysis inhibitor; TNF, tumor necrosis factor. *(Courtesy Eli Lilly and Company.)*

using histamine$_2$ (H$_2$) antagonists blockers or proton pump inhibitors and DVT prophylaxis are recommended for all patients with severe sepsis or septic shock. The SCC guidelines recommend against the use of sodium bicarbonate for lactic acidemia if the pH is equal to or greater than 7.15.[16] Low-dose dopamine infusion for renal protection is not beneficial and should not be used.[16]

The initiation of nutritional therapy is critical in the management of the patient in severe sepsis or septic shock. The goal is to improve the patient's overall nutritional status, enhance immune function, and promote wound healing. A daily caloric intake of 25 to 30 kcal/kg of usual body weight is recommended. The enteral route is preferred. The ideal nutritional supplement for the patient in septic shock should be high in protein because of the metabolic derangements that develop in the hypermetabolic state. The amount of protein calories given depends on the patient's nitrogen balance. In early sepsis, the mix of nonprotein calories may be divided evenly between carbohydrates and fats. In the later stages, significant alterations in fat metabolism occur, and the lipid content should be limited to 10% to 15% of the total nonprotein calories. Specific nutritional therapies to reduce the inflammatory and hypermetabolic responses associated with sepsis, such as antioxidant supplementation and feeding with long-chain n-3 polyunsaturated fatty acids, are the source of much debate and are being evaluated.[8,107-110] Glutamine is considered by some to be an essential amino acid in critically ill patients and has the most empirical support.[87,107-108,110] Arginine has produced negative outcomes and is not recommended.[109]

NURSING MANAGEMENT

Prevention of severe sepsis and septic shock is one of the primary responsibilities of the nurse in the critical care area. These measures include the identification of patients at risk

Nursing Diagnoses

Septic Shock

- Deficient Fluid Volume related to relative loss
- Decreased Cardiac Output related to alterations in preload
- Decreased Cardiac Output related to alterations in afterload
- Decreased Cardiac Output related to alterations in contractility
- Impaired Gas Exchange related to ventilation/perfusion mismatching or intrapulmonary shunting
- Imbalanced Nutrition: Less Than Body Requirements related to increased metabolic demands or lack of exogenous nutrients
- Risk for Infection
- Anxiety related to threat to biologic, psychologic, or social integrity
- Compromised Family Coping related to a critically ill family member

and reduction of their exposure to invading microorganisms. Hand washing, aseptic technique, and an understanding of how microorganisms can invade the body are essential components of preventive nursing care. Early identification allows for early treatment and decreases mortality.[79] Box 39-15 depicts a simple screening tool for identifying patients with severe sepsis.

The patient in septic shock may have any number of nursing diagnoses, depending on the progression of the process (see the Nursing Diagnoses feature on Septic Shock). Nursing interventions include administering prescribed fluids and medications, promoting comfort and emotional support, and maintaining surveillance for complications. Continual observation to detect subtle changes that indicate the progression of the septic process is also very important.

Evidence-based guidelines for the management of the patient with severe sepsis or septic shock are listed in the Evidence-Based Practice feature on Severe Sepsis and Septic Shock Management Guidelines.

BOX 39-15   SCREENING PATIENTS FOR SEVERE SEPSIS

A patient who meets the following three criteria has a positive screen result that suggests severe sepsis:

A. INFECTION: Does your patient have one or more of the following infection criteria?
- ☐ Documented or suspected: Does the patient have positive culture results (e.g., blood, sputum, urine)?
- ☐ Antiinfective therapy: Is the patient receiving antibiotic, antifungal, or other antiinfective therapy?
- ☐ Pneumonia: Is there documentation of pneumonia (e.g., radiograph)?
- ☐ WBCs: Have WBCs been found in normally sterile fluid (e.g., urine, CSF)?
- ☐ Perforated viscus: Does the patient have a perforated hollow organ (e.g., bowel)?

Did you check any boxes above?

B. SIRS: Does your patient have two or more of the following SIRS criteria?
- ☐ Temperature: Is the patient's temperature $\geq 38°$ C ($\geq 100.4°$ F) or $\leq 36°$ C ($\leq 96.8°$ F)?
- ☐ Heart rate: Is the patient's heart rate ≥ 90 beats/min?
- ☐ Respiratory rate: Is the patient's respiratory rate ≥ 20 breaths/min?
- ☐ WBC count: Is the patient's WBC count $\geq 12,000/mm^3$ or $\leq 4000/mm^3$, or are there $>10\%$ immature neutrophils (left shift)?

Did you check two or more boxes above?

C. ACUTE ORGAN DYSFUNCTION: Does your patient have one or more of the following organ dysfunction criteria?
- ☐ Cardiovascular criteria: Does the patient have a systolic BP ≤ 90 mm Hg or mean arterial pressure ≤ 70 mm Hg (for at least 1 hour despite fluid resuscitation) or require vasopressor support?
- ☐ Respiratory criteria: Does the patient have a Pao_2/Fio_2 ratio ≤ 250, PEEP >7.5, or require mechanical ventilation?
- ☐ Renal criteria: Does the patient have low urine output (e.g., <0.5 mL/kg/hr for 1 hour despite adequate fluid resuscitation), increased creatinine ($>50\%$ increase from baseline), or require acute dialysis?
- ☐ Hematologic criteria: Does the patient have a low platelet count ($<100,000/mm^3$) or PT/PTT > upper limit of normal?
- ☐ Metabolic criteria: Does the patient have a low pH with a high lactate level (e.g., pH <7.30 and plasma lactate $\geq$ upper limit of normal)?
- ☐ Hepatic criteria: Are the patient's liver enzymes ≥ 2 upper limit of normal?
- ☐ CNS criteria: Does the patient have altered consciousness or a reduced Glasgow Coma Scale score?

Did you check any boxes above?

Boxes checked under INFECTION (A) plus SIRS (B) plus ORGAN DYSFUNCTION (C) equals a positive screen result that suggests severe sepsis.

BP, blood pressure; CNS, central nervous system; CSF, cerebral spinal fluid; Fio_2, fraction of oxygen in inspired air; Pao_2, arterial partial pressure of oxygen; PEEP, positive end-expiratory pressure; PT, prothrombin time; PTT, partial thromboplastin time; SIRS, systemic inflammatory response syndrome; WBC, white blood cell.
Modified from a form provided courtesy Eli Lilly and Company, 2004.

Evidence-Based Practice: Collaborative

Severe Sepsis and Septic Shock Management Guidelines

The following recommendations are graded in terms of quality of evidence from high (grade A) to very low (D). A strong recommendation (1) indicates that the desirable effects of the intervention clearly outweigh its undesirable effects. A weak recommendation (2) indicates that the tradeoff between desirable and undesirable effects is less clear.

- Resuscitation should be initiated as soon as severe sepsis is recognized with the following goals as targets: central venous pressure (CVP) between 8 and 12 mm Hg (12 to 15 mm Hg if mechanically ventilated); mean arterial pressure (MAP) of 65 mm Hg or greater; urine output (UO) or 0.5 mL/kg/hr or greater; and central venous oxygen saturation ($Scvo_2$) of 70% or greater or mixed venous oxygen saturation ($S\bar{v}o_2$) of 65% or greater (1C).
- If the above $Scvo_2$ or $S\bar{v}o_2$ goals are not reached with fluid resuscitation to the CVP target, packed red blood cells should be transfused to hematocrit of at least 30% or dobutamine should be administered up to 20 µg/kg/min (2C).
- Norepinephrine and dopamine are the initial vasopressors of choice (1C).
- Begin intravenous antibiotics within 1 hour of severe sepsis (1D) or septic shock (1B). Reassess antibiotic regimen daily (1C).
- Do not use low-dose dopamine for renal protection (1A).
- Increasing cardiac index to increase oxygen delivery to supranormal levels is not recommended (1B).
- Consider recombinant human activated protein C in adult patients with sepsis-induced organ dysfunction at high risk for death if there are no absolute contraindications with consideration to relative contraindications (2B). Do not use recombinant human activated protein C in adult patient with severe sepsis and low risk of death (1A).

- After tissue hypoperfusion has resolved, red blood cell transfusions should be used only when hemoglobin decreases below 7 g/dL to a target hemoglobin level of 7 to 9 g/dL unless extenuating circumstances (e.g., acute hemorrhage) require higher values (1B).
- Erythropoietin for anemia is not recommended unless there is another accepted reason for its administration (1B).
- Do not use antithrombin therapy (1B).
- Maintain a tidal volume of 6 mL/kg and an end-inspiratory plateau pressure less than 30 cm H_2O while mechanically ventilated (1B).
- Daily spontaneous breathing trials should be used to gauge the patient's readiness for extubation (1A).
- A sedation protocol should be used to guide treatment of mechanically ventilated patients (1B).
- The sedation protocol should include daily interruption or lightening of sedation (1B).
- Avoid neuromuscular blockers when possible (1B).
- Keep blood glucose levels less than 150 mg/dL (1B).
- Continuous venovenous hemofiltration and intermittent hemodialysis are equally effective for the hemodynamically stable patient with acute renal failure. Continuous hemofiltration provides easier management of fluid balance in hemodynamically unstable patients (2B).
- Do not use bicarbonate therapy to improve hemodynamics when treating hypoperfusion-induced lactic acidemia with a pH of at least 7.15 (1B).
- Deep vein thrombosis and stress ulcer prophylaxis should be given to patients with severe sepsis (1A).

Data from Dellinger RP et al: Surviving Sepsis Campaign: international guidelines for management of severe sepsis and septic shock: 2008, *Crit Care Med* 36:296, 2008.

Summary

Shock

- Shock is an acute, widespread process of impaired tissue perfusion that occurs when an imbalance develops between cellular oxygen supply and cellular oxygen demand.
- Shock can be classified as hypovolemic, cardiogenic, or distributive (septic, anaphylactic, and neurogenic), depending on the pathophysiologic cause and hemodynamic profile.
- Shock evolves through four stages: initial, compensatory, progressive, and refractory.
- The patient with a MAP less than 60 mm Hg or with evidence of multisystem organ hypoperfusion is considered to be in a shock state.
- Management of the patient in shock focuses on supporting oxygen delivery.
- Prevention of shock is one of the primary responsibilities of the nurse in the critical care area.

Hypovolemic Shock

- Hypovolemic shock results from a loss of circulating or intravascular volume due to an absolute or relative fluid loss.
- Initial hemodynamic parameters include a decreased CO or CI, decreased CVP or PAOP, and increased SVR.
- Medical management focuses on identifying and stopping the source of fluid loss and administering fluid to replace circulating volume.
- Nursing interventions include minimizing fluid loss, administering volume replacement, providing comfort and emotional support, and maintaining surveillance for complications.

Cardiogenic Shock

- Cardiogenic shock results from the impaired ability of the heart to pump due to primary ventricular ischemia, structural problems, or dysrhythmias.
- Initial hemodynamic parameters include a decreased CO or CI, increased PAOP or CVP (or both), and increased SVR.
- Medical management focuses on identifying the etiologic factors of pump failure and administering pharmacologic agents to enhance CO.
- Nursing interventions include limiting myocardial oxygen demand, enhancing myocardial oxygen supply, providing comfort and emotional support, and maintaining surveillance for complications.

Anaphylactic Shock

- Anaphylactic shock results from activation of mast cells and the release of biochemical mediators due to a severe antibody-antigen reaction.
- Hemodynamic parameters include decreased CO or CI, decreased RAP or PAOP, and decreased SVR.
- Medical management focused on removing the offending antigen, reversing the effects of the biochemical mediators, and promoting adequate tissue perfusion.
- Nursing interventions include facilitating ventilation, administering volume replacement, providing comfort and emotional support, and maintaining surveillance for complications.

Neurogenic Shock

- Neurogenic shock results from the loss of sympathetic tone due to interrupted impulse transmission or blockage of sympathetic outflow from the vasomotor center in the brain.
- Hemodynamic parameters include decreased CO or CI, decreased RAP or PAOP, decreased SVR, and decreased heart rate.
- Medical management focuses on preventing cardiovascular stability and promoting tissue perfusion.
- Nursing interventions include treating hypovolemia, maintaining normothermia, monitoring for dysrhythmias, promoting comfort and emotional support, and maintaining surveillance for complications.

Septic Shock

- Septic shock results from the initiation of the systemic inflammatory response due to microorganisms entering the body.
- Hemodynamic parameters include decreased CO or CI, decreased RAP or PAOP, decreased SVR, and increased heart rate.
- Medical management focuses on reversing the pathophysiologic responses, controlling the infection, and promoting metabolic support.
- Nursing interventions include administering prescribed fluids and medications, promoting comfort and emotional support, and maintaining surveillance for complications.

Case Study: Patient in Shock

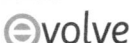 Answers to the Case Study Questions can be found on the Evolve web site at http://evolve.elsevier.com/Urden/.

Brief Patient History

Ms. B is a 76-year-old woman who has been in the surgical intensive care unit for the past 2 days after abdominal surgery for stage III ovarian cancer. Her thrombosed central line needs to be replaced. She has a history of allergy to kiwi and avocados but no known allergy to latex.

Clinical Assessment

Approximately 10 minutes after the central line insertion, Ms. B complains of feeling flushed, and she loses consciousness.

Diagnostic Procedures

Ms. B is unconscious and unresponsive to verbal or physical stimuli. Audible wheezing can be heard at the bedside. Her skin is visibly flushed and clammy to touch. Vital signs include the following: blood pressure of 60 mm Hg (determined by Doppler), heart rate of 160 beats/min (atrial tachycardia), respiratory rate of 30 breaths/min, and temperature of 99° F.

Medical Diagnosis

Ms. B is diagnosed with anaphylactic shock resulting from a latex allergy.

Questions

1. What major outcomes do you expect to achieve for this patient?
2. What problems or risks must be managed to achieve these outcomes?
3. What interventions must be initiated to monitor, prevent, manage, or eliminate the problems and risks identified?
4. What interventions should be initiated to promote optimal functioning, safety, and well-being of the patient?
5. What possible learning needs do you anticipate for this patient?
6. What cultural and age-related factors may have a bearing on the patient's plan of care?

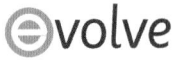 Be sure to check out the bonus material, including free self-assessment exercises, on the Evolve web site at http://evolve.elsevier.com/Urden/.

References

1. Maier RV: Approach to the patient with shock. In Fauci AS et al, editors: *Harrison's internal medicine*, ed 17, New York, 2008, McGraw-Hill.
2. Deitch EA et al: Role of the gut in the development of injury and shock induced SIRS and MODS: The gut-lymph hypothesis, a review, *Front Biosci* 11:520, 2006.
3. Heyland DK, McClave S: Nutrition in the critically ill. In Hall JB, Schmidt GA, Wood LDH, editors: *Principles of Critical Care*, ed 3, New York, 2005, McGraw-Hill.
4. Hameed SM et al: Oxygen delivery, *Crit Care Med* 31:S658, 2003.
5. Walley KR: Shock. In Hall JB, Schmidt GA, Wood LDH, editors: *Principles of Critical Care*, ed 3, New York, 2005, McGraw-Hill.
6. Parks JK et al: Systemic hypotension is a late marker of shock after trauma: A validation study of advanced trauma life support principles in a large national sample, *Am J Surg* 19:727, 2006.
7. Wilson M et al: Diagnosis and monitoring of hemorrhagic shock during the initial resuscitation of multiple trauma patients: a review, *J Emerg Med* 24:413, 2003.
8. Tappy L, Chioléro R: Substrate utilization in sepsis and multiple organ failure, *Crit Care Med* 35:S531, 2007.
9. Englehart MS, Schreiber MA: Measurement of acid-base resuscitation endpoints: lactate, base deficit, bicarbonate or what, *Curr Opin Crit Care* 12:569, 2006.
10. Husain FA et al: Serum lactate and base deficit as predictors of mortality and morbidity, *Am J Surg* 185:485, 2003.
11. Kruse JA: Lactic acidosis. In Kruse JA et al, editors: *Saunders Manual of Critical Care*, Philadelphia, 2003, Saunders.
12. FitzSullivan E et al: Serum bicarbonate may replace the arterial base deficit in the trauma intensive care unit, *Am J Surg* 190:961, 2005.
13. Martin MJ et al: Use of serum bicarbonate measurement in place of arterial base deficit in the surgical intensive care unit, *Arch Surg* 140:745, 2005.
14. Guzman JA: Monitoring oxygen transport. In Kruse JA et al, editors: *Saunders Manual of Critical Care*, Philadelphia, 2003, Saunders.
15. Dellinger RP et al: Surviving Sepsis Campaign guidelines for management of severe sepsis and septic shock, *Crit Care Med* 32:858, 2004.
16. Dellinger RP et al: Surviving sepsis campaign: International guidelines for management of severe sepsis and septic shock: 2008, *Crit Care Med* 36:296, 2008.
17. Collaborative Study Group on Perioperative Scvo2 Monitoring: Multicentre study on peri- and postoperative central venous oxygen saturation in high-risk surgical patients, *Crit Care* 10:R158, 2006.
18. Ho KM et al: The impact of arterial oxygen tension on venous oxygen saturation in circulatory failure, *Shock* 29:3, 2008.
19. Pearse R et al: Changes in central venous saturation after major surgery, and association with outcome, *Crit Care* 9:R694, 2005.
20. Pearse RM, Hinds CJ: Should we use central venous saturation to guide management in high-risk surgical patients, *Crit Care* 10:181, 2006.
21. Vallet B et al: Physiologic transfusion triggers, *Best Pract Res Clin Anaesthesiol* 21:173, 2007.
22. Bunn F et al: Colloid solutions for fluid resuscitation, *Cochrane Database Syst Rev* Jan 23(1):CD001319, 2008.
23. Alam HB, Rhee P: New developments in fluid resuscitation, *Surg Clin North Am* 87:55, 2007.
24. Cotton BA et al: The cellular metabolic and systemic consequences of aggressive fluid resuscitation strategies, *Shock* 26:115, 2006.
25. Stapleton RD et al: Feeding critically ill patients: what is the optimal amount of energy, *Crit Care Med* 35:S535, 2007.
26. Finfer S et al: A comparison of albumin and saline for fluid resuscitation in the intensive care unit, *N Engl J Med* 350:2247, 2004.
27. Finfer S et al: Effect of baseline serum albumin concentration on outcome of resuscitation with albumin or saline in patients in intensive care units: analysis of data from the saline versus albumin fluid evaluation (SAFE) study, *BMJ* 333:1044, 2006.
28. Gould S et al: Packed red blood cell transfusion in the intensive care unit: limitations and consequences, *Am J Crit Care* 16:39, 2007.

29. Dennison CA: Transfusion-related acute lung injury: a clinical challenge, *Dimens Crit Care Nurs* 27:1, 2008.

30. Kleinman S et al: Promoting recognition and prevention of transfusion-related acute lung injury, *Crit Care Nurse* 27:49, 2007.

31. Toy P et al: Transfusion-related acute lung injury: definition and review, *Crit Care Med* 33:721, 2005.

32. Dellinger RP: Cardiovascular management of septic shock, *Crit Care Med* 31:946, 2003.

33. Gehlbach BK, Schmidt GA: Bench-to-bedside review: treating acid-base abnormalities in the intensive care unit—the role of buffers, *Crit Care* 8:259, 2004.

34. Barr J et al: Outcomes in critically ill patients before and after the implementation of an evidence-based nutritional management protocol, *Chest* 125:1446, 2004.

35. Bistrian BR, McCowen KC: Nutritional and metabolic support in the adult intensive care unit: key controversies, *Crit Care Med* 34:1525, 2006.

36. Dhaliwal R et al: Combination enteral and parenteral nutrition in critically ill patients: harmful or beneficial? A systematic review of the evidence, *Intensive Care Med* 30:1666, 2004.

37. Kattelmann KD et al: Preliminary evidence for a medical nutrition therapy protocol: enteral feedings for critically ill patients, *J Am Diet Assoc* 106:1226, 2006.

38. American Diabetes Association: Standards of medical care in diabetes—2007, *Diabetes Care* 30:S4, 2007.

39. The ACE/ADA Task Force on Inpatient Diabetes: American College of Endocrinology and American Diabetes Association consensus statement on inpatient diabetes glycemic control: a call to action, *Diabetes Care* 29:1955, 2006.

40. Schetz M et al: Tight blood glucose control is renoprotective in critically ill patients, *J Am Soc Nephrol* 19:571, 2008.

41. Langouche L et al: Intensive insulin therapy protects the endothelium of critically ill patients, *J Clin Invest* 115:2277, 2005.

42. Van den Berghe G et al: Intensive insulin therapy in the critically ill patients, *N Engl J Med* 345:1359, 2001.

43. Davidson JE et al: Clinical practice guidelines for support of the family in the patient-centered intensive care unit, *Crit Care Med* 35:605, 2007.

44. American Association of Critical-Care Nurse Practice Alert: Family presence during CPR and invasive procedures, 2004. Available at www.aacn.org/AACN/practiceAlert.nsf/Files/FAMILY/$file/Family%20Presence%20During%20CPR%2011-2004.pdf (accessed May 2009).

45. Duran CR et al: Attitudes toward and beliefs about family presence: a survey of healthcare providers, patients' families, and patients, *Am J Crit Care* 16:270, 2007.

46. Hemila MR, Wahl WL: Management of the injured patient. In Doherty GM, Way LW, editors: *Current surgical diagnosis and treatment*, ed 12, New York, 2006, McGraw-Hill.

47. Kwan I et al: Timing and volume of fluid administration for patients with bleeding, *Cochrane Database Syst Rev* (3):CD002245, 2003.

48. Revell M et al: Endpoints for fluid resuscitation in hemorrhagic shock, *J Trauma* 54:S63, 2003.

49. Roberts K et al: Hypotensive resuscitation in patients with ruptured abdominal aortic aneurysm, *Eur J Vasc Endovasc Surg* 31:339, 2006.

50. Bulger EM et al: Hypertonic resuscitation modulates the inflammatory response in patients with traumatic hemorrhagic shock, *Ann Surg* 245:635, 2007.

51. Bulger EM et al: Hypertonic resuscitation of hypovolemic shock after blunt trauma: a randomized controlled trial, *Arch Surg* 143:139, 2008.

52. Mizushima Y et al: Fluid resuscitation of trauma patients: how fast is the optimal rate, *Am J Emerg Med* 23:833, 2005.

53. Ashby DT et al: Cardiogenic shock in acute myocardial infarction, *Catheter Cardiovasc Interv* 59:34, 2003.

54. Topalian S et al: Cardiogenic shock, *Crit Care Med* 36:S66, 2008.

55. Hochman JS: Cardiogenic shock complicating acute myocardial infarction: expanding the paradigm, *Circulation* 107:2998, 2003.

56. Menon V, Fincke R: Cardiogenic shock: a summary of the randomized SHOCK trial, *Congest Heart Fail* 9:35, 2003.

57. Reynolds HR, Hochman JS: Cardiogenic shock: current concepts and improving outcomes, *Circulation* 117:686, 2008.

58. Lim N et al: Do all nonsurvivors of cardiogenic shock die with a low cardiac index, *Chest* 124:1885, 2003.

59. Kohsaka S et al: Systemic inflammatory response syndrome after acute myocardial infarction complicated by cardiogenic shock, *Arch Intern Med* 165:1643, 2005.

60. Okuda M: A multidisciplinary overview of cardiogenic shock, *Shock* 25:557, 2006.

61. Hochman JS et al: Early revascularization and long-term survival in cardiogenic shock complicating acute myocardial infarction, *JAMA* 295:2511, 2006.

62. Magliato KE et al: Biventricular support inpatient with profound cardiogenic shock: a single center experience, *ASAIO J* 49:475, 2003.

63. Meyns B et al: Initial experiences with the Impella device in patients with cardiogenic shock—Impella support for cardiogenic shock, *Thorac Cardiovasc Surg* 51:312, 2003.

64. Ellis AK, Day JH: Diagnosis and management of anaphylaxis, *CMAJ* 169:307, 2003.

65. Tang A: A practical guide to anaphylaxis, *Am Fam Physician* 38:1325, 2003.

66. Lieberman P et al: Epidemiology of anaphylaxis: Findings of the American College of Allergy, Asthma and Immunology Epidemiology of Anaphylaxis working group, *Ann Allergy Asthma Immunol* 97:596, 2006.

67. Simons FER: Anaphylaxis, *J Allergy Clin Immunol* 121:S402, 2008.

68. American Heart Association: 2005 American Heart Association Guidelines for cardiopulmonary resuscitation and emergency cardiovascular care. Part 10.6: Anaphylaxis, *Circulation* 112:IV-143, 2005.

69. McLean APC et al: Adrenaline in the treatment of anaphylaxis: what is the evidence, *BMJ* 327:1332, 2003.

70. Sampson HA et al: Second symposium on the definition and management of anaphylaxis: summary report—second National Institute of Allergy and Infectious Disease/Food Allergy and Anaphylaxis Network symposium, *J Allergy Clin Immunol* 117:391, 2006.

71. Sicherer SH: Advances in anaphylaxis and hypersensitivity reactions to foods, drugs, and insect venom, *J Allergy Clin Immunol* 111:S829, 2003.

72. Lieberman P et al: The diagnosis and management of anaphylaxis: an updated practice parameter, *J Allergy Clin Immunol* 115:S483, 2005.

73. Bilello JF et al: Cervical spinal cord injury and the need for cardiovascular intervention, *Arch Surg* 138:1127, 2003.

74. Guly HR et al: The incidence of neurogenic shock in patients with isolated spinal cord injury in the emergency department, *Resuscitation* 76:57, 2008.

75. Stevens RD et al: Critical care and perioperative management in traumatic spinal cord injury, *J Neurosurg Anesthesiol* 15:215, 2003.

76. Ditunno JF et al: Spinal shock revisited: a four-phase model, *Spinal Cord* 42:383, 2004.

77. Krassioukov A, Claydon VE: The clinical problems in cardiovascular control following spinal cord injury: an overview, *Prog Brain Res* 152:223, 2006.

78. Young WF: Shock. In Stone CK, Humphries RL, editors: *Current diagnosis & treatment: emergency medicine*, ed 6, New York, 2008, McGraw-Hill.

79. Ely EW et al: Advances in the understanding of clinical manifestations and therapy of severe sepsis: an update for critical care nurses, *Am J Crit Care* 12:120, 2003.

80. Martin GS et al: The epidemiology of sepsis in the United States from 1979 through 2000, *N Engl J Med* 348:1546, 2003.

81. Dombrovskey VY et al: Rapid increase in hospitalization and mortality rates for severe sepsis in the United States: a trend analysis from 1993-2003, *Crit Care Med* 35:1244, 2007.

82. Guidet B et al: Incidence and impact of organ dysfunctions associated with sepsis, *Chest* 127:942, 2005.

83. Leone M, et al: Empirical antimicrobial therapy of septic shock patients: adequacy and impact on the outcome, *Crit Care Med* 31:462, 2003.

84. Levy MN et al: 2001 SCCM/ESICM/ACCP/ATS/SIS International sepsis definitions conference, *Crit Care Med* 31:1250, 2003.

85. American College of Chest Physicians/Society of Critical Care Medicine Consensus Conference Committee: Definitions for sepsis and organ failure and guidelines for the use of innovative therapies in sepsis, *Crit Care Med* 20:864, 1992.

86. Ahrens T, Vollman K: Severe sepsis management: are we doing enough, *Crit Care Nurs* 23(Suppl):2, 2003.

87. Cinel I, Dellinger RP: Advances in pathogenesis and management of sepsis, *Curr Opin Infect Dis* 20:345, 2007.

88. Groeneveld AB et al: Circulating inflammatory mediators predict shock and mortality in febrile patients with microbial infection, *Clin Immunol* 106:106, 2003.

89. Rivers EP, et al: The influence of early hemodynamic optimization on biomarker patterns of severe sepsis and septic shock, *Crit Care Med* 35:2016, 2007.

90. Singer M: Mitochondrial function in sepsis: Acute phase versus multiple organ failure, *Crit Care Med* 35:S441, 2007.

91. Angus DC, Crowther MA: Unraveling severe sepsis: why did OPTIMIST fail and what's next, *JAMA* 290:256, 2003.

92. Sharma S, Kumar A: Septic shock, multiple organ failure, and acute respiratory distress syndrome, *Curr Opin Pulm Med* 9:199, 2003.

93. Levi M: Disseminated intravascular coagulation, *Crit Care Med* 35:2191, 2007.

94. Elbers PWG, Ince C: Bench-to-bedside review: mechanisms of critical illness—classifying microcirculatory flow abnormalities in distributive shock, *Crit Care* 10:221, 2006.

95. Tzeciak S et al: Early microcirculatory perfusion derangements in patients with severe sepsis and septic shock: relationship to hemodynamics, oxygen transport, and survival, *Ann Emerg Med* 49:88, 2007.

96. Tamion F et al: Gastric mucosal acidosis and cytokine release in patients with septic shock, *Crit Care Med* 31:2237, 2003.

97. Baumgart K et al: Pathophysiology of tissue acidosis in septic shock: block microcirculation or impaired cellular respiration, *Crit Care Med* 36:640, 2008.

98. Uzzan B et al: Procalcitonin as a diagnostic test for sepsis in critically ill adults and after surgery or trauma: a systematic review and meta-analysis, *Crit Care Med* 34:1996, 2006.

99. Rivers E et al: Early goal-directed therapy in the treatment of severe sepsis and septic shock, *N Engl J Med* 345:1368, 2001.

100. Kumar A et al: Duration of hypotension before initiation of effective antimicrobial therapy is the critical determinant of survival in human septic shock, *Crit Care Med* 43:1589, 2006.

101. The ARDS Network: Ventilation with lower tidal volumes as compared with traditional tidal volumes for acute lung injury and the acute respiratory distress syndrome, *N Engl J Med* 342:1301, 2000.

102. Bernard GR et al: Efficacy and safety of recombinant human activated protein C for severe sepsis, *JAMA* 344:699, 2001.

103. Vincent JL et al: Drotrecogin alfa (activated) treatment in severe sepsis from the global open-label trial ENHANCE: further evidence for survival and safety and implications for early treatment, *Crit Care Med* 33:2266, 2005.

104. Powers J, Jacobi J: Treatment of severe sepsis with Xigris: implications for the clinical nurse specialist, *Clin Nurse Spec* 17:128, 2003.

105. Dellinger RP, Parrillo JE: Mediator modulation therapy of severe sepsis and septic shock: does it work, *Crit Care Med* 32:282, 2004.

106. Annane D et al: Effect of treatment with low doses of hydrocortisone and fludrocortisone on mortality in patients with septic shock, *JAMA* 288:862, 2002.

107. Beale RJ et al: Early enteral supplementation with key pharmaconutrients improves sequential organ failure assessment score in critically ill patients with sepsis: outcome of a randomized, controlled, double-blind trial, *Crit Care Med* 36:131, 2008.

108. Berger MM, Chioléro RL: Antioxidant supplementation in sepsis and systemic inflammatory response syndrome, *Crit Care Med* 35:S584, 2007.

109. Bristrian B, McCowen KC: Nutritional and metabolic support in the adult intensive care unit: key controversies, *Crit Care Med* 34:1525, 2006.

110. Vincent JL: Metabolic support in sepsis and multiple organ failure: more questions than answers, *Crit Care Med* 35:S436, 2007.

Systemic Inflammatory Response Syndrome and Multiple Organ Dysfunction Syndrome

*A*dvanced cardiopulmonary life support techniques and technology have allowed the survival of some critically ill or injured patients who previously would have died of an initial insult such as trauma, infection, shock, or other acute process. However, continued patient survival and long-term quality of life are threatened by two clinical syndromes—systemic inflammatory response syndrome (SIRS) and multiple organ dysfunction syndrome (MODS)—that may result in death or profound disability. SIRS is characterized by generalized systemic inflammation in organs remote from an initial insult. MODS results from SIRS and describes progressive physiologic failure of several interdependent organ systems; it is the major cause of death of patients cared for in critical care units.[1,2]

In 1992, the American College of Chest Physicians and the Society of Critical Care Medicine adopted a framework that described the interrelationships among the systemic inflammatory response, sepsis, bacteremia, and infection (Fig. 40-1) and multiple organ dysfunction (Fig. 40-2).[3] New terminology was proposed to describe the clinical manifestations of SIRS and its relationship to sepsis and MODS. Critical care professionals were urged to standardize terminology used in diagnosis, intervention, and research protocols.[3] In the past, terms such as *multiple systems organ failure, multiple organ failure syndrome*, and *progressive* or *sequential organ failure* were used to describe clinical syndromes of organ failure in critically ill patients. Because these terms imply organ failure rather than the dynamic process of organ dysfunction, the name of the syndrome was changed to *multiple organ dysfunction syndrome*.[3]

In 2001, the Society of Critical Care Medicine, the European Society of Intensive Care Medicine, the American College of Chest Physicians, the American Thoracic Society, and the Surgical Infection Society revisited the definitions for SIRS and sepsis, and they attempted to identify methodologies for improving the accuracy and reliability of the diagnosis. No changes to the proposed definitions from 10 years earlier were made; however, an expansion of the list of signs and symptoms of sepsis based on experienced clinical observations was established.[4]

This chapter provides information regarding the pathogenesis of SIRS and MODS. Current clinical management, select investigational therapies, and appropriate nursing diagnoses are addressed.

THE INFLAMMATORY RESPONSE

Acute inflammation is a biochemical and cellular process that only occurs in vascularized tissue in response to an insult or invasion.[5] During inflammation, the body creates a lethal microenvironment to localize the injury and kill microorganisms. Normally, the inflammatory process is contained within a restricted environment. If it is not contained, a systemic, widespread response (SIRS) occurs that is deleterious to organ function.[5] Fortunately, the body normally has a complex system of checks and balances to localize inflammation.

LOCAL INFLAMMATORY RESPONSE

The acute inflammatory response is a self-limiting (8 to 10 days), nonspecific response that usually occurs in an identical manner regardless of the cause. The response usually starts within seconds of the insult. Cell injury or death initiates the acute inflammatory response. Cellular injury occurs from several mechanisms, including tissue trauma, hypoxia, ischemia, infectious microorganisms, nutrient deprivation, genetic or immune defects, temperature extremes, chemical agents, and ionizing radiation.[5]

Mediators, which are facilitators of the local inflammatory response, are housed in the circulatory system and enhance the movement of plasma and blood cells from the circulation into the tissue around the injury. Mediators of the vascular response include leukocytes; plasma protein cascades (e.g., complement, coagulation, kinin-kallikrein system); platelets; and other inflammatory biochemicals, such as arachidonic acid (AA) metabolites (e.g., prostaglandins [PGs], leukotrienes [LTs]), interleukins (ILs), and tumor necrosis factor-α(TNF-α).[5]

Vascular Response. The local vascular effects of inflammation start immediately and sustain increased vascular permeability that lasts through acute inflammation. Several mechanisms are operable. Arterioles near the injury constrict briefly and then dilate to increase blood flow to the injured area and allow exudation of plasma and cells into tissues. Exudation causes interstitial edema and slows the microcirculation, making it more viscous. Concurrently, mediators such as bradykinin stimulate capillary and venule endothelial cells to retract, creating spaces at junctions between cells. Endothelial cell retraction allows leukocytes to squeeze out of the cell. The net effect is the movement of blood cells and plasma proteins into the inflamed tissue.[5]

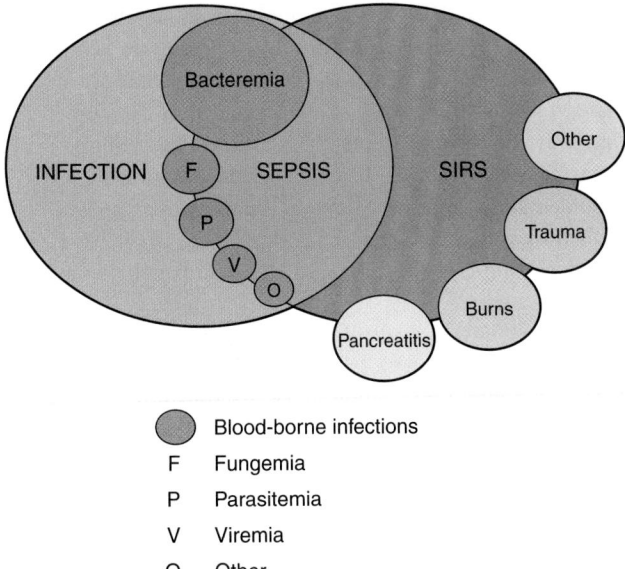

Figure 40-1 Interrelationships among systemic inflammatory response syndrome (SIRS), sepsis, and infection. *(From American College of Chest Physicians/Society of Critical Care Medicine Consensus Conference Committee, Crit Care Med 20:865, 1992.)*

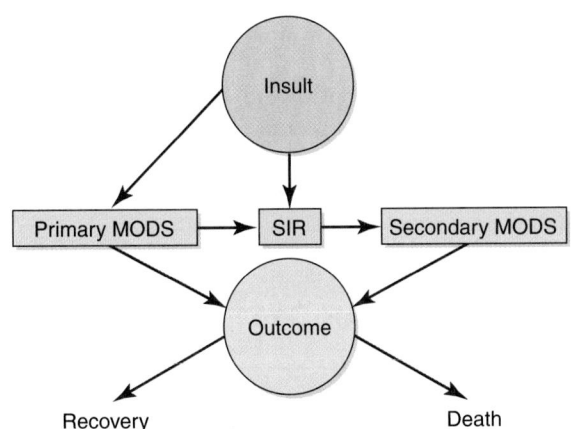

Figure 40-2 Causes and results of primary and secondary multiple organ dysfunction syndrome (MODS). SIR, systemic inflammatory response. *(From American College of Chest Physicians/ Society of Critical Care Medicine Consensus Conference Committee, Crit Care Med 20:868, 1992.)*

Neutrophil Response. Neutrophils engage in four functions related to inflammation: margination, diapedesis, chemotaxis, and phagocytosis. Many neutrophils normally adhere to the inside of blood vessel walls until needed (margination). On activation, neutrophils move to the area of injury by squeezing through the pores of blood vessels (diapedesis), are attracted to microbials or debris by chemical substances (chemotaxis), phagocytose bacteria or cellular debris, and then die. Monocytes and macrophages perform similar functions in a later stage of the inflammatory process.[5]

Plasma Protein Response. Three major plasma protein systems—the complement, kinin-kallikrein, and coagulation systems—participate in the acute inflammatory response.

Complement System. The complement system, a complex cascade of more than 20 serum proteins, is involved in inflammatory and immune processes that destroy bacteria and contribute to vascular changes. Activation of the complement cascade occurs through three pathways: classic, lectin, and alternative. The classic pathway is activated by proteins (antibodies) bound to the specific antigen.[5] The lectin pathway is similar to the classic pathway except that it is activated by bacterial carbohydrates. Polysaccharides from bacterial cell walls (e.g. gram-negative bacteria, fungi) initiate the alternative pathway.[5] The terminal pathway for each of these pathways results in lysis of the target cell. The effects of complement during inflammation are outlined in Box 40-1.[5] Activation of complement proteins stimulates coagulation, mast cells, and platelets.[6] Complement proteins are considered to be the most potent defenders against bacterial infection.[5]

Kinin-Kallikrein System. The kinin-kallikrein system controls vascular tone and permeability and is activated by stimulation of the plasma kinin cascade. Hageman factor (factor XII) of the coagulation cascade is also directly involved in kinin activation. Kinins are biochemicals that are controlled by kinases, enzymes present in the plasma and tissues. The end result of kinin activation is the production of bradykinin. Bradykinin has profound effects, including vasodilation at low doses, pain, extravascular smooth muscle contraction, increased vascular permeability, and leukocyte chemotaxis. Bradykinin facilitates endothelial retraction and increased vascular permeability processes involved in acute inflammation.[5]

Coagulation System. The coagulation system traps bacteria in injured tissue to prevent the spread of infection and together with platelets functions to control excessive bleeding. The human body normally maintains a balance between clot formation (thrombosis), which is needed to minimize blood loss and to repair wounds, and clot lysis (fibrinolysis), which maintains the patency of blood vessels.[5] Like the complement cascade, the coagulation system is a plasma protein system that can be activated through two pathways. The intrinsic pathway is activated when damaged endothelial cells come into direct contact with circulating blood. In this contact phase, proteins activate additional coagulation factors (XII, XI, IX, and VIII). The extrinsic pathway is activated by damaged tissue, which releases tissue factor and activates coagulation factor VII. Both pathways converge at factor X and proceed to fibrin polymerization and clot formation. Thirteen plasma proteins (factors I to XIII), produced primarily in the liver, participate in the coagulation cascade. The fibrinolytic system lyses fibrin clots through the actions of proteolytic and lysosomal enzymes. Plasmin splits fibrin and fibrinogen into fibrin degradation products, and consequently, the clots dissolve. This delicate balance between thrombin and plasmin in the circulation maintains normal coagulation and lysis during the inflammatory process. The end result of these complex interactions is a lesion that is ready to heal.[5-7] The coagulation system is discussed further in Chapter 43.

Platelets. Platelets normally circulate in the bloodstream until vascular injury occurs. Immediately after cellular injury, platelets work synergistically with the coagulation cascade to stop bleeding. Platelets degranulate and release biochemical mediators, which have profound vascular effects. Normally, complex systems work together to limit and localize the inflammatory response, thus limiting and confining the potentially destructive effects of uncontrolled mediator activity. Antiproteases, circulating albumin, vitamins C and E, red blood cells, and phagocytic cells limit the inflammatory response by inhibiting proteolytic enzyme activity, scavenging reactive oxygen metabolites, and removing the stimulus by phagocytosis.[5-8]

SYSTEMIC INFLAMMATORY RESPONSE

The systemic inflammatory response is an abnormal host response characterized by generalized inflammation in organs remote from the initial insult. SIRS is widespread inflammation or clinical responses to inflammation that occurs in patients suffering a variety of insults. Clinical conditions and manifestations associated with SIRS are listed in Box 40-2. These insults produce similar or identical systemic inflammatory responses, even in the absence of infection. SIRS is diagnosed when at least

---

| BOX 40-2 | CLINICAL CONDITIONS AND MANIFESTATIONS ASSOCIATED WITH SYSTEMIC INFLAMMATORY RESPONSE SYNDROME |

CLINICAL CONDITIONS
- Infection
- Infection of vascular structures (heart and lungs)
- Pancreatitis
- Tissue ischemia or hypoxia
- Multiple trauma with massive tissue injury
- Hemorrhagic shock
- Immune-mediated organ injury
- Exogenous administration of tumor necrosis factor or other cytokines

- Aspiration of gastric contents
- Massive transfusion
- Host defense abnormalities

CLINICAL MANIFESTATIONS
- Temperature >38° C or <36° C
- Heart rate >90 beats/min
- Respiratory rate >20 breaths/min or $Paco_2$ <32 mm Hg
- WBC >12,000 cells/mm³ or <4000 cells/mm³ or >10% immature (band) forms

WBC, white blood cell count.

---

two of four clinical manifestations occur in the high-risk patient. Manifestations of SIRS must represent an acute alteration from the patient's normal baseline and must not be related to other causes (e.g., neutropenia from chemotherapy). Organ dysfunction or failure, such as acute lung injury (ALI), acute renal failure, and MODS, is a complication of SIRS.[1-4] In epidemiologic studies, SIRS was found to occur in one third of all hospitalized patients, in 50% to 93% of all patients in critical care units, and in about 80% of all patients in surgical critical care units.[9-14]

When SIRS is a result of infection, the term *sepsis* is used. Severe sepsis is sepsis with hypoperfusion or systemic manifestations of hypoperfusion. Septic shock is sepsis-induced hypotension despite fluid resuscitation. SIRS, sepsis, severe sepsis, and septic shock represent a hierarchical continuum of the inflammatory response to infection.[15] Although infection and shock remain the most common precipitating factors, any disease that can induce a major inflammatory response is capable of initiating the events that lead to MODS.[2]

When SIRS is not contained locally, several consequences occur that lead to organ dysfunction, including intense, uncontrolled activation of inflammatory cells; direct damage of vascular endothelium; disruption of immune cell function; persistent hypermetabolism; and maldistribution of circulatory volume to organ systems.[1,2] Inflammation becomes a systemic, self-perpetuating process that is inadequately controlled and results in organ dysfunction.[2,5,16]

Not all patients develop MODS from SIRS. The development of MODS appears to be associated with failure to control the source of inflammation or infection, persistent hypoperfusion, flow-dependent oxygen consumption ($\dot{V}O_2$), or the continued presence of necrotic tissue.[2,17]

MULTIPLE ORGAN DYSFUNCTION SYNDROME

MODS results from progressive physiologic failure of two or more separate organ systems. It is defined as the "presence of altered organ function in an acutely ill patient such that homeostasis cannot be maintained without intervention."[3] Dysfunction of one organ may amplify dysfunction in another. Organ dysfunction may be absolute or relative and is a leading cause of late mortality after trauma.[16,18]

INCIDENCE

Lack of consensus regarding definitions for organ dysfunction, the number of organs involved, and the duration of organ dysfunction have hampered an accurate account of organ dysfunction in critically ill patients. Despite some variations in how previous researchers have defined organ dysfunction, mortality has been closely linked to the number of organ systems involved. Impairment of two or more organs is associated with an estimated mortality rate of 45% to 55%. This may increase to 80% with three or more organ systems and to 100% if three or more organ systems are severely compromised for longer than

4 days.[1,18] In a study of 869 trauma patients, mortality rates were 4.3% for single organ failure, 32% for two, 67% for three, and 90% for four or more.[18] Patient outcome is directly related to the number of organs involved.

HIGH-RISK PATIENTS

Although various patient populations are at risk for organ dysfunction, trauma patients are particularly vulnerable because they often experience ischemia-reperfusion events resulting from hemorrhage, blunt trauma, or sympathetic nervous system–induced vasoconstriction.[17-19] Other high-risk patients include those who have experienced infection, a shock episode, various ischemia-reperfusion events, acute pancreatitis, sepsis, burns, aspiration, multiple blood transfusions, or surgical complications. Patients age 65 years or older are at increased risk because of their decreased organ reserve and comorbidities.[20]

CLINICAL COURSE AND PROGRESSION

Organ dysfunction may be a direct consequence of the insult (primary MODS) or can manifest latently and involve organs not directly affected in the initial insult (secondary MODS) (see Fig. 40-2). Patients can experience both primary and secondary MODS (Fig. 40-3).

Primary Multiple Organ Dysfunction Syndrome. Primary MODS "directly results from a well-defined insult in which organ dysfunction occurs early and is directly attributed to the insult itself"[3] and accounts for only a small fraction of MODS cases. Direct insults initially cause localized inflammatory responses. Examples of primary MODS include the immediate consequences of posttraumatic pulmonary failure, thermal injuries, acute tubular necrosis, or invasive infections.[2] These cellular or microcirculatory events may lead to a loss of critical organ function induced by failure of delivery of oxygen and substrates, coupled with the inability to remove end-products of metabolism.[1,2,21] The inflammatory response in primary MODS has a less apparent presentation and may resolve without long-term implications. This primary dysfunction is thought to set the system up for a more observable inflammatory response leading to secondary MODS.[1]

Secondary Multiple Organ Dysfunction Syndrome. Secondary MODS is a consequence of widespread systemic inflammation that results in dysfunction of organs not involved in the initial insult.[3,4] The following discussion focuses on the relationship between SIRS and secondary MODS.

Secondary MODS develops latently after an initial insult. The early impairment of organs normally involved in immunoregulatory function, such as the liver and the gastrointestinal tract, intensifies the host response to the insult. It is postulated that the initial insult "primes" the inflammatory system in such a way that a mild second insult may perpetuate a hyperinflammatory response.[22] SIRS or sepsis is a common initiating event in the development of secondary MODS. Severe sepsis appears to initiate a period of circulatory instability and relative physiologic shock that is perpetuated by a cascade of inflammatory mediators, endothelial injury, bacterial insult, and microcirculatory

failure.[16] Noninfectious stimuli (e.g., inflammation, perfusion deficit, dead tissue) initiate similar cellular consequences. Interruption of tissue perfusion may ensue as a result of mismatched oxygen supply and demand, setting the stage for activation of SIRS and MODS.[23]

The definitive clinical course of secondary MODS has not been completely identified. One theory suggests that organ dysfunction may occur in a sequential or progressive pattern. This pattern begins with the lungs, the most commonly affected major organ, and then goes on to involve the liver, gut, and kidneys. A late component is cardiac and, sometimes, bone marrow dysfunction. Neurologic and autonomic system impairment may occur and propagate the progression of organ failure and is associated with illness severity and mortality.[24,25] Organs may fail simultaneously; for example, renal dysfunction may take place concurrently with hepatic dysfunction. After the initial insult and resuscitation, patients develop persistent hypermetabolism, a metabolic consequence of sustained systemic inflammation and physiologic stress, followed closely by pulmonary dysfunction, manifested as ALI.

Hypermetabolism accompanies SIRS but may not occur immediately after insult. Hypermetabolism generally lasts 7 days to more than 3 weeks and may be defined as resting energy expenditure greater than 115% of the predicted basal energy expenditure and oxygen consumption.[26] During hypermetabolism, changes occur in cellular anabolic and catabolic function, resulting in autocatabolism. Autocatabolism manifests as a severe decrease in lean body mass, severe weight loss, anergy, and increased cardiac output and $\dot{V}o_2$ resulting from profound alterations in carbohydrate, protein, and fat metabolism.[1,26] Concurrently, gastrointestinal, hepatic, and immunologic dysfunction may occur, which intensifies the SIRS.[27] Clinical consequences may affect gut function, wound healing, muscles wasting, host response, respiratory function, and continued promotion of the hypermetabolic response.[26]

A significant predictor of 28- to 30-day mortality for patients with MODS is a change in organ system dysfunction early in the course of illness. Russell and colleagues observed that worsening neurologic, renal, and hematologic function are specific to an increased mortality over the first 3 days of critical illness.[24] Levy and colleagues determined that stability or deterioration in respiratory, cardiovascular, or renal function in the first post-baseline day is indicative of increased mortality risk.[28] The development of renal and hepatic failure is a preterminal event in MODS, with death usually occurring approximately 14 to 21 days after the initial insult.[8] Patients with decreased physiologic organ reserve may present with signs and symptoms of organ dysfunction earlier than previously healthy patients.[16] Survivors may develop generalized polyneuropathy and a chronic form of pulmonary disease from ALI, complicating recovery. These patients often require prolonged, expensive rehabilitation.

PATHOPHYSIOLOGIC MECHANISMS

Secondary MODS results from altered regulation of the patient's acute immune and inflammatory responses. Dysregulation, or failure to control the host inflammatory response, leads to the

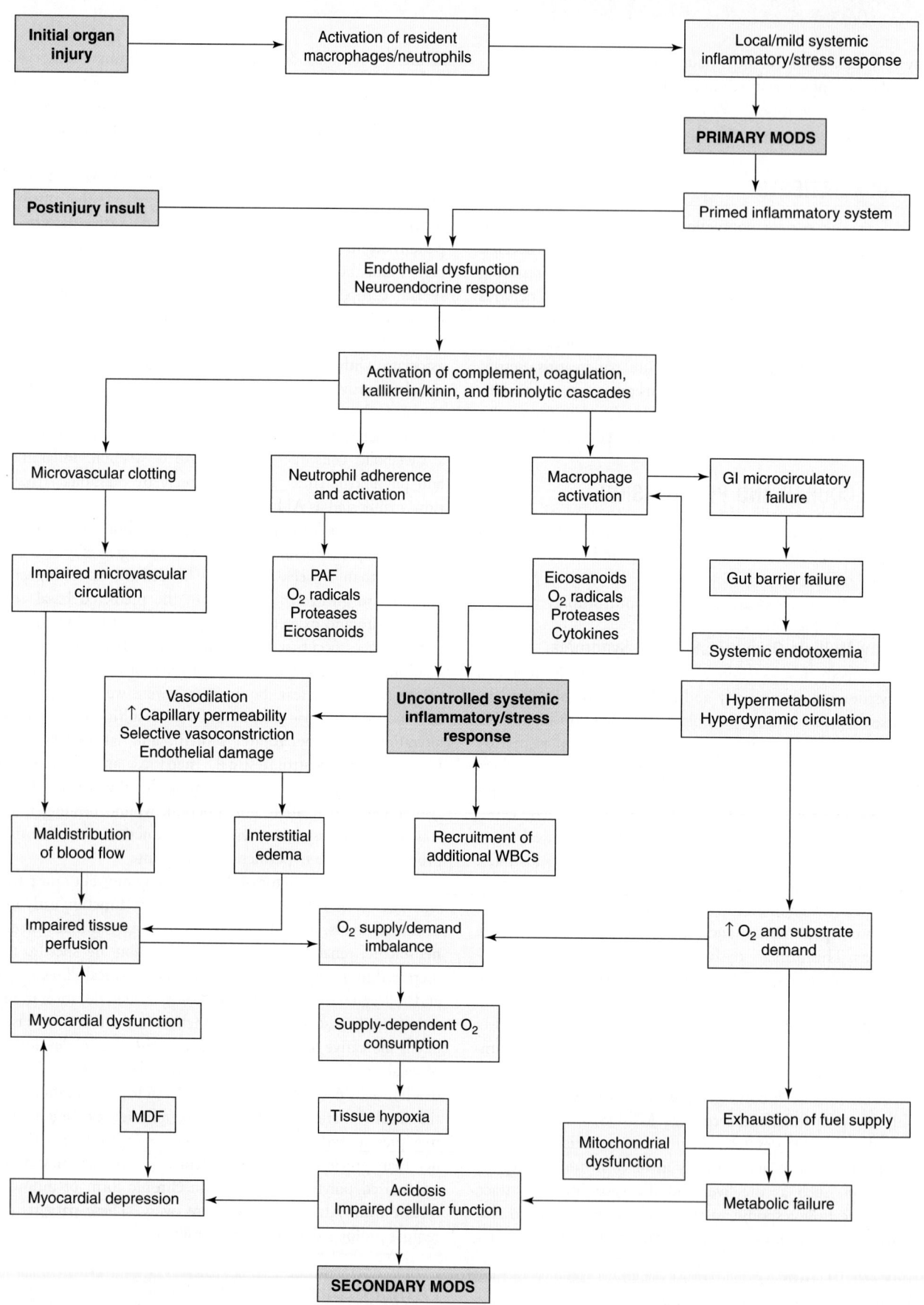

Figure 40-3 Pathogenesis of multiple organ dysfunction syndrome. GI, gastrointestinal; MDF, myocardial depressant factor; MODS, multiple organ dysfunction syndrome; PAF, platelet activating factor; WBCs, white blood cells. *(From Baldwin KM, Cheek DJ, Morris SE: Shock, multiple organ dysfunction syndrome, and burns in adults. In McCance KL, Huether SE, editors:* Pathophysiology: the biological basis for disease in adults and children, *ed 5, St Louis, 2006, p 1637, Mosby.)*

excessive production of inflammatory cells and biochemical mediators that cause widespread damage to vascular endothelium and organ damage.[1,2,5] The critically ill patient's compromised immune state also fosters an environment conducive to organ failure.

Certain cellular and biochemical activity evoke the inflammatory and immune responses implicated in SIRS and MODS. The mediators associated with SIRS and MODS can be classified as inflammatory cells, biochemical mediators, or plasma protein systems (outlined in Box 40-3). Activation of one mediator often leads to activation of another. The biologic activity of inflammatory cells, biochemical mediators, and plasma protein systems and how they work in concert to cause SIRS and MODS have not been totally determined. Plasma protein systems were discussed in the "Local Inflammatory Response" section.

Inflammatory Cells. Neutrophils, macrophages, monocytes, mast cells, platelets, and endothelial cells are inflammatory cells that mediate SIRS through their production of cytokines (biochemical mediators). Along with proinflammatory biochemicals released from damaged or necrotic tissue and circulating catecholamines (stress response), these inflammatory cells create a hypermetabolic state, cause maldistribution of circulatory volume, and alter inflammatory and immune functions.[1,21]

Neutrophils. During SIRS and MODS, neutrophils overreact systemically and damage normal cells in addition to killing bacteria. Neutrophils adhere to vascular endothelium and release cytotoxic biochemicals, including platelet-activating factor (PAF), TNF-α, AA metabolites, and toxic oxygen metabolites.[1,2,5,6,9] These substances cause tissue damage, vascular injury, edema, thrombosis, and hemorrhage in multiple organ systems. During SIRS or sepsis, neutrophilic function is modulated by other circulating mediators that intensify its inflammatory response particularly in the liver and the lungs.[5,29]

Monocytes and Macrophages. Monocytes and macrophages normally perform three major functions relative to inflammation: antigen processing and presentation, bacterial phagocytosis, and mediator production. Monocytes and macrophages detect, process, and present antigen to lymphocytes for initiation of the humoral and cellular components of the lymphocytic immune response. Macrophages play a significant role in organ injury by producing oxygen metabolites, initiating procoagulant activity, and releasing IL-1 and TNF-α.[1,6] TNF-α and IL-1 stimulate neutrophils and lymphocytes to activate the AA cascade. AA metabolites are vasoactive and cause vascular instability and altered organ blood flow. In the lungs, alveolar macrophages produce toxic oxygen metabolites and proteolytic enzymes that destroy alveolar epithelial cells. The role of macrophages and monocytes in organ dysfunction is most directly linked to their production of TNF-α and IL-1.[1,5,6]

Mast Cells. Mast cells are found in all body tissues, especially those adjacent to blood vessels. Physical injury, chemical agents, and immunologic or infectious causes activate mast cells and produce mediators through mast cell degranulation and new synthesis that have systemic and local effects.[1,5] Mast cell–regulated mediators from either process include histamine, TNF-α, interleukins, prostaglandins, and various other AA metabolites.[5]

Lymphocytes. Lymphocytes adhere to and are sequestered in the microvascular endothelium. Stimulated T and B lymphocytes produce cytokines such as IL-1 and IL-2, which activate other inflammatory cells.[30]

Endothelial Cells. The endothelium is a unicellular layer that lines the entire vascular system. Normally, little interaction occurs between the endothelium and leukocytes. However, during SIRS and MODS, endothelial cells become targets for leukocyte-derived mediators, and they become dysfunctional and release prothrombotic, proinflammatory, and vasoactive mediators. Endothelial damage results in the production of procoagulants such as tissue factor (TF), plasminogen-activating inhibitor (PAI), and prostacyclin (PGI$_2$), leading to the introduction of thrombin in the microvasculature.[31] Endothelial cells manufacture chemotactic agents that attract neutrophils to areas of inflammation and endothelial injury. Collectively, these processes cause widespread endothelial destruction, intravascular coagulation, vascular instability and permeability, which are key elements in SIRS and sepsis.

Inflammatory mediators that cause endothelial damage include endotoxin, TNF-α, IL-1, and PAF. These mediators also recruit and activate neutrophils, activate complement, and perpetuate destruction of the endothelium.[32] Endothelial cells produce and maintain a physiologic equilibrium between endothelin (the most potent vasoconstrictor known) and endothelial cell–derived relaxant factor (nitric oxide), a vasodilator.[5,31,32] An alteration in this balance leads to vascular instability, vasodilation, and the perfusion abnormalities commonly seen in patients with SIRS and MODS.

Biochemical Mediators. Multiple biochemical inflammatory mediators play a role in SIRS and MODS, including proteases, TNF-α, interleukins, PAF, AA metabolites, and oxygen metabolites. TNF-α, IL-1, and IL-6 appear to be the most important cytokines associated with SIRS, sepsis, and MODS.[33,34]

BOX 40-3 **INFLAMMATORY MEDIATORS ASSOCIATED WITH SYSTEMIC INFLAMMATORY RESPONSE AND MULTIPLE ORGAN DYSFUNCTION SYNDROMES**

INFLAMMATORY CELLS
- Neutrophils
- Macrophages or monocytes
- Mast
- Lymphocytes
- Endothelial

BIOCHEMICAL MEDIATORS
- Reactive oxygen species
  - Superoxide radical
  - Hydroxyl radical
  - Hydrogen peroxide
- Tumor necrosis factor

- Interleukins
- Platelet activating factor
- Arachidonic acid metabolites
  - Prostaglandins
  - Leukotrienes
  - Thromboxanes
- Proteases

PLASMA PROTEIN SYSTEMS
- Complement
- Kinin
- Coagulation

Reactive Oxygen Species. Reactive oxygen species are produced in excessive amounts during critical illness and have been implicated in MODS.[19,35] Oxygen metabolites are normally produced as the result of many physiologic processes. However, the body has numerous antioxidant and enzyme systems to convert free oxygen radicals to nontoxic substances to prevent tissue injury. Excessive oxygen metabolites cause lipid peroxidation and damage to the cell membrane, activate the complement and coagulation cascades, and cause deoxyribonucleic acid (DNA) damage.[8,36] Inflammatory neutrophils cause tissue injury by producing excessive numbers of reactive oxygen metabolites. Reperfusion organ injury is partially attributed to excessive oxygen metabolites. During reperfusion, severe tissue injury follows the massive production of oxygen free radicals. The organs most susceptible to injury include the small intestines, liver, lungs, heart, brain, stomach, muscle, and skin. In the future, antioxidant drug therapy may be effective in preventing organ dysfunction.[8,37,38]

Tumor Necrosis Factor-α. TNF-α is a polypeptide that is released from macrophages and lymphocytes in response to endotoxin, tissue injury, viral agents, and interleukins. When present in excessive amounts, TNF-α causes widespread destruction in most organ systems and is responsible for the pathophysiologic changes in SIRS and septic shock, including fever, hypotension, decreased organ perfusion, and increased capillary permeability.[16,39] TNF-α may precipitate organ injury by causing generalized endothelial injury, fibrin deposition, and a procoagulant state. TNF-α causes disseminated intravascular coagulation (DIC); interstitial pneumonitis; acute tubular necrosis; and necrosis of the gastrointestinal tract, liver, and adrenal glands. TNF-α stimulates AA metabolism, the clotting cascade, and the production of PAF. Metabolically, excessive TNF-α causes hyperglycemia that progresses to hypoglycemia and hypertriglyceridemia. The destructive effects of TNF-α are exacerbated by AA metabolites and stress hormones.[16,26,40] TNF-α has numerous biologic effects, which are outlined in Box 40-4.

Interleukins. Produced mainly by macrophages and lymphocytes, the interleukins are a class of cytokines that have biologic responses similar to that of TNF-α. Fourteen interleukins have been identified. Interleukin-1 (IL-1) has two known forms that cause organ dysfunction synergistically (Box 40-4). However, the effects of TNF-α are more destructive. Macrophages secrete substantial amounts of IL-1, whereas endothelial cells, epithelial cells, neutrophils, and B lymphocytes produce less. IL-1 causes vascular congestion, capillary leakage, and increased coagulation, all of which are associated with SIRS and sepsis. Like TNF-α, IL-1 has profound vascular endothelial effects. IL-1 stimulates the production of procoagulants by endothelial cells, increases catabolism of muscle tissue, and causes neutrophilia.[5,40] IL-1 and other immune cells enhance the production of IL-2, which amplifies the cardiovascular responses. IL-6 is released by lymphocytes, macrophages, and fibroblasts; it mediates the acute-phase protein response to injury and stimulates the proliferation of B cells.[40] IL-8 is a potent leukocyte activator, specifically for neutrophilic, chemotactic recruitment.[40,41] Raised levels of IL-8 have been detected soon after IL-6 is identified after insult. The influences of IL-8 on leukocyte activities and attraction suggest that IL-8 is important in the development of MODS and ALI.[40,41]

Platelet-Activating Factor. PAF, a potent proinflammatory phospholipid, is released from inflammatory and immune cells in response to a multitude of factors or stimuli.[42] PAF is released by platelets, mast cells, monocytes, macrophages, neutrophils, and endothelial cells. PAF has widespread effects on the heart, the vascular system, procoagulation, platelets, and the lungs. Effects of PAF include platelet aggregation, with

---

BOX 40-4   SELECTED EFFECTS OF TUMOR NECROSIS FACTOR AND INTERLEUKIN-1

VASCULAR EFFECTS
- Endothelial permeability
- Increased procoagulant activity
- Local vasodilation
- Release of platelet-activating factor (PAF)
- Release of endothelial cytokines
- Disseminated intravascular coagulation (DIC)
- Leukocyte adherence

HEMATOLOGIC EFFECTS
- Chemotaxis
- Release of leukocyte arachidonic acid metabolites
- Initial neutropenia
- Stimulation of polymorphonuclear leukocytes

HEPATIC EFFECTS
- Increased triglycerides caused by suppression of lipoprotein lipase

- Decreased synthesis of plasma proteins: albumin and transferrin
- Increased synthesis of acute-phase proteins
- Production of complement components
- Synthesis of clotting factors

CENTRAL NERVOUS SYSTEM EFFECTS
- Prostaglandin release in the brain
- Fever
- Headache
- Anorexia

CARDIOVASCULAR SYSTEM EFFECTS
- Tachycardia
- Increased cardiac output
- Decreased systemic vascular resistance
- Hypotension

Modified from Zimmerman JJ, Ringer RV: Inflammatory host responses in sepsis, *Crit Care Clin* 8:163, 1992.

resultant microvascular stasis and ischemia in the microvascular bed; platelet release of serotonin, which increases vascular permeability; and increased vasoconstriction from increased production of thromboxane A_2, an AA metabolite.[42,43]

Arachidonic Acid Metabolites. AA is a highly metabolic fatty acid that is a precursor of many biologically active substances known as *eicosanoids*. Lipid peroxidation of neutrophil cell membranes induces a release of these metabolites.[1] Select eicosanoids are implicated in the pathogenesis of SIRS and MODS. Eicosanoids contribute to organ failure by altering vascular reactivity and permeability and by fostering the accumulation and activation of inflammatory cells.[44] Activation of the AA cascade by hypoxia, ischemia, endotoxin, catecholamines, and tissue injury produces metabolites from the cyclooxygenase and lipoxygenase pathways. AA metabolites produced through the cyclooxygenase pathway are called *prostaglandins* (PGs) and *thromboxanes* (TXs), whereas those from the lipoxygenase pathway are called *leukotrienes* (LTs). AA metabolites have profound effects on vasculature and cause vascular instability and maldistribution of blood flow. Some eicosanoids (e.g., PGH_2, TXA_2, LTD_4) are vasoconstrictors, and others (e.g., PGE_2, PGI_2) have potent vasodilatory properties. All leukotrienes and TXA_2 enhance capillary membrane permeability and increase vascular leakage. TXA_2, PGH_2, and PGF_2 are potent platelet aggregators.[44]

Proteases. Proteases are proteolytic (protein-digesting) enzymes released from neutrophils. Proteases damage endothelium and contribute to vascular permeability and organ dysfunction.[1] One such protease, neutrophil elastase, damages lung tissue by inducing IL-8 production, attracting additional neutrophils, and stimulating mucus secretion.

ORGAN-SPECIFIC MANIFESTATIONS

Secondary MODS is a systemic disease with organ-specific manifestations. Organ dysfunction is influenced by numerous factors, including organ host defense function, response time to the injury, metabolic requirements, organ vasculature response to vasoactive drugs, organ sensitivity to damage, and physiologic reserve. The responses of the gastrointestinal, hepatobiliary, cardiovascular, pulmonary, renal, and hematologic systems are discussed in the following paragraphs. Clinical manifestations of organ dysfunction are outlined in Box 40-5.

Gastrointestinal Dysfunction. The gastrointestinal tract plays an important role in MODS. Gastrointestinal organs normally have immunoregulatory functions, and the gastrointestinal tract contains about 70% to 80% of the immunologic tissue of the entire body. A normally functioning gastrointestinal tract prevents bacteria from entering the systemic circulation.[1] Normal gut flora and gut environment are altered in patients with severe SIRS.[27] With microcirculatory failure to the gastrointestinal tract, the gut's barrier function may be lost. Consequently, gastrointestinal dysfunction amplifies SIRS and gut damage, which may lead to bacterial translocation and endogenous endotoxemia.[1,5]

Three specific mechanisms link the gastrointestinal tract and latent organ dysfunction. First, hypoperfusion and shocklike states damage the normal gastrointestinal mucosa barrier by decreasing mesenteric blood flow, leading to hypoperfusion of the villi, mucosal edema, ischemic necrosis, sloughing of the mucosa, and malabsorption. The gastrointestinal tract is extremely vulnerable to oxygen metabolite–induced reperfusion injury. Endothelial injury and gastrointestinal lesions occur in response to mediator-induced tissue damage. Ischemic events and the absence of feedings can disrupt the normal metabolism of the gastric or intestinal lumen and the normal protective function of the gut barrier.[45-47]

Second, the translocation of normal gastrointestinal bacteria through a "leaky gut" into the systemic circulation initiates and perpetuates an inflammatory focus in the critically ill patient.[46] The gastrointestinal tract harbors organisms that present an inflammatory focus when translocated from the gut into the portal circulation and inadequately cleared by the liver. Healthy probiotics (e.g., *Bifidobacterium, Lactobacillus*) are decreased in a SIRS state, and pathogenic organisms (e.g., *Staphylococcus, Pseudomonas*) proliferate.[27,48,49] Hepatic macrophages respond to the presence of enteric organisms by producing tissue-damaging amounts of TNF-α, which further propagates the inflammatory mechanisms. The primary mechanism of bacterial translocation has been associated with intestinal bacterial overgrowth.[27,48]

The third mechanism linking the gastrointestinal tract and organ dysfunction is colonization. The oropharynx of the critically ill patient becomes colonized with potentially pathogenic organisms from the gastrointestinal tract.[49] Pulmonary aspiration of colonized secretions presents an inflammatory focus that can contribute to concomitant pulmonary dysfunction.

Hepatobiliary Dysfunction. The liver plays a vital role in host homeostasis related to the acute inflammatory response. The liver responds to SIRS by selectively changing carbohydrate, fat, and protein metabolism. Consequently, hepatic dysfunction after a critical insult threatens the patient's survival.[50]

The liver normally controls the inflammatory response by several mechanisms. Kupffer cells, which are hepatic macrophages, detoxify substances that may normally induce systemic inflammation and vasoactive substances that cause hemodynamic instability. Failure to detoxify gram-negative bacteria translocated from the gastrointestinal tract causes endotoxemia, perpetuates SIRS, and may lead to MODS. The liver also produces proteins and antiproteases to control the inflammatory response; however, hepatic dysfunction limits this response.[23,50]

The liver and gallbladder are extremely vulnerable to ischemic injury. Ischemic hepatitis occurs after a prolonged period of physiologic shock and is associated with centrilobular hepatocellular necrosis.[51] The degree of hepatic damage is related directly to the severity and duration of the shock episode. Terms such as *shock liver* and *posttraumatic hepatic insufficiency* have been used to describe ischemic hepatitis. Anoxic and reperfusion injuries damage hepatocytes and the vascular endothelium.[15,29,52] Patients at high risk for ischemic hepatitis after a hypotensive event include those with a history of

BOX 40-5   CLINICAL MANIFESTATIONS OF ORGAN DYSFUNCTION

GASTROINTESTINAL
- Abdominal distention
- Intolerance to enteral feedings
- Paralytic ileus
- Upper or lower gastrointestinal bleeding
- Diarrhea
- Ischemic colitis
- Mucosal ulceration
- Decreased bowel sounds
- Bacterial overgrowth in stool

HEPATIC
- Jaundice
- Increased serum bilirubin (hyperbilirubinemia)
- Increases serum ammonia
- Decreased serum albumin
- Decreased serum transferrin

GALLBLADDER
- Right upper quadrant tenderness or pain
- Abdominal distention
- Unexplained fever
- Decreased bowel sounds

METABOLIC AND NUTRITIONAL
- Decreased lean body mass
- Muscle wasting
- Severe weight loss
- Negative nitrogen balance
- Hyperglycemia
- Hypertriglyceridemia
- Increased serum lactate
- Decreased serum albumin, serum transferrin, prealbumin
- Decreased retinol-binding protein

IMMUNE
- Infection
- Decreased lymphocyte count
- Anergy

PULMONARY
- Tachypnea
- Acute lung injury pattern of respiratory failure (dyspnea, patchy infiltrates, refractory hypoxemia, respiratory acidosis, abnormal O_2 indexes)
- Pulmonary hypertension

RENAL
- Increased serum creatinine, blood urea nitrogen levels
- Oliguria, anuria, or polyuria consistent with prerenal azotemia or acute tubular necrosis
- Urinary indexes consistent with prerenal azotemia or acute tubular necrosis

CARDIOVASCULAR
Hyperdynamic
- Decreased pulmonary capillary occlusion pressure
- Decreased systemic vascular resistance
- Decreased right atrial pressure
- Decreased left ventricular stroke work index
- Increased oxygen consumption
- Increased cardiac output, cardiac index, heart rate

Hypodynamic
- Increased systemic vascular resistance
- Increased right atrial pressure
- Increased left ventricular stroke work index
- Decreased oxygen delivery and consumption
- Decreased cardiac output and cardiac index

CENTRAL NERVOUS SYSTEM
- Lethargy
- Altered level of consciousness
- Fever
- Hepatic encephalopathy

COAGULATION OR HEMATOLOGIC
- Thrombocytopenia
- Disseminated intravascular coagulation pattern

cardiac failure or cardiac dysrhythmias. Clinical manifestations of hepatic insufficiency are evident 1 to 2 days after the insult. Jaundice and transient elevations in serum transaminase and bilirubin levels occur. Hyperbilirubinemia, possibly the most reliable measure of hepatic dysfunction, results from hepatocyte anoxic injury and an increased production of bilirubin from hemoglobin catabolism.[15] Ischemic hepatitis may resolve spontaneously or progress to fulminant hepatic failure. Although ischemic hepatitis is not a life-threatening complication, it can contribute to morbidity and mortality as a component of MODS.[52] Researchers have proposed that serum bilirubin is a valid indicator of hepatic dysfunction in MODS because it significantly differentiates MODS survivors from

nonsurvivors.[50,51] Fulminant hepatic failure is discussed further in Chapter 34.

Acalculous cholecystitis manifests 3 to 4 weeks after an insult. Its pathogenesis is unclear, but it may be related to ischemic reperfusion injury, positive end-expiratory pressure (PEEP) greater than 5 cm H_2O, volume depletion, total parenteral nutrition, narcotics, and cystic duct obstruction as a result of hyperviscous bile.[53] Visceral hypotension and vasoactive medication use may decrease perfusion of the gallbladder mucosa contributing to ischemia. Bacterial invasion may stimulate activation of factor XII and initiate the coagulation pathway.[53] Clinical manifestations of acalculous cholecystitis may mimic acute cholecystitis with gallstones. However, patients may demonstrate vague symptoms, including right upper quadrant pain and tenderness. Critical to the detection of acalculous cholecystitis is the recognition of abdominal distention, unexplained fever, loss of bowel sounds, and a sudden deterioration in the patient's condition. About 50% of patients with acalculous cholecystitis have gallbladder gangrene, and 10% have gallbladder perforation, requiring a cholecystectomy.[54]

Hypermetabolism accompanies SIRS and is commonly referred to as the *metabolic response to injury*. During hypermetabolism and SIRS, the liver perpetuates selected changes in metabolism, including increased gluconeogenesis, glucogenesis, lipogenesis, and increased production of positive acute-phase reactant proteins (e.g., C-reactive protein).[23] Conversely, the liver decreases synthesis of other negative acute-phase proteins, particularly albumin and transferrin.[55] This metabolic response is partially mediated by IL-1, TNF-α, selected AA metabolites, and the stress hormones.[1,29,50]

Pulmonary Dysfunction.
The lungs, which are frequent and early target organs for mediator-induced injury, are usually the first organs affected in the progression of SIRS to MODS.[56] ALI or ARDS is the pulmonary manifestation of the systemic condition of MODS.[15] Patients who develop MODS usually have pulmonary symptoms; however, not all patients with ALI develop secondary MODS. ALI or ARDS patients who develop SIRS or sepsis concurrently with acute respiratory failure are at the greatest risk for MODS.[24,57]

ALI associated with MODS usually occurs 24 to 72 hours after the initial insult. Patients initially exhibit a low-grade fever, tachycardia, dyspnea, and mental confusion. As dyspnea, hypoxemia, and the work of breathing increase, intubation and mechanical ventilation are required. Acute pulmonary dysfunction results in refractory hypoxemia caused by intrapulmonary shunting, decreased pulmonary compliance, and altered airway mechanics; there usually is radiographic evidence of noncardiogenic pulmonary edema.[26,58]

Mediators associated with ALI include inflammatory cells such as polymorphonuclear cells, macrophages, monocytes, endothelial cells, and mast cells; and biochemical mediators such as AA metabolites, toxic oxygen metabolites, proteases, TNF, PAF, and interleukins.[58] Intense mediator activity damages the pulmonary vascular endothelium and the alveolar epithelium, resulting in surfactant deficiency, mild pulmonary hypertension, and increased pulmonary capillary permeability leading to increased lung water (noncardiogenic pulmonary edema). ALI is discussed further in Chapter 24.

Renal Dysfunction.
Acute renal failure is a common manifestation of MODS. The kidney is highly vulnerable to reperfusion injury. Consequently, renal ischemic-reperfusion injury may be a major cause of renal dysfunction in MODS. The patient may demonstrate oliguria or anuria resulting from decreased renal perfusion and relative hypovolemia. Early oliguria is likely caused by decreases in renal perfusion related to shocklike states; late oliguria is typically a sign of evolving renal injury and ischemia.[15] The condition may become refractory to diuretics, fluid challenges, and dopamine. Prerenal

oliguria may progress to acute tubular necrosis, necessitating hemodialysis or other renal therapies.[26,59] The frequent use of nephrotoxic drugs during critical illness also intensifies the risk of progressive renal impairment. An elevated serum creatinine level is usually a late sign, but it is typically accepted as the index for renal dysfunction.[15] Researchers have proposed that the serum creatinine level is a valid indicator of renal function because it significantly differentiates MODS survivors from nonsurvivors.[60] Additional signs of renal impairment may include decreased erythropoietin induced anemia, vitamin D malabsorption, and altered fluid and electrolyte balance. Acute renal failure is discussed further in Chapter 31.

Cardiovascular and Hematologic System Dysfunction.
The initial cardiovascular response in SIRS or sepsis is myocardial depression; decreased right atrial pressure and systemic vascular resistance (SVR); and increased venous capacitance, $\dot{V}O_2$, cardiac output (CO), and heart rate. Despite an increased CO, myocardial depression occurs and is accompanied by decreased SVR, increased heart rate, and ventricular dilation.[33] These compensatory mechanisms help maintain CO during the early phase of SIRS or sepsis. An inability to increase CO in response to a low SVR may indicate myocardial failure or inadequate fluid resuscitation, and it is associated with increased mortality. Oxygen consumption may be twice that of normal and may be flow dependent.

As MODS progresses, cardiac failure develops. Cardiac dysfunction is characterized by ventricular dilation, decreased diastolic compliance, and decreased systolic contractile function. Cardiovascular function becomes vasopressor dependent. Cardiac failure may be caused by immune mediators, TNF-α, acidosis, or myocardial depressant factor, a substance secreted by the pancreas. TNF-α has a myocardial-depressant effect and is associated with myocardial depression during septic shock.[61] Myocardial depression is exacerbated by myocardial hypoperfusion from a low CO state and persistent lactic acidosis. Cardiogenic shock and biventricular failure occur and lead to death.[62] Cardiac failure is discussed further in Chapter 19, and more information on cardiogenic shock can be found in Chapter 39.

The most common manifestations of hematologic dysfunction in sepsis or MODS are thrombocytopenia, coagulation abnormalities, and anemia.[15,63] The most severe is coagulation system dysfunction manifesting as DIC. DIC is a complex, consumptive coagulopathy that occurs in patients with a variety of disorders, including sepsis, tissue injury, and shock; it is overstimulation of the normal coagulation process. DIC results simultaneously in microvascular clotting and hemorrhage in organ systems, leading to thrombosis and fibrinolysis in life-threatening proportions. Clotting factor derangement leads to further inflammation and further thrombosis. Microvascular damage leads to further organ injury. Cell injury and damage to the endothelium activate the intrinsic or extrinsic coagulation pathways.[16,56] Low platelet counts and elevated D-dimer concentrations and fibrinogen degradation products are clinical indicators of DIC. DIC is discussed further in Chapter 43.

COLLABORATIVE MANAGEMENT OF HIGH-RISK PATIENTS

Caring for the high-risk SIRS or MODS patient requires astute assessments to detect early organ manifestations of this syndrome. Patients who continue to experience sites of inflammation, septic foci, and inadequate tissue perfusion may be at higher risk. Nursing diagnoses applicable to this patient population are outlined in the Nursing Diagnoses feature on Multiple Organ Dysfunction Syndrome.

The patient with MODS requires multidisciplinary collaboration in clinical management, including fluid resuscitation and hemodynamic support (when appropriate), prevention and treatment of infection, maintenance of tissue oxygenation, nutritional and metabolic support, comfort and emotional support, and support for individual organ function.[3,21,56] The use of investigational therapies may be part of the patient's clinical management. Collaborative management of the patient with MODS is outlined in Box 40-6.

PREVENTION, DETECTION, AND TREATMENT OF INFECTION

Identification and treatment of the underlying source of inflammation or infection are the most important ways to reduce mortality. Medical and surgical intervention to remove sources of infection or contamination may limit the inflammatory response and improve chances of recovery.[56] Surgical procedures such as early fracture stabilization, removal of infected organs or tissue, and burn excision are helpful. Appropriate antibiotics are needed if the cause cannot be removed by surgical débridement or incision and draining.[56,64] Other timely interventions, such as prevention of skin ulceration and early nutritional support, can improve outcomes.[16] Risk for Infection

is a highly relevant nursing diagnosis during this period. Nursing management includes strict adherence to standards of practice to prevent infection. Practices related to infection control with invasive hemodynamic monitoring, urinary catheters, mechanical ventilators, endotracheal tubes, intracranial pressure monitoring devices, total parenteral nutrition, and wound care must be stringent to prevent further infection. Prevention of a concomitant ventilator-associated pneumonia or aspiration pneumonia is a priority.[65,66] Regardless of the identification of potential risk factors, clinical markers, bacterial contaminants, and investigative approaches for detection and prevention, treatment remains largely supportive and little improvement in the mortality rate has been appreciated.[9,64]

MAINTENANCE OF TISSUE OXYGENATION

Normally, under steady state conditions, $\dot{V}O_2$ is relatively constant and independent of oxygen delivery (DO_2) unless delivery becomes severely impaired. The relationship is called *supply-independent oxygen consumption* ($\dot{V}O_2$ is about 25% of DO_2). Consequently, a percentage of oxygen is not used (physiologic reserve). Patients with SIRS/MODS often develop supply-dependent oxygen consumption in which $\dot{V}O_2$ becomes

---

Nursing Diagnoses

Multiple Organ Dysfunction Syndrome

- Decreased Cardiac Output related to alterations in preload
- Decreased Cardiac Output related to alterations in afterload
- Decreased Cardiac Output related to alterations in contractility
- Impaired Gas Exchange related to ventilation/perfusion mismatching or intrapulmonary shunting
- Ineffective Renal Tissue Perfusion related to decreased renal blood flow
- Ineffective Cardiopulmonary Tissue Perfusion related to decreased coronary blood flow
- Imbalanced Nutrition: Less Than Body Requirements related to increased metabolic demands or lack of exogenous nutrients
- Risk for Infection
- Acute Pain related to transmission and perception of cutaneous, visceral, muscular, or ischemic impulses
- Acute Confusion related to sensory overload, sensory deprivation, and sleep pattern disturbance
- Anxiety related to threat to biologic, psychologic, or social integrity
- Compromised Family Coping related to a critically ill family member

---

BOX 40-6   COLLABORATIVE MANAGEMENT: MULTIPLE ORGAN DYSFUNCTION SYNDROME

- Support oxygen transport:
  - Establish a patent airway.
  - Initiate mechanical ventilation.
  - Administer oxygen.
  - Administer fluids (crystalloids, colloids, blood and other blood products).
  - Administer vasoactive medications.
  - Administer positive inotropic medications.
  - Administer antidysrhythmic medications.
  - Ensure sufficient hemoglobin and hematocrit.
- Support oxygen use:
  - Identify and correct cause of lactic acidosis.
  - Ensure adequate organ and extremity perfusion.
- Decrease oxygen demand:
  - Administer sedation or paralytics.
  - Administer antipyretics and external cooling measures.
  - Administer pain medications.
- Identify the underlying cause of inflammation and treat accordingly:
  - Remove infected organs or tissue.
  - Administer antibiotics.
- Initiate nutritional support.
- Treat individual organ dysfunction:
  - Gastrointestinal
  - Hepatobiliary
  - Pulmonary
  - Renal
  - Cardiovascular
  - Coagulation system
- Maintain surveillance for complications, including infection.
- Provide comfort and emotional support.

dependent on DO_2, rather than demand, at a normal or high DO_2.[52] When $\dot{V}O_2$ does not equal demand, a tissue oxygen debt develops, subjecting organs to failure.[23,56]

Hypoperfusion and resultant organ hypoxemia often occur in patients at high risk for MODS, subjecting essential organs to failure. Effective fluid resuscitation and early recognition of flow-dependent $\dot{V}O_2$ is essential, and patients at risk for MODS require hemodynamic monitoring, frequent measurements or surrogate measurements of DO_2 and $\dot{V}O_2$, and serum lactate levels to guide therapy. Serum lactate levels provide information regarding the severity of impaired perfusion and the presence of lactic acidosis and differ significantly in MODS survivors and nonsurvivors.[26,66] Failure to maintain adequate oxygenation to vital organs results in organ dysfunction. Despite adequate DO_2, $\dot{V}O_2$ may not meet the needs of the body during MODS.

Patients with ALI, ARDS, MODS, or sepsis frequently manifest supply-dependent oxygen consumption and are unable to use oxygen appropriately despite normal delivery.[20,23,56] Interventions that decrease oxygen demand and increase oxygen delivery are essential. Sedation, mechanical ventilation, temperature and pain control, and rest may be able to decrease oxygen demand.[56] Oxygen delivery may be increased by maintaining normal hematocrit and PaO_2 levels, using PEEP, increasing preload or myocardial contractility to enhance CO, or reducing afterload to increase CO. Various methods of kinetic or prone therapies are available and may enhance alveolar recruitment, improve oxygenation delivery, and decrease other potential complications.

NUTRITIONAL AND METABOLIC SUPPORT

Hypermetabolism in SIRS or MODS results in profound weight loss, cachexia, and loss of organ function. The goal of nutritional support is the preservation of organ structure and function. Although nutritional support may not alter the course of organ dysfunction, it prevents generalized nutritional deficiencies and preserves gut integrity. The enteral route is preferable to parenteral support.[67,68] Enteral feedings are given distal to the pylorus to reduce the risk pulmonary aspiration. Enteral feedings may limit bacterial translocation. In addition to early nutritional support, the pharmacologic properties of enteral feeding formulas may limit SIRS for selected critical care populations. Supplementation of enteral feedings with glutamine may be beneficial; however, arginine, a precursor to nitric oxide, should be avoided in critically ill patients.[69-71] Enteral feedings with omega-3 fatty acids may lessen the development of SIRS and improve outcomes.[67,69] Guidelines for nutritional support during SIRS for trauma patients are outlined in the Evidence-Based Practice feature on Nutritional Support During SIRS for Trauma Patients. Nutritional support is discussed further in Chapter 8.

EXPERIMENTAL APPROACHES IN SYSTEMIC INFLAMMATORY RESPONSE AND MULTIPLE ORGAN DYSFUNCTION SYNDROMES

Neither organ-specific nor pharmacologic interventions have been highly effective in improving survival in patients with MODS. The focus remains improvement of the host response to inflammation by targeting and controlling the effects of mediators that cause SIRS and MODS. Animal model studies continue to provide information regarding the efficacy of drugs that prevent organ dysfunction. Experimental treatments and drugs are being tested in human clinical trials. However, the initial enthusiasm about inflammatory therapies has been dampened, with many clinical trials reporting negative findings.[72]

Although conceptually hypothesized, the efficacy of continuous venovenous hemofiltration as a method of removing inflammatory mediators remains unsubstantiated.[73] Although filtration of large leukocytes has been successful, the inflammatory response has not been halted. Hemofiltration will remain as an organ-specific therapy to improve survival for the MODS patient with acute renal failure.

Evidence-Based Practice: Collaborative

Nutritional Support During SIRS for Trauma Patients

- Parenteral nutrition should be avoided in patients who tolerate enteral feedings.
- There is no difference in efficacy between jejunal and gastric feeding.
- Patients should receive 20 to 25 kcal/kg/day during the acute phase.
- The respiratory quotient is monitored and maintained at less than 0.9.
- Fat emulsions are limited to 0.5 to 1 g/kg/day to prevent iatrogenic immunosuppression associated with lipids and fat overload syndromes.

- Plasma transferrin and prealbumin levels are used to monitor hepatic protein synthesis. Efficient protein use must be assessed with nitrogen balance studies.
- Omega-3, glutamine, and arginine supplementation is recommended. Arginine should be strictly avoided in septic patients.

Data from Orr PA, Case KO, Stevenson JJ: Metabolic response and parenteral nutrition in trauma, sepsis, and burns, *J Infus Nurs* 25:45, 2002; Todd SR, Kozar RA, Moore FA: Nutrition support in adult trauma patients, *Nutr Clin Pract* 21:421, 2006; Kreymann KG et al: ESPEN Guidelines on enteral nutrition: intensive care, *Clin Nutr* 25:210, 2006.

BOX 40-7 EXPERIMENTAL PHARMACOLOGIC APPROACHES IN SYSTEMIC INFLAMMATORY RESPONSE AND MULTIPLE ORGAN DYSFUNCTION SYNDROMES

- Neutrophil inhibitors (pentoxifylline, adenosine, aminophylline, terbutaline, dibutyl-cAMP, caffeine, forskolin)
- White blood cell adherence inhibitors
- Antioxidants or oxygen radical scavengers
- Arachidonic acid metabolite modulators
  - Monoclonal antibodies to phospholipase A_2
  - Cyclooxygenase inhibitors (ibuprofen, indomethacin)
  - Thromboxane synthetase inhibitors
  - Thromboxane receptor blockers
- Lipoxygenase inhibitors
- Leukotrienes antagonists
- Platelet-activating factor (PAF) inhibitors
- Monoclonal antibodies to decrease adhesion of neutrophils to the endothelium
- Protease inhibitors
- Modulation of macrophage function (n-3 polyunsaturated fatty acids)
- Stimulation of lymphocyte function (arginine, n-3 polyunsaturated fatty acids)
- Antiendorphin therapy
- Antihistamines
- Glucocorticoids

Immunomodulatory strategies should theoretically prevent the conversion from SIRS to bacterial sepsis, septic shock, and MODS. Clinical trials with anti-TNF-α antibodies, IL-1 receptor antagonists, and anti-lipopolysaccharide monoclonal antibodies have been carried out, but no significant effects on systemic inflammation were discerned; however, research continues on genetic silencing of inflammatory cytokines.[74] Using genetic transfer of antiinflammatory IL-10, sepsis-induced organ failure was attenuated in a mice through modulation of the proinflammatory cytokines, particularly TNF-α.[75]

Pharmacologic approaches that inhibit neutrophil function may be beneficial in SIRS and are listed in Box 40-6. As immunomodulators, these drugs moderate neutrophil-induced injury in endothelial cells. Pentoxifylline reduces the adhesiveness of activated neutrophils to the endothelium and the release of toxic oxygen metabolites and lysosomal enzymes, and it inhibits neutrophil activation by endotoxin, TNF-α, and IL-1. Adenosine, another potential neutrophil inhibitor, reduces granulocyte adherence, inhibits superoxide ion formation, limits the effects of reperfusion injury, and protects endothelial cells.[72] Naturally occurring substances, including some interleukins, inhibit the adherence of neutrophils to the endothelium. Monoclonal antibodies may be available to decrease the adhesion of neutrophils to the endothelium. Antioxidants, drugs that scavenge oxygen radicals or bind free

oxygen radicals, and protease inhibitors may be effective in managing SIRS or sepsis and shock.[72,76]

Eicosanoid modulation involves the use of pharmacologic agents to negate the destructive effects of AA metabolites. Agents that may inhibit the release or destructive activity of AA metabolites are listed in Box 40-7. The effectiveness of these agents in modulating the response to sepsis is being investigated. In contrast to AA metabolites that have damaging effects, the administration of PGI_2 may be effective in limiting the systemic inflammatory response because of its local vasodilatory effects and antiplatelet properties.[72]

Recent investigational emphasis has been placed on anticytokine therapy in the treatment of SIRS and MODS. Several cytokines play an important role in uncontrolled inflammation, including TNF-α and IL-1. The TNF-α inhibitors, anti–TNF-α antibody agents, and IL-1 receptor antagonists may demonstrate efficacy in the future.[72] It is highly likely that a combination of drugs will be needed to suppress SIRS and to prevent MODS.

Summary

Inflammatory Response

- Acute inflammation is a biochemical and cellular process that occurs only in vascularized tissue in response to an insult or invasion.

Systemic Inflammatory Response

- The systemic inflammatory response is an abnormal host response characterized by generalized inflammation in organs remote from the initial insult.
- Consequences include uncontrolled activation of inflammatory cells, damage of vascular endothelium, disruption of immune cell function, hypermetabolism, and maldistribution of circulatory volume.

Multiple Organ Dysfunction Syndrome

- MODS results from progressive physiologic failure of two or more separate organ systems.
- Organ dysfunction is influenced by numerous factors, including organ host defense function, response time to the injury, metabolic requirements, organ vasculature response to vasoactive drugs, and organ sensitivity to damage and physiologic reserve.
- Collaborative management focuses on fluid resuscitation and hemodynamic support, prevention and treatment of infection, maintenance of tissue oxygenation, nutritional and metabolic support, comfort and emotional support, and preservation of individual organ function.

Case Study: Patient with Systemic Inflammatory Response Syndrome

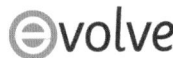 Answers to the Case Study Questions can be found on the Evolve web site at http://evolve.elsevier.com/Urden/.

Brief Patient History

Mr. Z is a 38-year-old, Hispanic construction worker who sustained a liver laceration after falling from a roof. He required an exploratory laparotomy for splenectomy and repair of the liver laceration 4 days earlier. His medical history reveals no chronic health problems, although he smokes 20 packs of cigarettes per year.

Clinical Assessment

Mr. Z is admitted to the medical intensive care unit from the telemetry unit with acute respiratory insufficiency and hypotension. He is using his accessory muscles to breathe. He is speaking Spanish. Mr. Z's abdomen is distended, and there are no bowel sounds. Small amounts of dark green drainage are visible in the nasogastric tube. There is no sign of redness or drainage around his surgical wound.

Diagnostic Procedures

Vital signs were as follows: blood pressure of 78/55 mm Hg, heart rate of 142 beats/min (sinus tachycardia), respiratory rate of 35 breaths/min, temperature of 103.1° F, and urine output of 20 mL over the past 8 hours. Arterial blood gas values on a 100% non-rebreather mask were as follows: pH of 7.22, PaO_2 of 54 mm Hg, $PaCO_2$ of 69 mm Hg, HCO_3^- level of 18 mEq/L, and O_2 saturation of 88%. The chest radiograph revealed infiltrates in the right lower lobe. Laboratory data revealed a hemoglobin level of 9.8 g/dL, hematocrit of 25%, and white blood cell count of 18,000/mm^3.

Medical Diagnosis

Mr. Z is diagnosed with severe sepsis.

Questions

1. What major outcomes do you expect to achieve for this patient?
2. What problems or risks must be managed to achieve these outcomes?
3. What interventions must be initiated to monitor, prevent, manage, or eliminate the problems and risks identified?
4. What interventions should be initiated to promote optimal functioning, safety, and well-being of the patient?
5. What possible learning needs do you anticipate for this patient?
6. What cultural and age-related factors may have a bearing on the patient's plan of care?

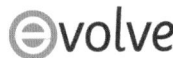 Be sure to check out the bonus material, including free self-assessment exercises, on the Evolve web site at http://evolve.elsevier.com/Urden/.

References

1. Baldwin KM et al: Shock, multiple organ dysfunction syndrome, and burns in adults. In McCance KL, Huether SE, editors: *Pathophysiology: the biological basis for disease in adults and children*, ed 5, St Louis, 2006, Mosby.
2. Fry DE: Systemic inflammatory response and multiple organ dysfunction: biologic domino effect. In Baue AE et al, editors: *Multiple organ failure: pathophysiology, prevention, and therapy*, New York, 2000, Springer-Verlag.
3. American College of Chest Physicians/Society of Critical Care Medicine Consensus Conference: Definitions for sepsis and organ failure and guidelines for the use of innovative therapies in sepsis, *Crit Care Med* 20:864, 1992.
4. Levy MM et al: 2001 SCCM/ESICM/ACCP/ATS/SIS International Sepsis Definitions Conference, *Crit Care Med* 31:1250, 2003.
5. Trask BC et al: Innate immunity: inflammation. In McCance KL, Huether SE, editors: *Pathophysiology: the biological basis for disease in adults and children*, ed 5, St Louis, 2006, Mosby.
6. Fry DE: Microcirculatory arrest theory of SIRS and MODS. In Baue AE et al, editors: *Multiple organ failure: pathophysiology, prevention, and therapy*, New York, 2000, Springer-Verlag.
7. Nimah M, Brilli RJ: Coagulation dysfunction in sepsis and multiple organ system failure, *Crit Care Clin* 19:441, 2003.
8. Nathan A, Singer M: Reactive oxygen species in clinical practice. In Baue AE et al, editors: *Multiple organ failure: pathophysiology, prevention, and therapy*, New York, 2000, Springer-Verlag.
9. Brun-Buisson C: The epidemiology of the systemic inflammatory response, *Intensive Care Med* 26(suppl 1):S64, 2000.
10. Sprung CL et al: An evaluation of systemic inflammatory response syndrome signs in the Sepsis Occurrence in Acutely Ill Patients (SOAP) study, *Intensive Care Med* 32:421, 2006.
11. Dulhunty JM et al: Does severe non-infectious SIRS differ from severe sepsis? Results from a multi-centre Australian and New Zealand intensive care unit study, *Intensive Care Med* 34(9):1654, 2008.
12. Sankoff JD et al: Validation of the Mortality in Emergency Department Sepsis (MEDS) score in patients with the systemic inflammatory response syndrome (SIRS), *Crit Care Med* 36:421, 2008.
13. Muckart DJ, Bhagwanjee S: American College of Chest Physicians/Society of Critical Care Medicine Consensus Conference definitions of the systemic inflammatory response syndrome and allied disorders in relation to critically injured patients, *Crit Care Med* 25:1789, 1997.
14. Hoover L et al: Systemic inflammatory response syndrome and nosocomial infection in trauma, *J Trauma* 61:310, 2006.
15. Khadaroo RG, Marshall JC: ARDS and the multiple organ dysfunction syndrome. Common mechanisms of a common systemic process, *Crit Care Clin* 18:127, 2002.
16. Ely EW et al: Advances in the understanding of clinical manifestations and therapy of severe sepsis: an update for critical care nurses, *Am J Crit Care* 12:120, 2003.
17. Cohn SM et al: Tissue oxygen saturation predicts the development of organ dysfunction during traumatic shock resuscitation, *J Trauma* 62:44, 2007.
18. Durham RM et al: Multiple organ failure in trauma patients, *J Trauma* 55:608, 2003.
19. Motoyama T et al: Possible role of increased oxidant stress in multiple organ failure after systemic inflammatory response syndrome, *Crit Care Med* 31:1048, 2003.
20. Epstein CD et al: Oxygen transport and organ dysfunction in the older adult trauma, *Heart Lung* 31:315, 2002.
21. Walsh C: Multiple organ dysfunction syndrome after multiple trauma, *Orthop Nurs* 24:324, 2005.

22. Tschoeke SK et al: The early second hit in trauma management augments the proinflammatory immune response to multiple injuries, *J Trauma* 62:1396, 2007.

23. Kim PK, Deutschman CS: Inflammatory responses and mediators, *Surg Clin North Am* 80:885, 2000.

24. Russell JA et al: Changing pattern of organ dysfunction in early human sepsis is related to mortality, *Crit Care Med* 28:3405, 2000.

25. Schmidt H et al: The alteration of autonomic function in multiple organ dysfunction syndrome, *Crit Care Clin* 24:149, 2008.

26. Majetschak M, Waydhas C: Infection, bacteremia, sepsis, and the sepsis syndrome: metabolic alterations, hypermetabolism, and cellular alterations. In Baue AE et al, editors: *Multiple organ failure: pathophysiology, prevention, and therapy*, New York, 2000, Springer-Verlag.

27. Shimizu K et al: Altered gut flora and environment in patients with severe SIRS, *J Trauma* 60:126, 2006.

28. Levy MM et al: Early changes in organ function predict eventual survival in severe sepsis, *Crit Care Med* 33:2194, 2005.

29. Szabo G et al: Liver in sepsis and systemic inflammatory response syndrome, *Clin Liver Dis* 6:1045, 2002.

30. Rote NS, Trask BC: Adaptive immunity. In McCance KL, Huether SE, editors: *Pathophysiology: the biological basis for disease in adults and children*, ed 5, St Louis, 2006, Mosby.

31. Joist J: Disseminated intravascular coagulation. In Baue AE et al, editors: *Multiple organ failure: pathophysiology, prevention, and therapy*, New York, 2000, Springer-Verlag.

32. Jones A, Kline J: Shock. In Marx J, editor: *Rosen's emergency medicine: concepts and clinical practice*, ed 6, Philadelphia, 2006, Mosby.

33. Shapiro N et al: Sepsis syndromes. In Marx J, editor: *Rosen's emergency medicine: concepts and clinical practice*, ed 6, Philadelphia, 2006, Mosby.

34. Bengmark S: Bioecologic control of inflammation and infection in critical illness, *Anesthesiol Clin* 24:299, 2006.

35. Abraham E, Singer M: Mechanisms of sepsis-induced organ dysfunction, *Crit Care Med* 35:2408, 2007.

36. Cunneen J, Cartwright M: The puzzle of sepsis: fitting the pieces of the inflammatory response with treatment, *AACN Clin Issues* 15:18, 2004.

37. Biesalski HK, McGregor GP: Antioxidant therapy in critical care—is the microcirculation the primary target? *Crit Care Med* 35:S577, 2007.

38. Heyland DK et al: Reducing Deaths due to OXidative Stress (the REDOXS study): rationale and study design for a randomized trial of glutamine and antioxidant supplementation in critically ill patients, *Proc Nutr Soc* 65:250, 2006.

39. Menges T et al: Sepsis syndrome and death in trauma patients are associated with variation in the gene encoding tumor necrosis factor, *Crit Care Med* 36:1456, 2008.

40. Rumalla V, Lowry SF: Counterregulation of severe inflammation: when more is too much and less is inadequate. In Baue AE et al, editors: *Multiple organ failure: pathophysiology, prevention, and therapy*, New York, 2000, Springer-Verlag.

41. Sablotzki A et al: The systemic inflammatory response syndrome following cardiac surgery: different expression of proinflammatory cytokines and procalcitonin in patients with and without multiorgan dysfunctions, *Perfusion* 17:103, 2002.

42. Stafforini DM et al: Platelet-activating factor, a pleiotropic mediator of physiological and pathological processes, *Crit Rev Clin Lab Sci* 40:643, 2003.

43. Poeze M et al: Platelet-activating factor. In Baue AE et al, editors: *Multiple organ failure: pathophysiology, prevention, and therapy*, New York, 2000, Springer-Verlag.

44. Manley FT et al. Eicosanoids. In Baue AE et al, editors: *Multiple organ failure: pathophysiology, prevention, and therapy*, New York, 2000, Springer-Verlag.

45. Beale RJ et al: Early enteral supplementation with key pharmaconutrients improves Sequential Organ Failure Assessment score in critically ill patients with sepsis: outcome of a randomized, controlled, double-blind trial, *Crit Care Med* 36:131, 2000.

46. Clark JA, Coopersmith CM: Intestinal crosstalk: a new paradigm for understanding the gut as the "motor" of critical illness, *Shock* 28:384, 2007.

47. Kattelmann KK et al: Preliminary evidence for a medical nutrition therapy protocol: enteral feedings for critically ill patients, *J Am Diet Assoc* 106:1226, 2006.

48. Deitch EA et al: Intestinal bacterial overgrowth induces the production of biologically active intestinal lymph, *J Trauma* 56:105, 2004.

49. Marshall JC et al: The gastrointestinal tract. The "undrained abscess" of multiple organ failure, *Ann Surg* 218:111, 1993.

50. Dhainaut JF et al: Hepatic response to sepsis: interaction between coagulation and inflammatory processes, *Crit Care Med* 29:S42, 2001.

51. Baue A: Liver: multiple organ dysfunction and failure. In Baue A et al, editors: *Multiple organ failure: pathophysiology, prevention, and therapy*, New York, 2000, Springer-Verlag.

52. Wong F: Liver and kidney diseases, *Clin Liver Dis* 6:981, 2002.

53. Puc MM et al: Ultrasound is not a useful screening tool for acute acalculous cholecystitis in critically ill trauma patients, *Am Surg* 68:65, 2002.

54. Proctor DD: Critical issues in digestive diseases, *Clin Chest Med* 24:623, 2003.

55. Ananian P et al: Serum acute-phase protein level as indicator for liver failure after liver resection, *Hepatogastroenterology* 52:857, 2005.

56. Krau SD: Making sense of multiple organ dysfunction syndrome, *Crit Care Nurs Clin North Am* 19:87, 2007.

57. Vincent JL, Zambon M: Why do patients who have acute lung injury/acute respiratory distress syndrome die from multiple organ dysfunction syndrome? Implications for management, *Clin Chest Med* 27:725, 2006.

58. Gurka D, Balk R: Acute respiratory failure, including acute lung injury and ARDS. In Parrillo J, Dellinger R, editors. *Critical care medicine: principles of diagnosis and management in the adult*, ed 2, St Louis, 2002, Mosby.

59. Gray M et al: Alterations of renal and urinary tract function. In McCance KL, Huether SE, editors: *Pathophysiology: the biological basis for disease in adults and children*, ed 5, St. Louis, 2006, Mosby.

60. Mullins R: Renal function and dysfunction in multiple organ failure. In: Baue AE et al, editors: *Multiple organ failure: pathophysiology, prevention, and therapy*, New York, 2000, Springer-Verlag.

61. Kumar A et al: Myocardial dysfunction in septic shock. Part II. Role of cytokines and nitric oxide, *J Cardiothorac Vasc Anesth* 15:485, 2001.

62. Vincent JL: Circulation. In Baue A et al, eds. *Multiple organ failure: pathophysiology, prevention, and therapy*, New York, 2000, Springer-Verlag.

63. Dhainaut JF et al: Dynamic evolution of coagulopathy in the first day of severe sepsis: relationship with mortality and organ failure, *Crit Care Med* 33:341, 2005.

64. Richards M et al: Epidemiology, prevalence, and sites of infections in intensive care units, *Semin Respir Crit Care Med* 24:3, 2003.

65. Grap MJ, Munro CL: Preventing ventilator-associated pneumonia: evidence-based care, *Crit Care Nurs Clin North Am* 16:349, 2004.

66. Dellinger RP et al: Surviving Sepsis Campaign: international guidelines for management of severe sepsis and septic shock: 2008, *Crit Care Med* 36:296, 2008.

67. Fitzsimmons L, Hadley SA: Nutritional management of the metabolically stressed patient, *Crit Care Nurs Q* 17:79, 1995.

68. Heyland DK et al: Validation of the Canadian clinical practice guidelines for nutrition support in mechanically ventilated, critically ill adult patients: results of a prospective observational study, *Crit Care Med* 32:2260, 2004.

69. Heyland DK et al: Canadian clinical practice guidelines for nutrition support in mechanically ventilated, critically ill adult patients, *JPEN J Parenter Enteral Nutr* 27:355, 2003.

70. Todd SR et al: Nutrition support in adult trauma patients, *Nutr Clin Pract* 21:421, 2006.

71. Kreymann KG et al: ESPEN Guidelines on enteral nutrition: intensive care, *Clin Nutr* 25:210, 2006.

72. Orr PA et al: Metabolic response and parenteral nutrition in trauma, sepsis, and burns, *J Infus Nurs* 25:45, 2002.

73. Ronco C et al: Interpreting the mechanisms of continuous renal replacement therapy in sepsis: the peak concentration hypothesis, *Artif Organs* 27:792, 2003.

74. McCall CE, Yoza BK: Gene silencing in severe systemic inflammation, *Am J Respir Crit Care Med* 175:763, 2007.

75. Kabay B et al: Interleukin-10 gene transfer: prevention of multiple organ injury in a murine cecal ligation and puncture model of sepsis, *World J Surg* 31:105, 2007.

76. Cuzzocrea S et al: Potential therapeutic effect of antioxidant therapy in shock and inflammation, *Curr Med Chem* 11:1147, 2004.

Since the late 1980s, trends of burn incidence, hospitalization, and death have all decreased.[1,2] These decreases are attributed to fire and burn prevention education, management of burn patients in specialized burn centers, regulation of consumer products, and implementation of occupational safety standards. Many programs and organizations are dedicated to the prevention of burn injury. Societal changes involving decreased smoking and alcohol abuse, changes in home cooking practices, and reduced industrial employment also have contributed to the decline in burn incidence.

Burn injuries that require medical treatment annually number 500,000 per year.[2] Burn injuries requiring hospitalization total approximately 40,000 per year, and 60% of these patients are admitted to one of the 125 specialized burn centers in the United Sates.[2]

Great advances have been made in the care of burn patients. In the mid-twentieth century, burn shock claimed many patients' lives. If shock did not cause death, infection or respiratory insufficiency did. With improvements in fluid resuscitation, better critical care management, and the trend toward early excision and grafting, mortality rates have decreased.[3] "Increased survival has led to a shift in focus from mortality to more intermediate- and long-term outcome measures such as rehabilitation, reconstruction, and reintegration into society."[3]

To provide comprehensive, holistic care for burn patients, close collaboration is required among members of the multidisciplinary team. The burn team comprises nurses, physicians, physical therapists, occupational therapists, recreational therapists, nutritionists, psychologists, social workers, family, and spiritual support staff members. The burn patient is characterized as the universal trauma model. The patient's response to a major burn injury is dramatic and involves multisystem alterations. Knowledge of local and systemic changes associated with patient needs is essential in providing care, which places extraordinary demands on the nurse in a burn practice who must be both a specialist and a broadly based generalist. The purpose of this chapter is to provide a basic understanding of the complexities of burn care and the patient's response to burn injury.

ANATOMY AND FUNCTIONS OF THE SKIN

The skin is the largest organ of the human body, ranging from 0.2 m^2 in the newborn to more than 2 m^2 in the adult. The integumentary system consists of two major layers: the epidermis and the dermis (Fig. 41-1).

The outermost layer of epidermis is 0.07 to 0.12 mm thick, with the deepest layer found on the soles of the feet and the palms of the hands. The epidermis is composed of dead, cornified cells that act as a tough protective barrier against the environment. From the surface inward, its five layers are stratum corneum, stratum lucidum, stratum granulosum, stratum spinosum, and stratum germinativum. The deepest layer of epidermis contains fibronectin, which adheres the epidermis to the basement membrane. The epidermis regenerates every 2 to 3 weeks. The second, thicker layer, the dermis, is 1 to 2 mm thick and lies below the epidermis, and it continuously regenerates. The dermis is composed of two layers: the more superficial, papillary layer next to the stratum germinativum and the deeper, reticular layer. The dermis, composed primarily of connective tissue and collagenous fiber bundles made from fibroblasts, provides nutritional support to the epidermis. The dermis contains the blood vessels; sweat and sebaceous glands; hair follicles; nerves to the skin and capillaries that nourish the avascular epidermis; and sensory fibers for pain, touch, and temperature. Mast cells in the connective tissue perform the functions of secretion, phagocytosis, and production of fibroblasts. Beneath the dermis is the hypodermis, which contains the fat, smooth muscle, and areolar tissue. The hypodermis acts as a heat insulator, shock absorber, and nutritional depot.[4]

The skin provides functions crucial to human survival. They include maintenance of body temperature; a barrier to evaporative water loss; metabolic activity (vitamin D production); immunologic protection by preventing microbes from entering the body; protection against the environment through the sensations of touch, pressure, and pain; and overall cosmetic appearance.

PATHOPHYSIOLOGY AND ETIOLOGY OF BURN INJURY

A burn is an injury resulting in tissue loss or damage. Injury to tissue can be caused by exposure to thermal, electrical, chemical, or radiation sources. The temperature or causticity of the burning agent and duration of tissue contact with the source determine the extent of tissue injury. Tissue damage can occur at various temperatures, usually between 40° C and 44° C.

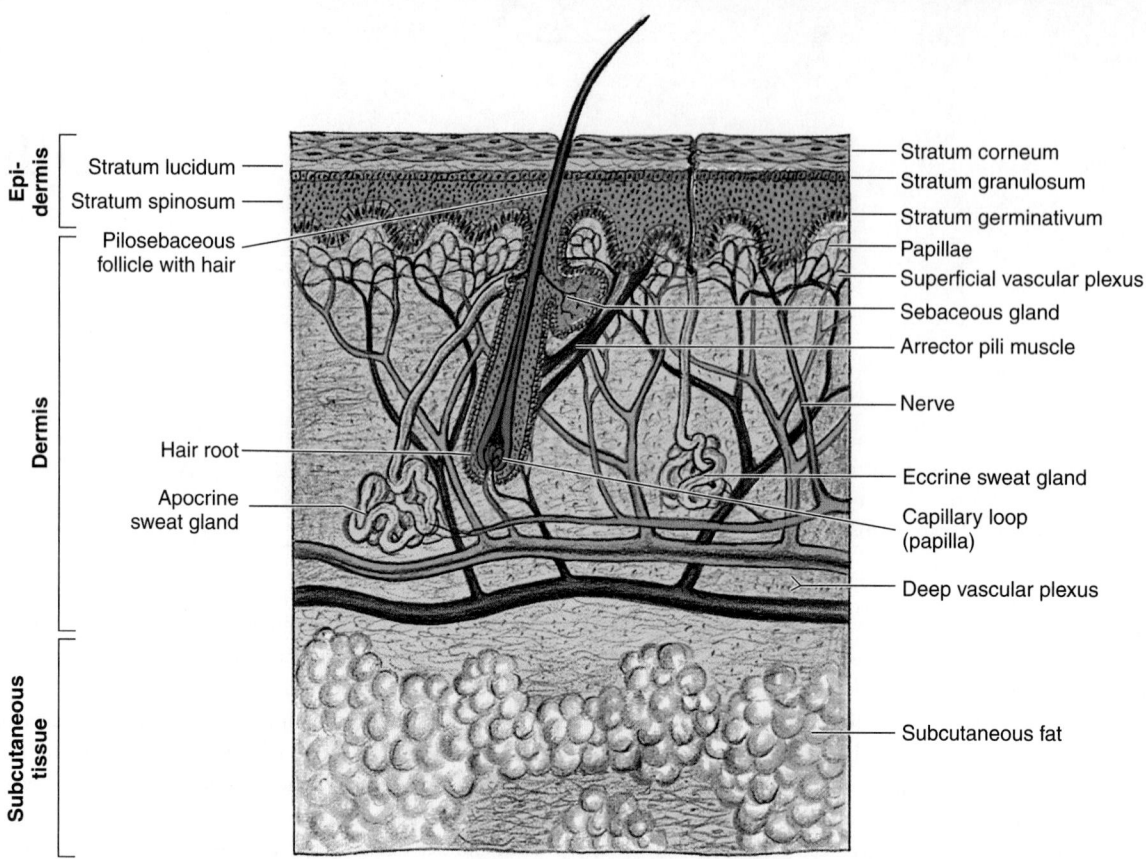

Figure 41-1 Anatomy of the skin. *(From Dains JE: Integumentary system. In Thompson JM et al: Mosby's clinical nursing, ed 5, St Louis, 2002, Mosby.)*

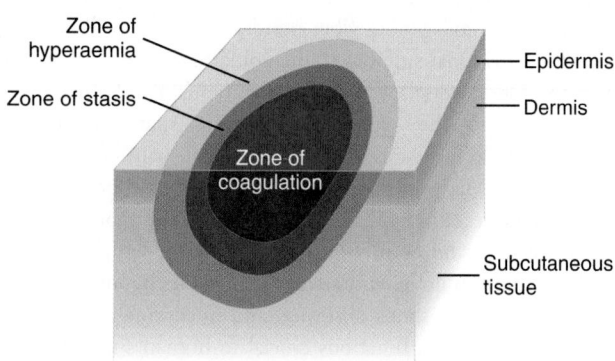

Figure 41-2 Zones of burn injury.

The burn wound itself is responsible for the local and systemic effects seen in the burned patient.[5] Tissue damage is caused by enzyme malfunction and denaturation of proteins. Prolonged exposure or higher temperatures can lead to cell necrosis and a process known as *protein coagulation*. The areas extending outward from this central area of injury sustain various degrees of damage and are identified by zones of injury.[6]

ZONES OF INJURY

Three concentric zones are present in burn injury: *zone of coagulation*, *zone of stasis*, and *zone of hyperemia* (Fig. 41-2). The central zone is the site of most severe damage, the peripheral

zone has the least. The central portion, or zone of coagulation, is usually the site of greatest heat transfer and where irreversible skin death occurs. This area is surrounded by the zone of stasis, which is characterized by impaired circulation that can lead to cessation of blood flow caused by a pronounced inflammatory reaction. This area is potentially salvageable; however, local or systemic factors can convert it into a full-thickness injury. Some of the factors that can lead to deeper wound conversion are toxic mediators of the inflammatory process, infection, inappropriate volume resuscitation, malnutrition, chronic illness, or the local wound care provided. It may take 48 to 72 hours to determine the full extent of injury in this area. The outermost area is the zone of hyperemia, where there is vasodilation and increased blood flow but minimal cell involvement. Early spontaneous recovery can occur in this area.[5,7]

CLASSIFICATION OF BURN INJURY

Burns are classified primarily according to size and depth of the injury. However, the type and location of the burn and the patient's age and medical history are also significant considerations. Recognition of the magnitude of burn injury, which is based on the depth and size of the burn and the prior health of the patient, is of crucial importance in the overall plan of care. Decisions concerning patient management and appropriate referral to a burn center are based on this assessment

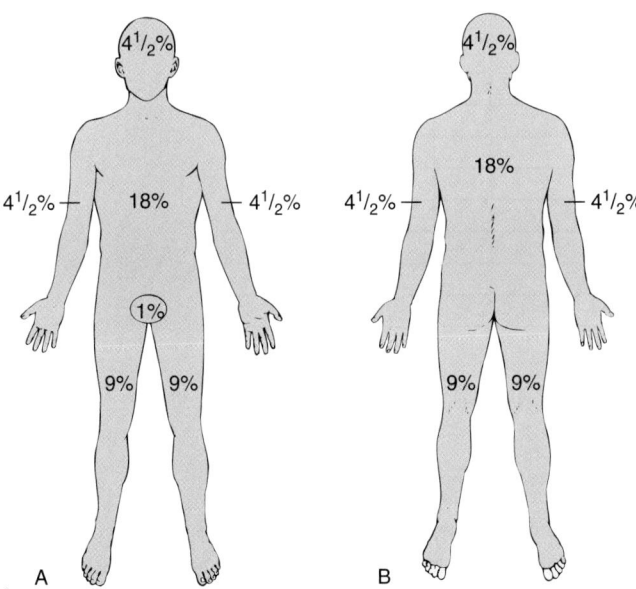

Figure 41-3 Estimation of adult burn injury: rule of nines. *A,* Anterior view. *B,* Posterior view. *(From Marx J et al: Rosen's emergency medicine concepts and clinical practice, ed 5, St Louis, 2002, Mosby.)*

(Box 41-1).[2] The patient's age and burn size are the cardinal determinants of survival.[8-10]

SIZE OF INJURY

Several different methods can be used to estimate the size of the burn area. A quick and easy method is the *rule of nines*, which often is used in the prehospital setting for initial triage of the burn patient (Fig. 41-3). With this method, the adult body is divided into surface areas of 9%. This method is modified for assessing infants and very small children. In the adult, the head and the anterior and posterior surfaces of the trunk are each 18% of the total body surface area (TBSA), each arm is 9%, each leg is 18%, and the perineum is 1%. Another method uses the measure of the palmar surface of the victim's hand as a gauge for estimating burn area. The palmar surface, which represents 1% of the TBSA, also can be useful for making burn estimates in the prehospital setting or for estimating the percentage of involvement in small and scattered areas of burn.

In the hospital setting, the Lund and Browder method (Fig. 41-4) is the most accurate and accepted method for determining the percentage of burn. Surface area measurements are assigned to each body part in terms of the age of the patient. This method is highly recommended for use with children younger than 10 years because it corrects for smaller surface areas of the lower extremities. It is also recommended for adult burn victims because of its accuracy.

The Berkow method also can be used to estimate burn size for infants and children because it accounts for the proportionate growth. This method requires special charts provided by the National Burn Institute, which are not always available in local hospitals but may be at hand in a designated burn center.

DEPTH OF BURN INJURY

Traditionally, burn depth has been classified in degrees of injury based on the amount of injured epidermis or dermis, or both: first-, second-, or third-degree burns. However, these terms are not descriptive of the burn surface. The depth of the burn is defined by how much of the skin's two layers are destroyed by the heat source.[11]

Burns are classified as *superficial, partial-thickness,* or *full-thickness burns.* These descriptions are based on the surface appearance of the wound. Superficial burns include first-degree burns. Partial-thickness wounds include various stages of second-degree burns, and full-thickness burns include third-degree burns. Some authorities further separate partial-thickness burns as *superficial, mid-dermal* or *deep-dermal partial-thickness burns.* Wound assessment involves recognition of the depth of injury and the size of burn, and it can be challenging even for experienced caregivers. Because the management of burn wounds is closely tied to the correct assessment of wound severity, some newer strategies, other than observation, are being investigated. Some of these techniques include burn wound biopsy and tissue histology, ultrasound, use of the laser Doppler flowmeter, thermography, light reflectance, and magnetic resonance imaging (MRI). Research with these techniques is ongoing, but they are currently limited by their clinical usefulness at the bedside.[6]

A *superficial (first-degree) burn* involves only the first two or three of the five layers of the epidermis. Erythema and mild discomfort characterize superficial partial-thickness wounds. Pain, the chief symptom, usually resolves in 48 to 72 hours. Common examples of these burn injuries are sunburns and minor steam burns such as those that may occur while a person is cooking. These wounds usually heal in 2 to 7 days and do not require medical intervention aside from pain relief, management of

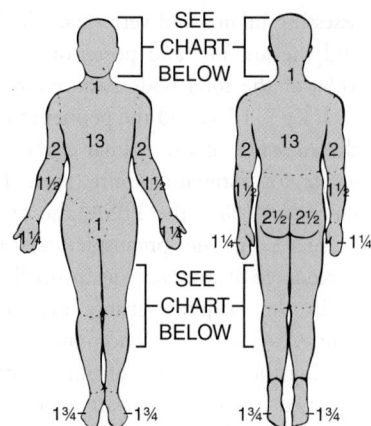

AREA	Inf.	1-4	5-9	10-14	15	Adult	Part.	Full	Total	Donor areas
HEAD	19	17	13	11	9	7				
NECK	2	2	2	2	2	2				
ANT. TRUNK	13	13	13	13	13	13				
POST. TRUNK	13	13	13	13	13	13				
R. BUTTOCK	2½	2½	2½	2½	2½	2½				
L. BUTTOCK	2½	2½	2½	2½	2½	2½				
GENITALIA	1	1	1	1	1	1				
R.U. ARM	4	4	4	4	4	4				
L.U. ARM	4	4	4	4	4	4				
R.L. ARM	3	3	3	3	3	3				
L.L. ARM	3	3	3	3	3	3				
R. HAND	2½	2½	2½	2½	2½	2½				
L. HAND	2½	2½	2½	2½	2½	2½				
R. THIGH	5½	6½	8	8½	9	9½				
L. THIGH	5½	6½	8	8½	9	9½				
R. LEG	5	5	5½	6	6½	7				
L. LEG	5	5	5½	6	6½	7				
R. FOOT	3½	3½	3½	3½	3½	3½				
L. FOOT	3½	3½	3½	3½	3½	3½				
						TOTAL				

Figure 41-4 The Lund and Browder burn estimate diagram. *(Modified from Cardona VD:* Trauma nursing from resuscitation through rehabilitation, *Philadelphia, 1995, Mosby.)*

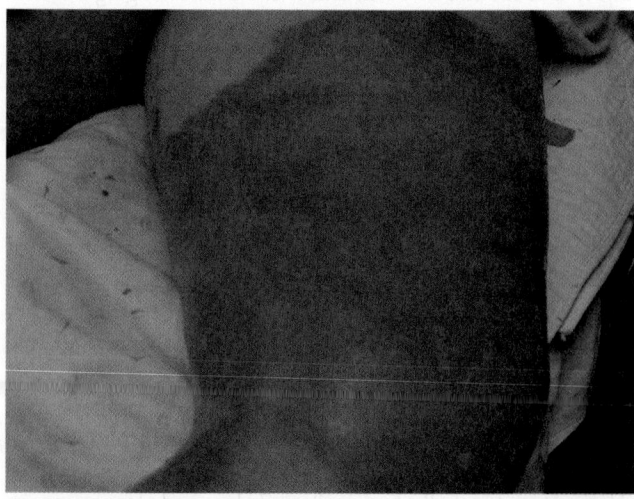

Figure 41-5 Partial-thickness burn to the left thigh.

pruitis (itching), and oral fluids. Swelling can be a common complication that may require intervention. Superficial burns are not included in the calculation of percent burn.

A *partial-thickness* or *superficial dermal (second-degree) burn* involves the upper third of the dermis. These burns usually are caused by brief contact with flames, hot liquid, or exposure to dilute chemicals (Fig. 41-5). A light to bright red or mottled appearance characterizes superficial second-degree burns. These wounds may appear wet and weeping, may contain bullae, and are extremely painful and sensitive to air currents. The microvessels that perfuse this area are injured, and permeability is increased, resulting in leakage of large amounts of plasma into the interstitium. This fluid lifts off the thin, damaged epidermis, causing blister formation. Despite the loss of the entire basal layer of the epidermis, a burn of this depth will heal in 7 to 21 days. Minimal scarring can be expected. Mid-dermal partial-thickness wounds commonly take 4 to 6 weeks to heal.

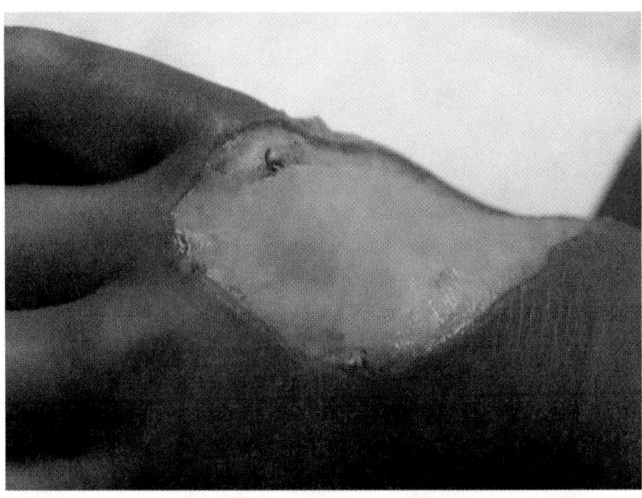

Figure 41-6 Full-thickness burn to the back of the hand.

Deep-dermal partial-thickness (second-degree) burns involve the entire epidermal layer and part of the dermis. These burns often result from contact with hot liquids or solids or with intense radiant energy. A deep-dermal partial-thickness burn usually is not characterized by blister formation. Only a modest plasma surface leakage occurs because of severe impairment in blood supply. The wound surface usually is red with patchy white areas that blanch with pressure. The appearance of the deep-dermal wound changes over time. Dermal necrosis and surface coagulated protein turn the wound from white to yellow. These wounds have a prolonged healing time. They can heal spontaneously as the epidermal elements germinate and migrate until the epidermal surface is restored, or they may require a skin substitute or surgical excision and grafting for wound closure. This process of healing by epithelialization can take up to 6 weeks. Left untreated, these wounds can heal primarily with unstable epithelium, late hypertrophic scarring, and marked contracture formation. Partial-thickness injuries can become full-thickness injuries if they become infected, if blood supply is diminished, or if further trauma occurs to the site. The treatment of choice is surgical excision and skin grafting.

A *full-thickness (third-degree) burn* involves destruction of all the layers of the skin down to and including the subcutaneous tissue (Fig. 41-6). The subcutaneous tissue is composed of adipose tissue, includes the hair follicles and sweat glands, and is poorly vascularized. A full-thickness burn appears pale white or charred, red or brown, and leathery. The surface of the burn may be dry, and if the skin is broken, fat may be exposed. Full-thickness burns usually are painless and insensitive to palpation. Because all epithelial elements are destroyed, the wound will not heal by reepitheliazation. Wound closure of small full-thickness burns (<4 cm^2 area) can be achieved with healing by contraction. All other full-thickness wounds require skin grafting for closure. Extensive full-thickness wounds leave the patient extremely susceptible to infections, fluid and electrolyte imbalances, alterations in thermoregulation, and metabolic disturbances.

The exact depth of many burn wounds cannot be clearly defined on the first inspection, and many burn wounds may contain superficial, mid-dermal, and deep-dermal wounds. A major difficulty is distinguishing deep-dermal partial-thickness from full-thickness injury. It is important to identify the depth of injury for appropriate treatment. Deep, partial-thickness wounds that will not heal within a relatively short time are treated with wound excision and grafting. Burn wounds can evolve over time, and they require frequent reassessment. Special consideration must always be given to very young and older patients because of their thin dermal layer. Older adults may also have reduced sensation and blood supply, causing them to be more susceptible to a full-thickness injury. Burn injuries in these age groups may be more severe than they initially appear.[12]

At the same time that assessment for wound depth occurs, the total percentage, or TBSA, of the burn is calculated. This calculation provides the basis for determining the amount of fluid required for treatment. All burn wound surface area percentages, except for superficial burns, are used to calculate the patient's fluid requirements.

TYPES OF INJURY

Thermal Burns. The most common type of burn is a thermal burn caused by steam, scalds, contact with heat, and fire injuries. "About 70% of burns in children are caused by scalds."[7] Toddlers are most often affected by scalding burns. Contact burns are also common. The length of time the hot object is in contact with the skin determines the depth of injury. Flame injuries are often associated with other trauma to the patient. The highest incidence of flame injuries occurs among people 15 to 29 years old.[4] Contact and flame burns tend to be deep-dermal or full-thickness injuries.

Electrical Burns. Electrical and lightning injuries result in 1000 deaths per year in the United States.[13] Low-voltage (alternating) current or high-voltage (alternating or direct) current can cause electrical burns. Children have the highest incidence of electrical injury. These accidents occur as a result of insertion of an object into an outlet or by biting or sucking electrical cords. Common situations that may increase the risk for electrical injuries include occupational exposure and accidents involving household current. Lightning causes approximately 80 deaths each year in the United States; the incidence is seven times greater among men than women.[13]

Chemical Burns. Acids and alkalis cause chemical burns. Alkalis commonly result in more severe injuries than do acid burns. Acid and alkali agents are found in many household and industrial substances, such as liquid concrete. The concentration of the chemical agent and the duration of exposure are the key factors that determine the extent and depth of damage. Progression of injury from chemical burns to their complete depth may be delayed, and the full extent of the injury may not be apparent until up to 48 hours after injury. Time must not be wasted in looking for the specific neutralizing agents because the injury is related directly to the concentration of the chemical and the duration of the exposure, and the heat of neutralization can extend the injury. Tar and asphalt burns are common and serious injuries.[9] Approximately 70% of chemical burns affect the hands.

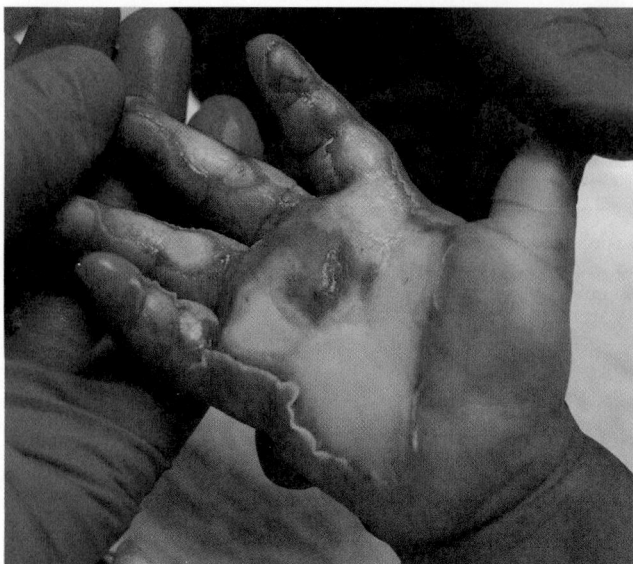

Figure 41-7 Full-thickness palm burn.

Radiation Burns. Burns associated with radiation exposure are uncommon. Radiation burns usually are localized and indicate high radiation doses to the affected area. Radiation burns may appear identical to thermal burns. The major difference is the time between exposure and clinical manifestation; it can be days to weeks, depending on the level of the radiation dose. Radiation injury can occur with exposure to industrial equipment, such as accelerators and cyclotrons, and equipment used for medical treatment.

LOCATION OF INJURY

Location of injury can be a determining factor in differentiating the level of care required. According to triage criteria from the American College of Surgeons, burns on the face, hands, feet, genitalia, major joints, and perineum are best treated in a burn center (Fig. 41-7). These burns involve functional areas of the body and often require specialized intervention. Injuries to these areas can result in significant long-term morbidity from impaired function and altered appearance.

PATIENT AGE AND HISTORY

Age and history are significant determinants of survival. Patients considered most at risk are those younger than 2 years and those older than 60 years. History of inhalation injury and electrical burns and all burns complicated by trauma and fractures (considered major injuries) significantly increase the risk for death. Obtaining the patient's medical history is important, particularly a history related to cardiac, pulmonary, and kidney dysfunction; diabetes; and central nervous system disorders. In evaluating the pediatric patient, it is essential to obtain a thorough history, especially for the nonverbal patient. Attention should be paid to the description of the burn event to rule out nonaccidental trauma (Fig. 41-8). Social services, such as child protective services and the police, should be consulted if abuse or neglect is suspected.

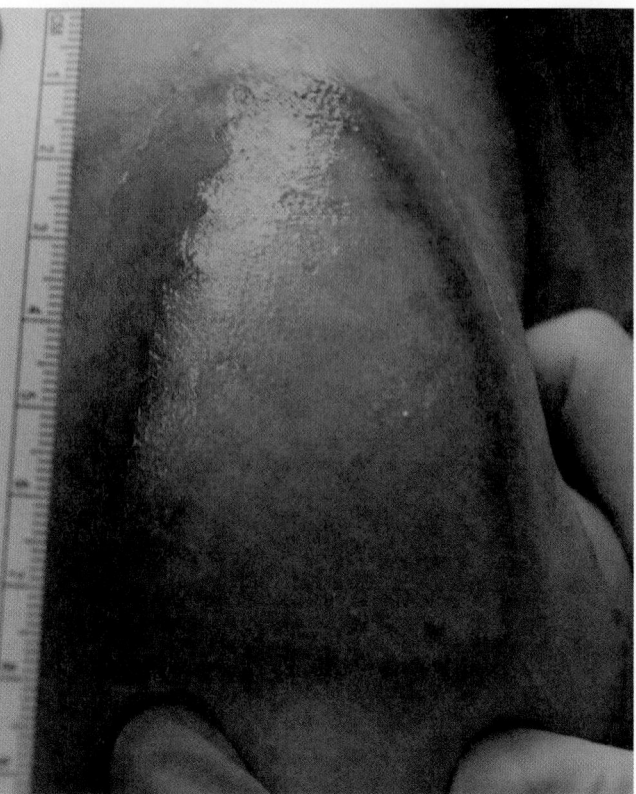

Figure 41-8 Partial-thickness iron burn to the right buttock from nonaccidental trauma.

INITIAL EMERGENCY BURN MANAGEMENT

The goals of acute care of the patient with thermal injuries are to save life, minimize disability, and prepare the patient for definitive care. The burn injury may involve multiple organ systems, and the approach to the injured patient should be expeditious and methodical in identifying problems and establishing priorities of care.[14]

The resuscitation phase begins immediately after the burn insult has occurred; therefore, the nurse is concerned with patient management at the scene until admission to an appropriate medical facility. As with any major trauma, the first hour after injury is crucial, but the first 24 to 36 hours after injury also are important in burn patient management. Management during this period has a major impact on the patient's survival and ultimate rehabilitation.

Obtaining a history regarding the nature of the injury is important in the management of the burn patient. Water heater, propane gas, grain elevator, and other types of explosions often throw the patient some distance and may result in concomitant orthopedic, neurologic, and internal trauma. It is valuable to know the specific agents involved if the burns are chemical. It also helps to know what substance was burned or inhaled and how long the patient was exposed to smoke or superheated air. A detailed patient history should include the mechanism of injury, patient's age, location and size of burn, type and amount of fluid already administered, known allergies, status of tetanus immunization, and significant medical history. All rings, watches, and jewelry are removed from injured limbs to avoid a tourniquet effect when edema occurs as a result of fluid shifts and fluid resuscitation.

AIRWAY MANAGEMENT

The first priority of emergency burn care is to secure and protect the airway. If there is any possibility of underlying cervical instability, cervical precautions must be initiated.[14] For patients with facial burns or exposure to fire in an enclosed space, or both, inhalation injury should be suspected. Carbon monoxide (CO) poisoning is associated with high mortality rates. Carboxyhemoglobin levels are obtained, and oxygen therapy is initiated. All patients with major burns or suspected inhalation injury are initially administered 100% oxygen.[14] The nurse should continue to observe the patient for clinical manifestations of impaired oxygenation, such as tachypnea, agitation, anxiety, and upper airway obstruction (e.g., hoarseness, stridor, wheezing). Early intubation may save the life of the patient who has an inhalation injury, because it may be impossible to perform this procedure later, when edema has obstructed the larynx. The need for frequent blood sampling and the benefit of continuous blood pressure monitoring may necessitate placement of an arterial line.

RESPIRATORY MANAGEMENT

Circumferential, full-thickness burns to the chest wall can lead to restriction of chest wall expansion and decreased compliance. Decreased compliance requires higher ventilatory pressures to provide the patient with adequate tidal volumes. In the patient who has not undergone intubation, clinical manifestations of chest wall restriction include rapid, shallow respirations; poor chest wall excursion; and severe agitation. Arterial blood gas analysis reveals a decrease in oxygen tension and an increasing partial pressure of carbon dioxide ($PaCO_2$) level. Patients receiving mechanical ventilation have increasing peak airway pressure values.

Escharotomies (burn eschar incisions) may be needed immediately to increase compliance and thereby lead to improved ventilation. These incisions usually are made bilaterally along the anterior axillary lines and are connected by a transverse incision at the costal margin (Fig. 41-9).

CIRCULATORY MANAGEMENT

The extent and depth of the burn are assessed. The extent of TBSA of the burn is calculated for estimation of fluid resuscitation requirements (Table 41-1); the Parkland formula is the most widely used method of calculation (see Case Study). Burn shock is caused by the loss of fluid from the vascular compartment into the area of injury, resulting in hypovolemia. The larger the percentage of burn area, the greater the potential for development of shock. Lactated Ringer's solution is infused

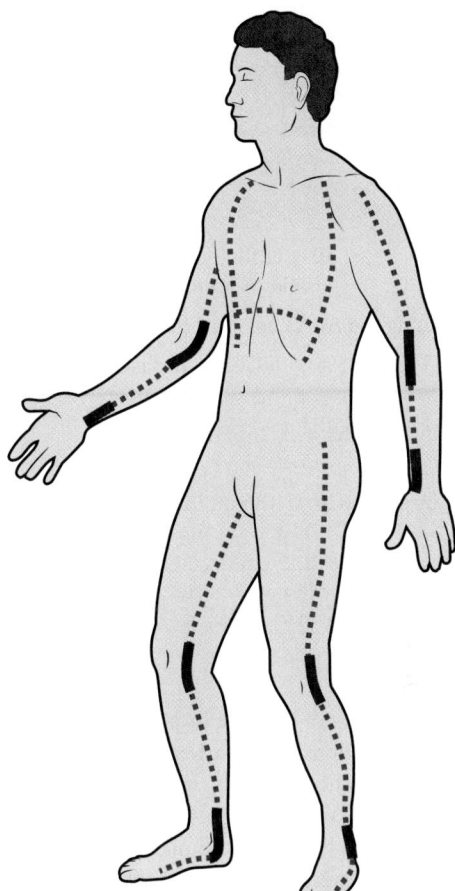

Figure 41-9 Preferred sites of escharotomy incisions. *(From Carrougher GJ: Burn care and therapy, St Louis, 1998, Mosby.)*

through a large-bore cannula (≥ 16 gauge) in a peripheral vein. Lactated Ringer's solution, an isotonic crystalloid, is the resuscitation fluid used most often. Given in large amounts, it can restore cardiac output to normal in most patients. It is preferred over normal saline because it most closely matches extracellular fluid. Because isotonic salt solutions generate no difference in osmotic pressure between plasma and interstitial space, the entire extracellular space must be expanded to replace intravascular losses. Diuretics should not be given during the resuscitative phase of burn care.

According to the Parkland formula (see Table 41-1), half of the calculated amount of fluid is administered to the patient in the first 8 hours after injury; 25% is given in the second 8 hours, and 25% is given in the third 8 hours. It is important to remember that calculated fluid requirements are guidelines. Fluid resuscitation is a dynamic process. The rate of fluid administration is adjusted according to the individual's response, which is determined by monitoring urine output, heart rate, blood pressure, and level of consciousness. Meticulous attention to the patient's intake and output is imperative to ensure that he or she is appropriately resuscitated. Underresuscitation may result in inadequate cardiac output, leading to inadequate organ perfusion and the potential for wound conversion from a partial- to full-thickness injury. Overresuscitation may lead to moderate to severe pulmonary edema, to excessive

TABLE 41-1 Formulas for Fluid Replacement or Resuscitation in First 24 Hours

Fluid and Dose Rate	ABA Consensus	Parkland	Modified Brooke	Brooke	Hypertonic
Electrolyte Solution	Ringer's lactate	Ringer's lactate	Ringer's lactate	Ringer's lactate	Hypertonic lactated saline (sodium, 250 mEq/L)
Dose: mL/kg/% burned*	2-4 50% of fluid over first 8 hr; 50% of fluid over next 16 hr	4	2	1.5	Rate based on urine output of 30-50 mL/hr
Examples using the ABA consensus formula: an 85-kg patient with 35% TBSA burn					
2 mL × 85 kg × 35% = 5950 mL in first 24 hours		3 mL × 85 × 35% = 8925 mL		4 mL × 85 × 35% = 11,900 mL	
2975 mL in first 8 hr = 372 mL/hr		4462 mL in first 8 hr = 558 mL/hr		5950 mL in first 8 hr = 744 mL/hr	
2975 mL in next 16 hr = 186 mL/hr		4462 mL in next 16 hr = 279 mL/hr		5950 mL in next 16 hr = 372 mL/hr	

*Adjust these rates to maintain a urine output > 30 mL/hr in adults or 1 mL/kg/hr in children.
ABA, American Burn Association; TBSA, total body surface area.

wound edema causing a decrease in perfusion of unburned tissue in the distal portions of the extremities, or to edema inhibiting perfusion of the zone of stasis, resulting in wound conversion.[10] Fluid requirements may be much higher than estimated using the Parkland formula. The recommendations for these situations are included later in this chapter.

Continuous monitoring with electrocardiograms (ECGs) should be used for serious thermal burn-injured patients, and in the presence of electrical burns, inhalation injury, or associated traumatic injury. ECG lead placement may present a challenge with extensive burns, and nontraditional locations on nonburned skin should be selected instead.

PATHOPHYSIOLOGY OF BURN SHOCK

Burn injuries greater than 35% of TBSA can result in burn shock.[8] Shock is defined as inadequate cellular perfusion. Significant burn injury results in hypovolemic shock and tissue trauma. Both cause the production and release of several local and systemic mediators. Burn shock can occur even when hypovolemia is corrected.

The first component of burn shock is hypovolemic shock. At the cellular level, the burning agent produces dilation of the capillaries and small vessels, increasing the capillary permeability. Plasma seeps out into the surrounding tissue, producing blisters and edema. The type, duration, and intensity of the burn all affect the amount and extent of fluid loss. This progressive fluid loss in extensive burns results in significant intravascular fluid volume deficit. Edema occurs locally in the burn wound and systemically in unburned tissues. Edema formation is unique to thermal injury.

Burn edema has been attributed to several factors. Barrier property changes of the capillary wall occur by direct injury and indirect mediator-modulated changes. Increases in permeability of protein and water occur, resulting in edema. In most

forms of shock, capillary pressure decreases as a result of arteriolar vasoconstriction. However, after burn injury, an increase in capillary pressure has been found in the burned tissue in the first minutes to hours after injury.[8] Coupled with this increase in capillary pressure is a negative interstitial hydrostatic pressure that occurs in the dermis layer of burned skin after thermal injury.[15] This negative interstitial hydrostatic pressure represents an edema-generating mechanism that occurs for approximately 2 hours after injury. Plasma colloid osmotic pressure is decreased as a result of protein leakage into the extravascular space. Plasma is then further diluted with fluid resuscitation. The osmotic pressure is decreased, and further fluid extravasation can occur.

In addition to leaking capillaries, local and systemic mediators cause edema and the cardiovascular problems seen in burn patients. These mediators include histamine, prostaglandins, kinins, and oxygen radicals, they increase arteriolar vasodilation. Manipulation of these mediators to stop the cascade of burn edema and burn shock is being researched.

The intravascular fluid changes combined with the action of inflammatory mediators and vasoconstricting mediators result in hemodynamic consequences in the burn patient. The hemodynamic alterations include decreased myocardial contractility and cardiac output despite adequate volume resuscitation, increased systemic vascular resistance (SVR), and increased pulmonary vascular resistance (PVR).[8] Increased PVR can lead to pulmonary edema. Large but judicious volumes of resuscitation fluids are required to maintain the vascular volume during the first few hours after a large burn injury to provide optimal resuscitation. Early and full fluid resuscitation can prevent the complications of acute renal failure, cardiovascular collapse, and death from shock. However, overresuscitation increases edema formation, which can further impair tissue oxygen diffusion. The nurse must assess the patient's fluid status and response to resuscitation to obtain the optimal response.

KIDNEY MANAGEMENT

If fluid resuscitation is inadequate, acute kidney injury (AKI) and acute renal failure (ARF) may occur. An indwelling urinary catheter should be placed for burns greater than 15% to 20% of TBSA in the emergency department to monitor urine output and the effectiveness of fluid resuscitation. A catheter may be necessary if the burn extends into the perineal area due to the presence or development of edema. Urinary catheters with temperature probes should be used whenever possible. The nurse measures urine output hourly. Adequate urine output for adults is 0.5 to 1 mL/kg/hr, or 30 to 50 mL/hr; for children, it is 1 mL/kg/hr.[10]

GASTROINTESTINAL MANAGEMENT

Patients with burns of more than 20% of TBSA are prone to gastric dilation as a result of paralytic ileus. Nasogastric or orogastric tubes are placed in these patients to prevent abdominal distention, emesis, and potential aspiration. This decrease in gastrointestinal function is caused by the effects of hypovolemia and the neurologic and endocrine response to injury. Gastrointestinal activity usually returns in 24 to 48 hours. Gastric prophylaxis with histamine₂ (H_2)-blockers or sucralfate is initiated, because burn patients are prone to *Curling stress ulcers*. These acute ulcerations of the duodenum are caused by sloughing of the gastric mucosa resulting from loss of plasma volume after severe burns. Enteral nutrition has been shown to be protective of gastric mucosal integrity and to improve intestinal flow and gastric motility in burned pateints.[16] Enteral nutrition should be started as soon as possible.[16]

PAIN MANAGEMENT

Burn injuries are very painful. Pain management must be addressed early and frequently reassessed to determine adequacy of interventions.[11] Intravenous opiates, such as morphine sulfate and fentanyl are indicated and are titrated to effect. Intravenous benzodiazepines for anxiolysis should also be administered and titrated to effect. Intramuscular or subcutaneous injections must not be administered, because absorption by these routes is unpredictable because of the fluid shifts that occur with burn injury. After a diet is tolerated, transition to oral medications should be undertaken. Pain management guidelines for administration and monitoring of patients are helpful and recommended.[17]

Pain results from the acute burn injury and throughout the phases of healing; procedural pain related to wound débridement, and surgical pain from skin grafting also occurs.[11] In the rehabilitation phase, *pruritus* (itch) may replace pain as a stressful symptom.[11] Antihistamine (H_1-blockers) are prescribed for the itching.[11]

EXTREMITY PULSE ASSESSMENT

Edema formation may cause neurovascular compromise to the extremities; frequent assessments are necessary to evaluate pulses, skin color, capillary refill, and sensation. Arterial circulation is at greatest risk with circumferential burns. If not corrected, reduced arterial flow causes ischemia and necrosis. The Doppler flow probe is one of the best ways to evaluate arterial pulses. An escharotomy may be required to restore arterial circulation and to allow for further swelling. The escharotomy can be performed at the bedside with a sterile field and scalpel. Care must be taken to avoid major nerves, vessels, and tendons. The incision extends through the length of the eschar, over joints, and down to the subcutaneous fat. The incision is placed laterally or medially on the extremity. If a single incision does not restore circulation, bilateral incisions are required (see Fig. 41-8).[9] If escharotomy is required before the patient is transferred to a burn center, consultation with the receiving physician is advised.

LABORATORY ASSESSMENT

Initial laboratory studies are performed: complete blood cell count, electrolytes, blood urea nitrogen (BUN), creatine, urinalysis, and blood screening. Special situations, such as inhalation injury, warrant arterial blood gas measurements, carboxyhemoglobin level determination, cultures, and alcohol and drug screens. A baseline assessment of nutritional status, including albumin and prealbumin, is helpful in monitoring future nutritional needs. An ECG is obtained for all patients with electrical burns or preexisting heart disease.

WOUND CARE

After the wounds have been assessed, topical antimicrobial therapy is not a priority during emergency care. However, the wounds must be covered with clean, dry dressings or sheets. Every attempt must be made to keep the patient warm because of the high risk of hypothermia. The administration of tetanus prophylaxis is recommended for all burns covering more than 10% of the TBSA and for patients with a questionable immunization history.

BURN CENTER REFERRAL

After initial treatment and stabilization at an emergency department, referral to a burn center is considered (see Box 41-1). A burn center must be able to deliver all therapy required, including rehabilitation, and must perform personnel training and burn research.[14] Patients meeting the criteria for referral need the expertise of a multidisciplinary team. Referring hospitals must always contact the burn center in their region.[4] Providers in the field should cover the burns with clean, dry cloth until arrival at the burn center. Early communication between the initial provider and the burn center is encouraged by the American Burn Association (ABA).[18]

SPECIAL MANAGEMENT CONSIDERATIONS

INHALATION INJURY

Inhalation injury can occur in the presence or absence of cutaneous injury. Inhalation injuries are strongly associated with burns sustained in a closed space, and they constitute the leading cause of fire-related deaths.[19] Inhalation injury appears in three basic forms, alone or in combination: carbon monoxide (CO) poisoning, direct heat injury, and chemical damage. The three types of inhalation injury are CO poisoning, upper airway injury, and lower airway injury.

Immediate measures to save the life of the burn patient include management of the airway. The burn patient may exhibit few or no signs of airway distress; however, thermal injury to the airway must be anticipated if facial burns, singed eyebrows and nasal hair, carbon deposits in the oropharynx, or carbonaceous sputum is present or if the history suggests confinement in a burning environment. Any of these findings indicates acute inhalation injury and requires immediate and definitive care. To prevent the necessity of tracheostomy or cricothyrotomy, the use of early intubation and respiratory support must be considered before tracheal edema occurs. Inhalation injury predisposes the patient to the development of pneumonia and acute lung injury.[19] Management of acute lung injury necessitates mechanical ventilatory support and, in extreme cases, high-frequency oscillatory ventilation or extracorporeal membrane oxygenation. The occurrence of inhalation injury with cutaneous burns increases the fluid requirements during resuscitation to a higher level than would be predicted by the cutaneous burn alone.

Carbon Monoxide Poisoning. Persons found dead at the scene of a fire may have few or no cutaneous thermal injuries, but they died of CO poisoning. CO is a colorless, odorless, and tasteless gas. Inhalation of CO, a by-product of the incomplete combustion of carbon, results in its bonding to available hemoglobin, producing carboxyhemoglobin (HbCO), which effectively decreases oxygen saturation of hemoglobin. The affinity of hemoglobin molecules for CO is approximately 200 times greater than that for oxygen.[20] Carboxyhemoglobin binds poorly with oxygen, reducing the oxygen-carrying capacity of blood and causing hypoxia. The shortage of oxygen at the tissue level is worsened by a shift to the left of the oxyhemoglobin dissociation curve, reflecting the fact that the oxygen in the hemoglobin is not readily given up to the cells.

Arterial oxygen saturation measurement is of limited value because oxygen saturation may be quite high despite dangerously low levels of oxygen content. Because the pulse oximeter cannot distinguish between oxyhemoglobin and carboxyhemoglobin, it is unreliable during the initial stages of CO poisoning. Arterial blood gas determinations and oxygen saturation are used to accurately assess the hemoglobin oxygen saturation level. A serum carboxyhemoglobin level is obtained the diagnosis. Normal carboxyhemoglobin levels are less than 2%. Carboxyhemoglobin levels of 40% to 60% often produce unresponsiveness or obtundation; levels of 15% to 40% may result in various degrees of central nervous system dysfunction. Levels of 10% to 15%, which can be found in cigarette smokers, rarely produce serious symptoms but may cause a headache.

The major clinical manifestations of severe CO poisoning are related to the central nervous system and the heart. Symptoms associated with CO poisoning include headache, dizziness, nausea, vomiting, dyspnea, and confusion. In severe cases, CO poisoning may lead to myocardial ischemia and central nervous system complications caused by lowered oxygen delivery and the already compromised circulatory system. Early signs of CO poisoning may include tachycardia, tachypnea, confusion, and lightheadedness. As the CO level rises, patients exhibit a decreased level of responsiveness, which may progress to unresponsiveness and respiratory failure.

The treatment of choice for CO poisoning is high-flow oxygen administered at 100% through a tight-fitting nonrebreathing mask or endotracheal intubation. The half-life of CO in the body is 4 hours at room air (21% oxygen), 2 hours at 40% oxygen, and 40 to 60 minutes at 100% oxygen.[20] The half-life of CO is 30 minutes in a hyperbaric oxygen chamber at three times atmospheric pressure. The use of hyperbaric oxygen is controversial in the care of the burn patient. Because of the rapid removal of CO with the administration of 100% oxygen, the time required to transport a patient who has received oxygen in the field should always be considered to avoid possible underestimation of inhalation injury.

Upper Airway Injury. Burns of the upper respiratory tract include those involving the pharynx, larynx, glottis, trachea, and larger bronchi. Injuries are caused by direct heat or by chemical inflammation and necrosis. Respiratory injury is most often confined to the upper airway. The heat exchange capability is so efficient that most heat absorption and damage occur in the pharynx and larynx above the true vocal cords.

Heat damage may be severe enough to cause upper airway obstruction at any time, beginning from moment of injury through the resuscitation period. Caution is taken for patients with severe hypovolemia, because supraglottic edema may be delayed until fluid resuscitation is under way. Patients must be monitored for hoarseness, stridor, audible airflow turbulence, and the production of carbonaceous sputum. Maximal edema occurs 24 hours after injury with upper airway injuries, and these patients should be observed in the intensive care unit for a minimum of 24 hours.[6]

The prediction of an upper airway obstruction is based on consideration of several variables: extent of injury to the face and neck, the presence of blisters on or redness of the posterior pharynx, signs of singed nasal hair, increased carboxyhemoglobin levels, increased rate and decreased depth of breathing, hoarseness (which indicates a significant decrease in the diameter of the airway), increased amount of sputum, and the circumstances of the burn event (whether it occurred in an enclosed space or involved superheated gases or steam). Steam has a heat-carrying capacity many times that of dry air, and it is capable of overwhelming the extremely efficient heat-dissipating capabilities of the upper airway.

Intubation is recommended whenever airway patency is questionable, rather than delaying intubation until airway obstruction is so severe that intubation becomes a challenge. After the airway is secure, priority is given to minimizing airway edema, maintaining pulmonary toilet, and treating bronchospasm. Elevating of the head of the bed to 30 degrees or higher decreases airway edema. Therapeutic deep breathing and coughing, early mobility, suctioning, and bronchodilators assist in mobilizing and removing secretions. Fiberoptic bronchoscopy may be required to remove secretions in some patients. Mechanical ventilatory support is necessary when respiratory fatigue or failure occurs. Precautions to prevent ventilator-associated pneumonia (VAP) should be implemented to avoid secondary infection. When prolonged ventilatory failure is expected because of severe inhalation, a tracheostomy is performed.[6]

Lower Airway Injury. Heated air rarely causes lower airway injury. If it does, it usually is associated with death at the scene. Lower airway injuries are typically caused by chemical damage to mucosal surfaces. Tracheobronchitis with severe spasm and wheezing may occur in the first minutes to hours after injury. Historically, the most accurate method of documenting lower airway injury is the xenon ventilation/perfusion lung scan. Prolonged retention or symmetry of washout of the radioisotope indicates pulmonary parenchymal injury on the side of the retained emissions. The onset of symptoms is unpredictable following smoke inhalation and patients at risk must be closely monitored for at least 24 to 48 hours after injury.

Research into optimal ventilator management strategies for patients with inhalation injury is a high priority.[21] In addition to thermal damage, secondary effects from massive fluid resuscitation and high-volume, high-pressure ventilator settings can precipitate acute lung injury (ALI) and acute respiratory distress syndrome (ARDS).[21] The use of lung protective ventilation with low tidal volumes, higher levels of positive end-expiratory pressure (PEEP) and plateau pressures maintained below 30 mm Hg are increasingly employed.[21] Other ventilator modes such as high-frequency oscillatory ventilation early in the care of patients with inhalation injury has also shown promising results.[22,23] Benefits include decreased rates of pneumonia and increased survival.[24] Treatment of lower airway injury is largely symptomatic. As with upper airway injury management, removal of secretions, ventilatory support, and tracheostomy may be required.

NONTHERMAL BURNS

Chemical Burns. Chemical burns can be caused by a variety of products. Acids, alkalis, and organic and inorganic compounds cause chemical burns. The acid or base quality determines the injurious nature of a product. The injury is caused by the pH of the product or by the concentration of the product. In the past, irrigation with neutralizing solutions was recommended to limit the extent and depth of chemical burns. This practice is no longer advocated because neutralizing agents may cause reactions that are exothermic (produce heat), thereby increasing the extent and depth of the burn. It also is possible that the neutralizing agent is neither immediately known nor available. Instead, large amounts of water should be used to flush the area. Clothing and shoes should be removed if they have been in contact with the chemical. Alkali burns of the eyes require continuous irrigation for many hours after the injury. Removal of contact lenses is necessary before irrigation.

Treatments for chemical burns vary. Phenol burns are first diluted, and then the skin is wiped quickly with polyethylene glycol or vegetable oil to decrease the severity of the burn. Areas exposed to hydrofluoric acid must be copiously irrigated with water; the burned area then can be treated with 2.5% calcium gluconate gel. The patient may need calcium gluconate supplements because the fluoride ion precipitates serum calcium, causing hypocalcemia. White phosphorus can ignite if kept dry, and these wounds must be covered with a moist dressing. After a tar or asphalt injury, the removal of tar or asphalt is best accomplished with the use of petroleum-containing distillates. One such product is Detachol (Ferndale Laboratories, Inc., Ferndale, MI). The solution can be placed directly on the wound and gently wiped off. Routine débridement of loose skin is initiated after tar removal. Topical antimicrobial therapy is then applied.

Electrical Burns. In electrical burns, the type and voltage of the circuit, resistance, pathway of transmission through the body, and duration of contact are considered in determining the amount of damage sustained. In these situations, the rescuer also may be injured if he or she becomes part of the electrical circuit. The rescuer must disconnect the electrical source to break the circuit or must know how to avoid becoming part of the circuit. The use of appropriately insulated equipment that diverts the circuit elsewhere is essential. Extreme caution must be used in the rescue of victims.

Electricity always travels toward the ground. The body conducts electrical current as a whole, as opposed to the earlier belief that it traveled most quickly through the nerves and circulatory system. Electrical burns often are much more serious than the surface appearance of the wound suggests.[24] As the electrical current passes through the body, it damages the inner tissues and may leave little evidence of a burn on the skin surface.

The electrical burn process can result in a profound alteration in acid-base balance and rhabdomyolysis resulting in myoglobinuria, which poses a serious threat to kidney function. Myoglobin is a normal constituent of muscle. With extensive muscle destruction, it is released into the circulatory system and filtered by the kidneys. It can be highly toxic and can lead to acute renal failure. Fluid resuscitation for the electrical burn patient does not correlate with the Parkland formula, and the fluid is adjusted according to the patient's urine output. If myoglobin is present in the urine, a urine output greater than 100 mL/hr in adults[24] and 2 mL/kg/hr in children is established until the urine is clear of all myoglobin pigment.

If hemoglobinuria is identified, the clinician should assume that the patient has myoglobinuria and acidosis. Sodium bicarbonate may be administered to bring the pH level into the normal range, to correct a documented acidosis, or to alkalize urine to promote myoglobin excretion. Diuretics also may be administered intravenously until myoglobinuria resolves. Sodium bicarbonate infusions and diuretic therapy are called *forced alkaline diuresis*. A baseline ECG and myocardial biomarker levels are obtained while the patient is in the emergency department. The following criteria are used for monitoring the cardiac status of burned patients:

- A history of loss of consciousness or cardiac arrest
- Documentation of cardiac dysrhythmia at the scene of the accident or in the emergency department

- Abnormal ECG findings on admission
- TBSA burns of more than 20%
- Very young age or advanced age
- Prior history of heart disease

Other burn patients may be admitted to nonmonitored settings and observed closely. Cardiac dysrhythmias must be treated promptly, and a protocol to rule out myocardial infarction must be followed.[7]

BURN NURSING DIAGNOSES AND MANAGEMENT

The clinical course of a burn injury has three phases: resuscitative, acute care, and rehabilitative. Each phase has a unique set of actual and potential problems. The resuscitative phase begins with initial hemodynamic response to the injury and lasts until capillary integrity is restored and the repletion of plasma volume by fluid replacement occurs. Spontaneous diuresis demonstrates that capillaries have regained their integrity. The acute phase begins with the onset of diuresis of fluid mobilized from the interstitial space and ends with the closure of the burn wound. The major focus of the acute phase is wound healing, wound closure, and prevention of infection. The rehabilitative phase begins when the patient is admitted to the hospital, with correction of functional deficits and scar management being major considerations. The rehabilitative phase may last months to years, depending on the severity of injury. The rehabilitation phase focuses on support for adequate wound healing, prevention of scarring and contractures, and psychological support of the patient and family.[25]

RESUSCITATION PHASE

Life-threatening airway and breathing problems, cardiopulmonary instability, and hypovolemia characterize the resuscitation phase, or shock phase. Every organ is involved in the physiologic response that occurs with thermal injury of greater than 20% of TBSA. The magnitude of this pathophysiologic response is proportional to the extent of cutaneous injury. The goal of the resuscitation phase is to maintain vital organ function and perfusion. Emergent interventions for inhalation injury, airway management, and hypovolemia are concurrently addressed.

Oxygenation Alterations. Inhalation injuries have emerged as the most common cause of death in burn patients, whereas 40 to 50 years ago, burn shock and then burn sepsis accounted for most burn-related deaths. Early diagnosis of inhalation injury is essential to minimize complications and to decrease the mortality rate. Three oxygenation complications are associated with smoke inhalation during the resuscitation phase: *CO poisoning, upper airway obstruction*, and *chemical pneumonitis*. Evaluation of a patient for inhalation injury includes physical assessment (e.g., singed facial hairs, mucosal burns of nose or mouth, carbonaceous sputum), arterial blood gas analysis, carboxyhemoglobin levels, chest radiography, flexible fiberoptic bronchoscopy, xenon 133 lung scan, and pulmonary function

tests.[19,26] Critical care nursing management includes the following:

- Assess breath sounds and the rate and quality of respirations.
- Administer oxygen as prescribed.
- Monitor carboxyhemoglobin levels.
- Elevate the head of the bed and implement VAP precautions.
- Assess and assist with pulmonary secretion suctioning.
- Observe for signs of airway obstruction (e.g., increased respiratory rate and heart rate, increased work of breathing, use of accessory muscles, stridor, wheezing, hoarseness, crackles).
- Prepare for endotracheal intubation and mechanical ventilation.
- Maintain accurate and timely documentation.

Impaired Gas Exchange. The most common pulmonary burn complication is CO poisoning. High-flow oxygen should be administered at 100% through a non-rebreathing mask or endotracheal intubation until the carboxyhemoglobin level is less than 10% to 15%.

Chemical pneumonitis is caused by inhalation of the by-products of combustion of substances such as cotton, aldehydes, oxides of sulfur, and nitrogen. Burning polyvinylchloride yields at least 75 potentially toxic compounds, including hydrochloric acid and CO. Within days after a burn, acute respiratory distress syndrome (ARDS) commonly develops in patients with chemical pneumonitis. The primary clinical manifestation of ARDS is hypoxemia that is refractory to oxygen therapy.[26] Early signs include increased pH, decreased $PaCO_2$, and an increased respiratory rate. Ventilatory support with the use of positive end-expiratory pressure (PEEP) is the treatment of choice.

Ineffective Airway Clearance. Laryngeal swelling and upper airway obstruction may occur at any time during the first 24 hours after the burn injury. Endotracheal intubation must be accomplished early because this simple procedure can become extremely difficult in the presence of laryngeal edema. There usually is time to intervene after obtaining the history and transporting the patient to the primary hospital. Edema may continue to develop for 72 hours after the burn incident. The patient who has not initially undergone intubation must be carefully monitored during this critical period. When prolonged ventilatory failure is expected as a result of severe inhalation, a tracheostomy is performed.[6]

Extubation should occur only if the patient can meet extubation criteria: level of consciousness assessed as *awake*, intact cough and gag reflexes, inspiratory effort greater than −25 cm H_2O in adults, vital capacity of 10 mL/kg, and decreased volume and tenacity of the sputum. Resolution of airway edema can be assessed by deflating the endotracheal cuff and observing the patient's ability to breathe around the endotracheal tube.

Although uncommon, laryngospasm must be addressed. It usually is brought on by airway irritation from the inhalation of noxious agents.

Ineffective Breathing Pattern. Circumferential, full-thickness burns to the chest wall are the most common cause of ineffective breathing patterns. Escharotomies should be performed in this situation, which will lead to improved chest wall compliance and breathing efficiency.

Fluid Resuscitation. Current resuscitation protocols emphasize fluid delivery rates based on the extent of burn and the patient's weight. The patient's weight measured in kilograms must be obtained on admission to the hospital. The extent of the burn is calculated by using one of the methods previously described. Several formulas are available to guide fluid resuscitation and should be used to assist in the management of fluid replacement (see Table 41-1). The formulas differ primarily in terms of administration, volume, and sodium content. The actual amount of fluid given to any patient must be based on that individual's response.

The type of fluid used in resuscitation and at what point a switch should be made to a colloid solution are controversial topics. There are no clear-cut guidelines for resuscitation. The administration of crystalloid fluid (lactated Ringer's solution) for the first 24 to 36 hours after the burn is the most common practice. Lactated Ringer's solution is the crystalloid solution of choice because of its physiologic similarity to the composition of extracellular fluid. For the pediatric population, the addition of lactated Ringer's solution with 5% dextrose (D_5LR) should be considered as maintenance fluid, especially in the first 24 hours. Assessment for secondary injuries that would affect the choice of fluid should be performed. Ideally, the capillary leak seals approximately 24 hours after the injury, making it possible to give colloid without leakage of protein into the interstitium. Colloid deficits are replaced in the next 24 hours with salt-free albumin or dextran at 0.3 to 1 mL/kg/% TBSA burn. In addition to colloid, maintenance fluids are given to replace evaporative losses, and the amount is adjusted according to the patient's serum electrolyte levels, urine output, weight, volume status, and clinical assessment.

The proposed benefit of colloid use is that less burn edema occurs, resulting in increased hemodynamic stability. Arguments have been made that colloid administration shows no more benefit than crystalloid and should be used judiciously because the cost is high. Hypertonic saline (lactated Ringer's solution with various concentrations of sodium lactate) also is used. The controversial benefit of hypertonic saline is an overall decrease in total fluid requirements. Serum sodium levels should be monitored routinely, and hypertonic saline should be stopped for sodium levels of 160 mEq/dL or greater.

Deficient Fluid Volume. Physiologic effects of the burn complicate the tissue damage that occurs after the burn insult. Coagulation factors are affected, protein is denatured, and cellular content is ionized. These factors, coupled with the dilation of capillaries and small vessels, lead to increased capillary permeability and fluid shifts from the intravascular space to the interstitial space. The lymphatic system, which normally carries away the increased interstitial fluid, may be damaged or overloaded and unable to function to its normal capacity.

In addition to the protein and electrolyte shift, an increased insensible water loss occurs. In the healthy adult, this loss is estimated to be 35 to 50 mL/hr. The burn patient's insensible water loss may be as much as 300 to 3000 mL/day. This increase may be related to temperature elevation, tracheostomy, and the size of the burn.

Burn shock is proportional to the extent and depth of injury. The loss of plasma begins almost immediately after the injury and reaches its peak within the first 48 hours. Desired clinical responses to fluid resuscitation include a urinary output of 0.5 to 1 mL/kg/hr, a heart rate lower than 120 beats/min, blood pressure in the normal to high range, a central venous pressure less than 12 cm H_2O or a pulmonary artery occlusion pressure (PAOP) less than 18 mm Hg, clear lung sounds, clear sensorium, and the absence of intestinal events, such as nausea and paralytic ileus. Heart rate, blood pressure, and central venous pressure values are not always accurate or reliable predictors of successful fluid resuscitation.

Potassium and sodium, the two electrolytes of concern during the resuscitation period, must be monitored carefully. *Hyperkalemia* can occur during this phase because of the release of potassium from damaged cells, because of metabolic acidosis, and because of impaired kidney function caused by hemoglobinuria, myoglobinuria, or decreased renal perfusion. The patient must be assessed for the clinical manifestations of hyperkalemia. Treatment includes correction of acidosis. During the resuscitation phase, using cation-exchange resins or intravenously administered insulin and hypertonic dextrose to transport potassium back into the cell is not recommended because of the unpredictable nature of fluid shifts that occur.

Hypokalemia can occur during the resuscitation phase because of the massive loss of fluids and electrolytes through the burn wounds or because of hemodilution. During the acute phase, it may be related to hemodilution; inadequate replacement; loss associated with diuresis, diarrhea, vomiting, nasogastric drainage, and long hydrotherapy sessions; or the shift of potassium from the intravascular space to the cell after the acidosis has been corrected. Nursing interventions include treating nausea and vomiting, limiting immersive hydrotherapy sessions to less than 30 minutes, preventing fluid volume excess, and judicious replacement of potassium.

Hyponatremia is not uncommon during the resuscitation phase because of the loss of sodium through the burn wound, the shift of fluid into the interstitial space, vomiting, nasogastric drainage, diarrhea, and the use of hypotonic salt solutions during the early phase of resuscitation. During this phase, it may be necessary to monitor serum sodium levels every 4 to 8 hours. Hyponatremia also may occur during the acute phase because of hemodilution and loss through the wound, lengthy hydrotherapy sessions, and excessive diuresis resulting from the fluid shift back into the intravascular space. Interventions are followed for treating nausea and vomiting, hydrotherapy sessions are limited, and intravenous replacement of sodium is considered. During diuresis, which occurs during the acute phase, restricting free water intake usually is the only required intervention to increase the serum sodium level.

Risk for Infection. Preventing infection in the burn patient is a true challenge and involves complex decision making. Infection leading to sepsis and multisystem organ failure is the most common cause of death after the initial resuscitation period.

There has been considerable debate about the infection control precautions to use with burn patients. The burn wound is the most common source of infection in the burn patient.

The loss of the protective mechanism of the skin and contamination from the patient's own bacterial flora can lead to bloodstream infections.[27] Some centers advocate routine wound surveillance cultures and wound biopsy to identify infection early.[27] Daily wound inspection for changes in appearance, such as an increase in exudate, odor, or color, is necessary to minimize the risk of bacteremia. Patients should not be treated with antibiotics prophylactically; rather, treatment should be tailored to positive culture results.

Cross-contamination by direct contact is a significant source of infection and a subsequent cause of sepsis.[27,28] Effective hand-washing technique cannot be overemphasized. Nurses must wash their hands and change gloves when moving from area to area on the same patient. For example, after changing the chest dressing, which may be contaminated with sputum from the tracheostomy, hands must be washed and gloves changed before the nurse moves to the legs. Gowns, gloves, and masks should be worn whenever there is contact with body fluids. These garments also must be changed and hands washed before caring for a different patient. Maintaining patient-specific dressings and topical agents is recommended. Equipment such as thermometers, intravenous pumps, and stethoscopes should be designated for each patient or, when shared, should be cleaned with appropriate bactericidal cleansers between patients. Some centers advocate the practice of protective isolation for all burn patients.[27]

Whichever precautions are used, everyone coming in contact with the patient, including the family and visitors, must be knowledgeable about the standard for infection control. These precautions should be strictly followed by all. Precautions should have sound rationale and should not increase the workload or the frustration of the burn team. Otherwise, compliance and consistent application of the standard will not occur, increasing the risk of infection and sepsis for the burn patient.

TISSUE PERFUSION

Ineffective Kidney Tissue Perfusion. Urinalysis to determine the myoglobin level may be performed soon after burn injury. Myoglobinuria can be detected grossly by the dark, port-wine color of the urine. Myoglobin is extremely toxic to the kidneys and can cause massive tubular destruction. It is best treated with rapid fluid administration and forced diuresis with diuretics such as mannitol, an osmotic diuretic. The goal is an hourly urine output that is at least double the general recommendations to flush the renal tubules. All other diuretics are avoided because they will deplete the already compromised intravascular volume. Sodium bicarbonate is sometimes given intravenously to alkalinize the urine and assist in the elimination of heme pigments.

Maintaining and monitoring the renal system is vital in burn patient management. Impairment of the renal system may be related to hemoglobinuria, myoglobinuria, hypoperfusion, and hypovolemia. Urinary output must be monitored every hour for the first 48 to 72 hours, and specific gravity values can be used to determine the adequacy of hydration status and renal competency. The urine glucose concentration is monitored, as are urine sodium, creatinine, and BUN levels. Use of an indwelling urinary catheter is appropriate for the first 48 to 72 hours. Because of the tremendous risk of infection related to indwelling catheters, they are removed as soon as possible. However, leaving the catheter in place may be necessary if perineal burns are involved. Oliguria is usually related to inadequate fluid resuscitation but may be associated with acute renal failure. Other signs of renal failure include increasing creatinine, BUN, phosphorus, and potassium levels; excessive fluid-weight gain; excessive edema; elevated blood pressure; lethargy; and confusion.

The presence of glucose in the urine causes osmotic diuresis. In this clinical situation, urine output is an unreliable estimate of volume status. Because of the increased loss of fluid through the kidneys, glucosuria may suggest the need for additional fluid beyond the original estimates.

Ineffective Cerebral Tissue Perfusion. The patient's neurologic status is assessed frequently during the first few days. Changes may be related to an associated head injury that occurred at the time of burn injury, hypoperfusion related to hypovolemia, hypoxemia associated with inadequate ventilation, CO poisoning, or electrolyte imbalances. Patients with electrical burns or major thermal burns may have peripheral neurologic injuries, which may not become evident for several days after the injury. The neurologic assessment includes use of the Glasgow Coma Scale. It is not unusual for the patient to be agitated, restless, and extremely anxious during the resuscitation phase of burn injury as a result of hypovolemia, pain, and the fear of disfigurement or death. However, the possibility of neurologic involvement must not be overlooked. Maintaining an adequate mean arterial pressure is essential to ensure adequate cerebral perfusion pressure.

Ineffective Peripheral Tissue Perfusion. Ineffective peripheral tissue perfusion results from third spacing of fluid during the resuscitation phase, which restricts blood flow to extremities. As hypovolemia ensues, vasoconstriction increases, which can be potentiated by the loss of body temperature. Peripheral tissue perfusion must be monitored carefully in all burn patients. Burned and unburned areas are carefully assessed for warmth, color, and peripheral pulses. Capillary refill time should be less than 3 seconds in unburned areas. Any clinical manifestation of diminished systemic tissue perfusion must be reported immediately. Nursing actions are taken to minimize any compromise of peripheral circulation. Close monitoring of appropriate fluid resuscitation and careful positioning of the patient are necessary to prevent compromised blood flow. Crossed legs, dependent positions, and pillows under the patient's knees should be avoided. Specialty mattresses and beds may be helpful to prevent secondary skin breakdown and assist with positioning and pulmonary toilet. The limbs should be elevated above the heart to decrease peripheral edema and enhance venous return.[10] Assisted range-of-motion exercises can help to decrease edema.

Monitoring the peripheral circulation is crucial in the burn patient with circumferential, full-thickness burns of the extremities. The resulting edema may severely compromise the venous system and then the arterial system. Neurovascular integrity of extremities with circumferential burns must be assessed every hour for the first 24 to 48 hours using the six Ps: *pulselessness, pallor, pain, paresthesia, paralysis,* and *poikilothermy.* Careful, ongoing assessment is necessary, especially for patients who are intubated and may not be able to communicate pain or paresthesia. The use of a Doppler flowmeter may be necessary. Loss of pulses is a late sign of compromised vascular flow. If any changes are noticed, the physician must be notified immediately. Numbness and paresthesia may occur only 30 minutes before loss of pulses. Irreversible nerve ischemia resulting in loss of function may begin after 12 to 24 hours. An escharotomy may become necessary to allow the underlying tissue to expand. In deeper wounds, a fasciotomy, which involves incision into the fascia, may be necessary.

An unfortunate scenario results when the patient's reports of ischemic pain and paresthesia in a circumferentially burned extremity go unheeded and neurovascular compromise is allowed to persist. Sensory nerve fibers become damaged, and altered sensations cease, which may be misinterpreted as improvement in neurovascular status. Permanent disability and possible loss of limb are eventual outcomes.

Ineffective Gastrointestinal Tissue Perfusion. Paralytic ileus is a common gastrointestinal complication that can occur during resuscitation or when sepsis develops. The abdomen and bowel sounds should be assessed every 2 hours during the initial phase and every 4 hours thereafter. If clinical manifestations of a paralytic ileus occur, oral intake is withheld, and a nasogastric tube is inserted and placed on low to medium suction. Paralytic ileus can be related to hypokalemia, the sympathetic response to severe trauma, or decreased tissue perfusion related to hypovolemia.

A stress ulcer (Curling ulcer) may develop as a result of decreased tissue perfusion to the gastrointestinal tract, a change in the quantity or quality of mucus (which has a pH of 1), or an increase in gastric acid secretion resulting from the stress response. Gastric acid should be maintained above a pH of 5 through the administration of antacids, H_2-blockers, or proton pump inhibitors to prevent the development of these ulcers. The patient should be carefully monitored for gastrointestinal bleeding. All stools and gastric content are tested for occult blood. The patient should be observed for epigastric discomfort or fullness, decreased blood pressure, or increased pulse. Advances in burn care such as early fluid resuscitation, early gastric feeding, and antacid therapy have decreased the reported incidence of stress ulcers to 2%.[29]

Invasive Monitoring. The decision to use invasive monitoring techniques requires careful consideration of the potential risk factors and how the data collected will influence the course of treatment. Invasive monitoring should be considered if treatment seems ineffective or if complicating factors occur, such as severe respiratory involvement, major life-threatening injuries, head injuries, or pneumothorax. Patients with preexisting medical conditions such as chronic obstructive pulmonary disease (COPD), congestive heart failure, and renal failure also may require invasive monitoring.[30]

Invasive monitoring includes direct measurement of central venous pressure, pulmonary artery pressure, arterial pressure, core temperature, cardiac output, SVR, and PVR. The use of an arterial line is considered if serial and frequent arterial blood gas values are required for respiratory management or for hemodynamic instability requiring the titration of vasoactive drugs. Central venous catheters can be helpful in the early stages of fluid resuscitation to deliver the massive amount of fluids required. The physician selects the catheter insertion site based on burn location and the purpose of the catheter. It is preferable not to insert catheters through burned skin. It may be appropriate to use a multilumen catheter that can serve as a route for fluid resuscitation, maintenance fluids, antibiotic therapy, and vasoactive drugs. The risks involved include the increased chance of infection, potential for pneumothorax, and difficulty with insertion if hypovolemia is present.

Pulmonary artery catheters are placed only when necessary for optimal care. They may be essential to the survival of the septic patient despite the risks involved. Pulmonary artery catheters can provide data about pulmonary artery occlusion pressure, cardiac output, stroke volume, SVR and PVR, core temperature, and mixed venous oxygen saturation levels.

Centrally placed intravascular catheters require meticulous care. Strict guidelines should be established and monitored. Catheters are inserted under sterile conditions, and the dressings are changed under the same conditions. Because infection is such a major concern, all invasive catheters are removed as early as possible.[28]

Hypothermia. Thermoregulation maintenance is a nursing challenge. The patient with extensive burn injury is at high risk for hypothermia. Hypothermia is especially problematic during initial treatment, during hydrotherapy, and immediately after surgery. Heat is lost through open burn wounds by means of evaporation and radiation. The patient's core temperature should be maintained between 99.6° F and 101° F. Heat shields or lamps, hypothermia blankets, and fluid warmers can be individually or simultaneously used to maintain body temperature.

Laboratory Assessment. Laboratory assessment is another important aspect of burn care. Because of the invasive nature of drawing blood, it is done only if absolutely indicated. Consideration should be given to the age of the patient, the size of the burn, the time since injury, and any underlying disease process.

White blood cell (WBC) counts usually are monitored for elevation, a sign of sepsis. It is not unusual, however, for the WBC count to fall below 5000/mm^3 within 48 hours after injury. The value may drop even lower—1500/mm^3 to 2000/mm^3—with the use of silver sulfadiazine. If the WBC count stays in this range for more than 12 hours, the use of a different topical agent is recommended. The WBC count usually becomes normal again after the switch. At this point, the use of silver sulfadiazine can be tested again by applying it to a small area. If the WBC count does not drop again within 12 hours, the use of silver sulfadiazine can be resumed. In practice, the need for discontinuation of silver sulfadiazine is not common, but it must be considered if the WBC count continues to fall.

Hemoglobin and hematocrit data can be useful in the resuscitative phase to guide fluid administration. If surgical débridement is required, monitoring blood counts in the postoperative period is important. Serum chemistry information is helpful for ongoing assessment of kidney function and electrolyte balance. The myriad tests available should be used appropriately and as indicated by individual patient needs.

ACUTE CARE PHASE

The acute care phase of burn management begins after resuscitation and lasts until complete wound closure is achieved. The early postresuscitation phase is a period of transition from the shock phase to the hypermetabolic phase. Major cardiopulmonary and wound changes occur that substantially alter the manner of patient care from that given during resuscitation. Cardiopulmonary stability is optimal during this period because wound inflammation and infection have not developed. Hypermetabolic changes can be complicated with the onset of wound infection and sepsis. Early wound excision and skin grafting procedures, local wound care, nutritional support, and infection control characterize this phase.

Critical care nurses play a major role in promoting the healing process. Nurses, as skilled clinicians of the burn team, provide daily wound assessment, hydrotherapy, débridement, preoperative and postoperative management, and pain management. Appropriate treatment results in critical differences in patient care and outcomes.

Immediately after injury, the body responds by initiating a series of physiologic changes to restore skin integrity. These physiologic changes include the inflammatory phase, the proliferative phase, and the maturation phase.

The Inflammatory Phase.
The inflammatory phase begins immediately after injury. Vascular changes and cellular activity characterize this period. Changes in the severed vessels occur in an attempt to wall off the wound from the external environment. Platelets, activated as a result of vessel wall injury, aggregate; blood coagulation is initiated; and in larger vessels, smooth muscle tissue contraction occurs, resulting in a reduction in the diameter of the vessel lumen. These brief but important compensatory mechanisms protect the individual from excessive blood loss and increased exposure to bacterial contamination. As vasodilation occurs, vascular permeability and blood supply to the wound site increase. As extravascular volume increases, signs of erythema, edema, and tenderness become apparent. Granulocytes invade the wound within 24 hours and initiate the phagocytosis of necrotic tissue and bacteria. Fibroblasts migrate to the wound and multiply, producing a bed of collagen. This phase of healing lasts from the moment of injury to day 3 or 4 after the traumatic event.[31]

The Proliferative Phase.
The proliferative phase of healing occurs approximately 4 to 20 days after injury. The key cell in this phase of healing, the fibroblast, rapidly synthesizes collagen. Collagen synthesis provides the needed strength for a healing wound. Epithelial cells migrate across the wound bed. After these cells contact each other, the wound is covered. This process is known as *epithelialization*. Myofibroblasts also play a role in healing by pulling down the wound edge toward the center in an effort to close the wound; this process is known as *wound contraction*.[31]

The Maturation Phase.
The maturation phase of healing occurs from approximately 20 days after injury to longer than 1 year after injury. During this period, the wound develops tensile strength as collagen deposits form scar tissue. Regardless of how well collagen realigns itself, the tissue of the wound will never regain the degree of strength or intactness inherent in uninjured tissue. Over time, scar tissue matures and becomes smaller and less bulky, and pigmentation returns.[31]

IMPAIRED TISSUE INTEGRITY

Management of the burn wound is the top priority after the resuscitation phase. The depth of the burn wound is the principal determinant of wound management. Expedient closure of the wounds decreases the potential for many complications, such as fluid and electrolyte imbalances, loss of proteins and nitrogen, and infection. The major goal of burn wound care is wound closure. Initial débridement is done by removal of blisters and loose skin. The assessment of wound depth by the clinician guides the treatment based on whether the wound will close in a reasonable time with daily dressings or will require surgical débridement. The assessment of wound depth can be a difficult challenge. There are many alternative dressing regimens for wound closure that are temporary, semipermanent, or permanent (discussed later). Several objectives must be met for optimal wound closure: control of infection through meticulous cleansing and débridement, promotion of reepithelialization, and preparation of the wound for grafting and closure. Other goals are reduction of scarring and contracture formation and providing patient comfort with appropriate psychological support and pharmacologic intervention.

Factors Affecting Healing of the Burn Wound.
Prompt application of topical antimicrobial therapy is important to prevent bacterial contamination, and the agent is selected based on the depth and location of burn injury. Sources of contamination include the patient's endogenous flora found on the skin, the upper respiratory tract, and the gastrointestinal tract. Exogenous flora found in the patient care setting include bacteria carried by staff members and present in the environment. Patient-specific factors that predispose the patient to infection include age, diabetes, steroid therapy, extreme obesity, severe malnutrition, and infections in remote sites. Because wound healing and clinical infection are inflammatory responses, it is essential to differentiate between normal wound inflammation in the presence of colonization of microorganisms and that of invading organisms. In diagnosing infection, the importance of microbiologic results must be evaluated in conjunction with clinical findings such as excessive erythema, edema, pain, and purulence. "Wound infection may lead to septicemia that may not only consume additional resources but may be associated with significant morbidity and mortality despite the advances in burn care."[32] Clinical findings in conjunction with burn wound biopsy or culture results determine the diagnosis of wound sepsis. Other factors that affect wound healing are tissue hypoxia from low blood flow to the burn wound, presence of eschar that will require débridement, exudate on the wound that can be harmful to the granulating wound or consume

oxygen in the wound, and trauma to the wound from daily dressing changes or lack of protection from the outside environment.

Wound Cleansing. A variety of equally appropriate methods can be used to cleanse burn wounds (e.g., sterile normal saline at the bedside, tap water in a hydrotherapy room). At some centers, a mild antimicrobial cleansing agent is used, such as chlorhexidine (Hibiclens). Wounds are gently cleansed with a gauze dressing or washcloth and patted dry before application of topical agents. Hydrotherapy facilitates the removal of debris and loose eschar. Denatured protein–rich pseudoeschar should be cleansed daily because it can slow healing and limit the innate ability of growth factors.[33] Daily cleansing and inspection of the wound and unburned skin are performed to assess for signs of healing and local infection. Wound care exposure is limited as much as feasible to prevent hypothermia and decrease exposure to bacteria. Measures to reduce pain and hypothermia are used. Patients must receive adequate premedication with analgesics, opiates, and sedatives.[17,18] The patient's vital signs are carefully monitored during this time, especially body temperature and blood pressure. Spray tables and specially designed upright and chair showers are the most commonly used methods to assist in the removal of topical agents and débridement.[9]

Wound Care. Although many options for burn wound care are available, the basic principle of maintaining a moist wound environment while preventing wound infection is the standard of care. Benefits include preventing wound desiccation, optimal function of local wound growth factors and proteolytic enzymes to remove dead tissue, increased reepitheliazation and collagen synthesis, and decreased wound fluid loss. The most common regimen for burn wound care continues to involve the application of a topical antimicrobial agent, followed by a primary gauze dressing to absorb burn wound drainage and an outer layer to provide increased absorption, compression, and occlusion.[4]

Another method consists of covering the wound with a thin layer of gauze or nonadherent dressing that can be impregnated with a petroleum product, with or without a topical antimicrobial. This method is useful for less severe wounds when the amount of drainage has decreased and wound closure has almost been achieved.

A third method consists of the application of topical agents covered with gauze or a nonadherent dressing, followed by a woven gauze dressing to secure the dressing in place. Advantages to this method include (1) greater ease of patient mobility, (2) decreased likelihood that the agent will be wiped off with movement, (3) decreased risk of infection from outside contamination, and (4) easier positioning of the patient. Disadvantages of this method include (1) the significant amount of nursing time required to change these dressings, (2) the inability to assess the wound directly except during the dressing change, (3) the increased risk of impaired peripheral circulation,[9] (4) increased costs for dressings, and (5) the length of sedation.

Topical Antibiotic Therapy. Burn injuries destroy the function of the skin's protective mechanism, including that of the sebaceous glands. Sebaceous glands normally secrete sebum, which contains fatty acids, including oleic acid. In addition to lubricating the skin, sebum is believed to help destroy some microorganisms, such as streptococci and some strains of staphylococci. Serum is lost from damaged capillaries, providing a rich nutritional medium for bacterial colonization. Topical antibiotic agents are used to control this colonization. Effective antibacterial agents should control colonization so that specimens for wound biopsy reveal fewer than 10^{23} microorganisms per gram of tissue. More than 10^{23} microorganisms per gram of tissue makes control of wound sepsis with topical antibiotics questionable. Oral or intravenous therapy may then be considered. Topical antibiotics selected must meet several criteria; side effects must be minimal; resistant strains must not develop with use; application must be easy and rapid; and use must be relatively economical. The most commonly used topical antibiotics are silver sulfadiazine (SSD), mafenide acetate cream (Sulfamylon), bacitracin ointment, and silver impregnated into the primary dressing[4,33,34] (Table 41-2).

SSD (Silvadene cream) is a broad-spectrum antimicrobial agent with bactericidal action against many gram-negative and gram-positive bacteria associated with burn-wound infection. It is a thick white cream that is applied once or twice daily to a wound that has not been grafted, according to the burn unit protocol.[34] To provide antimicrobial benefit, sustained release of silver is necessary. This is achieved with moisture provided by the wound exudate that may give the SSD cream layer a yellow-gray pseudo-eschar.[34] The old SSD layer must be removed by mechanical friction by a clean washcloth, soft bristle brush or sterile tongue-blade, prior to a new application.[34] The SSD cream removal is often painful for the patient, although reapplication of a new SSD layer is not. SSD does not penetrate eschar as readily as mafenide acetate.[34] A common side effect of silver sulfadiazine is leukopenia resulting from bone marrow suppression, which may develop 24 to 72 hours after application. SSD is indicated for use with partial- and full-thickness wounds and is the most commonly used topical antimicrobial agent used to treat burn wounds.[4]

Mafenide acetate cream penetrates through burn eschar and is bacteriostatic against many gram-negative and gram-positive organisms.[34] Its use is limited because the application is uncomfortable for the patient as it creates a burning sensation, and it is rapidly absorbed, requiring dressing changes two or three times daily. It is used routinely for coverage of small wounds involving anatomic areas that contain cartilage, such as the ears and nose.[34] Metabolic acidosis can result from the use of mafenide acetate. The patient must be observed closely for hyperventilation (see Table 41-2).

A 5% mafenide acetate solution is less painful on application than cream, and it is iso-osmolar and less desiccating to the burn wound. Gauze dressings are saturated with the solution and then applied over the burn wound and remoistened as needed. The eschar penetration of the solution and the antimicrobial benefits are superior to SSD, but it does not provide fungal coverage.

Bacitracin ointment is a topical agent applied to superficial burns and facial burns. Bacitracin is effective against gram-positive organisms but not gram-negative organisms or fungus. The open method of wound care is required with the use of bacitracin to prevent yeast overgrowth. One benefit of the open method is better visualization.

Silver ions are antimicrobial and silver coated dressings are recent additions to the topical wound care arsenal.[34,35] Specialist products include the Acticoat dressings that deliver nanocrysatlline-silver and remain in place for several days. The dressngs are moistened at least once each day as the moisture causes the release of silver ions into the burn wound, and the Acticoat dressings are changed only every three to four days.[34] Aquacel Ag, fiber dressings with silver are changed every other day or when nonadherent to the burn wound.[34,35] Other options are Contreet hydrocolloid dressing with silver, and foam dressing with silver.[35] These treatments provide a means to optimize burn wound healing while decreasing the frequency of dressing changes and associated pain for burned pateints.[34,35]

A Cochrane systematic review of dressing products for superficial and partial thickness burn wounds reported a shorter wound healing time, fewer dressing changes and consequently fewer pain-experience opportunities with hydrocolloid dressings, antimicrobial dressings with silver as the active ingredient, silicon dressings, nylon polyurethane film and biosynthetic dressings

compared to SSD cream.[35] The conclusion was that SSD cream use needs to be reconsidered as a treatment for superficial and partial thickness burn wounds as it was associated with delayed time to healing and more dressing changes than other products reviewed.[35]

Wound Débridement. Mid-dermal and deep-dermal wounds require removal of eschar for wound healing and closure. *Eschar* is the nonviable tissue that forms after the burn injury. This tissue has no blood supply, and polymorphonuclear leukocytes, antibodies, and systemic antibodies cannot reach these areas. Eschar provides an excellent medium for bacterial growth, and it is vital that burn wounds be cleansed daily and loose eschar débrided as necessary. Débridement has two major aims: (1) removal of tissue contaminated by foreign bodies and bacteria, thereby protecting patients from invasive infection, and (2) removal of devitalized tissue. The three types of débridement are mechanical, enzymatic, and surgical.

Mechanical Débridement. Mechanical débridement involves the use of scissors and forceps to gently lift and trim loose, necrotic tissue (Fig. 41-10). Experienced nurses and physicians

TABLE 41-2 Pharmacologic Management: Topical Antimicrobial Agents

AGENT	ADVANTAGES	DISADVANTAGES	IMPLICATIONS
Silver sulfadiazine	Painless application Broad spectrum Easy application Rare sensitivities	May produce transient leukopenia by bone marrow suppression Minimal eschar penetration Some gram-negative resistance	Monitor white cell count Observe wounds for tunneling and subeschar infection Monitor culture reports
Mafenide acetate cream	Broad spectrum (esp. *Pseudomonas* coverage) Easy application Penetrates eschar	Painful application Rare acid-base imbalance Frequent sensitivities	Provide adequate analgesia Monitor arterial blood gases Observe for hyperventilation Observe for rashes
Bacitracin	Painless application Nonirritating Transparent Nontoxic	No eschar penetration No gram-negative or fungal coverage	
Pure silver	Painless application Broad spectrum, including fungus and resistant organisms Rare sensitivity Less frequent dressing changes	Keep moist with sterile water, not saline	Maintain dry linens No reported side effects

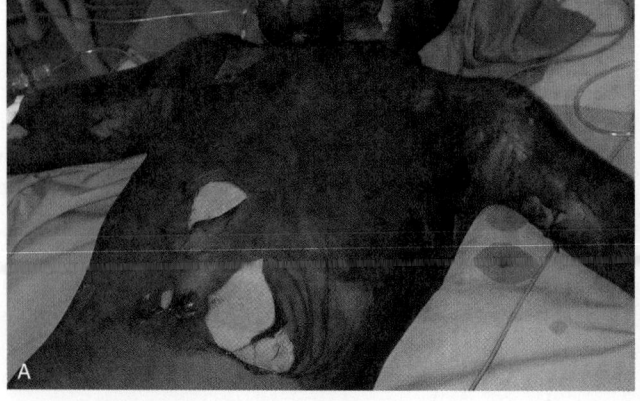
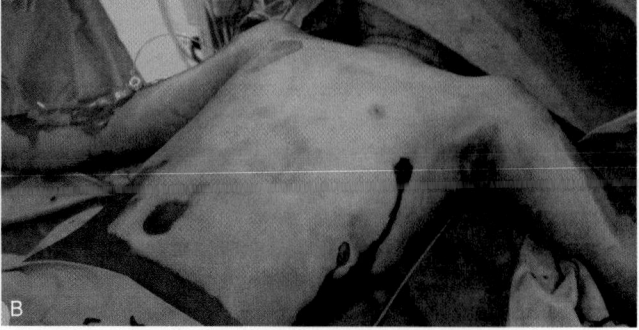

Figure 41-10 Anterior trunk and bilateral arm burn. *A,* Before mechanical débridement. *B,* After mechanical débridement.

perform this procedure. Sterile gauze may be used in the form of a wet-to-dry or wet-to-wet dressing to further débride the wound bed.

Enzymatic Débridement. Enzymatic débridement involves the topical application of proteolytic substances to the wound bed. These agents are useful in softening eschar and dissolving devitalized tissue. They promote the separation of eschar, which can lead to earlier wound closure.

Surgical Débridement. An experienced surgeon performs surgical débridement in the operating room. The goal of débridement is to remove nonviable tissue down to bleeding viable tissue with an electric dermatome or surgical knife.

Skin Substitutes. To assist in wound closure, many temporary and permanent skin substitute dressings have gained popularity throughout the United States. A wide variety of products is available. Each dressing has specific indications for use. Temporary substitutes are designed for placement on partial-thickness or clean, excised wounds, and permanent substitutes provide a permanent skin replacement.

Skin substitutes must possess properties that mimic the native epidermis and dermis. This involves a bilayer that has a collagen network that adheres to the wound bed with a protective synthetic outer layer. They are made from a variety of synthetic materials such as nylon, polyurethane, or solid silicone polymers. Skin barrier substitutes must possess several properties to accomplish their desired effect as a temporary wound covering to protect the granulating tissue and to preserve a clean, viable wound surface for future autografting (Box 41-2). The most important property of these materials is adherence so that the skin substitute can simulate the function of the skin. Adherence must be uniform to prevent fluid accumulation beneath the surface of the substitute, which can lead to bacterial proliferation.

For application of skin substitutes, the wound must be clean, and ideally, it should have a bacterial count of less than 10^5 organisms per gram of tissue. The burn wound must be free from eschar, and hemostasis must exist. Eschar and blood provide an excellent medium for bacterial proliferation, and the presence of blood may interfere with adherence. The surface is cleaned and rinsed with saline solution, and the skin barrier substitutes must be applied according to established procedures using sterile techniques.

BOX 41-2   IDEAL PROPERTIES OF SKIN SUBSTITUTES

- Adherence
- Decreased pain
- Easy application and removal
- Intact bacterial barrier
- Shelf storage capability
- Inexpensive in relation to alternatives
- Nonantigenic
- Similar to normal skin in transport of water vapor
- Elastic and durable
- Hemostatic
- Decreased protein and electrolyte loss
- Enhanced natural healing processes

Temporary Skin Substitutes

Polyurethane Film. A transparent adhesive-coated dressing that is applied directly to the burn wound, and is impermeable to bacteria and liquid. Polyurethane film is used primarily to cover donor sites, but some practitioners report using it over some partial-thickness burn wounds. It is suitable for light exudate wounds.[35] However, fluid can collect under the dressing in large quantities. When fluid collects, it often leaks and decreases the adherence of the dressing. The fluid can be removed with a needle and syringe, but the needle puncture must be patched afterward with a small piece of polyurethane film.

Biosynthetic Dressing. A semipermeable, biosynthetic, temporary wound dressing that is composed of nylon and a Silastic membrane combined with a collagen derivative can be used on several types of wounds, including partial-thickness burns and wounds, granulating wounds, and donor sites, and over split-thickness grafts. These wounds must be clean or débrided to healthy tissue before application.

A biosynthetic dressing has elasticity in all directions and conforms well to surfaces that are difficult to dress, such as the face, breasts, joints, and axilla. Because of its porosity, it allows the passage of some topical antibiotics to penetrate its membrane, reducing the bacterial count of the burn wound. A biosynthetic dressing may be applied after daily cleaning at the bedside or in the operating room. It is applied with the dull or nylon mesh side facing the wound. It can be held in place with a gauze dressing, and the area is immobilized for 24 to 48 hours, depending on the site, until adherence occurs. If fluid or air accumulates under the biosynthetic skin, it may be slit and the fluid expressed. If a large amount of fluid accumulates, the biosynthetic skin is removed and replaced. Biosynthetic skin initially adheres to the wound fibrin, which binds to the collagen and nylon backing of the material. Later, the cells migrate into the nylon mesh and further bind to the wound. As the wound heals, the dressing turns opaque and should be trimmed or peeled back. If bleeding occurs on removal, the dressing should be left in place and reevaluated for removal in a few days.

Hydrocolloidal Dressings. Hydrocolloidal dressings are oxygen-impermeable, waterproof occlusive dressings that are composed of an outer layer of polyurethane foam and an inner layer of hydrocolloid polymer complex. Hydrocolloid dressings are indicated for use on partial-thickness wounds. The dressing does not adhere to the wound bed; therefore, it does not damage new epithelium and decreases pain. Hydrocolloid dressings can absorb large amounts of exudate that produces an odor. Advantages of hydrocolloid dressings include rapid healing times and decreased pain. A disadvantage is the inability to visualize the wound bed.

Fear of bacterial proliferation limits the use temporary skin substitutes. None of these skin substitutes has antimicrobial properties. However, they can be used in conjunction with an antimicrobial agent.

DEFINITIVE BURN WOUND CLOSURE

The primary goal of burn wound management is wound closure during the acute phase. Full thickness (third-degree) burns are most often treated by excision and grafting.[36] If a burn wound does not heal in 10 to 14 days, excision should be undertaken to improve functional and cosmetic results, to decrease in-hospital time, and to reduce the cost of burn care.[4,36,37] Surgical débridement may begin as early as 3 to 5 days after the burn insult,[34] as soon as hemodynamic stability has been achieved. Some physicians operate within 24 hours of admission if the patient is hemodynamically stable. Typically, excision procedures are limited to 20% of the body surface or 2 hours of operating time. In patients with massive burns, excision procedures are commonly staged, requiring the patient to return to the operating room every 2 to 3 days until all wounds have been excised. This technique helps avoid excessive transfusions and limits the physiologic stress.[34]

Autografting with the patient's own skin from a donor site, is the preferred choice for wound closure. However, with large TBSA burns, availability of donor sites can be problematic. When an autograft is not available, many alternate methods are used to achieve this goal. Creative attempts have been initiated to establish a skin substitute that permanently closes the wound in a cosmetically and functionally acceptable fashion. Temporary skin substitutes may be used to provide permanent wound closure, but the process is complex. These bilayer products, such as Integra, involve application to a clean, excised burn wound. After 14 to 21 days, a neodermis is formed, and a thin epidermal autograft is placed. This is an area of evolving technology. These materials temporarily restore the protective barrier that the skin provides naturally. Skin substitutes can be used until the patient's own skin is available for harvesting. Previously used and healed donor sites can be used again in later return visits to the operating room.[36] Table 41-3 reviews advantages and disadvantages of different graft types.

Autograft. An autograft is a skin graft harvested from a healthy, uninjured donor site on the burn patient and then placed over the patient's burn wound to provide permanent coverage of the wound. Autografts are the only grafts that provide permanent wound coverage. Preferred sites for obtaining these grafts are the thighs, back, and abdomen; however, grafts can be harvested from almost anywhere on the body.

Surgical excision is performed to mechanically remove necrotic tissue from the burn wound; it may be performed tangentially or fascially. Tangential excision involves sequentially excising the eschar down to bleeding, viable tissue and then placing a split-thickness skin graft over the wound. Fascial excision is used when the wounds are deep and the fat does not appear viable.[36] Surgical intervention with split-thickness skin grafts often yields a better cosmetic result than does the natural healing process in deep, partial- and full-thickness injuries.

Sheets of the patient's epidermis and a partial layer of the dermis are harvested with use of a dermatome. These grafts are referred to as *split-thickness skin grafts* and can be applied to the wound bed as a sheet or in meshed form (Fig. 41-11).

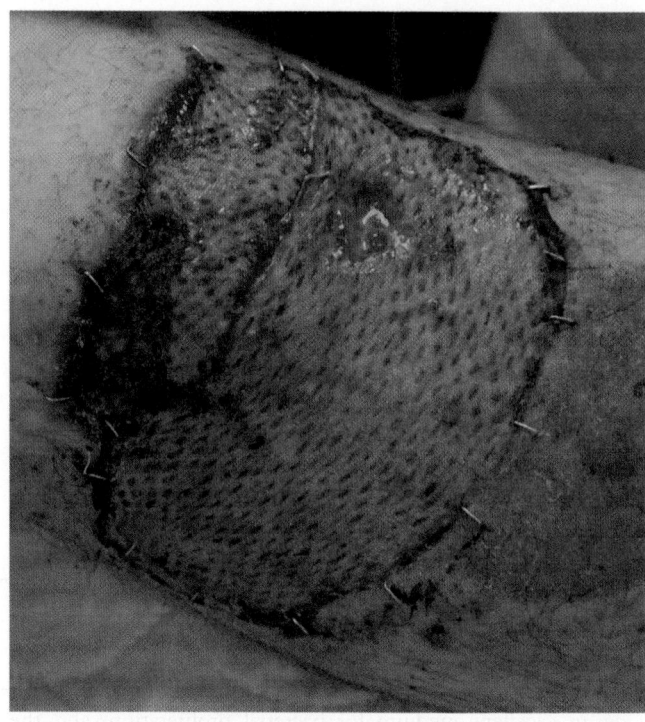

Figure 41-11 Split-thickness skin graft applied to the left thigh with staples.

TABLE 41-3 **Types of Grafts**			
Graft	**Use**	**Advantages**	**Disadvantages**
Autograft	Provides permanent coverage of burn wounds Used in sheets or meshed form	Permanent coverage Nonantigenic Least expensive Meshing allows a small amount of tissue to cover a large area	Lack of available donor sites, which may delay wound coverage Donor sites are painful partial-thickness wounds Must be done in surgical suite
Homograft (allograft)	Temporary wound coverage	Can be placed at bedside or in operating room Allows for vascularization over deep wound Provides better control over bacterial growth than xenograft	Possibility of disease transmission Antigenic; body rejects in approximately 2 weeks Not readily available to all burn centers Expensive Requires rigorous quality controls
Heterograph (xenograft)	Temporary wound coverage	Longer shelf life than allograft Can be meshed or comes in a variety of sizes	Antigenic; body rejects in 3 to 4 days Potential for digestion by wound collagenase, leading to increased chance of infection

The split-thickness skin grafts harvested are approximately twelve thousandths of an inch thick. The split-thickness skin graft can be meshed 1.5:1 to 4:1 in a mesher and then placed on the wounds.[4] The size of the mesh is based on the areas requiring grafting and the availability of donor skin. This meshing prevents serum accumulation under the graft and permits coverage of a surface area larger than its original surface. Grafts that are placed on the face, neck, lower portions of the arms, and hands are sheet grafts when possible. Grafts that are meshed can cover more area but may not produce the cosmetic appearance desired, and they therefore usually are placed on areas covered by clothing.

The grafts can be secured with sutures, fibrin glue, or staples. The choice of dressing that is placed over the graft varies widely based on physician and institution preference. One choice is fine mesh gauze impregnated with an emollient. It is placed over the graft, covered with a heavy gauze dressing, and secured to the patient with or without a splint, depending on the anatomic area of the graft. A vacuum-assisted closure (VAC) device provides a safe and effective method for securing split-thickness skin grafts, and it is associated with improved graft survival.[38] Negative wound pressure therapy can be used to secure the autograft in place. Trained nursing professionals or physicians remove the dressings on postoperative day 3 to 5 for assessment. Graft adherence and survival can be assessed in 48 to 72 hours. Autograft sites are assessed for adherence, presence of infection, and closure of interstices. Nurses, in collaboration with the multidisciplinary team, provide proper positioning, splinting, and pain management in the postoperative period.

Care of the donor site is equally important because it represents a wound similar to that of a partial-thickness injury. Donor sites can be covered with many different types of dressings. Some examples of donor site dressings include fine mesh gauze, Tegaderm, Acticoat, and Xeroform. The gauze is trimmed as it separates from the healing donor site over the next 10 days. These dressings should not be removed forcibly, because this would interfere with the reepitheliazation process and cause considerable pain.

Great care must be taken not to disturb the graft. Mobilization of the graft area usually occurs around the first dressing change on postoperative day 3 to 5 according to the surgeon's preference.

Biosynthetic Skin Substitutes. Skin substitutes include homografts (allografts) and heterografts (xenografts). *Homograft skin* can be obtained from live or deceased donors (cadaver skin). The homograft is harvested from cadaver skin and, with advances in cryopreservation, can be frozen and stored in a tissue bank. Because it is possible to transmit disease through the application of a homograft, tissue banks must adhere to strict guidelines. Before application, homograft skin is tested for a variety of transmissible diseases, including the human immunodeficiency virus (HIV) and hepatitis B surface antigens. Homograft skin can be applied as a biologic dressing for débridement at the bedside or as temporary wound coverage on excised burn wounds. The patient's wound readily accepts the homograft. Vascular ingrowth occurs, and the homograft seals the wound and protects it from bacterial invasion; however, it is rejected

approximately 2 weeks after its application. Homografts must be handled and applied very carefully. They must be placed with the shiny surface down and must be wrinkle-free. They must neither overlap each other nor lap over infected areas or uninjured areas. The grafts can be dressed with a nonadherent agent that usually is not changed for 24 to 48 hours.

Disadvantages include the homograft antigenicity, lack of accessibility, difficulties with storage and quality control, expense of procurement, and possibility of disease transmission from the donor. The microbiologic cleanliness of the cadaver skin is of extreme concern because of the burn patient's debilitated immunologic condition. Homografts are harvested during the first 4 hours after death, and they are taken from the abdomen, thighs, and back. Partial-thickness grafts are obtained, leaving the graft sites looking as if they were sunburned. Homografts usually are available only in centers in which the rigorous processing procedure can be achieved. These centers usually have skin and tissue bank facilities. Procurement of the allograft is much the same as for any other donated organ. The public, however, is not as well educated about the need for this organ as it is about eyes, liver, lung, kidneys, and hearts.

The *xenograft* (heterograft) is a graft transferred between two different species to provide temporary wound coverage. The most common and widely accepted xenograft is pigskin (porcine skin). Pigskin is available in frozen and shelf forms, with each type having a much longer storage life than an allograft. Depending on how the pigskin was prepared, it can have a shelf life of 1 month to 1 year. The pigskin is packaged in a variety of ways and in various sizes. It can be treated with silver sulfadiazine and can be meshed or nonmeshed. Pigskin can be used for temporary coverage of full- and partial-thickness wounds, burn wounds, and donor sites. It meets many of the ideal skin substitute properties mentioned previously. It has two disadvantages; it is antigenic, and it has the potential for being digested by the wound collagenase, possibly leading to infection.

Pigskin is applied in the same manner as a homograft. If the pigskin was frozen, it is thawed in a warm bath of saline solution. If it has been treated with silver sulfadiazine, it is thawed in water. The pigskin is placed on the wound with the dermal side down (the dermal side faces the center of the roll); it may be distinguished by its tendency to curl toward the dermal surface when held up at one end. Shelf-stored pigskin may be applied with either side to the wound. After the pigskin is in place, it may be dressed with antibacterial-impregnated dressings or other forms of dressings. Pigskin usually is removed or dissolves because of lack of blood supply in 5 to 7 days. If sloughing or purulent drainage occurs, the xenograft is removed (see Table 41-3).

Synthetic Skin. The lack of available donor sites for major burn injury often delays wound closure. In an effort to minimize infection and to promote healing, many attempts have been made to develop skin substitutes that will seal the wound in a functional and cosmetically acceptable fashion. Integra with a ultrathin layer of epidermal autograft has been used successfully.[40] A technique that involves the growth and subsequent graft placement of cultured epithelial autograft (CEA) has become an adjunct to the treatment of burn wounds.

A complex process that allows for separation of keratinocytes is performed. The CEA is grown over a period of 2 to 3 weeks to achieve a graft size of 25 cm². This represents an expansion of 50 to 70 times the original specimen. These confluent sheets of cultured epithelial cells are attached to a gauze backing and placed on the wound. The published results reveal that graft acceptance is unpredictable because the CEA lacks dermis. Even when grafts take initially, graft loss can occur later. Compared with other methods, the CEA also is more fragile, and the technique is quite costly. This therapy is being recommended as an adjunct for traditional split-thickness skin graft, and it continues to be investigated and combined with newer dermal skin substitutes.

Long-Term Postgraft Wound Care. Tiny water blisters often form 2 to 6 weeks after wound closure. These blisters usually open and heal without incident in 3 to 5 days. These areas must be kept clean with mild soap and covered with a bland ointment. For 6 to 8 weeks, a mild, nonalcohol-based skin cream is applied every 4 hours to these areas to lubricate the skin until natural lubrication occurs. Pruritus is common in the maturing burn wound. Patients can be relieved of this discomfort by the administration of an antipruritic agent, such as diphenhydramine hydrochloride, doxepin hydrochloride (5%), or hydroxyzine and by the application of moisturizing creams.

Another concern in burn wound healing is the prevention or reduction of hypertrophic scarring. Its prevention or reduction depends on the timely application of uniform pressure. Hypertrophic scarring can be controlled with the use of tubular support bandages applied within 5 to 7 days after the graft. Bandages are available in a variety of sizes and have the advantage of applying pressure to selected body areas while allowing the remaining burned area to heal sufficiently. They are readily available for immediate use during the wait for the commercial manufacture of the customized elastic pressure garment for long-term use, which can take up to 3 or 4 weeks.

Tubular support bandages apply tension in the medium range of 10 to 20 mm Hg. Tensions lower than this do not exert adequate pressure to control scarring, and higher tensions tend to cause edema in the distal parts of the extremities and may be too abrasive for newly grafted skin. Tension can be elevated if needed by placing silicone foam under the tubular support bandages over areas such as the axilla and knees.

Custom-made elastic pressure garments are worn for 6 months to 1 year after grafting. It is important to assess children for pressure points as weight is gained and as growth occurs. It is necessary to assess the garment for elasticity over time, because elasticity decreases with washing.

ACUTE PAIN

Pain is an individualized and subjective phenomenon, and it has physiologic and psychological components. A guideline-based approach can be helpful in properly recognizing and treating the pain related to burn injury.[17] Pain after burn injury is complex and includes background pain, breakthrough pain, and procedural pain.[41] Background pain is related to the physiologic changes associated with the burn injury and includes the damage or exposure of the nerve endings within partial-thickness burns and donor sites. Range of motion of the affected limbs and routine activities contribute to background pain. Breakthrough pain is described as episodes of pain more severe than background pain, and it is not relieved by routine pain medications. Procedural pain includes pain caused by interventions such as daily wound care, arterial punctures, chest physical therapy, and the use of splints.[41]

Loss of control, forced dependence, loneliness, and separation from home and family can contribute to anxiety, which heightens the patient's perception of pain. The patient's fears abound in thoughts of disfigurement and loss of love, function, and job. The psychological experience or subjective component may be related to past experiences, anxiety, and altered coping mechanisms. Attention to the psychological component of the patient's pain may lead to useful strategies that decrease perceived pain. If possible, past experiences with pain, hospitalization, and successful coping strategies should be explored. Pain is a psychological and physical experience that accumulates over time and becomes part of the individual's deepest psychology.[42]

Patients with partial-thickness burns experience extreme discomfort. The slightest air current over the surface of the burn may stimulate pain. Covering wounds with topical agents, dressings, and linen significantly decreases the pain. The nerve endings that have been completely destroyed by full-thickness burns are initially insensate but do transmit pain sensation when they regenerate. It is a common misconception that these wounds are painless. Patients may experience deep somatic pain from ischemia or inflammation. Not all wounds are full-thickness injuries; a combination of various wound depths is more common. Wound edges, which transition to less severely burned areas, are hypersensitive.

Pain continues even after healing; some patients describe the itching, tingling, and paresthesias as being as uncomfortable as the initial injury.[41] Paresthesias are abnormal neurologic sensations of numbness, tingling, or burning that can last 1 year or more after injury. It may be a false assumption to believe burn pain decreases over time.[41]

Inadequate pain management is an issue in many burn units because of the fear of opioid side effects and opioid addiction and the lack of pain evaluation or treatment protocols. Initially after burn injury, narcotics are administered intravenously in small doses and titrated to effect. The constant background pain may be addressed with the use of a patient-controlled analgesia device. After hemodynamic stability has occurred and gastrointestinal function has returned, oral narcotics can be useful. Additional premedication and analgesics are necessary during therapeutic procedures. The use of acetaminophen and nonsteroidal antiinflammatory drugs can be useful in patients who are not at risk for bleeding. Anxiolytics and antidepressants also should be considered and used appropriately. The nurse must be flexible with dosing and should assess the effectiveness of medication by using a numerical or visual analog scale. The nurse should assure the patient that pain control issues will be continually addressed.

Nonpharmacologic techniques, such as imagery, hypnosis, distraction, and methods adapted from some of the popular childbirth techniques, can be effective in reducing anxiety and the pain experience. Giving the patient some management control also can reduce anxiety and the perception of pain. The perception of pain often is increased in the patient who is anxious and lacks control of the situation.[36]

Treatment strategies need to be individualized. Failure to adequately treat pain can increase burn hypermetabolism, result in loss of confidence between the burn team and patient, and lead to the development of psychiatric disorders. The nurse should assess and discuss on a regular basis the patient's psychological status and avoid using psychotropics for analgesia and narcotics for anxiety and depression.

A multidisciplinary approach to burn treatment is integral in providing quality care. The burn team should work together to address all needs of the patient and family. The team should meet frequently to review patient care and maximize patient and family support.

IMBALANCED NUTRITION: LESS THAN BODY REQUIREMENTS

The basal metabolic rate of a burn patient may be elevated 40% to 100% above the normal rate, depending on the amount of TBSA involved. The metabolic rate is influenced by the amount of protein and albumin lost through the wounds, the catabolic response associated with stress, associated injuries, fluid loss, fever, infection, immobility, gender, and the height and weight of the patient before the injury.[38]

The goal in nutritional management of the burn patient is to provide adequate calories to enhance wound healing. To achieve this goal, nutritional support and a reduction of energy demand are imperative. Every effort should be made to reduce the release of catecholamines, which increase metabolic rate. Pain, fear, anxiety, and cold stimulate release of catecholamine stores. Appropriate interventions for each of these stimuli must be performed. Examples of nonpharmacologic interventions include early excision and burn wound closure, elevation of the environmental temperature to thermal neutrality (31.5° ± 0.7° C), and high-carbohydrate, high-protein feeds. Pharmacologic interventions include the administration of recombinant human growth hormone, low-dose insulin infusion, and the use of the synthetic testosterone analogue oxandrolone and beta-blockade with propranolol.[41]

The use of enteral and oral routes is preferred in the management of burn patients.[39] Because of the increased nutritional needs of the burn patient, oral feedings are usually inadequate, and supplemental enteral feedings are necessary. Caloric requirements are calculated on the basis of the size of the burn; the age, height, and weight of the patient; and stress factors. Protein and caloric requirements for the burn patient are elevated by a negative nitrogen balance. The daily protein requirement may increase to two to four times the normal 0.8 grams per kilogram of body weight. Carbohydrates and fat are used for energy and to spare proteins required for wound healing.

Daily caloric intake can be 2 to 20 times higher than normal. Vitamins and minerals usually are given in doses higher than normal. Serum albumin, prealbumin, iron, zinc, calcium, phosphate, and potassium values are monitored, and supplements given as indicated by results.[38]

REHABILITATION PHASE

The rehabilitation phase is one of recuperation and healing physically and emotionally. The patient is not acutely ill but may or may not be ready for discharge. This phase can last several years. The patient may require extensive reconstructive surgery. Psychologically, the patient focuses on attaining specific personal goals related to achieving as much preburn function as possible.[25] Minor and major accomplishments must be praised. This phase is characterized by scar management techniques and by physical and occupational therapy.

The burn team and the patient prepare for the transition to the outside world. The use of group therapy is a valuable tool used at many burn centers. Patients, family members, and health care providers express ideas and feelings. Often, burn patients establish priorities and make realistic decisions about their lives. Staff intervention during this phase is primarily one of support.

Impaired Physical Mobility. Tremendous advances have been made during the past 10 to 15 years in the physical care of the burn patient. The survival rate of patients with full-thickness burns greater than 40% of TBSA has increased significantly. Survival of patients with burns greater than 90% of TBSA is not impossible. As patients with larger and deeper burns survive, the challenge to maintain their optimal mobility and cosmetic appearance has been met with increased success. Rehabilitation needs must be addressed early in burn care. Nursing prescriptions for range-of-motion exercises, positioning, splinting, ambulation, and activities of daily living are initiated within the first 48 hours of hospitalization.

Despite the advances in other areas of burn care, contractures still develop after a burn injury. Contractures develop because of a variety of factors: the extent, depth, location, and configuration of the burn; the position of comfort the patient most frequently assumes; the relative underlying muscle strength; and the patient's motivation and compliance. The affected body parts should be positioned to prevent long-term deformity. Frequent change of position also is important and may need to be performed as often as every hour. Burn patients are at greater risk for pressure sores than the general hospital population, as well as the possible conversion of their partial-thickness burns to full-thickness burns.

Splints can be used to prevent or correct contracture or to immobilize joints after grafting. If splints are used, they must be checked daily for proper fit and effectiveness. Splints that are used to immobilize body parts after grafting must be left on at all times, except to assess the graft site for pressure points during every shift. Splints to correct severe contracture may be off for 2 hours per shift to allow burn care and range-of-motion exercises. Mild contracture may be kept in splints for 4 hours and out of splints for 4 hours to promote exercise and mobility.

Active exercise is encouraged and is preferred, although active-assisted or gentle-passive exercises also may be an important part of the rehabilitation program. Active exercise maintains muscle mass, aids in restoring protein structures within the muscle tissue, aids in venous and lymphatic return, and reduces the risk of pulmonary embolus and deep vein thrombosis. The patient's tolerance must be carefully evaluated. The number of repetitions of an exercise is proportional to the degree of anticipated contracture and the patient's tolerance. Anticipation of the patient's pain also must be carefully considered. Before range-of-motion exercises and activities of daily living are performed, the need for pain medication must be assessed.[12] Nursing diagnoses for the burn patient are summarized in the Nursing Diagnoses feature on Burn Injury.

Outpatient Burn Care. Outpatient burn care must be considered for minor burns. It is cost-effective and removes the potential for a wound infection by endemic, drug-resistant microorganisms within the hospital environment. The hospital environment also changes many of the self-care routines, such as diet, family contact, hygiene, and coping mechanisms. However, patients considered for outpatient burn care must be screened carefully. Nursing evaluation of the patient or family, or both, includes consideration of motivation, willingness to participate in care, ability to understand and perform the necessary procedures, potential aversions to wound care or dressing changes, and reliability of transportation. Medical considerations include hemodynamic stabilization, nutritional status, fluid and electrolyte balance, adequate pain control, and ruling out complications.[42]

A clean, synthetic antimicrobial agent can be applied to help reduce dressing change frequency. Home health nurses are helpful in monitoring these patients. If epithelialization of these wounds has not occurred in 2 to 3 weeks, use of primary excision and grafting must be considered.

To check for evidence of scarring, partial-thickness injuries must be monitored until epithelialization has occurred. If scarring occurs, compression dressings must be fitted and worn until the wound becomes quiescent, which requires 12 to 18 months.

Support of the Burn Patient. Burn injuries are physically and psychologically traumatic and life altering for the patient. The family of the burn patient is also affected, and their needs should be remembered during the healing process. There is often guilt associated with burn injuries, especially when the victim is a child. It is important for the clinical providers to support the burn patient in all aspects. As health care providers, we heal and support the patient throughout the hospital stay but often forget that the survivor's biggest challenges may still lie ahead after hospitalization. Many survivors have stated that they wish they could take the hospital staff home with them to help them transition into the community.[26]

Many resources are available to help the burn survivor cope after they are home and should be provided by the hospital team during their inpatient stay. Programs exist to help with issues such as social and school reentry, support for sexual considerations, and dealing with scars. These resources are needed at different times of the recovery process.[26] The clinical team and the community must collaborate to improve burn survivor transition and support.

STRESSORS OF BURN NURSING

Burn units are fascinating environments in which to work. They offer the fast-paced, high-technology atmosphere of any critical care setting; the complexity of advanced nursing management; and the dynamics of an interdisciplinary, collaborative model of practice. However, all of these elements combined contribute to a potentially stressful work environment for the nurse. The physical environment can be a difficult one in which to work for a variety of reasons. The amount of equipment necessary to maintain the patient can be overwhelming and can limit the workspace dramatically. The temperature of the room usually is kept at approximately 85° F and can become much warmer, depending on the amount of equipment in the room. Odors vary and can be very unpleasant. Noise levels within a unit also are distressing. Self-care and care of other nurses and staff are issues just as important as care of the patient and family. The decision to specialize in burn nursing is a meaningful and an important one.

Nursing Diagnoses

Burn Injury

- Impaired Gas Exchange related to ventilation/perfusion mismatching
- Ineffective Airway Clearance related to excessive secretions or abnormal viscosity of mucus
- Deficient Fluid Volume related to relative loss
- Risk for Infection risk factors: invasive lines, immunodeficiencies
- Acute Confusion related to sensory overload, sensory deprivation, sleep pattern disturbance
- Disturbed Body Image related to actual change in body structure, function, or appearance
- Powerlessness related to physical deterioration despite compliance

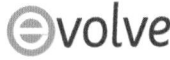

Brief Patient History

Ms. J is a 23-year-old victim of a house fire. She jumped out of a window approximately 6 feet off the ground to get out of the burning house. The paramedics at the scene reported she was alert and oriented but hysterical. She has a 4-year-old son who was rescued by firefighters and is not injured. She is allergic to penicillin but has no other medical or surgical history.

Clinical Assessment

Ms. J is sent from the emergency department to your trauma unit. She is intubated and sedated on arrival. Her face, ears, upper chest, arms, and back have partial-thickness burns, and she has a full-thickness burn to her forehead. Her breath sounds are auscultated as present bilaterally, but she is wheezing, and her sputum has a dark carbon appearance. She has a triple-lumen catheter in her right femoral vein with good blood return to all ports.

Diagnostic Procedures

Ms. J has a carboxyhemoglobin level of 3.4% and arterial blood gas values as follows: pH of 7.27, $Paco_2$ of 29 mm Hg, Pao_2 of 313 mm Hg, HCO_3^- of 14 mEq/L (mmol/L), and O_2 saturation of 88% on 100% Fio_2. Her serum cyanide level is 45 mmol/L. The chest radiograph obtained on arrival in the emergency department was normal. Her blood pressure is 85/50 mm Hg, heart rate is 136 beats/min (sinus tachycardia), respiratory rate is 14 breaths/min, and temperature is 96.3° F.

Medical Diagnosis

Ms. J is diagnosed with burns covering 50% of her total body surface area (TBSA), inhalation injury, and cyanide toxicity.

Questions

1. What major outcomes do you expect to achieve for this patient?
2. What problems or risks must be managed to achieve these outcomes?
3. What interventions must be initiated to monitor, prevent, manage, or eliminate the problems and risks identified?
4. What interventions should be initiated to promote optimal functioning, safety, and well-being of the patient?
5. What possible learning needs do you anticipate for this patient?
6. What cultural and age-related factors may have a bearing on the patient's plan of care?

Summary

- Burn care is highly complex, and decisions regarding appropriate management of burn injuries are best managed by certified burn centers. At a certified burn center, the most accurate burn size estimates can be made. Burn size, types of injury, location of the burn, and the patient's age and history are all determinants of survival.

- Size and depth of burns are divided into four main categories: (1) superficial (first-degree) burns, which are injuries to epidermis; (2) partial-thickness (second-degree) burns, which involve the epidermis and dermis of the skin; (3) deep-dermal, partial thickness (second-degree) burns, which involve the entire epidermal layer of the skin and part of the dermis; and (4) full-thickness (third-degree) burns, which involve destruction of skin layers from the epidermis down to and including the subcutaneous tissue.

- Accurate fluid resuscitation of a burn patient for more severe burn injuries (>10% of TBSA) is crucial in to prevent acute kidney injury that may result in acute kidney failure, cardiovascular collapse, and death from burn shock. The Parkland formula is a guide for determining resuscitation fluid (Ringer's lactate) volume. Overresuscitation is also a concern, because it can lead to increased edema formation. Careful assessment of the burn patient's intake and output is critical to achieve the optimal patient response to fluid resuscitation.

- After the resuscitative phase of burn patients, the acute care phase of wound healing, wound closure, and prevention of infection begins. This hypermetabolic phase can be complicated by wound infection and sepsis. Careful assessment for early wound excision and possibly skin grafting procedures versus local wound care, nutritional support needs, and infection control practices during admission affect the outcomes of the burn patient in this phase. The nutritional needs of burn patients are one to two times the normal calorie and protein needs, and supplements and supplemental tube feedings are often needed for these patients.

- The gold standard of burn wound care includes the application of a topical antimicrobial agent, followed by a gauze dressing to absorb excess drainage, with an outer layer to provide increased absorption, compression, and occlusion. Silver dressings have shown positive results in the prevention of bacterial growth without silver toxicity.

- The rehabilitative phase of the burn patient care starts from admission of the burn-injured patient and may last years, depending on future surgical procedures, therapy needs, contracture prevention, and psychological or emotional needs of the patient. Support of the patient is provided over the long term by local support groups, written information on handling of stress or anxiety, and visits from past burn survivors. All of the multidisciplinary needs of burn-injured patients need to be addressed for them to be able to perform in and feel accepted back into society.

References

1. Lancaster BA et al.: National Burn Repository 2006: A ten year review, *J Burn Care Res* 28(5):635-658, 2007.
2. American Burn Association: Fact sheet (2007). Available at www.ameriburn.org (accessed May 2009).
3. Pereira C et al.: Outcome measures in burn care: is mortality dead? *Burns* 30(8) 2004.
4. Edlich R et al.: Burns, thermal (2008). Available at http://emedicine.medscape.com/article/1278244-overview (accessed May 2009).
5. Demling RH et al: Burn wound module. Part IV. Burn wound: histological assessment (zones of injury). Available at www.burnsurgery.org (accessed May 2009).
6. Williams WG, Phillips LG: Pathophysiology of the burn wound. In Herndon DN, editor: *Total burn care*, ed 2, London, Saunders, 2002.
7. Hettiaratchy S, Dziewulski P: ABC of burns: pathophysiology and types of burns, *BMJ* 328(7453):1427-1429, 2004.
8. Kramer GC, Nguyen, TT: Pathophysiology of burn shock and burn edema. In Herndon DN, editor: *Total burn care*, ed 2, London, Saunders, 2002.
9. Still JM, Law EJ: Primary excision of the burn wound, *Clin Plast Surg* 27(1):23, 2000.
10. Larson K: Initial evaluation and management of the critically burned patient, *Mo Med* 100(6):582, 2003.
11. DeSanti L: Pathophysiology and current management of burn injury, *Adv Skin Wound Care* 18(5),2005.
12. Davidge K, Fish J MD: Classification of burn depth, *Geriatr Aging* 11(5):270-275, 2008.
13. Pruitt BA, Mason AD: Epidemiological, demographic and outcome characteristics of burn injury. In Herndon DN, editor: *Total burn care*, ed 2, London, 2002, Saunders.
14. Prem, SC et al: Initial evaluation and management of the burn patient (2008). Available at http://emedicine.medscape.com/article/435402-overview (accessed May 2009).
15. Lund T: Edema generation following thermal injury: an update, *J Burn Care Rehabil* 20:445, 1999.
16. Lee JO et al: Nutrition support strategies for severely burned patients, *Nutr Clin Pract* 20(3):325-330, 2005.
17. Ulmer JF: Burn pain management: a guideline-based approach, *J Burn Care Rehabil* 19:151, 1998.
18. White CE, Renz E: Advances in surgical care: management of severe burn injury, *Crit Care Med* 36(7), 2008.
19. Endorf FW, Gamelli RL: Inhalation injury, pulmonary perturbations, and fluid resuscitation, *J Burn Care Res* 28(1):80-83, 2007.
20. Traber DL et al: The pathophysiology of inhalation injury. In Herndon DN, editor: *Total burn care*, ed 2, London, 2002, Saunders.
21. Dries DJ: Key questions in ventilator management of the burn-injured patient, *J Burn Care Res* 30(1):128-138, 2009.
22. Cartotto R et al: Use of high-frequency oscillatory ventilation in burn patients, *Crit Care Med* 33(suppl 3):S175-S181, 2005.
23. Yowler CJ, Fratianne RB: Current status of burn resuscitation, *Clin Plast Surg* 27:1, 2000.
24. Pham TN, Gibran NS: Thermal and electrical injuries, *Surg Clin N Am* 87(1):185-206, 2007.
25. Blakeney PE et al: Psychosocial care of persons with severe burns, *Burns* 34(4):433-440, 2008.
26. Acton AR et al: The burn survivor perspective, *J Burn Care Res* 28(4), 2007.
27. Church D et al: Burn wound infections, *Clin Microbiol Rev* 19(2):403-434, 2006.
28. Weber J et al: Infection control in burn patients, *Burns* 30(8):A16-A24, 2004.
29. Robie DK, Herndon DN: Surgical management of complications of burn injury. In Herndon DN, editor: *Total burn care*, ed 2, London, 2002, Saunders.
30. Ansermino M, Hemsley C: ABC of burns: Intensive care management and control of infection, *BMJ* 329(7459): 220-223, 2004.
31. Stipcevic T, Piljac A, Piljac G: Enhanced healing of full-thickness burn wounds using rhamnolipid, *Burns* 32(1):24-34, 2007.
32. Sharma B: Infection in Patients with Severe Burns: Causes and Prevention Thereof, *Infect Dis Clin North Am* 21(3):745-759, 2007.
33. Demling RH et al: Burn wound module, part III: managing the burn wound. Available at www.burnsurgery.org/ (accessed May 2009).
34. Connor-Ballard PA: Understanding and managing burn pain: Part 2, *Am J Nurs* 109(5):54-62, 2009.
35. Wasiak J, Cleland H, Campbell F: Dressings for superficial and partial thickness burns. *Cochrane Database of Systematic Reviews* 2008, Issue 4. Art. No.: CD002106, 2008.
36. Orgill DP: Excision and skin grafting of thermal burns, *N Engl J Med* 360 (9):893-901, 2009.
37. Xiao-Wu et al: Effects of delayed wound excision and grafting in severely burned children, *Arch Surg* 137:1049-1054. 2002.
38. Wolf SE: The year in burns 2007, *Burns* 34(8):1059-1071, 2008.
39. Pereira CT et al: Altering metabolism, *J Burn Care Rehabil* 26(3):194-199, 2005.
40. Scherer LA et al: The vacuum assisted closure device: a method of securing skin grafts and improving graft survival, *Arch Surg* (137):930-934, 2002.
41. Summer GJ et al: Burn injury pain: the continuing challenge, *J Pain* 8(7):533-548, 2007.
42. Di Pasquale A et al: Model of psychological support for burn patients: analysis of the results of eight years experience, *Ann Burns Fire Disasters* 15(2):83-89, 2002.

Chapter 42

Organ Donation and Transplantation

Major advances in transplantation have been achieved since the first cadaver organs were transplanted in the 1960s. Transplantation has become an accepted form of therapy for end-stage organ failure. The field of transplantation is highly specialized and requires expert teams of surgeons, immunologists, and medical and nurse specialists to achieve successful outcomes.

Many problems are yet to be solved in the field of transplantation. Organs remain a scarce commodity, and a lack of available organs restricts the availability of transplantation for many individuals. Safe and efficacious control of the immune system remains elusive. Rejection and infection resulting from immunosuppression persist as the major causes of death in recipients. Chronic rejection is still not well understood. This type of rejection results in eventual graft failure and limits long-term survival in many types of organ recipients.

This chapter provides an overview of the specialized areas of organ donation, the immune system, immunosuppressant medications used to prevent rejection, and solid organ transplantation.

ORGAN DONATION

The evolution of organ donation has moved in tandem with the development of transplantation since the 1950s. With the evolution of *organ procurement organizations* (OPO), organ donation has developed as an entity separate and distinct from transplantation.

Animal research was used to establish kidney transplantation procedures for related and nonrelated donor organs. These investigational procedures led to the recovery of kidneys from donors before autopsy—the original source of organs for transplantation.

BRAIN DEATH

The first organ recovered for transplantation from a "dead" donor was in 1962. The recovery (procurement) of organs from a "dead body" led to the evolution of the concept of *brain death,* as distinguished from the cessation of the heart's beating (death). Initially, the belief in medicine was that a person was alive until the heart stopped beating. Before the use or definition of brain death and the establishment of brain death criteria, patients with an "irreversible" head injury were used for the recovery of kidneys for transplantation. The ventilator was removed, and the recovery procedure was initiated with the cessation of the heartbeat. In essence, the early donors were the same or similar to what is now referred to as *donation after cardiac death* (DCD) donors.

Brain Death Criteria. The criteria for brain death were developed late in the 1960s,[1] soon after the proposal of a brain death standard of death. The debate began as to how much of the brain must be destroyed for a patient to be declared dead. As a result, a nonsurvivable injury was defined as a head injury that results in an individual devoid of cerebral and brainstem function. This includes loss of cellular function, which is not congruent with the heart's not beating. These decisions provide the basis for the conclusion that an individual is dead when the requirements for brain death are met and not when the heart stops beating. This information resulted in passage of the Uniform Determination of Death Act of 1982.[2]

Source of Organ Donors. There are several sources of donor organs for transplantation. Transplant centers with kidney and liver organ transplant programs have living donors as a part of their program. Organ donation from a living donor predominantly involves donation of a single kidney (5,968 donations in 2008) or the lobe of a liver (249 donations in 2008).[3]

OPOs are responsible for the recovery of organs from brain dead and DCD donors. Specific descriptions of the categories of living and deceased donors are provided in Table 42-1. For the year 2008, the Organ Procurement and Transplant Network (OPTN) reported the following numbers of donors in the United States[3]:

Total donors: 14,202
Living donors: 6,218
Deceased donors: 7,984 (includes both brain death and DCD donors)

THE NEED

National Organ Transplant Act. With the passage of the National Organ Transplant Act (NOTA) in 1984,[4] the federal government began the process of establishing a comprehensive framework for the development and administration of a national transplantation system. During the succeeding years,

TABLE 42-1 Categories of Organ Donors

Donor	Definition
Deceased donor (brain dead donor)	A person who has been declared brain dead
Deceased after cardiac death (DCD) donor	Donor whose death is determined by cessation of heart and respiratory functions (not brain death)
Living, related donor	A family member who donates a kidney part of a liver, lung or pancreas to another family member that is related by blood
Living, unrelated donor	A person not related by blood who donates a kidney, part of a liver, lung or pancreas to a family member not related by blood (e.g., spouse, in-law, adopted child), friend, or stranger

more than 421,000 patients received organ transplants. Today, more than 102,000 patients await an organ for transplantation,[3] and approximately 50% will die while on the waiting list (Fig. 42-1).

Organ Donation and Recovery Improvement Act. The Organ Donation and Recovery Improvement Act (ODRIA) of 2004[5] is the first federal legislation since 1990 to amend the NOTA. The act focuses on strengthening efforts to increase organ donation rates. There are three important aspects of the legislation:

1. The federal government's role in educating the public about organ donation
2. The importance of discussing organ and tissue donation as a family
3. The contribution of living donors and the advancements in medical technology that make living donation possible

The key provisions of the act concern the following:

1. Assistance for living organ donation
2. Public awareness, studies, and demonstrations
3. Funds for states' efforts
4. Grants for hospital donor coordinators
5. Studies relating to organ donation and the recovery, preservation, and transplantation of organs
6. Organ procurement organizations

The realization that organs from donors could be successfully transplanted into other individuals created the awareness that there was a need to develop a process to establish this organ source. The development of OPOs was a natural result of the increased demand for organs to transplant. There has been a slow evolution of the use of health care professionals to assist in the organ recovery process and development of organ procurement as a function within the hospital.

National Transplant Act. The passage of the NOTA resulted in the formation of the Organ Procurement and Transplant Network (OPTN),[6] which has oversight for transplantation and organ donation. The Centers for Medicare and Medicaid Services (CMS), previously known as the Health Care Financing Administration, has the authority under legislative provisions to certify OPOs.

Organ Procurement Organizations. There are 58 OPOs.[3] All OPOs are nonprofit corporations; they serve organ donation needs in the United States, Puerto Rico, Guam, and Bermuda. Each OPO provides organ donation services to a designated service area. The service areas vary significantly according to populations served, geographic coverage, transplant centers served, and number of donor hospitals. The OPO is a complex health care business that is the frontline constituent for organ donation. OPOs are central in bringing together the acquisition, placement, and transport of organs for transplantation. The OPO is responsible for numerous activities, which are listed in Box 42-1.

Uniform Anatomical Gift Act. The Uniform Anatomical Gift Act (UAGA) was initially passed in 1968, after the first

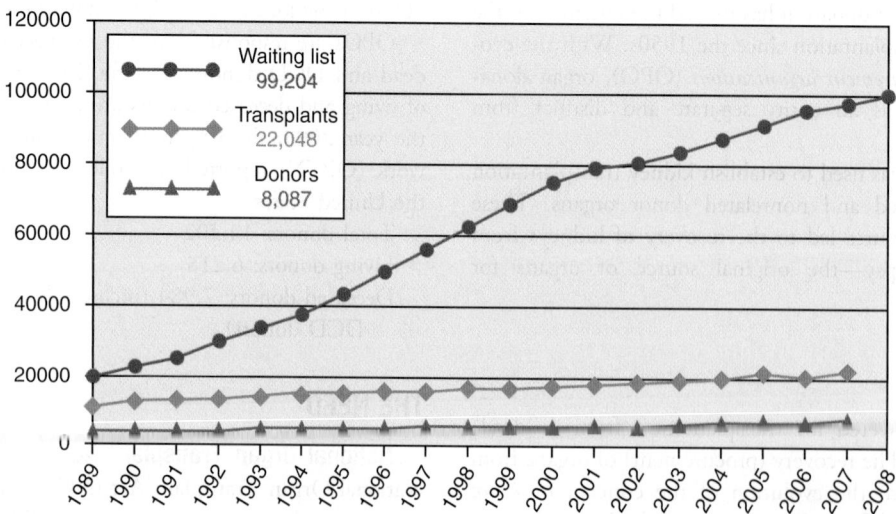

Figure 42-1 Comparison of the number of available donors, transplantations performed, and waiting list for transplantation. *(Data from the United Network for Organ Sharing [UNOS]: Available at www.unos.org [accessed August 2008].)*

BOX 42-1   ROLE OF THE ORGAN PROCUREMENT ORGANIZATION

1. Coordinate and manage the donation process, including all activities from initial donor referral and screening to distribution of the recovered organs.
2. Provide bereavement care and additional support services to donor families.
3. Provide public education, volunteer services, and development and implementation of media campaigns.
4. Provide professional education and hospital development, including education and training of nurses, physicians, and allied health professionals; compliance with hospital regulatory agencies, the Joint Commission, and the Center for Medicare and Medicaid Services; and implementation of donation policies and procedures.
5. Manage and distribute data and information to various clients.
6. Manage of a publicly responsible financial program that provides the support to successfully maintain various donation and donation-related services.

BOX 42-2   COLLABORATION BETWEEN ORGAN PROCUREMENT ORGANIZATION AND HOSPITALS

1. All hospitals must have an agreement with the designated organ procurement organization (OPO) and at least one tissue bank and one eye bank.
2. The hospital will contact the OPO in a timely manner about individuals who die or whose death is imminent in the hospital.
3. The OPO will then determine the medical suitability for donation.
4. The hospital must ensure, in collaboration with the OPO, that the family of each potential donor is informed of its option to donate organs or tissues.
5. Hospitals must work with the OPO, tissue bank, and eye bank in educating staff on donation, reviewing death records to improve identification of potential donors, and maintaining physiologic organ and tissue function of donors.

---

successful heart transplant in 1967. The UAGA created the power, not yet recognized as common law, to donate organs, eyes, and tissue in an immediate gift to a known recipient or to any recipient who might need an organ to survive. In 1987, the National Conference of Commissioners on Uniform State Laws revised the 1968 act to address circumstances and practice. However, only 26 states enacted the revised 1987 version, and other revisions were enacted on a state-by-state basis, so that individual states varied in their legal approach to organ and tissue donation. Neither the 1968 nor the 1987 UAGA recognized the system of organ procurement that was developed partly under federal law.

In 2006, the National Conference attempted to remedy this situation by promulgating a further revision of the UAGA attempted to resolve perceived inconsistencies and to increase the efficiency of the organ procurement system. The current mechanism for organ donation is a document of gift that an individual executes before death. The 2006 UAGA strengthened prior language to prevent others from overriding an individual's prior decision to make (or to refuse to make) an anatomical gift.

Uniformity among states is essential to effectively and efficiently carry out the process of organ donation. Thirty-five states have enacted the 2006 UAGA or have an updated version of the Act. Eleven states have the initiated the process to update the UAGA.[7]

ADDITIONAL FACTORS IN DONATION AND TRANSPLANTATION

Conditions of Participation. The current regulatory environment for hospitals is the result of implementation of the Conditions of Participation for organ donation[8] by the CMS (August 1998; revised January 2003). The Conditions of Participation impose requirements that a hospital must meet (Box 42-2) and are designed to increase organ donation.

Donation Outcomes. As stated in one study of best practices for organ donation,[9] "Outcome is measured in terms of consent rate, conversion rate, and referral rate. It is not good enough for hospitals to point to an obligatory policy and procedure for donation. Critical care nurses are the key ingredients in a hospital's successful donation program. They must work closely, collaboratively, and effectively with OPO staff if the ever-widening gap between organ supply and organ demand is to be decreased."

Informed Consent. The consent process for donation has changed since the early days of recovery of kidneys for transplantation. Adequate information and certain facts were rarely provided to families then. With the advances and prevalence of donation and transplantation, the consent process has become more complex. Consent in the United States has now advanced to two processes: family consent for donation and donor designation (donor consent for donation).

Informed consent is the process of reaching an agreement based on a full disclosure and full understanding of what will take place. Informed consent has components of disclosure, comprehension, competence, and voluntary response.[9] Consistent with other consent processes for medical procedures, there remains an ongoing debate as to how much information constitutes "informed consent." In 1998, Verble and Worth stated, "We believe that hospital personnel and procurement professionals would do well to adhere to what in legal circles is termed 'the minority point of view of disclosure'" (i.e., what a reasonable person would want to know).[10]

Presumed Consent. Presumed consent (opt-out system) is practiced in some other countries, including the United Kingdom. Presumed consent provides every adult the opportunity to express his or her refusal to be a donor of solid organs and tissues and to have this refusal recorded by publicly accountable authorities. A clinically and legally identified candidate for deceased organ and tissue donation is presumed to have consented to organ and tissue recovery unless he or she had registered a refusal.

Obtaining consent for donation has changed from a task predominantly for hospital personnel to one for OPO personnel using a team approaching collaboration with hospital personnel such as critical care nurses, hospital clergy, and physicians. This process has improved the problem areas identified by Verble and Worth in 1998[10]:

- Lack of knowledge of what constitutes an adequate consent
- Provision of inadequate information to provide a basis for the donation decision
- Inadequate management of family anxieties
- Improper introduction of the donation subject (Questions asked without skill in the consent process often evoke negative responses.)

Each consent for donation from the family has variables that result from a variety of factors, such as

- The circumstances of the death of the potential donor
- Prior discussion regarding intent to donate
- The care provided and experienced by the family from hospital personnel
- Religious and cultural beliefs
- Misinformation and inadequate information
- Lack of understanding or acceptance of the death, especially brain death
- The relationship or approach of hospital personnel and OPO professionals regarding donation

For legal and ethical reasons, it is necessary that the public be properly informed regarding organ and tissue donation before individuals decide to become donors. Assurance that an informed consent process is in place strengthens the ability to use donor documentation as consent.

Medical Examiners and Coroners. Consistent and respectful working relationships between medical examiners and coroners and organ and tissue donation agencies are essential to prevent the loss of organs and tissues for donation. In the United States, death investigators may be medical examiners, coroners, or a combination of both. Each state and the District of Columbia had legislation outlining its death investigation system. In some instances, states have specific language regarding the investigational process for deceased potential donors.

Medical examiners and coroners play an integral role in organ and tissue donation. They are responsible for investigating and determining the cause of deaths that occur in unexpected and violent circumstances. These deaths often engender organ and tissue donor candidates. Release of these patients' remains for donation is essential to increasing the number of organs available for transplantation.

Needs of Donor Families. The importance of the care provided to grieving families before and after organ and tissue donation should not be overlooked amid the clinical, technical, and legal aspects of donation. These families have special needs that result from their decision, which involves life (donation) and death (loss of a loved one).

The care of the donor family usually begins in an intensive care unit with hospital and OPO professionals. As stated by Riley and Coolican,[11] "The influence of the nurse's sensitivity at the time of the family's agonizing decisions and emotional upheaval is critical to the family's long-term response to grief." The critical care nurse and the OPO professional establish a unique relationship with the grieving family. They are part of the donation process with the family, and they are entrusted to carry out the specific wishes of the deceased and the family. For this reason, they make a difference in the lives of the families at a time when their actions make an enduring impression.

Bereavement and family support mechanisms are an integral part of most OPOs. Trained personnel from the OPO provide support to families approached about donation, whether the donation becomes a reality or not. Trained family support personnel can also assist with families during the actual donation process. The support services provided are intended to assist the family through the early grieving period. This "support" is not directed at actual family counseling. If other sources of professional counseling are needed, families are provided with resource contacts. The services provided by the family support personnel are varied; examples are listed in Box 42-3.

Not infrequently, the family of the donor and that of the recipient (or recipients) of donated organs communicate with each other. Their interaction can be facilitated with mutual concurrence, including the support of the OPO and the transplant center. This interaction can range from exchanging letters to actually meeting each other.

OPOs believe that providing donor families with personalized support is fundamental to their healing process. Various donor family surveys are conducted by OPOs; most frequently, families report that the ongoing support and follow-up by family support personnel facilitates their healing and helps reaffirm their lack of regret about the decision for donation. Giving compassionate and appropriate support to donor families assists them, and as a result, they become advocates for donation in the community.

Fears and Concerns about Donation. Fears and concerns about donation do affect the outcome for consent to donation. Research into these and other issues at the time of donation spans a quarter of a century.[12] Examples of these fears and concerns are

- Potential disfigurement or mutilation of the donor
- That the funeral for the donor will not allow for an open casket
- That the potential donor will be given inferior medical treatment

---

BOX 42-3 FAMILY SUPPORT DURING AND AFTER ORGAN DONATION

- Follow up with telephone calls and letters.
- Answer questions.
- Provide basic information regarding the outcome for the organs and tissues transplanted.
- Provide reference materials such as books, newsletters, and cards.
- Provide keepsakes, such as a lock of hair or a handprint from the donor.
- Present a donor medal.

- That the potential donor may not really be dead
- That the family will have to pay for the donation process

Because of these fears and concerns, which do not change over time, and the numerous individualized variables affecting families of potential donors, there may be no single right way to support and communicate with each family. These variables are not dissimilar from those that affect families of other critically ill patients in a critical care unit, such as the following:

- Timing (i.e., suddenness)
- Circumstances (e.g., attempted suicide)
- Death of a child versus an adult
- Loss of control
- Unknown environment
- Feelings of blame or responsibility
- Disbelief

Studies by Verble and Worth indicate that strategies for communication and support can be taught and planned for by the OPO personnel in collaboration with the hospital staff.[12] Their research provides recommendations such as the use of gentle, probing questions. A question can lead to the family's real concerns. Targeted strategies by trained requestors, who can provide immediate reassurance, may successfully address many fears and concerns.

Families in these circumstances need information to be provided many times. Assist the family by providing as much clarity as possible. Families need time—time to work their way through all that has happened, what is happening, and what is about to happen. They need to have access to their loved one; easy access can be reassuring, and they need to say goodbye.

As stated by Riley and Colican, "Critical care nurses do make a difference in the lives of those entrusted to their care. Professionals in the field of transplantation emphasize the value of critical care nurses in determining which patients are potential donors and introducing the topic of donation."[11] The current strategies for these discussions are the result of the collaborative work provided by the critical care nurse and the OPO professional. This team approach offers the family the benefit of a process that includes professionals who are trained to support them and who have the collective ability to make the appropriate connections during times of significant grief and loss.

TISSUE DONATION

The critical care nurse may be more familiar with organ donation than with tissue donation. For tissue donation, the critical care nurse should consider organ donor candidates and deceased patients who may contribute other tissues, such as bone, skin, vessels, heart valves, and corneas.

Organs donated save lives. Tissue donation, although not specifically life-saving, does significantly improve the quality of life for multitudes of people. Organ transplants such as hearts, livers, and kidneys usually attract media attention because of the drama associated with life-saving operations. However, more than 1 million people benefit from tissue donation each year. One tissue donor can potentially benefit as many as 50 people. Tissue transplants make possible the following:

- Skin grafts and reconstructive therapy for thousands of critically burned patients
- Donated corneas that avert or correct blindness
- Cardiovascular tissues, including heart valves to help repair cardiac defects or damage, pericardium to repair damaged dura, and saphenous veins for vascular repair
- Bone, cartilage, and tendon grafts to help restore function in people who would otherwise be incapacitated or disabled

Each hospital must have a formalized arrangement with one or more tissue banks and eye banks for the referral of potential tissue donors. The standards and procedures have some similarities to those for organ donors (e.g., identification of a potential donor and referrals). The most significant difference is the status of the potential donor. Whereas there are significant physiologic support factors to consider for organ donors, such as mechanical ventilation, any deceased patient has the potential to be considered for tissue donation. The consent process for the family of the deceased is the same as for organ donation. There are different screening requirements for tissue donors, and each tissue bank provides these specific details.

CHANGES IN ORGAN AND TISSUE DONATION

Donor Designation. Statistics for donation point to the reality that there continue to be barriers to higher donation rates. These include low rates of family consent to donation and missed opportunities to identify and refer all potential donors to OPOs so that families may be approached.

Many surveys spanning the past 20 years have indicated that 85% of Americans support organ donation, but only about 50% of families consent to donating a loved one's organs when presented with the opportunity. Polls also indicate that knowledge of a decedent's wish to be a donor would positively influence the family's decision to consent to donation. Often, however, potential organ donors in hospitals are not consistently identified, or no request is made to the family.

For more than 30 years, efforts to increase donation have included legislation, professional education and development, public education, training of donation requestors, media campaigns, and donor registries. In the past, health care professionals and organ and tissue procurement organizations were hesitant to honor donor designation. However, the public has now come to expect that the donor designation will be honored and that family consent will be sought if there is no donor designation. Forty-nine states now have donor registries. The primary issue for donor registries is the ability to demonstrate that the designated donor has been adequately informed regarding the decision.

With donor designation for organ and tissue donation, the family is informed of the decedent's wishes rather than being asked to consent. The OPO accepts a signed donor card or related document for donation, with or without a donor registry. Donor designation is changing the long-standing process for family consent and requires an even stronger and more cohesive working relationship between the critical care nurse and OPO professionals.

Donation after Cardiac Death Donor. A potential donation after cardiac death (DCD) donor is identified by cessation of heart and respiratory functions (not brain death). DCD donors were previously called *non–heart-beating* or *asystolic* donors.

In December 1997, the Institute of Medicine published a report entitled, *Non–Heart-Beating Organ Transplantation: Medical and Ethical Issues in Procurement.*[13] The findings and recommendations of that study defined the ethical and scientific recommendations for non–heart-beating organ donation and transplantation. The study concluded, "The recovery of organs from [non–heart-beating donors] is an important, medically effective, and ethically acceptable approach to reducing the gap between the demand for and the available supply of organs for transplantation."[13] A later study was published in 2000.[14]

After publication of the Institute of Medicine study, the U.S. Department of Health and Human Services requested a follow-up study to promote DCD donation. The study supported a patient- and family-centered approach to organ and tissue donation.[13]

The renewed interest in DCD donation comes from two central themes: (1) patient and family interest in organ donation in cases in which neurologic criteria for death cannot be met but the decision has been made to withdraw life-sustaining treatment, and (2) the potential for increasing the supply of organs for transplantation.[12] Predominantly kidneys and liver are recovered from DCD donors. Overall, the numbers of organs recovered per donor for transplantation are fewer with DCD donors. As technical expertise has increased, the inclusion of thoracic organ recoveries is on the rise.

A patient can become a DCD donor when medical intervention is stopped, cardiac and respiratory functions cease, death is declared, and organs are removed. This process occurs in the critical care unit or in the operating room (depending on institutional protocol) and must be carried out rapidly so that organs can be removed before they become unsuitable for transplantation.

There are two types of DCD donors from whom organs can be recovered: controlled and uncontrolled. In uncontrolled recovery, the organs are removed after the patient suffers a sudden cardiopulmonary arrest. In controlled recovery, a decision is made by the family or authorized person to discontinue life-sustaining medical intervention. Life-sustaining treatment is discontinued, but interventions to maintain the quality of the organs may be undertaken, such as placement of cannulas and administration of fluid or medication. Death is declared when cardiopulmonary function ceases. Organs are removed after death has been declared.

The critical care nurse, in collaboration with the local OPO, plays a key role in DCD donation. The decision pathway involves the patient's care team and the OPO team. Each team has separate but intersecting responsibilities regarding medications, procedures, family support, withdrawal of life support, and declaration of death. Each decision point involves cooperation between the OPO and the hospital representatives, typically the critical care nurse and the attending physician. Important features include the following:

- Family support and communication when the option is to withdraw life-sustaining treatment or stop cardiopulmonary resuscitation
- Assistance in establishing an environment of confidence with the family considering DCD donation by assuring family members that the decision to stop aggressive treatment has been made based on appropriately communicated information
- Early notification of, referral to, and involvement of the local OPO
- Participation in the timing and content of interactions between the OPO and the family

Barriers to Organ Donation after Cardiac Death. As this additional type of organ availability evolves, certain issues or barriers become prevalent (Table 42-2).[13] There were only 793 DCD donors in the United States in 2007, and the number of hospitals and OPOs participating in a DCD program continues to be relatively small. Since the 2004 emphasis on DCD programs, more OPOs have put DCD programs in place, but not at the rate previously expected. The reasons are not documented, but it is speculated that resistance to DCD programs on the part of health care professionals remains and that the outcomes from these donated organs have been inconsistent. Although an increase in DCD donors will not eliminate the gap between supply and demand, DCD donors are providing additional organs for transplantation.

DETERMINING BRAIN DEATH

Brain death is the term used to describe complete, irreversible cessation of function of the entire brain and brainstem. Spinal reflexes may continue to be present. At the point at which brain death

TABLE 42-2 Barriers to Organ Donation

Issue Source	Examples
Hospital factors	Lack of interest
	Resistance
	Failure to approve protocols
	Rapid decisions to terminate life-sustaining medical interventions
OPO factors	Limited resources
	Lack of resource skill for recovery process
	Low priority
	Resistance
Organs	Unknown outcomes over time
Adverse publicity	Media and public misunderstandings and anxiety
Ethics	Resistance to discontinuing life-sustaining medical interventions
	Perceived association with physician aid-in-dying
	Medical interventions
	Determinations of death

OPO, organ procurement organization.

occurs, the patient is dead, regardless of the presence of a heartbeat, maintenance of respiration by mechanical means, or functioning of other vital organs. The diagnosis of brain death is made by physical examination of the patient, usually by a neurologist, neurosurgeon, or neurointensivist. Absence of hypothermia and any central nervous system–depressant drugs in the blood is necessary to make the diagnosis of brain death. Several diagnostic procedures may be used to confirm the clinical diagnosis, although they usually are not mandatory. Transcranial Doppler ultrasonography, angiography, or positron emission tomography can confirm cessation of cerebral blood flow. Cessation of electrophysiologic function can be confirmed by an electroencephalogram (EEG) or evoked potential testing.[1] EEG is not the preferred diagnostic procedure of choice because of the potential for artifact.

The following guidelines reflect generic, scientifically based recommendations that may vary across practice settings and states according to institutional policy and local legislation. Box 42-4 describes the initial requirements for clinical determination of brain death.[15] Clinical determinants of brain death include coma or unresponsiveness, absence of cerebral motor responses to pain in all extremities, absence of brainstem reflexes, and apnea. For patients who are in a coma, the cause of the condition may determine what is visualized on neuroimaging studies. In most patients with brain death, studies will show abnormalities that are consistent with loss of brain and brainstem function. However, in some conditions such as hangings, patients have normal neuroimaging results even though they have sustained ischemic-anoxic cerebral injury.[15] In these patients, the determination of brain death must be made through appropriate observation and application of the clinical criteria.

Cerebral Motor Responses. Cerebral motor responses to pain in all extremities are absent in brain death. These motor responses can be stimulated by the application of pressure to the nail beds or the supraorbital ridge. Some motor responses may occur spontaneously during apnea testing because of the presence of hypoxia or hypotension and are considered spinal cord reflexes. These may also be elicited in the presence of respiratory acidosis and can include spontaneous flexion and muscle stretch reflexes in arms and legs that can resemble grasping movements. It is important to determine whether the patient has been given neuromuscular blocking agents that may induce pharmacologic motor weakness.

Brainstem Reflexes. Brainstem reflexes that will be tested include pupillary signs, ocular movements, facial sensory and motor responses, and pharyngeal and tracheal reflexes.

BOX 42-4 **INITIAL REQUIREMENTS FOR CLINICAL DETERMINATION OF BRAIN DEATH**

- Clinical or neuroimaging evidence of an acute catastrophic cerebral event consistent with the clinical diagnosis of brain death
- Exclusion of conditions that may confound clinical assessment of brain death, such as acute metabolic or endocrine derangements
- Confirmation of the absence of drug intoxication or poisoning
- Core body temperature higher than 32° C (90° F)

Pupillary Signs. Pupillary signs are evaluated by absence of the light reflex, which is consistent with brain death. Most often, the pupils are round, oval, or irregularly shaped, although dilated pupils may remain even after brain death has occurred. This dilation may exist if the sympathetic cervical pathways to the pupillary dilator muscle are intact. Medications do not normally alter pupil response, although the application of topical drugs or severe trauma to the eye may affect pupil reactivity.

Ocular Movements. Ocular movements, also described as "doll's eyes," and vestibulo-ocular ("cold caloric") reflexes are not present in brain death. A description of the method of testing for each of these reflexes is included in Chapter 27. The so-called doll's eyes are elicited by rapid turning of the head to 90 degrees laterally on both sides. The normal response is for the eyes to deviate opposite to the direction of head turning. In brain death, no eye movements occur in response to head movement (see Fig. 27-6 in Chapter 27).

The vestibulo-ocular reflex is elicited by elevating the patient's head 30 degrees and irrigating both tympanic membranes with 50 mL of iced saline or water (see Fig. 27-7 in Chapter 27). In brain death, no deviation of the eyes occurs in response to ear irrigation. It is recommended that the patient be observed for up to 1 minute after each ear irrigation; 5 minutes should be allowed before testing the opposite ear. It is important to state that several classes of drugs can influence the vestibulo-ocular reflex, including sedatives, aminoglycosides, tricyclic antidepressants, anticholinergics, and antiseizure medications.

Facial Sensory and Motor Responses. Facial sensory and motor responses are elicited by testing for corneal and jaw reflexes. Corneal reflexes can be tested by stroking a cotton-tipped swab across the cornea. Grimacing in response to pain can be demonstrated by applying deep pressure to the nail beds, the supraorbital ridge, or the temporomandibular joint. Severe trauma within these areas could inhibit interpretation of facial brainstem reflexes.

Pharyngeal and Tracheal Reflexes. Pharyngeal and tracheal reflexes are absent in patients with brain death. The gag reflex can be evaluated by stimulating the posterior part of the pharynx with a tongue blade. The cough reflex can be tested by using bronchial suctioning.

Apnea Testing. The loss of brainstem function results in loss of centrally controlled breathing, with resulting apnea. The respiratory neurons are controlled by central chemoreceptors that sense changes in the partial pressure of carbon dioxide ($PaCO_2$) and pH of the cerebrospinal fluid, which accurately reflect changes in plasma $PaCO_2$. The exact level of $PaCO_2$ necessary to maximally stimulate the chemoreceptors of central respiratory centers remains unknown in conditions consistent with hyperoxygenation and brainstem destruction. Target $PaCO_2$ levels have been derived on the basis of clinical observations and research involving apnea testing in brain death. Guidelines for determination of death based on these clinical and research data recommend achieving $PaCO_2$ levels greater than 60 mm Hg for maximal stimulation of brainstem respiratory centers.[15] Box 42-5 describes the procedure for apnea testing.

BOX 42-5 APNEA TESTING PROCEDURE

1. Disconnect the ventilator.
2. Deliver 100% oxygen at a rate of 6 L/min through the endotracheal tube. The oxygen cannula can be placed at the level of the carina.
3. Observe the patient closely for respiratory movements (abdominal or chest excursions that produce adequate tidal volumes).
4. Measure Pao_2, $Paco_2$, and pH after approximately 8 minutes, and reconnect the ventilator.

BOX 42-6 PRECAUTIONS TO OBSERVE DURING APNEA TESTING

- Maintain patient's core body temperature at more than 36.5° C.
- Maintain patient's systolic blood pressure at 90 mm Hg or greater.
- Establish euvolemia (normal volume) in the patient.
- Establish eucapnia ($Paco_2$ approximately 40 mm Hg) in the patient.
- Maintain or achieve normal oxygen levels (option: Pao_2 of approximately 200 mm Hg) in the patient.

To avoid cardiac dysrhythmias and the systemic hypotension that may occur during the apnea test, clinicians should follow the precautions outlined in Box 42-6. Finally, the interpreted results of an apnea test are shown in Table 42-3. Apnea test results can be (1) positive, (2) negative, (3) demonstrative of cardiovascular or pulmonary instability, or (4) inconclusive.

Brain death policies vary by institution and may also be defined by statutes in each state. In some patients, confirmatory tests are necessary to determine brain death. Table 42-4 provides a reference to the types of confirmatory testing most frequently used in declaring brain death. All clinical tests of cardinal findings are equally essential in declaring brain death.

Communication with Family. The nurse caring for a potential organ donor and his family may find confusion and misconceptions associated with the topic of brain death. Family members of patients who are being evaluated for brain death may believe that their loved one is being "kept alive" by the ventilator because he is warm, his coloring indicates adequate perfusion to vital organs, and he appears to have respirations. It is important to establish with families that brain death is irreversible and is not the same as a comatose state. The patient will not recover or get better through additional medical treatment or a prolonged rehabilitation. Critical care nurses benefit from becoming familiar with the concept of brain death and its medical and legal criteria, because they may need to explain brain death to families who are confused and in crisis.[15]

The terminology used in cases in which patients are pronounced dead on the basis of neurologic criteria can be confusing for families. The term *brain death* can mean to some that only the brain is dead but the other organs are alive. Similarly, the term *life support* can imply that the patient is not truly dead. Use of terms such as *artificial respiration* or *mechanical ventilation* may create less confusion. There may also be confusion about when death is to be recorded for a patient who is declared brain dead. When death is pronounced on the basis of neurologic criteria, the time of death is established as the time of pronouncement, rather than the time at which the patient is withdrawn from mechanical support.[16]

MANAGEMENT OF THE ORGAN DONOR

After the potential organ donor has been officially declared brain dead, management shifts to provide care of the patient that preserves and promotes organ function and viability. Referred to as donor management, this is a process that focuses on maintaining hemodynamic stability and normative laboratory parameters, ultimately resulting in optimal organ function. The care of the donor in this phase may last for several hours, and it is generally done under the direction of the OPO professional working collaboratively with the attending physicians and critical care nursing staff.

A standardized set of orders is most often used by the OPO professional to initiate treatment and to provide a continuing evaluation tool that can be used to address management concerns as they arise. It provides a baseline to indicate significant

TABLE 42-3 Apnea Test Results

Result	Findings
Positive	Respiratory movements are absent; posttest arterial $Paco_2$ is ≥60 mm Hg. Result supports clinical determination of brain death.
Negative	Respiratory movements occur regardless of arterial $Paco_2$ level. Result does not support clinical determination of brain death; apnea test can be repeated.
Occurrence of cardiovascular or pulmonary instability	Systolic blood pressure decreases to <90 mm Hg; arterial oxygen desaturation occurs; cardiac dysrhythmia occurs. The nurse should immediately obtain a blood sample for arterial blood gas analysis and reconnect the ventilator. Confirmatory test to finalize clinical determination of brain death may be performed at discretion of physician.
Inconclusive	No respiratory movements are observed; posttest arterial $Paco_2$ is <60 mm Hg without marked cardiovascular instability.

TABLE 42-4 Confirmatory Tests of Brain Death

Test	Results
Cerebral angiography	No intracerebral filling at level of carotid bifurcation or circle of Willis Patent external carotid circulation
Electroencephalography	No electrical activity during a period of a least 30 minutes of recording
Transcranial Doppler sonography	No diastolic or reverberating flow Systole-only or retrograde diastolic flow Small systolic peaks in early systole
Somatosensory and brainstem auditory evoked potentials testing	No responses
Technetium Tc 99m brain scan (cerebral blood flow scan)	No uptake of radionuclide in brain parenchyma ("hollow skull" phenomenon)
Magnetic resonance imaging	Not yet determined

trends or shifts in the donor's status. These standardized orders should emphasize the following treatment guidelines[17]:

- Hypertension and hypotension
- Glucose management
- Temperature management
- Anemia
- Coagulopathy and thrombocytopenia
- Mechanical ventilation
- Fluid and electrolytes
- Polyuria
- Acid-base management

Usually, the OPO donor coordinator is the person who writes the orders for the hospital chart to initiate standard donor care, as listed in Box 42-7.

The OPO professional also initiates a thorough physical examination of the patient and completes an extensive medical and social history. It is critical that events leading to the hospitalization, extent and duration of any cardiac arrest, cardiopulmonary resuscitation efforts, drugs administered, and signs of chest and abdominal trauma be identified. In addition to initiating the treatment guidelines, the OPO professional is responsible for ordering serologic testing to screen the patient for a variety of transmissible diseases including, but not limited to, human immunodeficiency virus (HIV), hepatitis, cytomegalovirus (CMV), and syphilis.

The medical behavioral history is sensitive for identification of high-risk behaviors of the donor (e.g., intravenous drug use, male-to-male sexual contact, incarceration). The completion of these

---

BOX 42-7 DONOR MANAGEMENT PLAN OF CARE

- Transfer care to the organ procurement organization (OPO).
- Discontinue all previous orders.
- Measure blood pressure, heart rate, temperature, urine output, central venous pressure (CVP; if central venous catheter is present), and pulmonary artery occlusion pressure (PAOP; if pulmonary artery catheter is present) every hour.
- Reorder mechanical ventilator parameters as previously set.
- Maintain head of bed at 30 to 40 degrees of elevation.
- Continue routine pulmonary suctioning and side-to-side body positioning.
- Use warming blanket to maintain body temperature higher than 36.5° C.
- Maintain sequential compression devices.
- Continue chest tube suction or water seal (if present) as previously ordered.
- Set nasogastric or orogastric tube (if present) to low intermittent suction.
- Administer intravenous fluid: 5% dextrose in 0.45% sodium chloride solution plus 20 mEq/L (mmol/L) potassium chloride at 75 mL/hr.
- Call the OPO coordinator if any of the following occurs:
  - Mean arterial pressure is less than 70 mm Hg
  - Systolic pressure is greater than 170 mm Hg
  - Heart rate is less than 60 or more than 130 beats/min
  - Temperature is less than 36.5° C or more than 37.8° C
  - Urine output is less than 75 or more than 250 mL/hr
  - CVP or PAOP is less than 8 or more than 18 mm Hg

- Administer pantoprazole 40 mg intravenously every 24 hours, giving the first dose immediately; give artificial tears every hour and as needed to prevent corneal drying.
- Administer albuterol and Atrovent unit dose (500 mcg) per aerosol every 4 hours.
- Continue antibiotics previously ordered at same dose and frequency.
- Continue vasoactive drug infusions (e.g., dopamine, norepinephrine) at previously ordered concentrations and infusion rates.
- Review all medications previously ordered. Most medications (anticonvulsant agents, pain medications, laxatives, gastrointestinal motility agents, subcutaneous heparin, osmotic agents [mannitol], and diuretic agents) are unnecessary during donor care and will be discontinued automatically as the care is transferred to the OPO. Review any other medications in question with the physician.
- Send blood samples to the laboratory immediately for measurement of electrolytes, magnesium, ionized calcium, complete blood cell count, platelets, glucose, blood urea nitrogen, creatinine, phosphorous, arterial blood gas values, prothrombin time, and activated partial thromboplastin time; resample every 4 hours.
- Send blood for type and screen with the preceding blood sample (if not previously done).
- Obtain finger-stick glucose values every 2 hours; contact the OPO if the glucose level is less than 5.0 mmol/L (90 mg/dL) or greater than 10.0 mmol/L (180 mg/dL).
- Obtain an electrocardiogram at initial donor evaluation.
- Add other orders for specific organ evaluation as indicated.

tests and the accompanying medical and social history is necessary to determine the suitability of the donor and the subsequent allocation and recovery of the organs for transplantation.

NURSING MANAGEMENT

The primary goals of nursing management of the donor are to oxygenate the organs, to maintain hemodynamic stability, to maintain fluid and electrolyte balance, and to maintain temperature regulation. These goals can be accomplished by the use of treatment guidelines such as standard orders provided by the OPO and the Critical Pathway for the Organ Donor (Table 42-5). This tool, developed by the United Network for Organ Sharing (UNOS), is a multidisciplinary approach to identifying key events, processes, and timelines that may be anticipated in the care of an organ donor. It also promotes more efficient care of the donor by eliminating unnecessary and expensive tests while adopting a standard of care that maximizes organ recovery and transplantation. Although hospitals and OPOs vary in their standing orders or guidelines, the basic principles reflected in the pathway are universally recognized as effective donor care and management.

The role of the critical care nurse in continuing care of the donor is complex. Tools such as the standing orders provided by the OPO professional are focused on managing the circumstances presented by a brain dead patient. However, it is important that physicians and other health care workers, such as respiratory therapists, also assist in the management of the potential donor. The nursing goals for care of the potential donor focus on maintaining the donor in a state of hemodynamic stability that supports organ function. The complications that arise from brain death lead to a lack of autoregulation of the brain and create intense vasodilation and, potentially, cardiac dysrhythmias. The lack of blood flow in the brain forces a loss of temperature regulation and a lack of antidiuretic hormone, which causes diabetes insipidus and resultant fluid and electrolyte disorders. Donor management may require from several hours up to 36 hours to optimize organ function for the recipient.

RECOVERY OF ORGANS

The donor management phase continues into the operating room setting after the OPO professional has successfully identified potential recipients for the organs that have been donated. A time is set with the operating room, and the recovery and transplantation teams are activated. The role of the OPO professional continues to ensure that the patient remains in a stable condition during transport to the operating room and through the recovery procedure. Donors are transferred to the operating room with ongoing monitoring of heart rate, blood pressure, and any intravenous medications. Ventilator support is continued, and a nurse anesthetist or anesthesiologist supports the patient to ensure maximum stability. The OPO professional serves as a vital part of the recovery team and ensures that ongoing monitoring and documentation is completed. The OPO professional also provides communication back to the critical care staff and to the donor's family after the case is completed and organs are recovered. At the completion of the donor case, the critical care nurse may still be providing support to the donor family in the critical care unit, or the family may have decided to leave the hospital and return home. The OPO professional provides immediate feedback to the nursing and medical staff who have been an integral part of the donation process.

ROLE OF THE CRITICAL CARE NURSE IN ORGAN DONATION

The role of the critical care nurse in organ donation is one that is complex and challenging and contributes to saving lives. Critical care nurses provide the link between the OPO, donor families, and potential organ transplant recipients. As the health care provider responsible for the care of a critically ill patient, the nurse is also often in the role of providing support to the donor family. The nurse may be involved in helping the family to understand the diagnosis of brain death and in answering questions and concerns that arise. This unique role is instrumental in ensuring that a potential organ donor and his or her family are offered the opportunity to donate organs for transplantation. Nurses must be familiar with the criteria for brain death and the applicable protocols for their institutions, and they may also be involved in obtaining consent for donation.

In accordance with the federal government and the CMS Conditions of Participation, all patients who meet the criteria for brain death must be referred to the local OPO and considered potential organ donors. The local OPO is consulted when it is believed that the patient's brain death is imminent.[18] This call sets into motion the referral process, and involves the nurse and the OPO working together while the patient is evaluated for medical suitability.

As the patient's condition is identified as meeting criteria for brain death, the focus of care the nurse has been providing shifts from that of saving the patient to that of promoting optimal physiologic status to preserve organ function. The critical care nurse works with the OPO professional to assume responsibility for the medical management of the donor. The OPO professional is generally not an employee of the hospital and therefore depends on the support and involvement of the bedside nurse. Together, they work to keep the patient hemodynamically stable while the various organs are evaluated for suitability for transplantation. The nurse coordinates with the OPO professional to obtain a variety of evaluative tests, such as electrocardiograms, chest radiographs, and echocardiograms, along with tests that determine the function of the liver, the kidney, and the pancreas. The standing orders provided by the OPO professional assist the critical care nurse in the management of the donor, a process that can be challenging and may last for several hours until the patient is taken to the operating room.

The role of the critical care nurse is vital to the successful recovery of transplantable organs. Research indicates that the attitude of health care professionals toward donation affects donation rates.[19] If a health care professional is not supportive of organ donation, the family is denied the autonomy to make its own decision, and a potential transplant recipient is denied a chance at life.[19] Although the process is complex and

TABLE 42-5 Critical Pathway for the Organ Donor

Patient name: _____
ID number: _____

Collaborative Practice	Phase I Referral	Phase II Declaration of Brain Death and Consent	Phase III Donor Evaluation	Phase IV Donor Management	Phase V Recovery Phase
The following professionals or departments may be involved in the donation process; check all that apply: Physician Critical care RN **Organ procurement organization (OPO)** **Organ procurement coordinator (OPC)** Medical examiner (ME)/coroner Respiratory Laboratory Pharmacy Radiology Anesthesiology OR/surgery staff Clergy Social worker	Notify physician regarding OPO referral Contact OPO referral: potential donor with severe brain insult **OPC on site and begins evaluation*** **Time** ___ **Date** ___ **Height** ___ **Weight** ___ **as documented** **ABO as documented** Notify house supervisor/charge nurse of presence of OPC unit	Brain death documented Time ___ Date ___ **Patient accepted as potential donor** Physician notifies family of death Plan family approach with OPC Offer support services to family (e.g., clergy) **OPC/hospital staff talks to family about donation** Family accepts donation **OPC obtains signed consent and medical/social history** **Time** ___ **Date** ___ ME/coroner notified ME/coroner releases body for donation *Family/ME/coroner denies donation—stop pathway, initiate postmortem protocol, support family*	**Obtain pre/post- transfusion blood for serology testing (e.g, HIV, hepatitis, VDRL, CMV)** **Obtain lymph nodes and/or blood for tissue typing** **Notify house supervisor of pending donation** **Measure chest and abdominal circumferences** **Lung measurements per CXR** **Cardiology consult as requested by OPC** *Donor organs unsuitable for transplant—stop pathway, initiate postmortem protocol, support family*	**OPC writes orders** **Organ placement** **OPC sets tentative OR time** Insert arterial line/ 2 large-bore IV lines Possibly insert central venous catheter	**Checklist for OR** **Supplies given to OR** Prepare patient for transport to OR IVs, pumps O₂ Ambu bag PEEP valve Transport to OR Date ___ Time ___ OR nurse: ___ Reviews consent form Reviews brain death documentation Checks patient's ID band

Continued

TABLE 42-5   Critical Pathway for the Organ Donor—cont'd

Patient name: _____
ID number: _____

Collaborative Practice	Phase I Referral	Phase II Declaration of Brain Death and Consent	Phase III Donor Evaluation	Phase IV Donor Management	Phase V Recovery Phase
Laboratory, diagnostics		**Review previous laboratory results** **Review previous hemodynamics**	Blood and chemistry CBC + differential UA C&S PT, PTT ABO A subtype Liver function test Blood culture × 2, 15 minutes to 1 hour apart Sputum Gram stain and C&S Type and crossmatch ___ (#) units PRBCs CXR, ABGs, ECG, Echo **Consider cardiac death** **Consider bronchoscopy**	**Determine need for additional laboratory testing** CXR after line placement (if done) Serum electrolytes Hct and Hgb after PRBC Rx PT, PTT BUN, serum, creatinine after correcting fluid deficit Notify OPC for ___ PT >14 sec ___ aPTT <28 sec ___ Urine output ___ <1 mL/kg/hr ___ >3 mL/kg/hr HCt ↓30 Hgb ↓10 Na ↑150 mmol/L	Samples for laboratory test obtained in OR per surgeon or OPC request **Communicate with pathology: biopsy liver and/or kidney as indicated**
Respiratory	Patient on ventilator Suction q2hr Reposition q2hr	Prepare for apnea testing; set FiO₂ at 1.00, and anticipate need to decrease rate if PCO₂ ↓ 45 mm Hg	**Maximize ventilator settings to achieve SaO₂ of 98%-99%** **PEEP = 5 cm H₂O** **Challenge for lung placement: FiO₂ at 1.00, PEEP at 5 cm H₂O × 10 min** **ABGs as ordered** **VS q1hr**	Notify OPC for ___ BP <90 mm Hg systolic ___ HR <70 or >120 beats/min ___ CVP <4 or >11 ___ PaO₂ <90 mm Hg or ___ SaO₂ <95%	Portable O₂ at FiO₂ of 1.00 for transport to OR Ambu bag and PEEP valve Move to OR
Treatments, ongoing care	Use warming or cooling blanket to maintain temperature at 36.5° C to 37.5° C. NG tube to low intermittent suction	Check NG tube placement and output. Obtain actual height ___ and weight ___ if not previously obtained.	Set OR temperature as directed by OPC Postmortem care at conclusion of case		

Medications	Medication as requested by OPC	**Fluid resuscitation:** consider crystalloids, colloids, blood products / **Discontinue meds** except vasopressors and antibiotics / **Broad-spectrum antibiotic if not previously ordered** / **Vasopressor support to maintain BP >90 mm Hg systolic** / **Electrolyte K, Ca²⁺ PO₄, Mg²⁺ replacement** / **Hyperglycemia: consider insulin infusion** / **Oliguria: consider diuretics** / **Diabetes insipidus: consider antidiuretics** / **Paralytic as indicated for spinal reflexes**		**Discontinue antidiuretics** / **Diuretics as needed** / **Heparin, 350 units/kg or as directed by surgeon**
Optimal outcomes	The potential donor is identified, and a referral is made to the OPO.	The family is offered the option of donation, and their decision is supported.	The donor is evaluated and found to be a suitable candidate for donation.	Optimal organ function is maintained.	All potentially suitable organs for which consent obtained are recovered for transplantation.

*Areas in **bold** indicate organ procurement coordinator (OPC) activities.*

ABGs, arterial blood gases; ABO, blood types; aPTT, activated partial thromboplastin time; BP, blood pressure; BUN, blood urea nitrogen; C&S, culture and sensitivities; CBC, complete blood cell count; CMV, cytomegalovirus; CVP, central venous pressure; CXR, chest radiograph; DC, discontinue; ECG, electrocardiogram; Echo, echocardiogram; Hct, hematocrit; Hgb, hemoglobin; HIV, human immunodeficiency virus; HR, heart rate; ID, identification; NG, nasogastric; OR, operating room; PaO₂, partial pressure of oxygen; PEEP, positive end-expiratory pressure; PRBC, packed red blood cells; PT, prothrombin time; PTT partial thromboplastin time; RN, registered nurse; SaO₂, oxygen saturation; UA, urinalysis; VDRL, Venereal Disease Research Laboratories; VS, vital signs.

From the United Network for Organ Sharing.

challenging, it is also unique in that lives are saved as a result of the family's decision to donate and the care provided to the donor.

IMMUNOLOGY OF TRANSPLANT REJECTION

Organ transplantation has become a commonly practiced procedure for end-stage cardiac, pulmonary, liver, kidney, and pancreatic disease. Major advances have been made in organ procurement and preservation, surgical techniques, and identification and treatment of rejection. The ultimate long-term success of any transplantation depends on the immune system's tolerance of the transplanted graft. Virtually every body cell carries distinctive molecules that enable the immune system to distinguish self from non-self. A normally functioning immune system is designed to eliminate the foreign invader recognized as nonself. Only suppression or regulation of this normal immune response to the foreign organ can achieve tolerance of the transplanted organ. To understand the principles of immunosuppressive therapy, it is important to have some understanding of the cells of the immune system, the immune response, and the process of organ rejection.

IMMUNE MECHANISM

Whenever the body is confronted with any substance that is nonself, a *primary immune response* is elicited. There are three phases of any primary immune response: (1) recognition of the substance as nonself, (2) proliferation of immunocompetent cells, and (3) action against the foreign substance (effector phase). During the primary response, immunologic memory is established, and any subsequent encounter with the same

substance induces a more rapid and intense immune response. Subsequent encounters are called *secondary immune responses*.

An antigen is a substance that is capable of eliciting an immune response. Each cell has antigens on its surface that are determined by a series of linked genes known as the *major histocompatibility complex (MHC)*. If tissue from one person is transplanted into a genetically different person, the antigens on the transplanted tissue cells are immediately recognized as nonself, and rejection occurs. MHC determines the antigens to which the immune system should respond. The human MHC is called *human leukocyte antigen* (HLA), because these markers were first discovered on lymphocytes. The HLA gene complex is located on chromosome 6, and it is genetically determined by the two haplotypes inherited from an individual's biologic parents.

HLA antigens are further divided into two classes. Class I antigens consist of HLA-A, HLA-B, HLA-C, and HLA-D loci and are expressed on the plasma membranes of all nucleated cells. Class II antigens consist of HLA-DR, HLA-DQ, and HLA-DP loci; they are expressed on activated immune cells.[20] Because of the potential for millions of different arrangements of these antigens, the chances of finding a donor organ with the same histocompatibility genes as a recipient are almost nil unless the donor and recipient are identical twins.

CELLS OF THE IMMUNE SYSTEM

The immune system houses a vast number of cells responsible for general defense and for very specific immune responses. Only a few of each specific cell type are stored. When a particular antigen (foreign protein) appears, those few cells are stimulated to multiply and mount a response. Immune cells are originally produced in the bone marrow as stem cells; their descendants become lymphocytes or phagocytes (Fig. 42-2).

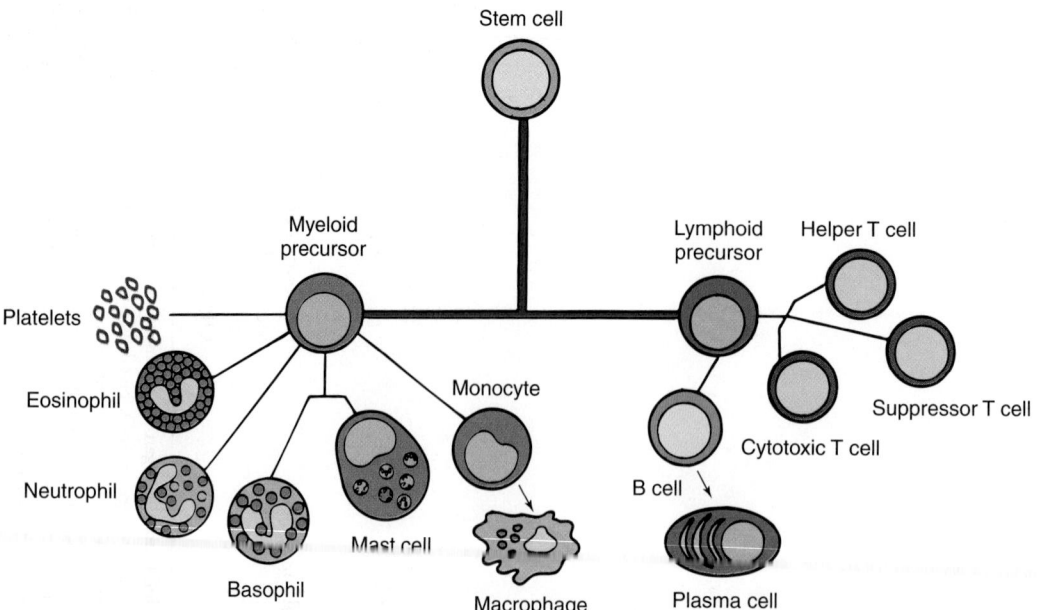

Figure 42-2 All cells of the immune system originate from stem cells in the bone marrow. *(From Schindler LW:* Understanding the immune system, NIH *publication no. 90-529, Bethesda, 1990, U.S. Department of Health and Human Services.)*

The two major classes of lymphocytes are *B cells* and *T cells.* B cells remain in the bone marrow to complete their maturation. The T cells migrate to the thymus gland and mature there. In the thymus, T cells acquire the ability to distinguish self from nonself. After they are mature, some B and T cells are housed in the lymph nodes, whereas others circulate in the blood and lymph systems.

Humoral Immunity. Humoral immunity is mediated by B cells. They are responsible for the production of antibody or immunoglobulin. When a B cell encounters an antigen to which it is specifically coded to respond, the B cell enlarges, divides, and differentiates into a *plasma cell.* It is the plasma cell that actually produces and secretes antigen-specific *antibody* (Fig. 42-3). After exposure to an antigen, the immune system retains a memory of that antigen. Subsequent exposure stimulates the B cell memory cells, resulting in a rapid mobilization of antibody-secreting cells. Antibodies work in several ways, but their primary purpose is to mark an antigen for destruction by the immune system. Other antibodies are capable of neutralizing toxins produced by bacteria, or they can trigger the release of serum proteins known as *complement.*

Cell-Mediated Immunity. Cell-mediated immunity is determined by T cells that are specifically sensitized. Approximately 65% to 80% of all lymphocytes are T cells, of which there are three basic types: cytotoxic T cells, helper T cells, and suppressor T cells.

Cytotoxic T cells. Cytotoxic T cells are cells capable of killing invading cells. Their primary role is to rid the body of cells that have become infected, have been transformed by cancer, or are nonself (e.g., transplanted tissue). They are also called *T8* or *CD8 lymphocytes,* referring to a marker that distinguishes cytotoxic T cells from other T cells. Cytotoxic T cells are activated by macrophages that present the foreign antigen to immature cytotoxic T cells. With the assistance of helper T cells and their release of chemical mediators, the cytotoxic T cells mature and kill foreign cells that carry that specific antigen (Fig. 42-4).

Helper T Cells. Helper T cells upregulate the immune response by stimulating B cells to differentiate into plasma cells and begin antibody production, by activating cytotoxic T cells, and by stimulating natural killer (NK) cells and macrophages. Helper T cells are identified by their T4 or CD4 marker. Figure 42-5 illustrates the process responsible for activating helper T cells. *Macrophages* present processed antigen to the immature helper T cells. With the assistance of chemical mediators (interleukins) released by the macrophages, the helper T cells mature and begin to activate other cells of the immune system previously described.

Suppressor T Cells. A third type of T cell is the *suppressor T cell.* These cells suppress, or downregulate, the immune response. They play an important role in keeping the immune response controlled and in turning off the response after the antigenic threat is no longer present.

Other Immune System Defenses. T and B cells work with other parts of the immune system, notably NK cells, phagocytic cells, and complement, to enhance the immune response.

Natural Killer Cells. NK cells are another type of lymphocyte. They are not targeted for any specific antigen but will

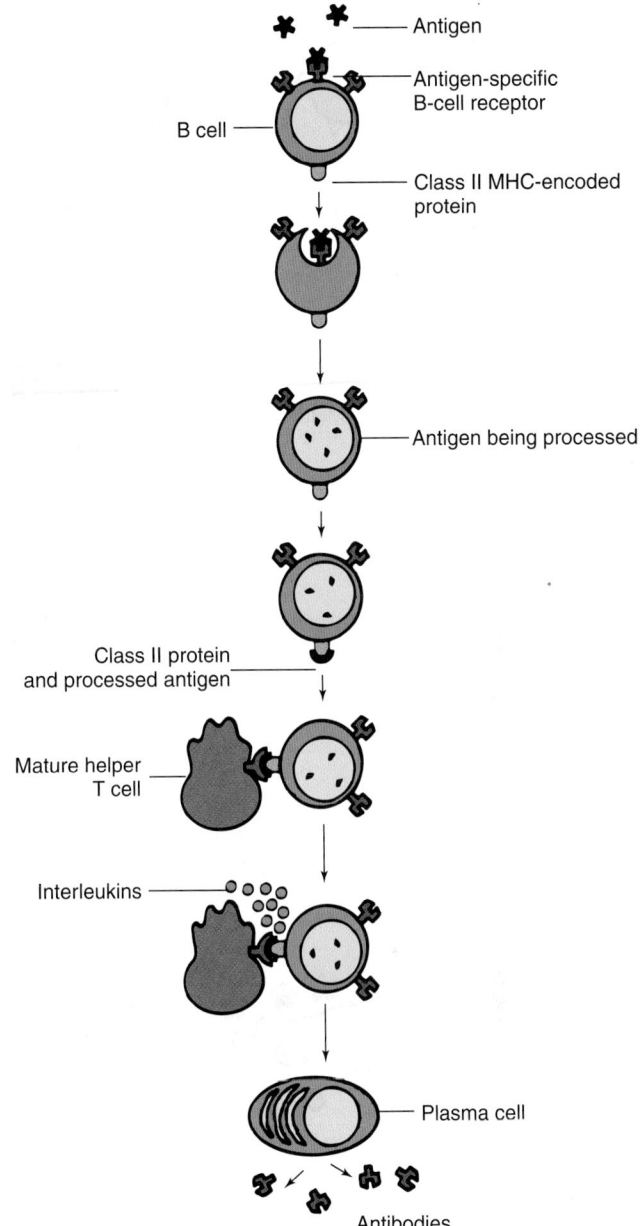

Figure 42-3 Foreign antigen is processed by the B cell and displayed with its major histocompatibility complex (MHC) class II antigen (protein), which attracts helper T cells. The release of interleukins by the helper T cell stimulates differentiation of the B cell into a plasma cell, which begins to produce antibody. *(From Schindler LW: Understanding the immune system, NIH publication no. 90-629, Bethesda, 1990, U.S. Department of Health and Human Services.)*

attack and destroy any cell that is identified as nonself. NK cells contain granules filled with potent chemicals that are released when they bind to the targeted nonself cell. These chemicals are capable of lysing the cell membrane and causing the cell's death. NK cells can also cause tissue inflammation through the release of proinflammatory cytokines.[21]

Phagocytes. Phagocytes are a major category of immune cells capable of destroying alien cells. Critical phagocytes include monocytes, macrophages, neutrophils, eosinophils,

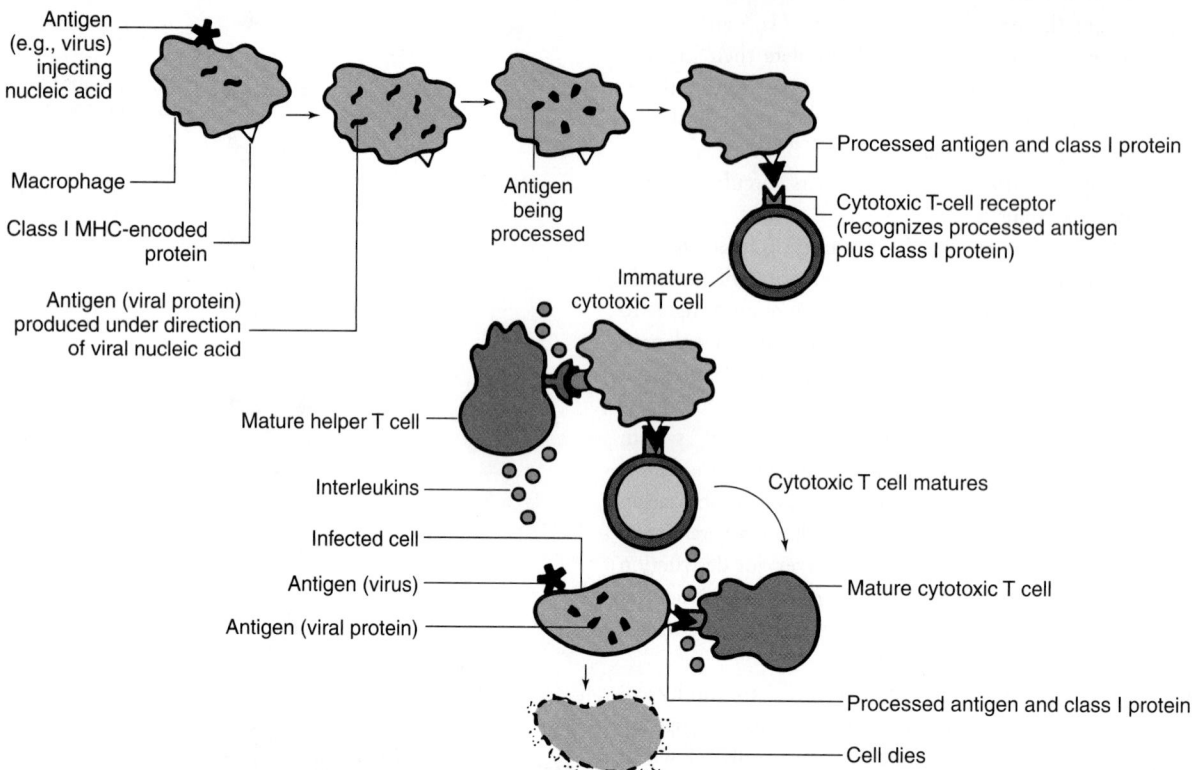

Figure 42-4 The macrophage presents the processed antigen from the foreign organism on the major histocompatibility complex (MHC) class I protein to the cytotoxic and helper T cells. Aided by the release of interleukins from the helper T cell, the cytotoxic T cell matures and kills the foreign cell. *(From Schindler LW: Understanding the immune system, NIH publication no. 90-629, Bethesda, 1990, U.S. Department of Health and Human Services.)*

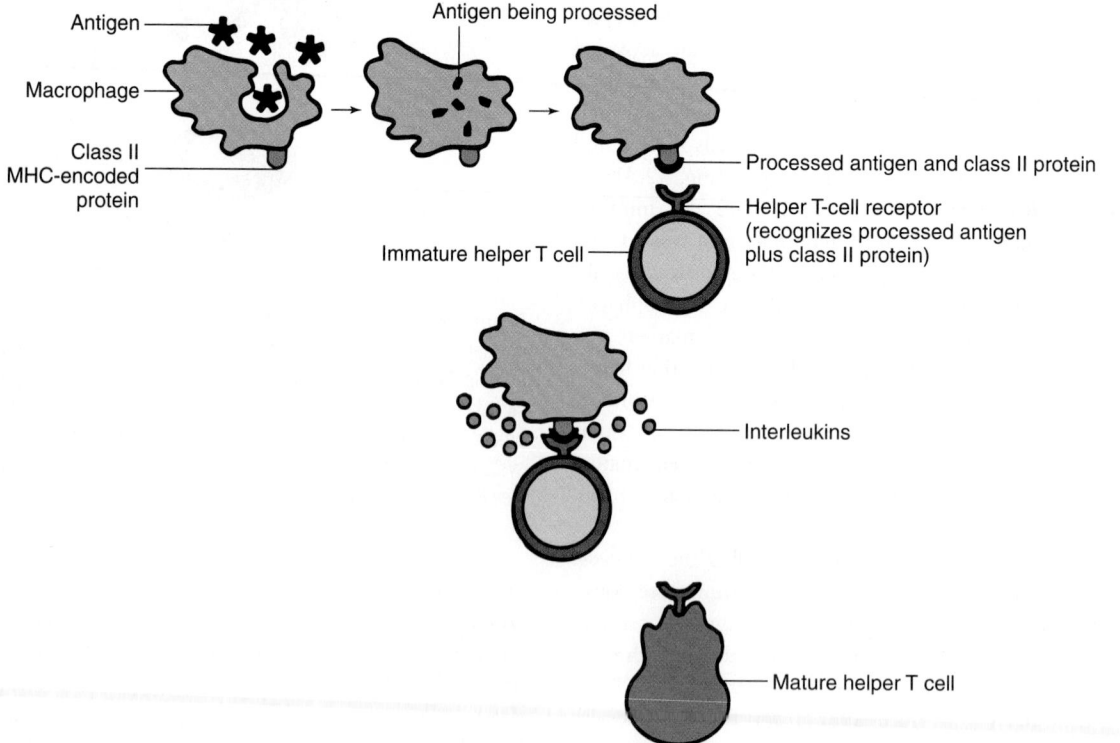

Figure 42-5 The helper T cell is activated by the presence of processed antigen in combination with the major histocompatibility complex (MHC) class II antigen (protein) on the surface of a macrophage. It matures with the stimulus from interleukins. *(From Schindler LW: Understanding the immune system, NIH publication no. 90-629, Bethesda, 1990, U.S. Department of Health and Human Services.)*

TABLE 42-6 Phagocytes and Their Functions

Phagocyte	Function
Monocytes	Migrate from blood tissues to become macrophages Act as scavenger cells in tissues Present antigen to T cells
Macrophages	Secrete enzymes, complement proteins, and immune regulatory factors (cytokines) Activated by lymphokines
Neutrophils	Contain granules capable of destroying alien organisms Key role in inflammatory reactions
Eosinophils	Contain granules capable of destroying alien organisms Weaker phagocyte
Basophils	Contain granules capable of destroying alien organisms Key role in allergic reaction

and basophils. Table 42-6 outlines the primary functions of these cells. Macrophages are vitally important to the immune response because of their role in "presenting" antigens to the helper and cytotoxic T cells. This presentation alerts T cells to the presence of antigen. Macrophages also produce chemical regulators, or interleukins, that stimulate the maturation of helper and cytotoxic T cells.

Complement. An important system in the immune response is complement. Complement consists of a series of 25 proteins, and when activated, they develop into powerful enzymes capable of lysing alien cell walls. Complement is triggered by the presence of antibody bound to an alien cell or antigen (antigen-antibody complex). Complement also stimulates basophils, attracts neutrophils, and coats alien cells to make them more attractive to phagocytes. The latter action is called *opsonization*.

GRAFT REJECTION

Rejection of any transplanted organ occurs when the transplanted tissue is recognized as nonself by the immune system. Cellular-mediated rejection occurs when HLA class I antigens, displayed on donor cells, activate helper T cells that promote the expansion of cytotoxic T cells and recruitment of macrophages into the transplanted tissue. NK cells also begin to attack any cell with foreign HLA class I antigens. As a result, the transplanted organ becomes infiltrated with these cells, which proceed to destroy the foreign graft tissue.

At the same time, antibody-mediated or humoral-mediated rejection occurs as antigen-antibody complexes form. These complexes are present in the transplanted organ and release complement that is capable of cell destruction. Complement plays a role in recruiting basophils and tissue-destroying neutrophils to the site. Antibody also coats the foreign cells, making them more attractive to macrophages.

Graft rejection can occur at different time intervals and has different injury patterns. The three types of rejection patterns are hyperacute rejection, acute rejection, and chronic rejection.

Hyperacute Rejection. Hyperacute rejection occurs within hours after transplantation and results in immediate graft failure. The primary mechanism triggering this response is activation of humoral-mediated rejection. Such an immediate response by the immune system is caused by the presence of preformed reactive antibodies as a consequence of previous exposure to antigens. Presensitization can be the result of previous blood transfusions, multiple pregnancies, or previous organ transplantation.[20] Left ventricular assist devices, which are used as a bridge in patients who are to undergo heart transplantation, can also sensitize potential recipients because of the physical properties of the device itself, activation of the immune system, and increased production of antibodies.[21,22] Transplantation of an organ from a donor with an incompatible blood type can have the same effect. Hyperacute rejection is prevented by testing for the presence of preformed antibodies in the recipient and by selecting donors with compatible blood types.

Acute Rejection. Acute rejection occurs weeks to months after transplantation. Class I or II antigens on the cells of the transplanted graft activate cellular-mediated rejection.

Chronic Rejection. Chronic rejection occurs at varying times after transplantation and progresses for years until the ultimate deterioration of the transplanted organ. Chronic rejection is the result of humoral-mediated and cellular-mediated immune responses. Chronic inflammation results in diffuse scarring of tissue and stenosis of the organ's vasculature, ultimately leading to ischemia and necrosis of tissue. Chronic lung rejection results in small airway destruction, and chronic liver rejection causes diminution of bile ducts.

IMMUNOSUPPRESSIVE THERAPY

Immunosuppressive protocols vary among institutions and according to the type of organ transplanted. The primary goal of all protocols is to suppress the activity of helper and cytotoxic T cells. Therapy ideally interferes with the secretion of interleukins, which stimulate the immune response. In general, most protocols combine high-dose corticosteroids with a *calcineurin inhibitor* such as cyclosporine or tacrolimus in addition to mycophenolate mofetil, sirolimus, and occasionally azathioprine. These *triple-drug regimens* are designed to prevent rejection while reducing the toxicity of the individual drugs. In addition to these primary agents, cytolytic therapy is often used in an attempt to induce graft tolerance and prevent early rejection. Cytolytic agents include antilymphocyte globulins, antithymocyte globulins, and OKT3 monoclonal antibody (discussed later). Table 42-7 summarizes immunosuppressive drugs. Absolute care must be taken to monitor the effectiveness of drug therapy and to minimize unnecessarily high doses of these agents, which could predispose patients to greater risks for infection, malignancy, or other toxic effects.

Corticosteroids. Corticosteroids—intravenous methylprednisolone (Solu-Medrol) and oral prednisone—have complex and diverse effects on the immune system. They are used for

TABLE 42-7 Pharmacologic Management: Organ Transplantation

DRUG	DOSAGE*	ACTIONS	SPECIAL CONSIDERATIONS
Azathioprine	Titrate to WBC count of 3000-6000 cells/mm^3	Inhibits purine synthesis	Monitor for bone marrow depression
Cyclosporine gelatin (Neoral),† oral solution and capsules	Therapeutic range: 100-400 ng/mL Standard dose ranges for specific organs (all split bid): Liver, 14-18 mg/kg/day Kidney, 10-14 mg/kg/day, tapered to 5-10 mg/kg/day Heart, 4-6 mg/kg/day	Suppresses T lymphocytes	Hold for elevated levels Watch for nephrotoxicity, HTN, hepatotoxicity, tremors, and seizures Watch for drugs that exhibit nephrotoxic synergy (e.g., gentamicin, tobramycin, vancomycin, amphotericin B, ketoconazole, cimetidine, ranitidine)
Daclizumab (Zenapax)	1 mg/kg	Blocks interleukin-2 receptor sites	Used as induction therapy No pretreatment needed
Muromonab-CD3 (Orthoclone OKT3)	5 mg/day for 5-7 days (less in some centers)	Suppresses circulating T lymphocytes	Watch for reactions For initial doses, pretreat with Acetaminophen (Tylenol) Diphenhydramine (Benadryl) Hydrocortisone, 50 mg
Mycophenolate mofetil (CellCept)	2-3 g/day split bid	Similar to azathioprine but less toxic to bone marrow	Increased blood level concentrations when used with other drugs excreted through the renal tubules
Prednisone	1 mg/kg/day, tapered to 0.3 mg/kg/day or off, if tolerated	Suppresses inflammatory response	Tapered to as low a dose as tolerated Dose is increased with rejection
Rabbit antithymocyte globulin (Thymoglobulin, RATG)	2.5 mg/kg for 1-7 days May be given once daily initially then every other day	Suppresses circulating T lymphocytes	Used in lung transplantation for induction therapy Used as rescue therapy for other transplantation procedures Watch for reactions Pretreatment may be used
Sirolimus (Rapamycin, Rapamune)	10 mg/day, tapered to trough level of 12-20 mg/mL (depending on organ and center)	Blocks ability of cytokines to activate T and B lymphocytes	Synergistic effects when used with cyclosporine or tacrolimus Watch for thrombocytopenia Used in place of azathioprine or mycophenolate mofetil
Tacrolimus (Prograf, FK506)	0.1-0.3 mg/kg/day split bid Therapeutic range: 5-20 ng/mL	Inhibition of interleukin release	Nephrotoxicity with high doses Hyperkalemia

*These dosage ranges are general guidelines. Significant variations in dosages occur based on institutional practices, other drugs being used in combination, type of transplantation, and patient response to the drugs.
†The cyclosporine preparations Neoral and Sandimmune are not bioequivalent and cannot be used interchangeably; Gengraf and Neoral are bioequivalent.
HTN, hypertension; WBC, white blood cell.

maintenance therapy and to treat acute rejection. The antiinflammatory actions of steroids provide important protection of the transplanted organ against permanent damage from the rejection process. As maintenance therapy, steroids impair the sensitivity of T cells to antigen, decrease the proliferation of sensitized T cells, and impair the production of interleukins. Steroids also decrease macrophage mobility.

Chronic steroid therapy is associated with numerous adverse effects and predisposes the patient to an increased risk of infection (see Table 42-7). A primary goal of therapy is to titrate the drug dose to as low a level as possible. An ideal therapeutic regimen would allow for elimination of the drug altogether. Chronic use is associated with painful osteoporosis, avascular necrosis of joints, fragile skin that is easily traumatized, poor wound healing, susceptibility to skin cancers, steroid-induced acne, and problems with obesity. Elimination of these side effects would enhance the quality of life for many recipients.

Cyclosporine. Cyclosporine belongs to a class of immuno-suppressants called calcineurin inhibitors. Its primary mechanism of action is to suppress the activation of T lymphocytes, which inhibits the production of interleukin-2 (IL-2).[23] Because cyclosporine is specifically targeted for T cells, the patient's immune system is not totally impaired, and some ability to protect the body from infection is preserved.

Three preparations of cyclosporine are available. The first preparation to arrive on the market was Sandimmune (Novartis), followed by Neoral (Novartis). Neoral has demonstrated greater bioavailability and drug exposure than Sandimmune, with no significantly greater adverse events.[24,25] Neoral and Sandimmune are not bioequivalent and cannot be used interchangeably. Gengraf (Abbott Laboratories) is the latest form of cyclosporine to be introduced to the market. Gengraf is bioequivalent to Neoral, and because it is a generic formulation, it is less costly. Gengraf is also better tolerated by patients, who report that it is easier to swallow, tastes better, and has less impact on breath and body odor.[26] The most common side effects of cyclosporine are hypertension, hyperlipidemia, hirsutism, gingival hyperplasia, nephrotoxicity, hepatotoxicity, and seizures.[23]

Tacrolimus. Tacrolimus (Prograf, FK506) was first approved for use in clinical trials for liver transplant recipients in February 1989.[27] Tacrolimus is a calcineurin inhibitor similar to cyclosporine. It inhibits T-cell activation by inhibiting the formation of IL-2.[23] Tacrolimus is used in place of cyclosporine in the immunosuppressive regimen of some transplant programs because of its more favorable side effect profile. Tacrolimus is less likely than cyclosporine to cause hyperlipidemia, hypertension, and hirsuitism.[23] The most common side effects of Tacrolimus are diabetes mellitus,[28] electrolyte imbalances (hyperkalemia, hypophosphatemia, hypomagnesemia), nephrotoxicity, and tremor.[23]

Azathioprine. Azathioprine (Imuran) is an antimetabolite that interferes with purine synthesis, which is necessary for the production of antibodies and for the synthesis of nucleic acids in rapidly proliferating cells, such as the cells of the immune system. Azathioprine is used as a maintenance drug to prevent the activation and rapid proliferation of T cells responding to an antigen. A common adverse effect is suppression of other rapidly proliferating cells; this results in leukopenia, thrombocytopenia, and anemia. The dose of the drug is adjusted to keep the white blood cell count between 3000 and 5000 cells/mm^3, thereby protecting the patient from an increased risk of infection. The actual minimum acceptable white blood cell count varies with institutional preferences and the type of organ transplanted. Many centers have abandoned the use of azathioprine in favor of mycophenolate mofetil.

Mycophenolate Mofetil. Mycophenolate mofetil (CellCept) is a derivative of mycophenolic acid. Mycophenolic acid is a selective inhibitor of the enzyme inosine monophosphate dehydrogenase, which is crucial in the pathway for purine synthesis. Because this pathway is responsible for signaling lymphocyte proliferation, mycophenolate mofetil is a potent inhibitor of T and B lymphocyte proliferation.[29] This inhibition also disrupts antibody formation and the generation of cytotoxic T cells, effectively suppressing cellular-mediated and humoral-mediated immunity. The mechanism of action is similar to that of azathioprine except that mycophenolate mofetil selectively inhibits T and B cells.

The use of mycophenolate mofetil in heart transplant recipients was associated with significant reduction in mortality and graft loss, as well as a significant reduction in severe rejection requiring treatment.[30,31] Its use was also associated with delayed progression of coronary artery intimal thickening, a type of proliferative arteriopathy associated with chronic rejection in heart transplant recipients.[32] Side effects consist mainly of gastrointestinal symptoms such as nausea, vomiting, diarrhea, gastritis, and anorexia.[33] Leukopenia is sometimes seen, although not to the same extent as with azathioprine.

The gastrointestinal side effects of mycophenolate mofetil are sometimes difficult to tolerate for patients and may lead to dose interruptions or omissions. A newer and better tolerated formulation of mycophenolate, mycophenolate sodium, is now available. This is an enteric-coated tablet that can be given to patients who do not tolerate the traditional formulation of mycophenolate mofetil. Several studies have shown that mycophenolate sodium is therapeutically similar and has a comparable safety profile to mycophenolate mofetil.[34-36]

Sirolimus. Sirolimus (Rapamycin, Rapamune) is a newer immunosuppressive agent that is also a macrolide antibiotic known for its powerful antifungal properties. Whereas cyclosporine and tacrolimus inhibit cytokine production, the mechanism of action of sirolimus is to block the effect of cytokines on the proliferation of lymphoid cells (T and B lymphocytes) by inhibiting a protein (mTOR) that is essential for cytokine-driven T-cell proliferation.[37-39] This class of drugs are also known as *proliferation signal inhibitors*. Several large clinical trials in kidney transplant recipients found fewer cases of rejection among patients who received sirolimus compared to those who received azathioprine or placebo.[40] Studies have also shown that heart transplant recipients treated with sirolimus have lower rates of rejection and fewer total episodes of rejection, all without increased rates of infection.[39-41]

Sirolimus also inhibits the proliferation of nonlymphoid cells such as endothelial and smooth muscle cells, as well as fibroblasts.[39] Studies have shown that sirolimus slows the progression of graft vasculopathy in heart transplant recipients.[42,43] However, the fibroblasts and endothelial cells that are inhibited by sirolimus are also responsible for wound healing. Several studies found a significant increase in impaired wound healing among heart transplant recipients who received sirolimus compared with other immunosuppressants such as azathioprine or mycophenolate mofetil.[44-46] Many centers are now delaying the introduction of sirolimus into the immunosuppressant regimen until the recipient is several months from transplantation and has had the opportunity to heal any surgical wounds. Another immunosuppressant agent should be substituted for sirolimus for several weeks to months before any scheduled surgical procedure, to lessen the risk of delayed wound healing. Other primary side effects of the drug include hyperlipidemia and myelosuppression.[47,48] Most of the myelosuppressive effect is directed at platelets, and severe thrombocytopenias can result, making it necessary to discontinue the drug.

Although dosages vary among institutions, several administer a loading dose followed by a maintenance dose to achieve serum levels between 5 and 15 ng/mL. Because of its prolonged half-life, sirolimus is administered once daily. Sirolimus also been shown to have synergistic effects when combined with cyclosporine and tacrolimus, which can result in a lower dose requirement for these drugs. Because cyclosporine and tacrolimus can be nephrotoxic, lower doses of these two medications can be advantageous.[38,48] Sirolimus also specifically interacts with cyclosporine and must be administered 4 hours after cyclosporine.

Everolimus. Everolimus is an analogue of sirolimus with shorter half-life and a more rapid time to steady state. Everolimus is also more convenient to administer in that, unlike sirolimus, it can be given concomitantly with cyclosporine.[49-51] Like sirolimus, everolimus is a proliferation signal inhibitor and works by blocking IL-2 receptor signal transduction in activated lymphocytes.[52,53] Several studies have found that the synergistic effect of everolimus and calcineurin inhibitors such as cyclosporine and tacrolimus allows for lower doses of those drugs to be used.[54] Lower doses of calcineurin inhibitors have been shown to be beneficial in improving renal function in kidney transplant recipients.[55] Several trials are being conducted to study the safety and efficacy of everolimus in calcineurin inhibitor–free regimens.[55-57]

Side effects of sirolimus and everolimus are similar; both can cause hypertension, hypercholesterolemia, hypertriglyceridemia, thrombocytopenia, edema, acne, rash, and mouth sores.[23]

INDUCTION THERAPY

Induction therapy involves the intraoperative and/or postoperative use of an immunosuppressive agent for a limited period of time. The purpose of induction therapy is to induce tolerance to the transplanted graft. It is used by some, but not all, transplant centers, because there is ongoing debate regarding the need for and effectiveness of induction therapy.

Antilymphocyte Preparations. Muromonab-CD3 (Orthoclone OKT3) was one of the first drugs introduced to target distinct subpopulations of T cells. It is a monoclonal antibody produced in mice to specifically target cells with the T3 surface antigen found on mature T cells. Orthoclone OKT3 removes these cells from circulation by forming antibody-antigen complexes. Orthoclone OKT3 also interferes with T-cell recognition of foreign antigen, which renders the T cells incapable of responding.[23] OKT3 can be used as induction therapy or to treat and reverse severe rejection.

Because the drug is an animal protein, antibodies against it develop in some patients. Its initial adverse effects are caused by the massive destruction of T cells, which leads to cytokine release syndrome, resulting in fever, rigors, and pulmonary edema. Reactions usually subside with subsequent doses. As the T-cell population declines, the severity of the reaction diminishes. Orthoclone OKT3 usually is administered for 5 to 7 days and then stopped. The severity of reactions can be minimized by pretreatment of patients with acetaminophen

and diphenhydramine for the initial doses. A dose of 50 mg of hydrocortisone is often given with the first dose of Orthoclone OKT3. A greater concern regarding the use of Orthoclone OKT3 is the increased incidence of lymphoma in patients who have received the drug.[22,58] Incidence varies from center to center, probably related to the length of therapy in the different protocols.

Antithymocyte Preparations. Antithymocyte preparations are made by injecting human thymocytes into an animal, usually a horse, rabbit, or goat. The animal produces antibody in response to the foreign human antigen. Antibody to human thymocytes can then be extracted from the serum of the animal. Antithymocytes cause depletion of T cells by promoting T-cell clearance from the circulation and modulation of T-cell activation.[23] Depending on the protocol of the institution, antithymocyte preparations may be administered as induction therapy or to treat acute rejection. As with Orthoclone OKT3, patients are subject reactions caused by the release of pyrogens during the massive T-cell lysis and by the foreign animal protein contained in the preparation.

Antilymphocyte and antithymocyte preparations are cytolytic drugs. Use of cytolytic drugs has been associated with an increased incidence of malignancy,[22,58] most likely caused by the suppression of cytotoxic T cells, which normally play an important role in identifying and eliminating malignant cells. For that reason, many centers use these drugs only to reverse rejections that are unresponsive to conventional treatment with increased corticosteroids. However, a short (3-day) course of antihuman thymocyte immunoglobulin has been successfully used for induction therapy, with a demonstrated lower rate of early rejection and absence of a long-term cancer-promoting effect at 5 and 10 years of follow-up.[59]

Interleukin-2 Receptor Antagonists. There are two preparations of IL-2 receptor antagonist (IL-2Ra): daclizumab and basiliximab. Both are monoclonal antibodies, but basiliximab is a combination of human and murine antibodies, whereas daclizumab is 90% human.[60] IL-2Ra are antibodies to a receptor found on activated T lymphocytes. As discussed earlier, IL-2 mediates the activation of T lymphocytes; IL-2Ra competitively antagonizes this function.[61] Data from kidney transplant studies showed that patients who received daclizumab for induction therapy had the smallest risk of posttransplantation lymphoproliferative disease, compared with patients receiving antithymocyte and antilymphocyte induction agents.[62] Meta-analysis of IL-2Ra induction therapy after heart transplantation found no significant differences regarding mortality, infection, or malignancy.[63]

IL-2Ra are generally better tolerated than other induction agents, with fewer incidences of fever, leukopenia, thrombocytopenia, and other adverse reactions.[61]

Newer Induction Agents

Alemtuzumab (Campath 1H). Campath 1H is a humanized antibody targeted against the CD52 antigen that is present on the surface of lymphocytes; it causes depletion of peripheral lymphocytes, monocytes, and NK cells. Campath is used in the treatment of chronic lymphocytic leukemia and is being investigated for use in transplantation.[64-66]

BOX 42-8	NEW YORK HEART ASSOCIATION CLASS AND PHYSICAL MANIFESTATIONS OF HEART DISEASE

NYHA Class	Physical Manifestation
I	No limitation of physical activity; no dyspnea, fatigue, or palpitations with ordinary activity
II	Slight limitation of physical activity; patients have fatigue, palpitations, and dyspnea with ordinary physical activity but are comfortable at rest
III	Marked limitation of activity; less than ordinary physical activity results in symptoms, but patients are comfortable at rest
IV	Symptoms are present at rest, and any physical exertion exacerbates the symptoms

HEART TRANSPLANTATION

The first human heart transplantation was performed at the University of Capetown, South Africa, in 1967 by Christian Barnard; the patient survived 18 days. In 1968, Shumway and colleagues performed the first such in the United States, at Stanford University.[67] The number of heart transplantation procedures grew dramatically for the first few years and then rapidly declined because of poor results. It was not until 1972 to 1974 that clinical survival improved and interest was regenerated. The development of the endomyocardial biopsy in 1972 was a major milestone in the detection of allograft rejection. The introduction of T cell–specific agents, such as rabbit antithymocyte globulin, and the ability of laboratories to measure specific T cells (rosette counts) contributed to an increase in 1-year survival by approximately 20%. In 1981, the immunosuppressive drug cyclosporine was introduced in the clinical setting, improving survival at 1 year by about 20%. The number of transplantation procedures grew rapidly.[67]

INDICATIONS AND SELECTION

Heart transplantation is deemed necessary for an individual who suffers from cardiac disease if the symptoms of heart failure can no longer be managed with conventional medical therapy, if there are no surgical options offering a more favorable long-term outcomes, and if the individual's short-term prognosis is poor without transplantation.[68,69] The most common conditions necessitating heart transplantation are cardiomyopathies of various origins (idiopathic, viral, valvular) and coronary artery disease.[70] Other, less common etiologic factors include severe heart failure resulting from chemotherapy, radiation treatment, myocardial tumor, and complex congenital defects. Many centers grade the severity of heart failure by the classification developed by the New York Heart Association (NYHA) (Box 42-8), which is based on the amount of exertion required to cause symptoms. Most patients are categorized as NYHA class III to IV. The anticipated length of hospital stay is 7 to 14 days.

BOX 42-9	HEART TRANSPLANTATION CONTRAINDICATIONS

- Advanced age
- Significant systemic or multisystem disease
- Fixed severe pulmonary hypertension
- Active infection
- Recent pulmonary infarction
- Cachexia or obesity
- Psychiatric illness
- Drug or alcohol abuse

In addition to satisfying medical criteria, patients generally are evaluated for the presence of familial or social support, absence of chemical dependence, and commitment to adhering to a strict, lifelong medical regimen and follow-up. Specific contraindications to heart transplantation are listed in Box 42-9. Heart transplant recipients range from neonates to patients in their 60s; upper age limits vary among transplant institutions. Advanced age was once considered an absolute contraindication to transplantation, but it is now considered a relative contraindication, based on the findings of several studies that demonstrated excellent survival in carefully selected older recipients.[71,72]

Preexisting malignancy, once considered an absolute contraindication because of the potential for recurring cancer or development of second cancers due to therapeutic immunosuppression, is now considered only a relative contraindication if the potential recipient has been free of malignancy for a specific number of years and if there is no sign of metastasis.[73] Severe liver and kidney dysfunction that is not thought to be reversible by an increase in cardiac output is also a contraindication for transplantation. Diabetes mellitus is not an absolute contraindication if the hyperglycemia is adequately treated and there is no sign of end-organ damage such as nephropathy, neuropathy, or retinopathy. If the patient has an active infection, transplantation is delayed until the infection has cleared. Recent pulmonary infarctions increase the risk for postoperative infection and complicate oxygenation and ventilation; a recent history of infarction often precludes transplantation.

The active waiting list is prioritized by acuity, length of time on the waiting list, ABO blood group, and weight. Distribution of organs is regulated by a regional, state, and national network organized and managed by UNOS and contracted by the federal government.[3] Acuity is determined by the patient's need for inotropic support, mechanical ventilation, or mechanical assist devices. Patients who require this degree of assistance are listed as status 1A or 1B; all other heart transplantation candidates are listed as status 2.

HEART TRANSPLANTATION SURGICAL PROCEDURE

Biatrial Technique. The standard surgical procedure for orthotopic heart transplantation (OHT) was originally developed by Lower and Shumway in 1960.[74] A standard median sternotomy is used, the great vessels are cannulated, and cardiopulmonary bypass is instituted after anticoagulation and standard hypothermia are achieved. The donor heart is prepared by interconnecting the pulmonary veins to form a single left atrial cuff and by trimming the aorta and pulmonary artery to fit the recipient's anatomy. All of the recipient's heart is removed except the posterior walls of the atria that contain the orifices of the pulmonary veins and vena cava. Four major anastomoses are performed between the donor heart and the recipient's native atrial remnant; in order, they are those of the right and left atria, the aorta, and the pulmonary artery (Fig. 42-6).[75] The native atrial remnant remains innervated by the parasympathetic and sympathetic nerve fibers from the autonomic nervous system. The donor heart, however, is denervated, resulting in a faster resting heart rate of 90 to 100 beats/min. The rate of the transplanted heart is the normal intrinsic rate generated by the donor sinoatrial (SA) node located in the right atrium.

Although it was long regarded as the gold standard for heart transplantation, the standard biatrial technique had disadvantages related to anatomic abnormalities remaining after the surgical procedure. The anastomosis of the donor and recipient atria left large abnormal atrial cavities.[76] The loss of normal atrial anatomy increases the risk of mitral and tricuspid valve regurgitation, atrial septal aneurysms, atrial thrombus formation, and tachydysrhythmias.[77,78]

Bicaval Technique. The bicaval technique, an alternative to the standard surgical approach, was originally reported by Sievers and associates in 1991 and is now the most commonly used method for orthotopic heart transplantation.[75,79] The five anastomotic sites of the bicaval technique include the left atrial cuff, which contains the pulmonary veins, the superior and inferior vena cava, the aorta, and the main pulmonary artery. This technique leaves the recipient with more anatomically normal atria. Benefits of the bicaval technique include preserved SA node function with decreased incidences of atrial dysrhythmias and mitral and tricuspid regurgitation.[80,81] Though it is rare,

superior vena caval stenosis is a complication that has been reported in the literature.[80]

POSTOPERATIVE MEDICAL AND NURSING MANAGEMENT

Immediate postoperative management of the heart transplant recipient is similar to that of patients undergoing other heart surgery procedures. Nursing care of the transplant recipient involves several nursing diagnoses, as listed in the Nursing Diagnoses feature on Heart Transplantation. The most frequently used diagnosis is Decreased Cardiac Output. Possible causes for a decrease in cardiac output include dysrhythmias, hypothermia, myocardial depression, tamponade, and rejection.

Variables that influence myocardial performance include prolonged ischemic time (time from excision of the donor heart to removal of the aortic cross-clamp after implantation into the recipient); reperfusion injury; and hypothermia. Dysrhythmias may occur as a result of myocardial irritation, local ischemia, edema around the atrial suture line, and disruption of the SA nodal blood supply.[82]

An electrocardiogram abnormality unique to the transplanted heart is the presence of a second P wave, which is generated by the native SA node that has been left in the atrial cuff. Because this impulse does not cross the suture line, it is capable of conducting only through the remnant of the native recipient atria. This impulse is not seen in hearts transplanted with use of the bicaval technique, because the native right atrium and its SA node are removed.

Isoproterenol, a powerful β-adrenergic antagonist, is sometimes used in the postoperative period for chronotropic (heart rate) support. Its chronotropic and vasodilator properties effectively sustain the heart rate, increase cardiac output, and decrease pulmonary vascular resistance (PVR). PVR may be increased as a result of preexisting left ventricular failure and may be a cause of transient right ventricular dysfunction in the newly transplanted heart. Dopamine and epinephrine are often used for inotropic support in the postoperative period. However, the use of inotropic and chronotropic drugs is highly individualized based on institutional preference. Generally speaking, inotropic drugs

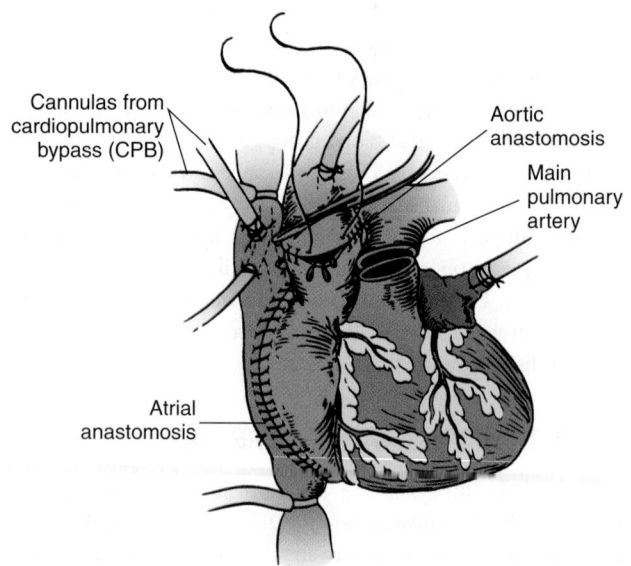

Figure 42-6 Surgical procedure for heart transplantation. *(Modified from Hurst JW et al: The heart, ed 7, New York, 1990, McGraw-Hill.)*

Cannulas from cardiopulmonary bypass (CPB)

Aortic anastomosis

Main pulmonary artery

Atrial anastomosis

Nursing Diagnoses

Heart Transplantation

- Decreased Cardiac Output related to alterations in preload
- Decreased Cardiac Output related to alterations in afterload
- Decreased Cardiac Output related to alterations in heart rate
- Risk for Infection: immunosuppressive drugs required to prevent rejection of transplanted organ
- Disturbed Body Image related to actual change in body structure, function, or appearance
- Anxiety related to threat to biologic, psychologic, and social integrity
- Readiness for Enhanced Knowledge: Posttransplantation Self-Care Regimen, immunosuppressive drugs, cardiac drugs, diuretics, and clinical manifestations of infection

are gradually discontinued over 24 to 48 hours as tolerated by the patient, and the need for isoproterenol decreases as the heart begins to maintain its normal intrinsic rate of approximately 100 beats/min. Temporary pacing is required only occasionally, and fewer than 10% of transplant recipients require a permanent pacemaker implant.[82]

Cardiac tamponade does not occur with greater frequency in heart transplantation compared with other cardiac surgeries, but it may occur insidiously as a result of an enlarged pericardial sac due to long-standing cardiomyopathy. Patients who have had chronic right ventricular failure, subsequent liver enlargement, and abnormal coagulation studies may benefit from preoperative administration of fresh plasma or fresh-frozen plasma. Plasma contains most clotting factors and is indicated for liver dysfunction. Administration of plasma may decrease the risk of bleeding and tamponade.

Rejection Surveillance. Rejection is the most common etiologic factor responsible for low cardiac output during the first 3 months after heart transplantation. Hyperacute rejection occurs only in the immediate postoperative period. It is a rare complication that necessitates retransplantation for survival. Acute rejection can occur at any time, although it is most likely to occur during the first 3 to 6 months after transplantation.

Diagnosis of rejection is determined by endomyocardial biopsy. A bioptome is percutaneously inserted through the right internal jugular vein and advanced through the right atrium to the right ventricle with the aid of fluoroscopy or echocardiography to obtain biopsy specimens. Four to five samples of myocardial tissue are obtained from the interventricular septum. The samples are microscopically evaluated for interstitial and perivascular infiltration. Cardiac biopsies are graded according to the severity of the interstitial infiltration of lymphocytes. The standardized cardiac biopsy grading scale ranges from 0 to 4 (Box 42-10).[83]

Surveillance for rejection is typically performed weekly for the first 4 to 6 weeks. The frequency of surveillance biopsies gradually decreases in relation to the patient's rejection history and institutional preference. A major but rare complication of biopsy is ventricular perforation, which results in cardiac tamponade. This emergency situation may require open heart surgical repair. Pneumothorax may result from perforation of the visceral pleura during cannulation of the jugular vein; its clinical

manifestations are a sudden onset of sharp pain in the affected side and dyspnea. Many institutions require heart transplant recipients to undergo biopsy monitoring for the rest of their lives.

Treatment of acute rejection episodes may require intravenously administered methylprednisolone. Recurrence of acute rejection is managed with various pharmacologic agents, depending on the clinical picture and institution. Strategies include augmenting current maintenance immunosuppression or switching to alternatives such as tacrolimus, mycophenolate mofetil, or rapamycin. Orthoclone OKT3, a monoclonal antibody, is used for recurrent rejection; it is used also as an induction immunosuppressive agent for the first 7 to 14 days after surgery. If Orthoclone OKT3 is being used for a second time, the patient must be tested for the presence of antibodies, which may contraindicate its use. Other agents used for recurrent rejection are polyclonal antibodies such as antilymphocyte globulin or antithymocyte globulin.

Salvage therapy for persistent rejection that has not responded to conventional immunosuppression, multiple steroid boluses, or anti–T-cell antibodies consists of total lymphoid irradiation. Low-dose ionizing radiation is used to treat the lymphoid tissue. Areas exposed to radiation are the axilla, the sternum, the clavicle, the paraaorta, the ilium, the inguinofemoral lymph nodes, and the spleen.[84]

Infection Surveillance. Infection surveillance is a high priority for the immunocompromised person. It is well known that immunosuppression predisposes the patient to infection by a multitude of opportunistic pathogens that cannot easily be prevented with infection control. Development of infection is encountered most often in the early postoperative period, when immunosuppression is maximized. Infection is one of the leading causes of death during this period (up to 2 years after surgery).[70] Great care must be taken to use aseptic technique for all intravenous line and dressing changes. Centers differ widely in their protective practices regarding the transplant recipient. Some use reverse isolation, whereas others put transplant recipients in rooms with other patients and simply use standard precautions.

Development of fever is aggressively investigated, with systematic blood, wound, and respiratory tract cultures, chest radiographs, and observation. Because steroids are known to suppress the body's inflammatory reaction, an elevated temperature generally is considered significant when it reaches 38° C (100.4° F). Nurses must be suspicious of any new productive cough, dry cough, change in type of secretions, or change in chest roentgenogram findings.

CMV is a particular threat to transplant recipients. CMV is a herpesvirus that can produce latent infection that persists throughout life. Between 50% and 80% of adults in the United States are infected with CMV by age 40 years.[85] The virus can be transmitted through organ and blood product donation; transplantation from a CMV-seropositive donor to a CMV-seronegative recipient poses the highest risk to the recipient for acquiring a primary infection. An antiviral agent, ganciclovir, can inhibit viral replication and ameliorate symptoms and is used in the prophylaxis and treatment of CMV infections.[86,87]

| BOX 42-10 | STANDARDIZED CARDIAC BIOPSY GRADING[83] |

Grade	Nomenclature
0	No evidence of acute rejection (NER)
1A	Focal, mild acute rejection (AR)
1B	Diffuse, mild AR
2	Focal, moderate AR
3A	Multifocal aggressive, low-moderate AR
3B	Diffuse borderline, severe AR
4	Diffuse aggressive, severe AR

CMV immune globulin is being used increasingly for the prevention of primary CMV disease and for treatment of CMV disease.[88-90]

PATIENT EDUCATION

As with all transplant recipients, postoperative care includes educating the patient regarding compliance and record keeping. Education is provided on the immunosuppressive medication regimen, risks and signs and symptoms of infection, myocardial biopsy, and symptoms of heart failure. Patients may be required to check their blood glucose, blood pressure, temperature, and daily weight at home. At first, frequent clinic visits are needed to monitor progress and adjust medications. As the patient progresses, a schedule is established for routine laboratory tests and clinic visits to ensure long-term success of the transplant.

LONG-TERM CONSIDERATIONS

Chronic immunosuppression results in significant morbidity. Steroid administration can result in osteoporosis, avascular necrosis of joints, fragile skin, and obesity. Cyclosporine can induce renal insufficiency, excessive hair growth, gingival hyperplasia, tremor, and hypertension necessitating pharmacologic control. Azathioprine can be hepatotoxic. Concomitant use of these immunosuppressants also leaves patients more susceptible to malignancies and late infections (see Table 42-7).

Graft vasculopathy, or coronary artery disease in the transplanted heart, is thought to develop as a result of chronic rejection and is a major cause of late morbidity and mortality.[70] It is a diffuse and rapidly progressive type of coronary disease that causes concentric narrowing of the coronary arteries. Because the lesions are discrete, they are not amenable to interventions such as angioplasty or bypass grafting.

Patients with denervated hearts cannot feel anginal pain, although reinnervation of transplanted hearts can occur over time and can allow patients to feel chest pain. More often, their symptoms of graft vasculopathy are ischemic injury, heart failure, or sudden death. The disease is recognized initially by angiographic screening and later in the course of the disease by the presence of silent infarctions on electrocardiography. Patients may have the disease and demonstrate no clinical sequelae. Many transplantation programs have initiated baseline and annual angiographic studies to look for the development and progression of graft vasculopathy. Proliferation signal inhibitors such as sirolimus and everolimus are sometimes used as prophylaxis against graft vasculopathy or to slow its progression. However, the only definitive treatment for advanced graft vasculopathy is retransplantation.

In general, heart transplant recipients report improvement in their quality of life.[91-94] Ninety percent report no activity limitations at 5 years after transplantation.[70] However, fewer than 35% return to full-time employment, and many who are able to work cannot find suitable employment because of employers' concerns about liability, lack of health insurance, and the need to qualify for medical disability.[95,96] From 1997 through 2004, the 1-, 3-, and 5-year survival rates after heart transplantation

were 87.7%, 79.1%, and 72.5%, respectively.[97] Leading causes of mortality 3 to 5 years after transplantation are malignancy (18.5%), graft vasculopathy (14.3%), and graft failure (14.7%).[70]

In 2005, 2209 heart transplants were performed in the United States. On May 1, 2009, there were 2799 people registered on waiting lists to receive a heart transplant.[97] The number of heart transplantation procedures performed is greatly influenced by the limited donor pool (see Fig. 42-1). The 1-year survival rate for heart transplant recipients, as reported by the UNOS Scientific Registry, is 87.7%.[97]

HEART-LUNG TRANSPLANTATION

Combined heart-lung transplantation (HLT) research has been built on the foundation established by heart transplantation through years of laboratory investigation. Interest in the procedure gained momentum with the introduction of cyclosporine, because it permitted the delay of high-dose steroid therapy (whose use impaired bronchial healing and favored early postoperative infections). In 1981 at Stanford University, Reitz and colleagues performed the first HLT resulting in long-term survival; the patient lived for more than 5 years.[98]

HLT, now in its third decade, is the therapy of choice for some cardiac and cardiopulmonary diseases. Research and laboratory investigations continue in the development of new immunosuppressants, preservation solutions, and techniques.

INDICATIONS AND SELECTION

HLT is an established treatment for selected patients with irreversible, progressively disabling, end-stage cardiopulmonary and pulmonary disease. The main indications for combined HLT are congenital heart disease and idiopathic pulmonary arterial hypertension; these have accounted for almost 60% of the reported HLTs since 1982.[99] Other indications include cystic fibrosis (14.0%), acquired heart disease (3.6%), chronic obstructive pulmonary disease and emphysema (3.8%), idiopathic pulmonary fibrosis (2.8%), and α_1-antitrypsin deficiency.[99]

Specific etiologic factors in pulmonary disease can be grouped according to the type of lung abnormality as pulmonary vascular disease, obstructive lung disease, and restrictive lung disease.[100,101] Box 42-11 lists indications for HLT. Optional single-lung (SLT) or double-lung (DLT) transplantation is discussed in a later section.

HLT is the operation of choice for patients whose pulmonary disease process has irreversibly disabled the heart. HLT is the preferential procedure because transplantation of the entire heart-lung block eliminates having to separate the pulmonary artery and veins, avoiding subsequent reanastomoses and decreasing bleeding complications. However, if the heart is judged to be only temporarily dysfunctional and can be expected to regain adequate function after transplantation of a healthy lung or lungs, the native heart may be left in place,[101,102] and SLT or DLT may be performed. Another option is to transplant the heart-lung block into such an individual and then donate the native heart to another recipient. This is referred to as the *domino procedure.*[103]

The evaluation of HLT candidates is similar to that for heart transplant recipients with respect to patient commitment to compliance with a strict, lifelong medical regimen. Contraindications to HLT are listed in Box 42-12. Systematic disease, active extrapulmonary infection, and other organ diseases are absolute contraindications. Cachexia and obesity are obstacles that can be eliminated by nutritional support and weight reduction. Truncal obesity is especially undesirable, because it significantly decreases diaphragmatic excursion, hinders postoperative mobilization, and may complicate recovery.[100] Preoperative use of corticosteroids has been implicated as a cause of tracheal and bronchial dehiscence in the early postoperative period.[100,101] Previous cardiothoracic surgery is a relative contraindication because of the risk of bleeding associated with the presence of pleural adhesions.[100] Removal of the native lung may precipitate pleural bleeding in the posterior pleural space, which can be particularly difficult to control because of the location.[104]

BOX 42-11 INDICATIONS FOR SINGLE-LUNG, DOUBLE-LUNG, AND HEART-LUNG TRANSPLANTATION

PULMONARY VASCULAR DISEASE
- Primary pulmonary hypertension
- Pulmonary hypertension due to secondary thromboembolic disease
- Eisenmenger's syndrome
- Cardiomyopathy with pulmonary hypertension

OBSTRUCTIVE LUNG DISEASE
- Emphysema
- α_1-Antitrypsin deficiency
- Cystic fibrosis

- Bronchiectasis
- Bronchopulmonary dysplasia
- Idiopathic or posttransplantation obliterative bronchiolitis
- Lymphangioleiomyomatosis

RESTRICTIVE LUNG DISEASE
- Idiopathic pulmonary fibrosis
- Sarcoidosis
- Asbestosis
- Histiocytosis X
- Bronchiolitis obliterans organizing pneumonia
- Desquamative interstitial pneumonitis

BOX 42-12 CONTRAINDICATIONS TO SINGLE-LUNG, DOUBLE-LUNG, AND HEART-LUNG TRANSPLANTATION

ABSOLUTE CONTRAINDICATIONS
- Significant systemic or multisystem disease
- Active intrapulmonary or extrapulmonary infection
- Cachexia or obesity
- Current cigarette smoking
- Psychiatric illness
- Drug or alcohol abuse
- Symptomatic osteoporosis
- Severe chest wall deformity
- Hepatitis B

- Malignancy precluding long-term survival

RELATIVE CONTRAINDICATIONS
- Corticosteroid therapy
- Previous cardiothoracic surgery
- Age (specific to transplant program)
- Kidney disease
- Liver disease
- Previous cardiothoracic surgery

HEART-LUNG TRANSPLANTATION SURGICAL PROCEDURE

Success of HLT depends in part on the selection and procurement of suitable donor organs. The lungs are particularly difficult to procure because they are vulnerable to complications related to brain death. Prolonged mechanical ventilation is required, which increases the risk of infection. Any infection usually precludes donation. Neurogenic pulmonary edema also may damage the lungs, making their donation impossible. Lungs have a limited ischemic time of about 4 hours, which restricts the geographic area for donor procurement.[104] Lung preservation has improved, and distant procurement with 2 to 3 hours of transport time has increased the donor pool.[105]

Before the removal of the heart-lung block, alprostadil (prostaglandin E_1 [PGE_1]) is administered gradually until a systemic effect is achieved. PGE_1 is used to ensure complete pulmonary vasodilatation for uniform cooling and distribution of pulmonoplegia.[105,106]

The operation for the recipient is performed through a median sternotomy or a bilateral thoracosternotomy (clamshell) incision. The patient is heparinized and placed on cardiopulmonary bypass, and the heart is excised. Care is taken to ensure preservation of the recipient's phrenic, vagus, and laryngeal nerves. The lungs are removed separately to decrease the risk of nerve damage. A left pneumonectomy is usually performed first, because it is technically easier. The pulmonary artery, pulmonary veins, and main stem bronchus are isolated and excised in that order.[107] The donor heart and lungs are then implanted as a block. The heart is put into the orthotopic position and anastomosed to the native aorta and remnant recipient atria. The tracheal anastomosis in HLT is performed just above the level of the carina (Fig. 42-7).[106]

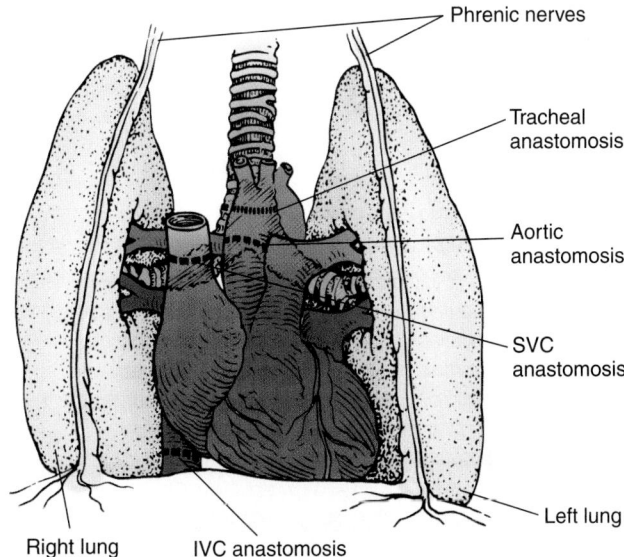

Figure 42-7 Surgical procedure for heart-lung transplantation. IVC, inferior vena cava; SVC, superior vena cava. *(Modified from Reitz BA et al: Heart and lung transplantation, J Thorac Cardiovasc Surg 80[3]:360, 1980.)*

POSTOPERATIVE MEDICAL AND NURSING MANAGEMENT

Immediate postoperative care of the heart-lung transplant recipient is similar to that for the heart transplant recipient. Several nursing diagnoses are associated with care of the heart-lung transplant recipient, as listed in the Nursing Diagnoses feature on Heart-Lung Transplantation. The most common complication is bleeding, because patients who have been cyanotic often have large bronchial vessels that cross behind the trachea and tend to be a source of bleeding. Achieving hemostasis at this site can be technically difficult because of the anatomic location. Patients who have had previous thoracic surgery require more surgical dissection because of scarring and therefore may have increased risk of bleeding.

Careful monitoring of bleeding and maintenance of the patency and function of mediastinal and pleural chest tubes are essential. Bleeding in amounts greater than 100 to 200 mL/hr for longer than 3 hours with normal coagulation studies is cause for concern about a surgical bleed. If bleeding of this nature persists, reexploration of the chest usually is indicated. The transplanted lung is susceptible to fluid overload because of the disruption of pulmonary lymphatics and the increase in extravascular lung water that is common after lung transplantation.[101] Replacement of blood loss with crystalloid or colloid therapy must be done carefully to minimize the risk of fluid overload in the transplanted lungs and the development of acute lung injury (see Chapter 24).

Patients are maintained on mechanical ventilation to support oxygenation for 12 to 48 hours. At least 5 cm H_2O of positive end-expiratory pressure (PEEP) is used routinely to prevent atelectasis, although high amounts of PEEP should be avoided to prevent barotrauma to the newly transplanted lungs. Endotracheal tube placement is monitored by auscultation and chest radiographic evaluation. The endotracheal tube must be well secured and movement must be minimized to protect the tracheal anastomosis. Suctioning must be gentle, and to avoid disruption of the suture line, the suction catheter is not advanced beyond the end of the tube. Small amounts of bloody secretions can be expected with suctioning, but overt hemoptysis can be a sign of dehiscence, which requires immediate attention. Patients are weaned from ventilatory support as soon as possible. The longer the period of intubation, the higher the risk of pneumonia.[101] After extubation, patients are encouraged to cough, deep-breathe, and get out of bed.

Pharmacologic support is similar to that used after heart transplantation. Isoproterenol may be given to augment the heart rate, and dopamine is used for inotropic support and vasodilation of the kidney. Additional inotropic support is achieved with epinephrine if necessary. PGE_1 is administered primarily for pulmonary vasodilation, and sodium nitroprusside is given for its systemic vasodilative properties (see "Vasodilator Drugs" in Chapter 20). Inhaled nitric oxide (iNO) is a potent vasodilator that selectively dilates pulmonary vessels; this improves gas exchange and decreases pulmonary artery pressures and PVR, thereby decreasing the workload of the newly transplanted heart. Inhaled nitric oxide is also protective against ischemia reperfusion injury of the lung after transplantation.[108,109]

Immunosuppression. As with other types of organ transplantation, the immunosuppressive protocols for HLT vary among institutions. Generally speaking, they include an initial triple-drug regimen comprising a calcineurin inhibitor such as cyclosporine or tacrolimus, mycophenolic acid or azathioprine, and corticosteroids. High-dose steroids must be used judiciously because of the deleterious effects of steroids on wound healing. This is especially concerning in HLT because of the decreased vascularity of the trachea and resultant delayed anastomotic healing. Induction therapy also varies, with approximately 30% of centers choosing to forego the use of induction agents and the remainder using an IL-2Ra such as daclizumab or basiliximab or polyclonal antibodies such as OKT-3 or rabbit antithymocyte globulin (RATG) as their agent of choice.[99]

Infection Surveillance. Surveillance for infection and rejection in the heart-lung transplant recipient is accomplished by bronchoscopy. This is performed initially at clinically determined or set intervals to monitor the tracheal anastomosis for evidence of healing, to obtain bronchoalveolar lavage washings for appropriate cultures, and to obtain biopsy specimens for the diagnosis of rejection. Bronchoscopic examination provides visual evidence of tracheal anastomosis healing, which can determine the introduction of maintenance corticosteroids to the immunosuppressive regimen.[110]

As in the heart transplant recipient, presence of fever is an indication for aggressive evaluation. Serial chest radiographic films are used to monitor for infiltrate. However, it is difficult to distinguish infection from rejection by this means. Radiographic changes are used with other clinical evidence, including the partial pressure of oxygen (PaO_2), O_2 saturation, presence or absence of fever, and culture reports, to determine the course of action. Documented infections are treated with appropriate antibiotics.

Nursing Diagnoses

Heart-Lung Transplantation

- Ineffective Airway Clearance related to excessive secretions or abnormal viscosity of mucus
- Ineffective Breathing Pattern related to decreased lung expansion
- Impaired Gas Exchange related to ventilation/perfusion mismatching or intrapulmonary shunting
- Decreased Cardiac Output related to alterations in preload
- Decreased Cardiac Output related to alterations in afterload
- Decreased Cardiac Output related to alterations in heart rate
- Risk for Infection: immunosuppressive drugs required to prevent rejection of transplanted organ
- Disturbed Body Image related to actual change in body structure, function, or appearance
- Anxiety related to threat to biologic, psychologic, and social integrity
- Readiness for Enhanced Knowledge: Posttransplantation Self-Care Regimen, immunosuppressive drugs, cardiopulmonary drugs, diuretics, and clinical manifestations of infection

Rejection Surveillance. Rejection, which can be definitively diagnosed only by transbronchial biopsy, is graded by histologic findings of acute and chronic lung rejection (Table 42-8).[111] Procedural complications after bronchoscopic examination are a transient fever, a fall in the PaO_2 level, infection, and pneumothorax. Chest radiographic examination must be done after each bronchoscopy to rule out pneumothorax.

Pulmonary rejection is treated by augmentation of maintenance immunosuppression, pulses of intravenously administered corticosteroid, or switching to alternative immunosuppressants. Augmentation may be in the form of increasing the cyclosporine or tacrolimus dose to achieve a higher drug level, increasing azathioprine or mycophenolate mofetil, increasing the maintenance prednisone dose, or some combination of these. Pulsing is the method of administering large doses of corticosteroids over a relatively short period. A commonly used pulse dose of steroid is 1 g of Solu-Medrol given once daily for 3 consecutive days. Quick resolution of radiographic changes after the administration of steroid pulses provides a retrospective confirmation of the diagnosis of rejection. Monoclonal and polyclonal antibodies also can be used to treat acute intractable rejection, as in the treatment of recurrent heart rejection.

Pulmonary function testing is a noninvasive method of assessing lung function and the presence of rejection. Lung denervation does not adversely affect the control of ventilation at rest or during exercise.[112] Pulmonary function testing uses a wide range of parameters to measure the functions of the lung at rest and during exercise. The functions are measured in percentages based on weight, gender, and age. The focus is usually on the forced expiratory volume in 1 second (FEV_1), forced vital capacity (FVC), forced expiratory flow rate between 25% and 75% of FVC ($FEF_{25\%-75\%}$), and arterial blood gases. These functions are sensitive to slight changes in oxygenation and ventilation caused by infection or rejection. Acute changes in pulmonary function test results and in PaO_2 are indications for transbronchial biopsy.[110]

Rejection of the heart occurs less often in heart-lung recipients. Endomyocardial biopsy is performed less often.[113] When required, the procedure is similar to that described earlier for heart transplant recipients.

PATIENT EDUCATION

Patient education should be provided to cover all aspects of the immunosuppressive medication regimen, signs and symptoms of infection, role of pulmonary function tests, myocardial biopsy, transbronchial biopsy, and clinical signs of cardiac and pulmonary failure. A discussion of lifestyle adjustments, long-term considerations, and follow-up visits is always included.

LONG-TERM CONSIDERATIONS

Chronic immunosuppression in the heart-lung transplant recipient carries the same consequences as in those receiving a heart alone. Accelerated graft atherosclerosis can be a late complication, and it follows a course similar to that in the heart recipient. A major long-term complication in lung transplantation is obliterative bronchiolitis, an inflammatory disorder of the small airways that leads to obstruction and destruction of pulmonary bronchioles.[111] Features of obliterative bronchiolitis are listed in Box 42-13. Obliterative bronchiolitis may represent a manifestation of chronic pulmonary allograft rejection.[112,114,115] The only definitive treatment for end-stage obliterative bronchiolitis is retransplantation. Retransplantation in heart-lung recipients carries a high risk for complications related to infection, delayed healing related to steroid therapy, renal insufficiency related to chronic cyclosporine use, and bleeding related to scarring from the previous surgery.

CMV is a significant threat to the lung transplant recipient. Prophylaxis and treatment of CMV disease are similar to those for heart recipients; however, institutions vary regarding the anti-CMV agents used and duration of prophylaxis and treatment.[86-90]

Thirty-one HLT procedures were performed in the United States in 2007.[97] As of May 1, 2009, there were 84 candidates on the national waiting list for HLT.[97] The restricted donor pool remains the major factor limiting the number of HLTs performed.

TABLE 42-8 Standardized Pulmonary Biopsy Grading

Category	Grade
A. Acute rejection	0 – None
	1 – Minimal
	2 – Mild
	3 – Moderate
	4 – Severe
B. Airway inflammation—lymphocytic bronchitis/bronchiolitis	0 – None
	1 – Minimal
	2 – Mild
	3 – Moderate
	4 – Severe
	X – Ungradable
C. Chronic airway rejection—bronchiolitis obliterans	a. Active
	b. Inactive
D. Chronic vascular rejection—accelerated graft vascular sclerosis	

Modified from Yousem SA et al: Revision of the working formulation for the classification of pulmonary allograft rejection: Lung Rejection Study Group, *J Heart Lung Transplant* 15:1, 1996.

BOX 42-13 FEATURES OF OBLITERATIVE BRONCHIOLITIS

- Rapid rate of development: several months to 1 to 2 years
- Bronchitic symptoms followed by early development of dyspnea
- Distinct infiltrative component on chest radiograph
- Severe obstructive and restrictive disease
- Decreased total lung capacity
- Largely irreversible with bronchodilator therapy

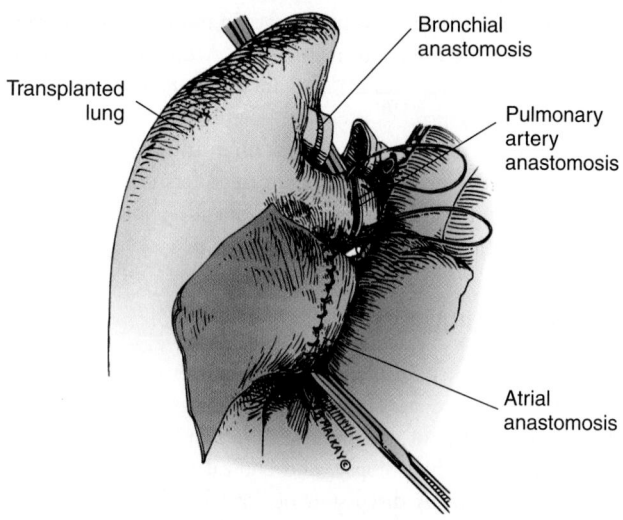

Figure 42-8 Surgical procedure of single-lung transplantation. *(Modified from Baumgartner WA et al: Heart and heart-lung transplantation, ed 2, Philadelphia, 2002, WB Saunders.)*

From 1997 to 2004, the 1-, 3-, and 5-year survival rates after HLT were 67.5%, 49.8%, and 40.1%, respectively.[97] The leading causes of mortality 3 to 5 years after transplantation were obliterative bronchiolitis (40%), graft failure (15.7%), and cardiovascular disease (11.4%).[116]

SINGLE-LUNG AND DOUBLE-LUNG TRANSPLANTATION

SINGLE-LUNG TRANSPLANTATION

Transplantation teams have explored, modified, and successfully pursued the development of pulmonary transplantation, building on the knowledge gained from HLT. Considerations in choosing lung transplantation include the specific disease process, the need for cardiac repair, and donor availability. SLT is an alternative to HLT in a selected group of patients. Generally speaking, SLT is most appropriate for patients with restrictive lung disease (e.g., idiopathic pulmonary fibrosis, sarcoidosis) or noninfectious obstructive lung disease (e.g., emphysema) in the absence of significant cardiac dysfunction.

SINGLE-LUNG TRANSPLANTATION SURGICAL PROCEDURE

Transplantation that is contralateral to (on the opposite side from) a previous thoracotomy is preferable to avoid adhesions that require further surgical dissection.[100] The left lung is sometimes preferred, because it is easier to expose and has a longer left main bronchus. The longer bronchus gives the surgeon more flexibility in trimming the suture site as needed for anastomosis (Fig. 42-8).[117] If there is a significant disproportion of ventilation and perfusion to one side, transplantation on the worse side may be the preferred option.[101] With SLT, the remaining native lung, which has restrictive or obstructive pathophysiology, will have a higher vascular resistance than the

transplanted lung. The blood flow is then automatically directed toward the new lung. Advantages to SLT are better use of donor resources, decreased operative risks, and decreased short-term and fewer long-term complications, as listed in Box 42-14. Contraindications to SLT are similar to those listed for the HLT candidate.

DOUBLE-LUNG OR BILATERAL-LUNG TRANSPLANTATION

Pulmonary diseases that typically are associated with chronic lung infections, such as cystic fibrosis or bronchiectasis, require transplantation of both lungs because of the risk of cross-infection from the native lung into the transplanted lung.

Double-Lung Transplantation Surgical Procedure. Use of cardiopulmonary bypass is becoming less common during lung transplantation. However, patients with moderate to severe pulmonary hypertension typically require cardiopulmonary bypass, because clamping of the pulmonary artery, necessary for removal of the diseased lung, may cause sudden right heart failure.[110] Inability to maintain adequate oxygenation and ventilation with a single lung, sudden increases in pulmonary artery pressure, poor right ventricular function, and hemodynamic compromise indicate the need for cardiopulmonary bypass.[118]

The surgical procedure is similar for SLT and DLT, with a few exceptions. DLT is usually performed as a bilateral, sequential SLT. The surgical incision for SLT can be an anterolateral or posterolateral thoracotomy at the level of the fourth or fifth intercostal space. DLT is performed through bilateral anterior thoracosternotomies extending from the midaxillary line and across the sternum at the fourth intercostal space (clamshell incision).[107] The clamshell incision is extremely painful for most patients, necessitating frequent pain assessment and intervention by the nurse. A median sternotomy or bilateral anterior thoracotomies are alternative surgical approaches.

The anastomotic sites for DLT include the back wall of the atria (containing the four pulmonary vein orifices), the bronchus, and the main pulmonary artery, as illustrated in Figure 42-9.[107] Donor and recipient arteries are trimmed to suitable lengths, and end-to-end anastomoses is performed. Bronchial anastomosis is performed with a running suture. After the atrial clamp is slowly removed, the patient is assessed for bleeding.[101,117] In some transplant centers, the omentum is brought through the diaphragm from the abdomen and wrapped around the bronchus

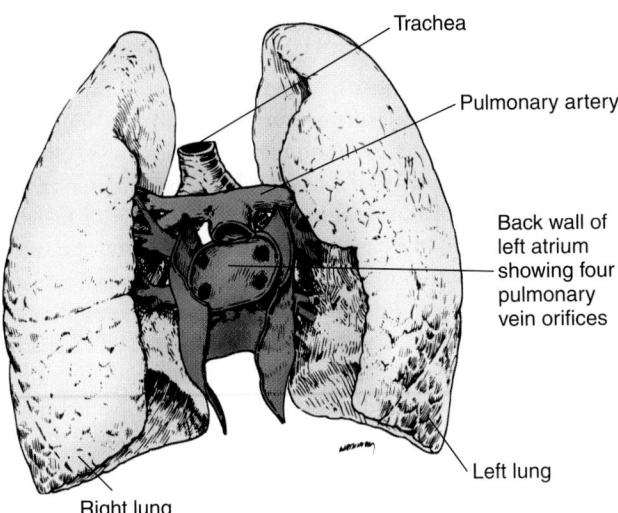

Figure 42-9 Double-lung transplant graft before implantation into a recipient. *(Modified from Baumgartner WA et al: Heart and heart-lung transplantation,* ed 2, Philadelphia, 2002, WB Saunders.)

Nursing Diagnoses

Single-Lung and Double-Lung Transplantation

- Ineffective Airway Clearance related to excessive secretions or abnormal viscosity of mucus
- Impaired Gas Exchange related to ventilation/perfusion mismatching or intrapulmonary shunting
- Risk for Infection: immunosuppressive drugs required to prevent rejection of transplanted organ
- Disturbed Body Image related to actual change in body structure, function, or appearance
- Anxiety related to threat to biologic, psychologic, and social integrity
- Readiness for Enhanced Knowledge: Posttransplantation Self-Care Regimen, immunosuppressive drugs, pulmonary drugs, diuretics, and clinical manifestations of infection

for added stability of the anastomosis and increased vascular supply. Disadvantages of this maneuver include a larger incision and involvement of the abdominal cavity.[107]

Lung Volume Reduction Surgery. Lung volume reduction is a surgical procedure that may be an option in candidates for lung transplantation. Although the procedure does not result in better lung function compared with transplantation, it does avoid complications related to immunosuppression and transplantation. It may be an early option for patients who could require lung transplantation in the future.[117,119]

Living Donor Lung Transplantation. Another alternative to traditional lung transplantation is living donor lung transplantation. In this procedure, the lungs are harvested not from a brain dead donor but from two living donors who each provide a right or left lower lobe to the recipient. The two donated lobes essentially function as new lungs. Recipients of this type of transplant tend to be patients with cystic fibrosis or other patients who are smaller in size. A smaller recipient increase the likelihood that two lobes will be able to provide adequate pulmonary function.[120] Living donor lung transplantation is still specialized and is not as commonly practiced as cadaveric lung transplantation. Only three living donor lung transplantations were performed in 2003.[97] The overall actuarial survival rates of 70%, 54%, and 45% at 1, 3, and 5 years, respectively,[121] are comparable to the rates reported from the International Society for Heart and Lung Transplantation 2003 registry for cadaveric bilateral lung transplantation.[122,123]

POSTOPERATIVE MEDICAL AND NURSING MANAGEMENT

Postoperative care of single-lung and double-lung transplant recipients is similar to that for HLT patients, as described earlier. Several nursing diagnoses are associated with care of SLT and DLT patients, as listed in the Nursing Diagnoses feature on Single-Lung and Double-Lung Transplantation.

SLT patients typically require mechanical ventilation for a shorter duration. Less bleeding can be anticipated because of the brevity of the surgical procedure. A single pleural chest tube usually is sufficient for drainage. A pulmonary artery catheter may be used to measure right ventricular response when significant ventilation/perfusion mismatching occurs. In the event of elevated pulmonary artery pressures, pharmacologic vasodilation or afterload reduction can be instituted. Patients with pulmonary hypertension may have a greater ventilation/perfusion mismatch, resulting in larger arteriolar-arterial gradient.[117,119]

Immunosuppression for lung recipients is essentially the same as for HLT patients. Initiation of steroids depends on institutional preference and healing of the bronchial anastomosis.

Surveillance for rejection and infection is similar to that in HLT. Pulmonary function testing is not initiated until the second or third postoperative week to allow for surgical recovery.[124] Decreased lung function caused by fluid shifts, microatelectasis, and splinting from incisional pain interferes with accurate testing. In unilateral lung transplantation, the transplanted lung functions in parallel with the native lung, which can be expected to retain any pathology.[125] The patient's condition must be measured by comparison with his or her own baseline and not with normal standards. This concept also can be applied to the evaluation of arterial blood gases during the immediate postoperative period of intubation. Oxygenation and ventilation occur in both diseased and transplanted lungs, and parameters for evaluation need to be adjusted accordingly.

PATIENT EDUCATION

Patient education should be provided to cover all aspects of the immunosuppressive medication regimen, signs and symptoms of infection, role of pulmonary function tests, transbronchial biopsy, and clinical signs of pulmonary failure. A discussion of lifestyle adjustments, long-term considerations, and follow-up visits is included.

LONG-TERM CONSIDERATIONS

Clinically, single-lung transplant recipients function as well as other patients who have only one lung. With physical exertion, some patients may complain of shortness of breath. A combination of chest roentgenography, bronchoscopic examination, and pulmonary function testing is used in the detection and diagnosis of rejection and infection. Long-term complications for single- and double-lung transplant recipients are similar to for heart transplant recipients. As in HLT, many of these patients experience obliterative bronchiolitis as a major long-term complication.

From 1997 to 2004, the 1-, 3-, and 5-year survival rates were 84%, 60.7%, and 44.1%, respectively, for SLT and 82.7%, 64.8%, and 50.3%, respectively, for DLT.[97] Leading causes of mortality at 3 to 5 years after transplantation were obliterative bronchiolitis (30%), graft failure (18.8%), and infection (18.3%).[116]

LIVER TRANSPLANTATION

Liver transplantation was first attempted in canine models in the 1950s. The outcomes were unsuccessful because of technical complications, infection, and graft failure.[126,127] The effort to improve surgical technique continued, and successful liver transplantation in dogs was achieved several years later by Moore and colleagues[128,129] and Starzl and coworkers.[130] In 1963, Starzl and colleagues[131] performed the first human liver transplantation operation. Although the patient died intraoperatively, this attempt pioneered the possibility of liver transplantation in human beings.

The first successful human liver transplantation was performed in 1967 by Starzl and his colleagues[132] in a patient with malignant hepatoma. The patient survived 1 year before succumbing to recurrent disease. Patient 1-year survival rates in the late 1960s and throughout the 1970s remained at less than 50% despite continued improvements in the surgical techniques. These early attempts were hindered by the difficulty of the surgery, poor methods of organ preservation, and inadequate immunosuppression.

Clinical trials of cyclosporine began in 1979 and revolutionized liver transplantation. One-year survival rates in the early 1980s increased to 70% and higher.[133,134] This prompted the National Institutes of Health to declare that liver transplantation was no longer experimental but rather an accepted therapeutic modality for patients with end-stage liver disease.[135] This position statement resulted in an increase in the number of liver transplant centers worldwide and in the number of liver transplantations performed. Fewer than 200 liver transplantations were performed in 1983, but almost 6500 were performed in 2007, including deceased and living donors combined. In 2007, patient survival rates after liver transplantation in 2007 were greater than 85% at 1 year and 70% to 75% at 5 years.[136]

INDICATIONS AND SELECTION

Liver transplantation must be considered for any patient who suffers from irreversible acute or chronic liver disease that is progressive and for which there is no therapy of established efficacy. Diseases of the liver may be categorized as chronic, vascular, fulminant or subfulminant and include inborn errors of metabolism and hepatic malignancies. Box 42-15 lists the most common diseases seen in patients who undergo liver transplantation. In the United States, the single most common indication for liver transplantation in adults is chronic viral hepatitis C.[137,138] Biliary atresia and metabolic disorders account for more than 70% of the diseases leading to transplantation in the pediatric population.[137,139]

Candidate selection is an important aspect of transplantation. Given the shortage of available organs, the transplantation team must have reasonable assurance of a successful outcome. The timing of transplantation is of utmost importance: The patient must not be so ill as to be unable to survive the surgery but yet is experiencing deterioration in the quality of life. Body mass index (BMI) plays a role in posttransplantation survival. Patients who are underweight (BMI <20) or morbidly obese (BMI >40) are at greater risk for death after transplantation.[140] In general, liver transplantation is not to be offered to persons in the following groups:

- Those who would not be likely to survive major surgery
- Those who would not survive the effects of long-term immunosuppression

---

BOX 42-15 END-STAGE LIVER DISEASES COMMONLY TREATED WITH LIVER TRANSPLANTATION

CHOLESTATIC LIVER DISEASES
- Biliary atresia
- Primary sclerosing cholangitis
- Primary biliary cirrhosis

CHRONIC HEPATOCELLULAR DISEASES
- Viral hepatitis (types A, B, C, D, E)
- Alcoholic liver disease (Laennec disease)
- Autoimmune hepatitis
- Cryptogenic cirrhosis
- Drug-induced liver disease

VASCULAR DISEASES
- Budd-Chiari syndrome
- Veno-occlusive disease

FULMINANT AND SUBFULMINANT HEPATIC FAILURE
- Viral hepatitis (types A, B, C, D, E)

- Drug-induced liver failure (acetaminophen, isoniazid overdoses)
- Fulminant Wilson's disease

INBORN METABOLIC DISORDERS
- Wilson's disease
- α_1-Antitrypsin deficiency
- Hemochromatosis
- Tyrosinemia
- Glycogen storage disease, types I and II

PRIMARY HEPATIC MALIGNANCIES
- Hepatocellular carcinoma
- Hemangioendothelioma
- Hepatoblastoma

- Those who have a disease that is likely to recur quickly and fatally after transplantation
- Those who are not willing to comply with long-term and sometimes difficult and demanding medical regimens

The absolute contraindications listed in Box 42-16 fall under these four specific categories.

Having one relative contraindication may not rule out transplantation, but having several predicts poor outcome. Chronologic age is less important than physiologic age. Reports of transplantation in older patients describe favorable results.[141] Certain diseases can recur after transplantation, including viral hepatitis,[142,143] sclerosing cholangitis,[144] and biliary malignancies.[145] In the case of viral hepatitis, serologic indicators of viral replication are monitored closely. In the presence of aggressively replicating virus and in certain malignancies, it is in the patient's best interest not to proceed to transplantation, because it would actually hasten death. Multicenter protocols are important in evaluating the outcomes and efficacies of transplantations in patients with diseases that recur. The decision to offer liver transplantation to any patient must be based on evaluation criteria, which vary among institutions and which are modified as advances in technical ability, immunosuppression, and perioperative management continue. In the absence of complications, the average hospital stay after liver transplantation is 7 to 14 days.[137]

Recipient Evaluation. The candidate for liver transplantation undergoes a thorough evaluation to determine the cause and severity of the liver disease, to establish the need for transplantation rather than other interventions, and to identify objective indications and contraindications. Evaluation begins with a carefully elicited patient history (Box 42-17). A comprehensive approach includes laboratory, radiographic, and diagnostic testing and multidisciplinary consultations (Box 42-18). Not every patient undergoes every test and consultation. Careful history taking and a good physical examination direct the initial diagnostic testing. For instance, a patient with a past history of malignancy would undergo extensive testing to rule out metastases, whereas a patient with fulminant hepatic failure may

have a more abbreviated workup that is focused on determining the cause and potential for hepatic recovery.

During the workup, the candidate's support systems are evaluated by the entire transplantation team, which includes the surgeon, the hepatologist, the clinical transplantation nurse coordinator, the social worker, the dietitian, and the financial counselor. Other services, such as cardiology, nephrology, psychiatry, gynecology, anesthesia, infectious disease, endocrinology, hematology, rheumatology, and oral surgery or dentistry, may also be included in the evaluation. Ideally, all immunizations are brought up to date in an attempt to minimize postoperative infections. The patient and family receive education regarding the evaluation, waiting list, surgery, postoperative management including immunosuppression, and long-term follow-up. At the conclusion of the evaluation, one of several outcomes is possible: (1) the patient is deemed a transplant candidate, (2) the patient is deemed not a candidate, or (3) the patient may be a candidate some time in the future if certain criteria are met. These criteria may be of a physical nature (e.g., it is too early in the disease process to list now, in which case the patient will be re-evaluated at set intervals), or they may be of a psychosocial nature (e.g., the patient must attend a formal alcohol or drug rehabilitation program or undergo treatment of depression).

After candidacy has been determined and the patient is ready for transplantation, his or her social security number is entered into the national computer system operated by UNOS. Objective criteria are used to place a patient on the waiting list. These data are used in a formula to determine the patient's score, which is directly associated with the patient's risk of death within 3 months (the higher the score, the higher the risk).

Model for End-Stage Liver Disease. The Model for End-Stage Liver Disease (MELD) formula is used in all U.S. transplant centers to calculate risk of mortality in patients 12 years old or older.[137] The MELD objective criteria include serum total bilirubin, serum creatinine, prothrombin time, and international normalized ratio.

Pediatric End-Stage Liver Disease Formula. The Pediatric End-Stage Liver Disease (PELD) formula is used for patients

---

BOX 42-16	CONTRADICTIONS TO LIVER TRANSPLANTATION

ABSOLUTE CONTRAINDICATIONS
- Brain death
- Metastatic malignancy
- Extrahepatic malignancy
- Active drug or alcohol abuse
- Advanced cardiopulmonary disease
- Acquired immunodeficiency syndrome
- Extrahepatic sepsis

RELATIVE CONTRAINDICATIONS
- Physiologic age
- Advanced renal disease
- Multiple hepatic malignancies
- Moderate cardiopulmonary disease
- Peripheral vascular disease
- Psychosocial behaviors indicating noncompliance with medical regimens
- Human immunodeficiency virus infection

BOX 42-17	PRETRANSPLANTATION HISTORY FOR A PATIENT WITH END-STAGE LIVER DISEASE

- Risk factors for viral hepatitis: transfusions, intravenous drug abuse, tattoos, other parenteral exposure
- Family history of liver disease
- Associated disorders: hypothyroidism, osteoporosis, infertility, arthritis
- Onset, duration, and description of symptoms and complications: jaundice, lethargy, bleeding disorders, pruritus, confusion, ascites, edema, melenic stools, abdominal pain, bone pain or fractures, chronic diarrhea, gynecomastia (in men), amenorrhea (in women)
- Current and past medical history: hospitalizations, surgeries
- Social history: exposure to alcohol, drugs, toxins, tobacco products
- Status of immunizations

BOX 42-18 SAMPLE EVALUATION BEFORE LIVER TRANSPLANTATION

LABORATORY TESTS

- Liver function profile: transaminases (AST, ALT, GGT), alkaline phosphatase, bilirubin, albumin, prothrombin time, partial thromboplastin time, clotting factors, cholesterol, triglycerides
- Kidney function profile with electrolytes: blood urea nitrogen, creatinine, sodium, potassium, carbon dioxide, chloride
- Hematology: CBC, reticulocytes, ESR
- Thyroid function: T_3RIA; T_4RIA; thyroid-stimulating hormone; T_4 and T_3 uptake
- Serology studies for hepatic viruses and other infectious diseases: viral hepatitis (A, B, C, D, E); cytomegalovirus, Epstein-Barr virus, herpesvirus I and II, parvovirus, HIV; RPR
- Blood type and antibody screen
- Immunologic profiles: antinuclear antibody; antimitochondrial antibody; anti–smooth muscle antibody; immunoglobulins (A, G, M)
- Nutritional profiles: vitamin levels (A, D, E, B_{12}, folate); iron studies with ferritin
- Tumor markers: α-fetoprotein, CEA, PSA,
- Miscellaneous: ceruloplasmin, α_1-antitrypsin level and phenotype

Urine

- 24-Hour protein and electrolytes, cultures, creatinine clearance, urinalysis, copper

Stool

- Ova, cysts, parasites, occult blood, 48-hour fecal fat, cultures

Gastrointestinal Workup

- Endoscopy, colonoscopy, endoscopic retrograde cholangiopancreatography, liver biopsy

Pulmonary Profile

- Arterial blood gases, pulmonary function studies

Radiographic and Diagnostic Tests

- Chest radiograph, ultrasound studies of liver including vascular studies

Optional Tests

- Doppler studies; sinus radiography; computed tomography (abdomen, chest, head); electrocardiography; echocardiography; cardiac stress test; cardiac catheterization; mammography; peripheral vascular studies; carotid ultrasonography; abdominal angiography; percutaneous cholangiography; bone mineral density

---

ALT, alanine aminotransferase; AST, aspartate transaminase; CBC, complete blood cell count; CEA, carcinoembryonic agents; ESR, erythrocyte sedimentation rate; GGT, γ-glutamyltransferase; HIV, human immunodeficiency virus; PSA, prostate-specific antigen; RPR, rapid plasma reagin; T_3RIA; serum triiodothyronine (T_3) radioimmunoassay; T_4RIA, serum triiodothyronine (T_4) radioimmunoassay.

---

11 years old or younger.[146] The PELD objective criteria include date of birth, gender, weight, height, serum albumin, serum total bilirubin, prothrombin time, and international normalized ratio.

Placement on the waiting list is determined by blood type, weight, and patient urgency. Patients with acute fulminant hepatic failure are considered to be in most urgent need and are placed at the top of the list. Patients with chronic end-stage liver disease are prioritized by their MELD or PELD score. Those with higher scores are placed higher on the list. The duration of waiting time is used only as a tie-breaker for patients with equal scores. Each UNOS region has special exception cases that must be voted on by the regional review board (comprising one member from each transplant center in the region). In these cases, the board may be asked to assign higher-than-calculated scores for patients with special problems that are not addressed by the use of only objective criteria, such as children with intractable pruritus, ascites, hemorrhage, or infectious complications[146] and patients with hepatocellular carcinoma.[147]

The frequency of recalculation of the MELD score is determined by the score itself. MELD scores greater than 25, between 19 and 24, and between 11 and 18 are evaluated every 7, 30, and 90 days, respectively.[148] A score of less than 10 is recalculated yearly[148] barring any exacerbation of the liver disease or patient condition.

Next, one of the most difficult phases begins: the waiting period. It is not possible to anticipate when an appropriate organ will become available. The patient may feel that his or her life is being put "on hold." Because of the shortage of donors, it is not uncommon for patients in critical care units to die while awaiting transplantation; this is especially true for pediatric recipients. And knowing that another person must die so that he or she may live can cause feelings of guilt as the patient hopes for a liver to become available. Patients with end-stage liver disease know that the only alternative to transplantation is death. By understanding the basic social processes that patients experience while awaiting transplantation, nurses can facilitate health promotion activities.[149] It is important for the patient and family to receive ongoing psychosocial assessment and to attend pretransplantation support groups, which are available at most transplant centers.

Pretransplantation Phase. The patient with end-stage liver disease who is awaiting a transplant may pose one of the greatest care challenges in the critical care unit. Hepatic encephalopathy, coagulopathies, portal hypertension, severe fluid and electrolyte imbalances, cardiac compromise, and renal deterioration are not uncommon. Frequent mental status assessments are important in determining the patient's continued candidacy for transplantation. Hepatic encephalopathy may improve with the administration of antibiotics and laxatives, or the patient may proceed to stage IV coma. Protection of the airway is especially important in an encephalopathic patient who is not intubated. In these circumstances, if hematemesis or vomiting occurs, intubation and use of paralytic agents may be necessary to protect the patient's airway. Diagnostic studies may be needed to evaluate the possibility of an intracranial bleed. The head of the patient's bed is maintained at 30 to 45 degrees to avoid even slight increases in intracranial pressure. Patients who have chronic liver disease also have nutritional deficits. They require supplements of the fat-soluble vitamins (A, D, E, and K), may be on protein restriction to reduce serum ammonia levels, and may experience severe muscle wasting.

Consequences of portal hypertension must be corrected. Gastrointestinal hemorrhage from varices may respond to administration of propranolol or to procedures such as banding and sclerotherapy. Portal hypertension may be reduced by transjugular intrahepatic portosystemic shunting (TIPS) in interventional radiology. Rarely, the patient may need to undergo surgical intervention with a vascular shunt created between the portacaval system and the mesangial, splenic, or renal vascular system. Patients with massive ascites usually have total body fluid overload but are intravascularly contracted and require sodium restriction and administration of colloidal fluids (e.g., albumin) along with diuretics. Careful documentation of fluid intake and output, daily weight determinations, and frequent measurement of vital signs are needed to monitor fluid status. Ascites can interfere with lung expansion and can compromise oxygenation. Patients with large, distended abdomens also find adequate oral nutrition difficult. Use of diuretics to control ascites is common but can compromise kidney function or even worsen hepatorenal syndrome. Paracentesis (removal of ascites) may be required for intractable ascites. However, frequent large-volume paracentesis procedures can contribute to renal demise and cardiovascular compromise related to fluid volume shifts.

Spontaneous bacterial peritonitis can be manifested in the patient with end-stage liver disease by an acute decline in the hepatic and renal function accompanied by fever, abdominal pain, and hepatic encephalopathy. The paracentesis fluid shows increased white blood cells with or without a positive culture. Patients are treated aggressively with antibiotics and are temporarily deferred from transplantation during treatment for and recovery from bacterial peritonitis.

Determining Donor Suitability. The two criteria necessary for matching a donor liver to a recipient are blood type and body size. HLA tissue typing is not used in the matching of donor livers, because it has not been shown to significantly affect patient outcomes. Donors are carefully screened for infectious diseases and metastatic carcinomas, because these can be transmitted to the recipient. The transplant center is notified by the regional OPO that a liver is available. If the organ is accepted, a member of the transplantation team contacts the patient.

In very urgent situations, the donor blood type (e.g., type A) may not be compatible with that of the recipient (e.g., type O). Despite this incompatibility, such liver transplantations can be successful. There may be some early postoperative complications, such as mild hemolysis, higher incidence of acute cellular rejection, and increased postoperative hepatic vascular and biliary complications, but innovative use of immunosuppressive regimens and plasmapheresis have improved graft survival of patients with recipient-donor ABO incompatibility.[150,151] Extended-criteria donor livers, such as those with a cold ischemia time longer than 12 hours or those from donors older than 60 years, that are otherwise unremarkable are expanding the donor pool and shortening waiting times.[152]

After a donor liver becomes available, it is necessary to expedite the preoperative preparation of the recipient. The use of University of Wisconsin preservation solution has allowed for longer cold ischemia time (i.e., the length of time from when the organ is removed from the donor, flushed, and packed in ice for storage until the time when it is transplanted). However, cold ischemia times of longer than 12 hours are correlated with increased recipient morbidity and mortality.[137]

Living Donor Liver Transplantation. Since 1985, approximately 23,000 people have died while registered and awaiting a liver from a deceased donor. About one half of the 127 liver transplant centers in the United States offer *living donor liver transplantation* (LDLT). The peak number of LDLT procedures, 522, occurred in 2001, after which there the incidence declined to a total of 266 procedures in 2007.[136]

LDLT began in 1989 with adult-to-child donations, commonly from a parent to his or her infant. The left lateral hepatic lobe is resected, leaving the donor with the larger mass of liver remaining.[153] In such cases, the risks to the healthy donor are thought to be outweighed by the benefits of having a healthy child.[154] Adult-to-adult LDLT donation began in the 1990s. The whole left hepatic lobe or right hepatic lobe is resected, taking 30% to 60% of the liver mass from the live donor.[153] Complications for the donor after partial hepatectomy are usually of low severity. The most common ones are bile leak, bacterial infection, incisional hernia, pleural effusion, neuropraxia (temporary nerve dysfunction), wound infection, and abdominal abcess.[148,154] More serious potential complications for the liver donor include portal vein thrombosis, inferior vena cava thrombosis, and death.[148,154,155] By 2006, there had been 14 deaths among living liver donors reported in the United States and Europe.[155] Critical care nurses play an important role in caring for these donors and must be vigilant in assessing for complications and initiating early interventions.

LIVER TRANSPLANTATION SURGICAL PROCEDURE

Liver transplantation surgery is lengthy and technically difficult, often lasting 4 to 12 hours. The procedure involves the combined efforts of surgeons, anesthesiologists, nurse anesthetists, operating room nurses and technicians, perfusionists, and personnel from the blood bank and laboratory and radiology departments, among others. The patient is taken to the operating room for anesthesia induction, insertion of large-bore intravenous catheters that allow high-volume fluid infusion, and insertion of a pulmonary artery catheter for hemodynamic monitoring. Continuous renal replacement may be continued or initiated in the operating room by a filter-trained critical care or dialysis nurse. Other devices, such as an arterial line, a nasogastric tube, and a urinary drainage catheter, are also inserted. The patient is positioned on the operating room table in such a way as to minimize pressure that could cause ischemia and chronic injury to tissue and peripheral nerves. Liver transplantation surgery can be divided into three stages: (1) recipient hepatectomy, (2) vascular anastomoses with donor liver, and (3) biliary anastomosis.

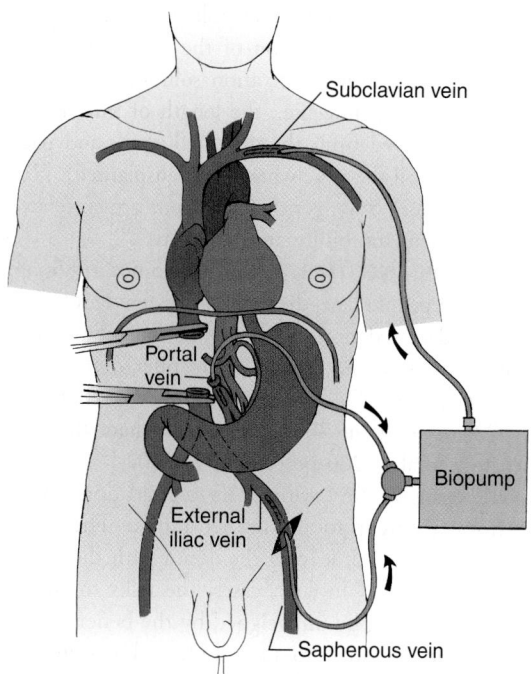

Figure 42-10 Venovenous bypass during removal of the native liver. The portal and iliac veins are cannulated, and blood is circulated by a centrifugal pump to the subclavian vein.

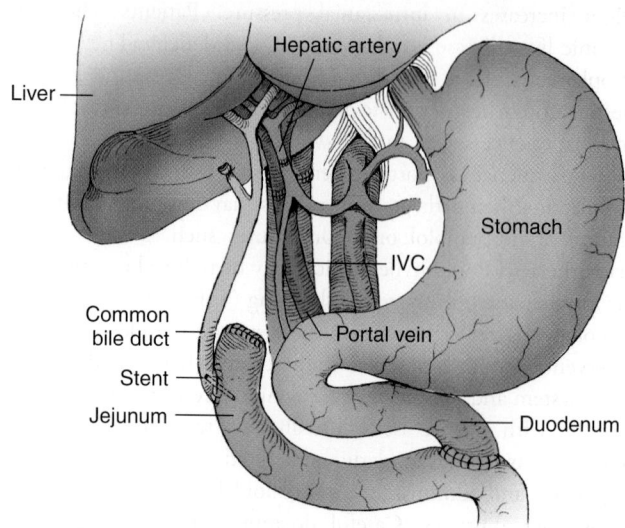

Figure 42-11 Roux-en-Y procedure (choledochojejunostomy). IVC, inferior vena cava.

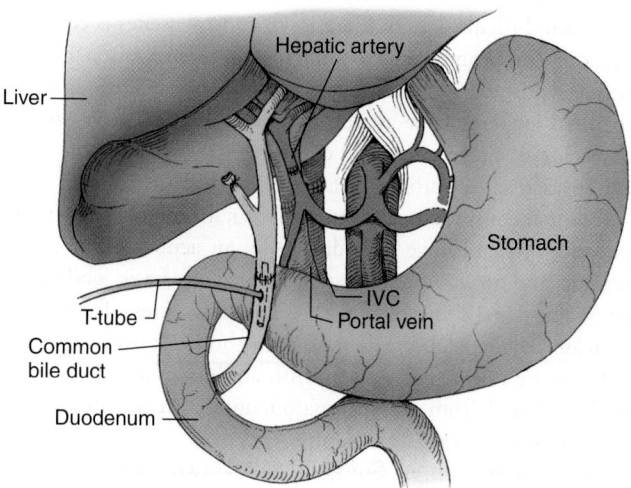

Figure 42-12 Choledochocholedochostomy procedure. IVC, inferior vena cava.

Recipient Hepatectomy. Stage 1 is the longest and most difficult part of the surgery, because it involves removal of the native liver. It is complicated even more by coagulopathies, adhesions, portal hypertension, and venous collaterals. Before completion of this stage, the patient may be placed on venovenous bypass (Fig. 42-10), although not all patients require this procedure. A centrifugal pump cycles the blood out through iliac and portal vein cannulas and returns it to the central circulation through the axillary or subclavian vein. Advances in surgical techniques, anesthesia, and fluid management have shortened the length of surgery enough to warrant elimination of venovenous bypass in some cases.

Vascular Anastomoses with a Donor Liver. Stage 2 comprises the four vascular anastomoses: suprahepatic inferior vena cava, infrahepatic vena cava, hepatic artery, and portal vein. Many variations and adaptations, such as vascular patches, may be used, depending on the anatomy of the donor and recipient. If venovenous bypass is used, it is removed after the infrahepatic vena cava anastomosis and before the hepatic artery anastomosis.

Biliary Anastomosis. Stage 3 can be achieved by *choledochojejunostomy* (bile duct to jejunum) or by *choledochocholedochostomy* (bile duct to bile duct). Choledochojejunostomy is performed in patients who have diseased bile ducts, such as those with biliary atresia or sclerosing cholangitis. It is also known as a *Roux-en-Y* procedure and is shown in Figure 42-11. The choledochocholedochostomy is performed in patients who have a healthy and intact common bile duct and is shown in Figure 42-12. The patient returns from surgery with or without an external stent or T-tube that is connected to a bag into which bile drains. Patients who do not have external biliary tubes may have an internal stent inserted in the bile duct across

the biliary anastomosis. Eventually, the internal stent moves and is passed with the stool.

POSTOPERATIVE MEDICAL AND NURSING MANAGEMENT

The common nursing diagnoses associated with liver transplantation are listed in the Nursing Diagnoses feature on Liver Transplantation. After surgery, some patients are extubated before they arrive in the critical care unit, but most arrive unreversed from anesthesia and remain intubated for 12 to 24 hours. Immediate goals include (1) reestablishment of normal body temperature, (2) hemodynamic stabilization, and (3) maintenance of an effective airway. Postoperative hypothermia is common after orthotopic liver transplantation (OLT). The critical care nurse must achieve rewarming safely by the use of methods such as warming blankets, heating lamps, and head covers.

Nursing Diagnoses

Liver Transplantation

- Risk for Infection: immunosuppressive drugs required to prevent rejection of the transplanted liver
- Imbalanced Nutrition: Less Than Body Requirements related to lack of exogenous nutrients or increased metabolic demand
- Deficient Fluid Volume related to absolute loss
- Disturbed Body Image related to actual change in body structure, function, or appearance
- Anxiety related to threat to biologic, psychologic, and social integrity
- Readiness for Enhanced Knowledge: Posttransplantation Self-Care Regimen, immunosuppressive drugs, and clinical manifestations of infection

---

BOX 42-19 COMMON COMPLICATIONS AFTER LIVER TRANSPLANTATION

PULMONARY COMPLICATIONS
- Pleural effusion
- Pulmonary edema
- Pneumonia
- Pneumothorax or hemothorax
- Atelectasis
- Paralysis of right diaphragm

BILIARY COMPLICATIONS
- Leaks
- Strictures
- Obstruction
- Infection (cholangitis)
- Breakdown of anastomosis

GASTROINTESTINAL COMPLICATIONS
- Bleeding and ulceration
- Gastrointestinal infections (cytomegalovirus, *Candida*, *Clostridium difficile*)
- Bowel perforations

VASCULAR COMPLICATIONS
- Hepatic artery thrombosis
- Portal vein thrombosis
- Vena caval thrombosis
- Peripheral and central line sepsis
- Hepatic vein thrombosis

Hemodynamics. Hemodynamic stabilization is a particular challenge, because the patient may arrive hypervolemic, euvolemic, or hypovolemic and may be hypertensive or hypotensive. Assessment of total body fluids compared with intravascular fluid status is important. Because of inherent presurgical problems with decreased serum albumin, some centers tend to keep the patient "dry." Hypervolemia often results in third spacing, with resultant ascites and a leaking wound. Accurate measurements of hemodynamic function, such as arterial blood pressure, peripheral blood pressure, central venous pressure, pulmonary artery pressure, PAOP or "wedge" pressure, urinary output, patency of drains, and bile totals are assessed frequently to evaluate true volume status. Choice of replacement fluids and pharmacologic agents for correction of volume and blood pressure abnormalities is specific to the transplant center. These protocols vary in their use of albumin or fresh-frozen plasma, and in the use of intravenous renal-dose dopamine or prostaglandin, as well as other agents and solutions. Still, the goals are the same: optimize tissue perfusion and deliver oxygen to all tissues, especially the newly transplanted graft.

Electrolytes. Electrolyte abnormalities can occur after OLT. Disturbances in potassium and magnesium levels are common. High serum levels of electrolytes are usually associated with renal impairment; low levels can be the result of drug side effects (e.g., diuretic therapy). The presence of hypernatremia or hyponatremia complicates the correction of volume status and fluid replacement.

Pulmonary Management. Ventilatory support of the patient is maintained until the anesthetic agent has been metabolized and cleared by the new liver and the patient awakens. Frequent measurement of arterial blood gas levels, continuous pulse oximetry, and assessment of breath sounds are needed. The patient may require changes in ventilatory settings, suctioning to remove secretions, or administration of pharmacologic agents to correct acid-base imbalances. Pulmonary complications are common, as listed in Box 42-19. While the patient is on ventilatory support, pneumonia can be avoided by maintaining the head of bed elevated at 30 degrees, turning the patient frequently, providing good oral care, and brushing the patient's teeth. After extubation, patients must be encouraged to perform incentive spirometry exercises and to turn, cough, and deep-breathe frequently to help prevent atelectasis and pneumonia. Respiratory treatments with bronchodilators, prophylactic antimicrobials, and chest physiotherapy also may be used.

Coagulopathy Risk. Management of coagulopathies is important in the early postoperative phase. Characterization and careful measurement of drain lines and drainage from incisions are needed along with other nursing assessments of blood loss, such as identifying signs of hypovolemia, tachypnea, tachycardia, or poor peripheral oxygenation. A sudden increase in abdominal girth, sanguineous nasogastric output, and black, tarry stools are hallmarks of bleeding problems and must be reported immediately. Laboratory monitoring during the first 24 hours after surgery is necessary to assess blood loss and coagulopathies and includes hematocrit, hemoglobin, platelet count, prothrombin time, partial thromboplastin time, fibrinogen, and fibrin split products. Reversal of coagulopathies is done judiciously, with consideration for the potential to thrombose newly anastomosed blood vessels in the liver. Blood products such as platelets, fresh-frozen plasma, and specific factors can be given along with pharmacologic agents such as vitamin K.

Neurologic Status. Neurologic assessment of the patient is important in the early postoperative phase to determine mental status and graft function. Patients who were encephalopathic preoperatively are usually slower to clear mentally. Nevertheless, with good liver function, the patient should be alert and oriented within 1 to 2 days: The improved mental status is a reflection of a functional new liver. Certain pharmacologic agents, including immunosuppressants, can cause peripheral and central neurologic side effects that may alter neurologic status. Induction therapy may be used to delay the initiation of immunosuppressant medications associated with neurologic and nephrogenic side effects.[156,157]

Pain Management. The critical care nurse must always be aware of the potential for intracranial bleeds in a patient who has coagulopathies, serum sodium imbalances, and hemodynamic instability. All of these conditions can interfere with pain management, because the pharmacologic agents used for pain can mask deterioration in mental status. Medications to relieve pain are administered, but other, nonpharmacologic nursing interventions also must be used.

Glucose Control. Intensive blood glucose control (<150 mg/dL) during liver transplantation surgery has been associated with a significant decrease in the infection rate at 30 days and in the mortality rate at 1 year.[158] In the intensive care setting, insulin therapy is used to support the newly transplanted liver during the fluctuations in blood glucose related to the patient's immunosuppressant regimen.

Kidney Function. Liver transplantation can alter kidney function by several mechanisms, including cyclosporine or tacrolimus administration, acute tubular necrosis, intrinsic kidney disease, and poor liver function. Some studies estimate that 21% to 73% of OLT patients develop renal failure.[159] Patients are managed with attention to fluid and electrolyte imbalances, by avoidance of nephrotoxic drugs, and occasionally with ultrafiltration, continuous renal replacement therapy, or intermittent hemodialysis. With good liver function, kidney function usually improves. However, certain immunosuppressive agents and antimicrobials can deleteriously affect kidney function. Adjustments in dose or avoidance of use must be balanced with assessment of kidney and liver function. Daily monitoring of cyclosporine or tacrolimus serum levels is vital to determining adequate immunosuppression, and daily serum creatinine levels are necessary to watch for renal impairment. As the patient's condition continues to improve, the frequency of laboratory testing may decrease.

Infection Risk. Immunosuppressive therapy places the transplant recipient at an increased risk for infection. Infectious complications are common and continue to be the leading cause of death among OLT patients.[160,161] The potential for infection is greatest when patients receive high doses of immunosuppressants. All persons who come into contact with the transplant recipient throughout the hospitalization must practice good hand-washing techniques and standard precautions to prevent the transmission of infection.[160] Infections are treated with appropriate antimicrobials specific to the invading organism. Prophylactic therapies are commonly used as well.[139,148,161]

Bile Drains. Careful attention to any external biliary drain line is important. If the patient has an external biliary drain, the critical care nurse documents color, character, and amount of drainage and reports any changes. Biliary complications can occur after OLT. Posttransplantation complications, including biliary ones, are listed in Box 42-19.

Nutrition. The nasogastric tube is removed when its output is minimal, bowel sounds have returned, and the patient is extubated. If the patient will be intubated longer than several days, total parenteral nutrition may be started. Consultation with a nutritionist (dietitian) should be sought after the patient is stable. Prealbumin levels may be measured to assess nutritional status.

Otherwise, nutrition may begin orally or through a feeding tube as soon as bowel function returns. The diet is slowly advanced as tolerated.

Liver Function Tests. The standard laboratory biomarkers used to monitor graft function are serum aspartate aminotransferase (AST), alanine aminotransferase (ALT), alkaline phosphatase, and γ-glutamyltransferase (GGT); serum bilirubin; and prothrombin time. The serum levels of these markers are measured frequently during the first few postoperative days and may continue to rise before peaking and subsequently falling. As liver function improves, the frequency of laboratory testing decreases, but the critical care nurse can anticipate performing these liver function tests daily after the initial postoperative period.

Liver Graft Nonfunction. The patient with suspected primary nonfunction of a liver graft demonstrates (1) hemodynamic instability, (2) progressive deterioration of kidney function, (3) coagulopathies and abnormal serum liver function laboratory tests, (4) hypoglycemia, (5) continued ventilatory dependence, and (6) an inability to awaken from anesthesia. Continued nonfunction of the graft necessitates relisting the patient for another donor liver. Early signs of optimal graft function include improving kidney function, mental alertness, a high to normal serum glucose concentration, and early extubation. The serum ALT, AST, GGT, and alkaline phosphatase levels may peak on the third or fourth day but later decrease. The serum bilirubin concentration may take a week before beginning to fall, and there may be a mild elevation when the external biliary drainage tube is clamped or after a blood transfusion. Early mobilization and physical therapy are encouraged.

Rejection Surveillance. Acute rejection in OLT is a cellular-mediated event and should be suspected if the serum liver function laboratory tests, especially AST and ALT, become elevated compared with previous levels. Such elevations usually precede any other sign of acute rejection of the liver allograft. Sometimes, the patient also exhibits fever, a drop in bile output (if a T-tube is still connected to a drainage bag), and a change in the color and viscosity of the bile. At first the patient may not have any other physical symptoms, but eventually late signs of rejection may occur, including malaise, dark urine, and clay-colored stools. Certain infections, such as CMV, can also cause liver function test values to increase.

Rejection is suspected when liver function test values increase, but other reasons for these elevations need to be ruled out. Mechanical and vascular complications are ruled out by Doppler ultrasonography and angiography. Endoscopic retrograde cholangiopancreatography, hepatobiliary iminodiacetic acid (HIDA) scanning, or transhepatic cholangiography may reveal biliary obstruction or leakage. A liver biopsy may be indicated to determine cause of liver dysfunction if the other tests are inconclusive. Acute rejection can occur at any time after transplantation, but most commonly it occurs during the first few months and even as early as the first week after surgery. Most liver transplant recipients experience at least one acute rejection episode. Treatment of acute rejection requires increasing immunosuppression (i.e., an increase in tacrolimus or steroid dose and possibly an addition of monoclonal or polyclonal antilymphocyte antibodies or other newer pharmacologic agents). Immunosuppressant protocols vary from center to center and are usually successful at reversing acute rejection.

Chronic rejection is a humoral event and is progressive and nonreversible. Chronic rejection in a liver transplant recipient usually requires retransplantation if the patient is still a candidate.

Transfer Out of Critical Care. After the patient is stable and the transplanted liver is functional, catheters and drains are removed before the patient is transferred out of the critical care unit. Central venous catheters and arterial lines are removed. The urinary catheter is removed as soon as the patient is awake enough to be continent. Drain lines are removed as drainage outputs become minimal. As the patient begins to participate in self-care, plans are made for transfer out of the critical care unit to the transplantation nursing unit.

On the transplantation unit, laboratory data and vital signs continue to be monitored on a routine basis. Self-care is promoted.[137] Increasing levels of physical therapy are encouraged, diet is advanced, and much of the nurse's effort is directed toward teaching the patient and family.

PATIENT EDUCATION

Considerable attention is focused on patient education and discharge planning.[137] Discharge booklets are helpful in the education process. It is important for the patient to learn how to self-administer medications, monitor vital signs, care for the incision and the T-tube (if present), prevent infections, and identify problems that must promptly receive medical attention. Because it is not uncommon for patients to be discharged within 2 weeks after OLT, it is important for discharge instructions to begin as soon as the patient is mentally alert. Patients discharged early may require home health nurse referrals to assist with follow-up of incision care, intravenous therapies, and other procedures. Education must be provided about rejection surveillance, signs and symptoms of infection, lifestyle changes as needed, long-term medication considerations, and the follow-up visit schedule.

LONG-TERM FOLLOW-UP

OLT patients who do not live in the same city in which their surgery was performed usually remain in the immediate area of the transplant center after discharge before returning home. During this period, they may be monitored by a home health nurse and be seen in clinic several times a week by the transplantation team. Continued serologic testing is done to monitor graft function, to determine blood levels of certain immunosuppressive agents, and to identify postoperative complications. Although many of these complications can be managed successfully in the outpatient setting, readmissions do occur. Because rejections, readmissions, grieving for the donor, and pharmacologic side effects can create anxiety for the family and the patient, they are encouraged to attend transplantation support groups if offered by the center. After patients return home, they are encouraged to resume a close relationship with their local primary care physician and gastroenterologist.

With the proliferation in the number of liver transplantations being performed, it is not unreasonable for these patients to be admitted to a non–tertiary care hospital for management of some long-term posttransplantation complications. Even nurses who work for hospitals that do not perform transplantations may have the opportunity to care for these patients. Nontransplantation nurses in these settings must become knowledgeable about the signs and symptoms of rejection, administration of immunosuppressant medications, and monitoring of drug levels.[162]

OLT patients need long-term follow-up surveillance for hypertension, kidney failure, obesity, dyslipidemias, biliary and infectious complications, and malignancies.[138,148] Early intervention affects the quality and length of life. Behavior modifications and therapeutic lifestyle changes should be frequently reinforced to positively affect long-term health. Financial concerns are a major source of stress in this patient population. Many transplant recipients suffered from chronic liver disease before their surgery. They often were disabled for some time and already have experienced financial stressors related to illness. As these patients live longer with liver transplants, issues of insurability, continued disability, and even the ability to obtain work will have to be addressed.[137,163]

Transplantation offers hope for survival, but at considerable expense. Many insurance providers, including Medicare, provide partial reimbursement for liver transplantation. The costs can be staggering. Liver transplantation surgery has been reported to be the single most costly procedure in health care.[164] In this age of managed health care, it becomes a challenge for institutions to provide this labor-intensive, life-saving procedure economically. In attempts to control costs and optimize outcomes, insurance companies are designating "centers of excellence." This means that more patients will be traveling some distance to receive a transplant. As competition for the health care dollar increases, workloads and the character of the work itself will change. Nurses can have a positive impact on cost containment[164] and must continue to provide research for cost-effective health care techniques.

Clinical trials are seeking to identify new drugs and to define improved treatment protocols.[165-167] With increasing choices of therapies, drugs will be selected for patients after other immunosuppressive therapies have failed or severe side effects have occurred.[143,168] Studies on tolerance and chimerism also may influence future immunosuppressive protocols.[137] As recipients spend more time on the waiting list, improved methods of medical management of end-stage liver disease and bridges to transplantation become more necessary, including transarterial chemoembolization (TACE) of hepatocellular cancer and TIPS.

A limiting factor in liver transplantation continues to be the shortage of organ donors (see Fig. 42-1).[169] Attention is being focused on ways to increase the number and availability of donor organs. Reduced-size organs are a common occurrence. A split-liver technique, in which one liver is divided and transplanted into two recipients, is possible. Studies are exploring the roles of xenografts and bioartificial liver devices that can support the patient who is awaiting a homograft.[170] Expanded criteria for deceased donors have led to changes in posttransplantation recipient therapies.[152,153,171] The use of living donors for pediatric and adult recipients will continue.[171-173] Recipient selection criteria also will continue to be redefined for diseases and conditions such as hepatic malignancies,[168,171] HIV positivity,[174] and alcoholism.[175] As recipients live longer and healthier lives, reproduction and pregnancy after transplantation will become more common.[176] These and other factors will influence the future of liver transplantation.

KIDNEY TRANSPLANTATION

The first successful kidney transplantation was performed in 1954 in Boston. Today, it is the treatment of choice for patients with end-stage kidney disease. It allows the recipient to lead a much less restricted lifestyle and provides a more cost-effective treatment method than long-term dialysis.[177] Advances in the study of the immune system and the development of new immunosuppressant medications have allowed for increased graft survival rates for deceased donor and living donor kidney transplants.

In the early years of transplantation, large doses of oral steroids were the immunosuppressant of choice for preventing graft rejection. Large doses or prolonged use of oral steroids can cause severe osteoporosis, decreased wound healing, and many of the symptoms of Cushing's syndrome. In the 1970s, cyclosporine was added to the list of immunosuppressive medications used to prevent rejection. Cyclosporin represented a breakthrough in immunosuppressive agents, and the graft survival rates soared.[170] There are now many agents to choose from. Most transplant centers use a combination of agents to prevent rejection, in an attempt to lower the doses of each agent so that the associated side effects can be minimized.

In 2006, a total of 16,646 kidney transplantations were performed in the United States. However, 78,611 patients were listed with the Scientific Registry of Transplant Recipients (SRTR) awaiting a donor kidney.[178] Finding new medications and ways to increase the number of donor organs recovered are two of the challenges that the transplantation community faces.

INDICATIONS AND SELECTION

Many disease processes can lead to end-stage kidney disease. For this reason, potential recipients must undergo numerous laboratory tests and some noninvasive physical testing before they can be approved as candidates (Box 42-20). Because, after transplantation, the patient's immune system will be purposely and controllably compromised, there are several contraindications to kidney transplantation (Box 42-21). If any of these risk factors is present, the patient's risk is determined to be too high for transplantation and the immunosuppressant regimen that follows. The alternative for such a patient is to decrease or eliminate the risk factors that can be controlled and be re-evaluated at a later date. If the candidate is unwilling to eliminate controllable high-risk behaviors, the only alternative for survival is to remain on dialysis.

BOX 42-20 EVALUATION BEFORE KIDNEY TRANSPLANTATION

- Chem 24 panel; human leukocyte antigen tissue typing; prothrombin time; partial thromboplastin time; complete blood count with differential; platelet count; human immunodeficiency virus; hepatitis; cytomegalovirus; Epstein-Barr virus; lipid profile; urine for analysis, culture, and sensitivities; 24-hour urine for creatinine clearance and protein (if patient still produces urine); dialysate fluid for culture and sensitivity (if patient is undergoing continuous ambulatory peritoneal dialysis)
- Kidney ultrasonography or spiral computed tomography; chest radiography (posteroanterior and lateral views); electrocardiography; stress test and cardiac catheterization (if indicated); weight management (if indicated); colonoscopy (if >55 years old); mammography (for women >35 years old); venography (for patients with diabetes)
- Consultants: psychologist or psychiatrist, urologist, transplantation surgeon or transplantation nephrologist, social worker, dietitian, chaplain, financial counselor

---

BOX 42-21 CONTRAINDICATIONS TO KIDNEY TRANSPLANTATION

- Malignancy during the past 3 years
- Active infectious process
- Advanced cardiopulmonary disease
- High risk for surgery
- Noncompliance with current medical regimen
- Recreational drug use
- Other serious contributing disease processes

KIDNEY TRANSPLANTATION SURGICAL PROCEDURE

When the kidney to be transplanted is procured from the donor, whether living or deceased, the ureter, renal vein, and renal artery are dissected, leaving as much length as possible.

Living Donor Kidney Transplantation. If the donor is living, the procurement can take place as a laparoscopic procedure or as an open procedure. After the kidney is secured, it is flushed with a cold electrolyte preservative solution until the venous return is clear.[179] This usually requires 100 to 200 mL of solution.[179] The kidney is then transported to operating room to be transplanted.

Deceased Donor Kidney Transplantation. If the kidney is from a deceased donor, it is flushed with a cold electrolyte preservative solution and simultaneously cooled externally as quickly as possible. It can be transported on a kidney perfusion machine or packed in an iced preservation solution. After it is procured and placed in the hypothermic solution, it can be maintained for 48 to 72 hours before it must be transplanted.[179] Most transplant centers attempt to transplant the

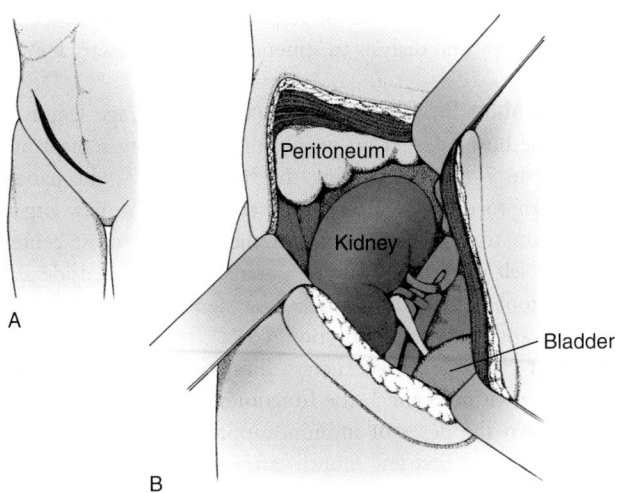

Figure 42-13 Placement of the renal graft into the iliac fossa. *A,* The incision in the right side of the abdomen is used for graft implantation in the right iliac fossa. *B,* The iliac vessels are exposed. *(Modified from Smith SL: AACN tissue and organ transplantation: implications for professional nursing practice, St Louis, 1990, Mosby.)*

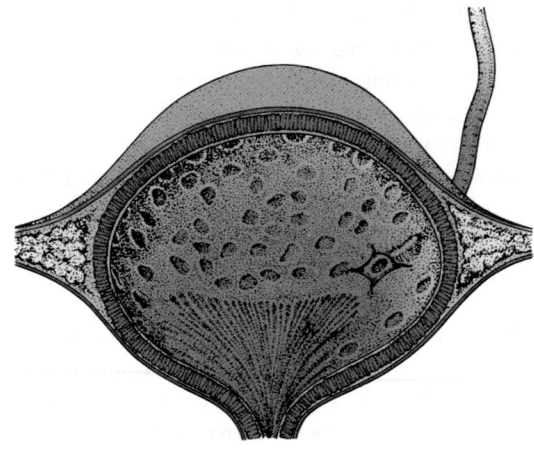

Figure 42-14 Ureteroneocystostomy reconstruction of the urinary tract. The donor ureter is passed through a posterior bladder wall tunnel and anastomosed to the bladder mucosa. *(From Smith SL: AACN tissue and organ transplantation: implications for professional nursing practice, St Louis, 1990, Mosby.)*

organ within 24 hours after procurement, to avoid cold ischemic injury and acute tubular necrosis.[179] At the time of procurement, the kidney is assessed in situ for color, shape, and form. It is palpated to determine firmness, and often a biopsy is taken to rule out undiagnosed kidney dysfunction.

Recipient Surgery. The patient is anesthetized in the usual manner, and a urinary catheter is placed. A curvilinear incision is made 3 to 4 cm above the symphysis pubis and extended to the iliac crest (Fig. 42-13A). The kidney is to be placed in the extraperitoneal space of the right or left iliac fossa. The muscles and fascia are divided and retracted medially to expose the iliac vessels. The renal artery is anastomosed to the external iliac artery, using an end-to-side or an end-to-end anastomosis, and the vein is sutured to the common iliac vein in a similar manner (see Fig. 42-13B).[179]

After the revascularization procedures are completed, the ureteral anastomosis is performed. The most common method used is *ureteroneocystostomy.* During this procedure, an incision is made in the dome of the recipient's bladder. The donor ureter is tunneled through the recipient's mucosal layer and sutured (end-to-side) to the mucosal opening (Fig. 42-14).[179] If the patient has a history of bladder surgeries, augmentations, or infections, a *ureteroureterostomy* can be done, in which the donor ureter is anastomosed to the recipient's ureter. If the patient has a history of ureteral reflux in his or her native kidneys, the *ureteroneocystostomy* is the procedure of choice. Tunneling of the ureter prevents reflux into the transplanted kidney with every bladder contraction.[179]

During the surgery, a central venous pressure ranging from 8 to 16 mm Hg must be maintained, and a systolic blood pressure at least as high as the patient's baseline value should be maintained to ensure adequate perfusion of the transplanted kidney.

POSTOPERATIVE MEDICAL MANAGEMENT AND NURSING CARE

After the transplantation is completed and the patient is stable and ready for discharge from the recovery room, most transplant centers admit the patient directly to the organ transplantation unit or to the critical care unit. Serious complications can occur in the immediate postoperative period, and sound knowledge base of medical/surgical nursing, kidney function, anatomy, and immunosuppressive medications is imperative. Relevant nursing diagnoses are listed in the Nursing Diagnoses feature on Kidney Transplantation.

Fluid Status. If the transplanted organ is working well, the patient's fluid status, as monitored by observations of central venous pressure, weight, and vital signs, must be regulated very closely. Adequate hydration is an absolute necessity for continued graft function in the immediate postoperative period. Hypovolemia can lead to compromised blood flow to the kidney, acute tubular necrosis, and possible graft failure. The new kidney will be producing large amounts of urine, and fluid replacement, usually maintained in a 1:1 ratio, must be sustained.

Electrolytes. Electrolyte balance is also of grave concern. Because of the large volumes of urine produced, the potential exists for hypokalemia, hypomagnesemia, and hypocalcemia, leading to possible cardiac compromise.[180] These electrolytes must be monitored at least every 4 to 6 hours and replaced as necessary. Assessment of the blood urea nitrogen and the creatinine concentration also is necessary every 4 to 6 hours to monitor graft function and determine the need for dialysis.

Postoperative Complications. The complete blood count and platelet count should be monitored every 4 to 6 hours. Blood loss during the operation is minimal, usually 500 mL or less. Abrupt decreases or continuously falling counts may indicate hemorrhage at an anastomosis site, which requires a return to the operating room for repair. Even with minimal blood loss during surgery, transfusion of blood products after the surgery is often necessary. Frequent observation and assessment of the surgical incision are needed to evaluate for drainage and swelling. Urine output volume and color should be monitored at least every 30 minutes. The bladder anastomosis is fragile, and it is not uncommon for clots to occlude the catheter. The bladder must remain decompressed for several days to promote proper healing. If clots occlude the end of the catheter, gentle irrigation or aspiration may be necessary. If the clot cannot be dislodged or aspirated out, it may be necessary to change the catheter. Painful bladder spasms also can occur, and opiates, usually in the form of a belladonna and opium suppository, may be required to relax the bladder.

Immunosuppression. Initiation of induction immunosuppressant therapy begins at the time of transplantation, usually in the form of a polyclonal antithymocyte/antilymphocyte intravenous compound or an intravenous monoclonal antibody compound. These compounds remove the lymphocytes from the patient's system, preventing rejection and suppressing the immune system until oral drugs can be safely administered and blood levels are sufficient to allow discontinuation of the intravenous agent. Because the patient is now immunocompromised, strict aseptic technique is required to prevent infection.

Infection Risk. Thorough hand washing, aseptic dressing changes, discontinuation of any unnecessary invasive lines, and limiting the number of visitors are necessary protective measures. Because of the patient's immunocompromised status, subtle changes in the temperature, white blood cell count, or wound drainage can signal an active infection. Patients also are susceptible to infection by opportunistic native organisms such as *Candida*, pneumocystis pneumonia, CMV, Epstein-Barr virus, and herpes simplex virus.

Kidney Graft Nonfunction. If the kidney is not functioning in the immediate postoperative period, the patient's fluid status must be monitored very closely. Hypervolemia in these patients may be so great that respiratory compromise occurs. Electrolyte dilution, resulting from the fluid overload, is a concern. Output monitoring and bladder decompression still must be maintained. If the kidney function is slow to recover, a continuous dopamine infusion may be initiated at a rate of 3 mcg/kg/min to increase urine output. However, closer observation of blood pressure then becomes necessary to observe for potentially serious hypertension that would require medical management.

If significant fluid overload or respiratory compromise occurs, oxygen therapy and dialysis treatments may be necessary for several days.

Preparation for Discharge Home. The average length of stay in the hospital after an uncomplicated kidney transplantation is 5 to 7 days.[177] During the first few days, the patient must learn to care for himself or herself and the new organ. Medication regimens are very complicated, and most centers initiate a self-medication program at the patient's bedside as a training tool. Patients are taught the signs and symptoms of infection and graft rejection (Box 42-22), the protocols of the transplant clinic, and new dietary limitations. Frequent transplant clinic visits to check the functioning of the organ and to adjust down the doses of immunosuppressant medications are necessary for the first few months after transplantation.[177]

LONG-TERM CONSIDERATIONS

Rejection of the transplanted kidney is an ongoing concern for all of these patients. The graft function is monitored closely, and if rejection is suspected, a biopsy is performed. If the biopsy reveals acute rejection, rescue therapy is initiated. This therapy can be in the form of high-dose intravenous steroids for mild rejection or intravenous monoclonal antibody for moderate to severe rejection. If the biopsy reveals chronic rejection, the oral immunosuppressant medications are increased or returned to the higher doses used immediately after transplantation. No two patients' immune systems are exactly alike, and the immunosuppressant medication regimen required to prevent rejection must be tailored to each patient individually. The goal is to create a balance among medications that allows the patient to fight off most infections but avoid rejection of the transplanted organ.

Patient adherence to the complicated medical regimen that is required to maintain a transplanted organ is of major concern. Adequate education of the patient and family as to the importance of taking the medications as instructed is of paramount importance. Patients are reluctant to take the medications appropriately if they are experiencing severe or disfiguring side effects. Decreasing the dose of the medications can often alleviate these side effects but may lead to a rejection episode.

Patients often have financial concerns. A 1-month supply of medications can cost more than $1200, and paying for the medications over the long term is too great a burden for

---

BOX 42-22 **SIGNS AND SYMPTOMS OF KIDNEY REJECTION**

- Increased tenderness over the transplanted kidney site
- Decreased urine output
- Increased serum creatinine levels, greater than patient's baseline level
- Fever
- Rapid weight gain (4 to 6 pounds in a 24-hour period)
- Swelling, usually in the hands and feet

some patients. The federal government helps to pay for the immunosuppressant medications for 30 months after transplantation.[181] After that time, the patient is considered cured, and the government assistance ends. This forces the patient to assume the full financial responsibility for the medications that are required to maintain the transplant.

Kidney transplantation has changed a great deal during the past 40 years. Continuing research with new immunosuppressant medications is the key to continued advances in this dynamic field. Increasing public awareness of the need for donor organs is one strategy to increase the donor pool. Combating rumors and false information with good public education campaigns is important. Consideration of older donors and non–heart-beating donors is an additional strategy. Transplanting donor organs into more patients and helping patients keep their transplanted kidneys functional are the primary goals of all kidney transplant centers around the world.

PANCREAS TRANSPLANTATION

One of the most common causes of chronic kidney disease is insulin-dependent diabetes mellitus (type 1). Despite meticulous glycemic control, dietary restrictions, healthy exercise programs, and advances in disease-modifying medication regimens, many patients with type 1 diabetes mellitus develop chronic kidney disease requiring long-term dialysis treatments. The first pancreas transplantation procedures were performed in 1966, with little success. Advances in immunosuppressive medications, diagnosis of rejection, management of the exocrine secretions, and improved surgical techniques have dramatically improved the success rate of pancreas transplantation.[179] A total of 914 kidney-pancreas and 390 pancreas-only transplantations were performed in 2006; however, the number of patients on the waiting list for these operations was 4032.[178] The advances in immunosuppressant medications and in diagnosis of rejection have resulted in 1-year patient and graft survival rates of 92% and 80%, respectively.[182]

INDICATIONS AND SELECTION

Patients who are selected for pancreas transplantation must undergo a thorough evaluation similar to that for other transplantation candidates (Box 42-23). The disease processes

---

BOX 42-23 EVALUATION BEFORE PANCREAS TRANSPLANTATION

- Blood chemistries, tissue typing, and viral studies similar to those for kidney transplantation candidates
- Complete cardiovascular workup, including cardiac catheterization
- Complete vascular studies, particularly of the lower extremities, to ensure proper vascularization of the graft
- Nerve conduction studies to evaluate for neuropathy
- Urologic and bladder function studies
- Consultations as required for all transplantation candidates

---

involved in diabetes mellitus and their effects on all major body systems require that special care be taken to ensure the candidate is in the best possible condition before transplantation. Severe and often life-threatening complications can occur after transplantation if the major body systems have not been properly evaluated beforehand.

PANCREAS TRANSPLANTATION SURGICAL PROCEDURE

The surgical techniques for pancreas transplantation are diverse, and different programs use different methods. The principles are consistent, however, and include three concepts: (1) providing adequate arterial blood flow to the pancreas and duodenal segment, (2) providing adequate venous outflow from the pancreas through the portal vein, and (3) providing management of the pancreatic exocrine secretions. The native pancreas is not removed.[182]

Arterial and Venous Revascularization. Pancreas graft arterial revascularization typically is accomplished using the recipient's right common or external iliac artery. The Y-graft of the pancreas is anastomosed end-to-side to the chosen artery. The entire iliac vein is dissected from the vena cava to the distal external iliac vein, and all the deep internal iliac venous branches are divided. The portal vein is then anastomosed end-to-side to the common iliac vein, and the donor iliac Y extension graft is anastomosed end-to-side to the common iliac artery.

Exocrine Drainage. The exocrine drainage of the pancreas presents one of the most challenging aspects of the transplantation procedure. Pancreatic exocrine drainage is handled by means of anastomosis of the duodenal segment to the bladder or to the small intestine. Approximately 75% of pancreas transplantations are performed with enteric (bowel) drainage (Fig. 42-15), with urinary diversion (bladder drainage) being used in 25% (Fig. 42-16).

Enteric drainage is the draining of exocrine secretions into the bowel. The pancreas and a segment of the donor duodenum are transplanted onto the recipient's small bowel. All of the enzymes are drained into the bowel and excreted with the stool. Drainage to the bowel offers the most physiologic way of handling the exocrine secretions. The graft is usually placed intraperitoneally. The abdomen is entered through a midline incision. The peritoneum is incised over the common iliac artery, from the aortic bifurcation to the distal portion of the external iliac artery. The native ureter is identified and preserved.

Enteric drainage of pancreas grafts is physiologic with respect to the delivery of pancreatic enzymes and bicarbonate into the intestines for reabsorption. Enteric drainage has the advantage of avoidance of metabolic, infectious, and dysfunctional bladder complications, and this is associated with lower reoperation and leakage rates. However, it has a major disadvantage because it does not allow, as bladder drainage does, for monitoring of pancreatic enzymes as a direct measure of pancreatic function. With successful application of the new immunosuppressant agents and reduction of the incidences of rejection, enteric drainage after pancreas transplantation has increased in popularity.

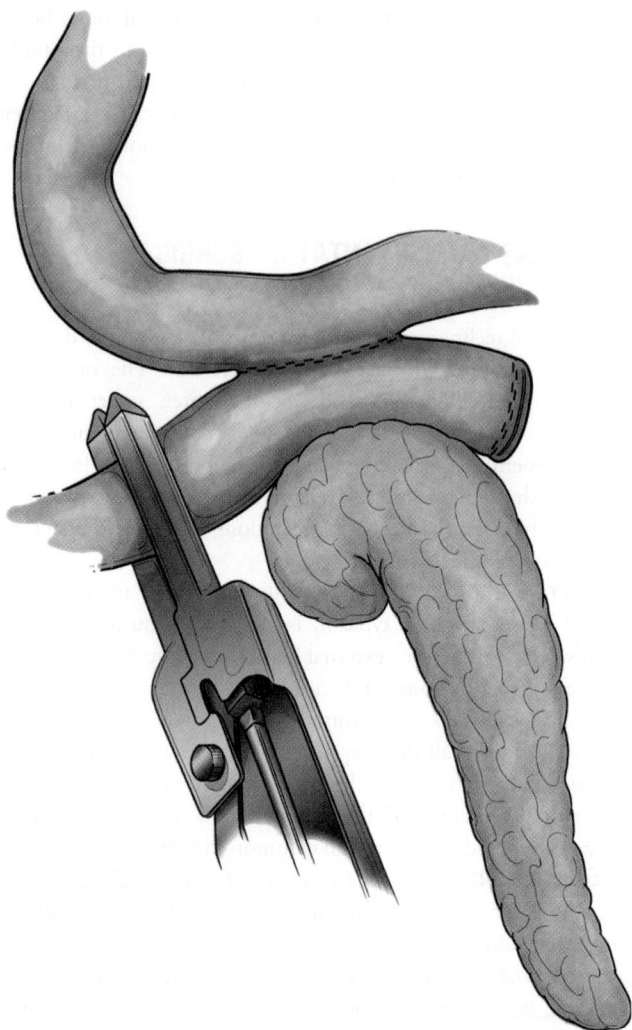

Figure 42-15 Exocrine management by bowel diversion. A segment of the donor bowel remains attached to minimize handling of pancreas.

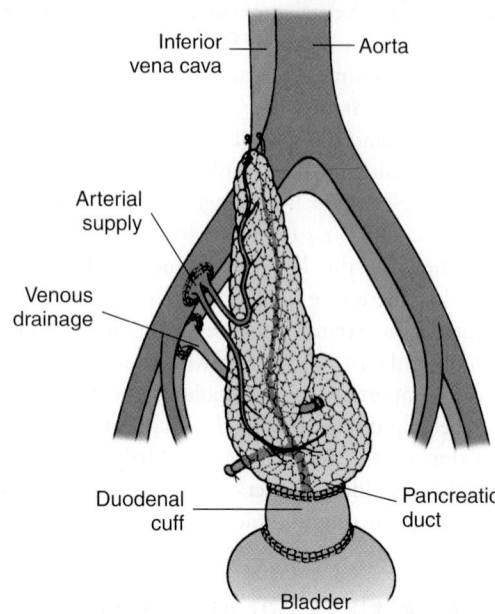

Figure 42-16 Exocrine management by urinary diversion. *(Modified from Smith SL: AACN tissue and organ transplantation: implications for professional nursing practice, St Louis, 1990, Mosby.)*

is associated with poorer graft outcomes. The characteristics of pancreas-after-kidney transplantation are lower technical complications, a better kidney, a lower risk of leakage, and the use of different donors, which may lead to immunologic complications.

POSTOPERATIVE MEDICAL MANAGEMENT AND NURSING CARE

After surgery, the patient is taken to the intensive care unit. Even though these patients now have a functioning pancreas, they are at high risk for surgical complications because of the long-term effects of diabetes. Oxygenation, hemodynamics, and cardiac status must be monitored closely. If a simultaneous kidney transplantation is performed, fluid and electrolyte management is indicated, including intravenous fluid replacement, monitoring of intake and output, and measurements potassium, blood urea nitrogen, and creatinine levels. A nasogastric tube is usually placed and remains for 24 to 48 hours after surgery. A continuous insulin drip may be used to rest the new graft and prevent hyperglycemia. Frequent blood glucose monitoring is essential for patient safety while on the continuous insulin infusion is in place.

The same aseptic techniques used for kidney transplant recipients are used for pancreas transplant recipients. An increased potential for urinary catheter occlusion exists for pancreas recipients who have undergone a urinary diversion procedure. The exocrine pancreatic enzymes make the urine more viscous, and they irritate the anastomosis site on the bladder, causing an increased risk of bleeding. The same gentle aspiration

Most transplantation centers place both organs on the right side, although some put the pancreas on the right and the kidney on the left. The cold-ischemia time of the pancreas before implantation should be minimized. Pancreas allografts do not tolerate cold ischemia as well as kidney allografts do. Ideally, the pancreas should be revascularized within 24 hours from the time of cross-clamping at procurement.

Simultaneous Pancreas-Kidney Transplantation. Simultaneous pancreas-kidney transplantation carries a risk of higher complications but is associated with better graft outcomes. The characteristics of simultaneous transplantation are higher technical complications, lower rejection rates, higher-risk patients, longer time on the waiting list, and for the patient undergoing continuous ambulatory peritoneal dialysis, a higher risk of intraabdominal infection and ascites.

Pancreas-after-Kidney Transplantation. Pancreas-after-kidney transplantation has a lower risk of complications but

Nursing Diagnoses

Pancreas Transplantation

- Risk for Infection: immunosuppressive drugs required to prevent rejection of pancreas
- Imbalanced Nutrition: Less Than Body Requirements related to lack of exogenous nutrients and increased metabolic demand
- Disturbed Body Image related to actual change in body structure, function, or appearance
- Anxiety related to threat to biologic, psychologic, and social integrity
- Activity Intolerance related to prolonged immobility or deconditioning
- Readiness for Enhanced Knowledge: Posttransplantation Self-Care Regimen, immunosuppressive drugs, and clinical manifestations of infection

techniques described earlier can be used to clear out the clots. Continuous bladder irrigation may be necessary to keep the catheter patent (see the Nursing Diagnoses feature on Pancreas Transplantation).

LONG-TERM CONSIDERATIONS

Rejection in this patient population can be very difficult to detect. Serum amylase levels after pancreas-only transplantation are not effective in monitoring graft function, and blood glucose levels become elevated only in the late stages of rejection. Urine amylase levels in patients with the urinary diversion are an effective means of monitoring for rejection. If a kidney transplantation has been performed simultaneously, an increase in the serum creatinine level is predictive of rejection. Because of the fragility of pancreas tissue, a pancreas biopsy is rarely performed. However, a kidney biopsy specimen may be obtained to determine rejection and treatment options. Treatment of pancreas rejection is the same as for all other types of organ rejection.

Adherence to the medication regimen is always a concern. It is very important that the patient take the immunosuppressants as prescribed by the physician. Patients with functional pancreas grafts continue to need glucose monitoring at home but often forget to continue this practice after they no longer require insulin. Continued monitoring with frequent clinic visits is required for several months after transplantation.

Islet Cell Transplantation. Islet cell transplantation continues to be investigational. Research studies being conducted in this dynamic field may allow for a nonsurgical means of transplantation in the future. As with all other organs, donors are in short supply. Finding ways to increase the number of donors, perfecting surgical techniques, and improving immunosuppressant medications will lead to an insulin-free treatment option and may one day represent the treatment of choice for patients with insulin-dependent diabetes mellitus.

Summary

- The fields of organ donation and solid organ transplantation have made dramatic progress in the past 50 years. There is every reason to believe that this trajectory will continue. As transplantation becomes more widespread, more nurses will encounter patients who have undergone solid organ transplantation. Even more likely is that critical care nurses will assist with the care of a potential organ donor. Knowledge of the rationales for care is essential to delivering safe and high-quality patient care.
- There are 58 OPOs in the United States, Puerto Rico, Guam, and Bermuda. They are nonprofit corporations that provide organ donation services to a designated regional area.
- There are many more individuals listed for transplants than the number of donor organs available (see Fig. 42-1).
- The recipient of an organ transplant is required to adhere to a strict regimen of immunosuppressive medications to avoid rejection of the organ by the own immune system, which recognizes the foreign graft as nonself. The immunosuppressants increase vulnerability to infection. The goal is to create a balance among medications that allows the patient to fight off most infections but avoid rejection of the transplanted organ.
- The transplanted heart must come from a deceased donor. Immediate postoperative management of the heart transplant recipient is similar to that for patients undergoing other heart surgery procedures.
- Transplanted lungs come from a deceased donor. Lungs have a limited ischemic time of about 4 hours, which limits the geographic area for donor procurement, and relatively few are available for donation.
- Liver transplants may come from a deceased donor or from a living donor who donates a section of the liver. Before transplantation, the severity of liver disease and level of placement on the transplantation waiting list is determined by the MELD score for anyone older than 12 years. The postoperative course is highly variable. Many liver transplant recipients were encephalopathic before transplantation and may have a complicated course afterward. Other patients who have a lower MELD score and receive a functional kidney may recover very quickly and should be alert and oriented within 1 to 2 days.
- Kidney transplants come from a decreased donor or from a living donor who donates one kidney. Postoperative management of fluid status is vital to ensure that the kidney is functional and to avoid volume overload. The bladder must remain decompressed by a urinary catheter for several days to promote effective healing.
- Pancreas transplantation is usually performed in tandem with kidney transplantation, because most recipients have type 1 diabetes mellitus that has caused their kidneys to fail.

Case Study: Patient with a Transplant

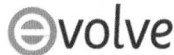 Answers to the Case Study Questions can be found on the Evolve web site at http://evolve.elsevier.com/Urden/.

Brief Patient History

Mr. V is a 42-year-old man with chronic viral hepatitis C. He has a Model for End-Stage Liver Disease (MELD) score greater than 25. Mr. V is in acute fulminant hepatic failure and is on the waiting list to receive a liver transplant. Mr. V was hospitalized 2 weeks ago with ascites, hepatorenal syndrome, and hepatic encephalopathy. He has been treated with diuretics, antibiotics, and laxatives. Before transplantation, he remained in the intermediate care unit and was not intubated. He is now undergoing liver transplantation.

Clinical Assessment

Mr. V is admitted to the intensive care unit from the operating room after receiving an orthotopic liver transplant. He is intubated and sedated. Mr. V moves all extremities but does not follow commands. He has a nasogastric tube, pulmonary artery catheter, arterial line, urinary catheter, abdominal drain (draining bright red blood), and external biliary drain in place. Continuous renal replacement is in progress.

Diagnostic Procedures

Baseline vital signs include the following: blood pressure of 100/60 mm Hg, heart rate of 118 beats/min (sinus tachycardia), respiratory rate of 20 breaths/min, temperature of 98.3° F, and O_2 saturation of 98%.

Urine output was 75 mL/hr and is now 15 mL/hr. Central venous pressure is 14 mm Hg, pulmonary artery pressure is 30/16 mm Hg, pulmonary artery occlusion pressure is 18 mm Hg, and intraabdominal pressure is greater than 25 mm Hg.

His current laboratory values include the following:
White blood cell count: 3100 cells/mm^3
Hematocrit: 25.3%

Hemoglobin: 8.6 g/dL
Platelet count: 47,000/microliter
Aspartate aminotransferase: 315 U/L
Aminotransferase: 230 U/L
Alkaline phosphatase: 380 U/L
γ-Glutamyltransferase: 1040 U/L
Total bilirubin: 12.5 mg/dL
Prothrombin time: 21.3 seconds
International normalized ratio: 2.5
Partial thromboplastin time: 69.9 seconds
Blood urea nitrogen: 39 mg/dL
Serum creatinine: 1.4 mg/dL
Potassium: 3.8 mEq/L (mmol/L)

Medical Diagnosis

Mr. V is diagnosed with intraabdominal hypertension and abdominal compartment syndrome.

Questions

1. What major outcomes do you expect to achieve for this patient?
2. What problems or risks must be managed to achieve these outcomes?
3. What interventions must be initiated to monitor, prevent, manage, or eliminate the problems and risks identified?
4. What interventions should be initiated to promote optimal functioning, safety, and well-being of the patient?
5. What possible learning needs do you anticipate for this patient?
6. What cultural and age-related factors may have a bearing on the patient's plan of care?

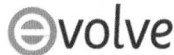 Be sure to check out the bonus material, including free self-assessment exercises, on the Evolve web site at http://evolve.elsevier.com/Urden/.

References

1. Beecher HK: A definition of irreversible coma: report of the Harvard Medical School committee to examine the definition of brain death, *JAMA* 205(6):337, 1968.
2. Uniform Brain Death Act, 12 Uniform Law Annotated (ULA) 15 (1978), superseded by Uniform Determination of Death Act, 12 ULA 236 (Suppl 1982).
3. Organ Procurement and Transplantation Network (OPTN).. Donors recovered in the U.S. by donor type. Available at http://optn.transplant.hrsa.gov (accessed May 2009).
4. National Organ Transplant Act of 1984, Pub. L. No. 98-507, 98 Stat 2339 (1984)
5. Organ Donation and Recovery Improvement Act of 2004, Pub. L. No. 108-216.
6. National Transplant Act of 1984, 42 USC, beginning §273.
7. The National Conference of Commissioners on Uniform State Laws: Uniform Anatomical Gift Act. Available at http://www.anatomicalgiftact.org (accessed May 2009).
8. Title 42, Public Health. Chapter IV, Part 482, Subpart C, Section 482.45.
9. Ehrle R et al: Referral, request, and consent for organ donation: best practice—a blueprint for success, *Crit Care Nurse* 19(2):32, 1999.
10. Verble M, Worth J: Adequate consent: its content in the donation discussion, *J Transplant Coordination* 8(2):101, 1998.
11. Riley L, Coolican M: Needs of families of organ donors: facing death and life, *Crit Care Nurse* 19(2):53, 1999.
12. Verble M, Worth J: Overcoming families' fears and concerns in the donation discussion, *Prog Transplant* 10(3):155, 2000.
13. Division of Health Care Services, Institute of Medicine: *Non–heart-beating organ transplantation: medical and ethical issues in procurement*, Washington, DC, 1997, National Academies Press.
14. Division of Health Care Services, Institute of Medicine. *Non–heart beating organ transplantation: practice and protocols*, Washington, DC, 2000, National Academies Press.
15. Sullivan J et al: Determining brain death, *Crit Care Nurse* 19(2):37, 1999.
16. Wijdicks EFM: Determining brain death in adults, *Neurology* 45:1003, 1995.

17. Powner DJ et al: Proposed treatment guidelines for donor care, *Progr Transplantation* 14(1):16, 2004.

18. Department of Health and Human Services, Health Care Financing Administration: Medicare and Medicaid programs: hospital conditions of participation; identification of potential organ, tissue, and eye donors and transplant hospitals; provision of transplant-related data. Final rule, *Fed Reg* 63(119):33856, 1998.

19. McCoy J, Argue P: The role of critical care nurses in organ donation: a case study, *Crit Care Nurse* 19(2):48, 1999.

20. Van Gelder FEL, Ohler L: Basics in transplant immunology. In Ohler L, Cupples S, editors: *Core curriculum for transplant nurses*, Philadelphia, 2008, Mosby Elsevier.

21. Kroemer A et al: The innate natural killer cells in transplant rejection and tolerance induction, *Curr Opin Organ Transplant* 13:339, 2008.

22. Schuster M et al: B-cell activation and allosensitization after left ventricular assist device implantation is due to T-cell activation and CD40 ligand expression, *Human Immunol* 63:211,2002.

23. Costello A, Pearson GJ: Transplant pharmacology. In Ohler L, Cupples S, editors: *Core curriculum for transplant nurses*, Philadelphia, 2008, Mosby Elsevier.

24. White M et al: Pharmacokinetic, hemodynamic, and metabolic effects of cyclosporine Sandimmune versus the microemulsion Neoral in heart transplant recipients, *J Heart Lung Transplant* 16:787, 1997.

25. Meulle EA et al: Pharmacokinetics and tolerability of a microemulsion formulation of cyclosporine in renal allograft recipients: a concentration-controlled comparison with the commercial formulation, *Transplantation* 57:1178, 1994.

26. Steinberg SM et al: Randomized, open label preference study of two cyclosporine capsule formulations (USP modified) in stable solid-organ transplant recipients, *Clin Ther* 25(7):2037, 2003.

27. Staschak SM, Zamberlan K: Recent development: FK506. In Sigardson-Poor KM, Haggerty LM, editors: *Nursing care of the transplant recipient*, Philadelphia, 1990, WB Saunders.

28. Vincenti F et al: Results of an international randomized trial comparing glucose metabolism disorders and outcome with cyclosporine versus tacrolimus, *Am J Transplant* 7:1506, 2007.

29. Bullingham RE et al: Clinical pharmacokinetics of mycophenolate mofetil, *Clin Pharmacokinet* 34:429,1998.

30. Eisen HJ et al: Three year results of a randomized double blind controlled trial of mycophenolate mofetil versus azathioprine in cardiac transplant recipients, *J Heart Lung Transplant* 24:5, 2005.

31. Kobashigawa JA et al: A randomized active-controlled trial of mycophenolate mofetil in heart transplant recipients. Mycophenolate mofetil investigators, *Transplantation* 66:4, 1998.

32. Kobashigawa JA et al: Mycophenolate mofetil reduces intimal thickness by intravascular ultrasound after heart transplant: reanalysis of the multicenter trial, *Am J Transplant* 6:5, 2006.

33. Behrend M: Adverse gastrointestinal effects of mycophenolate mofetil, *Drug Safety* 24:645, 2001.

34. Budde K et al: Enteric coated mycophenolate sodium can be safely administered in maintenance renal transplant patients: results of a 1 year study, *Am J Transplant* 4:237, 2004.

35. Salvadori M et al: Enteric coated mycophenolate sodium is therapeutically equivalent to mycophenolate mofetil in de novo renal transplant patients, *Am J Transplant* 4:231, 2004.

36. Kobashigawa JA et al: Similar efficacy and safety of enteric coated mycophenolate sodium compared with mycophenolate mofetil in de novo heart transplant recipients: results of a 12 month single blind randomized parallel group multicenter study, *J Heart Lung Transplant* 25:935, 2006.

37. Ingle GT et al: Sirolimus: continuing the evolution of transplant immunosuppression, *Ann Pharmacother* 34:1044, 2000.

38. McAlister VC et al: Sirolimus-tacrolimus combination immunosuppression, *Lancet* 355:376, 2000.

39. Radovancevic B, Vrtovec B: Sirolimus therapy in cardiac transplantation, *Transplant Proc* 35:171S, 2003.

40. Machado PG et al: An open-label randomized trial of the safety and efficacy of sirolimus vs. azathioprine in living related renal allograft recipients

41. Keogh A et al: Sirolimus in de novo heart transplant recipients reduces acute rejection and prevents coronary artery disease at 2 years: a randomized clinical trial, *Circulation*, 110: 2694, 2004.

42. Mancini D et al: Use of rapamycin slows progression of cardiac transplantation vasculopathy, *Circulation* 108:48, 2003.

43. Eisen H et al: Everolimus for the prevention of allograft rejection and vasculopathy in cardiac transplant recipients, *N Engl J Med* 349:847, 2003.

44. Keogh A et al: Sirolimus in de novo heart transplant recipients reduces acute rejection and prevents coronary artery disease at 2 years: a randomized clinical trial, *Circulation* 110:2694, 2004.

45. Kobashigawa JA et al: Tacrolimus with mycophenolate mofetil (MMF) or sirolimus vs. cyclosporine with MMF in cardiac transplant patients: 1-year report, *Am J Transplant* 6:1377 2006.

46. Kuppahally S et al: Wound healing complications with de novo sirolimus versus mycophenolate mofetil-based regimen in cardiac transplant recipients, *Am J Transplant* 6:986, 2006.

47. Kahan BD et al: Immunosuppressive effects and safety of a sirolimus/cyclosporine combination regime for renal transplantation, *Transplantation* 66:1040, 1998.

48. Watson CJE et al: Sirolimus: a potent new immunosuppressant for liver transplantation, *Transplantation* 67: 505, 1999.

49. Pascual J: Everolimus (Certican) in renal transplantation: a review of clinical trial data, current usage and future directions, *Transplant Rev* 20:1, 2006.

50. Ferron GM et al: Population pharmacokinetics of sirolimus in kidney transplant patients, *Clin Pharmacol Ther* 61:416, 1997.

51. MacDonald A et al: Clinical pharmacokinetics and therapeutic drug monitoring of sirolimus, *Clin Ther* 22:B101, 2000.

52. Böhler T et al: Pharmacodynamic effects of everolimus on anti-CD3 antibody-stimulated T-lymphocyte proliferation and interleukin-10 synthesis in stable kidney-transplant patients, *Cytokine* 42:306, 2008.

53. Valantine H et al: From clinical trials to clinical practice: an overview of Certican (everolimus) in heart transplantation, *J Heart Lung Transplant* 24:S185, 2005.

54. Pascual J: Concentration controlled everolimus (Certican): combination with reduced dose calcineurin inhibitors, *Transplantation* 79:S76, 2005.

55. Vitko S et al: Everolimus (Certican) 12 months safety and efficacy versus mycophenolate mofetil in de novo renal transplant recipients, *Transplantation* 78:1532, 2004.

56. Chapman HR et al: Proliferation signal inhibitors in transplantation: questions at the cutting edge of everolimus therapy, *Transplant Proc* 39:2937, 2007.

57. Rothenburger M et al: Calcineurin inhibitor free immunosuppression using everolimus (Certican) in maintenance heart transplant recipients: 6 months follow up, *J Heart Lung Transplant* 26:250, 2007.

58. Carrier M et al: Value of monoclonal antibody OKT3 in solid organ transplantation: a meta-analysis, *Transplant Proc* 24:2586, 1992.

59. Van Gelder T et al: A randomized trial comparing safety and efficacy of OKT3 and a monoclonal anti-interleukin-2 receptor antibody (BT563) in the prevention of acute rejection after heart transplantation, *Transplantation* 62:51, 1996.

60. Pascual J et al: Anti-interleukin-2 receptor antibodies: basiliximab and daclizumab, *Nephrol Dialysis Transplant* 16:1756, 2001.

61. Webster A et al: Interleukin 2 receptor antagonists for renal transplant recipients: a meta-analysis of randomized trials, *Transplantation* 77:166, 2004.

62. Cherikh WS et al: Association of the type of induction immunosuppression with posttransplant lymphoproliferative disorder, graft survival, and patient survival after primary kidney transplantation, *Transplantation* 76:1289, 2003.

63. Møller CH et al: Interleukin-2 receptor antagonists as induction therapy after heart transplantation: systematic review with meta-analysis of randomized trials, *J Heart Lung Transplant*, 27:835, 2008.

64. Kirk AD et al: Results from a human renal allograft tolerance trial evaluating the humanized CD52-specific mono-clonal antibody alemtuzumab (CAMPATH-1H), *Transplantation* 76:120, 2003.

65. Knechtle SJ et al: Campath-1H induction plus rapamycin monotherapy for renal transplantation: results of a pilot study, *Am J Transplant* 3:722, 2003.

66. Vincenti F: Current use and future trends in induction therapy, *Saudi J Kidney Dis Transplant* 16:506, 2005.

67. Reitz B: The history of heart and heart-lung transplantation. In Baumgartner WA et al, editors: *Heart and heart-lung transplantation*, Philadelphia, 1990, WB Saunders.

68. Hartley C et al: Heart transplantation. In Ohler L, Cupples S, editors: *Core curriculum for transplant nurses*, Philadelphia, 2008, Mosby Elsevier.

69. Horvath KA, Fullerton DA: Heart transplantation. In Stuart FP et al, editors: *Organ transplantation*, Georgetown, TX, 2003, Landes Bioscience.

70. Taylor DO et al: Registry of the International Society for Heart and Lung Transplantation: twenty-fourth official adult heart transplant report—2007, *J Heart Lung Transplant* 26:769, 2007.

71. Aliabadi AZ et al: Immunosuppressive therapy in older cardiac transplant patients, *Drugs Aging* 24:913, 2007.

72. McCarthy PM et al: Evolving strategies for surgical management of patients with severe left ventricular dysfunction, *Heart Lung Circ* 12:31, 2003.

73. Oechselin E et al: Pretransplant malignancy in candidates and posttransplant malignancy in recipients of cardiac transplantation, *Ann Oncol* 7:1059, 1996.

74. Lower RR, Shumway NE: Studies on the orthotopic homotransplantations of the canine heart, *Surg Forum* 11:18, 1960.

75. Aziz TM et al: Orthotopic cardiac transplantation technique: a survey of current practice, *Ann Thorac Surg* 68:1242, 1999.

76. Rees AP et al: Valvular regurgitation and right-side cardiac pressures in heart transplant recipients by complete Doppler and color flow evaluation, *Chest* 104:82, 1993.

77. Angerman CE et al: Anatomic characteristics and valvular function of the transplanted heart: thoracic versus transesophageal echocardiographic findings, *J Heart Transplant* 9:331, 1990.

78. Jacquet L et al: Cardiac rhythm disturbance early after orthotopic heart transplantation: prevalence and clinical importance of observed abnormality, *J Am Coll Cardiol* 16:832, 1990.

79. Sievers HH et al: An alternative technique for orthotopic cardiac transplantation with preservation of the normal anatomy of the right atrium, *Thorac Cardiovasc* 39:70, 1991.

80. Miniati DH, Robbins RC: Techniques in orthotopic cardiac transplantation: a review, *Cardiol Rev* 9131, 2001.

81. Brandt M: Influence of bicaval anastomoses on late occurrence of atrial arrhythmia after heart transplantation, *Ann Thorac Surg* 64:70, 1997.

82. Dibiase A et al: Frequency and mechanism of bradycardia in cardiac transplant recipients and need for pacemakers, *Am J Cardiol* 67:1385, 1991.

83. Stewart S et al: Revision of the 1990 working formulation for the standardization of nomenclature in the diagnosis of heart rejection, *J Heart Lung Transplant* 24:1710, 2005.

84. Hunt SA et al: Total lymphoid irradiation for treatment of intractable cardiac allograft rejection, *J Heart Lung Transplant* 10:211, 1991.

85. Centers for Disease Control and Prevention (CDC): Cytomegalovirus (CMV): About CMV 2008. Available at www.cdc.gov/cmv/facts.htm (accessed May 2009).

86. Merigan TC et al: A controlled trial of ganciclovir to prevent cytomegalovirus disease after heart transplantation, *N Engl J Med* 326:1182, 1992.

87. Patel R et al: Cytomegalovirus prophylaxis in solid organ transplant recipients, *Transplantation* 61:1279, 1996.

88. Snydman DR et al: Final analysis of primary cytomegalovirus disease prevention in renal transplant recipients with a cytomegalovirus-immune globulin: comparison of the randomized and open label trials, *Transplant Proc* 23:1357, 1991.

89. George MJ et al: Use of ganciclovir plus cytomegalovirus immune globulin to treat CMV pneumonia in orthotopic liver transplant recipients, *Transplant Proc* 25:22, 1993.

90. Bonaros N et al: CMV-hyperimmune globulin for preventing cytomegalovirus infection and disease in solid organ transplant recipients: a meta-analysis, *Clin Transplant* 22(1):89, 2008.

91. Decampli WM et al: Characteristics of patients surviving more than ten years after cardiac transplantation, *J Thoracic Cardiovasc Surg* 109:1103, 1995.

92. Lough ME et al: Impact of symptom frequency and symptom distress on self-reported quality of life in heart transplant recipients, *Heart Lung* 16:193, 1987.

93. Packa RD: Quality of life of adults after a heart transplant, *J Cardiovasc Nurs* 13:12, 1989.

94. Burra P et al: Quality of life following organ transplantation, *Transplant Int* 20:397, 2006.

95. Evans RW et al: *The National Heart Transplantation Study: final report*, Seattle, 1984, Batelle Human Affairs Research Centers.

96. Lough ME: Quality of life issues following heart transplantation, *Prog Cardiovasc Nurs* 1:17, 1986.

97. United Network of Organ Sharing. US Transplantation Data, Available at www.unos.org/data (accessed May 2009).

98. Reitz B: The history of heart and heart-lung transplantation. In Baumgartner WA et al, editors: *Heart and heart-lung transplantation*, Philadelphia, 1990, WB Saunders.

99. Christie JD et al: Registry of the International Society for Heart and Lung Transplantation: twenty-fifth official adult lung and heart/lung transplantation report—2008, *J Heart Lung Transplant* 9:957, 2008.

100. Marshall SE et al: Selection and evaluation of recipients for heart-lung and lung transplantation, *Chest* 98:1488, 1990.

101. Egan TM et al: Lung transplantation, *Curr Probl Surg* 10:673, 1989.

102. Hutter JA: Heart-lung transplantation: better use of resources, *Am J Med* 85:4, 1988.

103. Klepetko W et al: Domino transplantation of heart-lung and heart: an approach to overcome the scarcity of donor organs, *J Heart Lung Transplant* 10:129, 1991.

104. Theodore J, Lewiston N: Lung transplantation comes of age, *N Engl J Med* 322:772, 1991.

105. Hakim M et al: Selection and procurement of combined heart and lung grafts for transplantation, *J Thorac Cardiovasc Surg* 95:474, 1988.

106. Starnes V: Heart-lung transplantation: an overview, *Cardiol Clin* 8:159, 1990.

107. Conte JV, Reitz B: Operative technique of single-lung, bilateral lung, and heart-lung transplantation. In Baumgartner WA et al, editors: *Heart and heart-lung transplantation*, Philadelphia, 1990, WB Saunders.

108. Thabut G et al: Preventive effect of inhaled nitric oxide and pentoxifylline on ischemia reperfusion injury after lung transplantation, *Transplantation* 71:1295, 2001.

109. George I et al: Clinical indication for use and outcomes after inhaled nitric oxide therapy, *Ann Thorac Surg* 82:2161, 2006.

110. Valentine VG et al: Clinical diagnosis in heart and lung allograft rejection. In Solez K et al, editors: *Solid organ transplant rejection*, New York, 1996, Marcel Dekker.

111. Yousem SA et al: A working formulation for the standardization of nomenclature in the diagnosis of heart and lung rejection: lung rejection study group, *J Heart Lung Transplant* 9:593, 1990.

112. Theodore J: Pulmonary function in the uncomplicated human transplanted lung, *ACP* 2:301, 1987.

113. Baldwin JC: Comparison of cardiac rejection in heart and heart-lung transplantation, *J Heart Transplant* 6:352, 1987.

114. Theodore J et al: Obliterative bronchiolitis, *Clin Chest Med* 11:309, 1998.

115. Glanville AR et al: Obliterative bronchiolitis after heart-lung transplantation: apparent arrest by augmented immunosuppression, *Ann Intern Med* 107:300, 1987.

116. Trulock EP et al: Registry of the International Society for Heart and Lung Transplantation: twenty-fourth official adult lung and heart-lung transplantation report—2007, *J Heart Lung Transplant* 26:782, 2007.

117. Starnes VA et al: Current trends in lung transplantation: lobar transplantation and expanded use of single lungs, *J Thorac Cardiovasc Surg* 104:1060, 1992.

118. Meyers BF, Patterson A: Lung transplantation: current status and future prospects, *World J Surg* 23:1156, 1999.

119. Cooper JD et al: Bilateral pneumectomy (volume reduction) for chronic obstructive pulmonary disease, *J Thorac Cardiovasc Surg* 109:116, 1995.

120. Cohen RG, Starnes VA: Living donor lung transplantation, *World J Surg* 25:244, 2001.

121. Starnes VA et al: A decade of living lobar lung transplantation: recipient outcomes, *J Thorac Cardiovasc Surg* 127:114, 2004.

122. Trulock EP et al: The registry of the International Society for Heart and Lung Transplantation: twentieth official adult lung and heart-lung transplant report—2003, *J Heart Lung Transplant* 22:625, 2003.

123. Date M et al: Improved survival after living-donor lung transplantation, *J Thorac Cardiovasc Surg* 128:933, 2004.

124. Marshall SE et al: Prospective analysis of serial pulmonary function studies, transbronchial biopsies in single-lung transplant recipients, *Transplant Proc* 23:1217, 1991.

125. Gaissert HA et al: Comparison of early functional results after volume reduction or lung transplantation for chronic obstructive pulmonary disease, *J Thoracic Cardiovasc Surg* 111:296, 1996.

126. Welch CS: A note on transplantation of the whole liver in dogs, *Transplant Bull* 2(2):54, 1955.

127. Cannon GA: Organs, *Transplant Bull* 3(1):7, 1956.

128. Moore FD et al: One-stage homotransplantation of the liver following total hepatectomy in dogs, *Transplant Bull* 6:103, 1959.

129. Moore FD et al: Experimental whole organ transplantation of the liver and of the spleen, *Ann Surg* 152(3):374, 1960.

130. Starzl TE et al: Reconstructive problems in canine homotransplantations with special reference to the postoperative role of hepatic vein flow, *Surg Gynecol Obstet* 111(6):733, 1960.

131. Starzl TE et al: Homotransplantation of the liver in humans, *Surg Gynecol Obstet* 117(6):659, 1963.

132. Starzle TE et al: Orthotopic homotransplantation of the human liver, *Ann Surg* 168(3):392, 1968.

133. Cosimi AB: Update on liver transplantation, *Transplant Proc* 23(4):2083, 1991.

134. Starzl TE et al: Liver transplantation with the use of cyclosporin A and prednisone, *N Engl J Med* 305:266, 1981.

135. National Institutes of Health: National Institutes of Health Consensus Development Conference Statement: liver transplantation—June 20-23, 1983, *Hepatology* 4(1S):107S, 1984.

136. United States Department of Health and Human Services. 2007 OPTN/SRTR Annual Report, Table 1.13, Unadjusted Graft and Patient Survival at 3 Months, 1 Year, 3 Years, 5 Years, and 10 Years Survival (%). Available at www.ustransplant.org/annual_reports/current/default.htm (accessed May 2009).

137. Cupples SA, Ohler L: *Transplantation nursing secrets*, Philadelphia, 2003, Hanley & Belfus.

138. Terrault NA: Hepatitis C virus and liver transplantation, *Semin Gastrointest Dis* 11(2):96, 2000.

139. Cupples SA, Ohler L, editors: *Solid organ transplantation: a handbook for primary care providers*, New York, 2002, Springer.

140. Pelletier SJ et al: Effect of body mass index on the survival benefit of liver transplantation, *Liver Transpl* 13(12):1678, 2007.

141. Lipschutz GS, Busuttil RW: Liver transplantation in those of advancing age: the case for transplantation, *Liver Transpl* 13(10):1355, 2007.

142. Lake JR: Transplantation for chronic viral hepatitis. In Busittil RW, Klintmalm GB, editors: *Transplantation of the liver*, Philadelphia, 1996, WB Saunders.

143. Chalasani N: Peginterferon alfa2 for hepatitis C after liver transplantation: 2 randomized controlled trials, *Hepatology* 41(2):289, 2005.

144. Crippen J: Transplantation for sclerosing cholangitis. In Busittil RW, Klintmalm GB, editors: *Transplantation of the liver*, Philadelphia, 1996, WB Saunders.

145. Rosen CB et al. Surgery for cholangiocarcinoma: the role of liver transplantation, *HPB Surg* 10(3):186, 2008.

146. Barshes NR et al: Pediatric end-stage liver disease (PELD) model as a predictor of survival benefit and posttransplant survival in pediatric liver transplant recipients, *Liver Transpl* 12(3):475, 2006.

147. Varela M et al: Hepatocellular carcinoma in the setting of liver transplantation, *Liver Transpl* 12:1028, 2006.

148. Bufton S et al: Liver transplantation. In Ohler L, Cupples S: *Core curriculum for transplant nurses*, St. Louis, 2008, Mosby Elsevier.

149. Baker M, McWilliams C: How patients manage life and health while waiting for a liver transplant, *Prog Transplant* 13(1):47, 2003.

150. Farges O et al: Long-term results of ABO-incompatible liver transplantation, *Transplant Proc* 27:1701, 1995.

151. Heffron T et al: Successful ABO-incompatible pediatric liver transplantation utilizing standard immunosuppression with selective postoperative plasmapheresis, *Liver Transpl* 12(6):972, 2006.

152. Barshes NR et al: Waitlist mortality decreases with increased use of extended criteria donor liver grafts at adult liver transplant centers, *Liver Transpl* 7(5)2007, 1265.

153. Lapointe-Rudow D, Goldstein MJ: Critical care management of the liver transplant recipient, *Crit Care Nurs Q* 31(3):232, 2008.

154. Ghobrial RM et al: Donor morbidity after living donation for liver transplantation, *Gastroenterology* 135(2):468, 2008.

155. Bramstedt KA: Living liver donor mortality: where do we stand? *Am J Gastroenterol* 101(4):755, 2006.

156. Tector AJ et al: Promising early results with immunosuppression using rabbit antithymocyte globulin and steroids with delayed introduction of tacrolimus in adult liver recipients, *Liver Transpl* 10:404, 2004.

157. Shah A: Induction immunosuppression with rabbit antithymocyte globulin in pediatric liver transplantation, *Liver Transpl* 12(8):1210, 2006.

158. Ammori JB et al: Effect of intraoperative hyperglycemia during liver transplantation, *J Surg Res* 140(2):227, 2007.

159. Ojo A et al: Chronic renal failure after transplantation of a non-renal organ, *N Engl J Med* 349(10):931, 2003.

160. Preksaitis J et al editors: *American Society of Transplantation Infectious Disease Community of Practice infectious disease guidelines*, Mt. Lauren, NJ, 2004, American Society of Transplantation.

161. Hoffman FM et al: Caring for transplant recipients in a nontransplant setting, *Crit Care Nurse* 26(2), 2006.

162. Thomas DJ: The lived experience of people with liver transplants, *J Transplant Coord* 5:65, 1995.

163. Morrissey M, Rustand L: Financial consideration in liver transplantation. In Busittle RW, Klintmalm GB, editors: *Transplantation of the liver*, Philadelphia, 1996, WB Saunders.

164. Eckhoff DE: Liver transplantation in the era of cost constraints, *South Med J* 93(4):392, 2000.

165. Eason J et al: Steroid-free liver transplantation using rabbit antithymocyte globulin and early tacrolimus therapy, *Transplantation* 75(8):1396, 2003.

166. Kato T et al. Pediatric liver transplant with campath 1H induction: preliminary report, *Transplant Proc* 38(10):3609, 2006.

167. Nair S et al: Sirolimus monotherapy in nephrotoxicity due to calcineurin inhibitors in liver transplant recipients, *Liver Transpl* 9(2):126, 2003.

168. Varela M et al: Hepatocellular carcinoma in the setting of liver transplantation, *Liver Transpl* 12:1028, 2006.

169. Prince M, Hudson J: Liver transplantation for chronic liver disease: advances and controversies in an era of organ shortage, *Postgrad Med J* 78:135, 2002.

170. Stuart F et al: *Organ transplantation*, ed 2, Georgetown, TX, 2003, Landes Bioscience.

171. Said A, Lucey R: Liver transplantation: an update 2008, *Curr Opin Gastroenterol* 24:339, 2008.

172. Campsen J et al. Outcomes of living donor liver transplantation for acute liver failure: the Adult-to-adult Living Liver Transplantation Cohort Study, *Liver Transpl* 14(9):1273, 2008.

173. Berg C et al: Improvement in survival associated with adult-to-adult living donor liver transplantation, *Gastroenterology* 133:1806, 2007.

174. Kuo P, Stock P: Transplantation in the HIV⁺ patient, *Am J Transplant* 1(1):13, 2001.

175. Bramstedt KA: Alcohol abstinence criteria for living liver donors and their organ recipients, *Curr Opin Organ Transpl* 132:207, 2008.

176. Bonanno C, Dove L: Pregnancy after liver transplantation, *Semin Perinatol* 31(6):348, 2007.

177. Danovich GM: *Handbook of kidney transplantation*, ed 4, Philadelphia, 2005, Lippincott Williams & Wilkins.

178. United States Department of Health and Human Services. OPTN/SRTR Annual Report,: Kidney and Pancreas Transplantation in the United States, 1997-2006: The HRSA Breakthrough Collaboratives and the 58 DSA Challenge Available at www.ustransplant.org/annual_Reports/current/chapter_iv_AR_cd.htm?cp=5#0 (accessed May 2009).

179. Forsythe LR, editor: *Transplantation: a companion to specialist surgical practice*, ed 3, Philadelphia, 2005, Elsevier.

180. Holechek MJ, Armstrong G: Kidney transplantation. In Ohler L, Cupples S, editors: *Core curriculum for transplant nurses*, Philadelphia, 2008, Mosby Elsevier.

181. St Peter WL: Chronic kidney disease and Medicare, *JMCP J Manag Care Pharm* 13(9):S13, 2007.

182. Blakely MD et al: Pancreas and kidney-pancreas transplantation. In Ohler L, Cupples S, editors: *Core curriculum for transplant nurses*, Philadelphia, 2008, Mosby Elsevier.

Hematologic Disorders and Oncologic Emergencies

$\mathcal{U}$nderstanding the pathology of a disease, the areas of assessment on which to focus, and the usual medical management allows the critical care nurse to more accurately anticipate and plan nursing interventions. This chapter focuses on hematologic and oncologic disorders commonly seen in the critical care environment.

OVERVIEW OF COAGULATION AND FIBRINOLYSIS

Hemostasis, the ability of the body to control bleeding and clotting, is an intricate balancing act between the coagulation mechanism and fibrinolysis. Four major actions are involved in achieving hemostasis: (1) local vasoconstriction to reduce blood flow; (2) platelet aggregation at the injury site and formation of a platelet plug; (3) formation of a fibrin mesh to strengthen the plug; and (4) dissolution of the clot after tissue repair is complete.[1] Disruption of the normal hemostatic balance can result in devastating hemorrhagic or thrombotic conditions.

COAGULATION MECHANISM

The coagulation mechanism consists of 13 factors that work together through a series of feedback loops to achieve hemostasis (Table 43-1 and Fig. 43-1). Depending on the initial triggering event, the extrinsic or intrinsic coagulation pathway is intiated.[1,2] The extrinsic pathway begins when vascular injury occurs, resulting in release of tissue factor and activation of coagulation factor VII. The intrinsic pathway is activated when the damaged subendothelium comes into direct contact with circulating blood. In this contact phase, proteins activate additional coagulation factors (XII, XI, IX, and VIII).[1] At this point, the two pathways converge into a common pathway, and prothrombin and fibrinogen are converted to their active forms, resulting in clot formation.[3,4]

CLOT FORMATION

Platelets are activated by the arrival of thrombin at the site of injury (Fig. 43-2).[2] Local platelets change shape, become sticky, and begin to aggregate along the vessel wall. Activated platelets undergo degranulation, releasing several factors to assist in clot formation. Serotonin and histamine, two potent vasoconstrictors, help limit blood loss while the clot is forming. The prostaglandin thromboxane A_2 (TXA_2) contributes to vasoconstriction and promotes further platelet degranulation. Adenosine diphosphate (ADP) recruits platelets by increasing adherence and degranulation,[2,3] and the process continues.

At the convergence of the intrinsic and extrinsic pathways, factor X is converted into its active form, thereby enabling the conversion of prothrombin to thrombin. Thrombin then converts fibrinogen to fibrin. Strands of fibrin form and radiate around the newly formed clot, essentially creating a net in which platelets, red blood cells (RBCs), and white blood cells (WBCs) are trapped.[1] The clot is further secured to the site as platelet actomyosin causes it to contract and consolidate.[2]

REGULATORY MECHANISMS

Under normal conditions, feedback systems prevent the coagulation process from spinning out of control. Prostacyclin I_2 (PGI_2) is a prostaglandin released from damaged endothelial cells. It counteracts the effects of TXA_2, serotonin, and histamine through vasodilation and inhibition of platelet degranulation.[1-3] Another means of regulating clot formation is through inhibition of enzymes necessary for activation of coagulation factors along the intrinsic and extrinsic pathways, preventing the conversion of prothrombin to thrombin. The most important of these regulators is antithrombin III; however, protein C and protein S also play a role in thrombin inhibition.[5]

FIBRINOLYSIS

The process of fibrinolysis promotes dissolution and remolding of the clot to promote repair of the vessel wall and maintain flow through the vessel lumen (Fig. 43-2D).[2] Fibrinolysis begins as soon as the fibrin clot is formed. Circulating plasminogen, a precursor to the powerful enzyme plasmin, binds to fibrin and is trapped within the newly formed clot. The injured epithelial wall releases tissue-type plasminogen activator (tPA), which converts plasminogen to its active state, plasmin. The plasmin begins to digest the fibrin, rapidly breaking down the clot.[2,4] When fibrin is broken down, the fibrin degradation products released act as anticoagulants.

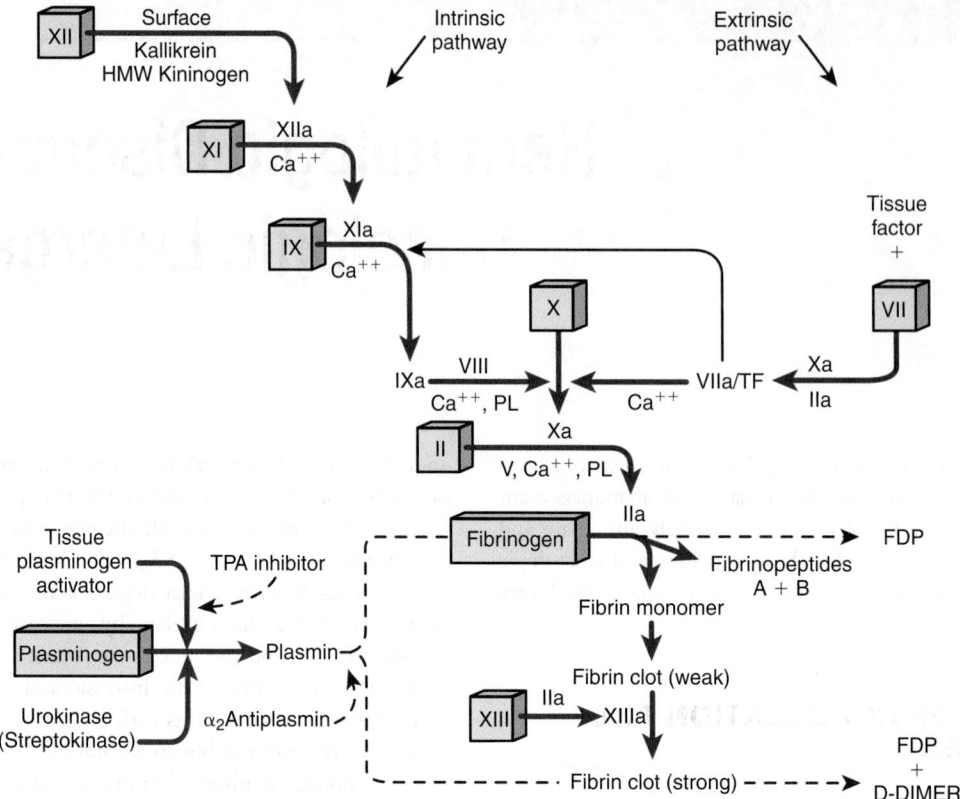

Figure 43-1 Coagulation cascade. Fibrin clot formation results from the generation of thrombin, which depends on the sequential interaction of proenzymes and activated coagulation factors in the intrinsic, extrinsic, and common pathways of coagulation. Ca⁺⁺, calcium; FDP, fibrin degradation product; HMW, high-molecular-weight; PL, phospholipids; TPA, tissue-type plasminogen activator. *(From Noble J:* Textbook of primary care medicine, *ed 3, St Louis, 2001, Mosby.)*

TABLE 43-1	Coagulation Factors and Common Names
Factor	**Common Name**
I	Fibrinogen
II	Prothrombin
III	Tissue factor
IV	Calcium
V	Proaccelerin
VI	Accelerin
VII	Proconvertin
VIII	Antihemophilic
IX	Christmas factor
X	Stuart
XI	Plasma thromboplastin antecedent
XII	Hageman factor
XIII	Fibrin stabilizing factor

DISSEMINATED INTRAVASCULAR COAGULATION

DESCRIPTION

Disseminated intravascular coagulation (DIC) is a syndrome that arises as a complication of other serious or life-threatening conditions. Although DIC is not seen often, it can seriously hamper diagnostic and treatment efforts for the critically ill patient. An understanding of the etiologic and pathophysiologic mechanisms of DIC can assist in anticipating the syndrome's occurrence, recognizing its signs and symptoms, and prompting intervention. Also known as consumptive *coagulopathy*, DIC is characterized by bleeding and thrombosis, both of which result from depletion of clotting factors, platelets, and RBCs. If not treated quickly, DIC will progress to multiple organ failure and death.[6]

ETIOLOGY

Many clinical events can prompt the development of DIC in the critically ill patient, but the exact underlying trigger may not be identifiable (Box 43-1). There are, however, some commonly known conditions associated with the development of DIC.

Sepsis, particularly that caused by gram-negative organisms, can be identified as the culprit in as many as 20% of cases, making it the most common cause of DIC. In this instance, endotoxins serve as a trigger for activation of tissue factor and the extrinsic coagulation pathway. Metabolic acidosis and hypoperfusion associated with shock syndromes can result in increased formation of free radicals and damage to tissues. Tissue factor is activated, resulting in DIC. Massive trauma or burns are frequently associated with DIC. Direct tissue damage activates the extrinsic coagulation pathway, and damage to endothelial surfaces activates the intrinsic pathway.[3] Obstetric

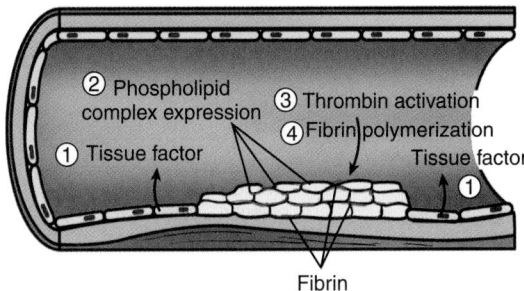

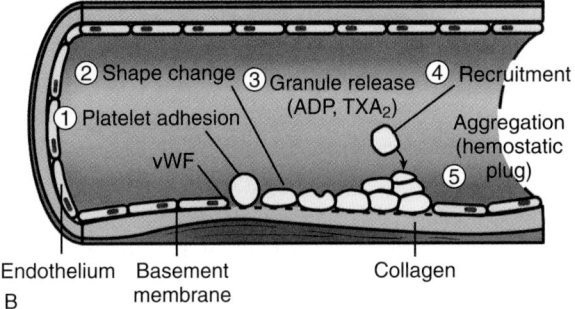

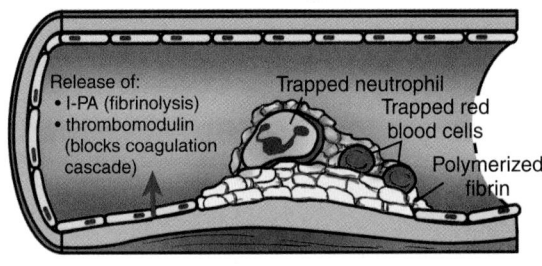

Figure 43-2 Diagrammatic representation of the normal hemostatic process. *A,* After vascular injury, local neurohumoral factors induce a transient vasoconstriction. *B,* Platelets adhere to exposed extracellular matrix (ECM) by means of von Willebrand factor (vWF) and are activated, undergoing a shape change and granule release. Released adenosine diphosphate (ADP) and thromboxane A_2 (TXA₂) lead to further platelet aggregation to form the primary hemostatic plug. *C,* Local activation of the coagulation cascade (involving tissue factor and platelet phospholipids) results in fibrin polymerization, "cementing" the platelets into a definitive secondary hemostatic plug. *D,* Counterregulatory mechanisms, such as release of tissue-type plasminogen activator (t-PA) (fibrinolytic) and thrombomodulin (interfering with the coagulation cascade), limit the hemostatic process to the site of injury. *(From Cotran RS et al: Robbins pathologic basis of disease, ed 6, Philadelphia, 1999, Saunders.)*

BOX 43-1 CAUSES OF DISSEMINATED INTRAVASCULAR COAGULATION

OBSTETRIC COMPLICATIONS
- Abruptio placentae
- Retained dead fetus
- Septic abortion
- Amniotic fluid embolism
- Toxemia

INFECTIONS
- Gram-negative sepsis
- Meningococcemia
- Rocky Mountain spotted fever
- Histoplasmosis
- Aspergillosis
- Malaria

NEOPLASMS
- Carcinomas of pancreas, prostate, lung, and stomach
- Acute promyelocytic leukemia

MASSIVE TISSUE INJURY
- Traumatic
- Burns
- Extensive surgery

MISCELLANEOUS
- Acute intravascular hemolysis
- Snakebite
- Giant hemangioma
- Shock
- Heat stroke
- Vasculitis
- Aortic aneurysm
- Liver disease

emergencies, such as abruptio placenta, retained placenta, or incomplete abortion, are also associated with the development of DIC. Tissue factor is concentrated in the placenta, and damage or disruption of this structure can activate coagulation pathways, resulting in coagulopathy.[7]

PATHOPHYSIOLOGY

Regardless of the cause, the common thread in the development of DIC is damage to the endothelium that results in activation of the coagulation mechanism (Fig. 43-3). The extrinsic coagulation pathway plays a major role in the development of DIC. Direct damage to the endothelium results in the release of tissue factor and activation of this pathway. The secondary surge of thrombin formation as a result of activation of the intrinsic coagulation pathway leads to the massive disruption of the delicate balance that is hemostasis. Excessive thrombin formation results in rapid consumption of coagulation factors and depletion of regulatory substances—protein C, protein S, and antithrombin.[5] With no checks and balances, thrombi continue to form along damaged epithelial walls, resulting in occlusion of the vessels. As occlusion reaches a critical level, tissue ischemia ensues, leading to further tissue damage and perpetuating the process. Eventually, end-organ function is affected by the ischemia, and failure is evident.[11]

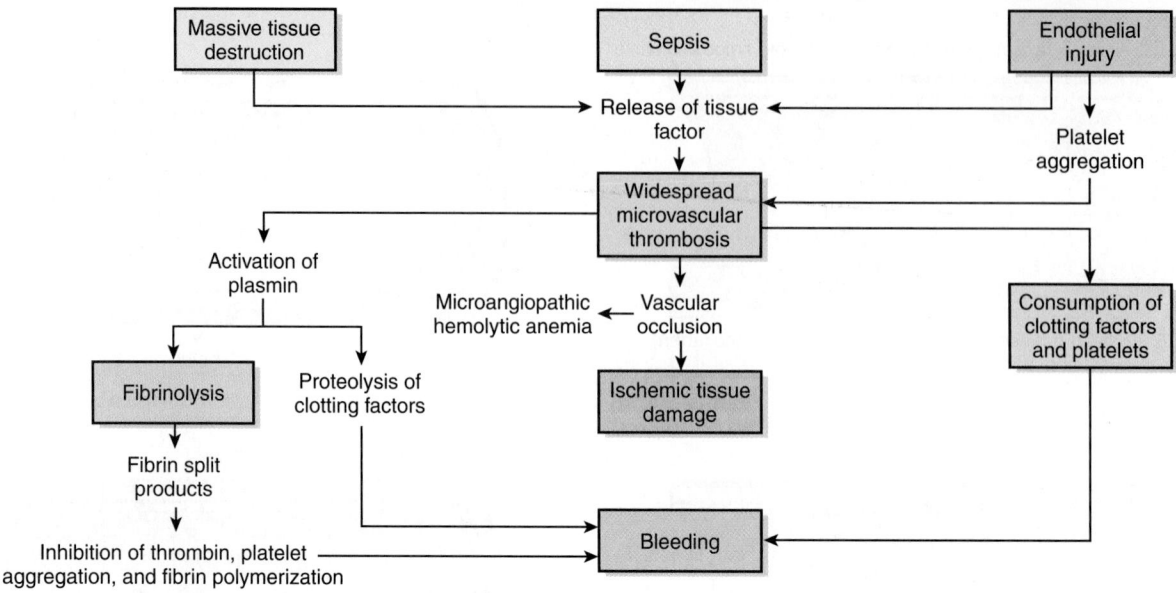

Figure 43-3 Pathophysiology of disseminated intravascular coagulation. *(From Cotran RS et al:* Robbins pathologic basis of disease, *ed 6, Philadelphia, 1999, Saunders.)*

In response to the formation of clots, the fibrinolytic system is activated. As plasmin breaks down the fibrin clots, fibrin split products are released, and they act as anticoagulants.[3,7] Coupled with depletion of circulating clotting factors, activation of fibrinolysis results in excessive bleeding. The end result is shock and further tissue ischemia that aggravate end-organ dysfunction and failure. Death is imminent if this destructive cycle is not interrupted.[8]

ASSESSMENT AND DIAGNOSIS

Favorable outcomes for patients with DIC depend on accurate and timely diagnosis of the condition. Realization of the role underlying pathology plays, recognition of clinical manifestations, and assessment of appropriate laboratory values are key steps in this process.

Clinical Manifestations. Clinical manifestations are related to the two primary pathophysiologic mechanisms of DIC: the formation of thrombi and bleeding. Thrombi in peripheral capillaries can lead to cyanosis, particularly in the fingers, toes, ears, and nose. In severe, untreated cases, this peripheral ischemia may progress to gangrene.[3,5,6,9,10] As the condition progresses, ischemia worsens,

and end organs are affected. The result of this more central ischemia can be respiratory insufficiency and failure, acute tubular necrosis, bowel infarction, and ischemic stroke. The tissue damage that results perpetuates the anomalies of DIC.

As coagulation factors are depleted, bleeding from intravenous and other puncture sites is observed. Ecchymoses may result from even routine interventions such as the use of a manual blood pressure cuff, bathing, or turning.[3] Bloody drainage may also occur from surgical sites, drains, and urinary catheters. With progression of DIC, the patient is at risk for severe gastrointestinal or subarachnoid hemorrhage.[3,6] Table 43-2 lists many of the common signs and symptoms of DIC.

Laboratory Findings. Laboratory tests used to diagnose DIC essentially assess the four basic characteristics of this syndrome: (1) increased coagulant activity, (2) increased fibrinolytic activity, (3) impaired regulatory function, and (4) end-organ failure.

Continuous activation of the coagulation pathways results in consumption of coagulation factors. Because of this, the prothrombin time (PT), the activated partial thromboplastin time (aPTT), and the international normalized ratio (INR) values are elevated. Although the platelet count may fall within normal

TABLE 43-2 Common Signs and Symptoms of Disseminated Intravascular Coagulation

System	Signs Related to Hemorrhage	Signs Related to Thrombi
Integumentary	Bleeding from gums, venipunctures, and old surgical sites; epistaxis; ecchymoses	Peripheral cyanosis, gangrene
Cardiopulmonary	Hemoptysis	Dysrhythmias, chest pain, acute myocardial infarction, pulmonary embolus, respiratory failure
Renal	Hematuria	Oliguria, acute tubular necrosis, renal failure
Gastrointestinal	Abdominal distention, hemorrhage	Diarrhea, constipation, bowel infarct
Neurologic	Subarachnoid hemorrhage	Altered level of consciousness, ischemic stroke

ranges, serial examination reveals a declining trend in values. An unexpected drop of at least 50% in the platelet count, particularly in the presence of known contributing factors and associated signs and symptoms, strongly indicates DIC.[1] Fibrinogen levels drop as more and more clots are formed. Thrombus formation in small vessels narrows the vessel lumen, forcing RBCs to squeeze through. The resulting damage and fragmentation of these cells can be seen on microscopic examination of blood samples. Damaged, fragmented RBCs are called *schistocytes.*[3,6,11]

In response to the excess clotting activity, the fibrinolytic process accelerates, and levels of by-products increase. This is reflected in markedly elevated levels of fibrin degradation products. Another key laboratory test used to evaluate the degree of clot dissolution—and therefore the severity of the coagulopathy—is the D-dimer level.[1] D-dimers exclusively indicate clot degradation because, unlike fibrin degradation products, which also result from the breakdown of free circulating fibrin, D-dimers result only from dissolution of clots.[3] With progression of the coagulopathy, normal regulatory mechanisms are disrupted, as reflected in decreasing levels of inhibitory factors such as protein C, factor V, and antithrombin III.[3,6]

Unchecked DIC resulting in occlusion of vessels and tissue ischemia leads to end-organ dysfunction. Respiratory failure, indicated by abnormal arterial blood gas (ABG) levels; liver failure, indicated by increasing liver enzymes; and renal impairment, indicated by rising blood urea nitrogen (BUN) and creatinine levels are common findings in advanced DIC.

No single laboratory study can confirm the diagnosis of DIC, but several key results are strong indicators of the condition (Table 43-3). The International Society of Thrombosis and Hemostasis emphasizes early detection of DIC through observation of abnormal trends in laboratory values.[5]

MEDICAL MANAGEMENT

Without question, the primary intervention in DIC is prevention. Being aware of the conditions that commonly contribute to the development of DIC and treating them vigorously and without delay provide the best defense against this devastating condition.[3,5,6,9,11] After DIC is identified, maintaining organ perfusion and slowing consumption of coagulation factors are paramount to achieving a favorable outcome.[3]

Multiple organ dysfunction syndrome (MODS) frequently results from DIC and exacerbates the underlying pathology. It is essential to prevent end-organ ischemia and damage by supporting blood pressure and circulating volume. Administration of intravenous fluids and inotropic agents and, if overt hemorrhaging is evident, infusion of packed RBCs are appropriate interventions to replace blood volume and essential, oxygen-carrying RBCs.

In the presence of severe platelet depletion ($<50,000/mm^3$) and severe hemorrhage, platelet transfusions are often indicated.[5,6] However, caution must be used when administering platelets because antiplatelet antibodies may be formed. These antibodies may become activated during future platelet transfusions and elicit DIC.[3]

Replacement of clotting factors in the patient with DIC is thought by some authorities to perpetuate the coagulopathy; however, there is little scientific evidence to support this theory.[1] Fibrinogen levels less than 100 mg/dL indicate the appropriateness of administering cryoprecipitate. A prolonged PT indicates the need for fresh-frozen plasma.[3,5,6]

Slowing consumption of coagulation factors by inhibiting the processes involved in clot formation is another strategy used in treating DIC. The use of heparin, particularly low-molecular-weight heparin, to prevent formation of future clots is controversial. It is contraindicated in patients with DIC associated with recent surgery or with gastrointestinal or central nervous system (CNS) bleeding. However, heparin has been beneficial in obstetric emergencies such as retained placenta or incomplete abortion, severe arterial occlusions, or MODS caused by microemboli.[3,6] Inhibitors such as aminocaproic acid may be used in conjunction with heparin.[6]

The use of recombinant human protein C is gaining popularity in treating DIC, especially in the setting of severe sepsis. Protein C acts as an anticoagulant and works to restore normal inhibition of coagulation pathways. However, it has been associated with an increased incidence of intracerebral bleeding and must be used with caution in patients with severely decreased platelets.[3,5]

Thrombin production in DIC surpasses that of antithrombins and other regulatory factors that would normally be present to inactivate thrombin and its subsequent actions. The use of antithrombin III has recently been approved in the United States. Ongoing research is yielding promising results in the treatment of DIC. One interesting area of research is the use of protease inhibitors. Protease molecules normally inhibit the conversion of fibrinogen to fibrin in the coagulation mechanism, but in DIC, this inhibitory mechanism is impaired. The introduction of protease inhibitors by intravenous infusion may be advantageous in arresting DIC.[3]

NURSING MANAGEMENT

Nursing management of the patient with DIC incorporates a variety of nursing diagnoses (see the Nursing Diagnoses feature on Disseminated Intravascular Coagulation). Assessment and

---

TABLE 43-3 Key Laboratory Studies in Disseminated Intravascular Coagulation

Test	Value
Prothrombin time (PT)	>12.5 sec
Platelets	$<50,000/mm^3$, or at least 50% drop from baseline
Activated partial thromboplastin time (aPTT)	>40 sec
D-dimer	>250 ng/mL
Fibrin degradation products (FDP)	>40 µg/mL
Fibrinogen	<100 mg/dL

Disseminated Intravascular Coagulation

- Deficient Fluid Volume related to active blood loss
- Decreased Cardiac Output related to alterations in preload
- Risk for Infection
- Anxiety related to threat to biologic, psychologic, and/or social integrity
- Compromised Family Coping related to a critically ill family member

monitoring are the primary weapons in the critical care nurse's arsenal against DIC. Knowing the diseases and conditions that are most often associated with DIC and understanding the pathophysiologic mechanisms involved enables the critical care nurse to anticipate its development and intervene quickly.

Frequent assessments should include parameters for neurologic status, renal function, cardiopulmonary function, and skin integrity that indicate impaired tissue or organ perfusion. Particular parameters to include are mental status, BUN and creatine levels, urine output, vital signs, hemodynamic values, cardiac rhythm, arterial blood gas and pulse oximetry values, skin breakdown, ecchymoses, or hematomas.[6]

The critical care nurse must recognize and support the patient's vital physiologic functions. Administration of intravenous fluids, blood products, and inotropic agents to provide adequate hemodynamic support and tissue oxygenation is essential in preventing or combating end-organ damage. Close monitoring of vital signs, hemodynamic parameters, intake and output, and appropriate laboratory values assists the critical care nurse in administering and titrating appropriate agents.

Awareness of the patient's bleeding potential necessitates adjustments to normal nursing interventions (see the Nursing Interventions Classification feature on Bleeding Precautions). The nurse avoids unnecessary venipunctures that may result in bleeding, bruising, or hematomas by drawing blood from and administering medications through existing arterial or venous lines. The use of manual or automatic blood pressure cuffs is avoided whenever possible. If tracheal or oral suctioning is necessary, the use of low-level suction is recommended.[6] Meticulous skin care is advised, keeping the skin moist and using specialty mattresses and beds as appropriate to prevent breakdown. Gentle care should be used when bathing or turning the patient to prevent bruising or hematoma formation.

The development of DIC in the already critically ill patient can be stressful for the patient and his or her significant others. It is imperative to provide psychosocial support throughout this crisis. Calm reassurance and uncomplicated explanations of the care the patient is receiving can help to allay much of the anxiety experienced. The critical care nurse must answer all questions and provide information in terms best understood by all parties. The use of an interpreter when English is not the primary language can enhance understanding and help avoid misconceptions. Providing spiritual support as requested may also be of assistance. Collaborative management of the patient with DIC is outlined in Box 43-2.

THROMBOCYTOPENIA

DESCRIPTION

Thrombocytopenia is defined as a platelet count less than $140,000/mm$.[12,13] Similar to DIC, thrombocytopenia often results from another underlying condition that affects the platelet count. Thrombocytopenia is more common in women than in men, affecting adults most often between the ages of 20 and 50 years.[14,15]

Bleeding Precautions

Definition
Reduction of stimuli that may induce bleeding or hemorrhage in at-risk patients

Activities
Monitor the patient closely for hemorrhage.
Note hemoglobin/hematocrit levels before and after blood loss, as indicated.
Monitor for signs and symptoms of persistent bleeding (e.g., check all secretions for frank or occult blood).
Monitor coagulation studies, including prothrombin time (PT), partial thromboplastin time (PTT), fibrinogen, fibrin degradation/split products, and platelet counts, as appropriate.
Monitor orthostatic vital signs, including blood pressure.
Maintain bed rest during active bleeding.
Administer blood products (e.g., platelets, fresh-frozen plasma), as appropriate.
Protect the patient from trauma, which may cause bleeding.
Avoid injections (IV, IM, or SQ), as appropriate.

Instruct the ambulating patient to wear shoes.
Use soft toothbrush or toothettes for oral care.
Use electric razor, instead of straight-edge, for shaving.
Tell patient to avoid invasive procedures; if they are necessary, monitor closely for bleeding.
Coordinate timing of invasive procedures with platelet or fresh-frozen plasma transfusions, if appropriate.
Refrain from inserting objects into a bleeding orifice.
Avoid taking rectal temperatures.
Tell patient to avoid lifting heavy objects.
Administer mediations (e.g., antacids), as appropriate.
Instruct patient to avoid aspirin and other anticoagulants.
Instruct patient to increase intake of foods rich in vitamin K.
Use therapeutic mattress to minimize skin trauma.
Prevent constipation (e.g., encourage fluid intake and stool softeners), as appropriate.
Instruct the patient and/or family on signs of bleeding and appropriate actions (e.g., notify the nurse), should bleeding occur.

From Bulechek GM et al: *Nursing interventions classification (NIC)*, ed 5, St Louis, 2008, Mosby.
IM, intramuscular; IV, intravenous; SQ, subcutaneous.

BOX 43-2 COLLABORATIVE MANAGEMENT: DISSEMINATED INTRAVASCULAR COAGULATION

- Identify and eliminate the underlying cause.
- Provide hemodynamic support to prevent end-organ ischemia.
  - Intravenous fluids
  - Positive inotropic agents
- Administer blood and blood components.
  - Fresh-frozen plasma
  - Platelets
  - Cryoprecipitate
  - Antithrombin III
- Administer medications.
  - Heparin
- Aminocaproic acid
- Protein C
- Antithrombin III
- Initiate bleeding precautions.
- Maintain surveillance for complications.
  - Hypovolemic shock
  - Peripheral ischemia
  - Central ischemia
  - Multiple organ dysfunction syndrome (MODS)
- Provide comfort and emotional support.

TABLE 43-4 Idiopathic Thrombocytopenia Purpura: Signs, Symptoms, and Laboratory Data

System or Study	Signs and Symptoms
Integumentary	Petechial hemorrhage of lower extremities, ecchymoses, gingival bleeding, spontaneous epistaxis
Neurologic	Sudden, severe headache; nausea and vomiting; seizures; focal neurologic deficits; decreased level of consciousness
Renal	Hematuria
Gastrointestinal	Hematemesis, melena, hematochezia
Other	Heavy menses in women, retinal hemorrhage
Laboratory	Decreased platelet count, often $<30,000$ mm^3

ETIOLOGY

Onset of thrombocytopenia often follows a viral infection, pregnancy, administration of certain medications (e.g., heparin, thiazide diuretics, chemotherapeutic agents), malignancies, splenomegaly, blood transfusions, or alcoholism.[8,14] Regardless of the precipitating condition, the development of thrombocytopenia occurs by means of one of four mechanisms: (1) decreased platelet production, (2) increased platelet destruction, (3) splenic sequestration of platelets, and (4) platelet dilution.[12] The most common form of thrombocytopenia seen in the critical care unit is idiopathic thrombocytopenic purpura (ITP).[13]

PATHOPHYSIOLOGY

In ITP, lymphocytes produce antibodies that begin to destroy existing platelets. The cause of this autoimmune response is unknown.[16,17] With insufficient platelets available, the normal coagulation pathways are disrupted. Inadequate hemostasis ensues, and bleeding results. Although life-threatening gastrointestinal or intracerebral bleeding can occur, the bleeding seen in ITP does not result in deep visceral hemorrhage and hematoma.[12]

ASSESSMENT AND DIAGNOSIS

Idiopathic thrombocytopenic purpura is characterized by the gradual onset of signs and symptoms.[16] The diagnosis is primarily based on findings in the patient's history and physical examination.

Clinical Manifestations. Petechial hemorrhages, which manifest as small, red spots primarily on legs and oral mucosa, are most indicative of a platelet disorder, unlike larger hematomas, which are most commonly associated with coagulation disorders.[13,17] Bruising unrelated to trauma is another common sign of ITP.[14] The signs and symptoms of ITP are listed in Table 43-4.

Unusual bleeding is a hallmark of ITP. Excessive bleeding from the gums after dental work, spontaneous epistaxis, blood in the urine or stool, and in women, unusually heavy menses

are typical features of ITP. Rarely, retinal hemorrhage or intracerebral bleeding may be observed.[16,17]

Laboratory Findings. A complete blood cell count reveals a severely diminished platelet count, often falling below 30,000/mm^3 for a patient with ITP.[14] However, the numbers of RBCs and WBCs, the hemoglobin level, results of coagulation studies, and bleeding times are normal.

MEDICAL MANAGEMENT

In most cases, ITP resolves spontaneously, and treatment is not necessary. In mild cases in which diminished platelets counts result in symptoms, administration of oral corticosteroids is appropriate.[12,15] Platelet counts will increase to normal levels with 2 to 6 weeks, and dosages can then be tapered.

In patients exhibiting life-threatening hemorrhage, rapid intervention is necessary. Administration of intravenous immunoglobulin suppresses the platelet-destroying antibody response. This therapy is extremely expensive and is reserved for the most severe manifestations of ITP.[18] High-dose methylprednisolone can be given intravenously and is very effective in treating ITP.[13] Platelet transfusion is recommended after administration of intravenous immunoglobulin or methylprednisolone. When steroid therapy fails to arrest the condition, surgical removal of the spleen is considered.[15,17,19]

NURSING MANAGEMENT

Nursing management of the patient with ITP incorporates a variety of nursing diagnoses (see the Nursing Diagnoses feature on Idiopathic Thrombocytopenia Purpura). Nursing interventions are directed toward bleeding prevention (see the NIC feature on Bleeding Precautions) and supportive measures. Recognizing potential hazards and providing a safe care environment is of utmost concern. For example, padding bed rails can protect the patient from bruising. Substituting sponge-tipped oral care devices for firm-bristled toothbrushes can help minimize mucosal trauma and bleeding, and the patient is instructed on to blow the nose gently to avoid instigating epistaxis. When shaving patients, the use of an electric razor is preferred to reduce the risk of laceration associated with a blade. Venipuncture and intramuscular injections are avoided.[20] In the event venipuncture is required, prolonged pressure on the site may be necessary to arrest bleeding. The critical care nurse must carefully administer prescribed medications, monitor for adverse effects of platelet transfusions, and monitor for complicating or contributing factors, such as hemorrhage and infection. Collaborative management of the patient with ITP is outlined in Box 43-3.

HEPARIN-INDUCED THROMBOCYTOPENIA

DESCRIPTION

Another form of thrombocytopenia seen in critical care patients is heparin-induced thrombocytopenia (HIT). There are two distinct types of HIT. The most common form is non–immune-mediated HIT, formally known as type 1 HIT.[21] Seen in up to 30% of patients receiving heparin therapy, this nonautoimmune condition manifests within a few days of initiation of therapy. Platelet depletion is moderate, counts are usually less than 100,000/mm^3, and the condition is transient, often resolving spontaneously. Discontinuation of heparin is not required. The second form is type 2 HIT, or immune-mediated HIT,[21] which is less commonly encountered but has more severe consequences.[22-24] This discussion is limited to immune-mediated HIT.

Nursing Diagnoses

Idiopathic Thrombocytopenia Purpura

- Deficient Fluid Volume related to active blood loss
- Powerlessness related to lack of control over the current situation and/or disease progression
- Disturbed Body Image related to actual change in body structure, function, or appearance

---

BOX 43-3 COLLABORATIVE MANAGEMENT: IDIOPATHIC THROMBOCYTOPENIA PURPURA

- Administer medications.
  - Glucocorticoids
  - Intravenous immunoglobulin
- Prepare patient for splenectomy if unresponsive to medication therapy.
- Administer platelets.
- Initiate bleeding precautions.
- Maintain surveillance for complications.
  - Intracranial or other major hemorrhage
  - Severe blood loss
- Provide comfort and emotional support.

ETIOLOGY

Immune-mediated HIT is a response to the administration of heparin therapy. It has been observed in 0.5% to 5% of patients treated with unfractionated heparin and has occurred after exposure to low-molecular-weight heparin (LMWH), although to a lesser degree.[25] The disorder is characterized by severe thrombocytopenia during heparin therapy. Diagnostically it is identified by a platelet count less than 50,000/mm^3 or at least a 50% decrease from the baseline platelet count from the initiation of therapy. Onset usually occurs 5 to 14 days from the first exposure to heparin, but the onset can occur within hours of a reexposure to heparin.[23,24,27] Depending on the source of the disorder, reported mortality rates are as high as 30%.[26,27]

PATHOPHYSIOLOGY

The thrombocytopenia that occurs with immune-mediated HIT is related to the formation of heparin-antibody complexes. These complexes release a substance known as platelet factor 4 (PF4). PF4 attracts heparin molecules, forming immunogenic complexes that adhere to platelet and endothelial surfaces (Fig. 43-4).

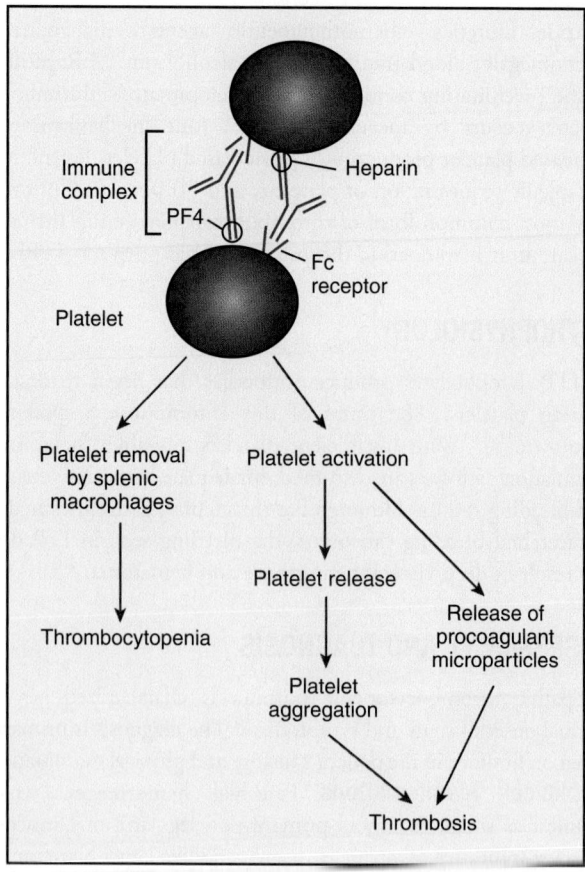

Figure 43-4 Pathophysiology of heparin-induced thrombocytopenia. Heparin binds to platelet factor 4 (PF4), forming a highly reactive antigenic complex on the surface of platelets. Susceptible patients then develop an antibody (IgG) to the heparin/PF4 antigenic complex. The IgG then activates the platelets through their F$_C$ receptors. Thrombocytopenia develops as the reticuloendothelial system consumes activated platelets, platelet microaggregates, and IgG-coated platelets. *(Courtesy GlaxoSmithKline, Philadelphia, PA.)*

Activation of platelets stimulates the release of thrombin and the subsequent formation of platelet clumps.[21,22,25]

Patients with immune-mediated HIT are at greater risk for thrombosis than bleeding. Vessel occlusion can result in the need for limb amputation, stroke, acute myocardial infarction, and even death.[12,22-24,27] The resultant formation of fibrin-platelet–rich thrombi is the primary characteristic of HIT that distinguishes it from other forms of thrombocytopenia and gives rise to its more descriptive name: white clot syndrome.[22]

ASSESSMENT AND DIAGNOSIS

HIT can be associated with severe consequences. Rapid recognition of risk factors and subsequent development of signs and symptoms is essential in treating this condition.

Clinical Manifestations. Common signs and symptoms are listed in Table 43-5. The clinical manifestations of HIT are related to the formation of thrombi and subsequent vessel occlusion.[21] Most thrombotic events are venous, although venous and arterial thrombosis can occur. Thrombotic events typically include deep vein thrombosis, pulmonary embolism, limb ischemia thrombosis, thrombotic stroke, and myocardial infarction.[21] The presence of blanching and the loss of peripheral pulses, sensation, or motor function in a limb indicate peripheral vascular thrombi. Neurologic signs and symptoms such as confusion, headache, and impaired speech can signal the onset of cerebral artery occlusion and stroke. Acute myocardial infarction may be heralded by dyspnea, chest pain, pallor, and alterations in blood pressure. Thrombi in the pulmonary vasculature may be evidenced by pleuritic pain, rales, and dyspnea.[12,21,22,26]

Laboratory Findings. The key indicator for identifying HIT is the platelet count. General consensus in the literature considers a platelet count of less than 100,000/mm^3 or a sudden drop of 50% from the patient's baseline after initiation of heparin therapy to strongly indicate HIT.[21,25]

Two types of assays have become available to assist in confirming the diagnosis of HIT: activation assays, based on platelet aggregation or the release of granular contents such as serotonin, and assays that identify the HIT antigen. Activation assays are highly sensitive in detecting the presence of HIT. The most common assay used is heparin-induced platelet aggregation (HIPA). Serotonin release assay (SRA) is used by a few institutions. The enzyme-linked immunosorbent assay (ELISA) identifies the presence of the HIT antigen.[22]

MEDICAL MANAGEMENT

Early identification is critical to managing the effects of immune-mediated HIT. The College of American Pathologists recommendations include obtaining a baseline platelet count before initiation of therapy and routine monitoring during the highest risk period, which is 5 to 10 days after initiation.[34] When a decrease in the platelet count is detected, heparin therapy should be discontinued immediately, and the patient should be tested for the presence of heparin antibodies.[12,22,24,27] If the original indication for heparin still exists or new thromboses occur, an alternative form of anticoagulation is usually necessary.[25]

Direct thrombin inhibitors (DTIs) are being used with increasing frequency to treat HIT. DTIs bind directly to the thrombin molecule, thereby inhibiting its action.[21,25] The U.S. Food and Drug Administration (FDA) has approved two such drugs for use in the United States: lepirudin and argatroban. Warfarin, although commonly used to treat deep vein thrombosis, is not indicated as a sole agent in treating HIT because of its prolonged onset of action. Studies have shown that the use of warfarin without concomitant use of DTIs can significantly increase the incidence of thrombosis in patients with HIT. Comparative information on these medications is provided in Table 43-6.[22,25] The optimal duration of anticoagulation in patients with HIT is not known.[27]

TABLE 43-5 Heparin-Induced Thrombocytopenia: Signs, Symptoms, and Laboratory Data

System or Study	Signs and Symptoms
Cardiac	Chest pain, diaphoresis, pallor, alterations in blood pressure, dysrhythmias
Vascular	Arterial: pain, pallor, pulselessness, paresthesia, paralysis Venous: pain, tenderness, unilateral leg swelling, warmth, erythema, a palpable cord, pain on passive dorsiflexion of the foot, and spontaneous maintenance of the relaxed foot in abnormal plantar flexion (Homans' sign)
Pulmonary	Dyspnea, pleuritic pain, rales, chest pain, chest wall tenderness, back pain, shoulder pain, upper abdominal pain, syncope, hemoptysis, shortness of breath, wheezing
Renal	Thirst, decreased urine output, dizziness, orthostatic hypotension.
Gastrointestinal	Abdominal pain, vomiting, bloody diarrhea, abnormal bowel sounds
Neurologic	Confusion, headache, impaired speech patterns, hemiparesis or hemiplegia, vision disturbances, dysarthria, aphasia, ataxia, vertigo, nystagmus, sudden decrease in consciousness
Laboratory	Platelets <50,000/mm^3 or sudden drop of 30% to 50% from baseline; positive results for HIPA, SRA, ELISA

ELISA, enzyme-linked immunosorbent assay; HIPA, heparin-induced platelet aggregation; SRA, serotonin release assay.

TABLE 43-6 Pharmacologic Management: Heparin-Induced Thrombocytopenia

DRUG	DOSAGE	ACTIONS	SPECIAL CONSIDERATIONS
Lepirudin (Refludan)	Loading dose: 0.4 mg/kg IV bolus IV infusion: 0.15 mg/kg/hr	Used to inhibit free and clot-bound thrombin; a recombinant form of leech-derived hirudin	Monitor aPTT; maintain INR 1.5-2.5 times normal Reduce dosage in patients with known or suspected renal insufficiency Side effects include bleeding Can develop antilepirudin antibodies that enhance anticoagulant effect
Argatroban	Loading dose: None IV infusion: 2 mcg/kg/min not to exceed 10 mcg/kg/min	Used to inhibit thrombin	Obtain baseline aPTT 2 hr after therapy started Monitor aPTT; maintain INR 1.5-3.0 times initial baseline Reduce dosage in patients with known or suspected hepatic impairment
Bivalirudin	Loading dose: 0.75 mg/kg IV bolus IV infusion: 1.75-2.0 mg/kg/hr	Used to inhibit thrombin	Monitor aPTT, maintain INR 1.5-2.5 times initial baseline Adjust dose in presence of renal failure
Warfarin	5 mg/day	Depletes vitamin K and protein C	Overlap administration with DTI for minimum of 4-5 days, maintain INR >2.3 in combination with lepirudin and >4.0 in combination with argatroban

aPTT, activated partial thromboplastin time; DTI, direct thrombin inhibitor; INR, international normalized ratio; IV, intravenous.

NURSING MANAGEMENT

Nursing management of the patient with HIT incorporates a variety of nursing diagnoses (see the Nursing Diagnoses feature on Heparin-Induced Thrombocytopenia). Nursing interventions include monitoring all patients on heparin for signs and symptoms of HIT, ensuring that all heparin is discontinued, maintaining surveillance for complications, and providing comfort and emotional support. The critical care nurse plays a pivotal role in prevention and detection of heparin-induced thrombocytopenia. Initial assessment is crucial to identifying those patients at risk for HIT. Ascertaining a medical history that includes previous heparin therapy, deep vein thrombosis, or cardiovascular surgery that included the use of cardiopulmonary bypass can alert the nurse to potential problems. Patients with HIT remain at high risk for thrombotic complications for several days or weeks after cessation of heparin. Vigilant monitoring, early recognition of signs and symptoms, deep vein thrombosis prevention strategies, and prompt notification of the physician are key roles of the critical care nurse. Ensuring that all heparin has been removed from the patient's hemodynamic pressure monitoring system, avoiding the use of heparin-coated catheters, and discontinuing heparin flushes to maintain the patency of other intravenous lines are essential elements of nursing management.[21]

Nursing Diagnoses

Heparin-Induced Thrombocytopenia

- Ineffective Cardiopulmonary Tissue Perfusion related to decreased coronary blood flow
- Ineffective Peripheral Tissue Perfusion related to decreased peripheral blood flow
- Ineffective Renal Tissue Perfusion related to decreased renal blood flow
- Ineffective Gastrointestinal Tissue Perfusion related to decreased gastrointestinal blood flow
- Ineffective Cerebral Tissue Perfusion related to decreased cerebral blood flow
- Powerlessness related to lack of control over the current situation or disease progression
- Deficient Knowledge related to lack of previous exposure to information (see the Patient Education feature on Heparin-Induced Thrombocytopenia)

Patient Education. Prevention of subsequent episodes in patients sensitized to heparin includes education of the patient and family (see the Patient Education feature on Heparin-Induced Thrombocytopenia). The use of medical alert bracelets and listing heparin allergies in the medical record are necessary to avoid this serious complication in the future.

Collaborative management of the patient with immune-mediated HIT is outlined in Box 43-4.

Patient Education: Heparin-Induced Thrombocytopenia

- Pathophysiology of disease
- Purpose of heparin
- Measures to avoid future exposure to heparin
  - Identify different types of heparin (unfractionated and low-molecular-weight forms).
  - Encourage purchase of medical alert bracelet or similar type of warning device.
  - Tell any new health care provider about the heparin allergy and previous reaction.

BOX 43-4 COLLABORATIVE MANAGEMENT: HEPARIN-INDUCED THROMBOCYTOPENIA

- Stop all heparin exposure.
  - Unfractionated and low-molecular-weight heparins by any route
  - Heparin flushes
  - Heparin-coated vascular access devices
- Begin therapy with an alternative anticoagulant.
  - Lepirudin
  - Argatroban
- Maintain surveillance for complications.
  - Deep vein thrombosis
- Pulmonary emboli
- Acute limb ischemia
- Ischemic stroke
- Acute myocardial infarction
- Administer antifibrinolytic therapy (as indicated) if thrombosis occurs.
- Prepare patient for surgical embolectomy (as indicated) if thrombosis occurs.
- Provide comfort and emotional support.

TUMOR LYSIS SYNDROME

DESCRIPTION

Tumor lysis syndrome (TLS) refers to a variety of metabolic disturbances that may be seen with the treatment of cancer. A potentially lethal complication of various forms of cancer treatment, TLS occurs when large numbers of neoplastic cells are rapidly killed, resulting in the release of large amounts of potassium, phosphate, and uric acid into the systemic circulation. It is most commonly seen in patients with lymphoma, leukemia, or multiple metastatic conditions.[28,29]

ETIOLOGY

Although most often associated with the use of chemotherapeutic drugs, biological agents, and irradiation used in the treatment of malignant disorders, TLS can in rare instances occur spontaneously. The development of TLS has been linked to other pathophysiologic conditions such as elevated WBC counts, large tumors, multiple organ involvement by malignancy, and renal insufficiency.[20,30,31]

PATHOPHYSIOLOGY

The primary mechanism involved in the development of TLS is the destruction of massive numbers of malignant cells by chemotherapy or radiation therapy. Massive destruction of cells releases large amounts of potassium, phosphorus, and nucleic acids, leading to severe metabolic disturbances, such as hyperuricemia, hyperkalemia, hyperphosphatemia, and hypocalcemia (Table 43-7). Vomiting, diarrhea, and other insensible fluid losses from fever or tachypnea also contribute to these electrolyte disturbances.[29] Death of patients with TLS is most often caused by complications of renal failure or cardiac arrest.[28]

TABLE 43-7 Electrolyte Abnormalities Encountered in Tumor Lysis Syndrome and Their Clinical Consequences

Electrolyte	Pathophysiology	Clinical Consequence	Treatment Options
Potassium	Rapid expulsion of intracellular K^+ into the circulation due to cell lysis	Adverse skeletal and cardiac manifestations (e.g., ventricular dysrhythmias, weakness, paresthesias)	Insulin/glucose, sodium bicarbonate, inhaled beta-agonist, K^+-binding resins, dialysis, calcium gluconate
Phosphate	Release of intracellular PO_4^- due to cell lysis. May be compounded by renal dysfunction	Muscle cramps, tetany, dysrhythmias, seizures	Dialysis, phosphate binders
Calcium	Precipitation of the calcium phosphate complex because of the rapid increase in the phosphorous concentration	Muscle cramps, tetany, dysrhythmias, seizures, renal failure (acute nephrocalcinosis)	Calcium gluconate (treatment should be reserved for those with neuromuscular irritability)
Uric acid	Cell lysis leads to increased levels of purine nucleic acids into the circulation that are metabolized to uric acid	Renal failure (uric acid nephropathy)	Hydration, dialysis, xanthine oxidase inhibitors, alkalization of urine, urate oxidase

Hyperuricemia. Hyperuricemia occurs 48 to 72 hours after the initiation of anticancer therapy.[29] Tumor cells undergo rapid growth and development, and large amounts of nucleic acids are present within them. When therapy is initiated, tumor cell destruction releases nucleic acids, which are metabolized into uric acid. Metabolic acidosis ensues, resulting in crystallization of the uric acid in the distal tubules of the kidney and leading to obstruction of urine flow. Glomerular filtration rates drop as the kidneys are unable to clear the increasing amounts of uric acid. Consequently, renal insufficiency and acute renal failure eventually occur. Acute renal failure is discussed further in Chapter 31.

Hyperuricemia associated with TLS can be potentiated by several other factors, including elevated uric acid levels before the initiation of therapy. Other causes of increased uric acid production are elevated WBC counts, destruction of WBCs, and enlargement of the lymph nodes, spleen, or liver.[28-30]

Hyperkalemia. Hyperkalemia occurs within 6 to 72 hours after the initiation of chemotherapy. This is the most deleterious of all the manifestations of TLS.[29] In addition to the release of nucleic acids, tumor cell destruction also results in the release of potassium. Renal insufficiency related to hyperuricemia prevents adequate excretion of potassium, and levels rise. The resultant hyperkalemia may have a profound effect on intracellular and extracellular fluid levels.[28] Left untreated, hyperkalemia can have devastating consequences, including cardiac arrest and death.[28,29]

Hyperphosphatemia and Hypocalcemia. Hyperphosphatemia and hypocalcemia occur 24 to 48 hours after the initiation of therapy.[29] Phosphorus levels also rise as a consequence of tumor cell destruction. Calcium ions then bind with the excess phosphorus, creating calcium phosphate salts and bringing about hypocalcemia. These salts precipitate in the kidney tubules, worsening renal insufficiency. Hypocalcemia causes tetany and cardiac dysrhythmias, which can result in cardiac arrest and death.[28,29]

ASSESSMENT AND DIAGNOSIS

Detection and recognition of TLS is accomplished through assessment of clinical manifestations, evaluation of laboratory findings, and other diagnostic tests. Table 43-8 summarizes common findings in TLS.[28-30]

Clinical Manifestations. Clinical manifestations are related to the metabolic disturbances associated with TLS. The patient's history reveals an unexplained weight gain after initiation of chemotherapy or radiation therapy. The weight gain is associated with fluid retention due to electrolyte disturbances. Other early signs heralding the onset of TLS include diarrhea, lethargy, muscle cramps, nausea, vomiting, paresthesias, and weakness.

Laboratory Findings. Laboratory findings demonstrate electrolyte disturbances such as elevated potassium and phosphorus levels and a decreased calcium level. Uric acid levels are increased. Elevated levels of BUN and creatinine and a decreased creatinine clearance also indicate TLS. Metabolic acidosis is confirmed by the presence of decreased pH, bicarbonate levels, and partial pressure of carbon dioxide ($PaCO_2$) on arterial blood gas measurements.[32]

Other Diagnostic Tests. Physical examination reveals positive Chvostek's and Trousseau's signs related to hypocalcemia.

Hyperactive deep tendon reflexes indicate hyperkalemia and hypocalcemia.[28] Potassium and calcium disturbances result in changes that can be seen on the electrocardiogram (ECG), such as peaked or inverted T waves, altered QT intervals, widened QRS complexes, and dysrhythmias.[28-30]

MEDICAL MANAGEMENT

Medical interventions are aimed at maintaining adequate hydration, treating metabolic imbalances, and preventing life-threatening complications (see Table 43-7).[28,29,31] Administration of intravenous fluids may be necessary early in the course of treatment if inadequate hydration exists. The administration of isotonic saline (0.9% normal saline) reduces serum concentrations of uric acid, phosphate, and potassium.[29] The use of nonthiazide diuretics to maintain adequate urine output may be required. If renal failure occurs, hemodialysis should be considered.[29]

Electrolytes and arterial blood gases are closely monitored. Dietary restrictions of potassium and phosphorus may be necessary. The goals in treating hyperuricemia are to inhibit uric acid formation and to increase renal clearance.[29] This can be accomplished through the administration of sodium bicarbonate to increase the pH of the urine to above 7.0, which increases the solubility of uric acid, preventing subsequent crystallization. Allopurinol administration can also inhibit uric acid formation.[28]

If potassium levels rise dangerously, Kayexalate (sodium polystyrene sulfonate) may be given orally, or if the patient is unable to tolerate oral medications due to nausea and vomiting, rectal instillation may be used. If the patient is oliguric, glucose and insulin infusions may be given to facilitate lowering the potassium levels. A 10% solution of calcium gluconate may be administered to stabilize cardiac tissue membranes to prevent life-threatening dysrhythmias.[33] Phosphorus-binding antacids can be used for treating hyperphosphatemia. Stool softeners may be necessary to treat the constipation often associated with the administration of these antacids. Calcium gluconate may be required to replace calcium, but it should be used judiciously.[28]

TABLE 43-8	Common Findings in Tumor Lysis Syndrome
Diagnostic Parameter	Findings
Clinical	Weight gain, edema, diarrhea, lethargy, muscle cramps, nausea and vomiting, paresthesia, weakness, oliguria, uremia, seizures
Laboratory	↑Potassium, phosphorus, uric acid, BUN, Cr ↓Calcium, creatinine clearance, pH, bicarbonate, $PaCO_2$
Diagnostic	Positive Chvostek's and Trousseau's signs, hyperactive deep tendon reflexes, dysrhythmias, ECG changes

BUN, blood urea nitrogen; Cr, creatinine; ECG, electrocardiogram; $PaCO_2$, partial pressure of carbon dioxide; ↑, increased; ↓, decreased.

NURSING MANAGEMENT

Nursing management of the patient with TLS incorporates a variety of nursing diagnoses (see the Nursing Diagnoses feature on Tumor Lysis Syndrome). Assessment and continued monitoring of the patient is an important role of the critical care nurse when caring for the patient with TLS. Recognizing critical laboratory changes or development of symptoms and notifying the physician in a timely manner are essential.[33] Insertion of a urinary catheter and maintenance of the intravenous line site are necessary to ensure adequate intake and output. Vital signs should be monitored frequently, and weight should be monitored daily.[28]

Nursing interventions are aimed at preventing complications. Seizure precautions should be instituted, especially if calcium levels are disrupted. Insertion of a nasogastric tube is appropriate if nausea or vomiting occurs. Dietary adjustments are necessary, such as potassium and phosphorus restrictions in the presence of elevated serum levels and providing additional fiber to combat the constipation associated with the administration of antacids.

Education of the patient and family is a primary role of the critical care nurse. All treatments and interventions should be explained before carrying them out, and questions should be answered at a level understandable to the patient and family. Before discharge, potential risk factors and identification of early signs and symptoms should be reviewed.[32]

Collaborative management of the patient with TLS is outlined in Box 43-5.

Nursing Diagnoses

Tumor Lysis Syndrome

- Excess Fluid Volume related to renal dysfunction
- Decreased Cardiac Output related to alterations in contractility
- Anxiety related to threat to biologic, psychologic, and/or social integrity
- Ineffective Coping related to a situational crisis and personal vulnerability

---

BOX 43-5 COLLABORATIVE MANAGEMENT: TUMOR LYSIS SYNDROME

- Facilitate adequate renal function.
  - Volume hydration with 0.9% normal saline
  - Nonthiazide diuretics
- Treat hyperkalemia.
  - Kayexalate
  - Glucose and insulin
- Treat hyperuricemia.
  - Sodium bicarbonate
  - Allopurinol
- Treat hyperphosphatemia.
  - Dietary restrictions
  - Phosphorus-binding antacids
- Treat hypocalcemia.
  - Calcium gluconate
- Maintain surveillance for complications.
  - Acute renal failure
  - Cardiac dysrhythmias
- Provide comfort and emotional support.

HOSPITAL-ACQUIRED ANEMIA

DESCRIPTION AND ETIOLOGY

Hospital-acquired anemia is commonly seen in critically ill patients, and it demonstrates many of the same characteristics as those encountered in chronic disease. Much research has been focused on identifying the contributing factors and interventions related to this issue. Frequent phlebotomy, coagulopathies, and nutritional deficits are just a few reasons for this increasing problem.[34] The demand for human blood products is outstripping current and projected supplies, and public confidence in the safety of our blood supply is deteriorating.[35] For these reasons, research has been focused on determining ways to minimize iatrogenic blood losses, improve blood salvage techniques, and develop alternatives to traditional blood transfusion therapy.

Risks Associated with Blood Transfusions. Studies have shown that as many as 50% of transfusions administered in the intensive care unit (ICU) are related to nosocomial anemia.[34,36] Although the risks associated with transfusions have significantly decreased with the advent of better screening techniques and safer storage mechanisms, it is highly unlikely that the risks will be eradicated completely.

Transmission of Infection. Protecting our blood supply from viral contamination depends on the appropriate selection of donors and meticulous screening of the donated blood for contaminants. Current methods for detecting contaminants in blood are quite sophisticated, but they are not able to detect viruses when the donor is in the seroconversion period. Viruses that can be transmitted through blood transfusion include hepatitis B and C, human immunodeficiency virus (HIV), and cytomegalovirus.[34,35,37]

Less commonly, bacterial contamination may occur. It most often results from inadequate skin disinfection at the phlebotomy site, an undetected bacteremia in the donor, or minute leaks in the blood storage container itself. Common bacterial contaminants include *Serratia, Yersinia, Pseudomonas,* and *Campylobacter* species.[35]

Immunosuppression. Among other studies, Project Impact, sponsored by the Society for Critical Care Medicine, has produced data that link blood transfusions in the critically ill with an increase in the rate of hospital-associated infections such as pneumonia and surgical site infections.[34] This increased hospital-associated infection rate may be linked to immunosuppression related to the transfusion itself.[35] Decreased lymphocytes, changes in T-cell ratios, dysfunctional B cells, and activation of immune cells have been attributed to blood transfusions.

Circulatory Overload. The introduction of increased volume during blood transfusions may be related to fluid volume overload problems. The delicate balance necessary to maintain stability in the critically ill patient can be disrupted by the introduction of blood volume and necessary flush solutions. The inability of compromised renal and cardiovascular systems to handle the additional fluid load may result in pulmonary edema or heart failure.[34,37]

Stored Blood. The average shelf life of a unit of blood is 21 to 42 days.[34,35] This period depends on the storage solution, the type of processing used, and the storage system itself. As blood ages during storage, changes take place that contribute to blood-related complications.[34,36] RBCs break down, releasing potassium and bilirubin, which may result in dangerous elevations of these substances in the patient receiving the transfusion. The breakdown of the RBCs also results in depletion of oxygen-carrying capacity of the transfused blood. Citrate, which is used as a preservative, can bind with calcium released from damaged RBCs, resulting in hypocalcemia.[34]

Clerical Risk Factors. The process of blood transfusion from donor to recipient requires a tremendous amount of documentation; nonetheless, there is room for error, which can lead to mismatching of patient and donor blood types. Hemolytic reactions are the unfortunate and often deadly consequence of these preventable errors (see Patient Safety Alert).

BLOOD CONSERVATION STRATEGIES

As more patients and clinicians opt for the limited use of blood products, strategies for conserving blood and preventing unnecessary loss become an important part of the critical care nurse's standard of care. These strategies include minimizing blood loss, managing oxygen delivery and consumption, stimulating production of RBCs, and understanding transfusion safety and alternative agents.

Minimizing Blood Loss. Frequent laboratory tests have been shown to be a major culprit in the development of hospital-acquired anemia in critically ill patients.[38] Blood losses correspond to actual volume of samples and discards when drawing from venous access lines. Critical care nurses can be instrumental in significantly decreasing blood loss in this arena. The use of pediatric collection tubes and point-of-care testing are techniques that yield valid diagnostic results but require smaller blood samples. Closed-loop vascular devices that retain the sterility of the potential discard and allow its return to the patient are also being used.

Patient Safety Alert

National Patient Safety Goal (NPSG).01.03.01

Eliminate transfusion errors related to patient misidentification.

Elements of Performance for NPSG.01.03.01

1. Before initiating a blood or blood component transfusion, the patient is objectively matched to the blood or blood component during a two-person bedside or chair-side verification process. At least two unique identifiers are used in the process, and it is conducted after the blood or blood component that matches the order has been issued or dispensed.

   Note: If two individuals are not available, an automated identification technology (e.g., bar coding) may be used in place of one of the individuals.

2. When using a two-person bedside or chair-side verification process, one individual conducting the identification verification must be the qualified transfusionist who will administer the blood or blood component to the patient.

3. When using a two-person bedside or chair-side verification process, the second individual conducting the identification verification must be qualified to participate in the process.

Noninvasive monitoring devices such as pulse oximetry and capnography can reduce the need for arterial blood gas analysis.

The critical care nurse plays a key role in preventing and managing hemorrhagic blood loss in the critically ill patient. Control of hypertension, which can contribute to significant hemorrhage, can be accomplished through fluid management and the administration of antihypertensive and vasodilatory medications as needed. Blood salvage devices can be employed to collect shed blood and return it to the patient. Several pharmacologic agents can assist in achieving hemostasis and can prevent further blood loss. Desmopressin is a potent vasoconstrictor that also affects clotting factor VIII.[37] Aminocaproic acid (Amicar) inhibits activation of plasminogen.[39] All of these agents and devices work to control bleeding.

Managing Oxygen Delivery and Consumption. Illness-related stress, blood loss from surgery, infection, pain, and anxiety contribute to the higher than normal demand for oxygen by the critically ill patient.[36] Monitoring pulse oximetry is useful in identifying activities and interventions that can contribute to the imbalance between supply and demand. Supplemental oxygen therapy assists in maintaining available oxygen supplies. Promoting a restful environment through modulation of nursing care activities and providing pain and sedation control can assist in decreasing the demand for oxygen. It is important to monitor cardiac output and other hemodynamic parameters to manage interventions that optimize oxygen delivery. Administration of fluids and inotropic agents optimizes blood pressure and cardiac output, and vasodilators are used to decrease afterload and improve efficiency of cardiovascular function.

Stimulating Production of Red Blood Cells. Insufficient erythropoiesis can contribute to anemia in the critically ill patient. The administration of epoetin alpha can stimulate the production of RBCs, reducing the need for transfusions.[36-39] Iron preparations such as ferrous sulfate, iron sucrose, or iron gluconate may be administered to provide necessary iron stores for the increased erythropoiesis.

Encouraging Safer Transfusions and Alternative Agents. Finding ways to decrease the risks associated with blood transfusions and make the blood supply safer for patients is a high priority. Better, more sensitive screening tests, irradiation, and removal of leukocytes are a few of the current methods in use. Plasma expanders manufactured from nonhuman sources are also available. Autologous transfusions, for which the patient donates his or her own blood before a surgical procedure or other anticipated need, has also been a common practice for many years. Recombinant DNA technology is being used to develop safe alternatives to blood transfusions. The use of blood from other species is being researched in the quest to provide safe and effective products for use in severe anemia.[40]

SPECIAL CONSIDERATIONS FOR THE SURGICAL PATIENT

The surgical patient who wants to avoid the use of blood transfusions presents special problems. However, several strategies can be used during surgery to minimize the need for transfusions.

Pharmacologic Agents. Antifibrinolytic agents such as tranexamic acid (cyklokapron) and aminocaproic acid (Amicar) can be administered to promote hemostasis. Vasopressin or desmopressin (DDAVP) are potent vasoconstrictors that can slow blood leakage from small vessels.[37,41,42]

Autologous Blood Donation. The patient undergoing surgery who wants to avoid blood transfusions may choose to donate his or her own blood several weeks before surgery. Autologous donation can also be accomplished intraoperatively. This technique provides the patient with fresh, whole blood to be used during surgery. Intraoperative autologous donation is used most often in emergency or traumatic surgery.[40,41]

Platelet Sequestration. Like intraoperative autologous blood donation, plateletpheresis may be performed just before beginning surgery. The platelets are then reinfused when necessary.[40,41] Although controversial, this procedure has been shown to be effective in decreasing chest tube drainage after cardiovascular bypass surgery.[41]

Blood Salvaging. For autotransfusion, blood salvage devices collect blood from the operative site, separate and wash the RBCs, and return them to the patient. Similar to autologous donation, the patient receives his or her own blood and avoids the risks associated with nonautologous blood transfusions.[40]

Anesthesia-Induced Hypotension. The use of induced hypotension is controversial, and results have been inconsistent. Hypotension can lead in tissue ischemia and result in cardiac dysrhythmias, acute myocardial infarction, stroke, and damage to renal or hepatic cells. However, controlled mild hypotension may be useful when a large blood loss is anticipated, such as in the context of orthopedic procedures.[43]

Surgical Techniques and Instruments. Technology has provided many tools that have made it possible to significantly decrease surgical blood loss and the need for blood transfusions. Minimally invasive procedures such as laparoscopic and endoscopic approaches and advances in interventional radiologic techniques have made a significant contribution. The gamma knife, the argon beam coagulator, and the harmonic scalpel are examples of tools that have also been instrumental in decreasing the need for postoperative transfusions.

Summary

Coagulation and Fibrinolysis

- Hemostasis is the ability of the body to control bleeding and clotting.
- Four actions are involved in achieving hemostasis: local vasoconstriction to reduce blood flow; platelet aggregation at the injury site and formation of a platelet plug; formation of a fibrin mesh to strengthen the plug; and dissolution of the clot after tissue repair.

Disseminated Intravascular Coagulation

- DIC is characterized by bleeding and thrombosis, which result from depletion of clotting factors, platelets, and RBCs and, if left untreated, will result in death.

- Medical management focuses on identification of the underlying cause, provision of hemodynamic support to preserve end-organ function, and administration of blood, blood components, and medications to interrupt the process.
- Nursing actions include initiating bleeding precautions, providing comfort and emotional support, and maintaining surveillance for complications (e.g., hypovolemic shock, ischemia, multiple organ dysfunction syndrome).

Idiopathic Thrombocytopenia Purpura

- Idiopathic thrombocytopenia purpura is caused by an autoimmune response that results in the destruction of existing platelets.
- Medical management focuses on administration of glucocorticoids, immunoglobulin, and platelets.
- Nursing actions include initiating bleeding precautions, providing comfort and emotional support, and maintaining surveillance for complications (e.g., intracranial hemorrhage, severe blood loss).

Heparin-induced Thrombocytopenia

- There are two forms of heparin-induced thrombocytopenia: type 1 and type 2. Type 1 is more common, milder, and transient. Type 2 is the result of an autoimmune response to the administration of heparin and is more severe than type 1.
- Medical management focuses discontinuation of all heparin, initiation of anticoagulation with an alternative anticoagulant, and treatment of thrombosis.
- Nursing actions include providing comfort and emotional support and maintaining surveillance for complications (e.g., deep vein thrombosis, pulmonary emboli, limb ischemia, ischemic stroke, acute myocardial infarction).

Tumor Lysis Syndrome

- Tumor lysis syndrome occurs when a large number of neoplastic cells are rapidly killed, resulting in the release of large amounts of potassium, phosphate, and uric acid in the systemic circulation.
- Medical management focuses on preservation of renal function and treatment of electrolyte disorders (hyperkalemia, hyperuricemia, hyperphosphatemia, and hypocalcemia).
- Nursing actions include providing comfort and emotional support and maintaining surveillance for complications (e.g., acute renal failure, dysrhythmias).

Hospital-Acquired Anemia

- Risks associated with blood transfusions include transmission of infection, immunosuppression, and circulatory overload.
- Blood conservation strategies include minimizing blood loss, managing oxygen delivery and consumption, and stimulating production of RBCs.

Case Study: Patient with Hematologic Disorders and Oncologic Emergencies

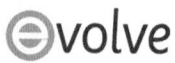 Answers to the Case Study Questions can be found on the Evolve web site at http://evolve.elsevier.com/Urden/.

Brief Patient History

Mr. L is an otherwise healthy, 23-year-old, African American man who presents with a week-long history of diarrhea, nausea, and vomiting after attending a barbecue last weekend.

Clinical Assessment

Mr. L is admitted to the intensive care unit from the emergency department with hypotension, fever, and leukocytosis.

Diagnostic Procedures

His vital signs are as follows: blood pressure of 65/42 mm Hg, heart rate of 145 beats/min (sinus tachycardia), respiratory rate of 35 breaths/min, and temperature of 102.4° F. His white blood cell count is 25,000/mm^3 with 15% bands, lactate level is 7 mmol/L, prothrombin time is 25 seconds, and platelet count is 22,000/mm^3. Blood cultures reveal gram-negative bacilli.

Medical Diagnosis

Mr. L is diagnosed with severe sepsis and disseminated intravascular coagulation.

Questions

1. What major outcomes do you expect to achieve for this patient?
2. What problems or risks must be managed to achieve these outcomes?
3. What interventions must be initiated to monitor, prevent, manage, or eliminate the problems and risks identified?
4. What interventions should be initiated to promote optimal functioning, safety, and well-being of the patient?
5. What possible learning needs do you anticipate for this patient?
6. What cultural and age-related factors may have a bearing on the patient's plan of care?

---

evolve Be sure to check out the bonus material, including free self-assessment exercises, on the Evolve web site at http://evolve.elsevier.com/Urden/.

References

1. McCance KL: Structure and function of the hematologic system. In McCance KL, Huether SE, editors: *Pathophysiology: the biologic basis for disease in adults and children*, ed 5, St Louis, 2006, Mosby.
2. Furie B, Furie BC: Mechanisms of thrombus formation, *N Engl J Med* 359:938, 2008.
3. Geiter H: Disseminated intravascular coagulation, *Dimens Crit Care Nurs* 22:108, 2003.
4. Doshi SN, Marmur JD: Evolving role of tissue factor and its pathway inhibitor, *Crit Care Med* 30:S241, 2002.
5. Castoldi E, Hackeng TM: Regulation of coagulation by protein S, *Curr Opin Hematol* 15:529, 2008.
6. Bick RL: Disseminated intravascular coagulation: current concepts of etiology, pathophysiology, diagnosis, and treatment, *Hematol Oncol Clin North Am* 17:149, 2003.
7. Levi M: Disseminated intravascular coagulation, *Crit Care Med* 35:2191, 2007.
8. Wada H: Disseminated intravascular coagulation, *Clin Chim Acta* 344:13, 2004.
9. Slofstra SH et al: Disseminated intravascular coagulation, *Hematol J* 4:295, 2003.
10. Dressler DK: DIC: coping with a coagulation crisis, *Nursing2004* 34(5):58, 2004.
11. Zeerleder S et al: Disseminated intravascular coagulation in sepsis, *Chest* 128:2864, 2005.
12. George JN: Platelet disorders. In Beers MH et al, editors: *The Merck manual of diagnosis and therapy*, ed 18, Whitehouse Station, NJ, 2006, Merck Research Laboratories.
13. George JN: Thrombotic thrombocytopenic purpura, *N Engl J Med* 354:1927, 2006.
14. Noonan K: Introduction to B-cell disorders, *Clin J Oncol Nurs* 11:3, 2007.
15. Stasi R, Provan D: Management of immune thrombocytopenic purpura in adults, *Mayo Clin Proc* 79:504, 2004.
16. Crowther MA, George JN: Thrombotic thrombocytopenic purpura: 2008 update, *Cleve Clin J Med* 75:369, 2008.
17. Sadler JE et al: Recent advances in thrombotic thrombocytopenic purpura, *Hematology Am Soc Hematol Educ Program* 2004:407, 2004.
18. Ballow M: Clinical and investigational considerations for the use of IGIV therapy, *Am J Health Syst Pharm* 15:S12, 2005.
19. Kremer Hovinga JA, Meyer SC: Current management of thrombotic thrombocytopenic purpura, *Curr Opin Hematol* 15:445, 2008.
20. Otto SE: *Oncology nursing clinical reference*, St Louis, 2004, Mosby.
21. Levine RL, Cooney MF: Implications, management and prevention of heparin-induced thrombocytopenia in the critical care setting, *AACN News* November, 2006.
22. Warkentin TE: Heparin-induced thrombocytopenia, *Hematol Oncol Clin North Am* 21:589, 2007.
23. Selleng K et al: Heparin-induced thrombocytopenia in intensive care patients, *Crit Care Med* 35:1165, 2007.
24. Cooney MF: Heparin-induced thrombocytopenia, *Crit Care Nurse* 26(6):30, 2006.
25. Jang I, Hursting M: When heparins promote thrombosis: review of heparin-induced thrombocytopenia, *Circulation* 111:2671, 2005.
26. Arepally GM, Ortel, TL: Heparin-induced thrombocytopenia, *N Engl J Med* 355:809, 2006.
27. Warkentin TE, Greinacher A, editors: *Heparin-induced thrombocytopenia*, ed 3, New York, 2004, Marcel Dekker.
28. Menajovsky LB: Heparin-induced thrombocytopenia: clinical manifestations and management strategies, *Am J Med* 118(suppl 8A):21S, 2005.
29. Robison J: Metabolic emergencies: tumor lysis syndrome. In Newton S et al, editors: *Oncology nursing advisor: a comprehensive guide to clinical practice*, St Louis, 2009, Mosby.
30. Davidson MB et al: Pathophysiology, clinical consequences, and treatment of tumor lysis syndrome, *Am J Med* 116:546, 2004.

31. Higdon ML, Higdon JA: Treatment of oncologic emergencies, *Am Fam Physician* 74:1873, 2006.

32. Zobec A: Tumor lysis syndrome. In Gates RA, Fink RM, editors, *Oncology nursing secrets*, ed 3, St Louis, 2008, Mosby.

33. Shelton BK: Tumor lysis syndrome. In Chernecky CC, Murphy-Ende K, editors: *Acute care oncology*, ed 2, St Louis, 2009, Saunders.

34. Myers JS. Complications of cancer and cancer treatment. In Langhorne ME et al, editors, *Oncology nursing*, ed 5, St Louis, 2007, Mosby.

35. Raghavan M, Marik PE: Anemia, allogenic blood transfusion, and immunomodulation in the critically ill, *Chest* 127:295, 2005.

36. Gould S et al: Packed red blood cell transfusion in the intensive care unit: limitations and consequences, *Am J Crit Care* 16:39, 2007.

37. Thomas J, Martinez A: Blood conservation in the critically ill, *Am J Health Syst Pharm* 64:S11, 2007.

38. Vernon S, Pfeifer GM: Blood management strategies for critical care patients, *Crit Care Nurse* 23(6):34, 2003.

39. Tinmouth AT et al: Blood conservation strategies to reduce the need for red blood cell transfusion in critically ill patients, *CMAJ* 178:49, 2008.

40. Shermock KM et al: Erythropoietic agents for anemia of critical illness, *Am J Health Syst Pharm* 65:540, 2008.

41. Kirschman RA: Finding alternatives to blood transfusion, *Holist Nurs Pract* 18(6):277, 2004.

42. Putney LJ: Bloodless cardiac surgery: not just possible, but preferable, *Crit Care Nurs Q* 30:263, 2007.

43. Schaefer J: Advances and dilemmas in recombinant blood products, *J Infus Nurs* 25:305, 2002.

44. Degoute CS: Controlled hypotension: a guide to drug choice, *Drugs* 67:1053, 2007.

APPENDIX A

Nursing Management Plans of Care

NURSING MANAGEMENT PLAN: Activity Intolerance

Definition: Insufficient physiologic or psychologic energy to endure or complete required or desired daily activities

Activity Intolerance Related to Cardiopulmonary Dysfunction

Defining Characteristics

- Chest pain with activity
- Electrocardiographic changes with activity
- Heart rate is > 15 beats/min above baseline with activity for patients on beta-blockers or calcium channel blockers
- Heart rate remains elevated above baseline 5 minutes after activity
- Breathlessness with activity
- SpO_2 < 92% with activity
- Postural hypotension when moving from supine to upright position
- Patient reports fatigue with activity

Outcome Criteria

- Heart rate is < 20 beats/min above baseline with activity and is < 10 beats/min above baseline with activity for patients on beta-blockers or calcium channel blockers.
- Heart rate returns to baseline 5 minutes after activity.
- Chest pain with activity is absent.
- Patient reports tolerance to activity.

Nursing Interventions and Rationale

1. Encourage active or passive range-of-motion exercises while the patient is in bed *to keep joints flexible and muscles stretched.*
2. Teach patient to refrain from holding breath while performing exercises and *to avoid the Valsalva maneuver.*
3. Encourage performance of muscle-toning exercises at least three times daily, *because a toned muscle uses less oxygen when performing work than an untoned muscle.*
4. Progress ambulation *to increase tolerance to activity.*
5. Teach patient to take pulse *to determine activity tolerance:* Take pulse for a full minute before exercise and then for 10 seconds and multiply by 6 at exercise peak.

Activity Intolerance Related to Prolonged Immobility or Deconditioning

Defining Characteristics

- Decrease in systolic blood pressure is > 20 mm Hg;
- Increase in heart rate is > 20 beats/min with postural change
- Syncope with postural change
- Patient reports lightheadedness with postural change

Outcome Criteria

- Decrease in systolic blood pressure is < 10 mm Hg;
- Increase in heart rate is < 10 beats/min with postural change.
- Syncope or lightheadedness is absent with postural change.

Nursing Interventions and Rationale

1. Instruct the patient how to perform straight-leg raises, dorsiflexion or plantar flexion, and quadriceps-setting and gluteal-setting exercises *to increase muscular and vascular tone.*
2. Consult with physician regarding the administration of fluids to ensure that the patient is hydrated to 24-hour fluid requirements per body surface area (BSA) *to increase preload and thereby increase stroke volume and cardiac output.*
3. Reposition patient incrementally *to avoid syncope:*
   a. Head of bed to 45 degrees and hold until symptom free
   b. Head of bed to 90 degrees and hold until symptom free
   c. Dangle until symptom free
   d. Stand until symptom free and ambulate
4. Collaborate with physician regarding patient's activity level *to ensure patient's safety.*

NURSING MANAGEMENT PLAN: **Acute Confusion**

Definition: Abrupt onset of a cluster of global, transient changes and disturbances in attention, cognition, psychomotor activity, level of consciousness, and/or sleep/wake cycle

Acute Confusion Related to Sensory Overload, Sensory Deprivation, and Sleep Pattern Disturbance

Defining Characteristics

Early Symptoms

- Sudden onset of global cognitive function impairment (hours to days)
- Restlessness, agitation, and combative behavior
- Drowsiness (can lead to loss of consciousness)
- Slurring of speech, inappropriate statements or "word salad," mumbling, or inappropriate gestures
- Short attention span (needs questions repeated); inability to learn new material
- Disordered sleep/wake cycle
- Disorientation to person, time, place, and situation
- Difficulty in separating dreams from reality (may experience bizarre dreams or nightmares)
- Anger at staff for continued questions about his or her orientation

Later Symptoms

- Symptoms that tend to fluctuate throughout the day and night
- Continuations of early symptoms, which may be more frequent or of longer duration
- Illusions
- Hallucinations
- Extreme agitation (e.g., attempts to climb out of bed, pull out catheters, rip off dressings)
- Calling out in loud voice, swearing, or attempting to bite or hit people who approach patient

Nursing Interventions and Rationale

1. Determine and document the patient's dominant spoken language, his or her literacy, and the languages in which he or she is literate. *Sometimes, people are not literate in their spoken language, or, less commonly, they are literate only in their second language.*
2. Determine and document patient's premorbid degree of orientation, cognitive capabilities, and any sensory/perceptual deficits. *Assuming that the patients were or were not fully oriented before critical care admission bases the nurse's assessment on possibly erroneous assumptions.*

For Sensory Overload

1. Initiate each nurse/patient encounter by calling the patient by name and identifying yourself by name. *This fosters reality orientation and assists the patient in filtering irrelevant or impersonal conversation.*
2. Assess the patient's immediate physical environment from his or her viewpoint, and explain equipment, its sounds, and its therapeutic purpose. Demonstrate audible and visual alarms, and explain possible alarm conditions. *This decreases alienation of the patient from the technologic environment and reduces the inherent sense of fear and urgency accompanying alarm conditions.*
3. Provide preparatory sensory information by explaining procedures in relation to the sensations the patient will experience, including duration of sensations. *Preparatory sensory information enhances learning and lessens anticipatory anxiety.*
4. Limit noise levels. *Audible alarms cannot and must not be silenced, and many critical but noisy activities must take place in the critical care area. It has been shown, however, that noise levels produced by clinical personnel exceed those levels designated as acceptable and are often greater than those generated by technologic devices.* Keep staff conversations soft enough that they are inaudible to the patient whenever possible. Assume that everything said at or around a patient's bedside is intended for that patient's awareness and that it will be interpreted as pertaining to him or her. *As in the discussion that follows, conversations about the patient but not to him or her foster depersonalization and delusions of reference.*
5. Enforce nighttime noise limits.
6. Readjust alarm limits on physiologic monitoring devices as the patient's condition changes (improves or deteriorates) *to lessen unnecessary alarm states.*
7. Consider use of headphones and compact disk or digital music player with patient's favorite and/or subliminal or classical music. *This can effectively filter out assaultive noise of the critical care environment and supplant it with familiar, soothing sounds and rhythms.*
8. Modify lighting. *Day and night cycles need to be simulated with environmental lighting.* Never turn on overhead fluorescent lights abruptly without warning the patient, assisting him or her out of the supine position, and/or shielding his or her eyes with gauze or a face cloth. *Continuous bright lighting sustains anxiety and promotes circadian rhythm desynchronization.*
9. Shield patients from viewing urgent and emergent events in the critical care unit. *Resuscitation efforts, albeit difficult to conceal, engender fear in the patient and a sense of instability and vulnerability (e.g., "I'm next").* When such an event occurs, elicit the patient's cognitive and emotional reaction; thoughts, impressions, and feeling need to be shared and misconceptions clarified. A useful approach in this interchange is that of emphasizing the

NURSING MANAGEMENT PLAN: Acute Confusion—*cont'd*

differences between the patient at hand and the one resuscitated (e.g., "He was considerably older," "more unstable," "had serious lung disease").

10. Ensure patients' privacy, modesty, and dignity. *Physical exposure and nudity, although they seemingly pale in importance compared with priorities such as physiologic assessment and stabilization, are primal indignities for all individuals.* Keep the patient minimally exposed. When, in the course of assessment and intervention, it becomes necessary to expose the patient, verbally apologize for this necessity. *To be naked is to feel vulnerable; to be vulnerable is to feel fearful. In this regard, fear is an emotion that is preventable through nursing intervention.*

For Sensory Deprivation

1. Provide reality orientation in four spheres (personal, place, time, and situation) at more frequent intervals than when testing. Convey this information in the context of routine conversation. *Sample statements:* "Mr. Clark, this is Tuesday morning and you're in University Hospital. Your heart surgery was yesterday morning, and you're doing well. My name is Joe, and I'm your nurse today." *The patient is made to feel patronized by repetitions such as "Do you know where you are?" Given the effects of general anesthesia, opioid analgesics, sedatives, and sleep, it is expected that some degree of disorientation will exist normally.*

2. Ensure the patient's visual access to a calendar.

3. Apprise the patient of daily news events and the weather.

4. Touch patients for the express purpose of communicating caring. Hold their hands, stroke their brows, and rub the skin on an aspect of the arms. *Touch is the universal language of caring. In the setting of critical care, in which there is considerable physical body manipulation, it is useful and important to contrast assaultive touch with comforting touch. Touch can be used as a technique for distraction from painful stimuli when used in conjunction with uncomfortable procedures. (NOTE: See later discussion of the use of touch in management of the patient experiencing hallucinations.)*

5. Foster liberal visitation by family and significant others. Encourage significant others to touch the patient as consistent with their individual comfort level and cultural norms.

6. Structure and identify opportunities for the patient to exercise decision-making skills, however small. *Although not so designated, patients with sensory alterations also experience a type of cognitive deprivation.*

7. Assist patients to find meaning in their experiences. Explain the therapeutic purpose of all they are asked to do for themselves and all that is done with them and for them. Avoid statements such as "Will you turn to that side for me?" or "I need you to swallow this medication." *These statements implicitly convey that the maneuver has some*

value for the nurses instead of the patients. Similarly, use "thank you" judiciously. *This simple salutation, when used indiscriminately, suggests something was done to benefit the nurses, not the patients. Patients need to find meaning and to identify their roles in the experience of critical illness and critical care. The sensations that constitute this experience and those that do not are made bearable and intelligible when attached to a larger picture of their conditions, treatment, and progress.*

For Hallucinations

1. Approach the patient with a calm, matter-of-fact demeanor. *The goal of this interaction is for the nurse to demonstrate external control. This helps decrease the anxiety and fear that generally accompany hallucinations and allows the patient to feel safe. Anxiety is transferable.*

2. Address the patient by name. *This is a useful presentation of reality because self-identity is the last sphere of orientation to vanish.*

3. In responding to the patient's description of the hallucination, do not deny, argue, or attempt to disprove the existence of the perceived event. *Statements such as "There are no voices coming from that air vent" or "Look, I'm brushing my hand across the wall, and there are no bugs" confuse the patient further, because the hallucination, although frightening, is his or her perceived reality.*

4. Express to the patient that your experiences are dissimilar, and acknowledge how frightening his or hers must be. *Sample statements:* "I don't hear (see, etc.) what you do, but I know how frightening such an experience must be to you. I'm Joe, your nurse, and I'm going to stay with you until the voices (visions, etc.) go away." Remain with any patient who is experiencing a hallucination. *Feelings of fear and anxiety often accelerate when a patient is left alone. He or she needs someone to represent a nonthreatening reality. Validating the patient's feelings demonstrates acceptance and sensitivity to the experience and promotes trust.*

5. Do not explore the content of the hallucination with the patient by asking about its nature or character. *The nurse is the patient's link with reality. Pursuit of a detailed description of a hallucination may signify to the patient that the nurse accepts his or her sensory distortion as factual. This may further confuse the patient and distance him or her more from reality. (An exception is the patient who the nurse suspects is experiencing auditory hallucinations [i.e., hearing voice commands].* Ascertain that the voices are not telling the patient to harm himself or herself, by asking simply and concretely, "What are the voices saying?") *The nurse can help bridge the gap between the patient's misperception and reality by addressing the feelings (e.g., fear, anxiety) and/or meanings (e.g., danger, death) engendered by the*

Continued

NURSING MANAGEMENT PLAN: Acute Confusion—*cont'd*

hallucination. Determine how the misperception affects the patient emotionally, acknowledge those feelings, and use a calm, controlled, matter-of-fact approach to provide the trust and comfort the patient needs to tolerate this frightening experience. ***In other words, the nurse should deal with the intent more than the content of the hallucination. The resultant decrease in anxiety will enable the patient to focus more accurately on his or her immediate environment.***

6. Talk concretely with the patient about things that are really happening. *Sample statements:* "How does your chest incision feel this afternoon, Mr. Clark?" "Your sister Kate was here to see you, but you were sleeping. She went down to the cafeteria and will be back." "Your secretions are a little easier for you to cough up today." ***Interpretation of reality-based stimuli by the nurse encourages the patient to focus on actual circumstances and discourages a preoccupation with sensory misperceptions.***

7. Distract the patient by changing the topic. ***This tactic is useful in situations of escalating anxiety and confusion or when all else fails. Topics need to consist of basic themes that are universally understood and culturally congruent, such as music, food, or weather. They may also be topics of special interest to the patient, such as hobbies, crafts, or sports. Topics that evoke strong emotions, such as politics, religion, or sexuality, should be avoided with most patients. This is especially true of the patient with reality distortions; sometimes, hallucinations and delusions are expressions of repressed conflicts associated with religious, sexual, or aggressive issues. Pursuit of such subjects could increase confusion and anxiety.***

8. Consider the following regarding the use of touch. ***Touch presents a nonthreatening external reality and can therefore be useful in the management of patients with sensory alterations. However, for the patient experiencing hallucinations (as well as delusions and illusions), touch can be readily misinterpreted as, for instance, aggression or pain, or it can actually provide the basis for a tactile illusion.*** Avoid the use of touch as an intervention strategy for any patient who demonstrates escalating anxiety or paranoid, suspicious, or mistrustful thoughts.

9. For auditory hallucinations:
   a. *Patient behaviors:* Head cocked as if listening to an unseen presence; lips moving.
   b. *Therapeutic nurse responses:* "Mr. Clark, you appear to be listening to something." If the patient acknowledges voices: "I don't hear any voices, but I know this is troubling you. The voices will go away. Nothing is going to harm you. I'm Joe, your nurse, and I'll be here with you."
   c. *Nontherapeutic nurse responses:* "Tell me about your conversations with these voices." "To whom do these voices belong—anyone you know?"

10. For visual hallucinations:
    a. *Patient behaviors:* Staring into space as if focused on an unseen object; startled movements and anxious facial expression.
    b. *Therapeutic nurse responses:* "Mr. Clark, something seems to be troubling you. Tell me what it is." If patient states he visualizes people, images, or the devil in his environment and implies a sense of danger, respond, "There are only nurses and doctors here, Mr. Clark. I know this must be upsetting, but these images will go away. We're here with you in the hospital. Nothing will happen to you."
    c. *Nontherapeutic nurse responses:* "Describe the people you see. What are they wearing?" "What does the devil mean in your life? What about God?"

For Delusions

1. Explain all unseen noises, voices, and activity simply and clearly. ***They readily feed a delusional system.*** *Sample statements:* "That is Dr. Smith. He's come to see you and other patients here in the hospital." "The voices and activity you hear are from the bedside of the patient behind this curtain. He's being helped by one of the nurses."

2. Avoid the "negative challenge" of the patient's delusions (e.g., "Nobody here stole your belongings" or "Doctors and nurses do not harm people"). Similarly, avoid defending the referents of the patient's belief: "Nurses are good" and "Doctors mean well." ***A delusion is a belief, albeit false, that cannot be changed with logic. To attempt this change is to challenge the patient's belief system and thereby escalate his or her anxiety, further blurring the boundaries between reality and the patient's internally based "logic."***

3. For the patient with persecutory delusions who refuses food, fluids, or medications because of a belief that he or she has been poisoned or are tainted, permit the refusal unless it is a life/threatening event. Try again in 20 minutes; allow the patient to choose an alternative selection of food or to read the label on the unit's medication. ***Coercion, show of force, or engagement in complicated, logical justifications will only heighten the patient's suspiciousness and possibly reinforce the delusional belief. When the patient feels more in control, he or she need not rely on the "paradoxical" quality of the delusion to equip him or her with a false sense of power. His or her power instead is derived from making reality-based decisions.***

4. Staff members should be particularly careful not to engage in unnecessary laughter or whispering within view of the delusional patient. ***The delusional patient is hypervigilant, scanning the environment for evidence to corroborate or confirm his or her belief that staff members are colluding***

NURSING MANAGEMENT PLAN: **Acute Confusion**—*cont'd*

against him or her; laughter and whispers easily suggest this belief, this delusion of reference. This rationale also pertains to the patient experiencing hallucinations and/or illusions.

5. Observe the principles detailed in the third intervention in "For Hallucinations."

For Illusions

1. Interprets a reality/based stimulus for the patient in a calm, matter/of/fact manner. *Seen and unseen noises, voices, activity, and people can provide the stimulus for a sensory misinterpretation, an illusion.*

2. Minimize stimulation in the patient's immediate environment. *Nursing interventions detailed previously under "Sensory Overload" are especially relevant here.*

3. Address the feeling and meaning associated with the experience, not the content of the sensory misinterpretation.

a. *Patient behaviors:* Eyes darting, startled movements, frightened facial expression. "I know who you are. You're the devil come to take me to hell."

b. *Therapeutic nurse responses:* "I'm Joe, your nurse. I know this experience is troubling for you. You're in the hospital, and no one here will harm you."

c. Nontherapeutic nurse responses: "There are no such things as devils and angels." "Do you think the devil would be dressed in white?" **The first nontherapeutic nurse response carries a parental tone (i.e., "You know better than that."), infantilizing the patient and adding to his or her feelings of powerlessness over the environment. The second nontherapeutic response reflects obvious logic, which is not in the patient's sensory domain; it cannot be processed and only adds to his or her confused state.**

4. Observe the principles detailed in the fifth intervention of "For Hallucinations."

NURSING MANAGEMENT PLAN: Acute Pain

Definition: Unpleasant sensory and emotional experience arising from actual or potential tissue damage or described in terms of such damage (International Association for the Study of Pain); sudden or slow onset of any intensity from mild to severe with an anticipated or predictable end and a duration of less than 6 months

Acute Pain Related to Transmission of Perception of Cutaneous, Visceral, Muscular, or Ischemic Impulses

Defining Characteristics
Subjective
- Patient verbalizes presence of pain
- Patient rates pain on a scale of 1 to 10 using a visual analog scale

Objective
- Increase in blood pressure, heart rate, and respiratory rate
- Pupillary dilation
- Diaphoresis, pallor
- Skeletal muscle reactions (e.g., grimacing, clenching fists, writhing, pacing, guarding or splinting of affected part)
- Apprehension, fearful appearance
- May not exhibit any physiologic change

Outcome Criteria
- Patient verbalizes that pain is reduced to a tolerable level or is totally relieved.
- Patient's pain rating is lower on a scale of 1 to 10.
- Blood pressure, heart rate, and respiratory rate return to baseline 5 minutes after administration of an intravenous opioid analgesic or 20 minutes after administration of intramuscular opioid analgesic.

Nursing Interventions and Rationale
1. Modify variables that heighten the patient's experience of pain.
   a. Explain to the patient that frequent, detailed, and seemingly repetitive assessments will be conducted to allow the nurse to better understand the patient's pain experience, not because the existence of pain is in question.
   b. Explain the factors responsible for pain production in the individual. Estimate the expected duration of the pain if possible.
   c. Explain diagnostic and therapeutic procedures to the patient in relation to sensations the patient should expect to feel.
   d. Reduce the patient's fear of addiction by explaining the difference between drug tolerance and drug addiction. *Drug tolerance is a physiologic phenomenon in which a medication begins to lose effectiveness after repeated doses; drug dependence is a psychologic phenomenon in which opioids are used regularly for emotional, not medical, reasons.*
   f. Instruct the patient to ask for pain medication when pain is beginning and not to wait until it is intolerable.

   g. Explain that the physician will be consulted if pain relief is inadequate with the present medication.
   h. Instruct patient in the importance of adequate rest, especially when it reduces pain *to maintain strength and coping abilities and to reduce stress.*
2. Collaborate with physician regarding pharmacologic interventions.
   - **For postoperative or posttraumatic cutaneous, muscular, or visceral pain,** perform the following:
     a. Medicate with an opioid analgesic to break the pain cycles as long as level of consciousness and vital signs are stable: check patient's previous response to similar dosage and opioids.
       (1) Given a physician order for a range of doses of an opioid analgesic, start with the lowest dose *to evaluate the patient's individual response to medication.*
     b. Continuous pain requires continuous analgesia.
       (1) Establish optimal analgesic dose that brings optimal pain relief.
       (2) Offer pain medication at prescribed regular intervals rather than making patient ask for it *to maintain more steady blood levels.*
       (3) Consider waking patient to avoid loss of opiate blood levels during sleep.
     c. If administering medication on as-necessary (PRN) basis, give it when the patient's pain is just beginning, rather than at its peak. Advise patient to intercept pain, not endure it, or several hours and higher doses of opioid analgesics may be necessary to relieve pain, leading to a cycle of undermedication and pain alternating with overmedication and drug toxicity.
     d. Perform rehabilitation exercises (turn, deep breathe, leg exercises, ambulate) shortly before peak of drug effect *because this will be the optimal time for the patient to increase activity with the least risk of increasing pain.*
     e. When making the transition from one drug to another or from intramuscular or intravenous to oral medication, use an equianalgesic chart. *Equianalgesic means approximately the same pain relief. The patient's response should be closely monitored to determine if the right analgesic choice was made.*
     f. To assess effectiveness of pain medication, do the following:
       (1) Reevaluate pain 5 minutes after intravenous and 20 minutes after intramuscular medication administration, observe patient's behavior, and ask patient to rate pain on a scale of 1 to 10.
       (2) Collaborate with the physician to add or delete other medications that potentiate the action of analgesics, such as antiemetics, hypnotics, sedatives, or muscle relaxants.

NURSING MANAGEMENT PLAN: Acute Pain—*cont'd*

(3) Observe for indicators of undertreatment: report of pain not relieved; observed restlessness, sleeplessness, irritability, and anorexia; decreased activity level.

(4) Observe for indicators of overtreatment: hypotension or bradycardia; respiratory rate < 10/min; excessive sedation.

g. If patient-controlled analgesia (PCA) is used, perform the following:

(1) Instruct the patient on what the drug is, the dose, and how often it can be self-administered by pushing the button to activate the PCA machine. For example, "When you have pain, instead of asking the nurse to bring medication, push the button that activates the machine and a small dose of the pain medicine will be injected into your IV line. You can keep your pain under control by administering additional medicine as soon as your pain begins to return or increases. Push the button before undertaking a painful activity, such as ambulation. Try to balance your pain relief against sleepiness, and don't activate the machine if you start to feel sleepy. If your pain medicine seems to stop working despite pushing the button several times, call the nurse to check your IV. If you are not receiving adequate pain relief, the nurse will call your doctor."

(2) Monitor vital signs, especially blood pressure and respiratory rate, every hour for the first 4 hours, and assess postural heart rate and blood pressure before initial ambulation.

(3) Monitor respiratory rate every 2 hours while patient is on patient-controlled analgesia.

(4) If patient's respiratory rate decrease to < 10/min or if patient is overly sedated, anticipate administration of naloxone.

h. If epidural opioid analgesia is used, do the following:

(1) Keep patient's head elevated 30 to 45 degrees after injection *to prevent respiratory depressant effects.*

(2) Observe closely for respiratory depression up to 24 hours after injection. Monitor respiratory rate every 15 minutes for 1 hour; every 30 minutes for 7 hours; and every hour for the remaining 16 hours.

(3) Assess for adequate cough reflex.

(4) Avoid use of other central nervous system depressants, such as sedatives.

(5) Observe for reports of pruritus, nausea, and vomiting.

(6) Anticipate administration of naloxone for respiratory depression (and smaller doses of naloxone for pruritus).

(7) Assess for and treat urinary retention.

(8) Assess epidural catheter site for local infection. Keep the catheter taped securely *to prevent catheter migration.*

- **For peripheral vascular ischemic pain (hypothetic vascular occlusion of leg)**, do the following:

  a. Correctly identify and differentiate ischemic pain from other types of pain. (*NOTE: Ischemic pain is usually a burning, aching pain made worse by exercise and lessened or relieved by rest. Eventually, the pain occurs at rest. Coldness and pallor of extremity may be noted, especially if the limb is elevated above the heart level. Rubor and mottling of the skin may be evident from prolonged tissue anoxia and inability of damaged vessels to constrict. Eventually, cyanosis and gangrenous tissue will be evident. Chronic ischemia leads to visible changes in the limb, such as flaking skin, brittle nails and hair, leg ulcers, and cellulitis*).

  b. Administer pain medications, and evaluate their effectiveness as previously described. *Remember that the pain of ischemia is chronic and continuous and can make the patient irritable and depressed.*

  c. Treat the cause of the ischemic pain, and institute measures *to increase circulation to the affected part.*

3. Initiate nonpharmacologic interventions.

   a. Treat contributing factors; provide explanations (see intervention no. 2 at beginning of this nursing management plan).

   b. Apply comfort measures.

      (1) Use relaxation techniques, such as back rubs, massage, warm baths, music, and aroma therapy.

         (a) Use blankets and pillows *to support the painful part and reduce muscle tension.*

         (b) Encourage slow, rhythmic breathing.

      (2) Encourage progressive muscle relaxation techniques.

         (a) Instruct patient to inhale and tense (tighten) specific muscle groups and then relax the muscles as exhalation occurs.

         (b) Suggest an order for performing the tension and relaxation cycle (e.g., start with facial muscles and move down body, ending with toes).

      (3) Encourage guided imagery.

         (a) Ask patient to recall an experienced image that is very pleasurable and relaxing and involves at least two senses.

         (b) Have patient begin with rhythmic breathing and progressive relaxation and then travel mentally to the scene.

         (c) Have patient slowly experience the scene (e.g., how it looks, sounds, smells, feels).

         (d) Ask patient to practice this imagery in private.

         (e) Instruct patient to end the imagery by counting to three and saying, "Now I'm relaxed." If the person does not end the imagery and falls asleep, the purpose of the technique is defeated.

NURSING MANAGEMENT PLAN: Anxiety

Definition: Vague uneasy feeling of discomfort or dread accompanied by an autonomic response (the source often nonspecific or unknown to the individual); a feeling of apprehension caused by anticipation of danger. It is an alerting signal that warns of impending danger and enables the individual to take measures to deal with threat.

Anxiety Related to Threat to Biologic, Psychologic, or Social Integrity

Defining Characteristics
Subjective
- Verbalizes increased muscle tension
- Expresses frequent sensation of tingling in hands and feet
- Relates continuous feeling of apprehension
- Expresses preoccupation with a sense of impending doom
- Reports difficulty falling asleep
- Repeatedly expresses concerns about changes in health status and outcome of illness

Objective
- Psychomotor agitation (fidgeting, jitteriness, restlessness)
- Tightened, wrinkled brow
- Strained (worried) facial expression
- Hypervigilance (scans environment)
- Startles easily
- Distractibility
- Sweaty palms
- Fragmented sleep patterns
- Tachycardia
- Tachypnea

Outcome Criteria
- Patient effectively uses learned relaxation strategies.
- Patient demonstrates significant decrease in psychomotor agitation.
- Patient verbalizes reduction in tingling sensations in hands and feet.
- Patient is able to focus on the tasks at hand.
- Patient expresses positive, future-based plans to family and staff.
- Patient's heart rate and rhythm remain within limits commensurate with physiologic status.

Nursing Interventions and Rationale
1. Instruct the patient in the following simple, effective relaxation strategies:
   a. If not contraindicated for cardiovascular reasons, tense and relax all muscles progressively from toes to head. *Progressive toe-to-head relaxation releases the muscular tension that may be a stress-related effect resulting from the threat or change in the patient's health status and outcome of illness.*
   b. Perform slow deep-breathing exercises. *Deep-breathing exercises provide slow, rhythmic, controlled breathing patterns that relax the patient and distract him or her from the effects of his or her illness and hospitalization.*
   c. Focus on a single object or person in the environment. *Focusing on a single object or person helps the patient dismiss myriad disorienting stimuli from his or her visual-perceptual field, which can have a dizzying, distorted effect. A clear sensorium allows him or her to feel more in control of his or her environment.*
   d. Listen to soothing music or relaxation tapes with eyes closed. *Music or words expressed in soft, low tones tend to produce soothing, relaxing effects that counteract or inhibit escalating anxiety and provide respites from the patient's situational crisis. Closed eyes eliminate distracting visual stimuli and promote a more restful environment.*
2. Actively listen to and accept the patient's concerns regarding the threats from his or her illness, outcome, and hospitalization. *Active listening and unconditional acceptance validate the patient as a worthwhile individual and assure him or her that his or her concerns, no matter how great, will be addressed. Knowledge that he or she has an avenue for ventilation will assuage anxiety.*
3. Help the patient distinguish between realistic concerns and exaggerated fears through clear, simple explanations. *Sample statements:* "Your lab results show that you're doing okay right now." "The shortness of breath you're experiencing is not unusual." "The pain you described is expected, and this medication will relieve it." *A patient who is informed about his or her progress and is reassured about expected symptoms and management of care will be better equipped to maintain a more realistic perspective of his or her illness and its outcome. Anxiety emanating from imagined or exaggerated fears will likely be assuaged or averted.*
4. Provide simple clarification of environmental events and stimuli that are not related to the patient's illness and care. *Sample statements:* "That loud noise is coming from a machine that is helping another patient." "The visitor behind the curtain is crying because she's had an upsetting day." "That gurney is here to take another patient to x-ray." *Clarification of events and stimuli that are unrelated to the patient helps to disengage him or her from the extant anxiety-provoking situations surrounding him or her, avoiding further anxiety and apprehension.*
5. Assist the patient in focusing on building on prior coping strategies to deal with the effects of his or her illness and care. *Sample statements:* "What methods have helped you get through difficult times in the past?" "How can we help you

NURSING MANAGEMENT PLAN: **Anxiety**—*cont'd*

use those methods now?" (See the nursing management plan for Ineffective Coping for interventions that assist patients to use coping strategies effectively.) ***Use of previously successful coping strategies in conjunction with newly learned techniques arms the patient with an arsenal of weapons against anxiety, providing him or her with greater control over the situational crisis and decreased feelings of doom and despair.***

6. Give the patient permission to deny or suppress the effects of his or her illness and hospitalization with which he or she cannot cope or control. *Sample statements:* "It's perfectly okay to ignore things you can't handle right now." "How can we help ease your mind during this time?" "What are some things or tasks that may help distract you?" ***Adaptive denial can be helpful in reducing feelings of anxiety in patients with life-threatening illness.***

NURSING MANAGEMENT PLAN: Autonomic Dysreflexia

Definition: Life-threatening, uninhibited sympathetic response of the nervous system to a noxious stimulus after a spinal cord injury at T7 or above

Autonomic Dysreflexia Related to Excessive Autonomic Response to Noxious Stimuli (e.g., Distended Bladder, Distended Bowel, Skin Irritation)

Defining Characteristics

- Paroxysmal hypertension (sudden increase in both systolic and diastolic blood pressure > 20 mm Hg above patient's normal blood pressure); for many spinal cord injury patients, a normal blood pressure may be only 90/60 mm Hg
- Pounding headache
- Bradycardia (may be a relative slowing so the heart rate may still appear with in the normal range)
- Profuse sweating (above the level of the injury) especially in the face, neck, and shoulders
- Pilomotor erection (goose bumps) above the level of the injury
- Cardiac dysrhythmias (atrial fibrillation; premature ventricular contractions; and atrioventricular conduction abnormalities)
- Flushing of the skin (above the level of the injury) especially in the face, neck, and shoulders
- Blurred vision
- Appearance of spots in the visual fields
- Nasal congestion
- Feelings of apprehension or anxiety

Outcome Criteria

- Blood pressure returns to patient's baseline level
- Heart rate and rhythm returns to patient's baseline level
- Absence of headache
- Absence of sweating flushing, and piloerection above level of injury
- Absence of visual disturbances and nasal congestion
- Absence of feelings of apprehension or anxiety

Nursing Interventions and Rationale

1. Place the patient on cardiac monitor, and assess for bradycardia or other dysrhythmias. *Disturbances of cardiac rate and rhythm can occur because of autonomic dysfunction associated with dysreflexia.*
2. Check the patient's blood pressure every 3 to 5 minutes *as blood pressure may fluctuate very quickly.*
3. Sit the patient upright and lower their legs if possible *to decrease venous return and blood pressure.*
4. Loosen any clothing or constrictive devices *to decrease venous return and blood pressure.*

5. Investigate for and remove instigating cause of dysreflexia:
   a. Bladder
      (1) If indwelling catheter not in place, catheterize patient immediately.
         (a) Prior to inserting the catheter, instill 2% lidocaine jelly into the urethra and wait 2 minutes, if possible.
         (b) Drain 500 mL of urine, and recheck BP.
         (c) If BP still elevated, drain another 500 mL of urine.
         (d) If BP declines after the bladder is empty, serial BP must be monitored closely because the bladder can go into severe contractions causing hypertension to recur.
      (2) If indwelling catheter is in place, check the catheter and tubing for kinks, folds, constrictions, or obstructions, and for correct placement. If problem is found, correct it immediately.
      (3) If catheter is plugged, irrigate it gently with no more than 10-15 mL of sterile normal saline solution at body temperature.
      (4) If unable to irrigate catheter, remove it and prepare to reinsert a new catheter: proceed with its lubrication, drainage, and observation as outlined above.
      (5) Avoid manually compressing or tapping on the bladder.
   b. Bowel: if systolic blood pressure is ≥ 150 mm Hg, proceed to #6 prior to checking for a fecal impaction.
      (1) With a gloved hand, instill a topical anesthetic agent (2% lidocaine jelly), generously into the rectum *to decrease flow of impulses from bowel.*
      (2) Wait 2 minutes if possible *for sensation in area to decrease.*
      (3) With a gloved hand, insert a lubricated finger into the rectum and check for the presence of stool
      (4) If stool is felt, gently remove, if possible.
   c. Skin
      (1) Loosen clothing or bed linens as indicated.
      (2) Inspect skin for pimples, boils, pressure ulcers, and ingrown toenails, and treat as indicated.
6. If symptoms of dysreflexia do not subside, collaborate with physician regarding the administration of antihypertensive medications (e.g., nifedipine [immediate-release form], nitrates [sodium nitroprusside, isosorbide dinitrate, or nitroglycerin ointment], hydralazine, mecamylamine, diazoxide, phenoxybenzamine, captopril, prazosin).
   a. Administer medications, and monitor their effectiveness.
   b. Assess blood pressure and heart rate.
7. Instruct patient about causes, symptoms, treatment, and prevention of dysreflexia.
8. Encourage patient to carry medical bracelet or informational card to present to medical personnel in the event dysreflexia may be developing.

NURSING MANAGEMENT PLAN: Compromised Family Coping

Definition: Usually, supportive primary person (family member or close friend) provides insufficient, ineffective, or compromised support, comfort, assistance, or encouragement that may be needed by the patient to manage or master adaptive tasks related to his or her health challenge.

Compromised Family Coping Related to Critically Ill Family Member

Defining Characteristics

* Disruption of usual family functions and roles
* Inability to accept or deal with crisis situation; use of defense mechanisms (e.g., denial, anger); unrealistic expectations of patient's outcome and care provided; judgmental toward health care providers
* Nonrecognition that family is in state of crisis
* Inappropriate emotional outbursts; arguments among family and with others; inability to respond to each other's feelings or support each other
* Misinterpretation of information; short attention span with repeated questions about information already provided; members not sharing information with each other
* Inability to make decisions regarding changes in family structure or about course of care for ill member; noncooperation among family members
* Expressions of grief, hopelessness, powerlessness, and isolation; do not seek or respond to support services
* Hesitancy to spend time with ill person in the critical care unit, or inappropriate behavior when visiting (may upset patient)
* Neglect of own personal health; fatigue, apathy; refusal of offers for respite time

Outcome Criteria

* The family will express an understanding of course/prognosis of illness, therapies, and alternative measures.
* The family will diminish or resolve conflicts and cooperate in decision making.
* The family will develop trust and mutual support for each member and form a cohesive unit.
* The family will support ill person in making decisions (if capable) or respect prior wishes regarding provision of health care.
* Family efforts will be directed toward a purpose and readjust to changes in life patterns and role function. Members will accept responsibility for changes.
* The family will identify and use effective coping strategies.
* The family will identify and use available resources as needed to facilitate resolution of the crisis.
* The family will have a sense of control and confidence in meeting personal and collective needs.

Nursing Interventions and Rationale

1. Identify family's perception of the crisis situation. Determine family structure; roles' developmental phase; and ethnic, cultural, and belief factors that may affect communication with family and the plan of care. Identify strengths of the family. *All initial nursing interventions should be directed toward resolving the crisis situation. Understanding and using family theory principles will facilitate this process and individualize care.*
2. Provide honest and accurate information in language persons can understand. Give updated information as appropriate. Listen! *This facilitates open communication among family and health care providers, projects a caring attitude and concern for them and patient, and assists family in making decision and being involved with the plan and goals of care.*
3. Encourage liberal visitation with patient. Before the visit, prepare family members for what they will observe in a technical environment. Inform them about patient's appearance, behaviors (etc.) that may be distressing to them. Explain the etiology of patient responses to stimuli (e.g., pain, trauma, surgery, medication), and explain that these behaviors are being monitored and are usually temporary. Encourage them to touch the patient and let the patient know of their presence. *This prevents a strong emotional reaction to an unfamiliar and frightening situation, involves family as support to each other and to the patient, demonstrates the nurse's concern for them as persons, and facilitates satisfaction with care being provided for their loved one.*
4. Identify and support effective coping behaviors. *This aids in the family's sense of control and resolution of helplessness/powerlessness.*
5. Observe for signs of fatigue and the need for emotional/spiritual support and respite from hospital waiting routine. Encourage family to verbalize feelings. Provide information on available resources. Alert interdisciplinary team members (social, psychologic, spiritual) to family needs. Provide pager device (if available), or obtain phone numbers when family leaves the hospital premises. *This provides support and comfort, facilitates hope, resolves sense of isolation, gives sense of security, and diminishes guilt feeling for attending to personal needs.*
6. Instruct family in simple care-giving techniques, and encourage participation in patient's care. *This facilitates giving a sense of normalcy to the experience, self-confidence, and assurance that good care is being provided.*

Continued

NURSING MANAGEMENT PLAN: Compromised Family Coping—*cont'd*

7. Serve as advocate for patient and family. Teach family how to negotiate with the health care delivery system, and include them in health care team conferences when appropriate. *This facilitates informed decision making, promotes control and satisfaction, and permits mutual goal-setting.*

8. Consider nonbiologic or nonlegal family relationships. Encourage contact with patient and participation in care. *This facilitates holistic care and support of emotional ties and demonstrates respect for the family unit and relationships.*

9. Provide emotional support and compassion when patient's condition worsens or deteriorates. *The use of touch and expression of concern for the patient and family convey comfort and trust in the health care provider and respect and assurance that the family's loved one will receive appropriate care and attention.*

NURSING MANAGEMENT PLAN: Decreased Cardiac Output

Definition: Inadequate blood pumped by the heart to meet the metabolic demands of the body

Decreased Cardiac Output Related to Alterations in Preload

Defining Characteristics

- Cardiac output is < 4.0 L/min
- Cardiac index is < 2.5 L/min/m^2
- Heart rate is > 100 beats/min
- Urine output is < 30 mL/hr or 0.5 mL/kg/hr
- Decreased mentation, restlessness, agitation, confusion
- Diminished peripheral pulses
- Blue, gray, or dark purple tint to tongue and sublingual area
- Systolic blood pressure is < 90 mm Hg
- Subjective complaints of fatigue

Reduced Preload
- Right atrial pressure is < 2 mm Hg
- Pulmonary artery occlusion pressure is < 6 mm Hg

Excessive Preload
- Right atrial pressure is > 8 mm Hg
- Pulmonary artery occlusion pressure is > 12 mm Hg

Outcome Criteria

- Cardiac output is 4-8 L/min
- Cardiac index is 2.5-4 L/min/m^2
- Right atrial pressure is 2-8 mm Hg
- Pulmonary artery occlusion pressure is 6-12 mg Hg

Nursing Interventions and Rationale

1. Collaborate with physician regarding the administration of oxygen to maintain an SpO$_2$ > 92% *to prevent tissue hypoxia.*
2. Maintain surveillance for signs of decreased tissue perfusion and acidosis *to facilitate the early identification and treatment of complications.*
3. Monitor fluid balance and daily weights to facilitate regulation of the patient's fluid balance.

For Reduced Preload Resulting from Volume Loss
1. Collaborate with physician regarding the administration of crystalloids, colloids, blood, and blood products *to increase circulating volume.*
2. Limit blood sampling, observe intravenous lines for accidental disconnection, apply direct pressure to bleeding sites, and maintain normal body temperature *to minimize fluid loss.*
3. Position patient with legs elevated, trunk flat, and head and shoulders above the chest *to enhance venous return.*

4. Encourage oral fluids (as appropriate), administer free water with tube feedings, and replace fluids that are lost through wound or tube drainage *to promote adequate fluid intake.*
5. Maintain surveillance for signs of fluid volume excess and adverse effects of blood and blood product administration *to facilitate the early identification and treatment of complications.*

For Reduced Preload Resulting from Venous Dilation
1. Collaborate with physician regarding the administration of vasoconstrictors *to increase venous return.*
2. Maintain surveillance for adverse effects of vasoconstrictor therapy *to facilitate the early identification and treatment of complications.*
3. If patient is hyperthermic, administer tepid bath, hypothermia blanket, and/or ice bags to axilla and groin *to decrease temperature and promote vasoconstriction.*

For Excessive Preload Resulting from Volume Overload
1. Collaborate with physician regarding the administration of the following:
   a. Diuretics to remove excessive fluid.
   b. Vasodilators to decrease venous return.
   c. Inotropes to increase myocardial contractility.
2. Restrict fluid intake and double concentrate intravenous drips *to minimize fluid intake.*
3. Position patient in semi-Fowler's or high-Fowler's position *to reduce venous return.*
4. Maintain surveillance for signs of fluid volume deficit and adverse effects of diuretic, vasodilator, and inotropic therapies *to facilitate the early identification and treatment of complications.*

For Excessive Preload Resulting from Venous Constriction
1. Collaborate with physician regarding the administration of vasodilators *to promote venous dilation.*
2. Maintain surveillance for adverse effects of vasodilator therapy *to facilitate the early identification and treatment of complications.*
3. If patient is hypothermic, wrap him or her in warm blankets or administer hyperthermia blanket *to increase temperature and promote vasodilation.*

Decreased Cardiac Output Related to Alterations in Afterload

Defining Characteristics

- Cardiac output is < 4 L/min
- Cardiac index is < 2.5 L/min/m^2
- Heart rate is > 100 beats/min
- Urine output is < 30 mL/hr

Continued

NURSING MANAGEMENT PLAN: Decreased Cardiac Output—*cont'd*

- Decreased mentation, restlessness, agitation, confusion
- Diminished peripheral pulses
- Blue, gray, or dark purple tint to tongue and sublingual area
- Systolic blood pressure is < 90 mm Hg
- Subjective complaints of fatigue

Reduced Afterload
- Pulmonary vascular resistance is < 100 dyn·sec·cm^{-5}
- Systemic vascular resistance is < 800 dyn·sec·cm^{-5}

Excessive Afterload
- Pulmonary vascular resistance is > 250 dyn·sec·cm^{-5}
- Systemic vascular resistance is > 1200 dyn·sec·cm^{-5}

Outcome Criteria
- Cardiac output is 4-8 L/min
- Cardiac index is 2.5-4 L/min/m^2
- Pulmonary vascular resistance is 80-250 dyn·sec·cm^{-5}
- Systemic vascular resistance is 800-1200 dyn·sec·cm^{-5}

Nursing Interventions and Rationale
1. Collaborate with physician regarding the administration of oxygen to maintain an SpO_2 > 92% *to prevent tissue hypoxia.*
2. Maintain surveillance for signs of decreased tissue perfusion and acidosis *to facilitate the early identification and treatment of complications.*

For Reduced Afterload:
1. Collaborate with physician regarding the administration of vasoconstrictors *to promote arterial vasoconstriction and prevent relative hypovolemia.* If decreased preload is present, implement nursing management plan of care, Decreased Cardiac Output Related to Alterations in Preload.
2. Maintain surveillance for adverse effects of vasoconstrictor therapy *to facilitate the early identification and treatment of complications.*
3. If patient is hyperthermic, administer tepid bath, hypothermia blanket, and/or ice bags to axilla and groin *to decrease temperature and promote vasoconstriction.*

For Excessive Afterload:
1. Collaborate with physician regarding the administration of vasodilators *to promote arterial vasodilation.*
2. Collaborate with physician regarding initiation of intraaortic balloon pump *to facilitate afterload reduction.*
3. Promote rest and relaxation and decrease environmental stimulation *to minimize sympathetic stimulation.*
4. Maintain surveillance for adverse effects of vasodilator therapy *to facilitate the early identification and treatment of complications.*

5. If patient is hypothermic, wrap patient in warm blankets or administer hyperthermia blanket *to increase temperature and promote vasodilation.*
6. If patient is in pain, treat pain *to reduce sympathetic stimulation.* Implement nursing management plan of care, Acute Pain Related to Transmission and Perception of Cutaneous, Visceral, Muscular, or Ischemic Impulses.

Decreased Cardiac Output Related to Alterations in Contractility

Defining Characteristics
- Cardiac output is < 4 L/min
- Cardiac index is < 2.5 L/min/m^2
- Heart rate is > 100 beats/min
- Urine output is < 30 mL/hr
- Decreased mentation, restlessness, agitation, confusion
- Diminished peripheral pulses
- Blue, gray, or dark purple tint to tongue and sublingual area
- Systolic blood pressure is < 90 mm Hg
- Subjective complaints of fatigue
- Right ventricular stroke work index is < 7 g/m^2/beat
- Left ventricular stroke work index is < 35 g/m^2/beat

Outcome Criteria
- Cardiac output is 4-8 L/min
- Cardiac index is 2.5-4 L/min/m^2
- Right ventricular stroke work index is 7-12 g/m^2/beat
- Left ventricular stroke work index is 35-85 g/m^2/beat

Nursing Interventions and Rationale
1. Collaborate with physician regarding the administration of oxygen to maintain an SpO_2 > 92% *to prevent tissue hypoxia.*
2. Maintain surveillance for signs of decreased tissue perfusion and acidosis *to facilitate the early identification and treatment of complications.*
3. Ensure preload is optimized. If preload is reduced or excessive, implement nursing management plan of care, Decreased Cardiac Output Related to Alterations in Preload.
4. Ensure afterload is optimized. If afterload is reduced or excessive, implement nursing management plan of care, Decreased Cardiac Output Related to Alterations in Afterload.
5. Ensure electrolytes are optimized. Collaborate with physician regarding the administration of electrolyte replacement therapy *to enhance cellular ionic environment.*
6. Collaborate with physician regarding the administration of inotropes *to enhance myocardial contractility.*
7. Monitor ST segment continuously *to determine changes in myocardial tissue perfusion.* If myocardial ischemia present, implement nursing management plan of care, Ineffective Cardiopulmonary Tissue Perfusion.

NURSING MANAGEMENT PLAN: Decreased Cardiac Output—*cont'd*

Decreased Cardiac Output Related to Alterations in Heart Rate or Rhythm

Defining Characteristics

- Cardiac output is < 4 L/min
- Cardiac index is < 2.5 L/min/m^2
- Heart rate is > 100 beats/min or < 60 beats/min
- Urine output is < 30 mL/hr or 0.5 mL/kg/hr
- Decreased mentation, restlessness, agitation, confusion
- Diminished peripheral pulses
- Blue, gray, or dark purple tint to tongue and sublingual area
- Systolic blood pressure is < 90 mm Hg
- Subjective complaints of fatigue
- Dysrhythmias

Outcome Criteria

- Cardiac output is 4-8 L/min
- Cardiac index is 2.5-4 L/min/m^2
- Absence of dysrhythmias or return to baseline
- Heart rate is > 60 beats/min or < 100 beats/min

Nursing Interventions and Rationale

1. Collaborate with physician regarding the administration of oxygen to maintain an SpO$_2$ > 92% *to prevent tissue hypoxia.*
2. Ensure electrolytes are optimized. Collaborate with physician regarding the administration of electrolyte therapy *to enhance cellular ionic environment and avoid precipitation of dysrhythmias.*
3. Collaborate with physician and pharmacist regarding patient's current medications and their effect on heart rate and rhythm *to identify any prodysrhythmic or bradycardic side effects.*
4. Maintain surveillance for signs of decreased tissue perfusion and acidosis *to facilitate the early identification and treatment of complications.*
5. Monitor ST segment continuously *to determine changes in myocardial tissue perfusion.* If myocardial ischemia is present, implement nursing management plan of care, Altered Cardiopulmonary Tissue Perfusion.

For Lethal Dysrhythmias or Asystole

1. Initiate Advanced Cardiac Life Support interventions and notify physician immediately.

For Nonlethal Dysrhythmias

1. Collaborate with physician regarding administration of antidysrhythmic therapy, synchronized cardioversion, and/or overdrive pacing *to control dysrhythmias.*
2. Maintain surveillance for adverse effects of antidysrhythmic therapy *to facilitate the early identification and treatment of complications.*

For Heart Rate < 60 Beats/Min

1. Collaborate with physician regarding the initiation of temporary pacing *to increase heart rate.*

Decreased Cardiac Output Related to Sympathetic Blockade

Defining Characteristics

- Decreased cardiac output and cardiac index
- Systolic blood pressure is < 90 mm Hg or below patient's baseline
- Decreased right atrial pressure and pulmonary artery occlusion pressure
- Decreased systemic vascular resistance
- Bradycardia
- Cardiac dysrhythmias
- Postural hypotension

Outcome Criteria

- Cardiac output and cardiac index are within normal limits.
- Systolic blood pressure is > 90 mm Hg or returns to baseline.
- Right atrial pressure and pulmonary artery occlusion pressure are within normal limits.
- Systemic vascular resistance is within normal limits.
- Sinus rhythm is present.
- Dysrhythmias are absent.
- Fainting or dizziness with position change is absent.

Nursing Interventions and Rationale

1. Implement measures to prevent episodes of postural hypertension:
   a. Change patient's position slowly *to allow the cardiovascular system time to compensate.*
   b. Apply pneumatic compression stockings *to promote venous return.*
   c. Perform range-of-motion exercises every 2 hours *to prevent venous pooling.*
   d. Collaborate with the physician and physical therapist regarding the use of a tilt table *to progress the patient from supine to upright position.*
2. Collaborate with the physician regarding the administration of the following:
   a. Crystalloids and/or colloids to increase the patient's circulating volume, *which increases stroke volume and subsequently cardiac output.*
   b. Vasopressors if fluids are ineffective to constrict the patient's vascular system, *which increases resistance and subsequently blood pressure.*
3. Monitor cardiac rhythm for bradycardia and/or dysrhythmias, *which can further decrease cardiac output.*
4. Avoid any activity that can stimulate the vagal response *because bradycardia can result.*
5. Treat symptomatic bradycardia and symptomatic dysrhythmias according to unit's emergency protocol or advanced cardiac life support (ACLS) guidelines.

NURSING MANAGEMENT PLAN: Decreased Intracranial Adaptive Capacity

Definition: Intracranial fluid dynamic mechanisms that normally compensate for increases in intracranial volumes are compromised, resulting in repeated disproportionate increases in intracranial pressure (ICP) in response to a variety of noxious and non-noxious stimuli.

Decreased Intracranial Adaptive Capacity Related to Failure of Normal Intracranial Compensatory Mechanisms

Defining Characteristics
- Intracranial pressure is > 15 mm Hg, sustained for 15-30 minutes
- Headache
- Vomiting, with or without nausea
- Seizures
- Decrease in Glasgow Coma Scale score of 2 or more points from baseline
- Alteration in level of consciousness, ranging from restlessness to coma
- Change in orientation: disoriented to time and/or place and/or person
- Difficulty or inability to follow simple commands
- Increasing systolic blood pressure of more than 20 mm Hg with widening pulse pressure
- Bradycardia
- Irregular respiratory pattern (e.g., Cheyne-Stokes, central neurogenic hyperventilation, ataxic, apneustic)
- Change in response to painful stimuli (e.g., purposeful to inappropriate or absent response)
- Signs of impending brain herniation:
    Hemiparesis or hemiplegia
    Hemisensory changes
    Unequal pupil size (1 mm or more difference)
    Failure of pupil to react to light
    Disconjugate gaze and inability to move one eye beyond
        midline if third, fourth, or sixth cranial nerves involved
    Loss of oculocephalic or oculovestibular reflexes
    Possible decorticate or decerebrate posturing

Outcome Criteria
- Intracranial pressure is ≤ 15 mm Hg.
- Cerebral perfusion pressure is > 60 mm Hg.
- Clinical signs of increased intracranial pressure are absent.

Nursing Interventions and Rationale
1. Maintain adequate cerebral perfusion pressure.
    a. Collaborate with physician regarding the administration of volume expanders, vasopressors, or antihypertensives *to maintain the patient's blood pressure within normal range.*
    b. Implement measures to reduce intracranial pressure.
        (1) Elevate head of bed 30 to 45 degrees *to facilitate venous return.*
        (2) Maintain head and neck in neutral plan (avoid flexion, extension, or lateral rotation) *to enhance venous drainage from the head.*
        (3) Avoid extreme hip flexion.
        (4) Collaborate with the physician regarding the administration of steroids, osmotic agents, and diuretics and need for drainage of cerebrospinal fluid if a ventriculostomy is in place.
        (5) Assist patient to turn and move self in bed (instruct patient to exhale while turning or pushing up in bed) *to avoid isometric contractions and Valsalva maneuver.*
2. Maintain patent airway and adequate ventilation and supply oxygen *to prevent hypoxemia and hypercarbia.*
3. Monitor arterial blood gas values and maintain PaO_2 > 80 mm Hg, $PaCO_2$ > 35 mm Hg, and pH at 7.35-7.45 *to prevent cerebral vasodilation.*
4. Avoid suctioning beyond 10 seconds at a time; hyperoxygenate and hyperventilate before and after suctioning.
5. Plan patient care activities and nursing interventions around patient's intracranial pressure response. Avoid unnecessary additional disturbances, and allow patient up to 1 hour of rest between activities as frequently as possible. *Studies have shown the direct correlation between nursing care activities and increases in intracranial pressure.*
6. Maintain normothermia with external cooling or heating measures as necessary. Wrap hands, feet, and male genitalia in soft towels before cooling measures *to prevent shivering and frostbite.*
7. With physician's collaboration, control seizures with prophylactic and as-necessary (PRN) anticonvulsants. *Seizures can greatly increase the cerebral metabolic rate.*
8. Collaborate with the physician regarding the administration of sedatives, barbiturates, or paralyzing agents *to reduce cerebral metabolic rate.*
9. Counsel family members to maintain calm atmosphere and avoid disturbing topics of conversation (e.g., patient condition, pain, prognosis, family crisis, financial difficulties).
10. If signs of impending brain herniation are present, implement the following:
    a. Notify the physician at once.
    b. Ensure that head of bed is elevated 45 degrees and that patient's head is in neutral plane.
    c. Administer mainline intravenous infusion slowly to keep-open rate.
    d. Drain cerebrospinal fluid as ordered if a ventriculostomy is in place.
    e. Prepare to administer osmotic agents and/or diuretics.
    f. Prepare patient for emergency computed tomography head scan and/or emergency surgery.

NURSING MANAGEMENT PLAN: Deficient Fluid Volume

Definition: Decreased intravascular, interstitial, and/or intracellular fluid. This refers to dehydration, water loss alone without a change in sodium concentration.

Deficient Fluid Volume Related to Absolute Loss

Defining Characteristics
- Cardiac output is < 4 L/min
- Cardiac index is < 2.2 L/min
- Pulmonary artery occlusion pressure is < 6 mm Hg
- Right atrial pressure is < 2 mm Hg
- Tachycardia
- Narrowed pulse pressure
- Systolic blood pressure is < 100 mm Hg
- Urinary output is < 30 mL/hr
- Pale, cool, moist skin
- Apprehensiveness

Outcome Criteria
- Cardiac output is > 4 L/min, and cardiac index is > 2.2 L/min.
- Pulmonary artery occlusion pressure is > 6 mm Hg or returns to baseline level.
- Right atrial pressure is > 2 mm Hg or returns to baseline level.
- Heart rate is normal or returns to baseline level.
- Systolic blood pressure is > 90 mm Hg.
- Urinary output is > 30 mL/hr.

Nursing Interventions and Rationale
1. Secure airway, and administer high-flow oxygen.
2. Place patient in supine position with legs elevated *to increase preload.* For patient with head injury, consider using low-Fowler's position with legs elevated.
3. For fluid repletion, use the 3:1 rule, replacing three parts of fluid for every unit of blood lost.
4. Administer crystalloid solutions using the fluid challenge technique: infuse precise boluses of fluid (usually 5 to 20 mL/min) over 10-minute periods; monitor hemodynamic pressures serially *to determine successful challenging.* If the pulmonary artery occlusion pressure elevates more than 7 mm Hg above beginning level, the infusion should be stopped. If the pulmonary artery occlusion pressure rises only to 3 mm Hg above baseline or falls, another fluid challenge should be administered.
5. Replete fluids first before considering use of vasopressors, *because vasopressors increase myocardial oxygen consumption out of proportion to the reestablishment of coronary perfusion in the early phases of treatment.*
6. When blood replacement is indicated, replace it with fresh packed red cells and fresh frozen plasma *to keep clotting factors intact.*
7. Move or reposition patient minimally to decrease or limit tissue oxygen demands.

8. Evaluate patient's anxiety level, and intervene through patient education or sedation *to decrease tissue oxygen demands.*
9. Maintain surveillance for signs and symptoms of fluid overload.

Deficient Fluid Volume Related to Decreased Secretion of Antidiuretic Hormone (ADH)

Defining Characteristics
- Confusion and lethargy
- Decreased skin turgor
- Thirst
- Weight loss over short period
- Decreased pulmonary artery occlusion pressure
- Decreased right atrial pressure
- Urinary output is > 6 L/day
- Serum sodium is > 148 mEq/L
- Serum osmolality is > 295 mOsm/kg
- Urine osmolality is <100 mOsm/kg
- Urine specific gravity is < 1.005

Outcome Criteria
- Weight returns to baseline.
- Urinary output is >30 mL/hr and < 200 mL/hr.
- Serum osmolality is 280-295 mOsm/kg.
- Urine specific gravity is 1.010-1.030.

Nursing Interventions and Rationale
1. Record intake and output every hour, noting color and clarity of urine *because color and clarity are an indication of urine concentration.*
2. Monitor cardiac rhythm continuously for dysrhythmias *caused by electrolyte imbalance.*
3. Collaborate with physician regarding administration of vasopressin or desmopressin *to replace ADH.*
   a. Monitor patient for adverse effects of medications (e.g., headache, chest pain, abdominal pain) *caused by vasoconstriction.*
   b. Report adverse effects to physician immediately.
4. Collaborate with physician regarding intravenous fluid and electrolyte replacement therapy *to restore fluid balance, correct dehydration, and maintain electrolyte balance.*
   a. Administer hypotonic saline *to replace free water deficit.*
5. Provide oral fluids low in sodium such as water, coffee, tea, or orange juice *to decrease sodium intake.*
6. Weigh patient daily (at same time, in same amount of clothing, and preferably with same scale) *to ensure accuracy of readings.*
7. Reposition patient every 2 hours to prevent skin integrity issues caused by dehydration.
8. Provide mouth care every 4 hours to prevent breakdown of oral mucous membranes.

Continued

NURSING MANAGEMENT PLAN: Deficient Fluid Volume—*cont'd*

9. Collaborate with physician regarding administration of medications to prevent constipation *caused by dehydration.*
10. Maintain surveillance for symptoms of hypernatremia (muscle twitching, irritability, seizures), hypovolemic shock (hypotension, tachycardia, decreased CVP and PAOP), and deep vein thrombosis (calf pain, tenderness, swelling).

Deficient Fluid Volume Related to Relative Loss

Defining Characteristics
- Pulmonary artery occlusion pressure is < 6 mm Hg
- Right atrial pressure is < 2 mm Hg
- Tachycardia
- Narrowed pulse pressure
- Systolic blood pressure is < 100 mm Hg
- Urinary output is < 30 mL/hr
- Increased hematocrit level

Outcome Criteria
- Pulmonary artery occlusion pressure is > 6 mm Hg or returns to baseline level
- Right atrial pressure is > 2 mm Hg or returns to baseline level
- Systolic blood pressure is > 90 mm Hg.
- Urinary output is > 30 mL/hr.
- Hematocrit level is normal.

Nursing Interventions and Rationale

1. Collaborate with the physician regarding the administration of intravenous fluid replacements (usually normal saline solution or lactated Ringer's solution) at a rate sufficient to maintain urinary output >30 mL/hr. Colloid solutions are avoided in the initial phases (but can be used later) because of the possibility of increased edema formation *as a result of the increased capillary permeability.*

NURSING MANAGEMENT PLAN: **Deficient Knowledge**

Definition: Absence or deficiency of cognitive information related to a specific topic

Deficient Knowledge Related to Cognitive or Perceptual Learning Limitations: Sensory Overload, Sleep Deprivation, Medications, Anxiety, Sensory Deficits, or Language Barrier

Defining Characteristics
- Verbalized statement of inadequate knowledge of skills
- Verbalization of inadequate recall of information
- Verbalization of inadequate understanding of information
- Evidence of inaccurate follow-through of instructions
- Inadequate demonstration of a skill
- Lack of compliance with prescribed behavior

Outcome Criteria
- Patient participates actively in necessary and prescribed health behaviors.
- Patient verbalizes adequate knowledge or demonstrates adequate skills.

Nursing Interventions and Rationale
1. Determine specific cause of patient's cognitive or perceptual limitation.
2. Provide uninterrupted rest period before teaching session to decrease fatigue and encourage optimal state for learning and retention.
3. Manipulate environment as much as possible to provide quiet and uninterrupted learning sessions.
   a. Ensure that lights are bright enough to see teaching aids but not too bright.
   b. Schedule care and medications to allow uninterrupted teaching periods.
   c. Move patient to quiet, private room for teaching if possible.
4. Adapt teaching sessions and materials to patient's and family's levels of education and ability to understand.
   a. Provide printed material appropriate to reading level.
   b. Use terminology understood by the patient.
   c. Provide printed materials in patient's primary language if possible.
   d. Use interpreters during teaching sessions *when necessary.*
5. Teach only present-tense focus during periods of sensory overload.
6. Determine potential effects of medications on ability to retain or recall information. Avoid teaching critical content while patient is taking sedatives, analgesics, or other medications that affect memory.

7. Reinforce new skills and information in several teaching sessions. Use several senses when possible in teaching session (e.g., see a film, hear a discussion, read printed information, demonstrate skills related to self-injection of insulin).
8. Reduce patient's anxiety.
   a. Listen attentively, and encourage verbalization of feelings.
   b. Answer questions as they arise in a clear and succinct manner.
   c. Elicit patient's concerns, and address those issues first.
   d. Give only correct and relevant information.
   e. Continually assess response to teaching session, and discontinue if anxiety increases or physical condition becomes unstable.
   f. Provide nonthreatening information before more anxiety-producing information is presented.
   g. Plan for several teaching sessions so information can be divided into small, manageable packages.

Deficient Knowledge Related to Lack of Previous Exposure to Information

Defining Characteristics
- Verbalized statement of inadequate knowledge or skills
- New diagnosis or health problem requiring self-management or care
- Lack of prior formal or informal education about the specific health problem
- Demonstration of inappropriate behaviors related to management of health problem

Outcome Criteria
- Patient verbalizes adequate knowledge about or performs skills related to disease process, its causes, factors related to onset of symptoms, and self-management of disease or health problem.
- Patient actively participates in health behaviors required for performance of a procedure or in those behaviors enhancing recovery from illness and preventing recurrence or complications.

Nursing Interventions and Rationale
1. Determine existing level of knowledge or skill.
2. Assess factors that affect the knowledge deficit:
   a. Learning needs, including patient's priorities and the necessary knowledge and skills for safety.
   b. Learning ability of patient, including language skills, level of education, ability to read, preferred learning style.

Continued

NURSING MANAGEMENT PLAN: Deficient Knowledge—cont'd

c. Physical ability to perform prescribed skills or procedures; consider effect of limitations imposed by treatment such as bedrest, restriction of movement by intravenous or other equipment, or effect of sedatives or analgesics.

d. Psychologic effect of stage of adaptation to disease.

e. Activity tolerance and ability to concentrate.

f. Motivation to learn new skills or gain new knowledge.

3. Reduce or limit barriers to learning:

a. Provide consistent nurse-patient contact to encourage development of trusting and therapeutic relationship.

b. Structure environment to enhance learning; control unnecessary noise, interruptions.

c. Individualize teaching plan to fit patient's current physical and psychologic status.

d. Delay teaching until patient is ready to learn.

e. Conduct teaching sessions during period of day when patient is most alert and receptive.

f. Meet patient's immediate learning needs as they arise (e.g., give brief explanation of procedures when they are performed).

4. Promote active participation in the teaching plan by the patient and family:

a. Solicit input during development of plan.

b. Develop mutually acceptable goals and outcomes.

c. Solicit expression of feelings and emotions related to new responsibilities.

d. Encourage questions.

5. Conduct teaching sessions, using the most appropriate teaching methods.

6. Repeat key principles, and provide them in printed form *for reference at a later time.*

7. Give frequent feedback to patient when practicing new skills.

8. Use several teaching sessions when appropriate. New information and skills should be reinforced several times after initial learning.

9. Initiate referrals for follow-up if necessary:

a. Health educators

b. Home health care

c. Rehabilitation programs

d. Social services

10. Evaluate effectiveness of teaching plan, based on patient's ability to meet preset goals and objectives *to determine need for further teaching.*

NURSING MANAGEMENT PLAN: Disturbed Body Image

Definition: Confusion in mental picture of one's physical self

Disturbed Body Image Related to Actual Change in Body Structure, Function, or Appearance

Defining Characteristics

- Actual change in appearance, structure, or function
- Avoidance of looking at body part
- Avoidance of touching body part
- Hiding or overexposing body part (intentional or unintentional)
- Trauma to nonfunctioning part
- Change in ability to estimate spatial relationship of body to environment
- Verbalization of the following:
  Fear of rejection or reaction by others
  Negative feeling about body
  Preoccupation with change or loss
  Refusal to participate in or to accept responsibility for self-care of altered body part
- Personalization of part or loss with a name
- Depersonalization of part or loss by use of impersonal pronouns
- Refusal to verify actual change

Outcome Criteria

- Patient verbalizes the specific meaning of the change to him or her.
- Patient requests appropriate information about self-care.
- Patient completes personal hygiene and grooming daily with or without help.
- Patient interacts freely with family or other visitors.
- Patient participates in the discussions and conferences related to planning his or her medical and nursing management in the critical care unit and transfer from the unit.
- Patient talks with trained visitors (support-group representatives) at least twice about his or her loss.

Nursing Interventions and Rationale

1. Evaluate patient's mental, physical, and emotional state; recognize assets, strengths, response to illness, coping mechanisms, past experience with stress, and support system.
2. Appraise the response of family and significant others. *Body image is derived from the "reflected appraisals" of family and significant others.*
3. Determine the patient's goals and readiness for learning.
4. Provide the necessary information to help the patient and family adapt to the change. Clarify misconceptions about future limitations.
5. Permit and encourage the patient to express the significance of the loss or change; note nonverbal behavior responses.
6. Allow and encourage the patient's expression of anxiety. *Anxiety is the most predominant emotional response to a body image disturbance.*

7. Recognize and accept the use of denial as an adaptive defense mechanism when used early and temporarily.
8. Recognize maladaptive denial as that which interferes with the patient's progress and/or alienates support systems. Use confrontation.
9. Provide an opportunity for the patient to discuss sexual concerns.
10. Touch the affected body part *to provide the patient with sensory information about altered body structure and/or function.*
11. Encourage and provide movement of altered body part *to establish kinesthetic feedback. This enables the person to know his or her body as it now exists.*
12. Prepare the patient to look at the body part. Call the body part by its anatomic name (e.g., stump, stoma, limb) as opposed to "it" or "she." *The use of impersonal pronouns increases a sense of fantasy and depersonalization of the body part.*
13. Allow the patient to experience excellence in some aspect of physical functioning—walking, turning, deep breathing, healing, self-care—and point out progress and accomplishment. *This helps to balance the patient's sense of dysfunction with function.*
14. Avoid false reassurance. Acknowledge the difficulty of incorporating the altered body part or function into one's body image. *This evidences the nurse's sensitivity and promotes trust.*
15. Talk with the patient about his or her life, generativity, and accomplishments. *Patients with disturbances in body image frequently see themselves in a distortedly "narrow" sense. Encouraging a wider focus of themselves and their life reduces this distortion.*
16. Help the patient explore realistic alternatives.
17. Recognize that incorporating a body change into one's body image takes time. Avoid setting unrealistic expectations and *thereby inadvertently reinforcing a low self-esteem.*
18. Suggest the use of additional resources such as trained visitors who have mastered situations similar to those of the patient. Refer the patient to a psychiatric liaison nurse or psychiatrist if needed.

Disturbed Body Image Related to Functional Dependence on Life-Sustaining Technology, Including a Ventilator, Dialysis, IABP, or Halo Traction

Defining Characteristics

- Actual change in function requiring permanent or temporary replacement
- Refusal to verify actual loss
- Verbalization of the following: feelings of helplessness, hopelessness, powerlessness, fear of failure to wean from technology

Continued

NURSING MANAGEMENT PLAN: **Disturbed Body Image**—*cont'd*

Outcome Criteria

- Patient verifies actual change in function.
- Patient does not refuse or fight technologic intervention.
- Patient verbalizes acceptance of expected change in lifestyle.

Nursing Interventions and Rationale

1. Evaluate patient's response to the technologic intervention.
2. Assess responses of family and significant others. *Body image is derived from the "reflected appraisals" of family and significant others.*
3. Provide information needed by patient and family.
4. Promote trust, security, comfort, and privacy.
5. Recognize anxiety. Allow and encourage its expression. *Anxiety is the most predominant emotion accompanying body image alterations.* Implement nursing management plan of care, Anxiety Related to Threat to Biologic, Psychologic, or Social Integrity
6. Assist patient to recognize his or her own functioning and performance in the face of technology. For example, assist patient to distinguish spontaneous breaths from mechanically delivered breaths. *The activity will assist in weaning patient from the ventilator when feasible. To establish realistic, accurate body boundaries, a patient needs help to separate himself or herself from the technology that is supporting his or her functioning. Any participation or function on the part of the patient during periods of dependency is helpful in preventing and/or resolving an alteration in body image.*
7. Plan for discontinuation of the treatment (e.g., weaning from ventilator). Explain procedure that will be followed, and be present during its initiation.
8. Plan for transfer from the critical care environment.
9. Document care, ensuring an up-to-date management plan is available to all involved caregivers.

NURSING MANAGEMENT PLAN: **Disturbed Sleep Pattern**

Definition: Time-limited disruption of sleep (natural, periodic suspension of consciousness) amount and quality

Disturbed Sleep Pattern Related to Fragmented Sleep

Defining Characteristics
- Decreased sleep during one block of sleep time
- Daytime sleepiness
- Decreased sleep
  Less than one half of normal total sleep time
  Decreased slow-wave or rapid-eye-movement (REM) sleep
- Anxiety
- Fatigue
- Restlessness
- Disorientation and hallucinations
- Combativeness
- Frequent awakenings

Outcome Criteria
- Patient's total sleep time approximates patient's normal.
- Patient can complete sleep cycles of 90 minutes without interruption.
- Patient has no delusions or hallucinations.
- Patient has reality-based thought content.

Nursing Interventions and Rationale
1. Assess normal sleep pattern on admission and any history of sleep disturbance or chronic illness that may affect sleep or sedative/hypnotic use. Promote normal sleep activity while patient is in critical care unit. Assess sleep effectiveness by asking patient how his or her sleep in the hospital compares with sleep at home. *The best treatment for sleep pattern disturbance is prevention.*
2. Promote comfort, relaxation, and a sense of well-being. Treat pain; change, smooth, or refresh bed linens at bedtime; and provide oral hygiene. Eliminate stressful situations before bedtime. Use relaxation techniques, imagery, music, massage, or warm blankets. Have a close family member sit beside the bed and provide the patient with his or her own garments or coverings. Provide quiet or background noise of the television or music (patient preference) *to best promote sleep.* Provide a comfortable room temperature.
3. Minimize noise, particularly that of the staff and noisy equipment. Reduce the level of environmental stimuli. Dim the lights at night.
4. Foods containing tryptophan (e.g., milk, turkey) may be appropriate *because these promote sleep.*
5. Plan nap times to assist in approximating the patient's normal 24-hour sleep time.
6. Minimize awakenings *to allow for at least 90-minute sleep cycles.* Continually assess the need to awaken the patient, particularly at night. Distinguish between essential and nonessential nursing tasks. Organize nursing management to allow for maximal amount of uninterrupted sleep while ensuring close monitoring of the patient's condition. Whenever possible, monitor physiologic parameters without waking the patient. Coordinate awakenings with other departments, such as respiratory therapy, laboratory, and radiography, *to minimize sleep interruptions.*
7. Be aware of the effects of commonly used medications on sleep. *Many sedative and hypnotic medications decrease REM sleep.* Sedative and analgesic medications should not be withheld, but rather, medications that minimally disrupt sleep should be used to complement comfort measures, with dosages reduced gradually as the medication is no longer necessary. Do not abruptly withdraw REM-suppressing medications *because this can result in REM rebound.*
8. Document amount of uninterrupted sleep per shift, especially sleep episodes lasting longer than 2 hours. *Sleep pattern disturbance is diagnosed, treated, and resolved more efficiently when formally documented in this manner.*

NURSING MANAGEMENT PLAN: Dysfunctional Ventilatory Weaning Response

Definition: Inability to adjust to lowered levels of mechanical ventilator support that interrupts and prolongs the weaning process

Dysfunctional Ventilatory Weaning Response (DVWR) Related to Physical, Psychosocial, or Situational Factors

Defining Characteristics

Mild DVWR

- Responds to lowered levels of mechanical ventilator support with

  Restlessness

  Slightly increased respiratory rate from baseline

  Expressed feelings of increased need for oxygen; breathing discomfort; fatigue; warmth

  Queries about possible machine malfunction

  Increased concentration on breathing

Moderate DVWR

- Responds to lowered levels of mechanical ventilator support with

  Slight baseline increase in blood pressure is < 20 mm Hg

  Slight baseline increase in heart rate is < 20 beats/min

  Baseline increase in respiratory rate is < 5 breaths/min

  Hypervigilance to activities

  Inability to respond to coaching

  Inability to cooperate

  Apprehension

  Diaphoresis

  Eye widening ("wide-eyed look")

  Decreased air entry on auscultation

  Color changes: pale, slight cyanosis

  Slight respiratory accessory muscle use

Severe DVWR

- Responds to lowered levels of mechanical ventilator support with

  Agitation

  Deterioration in arterial blood gases from current baseline

  Baseline increase in blood pressure is >20 mm Hg

  Baseline increase in heart rate is >20 beats/min

  Respiratory rate increases significantly from baseline

  Profuse diaphoresis

  Full respiratory accessory muscle use

  Shallow, gasping breaths

  Paradoxic abdominal breathing

  Discoordinated breathing with the ventilator

  Decreased level of consciousness

  Adventitious breath sounds, audible airway secretions

  Cyanosis

Outcome Criteria

- Airway is clear.
- Underlying disorder is resolving.
- Patient is rested, and pain is controlled.
- Nutritional status is adequate.
- Patient has feelings of perceived control, situational security, and trust in the nurses.
- Patient is able to adapt to selected levels of ventilator support without undue fatigue.

Nursing Interventions and Rationale

1. Communicate interest and concern for the patient's well-being, and demonstrate confidence in ability to manage weaning process *to instill trust in the patient.*
2. Use normalizing strategies (e.g., grooming, dressing, mobilizing, social conversation) *to reinforce the patient's self-esteem and feeling of identity.*
3. Identify parameters of the patient's usual functioning before the weaning process begins *to facilitate early identification of problems.*
4. Identify the patient's strengths and resources that can be mobilized *to enhance the patient's coping and maximize weaning effort.*
5. Note concerns that adversely affect the patient's comfort and confidence, and manage them discreetly *to facilitate the patient's ease.*
6. Praise successful activities, encourage a positive outlook, and review the patient's positive progress *to increase the patient's perceived self-efficacy.*
7. Inform the patient of his or her situation and weaning progress *to permit the patient as much control as possible.*
8. Teach the patient about the weaning process and how he or she can participate in the process.
9. Negotiate daily weaning goals with the patient *to gain cooperation.*
10. Position the patient with the head of the bed elevated *to optimize respiratory efforts.*
11. Coach the patient in breath control by regular demonstrations of slow, deep, rhythmic patterns of breathing *to assist with dyspnea.*
12. Remain visible in the room and reassure the patient that help is immediately available if needed *to reduce the patient's anxiety and fearfulness.*
13. Encourage the patient to view weaning trials as a form of training, regardless of whether the weaning goal is achieved *to avoid discouragement.*
14. Encourage the patient to maintain emotional calmness by reassuring, being present, comforting, talking down if emotionally aroused, and reinforcing the idea that he or she can and will succeed.

NURSING MANAGEMENT PLAN: **Dysfunctional Ventilatory Weaning Response**—*cont'd*

15. Monitor the patient's status frequently *to avoid undue fatigue and anxiety.*
16. Provide regular periods of rest by reducing activities, maintaining or increasing ventilator support, and providing oxygen as needed before fatigue advances.
17. Provide distraction (e.g., visitors, radio, television, conversation) when the patient's concentration starts to create tension and increases anxiety.
18. Ensure adequate nutritional support, sufficient rest and sleep time, and sedation or pain control *to promote the patient's optimal physical and emotional comfort.*
19. Start weaning early in the day *when the patient is most rested.*
20. Restrict unnecessary activities and visitors who do not cooperate with weaning strategies *to minimize energy demands on the patient during the weaning process.*
21. Coordinate necessary activities to promote adequate time for rest and relaxation.
22. Monitor the patient's underlying disease process *to ensure it is stabilized and under control.*
23. Advocate for additional resources (e.g., sedation, analgesia, rest) needed by the patient *to maximize comfort status.*
24. Develop and adhere to an individualized plan of care *to promote the patient's feelings of control.*

NURSING MANAGEMENT PLAN: Excess Fluid Volume

Definition: Increased isotonic fluid retention

Excess Fluid Volume Related to Increased Secretion of Antidiuretic Hormone (ADH)

Defining Characteristics
- Headache
- Decreased sensorium
- Weight gain over short period
- Intake greater than output
- Increased pulmonary artery occlusion pressure
- Increased right atrial pressure
- Urine output is < 30 mL/hr
- Serum sodium is < 120 mEq/L
- Serum osmolality is < 275 mOsm/kg
- Urine osmolality greater than serum osmolality
- Urine sodium is > 200 mEq/L
- Urine specific gravity is > 1.03

Outcome Criteria
- Weight returns to baseline.
- Urine output is > 30 mL/hr.
- Serum sodium is 135-145 mEq/L.
- Urine specific gravity is 1.005-1030.

Nursing Interventions and Rationale
1. Monitor cardiac rhythm continuously for dysrhythmias *caused by electrolyte imbalance.*
2. Restrict patient's fluids to 500 mL less than output per day *to decrease fluid retention.*
3. Provide patient chilled beverages high in sodium content such as tomato juice or broth *to increase sodium intake.*
4. Collaborate with physician regarding administration of demeclocycline, lithium, and/or opioid agonists *to inhibit renal response to ADH.*
5. Collaborate with physician regarding administration of hypertonic saline and furosemide *for rapid correction of severe sodium deficit and diuresis of free water.*
   a. Administer hypertonic saline at a rate of 1 to 2 mL/kg/hr until the patient's serum sodium is increased no greater than 1 to 2 mEq/L/hr.
6. Weigh patient daily (at same time, in same amount of clothing, and preferably with same scale) *to ensure accuracy of readings.*
7. Provide frequent mouth care to prevent breakdown of oral mucous membranes.
8. Initiate seizure precautions because patient is at high risk as a result of hyponatremia.
   a. Pad side rails of bed to protect patient from injury.
   b. Remove any objects from immediate environment that could injure patient in the event of a seizure.
   c. Keep appropriate-size oral airway at bedside to assist with airway management after the seizure.
9. Collaborate with physician regarding administration of medications to prevent constipation *caused by decreased fluid intake and immobility.*
10. Maintain surveillance for symptoms of hyponatremia (e.g., headache, abdominal cramps, weakness) and congestive heart failure (e.g., dyspnea, rales, increased central venous pressure and pulmonary artery occlusion pressure).

Excess Fluid Volume Related to Renal Dysfunction

Defining Characteristics
- Weight gain that occurs during a 24- to 48-hour period
- Dependent pitting edema
- Ascites in severe cases
- Fluid crackles on lung auscultation
- Exertional dyspnea
- Oliguria or anuria
- Hypertension
- Engorged neck veins
- Decrease in urinary osmolality as renal failure progresses
- Right atrial pressure is > 8 mm Hg
- Pulmonary artery occlusion pressure is > 12 mm Hg

Outcome Criteria
- Weight returns to baseline.
- Edema or ascites is absent or reduced to baseline.
- Lungs are clear to auscultation.
- Exertional dyspnea is absent.
- Blood pressure returns to baseline.
- Heart rate returns to baseline.
- Neck veins are flat.
- Mucous membranes are moist.

Nursing Interventions and Rationale
1. Promote skin integrity of edematous areas by frequent repositioning and elevation of areas where possible. Avoid massaging pressure points or reddened areas of skin *because this results in further tissue trauma.*
2. Plan patient care to provide rest periods *to not heighten exertional dyspnea.*
3. Weigh patient daily (at same time, in same amount of clothing, and preferably with same scale).
4. Instruct the patient about the correlation between fluid intake and weight gain, using commonly understood fluid measurements; for example, ingesting 4 cups (1000 mL) of fluid results in an approximate 2-pound weight gain in the anuric patient.

NURSING MANAGEMENT PLAN: **Hyperthermia**

Definition: Body temperature elevated above normal range

Hyperthermia Related to Increased Metabolic Rate

Defining Characteristics
- Increased body temperature above normal range
- Seizures
- Flushed skin
- Increased respiratory rate
- Tachycardia
- Skin warm to touch
- Diaphoresis

Outcome Criteria
- Temperature is within normal range.
- Respiratory rate and heart rate are within patient's baseline range.
- Skin is warm and dry.

Nursing Interventions and Rationale
1. Monitor temperature every 15 minutes to 1 hour until within normal range and stable and then every 4 hours *to maintain close surveillance for temperature fluctuations and evaluate effectiveness of interventions.*
   a. Use temperature taken from pulmonary artery catheter or bladder catheter if available *because these methods closely reflect core body temperature.*
   b. Use tympanic membrane temperature if core body temperature devices are unavailable.
   c. Use rectal temperature if none of the methods listed above are available.
2. Collaborate with physician regarding administration of antithyroid medications *to block the synthesis and release of thyroid hormone.*
3. Collaborate with physician regarding the use of cooling blanket *to facilitate heat loss by conduction.*
   a. Wrap hands, feet, and genitalia to protect them from maceration during cooling and decrease chance of shivering.
   b. Avoid rapidly cooling the patient and overcooling the patient because this initiates the heat-conserving response (i.e., shivering).
4. Place ice packs in patient's groin and axilla *to facilitate heat loss by conduction.*
5. Maintain patient on bedrest *to decrease the effects of activity on the patient's metabolic rate.*
6. Provide tepid sponge baths *to facilitate heat loss by evaporation.*
7. Decrease the patient's room temperature *to facilitate radiant heat loss.*
8. Place fan near patient to circulate cool air *to facilitate heat loss by convection.*
9. Provide patient with nonrestrictive gown and lightweight bed coverings *to allow heat to escape from the patient's trunk.*
10. Collaborate with physician and respiratory therapist on the administration of oxygen to maintain $SpO_2 > 90\%$ *because patient has increased oxygen consumption resulting from an increased metabolic rate.*
11. Collaborate with physician regarding use of antipyretic medications *to facilitate patient comfort.*
12. Collaborate with physician regarding use of intravenous and oral fluids *to maintain adequate hydration of the patient.*

Hyperthermia Related to Pharmacogenic Hypermetabolism (Malignant Hyperthermia)

Defining Characteristics
Early Signs
- Blood pressure is > 140/90 mm Hg
- Profuse diaphoresis
- Heart rate is > 100 beats/min
- Masseter and general skeletal muscle rigidity and fasciculations
- Tachypnea
- Decreased level of consciousness
- Increased end-tidal carbon dioxide pressure (P_{ETCO_2})

Late Signs
- Increasing core body temperature up to 42° to 43° C (107.6° to 109.4° F)
- Hot skin
- Systolic blood pressure is < 90 mm Hg
- Heart rate is > 100 beats/min and ventricular dysrhythmias
- Cardiac index is > 4.0 L/min/m^2
- Pulmonary artery occlusion pressure is > 12 mm Hg
- Continued skeletal muscle rigidity and fasciculations
- PaO_2 is < 80 mm Hg
- Respiratory and metabolic acidosis
- Fixed, dilated pupils
- Seizures, coma, or decerebrate posturing
- Urinary output is < 30 mL/hr; urine color reddish brown (myoglobinuria)
- Prolonged bleeding (disseminated intravascular coagulation [DIC])

Outcome Criteria
- Core body temperature is below 38.3° C (101° F).
- Muscle rigidity and fasciculations are absent.
- Patient is alert and oriented.
- Pupils are normoreactive.

Continued

Nursing Interventions and Rationale

1. Obtain the emergency kit for malignant hyperthermia. It is recommended that health care institutions have an emergency malignant hyperthermia kit available that contains the items mentioned in the following plan. Call the malignant hyperthermia hotline for more information (1-800-644-9737).

2. Collaborate with the physician to implement measure to rapidly decrease metabolism:
   a. Administer dantrolene (Dantrium) at a dose of 2.5 mg/kg rapidly through a large-bore intravenous (IV) line, *which relaxes skeletal muscles by reducing the release of calcium from the sarcoplasmic reticulum.*
   b. Observe for infiltration of dantrolene into surrounding tissues. *Dantrolene is very alkaline and irritating to tissues.*

3. Collaborate with the physician to initiate cooling measures:
   a. Administer cold IV solutions (IV bag has been submerged in ice bath before solution is administered).
   b. Provide cool-water sponge bath.
   c. Apply cooling blanket until temperature is within 1° to 3° F of desired level *to avoid "overshoot," in which excessive cooling lowers the body temperature below the desired range.*
   d. Institute iced saline lavages of stomach, rectum, and bladder.
   e. Monitor core temperature continuously *to avoid overcooling.*

4. Collaborate with physician to implement interventions to reverse metabolic and respiratory acidosis:
   a. Administer sodium bicarbonate at a dose of 1-2 mEq/kg IV as necessary *to treat metabolic acidosis and hyperkalemia.*
   b. Hyperventilate patient with 100% oxygen; then ventilate with 15-20 mL/kg tidal volume at 15-20 breaths/min.
   c. Assess arterial blood gas values frequently, and make ventilatory adjustments as necessary *to remedy hypoxemia and hypercarbia.*

5. Collaborate with physician to provide adequate nutrients to the tissues, and correct electrolyte imbalances:
   a. Administer 50% dextrose and regular insulin *to increase glucose uptake into liver to meet hypermetabolic needs of body and enhance the movement of potassium from extracellular fluid back into the cells.*
   b. Administer calcium chloride at a dose of 10 mg/kg IV or calcium gluconate at a dose of 10-50 mg/kg *for life-threatening hyperkalemia.*
   c. Monitor serum electrolytes *to assess efficacy of previously mentioned action.*
   d. Monitor blood urea nitrogen (BUN) and creatinine levels *to evaluate for renal failure.*
   e. Monitor serum enzyme levels, particularly creatine phosphokinase (CPK) elevations *for indication of degree of muscle hyperactivity.*

6. Collaborate with physician to correct cardiovascular instability and dysrhythmias:
   a. Titrate vasoactive and inotropic drips per protocol to desired systemic blood pressure, pulmonary artery occlusion pressure, and/or pulmonary artery diastolic pressure.
   b. Follow critical care emergency standing orders about the administration of antidysrhythmic agents.
   c. Do not administer calcium channel blockers *as they may cause hyperkalemia and cardiac arrest in the presence of dantrolene.*

7. Collaborate with physician to maintain a high urinary output (>50 mL/hr):
   a. Administer osmotic agents (mannitol) *for excretion of excess fluid load and to increase urinary output to prevent renal failure.*
   b. Administer diuretics (furosemide) *to enhance secretion of myoglobin, potassium, sodium, and magnesium.*
   c. Administer supplemental potassium chloride as indicated by serum potassium levels.
   d. Administer steroids (e.g., Solu-Cortef) *for its mineralocorticoid effect of potassium excretion, to increase glomerular filtration rate, and to reduce cerebral edema.*

8. Maintain surveillance for hematologic abnormalities:
   a. Monitor coagulation studies *for indications of DIC and for efficacy of heparin therapy.*
   b. Assess stool, urinary, and nasogastric (NG) drainage for occult blood.

9. Weigh patient daily (at same time, in same amount of clothing, and preferably with same scale) *to assist in assessment of hydration status.*

NURSING MANAGEMENT PLAN: Hypothermia

Definition: Body temperature below normal range

Hypothermia Related to Decreased Metabolic Rate

Defining Characteristics
- Reduction in body temperature below normal range
- Shivering
- Pallor
- Piloerection
- Hypertension
- Skin cool to touch
- Tachycardia
- Decreased capillary refill

Outcome Criteria
- Temperature is within normal range.
- Heart rate is within patient's baseline range.
- Skin is warm and dry.
- Capillary refill is normal.

Nursing Interventions and Rationale
1. Monitor temperature every 15 minutes to 1 hour until within normal range and stable and then every 4 hours *to maintain close surveillance for temperature fluctuations and evaluate effectiveness of interventions.*
   a. Use temperature taken from pulmonary artery catheter or bladder catheter if available *because these methods closely reflect core body temperature.*
   b. Use tympanic membrane temperature *if core body temperature devices are unavailable.*
   c. Use rectal temperature if none of the methods listed above are available.
2. Collaborate with physician regarding administration of thyroid medications *to replace lacking thyroid hormone.*
3. Collaborate with physician regarding the use of fluid-filled heating blanket *to facilitate rewarming by conduction.*
4. Initiate forced air-warming therapy *to facilitate convective heat gain.*
5. Provide patient with warm blankets *to facilitate heat transfer to the patient.*
6. Increase the patient's room temperature *to decrease radiant heat loss.*
7. Replace wet patient gown and bed linen promptly *to decrease evaporative heat loss.*
8. Warm intravenous fluids and blood products *to facilitate rewarming by conduction.*

Hypothermia Related to Exposure to Cold Environment, Trauma, or Damage to the Hypothalamus

Defining Characteristics
- Core body temperature below 35° C (95° F)
- Skin cold to touch
- Slurred speech, incoordination
- At temperature below 33° C (91.4° F):
  Cardiac dysrhythmias (atrial fibrillation, bradycardia)
  Cyanosis
  Respiratory alkalosis
- At temperatures below 32° C (89.6° F):
  Shivering replaced by muscle rigidity
  Hypotension
  Dilated pupils
- At temperatures below 28° to 29° C (82.4° to 84.2° F):
  Absent deep tendon reflexes
  3 to 4 breaths/min to apnea
  Ventricular fibrillation possible
- At temperatures below 26° to 27° C (78.8° to 80.6° F):
  Coma
  Flaccid muscles
  Fixed, dilated pupils
  Ventricular fibrillation to cardiac standstill
  Apnea

Outcome Criteria
- Core body temperature is greater than 35° C (95° F).
- Patient is alert and oriented.
- Cardiac dysrhythmias are absent.
- Acid-base balance is normal.
- Pupils are normoreactive.

Nursing Interventions and Rationale
1. Monitor core body temperature continuously.
2. Collaborate with the physician regarding the need for intubation and mechanical ventilation.
   a. Heated air or oxygen can be added *to help rewarm the body core.*
   b. Do not hyperventilate the hypothermic patient because carbon dioxide production is low and this action may induce severe alkalosis and precipitate ventricular fibrillation.
3. Maintain cardiopulmonary resuscitation and advanced cardiac life support (ACLS) until core body temperature

Continued

NURSING MANAGEMENT PLAN: **Hypothermia**—*cont'd*

is up to at least 29.5° C (85.1° F) before determining that patients cannot be resuscitated. *Electrical defibrillation is usually successful in terminating ventricular fibrillation if the temperature is greater than 28° C (82.4° F).*

4. Administer cardiac resuscitation drugs sparingly *because as the body warms, peripheral vasodilation occurs. Drugs that remain in the periphery are suddenly released, leading to a bolus effect that may cause fatal dysrhythmias.*

5. Monitor arterial blood gas values *to direct further therapy,* and ensure that the pH, PaO_2, and $PaCO_2$ are corrected for temperature.

6. Rewarm patient rapidly *because the pathophysiologic changes associated with chronic hypothermia have not had time to evolve.*

a. Institute rapid, active rewarming by immersion in warm water (38° to 43° C) (100.4° to 109.4° F).

b. Apply thermal blanket at 36.6° to 37.7° C (97.9° to 99.9° F). Some researchers suggest rewarming only the torso or trunk first, leaving the extremities exposed to room temperature. *This is done to prevent early peripheral vasodilation with abrupt redistribution of intravascular volume. This also prevents colder blood trapped in the extremities from returning to the body core before the heart is rewarmed.*

c. Perform rapid core rewarming with heated (37° to 43° C; 98.6° to 109.4° F) intravenous infusion, hemodialysis, peritoneal dialysis, and colonic or gastric irrigation fluids.

7. Monitor peripheral circulation because gangrene of the fingers and toes is a common complication of accidental hypothermia.

NURSING MANAGEMENT PLAN: Imbalanced Nutrition: Less Than Body Requirements

Definition: Intake of nutrients insufficient to meet metabolic needs

Imbalanced Nutrition: Less than Body Requirements Related to Lack of Exogenous Nutrients and Increased Metabolic Demand

Defining Characteristics

- Unplanned weight loss of 20% of body weight within the past 6 months
- Serum albumin is < 3.5 g/dL
- Total lymphocytes are < 1500/mm^3
- Anergy
- Negative nitrogen balance
- Fatigue; lack of energy and endurance
- Nonhealing wounds
- Daily caloric intake less than estimated nutritional requirements
- Presence of factors known to increase nutritional requirements (e.g., sepsis, trauma, multiple organ dysfunction syndrome)
- Maintenance of nothing by mouth (NPO) status for > 7-10 days
- Long-term use of 5% dextrose intravenously
- Documentation of suboptimal calorie counts
- Drug or nutrient interaction that might decrease oral intake (e.g. chronic use of bronchodilators, laxatives, anticonvulsives, diuretics, antacids, opioids)
- Physical problems with chewing, swallowing, choking, and salivation and presence of altered taste, anorexia, nausea, vomiting, diarrhea, or constipation

Outcome Criteria

- Patient exhibits stabilization of weight loss or weight gain of one-half pound daily.
- Serum albumin is > 3.5 g/dL.
- Total lymphocytes are < 1500/mm^3.
- Patient has positive response to cutaneous skin antigen testing.
- Patient is in positive nitrogen balance.
- Wound healing is evident.
- Daily caloric intake equals estimated nutritional requirements.
- Increased ambulation and endurance are evident.

Nursing Interventions and Rationale

1. Inquire if patient has any food allergies and food preferences *to ensure the food provided to the patient is not contraindicated.*
2. Monitor patient's caloric intake and weight daily *to ensure adequacy of nutritional interventions.*
3. Collaborate with dietitian regarding patient's nutritional and caloric needs *to determine the appropriateness of the patient's diet to meet those needs.*
4. Monitor patient for signs of nutritional deficiencies *to facilitate evaluation of extent of nutritional deficient.*
5. Provide patient with oral care before eating *to ensure optimal consumption of diet.*
6. Assist patient to eat as appropriate *to ensure optimal consumption of diet.*
7. Collaborate with physician regarding the administration of parenteral and enteral nutrition as needed.

NURSING MANAGEMENT PLAN: Impaired Gas Exchange

Definition: Excess or deficit in oxygenation and/or carbon dioxide elimination at the alveolar-capillary membrane

Impaired Gas Exchange Related to Alveolar Hypoventilation

Defining Characteristics

- Abnormal arterial blood gas values (decreased PaO_2, increased $PaCO_2$, decreased pH, decreased SaO_2)
- Somnolence
- Neurobehavioral changes (e.g., restlessness, irritability, confusion)
- Tachycardia or dysrhythmias
- Central cyanosis

Outcome Criteria

- Arterial blood gas values are within patient's baseline.
- Central cyanosis is absent.

Nursing Interventions and Rationale

1. Initiate continuous pulse oximetry or monitor SpO_2 every hour.
2. Collaborate with physician on the administration of oxygen to maintain an $SpO_2 > 90\%$.
   a. Administer supplemental oxygen by an appropriate oxygen-delivery device *to increase driving pressure of oxygen in the alveoli.*
   b. If supplemental oxygen alone is not effective, administer continuous positive airway pressure (CPAP) by noninvasive positive pressure ventilation (NPPV) or positive end-expiratory pressure (PEEP) by invasive positive pressure mechanical ventilation *to open collapsed alveoli and increase the surface area for gas exchange.*
3. Prevent hypoventilation.
   a. Position patient in high-Fowler's position or semi-Fowler's position *to promote diaphragmatic descent and maximal inhalation.*
   b. Assist with deep-breathing exercises and/or incentive spirometry with sustained maximal inspiration 5 to 10 times/hr *to help reinflate collapsed portions of the lung.* See the nursing management plan for Ineffective Breathing Pattern Related to Decreased Lung Expansion for further instructions.
   c. Treat pain, if present, *to prevent hypoventilation and atelectasis.* Implement the nursing management plan of care, Acute Pain Related to Transmission and Perception of Cutaneous, Visceral, Muscular, or Ischemic Impulses.
4. Assist physician with intubation and initiation of mechanical ventilation as indicated.

Impaired Gas Exchange Related to Ventilation/Perfusion Mismatching or Intrapulmonary Shunting

Defining Characteristics

- Abnormal arterial blood gas values (decreased PaO_2, decreased SaO_2)
- Somnolence
- Neurobehavioral changes (restlessness, irritability, confusion)
- Central cyanosis

Outcome Criteria

- ABG values are within patient's baseline.
- Central cyanosis is absent.

Nursing Interventions and Rationale

1. Initiate continuous pulse oximetry, or monitor SpO_2 every hour.
2. Collaborate with physician on the administration of oxygen to maintain an $SpO_2 > 90\%$.
   a. Administer supplemental oxygen by an appropriate oxygen-delivery device *to increase driving pressure of oxygen in the alveoli.*
   b. If supplemental oxygen alone is not effective, administer continuous positive airway pressure (CPAP) by noninvasive positive pressure ventilation (NPPV) or positive end-expiratory pressure (PEEP) by invasive positive pressure mechanical ventilation *to open collapsed alveoli and increase the surface area for gas exchange.*
3. Position patient to optimize ventilation/perfusion matching.
   a. For patient with unilateral lung disease, position with the good lung down *because gravity will improve perfusion to this area, and this will best match ventilation with perfusion.*
   b. For patient with bilateral lung disease, position with the right lung down *because this lung is larger than the left and affords a greater area for ventilation and perfusion,* or change position every 2 hours, favoring positions that improve oxygenation.
   c. For patient with diffuse bilateral disease, collaborate with the physician regarding the use of prone positioning *to encourage perfusion to the anterior region of the lungs, which are usually less damaged than the posterior region.*
   d. Avoid any position that seriously compromises oxygenation status.
4. Perform procedures only as needed and provide adequate rest and recovery time in between *to prevent desaturation.*
5. Collaborate with the physician regarding the administration of the following:
   a. Sedatives *to decrease ventilator asynchrony and facilitate patient's sense of control.*
   b. Neuromuscular blocking agents *to prevent ventilator asynchrony and decrease oxygen demand.*
   c. Analgesics *to treat pain if present.* Implement the nursing management plan of care, Acute Pain Related to Transmission and Perception of Cutaneous, Visceral, Muscular, or Ischemic Impulses.
6. Evaluate patient for the presence of secretions. If present, implement the nursing management plan of care, Ineffective Airway Clearance Related to Excessive Secretions or Abnormal Viscosity of Mucus.

NURSING MANAGEMENT PLAN: **Impaired Spontaneous Ventilation**

Definition: Decreased energy reserves results in an individual's inability to maintain breathing adequate to support life

Impaired Spontaneous Ventilation Related to Respiratory Muscle Fatigue or Metabolic Factors

Defining Characteristics

- Dyspnea and apprehension
- Increased metabolic rate
- Increased restlessness
- Increased use of accessory muscles
- Decreased tidal volume
- Increased heart rate
- Abnormal arterial blood gas values (decreased PaO_2, increased $PaCO_2$, decreased pH, decreased SaO_2)
- Decreased cooperation

Outcome Criteria

- Metabolic rate and heart rate are within patient's baseline.
- Patient experiences eupnea.
- ABG values are within patient's baseline.

Nursing Interventions and Rationale

1. Collaborate with the physician regarding the application of pressure support to the ventilator *to assist patient in overcoming the work of breathing imposed by the ventilator and endotracheal tube.*
2. Carefully snip excess length from the proximal end of the endotracheal *tube to decrease dead space and thereby decrease the work of breathing.*
3. Collaborate with the physician and dietitian to ensure that at least 50% of the diet's nonprotein caloric source is in the form of fat rather than carbohydrates *to prevent excess carbon dioxide production.*
4. Collaborate with the physician and respiratory therapist regarding the best method of weaning for individual *patients because each situation is different and a variety of weaning options are available.*
5. Collaborate with the physician and physical therapist regarding a progressive ambulation and conditioning plan *to promote overall muscle conditioning and respiratory muscle functioning.*
6. Determine the most effective means of communication for the patient *to promote independence and reduce anxiety.*
7. Develop a daily schedule and post it in patient's room *to coordinate care and facilitate patient's involvement in the plan.*
8. Treat pain, if present, *to prevent respiratory splinting and hypoventilation.* Implement the nursing management plan of care, Acute Pain Related to Transmission and Perception of Cutaneous, Visceral, Muscular, or Ischemic Impulses.
9. Ensure that patient receives at least 2- to 4-hr intervals of uninterrupted sleep in a quiet, dark room. Collaborate with the physician and respiratory therapist regarding the use of full ventilatory support at night *to provide respiratory muscle rest.*
10. Place patient in semi-Fowler's position or in a chair at the bedside *for best use of ventilatory muscles and to facilitate diaphragmatic descent.*
11. Explain the weaning procedure to the patient before the trial *so that patient will understand what to expect and how to participate.*
12. Monitor patient during the weaning trial for evidence of respiratory muscle fatigue *to avoid overtiring the patient.*
13. Provide diversional activity during the weaning trial *to reduce the patient's anxiety.*
14. Collaborate with physician and respiratory therapist regarding the removal of the ventilator and artificial airway *when patient has been successfully weaned.*

NURSING MANAGEMENT PLAN: **Impaired Swallowing**

Definition: Abnormal functioning of the swallowing mechanism associated with deficits in oral, pharyngeal, or esophageal structure or function

Impaired Swallowing Related to Neuromuscular Impairment, Fatigue, and Limited Awareness

Defining Characteristics
- Evidence of difficulty swallowing
  - Drooling
  - Difficulty handling oral secretions
  - Absence of gag, cough, and/or swallow reflex
  - Moist, wet, gurgling voice quality
  - Decreased tongue and mouth movements
  - Presence of dysarthria
- Difficulty handling solid foods:
  - Uncoordinated chewing or swallowing
  - Stasis of food in the oral cavity
  - Wet-sounding voice or change in voice quality
  - Sneezing, coughing, or choking with eating
  - Delay in swallowing of more than 5 seconds
  - Change in respiratory patterns
- Difficulty handling liquids:
  - Momentary loss of voice or change in voice quality
  - Nasal regurgitation of liquids
  - Coughing with drinking
- Evidence of aspiration
  - Hypoxemia
  - Productive cough
  - Frothy sputum
  - Wheezing, crackles, or rhonchi
  - Temperature elevation

Outcome Criteria
- Evidence of swallowing difficulties is absent.
- Evidence of aspiration is absent.

Nursing Interventions and Rationale
1. Collaborate with physician and speech therapist regarding swallowing evaluation and rehabilitation program *to decrease the incidence of aspiration.*
2. Collaborate with physician and dietitian regarding a nutritional assessment and nutritional plan *to ensure that the patient is receiving enough nutrition.*
3. Place the patient in an upright position with the head midline and the chin slightly down *to keep food in the anterior portion of the mouth and to prevent it from falling over the base of the tongue into the open airway.*
4. Provide patient with single-textured soft foods (e.g., cream cereals) that maintain their shape *because these foods require minimal oral manipulation.*
5. Avoid particulate foods (e.g., hamburger) and foods containing more than one texture (e.g., stew) *because these foods require more chewing and oral manipulation.*
6. Avoid dry foods (e.g., popcorn, rice, crackers) and sticky foods (e.g., peanut butter, bananas) *because these foods are difficult to manipulate orally.*
7. Provide patient with thick liquids (e.g., fruit nectar, yogurt) *because thick liquids are more easily controlled in the mouth.*
8. Thicken thin liquids (e.g., water, juice) with a thickening preparation or avoid them *because thin liquids are easily aspirated.*
9. Place foods in the uninvolved side of the mouth *because oral sensitivity and function are greatest in this area.*
10. Avoid the use of straws *because they can deposit the liquid too far back in the mouth for the patient to handle.*
11. Serve foods and liquids at room temperature *because the patient may be overly sensitive to heat or cold.*
12. Offer solids and liquids at different times *to avoid swallowing solids before being properly chewed.*
13. Provide oral hygiene after meals *to clear food particles from the mouth that could be aspirated.*
14. Collaborate with physician and pharmacist regarding oral medication administration *to adjust medication regimen to prevent aspiration and choking and to ensure all prescribed medications are swallowed.*
15. Crush tablets (if appropriate) and mix with food that is easily formed into a bolus, use thickened liquid medications (if available), and/or embed small capsules into food *to facilitate oral medication administration.*
16. Inspect mouth for residue after all medication administration *to ensure medication has been swallowed.*
17. Educate patient and family on the swallowing problem, rehabilitation program, and emergency measures for choking.

NURSING MANAGEMENT PLAN: **Impaired Verbal Communication**

Definition: Decreased, delayed, or absent ability to receive, process, transmit, and use a system of symbols

Impaired Verbal Communication Related to Cerebral Speech Center Injury

Defining Characteristics
- Inappropriate or absent speech or responses to questions
- Inability to speak spontaneously
- Inability to understand spoken words
- Inability to follow commands appropriately through gestures
- Difficulty or inability to understand written language
- Difficulty or inability to express ideas in writing
- Difficulty or inability to name objects

Outcome Criterion
- Patient is able to make basic needs known.

Nursing Interventions and Rationale
1. Consult with physician and speech pathologist *to determine the extent of the patient's communication deficit (e.g., whether fluent, nonfluent, or global aphasia is involved).*
2. Have the speech therapist post a list of appropriate ways to communicate with the patient in the patient's room *so that all nursing personnel can be consistent in their efforts.*
3. Assess the patient's ability to comprehend, speak, read, and write.
   a. Ask questions that can be answered with "yes" or "no." If a patient answers "yes" to a question, ask the opposite (e.g., "Are you hot?" "Yes." "Are you cold?" "Yes."). *This may help determine whether the patient understands what is being said.*
   b. Ask simple, short questions, and use gestures, pantomime, and facial expressions to give the patient additional clues.
   c. Stand in the patient's line of vision, giving a good view of your face and hands.
   d. Have the patient try to write with a pad and pencil. Offer pictures and alphabet letters at which to point.
   e. Make flash cards with pictures or words depicting frequently used phrases (e.g., glass of water, bedpan).
4. Maintain an uncluttered environment, and decrease external distractions *to enhance communication.*
5. Maintain a relaxed and calm manner, and explain all diagnostic, therapeutic, and comfort measures before initiating them.
6. Do not shout or speak in a loud voice. *Hearing loss is not a factor in aphasia, and shouting will not help.*
7. Have only one person talk at a time. *It is more difficult for the patient to follow a multisided conversation.*
8. Use direct eye contact, and speak directly to the patient in unhurried, short phrases.
9. Give one-step commands and directions, and provide cues through pictures and gestures.
10. Try to ask questions that can be answered with a "yes" or a "no," and avoid topics that are controversial, emotional, abstract, or lengthy.
11. Listen to the patient in an unhurried manner, and wait for his or her attempt to communicate.
    a. Expect a time lag from when you ask the patient something until the patient responds.
    b. Accept the patient's statement of essential words without expecting complete sentences.
    c. Avoid finishing the sentence for the patient if possible.
    d. Wait approximately 30 seconds before providing the word the patient may be attempting to find (except when the patient is very frustrated and needs something quickly, such as a bedpan).
    e. Rephrase the patient's message aloud *to validate it.*
    f. Do not pretend to understand the patient's message if you do not.
12. Encourage the patient to speak slowly in short phrases and to say each word clearly.
13. Ask the patient to write the message, if able, or draw pictures if only verbal communication is affected.
14. Observe the patient's nonverbal clues for validation (e.g., answers "yes" but shakes head "no").
15. When handing an object to the patient, state what it is *because hearing language spoken is necessary to stimulate language development.*
16. Explain what has happened to the patient, and offer reassurance about the plan of care.
17. Verbally address the problem of frustration over the inability to communicate, and explain that both the nurse and the patient need patience.
18. Maintain a calm, positive manner, and offer reassurance (e.g., "I know this is very hard for you, but it will get better if we work on it together").
19. Talk to the patient as an adult. Be respectful, and avoid talking down to the patient.
20. Do not discuss the patient's condition or hold conversations in the patient's presence without including him or her in the discussion. *This may be the reason some aphasic patients develop paranoid thoughts.*

Continued

NURSING MANAGEMENT PLAN: Impaired Verbal Communication—*cont'd*

21. Do not exhibit disapproval of emotional utterances or spontaneous use of profanity; instead, offer calm, quiet reassurance.
22. If the patient makes an error in speech, do not reprimand or scold but try to compliment the patient by saying, "That was a good try."
23. Delay conversation if the patient is tired. *The symptoms of aphasia worsen if the patient is fatigued, anxious, or upset.*

24. Be prepared for emotional outbursts and tears from patients who have more difficulty in expressing themselves than with understanding. *The patient may become depressed, refuse treatment and food, ignore relatives, and push objects away.* Comfort the patient with statements such as, "I know it's frustrating and you feel sad, but you are not alone. Other people who have had strokes have felt the way you do. We will be here to help you get through this."

NURSING MANAGEMENT PLAN: Ineffective Airway Clearance

Definition: Inability to clear secretions or obstructions from the respiratory tract to maintain a clear airway

Ineffective Airway Clearance Related to Excessive Secretions or Abnormal Viscosity of Mucus

Defining Characteristics
- Abnormal breath sounds (displaced normal sounds, adventitious sounds, diminished or absent sounds)
- Ineffective cough with or without sputum
- Tachypnea, dyspnea
- Verbal reports of inability to clear airway

Outcome Criteria
- Cough produces thin mucus.
- Lungs are clear to auscultation.
- Respiratory rate, depth, and rhythm return to baseline.

Nursing Interventions and Rationale
1. Assess sputum for color, consistency, and amount.
2. Assess for clinical manifestations of pneumonia.
3. Provide for maximal thoracic expansion by repositioning, deep breathing, splinting, and pain management **to avoid hypoventilation and atelectasis.** If hypoventilation is present, implement the nursing management plan of care, Ineffective Breathing Pattern Related to Decreased Lung Expansion.
4. Maintain adequate hydration by administering oral and intravenous fluids (as ordered) **to thin secretions and facilitate airway clearance.**
5. Provide humidification to airways by an oxygen-delivery device or artificial airway **to thin secretions and facilitate airway clearance.**
6. Administer bland aerosol every 4 hours **to facilitate expectoration of sputum.**
7. Collaborate with the physician regarding the administration of the following:
   a. Bronchodilators **to treat or prevent bronchospasms and facilitate expectoration of mucus.**
   b. Mucolytics and expectorants **to enhance mobilization and removal of secretions.**
   c. Antibiotics **to treat infection.**
8. Assist with directed coughing exercises **to facilitate expectoration of secretions.** If patient is unable to perform cascade cough, consider using huff cough (patients with hyperactive airways), end-expiratory cough (patient with secretions in distal airway), or augmented cough (patient with weakened abdominal muscle).
   a. Cascade cough—instruct patient to do the following:
      (1) Take a deep breath, and hold it for 1 to 3 seconds.
      (2) Cough out forcefully several times until all air is exhaled.
      (3) Inhale slowly through the nose.
      (4) Repeat once.
      (5) Rest, and then repeat as necessary.
   b. Huff cough—instruct patient to do the following:
      (1) Take a deep breath, and hold it for 1 to 3 seconds
      (2) Say the word "huff" while coughing out several times until air is exhaled
      (3) Inhale slowly through the nose
      (4) Repeat as necessary
   c. End-expiratory cough—instruct patient to do the following:
      (1) Take a deep breath, and hold it for 1 to 3 seconds.
      (2) Exhale slowly.
      (3) At the end of exhalation, cough once.
      (4) Inhale slowly through the nose.
      (5) Repeat as necessary, or follow with cascade cough.
   d. Augmented cough—instruct patient to do the following:
      (1) Take a deep breath, and hold it for 1 to 3 seconds.
      (2) Perform one or more of the following maneuvers to increase intraabdominal pressure:
         (a) Tighten knees and buttocks.
         (b) Bend forward at the waist.
         (c) Place a hand flat on the upper abdomen just under the xiphoid process and press in and up abruptly during coughing.
         (d) Keep hands on the chest wall and press inward with each cough.
      (3) Inhale slowly through the nose.
      (4) Rest and repeat as necessary.
9. Suction nasotracheally or endotracheally as necessary **to assist with secretion removal.**
10. Reposition patient at least every 2 hours or use kinetic therapy **to mobilize and prevent stasis of secretions.**
11. Allow rest periods between coughing sessions, suctioning, or any other demanding activities **to promote energy conservation.**

NURSING MANAGEMENT PLAN: **Ineffective Breathing Pattern**

Definition: Inspiration and/or expiration that does not provide adequate ventilation

Ineffective Breathing Pattern Related to Decreased Lung Expansion

Defining Characteristics

- Abnormal respiratory patterns (hypoventilation, hyperventilation, tachypnea, bradypnea, obstructive breathing)
- Abnormal arterial blood gas values (increased $Paco_2$, decreased pH)
- Unequal chest movement
- Shortness of breath, dyspnea

Outcome Criteria

- Respiratory rate, rhythm, and depth return to baseline.
- Minimal or absent use of accessory muscles.
- Chest expands symmetrically.
- Arterial blood gas values return to baseline.

Nursing Interventions and Rationale

1. Treat pain, if present, **to prevent hypoventilation and atelectasis.** Implement the nursing management plan of care, Acute Pain Related to Transmission and Perception of Cutaneous, Visceral, Muscular, or Ischemic Impulses.
2. Position patient in high-Fowler's or semi-Fowler's position **to promote diaphragmatic descent and maximal inhalation.**
3. Assist with deep-breathing exercises and incentive spirometry with sustained maximal inspiration 5 to 10 times/hr **to help reinflate collapsed portions of the lung.**
   a. Deep breathing—instruct patient to do the following:
      (1) Sit up straight or lean forward slightly while sitting on edge of bed or chair (if possible).
      (2) Take in a slow, deep breath.
      (3) Pause slightly, or hold breath for at least 3 seconds.
      (4) Exhale slowly.
      (5) Rest, and repeat.
   b. Incentive spirometry—instruct patient to do the following:
      (1) Exhale normally.
      (2) Place lips around the mouthpiece, and close mouth tightly around it.
      (3) Inhale slowly and as deeply as possible, noting the maximal volume of air inspired.
      (4) Hold maximal inhalation for 3 seconds.
      (5) Take the mouthpiece out of mouth, and slowly exhale.
      (6) Rest, and repeat.

4. Assist physician with intubation and initiation of mechanical ventilation as indicated.

Ineffective Breathing Pattern Related to Musculoskeletal Fatigue or Neuromuscular Impairment

Defining Characteristics

- Unequal chest movement
- Shortness of breath, dyspnea
- Use of accessory muscles
- Tachypnea
- Thoracoabdominal asynchrony
- Abnormal arterial blood gas values (increased $Paco_2$, decreased pH)
- Nasal flaring
- Assumption of 3-point position

Outcome Criteria

- Respiratory rate, rhythm, and depth return to baseline.
- Use of accessory muscles is minimal or absent.
- Chest expands symmetrically.
- Arterial blood gas values return to baseline.

Nursing Interventions and Rationale

1. Prevent unnecessary exertion **to limit drain on patient's ventilatory reserve.**
2. Instruct patient in energy-saving techniques **to conserve patient's ventilatory reserve.**
3. Assist with pursed-lip and diaphragmatic breathing techniques **to facilitate diaphragmatic descent and improved ventilation.**
   a. Diaphragmatic breathing—instruct the patient to do the following:
      (1) Sit in the upright position.
      (2) Place one hand on the abdomen just above the waist and the other on the upper chest.
      (3) Breathe in through the nose, and feel the lower hand push out; the upper hand should not move.
      (4) Breathe out through pursed lips, and feel the lower hand move in.
4. Position patient in high-Fowler's or semi-Fowler's position **to promote diaphragmatic descent and maximal inhalation.**
5. Assist physician with intubation and initiation of mechanical ventilation as indicated.

NURSING MANAGEMENT PLAN: **Ineffective Cardiopulmonary Tissue Perfusion**

Definition: Decrease in oxygen resulting in the failure to nourish the tissues at the capillary level

Ineffective Cardiopulmonary Tissue Perfusion Related to Decreased Coronary Blood Flow

Defining Characteristics
- Chest discomfort with or without radiation to the arms, back, neck, jaw, or epigastrium
- Shortness of breath
- Weakness
- Diaphoresis
- Nausea
- Lightheadedness
- ST-segment elevation on 12-lead electrocardiogram (ECG)
- Elevated troponin I
- Elevated CK-MB enzymes
- Elevated myoglobin

Outcome Criteria
- Systolic blood pressure is > 90 mm Hg.
- Mean arterial pressure is > 60 mm Hg.
- Heart rate is < 100 beats/min.
- Pulmonary artery pressures are within normal limits or back to baseline.
- Cardiac index is > 2.2 $L/min/m^2$.
- Urine output is > 0.5 mL/kg/hr or > 30 mL/hr.
- 12-lead ECG is normalized without new Q waves.
- Chest pain is absent.
- CK-MB enzymes, troponin I, and myoglobin levels are within normal range.

Nursing Interventions and Rationale
1. Collaborate with the physician regarding the administration of fibrinolytic therapy or the preparation of the patient for percutaneous coronary intervention (PCI) *to restore myocardial blood flow.*
2. Collaborate with physician regarding the administration of oxygen at 2 L/min to achieve SpO_2 > 90% *to maximize myocardial oxygen supply.*
3. Collaborate with physician regarding the administration of sublingual nitroglycerin and/or intravenous nitroglycerine infusion *to augment coronary blood flow and reduce cardiac work by decreasing preload and afterload.*

   a. Do not administer nitrates to patients who have taken phosphodiesterase inhibitors for erectile dysfunction within the last 24 or 48 hours (depending the medication). *as severe hypotension may occur.*

4. Collaborate with physician regarding the administration of morphine *to control pain.*
5. Collaborate with the physician regarding the administration of aspirin, antiplatelet therapy, and heparin *to prevent recurrent thrombosis and inhibit platelet function.*
6. Collaborate with the physician regarding the administration of beta-blockers *to decrease myocardial oxygen demand and prevent recurrent ischemia.*
7. Collaborate with the physician regarding the administration of angiotensin-converting enzyme (ACE) inhibitors *to block the conversion of angiotensin I to angiotensin II, a potent vasoconstrictor.*
8. Maintain the patient on bed rest with bedside commode privileges *to minimize myocardial oxygen demand.*
9. Monitor patient's hemodynamic and cardiac rhythm status:
   a. Select cardiac monitoring leads based on infarct location and rhythm to obtain the best rhythm for monitoring.
   b. Evaluate cardiac rhythm for presence of dysrhythmias, which are common complications of myocardial ischemia.
   c. Collaborate with physician regarding the administration of antidysrhythmic medications.
   d. Assess serum electrolytes (potassium and magnesium) and arterial blood gases.
   e. Collaborate with physician regarding the administration of electrolytes to correct any imbalances.
   f. Monitor ST segment continuously to determine changes in myocardial tissue perfusion.
   g. Monitor patient's blood pressure at least every hour as many conditions (e.g., drugs, dysrhythmias, myocardial ischemia) may cause hypotension (systolic blood pressure < 90 mm Hg).
   h. Treat symptomatic dysrhythmias according to unit's emergency protocol or advanced cardiac life support (ACLS) guidelines.
10. Instruct patient to avoid the Valsalva maneuver as forced expiration against a closed glottis causes sudden and intense changes in systolic blood pressure and heart rate.

NURSING MANAGEMENT PLAN: **Ineffective Cerebral Tissue Perfusion**

Definition: Decrease in oxygen resulting in the failure to nourish the tissues at the capillary level

Ineffective Cerebral Tissue Perfusion Related to Decreased Blood Flow

Defining Characteristics
- Decreased level of consciousness
- Hemiparesis or hemiplegia
- Visual changes
- Aphasia
- Dysphagia
- Facial droop
- Cognitive deficits
- Ataxia

Outcome Criteria
- Absence of neurologic deficits
- Blood pressure within ordered parameters

Nursing Interventions and Rationale
1. Collaborate with physician regarding the administration of fibrinolytic therapy *to facilitate lysis of the clot and restoration of blood flow to affected area.*
2. Monitor the patient for alterations in blood pressure, oxygenation, temperature, rhythm, and glucose levels.
3. Collaborate with physician regarding the administration vasodilators for hypertension *to maintain the patient's blood pressure within desired range.* Use caution in lowering blood pressure *as hypotension decreases cerebral blood flow.*
   a. Patients receiving fibrinolytic therapy—keep systolic blood pressure < 185 mm Hg and diastolic blood pressure < 110 mm Hg.
   b. Patients not receiving fibrinolytic therapy—keep systolic blood pressure < 220 mm Hg and diastolic blood pressure < 120 mm Hg
4. Collaborate with physician regarding the administration of intravenous fluids and vasoconstrictors for hypotension *as hypotension decreases cerebral blood flow.*
5. Collaborate with physician regarding the administration of oxygen to maintain SpO_2 > 95% *to prevent hypoxemia and potential worsening of the neurologic injury.*
6. Collaborate with physician regarding administration of acetaminophen for elevated temperature *because hyperthermia is associated with increase morbidity in the stroke patient.*
7. Collaborate with the physician regarding the treatment of dysrhythmias *due to increased sympathetic nervous system stimulation.*

8. Collaborate with the physician regarding the administration of insulin for hyperglycemia *as elevated blood glucose as been linked to an increase the area of infarct.*
9. Collaborate with the speech therapist regarding the patient's ability to swallow before initiating oral feedings *to ensure patient is not at risk for aspirating.*
10. Collaborate with the physical therapist to assess the patient's ability to ambulate safely *to ensure the patient is not at risk for falling* and ability to perform activities of daily living *to facilitate discharge home.*
11. Maintain surveillance for complications such as increased intracranial pressure, seizures, and acute respiratory failure.
12. Collaborate with the physician and rehabilitation specialist regarding the patient's need for rehabilitation *to maximize the patient's independence.*

Ineffective Cerebral Tissue Perfusion Related to Hemorrhage

Defining Characteristics
Intracerebral Hemorrhage
- Alteration in level of consciousness
- Nausea and vomiting
- Headache
- Seizures
- Hypertension
- Focal neurologic deficits

Subarachnoid Hemorrhage
- Sudden onset of severe headache, nausea, and/or vomiting
- Symptoms of meningeal irritation:
  - Nuchal rigidity and pain
  - Back pain
  - Bilateral leg pain
  - Kernig's sign: resistance to full extension of the leg at the knee when the hip is flexed
  - Brudzinski's sign: flexion of the hip and knee during passive neck flexion
- Photophobia and visual changes
- Sudden loss of consciousness
- Altered level of consciousness
- Seizures
- Focal neurologic deficits

Outcome Criteria
- Patient is oriented to time, place, person, and situation.
- Pupils are equal and normoreactive.
- Blood pressure is within baseline.

NURSING MANAGEMENT PLAN: **Ineffective Cerebral Tissue Perfusion**—*cont'd*

- Motor function is bilaterally equal.
- Headache, nausea, and vomiting are absent.
- Patient verbalizes importance of and displays compliance with reduced activity.

Nursing Interventions and Rationale

1. Assess for indicators of increased intracranial pressure and brain herniation (see the nursing management plan Decreased Intracranial Adaptive Capacity Related to Failure of Normal Intracranial Compensatory Mechanism).

2. Collaborate with the physician regarding the administration of anticonvulsant medications *to prevent the onset of seizures or to control seizures.*

3. Collaborate with physician regarding the administration vasodilators for hypertension *to avoid further bleeding.* Use caution in lowering blood pressure *as hypotension decreases cerebral blood flow.*

   a. If systolic blood pressure is > 200 mm Hg or mean arterial pressure is > 150 mm Hg, aggressive reduction in blood pressure is indicated.

   b. If systolic blood pressure is > 180 mm Hg or mean arterial pressure is > 130 mm Hg in the presence of increased intracranial pressure, cautious reduction in pressure is indicated maintaining cerebral perfusion pressure > 60-80 mm Hg.

   c. If systolic blood pressure is > 180 mm Hg or mean arterial pressure is > 130 mm Hg in the absence of elevated intracranial pressure, reduction in blood pressure is indicated with a target of 160/90 mm Hg.

4. Collaborate with the physician regarding the administration of insulin for hyperglycemia *as elevated blood glucose as been linked to an increase the area of infarct.*

5. Collaborate with physician regarding administration of acetaminophen for elevated temperature *because hyperthermia is associated with increased morbidity in the stroke patient.*

6. Initiate precautions *to prevent rebleeding.*

   a. Ensure bed rest in a quiet environment *to lessen external stimuli.*

   b. Maintain a darkened room to lessen symptoms of photophobia.

   c. Restrict visitors, and instruct them to keep conversation as nonstressful as possible.

   d. Administer prescribed sedatives as prescribed *to reduce anxiety to promote rest.*

   e. Administer analgesics as prescribed *to relieve or lessen headache.*

   f. Provide a soft, high-fiber diet and stool softeners to prevent constipation, which can lead to straining and increased risk of rebleeding.

   g. Assist with activities of daily living (feeding, bathing, dressing, toileting).

   h. Avoid any activity that could lead to increased intracranial pressure; ensure that patient does not flex hips beyond 90 degrees and avoids neck hyperflexion, hyperextension, or lateral hyperrotation *that could impede jugular venous return.*

7. Collaborate with the physical therapist to assess the patient's ability to ambulate safely *to ensure the patient is not at risk for falling* and ability to perform activities of daily living *to facilitate discharge home.*

8. Collaborate with the physician and rehabilitation specialist regarding the patient's need for rehabilitation *to maximize the patient's independence.*

NURSING MANAGEMENT PLAN: Ineffective Coping

Definition: Inability to form a valid appraisal of the stressors, inadequate choices of practiced responses, and/or inability to use available resources

Ineffective Coping Related to Situational Crisis and Personal Vulnerability

Defining Characteristics

- Verbalization of inability to cope. *Sample statements:* "I can't take this anymore." "I don't know how to deal with this."
- Ineffective problem solving (problem lumping). *Sample statements:* "I have to eliminate salt from my diet. They tell me I can no longer mow the lawn. This hospitalization is costing a mint. What about my kids' future? Who's going to change the oil in the car? This is an incredible amount of time away from work."
- Ineffective use of coping mechanisms
  Projection: blames others for illness or pain
  Displacement: directs anger and/or aggression toward family. *Sample statements:* "Get out of here. Leave me alone." Cursing, shouting, or demanding attention; striking out or throwing objects
  Denial: of severity of illness and need for treatment
- Noncompliance. *Examples:* activity restriction; refusal to allow treatment or to take medications
- Suicidal thoughts (verbalizes desire to end life)
- Self-directed aggression. *Examples:* disconnects or attempts to disconnect life-sustaining equipment; deliberately tries to harm self
- Failure to progress from dependent to more independent state (refusal or resistance to care for self)

Outcome Criteria

- Patient verbalizes beginning ability to cope with illness, pain, and hospitalization. *Sample statements:* "I'm trying to do the best I can." "I want to help myself get better."
- Patient demonstrates effective problem solving (lists and prioritizes problems from most to least urgent).
- Patient uses effective behavioral strategies to manage the stress of illness and care.
- Patient demonstrates interest or involvement in illness or environment. *Examples:* patient does the following:
  Requests medications when anticipating pain
  Questions course of treatment, progress, and prognosis
  Asks for clarification of environmental stimuli and events
  Seeks out supportive individuals in his or her environment
  Uses coping mechanisms and strategies more effectively to manage situational crisis
  Demonstrates significant reduction in impulsive, angry, or aggressive outbursts (projection, shouting, cursing) directed toward family

Verbalizes future-based plans, with cessation of self-directed aggressive acts and suicidal thoughts
Willingly complies with treatment regimen
Begins to participate in self-care

Nursing Interventions and Rationale

1. Actively listen and respond to patient's verbal and behavioral expressions. *Active listening signifies unconditional respect and acceptance for the patient as a worthwhile individual. It builds trust and rapport, guides the nurse toward problem areas, encourages the patient to express concerns, and promotes compliance.*
2. Offer effective coping strategies to help the patient better tolerate the stressors related to his or her illness and care. Give permission to vent feelings in a safe setting. Sample statements: "I don't blame you for feeling angry or frustrated." "Others who are ill like you have expressed similar feelings." "I will listen to anything you want to share with me." "We don't have to talk; I'd like to sit here with you." "It's perfectly okay to cry." *Individuals who are provided with opportunities to express their feelings will be better able to release pent-up emotions and derive a greater sense of relief and comfort. They are less likely to resort to overly impulsive, aggressive acts, which may harm self or others.*
3. Inform the family of the patient's need to displace anger occasionally but that you will be working with the patient to help him or her release his or her feelings in a more constructive, effective way. *Family members who are well informed are better equipped to cope with their loved one's emotional anguish and outbursts. They are less likely to waste energy on feelings of guilt, fear, anger, or despair and can use their strength to help the patient in more constructive ways. The knowledge that their loved one is being cared for emotionally as well as physically provides family members with a greater sense of comfort and understanding. They will feel nurtured and respected by the nurse's attempt to include them in the process.*
4. With the patient, list and number problems from the most to least urgent. Assist him or her in finding immediate solutions for most urgent problems; postpone those that can wait; delegate some to family members; and help him or her to acknowledge problems that are beyond his or her control. *Listing and numbering problems in an organized fashion help to break them down into more manageable "pieces" so that the patient is better able to identify solutions for those that are solvable and to suppress those that are less relevant or not amenable to interventions.*
5. Identify individuals in the patient's environment who best help him or her to cope, and identify those who do not.

NURSING MANAGEMENT PLAN: **Ineffective Coping**—*cont'd*

Validate your observations with the patient. Sample statements: "I notice you seemed more relaxed during your daughter's visit." "After the clergy left, you were able to sleep a bit longer than usual; would you like to see him more often?" "Your grandson was a bit upset today; I'll be glad to talk to him if you like." ***Supportive persons can invoke a calming effect on the patient's physiologic and psychologic states. Conversely, well-meaning but nonsupportive individuals can have a deleterious effect on the patient's ability to cope and must be carefully screened and counseled by the nurse.***

6. Teach the patient effective cognitive strategies to help him or her better manage the stress of critical illness and care. Help him or her construct pleasant thoughts, situations, or images that can simultaneously inhibit unpleasant realities. Examples: a day at the beach, a walk in the park, drinking a glass of wine, or being with a loved one. ***Pleasant thoughts and images constructed during critical illness and care tend to inhibit or reduce the intensity of the unpleasant, stressful effects of the experience.***

7. Assist the patient in using coping mechanisms more effectively so he or she can better manage his or her situational crisis.
   a. Suppression of problems beyond his or her control
   b. Compensation for illness and its effects; focusing on his or her strengths, interests, family, and spiritual beliefs
   c. Adaptive displacement of anger, fear, or frustration through healthy, verbal expressions to staff. ***Effective use of coping mechanisms helps to assuage the patient's***

painful feelings in a safe setting. The patient is strengthened and need not resort to the use of more ineffective defenses to eliminate anxiety.

8. Initiate a suicidal assessment if the patient verbalizes the desire to die, states that life is not worth living, or exhibits self-directed aggression. *Sample statement:* "We know that this is a bad time for you. You're saying repeatedly that you want to die. Are you planning to harm yourself?" If the response is "yes," remain with the patient, alert staff members, and provide for psychiatric consultation as soon as possible. Continue to express concern to the patient and protect him or her from harm. ***Suicidal thoughts as a result of ineffective coping or exhaustion of coping devices are not an uncommon occurrence in critically ill patients. If the mood state is distressing enough, a patient may seek relief by attempting a self-destructive act. Although the patient may not imminently have the energy to succeed in his or her attempt, voicing a specific plan signifies a depressed mood state and depletion of coping strategies. Immediate intervention is needed, because the attempt may be successful when the patient's energy is restored.***

9. Encourage the patient to participate in self-care activities and treatment regimen in accordance with his or her level of progress. Offer praise for his or her efforts toward self-care. ***Patients who take an active role in their own treatment and progress are less apt to feel like helpless or powerless victims. This greater sense of control over their illness and environment will guide them more swiftly toward becoming as independent as possible.***

NURSING MANAGEMENT PLAN: Ineffective Gastrointestinal Tissue Perfusion

Definition: Decrease in oxygen resulting in the failure to nourish the tissues at the capillary level

Ineffective Gastrointestinal Tissue Perfusion Related to Decreased Gastrointestinal Blood Flow

Defining Characteristics
- Abdominal pain
- Melena
- Abdominal distention
- Hyperactive to absent bowel sounds range from hyperactive to absent
- Guarding
- Fever
- Hypotension
- Tachycardia
- Altered mental status
- Urine output is < 30 mL/hr

Outcome Criteria
- Normal bowel sounds
- Absence of abdominal pain, distention, and guarding
- Urinary output is > 30 mL/hr.
- Vital signs at baseline
- Normal mentation

Nursing Interventions and Rationales

1. Collaborate with physician regarding the administration of crystalloids, colloids, blood, and blood products *to maintain adequate circulating volume.* Implement the nursing management plan, Deficit Fluid Volume Related to Absolute Loss.
2. Collaborate with physician regarding pain management. Implement the nursing management plan, Acute Pain Related to Transmission and Perception of Cutaneous, Visceral, Muscular, or Ischemic Impulses.
3. Collaborate with physician regarding the administration of oxygen to maintain SpO_2 > 92% *to prevent hypoxemia and potential worsening of the gastrointestinal injury.*
4. Collaborate with physician regarding the administration of electrolyte replacement therapy *to maintain adequate electrolyte balance.*
5. Collaborate with dietitian regarding administration of nutrition *because patient will be unable to eat.* Implement the nursing management plan, Imbalanced Nutrition: Less Than Body Requirements.
6. Maintain surveillance for complications such as gastrointestinal hemorrhage, hypovolemic shock, and septic shock.
7. Collaborate with physician regarding preparation for surgery *to remove infarcted bowel.*

NURSING MANAGEMENT PLAN: **Ineffective Peripheral Tissue Perfusion**

Definition: Decrease in oxygen resulting in the failure to nourish the tissues at the capillary level

Ineffective Peripheral Tissue Perfusion Related to Decreased Peripheral Blood Flow

Defining Characteristics

- Weak and/or unequal peripheral pulses
- Delayed capillary refill
- Ischemic pain from extremity
- Cool skin on extremity
- Pale extremity
- Paresthesias from extremity

Outcome Criteria

- Peripheral pulses are full and equal bilaterally.
- Capillary refill is equal bilaterally.
- Ischemic pain is absent.
- Skin temperature is equal in both extremities.
- Skin is pink and warm in both extremities.
- Paresthesias are absent.

Nursing Interventions and Rationale

1. Collaborate with physician regarding the administration of antiplatelet, anticoagulant, and/or fibrinolytic therapy.
2. Collaborate with physician regarding pain management. Implement the nursing management plan of care, Acute Pain Related to Transmission and Perception of Cutaneous, Visceral, Muscular, or Ischemic Impulses.
3. Ensure patient is adequately hydrated *to decrease blood viscosity.*
4. Maintain affected extremity in dependent position if possible *to enhance blood flow.*
5. Keep affected extremity warm and protect it from injury. *Do not apply heat directly to the affected extremity because this can result in injury.*
6. Maintain surveillance for pain, pallor, pulselessness, paresthesia, paralysis, and poikilothermia *as indicators of abrupt change in blood flow.*
7. Maintain surveillance for tissue breakdown and arterial ulcers *as indicators of injury.*
8. Prepare patient for possible surgery or interventional procedure to restore blood flow.

NURSING MANAGEMENT PLAN: Ineffective Renal Tissue Perfusion

Definition: Decrease in oxygen resulting in the failure to nourish the tissues at the capillary level

Ineffective Renal Tissue Perfusion Related to Decreased Renal Blood Flow

Defining Characteristics
- Anuria or oliguria
- Decreased urinary creatinine clearance
- Increased serum creatinine
- Increased blood urea nitrogen (BUN)
- Electrolyte abnormalities: potassium, sodium
- Increased mean arterial pressure, pulmonary artery occlusion pressure, and right atrial pressure
- Sinus tachycardia
- Metabolic acidosis
- Crackles on lung auscultation
- Engorged neck veins
- Fluid weight gain
- Pitting edema
- Mental status changes
- Anemia

Outcome Criteria
- Cardiac output is > 4.0 L/min.
- Cardiac index is > 2.2 L/min/m^2.
- Mean arterial pressure, pulmonary artery occlusion pressure, and right atrial pressure are within normal limits for patient.
- Electrolytes are within normal range.
- Serum creatinine and BUN are within normal range.
- Normal acid-base balance.
- Level of consciousness is normal.
- Lungs are clear on auscultation.
- Urinary output is within normal limits, or patient is stable on dialysis.
- Hemoglobin and hematocrit values are stable.

Nursing Interventions and Rationale
1. Monitor intake and output, urine output, and patient weight.
2. Collaborate with physician regarding the administration of crystalloids, colloids, blood, and blood products *to increase circulating volume and maintain mean arterial pressure > 70 mm Hg.*
3. Collaborate with physician regarding the administration of inotropes *to enhance myocardial contractility and increase cardiac index to > 2.5 L/min.*
4. Collaborate with physician regarding the administration of diuretics to the oliguric patient *to flush out cellular debris and increase urine output.*
5. Minimize the patient's exposure to nephrotoxic drugs *to decrease damage to kidneys.*
6. Monitor blood levels of drugs cleared by kidneys *to avoid accumulation.*
7. Monitor patient for signs of electrolyte imbalance *due to impaired electrolyte regulation.*
8. Maintain surveillance for signs and symptoms of fluid overload.
9. Monitor patient's clinical status and response to dialysis therapy *to ensure the patient is receiving safe and effective dialytic therapy.*

NURSING MANAGEMENT PLAN: **Powerlessness**

Definition: Perception that one's own action cannot significantly affect an outcome; a perceived lack of control over a current situation or immediate happening

Powerlessness Related to Lack of Control Over Current Situation or Disease Progression

Defining Characteristics
Severe
- Verbal expressions of having no control or influence over situation
- Verbal expressions of having no control or influence over outcome
- Verbal expressions of having no control over self-care
- Depression over physical deterioration that occurs despite patient's compliance with regiments
- Apathy

Moderate
- Nonparticipation in care or decision making when opportunities are provided
- Expressions of dissatisfaction and frustration about inability to perform previous tasks and/or activities
- Lack of progress monitoring
- Expressions of doubt about role performance
- Reluctance to express true feelings, fearing alienation from caregivers
- Passivity
- Inability to seek information about care
- Dependence on others that may result in irritability, resentment, anger, and guilt
- No defense of self-care practices when challenged

Low
- Passivity

Outcome Criteria
- Patient verbalizes increased control over situation by wanting to do things his or her way.
- Patient actively participates in planning care.
- Patient requests needed information.
- Patient chooses to participate in self-care activities.
- Patient monitors progress.

Nursing Interventions and Rationale
1. Evaluate the patient's feelings and perception of the reasons for lack of power and sense of helplessness.
2. Determine as far as possible the patient's usual response to limited control situations. Determine through ongoing assessment the patient's usual locus of control (i.e., believes that influence over his or her life is exerted by luck, fate, powerful persons [external locus of control] or that influence is exerted through personal choices, self-effort, self-determination [internal locus of control]).
3. Support patient's physical control of the environment by involving him or her in care activities; knock before entering room if appropriate; ask permission before moving personal belongings. Inform the patient that, although an activity may not be to his or her liking, it is necessary. *This gives the patient permission to express dissatisfaction with the environment and the regimen.*
4. Personalize the patient's care using his or her preferred name. *This supports the patient's psychologic control.*
5. Provide therapeutic rationale for all the patient is asked to do for himself or herself and for all that is being done for and with him or her. Reinforce the physician's explanations; clarify misconceptions about the illness situation and treatment plans. *This supports the patient's cognitive control.*
6. Include the patient in care planning by encouraging participation and allowing choices wherever possible (e.g., timing of personal care activities; deciding when pain medicines are needed). Point out situations in which no choices exist.
7. Provide opportunities for the patient to exert influence over himself or herself and his or her body, thereby affecting an outcome. For example, share with the patient the nurse's assessment of his or her breath sounds and explain that they can be improved by self-initiated deep-breathing exercises. *Feedback that the patient has been successful in helping clear his or her lungs reinforces the influence he or she does retain.*
8. Encourage family to permit patient to do as much independently as possible *to foster perception of personal power.*
9. Assist the patient to establish realistic short-term and long-term goals. *Setting unrealistic or unattainable goals inadvertently reinforces the patient's perception of powerlessness.*
10. Document care to provide for continuity *so that the patient can maintain appropriate control over the environment.*
11. Assist the patient to regain strength and activity tolerance as appropriate, *increasing a sense of control and self-reliance.*
12. Increase the sensitivity of the health team members and significant others to the patient's sense of powerlessness. Use power over the patient carefully. Use the words *must, should,* and *have to* with caution *because they communicate coercive powers and imply that the objects of "musts" and "shoulds" are of benefit to the nurse instead of the patient.*
13. Plan with the patient for transfer from the critical care unit to the intermediate unit and eventually to home.

NURSING MANAGEMENT PLAN: Relocation Stress Syndrome

Definition: Physiologic and/or psychological disturbances after transfer from one environment to another

Relocation Stress Syndrome Related to Transfer Out of the Intensive Care Unit

Defining Characteristics
- Alienation
- Aloneness
- Anger
- Anxiety
- Concern over relocation
- Dependency
- Depression
- Fear of an unknown environment
- Frustration
- Increased illness
- Increased physical symptoms
- Increased verbalization of needs
- Insecurity
- Loneliness
- Loss of identify
- Loss of self-esteem
- Loss of self-worth
- Move from intensive care unit to another environment
- Pessimism
- Sleep disturbance
- Unwillingness to move
- Withdrawal
- Worry

Outcome Criteria
- Patient will express willingness to move to new environment.
- Absence of anxiety

Nursing Interventions and Rationale
1. Initiate pretransfer teaching as soon as appropriate during the patient's stay in the intensive care unit *to ease the transition from the intensive care to the next environment.* Teaching should focus on the on differences in the environment and the care they would receive.
2. Provide the patient and family written information regarding the transfer (if available) *to enhance effectiveness of teaching.*
3. Help the patient see that progress is being made *in preparation for transfer.* Each time a tube is removed or a treatment frequency is decreased, reinforce with the patient and family that the patient is progressing.
4. Remove monitoring and supportive equipment from the patient's room when no longer needed *to allow the patient to experience the loss of technology while still in the intensive care unit.*
5. Encourage patient and family to discuss concerns regarding relocation.
6. Assist patient and family members to develop and maintain a positive perception of the transfer.
7. Arrange for the patient's family to have a tour of the new unit *as a means of familiarizing them with the unit before the patient's transfer.*

NURSING MANAGEMENT PLAN: Risk for Aspiration

Definition: At risk for entry of gastrointestinal secretions, oropharyngeal secretions, solids, or fluids into tracheobronchial passages

Risk Factors

- Impaired laryngeal sensation or reflex
  - Reduced level of consciousness
  - Extubation
- Impaired pharyngeal peristalsis or tongue function
  - Neuromuscular dysfunction
  - Central nervous system dysfunction
  - Head or neck injury
- Impaired laryngeal closure or elevation
  - Laryngeal nerve dysfunction
  - Artificial airways
  - Gastrointestinal tubes
- Increased gastric volume
  - Delayed gastric emptying
  - Enteral feedings
  - Medication administration
- Increased intragastric pressure
  - Upper abdominal surgery
  - Obesity
  - Pregnancy
  - Ascites
- Decreased lower esophageal sphincter pressure
  - Increased gastric acidity
  - Gastrointestinal tubes
- Decreased antegrade esophageal propulsion
  - Trendelenburg or supine position
  - Esophageal dysmotility
  - Esophageal structural defects or lesions

Outcome Criteria

- Breath sounds are normal, or there is no change in patient's baseline breath sounds.
- Arterial blood gas values remain within patient's baseline.
- There is no evidence of gastric contents in lung secretions.

Nursing Interventions and Rationale

1. Assess gastrointestinal function *to rule out hypoactive peristalsis and abdominal distention.*
2. Position patient with head of bed elevated 30 degrees *to prevent gastric reflux through gravity.* If head elevation is contraindicated, position patient in right lateral decubitus position *to facilitate passage of gastric contents across the pylorus.*
3. Maintain patency and functioning of nasogastric suction apparatus *to prevent accumulation of gastric contents.*
4. Provide frequent and scrupulous mouth care *to prevent colonization of the oropharynx with bacteria and inoculation of the lower airways.*
5. Ensure that the endotracheal or tracheostomy cuff is properly inflated *to limit aspiration of oropharyngeal secretions.*
6. Treat nausea promptly; collaborate with physician on an order for antiemetic *to prevent vomiting and resultant aspiration.*

Additional Interventions for Patient Receiving Continuous or Intermittent Enteral Tube Feedings

7. Position patient with head of bed elevated 45 degrees *to prevent gastric reflux.* If a head-down position becomes necessary at any time, interrupt the feeding 30 minutes before the position change.
8. Check placement of feeding tube by auscultation or radiographically at regular intervals (e.g., before administering intermittent feedings and after position changes, suctioning, coughing episodes, or vomiting) *to ensure proper placement of the tube.*
9. Monitor patient for signs of delayed gastric emptying *to decrease potential for vomiting and aspiration.*
   a. For large-bore tubes, check residuals of tube feedings before intermittent feedings and every 4 hours during continuous feedings. Consider withholding feedings for residuals greater than 150% of the hourly rate (continuous feeding) or greater than 50% of the previous feeding (intermittent feeding).
   b. For small-bore tubes, observe abdomen for distention, palpate abdomen for hardness or tautness, and auscultate abdomen for bowel sounds.

NURSING MANAGEMENT PLAN: Risk for Infection

Definition: At increased risk for being invaded by pathogenic organisms

Risk Factors

- Inadequate primary defenses (e.g., broken skin, traumatized tissue, decreased ciliary action, stasis of body fluids, change in pH secretions, altered peristalsis)
- Inadequate secondary defenses (e.g., decreased hemoglobin, leukopenia, suppressed inflammatory or immune response)
- Immunocompromise
- Inadequate acquired immunity
- Tissue destruction and increased environmental exposure
- Chronic disease
- Invasive procedures
- Malnutrition
- Pharmacologic agents (e.g., antibiotics, steroids)

Outcome Criteria

- Total lymphocyte count is > 1000/mm^3.
- White blood cell count is within normal limits.
- Temperature is within normal limits.
- Blood, urine, wound, and sputum culture results are negative.

Nursing Interventions and Rationale

1. Perform proper hand hygiene before and after patient care *to reduce the transmission of microorganisms.*
2. Use appropriate personal protective equipment in accordance with CDC guidelines.
3. Use aseptic technique for insertion and manipulation of invasive monitoring devices, intravenous (IV) lines, and urinary drainage catheters *to maintain sterility of environment.*
4. Stabilize all invasive lines and catheters *to avoid unintentional manipulation and contamination.*
5. Use aseptic technique for dressing changes *to prevent contamination of wounds or insertion sites.*
6. Change any line placed under emergent conditions within 24 hours *because aseptic technique is usually breached during an emergency.*
7. Collaborate with the physician to change any dressing that is saturated with blood or drainage *because these are mediums for microorganism growth.*
8. Minimize use of stopcocks and maintain caps on all stopcock ports *to reduce the ports of entry for microorganisms.*
9. Avoid the use of nasogastric tubes, nasotracheal tubes, and nasopharyngeal suctioning in the patient with a suspected cerebrospinal fluid leak *to decrease the incidence of central nervous system infection.*
10. Change ventilator circuits with humidifiers no more often than every 48 hours *to avoid introducing microorganisms into the system.*
11. Provide the patient with a clean manual resuscitation bag *to avoid cross-contamination between patients.*
12. Provide oral care to patient with artificial airway or unresponsive patient every 2 to 4 hours and PRN *to decrease the incidence of hospital acquired pulmonary infections.*
    a. Swab mouth and moisten lips every 4 hours.
    b. Brush teeth with inline suction toothbrush every 12 hours.
    c. Suction subglottic secretions (secretions pooling above the cuff of the endotracheal (ET) or tracheostomy tube) every 12 hours and before repositioning the tube or deflation of the cuff.
    d. Provide lip moistener to keep patient's lips moistened PRN during each shift.
13. Cleanse in-line suction catheters with sterile saline according to the manufacturer's instructions *to avoid accumulation of secretions within the catheter.*
14. Maintain the head of the bed elevated at 30 to 45 degrees in patients with an artificial airway *to decrease the incidence of aspiration.*
15. Use disposable sterile scissors, forceps, and hemostats *to reduce the transmission of microorganisms.*
16. Maintain a closed urinary drainage system *to decrease incidence of urinary infections.*
17. Keep the urinary drainage tubing and bag below the level of the patient's bladder *to prevent the backflow of urine.*
18. Assess the urinary drainage tubing for kinks *to prevent stasis of urine.*
19. Protect all access device sites from potential sources of contamination (nasogastric reflux, draining wounds, ostomies, sputum).
20. Refrigerate parenteral nutrition solutions and opened enteral nutrition formulas *to inhibit bacterial growth.*
21. Maintain daily surveillance of invasive devices for signs and symptoms of infection.
22. Notify physician of elevated temperature or if any signs or symptoms of infection are present.

Additional Interventions for Patient Receiving Immunosuppressive Drugs

23. Obtain blood, urine, and sputum cultures for temperature elevations > 38° C (100.4° F) *inasmuch as elevation likely is caused by bacteremia or bladder or pulmonary infection.*
24. Auscultate breath sounds at least every 6 hours. *Pulmonary infection is the most common type of infection, and changes in breath sounds might be an early indication.*
25. Inspect wounds at least every 8 hours for redness, swelling, and/or drainage, *which may indicate infection.*
26. Inspect overall skin integrity and oral mucosa for signs of breakdown, *which place the patient at risk for infection.*

NURSING MANAGEMENT PLAN: **Risk for Infection**—*cont'd*

27. Notify physician of new-onset cough. ***Even a nonproductive cough may indicate pulmonary infection.***

28. Monitor white blood cell count daily, and report leukocytosis or sudden development of leukopenia, ***which may indicate an infectious process.***

29. Protect patient from exposure to any staff or family member with contagious lesion (e.g., herpes simplex) or respiratory infections.

30. Collaborate with dietitian regarding the patient's nutritional status and need for augmentation of nutritional intake as necessary ***to prevent debilitation and increased susceptibility to infection.***

31. Collaborate with physician to remove invasive lines and catheters as soon as possible ***to decrease potential portals of entry.***

32. Teach patient the clinical manifestations of infection. ***A knowledgeable patient will seek medical attention promptly, which will result in earlier treatment and a decreased risk that infection will become life threatening.***

NURSING MANAGEMENT PLAN: **Situational Low Self-Esteem**

Definition: Development of a negative perception of self-worth in response to a current situation

Situational Low Self-Esteem Related to Feelings of Guilt About Physical Deterioration

Defining Characteristics
- Inability to accept positive reinforcement
- Lack of follow-through
- Nonparticipation in therapy
- Not taking responsibility for self-care (i.e., self-neglect)
- Self-destructive behavior
- Lack of eye contact

Outcome Criteria
- Patient verbalizes feelings of self-worth.
- Patient maintains positive relationships with significant others.
- Patient manifests active interest in appearance by completing personal grooming daily.

Nursing Interventions and Rationale
1. Evaluate the meaning of health-related situation. How does the patient feel about himself or herself, the diagnosis, and the treatment? How does the present fit into the larger context of his or her life?
2. Assess the patient's emotional level, interpersonal relationships, and feeling about himself or herself. Recognize the patient's uniqueness (e.g., how the hair is worn, preference for name used).
3. Help the patient discover and verbalize feelings and understand the crisis by listening and providing information.
4. Assist the patient to identify strengths and positive qualities that increase the sense of self-worth. Focus on past experiences of accomplishment and competency. Help the patient with positive self-reinforcement. Reinforce the obvious love and affection of family and significant others.
5. Assess coping techniques that have been helpful in the past. Help the patient decide how to handle negative or incongruent feedback about the situation.
6. Encourage visits from family and significant others. Facilitate interactions, and ensure privacy. Help family members entering the critical care unit by explaining what they will see. Increase visitors' comfort with equipment; offer chairs and other courtesies.
7. Encourage the patient to pursue interest in individual or social activities, even though difficult in the critical care unit.
8. Reflect caring, concern, empathy, respect, and unconditional acceptance in nurse-patient relationships.
9. Remember that for the patient the nurse is a significant other who provides important appraisals of the patient and who can facilitate the change process.
10. Help the family support the patient's self-esteem.
11. Provide for continuity of nurse assignment to ensure consistent contacts that can ***facilitate support of the patient's self-esteem.***

NURSING MANAGEMENT PLAN: **Unilateral Neglect**

Definition: Lack of awareness and attention to one side of the body

Unilateral Neglect Related to Perceptual Disruption

Defining Characteristics

- Neglect of involved body parts and/or extrapersonal space
- Denial of existence of the affected limb or side of body
- Denial of hemiplegia or other motor and sensory deficits
- Left homonymous hemianopia
- Difficulty with spatial-perceptual tasks
- Left hemiplegia

Outcome Criteria

- Patient is safe and free from injury.
- Patient is able to identify safety hazards in the environment.
- Patient recognizes disability and describes physical deficits present (e.g., paralysis, weakness, numbness).
- Patient demonstrates ability to scan the visual field to compensate for loss of function or sensation in affected limbs.

Nursing Interventions and Rationale

1. Adapt environment to patient's deficits *to maintain patient safety.*
   a. Position the patient's bed with the unaffected side facing the door.
   b. Approach and speak to the patient from the unaffected side. If the patient must be approached from the affected side, announce your presence as soon as entering the room *to avoid startling the patient.*
   c. Position the call light, bedside stand, and personal items on the patient's unaffected side.
   d. If the patient will be assisted out of bed, simplify the environment *to eliminate hazards* by removing unnecessary furniture and equipment.
   e. Provide frequent reorientation of the patient to the environment.
   f. Observe the patient closely, and anticipate his or her needs. *In spite of repeated explanation, the patient may have difficulty retaining information about the deficits.*
   g. When patient is in bed, elevate his or her affected arm on a pillow *to prevent dependent edema and support the hand in a position of function.*
2. Assist the patient to recognize the perceptual defect.
   a. Encourage the patient to wear any prescriptive corrective glasses or hearing aids *to facilitate communication.*
   b. Instruct the patient to turn the head past midline *to view the environment on the affected side.*
   c. Encourage patient to look at the affected side and to stroke the limbs with the unaffected hand. Encourage handling of the affected limbs *to reinforce awareness of the affected side.*
   d. Instruct the patient to look for the affected extremity when performing simple tasks *to know where it is at all times.*
   e. After pointing to them, have the patient name the affected parts.
   f. Encourage the patient to use self-exercises (e.g., lifting the affected arm with the unaffected hand).
   g. If the patient is unable to discriminate between the concepts of *right* and *left*, use descriptive adjectives such as "the weak arm," "the affected leg," or "the good arm" to refer to the body. Use gestures, not just words, to indicate right and left.
3. Collaborate with the patient, physician, and rehabilitation team *to design and implement a beginning rehabilitation program for use during the critical care unit stay.*
   a. Use adaptive equipment (braces, splints, slings) as appropriate.
   b. Teach the patient the individual components of any activity separately, and then proceed to integrate the component parts into a completed activity.
   c. Instruct the patient to attend to the affected side, if able, and to assist with the bath or other tasks.
   d. Use tactile stimulation to reintroduce the arm or leg to the patient. Rub the affected parts with different textured materials to stimulate sensations (e.g., warm, cold, rough, soft).
   e. Encourage activities that require the patient to turn the head toward the affected side, and retrain the patient to scan the affected side and environment visually.
   f. If the patient is allowed out of bed, cue him or her with reminders to scan visually when ambulating. Assist and remain in constant attendance *because the patient may have difficulty maintaining correct posture, balance, and locomotion.* There may be vertical-horizontal perceptual problems, with the patient leaning to the affected side to align with the perceived vertical. Provide sitting, standing, and balancing exercises before getting the patient out of bed.
4. Assist patient with oral feedings.
   a. Avoid giving patient any very hot food items that could cause injury.
   b. Place the patient in an upright sitting position if possible.
   c. Encourage the patient to feed himself or herself; if necessary, guide the patient's hand to the mouth.
   d. If the patient is able to feed himself or herself, place one dish at a time in front of the patient. When the patient is finished with the first, add another dish. Tell the patient what he or she is eating.
   e. Initially, place food in patient's visual field; then gradually move the food out of the field of vision and teach the patient to scan the entire visual field.

Continued

NURSING MANAGEMENT PLAN: **Unilateral Neglect**—*cont'd*

f. When the patient has learned to visually scan the environment, offer a tray of food with various dishes.

g. Instruct the patient to take small bites of food and to place the food in the unaffected side of the mouth.

h. Teach the patient to sweep out pockets of food with the tongue after every bite *to eliminate retained food in the affected side of the mouth.*

i. After meals or oral medications, check the patient's oral cavity for pockets of retained material.

5. Initiate patient and family health teaching.

a. Assess to ensure that the patient and the family understand the nature of the neurologic deficits and the purpose of the rehabilitation plan.

b. Teach the proper application and use of any adaptive equipment.

c. Teach the importance of maintaining a safe environment, and point out potential environmental hazards.

d. Instruct family members how to facilitate relearning techniques (e.g., cueing, scanning visual fields).

APPENDIX B
Physiologic Formulas for Critical Care

HEMODYNAMIC FORMULAS

MEAN (SYSTEMIC) ARTERIAL PRESSURE (MAP)

$$MAP = \frac{(\text{Diastolic} \times 2) + (\text{Systolic} \times 1)}{3}$$

SYSTEMIC VASCULAR RESISTANCE (SVR)

$$\frac{MAP - RAP}{CO} = \begin{array}{l} \text{SVR in units} \\ \text{(Normal range is 10-18 units.)} \end{array}$$

$$\frac{MAP - RAP}{CO} \times 80 = \begin{array}{l} \text{SVR in dyn·sec·cm}^{-5} \\ \text{(Normal range is 800-1400} \\ \text{dyn·sec·cm}^{-5}.) \end{array}$$

SYSTEMIC VASCULAR RESISTANCE INDEX (SVRI)

$$\frac{MAP - RAP}{CI} \times 80 = \begin{array}{l} \text{SVR in dyn·sec·cm}^{-5}/\text{m}^2 \\ \text{(Normal range is 2000-2400} \\ \text{dyn·sec·cm}^{-5}/\text{m}^2.) \end{array}$$

PULMONARY VASCULAR RESISTANCE (PVR)

$$\frac{PAP \text{ mean} - RAP}{CO} = \begin{array}{l} \text{PVR in units} \\ \text{(Normal range is 1.2-3 units.)} \end{array}$$

$$\frac{PAP \text{ mean} - RAP}{CO} \times 80 = \begin{array}{l} \text{PVR in dyn·sec·cm}^{-5} \\ \text{(Normal range is 100-250} \\ \text{dyn·sec·cm}^{-5}.) \end{array}$$

PULMONARY VASCULAR RESISTANCE INDEX (PVRI)

$$\frac{PAP \text{ mean} - PAOP}{CI} \times 80 = \begin{array}{l} \text{PVR in dyn·sec·cm}^{-5}/\text{m}^2 \\ \text{(Normal range is 225-315} \\ \text{dyn·sec·cm}^{-5}/\text{m}^2.) \end{array}$$

LEFT CARDIAC WORK INDEX (LCWI)

Step 1. $MAP \times CO \times 0.0136 = LCW$

Step 2. $\dfrac{LCW}{BSA} = \begin{array}{l} LCWI \\ \text{(Normal range is 3.4-4.2 kg-m/m}^2.) \end{array}$

LEFT VENTRICULAR STROKE WORK INDEX (LVSWI)

Step 1. $MAP \times SV \times 0.0136 = LVSW$

Step 2. $\dfrac{LVSW}{BSA} = \begin{array}{l} LVSWI \\ \text{(Normal range is 50-62 g-m/m}^2.) \end{array}$

RIGHT CARDIAC WORK INDEX (RCWI)

Step 1. $PAP \text{ mean} \times CO \times 0.0136 = RCW$

Step 2. $\dfrac{RCW}{BSA} = \begin{array}{l} RCWI \\ \text{(Normal range is 0.54-0.66 kg-m/m}^2.) \end{array}$

RIGHT VENTRICULAR STROKE WORK INDEX (RVSWI)

Step 1. $PAP \text{ mean} \times SV \times 0.0136 = RVSW$

Step 2. $\dfrac{RVSW}{BSA} = \begin{array}{l} RVSWI \\ \text{(Normal range is 7.9-9.7 g-m/m}^2.) \end{array}$

CORRECTED QT INTERVAL (QTc)

$$\frac{QT}{\sqrt{(\text{RR interval})}} = QTc$$

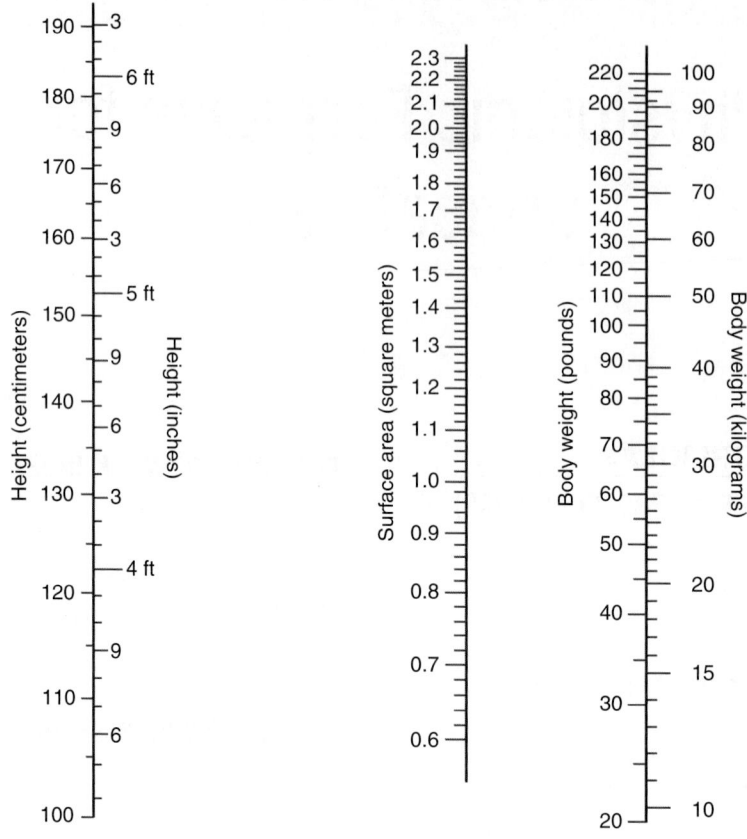

Figure B-1 Body surface area (BSA) nomogram.

BODY SURFACE AREA (BSA)

Many hemodynamic formulas can be indexed or adjusted to body size by use of a BSA nomogram (Fig. B-1). To calculate BSA:

1. Obtain height and weight.
2. Mark height on the left scale and weight on the right scale.
3. Draw a straight line between the two points marked on the nomogram.

The number where the line crosses the middle scale is the BSA value.

PULMONARY FORMULAS

CALCULATION OF THE SHUNT EQUATION (Qs/QT)

$$\frac{Qs}{Qt} = \frac{Cco_2 - Cao_2}{Cco_2 - Cvo_2}$$

Cco_2 = capillary oxygen content (calculated value)
Cao_2 = arterial oxygen content (calculated value)
Cvo_2 = venous oxygen content (calculated value)
Normal value is less than 5%.

CALCULATION OF THE PULMONARY CAPILLARY OXYGEN CONTENT (Cco_2)

$$Cco_2 = (Hgb \times 1.34 \times Sco_2) + (Pco_2 \times 0.003)$$

Hgb = hemoglobin (measured by laboratory sample or arterial blood gas)
Sco_2 = pulmonary capillary oxygen saturation
Pco_2 = partial pressure of oxygen in capillary blood
Normal value is greater than 19 mL/dL.

CALCULATION OF ARTERIAL OXYGEN CONTENT (Cao_2Cao_2)

$$Cao_2 = (Hgb \times 1.34 \times Sao_2) + (0.003 \times Pao_2)$$

Hgb = hemoglobin (measured by laboratory sample or arterial blood gas)
Sao_2 = arterial oxygen saturation (measured by arterial blood gas)
Pao_2 = partial pressure of oxygen in arterial blood (measured by arterial blood gas)
Normal range is 17 to 20 mL/dL.

CALCULATION OF VENOUS OXYGEN CONTENT (C_{VO_2})

$$C_{VO_2} = (Hgb \times 1.34 \times S\overline{v}O_2) + (0.003 \times P\overline{v}O_2)$$

Hgb = hemoglobin (measured by laboratory sample or arterial blood gas)
$S\overline{v}O_2$ = mixed venous oxygen saturation (measured by mixed venous blood gas or oximetric pulmonary artery catheter)
$P\overline{v}O_2$ = partial pressure of oxygen in mixed venous blood (measured by mixed venous blood gas)
Normal range is 12 to 15 mL/dL.

CALCULATION OF ALVEOLAR PRESSURE OF OXYGEN (P_{AO_2})

$$P_{AO_2} = F_{IO_2} \times (Pb - P_{H_2O}) - P_{aCO_2}/RQ$$

F_{IO_2} = fraction of inspired oxygen (obtained from oxygen settings)
Pb = barometric pressure (assumed to be 760 mm Hg at sea level)
P_{H_2O} = water pressure in the lungs (assumed to be 47 mm Hg)
P_{aCO_2} = partial pressure of carbon dioxide in arterial blood (measured by arterial blood gas)
RQ = respiratory quotient (assumed to be 0.8)
Normal range is 60 to 100 mm Hg.

CALCULATION OF PaO_2/F_{IO_2} RATIO

$$PaO_2/F_{IO_2} \text{ ratio} = \frac{PaO_2}{F_{IO_2}}$$

PaO_2 = partial pressure of oxygen in arterial blood (measured by arterial blood gas)
F_{IO_2} = fraction of inspired oxygen (obtained from oxygen settings)
Normal range is greater than 400 mm Hg.

CALCULATION OF ARTERIAL/ALVEOLAR RATIO

$$PaO_2/P_{AO_2} = \frac{PaO_2}{P_{AO_2}}$$

PaO_2 = partial pressure of oxygen in arterial blood (measured by arterial blood gas)
P_{AO_2} = partial pressure of oxygen in alveoli (calculated value)
Normal value is greater than 0.74.

CALCULATION OF ALVEOLAR-ARTERIAL GRADIENT

$$P(A - a)O_2 = P_{AO_2} - PaO_2$$

P_{AO_2} = partial pressure of oxygen in alveoli (calculated value)
PaO_2 = partial pressure of oxygen in arterial blood (measured by arterial blood gas)
Normal range is 25 to 65 mm Hg or 100% O_2.

CALCULATION OF THE DEAD SPACE EQUATION (V_D/V_T)

$$\frac{V_D}{V_T} = \frac{(P_{aCO_2} - P_{ETCO_2})}{P_{aCO_2}}$$

P_{aCO_2} = partial pressure of carbon dioxide in arterial blood (measured by arterial blood gas)
P_{ETCO_2} = partial pressure of carbon dioxide in exhaled gas (measured by end-tidal CO_2 monitor)
Normal range is 0.2 to 0.4 (20% to 40%).

CALCULATION OF STATIC COMPLIANCE (C_{ST})

This value is calculated for mechanically ventilated patients.

$$C_{ST} = \frac{V_T}{(PP - PEEP)}$$

V_T = tidal volume (obtained from ventilator)
PP = plateau pressure (measured by ventilator)
$PEEP$ = positive end-expiratory pressure (obtained from ventilator)
Normal range is 60 to 100 mL/cm H_2O.

CALCULATION OF DYNAMIC COMPLIANCE (C_{DY})

This value is calculated for mechanically ventilated patients.

$$C_{DY} = \frac{V_T}{(PIP - PEEP)}$$

V_T = tidal volume (obtained from ventilator)
PIP = peak inspiratory pressure (obtained from ventilator)
$PEEP$ = positive end-expiratory pressure (obtained from ventilator)
Normal range is 40 to 80 mL/cm H_2O.

NEUROLOGIC FORMULAS

CALCULATION OF CEREBRAL PERFUSION PRESSURE (CPP)

$$CCP = MAP - ICP$$

MAP = mean arterial pressure (measured by arterial line or blood pressure cuff)
ICP = intracranial pressure (measured by intracranial pressure monitoring device)
Normal range is 60 to 150 mm Hg.

CALCULATION OF ARTERIOJUGULAR OXYGEN DIFFERENCE ($AjDO_2$)

$$AjDO_2 = (SaO_2 - SjvO_2) \times 1.34 \times Hgb$$

SaO_2 = arterial oxygen saturation (measured by arterial blood gas)
$SjvO_2$ = jugular venous oxygen saturation (measured jugular blood gas or jugular venous catheter)
Hgb = hemoglobin (measured by laboratory sample or arterial blood gas)
Normal range is 5 to 7.5 mL/dL.

ENDOCRINE FORMULAS
CALCULATION OF SERUM OSMOLALITY

$$\text{Serum osmolality} = 2(\text{Na}^+ + \text{K}^+) + \frac{\text{Glucose}}{18} + \frac{\text{BUN}}{2.8}$$

Na^+ = sodium
K^+ = potassium
BUN = blood urea nitrogen
Normal range is 275 to 295 mOsm/kg of water.

ESTIMATION OF FLUID VOLUME DEFICIT IN LITERS

$$\text{Fluid volume deficit} = \frac{0.6(\text{kg/weight}) \times (\text{Na}^+ - 140)}{140}$$

Na^+ = sodium

RENAL FORMULA
CLEARANCE

$$\text{Clearance} = \text{U} \times \frac{(\text{V})}{(\text{P})}$$

U = concentration of substance in urine
V = time
P = concentration of substance in plasma
Normal range depends on substance measured.

NUTRITIONAL FORMULAS*
FORMULAS FOR ESTIMATING CALORIC NEEDS

Step 1. Calculate basal energy expenditure (BEE). This is the energy needed for basic life processes, such as respiratory function and maintenance of body temperature.

> *Women:* BEE = 795 + 7.18 × weight(kg)
> *Men:* BEE = 879 + 10.20 × weight(kg)

Step 2. Multiply by an appropriate stress factor to meet the needs of the ill or injured patient (see the following table). If the patient has more than one stressor (e.g., burn and pneumonia), use only the stress factor for the highest level of stress.

*Data from Deitch EA: Crit Care Clin 11:735, 1995; Owen OE et al: Am J Clin Nutr 4:1, 1986; Owen OE et al: Am J Clin Nutr 46:875, 1987; Garrel DR, Jobin N, de Jonge LH: Nutr Clin Pract 11:99, 1996.

Type of Stress	Multiply the Value from Step 2 by
Fever	1 + 0.13/1° C above normal (or 0.07/1° F)
Pneumonia	1.2
Major injury	1.3
Severe sepsis, burn of 15%-30% of BSA	1.5
Burn of 31%-49% of BSA content (calculated value)	1.5-2.0
Burn ≥ 50% of BSA	1.8-2.1

BSA, body surface area.

ESTIMATING PROTEIN NEEDS

Protein needs vary with the degree of malnutrition and stress (see the following table).

Condition	Multiply Desirable Body Weight (kg) by
Healthy individual or well-nourished elective surgery patient	0.8-1.0 g protein
Malnourished or catabolic state (e.g., sepsis, major injury)	1.2 to 2+ g protein
Burns	
15%-30% BSA	1.5 g protein
31%-49% BSA	1.5-2.0 g protein
50% or greater BSA	2.0-2.5 g protein

BSA, body surface area.

EXAMPLE OF A CALCULATION OF CALORIE AND PROTEIN NEEDS

A 28-year-old woman has a fracture of the left femur and burns to 40% of her BSA after a motor vehicle crash. Her height is 1.65 m (5 ft 5 in), and her weight is 59.1 kg (130 lb).

Energy Needs
1. BEE = 795 + 7.18 × 59.1 = 1219 calories/day
2. Energy needs for injury = 1219 calories × 1.75 = 2133 calories/day

Protein needs
Protein needs = 59.1 kg × 1.75 g = 103 g/day

Index

SPECIAL FEATURES